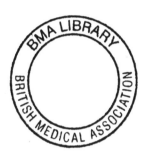

Critical Heart Disease in Infants and Children

Critical Heart Disease in Infants and Children

THIRD EDITION

Ross M. Ungerleider, MD, MBA

Director, Heart Center
Driscoll Children's Hospital
Corpus Christi, Texas

Jon N. Meliones, MD, MS, FCCM

Professor of Pediatrics Section Chief
Divisions of Critical Care and Hospitalists Medicine
Children's Memorial Herman Hospital
UT Health McGovern Medical School
Houston, Texas

Kristen Nelson McMillan, MD

Assistant Professor of Anesthesiology and Critical Care Medicine
and Pediatrics
Division of Pediatric Anesthesia and Critical Care Medicine
Director, Pediatric Cardiac Critical Care
Medical Director, Pediatric Ventricular Assist Device Program
The Johns Hopkins University School of Medicine
Baltimore, Maryland

David S. Cooper, MD, MPH

Medical Director, Cardiac Intensive Care Unit
The Heart Institute
Center for Acute Care Nephrology
Cincinnati Children's Hospital Medical Center
Cincinnati, Ohio

Jeffrey P. Jacobs, MD, FACS, FACC, FCCP

Professor of Surgery and Pediatrics
The Johns Hopkins University
Deputy Director, John's Hopkins All Children's Heart Institute
Surgical Director of Heart Transplantation
Johns Hopkins All Children's Hospital
Saint Petersburg, Florida

ELSEVIER

ELSEVIER

1600 John F. Kennedy Blvd.
Ste 1600
Philadelphia, PA 19103-2899

CRITICAL HEART DISEASE IN INFANTS AND CHILDREN,
THIRD EDITION   ISBN: 978-1-4557-0760-7
Copyright © 2019 by Elsevier, Inc. All rights reserved.

Notices

Libary of Congress Control Number: 2018949817

Previous editions copyrighted 2006 and 1995.

Content Strategist: Nancy Duffy
Senior Content Development Specialist: Deidre Simpson
Publishing Services Manager: Catherine Jackson
Senior Project Manager: Amanda Mincher
Design Direction: Amy Buxton

Printed in China

Last digit is the print number: 9   8   7   6   5   4   3   2   1

**To our readers, whose dedication to learning, commitment to caring,
and passion to constantly improving our profession gives us all great hope.**

****

*Dedicated to my children, Susan, Peter, Graham, Brynn, and Worth, without
whom I would never have been able to fully comprehend why we in this field often exhaust
ourselves making sure we do our best; and to my wife, Jamie, who has helped nourish and
nurture the spirit called by my name with love, knowledge, wisdom, and joy.*

RMU

*To my incredible wife, Christine—thank you for the love, advice, and support—and to all
my amazing children; you inspire me every moment of every day!*

JNM

*To my father, Lesley Nelson: Thank you for being my lifelong hero and for
always being there, supporting, encouraging, and loving me.
To my husband, William McMillan: Thank you for your service to our country
and for your endless and unwavering dedication and love to me and to our
families. You are what makes all of this possible every day.
To my siblings, Kathe and Jon: Thank you for your unwavering support and love.
To Dr. David Nichols: Thank you for your passion and tremendous ability to teach cardiac
critical care that started me on this amazing road and continues to inspire me and countless
others.
To all of my patients and their families: There are not enough words to say what a privilege it
has been to be a part of your lives. Thank you for all you have taught me.*

KNM

*In memory of my father, Hy, for teaching me the value of hard work. To my mother, Irene,
for imparting unto me a love of learning and teaching. To my wife, Lisa, for her love and
unwavering support. To my children, Michael, Adam, and Daniel, for reminding me why I
do what I do and inspiring me to be better than I am.*

DSC

*To my parents, David and Marilyn Jacobs, for giving me the opportunity; to my wife, Stacy,
for supporting and loving me; to my children, Jessica and Joshua, for making me proud and
motivated; and to my patients, who represent the rationale for this initiative.*

JPJ

Contributors

Mubbasheer Ahmed, MD
Assistant Professor of Pediatrics
Baylor College of Medicine
Texas Children's Hospital
Houston, Texas

Samuel M. Alaish, MD
Associate Professor of Surgery
The Johns Hopkins University School of Medicine
Surgical Director, THRIVE Center for Pediatric Intestinal
  Rehabilitation
The Johns Hopkins Children's Center
Baltimore, Maryland

Euleche Alanmanou, MD, FAAP
Clinical Professor of Anesthesiology
University of Texas Medical Branch
Galveston, Texas
Clinical Coordinator of Pediatric Cardiac Anesthesiology
Department of Anesthesiology and Critical Care
Driscoll Children's Hospital
Corpus Christi, Texas

Plato Alexander, MD, MBA
Associate Director
Cardiovascular Intensive Care Unit
Johns Hopkins All Children's Hospital
St. Petersburg, Florida

Alaa Aljiffry, MBBS
Assistant Professor of Pediatrics
Pediatric Cardiology
Emory University
Pediatric Cardiac Intensivist
Children's Health Care of Atlanta
Atlanta, Georgia

Melvin C. Almodovar, MD
University of Miami
Miami, Florida

Bahaaldin Alsoufi, MD
Professor of Surgery
University of Louisville School of Medicine
Director of Pediatric Cardiac Surgery
Norton Children's Hospital
Louisville, Kentucky

Marc M. Anders, MD
Assistant Professor of Pediatrics
Texas Children's Hospital
Houston, Texas

Nicholas D. Andersen, MD
Chief Resident, Congenital Cardiac Surgery
Department of Cardiac Surgery
Boston Children's Hospital
Boston, Massachusetts

Judith Ascenzi, DNP, APRN-CNS, RN, CCRN
Nurse Manager
Pediatric Intensive Care Unit
The Johns Hopkins Hospital
Baltimore, Maryland

Scott I. Aydin, MD
Assistant Professor of Pediatrics
Division of Pediatric Critical Care Medicine and Cardiology
Icahn School of Medicine
Kravis Children's Hospital at Mount Sinai
New York, New York

Matthew K. Bacon, MD
Assistant Professor of Pediatrics
UK Healthcare
University of Kentucky
Kentucky Children's Hospital
Lexington, Kentucky

David J. Barron, MD, FRCP, FRCS(CT)
Consultant Cardiac Surgeon
Department of Cardiac Surgery
Birmingham Children's Hospital
Birmingham, United Kingdom

Amy Basken, MS
Director of Programs
Pediatric Congenital Heart Association
Madison, Wisconsin

Kimberly D. Beddows, NP
Nurse Practitioner, Pediatric Heart Transplant
Pediatric Heart Center
The Children's Hospital at Montefiore
New York, New York

Melania M. Bembea, MD, MPH, PhD
Associate Professor of Anesthesiology and Critical Care
    Medicine
The Johns Hopkins University School of Medicine
Baltimore, Maryland

Alexis L. Benscoter, DO
Assistant Professor of Cardiology
Cincinnati Children's Hospital Medical Center
Cincinnati, Ohio

Charles P. Bergstrom, MD
Assistant Professor of Pediatric Critical Care Medicine
Medical College of Wisconsin
Milwaukee, Wisconsin

Meghan Bernier, MD
Instructor of Anesthesiology and Critical Care Medicine
The Johns Hopkins University School of Medicine
Baltimore, Maryland

Steve Bibevski, MD, PhD
Section of Pediatric and Congenital Cardiac Surgery
The Heart Institute
Joe DiMaggio Children's Hospital
Hollywood, Florida

David Bichell, MD
William S. Stoney Jr. Chair in Surgery
Professor of Surgery
Division of Cardiac Surgery
Vanderbilt University
Nashville, Tennessee

Geoffrey L. Bird, MD, MSIS
Assistant Professor of Pediatrics, Critical Care Medicine, and
    Anesthesiology
Cardiac Critical Care Medicine
Children's Hospital of Philadelphia
Philadelphia, Pennsylvania

Konstantinos Boukas, MD
Assistant Professor of Pediatrics
Division of Critical Care Medicine
UTHealth McGovern Medical School
Houston, Texas

Edward L. Bove, MD
Helen and Marvin Kirsh Professor of Surgery
Professor of Cardiac Surgery
Section of Pediatric Cardiovascular Surgery
University of Michigan Medical School
Ann Arbor, Michigan

Ken Brady, MD
Associate Professor of Pediatric Anesthesiology
Texas Children's Hospital
Houston, Texas

Craig S. Broberg, MD
Associate Professor of Cardiology and Radiology
Knight Cardiovascular Institute
Oregon Health and Science University
Portland, Oregon

Ronald A. Bronicki, MD, FCCM, FACC
Professor of Pediatrics
Sections of Critical Care Medicine and Cardiology
Baylor College of Medicine
Texas Children's Hospital
Houston, Texas

Julie A. Brothers, MD
Associate Professor of Pediatrics
Perelman School of Medicine
University of Pennsylvania
Attending Physician
Division of Cardiology
The Children's Hospital of Philadelphia
Philadelphia, Pennsylvania

Kristen M. Brown, DNP, CRNP, CPNP-AC
Acute Care Pediatric Nurse Practitioner
Anesthesia and Critical Care Medicine
The Johns Hopkins University School of Medicine
Instructor
Advanced Practice Simulation Coordinator
Acute and Chronic Care
The Johns Hopkins University School of Nursing
Baltimore, Maryland

John R. Brownlee, MD
Pediatric Cardiology
Driscoll Children's Health System
Corpus Christi, Texas

Roosevelt Bryant III, MD
Assistant Professor of Surgery
University of Cincinnati College of Medicine
Surgical Director, Pediatric Heart Transplant Services
The Heart Institute
Cincinnati Children's Hospital Medical Center
Cincinnati, Ohio

Amulya Buddhavarapu, MD
Resident
Department of Pediatrics
Driscoll Children's Hospital
Texas A&M University
Corpus Christi, Texas

Duke E. Cameron, MD
Professor of Surgery
Harvard Medical School
Division of Cardiac Surgery
Massachusetts General Hospital
Boston, Massachusetts

Paul J. Chai, MD
Associate Professor of Surgery
Department of Pediatric Cardiac Surgery
Columbia University Medical Center
Morgan Stanley Children's Hospital
New York, New York

Paul A. Checchia, MD, FCCM, FACC
Professor of Pediatrics
Sections of Critical Care Medicine and Cardiology
Baylor College of Medicine
Texas Children's Hospital
Houston, Texas

Ira M. Cheifetz, MD
Chief Medical Officer
Children's Services
Duke Children's Hospital
Associate Chief Medical Officer
Duke University Hospital
Division Chief, Pediatric Critical Care Medicine
Professor of Pediatrics and Anesthesiology
Duke University Medical Center
Durham, North Carolina

Clifford Chin, MD
Professor of Pediatrics
University of Cincinnati College of Medicine
Medical Director, Pediatric Heart Transplant Services
The Heart Institute
Cincinnati Children's Hospital Medical Center
Cincinnati, Ohio

Jill Marie Cholette, MD
Associate Professor of Pediatrics
University of Rochester
Rochester, New York

Charles R. Cole, MD
Fellow
Department of Cardiothoracic Surgery
University of Colorado
Aurora, Colorado

David S. Cooper, MD, MPH
Medical Director, Cardiac Intensive Care Unit
The Heart Institute
Center for Acute Care Nephrology
Cincinnati Children's Hospital Medical Center
Cincinnati, Ohio

John D. Coulson, MD
Clinical Associate
Assistant Professor, Part-Time Faculty
Department of Pediatrics
Division of Pediatric Cardiology
The Johns Hopkins University School of Medicine
Baltimore, Maryland

Ralph J. Damiano Jr., MD
Evarts A. Graham Professor of Surgery
Chief, Division of Cardiothoracic Surgery
Washington University School of Medicine
Barnes-Jewish Hospital
Saint Louis, Missouri

Miguel DeLeon, MD
Medical Director, Neonatal Intensive Care Unit
Department of Neonatology
Driscoll Children's Hospital
Medical Director, Neonatal Intensive Care Unit
Department of Neonatology
Corpus Christi Medical Center
Corpus Christi, Texas

Holly C. DeSena, MD
Assistant Professor
The Heart Institute
Cincinnati Children's Hospital
Cincinnati, Ohio

Nina Deutsch, MD
Associate Professor of Anesthesiology and Pediatrics
Children's National Medical Center
George Washington University
Washington, D.C.

Pirooz Eghtesady, MD, PhD
Emerson Chair in Pediatric Cardiothoracic Surgery
Chief, Section of Pediatric Cardiothoracic Surgery
Washington University School of Medicine
St. Louis Children's Hospital
St. Louis, Missouri

Branden Engorn, MD
Fellow
Department of Anesthesiology Critical Care Medicine
Children's Hospital Los Angeles
Fellow
Department of Anesthesiology Critical Care Medicine
Keck School of Medicine of the University of Southern
    California
Los Angeles, California

Allen Everett, MD
Professor of Pediatrics
Division of Pediatrics and Cardiology
The Johns Hopkins University
Baltimore, Maryland

Lloyd Felmly, MD
Resident Physician
Department of Surgery
Division of Cardiothoracic Surgery
Medical University of South Carolina
Charleston, South Carolina

Andrew C. Fiore, MD
Professor of Surgery
Division of Pediatric Cardiovascular Surgery
Cardinal Glennon Children's Hospital
Saint Louis University School of Medicine
St. Louis, Missouri

Gregory A. Fleming, MD, MSCI
Assistant Professor of Pediatrics
Division of Pediatric Cardiology
Duke University Medical Center
Durham, North Carolina

Saul Flores, MD
Assistant Professor of Pediatrics
Section of Critical Care
Texas Children's Hospital
Baylor College of Medicine
Houston, Texas

Rodney Franklin, MD
Department of Pediatric Cardiology
Royal Brompton Hosptal
London, United Kingdom

Charles D. Fraser III, MD
Resident
Department of Surgery
The Johns Hopkins Hospital
Baltimore, Maryland

Michael Gaies, MD, MPH, MS
Assistant Professor of Pediatrics and Communicable Diseases
University of Michigan
Ann Arbor, Michigan

James J. Gangemi, MD
Associate Professor of Surgery and Pediatrics
Division of Thoracic and Cardiovascular Surgery
University of Virginia Health System
Charlottesville, Virginia

Lasya Gaur, MD
Assistant Professor of Pediatric Cardiology
The Johns Hopkins Hospital
Baltimore, Maryland

Nancy S. Ghanayem, MD
Professor of Pediatrics (Critical Care)
Baylor College of Medicine
Texas Children's Hospital
Houston, Texas

Salil Ginde, MD
Assistant Professor of Internal Medicine and Pediatrics
  (Cardiology)
Medical College of Wisconsin
Milwaukee, Wisconsin

Katja M. Gist, DO, MSc
Assistant Professor
Department of Pediatrics
Heart Institute
Children's Hospital Colorado
Denver, Colorado

Allan Goldman, MRCP, MBBcH, MSc
Great Ormond Street Hospital for Children
NHS Foundation Trust
London, United Kingdom

Stuart L. Goldstein, MD
Director, Center for Acute Care Nephrology
Department of Pediatrics
The Heart Institute
Division of Nephrology and Hypertension
Cincinnati Children's Hospital Medical Center
Cincinnati, Ohio

Dheeraj Goswami, MD
Assistant Professor of Anesthesia and Critical Care Medicine
The Johns Hopkins Hospital
Baltimore, Maryland

Eric M. Graham, MD
Professor of Pediatrics
Chief, Division of Pediatric Cardiology
Medical University of South Carolina
Charleston, South Carolina

Michelle A. Grenier, MD
Director of Imaging
Pediatric Cardiology
Driscoll Children's Hospital
Corpus Christi, Texas

Stephanie S. Handler, MD
Assistant Professor of Pediatrics (Cardiology)
Medical College of Wisconsin
Milwaukee, Wisconsin

James R. Herlong, MD
Division Chief, Pediatric Cardiology
Sanger Heart and Vascular Institute
Charlotte, North Carolina

Kevin D. Hill, MD, MSCI
Associate Professor of Pediatrics
Division of Pediatric Cardiology
Duke University Medical Center
Durham, North Carolina

Jennifer C. Romano, MD, MS
Assistant Professor of Cardiac Surgery and Pediatrics
Section of Pediatric Cardiovascular Surgery
University of Michigan Medical School
Ann Arbor, Michigan

Siew Yen Ho, PhD
Cardiac Morphology Unit
Royal Brompton Hospital
Imperial College London
London, United Kingdom

George M. Hoffman, MD
Professor of Anesthesiology and Pediatrics
Medical Director, Pediatric Anesthesiology
Medical College of Wisconsin and Children's Hospital of
    Wisconsin,
Milwaukee, Wisconsin

Osami Honjo, MD, PhD
The Hospital for Sick Children
University of Toronto
Toronto, Canada

Christoph P. Hornik, MD, MPH
Associate Professor
Division of Pediatric Critical Care Medicine
Department of Pediatrics
Duke University
Durham, North Carolina

Daphne T. Hsu, MD
Professor of Pediatrics
Albert Einstein College of Medicine
Chief, Pediatric Cardiology
Co-Director, Pediatric Heart Center
The Children's Hospital at Montefiore
New York, New York

Charles B. Huddleston, MD
Professor of Surgery
Division of Pediatric Cardiology
Saint Louis University School of Medicine
St. Louis, Missouri

Christin Huff, MSN, CPNP-AC
Nurse Practitioner
Cardiac Critical Care
Cincinnati Children's Hospital Medical Center
Cincinnati, Ohio

Elizabeth A. Hunt, MD, MPH, PhD
Director, Johns Hopkins Medicine Simulation Center
Associate Professor of Anesthesiology and Critical Care
    Medicine
The Johns Hopkins University School of Medicine
Baltimore, Maryland

Salim F. Idriss, MD, PhD
Associate Professor
Departments of Pediatrics, Pediatric Cardiology, and Pediatric
    Electrophysiology
Duke University
Durham, North Carolina

Ilias Iliopoulos, MD, FRCPCH, FRCPC, FAAP
Cardiac Critical Care
The Heart Institute
Cincinnati Children's Hospital Medical Center
Assistant Professor
Department of Pediatrics
University of Cincinnati
Cincinnati, Ohio

Kimberly Ward Jackson, MD
Director, Pediatric Emergency Response
Assistant Professor of Pediatrics
Duke University
Durham, North Carolina

Jeffrey P. Jacobs, MD, FACS, FACC, FCCP
Professor of Surgery and Pediatrics
The Johns Hopkins University
Deputy Director, John's Hopkins All Children's Heart Institute
Surgical Director of Heart Transplantation
Johns Hopkins All Children's Hospital
Saint Petersburg, Florida

Marshall L. Jacobs, MD
Professor of Surgery
Division of Cardiac Surgery
The Johns Hopkins School of Medicine
Baltimore, Maryland

James Jaggers, MD
Chief, Congenital Cardiac Surgery
Professor of Surgery
Barton Elliman Chair of Pediatric Cardiac Surgery
University of Colorado
Aurora, Colorado

Laura N. Jansen, PA-C
Physician Assistant
Pediatric Cardiothoracic Surgery
Levine Children's Hospital
Charlotte, North Carolina

Christopher M. Janson, MD
Assistant Professor of Pediatrics
Children's Hospital of Philadelphia, Cardiac Center
The Children's Hospital of Philadelphia
Philadelphia, Pennsylvania

Robert Jaquiss, MD
Pogue Distinguished Chair in Pediatric Cardiac Surgery
    Research
Departments of Cardio Thoracic Surgery and Pediatrics
The University of Texas Southwestern Medical Center
Dallas, Texas

Emily Johnson, MSN, RN, CPNP-PC/AC
Nurse Practitioner
Pediatric Palliative Care
Bloomberg Children's Center
The Johns Hopkins Hospital
Baltimore, Maryland

Melissa B. Jones, MSN, APRN, CPNP-AC
Nurse Practitioner Team Lead for Critical Care
Cardiac Critical Care
Children's National Health System
Washington, D.C.

Lindsey Justice, DNP, RN, CPNP-AC
Cardiac Intensive Care Unit Nurse Practitioner
The Heart Institute
Cincinnati Children's Hospital Medical Center
Cincinnati, Ohio

Patricia L. Kane, MSN, CNS, CPNP
Lead Nurse Practitioner
Pediatric Cardiology/Cardiac Surgery
The Johns Hopkins Hospital
Baltimore, Maryland

Tara Karamlou, MD, MSc
Associate Professor of Surgery
Mayo Clinic
Cardiothoracic Surgeon
Western Regional Medical Center
Goodyear, Arizona

Vyas M. Kartha, MD, FAAP
Director, Pediatric Cardiac Anesthesia
Department of Anesthesiology
Johns Hopkins All Children's Hospital
St. Petersburg, Florida

Minoo N. Kavarana, MD, FACS
Associate Professor of Surgery
Medical University of South Carolina
Charleston, South Carolina

Abigail May Khan, MD
Assistant Professor of Medicine
Knight Cardiovascular Institute
Oregon Health and Science University
Portland, Oregon

Valerie King, BS
Parent as Collaborative Leader Educator
Parent Advocate
Yadkinville, North Carolina

Roxanne E. Kirsch, MD, MBE
Cardiac Intensivist
Department of Pediatric Critical Care and Anesthesiology
Critical Care Bioethics Associate
Department of Bioethics
The Hospital for Sick Children
Toronto, Ontario, Canada

Paul M. Kirshbom, MD
Chief, Pediatric Cardiac Surgery
Department of Surgery
Carolinas Healthcare System
Charlotte, North Carolina

Christopher J. Knott-Craig, MD
Professor of Surgery
Chief, Cardiovascular Surgery
Director, Heart Institute
University of Tennessee Health Sciences Center
Le Bonheur Children's Hospital
Memphis, Tennessee

Jeannie Koo, MSN, BSN
Nurse Practitioner
Pediatric Critical Care
Duke University Medical Center
Durham, North Carolina

Jennifer Kramer, MD
Pediatric Cardiology and Pediatric Critical Care Fellow
Department of Pediatrics
Division of Pediatric Cardiology
Department of Anesthesiology and Critical Care Medicine
Division of Pediatric Anesthesiology and Critical Care Medicine
The Johns Hopkins University School of Medicine
Baltimore, Maryland

Catherine D. Krawczeski, MD
Medical Director, Cardiovascular Intensive Care Unit
Department of Pediatrics
Division of Cardiology
Stanford University
Palo Alto, California

Ganga Krishnamurthy, MBBS
Garrett Isaac Neubauer Associate Professor of Pediatrics
Director of Neonatal Cardiac Intensive Care
Columbia University Medical Center
Morgan Stanley Children's Hospital
New York, New York

Sapna R. Kudchadkar, MD, PhD
Associate Professor
Department of Anesthesiology and Critical Care Medicine
The Johns Hopkins University School of Medicine
Baltimore, Maryland

Karan R. Kumar, MD
Pediatric Critical Care Fellow
Division of Pediatric Critical Care Medicine
Duke University
Durham, North Carolina

T.K. Susheel Kumar, MD
Assistant Professor
Pediatric Cardiothoracic Surgery
Le Bonheur Children's Hospital
Memphis, Tennessee

David M. Kwiatkowski, MD, MS
Assistant Professor
Department of Pediatrics
Division of Cardiology
Stanford University
Palo Alto, California

Jacqueline M. Lamour, MD
Professor of Pediatrics
Albert Einstein College of Medicine
Pediatric Heart Center
The Children's Hospital at Montefiore
Bronx, New York

Timothy S. Lancaster, MD
Fellow in Cardiothoracic Surgery
Washington University School of Medicine
St. Louis Children's Hospital
Barnes-Jewish Hospital
St. Louis, Missouri

Benjamin J. Landis, MD
Assistant Professor of Pediatrics and Medical and Molecular
    Genetics
Indiana University School of Medicine
Indianapolis, Indiana

Javier J. Lasa, MD, FAAP
Assistant Professor of Pediatrics
Sections of Critical Care Medicine and Cardiology
Baylor College of Medicine
Texas Children's Hospital
Houston, Texas

Matthew H.L. Liava'a, FRACS
Assistant Attending
Department of Pediatric Cardiac Surgery
Columbia University Medical Center
Morgan Stanley Children's Hospital
New York, New York

Daniel J. Licht, MD
Associate Professor of Neurology and Pediatrics
Department of Pediatrics
Division of Neurology
Children's Hospital, Philadelphia
Associate Professor
Department of Neurology
Perelman School of Medicine
The University of Pennsylvania
Philadelphia, Pennsylvania

Matthew T. Lisi, MD
Assistant Professor of Pediatric Cardiology
Wake Forest University School of Medicine
Winston Salem, North Carolina

Ryan Loftin, MD
Medical Director, Maternal Fetal Medicine
Driscoll Health System
Corpus Christi, Texas

Rohit S. Loomba, MD, MS
Clinical Fellow
Division of Cardiology
Cincinnati Children's Hospital Medical Center
Cincinnati, Ohio

Bradley S. Marino, MD, MPP, MSCE
Professor of Pediatrics and Medical Social Sciences
Northwestern University Feinberg School of Medicine
Co-Director, Research and Academic Affairs
Divisions of Cardiology and Critical Care Medicine
Ann and Robert H. Lurie Children's Hospital of Chicago
Chicago, Illinois

Thomas S. Maxey, MD
Pediatric Heart Surgeon
Levine Children's Hospital
Charlotte, North Carolina

Karen McCarthy, PhD
Cardiac Morphology Unit
Royal Brompton Hospital
Imperial College London
London, United Kingdom

Michael C. McCrory, MD, MS
Associate Professor of Anesthesiology and Pediatrics
Wake Forest School of Medicine
Winston-Salem, North Carolina

Inder D. Mehta, MD
Congenital Cardiovascular Surgeon
Driscoll Children's Hospital
Corpus Christi, Texas

Christopher Mehta, MD
Cardiothoracic Surgery Fellow
Department of Surgery
Northwestern University
Chicago, Illinois

Jon N. Meliones, MD, MS, FCCM
Professor of Pediatrics Section Chief
Divisions of Critical Care and Hospitalists Medicine
Children's Memorial Herman Hospital
UT Health McGovern Medical School
Houston, Texas

Christine Meliones, MSN, CPNP-AC/PC, FNP
Pediatric and Adult Congenital Electrophysiology Nurse
    Practitioner
Pediatric Cardiology/Electrophysiology
Duke University
Durham, North Carolina

Alison Miles, DO
Assistant Professor
Department of Pediatric Anesthesiology and Critical Care
    Medicine
Johns Hopkins Medicine
Baltimore, Maryland

Michael E. Mitchell, MD
Professor of Pediatric Cardiothoracic Surgery
Department of Surgery
Children's Hospital of Wisconsin
Professor of Surgery
Medical College of Wisconsin
Milwaukee, Wisconsin

Erica Molitor-Kirsch, MD
Medical Director, Cardiac Critical Care
Children's Mercy Hospital
Professor of Pediatrics
University of Missouri–Kansas City
Kansas City, Missouri

Jenny A. Montgomery, RN, MSN, CPNP-AC
Cardiovascular Nurse Practitioner Coordinator
Pediatric Heart Center
Driscoll Children's Hospital
Corpus Christi, Texas

Lisa Moore, RN, MSN, MHA, NEA-BC
Senior Director, Nursing
Heart Institute
Johns Hopkins All Childrens Hospital
St. Petersburg, Florida

David L.S. Morales, MD
Chief, Pediatric Cardiothoracic Surgery
Cincinnati Children's Hospital Medical Center
Cincinnati, Ohio

Cara Morin, MD, PhD
Clinical Fellow
Cincinnati Children's Hospital
Cincinnati, Ohio

Nicholas Morin, MD, PhD
Johns Hopkins Medicine
Baltimore, Maryland

Steven S. Mou, MD
Associate Professor of Anesthesiology and Pediatrics
Wake Forest School of Medicine
Winston-Salem, North Carolina

Ashok Muralidaran, MD
Assistant Professor of Surgery and Pediatrics
Oregon Health and Science University
Portland, Oregon

Raghav Murthy, MD, DABS, FACS
Assistant Clinical Professor of Cardiovascular Surgery
Rady Children's Hospital
University of California, San Diego
San Diego, California

Joseph R. Nellis, MD, MBA
Resident
Department of Surgery
Duke University
Durham, North Carolina

Jennifer S. Nelson, MD, MS
Associate Professor of Surgery
University of Central Florida College of Medicine
Department of Cardiovascular Services
Nemours Children's Hospital
Orlando, Florida

Kristen Nelson McMillan, MD
Assistant Professor of Anesthesiology and Critical Care
    Medicine and Pediatrics
Division of Pediatric Anesthesia and Critical Care Medicine
Director, Pediatric Cardiac Critical Care
Medical Director, Pediatric Ventricular Assist Device Program
The Johns Hopkins University School of Medicine
Baltimore, Maryland

Melanie Nies, MD
Department of Pediatric Cardiology
The Johns Hopkins University
Baltimore, Maryland

John Nigro, MD
Cardiothoracic Surgery
Rady Children's Hospital–San Diego
San Diego, California

Corina Noje, MD
Assistant Professor of Anesthesiology and Critical Care
    Medicine
The Johns Hopkins University
Medical Director, Pediatric Transport
The Johns Hopkins Hospital
Baltimore, Maryland

Sarah E. Norris, MD
Assistant Professor of Pediatrics
Albert Einstein College of Medicine
Pediatric Heart Center
The Children's Hospital at Montefiore
Bronx, New York

James O'Brien, MD
Co-Director, The Ward Family Heart Center
Chief, Cardiothoracic Surgery
Children's Mercy Hospital
Kansas City, Missouri

George Ofori-Amanfo, MD
Chief, Divsion of Pediatric Critical Care Medicine
Professor of Pediatrics
Icahn School of Medicine
Kravis Children's Hospital at Mount Sinai
New York, New York

Richard G. Ohye, MD, CS
Professor and Associate Chair of Cardiac Surgery
Head, Section of Pediatric Cardiovascular Surgery
University of Michigan Medical School
Ann Arbor, Michigan

Yoshio Ootaki, MD, PhD
Departments of Pediatric Cardiothoracic Surgery and Pediatric
  Cardiology
Wake Forest Baptist Health
Winston Salem, North Carolina

Caroline P. Ozment, MD
Assistant Professor
Department of Pediatrics
Division of Pediatric Critical Care Medicine
Duke University
Durham, North Carolina

Giles J. Peek, MD
Professor of Clinical Cardiovascular and Thoracic Surgery
Division of Pediatric Cardiac Surgery
Albert Einstein College of Medicine
Pediatric Heart Center
The Children's Hospital at Montefiore
Bronx, New York

Autumn K. Peterson, BSN, MSN, CPNP-AC
Critical Care Pediatric Nurse Practitioner
Pediatric Critical Care Medicine
Duke Children's Pediatric and Congenital Heart Center
Duke University Medical Center
Durham, North Carolina

Renuka E. Peterson, MD
Associate Professor of Pediatric Cardiology
Division of Pediatric Cardiology
Cardinal Glennon Children's Hospital
Saint Louis University School of Medicine
St. Louis, Missouri

John K. Petty, MD
Associate Professor of Surgery and Pediatrics
Wake Forest School of Medicine
Winston-Salem, North Carolina

Prashob Porayette, MD, MSc
Pediatric Cardiologist
Driscoll Children's Hospital
Adjunct Assistant Professor of Pediatrics
Texas A&M College of Medicine
Corpus Christi, Texas

David E. Procaccini, PharmD
Clinical Pharmacy Practitioner
Pediatric Intensive Care and Pediatric Cardiology/Heart
  Transplant
The Johns Hopkins Hospital
Baltimore, Maryland

James Quintessenza, MD
Professor and Chief of Pediatric Cardiac Surgery
Kentucky Children's Hospital, University of Kentucky
Lexington, Kentucky
Professor and Attending Pediatric Cardiac Surgeon
Cincinnati Children's Hospital Medical Center
University of Cincinnati
Cincinnati, Ohio

William S. Ragalie, MD
Cardiothoracic Surgery Resident
Ronald Regan UCLA Medical Center
Los Angeles, California

William Ravekes, MD
Assistant Professor of Pediatrics
Division of Pediatric Cardiology
The Johns Hopkins University School of Medicine
Baltimore, Maryland

Tia T. Raymond, MD
Pediatric Cardiac Intensivists of North Texas, PLLC
Congenital Heart Surgery Unit
Medical City Children's Hospital
Dallas, Texas

Andrew Redington, MD
Chief, Pediatric Cardiology
Executive Co-Director, The Heart Institute
Cincinnati Children's Hospital Medical Center
Cincinnati, Ohio

Kyle J. Rehder, MD
Associate Professor of Pediatrics
Duke Children's Hospital
Physician Quality Officer
Duke Patient Safety Center
Duke University Health System
Durham, North Carolina

Becky Riggs, MD
Assistant Professor of Pediatric Anesthesiology and Critical Care
  Medicine
The Johns Hopkins University School of Medicine
Baltimore, Maryland

Ramon Julio Rivera, MD
Associate Professor of Anesthesiology
University of Texas Medical Branch
Driscoll Children's Hospital
Corpus Christi, Texas

Jennifer Roark, MSN, FNP-C
Nurse Practitioner
Department of Pediatrics
Division of Pediatric Cardiology
Duke University Medical Center
Durham, North Carolina

Lewis H. Romer, MD
Professor of Anesthesiology and Critical Care Medicine, Cell
  Biology, Biomedical Engineering, and Pediatrics
Center for Cell Dynamics
The Johns Hopkins University School of Medicine
Baltimore, Maryland

Amy Ryan, MSN, RN, CPNP-AC
Nurse Practitioner
Cardiac Intensive Care Unit
Cincinnati Children's Hospital Medical Center
Cincinnati, Ohio

Thomas D. Ryan, MD, PhD
Assistant Professor of Pediatrics
University of Cincinnati College of Medicine
Director of Clinical Operations, Cardiomyopathy/Heart Failure
The Heart Institute
Cincinnati Children's Hospital Medical Center
Cincinnati, Ohio

Beth A. Rymeski, DO
Assistant Professor of General and Thoracic Surgery
Cincinnati Children's Hospital
Cincinnati, Ohio

Peter Sassalos, MD
Assistant Professor of Cardiac Surgery
Section of Pediatric Cardiovascular Surgery
University of Michigan Medical School
Ann Arbor, Michigan

Jaclyn E. Sawyer, PharmD
Clinical Pharmacy Specialist, Cardiology
Division of Pharmacy
Cincinnati Children's Hospital Medical Center
Cincinnati, Ohio

Frank Scholl, MD
Chief, Pediatric and Congenital Heart Surgery
Surgical Director, Pediatric Heart Transplant
Memorial Healthcare System
Joe DiMaggio Children's Hospital
Hollywood, Florida

Kevin Patrick Schooler, MD, PhD
Associate Professor of Anethesiology and Critical Care Medicine
Driscoll Children's Hospital
Corpus Christi, Texas

Jennifer Schuette, MD, MS
Program Director, Pediatric Critical Care Medicine Fellowship
Assistant Professor of Anesthesiology and Critical Care
  Medicine
The Johns Hopkins University School of Medicine
Baltimore, Maryland

Jamie McElrath Schwartz, MD
Section Chief, Pediatric Critical Care
Director, Pediatric Cardiac Anesthesia
Pediatric Anesthesia and Critical Care Medicine
The Johns Hopkins University School of Medicine
Batimore, Maryland

Daniel R. Sedehi, MD
Assistant Professor of Medicine
Knight Cardiovascular Institute
Oregon Health and Science University
Portland, Oregon

Priya Sekar, MD, MPH
Assistant Professor of Pediatrics
Division of Pediatric Cardiology
The Johns Hopkins University School of Medicine
Baltimore, Maryland

Donald H. Shaffner, MD
Associate Professor of Anesthesiology and Crtical Care Medicine
The Johns Hopkins University School of Medicine
Baltimore, Maryland

Sanket Shah, MD, MHS
Assistant Professor of Pediatrics
Department of Pediatric Cardiology
Children's Mercy Hospital
Kansas City, Missouri

Irving Shen, MD
Professor of Surgery and Pediatrics
Doernbecher Children's Hospital
Oregon Health and Science University
Portland, Oregon

Avinash K. Shetty, MD
Professor of Pediatrics
Associate Dean for Global Health
Wake Forest School of Medicine
Winston-Salem, North Carolina

Edd Shope, ADN
Staff Nurse
Duke Life Flight
Duke University Medical Center
Durham, North Carolina

Darla Shores, MD
Associate Professor of Pediatric Gastroenterology
The Johns Hopkins University
Baltimore, Maryland

Ming-Sing Si, MD
Assistant Professor of Cardiac Surgery
Section of Pediatric Cardiovascular Surgery
University of Michigan Medical School
Ann Arbor, Michigan

Nida Siddiqi, PharmD
Clinical Pharmacy Specialist
Pediatric Critical Care and Transplantation Sidra Medicine
Doha, Qatar

Leah Simpson, RD
Clinical Dietitian Specialist III
Pediatric Nutrition
The Johns Hopkins Hospital
Baltimore, Maryland

Zdenek Slavik, MD
Department of Pediatric Cardiology
Royal Brompton Hospital
London, United Kingdom

Heidi A.B. Smith, MD, FAAP, MSCI
Department of Anesthesiology and Pediatrics
Vanderbilt University Medical Center
Nashville, Tennessee

Zebulon Z. Spector, MD
Medical Instructor
Division of Pediatric Cardiology and Electrophysiology
Department of Pediatrics
Duke University
Durham, North Carolina

Allison L. Speer, MD
Assistant Professor of Pediatric Surgery
McGovern Medical School
The University of Texas Health Science Center at Houston
Houston, Texas

Philip Spevak, MD, MPH
Associate Professor of Pediatrics
Johns Hopkins Medicine
Baltimore, Maryland

Dylan Stewart, MD, FACS
Assistant Professor of Surgery
The Johns Hopkins University
Baltimore, Maryland

Robert D. Stewart, MD
Staff, Pediatric and Congenital Heart Surgery
Heart and Vascular Institute
Cleveland Clnic
Cleveland, Ohio

James St. Louis, MD
Professor of Surgery
Children's Mercy Hospital
Kansas City, Missouri

Matthew L. Stone, MD, PhD
Fellow
Department of Surgery
Division of Thoracic and Cardiovascular Surgery
University of Virginia School of Medicine
Charlottesville, Virginia

Erik Su, MD
Director, Critical Care Ultrasound
Department of Anesthesiology and Critical Care Medicine
The Johns Hopkins University School of Medicine
Baltimore, Maryland

Kelly A. Swain, MSN, CPNP-AC
Critical Care Pediatric Nurse Practitioner
Pediatric Critical Care Medicine
Duke Children's Pediatric and Congenital Heart Center
Duke University Medical Center
Durham, North Carolina

Cliff M. Takemoto, MD
Associate Professor
Department of Pediatrics
Division of Pediatric Hematology
The Johns Hopkins University School of Medicine
Baltimore, Maryland

Sarah Tallent, BSN, MSN, CPNP-AC
Division of Pediatric Critical Care Medicine
Duke University Hospital
Durham, North Carolina

Ravi R. Thiagarajan, MBBS, MPH
Senior Associate in Cardiology
Associate Professor of Pediatrics
Boston Children's Hospital
Boston, Massachusetts

Chani Traube, MD, FAAP, FCCM
Department of Pediatrics
Weill Cornell Medical College
Department of Pediatrics
Memorial Sloan Kettering Cancer Center
New York, New York

Ephraim Tropp
MPH Student
Department of Epidemiology and Biostatistics
Graduate School of Public Health and Health Policy
City University of New York
New York, New York

Rocky Tsang, MD
Department of Pediatrics
Baylor College of Medicine
Texas Children's Hospital
Houston, Texas

Sebastian C. Tume, MD
Assistant Professor of Pediatrics
Baylor College of Medicine
Houston, Texas

Joseph W. Turek, MD, PhD
Chief, Pediatric Cardiothoracic Surgery
Department of Surgery
Duke University
Durham, North Carolina

Jennifer L. Turi, MD
Associate Professor of Pediatric Critical Care Medicine
Duke Children's Pediatric and Congenital Heart Center
Medical Director, Pediatric Cardiac Intensive Care Unit
Duke University Medical Center
Durham, North Carolina

Immanuel I. Turner, MD
Pediatric and Congenital Heart Surgery
Cardiac Center at Joe DiMaggio Children's Hospital
Hollywood, Florida

James S. Tweddell, MD
Chair, Cardiothoracic Surgery
Cincinnati Children's Hospital Medical Center
Professor of Surgery and Pediatrics
University of Cincinnati
Cincinnati, Ohio

Chinwe Unegbu, MD
Assistant Professor of Anesthesiology and Pediatrics
Division of Cardiac Anesthesiology
Division of Anesthesiology, Sedation, and Perioperative
    Medicine
Children's National Medical Center
Washington, District of Columbia

Ross M. Ungerleider, MD, MBA
Director, Heart Center
Driscoll Children's Hospital
Corpus Christi, Texas

Jamie Dickey Ungerleider, MSW, PhD
Coach and Wellness Consultant
Driscoll Children's Hospital
Corpus Christi, Texas

Graham D. Ungerleider, MD
Resident
Cardiothoracic Surgery
Keck School of Medicine of the University of Southern
    California
Los Angeles, California

Luca A. Vricella, MD
Professor of Surgery and Pediatrics
Director, Pediatric Cardiac Surgery and Transplantation
The Johns Hopkins University School of Medicine
Baltimore, Maryland

Eric L. Vu, MD
Assistant Professor of Anesthesiology and Perioperative and Pain
    Medicine
Baylor College of Medicine
Texas Children's Hospital
Houston, Texas

Rajeev S. Wadia, MD
Assistant Professor
Pediatric Cardiac Anesthesiologist and Critical Care Intensivist
The Johns Hopkins University School of Medicine
Baltimore, Maryland

Michael J. Walsh, MD
Associate Professor of Pediatrics
Wake Forest School of Medicine
Winston-Salem, North Carolina

Kevin M. Watt, MD, PhD
Department of Pediatrics
Duke Clinical Research Institute
Duke University
Durham, North Carolina

Karl Welke, MD, MS
Congenital Cardiac Surgeon
Sanger Heart and Vascular Institute
Levine Children's Hospital
Charlotte, North Carolina

Renée Willett, MD
Pediatric Cardiology Fellow
Boston Children's Hospital
Boston, Massachusetts

Derek A. Williams, DO
Associate Professor of Pediatric Cardiology
Wake Forest Baptist Health–Brenner Children's Hospital
Winston-Salem, North Carolina

Ronald K. Woods, MD, PhD
Associate Professor of Surgery
Division of Pediatric Cardiothoracic Surgery
Medical College of Wisconsin
Children's Hospital of Wisconsin
Milwaukee, Wisconsin

Charlotte Woods-Hill, MD
Pediatric Critical Care Attending
Anesthesia and Critical Care Medicine
Children's Hospital of Philadelphia
Philadelphia, Pennsylvania

Tharakanatha R. Yarrabolu, MD
Adjunct Assistant Professor
Texas A&M Health Science Center College of Medicine
Pediatric Cardiologist
Driscoll Health System
Driscoll Children's Hospital
Corpus Christi, Texas

Preface

Ring the bells that still can ring
Forget your perfect ending
There's a crack in everything
That's how the light gets in
That's how the light gets in

–**LEONARD COHEN**

This third edition of *Critical Heart Disease in Infants and Children* is written for the learner in each of you. Your learning part is connected to your courage piece—the element in you that is curious and willing to admit that you might "not know," and that is open to struggle as you grapple with new ways of thinking that sometimes challenge your well-groomed paradigms. Learners know that there is no single CAPITAL T Truth—that the truth is actually the consensus of numerous perspectives. This book is designed to offer numerous perspectives and invites you to take the ones that fit and that expand your ability to take care of children with complex heart disease.

The last edition of *Critical Heart Disease in Infants and Children* was published in 2006. The book, which was originally developed by David Nichols (now chair of the American Board of Pediatrics) was successful beyond expectations. It has served as a major resource for medical students, residents, faculty physicians, nurses, and other important health care providers who comprise the team of multidisciplinary providers who have helped advance the profession of pediatric cardiac critical care. For those of us who have participated in the development of this textbook, it has been a joy to see it on the shelves and countertops of intensive care units around the world.

Over the past few years, several of us have been asked why we haven't created a third edition. As if anything has changed since 2006! During the preparation and planning of this edition, we wanted to honor the enormous progress in our profession by creating a textbook with attention to numerous new topics (this edition has 28 more chapters than the second edition) while still keeping the material manageable. The first section of the book is devoted to the evolution of our specialty with regard to big picture thinking—leadership, systems, evaluation of outcome data, safety and quality collaboratives, ethics and decision making, family needs and expectations, and even training and mentoring. These are all new and unique and alone may help distinguish the value of this edition. Throughout the textbook, all chapters have been updated and, in many cases, we have invited new authors (not because of dissatisfaction with the previous authors—whose contributions we greatly appreciate and value—but because we wanted to invite new and emerging perspectives from others). In addition to updates on previous chapters, we have included chapters on low-birth-weight infants; bridging the fetus with critical heart disease to delivery and care; common general surgery issues for children with critical heart disease; management of common postoperative complications; the use of bedside ultrasound; biomarkers, transport, and stabilization of the newborn with critical heart disease; and adult congenital heart disease.

We have also created access to an online component that will provide the reader with the opportunity to view more expanded bibliographies, additional information (in appendix format), and even videos and other expanded media content.

You picked up this book to fill some of the "cracks" in you hungering for knowledge, and we, the editors, hope we have compiled a feast of helpful and useful information. We hope you enjoy letting in some of the light.

RMU
JNM
KNM
DSC
JPJ

Contents

Video Contents

1

Whole Brain Leadership for Creating Resonant Multidisciplinary Teams

ROSS M. UNGERLEIDER, MD, MBA; JAMIE DICKEY UNGERLEIDER, MSW, PHD

The animals decided they must do something to distinguish themselves and meet the challenges of a "new world" that demanded perfection. After consultation with experts, it was determined that development of universal expertise would be in their best interests, so they formed a leadership academy and adopted a curriculum consisting of running, climbing, digging, swimming, and flying. In order to produce the kind of expertise that would lead to best outcomes, all animals were mandated to take all the courses.

The duck was excellent in swimming. In fact, better than his instructor. But he made only passing grades in running and was very poor in climbing. He felt ashamed of his inability to climb and practiced until his webbed feet and wings were torn to a point where his swimming began to suffer.

The rabbit started at the top of the class in running but after an accident trying to fly from the "green" level takeoff platform, he had to go to a veterinarian, who placed his hind legs in a cast, and he was no longer able to run.

The squirrel was excellent in climbing but nearly drowned in the beginner's swimming class and was ridiculed by the fish, who told him he would never be able to swim due to his short arms and fluffy tail (which they felt was a disability) that when wet got heavy and weighed him down.

The eagle had a behavioral issue for which he was disciplined severely. In the climbing class, he beat all the others to the top of the tree but insisted on using his own way to get there and did not follow the "rules."

The birds all did great in flying, but many of them broke their beaks in digging, became unable to eat, and almost starved.

At the end of the year an abnormal frog that could swim exceeding well and also run, climb, and fly a little had the highest average and was declared valedictorian and the leader.

Modified from original fable by George Reavis

None of us is as smart as all of us.

Kenneth Blanchard

The culture of health care creates important challenges for health care professionals. In particular, we work in a culture that is (1) *hierarchical,* (2) *competitive,* and (3) *perfectionistic.* Unfortunately, the tendency of acquiescing to those demands is contrary to promoting resonant teamwork,[1] and it is important

for leaders of multidisciplinary teams to understand how to create environments that flatten the hierarchy (by encouraging all members of the team to contribute and to genuinely seek the wisdom and knowledge of their colleagues); environments that encourage collaboration and cooperation (emphasizing collective "wins" and "losses" both for the immediate team and for all of us, as a profession); and environments that invite excellence (which is a process) versus expectation of perfection (which is an unrealistic outcome).

The concepts described in this brief chapter emanate from our work coaching health care leaders (both authors are certified professional coaches and specialize in leadership coaching); consulting for health care systems and working for a variety of hospitals, academic medical centers, and medical schools; and from our training and experience in medicine (one author is a practicing pediatric cardiac surgeon), business, psychology, and interpersonal neurobiology (the science of relationships). Where appropriate, we provide references. Also, many of these concepts are nicely depicted in videos that accompany our presentations (some of which are linked in this chapter), and we encourage readers to watch them as they read.

Whole Brain Leadership

There is an increasing amount of information linking leadership to a combination of task and relational skills.[2-4] Information about brain function would attribute task-oriented focus to *left-brain* function and relationship-oriented focus to *right-brain* function. Interestingly, this dichotomy has been alluded to in health care as the difference between mechanical (predictable, linear) systems versus complex adaptive (unpredictable, nonlinear) systems.[5] In mechanical systems, behavior (and expected outcomes) conforms to reproducible patterns, and emergent (innovative) behavior is discouraged. For example, a ventilator is a mechanical system, and if it does not perform according to its settings, a repair person is called to *interrogate, judge, and fix* the system. Complex adaptive systems are unpredictable, and emergent (creative and innovative) behaviors can be welcomed with enthusiasm. In complex adaptive systems, differences are *explored* to be *understood and connected* (joined). A growing body of literature on leadership (far too expansive to reference here, but virtually every issue of *Harvard Business Review* for the past several years has articles on leadership)

• BOX 1.1   Qualities Attributed to Leadership Skill

Ability to be logical and realistic	Invites possibilities
Big picture orientation	Intuitive
Relationship focused	Task focused
Strategic/past aware	Good with numbers
Detailed	Values stories as information
Values facts as information	Good with concepts
Imaginative/creative	Analytical

TABLE 1.1   Leadership Qualities From Box 1.1 Reorganized Into "Whole Brain" Capacity

Left Brain	Right Brain
Ability to be logical and realistic	Invites possibilities
Detailed	Big picture orientation
Task focused	Relationship focused
Values facts as information	Values stories as information
Analytical	Intuitive
Good with numbers	Good with concepts
Strategic/Past aware	Imaginative/Creative

offers a variety of leadership traits such as many listed in Box 1.1. These leadership traits can be reorganized (Table 1.1) to better demonstrate the importance of what we refer to as *whole brain leadership*.

To develop and promote this kind of leadership, this chapter will outline a few areas for leadership development.

Integration

We define integration as the linkage of differentiated parts. That is essentially what great leaders do—they link differentiated parts. Integration is a delicate process. It is a dynamic and ever-changing challenge. Dan Siegel describes an integrated state as FACES (Flexible, Adaptive, Coherent, Energized, and Stable). Coherence is in itself an acronym[6] (Connected, Open, Harmonious, Engaged, Receptive, Emergent [creative], Noetic [inviting spontaneity and newness], Compassionate, Empathic), and all of these are important characteristics for a whole brain leader. Using this concept of integration, it is helpful to think of integration as the flowing of a river. Integrated states (FACES) are found in the middle of the river. On one riverbank is rigidity (linkage without differentiation), and on the other is chaos (differentiation without linkage). In rigid systems there is no allowance or acceptance for individual differences. A mechanical system is rigid. It is predictable and linear. Protocols and checklists can be rigid, and there is a space for them in all health care practices. Protocols and checklists prevent errors of omission, but they will not prevent errors of commission, as well as technical errors or errors of judgment. Protocols and checklists create conformity for tasks that lend themselves to conformity, but they do not necessarily create safety. (For instance, if the system is so rigid that no one is allowed to speak up to challenge a protocol—even when they see something that concerns them or when they have an "emergent" idea that

might be better—because it challenges a well-ingrained protocol, then the system becomes less flexible, unadaptive, and unsafe.) The animal school parable at the beginning of this chapter is an example of rigidity—making one size fit all and abolishing the unique and variable experiences and abilities of the differentiated members of a group. In chaotic systems there is no conformity. Differentiation abounds, and there is nothing linking the group—no common purpose or goal, no common beliefs, leaving no one to lead. Chaotic systems can be rich with ideas and energy, but without linkage through integrated leadership, there is no way to harness this "collective wisdom." The eventual outcome for these teams is *dis-integration*.

Whole brain leaders possess knowledge and awareness of the allure of these two riverbanks and try to keep their teams flowing in the river of integration.

Whole brain leaders can integrate their systems and create resonance in many ways, and some of these are described in the following sections.

Avoid Dissonance

To describe whole brain leadership in practical terms, we like to imagine that whole brain leaders are integrating three primary elements: self, others, and context, and we have described this in previous publications.[7,8] The challenges faced on teams generally revolve around these three entities.

Self. What are my needs? What are my opinions? What do I think I know, and what am I very committed to? What are my fears, and do I have enough self-awareness and comfort to be able to acknowledge them? What are my biases? Can I access any potential "unconscious biases" (see Chapter 9)? There is voluminous literature citing the importance of leaders having impeccable self-awareness and willingness to learn and to grow, and some ways that this can be manifested are described later in this chapter. Self-awareness is the first element for emotional intelligence, and whole brain leaders are emotionally intelligent.

Others. Whole brain leadership is relational leadership and requires the ability and willingness to value the perspectives of others. Resonant, whole brain leaders understand that just like themselves, all individuals in the system have needs, opinions, knowledge, and commitments. Whole brain leaders create resonance by making it apparent to team members that their individual and collective needs, values, opinions, ideas, and information are also known and considered as important. Leaders can do this by asking questions, being curious, and simply caring about the needs of others. This ability to develop genuine caring for the members of the team is considered by many successful leaders to be the keystone of successful leadership,[9,10] and it is an essential cultivator for resonance within the system. Whole brain leaders *genuinely care,* and they also *care in general,* meaning that they understand the power of story. Everyone in the system has a "story," and when we can know the story, then the system and how people are behaving or what they are wanting makes more sense. A powerful example of "caring in general" was created by the Cleveland Clinic Foundation in their video on empathy (https://www.youtube.com/watch?v=cDDWvj_q-o8). Valuing and tapping into the needs, knowledge, and experience of others is what makes whole brain leaders powerful and resonant. Whole brain leaders genuinely care, and they do this by exhibiting four major qualities that drive connection: (1) perspective taking (inquiring with curiosity to try and understand the experiences of others); (2) avoiding judgment regarding someone else's "truth"; (3) recognizing emotion in other people (which requires being "present" to the felt experience of others—having a sense for what might be happening for them "below the surface" that might not be expressed by their words); and (4) communicating and validating the importance of those emotions. These traits can be both learned and developed and are essential for whole brain leadership. The difference between empathy and sympathy is also beautifully described by Brené Brown (https://www.youtube.com/watch?v=1Evwgu369Jw) as the difference between driving disconnection versus driving connection. Creating connection is an essential component of resonant teamwork. In resonant teams all members are important and valuable; the team is a single organism, and when one part is affected, the entire organism is affected. Whole brain leaders understand this and cultivate that oneness through genuine caring.

Context. Context is the elephant in the room for health care. Context is the patient, the situation, the reason for us working together, the ever-present "need" that drives our health care world. Context is huge and just like each of us, has needs that must be acknowledged and valued. Teamwork would be difficult enough if it simply required us to "get along" with each other; it becomes daunting when we have to do this in the shadow of urgent, life-threatening, win-or-lose situations that challenge all that we might know and be capable of doing. Add to that challenge the perceived need for perfection, and we have the perfect storm. It is no wonder that many health care teams dis-integrate into rigidity (there is a single answer, and, by the way, it is the one espoused by the leader) or chaos (there is no way we can work together because we all have different opinions about how to get better results). Resonant teams understand that outcomes are an *indicator* of process *drivers.* Paul Baltaldan states that "every system is perfectly designed to give you the results you get," and some systems fall into chaos when the individuals disconnect from process and begin to focus solely on outcome.[11] Outcomes derive from structure and process (well described by the Donabedian model for health care quality or the Balanced Scorecard[12] approach to best outcomes) (see Chapter 2).

In their book *Primal Leadership,*[9] Daniel Goleman, Richard Boyatzis, and Annie McKee describe the concept of *resonant leadership* and provide a few examples of both resonant and dissonant leadership styles. Boyatzis and McKee went on to write an entire book on resonant leadership,[13] and their work is incorporated in our concept of whole brain leadership for creating resonant teamwork.[1,8] (Our work is also based on contributions from *many* others we have studied [and in some cases worked with] over the course of almost two decades, including Dan Siegel, Virginia Satir, Jean McLendon, Sidney Dekker, Don Beck, John Gottman, Doug Silsbee, Brené Brown, and Richard Strozzi-Heckler to name just a few).[1,3,4,10,14-32]

Whole brain leaders create resonance by understanding that *rigid* adherence to certain styles might fail to integrate the competing needs of self, others, and context, and over time this will lead to dissonance within a system. When there is dissonance, there is lack of positive energy, and members of these teams describe their working environment as follows: "sucking the energy from me," "oppressive," "it feels unsafe," "there is no point to my being here because no one cares what I think," "I just show up and do what I'm told" (which is symptomatic of a system that has disregarded someone's potential for unique contribution), "I'm looking for another job somewhere" (I'm checking out), or "I just come to work to make money so I can have a life outside of here" (I've checked out). Any of these, and other

comments that we have collected and reported,[11] are indicative that the system (team) is dissonant. We have now "collected" seven behaviors that we have observed in health care leaders that are dissonant leadership styles when used exclusively and exhaustively over time. We have also observed these behaviors in health care professionals. They are human behaviors inherent not just to leaders (who are every bit as human as the people they lead). Each of these behaviors shares lack of integration of self, other, and context. They are briefly described in the following sections.

Dissonant Styles in Which the Leader Fails to Integrate Others as Valuable Contributors to the Team

Commanding. These leaders are typically always "in charge" and lack curiosity to explore the stories of others. They commonly blame others or circumstances when things go wrong, have difficulty accepting any accountability, and exhibit little capacity for listening, asking, inquiring. They already know. Commanding leaders simply say, "Do it because I say so." The Federal Aviation Administration created cockpit resource management[33] to counteract the potential damage that can be done by a commanding leader who is unable or unwilling to access ideas, opinions, or information from others. Likewise, Karl Weick has written about how High Consequence Organizations can become High Reliability Organizations[34] by "flattening the hierarchy" to protect against commanding leaders when there are unexpected and potentially catastrophic events. In Weick's model the most important person on a team, at any moment in time, is the person with the most important and relevant information. It is the role of the leader to access that information, wherever and in whomever it resides. An example of a commanding leader is nicely demonstrated in this video (https://www.youtube.com/watch?v=sYsdUgEgJrY).

Pacesetting. This term was suggested in *Primal Leadership,*[9] and we have found it to be especially prevalent in cardiac teams, where perfection is often the goal. Pacesetting can be extremely dangerous because it always seems to be motivated by a "noble" need to do things right. Ironically, many people who have trained in medicine have been taught that "if you want a job done right, do it yourself." That is pacesetting. (Actually, if you want a job done *your way,* do it yourself; if you want it done "right," then it can be done by many people as long as you can accept that the "right" way will look different, and often unique and innovative, when you can let go of only one way being "right.") Pacesetters discourage emergent behaviors because their way is the right way, and this ultimately creates an environment of *mistrust* (a general sense of unease with someone or something) or *distrust* (lack of trust based on experience with someone or something). Pacesetters demand perfection (meaning the outcome must be precisely their way), and it is often simply not possible to satisfy them, so team members simply stop trying (and this leads to the experience of being no longer valuable to the team because one's opinions, knowledge, experience, and ideas are simply not welcomed). Pacesetters see themselves as being indispensable leaders because without their expertise, everything would fall apart. Ironically, pacesetters often become blamers when things do fall apart, despite their best intentions. Pacesetting can be insidious. Although pacesetting might be manifested by open disregard for the ideas of others, it can also be conveyed by the leader who simply comes along and does everything their way, even after the team has already agreed on a different plan. See if you can recognize the pacesetting in this video (https://www.youtube.com/watch?v=ZZv1vki4ou4).

Manipulating. Manipulation is the ultimate creator of mistrust. Leaders who manipulate are typically dishonest and unable or unwilling to communicate their needs. They typically abuse their position of authority to simply "trick" people into giving in to what they, the leader, wants. Leaders can gain insight that they are possibly being motivated to manipulate when they approach a dialogue, conflict, or problem with a predetermined conclusion regarding what they want and they begin thinking of strategies to get their needs met without wanting to directly express those needs. Manipulators are master strategists, and they are often fairly remorseless about the impact of their strategies on others. Their end justifies their means. They are driven solely by making sure they get their needs met, and they are never transparent.[35]

Dissonant Styles in Which the Leader Fails to Integrate Self as a Valuable Contributor to the Team

Placating. Placaters are driven by the need to be liked and to also make people on the team happy. Ironically, they generally fail at both. They become nontrusted because they do not express genuinely consistent values that team members know the leader is committed to. Instead, they seem to be constantly influenced by the last person who has talked with them. They can be paralyzed from making critical decisions because they are constantly worried about how they might be perceived or judged by others, particularly if they fail (and failure is common because little that these leaders do is an expression of their authentic skill set). Placaters invite chaos because rather than knowing how to "link," they give in to the constant demands of unending differentiation in the system. In trying to keep everyone happy, they become exhausted and frustrated; a sign of placating is occasional emotional explosion as the exhausted placater erupts against the disorganized demands coming at the leader from every insatiable source. Unfortunately, our health care culture risks the development of placating as a cultural norm as we are constantly reminded "to put the needs of others before our own."[36] In fact, the Accreditation Council for Graduate Medical Education (ACGME) definition of professionalism uses those precise words as an example of what professionalism requires. The conundrum is that we are all human and we have needs, and sometimes those needs, when they are not appropriately acknowledged and valued, continue to express themselves "below the surface" until they simply come out sideways or explode out the top. The antidote for placating is unflinching self-awareness to know what is important to us; self-compassion[37-39] for ourselves as learners and as valuable members of the team; and to constantly develop mindfulness around our evolving selves. Whereas commanding, pacesetting, and manipulating eradicate others, placating eradicates the self; it creates a form of relational suicide, and it is simply nonsustainable. In our work with (and in our own development as) leaders, this insatiable need to please others has created a common challenge, and the solution is simply to gently reacquaint ourselves with our humanness, the validity of our needs (values, opinions, knowledge, and skills), and some tools for integrating ourselves into a culture that has normalized disregard of the self. The patient (our context) always comes first. And so do you. And so do others. Whole brain leaders recognize the challenge of linking those differentiated parts without excluding the part that is themselves. It is a constant challenge to hang on to the self, and it is necessary to simply know that, because your team needs YOU and all the unique and extraordinary features that an authentic YOU can bring to the team.

Dissonant Styles in Which the Leader Fails to Integrate Context as a Valuable Component of the Team

Super Reasonable. We have seen this dissonant style most frequently when we have measured dissonant styles in medical systems. It seems to be the most convenient style that satisfies the need for our systems to be predictable and reproducible. It is a mechanical style because it disregards our human needs and variables. Mechanical focus works for mechanical systems (ventilators, heart lung machines, elevators, airplanes) that can be interrogated (inspected) and fixed. Human systems are complex adaptive systems, and the beauty of complex adaptive systems is that they express emergent (innovative) and unique behaviors that are not always predictable. None of us wants to be "fixed." We would rather be "explored and understood." Super reasonable dissonance treats people like robots (https://www.youtube.com/watch?v=753eH92u2B0), and a machine cannot give you what a person can. When leaders treat people like machines, they essentially are devaluing and dismissing the importance of our human factor. The only thing that is important is the *context.* Context is ubiquitous. There is always a sick patient, a chapter that needs to be written, a lecture to prepare, teaching rounds to attend, a meeting for making an important decision … always something to occupy us and distract us from our humanness. (Ironically, in recent years, "human factor" has become a phrase that connects our human capacity for making mistakes to the risk of error in medical systems. However, it is also our human capability for innovating, observing, and preventing mistakes that can lead to extraordinary advances and safety in medical systems. We have found ways to measure the lives *lost* through "human error,"[5] but how do we measure the lives *saved* because of our incredible human contributions?)

The insidious impact of denying our humanness is commonplace in medicine when super reasonable becomes the driving force. This is beautifully and poignantly portrayed in the movie *The Doctor* with William Hurt. In this movie William Hurt is a heart surgeon (how ironic) who develops cancer, and when his physician is informing him that he can begin radiation therapy on Thursday, he states that he cannot do that because he "has a heart surgery scheduled for Thursday." It takes his wife, sitting next to him, to overrule that objection and state, "No, Thursday is fine." He has cancer. He is human. He is attentive to context. That is super reasonable. (A bit later in this movie, he comes home early from work, and his wife calls their son, Nick, to come down and say hi to his father. Nick runs downstairs and picks up the phone and says, "Hi Dad" without even noticing his father standing there in the room. Of course, there is no one on the phone, and Nick says, "Mom, we got disconnected." Then Nick looks up and is totally surprised to see his father, in the flesh.) Super reasonable is a sure way to disconnection.

In Chapter 9 the syndrome of physician burnout is described, and one of the factors associated with burnout is *depersonalization,* which is a measured consequence of our medical education process. We have recorded a progressive increase in depersonalization across 4 years of medical school education for one group of students at a nationally recognized medical school. The class cohort shows an increase of depersonalization from approximately 10% of students at the beginning of medical school—during orientation—to approximately 45% of students at the completion of 4 years of medical school. Most disturbingly, depersonalization, unlike feelings of depression, anxiety, and other factors linked to burnout (which exhibit phasic increases and decreases throughout medical education), progressively increases and does not regress once it occurs. From this one medical school, almost half the graduating physicians are depersonalized at the time they begin their medical residency training.[40] Depersonalized physicians have just as many needs as they had before they became depersonalized; they are simply less aware of and less compassionate toward them. Ultimately, they begin to treat all people in the system (including their patients) as they have learned to treat themselves. Depersonalized (super reasonable) systems are subject to an 11-fold increase in medical errors, as well as to unprofessional and immoral acts, in addition to ultimate dis-integration from people who want more for their lives than burnout. Systems with depersonalized leaders feel oppressive and dehumanized. It is not possible to exist in them over the long haul, and they exhibit frequent turnover. Team members find ways to "check out," and there have also been reported examples of some leaders who have committed suicide because they cannot be perfect.

Dissonant Styles in Which the Leader Fails to Integrate Self, Others, and Context—A Totally Chaotic and Differentiated Team That Has No Linkage

Irrelevant. Irrelevance occurs when people become overwhelmed and are no longer capable of accessing their own needs or being available to the needs of others or the context. Irrelevance is nonattuned leadership; it is not focused, and it fails to connect. These are simply leaders who have "checked out" and who are no longer available. Unlike invisible leaders (described in the next paragraph), these leaders are often distracting with their presence. An example might be the leader who continually cracks jokes even when things are falling apart and need their attention. Irrelevant leaders tend to try to "minimize" problems and are not available to hear the very real concerns of their team members. Likewise, they tend to minimize important context issues and might not respond appropriately. Charles Bosk[41] termed the kind of errors these leaders make as "normative errors," meaning they fail to perform the normal duties and responsibilities of their leadership role. Irrelevance creates dissonance because the members of the team become discouraged that their leader is not "available" to connect with them around their concerns and instead is a distracting presence when they need to have focus. At an extreme the irrelevant leader has given in to substance abuse as a form of escape from the demands of the job. Irrelevance might seem funny and creative to the leader, but the leader is not attuned to the needs of the team.[1]

Invisible. Invisible leaders are not present for their "leadership moments." This is nicely described by Sidney Dekker in his work on "Just Culture."[29] The members of the team become secondary victims of an unexpected or untoward event. There are times when the team needs a leader to "step up" and take accountability for the team or to make a critical decision or to simply be "the leader." Invisible leaders tend to hide at these times in the hope that the moment will pass (unnoticed) or that they might escape unscathed. Many years ago the national media covered an "error" at a major medical center.[42] The hospital leader was not visible on the newscasts. Ultimately, an individual on the team got the majority of the blame. How different it might have been had the leader been immediately present and made a statement such as "This was a terrible tragedy for this patient; AND (we find it is always useful to insert "and" in place of "but," so as not to diminish the value of the immediately preceding statement; try it sometime) this was also a terrible tragedy for our extraordinary health care team—some of the best doctors and nurses in the world; AND this was a terrible tragedy for our hospital that this happened, and we commit to trying to understand how these things happen so that we can,

TABLE 1.2	Beneficial Leadership Traits When Strengths Used Appropriately
Strength Overdone	**Strength Used Appropriately**
Dissonant version	Resonant version
Commanding	Assertiveness
Pacesetting	Competence
Manipulating	Strategic
Placating	Genuine caring
Super reasonable	Logical
Irrelevant	Creative and fun
Invisible	Self-protective

as a health care system—as a really exceptional health care system experiencing a terrible tragedy—help prevent this from happening again—here or elsewhere." But the leader was not visible. He was nowhere to be found, and the events unfolded differently. Some of the members of that team are still affected by that lack of leadership.

All of these styles become dissonant when they are used exclusively, over time, as the most predictable response by the leader to a problem. The dissonance is created by the lack of FACES that resonant, whole brain leaders require in order to navigate the river of integration. Ironically, leaders (all of us) have access to each of these styles and, when integrated into a complete repertoire of response, can create a more vibrant ability to adapt and perform effectively. Each of these styles actually exists on a *continuum* or *spectrum* of strengths. When the strengths are overdone, they can lead to dissonance, but a strength used appropriately can be a powerful tool or style. In Table 1.2 we demonstrate how the style might look along this spectrum, with the "strength overdone" being represented as the dissonant style and the strength being used when needed and at appropriate times representing the more resonant version.

Whole brain leaders create resonance through their ability to integrate the various and changing needs of self, others, and context into a dynamic and stable system. They access a wide range of possibilities that include tasks that need to be accomplished, problems that need to be solved, and the needs of the people in the system that need to be valued. An example of this is nicely portrayed in the story of a young surgeon on vacation with his wife published many years ago when the ACGME first introduced their duty hour restriction, and we recommend reading it now so that you can integrate the information about resonance into your understanding of the story.[7]

Avoid the Four Horsemen of the Apocalypse

Several decades ago, a (then) young researcher in Seattle began investigating how couples managed conflict and how their management styles were connected with the ultimate fate of their marriage. John Gottman was a mathematician who believed that he could find logical explanations for how relationships thrived or disintegrated. His first book, *Why Marriages Succeed or Fail,* was a seminal work and becomes particularly relevant to teams taking care of critically ill infants when the word *Teams* is inserted in place of the word *Marriages.* Gottman's extraordinary work (based on extensive quantitative and qualitative research) became nationally prominent when it was recognized that he could watch a couple in conflict for approximately 2 minutes and then predict (with 95% accuracy over 15-year follow-up) whether they would stay married or end up divorced. He could even predict whether they would divorce early (within 4 years) or late (after 8 years) with the same 95% accuracy. His work was mentioned by Malcolm Gladwell in his book, *Blink,* and it has long served an important role in our own work with resonance in medical teams and the development of whole brain leadership. In his book, Gottman described the "four horsemen of the Apocalypse," and what he noticed as destroyers of couples relationships are every bit as relevant for team relationships. Whole brain leaders need to be aware of these four destructive influences and acquainted with the antidotes for them. We briefly describe them in the following paragraphs (and recognize that there is a lot of information around these factors that cannot be covered in the scope of this chapter).

Criticism. Criticism is poison, and it is ubiquitous on medical teams. Criticism is personal, and it is designed to identify a culprit and let that person know how much he or she is to blame. Criticism is the finger pointing at someone, chastising the person for a mistake. (Notice that when you are pointing a finger at someone, where your other three fingers are pointing!) Criticism is a form of punishment doled out to the offending party, and research on punishment is consistent—punishment does not work in technical fields. It only creates more of the undesirable behavior as people begin to focus more on how to avoid punishment rather than engaging in the more challenging process of trying to understand the driving force for their behavior. Punishment creates fear of future punishment, and the undesirable consequences of this have been well described by others as creating a proclivity to "choke"[43] or to disengage from the team or simply to find clever ways to disguise action to avoid more punishment. Regardless, criticism is destructive, and it generally makes everyone on a team feel demoralized and either afraid that they may be next to be criticized or simply feel badly for their colleague and teammate who is the recipient of the criticism. Criticism rarely creates problem solving as much as it creates polarization into the people who are "right" versus the people who are "wrong." The antidote for criticism is *complaint.* A complaint is not personal, and it invites ALL team members to engage in problem solving. Problems do not have names—they are gender neutral. Imagine the difference between criticism and complaint as if the problem is represented as a soccer ball. Criticism is like putting the soccer ball inside someone and then kicking the person around. A complaint is like putting the soccer ball on the floor and letting everyone kick it around. The problem is not "why do *YOU* keep killing all my neonates with your poor management?" (personal—ouch!) The problem is "*WE* keep struggling with our neonatal outcomes. What kinds of things should *WE* try to do differently?"

Contempt. Of the four horsemen, contempt may be the most destructive. Contempt does not necessarily require words; contempt can be conveyed by an expression (such as a slight tilt of the head and a rolling of the eyes). Contempt is a total annihilation of an "other." Contempt is essentially a way of discrediting the value of another team member and minimizing that member's importance to the team. Whole brain leaders develop antennae for contempt, and they do everything they can to remove it. The antidote for contempt is appreciation for what others know and can bring to the system. It has been written that great leadership requires great followership, meaning there are times to stop pacesetting and commanding and let another team member do what that person does best. Pacesetting is a subtle form of contempt

because pacesetters have a belief that there is only one way to do a job—their way. When contempt is expressed openly as disdain for the abilities of someone in the system, the system will need intervention to heal or it will disintegrate. One way to create this anticontempt energy in a system is to have team members identify the strengths of each member of the team and to make sure that those strengths are expressed as appreciations publicly and openly. Quin Studer describes a process of "managing up,"[44] which is a way of spreading positive stories about other people on the team. Notice the times that contempt appears in your system, either subtlety or overtly. And imagine how it might be different if the perspective of the recipient of the contempt were understood.

Defensiveness. Defensiveness is the other side of "blame." It is in effect the same as saying, "I didn't do it. She did it." Defensiveness is often found in systems in which the leader has allowed punishment and criticism to exist, so defensiveness is expressed as a way to avoid these consequences. The problem with defensiveness is that it creates divisiveness. Defensiveness does not need to exist in resonant systems where accountability is a part of problem solving as opposed to a part of the blame-seeking process. The antidote to defensiveness is self-accountability. Next time you have a quality improvement conference (morbidity and mortality conference) and a difficult outcome is being examined, try going around the room and, instead of assigning blame (root cause analysis), have each team member courageously take accountability for some piece of the outcome. What would each member have done differently, in retrospect? Have each team member imagine something he or she might wish he or she could have done now that the team member knows what happened. This creates a culture that reinforces our connectedness and dependence on one another. This interconnectedness of random events—often seemingly unrelated—contributing to one single occurrence is important for us to understand as we try to make sense of the overwhelming nature of what we experience. It is beautifully portrayed in the accident scene from Benjamin Button (https://www.youtube.com/watch?v=mTDs0lvFuMc#t=32.076865449). In many of our programs, the taxi driver (often the surgeon) who is at the end of a series of events gets the "blame" for an event, but "life, being what it is, a series of interconnected events," can sometimes result in an outcome that is the result of so many small events along the line. The power of self (and shared) accountability is enormously helpful to us as we attempt to put these events into perspective so that we can create resonance; understand interconnectedness; and remove blame and defensiveness as blockades to team understanding, improvement, and growth.

Flooding. Flooding refers to emotional overload. When we get flooded, we simply want to shut down and not address the moment. This can leave others on the team feeling abandoned, unheard, or ignored. When I (RMU) finish a challenging operation and return to my office, I am sometimes "flooded," and if my administrative assistant bombards me with a lot of requests—phone calls to return, tasks that need attention—I just want to ignore them. She might take this personally, when actually the person with the immediate need is me. So I have told my assistant that when I come back from the operating room and close the door to my office, it has nothing to do with her—I simply need time to recenter myself so that I am ready to be available. We have found that this works well, and the antidote for flooding is "self-soothing," which can simply be acknowledging as a leader that people (including the leader) have needs to center and reconnect to their internal resources so that they can move on to the next demand. We have described internal resources in previous publications,[45] and they can serve as a useful source for resilience and integration.

In the Prochaska change model, growth and change occur as we move from unconscious incompetence to conscious incompetence. That is a huge move—we simply become aware of our limitations and challenges. For whole brain leaders, this is a necessary movement. Nothing really changes. We are still incompetent, AND we are now available to learn tools to move us, slowly but inexorably, toward conscious competence and eventually (with practice and mastery—internal integration) to unconscious competence—and that is transformational change from which we never go back.

The following sections describe, briefly, a few leadership tools to consider. There are many, and we are simply presenting a few.

Accept Influence

In his work with couples, Gottman described (for his interview with the *Harvard Business Review*) the ability to "accept influence" as one of the most important elements for creating healthy relationships.[46] We have found this to be especially effective for medical teams. Accepting influence invites all the members of the team to be engaged and valued and to participate. By nature, leaders who accept influence have found a way to abolish contempt and to "push the up button" as they create joy and resourcefulness for their team, as well as a culture that promotes learning, growth, and change.[1] Accepting influence is a cultural change as much as it is a leadership tool. Imagine that in your organization you have a saltshaker full of "yes" crystals that you can sprinkle around liberally: "Yes, that is a good idea. Let's try it." "Yes, please keep calling me when you have concerns." "Yes, that would be great if you would present that information at our next conference." "Yes, I appreciate your thoughts on this." "Yes." "Yes" creates a different culture than the more typical "No" culture, where the saltshaker sprinkles around: "No, we don't do things that way around here." "No, when I want your opinion, I'll ask for it." "No, that is not something we're going to try." "No, I don't want your help." "No, I don't really care what you think." Which culture would feel more attractive to you? Furthermore, when we hear (or even feel or sense) "no," it often invites implicit memories of not getting our needs met. Consistent "no" might lead members of a team to give up and stop trying because trying will only bring on another "no." Leaders who emphasize accepting influence can do this in numerous ways—allowing others in the system to make suggestions and then taking those suggestions, even (especially) when they are different than the cultural "norm." This indicates to the team members that change is valued and ideas are respected.

There is a very instructive scene in the movie *Master and Commander* with Russell Crowe. He is the captain of a ship and is called to the deck because the person on watch "thinks" he saw an enemy ship through his spyglass. "You think you saw it?" asks Crowe. "Yes, I think so. I can't be sure. It was only for a moment—through the fog." Crowe then asks another member of the crew if he saw it. "No, sir. I didn't." Now this is a situation that would be ripe for contempt (disdain) and dismissal of the experience of the person in the minority opinion—in this case the person who "thinks" he "might" have seen something. In some dissonant teams there might be a sneering diminishment of the crew member who "thought" he saw something "only for a moment," unconfirmed by a more "trusted" team member. But Crowe does not take the bait. Instead he says, "Well, you did the right thing." (That is a way of sprinkling a "yes.") "Go back to your posts. Thank you." (another "yes") Then he (the captain) begins looking to verify if

there is an enemy ship. He sees it and provides the warning in time to save the crew—all because he "accepted influence." We can all do this. In a presidential address to the Southern Thoracic Surgical Association, a virtually uninterpretable photo of a cow is displayed by the speaker.[47] Only a few members of the audience even recognize it for what it is. If the leader simply ignores their perspective because he or she does not see what they see, then he or she misses out on valuable information because when the photo is redisplayed without the confusing background, the cow is readily apparent and can be seen by everyone in the audience. Accepting influence is a powerful tool for a leader to introduce into the system. It gives permission for people to speak up without fear of being ridiculed, ignored, or dismissed, and it allows the system to be greater than the limitations of any one person. If only one person sees something and the rest of the team is willing to accept the reality that someone is seeing something they themselves have not seen and they become curious to know more about what was seen and how they, too, might be able to see it, then the entire team becomes more powerful. Whole brain leaders accept influence because they genuinely value the perspectives of others, and they make their teams powerful as a result.

Be Ratio Minded

In an elegant investigation of the role of positivity and connectivity for business teams, Losade and Heaphy, from the University of Michigan School of Business, described the interrelationship between a variety of parameters to quality of performance.[48] Connectivity (an essential trait for whole brain leaders) became a control parameter that was linked to various ratios that were associated with whether the teams performed at a high, medium, or low level. A graph of their findings is displayed in Fig.1.1.

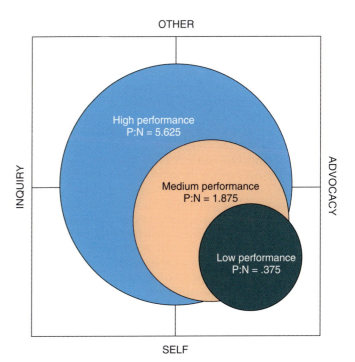

• **Figure 1.1** Emotional space projected over Inquiry/Advocacy and Other/Self. (Modified from Losade M, Heaphy E. The role of positivity and connectivity in performance of business teams: a nonlinear dynamic model. *Am Behav Sci.* 2004;47:740-765.)

TABLE 1.3	Team Function Ratios		
Ratio	High	Medium	Low
P:N	5.6:1	1.8:1	1:20
I:A	1:1	2:3	1:3
O:S	1:1	2:3	1:30

P:N, Positive versus Negative; *I:A,* Inquiry versus Advocacy; *O:S,* Other versus Self
From Losade M, Heaphy E. The role of positivity and connectivity in performance of business teams: a nonlinear dynamic model. *Am Behav Sci.* 2004;47:740-765.

What is remarkable about their findings is that the increasing ratio of positive to negative emotions (often referred to as essential for high performance) is interrelated to the ratio of "other-focus" versus "self-focus" and to the ratio of "inquiry" (curiosity about the perspectives of others) versus "advocacy" (fixed commitment to one's own perspective). The remarkable association of these three ratios to performance is displayed in Table 1.3.

Positive Versus Negative. The ratio and importance of positive to negative has long been emphasized by some organizations as crucial to high performance. What is more difficult to understand is that the relationship between positive and negative is very complex. Some teams have stated that it is easier to feel positive when things are going well and that therefore this ratio is really the result of how well the team is performing, not the other way around. However, Losade and Heaphy's research, as well as research by Gottman,[21,49] Fredrickson,[19,50,51] and others has demonstrated that it is actually the ability to create positivity that far exceeds negativity that leads to the better outcomes for teams. This is a ratio that is generated by whole brain leaders and in its most mature forms, is associated with high performance. The actual desired ratio varies from 3:1 (Fredrickson) to 5:1 (Gottman) to Losade and Heaphy's 5.6:1, likely depending on the type of team and what is being measured. However, three things are important to take away from this research. The first is the power of negativity. It takes much more positive to overcome the negative to produce high performance. The second is the absolute necessity for negativity to be present. Negative experience is important to acknowledge in a system. Without the negative there is a risk for false harmony,[52] and this would ultimately eradicate any credibility to positivity. Finally, from Losade and Heaphy's work is the critical interdependence of P:N with O:S and I:A. In the figure (see Fig. 1.1), P:N increases as the axis moves to the upper left quadrants ("other-focus" and "inquiry") and away from the lower right quadrant ("self-focus" and "advocacy"). High performance is a complex result of tools that whole brain leaders can employ to create more space for the perspectives of others (versus considering only their own self-perspective to have merit) as well as inquiring (with curious exploration, as one would for complex adaptive systems) to learn more about the opinions, perspectives, and knowledge of others rather than constantly advocating their own beliefs (and limiting the team to only what they know or believe). There are numerous techniques that leaders who are aware of these ratios can employ to improve performance of their teams.

Other Versus Self. A few things that leaders can do to improve the O:S ratio include cultivating connections among team members. One way to do this is to expand awareness of who the "others" are and appreciation for the wide array of talents, interests, and passions that we each bring to our teams. In our work with teams, we have sometimes referred to this as "attunement" (Dan Siegel would call this "mindsight").[1,28] Typically in our professional cultures, we refer to each other with titles (e.g., professor and chief of cardiothoracic surgery, nurse manager, director of in-patient services, lead perfusionist, assistant professor, staff nurse, chief executive officer, grand master), and these titles are often displayed on our name badges as if that defines who we really are. We have introduced to some teams the concept of slash IDs—that is, after our official title, there is a slash and then the rest of who we are, such as avid golfer, fisherman, reader, sports fanatic, and father of five children; or dog lover, cook, and stargazer—anything that tells our team we are more than a title. We have seen people actually inadvertently try to accomplish this when they have placed photos of their children or pets over their own on their name badge. The slash ID simply expands this to provide a larger window into the world of those wonderful "others" who are on our team. Another way whole brain leaders validate the perspectives of others is by accepting influence and cultivating a culture that invites engagement by all the members of the team. Finally, whole brain leaders validate the value of others by both "making" and "accepting" repair attempts. There has been a lot of work demonstrating that our most positive mentors have been the ones who have supported and nurtured us when we made mistakes. Mistakes made in an environment of support and caring are commensurate with learning.[53] In our systems we encounter errors, and sometimes this leads to "ruptured" relationships. One of the most powerful tools for healing these ruptures is to offer a repair attempt (a genuine, sincere apology), and more important than that (particularly for the leader to model) is to accept the repair attempt with compassion and understanding that ruptures and errors are a necessary part of our learning and growing processes. The power of an accepted repair is enormous, and the damage from a cursorily dismissed repair is equally important to appreciate. When a team member musters the courage to offer a repair, we serve our teams by stopping and simply noticing that this tender moment is an opportunity for us to heal (when we accept the repair with kindness and sensitivity) and with that healing, move forward to our next challenges.

Inquiry Versus Advocacy. There are many ways a leader can cultivate inquiry. One of the most powerful is to invite learning into the team. Carol Dweck has spent a lifetime describing the difference between learners (growth mindset) versus knowers (fixed mindset). Her work is beautifully portrayed in her book *Mindset,*[17] and we have referred to it in previous publications.[1,11,53] All of our teams are rich with talented, knowledgeable, capable, and passionate members who want the same thing: to do a great job taking care of sick patients. Each team member brings a unique set of information, experience, and ability. Whole brain leaders recognize that every one of us is an expert in something, so we are not afraid to ask for advice or for help. Inquiry is manifested as genuine, curious exploration to understand the perspectives and actions of another. Too often on medical teams, we observe inquiry as "inquisition"—the grilling of someone (who likely is about to be criticized, blamed, or disdained) to demonstrate that they are wrong—as opposed to genuine curious exploration to try and understand another's perspective. We can—should—imagine how to ask questions that help us understand rather than accuse, embarrass, or destroy. This is a difficult technique to learn. However, with commitment, training, and practice, whole brain leaders can achieve conscious competence and uncover new ways of connecting to their team member's ideas and to each other.

Learning is hard. We get stuck in schema (our strongly held belief in something), and then we evaluate information as either correct (it validates our belief) or as incorrect (it contradicts our belief). Ironically we can often find validation in the literature to support our strongly held beliefs; there is almost always a study to support or to contradict what we want to believe is true. Inquiry permits us to practice finding alternative information and other ways of managing a difficult problem. Inquiring leaders expand rather than contract the scope of their team's repository of possibilities and create opportunities that are flexible, adaptive, coherent, energized, and stable. In this sense, whole brain leaders promote the very nature of complex adaptive systems and permit growth, change, and learning, and with that, joy and positivity that lead to high performance.

Awareness of the impact of positivity, inquiry, and valuing the experience of others is a key ingredient for developing team resonance versus dissonance. Teams have an emotional culture[54] that whole brain leaders are attentive to. Emotional culture influences employee satisfaction, burnout, teamwork, and even hard measures such as financial performance and absenteeism. Positive emotions are consistently associated with better performance, quality, and customer service. Negative emotions such as group anger, sadness, fear, and the like usually lead to negative outcomes, including poor performance and high turnover.[54] Most people can generally distinguish as many as 135 different emotions, and even when this is occurring at a level below conscious awareness, these emotions can greatly affect how we feel or behave. We are all greatly influenced by what is happening around us through our mirror neurons.[55] Our ability to "attune" to the energy in our environment is what has helped to keep us "safe" through evolution. Notice your ability to be aware when you walk into a room of what the "energy" is in that room—is it safe, or tense, or joyful? Whole brain leaders remain attuned to and understand the importance of emotions such as joy, love, anger, fear, and sadness. These emotions become a valuable "dipstick" for team performance for leaders who are able to cultivate access to them.

Create Vision (Discover the "And")

Some of the best work we have encountered on teamwork relates to the importance of discovering the shared purpose and meaning for the team.[30] There are many ways for leaders to do this, and in the most effective circumstances, the shared mission is real and meaningful for all team members. This means that leaders cannot simply insert their vision as the team vision. The team vision needs to be crafted and constructed through exploration and understanding of what the organization is uniquely positioned to produce and what the team members value. All programs that deliver care to children with critical heart disease want to be "excellent," but excellence is a very general word and can manifest differently in a variety of programs. Some programs may define excellence as uniqueness, emphasizing techniques or procedures that they offer and in which they truly excel. Others may point to the volume of cases they perform and their outcomes for those cases (measured as Society of Thoracic Surgeons outcomes). Other programs may consider the nature of the procedures they perform and how they produce outcomes with best long-term quality of life. Finally, some programs may consider excellence to be manifested as being a truly great place in which to work (e.g., a J.D. Power top 100 place to work). Collins addresses this in his book, *Good to Great,* when he describes the "hedgehog principle." Basically, the hedgehog is really good at rolling up into a ball to protect itself. No animal is better at protecting itself in this manner from being eaten by

predators. Collins encourages organizations to also discover what they are uniquely positioned and resourced to be great at. Every organization, every team, can be exceptional at something, but discovering that something takes time, effort, and whole brain leadership. We like to think of it as "discovering the *and*" as portrayed in this link (https://www.youtube.com/watch?v=srHDgimlgTQ). We all want and expect to be excellent. Be aware that excellence is different than perfect. Excellence is a process that we can control. Perfection is an outcome that is not only out of our control but also impossible to attain. Wherever you see a commitment to perfection, as opposed to excellence, you will find shame and often the consequences of shame, which include blame, dishonesty, and unhappiness—all leading to poor performance. Discovering the "and" invites teams to be more than excellent and to encourage development of the team's "hedgehog product." It is a way for a team to develop uniqueness that is authentic and linked to its core strengths and talents. These teams discover how they are both "excellent at providing children's heart care" *and*. … The "and" is what else they do or offer that is unique and that distinguishes them. Great teams discover this additional area for performance around which they are able to be truly great. Whole brain leaders mine for uniqueness and authenticity to help craft organizational excellence by harnessing the strengths of the organization to a shared mission and purpose that is meaningful and achievable for the team. This generates *system esteem* and ultimately high performance.

Commitment

No matter where you work and what team you work with, the very nature of delivering care to neonates, infants and children, and adults with complex congenital heart disease is hard, unpredictable, and fraught with challenge. Plans do not always work out the way we hope, the team may encounter "clusters" of bad outcomes, or fractures in relationships from disagreements. The major difference between resonant and dissonant teams is that resonant teams find a way to work through these difficulties as a natural part of being in relationship. Members of resonant teams know—they have trust—that no matter what, their team will stand by them. Team members remain *committed* to the team and to each other, even (especially) when times are challenging. Ultimately, the best teams find ways to work through these times without destroying each other or disintegrating the team. They look at problems as challenges that all members can address, not as people who need to be "fixed" or removed. Research on relationships has emphasized the importance of commitment,[56,57] and teams are complex, adaptive relationships. There is likely no problem a team cannot solve if the team members view the problem as the challenge as opposed to each other as the challenge. Unfortunately, when caught up in the "amygdala hijacking" of intense difficulties, people tend to revert to some of their more primitive "survival" styles (exhibiting their strengths as overused) such as those outlined as dissonant styles earlier in this chapter, and most commonly this appears as blame (others do not count, "I need to protect myself") or super reasonable (people do not matter—only patients matter—which by the way is wrong. People do matter, and if we do not attend to our ability to work well together and support one another, the patients will suffer). However, you may recognize any or all of the dissonant coping styles, and simply being able to recognize them might be helpful. These styles tend to appear during times of stress, and they can also be simply termed "stress stances"—they are postures we exhibit when we become anxious and stressed.[26,58]

Whole brain leaders first need to recognize within themselves which of these coping styles they are most likely to adopt and simply acknowledge that when they are beginning to use this style, it is an indicator that they, too, are feeling stressed. It is a very useful *early warning sign*. They may also recognize these coping styles in members of the team and know that those team members are feeling stressed. If the team can become educated in this phenomenon, then the team can likely move from unconscious to conscious incompetence. (Nothing changes—the stress stances are still present—but they can now be named [what we name we tame] and acknowledged—not as something "wrong" with people, but rather as indicators that these team members feel stressed or anxious.) Tools for managing these situations are abundant and can be cultivated by whole brain leaders who appreciate the reality that their teams are composed of people and that people have needs and emotions and that people are not machines and cannot be managed like a mechanical system.

Among the tools that we have found helpful is to *solve the moment, not the problem*. It is often likely that the problem is bigger than the moment and will require an energized, engaged, and fully resourced team to be curious and open to potential solutions. (Dan Siegel refers to this state as COAL—Curious, Open, Accepting [the problem is the problem and it is here; the root of unhappiness is wanting things to be different than they are], and Loving [meaning have compassion for oneself and others on the team as learners, who, when they can, will try to do better].) The moment is more manageable and can be addressed with dialogue that simply acknowledges that the members of the team are wishing for something to be different.

One way to dialogue is to learn techniques for Nonviolent Communication.[25] These techniques can transform the way members of a team converse with one another around difficult situations. There are other methods for communicating that are taught in workshops on *Crucial Conversations, TeamSTEPPS, Cockpit Resource Management,* and a variety of communication tools. Regardless of which ones the team chooses, going through these trainings together is a growing and learning process that can be more valuable than the techniques themselves. Regardless of which techniques the team chooses to learn, however, the most important tool to implement is genuine caring and compassion for each member of the team.[59,60] Without this level of caring, tools are simply techniques that have no magic or soul.

Many problems that occur in our profession are unavoidable—patients bring us incredible challenges, and not all of these challenges are surmountable. All our team members come from differing backgrounds (cultural, family, and professional training). As leaders, we can help our team understand this and try not to take it personally. We can begin to see our organizations, not as problems to be solved, but rather as mysteries to be explored. When we fail, it is not because we are bad doctors. We simply had a bad outcome. This is how teams can try to stay connected. Commitment is staying connected as a team: through better and through worse, through sickness and in health, through paralyzed hemidiaphragm and recurrent arch obstruction.

Promote Work-Life Balance

Many of us trained in a time of relentless emphasis on work. It still is commonplace to attend a medical meeting and have a colleague ask, "Are you busy?" We rarely respond by saying, "No, I'm trying to spend more time with my family." It is a cultural value in our profession to be busy. How often do you think of taking a day off to spend doing something unrelated to work? And when you do, how do you feel about it? Guilty? Refreshed? Embarrassed? Secretive? Just notice. Whole brain leadership requires the ability to access emotions (attuning to both one's own emotions and the emotions of the team—mindsight) and to value them as important and meaningful. There is a younger generation arriving at our workplace—physicians and other health care professionals who may not share our cultural value of "busyness" as the proper spelling of our "business." Leadership for the future will likely need to find a way to tap into flexible, adaptive, coherent, energized, and stable ways to link this emerging culture with our goals for our teams. There is ample research documenting that work and life cannot be "balanced," but they can be *integrated* through *choice* into a life that is intentional, rewarding, and perfectly suited to how we want our individual lives to be. Leaders for the next generation of health care, particularly in the high-stakes, high-stress environment of managing patients with critical congenital heart disease will be obligated to emphasize ways to integrate work with life in some nonformulaic, individualized manner that attunes to the three elements demanding our attention mentioned at the beginning of this chapter: Self, Others, and Context. All three are valuable, important, and irrepressible. Honoring the needs of each creates balance, and ignoring any to the repeated exclusion of one over the others will create dis-ease. Whole brain leadership is a learning process that begins (and ends) with cultivation of the self, appreciation for others, and remarkable diligent attentiveness to context.

Selected References

A complete list of references is available on ExpertConsult.com.

1. Ungerleider RM, Ungerleider JD, da Cruz EM, Ivy D, Jaggers J, eds. *The Seven Practices of Highly Resonant Teams.* Vol. 6. 1st ed. Pediatric and Congenital Cardiology, Cardiac Surgery and Intensive Care. London: Springer-Verlag; 2014:3423–3450.
8. Dickey J, Ungerleider RM. Teamwork: a systems-based practice. In: Gravlee GP, et al, eds. *Cardiopulmonary Bypass: Principles and Practice.* Philadelphia: Lippincott, Williams and Wilkins; 2007:572–588.
11. Ungerleider JD, Ungerleider RM. Improved Quality and Outcomes Through Congruent Leadership, Teamwork and Life Choices. *Prog Pediatr Cardiol.* 2011;32:75–83.
29. Dekker S. *Just Culture: Balancing Safety and Accountability.* Dorchester: Dorset Press; 2012.
47. Ungerleider RM. Whom does the Grail serve? *Ann Thorac Surg.* 2007;83:1927–1933.
48. Losade M, Heaphy E. The Role of Positivity and Connectivity in Performance of Business Teams: A Nonlinear Dynamic Model. *Am Behav Sci.* 2004;47:740–765.
54. Barsade S, O'Neill OA. *Manage Your Emotional Culture.* Harvard Business Review; 2016(January-February): p. 58-66.

2

Optimizing Care Delivery: Quality and Performance Improvement

KYLE J. REHDER, MD; SARAH TALLENT, BSN, MSN, CPNP-AC;
JON N. MELIONES, MD, MS

With increased emphasis on tracking patient outcomes, reducing hospital-acquired conditions, promoting cost-conscious care, and inclusion of quality metrics as determinants of reimbursement, quality has become a major focus in health care. However, defining what *quality* means in any given health care setting can be challenging. An isolated decrease in patient mortality does not necessarily equate to quality care, nor does improvement in any one other metric, particularly if that improvement comes at the expense of another important outcome.

The Institute of Medicine (IOM) has provided six domains that define quality in the health care setting[1]:

- *Safe:* Avoiding harm to patients from the care that is intended to help them
- *Effective:* Providing services based on scientific knowledge to all who could benefit and refraining from providing services to those not likely to benefit (avoiding underuse and misuse, respectively)
- *Patient centered:* Providing care that is respectful of and responsive to individual patient preferences, needs, and values and ensuring that patient values guide all clinical decisions
- *Timely:* Reducing wait times and sometimes harmful delays for both those who receive and those who give care
- *Efficient:* Avoiding waste, including waste of equipment, supplies, ideas, and energy
- *Equitable:* Providing care that does not vary in quality because of personal characteristics such as gender, ethnicity, geographic location, and socioeconomic status

As health care providers, our primary goal is to deliver optimal outcomes to our patients, but this must be balanced with a fiscal responsibility to provide care that is both cost-conscious and sustainable. The primary tenet of medicine, "first do no harm," prioritizes patient safety in all that we do. In this manner the pursuit of quality care must consider not only singular patient outcomes but also other balancing measures, risk stratification and error proofing, and outcomes important to the greater populace. Similarly, attention must be paid to ensure this care is delivered in a consistent and equitable manner.

Quality Improvement/Performance Improvement

Determining the best medical treatments for patients has traditionally been driven by rigorous research in the form of basic science, translational research, and tightly controlled randomized clinical trials. Unfortunately, there is often a lag of more than a decade between new research defining a best practice and that practice becoming standard of care. Similarly, even when a best practice is known, it is commonly applied in an inconsistent fashion. This delivery gap is where quality improvement is an essential part of providing care (Fig. 2.1). Quality improvement methodologies are essential to ensuring consistent delivery of best care practices, particularly as patients' health issues have become more complicated and health care delivery systems have become more complex.

Although many of its concepts are relatively new to health care, the field and process of quality improvement should not be dismissed as a "soft science." Quality and performance improvement are built on proven strategies that have repeatedly enhanced patient care. Just as with traditional research, the best results in quality and performance improvement initiatives will be realized when rigorous methodology is applied.

Much of quality improvement science was developed and streamlined in business and manufacturing settings, with more recent introduction to the health care environment. The adaptation of these principles to the hospital setting may inherently lead to conflict and confusion, given the primary goal of business is to improve shareholder value, whereas the primary goal in medicine is to improve patient care. As a result, the direct translation of these business principles to health care can result in uncertainty as to the true focus of a given project, as well as which specific strategy is best suited for the problem being addressed. An added challenge to quality and performance improvement in the health care environment is the almost ubiquitous need for human factors management for successful project implementation. In the next several sections we describe some of the necessary strategies to achieve transformative care for patients.

Identifying Targets for Improvement

Health care is complex and constantly changing. Although providers and patients can typically identify many processes that either contribute to suboptimal outcomes or are substantial sources of dissatisfaction, determining specific targets for improvement can be challenging. It is also often unclear which improvement target should take priority at any given time and what resources might be available for the next improvement project.

The selection of improvement targets is generally achieved through the balance of two factors: those projects that can have

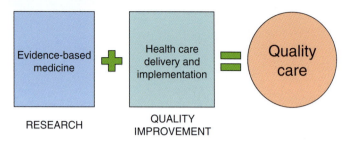

• **Figure 2.1** Combining evidence-based medicine and quality improvement to achieve optimal outcomes.

the greatest impact on patient care and those changes that can be easily made. The latter of these, often termed *low-hanging fruit,* often provide short-term projects with low resource requirements. Early "wins" with these projects can help bolster a culture of continuous improvement and gain momentum for those projects with the greatest potential impact. It is these impactful projects that will likely require greater resources and long-term commitment, and it is these projects where specific quality improvement methodologies and human factors engineering will be required to realize change.

Any quality improvement project should start with a clear statement of the project's goal. SMART statements are the generally accepted method for defining the aim and scope of the project:

Specific: Provide clear and unambiguous targets for improvement.
Measurable: Ensure that the outcome is objectively quantifiable and able to be tracked.
Achievable: Is the project goal attainable in terms of scope, resources, and time available?
Relevant: The "so-what" question. Is this an important initiative for the organization, the patients, or the staff? Is this the right intervention to affect the targeted outcome?
Time oriented: What time frame will this project span?

An example of a SMART statement with all the necessary elements might be: "We will reduce the number of pressure ulcers (grade 2 or higher) among patients in our unit to less than 2 ulcers per 1000 patient days by August 1st." This is a clearly measurable target with specific scope in terms of population and time frame. Of course, determination of "achievable" and "relevant" must be decided in collaboration with the unit leadership and with consideration for the current state as well as available resources for the project.

Leadership backing of quality improvement efforts is essential for several reasons. First, leadership can help prioritize those projects that are of greatest importance to the organization and, in the process, can also verify that necessary resources will be made available for project completion. The lack of such support can easily lead to project failure due to lack of means or inability to maintain momentum. Second, organizational leadership will be aware of other improvement initiatives that may be ongoing simultaneously. Coordinating these efforts can avoid confusion around institutional priorities and promote collaboration between medical teams. Finally, public affirmation by organizational leadership regarding the priority of an improvement project will help gain support from the staff and assist with sustainability after the initial intensive push for process change.

Early identification of key stakeholders and incorporation of these individuals into the planning process is essential to the success of any quality improvement effort. Building a multidisciplinary group of individuals with unique perspectives and priorities will help provide a clear and robust analysis of the problem at hand. Furthermore, inclusion of these individuals in development of interventions will bolster early multidisciplinary support for the project and potential solutions. Ideal project members are experienced frontline individuals with content expertise and strong teamwork skills who also hold significant influence in their work area (regardless of leadership titles or lack thereof). Paired with visible organizational leadership support, the buy-in of these influential frontline staff members will help garner widespread acceptance of new process flow or other solutions.

Defining project scope is another key ingredient to designing a successful improvement initiative. A natural tendency while assessing an array of issues in a given work area is to try to solve multiple problems at once. Unfortunately, this approach may lead to lack of clarity and spread resources too thin to accomplish project goals. Prioritization of a specific target outcome and use of a key driver diagram (Fig. 2.2) can help narrow the focus of the project to the most impactful interventions. Development of a SMART statement is then an ideal strategy to define clear boundaries and focus the scope of a given project.

Measurement/Metrics

Before starting any improvement project, it is essential to adequately capture the current state of the process or outcome of interest. Only by knowing the starting point will the project team know if change was achieved. Ideally, the outcome of interest should be easily measured, with high validity, and have a clear impact on patient outcomes.

Data collection efforts (i.e., accurate measurement and analysis) in health care typically lag behind similar efforts in industry. This is a function of multiple issues, including, but not limited to, lack of contemporary information technology (IT), lack of IT investment, noncomplementary IT (i.e., systems that do not "speak" to each other), and conflicting priorities. Increased use of electronic medical record systems has allowed for simplified tracking of certain key outcomes in many institutions, but these data sources may require careful monitoring to ensure validity.

Any process change may have unintended consequences; therefore it is essential to also monitor a balancing outcome that may be negatively affected by the proposed solution or process change. For example, if a new protocol is implemented providing prophylactic anticoagulation to a high-risk population, it would be important to monitor the incidence of bleeding in these patients. Balancing measures for process changes often include cost, time, or an outcome for a conflicting process.

Tracking improvement progress is best achieved through the use of control charts (Fig. 2.3), where the identified primary outcomes are tracked as a function of time, with notations on the chart for specific interventions or external changes that might influence the outcome of interest. These charts provide a clear visual representation of improvement over time and can facilitate statistical analysis of a process that lies within or drifts out of control parameters. Control charts also allow for ongoing monitoring of the outcome once the improvement initiative has concluded.

Improving Care

A variety of quality management and performance improvement (PI) methodologies are readily available for use in the hospital

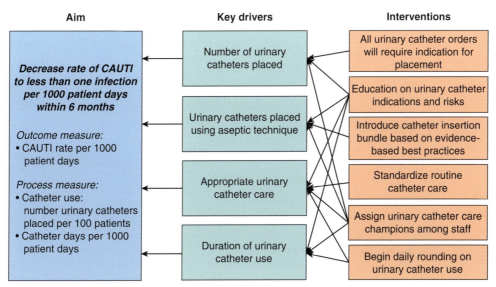

Figure 2.2 Example of a key driver diagram demonstrating an approach to reducing catheter-associated urinary tract infections *(CAUTIs)*. Once a project aim and primary outcome measure are identified, the key driver diagram identifies primary contributors to that outcome and potential interventions to promote change.

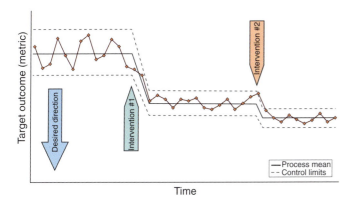

Figure 2.3 Sample control chart tracking impact of serial interventions on desired outcome.

setting. Most of these methodologies have been adapted from business and manufacturing and then successfully translated to health care.[1] Some of the more common quality improvement methodologies are summarized in Table 2.1, along with the tools commonly applied for each methodology. These methodologies often use similar tools, but each is suited for different aspects of process control or improvement across the continuum of health care delivery. Although an in-depth discussion of different methodologies is beyond the scope of this chapter, Table 2.1 highlights the primary utility of each strategy and principal strengths and weaknesses.

Not every process deficiency requires an intervention using in-depth quality improvement methodology. Many issues will have an obvious and simple solution and can best be addressed with a "just do it" approach. These changes are typically clearly needed and may not necessitate precise measurement of outcomes. However, if measurement is possible, the "just do it" approach may be the launching point for a series of Plan-Do-Study-Act cycles used in the Model for Improvement.[2]

Another strategy that will assist with acceptance of a new process is to make the "right" path the "easy" path. It is common for new initiatives to result in complex pathways to ensure the best outcome. However, the best-intentioned process will be ineffective if it is either too complex to follow or so onerous that staff develop work-arounds. Streamlining the new process, removing barriers to its implementation, or adding barriers to potential work-arounds can all act as forcing functions to help drive users of the process toward desired behaviors.

Following a period of intense focus on improvement, many processes and outcomes will drift back to their prior state, as attention is turned toward other issues and providers fall into old habits. During the development of improvement initiatives, attention must be paid to human factors that drive the process and potential strategies to increase sustainability. Six-Sigma methodology specifically addresses this issue with the "Control" phase of the DMAIC (Define, Measure, Analyze, Improve, and Control) model. Particular strategies that may be helpful include development of forcing functions that drive individuals to follow the desired process or protocol, hardwiring the new process into the existing work flow, making the desired process user friendly, and elimination of potential work-arounds. Continued monitoring of the outcomes of interest after conclusion of the improvement project will be important to confirm sustainability or to alert staff of process drift.

Given the detailed nature of improvement science, organizations or units looking to achieve real change will need to employ quality improvement experts or seek to attain quality improvement training for their staff. Identifying these quality leaders and supporting them with appropriate resources and data streams will be essential to achieving optimal patient outcomes.

Team Structure and Dynamics

Staffing models may vary widely among pediatric cardiac intensive care units (ICUs), and these staffing models may have significant effect on patient outcomes. Although many children are well cared for in combined medical-surgical units after congenital heart surgery,

TABLE 2.1	Common Quality Improvement Methodologies Used in Health Care			
Methodology	Primary Role	Key Strengths	Potential Limitations	Tools Commonly Utilized
Model for Improvement (Institute for Healthcare Improvement)	Rapid process improvement	• Simplicity • Swift implementation	• Superficial analysis • Reliance on trial and error	PDSA cycles, key driver diagrams, process mapping, cause and effect diagrams
Six Sigma	Minimize variability, reduce defects	• Thorough analysis with focus on statistical change • Focus on maintaining gains	• Complex methodology • Time intensive	DMAIC, process mapping, Pareto charts, cause-and-effect diagrams, value stream mapping
LEAN	Reduce waste, increase efficiency	• Focus on efficiency	• Limited scope	Value stream mapping, process mapping
Failure modes effect analysis (FMEA)	Error proofing	• Proactive risk identification • Increases process reliability	• Focus on major failures • Often not comprehensive • Complex methodology	Process mapping, error proofing, FMEA worksheets, SWIFT analysis
Root cause analysis	Error investigation	• Identification of previously unidentified risk	• Retroactive analysis; analysis may be limited by recall bias	Process mapping, error proofing

DMAIC, Define, Measure, Analyze, Improve, Control; *PDSA*, Plan-Do-Study-Act; *SWIFT*, structured what-if technique.

an increasing number of institutions have moved toward a model with a separate cardiac ICU, modeling what is commonplace in adult centers. This strategy allows for focused expertise among physician, nursing, respiratory therapy, and ancillary staff around the unique population of children with congenital and acquired heart disease and is supported by improved outcomes in high-volume centers and dedicated cardiac ICUs.[3-7]

Physician staffing of pediatric cardiac ICUs should include individuals with a strong understanding of the unique physiology of the congenital heart population and, when possible, prior training in both intensive care and cardiology. Inclusion of trainees, to be expected at most academic centers, is essential for the training of the next generation of cardiac ICU providers, as well as providing baseline management knowledge of this population to pediatric intensivists and cardiologists. Although cycling trainees through the unit for short rotations may add undesirable variability to staffing, these trainees may also provide unique perspective and offer partnering opportunities for research and improvement activities. Disruptions from the rotational nature of trainees can be minimized with a detailed and consistent orientation to the unit protocols and culture.

Advanced practice practitioners (nurse practitioners and physician assistants) may provide unique expertise in caring for children with congenital and acquired heart disease as a potential bridge between physicians and nursing staff. The addition of these practitioners as long-term members of the team allows for ongoing development of their skill set unique to this population. Advanced practice providers also foster ongoing relationship building within the team and may add continuity for patients with prolonged or recurrent hospitalizations.

Regardless of the unit structure or specific providers involved in care, patient outcomes will be optimized only if the medical team displays strong teamwork. This includes clear communication,

psychologic safety, and a culture of feedback. The latter directly ties into the capability of the team to continuously improve and is contingent on each of the former being in place. Specifically, use of debriefings as a feedback mechanism has been tied to improved outcomes in ICU patients. Proven team training strategies such as TeamSTEPPS[8] can be leveraged to teach other evidence-based tools to improve team behaviors and performance.

A growing body of evidence links local work culture to patient outcomes.[9-11] Teamwork scores, safety culture, staff burnout, and staff engagement scores have been linked to mortality, surgical complications, medical errors, and other hospital-acquired infections. To provide the best quality care to patients, unit leadership must recognize this link and foster a culture of strong teamwork and safety. In addition to focusing on optimal teamwork, Leadership WalkRounds is a specific tool that can be beneficial toward safety culture.[11] For WalkRounds, unit leaders circulate the unit on a biweekly or monthly basis during different shifts. During these rounds, they speak to as many frontline staff as possible, asking both "What is going well?" and "What could be better?" Feedback is then provided to all staff regarding findings, recognition of high points, and potential changes to address concerns. This interaction between leadership and staff builds psychologic safety, models effective feedback, proactively identifies issues before they affect patients, and highlights safety and quality as organizational priorities.

The impact of team dynamics and unit culture on patient outcomes demonstrates the comprehensive approach that must be taken to improve quality of care. Disease treatment must have a sound basis in evidence-based therapies, but enhancing health care delivery encompasses the entire process of caring for patients, including patients, providers, and staff, and the means by which care is supplied. This holistic approach to quality must be embraced to truly give our patients the pinnacle of care.

Monitoring Quality at a Unit and Organizational Level: The Balanced Scorecard

A common frustration of medical providers is the lack of meaningful feedback on their practice habits and a lack of transparency to organizational priorities. This lack of transparency often leaves providers feeling "kept in the dark" or asking "Is this the latest trend?" regarding strategic planning, quality management, and PI efforts.

To eliminate these questions and other impediments to success, clinical improvement strategies should be systematically implemented in a way that uses the advantages of each approach, while focusing on long-term goals. The balanced scorecard (BSC) can assist in aligning these goals.[12]

Originally developed to support PI in industry, the BSC has been touted as a strategic planning framework that consolidates multiple improvement projects into a single integrated platform.[12] As such, the scorecard is an integration of multiple interventions and keeps "score" of the success or failure of the strategic goals. This approach is fundamental to success, promotes balance in the organization, and aligns all disciplines around a focused strategic agenda.

BSC methodology starts with the development of the mission and strategic plan in conjunction with senior leadership.[1,2] Once the senior management team has defined the strategic goals, the key metrics that measure performance are developed. Finally, initiatives are developed to improve performance and support achievement of the strategic goals. As such, the scorecard functions as an important strategic platform that drives the integration of key initiatives, methodologies, and processes with focus on critical outcome measures. Although performance at the operational level frequently requires additional tools and techniques that bridge the gap between strategy and tactics, the BSC becomes the tool that identifies where initiatives should be focused and how these initiatives impact the whole organization.

The traditional health care BSC has the following perspectives: quality and safety, patient experience, work culture, and finance and growth (Table 2.2). In contrast to industry, which primarily focuses on financial performance, the quality and patient safety perspective is placed at the top of the health care BSC, indicating its priority importance.

Defining Goals Linking Performance Metrics

Once the strategic plan is defined, specific goals are determined by the team and linked to each strategic perspective. Limiting the goals to three or four per perspective is essential to maintaining focus on initiatives that will drive the strategic plan. After the goals are determined, specific metrics are defined and linked to each goal. The metrics must be measurable and collected at least quarterly. Performance targets are then defined and linked to each metric. It is best to pick targets from comparable institutions. If none are available, a modest improvement from baseline, such as 10% to 20% improvement is a good starting point. Many of the operational metrics that populate the BSC are derived from hospital operational and financial databases, patient safety data from internal safety reporting systems, patient satisfaction survey data, and work culture survey data. Validity of the data is key, and data accuracy must be ensured before presenting this to the team. Bad data will result in loss of confidence and can ruin the efforts before implementation.

Driving the Balanced Scorecard to Unit Levels

The performance on the scorecard rolls up to provide a single score for all goals and metrics. In this way it provides balance to the organization because the overall score will be low if the organization performs well in one perspective (e.g., finance and growth) and does poorly in another (e.g., quality and safety). The next step is to have individual scorecards at the service unit level and finally, at the individual operating unit level. This tiered approach encourages focused improvement efforts at the direct patient care level that are aligned with the strategic goals of the broader organization. Without this alignment, PI efforts are often reactionary and focused on local concerns that may have little impact on organizational outcomes. Aligning PI initiatives toward strategic goals provides a significant economy of scale and ensures that the entire organization benefits from collaborative efforts.

As an example, Duke Children's Hospital has used the BSC to drive systemic improvements in several areas.[13] Compared to the prior year in the quality and patient safety perspective, we witnessed a reduction in morbidity, a decrease in readmissions from 7% to 4%, a decrease in infection rates from 3% to 1%, and a decrease in length of stay by 0.6 days. These improvements were seen in conjunction with an increase in average daily census by 9% over the previous fiscal year.

In the finance and growth perspective, the patient flow team achieved a 26% improvement in discharge times and 10% improvement in pediatric ICU encounters. Multiple finance-based initiatives followed implementation of the BSC, resulting in an increase in the variable contribution margin by 240%. In the patient experience perspective, patient satisfaction scores have exceeded the set targets over the last fiscal year (Press Ganey overall mean score of 84). In the work culture perspective, independent observations of teamwork increased by 72% ($P < .001$) and overall perception of teamwork increased by 75% ($P < .001$). Surveys also demonstrated that 95% of participants believed that team training would improve the way they did business, and 100% of participants would recommend team training to coworkers.

The BSC is one methodology to ensure that strategy turns into action. Because of the wide variety of options available and the hospital staff's lack of experience, many providers find implementing clinical improvement programs in health care to be challenging.[12-14] To be successful, these programs must be supported by senior management, physicians, and caregivers. Physicians, as a group, often are difficult to engage. Improvement initiatives may require physicians to change their practice, yet they frequently do not include input from the physicians, resulting in a lack of physician support for improvement initiatives and placing physicians at odds with administrators.

Clinical improvement initiatives that involve a change in physician practice must engage physicians in the process. Engaging physicians is challenging because they typically lack a background in improvement science and perceive that they will have difficulty contributing to the mission. This reluctance can be overcome by developing a specific training program for physicians, identifying clear goals and areas of focus, and linking the physicians with current operational and clinical improvement teams. In this way the physicians can become an integral part of the process, and the organization can leverage their considerable influence to achieve success.

The BSC requires thoughtful, considered adjustments in goals and metrics to meet the changing strategic plan. For example, if an ICU expansion is planned, the BSC might be updated with

TABLE 2.2 Sample Balanced Scorecard

	TARGET[a]	Quarter Actual	YTD Actual
QUALITY AND PATIENT SAFETY			
Infection prevention: catheter associated bloodstream infection	0.0	0.00	0.00
Infection prevention: urinary catheter associated urinary tract infection	0.5	1.10	0.63
Infection prevention: hand hygiene	95%	100%	98%
Infection prevention: central venous line utilization ratio	80%	76.6%	79.2%
Infection prevention: urinary catheter utilization ratio	20%	18.1%	16.2%
Pressure injury: assessed patients with acquired pressure injuries	5%	7.2%	6.1%
Patient falls rate per 1000 inpatient days	0.0	0.00	0.32
Patient falls with injury per 1000 inpatient days	0.0	0.00	0.00
Preventable medication related SRS events with patient impact	0.3	1.5	0.45
Restraints: percent of patients restrained	4%	8.4%	3.6%
Transfusion deviations	0.0	0.0	0.0
FINANCE AND GROWTH			
Agency staff: percent of worked hours	0.0%	0.8%	0.6%
Flex expense percent variance	0.0%	−0.9%	0.7%
Flex FTE percent variance	0.0%	−1.3%	−0.4%
Nursing overtime: percent of paid hours	2.5%	1.1%	1.9%
Skill mix: RN nursing care hours as a percent of all nursing care hours	97.5%	98.1%	96.9%
WORK CULTURE			
Employee injury: rate of lost days of all inpatient nursing employees	0.0	0.0	0.0
Percent terminations annualized: overall	18%	23.1%	21.2%
Percent terminations annualized: RN	20%	24.5%	19.8%
RN staff: percent with BSN or above	80%	89.1%	84.7%
RN staff: percent with certification	50%	64.3%	59.6%
PATIENT EXPERIENCE			
Likelihood to recommend	90%	88%	94%
Responsiveness of hospital staff	80%	81%	84%
Acceptable noise levels at night	80%	63%	72%
Unit cleanliness	80%	82%	80%
Overall rating of unit	90%	91%	87%
Patient satisfaction: communication among team members	85%	82%	86%

[a]Note that "target" reflects an achievable metric, allowing the team to progress towards the overall goal (e.g., the overarching goal is to have zero infections and zero medication errors). Metrics highlighted in *blue* demonstrate areas where the team exceeds targets, while metrics highlighted in *orange* demonstrate performance below targets and potential focus areas for improvement efforts. *FTE*, Full-time equivalent; *SRS*, safety reporting system; *YTD*, year to date.

new goals and metrics tied to this project and reflected in the ICU scorecards. In this way the BSC functions as a living record of how performance is tracking against the strategic plan.

Benchmarking and Collaboration

Although the BSC allows for clear tracking of specific outcomes within an institution over time, it may not detail how that center's performance compares with other similar centers. Benchmarking against other centers is an important aspect of understanding the overall quality of care provided to patients. Outcomes databases like the Society of Thoracic Surgeons (STS) database allow institutions to follow their overall performance relative to peers. Beyond internally set targets, this benchmarking highlights strengths and weaknesses within a program and can help focus resources for areas needing further attention.

Even with comparative data, defining best practices within a single center can often be difficult, given small numbers of patients with heterogeneous disease processes and the lack of feasibility to try many different care strategies. Multi-institution quality improvement collaborations are a strategy to allow centers to learn from the experience of others, through shared evaluation of practice variability and the individual strengths of each institution. Several such collective efforts have led to improved care for children, including delivery of surfactant for preterm infants,[15] reductions of catheter-associated bloodstream infections through the National Association of Children's Hospitals and Related Institutions (NACHRI) collaborative,[16] and reductions of medical errors and other hospital-acquired conditions through the Solutions for Patient Safety collaborative.[17]

Within the congenital heart disease community, the National Pediatric Cardiology Quality Improvement Collaborative has successfully leveraged data from several large pediatric cardiac centers to highlight key areas of variability and identify best practices that may not have been successfully elucidated in prior smaller studies. With distribution of these best practices and increased focus on quality improvement at each individual site, the collaborative has seen a 40% decrease in mortality during the interstage period for hypoplastic left heart syndrome following the Norwood procedure among the participating institutions.[18] Similarly, the Pediatric Cardiac Critical Care Consortium (PC^4) is a large multicenter registry with robust data from 30 of the largest US children's hospitals.[19] PC^4 has delineated areas of substantial variability in care and outcomes[20-22] and provides participants benchmarking data and opportunities for collaborative quality improvement efforts.

Hallmarks of these collaborative efforts include transparency among center practices and the willingness to forego competition for the purposes of driving quality care. Centers must dedicate local resources not only to process improvement but also to data collection and validation. With these combined efforts, institutions can achieve better outcomes than any one center could achieve on its own, and for a larger number of patients.

Conclusion

Our primary goal as health care providers is to ensure that our patients get the best possible care. Quality improvement is the path by which we can achieve that promise in a consistent and reliable manner. Development of a robust quality framework for patient care will require:

- Validated and detailed data streams to effectively monitor processes and outcomes
- Application of proven quality improvement methodologies with dedicated resources that emphasize preserving progress in one process as new targets are identified
- Focus on safety and teamwork culture within units, including attention to human factors that affect execution of health care delivery
- Balancing priorities and strategic initiatives with careful consideration given to financial stability, growth, and sustainability
- Collaborative efforts between institutions to define and share best practices

Strong unit leadership will be needed to maintain the vision of the six domains of quality and to uphold patient-centered care and outcomes. With such leadership and combined with thoughtful application of improvement methodologies, it is possible to truly elevate the care we provide to our most vulnerable patients.

Selected References

A complete list of references is available at ExpertConsult.com.

1. Institute of Medicine (U.S.). Committee on Quality of Health Care in America. *Crossing the Quality Chasm: A New Health System for the 21st Century*. Washington, D.C.: National Academy Press; 2001.
4. Hornik CP, He X, Jacobs JP, et al. Relative impact of surgeon and center volume on early mortality after the Norwood operation. *Ann Thorac Surg*. 2012;93(6):1992–1997.
6. Pasquali SK, Li JS, Burstein DS, et al. Association of center volume with mortality and complications in pediatric heart surgery. *Pediatrics*. 2012;129(2):e370–e376.
7. Johnson JT, Tani LY, Puchalski MD, et al. Admission to a dedicated cardiac intensive care unit is associated with decreased resource use for infants with prenatally diagnosed congenital heart disease. *Pediatr Cardiol*. 2014;35(8):1370–1378.
19. Gaies M, Cooper DS, Tabbutt S, et al. Collaborative quality improvement in the cardiac intensive care unit: development of the Paediatric Cardiac Critical Care Consortium (PC4). *Cardiol Young*. 2015;25(5):951–957.

3

Streaming Analytics in Pediatric Cardiac Care

MELVIN C. ALMODOVAR, MD

Current-state computer and information technology allows extraction and aggregation of large volumes of diverse data types to support medical decision making in hospitalized patients.[1-3] With abundant and readily available data there has been growing interest and accumulating experience with advanced data analytics techniques such that there now exists both the demand *and* an opportunity for intensivists, among other clinicians, to pursue innovative information technology applications to benefit our fragile patients. But will we soon reach the "peak of inflated expectations" followed by a rapid descent to the "trough of disillusionment" before realizing the promises of precision medicine, big data analytics, and machine learning applications as some have suggested?[4] It is the author's belief that leveraging information technology and blending expertise from multiple disciplines such as medicine, engineering, mathematics, computer science, and even behavioral science will drive greater medical intelligence and more accurate and efficient health care across the range of clinical and nonclinical scenarios. The formal establishment of the field of biomedical informatics and growing experience with data science applications to support medical decision making and patient care delivery processes support this perspective.[5-7]

The purpose of this chapter is to describe basic principles of high-frequency data analytics and, specifically, how the streaming analytics approach may be applied in the pediatric cardiac intensive care unit (CICU) to enhance our understanding and management of the critically ill patient with cardiac disease.

Overview of Real-Time Data Analytics

Real-time data analytics involves the capture, processing, and analysis of data as data is entering the system. In the data-rich intensive care unit (ICU) environment, information and networking technology, the ready access to clinical information, and the application of mathematical modeling methods are beginning to support our ability to better manage multiparameter data streams in our assessment and treatment of patients.[8,9] Depending on the analytics platform and database structure, stored genetic and other patient-specific, structured, and unstructured historical data may also be included, thereby adding context for the population or circumstance of interest. At the same time, this would allow for growth of captured volumes of information for later use in research, quality, and outcomes analysis. Currently there is enthusiasm that robust data management capabilities will foster the development of predictive algorithms that may eventually support enhanced real-time decision making.[10,11] For example, in patients with borderline left heart structures being considered for or undergoing biventricular repair, preoperative and postoperative hemodynamic, imaging, laboratory, and historical data may be incorporated in a real-time analytics approach to support such decisions as (1) determining whether or not biventricular repair is feasible, (2) which targeted interventions may improve likelihood of success in attaining biventricular physiology, and (3) whether the intraoperative and postoperative data indicate a successful physiology or predict successful short- and long-term outcomes in this patient population. Population-based and patient-specific historical and real-time data are available in such scenarios and, ideally, would inform the decision-making approach during each management step over time. As one can see, such a scenario exemplifies a range of data analytics approaches that may be described to include the following major categories: descriptive analytics, predictive analytics, and prescriptive analytics. These categories may be viewed along a continuum that considers what *has happened,* what *could happen,* and what *should be done,* respectively. Descriptive analytics are familiar to all of us and involve the use of summary statistics that give insight into the past and are common in health care and non–health care industries. Predictive analytics employ the use of mathematical models to forecast the future or estimate data that are not yet in existence. Accurate prediction requires that certain conditions remain constant over time and that the correct or relevant data elements are included in the models.[12] There are a growing number of health care applications and numerous non–health care applications that are currently in existence as examples of predictive methods. The extent to which any of these applications is successful is highly dependent on its level of validation during algorithm development and testing, as well as a robust system of application evaluation and reengineering as needed. Prescriptive analytics incorporate the features of predictive modeling derived from historical and real-time data to achieve accurate near- or real-time prediction for the expressed purpose of driving actions. At this time, practical applications using this type of analytics in health care are relatively rare, at least in the live clinical setting because of limitations in extracting real-time data and a paucity of successfully validated predictive models. On the other hand, there are numerous non–health care applications that are successfully driven by prescriptive analytics methodology. Some examples of these include credit card fraud protection, cyber security monitoring, GPS location and guidance, and market data management to name a few.[13,14] Finally, from the capabilities afforded by predictive and prescriptive methods comes streaming analytics, or event stream processing, the basic foundation of which will be reviewed in the next section.

Streaming Analytics

Optimal care of critically ill cardiac patients requires thoughtful and accurate assessment of their physiologic state using a variety of data elements not just at a single point in time, but repetitively and in response to expected and unexpected events. Hence any care strategy must seek to achieve accurate diagnoses and to discern the patient's overall trajectory pattern with the paradigm that deviations from expected patterns or valid early warnings will be heeded and appropriate adjustments in care will be made.

Digital data stream analysis is not new, and, historically, high-frequency, high-volume data have been processed in batches and at periodic intervals (daily, weekly, or at longer intervals). Much of the impact of this work has been realized through automation of clerical tasks and standardization of routine decisions and actions. In commercial industries, stream analytics has resulted in improved business efficiency and customer satisfaction owing to data access, the Internet, and ubiquity of personal computers and mobile devices.[13,15,16] Unfortunately, many data management systems remain fragmented and struggle with the management of large volumes of high-variety data that may present rapidly, a major consequence of which is long latency periods for access to the right data to make timely and correct decisions. In contrast to batch processing, event stream processing involves the continuous analysis of flowing time series data with the primary goals of providing real-time insight about a situation and to allow early detection of anomalies. Importantly, there is an inverse relationship between response time latency (i.e., the time from event or data element capture to delivery of action) and tactical value, thus emphasizing the importance of timely data capture, analysis, and action within the streaming analytics process.[16] For such a system to be functional, it requires a complex architecture (Fig. 3.1) with the capability to support the swift collection and aggregation of highly variable data types, the ability to analyze that data in real time, and the ability to directly influence end users (or even automated computerized systems) to make and execute appropriate decisions and actions. Ideally, such a system would include measurable outcomes and similar events as input data elements from the data stream feedback loop. This enables a rapid-cycle process to assess system performance and to support system learning and refinement as needed, as would occur in a machine learning paradigm. An additional feature worth noting is the integration of historical data or low-frequency data elements that support this approach for patient-specific or population-based applications.

Development of a Real-Time Analytics Platform in the Cardiac Intensive Care Unit

In 2010 a team from the CICU at Boston Children's Hospital, led by P. Laussen and M. Almodovar began development of the T3 system to capture, display, store, and analyze physiologic data streams from bedside monitoring devices. The term "T3" arose from the primary functional elements of the system as initially conceived to include the ability to *track* relevant physiologic data, enable assessment of a patient's *trajectory* throughout the patient's course in the CICU, and to support the ability to *trigger* appropriate responses or actions. The T3 data collection and analytics platform was designed as a Web-based, vendor agnostic, and scalable software system with three main features: an interactive data visualization user interface, a robust data analytics engine, and high-volume data storage capability. Fig. 3.2 describes an overview of the T3 platform beginning with data stream capture and ending with the multiple interfaces between its main features and data use applications. Fig. 3.3 shows a simplified version of the system architecture, noting its relatively simple structure and the ability to add third-party algorithms plus access to cumulatively stored data. The primary goals of the technology were to improve visualization of data trends for CICU patients, to develop algorithms and predictive models driven by the real-time physiologic data to guide decision making, and to create a hosting platform for the development and testing of algorithms using large volumes of stored data.

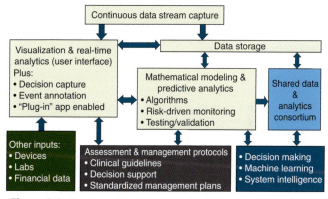

• **Figure 3.2** Overview of the T3 data collection and analytics platform.

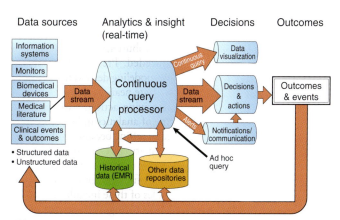

• **Figure 3.1** Stream processing architecture. *EMR,* Electronic medical record.

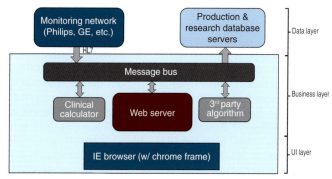

• **Figure 3.3** T3 software system architecture. *IE,* Internet Explorer; *UI,* user interface.

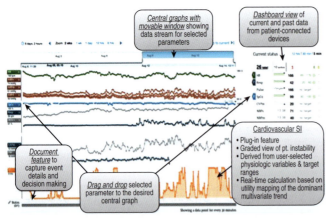

• **Figure 3.4** T3 user interface showing trend patterns for multiple physiologic parameters, including the cardiovascular stability index *(SI)*. Each data point represents 5-second averages of the continuously streamed data.

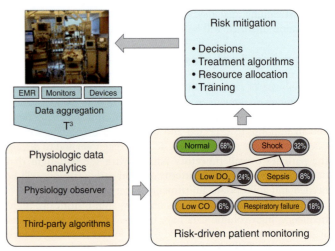

• **Figure 3.5** Risk-based monitoring process. *EMR,* Electronic medical record.

The T3 visualization user interface, as originally designed, is shown in Fig. 3.4 and demonstrates how multiple data streams are viewed simultaneously with trend patterns easily viewed in context with one another. The interactive interface allows selected parameters to be placed on the screen where desired and the ability to zoom in for higher resolution (down to 5-second interval averages between data points). The trend pattern can be examined along the timeline using a sliding, zoomable window for as long as the patient has been connected to a bedside monitor. The dashboard view in the upper right shows a sparkline summary of the recent data trends, the current parameter value, and user-determined boundary limits for each parameter. The user interface also allows for note entry or event annotation on the timeline (bottom) using free text entry or menu-driven options. This allows for decisions or other entries to be captured for easy querying and reporting at a later time.

Among the analytics features of the system is the ability to select a sample of multiparameter data from the live interface and display summary statistics in tabular form for each parameter. In addition, the first plug-in algorithm, the cardiovascular stability index (SI), was designed to represent a graded view of patient instability and is displayed along with the other parameters from which it is derived (see Fig. 3.4). The SI is generated from user-selected physiologic variables (for instance, oxygen saturation as measured by pulse oximetry [SpO_2], mean blood pressure [BP], and heart rate [HR]) and requires customized upper and lower target ranges for each included variable. The SI is a real-time calculation based on utility mapping of the dominant multivariate trend calculated from the streaming data; in essence the value is influenced by the rate of change and the extent to which the measured value deviates from the ideal range parameter for the selected variables. In the early experience with the algorithm, the predictive ability of the SI was evaluated in 28 neonates with hypoplastic left heart syndrome following stage I palliation. Using the variables SpO_2, HR, and mean arterial BP, the maximum SI within the first 6 to 48 hours postoperatively (SI >0.11) predicted an ICU length of stay greater than 12 days. All patients with SI less than 0.11 (*n* = 13) were discharged from the ICU within 12 days.

The most advanced analytics feature of the T3 platform involves a predictive analytics technique, termed *risk-based patient monitoring* or *risk analytics* (Etiometry, LLC, Brighton, Massachusetts), which involves signal processing methodology along with the application

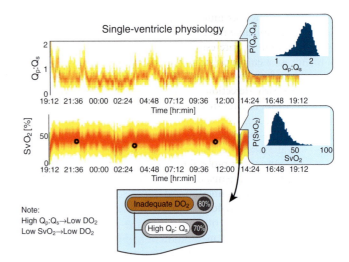

• **Figure 3.6** Panels showing probability density functions generated from streamed physiologic and intermittent laboratory data (SvO_2) for Q_p:Q_s and SvO_2. Note the trend pattern change in which a rise in Q_p:Q_s is associated with a decreased SvO_2 as would be expected in single-ventricle physiology with parallel circulations. *DO_2,* Oxygen delivery; *Q_p,* pulmonary blood flow; *Q_s,* systemic blood flow; *SvO_2,* mixed venous saturation.

of algorithms derived from physiology-based models to estimate the probability that a certain physiologic state exists. A key goal of this approach is to assist in the management of clinician data overload by processing multiparameter data streams and to account for the inherent uncertainty that exists in any clinical assessment or treatment decision.[10,11] A flow diagram depicting the risk-based monitoring process is shown in Fig. 3.5, where, as an example, the probability of shock is estimated given the quantitative assessment of its possible attributes. By signal processing methods, quantitative estimates that a condition exists (like shock or poor oxygen delivery) are generated from probability density functions for the relevant variables derived from the continuous physiologic data stream. Fig. 3.6 shows how the probability density functions for the attributes ratio of pulmonary to systemic blood flow (Q_p:Q_s) and mixed venous saturation (SvO_2) are viewed over time and how the data can be translated into a quantifiable risk of the condition, which in this case is inadequate oxygen delivery (IDO_2), using the single-ventricle physiology model. The analysis can be

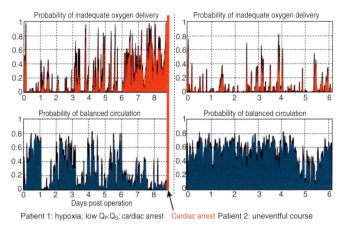

• **Figure 3.7** Risk-based analytics demonstration of the probability of inadequate oxygen delivery on two patients with single-ventricle physiology. $Q_P:Q_S$, Ratio of pulmonary to systemic blood flow.

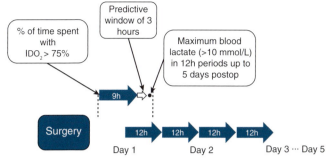

• **Figure 3.8** Test design scheme for the evaluation of the IDO_2 algorithm as a predictor of physiologic state as defined by lactate >10. IDO_2, Inadequate oxygen delivery.

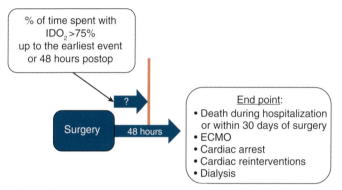

• **Figure 3.9** Test design scheme for the evaluation of the IDO_2 algorithm as a predictor of selected end point. *ECMO*, Extracorporeal membrane oxygenation; IDO_2, inadequate oxygen delivery.

computed at single or multiple time points or even continuously. Continuous real-time risk assessment reveals the trajectory pattern for a condition of interest that may evolve in due course or in response to therapeutic interventions. Taken further, if a given pattern can be shown to "predict" a certain outcome, then in theory the early detection of anomalies could be achieved from the data stream to alter treatment course to either achieve or avoid that outcome. Algorithm testing and proper validation is crucial for this to be adopted by clinicians and to be safely incorporated into clinical practice. In a simple but illustrative example, Fig. 3.7 shows the continuous probability assessments for IDO_2 and $Q_p:Q_s$ equal to 1 in two patients, one who experiences cardiac arrest and other experiencing an uneventful course. One can appreciate the difference in risk analytics trend pattern between the two patients experiencing different outcomes. One can also appreciate the sustained rise in IDO_2 probability and a simultaneously low risk of "imbalanced $Q_p:Q_s$" that occurred in patient 1 a few days leading up to the arrest, which might be attributable to the $Q_p:Q_s$ imbalance with low DO_2 as a cause of the event.

Since its initial creation, the IDO_2 algorithm has undergone further evaluation and testing in regard to its ability to predict a patient's physiologic state and outcomes.

In a retrospective study of a sample of 274 neonates undergoing cardiac surgery over a 4-year period, the risk analytics IDO_2 algorithm, derived from the continuous physiologic and periodic laboratory data parameters of SvO_2 value of 50% or less, SaO_2-SvO_2 difference of 50 or higher, and mean arterial blood pressure of 45 mm Hg or less, was evaluated as a predictor of blood lactate level greater than 10 mmol/L and separately as a predictor of poor outcome. Poor outcome was defined as experiencing cardiac arrest, dying by postoperative day 30, and the need for cardiac reintervention, mechanical circulatory support, or dialysis. The test design for predicting an abnormal physiologic state (lactate level greater than 10 mmol/L) involved identifying the percentage of time spent immediately postoperatively with IDO_2 probability greater than 75% over a 9-hour period leading up to a predictive window 3 hours before a maximum lactate value of greater than 10 mmol/L was measured. These 12-hour cycles occurred up to 5 days postoperatively as is shown diagrammatically in Fig. 3.8. In predicting poor outcome the test design involved identifying the percentage of time IDO_2 was greater than 75% up to the earliest event or 48 hours postoperatively. The schema for this design is shown in

Fig. 3.9. Receiver operating characteristic analysis revealed an area under the curve (AUC) for elevated blood lactate level prediction of 0.84 (0.75–0.9) and an AUC of 0.84 (0.77–0.89) in predicting poor outcome.

In a separate study the IDO_2 algorithm and thus the predictive analytics approach was evaluated in its ability to predict a measured SvO_2 value less than 40%. A low measured SvO_2 in high-risk postoperative cardiac patients has been widely accepted as a proxy for low cardiac output, a condition approaching a state of anaerobic metabolism, and high risk of poor clinical outcome.[17,18] In this multi-institutional study involving over 1500 cardiac surgical and nonsurgical cardiac patients less than 12 years of age, the IDO_2 algorithm (probability of IDO_2 value greater than 75%) driven off continuous physiologic data plus periodically measured SvO_2 by venous blood gas was shown to be a good predictor of SvO_2 less than 40% (AUC of 0.84). The test design was based off IDO_2 greater than 75% between 15 and 120 minutes leading up to SvO_2 measurement. In this study the relative risk of measuring a low SvO_2 level (<40%) increased with higher IDO_2 range, with the IDO_2 range 75% to 100% associated with a relative risk of 4 to 7 in this population of neonates, infants, and children with cardiac disease.

From these studies it is apparent that the IDO_2 algorithm provides real-time quantitative information about a patient's condition, and that the rise in IDO_2 value, even to modest levels, may signify an increased risk of inadequate DO_2, thus triggering some sort of action to potentially improve the patient's immediate course and subsequent outcome. To date neither the IDO_2 algorithm nor any of the work involving the T3 predictive analytics has been evaluated in relation to specific treatment actions. However, since its initial creation the T3 analytics platform has undergone modifications to the visualization user interface that enable its use as an always-on persistent display of the continuous data stream plus IDO_2 estimation, with the real-time incorporation of selected laboratory data in the same view. Body system and physiology-based views (i.e., respiratory and neurologic) have been developed with work on the incorporation of more diverse data elements ranging from static patient-specific information to digitally available waveform data.

Visual Analytics and Data Visualization

Visual analytics represents another area of science that is inherent to the streaming analytics approach. As described in the previous section, data visualization is an important component of the T3 analytics platform because it provides a graphical representation of data that identifies and communicates important patterns and concepts about the data. According to Alberto Cairo, a renowned data visualization expert, the goal of any visualization is to "assist the eyes and brain to perceive what lies beyond their natural reach." Thus data visualization seeks to integrate our visual perception capabilities with our cognitive abilities so that we can receive and process the information effectively.[19]

Ideally, a visualization should provide an intuitive, integrated view of relevant parameters while preserving situational context, support care management, and be interactive, allowing the end user to easily navigate and manipulate the data. Visual analytics involves analytic reasoning as facilitated by visualization interfaces and is believed to play a key role in supporting the effective use of data and information derived from big data analytics techniques.[20] When designing and implementing a data visualization tool, human factors principles should be considered to enhance the user experience and thus promote a higher likelihood of user adoption.[21] However, with any novel or evolving technology application, resistance to adoption may occur for a variety of reasons. This can be addressed with attention to potential or known barriers early in the design, testing, and implementation course. From the clinical safety perspective, simulation methods may be useful for training purposes and also to identify system glitches, through usability and heuristic evaluation, before and after the system is brought into production.[22]

Final Comments

Streaming analytics has made its way into the contemporary ICU, though this is not an entirely new phenomenon given the history of intensive monitoring and use of broad, though basic, types of clinical data since the early days of critical care medicine. What is different from previous eras are a number of factors related to the evolution of standards and expectations around outcomes, the growth in knowledge and information in medicine, advances in computer and information technology that bring massive volumes of information to us, and examples outside of health care that real-time analytics can be applied in profound and beneficial ways. Though limited to a few examples, this chapter highlights some of the early experience of streaming analytics in a critical care environment, specifically in a dynamic, high-volume pediatric CICU. The impetus to pursue high-frequency data analytics in this unit arose from the desire to better understand the trajectory patterns of critically ill patients in hopes of identifying anomalies in their course, affording the opportunity to proactively manage situations and avoid catastrophic events. In addition, it was recognized that the demands of the dynamic, data-rich, and resource-intensive CICU coupled with the potential for data overload among clinicians warranted pursuit of a system with T3's capabilities. It was also recognized that the electronic medical record and existing telemetry systems were not capable of providing an intuitive and integrated view of the data elements necessary to assist in the continuous and rapid assessment of a patient's trajectory or evolving pattern of deterioration. And lastly, without ready access to stored, aggregated data, extracting meaningful insight was onerous or impossible in some cases where event review was necessary. What has been achieved by the creation and implementation of the T3 system is summarized as follows:

1. High-frequency physiologic data from multiple sources are now captured, aggregated, and stored, then accessed and distributed.

2. Captured data can be organized and presented on an intuitive visual interface for efficient and effective processing by clinicians in the live clinical setting who must make timely assessments and interventions.

3. Streamed data can be analyzed in real time to produce a variety of metrics that help to quantitatively assess a patient's condition instantaneously or over time and allow for trend pattern assessment, including judgment of the response to treatment.

4. Predictive analytics using signal processing and mathematical modeling techniques from the combination of high-frequency data and intermittent data is achievable to estimate variables or a stream of relevant data that does not yet exist. With further development, testing, and validation, these streams may reduce data overload and improve the timeliness and effectiveness of care.

5. A robust data analytics platform can support integration of data that continuously grows and integrates elements from multiple sources, thus enhancing knowledge about the individual patient or groups of patients within a database and through data sharing across institutions and databases. Depending on the platform structure, databases can be leveraged to support benchmarking, protocol integration, and quality improvement and rapid-cycle research activity. Regardless of the system architecture, it is crucial that data privacy and security be achieved and maintained.

6. At the time of this writing, other systems with similar capabilities have been or are actively being developed at institutions around the world. Laussen and others at The Hospital for Sick Children in Toronto are expanding the data science approaches upon which the T3 platform is based, which now include waveform data. His colleagues in the neonatal ICU at the same institution have been working on big data applications using high-frequency analytics to enhance the monitoring and identification of important events in at-risk neonatal patients.[23] At Texas Children's Hospital, real-time high-frequency data were being used to develop an algorithm designed to identify subtle signs of clinical deterioration that may lead to cardiopulmonary arrest in complex neonatal patients with parallel circulations.[24] Finally, a group at Emory University Hospital, like others, has been working on the optimal engineering design to achieve the "smarter ICU," an important part of which involves the application of big data analytics to improve caregiver situation awareness for early identification of anomalies and prompt intervention.[25] From work described in this chapter, it appears that further technologic advances are likely and the achievement of automated intelligent early warning and patient management technology-driven processes involving streaming analytics are now within our reach.

Selected References

A complete reference list is available at ExpertConsult.com.

2. Frederick SA. Advanced Technology in Pediatric Intensive Care Units: Have They Improved Outcomes? *Pediatr Clin North Am.* 2016;63(2):293–301.
3. Celi LA, Csete M, Stone D. Optimal Data Systems: The Future of Clinical Predictions and Decision Support. *Curr Opin Crit Care.* 2014;20(5):8.
6. Simpao AF, Ahumada LM, Galvez JA, et al. A Review of Analytics and Clinical Informatics in Health Care. *J Med Syst.* 2014;38(45):7.
7. Suresh S. Big Data and Predictive Analytics. *Pediatric Clinics.* 2016;63(2):10.
10. Mcmanus M, Baronov D, Almodovar M, et al. *Novel Risk-based Monitoring Solution to the Data Overload in Intensive Care Medicine.* Paper presented at: IEEE 52nd Annual Conference on Decision and Control 2013.
11. Baronov D, McManus M, Butler E, et al. *Next Generation Patient Monitor Powered by In-Silico Physiology.* Paper presented at: Annual International Conference of the IEEE Engineering in Medicine and Biology Society 2015.
12. Davenport T. A Predictive Analytics Primer. *Harv Bus Rev.* 2014.
16. Pigni F, Piccoli G, Watson R. Digital Data Streams: Creating Value From the Real-Time Flow of Big Data. *Calif Manage Rev.* 2016;58(3).
20. Simpao A, Ahumada L, Rehman M. Big Data and Visual Analytics in Health Care. *Br J Anaesth.* 2015;115(3):7.
23. Khazaei H, Mench-Bressan N, McGregor C, et al. Health Informatics for Neonatal Intensive care Units: An Analytical Modeling Perspective. *IEEE.* 2015;3.

4

How to Interpret and Use Outcome Data

KARL WELKE, MD, MS; TARA KARAMLOU, MD, MSC; ROSS M. UNGERLEIDER, MD, MBA; JEFFREY P. JACOBS, MD

No concern is more important to parents than whether their child will be OK. For the team members who collaborate on the care of these children, "OK" can encompass many concerns, not simply "will the child survive surgery?" but "will he or she have a good quality of life?" and "what, if any, limitations might be expected?" These results may be measured as mortality, morbidity, length of stay, neurologic and functional outcomes, or quality of life, all of which are called *outcomes*. Our goal with this chapter is to simplify the complex science of the analysis of outcomes so that health care professionals can have a common language and shared concept of what is meant by the broad term *outcome*. Such understanding among providers will facilitate clear communication of accurate, relevant, and understandable information with each other and with the patient's family.

Relationship Between Structure, Process, and Outcome

In 1966 Avedis Donabedian described three domains of quality in medicine: structure, process, and outcomes.[1] Structure is the context in which care takes place, including the health care facilities, equipment, and personnel. Process is the action of taking care of the patients and can include protocols, as well as the organization of the delivery of health care. Outcomes are the results. Structure and process combine to influence outcome. If the outcomes being achieved are undesirable, modifiable structure and process measures should be investigated, for, as Paul Batalden stated, "Every system is perfectly designed to get the results it gets." The variation seen in outcomes across hospitals may be due to (1) differences in patient populations, (2) disparate structure and process, and (3) random variation or chance. If all hospitals had identical structure and processes, outcomes across these hospitals would be more similar.

Quality measures for congenital and pediatric heart surgery have been defined and sorted according to Donabedian's triad.[2] Intriguingly, the balanced scorecard principle propagated by Kaplan and Norton (described in Chapter 2) identifies outcomes as the result of specific process drivers. Many business models now employ the balanced scorecard approach to managing process drivers as the preferred method of influencing outcomes, or, stated in reverse, when the outcomes are not the ones that are desired—such as a high mortality, increased length of stay, or neurologic morbidity—then "what processes [or structures] need to be altered to improve the ultimate outcomes?" Structural measures include participation

in a national database, multidisciplinary rounds involving multiple members of the health care team, availability of a pediatric extracorporeal life support program, and surgical volumes. Process measures include the conduct of a multidisciplinary preoperative planning conference and a regularly scheduled quality assurance and improvement conference (also known as a mortality and morbidity or M and M conference), the interpretation of intraoperative transesophageal and epicardial echocardiography, the selection and time of administration of prophylactic antibiotics, and the use of preprocedural and postprocedural time-outs as well as handoff protocols. Outcomes measures include operative mortality and the occurrence of a variety of morbidities, including renal failure, neurologic deficits, arrhythmias, diaphragmatic paralysis, the need for postoperative mechanical circulatory support, and the need for unplanned reoperation or interventional catheterization. Although several of these structural and process measures have not been linked to outcomes by definitive research, they were chosen by experts as likely to be associated. Others are more complex than they may initially seem. For instance, the availability of intraoperative echocardiography is a structural measure; however, how well the team engages in a discussion of and responds to the echocardiographic findings in an operating room is part of the process of care. Multidisciplinary rounds, conferences, time-outs, and hand-offs present the same dilemma. The existence of these interactions could be considered a structural measure while the conduct of the meeting and the way in which information is exchanged are process measures. Part of the difficulty in selecting measures lies in the ability to describe them in ways that can be quantified.

Structural Measures

Volume is the most frequently cited structural measure associated with outcomes.[3-14] Volume has been defined in numerous ways, including all surgical cases performed, cases using or not using cardiopulmonary bypass, major or "index" cases, and cases sorted by level of surgical complexity or expected mortality risk. The definition of volume chosen should depend on the relationship being investigated. For example, if one wishes to know if the number of Norwood procedures performed by an institution is associated with mortality after that operation, the volume of Norwood operations performed should be used. If one is interested in whether or not the entire surgical experience of a program is associated with mortality after the Norwood operation, then the total surgical volume should be used. Volume is influenced by a number of factors. Alterations in program structure and process measures may attract referrals as might changes in outcomes.

Other structural measures include the number of health care providers and their experience and the physical attributes of the hospital. Markers of professional standing such as membership in a professional organization like the Congenital Heart Surgeons' Society may signal surgical expertise.[9] More recently, the addition of specialty boards in congenital heart surgery (the Congenital Heart Surgery Certificate of the American Board of Thoracic Surgery) provides an additional structural element—either the surgeon is board certified as a congenital heart surgeon or not. The physical layout of centers varies. In some centers the operating room, intensive care unit, and cardiac catheterization laboratory are in relative proximity, which facilitates transfer of patients from one environment to another. In other institutions, movement of patients between these environments requires an elevator transport. Likewise, having a dedicated cardiac intensive care unit is a structural element. When studying the influence of such structural elements, extra attention should be paid to those structures that are modifiable. Some structures are fixed and inherent to an institution, and although they may influence care, they cannot be altered. Current work in business circles tries to identify "process drivers" to better control outcomes.[15]

Process Measures

The *process* of care is critically important to the outcome. If a patient undergoes an operation in which technical errors are made, or if he or she is subjected to poor decision making related to the type or timing of surgical procedure or the conduct of perioperative care, they will be adversely affected. However, the associations between specific process measures related to congenital and pediatric cardiac surgery and subsequent outcomes have been poorly defined. This gap in knowledge may be for several reasons:

- First, it is difficult to distinguish between structural and process measures. For example, almost all programs now perform a preprocedural time-out and a handoff; however, the process of how that time-out or handoff is performed may vary between centers, including the actual safety for team members to "speak up" or the details of outlining the important specifics for (or of) the procedure to ensure that all equipment, supplies, personnel, and critical information are available. Furthermore, the relationship of this variation in the process to outcome may be impossible to determine because there are so many elements that factor into outcome. Likewise, most programs make multidisciplinary rounds, but the process for how these rounds are performed—how information is communicated or acted on—can be quite different between programs. It is very challenging to create a uniform process for some functions because there are so many important differences in people, structure, and even presentation of disease; nevertheless, variation in process may be critical in determining outcomes.

- Second, enthusiasm for process "mapping" has helped support the concept that process changes can result in improvement in outcomes. However, the uniqueness of our individual organizations and the wide variability in what processes need to be improved has led to considerable differences in process management across the spectrum of our varying structures. In other words, process management is far from "one size fits all." It may suffice to say that the presence of some attentiveness to process improvement may be the distinguishing feature of how outcomes are influenced, rather than applying a specific process across the profession.

- Third, the associations between process measure and outcomes can be confounded by structural measures. High surgical volume, a structural measure, may be associated with both a process of care that yields excellent results and superior outcomes.

- Fourth, few process measures are included in large databases. This limitation of many multi-institutional databases is in part due to the challenge of defining such measures of process and the burden of capturing these data and is also likely due to the lack of evidence supporting the relationship of most process measures to outcome.

- Fifth, if the outcome of interest occurs infrequently, the number of patients or operations in the study cohort may not allow for the power to detect a statistically significant association.

- Sixth, each individual component of the process acts in concert with the others in the continuum of care.

Therefore the link between a single process measure and an outcome may be difficult to discern. Although process measures are critically important to outcomes, additional work needs to be done to link process measures to outcome in congenital and pediatric cardiac surgery.

Outcome Measures

The outcome most commonly considered is mortality. First, it is a critically important outcome. Second, it is binary and relatively easy to measure. Third, mortality rates have been high for certain congenital cardiac operations, making it a variable that is not rare in appearance. Fourth, mortality as a discrete point of data is relatively easy to collect. Yet, even this seemingly straightforward concept is complex. The definition of mortality has varied over time. Definitions have included any death after surgery before discharge, any death within 30 days of surgery, death that can be definitively linked to the operation, and all deaths regardless of cause. Operative mortality is defined in all Society of Thoracic Surgeons (STS) databases as (1) all deaths, regardless of cause, occurring during the hospitalization in which the operation was performed, even if after 30 days (including patients transferred to other acute care facilities); and (2) all deaths, regardless of cause, occurring after discharge from the hospital but before the end of the 30th postoperative day.[16,17]

Given that the current mortality rate for all patients undergoing congenital cardiac surgery operations in the United States is under 4%, outcomes other than mortality are important to over 96% of patients. Perioperative morbidity is a group of outcome measures frequently collected in addition to mortality.[18] As with mortality, consistency of definition is critical. In addition, the data source may influence the apparent outcome by how complete or accurate the desired information is. For example, administrative data often does not differentiate between preexisting conditions and postoperative occurrences. As a result preexisting conditions may be linked to an operation as morbidities when in fact they were not.

Long-term functional and neurologic outcomes are increasingly important as more and more children who undergo cardiac surgery survive to adulthood. Yet these outcomes are infrequently collected due to cost and the logistical challenges. Several national quality collaboratives, including the National Pediatric Cardiology Quality Improvement Collaborative (NPC-QIC) and the Cardiac Neurodevelopmental Outcome Collaborative (CNOC), are now dedicated to the multi-institutional investigation of functional and neurodevelopmental outcomes among neonates and infants with congenital heart disease. These groups have also implemented cooperative practices among centers and practitioners, designed to improve care based on best practices.

Case-Mix Adjustment

Variation in medical and surgical outcomes may result from differences in severity of disease, differences in the effectiveness of treatment, or random chance.[19] Risk adjustment is necessary to account for differences in severity of disease, and data should be presented with confidence intervals to account for random chance. Adjusting for case mix in congenital and pediatric cardiac surgery is challenging because of the large numbers of diagnoses and procedures, as well as the large variety of potential risk factors, including chromosomal abnormalities, syndromes, noncardiac congenital anatomic abnormalities, and preoperative factors such as preoperative mechanical circulatory support, shock, preoperative mechanical ventilation, preoperative renal dysfunction, and preoperative neurologic deficit.

Risk Stratification

In pediatric and congenital cardiac surgery, risk stratification is a commonly used methodology to adjust for case mix. Risk stratification is a method of analysis in which the data are divided into relatively homogeneous groups (called strata). Methodologies of risk stratification evolved in pediatric and congenital cardiac surgery because, unlike other specialties such as adult cardiac surgery (in which a large numbers of individual operations, such as coronary artery bypass grafting and aortic valve replacement, are performed), congenital cardiac surgery consists of a wide variety of operations, each of which is performed in relatively small numbers. As a result, any one operation is not performed in large enough numbers to allow for meaningful comparison across hospitals. Therefore strategies were developed to group operations for analysis. In pediatric and congenital cardiac surgery, three methods of risk stratification have been used on a large multi-institutional basis:

1. **R**isk **A**djustment for **C**ongenital **H**eart **S**urgery-1 categories (RACHS-1 categories)[20-22]
2. **A**ristotle **B**asic **C**omplexity levels (ABC levels) and the Aristotle Comprehensive Complexity Score[22-27]
3. The **S**ociety of **T**horacic Surgeons (STS)–European **A**ssociation for Cardio-**T**horacic Surgery (EACTS) Congenital Heart Surgery Mortality Categories (STAT Mortality Categories)[28,29]

RACHS-1 categories were reported in 2002 and introduced into the STS Congenital Heart Surgery Database (STS CHSD) Feedback Report in 2006. The RACHS-1 methodology groups operations into six categories based on discharge mortality. With few exceptions, additional patient and disease specific factors are not considered. Operations with similar mortality rates were placed together so that operations with the lowest expected mortality are in category one and operations with the highest expected mortality are in category six. RACHS-1 was created using a combination of judgment-based and empirical methodology. RACHS-1 categories are used today in the analyses of administrative data because, unlike ABC levels and STAT Mortality Categories, the RACHS-1 methodology includes the linking of the International Classification of Diseases, Ninth Revision, Clinical Modification (ICD-9-CM) codes for the various operations to the mortality risk categories. A list of the RACHS-1 categories is provided in Online Appendix 1.

The ABC score and the ABC level were introduced into the STS CHSD Feedback Report in 2002. The ABC score and the ABC level are measures of procedural complexity based on the potential of mortality, the potential of morbidity, and technical difficulty of the operation. A listing of the ABC score and the ABC level values are provided in Online Appendix 2.

The Aristotle Comprehensive Complexity Score addressed a perceived limitation of RACHS-1 by adding patient- and disease-specific variables that were felt to increase the complexity of the operation and influence the outcome (particularly mortality) of a surgical repair.[16] Thus a 2.8-kg infant receiving complete repair of tetralogy of Fallot would have the additional patient-specific risk factor of young age and small weight compared to an elective tetralogy of Fallot repair on a 5-month-old. If a child received an aortopulmonary shunt in infancy because the child had an anomalous coronary artery, the anomalous coronary artery would be counted as a disease-specific risk factor in the Aristotle Comprehensive Complexity Score. Many of the patient-specific factors and disease-specific factors described in the Aristotle Comprehensive Complexity Score were ultimately incorporated into the STS CHSD Mortality Risk Model.[30-33]

The STAT Mortality Score and STAT Mortality Categories are an empirically derived methodology of complexity stratification based on statistical estimation of the risk of mortality from an analysis of objective data from the STS CHSD and the EACTS Congenital Heart Surgery Database. The STAT Mortality Score and STAT Mortality Categories were based on analysis of 77,294 operations entered in the STS CHSD and the EACTS Congenital Heart Surgery Database (EACTS, 33,360 operations; STS, 43,934 operations) and introduced into the STS CHSD Feedback Report in 2010. Procedure-specific mortality rate estimates were calculated using a Bayesian model that adjusted for small denominators. Operations were sorted by increasing risk and grouped into five categories that were designed to minimize within-category variation and maximize between-category variation. A listing of the STAT Mortality Categories is provided in Online Appendix 3.

Like RACHS-1 categories and ABC levels, the STAT Mortality Score and STAT Mortality Categories group operations based on the risk of in-hospital mortality. Unlike RACHS-1 and Aristotle, which use expert opinion (subjective probability) to group operations, operations were placed in the five STAT Mortality Categories based on actual objective mortality rates derived from the STS CHSD and the EACTS Congenital Heart Surgery Database.

STAT Mortality Categories include more operations and have better discrimination than either RACHS-1 categories or the ABC score. Regarding case inclusion, previously published data reveal that of the eligible cardiac index operations, 85.8% were eligible for analysis by the RACHS-1 method and 94.0% were eligible for analysis by the ABC approach.[22] Meanwhile, in the spring 2017 STS CHSD Feedback Report, 98.5% of all eligible cardiac index operations were eligible for analysis with STAT Mortality Categories. Regarding discrimination, the initial publication of STAT Mortality categories documented that the STAT Mortality Categories have better discrimination than RACH-1 or Aristotle.[28] In the subset of procedures for which RACHS-1 categories and ABC scores are defined, discrimination was highest for the STAT Mortality Score (C-index = 0.787), followed by STAT Mortality Categories (C-index = 0.778), RACHS-1 categories (C-index = 0.745), and ABC scores (C-index = 0.687). When patient covariates were added to each model, the C-index improved: STS-EACTS score (C-index = 0.816), STS-EACTS categories (C-index = 0.812), RACHS-1 categories (C-index = 0.802), and ABC scores (C-index = 0.795).

Importance of Disease- and Patient-Specific Factors

All four methods of risk stratification (RACHS-1, ABC score, STAT Mortality Score, and STAT Mortality Categories) classify patients by the operation performed. However, when analyzing outcomes, one must also account for unique features of a given patient: patient-specific factors and procedure-specific factors. Although RACHS-1, ABC score, STAT Mortality Score, and STAT Mortality Categories were all designed to be maximally homogeneous with respect to estimated mortality risk, residual variation still exists in risk across procedures within the same category.

Congenital heart disease is complicated. Moreover, every child is different. However, providers tend to group children into categories of heart defects and report outcomes according to these categories. Although this approach facilitates investigation of questions related to "outcomes science" and education, it may not necessarily direct the best treatment for each child. The concept of precision medicine, which is rapidly becoming the preferred approach, is based upon the concept of individualized care that integrates existing information but also accounts for the unique characteristics of any given patient.

A child with a specific heart defect may have *disease-specific* risk factors, and he or she may also have *patient-specific* risk factors. If these factors are associated with an outcome, it is important to know what these factors are so that children with and without such factors can be considered differently. It is also important to understand that many of these patient- and disease-specific factors can influence one another (interact) and therefore may behave differently in certain combinations or in specific patients. Examples of disease-specific risk factors are anatomic or physiologic variances that might be associated with a heart defect and that change the risk for that disease entity. For example, two babies with tetralogy of Fallot may be quite different if one has a left anterior descending artery from the right coronary artery crossing the right ventricular outflow tract or a very small or atretic pulmonary valve whereas the other does not. These anatomic subtypes may increase the risk or change the nature of surgery (thus leading to a different subset of potential complications or outcomes) compared to a child with a normal coronary pattern or a reasonably normal-sized pulmonary valve. Therefore simply compiling results for the defect tetralogy of Fallot will not account for the added incremental risk or differences conferred from these disease-specific features. Similarly, patients with hypoplastic left heart syndrome (HLHS) can be divided into four typical anatomic variants (aortic atresia with mitral atresia, aortic stenosis with mitral atresia, aortic atresia and mitral stenosis, and aortic stenosis with mitral stenosis). However, one of these (aortic atresia and mitral stenosis) has a higher prevalence of coronary abnormalities, which increases the risk of a poor outcome. If one investigates outcomes for all patients with HLHS without accounting for this specific characteristic, the results will not represent an accurate portrayal of the risk of an individual patient, and outcomes at institutions that include a high number of these "higher-risk" patients may be substantially different than institutions without patients with this anatomic subtype. Most outcome reports lump together all patients with HLHS; however, failure to distinguish important disease-specific risk factors may contribute to differences between institutional outcomes. Luckily, for most congenital heart defects, many of the unfavorable morphologic variants are known from past study, allowing the compilation of a fairly comprehensive list of common disease-specific factors that can influence the outcome and even the treatment strategy.

The ability to interpret outcome data is further complicated by patient-specific factors, such as patient age, weight, other noncardiac congenital anatomic abnormalities, chromosomal abnormalities, genetic syndromes, or concurrent illness. The STS CHSD defines and captures data about both procedure-specific factors and patient-specific factors, and these variables are included in the current STS CHSD data specifications and STS CHSD data collection forms,[34] as well as the current STS CHSD Mortality Risk Model.[30-33] These factors can have variable influence on both a preferred treatment strategy (including timing of intervention) and expected outcomes for the prescribed treatment strategy.

Risk Modeling

RACHS-1, ABC score, STAT Mortality Score, and STAT Mortality Categories all classify patients by the operation performed. In all three cases, mean mortality rates were used to determine to which category an operation was assigned. One patient who undergoes a certain operation may have a low expected mortality risk while another undergoing the same operation may have a high mortality risk; however, they are both in the same category because it is the mean mortality rate of all patients undergoing that operation that was considered for classification rather than individual situations. To account for patient-specific factors and procedure-specific factors, STS developed the STS CHSD Mortality Risk Model.[30-33] Variables included in the STS CHSD Mortality Risk Model are listed in Table 4.1.

Over the past 20 years the STS CHSD has expanded to include data from over 435,000 operations from 127 congenital heart surgery hospitals in North America—124 in the United States and 3 in Canada. Therefore the STS CHSD contains data from approximately 96% of pediatric heart surgery programs in the United States and approximately 98% of pediatric heart surgery operations performed in the United States. Because of the large amount of data submitted

TABLE 4.1	Variables Included in the Society of Thoracic Surgeons Congenital Heart Surgery Database Mortality Risk Model

Age[a]
Primary procedure[b]
Weight (neonates and infants)
Prior cardiothoracic operation
Any noncardiac anatomic abnormality (except "Other noncardiac congenital abnormality" with code value of 990)
Any chromosomal abnormality or syndrome (except "Other chromosomal abnormality" with code value of 310 and except "Other syndromic abnormality" with code value of 510)
Prematurity (neonates and infants)
Preoperative factors
- Preoperative/preprocedural mechanical circulatory support (IABP, VAD, ECMO, or CPS)
- Shock, persistent at time of surgery
- Mechanical ventilation to treat cardiorespiratory failure
- Renal failure requiring dialysis and/or renal dysfunction
- Preoperative neurologic deficit
- Any other preoperative factor (except "Other preoperative factors" with code value of 777)[c]

[a]Modeled as a piecewise linear function with separate intercepts and slopes for each STS-defined age group (neonate, infant, child, adult).
[b]The model adjusts for each combination of primary procedure and age-group. Coefficients obtained via shrinkage estimation with the Society of Thoracic Surgeons–European Association for Cardio-Thoracic Surgery (STS-EACTS [STAT]) Mortality Category[6] as an auxiliary variable.
[c]Any other preoperative factor is defined as any of the other specified preoperative factors contained in the list of preoperative factors in the data collection form of the STS Congenital Heart Surgery Database, exclusive of 777 = "Other preoperative factors."
CPS, Cardiopulmonary support; *ECMO*, extracorporeal membrane oxygenation; *IABP*, intraaortic balloon pump; *STS*, Society of Thoracic Surgeons; *VAD*, ventricular assist device.

to the STS CHSD and the nearly universal participation among congenital cardiac surgery centers in the United States, robust risk adjustment that accounts for a large number of influential patient- and disease-specific factors is possible.

The STS CHSD Mortality Risk Model was developed from an analysis of 52,224 index cardiac operations from 86 centers during the 4-year analytic window of January 1, 2010, to December 31, 2013. The 2014 STS-CHSD Risk Model has the highest c-index of any pediatric and congenital cardiac surgical risk model to date (c-index in developmental sample = 0.875, c-index in validation sample = 0.858) and is the state of the art in pediatric and congenital cardiac surgical risk adjustment. A c-index represents the likelihood that the results are more than random. For example, in a random model, such as a coin flip, the c-index is 0.5 because the likelihood of heads versus tails is 50/50. The model undergoes recalibration with updating of the coefficients in the model on a twice-yearly basis to coincide with the production of each STS CHSD Participant Feedback Report.

The following information is available in Table 16 of the STS CHSD Participant Feedback Report and is based on the STS CHSD Mortality Risk Model[35]:

- *Observed mortality rate* is a percentage calculated by dividing the number of observed deaths by the number of eligible patients included in the calculation. This percentage is often referred to as the "raw mortality rate" or the "unadjusted mortality rate."
- *Expected mortality rate* is a percentage that reports the number of expected deaths for the given case mix, using the STS CHSD Mortality Risk Model. The STS CHSD Mortality Risk Model is used to estimate the number of expected patient deaths when considering the unique case mix of an STS CHSD participant or the mix of patients treated as defined by all of the variables listed in Table 4.1.
- *Observed-to-expected (O/E) ratio* is the number of observed deaths divided by the number of expected deaths. An O/E ratio greater than 1 means that the STS CHSD participant had more deaths than expected based on the actual case mix of that STS CHSD participant. An O/E ratio of less than 1 means that the STS CHSD participant had fewer deaths than expected based on the actual case mix. Small differences in the O/E ratio are usually not statistically significant, which is why the O/E ratio is reported along with 95% confidence intervals.
- *Adjusted mortality rate (AMR)* is an estimate (based on the STS CHSD Mortality Risk Model) of what the hospital's mortality rate would be if its observed performance was extrapolated to the overall STS case mix (specifically, the mix of age, weight, procedure types, and other model-specific variables, including prior cardiothoracic operations, noncardiac congenital anatomic abnormalities, chromosomal abnormalities, syndromes, and preoperative risk factors). It is calculated by the following formula: AMR of hospital = O/E ratio of hospital × overall observed STS mortality rate. Small differences in the AMR are usually not statistically significant, which is why AMR is reported along with 95% confidence intervals.

Importance of Risk Adjustment

The importance of risk adjustment can be seen in the following example. The volume-mortality relationship in pediatric cardiac surgery was investigated using clinical data from the STS CHSD.[9] Average annual program case volumes were categorized into four groups: small (<150 cases per year), medium (150 to 249 cases per year), large (250 to 349 cases per year), and very large (>350

cases per year). When raw mortality rates were compared, there were no statistical differences in mortality between the four volume groups. However, this homogeneity was misleading. Small hospitals tended to operate on fewer neonatal patients and as a result fewer high-complexity patients. After adjustment for patient-level risk factors and surgical case mix, there was an inverse relationship between overall surgical volume as a continuous variable and mortality. Examined categorically, the mortality rate at small programs was significantly worse than that at very large programs. In addition, the volume-mortality relationship varied based on case difficulty. For low-difficulty operations, all four volume groups performed similarly. In contrast, for high-difficulty operations, small programs had substantially higher discharge mortality relative to very high-volume programs. For the Norwood procedure, very high-volume programs outperformed all other volume groups. In congenital cardiac surgery, volume alone is an imperfect discriminator of mortality. Patient and surgical case mix–adjusted data are essential for identifying better-performing, higher-quality hospitals. Furthermore, there are undoubtedly other factors that are not considered in databases and that exist besides volume, such as the experience or unique skills of individual members of the team or the ability of some groups to work as a team with higher performance than groups that are unable to work as an effective team regardless of volume.[36] This concept helps to explain how some small programs may perform consistently well and better than volume alone might predict.

Alternative Approaches

Most surgical registries, including the STS CHSD, are procedurally based. Patients are entered only if they receive surgery at a participating institution. Similarly, the STAT Mortality Categories are procedurally based. An alternative approach of analysis is the use of a diagnosis-based database, but the challenge for attaining these data from a variety of sources is quite daunting because it would require entering ALL patients born with congenital heart disease, regardless of what management strategy is employed (e.g., observation, medical management, catheter-based intervention, or surgery). On a less daunting scale, however, one could analyze outcomes of all patients treated with surgery stratified into diagnostic groups rather than procedural groups, and some of these diagnoses-based analyses are already present in the STS CHSD Participant Feedback Report.

No clinical database currently exists that includes all congenital cardiac patients regardless of whether or not they undergo surgery or transcatheter intervention. Such a diagnosis-based database would certainly be valuable. However, our current procedurally based database does provide a significant body of information upon which to try and understand the critically ill patients with congenital heart disease that have undergone surgery (who represent most of the patients we care for in our intensive care units). Together, the patient- and disease-specific factors, along with the risk-stratification algorithm, allow benchmarking of center-level performance compared to other national aggregate data.

Numerous factors impact a patient's risk of mortality. Although the focus of most assessments of mortality is on the performance of the congenital cardiac surgeon and the care provided by the congenital cardiac team, these elements are only part of the picture. The majority of a patient's mortality risk is determined by factors related to the patient themselves rather than the care they receive.[37] Karamlou and colleagues used the Congenital Heart Surgeons' Society data sets to analyze 2421 complex neonatal operations.

They found that institutional performance varied among groups and that institutional excellence in managing one particular group of patients did not translate into excellence in other groups. Moreover, surgeon and center volume (or other experience domains) influenced outcomes in only one of the defects studied (transposition of the great arteries [TGA]). Patient or disease factors, such as low birth weight or anatomy, were the most influential in all other complex groups. Risk stratification systems and mortality risk models are designed therefore to account for a portion of this risk. Most of the current models, as we have seen, are dominated by a variety of patient-specific and disease-specific factors such as anatomy or weight; some, however, might be improved by including management strategies or processes (including the date of surgery in relationship to admission or birth, or intubation or feeding status). Some of these factors are modifiable, and some are not. For example, a patient with an active respiratory illness who needs an operation requiring cardiopulmonary bypass will have a lower risk of mortality if the patient can wait until the illness has resolved. In other words, the patient's risk of death may be lowered by delaying the operation. A 3-year-old who undergoes elective repair of a secundum atrial septal defect has a lower mortality risk than a neonate undergoing a Norwood procedure regardless of the center where they undergo surgery. In this case the patient's risk cannot be modified because the patient's diagnosis cannot be changed. Patient outcomes may be improved by addressing modifiable risk factors so that patients arrive in the operating room in optimal condition for surgery. In addition, systemic factors or infrastructure that transcend the congenital cardiac surgical team may have an important impact on patient outcomes. This interdependence and shared resource necessity is highlighted in the paper by Caddell and colleagues,[38] which investigated the relationship between outcomes within complex pediatric surgical specialties. These authors concluded that "Hospitals with low mortality rates for 1 high-risk pediatric surgical specialty tended to have low rates for other specialties. This observation suggests that diverse surgical fields share institutional resources and processes that affect their mutual performance. Implementation of these common pillars may lead to broader improvements in quality than efforts focused on individual disciplines." The finding that rates of mortality for seemingly disparate pediatric surgical specialties (cardiac surgery, neurosurgery, general surgery) were correlated suggests that shared institutional resources and processes affect their mutual performance.

Utility of Benchmarking: National Quality Initiatives

A natural evolution of the expansion and refinement of participation in national registries is the use of the data to guide quality initiatives and to leverage benchmarking within collaborative learning models, thereby improving outcomes among all participating centers. These types of learning models and consortia have successful historical precedent, and are being used increasingly both nationally and regionally. Some examples of successful regional consortia include the Michigan Health and Hospital Association Keystone Center, the Blue Cross and Blue Shield of Michigan Cardiovascular Consortium (BMC2), and the Northern New England Cardiovascular Disease Study Group (NNECDSG).[39] The California Congenital Cardiac Consortium, is one of the first groups dedicated to congenital cardiac surgery, and this collaborative is focused on reducing and improving access to care through reducing socioeconomic and racial disparities. One of the most intriguing and potentially important aspects of collaborative learning was demonstrated by the observation that participation ALONE in the NNECDSG, even in the absence of adoption of prescribed care processes, resulted in improved outcomes at individual centers. This phenomenon suggests that enrollment of patients into a data repository represents a commitment to understanding one's own data, and this act alone translated into tangible and measureable quality improvement. In the current era, participation in the STS CHSD is considered to be a measureable quality factor.

Deconstructing Outcomes Data: Pitfalls and Caveats

The data available for the study of outcomes come from several sources. A local quality improvement initiative may rely solely on locally collected data. In this case the individual institutional database can be accessed to answer the specific question of interest. Multi-institutional databases can provide larger data sets for evaluation, but limitations of how the data are recorded and validity concerns may become more important. In general, databases can be classified as administrative and clinical.

Administrative databases were designed for billing purposes; however, due to their broad scope and ready availability, they have been used for the study of outcomes as well. The Kids' Inpatient Database, the National (Nationwide) Inpatient Sample, state inpatient databases, and Medicare and Medicaid databases are examples of administrative databases. These administrative databases are not specific to any one specialty and were not designed for the evaluation of outcomes but rather to capture basic information regarding the patients qualifying for data entry (e.g., patients admitted to a hospital, patients receiving a surgical intervention, patients over 65 years of age). In general they contain *some* of the information about *all* of the patients (who qualify for entry into the data set). Data are typically entered by nonclinicians who have little understanding of the various clinical entities they are coding. Furthermore, the data that might be required to distinguish variations in patients may not be recorded or available. However limited, they are a rich source of data and are valuable for describing patterns of care over large groups of patients and hospitals. They also contain data on patients who underwent treatment courses other than surgery, which allows for the creation of diagnosis-based cohorts and the comparison of surgical and nonsurgical treatment options. Administrative databases may capture a broader range of patients than clinical databases; however, coding limitations and concerns about accuracy limit their utility for congenital cardiac surgery quality assessment.

Clinical databases may be more detailed and are designed to capture information regarding certain subgroups of patients. In general, they tend to capture more details related to the management and treatment of certain groups of patients and are designed to provide access to more granular information that can help clinicians and researchers understand differences in various clinical strategies. Information is typically entered by clinicians who have more intimate knowledge of subtle clinical information that might influence data entry. In this sense, clinical databases tend to have *most* of the information about *some* of the patients (meaning those patients who are being specifically studied). Clinical databases are sometimes called "registries," and an example of this type of database for congenital heart disease is the Congenital Heart Surgeons' Society database. The STS CHSD is also a clinical database.

Several studies have examined the relative validity of administrative versus clinical nomenclature for the evaluation of quality of care for patients undergoing treatment for pediatric and congenital cardiac disease. Evidence from four recent investigations suggests that the capability of coding congenital cardiac lesions via the International Classification of Diseases (ICD) in administrative databases in the United States is poor[40-43]:

- First, in a series of 373 infants with congenital cardiac defects at Children's Hospital of Wisconsin, investigators reported that only 52% of the cardiac diagnoses in the medical records had a corresponding code in the administrative data in the hospital discharge database.[40]
- Second, the Hennepin County Medical Center discharge database in Minnesota identified all infants born during 2001 with a code for congenital cardiac disease using administrative data. A review of these 66 medical records by physicians was able to confirm only 41% of the codes contained in the administrative database.[41]
- Third, the Metropolitan Atlanta Congenital Defects Program of the Birth Defects branch of the Centers for Disease Control and Prevention of the U.S. government carried out surveillance of infants and fetuses with cardiac defects delivered to mothers residing in Atlanta during the years 1988 through 2003.[42] These records were reviewed and classified using both administrative coding and the clinical nomenclature used in STS CHSD. This study concluded that analyses-based administrative coding are likely to "have substantial misclassification" of congenital cardiac disease.
- Fourth, a study was performed using linked patient data (2004–2010) from the STS CHSD (clinical registry) and the Pediatric Health Information System (PHIS) database (administrative database) from hospitals participating in both in order to evaluate differential coding/classification of operations between data sets and subsequent impact on outcomes assessment.[43] The cohort included 59,820 patients from 33 centers. There was a greater than 10% difference in the number of cases identified between data sources for half of the benchmark operations. The negative predictive value of the administrative (versus clinical) data was high (98.8% to 99.9%); the positive predictive value was lower (56.7% to 88.0%). These differences translated into significant differences in assessment of outcome, ranging from an underestimation of mortality associated with truncus arteriosus repair by 25.7% in the administrative versus clinical data (7.01% versus 9.43%; $P = .001$) to an overestimation of mortality associated with ventricular septal defect (VSD) repair by 31.0% (0.78% versus 0.60%; $P = .1$). This study demonstrates differences in case ascertainment between administrative and clinical registry data for children undergoing cardiac operations, which translated into important differences in outcomes assessment.

Despite these limitations, administrative data may be the only source of information on programs that do not participate in voluntary clinical databases. Several potential reasons can explain the poor diagnostic accuracy of administrative databases:

- Miscoding is accidental.
- Coding is performed by medical records clerks who have never seen the actual patient.
- The medical record contains contradictory or poorly described information.
- There is lack of diagnostic specificity for congenital cardiac disease in the nomenclature used in administrative databases.
- The medical coders are inadequately trained.

- ICD-9 diagnostic codes do not capture much of the clinical detail useful for risk assessment.
- ICD-9 procedural codes are absent for key congenital cardiac operations such as the Norwood (stage 1) operation.

Although one might anticipate some improvement in diagnostic specificity with the adoption of ICD-10 by the United States, it is likely to still fall short from that currently achieved with clinical registries. (ICD-9 has only 29 congenital cardiac codes, and ICD-10 has 73 possible congenital cardiac terms.) It will not be until there is implementation of the pediatric and congenital cardiac components of ICD-11 that harmonization of clinical and administrative nomenclature will be achieved with the resolution therefore of many of these challenging issues.[44,45]

Clinical databases, such as the STS CHSD, the European Congenital Heart Surgeons Association (ECHSA) Congenital Database, the Extracorporeal Life Support Organization (ELSO) Registry, and the United Network for Organ Sharing (UNOS) Database, collect clinical data related to a specific niche within cardiac surgery. The basis for entry into STS CHSD and the ECHSA Congenital Database is having a coded congenital or pediatric cardiac operation. Several groups of patients do not appear in these surgical databases, including patients who:

- Present with congenital cardiac lesions and undergo interventional procedures or medical therapy
- Are referred to other institutions
- Die before planned treatment
- Are offered no treatment

As a result, one can only evaluate the outcomes of the subset of a center's patients who undergo surgery. Long-term follow-up data on patients are limited in short-term clinical registries like the STS CHSD.

The focus and scope of clinical databases are limited as well. As surgically focused registries, many details of the preoperative and postoperative course that may be relevant to short- and long-term outcomes may be omitted. Follow-up is truncated at discharge or 30 days after discharge depending on the measured outcome. Return visits for treatment of late complications as well as long-term morbidity, mortality, functional status, and neurologic status are not captured. The result is a helpful but limited view of the success of a center's treatment strategy for congenital cardiac lesions.

Clinical data may be more accurate with regard to data about preoperative factors and complications than administrative data. However, clinical data also contain a limited number of data elements and may suffer information bias from coding inaccuracies. The individuals who collect the data often have a stake in the outcomes of subsequent analyses, which could lead to gaming of the data. Data quality are also compromised when the financial and time commitments of data collection become too great, which is particularly a risk when data entry is added on to the task list of clinical personnel (as opposed to a knowledgeable data coordinator) with already overwhelming clinical responsibilities. Participation in most clinical databases is voluntary, which creates sampling biases. Smaller hospitals, hospitals with limited resources, and those with lower performance may abstain from participation. As a consequence, the results obtained may be more favorable than those achieved by the overall population of hospitals. In particular, hospitals that are interested enough to participate in a clinical database differ from nonparticipating hospitals in that they must at least have the infrastructure in place to collect data. Participation may be a marker for further differences in structure and process, including additional quality improvement initiatives. The STS CHSD has near universal participation in the United States, obviating some of these concerns about sampling bias. Furthermore, the STS CHSD has a robust process of data verification in place to ensure completeness and accuracy of the data, especially for the fields used in the publicly reported the STS CHSD Mortality Risk Model. STS CHSD data verification includes random site audits of 10% of centers per year, so that approximately half of the database is audited every 5 years. The 2016 STS CHSD audit of 2015 data revealed that in an analysis of general variables the rate of data completeness was 99.94% and the rate of data agreement (accuracy) was 98.05%. Meanwhile, in an analysis of mortality variables, the rate of data completeness was 100%, and the rate of data agreement (accuracy) was 99.09%.

As described earlier, an alternative strategy to procedurally based data collection and analysis is diagnosis-based data collection and analysis. With this strategy, rather than a surgical procedure, the entry criterion would be presentation with congenital cardiac disease. By capturing this denominator, outcomes of competing treatment modalities, such as surgical and interventional closure of ostium secundum atrial septal defects, could be compared. Institutional strategies and biases for care of patients with lesions such as HLHS, in which treatment and comfort care are options, could also be evaluated. By capturing patients when they are first identified, rather than when they undergo surgery, appropriate timing of procedures can be evaluated. In addition, the impact of local conditions, such as socioeconomic factors and regional infrastructure, on access to and quality of care can be appraised.

One deficiency in most of our clinical and administrative data sets is the lack of physiologic data. It is clear that even the inclusion of disease-specific and patient-specific factors does not tell the complete story. The presence of tricuspid insufficiency or right ventricular dysfunction in a patient with HLHS will dramatically increase the risk of any chosen strategy (both at the time of Norwood [stage 1] operation and at subsequent stages) regardless of surgeon or center experience. Furthermore, a patient with a high transpulmonary gradient or a high ventricular end-diastolic pressure undergoing a Fontan operation will likely have a very different convalescence compared to a patient with a low transpulmonary gradient and low ventricular end-diastolic pressure. It is likely that emerging technologies such as database linkages, so-called big data,[46] and machine learning/neural networking will provide a mechanism to include a comprehensive profile of a particular patient and allow the first steps toward understanding the risk of the individual patient and operationalizing precision medicine.

Ideally a congenital cardiac program should be evaluated on the short- and long-term outcomes of all patients it treats. The goal of the treatment of congenital cardiac disease is long-term survival with good quality of life. Data collection should mirror this objective. Outcomes other than operative mortality should be investigated. As short-term mortality continues to decline, long-term outcomes become more meaningful. In the long-term, morbidity and complications occur more frequently than mortality and may be more easily linked to processes of care. Functional status, patient-reported quality of life, and neurologic status can be investigated as continuous variables, making it possible to detect clinically significant differences with smaller sample sizes. The tracking of such outcomes is more costly than the extraction of mortality rates from existing databases but would lead to a more complete and patient-focused understanding of congenital and pediatric cardiac surgery and congenital and pediatric cardiac care.

Even if the source data are of excellent quality, comparison of cardiac surgery mortality rates among institutions is still problematic due to the combination of low case volumes and relatively low mortality rates. A study by Welke and colleagues[47] of national administrative data from the United States found that annual case volumes for individual pediatric cardiac surgical operations were too low to differentiate performance between hospitals on the basis of mortality. When operations were categorized into RACHS-1 categories, the results were similar. Even when all RACHS-1 categorized cases were aggregated, only 1.6% of hospitals had annual case volumes greater than the 525 cases needed to detect a doubling of mortality when compared with a hospital performing at the national mean (Fig. 4.1). The following example is based on the realistic assumption that the overall mortality rate for pediatric cardiac surgery in the United States is 4% and illustrates this predicament. One can try to answer the following question: Is a hospital that performs 200 operations per year and has a 4% mortality rate any different than a hospital that performs 200 operations per year and has an 8% mortality rate? For a sample size of 200, the 95% confidence intervals around a 4% mortality rate are 1% to 7%. For an 8% mortality rate, the confidence intervals are 4% to 11%. Because the 95% confidence intervals overlap, the mortality rates are not statistically different. This analysis concluded that pediatric cardiac surgical case volumes and mortality rates are too low to use mortality alone as the criterion to differentiate between hospitals.[47]

The problem of data representation becomes even more difficult when adjusting for sample size. A small-volume program may be doing an excellent job, but it may take years for them to demonstrate that excellence, simply due to the limitations of a small sample size. For example, if we flip a coin 10 times and it comes up heads 8 times, we may think we have a pretty good coin. But the only way to really know is to flip the coin 10,000 times and see how many times it comes up heads. Programs that publish exceptional results with small volume may simply have had what statisticians call a type II error created by the potential variance of small sample size. Likewise, a cluster of bad outcomes (the coin coming up tails) may dissipate when enough cases are performed to provide an adequate sample. Even more problematic is the fact that each coin is weighted by complexity of the procedure being performed and may have a greater likelihood to come up heads or tails so that we cannot simply expect predictable outcomes that lend themselves to easy comparison. Any evaluation of results needs to account for the likelihood of the coin to come up heads or tails (the difficulty of the case and the complexity of the patient's other problems). This concept is sometimes reported as "observed versus expected" mortality, as described earlier, with better centers having observed mortality lower than (better than) expected. In short, data on outcomes can be very complicated and difficult to interpret and can lend themselves to misrepresentation. Therefore when reporting data about outcomes, it is critical to report these data with risk adjustment to account for variations in case mix and also with confidence intervals to account for random variation or chance.

Interpretation of outcomes is further complicated by the variation in procedures that are performed by different surgeons. Some of the surgical options are dependent on the patient's unique anatomy, and some are related to surgeon's preference. Regardless, two patients with the "same" defect may receive entirely different procedures in the hands of two different surgeons, and the type of procedure may have important implications for long-term quality of life. Even if two centers have identical survival, complexity, and observed versus expected outcomes, they may still be extremely different centers depending on the procedures they decide to perform for each specific heart defect. For example, a small ductal-dependent 2.8-kg infant with pulmonary atresia/VSD and confluent pulmonary

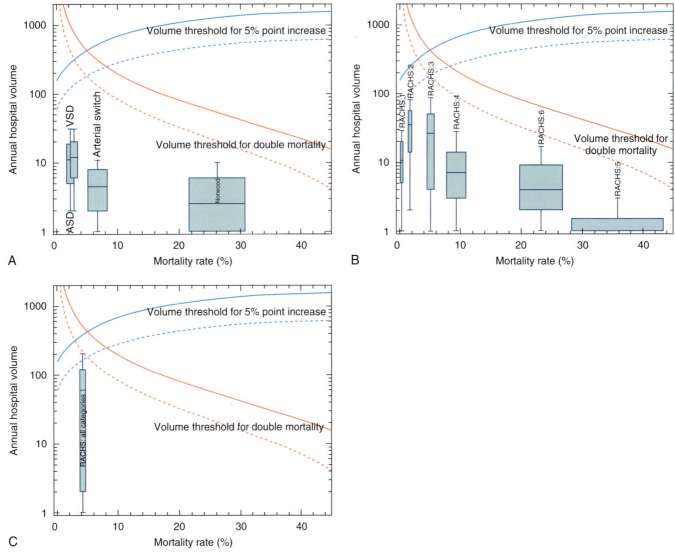

Figure 4.1 Actual hospital case volumes and threshold volumes necessary to detect a doubling of or 5 percentage point increase in the mortality rate. A, Selected operations. B, RACHS-1 cases by category. C, Hospital total RACHS-1 case volume. The height of each box ranges from the 25th to the 75th percentile of volume (for US hospitals), the whiskers are the 10th and 90th percentiles, and the median volume is depicted as a horizontal line. The width of each box represents the 95% confidence intervals of the mortality rate. As predicted mortality decreases, the volume for detecting a doubling increases. Operations with higher mortality require higher volume to detect a 5 percentage point difference in mortality. Threshold volumes for a one-tailed test, such as comparison of a hospital to a mean or benchmark, are depicted as dashed lines. Threshold volumes for a two-tailed test, such as comparison of two hospitals, are depicted as solid lines. *ASD,* Atrial septal defect closure; *RACHS:1,* Risk Adjustment for Congenital Heart Surgery, version 1; *VSD,* ventricular septal defect closure. (From Welke KF, Karamlou T, Ungerleider RM, et al. Mortality rate is not a valid indicator of quality differences between pediatric cardiac surgical programs. *Ann Thorac Surg.* 2010;89:139-144.)

arteries may receive palliation with an aortopulmonary shunt at one center, whereas another center may choose to perform a complete repair with VSD closure and right ventricular to pulmonary artery conduit. The baby receiving an aortopulmonary shunt may have ligation of the patent ductus arteriosus (PDA) at one center, whereas another center may choose to let the PDA close spontaneously after prostaglandins are discontinued. Each of these procedures are different; however, the reasons that drive these decisions are not standardized and cannot be evaluated with many databases. Another example might be the choice of aortic valve replacement for an 8-year-old. One center might choose to

use a mechanical prosthesis and another might decide to offer a Ross procedure (pulmonary autograft). Although short-term survival may be the same with either approach, long-term mortality and morbidity may be quite different. Such differences in long-term mortality and morbidity will be differentiated only with a database that functions as a platform for longitudinal follow-up.

Finally, a report of outcomes should include a description of the kinds of complications observed following surgery, as well as the likelihood of patients to die (fail to be "rescued") from these complications in the specific center. A report from the STS-CHSD[48] compared the incidence of complications from all centers that submitted data to STS CHSD, and the incidence of reported complications was remarkably similar for all institutions: approximately 40% of patients experience some type of complication after congenital or pediatric cardiac surgery. (These complications range from minor to major, but all can be measured and recorded by STS CHSD.) The manuscript then looked at the incidence of death (which was termed *failure to rescue*) for each center for patients with complications and was able to document a difference between institutions. Low-performing institutions had a rate of failure to rescue of 12.4%, whereas high-performing institutions had approximately 50% less failure to rescue (6.8%). There are also complications that patients may survive (be "rescued" from death) but that carry lifelong morbidity, such as the need for a permanent pacemaker, the need to replace an unrepairable valve with a mechanical valve (which requires anticoagulation) or a bioprosthetic valve (which will require re-replacement), the development of kidney failure that requires lifelong dialysis, or the presence of new significant neurologic (brain) disabilities. Other complications that do not generally carry lifelong implications, such as diaphragmatic paralysis, sternal infection, self-limited arrhythmias (such as junctional ectopic tachycardia), and chylothorax, may extend hospital length of stay, increase cost, and possibly result in another operation but should result in a good long-term outcome. In fact, a residual defect requiring reintervention (such as unplanned return to the operating room) is made worse by not being evaluated and managed appropriately (possibly trying to prevent recording it as a complication) rather than by doing what the patient needs. (Unplanned reoperation is a complication, but if the patient is discharged and returns at a later date for revision, the complication is no longer coded as such.) Similarly, although extracorporeal membrane oxygenation (ECMO) is considered a complication, the use of ECMO to support a patient so that his or her organs are adequately perfused may be preferable to avoiding ECMO, possibly increasing risk to the patient (from excessive inotropic therapy or impaired organ perfusion), in order to not have to record this complication. These examples speak to the complex nature and forces at play in reporting and evaluating outcomes for congenital and pediatric cardiac surgery.

Public Reporting

Public reporting is the disclosure of outcomes to the public. Although the practice has gained traction in recent years, it is not new. One of the earliest public reporting efforts was Florence Nightingale's publication in 1863 of hospital mortality rates in England.[49] In 1916 Ernest Amory Codman made public the outcomes of his End Result Hospital, which he had started after being fired from Massachusetts General Hospital for questioning the competency and commitment of his colleagues, as well as their refusal to disclose the results of their practices.[49,50] Public reporting was then essentially abandoned until the Health Care Financing Administration published hospital-specific mortality rates in 1986.[51] State-level initiatives began in 1990 in New York, and the STS began voluntary public reporting of adult cardiac surgery mortality in 2010.[52-57] The STS followed with voluntary public reporting of congenital heart surgery risk-adjusted operative mortality in 2015.[58-61] Currently a few states have public reporting initiatives for congenital heart surgery. These statewide initiatives consist of both mandatory and voluntary programs. In addition, many hospitals report pediatric cardiac surgical programmatic outcomes on their individual websites.

Public reporting efforts in congenital heart surgery focus almost exclusively on mortality. STS reports 4-year case volumes and outcomes for the overall pediatric and congenital cardiac program and for each STAT Mortality Category individually. Observed and expected mortality rates, O/E ratios, and AMR are reported for the same groupings.

To simplify publicly reported data for interpretation by patients and their families, STS also reports a one-, two-, or three-star rating for each hospital with three stars being the highest rating. Three-star programs are those for which the overall risk-adjusted operative mortality O/E ratio is less than 1 and the 95% confidence interval around overall risk-adjusted operative mortality O/E ratio does not overlap with 1. Two-star programs are those for which the 95% confidence interval around overall risk-adjusted operative mortality O/E ratio overlaps with 1. One-star programs are those for which the overall risk-adjusted operative mortality O/E ratio is greater than 1 and the 95% confidence interval around overall risk-adjusted operative mortality O/E ratio does not overlap with 1.

STS advocates rating of hospitals rather than ranking of hospitals. In contrast, U.S. News & World Report ranks hospitals. It collects structure and process measures, as well as a variety of outcome measures, including mortality as derived from the STS CHSD. In addition to surgical data, cardiology data and more systemic hospital measures are also included.

Unintended Consequences

Efforts to improve outcomes should focus on the surgeon and congenital cardiac team but should also investigate broader resources and practices within a hospital (as described in Chapters 1 and 2 of this textbook). Care must be taken in assigning importance to both structure and process, as well as to the subsequent outcomes. In most cases adherence to prescribed standards will lead to improved results; however, there may be exceptions. The setting of volume thresholds must be done with caution. Given that the mortality rates at hospitals of similar volumes vary widely, any chosen volume standard will exclude some excellent centers and some poor performers[8] (Fig. 4.2). If the continued existence of a program depends on its ability to meet a volume threshold, cases could be shifted or decision making altered to increase surgical volume. As a hypothetical example, a program that treats some fraction of patients with ostium secundum atrial septal defects by means of device closure in the cardiac catheterization laboratory (rather than by open-heart surgery) could shift to closing more or all of these defects surgically. Patients with ventricular septal defect and coarctation of the aorta could have their lesions treated in staged operations rather than one setting. Neonates born with tetralogy of Fallot could be treated initially with modified Blalock-Taussig shunts and later with full repairs, rather than neonatal repairs. None of these examples results in grossly inappropriate care, but they illustrate the idea that care may be driven (at least in part) by the economic necessity of the program to survive, by meeting a set volume standard, rather than entirely by what practitioners believe to be the most appropriate care for patients. Similarly, if a mortality standard is set that programs must meet for purposes of accreditation or reimbursement, the response from centers that see the need to meet the target as an economic necessity may be other than that which is intended. Upcoding, the entry of additional comorbidities into databases, may occur in an attempt to increase the expected mortality rate and thereby decrease the O/E mortality ratio. Alternatively, a lower-risk but less appropriate operation may be chosen to treat a given lesion. This potential disparity in how patients with congenital heart disease are managed contributes to the complexity of trying to compare (and rank) institutions. Because

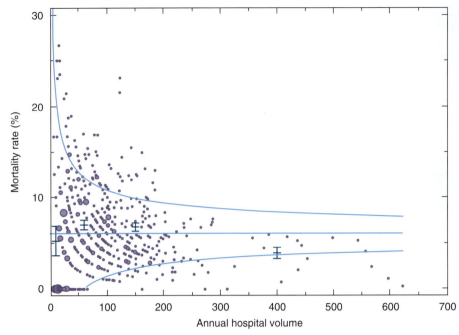

Figure 4.2 Individual hospital mortality rates are presented according to annual pediatric cardiac surgical volume. Not shown are 291 hospitals with fewer than 5 cases per year. The size of the circle at a given hospital annual volume and mortality rate represents the number of hospitals with that mortality rate at that volume. The horizontal line is the overall raw mortality rate (6.07%). The lines above and below this line represent the confidence intervals (CIs) of a hypothetical single institution at that volume and the average mortality rate; these give an idea of what mortality rates would be statistically different at that volume. The four marks with error bars are the collective mortality rates and 95% CIs for the four volume groups (<20 cases per year, 20 to 100 cases per year, 101 to 200 cases per year, and >200 cases per year). (From Welke KF, Diggs BS, Karamlou T, Ungerleider RM. The relationship between hospital surgical case volumes and mortality rates in pediatric cardiac surgery: a national sample 1988–2005. *Ann Thorac Surg.* 2008;86:889-896.)

the most commonly tracked outcome after congenital heart surgery is short-term mortality (in hospital and 30 days after discharge), the program may appear to be a high performer, whereas in actuality it is setting up patients for longer-term morbidity and suffering. Additionally, high-risk patients who were previously offered surgery may be denied treatment to keep the program mortality rate low. Patients with no other options may suffer or die for lack of treatment. For others, the decision to not operate or to be referred to another center may be appropriate. Again, however, it is the idea that program needs rather than patient needs could potentially drive clinical decision making that is inappropriate. Nevertheless, it is also a fact that some level of risk-averse behavior at some low-performing centers may actually be in the best interest of the patients.[56,57,61]

Conclusion

Our ability to assess quality in congenital cardiac surgery is constrained by the data and evidence available. The capacity of current metrics to differentiate high from low performers is limited by statistical constraints, as well as by challenges in recording differences between so many aspects of congenital cardiac care. Future efforts should be directed toward collecting and evaluating information that provides a broader picture of what makes a high-quality program (particularly structure or process measures that can be duplicated by other centers). Evaluating the surgical patient in the context of all patients with congenital cardiac disease will help determine the effectiveness of a program's broader approach. Tracking of long-term outcomes, including morbidity, mortality, neurologic status, and functional status, will help focus attention on the results and the timeline that matter most to patients and their families. Defining structural and process measures that affect outcome not only may improve the results of congenital cardiac surgery but may lead to improvement in other patient populations that share hospital resources. The result will be a more informative and patient-centered picture of the quality of care of the population of patients with congenital heart disease.

Reference

A complete list of references is available at ExpertConsult.

5

Pediatric Cardiac Intensive Care Unit Model

SCOTT I. AYDIN, MD; KONSTANTINOS BOUKAS, MD; JEANNIE KOO, CPNP-AC; JON N. MELIONES, MD; GEORGE OFORI-AMANFO, MD

Pediatric cardiac critical care medicine plays a central role in the care of patients with complex congenital and acquired heart disease. Over the last 20 years it has evolved into a distinct subspecialty with a clearly defined role in a congenital heart program. In most centers the pediatric cardiac intensive care unit (PCICU) forms the core of an integrated congenital heart program with a direct link to all the subspecialty services within the heart center (Fig. 5.1). The PCICU patient populations are heterogeneous in their demographics, anatomy, physiology, procedures, and outcomes, which results in an unpredictable environment where constant high-quality evaluation and management is essential. This resource-intensive environment not only stresses the people who work in the PCICU, but also consumes a lot of hospital resources

The concept of a PCICU originated from the unique challenges encountered in the preoperative and postoperative management of children with critical cardiac disease. In the early years of development of congenital heart surgery, pediatric cardiac surgeons were primarily responsible for the postoperative care. Over the last two decades, specialized cardiac intensive care units (ICUs) have emerged as a central component in the management of critically ill neonatal, pediatric, and adult patients with congenital and/or acquired heart disease. In addition, the scope of practice of the PCICU has grown to include patients with cardiac disease who have undergone noncardiac surgery or who are critically ill from noncardiac diseases such as acute respiratory failure. As a result of this specialization, outcomes have improved dramatically during this time period with patients surviving into adulthood as commonplace.[1,2] Although the reasons for this progress are multifactorial, advances in cardiac intensive care medicine have contributed to these improvements. The PCICU advances have been largely in the areas of clinical care model development and delivery, preoperative and early and late postoperative management strategies, patient monitoring, standardization of medical and nursing care pathways, development of quality and safety processes, nutrition, and multidisciplinary care delivery, including physical, occupational, and speech therapies.

Although data regarding the optimal method of care delivery to this specific patient population continue to emerge, there is significant center variation based on surgical volume, medical staff organization, and space allocation. The physician organization remains somewhat heterogeneous with units staffed with combinations of general intensivists, cardiac intensivists, cardiologists, and/or cardiac surgeons. Additionally, there may be differences in the protocols and best practices implemented in the care of the patients from unit to unit.[3,4] What seems to remain paramount in the care of this highly specialized patient population is that a dedicated team of professionals be tasked with the comprehensive care of critically ill pediatric and adult patients with congenital and/or acquired heart disease.

It is important to note that outcomes after cardiac surgery are now being reported transparently and publicly. Parents, colleagues, and referral groups should be able to know these data to help decide their plans for this high-stress situation. The role of the PCICU is paramount in achieving excellent outcomes. Two commonly used public recording databases that rank performance are the Society of Thoracic Surgeons–European Association for Cardio-Thoracic Surgery (STAT) score (Box 5.1) and the U.S. News & World Report Ranking (Table 5.1). As can be seen from both of these scorings, the PCICU is a major contributor to these important rankings and as such, an area of high focus. To achieve these goals a dedicated team specializing in children's heart care has been shown to improve outcome.[5]

Patient Population

The patient population in a PCICU can be stratified into three main categories:

1. Patients with congenital or acquired heart disease undergoing cardiovascular surgery (cardiac surgical patients)
2. Patients with congenital or acquired heart disease undergoing noncardiac surgery (noncardiac surgical patients)
3. Patients with congenital or acquired heart disease presenting with acute cardiorespiratory decompensation or other critical illnesses (cardiac medical patients)

Although the majority of patients fall into these three main categories, patient age may play a role in where they are ultimately admitted (e.g., extremely premature infant with hypoplastic left heart syndrome may be admitted to the neonatal intensive care unit [NICU]). Some centers adopt the approach of congenital cardiac critical care in which the unit provides care to patients of all ages from newborn to adulthood. Although this model provides a lifetime of continuity of care, the majority of the team is typically pediatric trained and may not have as much expertise in the management of comorbidities associated with aging, such as coronary artery disease, diabetes mellitus, obesity, and chronic obstructive

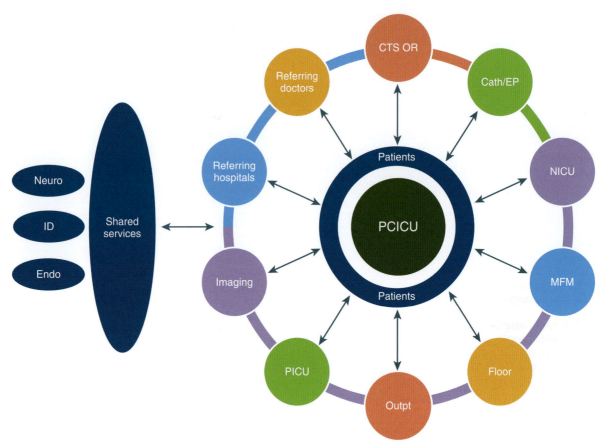

• **Figure 5.1** Role of the pediatric cardiac intensive care unit *(PCICU)* in a heart program. *Cath/EP,* Cardiac catheterization laboratory/electrophysiology; *CTS OR,* cardiothoracic operating room; *Endo,* endocrinology; *ID,* infectious disease; *MFM,* maternal fetal medicine; *Neuro,* neurology; *NICU,* neonatal intensive care unit; *Outpt,* outpatient.

pulmonary disease in adults with congenital heart disease (ACHD patients). The most commonly practiced model of PCICU in the larger heart centers is one that cares for patients from newborn up to 18 to 25 years of age. With such an approach the PCICU will capture up to 85% of critically ill patients with congenital heart disease (CHD) within a congenital heart program. Rarely the PCICU may take care of all postneonatal patients up to 18 to 25 years of age, whereas newborns with cardiac disease receive care in a NICU setting in the preoperative and postoperative periods. A growing model among small- to medium-sized programs is one in which all newborns receive their preoperative care in the NICU, and the immediate preoperative and post-operative management occurs in the PCICU. Finally, a model that has seen the most growth is one in which patient care, neonates included, preoperatively and postoperatively is delivered in the PCICU. One patient population, ACHD patients, remains a point of controversy as to where best to administer their care in the context of the complexities of their physiology and comorbidities, not to mention the social aspect of an adult cared for in a pediatric unit. Although each of these models has its merits and demerits (Table 5.2), there is an inherent tendency for variations in aspects of the patients' management. For instance, there may be some differences in fluid and electrolyte management of the newborn with CHD in the NICU versus the same newborn in the PCICU. To eliminate these care variations there is a strong need for multidisciplinary integration of care at both the nursing and physician levels and joint development of protocols and standardized care pathways to optimize

outcome. It is also essential to cross-train staff and develop specific metrics to assess protocol adherence.

Pediatric Cardiac Intensive Care Unit Care Model

Operational Components

The care model adopted by the PCICU is central to the overall function of the cardiac program. It is structured to be the core of an integrated care delivery system that supports both inpatient and outpatient areas of the cardiovascular program and plays a paramount role in the establishment of the continuum of care within the cardiovascular program. The successful PCICU positions itself to be readily available to provide immediate care to all critically ill cardiac patients in a calm, cordial, and efficient manner. It instills a culture of patient safety and multidisciplinary collaboration and delivers excellent clinical care while catering to the needs of the patients, their families, and referring physicians.

Philosophy and Approach

One of the central tenets of the evolution and maturation of cardiac intensive care has been the development of the multidisciplinary culture that includes all aspects of care, including pharmacy, dietary and nutrition, physical therapy, occupational therapy, speech

• BOX 5.1 The STAT Score

The STAT score is a tool designed to analyze the risk for mortality associated with congenital heart surgery procedures.

- *STAT Category 1* cases are less complex procedures that have a low risk of complications (e.g., closures of atrial septal defects and ventricular septal defects).
- *STAT Category 2* cases are procedures that have an increased risk of complications (e.g., coarctation of the aorta repair, congenitally corrected transposition of the great arteries, ventricular septal defect repair).
- *STAT Category 3* cases are complex procedures that have an increased risk of complications (e.g., hemi-Fontan and arterial switch operation).
- *STAT Category 4* cases are more complex procedures that have a higher risk of complications (e.g., tetralogy of Fallot repairs and truncus arteriosus repairs).
- *STAT Category 5* cases are the most complex procedures and have the highest risk of complications (e.g., Norwood procedure and heart-lung transplant).

Operative mortality is defined as (1) all deaths occurring during the hospitalization in which the procedure was performed, even after 30 days (including patients transferred to other acute care facilities), and (2) those deaths occurring after discharge from the hospital but within 30 days of the procedure.

The three categories of ratings are based on a participant's overall risk-adjusted O/E operative morality ratio:

- *One star:* higher-than-expected operative mortality; the 95% confidence interval (CI) for a participant's risk-adjusted O/E mortality ratio was entirely above the number 1.
- *Two stars:* as-expected operative mortality; the 95% CI for a participant's risk-adjusted O/E mortality ratio overlapped with the number 1.
- *Three stars:* lower-than-expected operative mortality; the 95% CI for a participant's risk-adjusted O/E mortality ratio was entirely below the number 1.

O/E, Observed-to-expected; STAT, Society of Thoracic Surgeons–European Association for Cardio-Thoracic Surgery.

TABLE 5.1 Metric for Children's Heart Center Performance *U.S. News & World Report Ranking*

Category	PCICU Role
Outcomes/Experience	
Survival post CHD surgery	Co-own
Survival post CHD complex surgery	Co-own
Survival post Norwood	Co-own
Survival post transplant	Co-own
Prevent infections	Co-own
Prevent ICU infections	Own
Prevent pressure ulcers	Own
Numbers	
Surgeries	None
Catheterizations	None
Norwood/hybrid	None
Program	
RN staffing	Co-own
CHD program	Co-own
Adult CHD	None
Heart transplant	None
Clinical services (OR)	Co-own
Clinical support services	Co-own
Advanced technology	Co-own
Specialized clinics/programs (balloon/stents)	Co-own
Full-time subspecialists	Own
Professional Recognition	
RN magnet	Co-own
MD reputation	Co-own
QI Efforts	
Best practices (M&M)	Own
QI efforts	Own
Health information technology	
Fellowship	Own
Clinical research	Own
Patient Support	
Family help	Own
Families in structuring care	Own

CHD, Congenital heart disease; ICU, intensive care unit; MD, physician; M&M, morbidity and mortality; OR, operating room; PCICU, pediatric cardiac intensive care unit; QI, quality improvement; RN, registered nurse.

therapy, social work, and child life. This approach allows for the recognition that each member of the team has ownership in the program and care of the patient. Ultimately, the expertise of each subspecialty is fully integrated in management algorithms for the benefit of the patient. A unique aspect of cardiac intensive care that sets it apart from general intensive care is the continuum of care provided. As noted earlier, some PCICUs provide preoperative management in the immediate postnatal period, postoperative management, and discharge planning and, in addition, play some role in aspects of interstage management of single-ventricle patients. The provision of such a continuum of care requires the understanding of preoperative and intraoperative management, which may facilitate the care of the patient in the postoperative period. Important as well are individualized and anticipatory approaches to the care of patients within the PCICU with continuous reevaluation of the management and the patients' response to interventions. Finally, the anticipatory culture is critical in the cardiac ICU for early recognition and timely response to changes in a patient's condition.

Patient Care

As much as possible, medical management of patients should be standardized with care pathways, protocols, and clearly delineated order sets. For effective implementation and tracking, the development of these tools require a multidisciplinary approach. As an

TABLE 5.2	Care Models: Pros and Cons	
	Pros	**Cons**
PICU model	When patient numbers low; provides consolidated ICU	Decentralized
PCICU model (NICU pre/post)	When patient numbers are higher and PCICU bed numbers are not enough, provides ICU level of care	Lack of preoperative and postoperative continuity of care Neonatal management differences Multiple transitions of care Dichotomized expertise in separate locations
PCICU model + IMU	Preoperative dedicated neonatal care Shared responsibilities Shared mental model Efficiencies in care Focused QI More established model Practical model for medium programs with limited ICU space More favorable model for research and training	Lack of preoperative and postoperative continuity of care Several transitions of care Dichotomized expertise in separate locations
PCICU model single stay	Continuity of care (preoperatively and postoperatively) Standardized preoperative and postoperative management More comprehensive approach to care involving all subspecialties More favorable model for research and training Fewer handoffs	Larger space requirements ICU less educated on D/C planning

DC, Discharge; *ICU,* intensive care unit; *IMU,* intermediate care unit; *NICU,* neonatal intensive care unit; *PCICU,* pediatric cardiac intensive care unit; *QI,* quality improvement.

example, an early extubation protocol cannot be successfully implemented without involvement of cardiac anesthesia providers. Also, the use of feeding protocols will need partnership with the dietary team and other providers outside the ICU. Such standardization not only minimizes errors but also alerts the team about patients who may have an unexpected course. For instance, a standardized postoperative inotrope regimen helps the PCICU team in early identification of patients who may have had an unexpected intraoperative course. Although most patients in the cardiac ICU have an uncomplicated course, the reported rate of significant complications ranges from 3% to 52%[3-9] depending on the complication examined. Some of these complications may be unavoidable, but the ability of the PCICU to recognize and promptly treat them is dependent on the quality of care delivered by the unit.

Organizational Structure. The complexity of the pediatric intensive care unit (PICU) and the high visibility/resource use, as well as the central role that the PCICU plays in the heart center, requires all stakeholders to have input. Managing these multiple factions requires the PCICU medical director, surgical director, and managers to develop a consistent and comprehensive strategy to monitor and improve performance and the team. We have suggested a group of standing meetings that we have found helpful (Table 5.3). These meetings will drive change as long as they have specific goals, data-driven agendas, follow-up, and communication back to the team. Several different challenges will be outlined in the following sections.

Performance Improvement. Performance improvement (PI) is the cornerstone for a successful PCICU. Databases are discussed in Chapter 3. Careful analysis and benchmarking of key data drives PI initiatives. Methodologies for performing PI are outlined in Chapter 2. However, to focus the PCICU team on key PI opportunities, we have included a list in Table 5.4. An example of this process

is outlined in Fig. 5.2. This PI process was used in performing chest closures in the PCICU. This is a process that is now done in the majority of ICUs around the country, yet there are many stakeholders in the process. To standardize this process we defined individual's roles, tasks, and quality measures and made a checklist for the procedure. The back of the checklist includes information that judges the quality of the process and possible opportunities for improvement. Another successful approach is to use a "cause-and-effect fish bone" approach. An example of how this is used in central line–associated bloodstream infection (CLABSI) is shown in Fig. 5.3. This approach helps to identify key areas of variability that are amendable to process improvement. Finally, PI should be a continuous process. One methodology to achieve this is continuously addressing high-risk conditions to determine opportunities for improvement. One such opportunity is "accidental extubations." Fig. 5.4 is a tool we use for continuous PI with accidental extubations. By continuously observing these high-risk conditions, we are able to identify opportunities early and ideally implement interventions before there is any patient harm.

Communication. Communication is paramount to the successful integration of care among the various disciplines involved in the management of the cardiac patient. Scripted handoff must be used when patients are transferred from one location to another and whenever there is a change in care teams. Some programs have used a "full-circle" handoff tool that involves the use of one comprehensive handoff sheet for patients leaving the PCICU for other locations, such as the cardiac catheterization laboratory or operating room, and returning to the PCICU.[10] This tool has improved information transfer between PCICU and anesthesia teams and has been particularly useful in cases in which the patient returns to the PCICU after shift change, when a new care team assumes management responsibility. Other modes of communication include routine multidisciplinary-psychosocial rounds involving

TABLE 5.3 Proposed Schedule for PCICU Meetings

Name	Goal	Members	Ownership	Frequency
Heart center leadership	Align all disciplines to achieve team goals	Senior clinicians, Ops	Heart center directors	Monthly
Surgical case conference	Discuss upcoming cases	All heart center clinicians	Cardiology/CV surgery	Weekly
PCICU safety	Identify opportunities to improve quality of care	PCICU faculty, CV surgery, cardiologists, RN management, staff and allied professionals	PCICU medical director/RN manager	Monthly
PCICU M&M	Review outcomes to determine systematic changes (e.g., CLABSI)	PCICU faculty, CV surgery, cardiologists, RN management, staff and allied professionals	PCICU medical director/RN manager	Monthly
PCICU Ops	Identify high-impact multidisciplinary areas for improvement and process improvement	PCICU medical director, RN manager, pharmacy, respiratory care	PCICU medical director/RN manager	Monthly
PCICU clinical case review	Review current/interesting cases to develop consensus	PCICU faculty/fellows/APP	PCICU faculty on service	Weekly
Code review	Review details of all codes/near code events	PCICU faculty, CV surgery, cardiologists, RN management, staff and allied professionals	PCICU code director	Monthly
Family meetings	Consolidate plans and identify communication concerns	PCICU attending/team/RN on service, social work, quality of care	PCICU clinical team	Done when needed or after 2 weeks in PCICU
Quality of care rounds	Identify barriers in care and care transitions	PCICU clinicians/staff, quality of care team, social work, transition of care teams	PCICU clinical team	Weekly
"Brain" rounds	Optimize neurologic outcomes	PCICU attending/team/on service, neurology	PCICU team	Weekly
Family advisory council	Identify family-directed initiatives to improve quality of care	Parents, PCICU clinicians, CV surgeons, cardiologists, PCICU nurse manager/staff	Family council lead/PCICU director/RN manager	Monthly

APP, Advanced practice provider; *CLABSI*, central line–associated bloodstream infection; *CV*, cardiovascular; *M&M*, morbidity and mortality; *Ops*, operations; *PCICU*, pediatric cardiac intensive care unit; *RN*, registered nurse.

the medical team, nursing, social work, physical therapy, occupational therapy, speech therapy, nutrition, and child life have greatly enhanced the ability of the PCICU to meet the needs of the family beyond medical treatment and to facilitate discharge planning.

Additional modes of communication include family-centered care, in which parents are allowed to be present at work rounds, during invasive procedures such as tracheal intubations, and during cardiopulmonary resuscitation.

Conflict Resolution. A simple strategy of shared decision making was described by Tom Karl and contemporized for health care by Jeff Jacobs and Dave Cooper.[11] Management for critically ill children with heart disease can elicit many different option and opinions. Jacobs and Cooper have described how when two health care providers disagree, each provider can classify the disagreement into three levels of decision (following the Karl-Jacobs [KJ] classification):

KJ level 1 decision: ''We disagree, but it really does not matter, so do whatever you desire!''
KJ level 2 decision: ''We disagree, and I believe it matters, but I am OK if you do whatever you desire!!''

KJ level 3 decision: ''We disagree, and I must insist (diplomatically and politely) that we follow the strategy that I am proposing!!!!!!''

The basis for a KJ level 1 decision is that both strategies are acceptable and neither strategy would likely increase the risk for the patient. When this discussion occurs, a reasonable response is, ''I do not need to weigh in on this decision.'' An example of a KJ level 1 decision is choosing a continuous furosemide infusion versus intermittent dosing in a postoperative patient with oliguria. For the patient it is likely that it really does not matter one way or the other, and the decision is based on "style."

A KJ level 2 decision implies that although there is a significant disagreement, it would be difficult to prove that one strategy is superior, and that either approach is unlikely to have an important effect on the outcome of the patient. In this decision scenario the conflict associated with and argument would outweigh the potential benefit of either strategy. In such a situation, a reasonable response would be, ''You have my opinion, but you are welcome to weigh the evidence and reach your own conclusion.'' An example of a KJ level 2 decision is choosing to use epinephrine (adrenaline)

TABLE 5.4	Performance Improvement Opportunities	
Area of Opportunities	Process Improvement Tool	Resources
ABG use	Just do it	
Accidental extubations	Just do it	
Blood use	Six Sigma	
Chest closure in unit	Just do it	
CLABSI	Six Sigma	Root cause analysis sheet
Feeding	Protocol/process control	Add
Goal agreement	Protocol/process control	
ICU-IMU/floor handoff	Six Sigma	
Laboratory usage	Just do it	
Nosocomial infections	Protocol/process control	
OR-ICU handoff	Six Sigma	See Fig. 5.3
PHTN strategy	Just do it	
Travel off unit	Protocol/process control	Add
Rounding efficiency	Protocol/process control	
Single-ventricle management	Protocol	
Ulcer	Just do it	

ABG, Arterial blood gas; *CLABSI,* central line–associated bloodstream infection; *ICU,* intensive care unit; *IMU,* intermediate care unit; *OR,* operating room; *PHTN,* pulmonary artery hypertension.

versus dopamine in a postoperative patient with hypotension and echocardiographic evidence of poor left ventricular contractility. In this example a given provider may truly believe that either epinephrine or dopamine is better; however, in the absence of evidence-based data the provider decides not to argue and instead agrees to use the treatment advocated by his or her colleague.

A KJ level 3 decision implies that there is significant disagreement, but based on scientific evidence as well as my own education, training, experience, and knowledge, I know that the only safe cause of action is the one that I am proposing. In such a situation a reasonable response would be, ''I have dealt with this in the past using various approaches, and I know that only strategy 'X' will be effective. The medical literature also supports this approach. Thus the risk for the patient will escalate if my strategy is not followed.'' An example of a KJ level 3 decision is deciding whether or not to return to the operating room to repair a residual lesion or perform a cardiac catheterization to determine the pathophysiology. In this case, either the surgeon or the intensivist may feel quite strongly that his or her opinion is true and correct and must be chosen. Many similar scenarios could be written for intensivists in their daily interactions with surgeons. In fact, similar scenarios could also be described that involve the daily interactions of any of the various members of the health care team. We all want to do what we have devoted our lives to learning. Abandoning the concept of ''patient ownership'' can create an environment that promotes this concept. Abdication of responsibility, micromanagement, or distancing oneself from a bad outcome will not help to achieve our goals. KJ level 1 decisions and KJ level 2 decisions

typically do not create stress on the team. KJ level 3 decisions are the real challenge. Occasionally the PCICU care team is faced with such level 3 decisions, and teamwork, shared decision making, and mutual respect may be challenged. Teamwork is a learned behavior, and mentorship is critical to achieve a proper balanced approach. If we agree to leave our egos at the door, then, in the final analysis, the team will benefit, and we will set the stage for optimal patient care. In the environment of strong disagreement, true teamwork and shared decision making are critical to preserve the unity and strength of the multidisciplinary team and simultaneously provide excellent health care. When these conditions arise, it is important to have these discussions in a nonthreatening environment (not at the bedside or potentially not in the unit), with the support of senior members of the team, and to avoid the need of decision making by a committee.

Care Delivery

Two predominant models of delivery of cardiac intensive care to patients with congenital and/or acquired heart disease exist in developed countries. The first model, which is also the historically older model, is one in which cardiac critical care is part of a general PICU. In this model the pediatric intensivist must understand normal and abnormal cardiopulmonary physiology, appreciate the anesthetic and surgical techniques used, apply appropriate monitoring, and supervise the hour-to-hour life support.[12] The second model, which has become increasingly prevalent, is one in which cardiac intensive care is delivered in a dedicated cardiac ICU by a distinct cardiac critical care team.[13] Services delivered in this setting are provided by a multidisciplinary group that includes pediatric cardiac intensivists, pediatric cardiologists, pediatric cardiac surgeons, cardiac nurses, respiratory therapists, and other specialized support staff who are specifically in tune with the needs of the patient with congenital and/or acquired heart disease.[14,15]

Regardless of which model is chosen or present, the pediatric general or cardiac intensive care physician needs to be familiar with selected cognitive areas unique to the care of these patients, such as cardiogenic shock, rhythm disturbances, basic echocardiographic interpretations, cardiomyopathies, and pulmonary hypertension to name a few.[16] What may become problematic in the assessment and management of patients with congenital and/or acquired heart disease is when the patient is viewed as a collection of organ system dysfunction. Rather, the goals of the pediatric cardiac intensivist along with the multidisciplinary team is to remain cognizant of how the heart may interact with other organs systems both in the normal and failing state. This aspect becomes vital when taking into account the frequent perturbations of physiology that exists in the postoperative period. The pediatric cardiac intensivist requires a unique skill set that goes beyond the typical intensivist or cardiologist. There must be proficient understanding of cardiac physiology (normal, developmental, and disease states), cardiac anatomy, and the multitude of surgical procedures and their indications. Furthermore, a strong understanding of the different imaging modalities, specifically as they relate to the heart and other organ systems, that are frequently used to diagnose patients with CHD and for continued assessment during their clinical course. A strong understanding of cardiac catheterization techniques is also critical, especially recognizing the information that may be learned that is otherwise not obtainable from standard ICU monitoring or noninvasive imaging. Another skill that is equally important, but at times more difficult to master, is determining the correct timing for referral for cardiac catheterization in

HCICU Bedside Procedure Checklist

One day prior: (RN)

☐	Notify charge RN of planned procedure date (time if known)
☐	Notify lead RT of planned procedure date (time if known)
☐	Order 1 unit RBCs for procedure

Day of procedure: (RT)

☐	Assess morning x-ray for ETT placement with HCICU team
☐	Assess tape integrity

Day of procedure: (RN)

☐	Bring headlight, Bovie, CV cart, and footstool to bedside
☐	Remove excess equipment from crib/bed space
☐	Clean off tray table and sanitize
☐	Have 1 unit RBCs checked and ready to give with filter in cooler at bedside
☐	Have 5 doses of epi spritzers at bedside (1 mcg/kg) (As previously ordered)
☐	Have CaCl at bedside (20 mg/kg) (As previously ordered)
☐	Have bottle of 5% albumin available at bedside (to be dosed 5 mL/kg)(As previously ordered)
☐	Request HCICU provider to input orders: Sedation/Analgesia/Paralytics and have ready at bedside as ordered
☐	Extend venous access line using a medline and a line with large bore tubing. Both labeled and accessible to HCICU Provider
☐	Extend art line with transducer tubing/stopcock and have labeled and accessible at base of bed
☐	Patient connected to temporary pacemaker cables with pacer box accessible at base of bed; MD to program accordingly to ensure appropriate settings
☐	Set up additional suction port for OR suction with tubing
☐	Monitor alarms accessible or accessible via remote monitor
☐	Change time scale on NIRS to 1 hour
☐	Notify 2nd nurse of planned procedure time

Upon OR team arrival: (RN, RT, and OR team)

☐	Position patient with right side to edge of bed; chest (shoulder) roll in place and patient lying flat; head turned to the side with ETT out of surgical field and supported
☐	Evaluate airway after positioning
☐	Airway suctioned and secretions cleared; free-flowing FiO_2 (Ambu bag) turned off at wall to prevent fire
☐	If patient on scheduled antibiotics, give dose within 30 minutes of skin incision if possible, otherwise continue as scheduled

Postprocedure: (HCICU provider)

☐	Order postprocedure blood gas frequency
☐	Evaluate postprocedure chest x-ray

Postprocedure: (RN)

☐	Reposition patient and remove shoulder/chest roll
☐	Obtain chest x-ray
☐	Return blood cooler to blood bank

Postprocedure: (RT)

☐	Turn ON free-flowing FiO_2 (Ambu bag)
☐	Reposition patient and remove shoulder/chest roll
☐	Evaluate airway after repositioning

Planned Date: _____

Time: _____

Surgery Attending:
☐ X   ☐ Y

HCICU Provider:

_____

Bedside RT: _____

2nd RN: _____

Day of procedure: (HCICU provider)

☐	Order sedation/analgesia/paralytics
☐	Program pacemaker accordingly to ensure appropriate settings if needed
☐	Keep PIP<30 with VT 6-10 mL/kg and $ETCO_2$ <45. If PIP >30 reassess airway position, atelectasis, etc
☐	Keep CVP <12-15 with good NIRS, HR, BP, and Epin ≤0.05. If CVP >15 and or NIRS, HR, BP abnl despite Epin = 0.05 consider leaving chest open

---

Fentanyl: _____ mcg/kg x _____ doses

Midazolam: _____ mg/kg x _____ doses

Ketamine _____ mg/kg x _____ doses

Rocuronium: _____ mg/kg x _____ doses

Unplanned extubation: ☐ Y   ☐ N

Line/Tube dislodgement: ☐ Y   ☐ N
Explain:

Significant change in clinical status: ☐ Y   ☐ N
Explain:

Obstacles to procedure or additional items not on checklist:

• **Figure 5.2** Protocol for closing chests in the pediatric cardiac intensive care unit (PCICU) with performance improvement component. *abnl*, Abnormal; *art*, arterial; *Bovie*, Bovie electrocautery; *BP*, blood pressure; *CV*, cardiovascular; *CVP*, central venous pressure; *epi/Epin*, epinephrine; *ETCO₂*, end-tidal carbon dioxide; *ETT*, endotracheal tube; *FiO₂*, fraction of inspired oxygen; *HCICU*, Heart Center Intensive Care Unit; *HR*, heart rate; *MD*, physician; *NIRS*, near-infrared spectroscopy; *OR*, operating room; *PIP*, peak inspiratory pressure; *RBC*, red blood cell; *RN*, registered nurse; *RT*, respiratory care; *VT*, tidal volume.

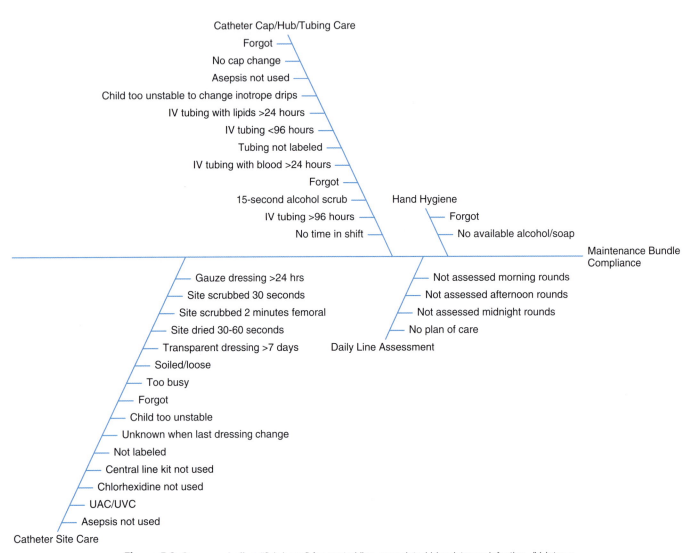

• **Figure 5.3** Cause-and-effect "fish bone" for central line–associated bloodstream infection. *IV,* Intravenous; *UAC,* umbilical artery catheter; *UVC,* umbilical venous catheter. (Courtesy Christine Meliones.)

Patient Data			

Patient Sticker

ETT Size:

Cuffed / Uncuffed

ETT Depth (pre-UPE):

# of days intubated:

Nursing Ratio:

RT Ratio:

Patient in restraints: Yes/No

If yes what kind:

Date:	Time:	Ventilator mode and settings prior to event:	
		Mode: Rate:	MAP:
Age:	Room #:	PIP/VT: I.T.:	AMP:
Weight:		PEEP: FiO2	Hz:

Adverse Events Due to Extubation:	CPR	Increased vent setting	Vital sign changes	Repeat diagnostic testing	Other:

Endotracheal tube tape/tube holder:

Was the tape completely adhered to the upper lip?	Yes	No
Was the tape/tube holder completely adhered to both cheeks?	Yes	No
Did the ETT slide through the tape?	Yes	No

Last known position of patient's body prior to event	Supine	Prone	L/R side lying

Patient's position at the time of the UPE (circle one of each):

Head (relative to body) Midline Left facing Right facing

Neck Neutral (sniffing) Extended (chin up) Flexed (chin to chest)

Body Supine Prone L/R side lying

Were any of the following used?

Z-Flow Blanket nest Neck rolls Other:

How was the ventilator tubing being supported?

Vent arm Bed arm None

Was there increased patient activity prior to the UPE?	Yes	No

Did the UPE occur during any of the following processes of direct care? *(circle all that apply)*

Retaping/Resecuring ETT Bathing Suctioning Weighing

RT Treatment Unknown Linen change/Bed change Repositioning Other:

Was the patient on vent wean?	Yes	No

Describe events that may have led to the extubation (e.g., ECHO, EEG, retaping ETT):

Time of last x-ray:

Was the tube in good position:

If no, when was it adjusted:

What continuous infusion sedation was the patient on prior to extubation?

Fentanyl: Versed:

Precedex: Paralytic:

Other:

# of Boluses in last hour:

Was the sedation weaned within the shift?	Yes	No

Patient's last Comfort B score:

Was reintubation necessary?	Yes	No

Patient's RT and RN:

Were any parents at the bedside at the time of the event?

• **Figure 5.4** A continuous evaluation process into "accidental extubations." Continuous performance improvement may involve constant observation of high-risk situations to provide early warning of potential risks. *AMP,* amplitude; *CPR,* cardiopulmonary resuscitation; *ECHO,* echocardiogram; *EEG,* electroencephalogram; *ETT,* endotracheal tube; *FiO₂,* fraction of inspired oxygen; *I.T.,* inspiratory time; *L,* left; *MAP,* mean airway pressure; *PEEP,* positive end-expiratory pressure; *PIP,* peak inspiratory pressure; *R,* right; *RN,* registered nurse; *RT,* respiratory therapist; *UPE,* unplanned extubation; *VT,* tidal volume.

the postoperative patient. Lastly, an understanding of cardiac electrophysiology (EP) is essential because life-threatening arrhythmias are not uncommon in the cardiac ICU setting. This includes proper arrhythmia identification and subsequent choice of therapy (antiarrhythmic medications, pacing/defibrillation modalities, and/or referral for EP study and/or ablation).[15] The use of a temporary pacemaker in the diagnosis and management of arrhythmias in the postoperative patient is also an essential skill for the cardiac intensivist.

The vast majority of ICUs delivering care to patients undergoing surgery for congenital and/or acquired heart disease exist within a university-affiliated freestanding children's hospital or a children's hospital within a hospital.[13] A recent survey of institutions demonstrated a nearly even split between centers providing cardiac intensive care within a general ICU setting and those with a dedicated cardiac ICU.[11,18] A factor that may be more important to the outcome of the critically ill cardiac patient may be the team caring for the patient rather than the physical location where the care is being delivered. To that point, the current distribution of physicians responsible for the care of these patients irrespective of their physical environment remains heterogeneous, with a combination of pediatric cardiologists, general intensivists, cardiothoracic surgeons, and dual-trained pediatric cardiology and critical care physicians assuming primary care roles.[13,17]

When examining the differences in care delivery characteristics that exist between the general PICU compared with the PCICU, the PCICU is much more frequently affiliated with a university and located within a freestanding children's hospital. In addition, dual-trained physicians in pediatric cardiology and critical care medicine, fellows, and physician extenders are the predominant providers to patients with congenital and/or acquired heart disease in the PCICU compared with similar patients cared for in the PICU. Furthermore, patients cared for in the PCICU are generally younger, smaller in size, and have longer preoperative length of stay.[13]

Outcomes

There is sparse evidence in pediatrics that cohorting and standardizing the care of patients with similar disease processes improves outcomes.[19-21] As mentioned previously, approximately half of the centers in the United States deliver cardiac intensive care services via a dedicated cardiac ICU, though there appears to be no statistically significant difference in morbidity and mortality.[23] However, there may be certain subpopulations of patients, such as transposition of the great arteries, that may benefit from receiving care in the cardiac ICU compared with the general PICU in regard to mortality and length of stay.[23] In addition, there may be instances when programs are in their infancy in which transition to or establishment of a dedicated cardiac ICU may drive improvements in outcomes. What may actually drive outcomes in patients after congenital and/or acquired heart disease surgery is the relationship of specific center factors, such as center volume, surgeon experience, and multidisciplinary specialized care. Several studies have demonstrated a correlation of outcomes and center volume, with the higher-complexity patient benefiting most from this relationship.[24-29] Furthermore, factors related to physician and staff training and expertise, as well as the presence of standardized protocols, may influence outcomes more than physical structure.[22,30] In the last several years there has been a rapid transition to a coverage model that consists of 24-hour 7-days-a-week in-house attending intensivist coverage. This model has demonstrated a potential for shorter lengths of stay and reduced morbidity and mortality.

Cost Containment. Resource use and cost containment are essential because the cost for PCICU care constitutes one-tenth to one-sixth of the total costs of congenital heart disease surgery.[31] The goal of a successful intensive care team is to optimize care while controlling costs. Cost-containment strategies in the PCICU should focus on the following:

1. Reducing length of ventilation/early extubation
2. Reducing length of stay/transfer of care
3. Reduction in laboratory, pharmacy, and radiology costs
4. Reducing blood product use
5. Improving enteral nutrition
6. Early deintensification of PCICU patients

Cardiac Step-Down and Intermediate Care Units

Children with congenital or acquired heart disease may require monitoring and intervention outside the critical care setting. Excellence in the care of the child with cardiac disease should extend beyond the intensive care setting. Strict criteria for admission to pediatric cardiac step-down and intermediate care units should be clearly defined to provide the most comprehensive and safest care for these complex patients. Such clear criteria are essential for transition of care and optimal timing of transfer and resource use. When a child transfers from the ICU setting to a step-down or intermediate care unit, a collaborative effort should be made to make the transition as seamless as possible. Redirection of care from critical illness to recovery or, frequently, chronic illness should employ a multidisciplinary approach with participation from pediatric critical care, cardiology, consulting services, specialized nursing, respiratory care, allied health professionals, social work, and family members.

Providers

Care coordination for children in cardiac step-down or intermediate care areas requires a variety of providers, each bringing his or her own expertise to facilitate a plan best suited for each patient. The team of providers should include representation from both pediatric cardiac critical care and cardiology. This may consist of attending physicians, advanced practice providers (e.g., nurse practitioner, physician assistant, clinical nurse specialist), and in academic institutions, fellows, residents, and interns. Although the cardiology team may lead care in this setting, input from the critical care service may be necessary for providing insight into ongoing critical care needs and past clinical course while in the ICU.

Multidisciplinary rounds provide a forum for those involved in a child's care to review past medical history, hospital course, recent events, and current problems to establish a plan of care. The use of standardized management plans has been considered useful and should be employed to determine normal convalescence and identify deviations from the expected clinical course. Although review of a patient's course and assessment traditionally is systems based, problem-based plans of care may be used for a comprehensive approach to management.

Nursing

The bedside nurse's role in step-down and intermediate care areas requires critical thinking and assessment skills. It incorporates family education and anticipatory guidance and discharge planning. Specialized nursing care for the child with congenital or acquired heart disease should extend through all levels of care from ICU to step-down and intermediate care areas. Rigorous nursing orientation, continued education, and skills development should be a priority to maintain high nursing standards. The development and retention of dedicated pediatric cardiac nurses is essential to a successful program. This may prove to be a challenge in shared model units where step-down and intermediate care areas incorporate a variety of subspecialties. The ratio of nurses to patients is typically 1:1 or 1:2 depending on patient acuity and the number of staff available per shift.

Nursing care in a PCICU is extremely specialized. Focusing on a rigorous orientation period and continued education is key for a successful program. A knowledge base of complex cardiac anatomy and physiology, monitoring, and interpretation of data is crucial for all care team members, but especially for the nurse at the bedside, where subtle changes and simple interventions can greatly impact patient outcomes.

Participation of the bedside nurse during daily rounds is integral for optimal patient care delivery. Although physical assessments are not performed as frequently outside the ICU, the bedside nurse is equipped to detect changes in a child's condition and should alert the team about any concerns for prompt evaluation and intervention and should therefore be exposed to similar education and orientation as the ICU nurse. The bedside nurse also plays an indispensable role in the coordination of inpatient services, discharge planning, and caregiver education.[15,32]

Allied Health Care Professionals

Comprehensive patient care requires the skills of allied health care staff and should be initiated early within the hospital stay. The nutritional needs of a child with a congenital or acquired heart defect are unique and require the specialized care of a registered dietitian. The dietitian can accurately assess and reassess a child's nutritional needs and growth parameters while an inpatient and, when needed, as an outpatient. Daily discussions of nutritional needs and growth should occur during rounds. For infants with cardiac disease, nutrition and feeding issues frequently prolong length of stay. The development of feeding protocols with a specialized team has been demonstrated to improve outcomes and potentially decrease hospital length of stay. The feeding team is composed of a registered dietitian, feeding therapists (occupational therapist and/or speech therapist), and a lactation specialist. Although feeding protocols and therapies are introduced in the ICU, progress continues while in step-down or intermediate care areas. The feeding team should have standardized documentation and communication with the provider team regarding oral feeding progress and the potential need for noninvasive or surgical feeding tube placement.

The neurodevelopment of children with CHD is another area that has gained attention over the course of the years. Neuroimaging and electroencephalography can be used for the evaluation of these patients, along with consulting pediatric neurologists. Given the fact that many patients develop neurodevelopmental problems, which carry a significant burden to the children, their caregivers, and families, more research is needed to identify interventions that could improve the outcomes.[33,34]

Infants with CHD often require long-term vascular access. It is imperative to avoid long-term central venous lines both for the increased risk of CLABSI and to avoid potential deep venous thrombosis of major vessels because of the need for future cardiac catheterizations. Peripherally inserted central catheter lines are an alternative, and for that reason specialized teams for vascular access have been created and used in mature heart centers, or interventional radiologists who specialize in the pediatric population are consulted. The PCICU owns the important role in identifying these patients early and organizing the process of vascular access.

Physical rehabilitation of the child with cardiac disease depends on the severity of illness and may be necessary to decrease hospital length of stay. Consistent and aggressive participation of occupational, physical, and speech therapists is essential for progress. Communication between providers and therapists about a child's advancement and potential therapy needs once he or she is an outpatient should occur on a regular basis.

Licensed clinical social workers are an integral member of the team and provide invaluable insight into patient and caregiver coping and stress management, home dynamics, and access-to-care issues essential for the eventual transition home.

Family-Centered Care

Family-centered care is vital in the ICU, step-down, and intermediate care areas. Families can provide a detailed medical history and help their child effectively cope with the hospitalization; they know the child best, and they can be an invaluable source of readily available, accurate information. Family-centered care empowers families to be advocates for their child's care and reinforces their invaluable contribution to the care of their child in the hospital. Introduction of the family as part of the care team begins on admission and when possible during prenatal visits for those patients whose diagnosis of a congenital heart defects occurs during the fetal period. Orientation to the physical space of the child's surroundings, as well as the medical team and support staff, and a review of what to expect all prepare and promote the patient and family to play an active role as part of the care team. Family presence during daily rounds should be encouraged and their concerns and questions addressed in a comforting and supportive manner.

Understanding how the family transitions through this process is difficult. A refined version of the PCICU Parental Stress Model has been developed; it outlined themes within the original model, time points of heightened stress, and expanded the categories of stressors by naming additional stressors within each category of infant, parent, and environment (Fig. 5.5).[35] This model is useful for elucidating the stress experience for parents with infants hospitalized in a PCICU for cardiac surgery and can be used to monitor interventions.

Although the transition from ICU care indicates improvement in a child's condition, it can be an extremely stressful time for patients and their caregivers. Caregivers should be encouraged to take a more active role in care once the child has transitioned out of the ICU to a step-down or intermediate care setting. This approach helps families to adapt to the care needs of their child before discharge. Implementation of a patient- or family-initiated rapid response system, commonly known as a Condition Help or Condition H, reinforces the patient's and caregiver's role as part of the medical team and can help to identify potential safety issues.[36] Incorporating Condition Help into an existing system is a relatively seamless process and does not necessarily increase the number of false calls but may improve overall outcome and patient satisfaction.[37,38]

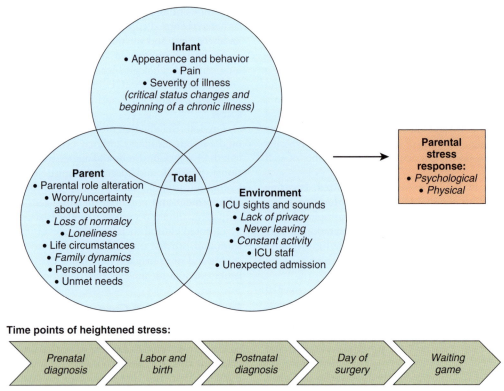

Time points of heightened stress:

Prenatal diagnosis → Labor and birth → Postnatal diagnosis → Day of surgery → Waiting game

• **Figure 5.5** The PCICU Parental Stress Model-Revised, with new themes/categories italicized. *ICU,* Intensive care unit; *PCICU,* pediatric cardiac intensive care unit. (From Lisanti AJ, Allen LR, Kelly L, Medoff-Cooper B. Maternal stress and anxiety in the pediatric cardiac intensive care unit. *Am J Crit Care.* 2017;26[2]:118-125.)

Escalation in Care

In the event that a child requires an increased level of care, a system must be in place for successful transfer back to the ICU. For planned transfers, as may occur after procedures (e.g., cardiac catheterization, surgical intervention, and procedural sedation), a standardized handoff should occur between the step-down/intermediate care team and the ICU team before transfer. Parents should be encouraged to be present for such handoffs to reinforce parental expectations and understanding of processes. For transfers prompted by acute decompensation a pediatric rapid response team should be urgently activated for immediate evaluation and management. Due to the fragile and clinically unpredictable nature of children with congenital and acquired heart defects, immediate assessment, monitoring and intervention by the cardiac critical care team is necessary.

Role for the Universal Care Model

The universal care model for pediatric cardiac care aims to minimize transitions of care from unit to unit and care team to care team by maintaining a patient within a single bed space from admission to discharge. This is an extension of the concept of acuity adaptable units, first introduced in the 1990s and most notable in the labor, delivery, recovery, postpartum care process. This model has been theorized to improve patient outcomes, decrease safety issues stemming from transfer of patient care, and increase patient and family comfort and satisfaction. For this care system to be successful, facility design and staffing plans must be developed to support this model. Units using this model employ single-patient rooms with the capability to provide technical support for the most critically ill child while creating a home-like environment for caregivers to room in. Collaboration of care between pediatric cardiology and pediatric cardiac critical care is continuous in the universal care model. Acuity-based staffing models can be challenging because nurse-to-patient ratios can range from 1:1 to 1:4 or 1:5; however, nursing staff is centralized to one location. Nursing skill sets will need to be broad, requiring specialized education and training.

Conclusion

Critically ill postoperative pediatric patients with congenital and/or acquired heart disease are best managed in the ICU structured to meet their unique needs. In addition, the ICU should be staffed with a multidisciplinary team of intensivists, cardiologists, surgeons, nurses, and other ancillary staff specifically trained to deliver the appropriate care to the patients. Ideally, the care would be delivered with specifically dedicated facilities, equipment, and strategies.

Selected References

A complete list of references is available at ExpertConsult.com.

2. Jacobs JP, He X, Mayer JE Jr, Austin EH 3rd, Quintessenza JA, Karl TR, et al. Mortality Trends in Pediatric and Congenital Heart Surgery: An Analysis of The Society of Thoracic Surgeons Congenital

Heart Surgery Database. *Ann Thorac Surg*. 2016;102(4):1345–1352.

9. Alten JA, Klugman D, Raymond TT, Cooper DS, Donohue JE, Zhang W, et al. Epidemiology and Outcomes of Cardiac Arrest in Pediatric Cardiac ICUs. *Pediatr Crit Care Med*. 2017;18(10):935–943.

11. Jacobs JP, Wernovsky G, Cooper DS, Karl TR. Principles of shared decision-making within teams. *Cardiol Young*. 2015;25(8):1631–1636.

13. Burstein DS, Rossi AF, Jacobs JP, Checchia PA, Wernovsky G, Li JS, et al. Variation in models of care delivery for children undergoing congenital heart surgery in the United States. *World J Pediatr Congenit Heart Surg*. 2010;1(1):8–14.

22. Srinivasan C, Sachdeva R, Morrow WR, Gossett J, Chipman CW, Imamura M, et al. Standardized management improves outcomes after the Norwood procedure. *Congenit Heart Dis*. 2009;4(5):329–337.

29. Hornik CP, He X, Jacobs JP, Li JS, Jaquiss RD, Jacobs ML, et al. Relative impact of surgeon and center volume on early mortality after the Norwood operation. *Ann Thorac Surg*. 2012;93(6):1992–1997.

6

Selection, Training, and Mentoring

SAUL FLORES, MD; MATTHEW K. BACON, MD; ROHIT S. LOOMBA, MD;
JENNIFER SCHUETTE, MD, MS

Over the last decade there has been a tremendous growth in the amount of medical and surgical advancements in the treatment of children and adults with congenital heart disease. Technologic improvements in extracorporeal cardiac support continue to decrease mortality rates in this group of patients.[1] Nonetheless, patients with complex forms of congenital heart disease often present significant management challenges for the cardiac intensive care unit (CICU) provider. In an attempt to understand and meet the demands of this patient population, cardiology, critical care, and anesthesiology providers have been tailoring their education and training to make steady improvements in the care provided to this group of patients.[2] Academic pediatric centers across the United States offer and provide additional time for education and training in pediatric subspecialties that encompass the fields of critical care, cardiology, and anesthesiology.[2,3] Available guidelines for training in pediatric cardiology, pediatric critical care, and pediatric anesthesiology exist,[4] but there is no consensus on the training pathway and duration or on the specifics of mentoring and recruitment for the next generation of CICU providers. These challenges, along with the continued transition nationally to dedicated pediatric cardiac critical care units and intensivists, have intensified the discussion to standardize the approach to pediatric cardiac intensivist training.

This chapter will provide historical background in the field of pediatric cardiac critical care, highlighting the development of the skills and expertise currently required to provide optimal care in the CICU. Description of current training pathways used by pediatric cardiac critical care providers will be reviewed. Introduction of a proposal for curriculum standardization and best practices to assess trainees in the field, focusing on the current graduate medical education paradigms of milestones and entrustable professional activities (EPAs), will be provided. A description for board certification, mentorship, and recruitment for CICU providers will also be presented.

History of the Cardiac Intensive Care Unit

Cardiac critical care developed out of the need to provide highly specialized care for children with complex congenital cardiac disease. The earliest pediatric cardiac surgeries were open procedures without the need for cardiopulmonary bypass, such as patent ductus arteriosus ligation (1938) and aortic coarctation repair (1945), and were performed by Robert Gross[5,6] with no substantial complications. However, later surgeries became more complex and required longer periods of recovery with a wider array of complications, and thus different groups of providers were enlisted to control and restore organ function.

In 1944 Alfred Blalock and Vivien Thomas performed a left subclavian artery to left pulmonary artery anastomosis on a 1-year-old child with tetralogy of Fallot.[7] This case was complicated by the onset of bilateral pneumothoraces during the postoperative course that required drainage and highlighted the care provided by pediatric house staff members.

In 1953 use of cardiopulmonary bypass for repair of cardiac defects by John Gibbon[8] heralded the development of the field of congenital cardiac surgery. Subsequently surgeries became more intricate as increasingly complex defects were repaired. In 1958 William Glenn[9] performed the superior vena cava to right pulmonary artery anastomosis on a 7-year-old patient with functionally univentricular anatomy, decreased pulmonary blood flow, and transposition of the great arteries. During surgery this case was complicated by cardiac arrest and atrial tachycardia that was later controlled with digitalis. In 1968 Francois Fontan performed the atriopulmonary connection in a 12-year-old patient with tricuspid atresia and normally related great vessels.[10] After surgery the child developed anuria requiring hemodialysis during postoperative day 1 and later a right pleural effusion requiring drainage.

By the 1970s complex congenital cardiac surgeries were mostly performed in older children. The use of prostaglandin E to maintain ductal patency, along with advances in cardiac catheterization and echocardiography, resulted in advances in neonatal cardiac surgery.[11] In 1974 Aldo Castaneda and the team at Boston Children's Hospital reported their experience performing open-heart surgery during the first 3 months of life and the postoperative management of these children.[12,13] These efforts, along with others, led to a revolution in neonatal congenital cardiac surgery and cardiac intensive care. In 1975 Adib Jatene performed the arterial switch operation that now bears his name. This case had substantial complications, characterized by renal failure and eventual death of the patient on postoperative day 3. Since then the arterial switch operation and the postoperative care for these patients has been optimized, and some centers report survival rates of up to 96% at 7 years.[14]

In the late 1970s hypoplastic left heart syndrome (HLHS) was almost invariably lethal. The surgical and clinical community was challenged by the lack of a feasible surgical repair and sustainable postoperative care. In 1977 William Norwood performed surgery on a 5-week-old infant with HLHS. The procedure consisted of an atrial septal defect enlargement, a cavopulmonary connection, a ductal ligation, left pulmonary artery banding, and side-to-side anastomosis of the aorta and main pulmonary artery. This case was complicated by desaturation, progressive acidosis, and the patient's eventual death. However, improvements in the surgical technique and postoperative care have largely improved outcomes, with some large studies reporting survival of over 75% after the stage I (Norwood) procedure.[15]

These procedures revolutionized and expanded the treatment of congenital cardiac disease and stimulated the development of pediatric CICUs focused on improving postoperative care. This ever-expanding field includes a steep learning curve and significant challenges for trainees. The 21st-century CICU provider must have a unique set of skills, characterized by in-depth knowledge of complex cardiac physiologies and understanding of the pathophysiology of critical illness and the unique ability to lead a multidisciplinary team capable of dealing with the most complex situations a patient with critical cardiac disease may encounter.

Cardiac Intensive Care Unit Staffing and Coverage

It is difficult to precisely determine staffing in the CICU with over 100 congenital surgery programs in the United States and many more across the world. A recent international survey of members of the Pediatric Cardiac Intensive Care Society (PCICS) provided demographic information regarding unit structure, staffing, and training of cardiac intensivists.[16] Based on this survey, the most frequent CICU staffing structure is composed of nurses and physicians independent from the general pediatric intensive care unit (PICU) (58%), followed by combined units (PICU/CICU) with dedicated CICU nurses and physicians (21%) and combined units (PICU/CICU) with no dedicated nurses and physicians (21%). In terms of staffing and training of CICU providers, the most common training background was critical care (51%), followed by cardiology (18%), dual training in critical care/cardiology (14%), and last, dual training in critical care/anesthesiology (10%).

Cardiac Intensive Care Training Pathways

Identifying the ideal education and training pathways for CICU providers is an area of active discussion. Currently most CICU providers are trained in critical care, cardiology, anesthesiology, or various combinations of the three. To understand the current training pathways, it is important to recognize the organization that oversees residency and fellowship training in the United States. The Accreditation Council for Graduate Medical Education (ACGME) is the governing body that sets the educational standards for the training of US physicians in residency and fellowship. The ACGME has instituted specific requirements for specialty and subspecialty training programs focused on ensuring the highest quality of training within these programs. The American Board of Pediatrics (ABP) is the entity that determines board certification eligibility for providers and has its own requirements that revolve around satisfactory development of clinical, professional, and academic skills. Although ABP board certification has long been established in pediatric cardiology and pediatric critical care, there currently is no certification offered in pediatric cardiac critical care.

Providers who seek board certification in pediatric critical care or cardiology must complete 3 years of training after pediatric residency. The ACGME and ABP do not have specific guidelines or requirements for CICU service duration; in fact, within pediatric critical care programs the ABP specifically limits time that can be spent in a "subspecialty ICU" to 6 months over the course of a pediatric critical care medicine (PCCM) fellow's 3 years of training. Fellowship programs in either specialty typically will have fellows rotate 3 to 4 months during the 3-year training program. Night coverage varies among centers based on the size of the program and the number of fellows available. For instance, large programs with more than five fellows per year in either specialty may have trainees cover four to seven overnight calls during their CICU rotation months, as well as additional night coverage throughout the duration of training. Other programs might use a night float system, resulting in fellows covering the cardiac patients for five or six nights at a stretch. Smaller programs may have much less cardiac exposure, and some fellows may train at a center where either pediatric cardiology fellows and/or PCCM fellows function mostly as observers in the CICU. Clearly there is marked inconsistency in the exposure of both cardiology and critical care trainees to care of CICU patients.

Dual training is available for board-eligible or board-certified providers in pediatric critical care or cardiology. Depending on the training background, trainees on this track must complete 2 years of additional training, of which at least 1 year must be broad-based clinical training. The training background generally determines the curriculum, and it is typically defined by the individual needs of the trainee and the program's need for service coverage. Typical rotation schedules for both a board-eligible cardiologist training in critical care and for a board-eligible intensivist training in cardiology are shown in Tables 6.1 and 6.2, respectively. Specific rotation requirements are not set forth by the ABP; therefore significant variations are possible depending on the training program

TABLE 6.1	Typical Rotation Schedule for a Fellow Previously Trained in Cardiology Who Is Training in Critical Care Over a 2-Year Period	
First Year	**Second Year**	
Pediatric ICU (7-8 months)	Pediatric ICU (4-5 months)	
Cardiac ICU (1 month)	Cardiac ICU (3-4 months)	
Anesthesia (1 month)	Elective/research (3-5 months)	
Elective/research (2-3 months)		

ICU, Intensive care unit.

TABLE 6.2	Typical Rotation Schedule for a Fellow Previously Trained in Critical Care Who Is Training in Cardiology Over a 2-Year Period	
First Year	**Second Year**	
Echocardiography (2-3 months)	Cardiac ICU (3-4 months)	
Cardiac catheterization (2-3 months)	Echocardiography (1 month)	
Inpatient cardiology (2 months)	Cardiac catheterization (1 month)	
Cardiac ICU (1-2 months)	Inpatient cardiology (1 month)	
Electrophysiology (1 month)	Electrophysiology (1 month)	
Heart failure (1 month)	Heart failure (1 month)	
Elective/research (1-2 months)	Elective/research (3-4 months)	

ICU, Intensive care unit.

and the previous training experience of an individual fellow. It should be noted that the ABP has no specific research requirement for fellows who undertake a second pediatric subspecialty fellowship, provided that the scholarly project from the initial subspecialty fellowship was approved by the appropriate ABP subboard and that the fellow has successfully passed that subboard examination. It is in the trainee's academic interest to continue moving forward with academic pursuits to better position himself or herself for a junior faculty position.

Although formal recognition by the ABP of programs for dual training in anesthesia and PCCM no longer exists, the board will, on a case-by-case basis, consider individual applications for dual training in both subspecialties. Stipulations for that training are as follows[17]:

- The pathway is available to those who have completed the required training for certification in general pediatrics.
- Both the anesthesiology and PCCM training must be completed in the same institution or in close geographic proximity in the same academic health system.
- Training in PCCM may precede or follow training in anesthesiology, or the training may be fully integrated.
- An individual in the pathway must be identified by the end of the first year of training or preferably before training begins in anesthesiology and PCCM.
- An outline of the 5-year plan that details how the training requirements of the ABP, the American Board of Anesthesiology (ABA), and the ACGME will be met must be submitted to both boards for approval. Individuals will be approved for this pathway on a case-by-case basis; programs will not be approved.
- Although double counting of scholarly activity/research experience is allowed, all clinical training requirements must be met in each discipline and may not be double counted.
- Six months of the scholarly activity required for PCCM certification will be completed during the 6 months of research time allowed during the anesthesiology residency. The trainee's scholarship oversight committee will oversee this training, as required by the ABP's General Criteria for Certification in the Pediatric Subspecialties.
- The 5 years of training will not confer eligibility for certification in pediatric anesthesiology by the ABA.
- Trainees in the pathway will be eligible for certification in both anesthesiology and PCCM upon the satisfactory completion of all 5 years of training. Certification in one discipline is not contingent upon certification in the other.

This wide range of training pathways and the conflicting opinions from experts in the field regarding the ideal training model[4,18] led to the development of an additional year of cardiac critical care training. This training is currently available for providers who have completed a pediatric critical care, cardiology, or neonatology fellowship, though currently there is no ACGME accreditation available for this additional clinical fellowship year. The curriculum of this additional year will depend on the provider's training background, but typically the initial months focus on the development of basic skills required in the CICU not covered during their previous training. For providers with pediatric critical care background, particular emphasis is placed on solidifying echocardiography, electrophysiology, and cardiac catheterization skills and interpretation, whereas providers with a pediatric cardiology background will focus on the stabilization and management of the critically ill child. The second part of the year will focus on the development of skills necessary to successfully lead a multidisciplinary team to provide care of a critically ill child

with congenital or acquired cardiac disease throughout the child's CICU stay.

Curriculum and Trainee Assessment

Curriculum

The multiple training pathways currently available to physicians who seek to practice in the CICU presents a challenge: how to ensure that each trainee acquires the necessary knowledge and skills to provide optimal, efficient, and safe care to this high-risk patient population regardless of the training pathway. Educators within pediatric cardiology have offered the most extensive expert analysis of what specifically should be required of trainees in their field who seek to practice in the CICU. While recognizing that core training in pediatric cardiology is not the same at all institutions and thus some modifications to postfellowship training might be required, Task Force 5 of the American College of Cardiology has twice published its recommendations regarding what constitutes an adequate fourth-year experience to prepare a board-eligible/board-certified pediatric cardiologist to practice in the CICU (see Table 6.1).[4,19] Not surprisingly, the response from those trained in critical care, many of whom had long practiced in the CICU, was to conclude that "all critically ill children are best cared for by a multidisciplinary team of clinicians with the intensivist as a team leader or co-leader."[18] These authors made the following additional points with regard to the adequacy of a fourth year of clinical training to prepare a cardiologist to lead a CICU team:

1. Abbreviated critical care rotations do not transform a cardiologist into an intensivist any more than a few clinical months of cardiology training would convert an intensivist into a cardiologist.
2. Training for any physician who wishes to practice PCCM or any other pediatric subspecialty should not be fast tracked.
3. Physicians who wish to fulfill both the cardiologist and the intensivist roles in the CICU should follow the 5-year training path outlined by the ABP for dual certification in PCCM and pediatric cardiology.

They concluded that "there should be no shortcuts in the care of critically ill children"—a point on which all who care for these high-risk patients can undoubtedly agree. The Task Force 5 authors reasonably countered that "efforts to gerrymander qualification boundaries to exclude able practitioners from practice work against, rather than foster, a culture of multidisciplinary collaborative care."

An expert panel composed of individuals of diverse training backgrounds was convened at the 10th annual meeting of the PCICS in 2014 to discuss the merits of the contribution of their field to the care of patients in the CICU.[11] One walks away from the opinions offered feeling quite uncertain that any single training pathway is the only right one:

From anesthesiology: The anesthesiologist is the intensivist of the operating room, and delivering care as the pediatric cardiac anesthesiologist is similar to delivering care in the CICU at two to three times the normal speed—albeit one patient at a time.

From cardiology: The practice of pediatric cardiac critical care goes beyond typical intensivist and cardiologist proficiencies. Extra time for skill acquisition in a mentored environment is advantageous. The completion of two fellowships is not necessary to function at a high level as a cardiac intensivist.

From critical care: Key elements of training are patient exposure, pattern recognition, reflection, collaboration, and humility; although working with providers of varying practice backgrounds can be frustrating, it is also an opportunity to evaluate the evidence and identify strategies that make sense.

From cardiology/critical care: These fields provide the advantage of exposure to diverse disease states and complex care of all organ systems in which communication with a wide variety of subspecialists is imperative, while also providing an advanced understanding of the complex physiology in the CICU patient population.

From neonatology: A background in neonatology adds expertise to the trainee in the preterm and very low-birth-weight population, as well as managing comorbidities specific to neonates.

Given the landscape of various training backgrounds that have lead people to practice in the CICU, it perhaps is the right time to take a step essentially backward to define the knowledge and skills that a CICU provider must have. Rather than focus on the path, developing a curriculum will allow us to focus on eliminating gaps in knowledge and abilities rather than highlighting them.

A proposed curriculum that stresses knowledge and skills is shown in Table 6.3. It is purposefully brief because it will hopefully stimulate discussion across the multiple specialties that have sent practitioners into the field of cardiac intensive care. Although it focuses on the specific clinical skills required to independently practice as a cardiac intensivist, additional abilities in the areas of professionalism, communication, team leadership, and academic pursuits will be equally important.

Assessment

Hand in hand with curriculum development is a need to construct a method of assessment and perhaps of accreditation and even board certification that would allow for systematic training—perhaps through multiple pathways—of CICU providers. To propose such a paradigm, an understanding of past and current rubrics for trainee assessment is needed.

In the 1970s and 1980s an initial push toward competency-based medical education failed to gain widespread support. Coincidentally, two events occurred in 1999 that again brought competency-based assessment to the forefront of postgraduate medical education: the Institute of Medicine released *To Err Is Human: Building a Safer Health System*, highlighting the deficiencies of care delivery in the United States; and the ACGME and American Board of Medical Subspecialties (ABMS) published a training rubric that focused on six core competencies of patient care, medical knowledge, practice-based learning and improvement, interpersonal and communication skills, professionalism, and systems-based practice. Work is currently underway to formally add two additional areas of competence—interprofessional collaboration and personal and professional development. Training programs across the landscape of graduate medical education were expected to create goals and objectives and to assess their trainees within this framework, and individual specialties identified subcompetencies under each of these six headings that were felt to encompass the critical abilities that a trainee in that specialty needed to acquire to provide care that met the following quality indicators: safe, effective, efficient, timely, patient centered, and equitable. Working groups within the ABP and the ACGME created 51 such subcompetencies for the specialty of pediatrics. Subsequently 21 pediatric subspecialty subcompetencies were selected from the original

51 to be used to assess fellowship trainees across all pediatric subspecialties.

In 2009 the ACGME and the ABMS partnered again to initiate the Milestone Project. Each specialty was asked to create, for each of the subcompetencies, a set of milestones that would allow supervising faculty and program directors to assess progression of the trainee through the stages shown in Fig. 6.1. Milestones were defined as skill- and knowledge-based developments that commonly occur by a specific time over the course of training. Although a number of studies have been undertaken to assess the effectiveness of this evaluation rubric, it is, by the admission of everyone involved, a work in progress. In fact, work on Milestones 2.0 is just getting underway within the ACGME—even as we await data on the effectiveness of the first version in meeting the stated goal: a physician who is competent to practice independently across all of the subcompetencies for his or her chosen specialty.

If one considers the competencies and subcompetencies to be the first layer of trainee assessment and the milestones to be the second, entrustable professional activities (EPAs) would be the third. The competencies and subcompetencies, although providing a systematic framework with which to evaluate trainees, suffer from what many consider to be a fatal flaw—they break down training and assessment into ever-smaller pieces that are amenable to being measured and to which a checklist can be applied without considering the trainee's ability to "pull it all together." The EPAs are designed to address the need for a broader assessment that incorporates the smaller pieces of the subcompetencies. As a broad example, one would want a cardiac intensivist who is ready for independent practice to not only be able to identify poor cardiac function on an echocardiogram and choose the right medications to support that failing heart, but also to demonstrate an ability to communicate with the family, to make the right decisions regarding consultation and additional studies needed for evaluation (in a cost-effective manner), and to orchestrate the care of the patient through effective team leadership—to name but a few pieces of the effective care puzzle. An EPA allows assessment of trainees across the continuum of knowledge, skills, and aptitudes needed to provide care to complex patients in the CICU. Although mapped to the subcompetencies, EPAs represent an attempt to evaluate a trainee's ability to successfully navigate every facet of care in a given clinical scenario. In fact, one could argue that a well-developed system of subcompetencies and EPAs is actually the ideal assessment rubric in a subspecialty in which practitioners have historically emerged from such a wide range of training backgrounds, given their focus on the application of well-rounded knowledge and skills rather than the training path taken to acquire them.

Because EPAs are currently being written across the graduate medical education community, much remains unknown regarding their application and effectiveness in providing actionable assessment information to trainees that results in providers who are able to effectively practice independently in the CICU. Fig. 6.2 depicts a common approach to documenting a trainee's performance with respect to a given EPA—a "grade," if you will. There are a number of unresolved issues related to EPAs, however, because they are in their relative infancy. Does a trainee need to attain the "competent" level for each subcompetency within the EPA to achieve a stage 3 assessment? Or should the assessment be more flexible? How many EPAs would be required to be completed over the course of training? How many would be needed to reach a defined assessment level before considering a trainee ready for independent practice? Given the current status of EPAs in the general graduate medical education community, all of these questions currently

TABLE 6.3	Proposed Curriculum for Practitioners in Pediatric Cardiac Critical Care
Patient care and medical knowledge: noncardiac	Endocrine • Recognize and manage adrenal insufficiency Hematology • Appropriately use pharmacologic agents and blood products to achieve and maintain hemostasis • Manage prophylactic and therapeutic anticoagulation Infectious disease • Recognize and manage sepsis and other serious infections • Recognize and manage hospital-acquired infections • Practice appropriate antibiotic stewardship Neurologic • Manage sedation and analgesia • Recognize and treat neurologic injury (seizure, stroke, hypoxic-ischemic injury) • Optimize neurocognitive outcomes Nutrition and fluid/electrolyte management • Provide adequate parenteral or enteral nutrition • Appropriately use diuretics to manage fluid balance Renal • Recognize, manage, and seek appropriate consultation for acute kidney injury • Institute renal replacement therapy when clinically indicated Respiratory • Manage mechanical ventilation (noninvasive and invasive, including nonconventional modes)
Patient care and medical knowledge: cardiac	Understand and apply the principles of cardiovascular physiology related to • Cardiac catheterization (indications for diagnostic evaluation and therapeutic intervention; interpretation of objective data) • Cardiopulmonary bypass • Cardiopulmonary interactions • Hemodynamic monitoring • Systolic and diastolic function • Vasoactive infusions Management of medical cardiac disease • Cardiac transplant • Cardiomyopathy • Dysrhythmia • Heart failure • Myocarditis • Pericardial disease • Pulmonary hypertension Preoperative and postoperative management, including the recognition and management of complications of anatomic cardiac disease • Shunt lesions (ASD, VSD, CAVC, PDA) • Anomalous pulmonary venous connections • Truncus arteriosus • Aortic stenosis • Coarctation of the aorta and interrupted arch • Pulmonary atresia/intact ventricular septum • Ebstein anomaly • Tetralogy of Fallot and its variants (tetralogy with pulmonary atresia, tetralogy/absent pulmonary valve) • Transposition of the great arteries and double-outlet right ventricle • Hypoplastic left heart syndrome and other single-ventricle variants
Procedural skills	Airway management, including management of the difficult airway and appropriate consultation Echocardiography (acquisition of images and interpretation) Management of mechanical circulatory support Cardiopulmonary resuscitation Pericardiocentesis Temporary pacemaker management Thoracostomy Vascular access (arterial and central venous)

ASD, Atrial septal defect; *CAVC,* complete atrioventricular canal; *PDA,* patent ductus arteriosus; *VSD,* ventricular septal defect.

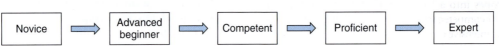

• **Figure 6.1** Performance progression in milestone-based subcompetencies.

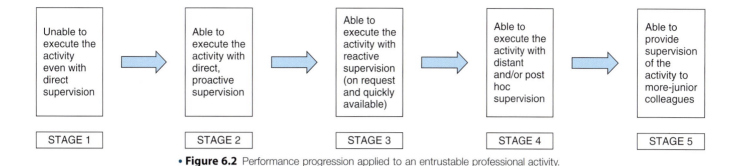

Unable to execute the activity even with direct supervision		Able to execute the activity with direct, proactive supervision		Able to execute the activity with reactive supervision (on request and quickly available)		Able to execute the activity with distant and/or post hoc supervision		Able to provide supervision of the activity to more-junior colleagues
STAGE 1		STAGE 2		STAGE 3		STAGE 4		STAGE 5

• **Figure 6.2** Performance progression applied to an entrustable professional activity.

• BOX 6.1 Proposed Entrustable Professional Activities for Pediatric Cardiac Intensive Care

- Preoperative and postoperative care of the neonate with congenital heart disease
- Preoperative and postoperative care of the infant/older child with congenital or acquired heart disease
- Preoperative and postoperative care of the adult with congenital heart disease
- Care of the patient with medical cardiac disease (heart failure, myocarditis, cardiomyopathy)
- Care of the patient with dysrhythmia
- Care of the patient requiring mechanical circulatory support
- Care of the patient at end of life

---

remain unanswered and will need to be addressed within our subspecialty.

Although it is well beyond the scope of this chapter to provide a detailed treatment of potential subcompetencies or EPAs that could be used for cardiac intensivist training, Box 6.1 lists a sample of seven possible EPAs for the cardiac intensivist. Although this could certainly be expanded upon based on consensus from educators in the field, we would caution that an excessive number of EPAs, especially if written to incorporate highly specific clinical situations, may result in loss of generalizability across programs and create an unrealistic expectation for completion in numbers that would be helpful. Table 6.4 provides sample EPA language, adapted from the Pediatric Milestones Project, that incorporates a majority of the current subspecialty competencies and their milestones.[20] Rather than providing a specific template from which the cardiac intensivist trainee would be assessed, this is presented to give the reader a sense of the language and construct of an EPA. A fully developed EPA would also include objectives and assessment strategies, which are not included here due to space limitations. As EPAs are developed, three key elements should be stressed: they should be manageable in number, built so that they are measurable and meaningful, and designed to measure what we really need to measure to assess readiness for independent practice.

The overarching goal of the EPA is to bring assessment into the authentic clinical environment and to align what we measure with what our trainees actually need to be able to do as clinicians. The EPA construct is meant to take a more holistic view of trainee assessment, embedding the context-independent subcompetencies and their milestones into a "real-world" clinical experience.[21,22] This "crosswalk" of competencies and EPAs should allow us, within the field of cardiac intensive care, to create a blueprint for curriculum and assessment that successfully determines a trainee's ability to

practice independently—regardless of the training pathway undertaken.[23] This rubric should assist our field in moving beyond the boilerplate but not terribly helpful mantras seen in many current evaluation comments, such as "needs to read more" and "great team player." Additionally, it should clarify for supervisors where a learner is on his or her progression to independent practice, ensuring both learner development and high-quality patient care.[24] Both undersupervision and oversupervision are problematic, either for the learner, for the patient, or both. Effective assessment tools within our subspecialty, and knowledgeable application of them by supervising faculty, should translate into trainees being appropriately challenged to work beyond the level at which they are entirely comfortable performing. The functional assessment of a given trainee shifts from being focused on trainee competence to instead being focused on required level of supervision.[25] This will perhaps make the transition to ever-increasing amounts of autonomy more transparent and smooth for all members of the multidisciplinary team.

Board Certification

The field of cardiac intensive care is now recognized as a discrete area of expertise and practice for which one can prepare through a variety of training pathways as previously discussed. What has not occurred, and is currently under discussion, is the creation of an official subspecialty recognized by the ABP and ABMS. Along with this would then come a process by which cardiac intensivists can receive board certification. The ABP is a member board of the ABMS, and thus all pediatric subspecialties wishing to be certified must undergo approval by the ABMS. This process must start with a desire for official creation of a subspecialty. The initiation of this process is no small task. It becomes imperative that a majority of those practicing in the subspecialty have voiced their approval and that enough of these members are available to actively participate in the application process itself.

If a subspecialty seeks to garner board certification status, the ABMS approval process is initiated by completion of a formal application. This detailed application requires the following information as a subspecialty is considered for certification:

- The purpose of the subspecialty
- Current status and identified need for the subspecialty
- Difference from current board-certified subspecialties
- General exposure of trainees to the subspecialty
- The number of current training positions available
- Sustainability of such training programs
- Proposed goals and objectives for training
- Projected cost of training in the proposed subspecialty
- Strategies for evaluation of both the subspecialty itself and of the trainees

TABLE 6.4   Proposed Entrustable Professional Activity Framework

Domain	Competency	Level 1	Level 2	Level 3	Level 4	Level 5
		DEVELOPMENTAL PROGRESSION OF MILESTONES				
Patient care	Gather essential and accurate information	Gathers too little or exhaustively gathers information	Begins to filter, prioritize, and synthesize information	Able to formulate real-time clinical conclusions as part of the information-gathering process	Gathers accurate and essential information, reaching precise clinical conclusions with ease	Unconscious gathering of essential and accurate information with appreciation of subtle differences based on clinical experience
	Provide transfer of care that ensures seamless transitions	Important content is missing or inaccurate, content is poorly organized	Fewer omissions/errors, receiver's needs still poorly addressed	Minimal errors, beginning to address potential issues for the receiver	Successfully adapts handoff based on level of complexity, ensures open communication	Handoffs are habitually efficient, complete, and error free and meet the receiver's needs
	Perform complete and accurate physical examinations	Unable to perform a physical examination tailored to the individual patient	Frequently misses or misinterprets critical findings	Performs a basic examination correctly, including recognition of abnormal findings	Performs, elicits, recognizes, and interprets examination findings correctly	Master clinician, recognizing and correctly interpreting even the most subtle findings
	Make informed diagnostic and therapeutic decisions; develop and carry out a management plan	Minimal ability to filter, reorganize, or synthesize data, leading to difficulty in developing a therapeutic plan; relies on directives from others for management plan	Excessive testing and interventions result in unfocused management plans; beginning to apply own knowledge but still heavily reliant on directives from others	Well-synthesized and organized assessment with a focused differential; theoretical knowledge and personal experience lead to independence in formulating plans in some situations	Able to practice early directed diagnostic hypothesis testing with well-established pattern recognition; uses experience and focused information gathering to formulate and carry out a plan	Uses clinical experience and knowledge base to synthesize information and make efficient interventions as a coordinated single process; easily formulates and carries out plans even when faced with unusual clinical scenarios
	Prescribe and perform all indicated medical procedures	Requires assistance with most/all invasive procedures required for the patient's care	Requires direct supervision with most invasive procedures required for the patient's care	Requires indirect supervision with most invasive procedures required for the patient's care	Requires indirect supervision for only highly complex procedures required for the patient's care	Able to perform all necessary procedures independently
	Counsel patients and families	Unable to meet the patient's/family's needs as a result of inadequate knowledge, excessive medical jargon, and/or inability to address patient's specific condition	Improved communication but does not allow for discussion or questions	Able to answer questions and foster a discussion but does not routinely ensure patient/family understanding	Family encouraged to engage in dialogue, questions answered, understanding checked	Forms a partnership with the family based on information sharing, ongoing dialogue, and mutually agreed-upon care plan
Medical knowledge	Demonstrate sufficient knowledge of the basic and clinically supportive sciences appropriate to provide appropriate care	Lacks basic knowledge of the anatomy, physiology, and pathophysiology of the patient	Demonstrates basic knowledge of the anatomy, physiology, and pathophysiology but is unable to apply it clinically	Demonstrates an understanding of the anatomy, physiology, and pathophysiology of the patient and applies it to the clinical situation in most situations	Applies past experience in addition to core knowledge to effectively provide care in most situations	Seamlessly applies past experience and incorporates vast fund of knowledge to provide effective care in even complex or unexpected situations

TABLE 6.4 Proposed Entrustable Professional Activity Framework—cont'd

Domain	Competency	DEVELOPMENTAL PROGRESSION OF MILESTONES				
		Level 1	Level 2	Level 3	Level 4	Level 5
Practice-based learning and improvement	Identify strengths, deficiencies, and limits in one's knowledge and expertise; incorporate formative feedback into daily practice	Demonstrates only superficial understanding of and insight into his or her performance; avoids feedback and/or is defensive	Increased insight but sees performance only as "right" or "wrong"; acknowledges feedback but little to no behavioral change	Actively seeks feedback and attempts to apply it in future situations	Proactively anticipates gaps and actively seeks resources to address them; improves daily practice based on both external feedback and personal insight	Self-directed in identifying, exploring, and addressing deficiencies
	Participate in the education of families, students, residents, and other health professionals	Gaps in knowledge and experience result in rigid, scripted education	Somewhat flexible in education approach, gaps in knowledge still exist	Solid breadth of knowledge and experience, able to modify teaching to meet needs of learner	Broad knowledge and experience supports learner-centered approach; empowers and motivates learner	Seamlessly, skillfully, and comfortably educates, ensuring learner understanding as a habit
Interpersonal and communication skills	Communicates effectively with families across a broad range of socioeconomic and cultural backgrounds	Relies on a standard approach to patients and families that does not vary	Begins to establish a rapport; identifies barriers to good communication but limited ability to manage them	Able to mitigate social and cultural barriers in most situations; promotes trust and understanding through verbal and nonverbal communication	Able to establish and maintain a therapeutic alliance; tailors communication to the recipient; makes appropriate ad hoc adjustments	Intuitively handles the gamut of difficult communication scenarios with grace and humility
	Communicates effectively with physicians and other health professionals	Rigid recitation of facts regardless of situation, audience, or context	Increased understanding of communication context, still errs on the side of inclusion of excessive detail	Tailors the communication strategy to the situation in most interactions, may struggle in unfamiliar situations	Has expanded strategies and can improvise in more difficult communication scenarios	Master of improvisation in any new or unusual communication scenario; sought out as a role model
Professionalism/ personal and professional development	Provide leadership that enhances team function and the learning environment	Does not clearly define roles/ expectations; disorganized and/or inefficient	Improved assignment of roles, manages mostly through direction rather than consensus building	Manages in an organized fashion, more emphasis on consensus building within the team	Organized, efficient, focused, and decisive; advocates for team and only rarely directive	Consensus building and empowerment of team members is the norm; inspires others to perform
	Recognize that ambiguity is part of clinical medicine and respond by using appropriate resources in dealing with uncertainty	Feels overwhelmed and inadequate when faced with uncertainty; rigid and authoritarian communication with families	Recognizes uncertainty and feels pressure from it; relies on rules and statistics in communicating with families	Anticipates and focuses on uncertainty and seeks additional information; minimal incorporation of family's perspective in balancing risk taking and goals of care	Balances delivery of information to the family with realism, hope, and exploration of patient goals	Flexible and committed to engagement with the family, acting as a resource to minimize uncertainty; able to accept what is truly unknown
Systems-based practice	Incorporate considerations of cost-awareness and risk-benefit analysis	Unaware of cost issues and frustrated by cost-containment measures	Uses externally provided information to inform cost-containing decisions, but application is not routinely appropriate	Able to apply risk-benefit analysis and cost awareness in most individual patient encounters	Recognizes the value in cost and risk-benefit analysis to guide decision making, and applies knowledge routinely	Integrates cost analysis into practice to minimize risk and optimize benefit across health delivery systems

The most contemporary example of a new pediatric subspecialty is that of pediatric hospital medicine (PHM). A petition was sent to the ABP in August 2014 asking for PHM to be considered a subspecialty of its own. In December 2015, after its own internal process, the ABP then informed the ABMS that PHM had the support of ABP in its application and recommended that the ABMS approve certification. Ultimately, in October 2016 PHM was officially recognized for subspecialty certification by ABMS. As demonstrated by this most recent example, this is both a time-consuming and labor-intensive process. Because discussion of seeking subspecialty certification for pediatric cardiac critical care has only arisen over the past few years, it will likely be several more years before the process unfolds in its entirety.

Tabbutt and Ghanayem[26] in 2016 made the case for a separate subboard in pediatric cardiac critical care. The proposition, formally presented in a white paper authored by six currently practicing pediatric cardiac intensivists, included the following:

- Eligible candidates would include those dually trained in pediatric critical care and pediatric cardiology and those trained primarily in either of these subspecialties who then complete a fourth year in an established pediatric cardiac critical care training program.
- Accreditation for programs offering a fourth year of training in pediatric cardiac critical care would be established through the ACGME.
- Once the board certification examination in pediatric cardiac critical care was established, current practitioners, regardless of training pathway, would have a 3-year grace period in which to sit for and pass the examination without the need for any additional training.

Although providing board certification in pediatric cardiac critical care would offer the advantage of establishing specific competencies to address the variation in knowledge and skill sets that occur when multiple training pathways exist, it also presents the following challenges: (1) which training pathways to include, (2) cost, (3) potential restriction of the pool of practitioners, and perhaps most importantly (4) unclear evidence that it would result in improved care.

A multicenter survey was conducted to determine the opinions that exist regarding board certification for pediatric cardiac critical care among pediatric cardiac intensivists. Using structured telephone interviews, this survey ultimately gathered data from 24 individuals. Of those interviewed, 7 (29%) were primarily cardiology trained, 8 (33%) were primarily critical care trained, another 8 (33%) had dual board certification, and 1 (5%) had another unspecified training pathway. Of these 24 responders, 13 (54%) definitely favored having formal board certification, 4 (16%) were in favor with some qualifiers, 4 (16%) were undecided, and 3 (12.5%) were not in favor. Operating under the assumption that a subspecialty is approved, all responders felt that those who have dual board certification in cardiology and critical care should be eligible for board certification, as well as those with board certification in critical care with an additional year of cardiac intensive care training. Nearly all (96%) felt that those with board certification in cardiology with an additional year of cardiac critical care training should be eligible for board certification. Only 50% felt that those who are board certified in anesthesia and have done additional cardiac intensive care training should be eligible, whereas less than 20% felt that those with either a neonatology or surgery board certification with additional cardiac critical care training should be board eligible.[27]

All 24 responders were surveyed regarding perceived benefits and potential concerns of board certification for the specialty.

When asked about perceived benefits, eight (33%) felt that this would lead to helpful formalization of the training curriculum. Similarly, seven (29%) felt that board certification would allow for the creation of a defined, specific knowledge base for those practicing in pediatric cardiac critical care. Other perceived benefits included legitimizing and/or increasing respect for the field and increasing objective measures of quality control/standardization for hiring.

The most common concern, voiced by nine (38%) responders, was that certification does not necessarily equate to clinical competence in the field. Six respondents (25%) felt that logistical issues would need to be overcome before starting the formal process to create a board-certified subspecialty. Additional concerns included fear that board certification would lead to a smaller pool of candidates from which to hire, the cost associated with taking additional board examinations, and concern that some training pathways may not be accepted as pathways to board eligibility.

Although a majority of cardiac intensivists appear to be in favor of board certification for the subspecialty, much work must be done within the subspecialty itself to identify and address issues pertinent to the process so that these can be detailed in the formal application and to ready the field for implementation if subspecialty certification is sought and ultimately received.

Recruitment

When faced with the task of recruitment of the next generation of cardiac intensivists, one might argue that the task should be easy given the multiple pathways described previously. The yearly applicant pool is vast, with routine exposure of cardiology, critical care, and anesthesia fellows to the CICU during their training. However, recruitment into careers in cardiac intensive care has not gone as smoothly as one might have predicted.

In 2004, survey results indicated a discrepancy between the growing need for cardiac intensivists and the number being formally trained.[28] At that time there were 12 cardiac intensive care programs offering a fourth year of clinical CICU-focused training in North America. Currently there are at least 23 such programs, with 2 in South America.[26,29] This obviously does not account for programs not listed or for the circumstance in which new faculty may choose to develop their own pathway with mentorship. Although opportunities for training have increased, many fourth-year fellowship openings continue to go unfilled. It is unknown at the current time if we are closer to closing the gap between physician demand and supply of adequately trained clinicians.

When we focus on recruitment it is important to consider on whom we should focus these efforts. As one might predict, this has also been a topic of much discussion. Should the focus be on medical school and resident trainees or on fellow trainees? What effort and resources should be dedicated to young faculty from the disciplines of pediatrics, pediatric cardiology, and pediatric critical care who have yet to define a specific clinical niche? Should recruitment also include trainees in anesthesia and/or neonatology?

In many situations the first introduction to a career in cardiac critical care may be after a trainee has made a preliminary career pathway decision. Many trainees leave residency having a clear career pathway, and at that time they likely have very little exposure to cardiac critical care. Adding to the complexity, the exposure that one critical care fellow gets at one institution can be vastly different than what he or she would get at another institution simply based on the organizational structure of the unit.

A proposed focus on recruiting is not to focus on specific people or trainees, but rather for current practitioners to identify the skills and qualities most valuable for a successful career in cardiac critical care. Once identified, these characteristics can be used as a backbone for identifying young trainees and early faculty members to begin the mentorship process. The focus should not be solely on the training pathway, but rather on the unique skill sets that predict success in the CICU—clinical acumen, the ability to lead a multidisciplinary team, procedural dexterity, and the ability to perform in a high-stress environment, to name just a few.

Focus should not be placed only on recruitment of fellow trainees because young faculty members are in a perfect position to transition into advanced training with support from their institution. Given the wide variance in training experience, it is reasonable to think that many young faculty do not appreciate their passion for cardiac critical care until they obtain their first faculty position. They may find themselves performing a job for which they feel inadequately prepared, or they may be excluded from caring for cardiac patients due to a perceived lack of training. We as cardiac critical care providers should seek to identify these faculty, and institutions should be open to supporting advanced training to provide the expertise needed at the bedside.

Mentorship

Mentorship is a highly personal experience, yet there are some underlying characteristics that are crucial to a successful mentorship relationship. Mentorship in its most general sense can be described as a long-term, mutual relationship between individuals wherein a person with more (or different) experience educates, guides, supports, and develops the less-experienced (or differently experienced) individual. Compared to the more formal experience of leadership, mentorship is a more organic experience, and it is important to recognize that the two are separate entities.[30-32] Mentorship is ubiquitous and of great importance in all of medicine, with pediatric cardiac critical care being no exception. Mentorship has been found to increase productivity and more importantly, satisfaction with work and the workplace.[33,34]

The notion of mentorship being organic is one that is important to most individuals seeking mentorship. A majority find that mentorship that has developed naturally without formal assignment of a mentor is more meaningful and effective.[35] This kind of mentorship forms naturally between two individuals who have a significant amount of interaction. Ungerleider and colleagues conducted a survey of cardiothoracic surgeons who were members of the Congenital Heart Surgeons Society (CHSS) or European Congenital Heart Surgeons Association (ECHSA) and found that most responders stated that a faculty member or surgical chief was most often their primary mentor. The next most frequently identified mentors were colleagues, followed by parents and spouses. Interestingly, a small proportion of responders shared that historical figures or even fictional characters served as mentors. Good mentors were often described as being knowledgeable, supportive, dedicated, able, and trustworthy.[30,36] Particularly in medicine, mentors may be different across different domains, and individuals may have different clinical, research, career planning, and personal mentors.[37]

Although mentorship overall has been demonstrated to be a highly positive experience, not all are entirely satisfied with their mentorship. Diekroger and colleagues conducted a survey of developmental-behavioral pediatrics fellows and found that 53% were not satisfied with the mentorship they were receiving. Those who reported being satisfied with their mentorship reported having mentors who were actively involved in several different domains of their career and lives.[37] But those not satisfied with their mentorship are not out of luck. Mentorships are dynamic, and mentors can enter one's career at any time.

Absence of a mentor is the most frequent reason cited for being dissatisfied with mentorship. Diekroger and colleagues found that 83% of those without a mentor wanted to have a mentor. Barriers to having a mentor included not having access to those with mentoring skills, incompatible personalities, lack of time among potential mentors, and lack of interest among potential mentors.

Although no pediatric cardiac critical care–specific data exist in the realm of mentorship, there is no reason to believe that the mentorship process should be any different in our subspecialty when compared to other areas of medicine. Certainly, there may be different nuances to mentorship within CICU practice, but the overall principles should not be vastly different. What is certain is that mentorship is critically important and can promote clinical, academic, and personal progress and improve overall morale in the unit.

Conclusion

The topics of training pathways, education, mentorship, and recruitment are vital to the continued growth of pediatric cardiac critical care as a specialty. With the enormous growth seen within the field in the last two decades, we are in an important era that will define the future of our subspecialty. Defining the end goals of training through the development of a subspecialty-specific curriculum, competencies, and EPAs are key steps toward optimizing the care delivered across institutions. We anticipate continued discussions on the benefits and risks of seeking a subspecialty board certification; regardless of the outcome of that debate, adequacy of training to support the delivery of high-quality care should remain our primary focus. This will help ensure that all children with congenital or acquired cardiac disease are cared for by physicians who are well trained to provide the complete scope of each patient's care.

References

A complete list of references is available at ExpertConsult.com.

7

Critical Care Databases and Quality Collaboratives

MICHAEL GAIES, MD, MPH, MS

Cardiac critical care has evolved into one of the cornerstones of successful congenital heart centers. Improvements in morbidity and mortality after pediatric and congenital heart surgery observed in the modern era[1] most likely resulted from several advances in perioperative care such as preoperative imaging, surgical techniques, anesthesia management, and mechanical circulatory support but are also due to increasingly specialized intensive care units (ICUs) and expert postoperative care. The degree to which any one of these domains impacts short- and long-term patient outcomes in children and adults with critical cardiovascular disease remains unclear, and this is particularly true when considering the role and contribution of critical care. A deeper understanding of critical care's impact on surgical outcomes represents crucial knowledge for efforts to continue improving the health of this patient population. Further, as the cohort of critically ill patients slowly shifts away from postoperative care to include more patients with end-stage heart failure (with or without underlying structural heart disease), multiorgan disease, and chronic device utilization (e.g., ventricular assist devices), measurement of critical care quality must account for this diversity.

Robust data infrastructures are essential to measuring cardiac critical care outcomes, assessing quality of care, and testing new treatment approaches or interventions. Multiple databases now exist that include practice and outcome information that could be used to measure the performance of critical care teams.[2] Finally, improving outcomes for children with critical cardiovascular disease depends upon converting these existing data into actionable information that drives practice change. Collaborative learning paradigms[3] are a means to such improvement, and burgeoning efforts within the field of pediatric cardiac critical care hold promise to achieve further reductions in morbidity and mortality for these vulnerable children.

This chapter begins with a framing of concepts and challenges in measuring critical care outcomes and quality, using risk-adjusted mortality as an illustrative example. We then describe the essential features of a clinical data repository for critical care quality and outcomes assessment. The breadth of existing data sources and registries for cardiac critical care data is described, with a subsequent focus on the two primary clinical databases used in North America: the Pediatric Cardiac Critical Care Consortium (PC[4]) clinical registry and the Virtual PICU System (VPS, LLC, Los Angeles, California) database. The chapter concludes with a discussion of collaborative quality improvement in the field of congenital cardiac care that involves interventions in the critical care environment.

Measuring Outcome and Quality of Critical Care

Defining Patient Outcomes and Quality Metrics

Outcome measures used for pediatric cardiac critical care quality assessment should ideally reflect the competence and performance of the cardiac intensive care unit (CICU) team and be independent of care provided and outcomes realized before and subsequent to the CICU admission. Hospital episode metrics (e.g., discharge mortality) are certainly most important to understanding patient-level outcomes, but these metrics do not inform improvement strategies because they do not necessarily provide granular information on the performance and quality of individual teams that separately care for a patient throughout the hospitalization. Congenital heart centers desiring to improve outcomes for hospitalized patients need quality metrics that disentangle teams' performance from one another. This is particularly true when considering the quality of care provided in the CICU.

Perioperative care is an illustrative example of the conundrum regarding team quality assessment; it is challenging to determine how the quality of intraoperative and postoperative care determines individual patient and aggregate population outcomes. For example, duration of mechanical ventilation after a particular operative procedure depends on ventilator management, administration of sedatives and analgesics, and weaning practices of the CICU team. However, despite any efforts made by the CICU to rapidly and safely extubate a postoperative patient, this metric is profoundly impacted by the preoperative physiology, presence of residual anatomic defects, anesthetic practices, and complicating surgical morbidities (e.g., phrenic nerve injury), which includes the quality of care provided by other provider teams. Thoughtful approaches to risk adjustment (see later) and outcome measurement are necessary to understand the unique impact of pediatric cardiac critical care team performance on surgical patients. Presenting existing data on overall program performance (e.g., hospital mortality after cardiovascular surgery) alongside CICU performance (e.g., CICU "attributable" mortality; see later discussion) may provide deeper insights to hospitals on where strengths and weaknesses lie in their overall perioperative care process.

Outcomes of medical (nonsurgical) CICU encounters may better reflect the interventions and quality of care provided by the CICU team. Establishing outcome benchmarks for commonly used quality metrics in general pediatric critical care (e.g., catheter-associated bloodstream infections, unplanned readmissions, frequency of cardiac arrest) is necessary for measuring performance in populations of patients with critical cardiovascular disease. Determining how to appropriately risk adjust outcomes specifically for surgical and medical patients in the CICU presents a challenge, but this approach also holds promise to provide useful, granular information to CICU providers; by measuring performance in these two distinct populations, CICUs may identify areas requiring improvement efforts that would not be elucidated by looking at the patient population as a whole.

Risk Adjustment in Critical Care Outcomes and Quality Assessment

Risk adjustment, broadly defined, is a methodologic approach to measuring outcomes while accounting for unique patient characteristics that impact those outcomes and are unrelated to the quality of care provided by the hospital or provider team.[4] In order for CICUs to understand their performance, adjusted quality metrics must reflect the unique patients they care for and the illness severity of those patients *at the time they assumed care of the patient* (Fig. 7.1). Multi-institutional clinical registries provide an excellent source of data for generating risk-adjustment models and for applying those models to calculate adjusted outcome measures that can be reported back to hospitals.

Risk adjustment after congenital heart surgery represents the most thorough and successful effort to date within the field of congenital cardiac care. The Society of Thoracic Surgeons Congenital Heart Surgery Database Mortality Risk Model[5] represents the current gold standard in surgical mortality risk adjustment. This empirically derived model accounts for patient characteristics and operative complexity before surgery. However, examination of two hypothetical patients undergoing the same operation highlights why additional tools are needed to assess CICU quality.

Consider two patients with no comorbidities or preoperative complications undergoing arterial switch operation for d-transposition of the great arteries. The first patient undergoes a straightforward operation and arrives at the CICU on low-dose inotropic support and mechanical ventilation. The second patient's intraoperative course is complicated by several bypass runs to revise the coronary buttons and arrives at the CICU with an open sternum and on extracorporeal membrane oxygenation (ECMO). Clearly the challenges to the CICU team differ significantly in these two patients, and operative mortality is much more likely in the second case than the first independent of the quality of care provided by the CICU team. According to the existing Society of Thoracic Surgeons (STS) risk-adjustment model, these patients would have identical predicted risk of mortality, reflecting none of the complexity faced by the second CICU patient. Measuring performance in the CICU must include markers of physiologic derangement and illness severity at the time of care transfer to the CICU team to understand how CICU care impacts eventual patient outcome. Thus complementary risk-adjustment approaches to disentangle quality of CICU care must be developed.

Existing risk-adjustment models used in general pediatric critical care outcomes assessment have proven insufficient for understanding the quality of pediatric CICU care, particularly in the setting of postoperative care.[6] Databases specifically designed to capture cardiac critical care outcomes have been used to develop new risk-adjustment methods that may solve this difficult problem of isolating CICU team performance. The first such attempt was performed using the VPS database cardiac module. Jeffries et al.[7] developed the Pediatric Index of Cardiac Surgical Intensive Care Mortality from a cohort of 16,574 cardiac surgery patients, and it predicted postoperative mortality in the ICU with an area under the curve of 0.87 and good calibration. However, important questions remained regarding this approach. The model included some postoperative variables that were collected up to 12 hours after admission from the operating room. Some of these predictor variables, such as use of ECMO within 12 hours of surgery, may be related more to CICU performance rather than baseline severity of illness upon arrival to the CICU and thus may lead to erroneous conclusions about quality. Further, this model is applied at the time of CICU admission, not when the patient returns from the operating room. Thus, in cases where patients are admitted preoperatively (e.g., neonates with ductal dependent circulations), illness severity is not assessed in the early postoperative period, and analysis of CICU postoperative care quality may be inaccurate.

To address remaining knowledge gaps and improve on existing methods, investigators from PC[4] developed a new risk-adjustment model to assess postoperative care quality in the CICU, again using mortality as the quality metric (personal communication of data under peer review). The important new features of this model include (1) that it is always applied at the time postoperative care begins in the CICU, providing a consistent assessment of patient illness severity at that time point, and (2) illness-severity measures are collected only within the first 2 postoperative hours, reducing the likelihood that variables like postoperative vasoactive support or ECMO utilization reflect the quality of CICU care. From a sample that included 8543 postoperative encounters across 23 dedicated CICUs, this model demonstrated excellent discrimination for CICU mortality with a c-statistic of 0.92. The model is being used to provide real-time information to PC[4] hospitals on adjusted CICU ("CICU attributable") surgical mortality for benchmarking and quality improvement purposes (see later discussion).

The approaches described earlier could and should be applied more widely to investigate CICU quality metrics that go beyond mortality. Several efforts are under way at the time of this writing within PC[4] to develop risk-adjustment models for cardiac arrest,[7a] duration of mechanical ventilation,[8] and CICU/hospital length of

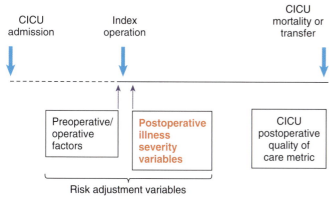

• **Figure 7.1** Conceptual model for assessment of postoperative quality of care by the cardiac critical care team. Accurate assessment of cardiac critical care quality requires measurement of illness severity at the time of postoperative transfer. This approach complements traditional risk-adjustment methods for measuring adjusted mortality after congenital heart surgery but focuses on critical care team performance. *CICU,* Cardiac intensive care unit.

stay accounting for illness severity at the time of CICU admission in postoperative encounters. It remains unclear whether new CICU-specific risk-adjustment models are necessary and will outperform existing methods[9-11] in use for general pediatric critical care in the measurement of outcomes for nonsurgical encounters.

Key Components of Effective Cardiac Critical Care Databases

The ideal cardiac critical care database for improving quality of care would manage the challenges described previously around heterogeneity of patients, separating CICU care from other domains, and risk adjustment. In addition, these databases should include two key components: a standard nomenclature and mechanisms that facilitate linkage between registries.

Common Nomenclature

Accurate measurement of clinical outcomes is dependent on a common nomenclature and standardized data collection. The International Society for Nomenclature of Paediatric and Congenital Heart Disease (ISNPCHD; http://www.ipccc.net/) and the Multi-Societal Database Committee for Pediatric and Congenital Heart Disease (MSDC), developed a consensus-based, comprehensive nomenclature for the diagnosis, procedures, and complications associated with the treatment of patients with pediatric and congenital cardiac disease.[12,13] This nomenclature has been adopted by several clinical databases, including most notably:

- The Society of Thoracic Surgeons (STS) Congenital Heart Surgery Database
- The European Association for Cardio-Thoracic Surgery (EACTS) Congenital Heart Surgery Database
- The IMPACT Interventional Cardiology Registry (**IM**proving **P**ediatric and **A**dult **C**ongenital **T**reatment) of the National Cardiovascular Data Registry of the American College of Cardiology Foundation and the Society for Cardiovascular Angiography and Interventions (SCAI)
- The Joint Congenital Cardiac Anesthesia Society–Society of Thoracic Surgeons Congenital Cardiac Anesthesia Database
- The Virtual PICU System (VPS)
- The Pediatric Cardiac Critical Care Consortium (PC[4])

A common nomenclature allows comparison of reported outcomes from different databases and registries and more importantly facilitates data sharing and integration across these sources.

Methods for Linking Databases

As is true in the clinical care of patients with pediatric and congenital cardiac disease, outcomes assessment benefits from multidisciplinary collaboration. Linking subspecialty databases (e.g., surgery and critical care) can facilitate sharing of longitudinal data across temporal, geographic, and subspecialty boundaries.[13-15] Clinical and administrative databases have been successfully linked using indirect identifiers,[16] and similar techniques could be used to link clinical databases. Innovative new software platforms can also facilitate direct sharing of data variables between registries and will promote more effective approaches to indirect linkage. Careful thought must be given during the design phase when new registries are developed to ensure the most efficient and seamless harmonization across databases.

Existing Critical Care Databases

A recent effort summarized the current scope of clinical registry projects in congenital cardiac care.[2] Three databases—the Paediatric Intensive Care Audit Network (PICANet, United Kingdom), VPS, and PC[4]—focus solely on critically ill patients, whereas many others include some data related to critical care (e.g., surgical databases). Other national and regional critical care databases—for example, the Australia and New Zealand Pediatric Intensive Care (ANZPIC) Registry—will include some cardiac-specific data on outcomes and practice. Of these, the PC[4] clinical registry is the only database exclusively dedicated to the cardiac critical care population.

Virtual PICU Systems Database

The VPS clinical database has been operated since 1997. The founders developed a repository to collect demographic, diagnostic, and severity of illness–adjusted outcome data from member units on all patients. The database has supported patient care, quality improvement, distance learning, and research initiatives. This platform provided a valuable resource of information to investigate how pediatric critical care was practiced across the United States. The database now includes several hundreds of thousands of cases from 120 member ICUs.

A separate cardiac module within the VPS database was created to provide more information on patients with critical cardiovascular disease. The VPS adopted the International Paediatric and Congenital Cardiac Code (http://www.ipccc.net/) nomenclature for cardiac diagnoses, cardiac surgical procedures and cardiac surgical complications. This cardiac module has been used to explore several outcomes related to cardiac critical care[17-19] and to develop risk-adjustment methods[7] for outcome reporting (see earlier discussion).

Pediatric Cardiac Critical Care Consortium Clinical Registry

In 2012, 12 children's hospitals formed the Pediatric Cardiac Critical Care Consortium (PC[4]; pc4quality.org) as a quality improvement collaborative for children with critical cardiovascular disease.[20] A granular, CICU-specific clinical registry was developed to be the data infrastructure for quality assessment and clinical research that would power improvement initiatives through collaborative learning (see later discussion). All CICU encounters from participating hospitals have been entered since 2013, and at the time of this writing more than 33,000 CICU encounters and 19,000 index surgical hospitalizations exist in the database. Since 2013 the number of hospitals submitting data to PC[4] has risen from 6 to now include over 30 from North America (Fig. 7.2).

The PC[4] clinical registry populates a real-time, Web-based analytics and reporting platform that participants use to view comparative reports on quality metrics and resource utilization (Fig. 7.3). This registry shares common variables with the Society of Thoracic Surgeons Congenital Heart Surgery Database and the IMPACT Registry; each hospital uses a software solution that ensures identical data on patient characteristics and anatomic and procedural variables across each of the three registries. The data in the PC[4] registry are rigorously audited, and this process has revealed excellent data integrity.[21] PC[4] investigators have published several reports from the clinical registry demonstrating variation in outcomes across hospitals, elucidating the epidemiology of cardiac

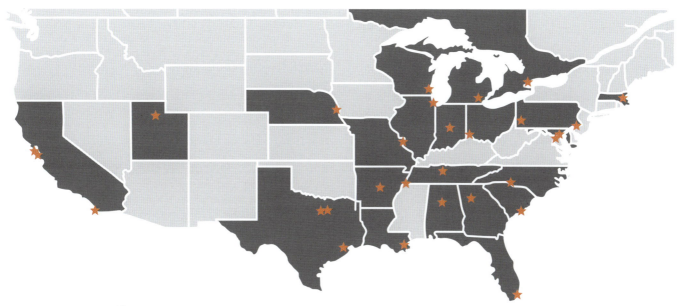

• **Figure 7.2** Hospitals participating in the Pediatric Cardiac Critical Care Consortium (PC⁴) in May 2017.

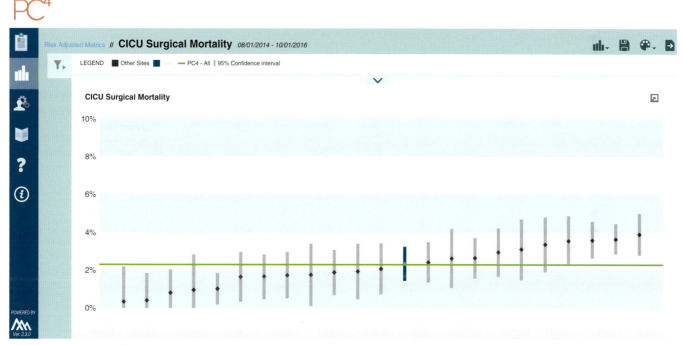

• **Figure 7.3** Example of real-time, adjusted benchmark reports for cardiac critical care units in PC⁴. Adjusted cardiac intensive care unit (CICU) mortality is shown in the figure. *(From pc4quality.org.)*

critical care outcomes and practice, and have developed new risk-adjustment methods to assess CICU quality.[8,22-27]

Quality Collaboratives in Pediatric Cardiac Critical Care

Clinical registries and databases should exist as repositories of outcomes data that are actively used to promote quality improvement. The core tenets of collaborative quality improvement are:
1. purposeful collection of granular clinical data,
2. providing timely performance feedback to clinicians, and

3. continuous quality improvement based on empirical analysis and collaborative learning.

Databases are necessary, but not sufficient, to facilitate quality improvement. An evolving body of literature demonstrates that merely submitting data to a clinical database does not result in improved clinical or resource utilization outcomes.[28,29] Share and colleagues[30] highlighted the benefits gained from participation in quality improvement collaboratives over and above participation in a national registry. Investigators showed greater improvement in rates of complications and mortality for adult patients undergoing general, vascular, and bariatric surgical procedures at hospitals that belonged to statewide quality collaborative programs for these specialties in Michigan compared to hospitals that submitted data to the National Surgical Quality Improvement Program (NSQIP) but were not part of any quality collaborative. This analysis highlights the gap between simply measuring and reporting outcomes versus an active infrastructure to promote quality improvement through collaboration.

Clinical registries and databases provide an essential foundation for improvement work because they contain high-quality patient and outcome data that can be used for comparative analysis of performance across hospitals. The next steps toward successful quality improvement include rigorous empirical analysis to identify high-performing hospitals with appropriately risk-adjusted data and uncovering the underlying features and practices of these hospitals that drive their outstanding outcomes. Finally, there must be a means to disseminate these findings across hospitals in a collaborative to inform participants how they might achieve better quality care and reduce preventable harm or unnecessary resource utilization. Transparency between hospitals in quality collaboratives has proven to be a very effective method for promoting quality improvement efforts.[31,32]

New collaborative learning approaches to congenital cardiac care have begun to permeate the field. The National Pediatric Cardiology Quality Improvement Collaborative (NPC-QIC) demonstrated success in achieving better weight gain and lower mortality during the interstage period for children undergoing stage 1 palliation for hypoplastic left heart syndrome (HLHS) and related diagnoses.[33,34] The NPC-QIC plans to implement a phase 2 improvement project that will be more focused on perioperative care in the CICU. In a project focused on the pediatric cardiac critical care environment, Mahle and colleagues from the Pediatric Heart Network used a collaborative learning intervention to successfully increase early extubation rates after repair of tetralogy of Fallot and coarctation in infants.[3,35] These successful examples illustrate that the core concepts presented earlier can lead to important improvements in the care of critically ill children and adults with pediatric and congenital cardiac disease:

both groups of investigators collected detailed data on practice and outcomes, identified the highest-performing hospitals in their collaborative, disseminated this information back to participants, and identified the practices at high-performing hospitals that could be implemented at lower-performing hospitals to improve outcomes.

As described earlier, PC⁴ has been developed and organized to promote collaborative learning among its participants. The collaborative uses its clinical registry to power a reporting platform that shows real-time benchmark data on critical care outcomes and resource utilization. The unique feature of the PC⁴ program is its transparency: hospitals can identify one another internally on the reporting platform by viewing outcome reports that are unblinded. This feature allows hospitals to directly identify high performers, thus facilitating conversations between clinicians and researchers at participating hospitals who desire to improve the quality of their care through reduction of complications or optimizing cost-effectiveness and efficiencies. This level of transparency is a condition of participation in PC⁴. In addition to providing the infrastructure for ad hoc local quality improvement efforts, PC⁴ has generated data suggesting opportunities for more far-reaching, multi-institutional collaborative learning projects. At the time of this writing, a collaborative-wide cardiac arrest prevention intervention is being implemented based on data showing wide variation in adjusted CICU rates of cardiac arrest across PC⁴ hospitals (Fig. 7.4).

Value of Quality Collaboratives

Despite the wealth of information contained in clinical registries managed by quality collaboratives and the potential to change practice and improve patient outcomes, many questions still exist regarding the true value of participation in these organizations. There is a clear business case for quality improvement collaboratives supported by a sizable body of literature[36-38]; these data illustrate the concept of "return on investment" (ROI) to hospitals that devote

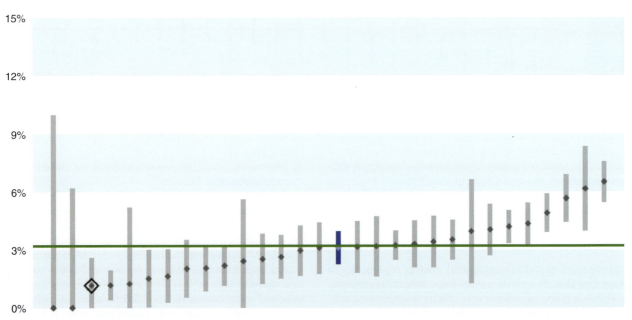

• **Figure 7.4** Adjusted cardiac arrest rate by cardiac intensive care unit. *(From pc4quality.org.)*

resources to participation in quality improvement collaboratives. There are several outcomes (or "returns") from collaborative quality improvement that could justify investment:

1. Better quality and outcomes consistent with a hospital's mission
2. Higher "ranking" on publicly available surveys or public outcome-reporting websites
3. Lower cost per case and better profit margin

Ultimately, it is incumbent on each collaborative to demonstrate that it can achieve one or more of these returns and furthermore to prove that the returns are directly attributable to participation in the collaborative. This demonstration of effectiveness depends upon sophisticated and impeccable scientific methods.

Finally, each collaborative must look for ways to reduce costs, to the degree possible, to maximize ROI. Limiting the personnel costs associated with data collection is probably the greatest lever for minimizing a hospital's investment, and capturing the data directly from the electronic health record is a means to this end. In doing so, hospitals and collaboratives will have to ensure that they can maintain the same level of data integrity that makes the information valuable in the first place.

Conclusion

Unique challenges exist in assessing and improving quality in the CICU, but several recent efforts prove that success is achievable. Robust databases exist to provide risk-adjusted outcome data and develop quality metrics for ongoing measurement of critical care performance. Thoughtful analytic approaches to isolate and identify quality of CICU care are under way. These data reveal high-performing CICUs, and with a collaborative spirit fueled by a commitment to transparent sharing of data on outcomes and practice, the pediatric cardiac critical care community can help improve the lives of children and adults with critical cardiovascular disease by learning from one another.

Selected References

A complete reference list is available at ExpertConsult.com.

2. Vener DF, Gaies M, Jacobs JP, Pasquali SK. Clinical databases and registries in congenital and pediatric cardiac surgery, cardiology, critical care, and anesthesiology worldwide. *World J Pediatr Congenit Heart Surg*. 2017;8:77–87.
12. Jacobs JP. Introduction–databases and the assessment of complications associated with the treatment of patients with congenital cardiac disease. *Cardiol Young*. 2008;18(suppl 2):1–37.
13. Jacobs JP, Jacobs ML, Mavroudis C, et al. Nomenclature and databases for the surgical treatment of congenital cardiac disease–an updated primer and an analysis of opportunities for improvement. *Cardiol Young*. 2008;18(suppl 2):38–62.
20. Gaies M, Cooper DS, Tabbutt S, et al. Collaborative quality improvement in the cardiac intensive care unit: development of the paediatric cardiac critical care consortium (PC4). *Cardiol Young*. 2015;25: 951–957.
29. Osborne NH, Nicholas LH, Ryan AM, Thumma JR, Dimick JB. Association of hospital participation in a quality reporting program with surgical outcomes and expenditures for Medicare beneficiaries. *JAMA*. 2015;313:496–504.
30. Share DA, Campbell DA, Birkmeyer N, et al. How a regional collaborative of hospitals and physicians in Michigan cut costs and improved the quality of care. *Health Aff (Millwood)*. 2011;30:636–645.
32. Forrest CB, Margolis P, Seid M, Colletti RB. PEDSnet: how a prototype pediatric learning health system is being expanded into a national network. *Health Aff (Millwood)*. 2014;33:1171–1177.
33. Anderson JB, Beekman RH 3rd, Kugler JD, et al. Improvement in interstage survival in a national pediatric cardiology learning network. *Circ Cardiovasc Qual Outcomes*. 2015;8:428–436.
35. Mahle WT, Nicolson SC, Hollenbeck-Pringle D, et al. Utilizing a collaborative learning model to promote early extubation following infant heart surgery. *Pediatr Crit Care Med*. 2016;17:939–947.

8

Improving Safety

CHARLOTTE WOODS-HILL, MD; GEOFFREY L. BIRD, MD, MSIS

In 2000 the Institute of Medicine's (IOM) landmark publication *To Err Is Human* made headlines around the nation with its assertion that nearly 100,000 people died each year in the United States due to medical errors.[1] *Crossing the Quality Chasm,* published 1 year later, identified safety as the first dimension of health care quality, without which the subsequent dimensions cannot be reliably achieved.[2] In the years since then, appreciation in the medical community of the real scope of preventable patient harm has only deepened. It truly is an epidemic—a 2013 study examining data from 2008 to 2011 suggests that 200,000 to 400,000 Americans experience death or premature death due to medical error each year.[3] Patient safety and preventable patient harm have become topics of the utmost importance to both the medical community and the general public, particularly as more institution-specific outcome metrics and adverse event data are readily accessible with a simple Internet search.[4]

The morbidity related to medical error in hospitalized pediatric patients is less certain, but most assuredly is not insignificant. In a retrospective review of 15 pediatric intensive care units (PICUs) across the United States, Agarwal et al.[5] found that over 60% of PICU patients experienced an adverse event, 45% of which were deemed preventable and 10% of which were either life threatening or permanent. Patients in a PICU are known to be at increased risk of nosocomial infection.[6] In addition, estimates of adverse drug events in PICU patients range from 22 to 59 per 1000 doses, with up to 11% of those events being of life-threatening severity.[7,8]

When specifically assessing the risk of preventable medical error for a child with cardiac disease, there is a relative paucity of incidence data. There is agreement that adverse events and medical errors do occur in cardiac surgery, owing to its high work load, complexity of involved tasks, and tendency of management plans to be uncertain and subject to change.[9] It is reasonable to suspect that given their fragile underlying physiology and the high-risk procedures they often require, pediatric cardiac intensive care unit (PCICU) patients are particularly vulnerable to medical error.[10] Jacques et al.[11] examined the clinical course of 191 patients with hypoplastic left heart syndrome (or physiologic equivalent) between 2001 and 2011 for errors that could impact patient outcome, and the most striking findings included the following: Errors were common overall, with nearly a quarter of patients experiencing a postoperative error (with delay in recognizing or managing a clinical scenario, error relating to airway management or extubation, and failure of attempted delayed sternal closure being most prevalent); the majority of postoperative errors were considered foreseeable; and postoperative errors were associated with increased risk of death or transplant.

Pediatric cardiac surgery clearly is a high-risk specialty with a very small margin for error, and the nature of the work—complex procedures taking place within a sophisticated organizational structure, dependent on frequent multidisciplinary collaboration, and tasking individuals with high-level technical and cognitive responsibilities—may lend itself to the human factors engineering and crew resource management approaches long used in aviation.[12] In this vein, Hickey et al.[13] took an innovative approach, applying the "threat and error" model of the National Aeronautics and Space Administration (NASA) to over 500 pediatric cardiac surgical admissions. This demonstrated that fully half of cases contained one or more errors and that cycles with multiple errors were very significantly associated with permanent harmful end states, including residual hemodynamic lesions, end-organ injury, and death.

Given the mounting evidence that hospitalized children are indeed at risk of medical error and its accompanying morbidity, it is paramount that every pediatric provider actively share in the responsibility to improve patient safety. There is perhaps no clinical environment in which this recognition—that improving patient safety is a shared, fundamental obligation—is more critical than in the perilous world of cardiac surgery. This chapter aims to introduce the reader to a selection of essential concepts and frameworks necessary to provide the safest possible care for pediatric cardiac patients, beginning with a review of key definitions and essential principles relating to patient safety and preventable patient harm, followed by a discussion of selected safety issues unique to a pediatric cardiac patient.

First, *error, adverse event,* and other key terms are defined and categorized in a useful taxonomy from original work by Kohn et al. in *To Err Is Human* (Table 8.1).[1]

In the years following the original IOM report, work by Reason and others has proposed that both human and nonhuman factors (i.e., systems), and the interaction of the two, are key in the origin of the majority of medical errors.[10] The concept of an organizational or systems-level analysis of adverse events in health care is fundamental to current approaches to increasing patient safety. Health care providers are likely familiar with Reason's famous "Swiss cheese" model of patient safety,[14] which is based on analysis showing that accidents are rarely the result of individual errors, but rather multiple errors within a fundamentally flawed system. In a complex system such as health care, both latent errors (due to organizational system or design failures) and active errors (due to an individual's failure) can occur, and the way to guarantee patient safety is to either prevent the error from occurring or prevent the error from causing harm through the application of multiple steps that function as a safety net.[15] The steps required to verify and dispense a medication

TABLE 8.1	Basic Language of Patient Safety
Patient Safety	Freedom from accidental injury; ensuring patient safety involves the establishment of operational systems and processes that minimize the likelihood of errors and maximize the likelihood of intercepting them when they occur.
Adverse Event	An injury resulting from a medical intervention.
Error	Failure of a planned action to be completed as intended or use of a wrong plan to achieve an aim; the accumulation of errors results in accidents.
Active Error	An error that occurs at the level of the frontline operator and whose effects are felt almost immediately.
Latent Error	Errors in the design, organization, training, or maintenance that lead to operator errors and whose effects typically lie dormant in the system for lengthy periods of time.
System	Set of interdependent elements interacting to achieve a common aim. These elements may be both human and nonhuman (equipment, technologies, etc.).
Human Factors	Study of the interrelationships between humans, the tools they use, and the environment in which they live and work.

From The Institute of Medicine. Kohn LT, Corrigan JM, Donaldson MS, eds. *To Err Is Human: Building a Safer Health System*. Washington, DC: The National Academies Press; 2000:26.

• BOX 8.1 Characteristics of High-Reliability Organizations

Preoccupation with failure (being highly aware of all error and potential for error)
Reluctance to simplify (understanding and appreciating the complexity of the work)
Sensitivity to operations (awareness of the work being done on the front lines)
Commitment to resilience (having the capacity to identify, contain, and improve from error)
Deference to expertise (allowing frontline workers to make decisions, avoid rigid hierarchies)

Modified from Hershey K. Culture of safety. Nurs Clin North Am. 2015;50:139-152; Weick KE, Sutcliffe KM. Managing the Unexpected: Assuring High Performance in an Age of Complexity. San Francisco: Jossey-Bass; 2001.

patient safety. As increasing attention has been paid to the frequency of adverse events in pediatric patients, it has become apparent that the definitions of *adverse event* and *preventable adverse event* and the ability of teams to consistently evaluate for "preventability" vary significantly.[17] Intriguing approaches to better define and identify adverse events using "trigger tool" methodology and targeted retrospective chart review have been piloted, but at this time much of what we know about incidence of preventable harm in hospitalized pediatric patients comes from incident reporting systems, which are subject to underreporting and other limitations.[17]

Embedding a Culture of Safety Into Pediatric Cardiac Intensive Care

Lessons From "High-Reliability Organizations"

Embracing the concept of a "culture of safety" is fundamental to institution- or unit-level efforts to reduce preventable patient harm. The Agency for Healthcare Research and Quality (AHRQ) reports that the term *culture of safety* first originated with high-reliability organizations (HROs)—organizations that operate with high potential for error but few adverse outcomes, typically used to mean nuclear or aviation industries.[18] In its current state, medicine is alarmingly far from establishing operating margins of safety comparable to these HROs. As a striking comparison from Weick and Sutcliffe,[19] the 400,000 people who die annually due to hospital-associated preventable harm is the equivalent of two 747 passenger jets crashing every day, every year—numbers that would bring air travel to a grinding halt, yet health care continues unaffected.

HROs are defined by Weick and Sutcliffe as sharing the core characteristics listed in Box 8.1, on a foundation of mutual trust.[18,19]

When evaluating if the concepts of HROs can translate fully to medicine, one should acknowledge one important limitation from the start. A core principle of the concept of reliability is to focus on defects (errors or adverse events) that can be measured as rates (defects as the numerator, population at risk as the denominator) and are free from reporting bias.[20] In applying reliability to health care, this focus translates well to problems with clear operational definitions and that occur at discrete points in time, such as central-line associated bloodstream infections. In truth, most patient safety issues do not lend themselves to

dose on an inpatient ward is a simple example of how medicine applies this safety net concept into daily work flow. Both the ordering clinician and a pharmacist independently verify the dose to be correct and appropriate for the patient and not in violation of the patient's medication allergy profile. A modern electronic medical record typically has built-in dose maximums and automatic warnings that notify a clinician if the chosen dose falls outside of typical prescribing norms. Often, two nurses also independently verify the medication name, dose, route, patient identifier, and infusion pump settings before administering the medication to the patient. These steps are designed not necessarily to prevent a clinician from ever inadvertently ordering an incorrect medication dose (which would represent a focus on active error) but to reduce the likelihood that an incorrect dose will ever reach and harm a patient via intentional system redundancies and double checks (a contrasting focus on latent error). This model has become hugely popular as a model of accident causation in many industries, including health care, and does offer useful constructs for understanding the constant interplay between individual humans and larger organizational systems, and how each may contribute to adverse events. There is, however, debate in the literature about its validity, particularly regarding its potential to oversimplify events and concern that it has swung the pendulum too far toward placing responsibility for accidents or errors on senior management, versus individuals at the "front lines."[16]

Although the definitions and mental models described earlier are a useful starting point, readers should also heed a note of caution about the imperfect standardization of the language of measurement in this manner.[20] This distinction may be part of why the success of efforts to transform medicine into an HRO has been somewhat limited to date.[21]

A great deal may be gained for health care, however, by understanding the organizational culture at the heart of HROs. Fundamentally, an HRO is a system that has developed a culture sensitive to safety that enables employees to maintain a low probability of adverse events despite unpredictable threats.[22] Within an HRO exists an expectation of employees to routinely question practices and search for anomalies that may create risk for error, to refuse to oversimplify safety issues, to work collaboratively and in deference to expertise rather than a rigid organizational hierarchy, and to create solutions when error does occur—essentially, to view reliability as a *continuous, ongoing,* and *active* pursuit rather than a simple numeric measure of past performance.[22,23] Embedding this culture into the practice of medicine has real potential to change patient outcomes for the better. Roberts et al.[24] published a compelling case report of a sustained decrease in mortality and serious safety events in a tertiary care PICU after adoption of HRO principles, followed by a recrudescence of such adverse events after a leadership change in the unit and abandonment of the HRO approach. Anesthesia may also be particularly suited for the introduction of the HRO model to reduce serious safety events.[24]

Clearly there are differences between aviation and health care that may require alterations in HRO-based methodology. Scheduled operation of a machine that is assumed to be functioning at peak performance is quite distinct from guiding an unexpectedly deteriorating human being from illness to health. However, the principle of high reliability—ability to perform with minimal adverse events despite high risk—is something that health care should certainly endeavor to embody. Indeed, if "the only realistic goal of safety management in complex health-care systems is to develop an intrinsic resistance to its operational hazards," HROs can provide a road map for building this intrinsic resistance.[25] The existing body of evidence for implementing HRO principles in the practice of medicine, though small, mandates our attention as we strive to reduce adverse outcomes for our patients.[24]

Defining and Building a Culture of Safety for Health Care

Specific to health care, the Joint Commission has defined safety culture as "the summary of knowledge, attitudes, behaviors, and beliefs that staff share about the primary importance of the well-being and care of the patients they serve, supported by systems and structures that reinforce the focus on patient safety."[26] Several key themes emerge when reviewing literature on how to construct a safety culture in health care.

First, there is a clear emphasis on examining medical errors through the lens of health care systems and how systems and individual workers intersect in ways that may be either predisposing to, or protective from, error. Returning back to Reason's foundational work, individual error is referred to as active error and is committed by a frontline health care worker at the so-called sharp end of health care, whereas systems error is latent error, originating from someone or something remote from direct patient care (such as managers, system designers, or administrators).[27] According to Reason, systems-based or latent errors are the greatest threat to complex industries like health care and are the root cause of most error.[27] There certainly is a growing body of evidence that nontechnical errors are more prevalent in health care delivery than technical errors and are driven the majority of the time by communication

breakdowns or by problematic team dynamics.[28] Catchpole et al.[29] found evidence that the primary threat to quality in pediatric cardiac surgery is error related to cultural and organizational failures. Indeed, some go so far as to suggest that "the need to implement effective health care organizing has become as pressing as the need to implement medical breakthroughs."[30] Health care is a dynamic system, with a basic structure and organization into which individual workers bring their own attitudes, behavior, and knowledge. Both parties impact the other continuously, and a focus solely on individual workers as the cause of medical error will be less effective than a strategy that acknowledges the critical interplay between systems and individuals that constantly occurs during patient care.

Second, Chassin and Loeb[31] propose three central attributes of a safety culture that reinforce one another: trust, report, and improve. Team members must trust their colleagues and their management structure to feel safe in speaking up about unsafe conditions that may endanger patients. Trust will be strengthened when frontline workers see that improvements have been made based on their concerns. Unfortunately, trust is not a given in all health care systems. The 2013 *National Healthcare Quality Report* found that many health care workers still believe that mistakes will be held against them, and in that same report, half of respondents reported no adverse events at their facility in the preceding year—a number that seems quite low, raising concern that fear of blame may lead to underreporting of medical error and continued risk to patients.[32] A culture of blame—one in which fear of criticism or punishment fosters an unwillingness to take risks or accept responsibility for mistakes—simply can no longer be tolerated in a health care system striving to improve patient safety.[29] A focus on blame perpetuates silence in the face of near misses and performance problems, ensuring that patients continue to be at risk of preventable harm; a *just culture,* in contrast, provides a supportive environment in which workers can question practices, express concerns, and admit mistakes without suffering ridicule or punishment.[33]

Underlying issues like trust and fear of blame is the larger construct of *communication* within health care systems. Communication barriers are one of the biggest safety challenges that critical care teams face.[34] As this fact has become increasingly studied and better understood, the old paradigm of the physician as the unquestioned captain of the team is, in safety-focused health care environments, gradually giving way to new communication strategies that prioritize care delivery over hierarchy. For example, family-centered rounds include parents/caregivers in daily discussions of progress and plans for the patient and have been shown to improve family satisfaction, discharge planning, and communication.[35] Including a daily goals sheet or checklist during rounds improves team cohesiveness, helps customize daily care plans to the specific needs of each patient, prompts regular review of simple but important safety items like central venous catheter duration or need for venous thromboembolism prophylaxis, and has been shown in some studies to decrease intensive care unit (ICU) length of stay.[35] Employing structured communication frameworks to convey changes in patient status or clinical concerns, such as the popular "SBAR" (situation, background, assessment, recommendations) tool, can improve situational awareness, reduce problems related to organizational hierarchy and experience, and improve collaboration between nurses and physicians.[36]

Finally, the concept of *accountability* is also fundamental to a safety culture in health care. Workers must feel empowered to hold not only themselves but also their coworkers to shared high standards in a manner that engenders transparency rather than attempts to assign blame. For example, the Joint Commission Center for Transforming Healthcare focuses on accountability as a key strategy to improve hand hygiene performance, a simple practice that is known to reduce incidence of hospital-associated infections yet one for which compliance rates are only around 40%.[37] Many hospitals have implemented programs that encourage any observer (including patients and families) to speak up if they note that hand hygiene was not performed before patient care. More broadly, safety event reporting systems discussed in the next section provide a method for concerned team members to report issues of various types for review. Actively giving and openly receiving feedback on issues relating to patient safety is an essential part of a safety culture in health care.

Safety Reporting Systems and Approaches to Analyzing Patient Safety Events

Patient safety incident reporting systems are now common in hospitals, increasingly embedded into electronic medical records or Web-based technology, and are fundamental to detecting safety events.[38] AHRQ proposes four key elements for an effective safety event reporting system (Box 8.2).[38]

Error-reporting systems can take many forms—voluntary or mandatory disclosures of events as they occur, automated surveillance, or chart review. Voluntary and mandatory reporting systems are common. Advantages of these kinds of systems are that they often permit any type of health care worker, regardless of position, to make a report, and that they may remove fear of punishment for speaking up by allowing reporting to be anonymous. Limitations include recall bias and underreporting—the latter often due to perception that little or no follow-up will occur after a report is made.[38]

This perception highlights that having a system in place for reporting safety events accomplishes little if not paired with a robust method for analyzing and addressing the content of the reports. A brief discussion of a select few approaches for safety event review with which the pediatric cardiac intensivist should be familiar follows.

Root cause analysis (RCA) and apparent cause analysis (ACA): RCA is a commonly used, formally structured approach to safety event analysis, originating in industrial accidents but now widely applied to health care. It is a retrospective, systems-based method to identify both active and latent error. RCAs typically start with data collection, then detailed reconstruction of how the events leading to the event in question occurred (the active errors), why the events occurred (the latent errors), with the end goal of eliminating the latent errors to prevent the adverse outcome from recurring.[39]

The Joint Commission has mandated RCAs be done for sentinel events since 1997. Although RCAs are widely used, evidence for RCA effectiveness is fairly limited, and there is concern that the significant resources required to carry out RCAs is not balanced by the results they yield, given that follow-up and corrective actions are often inconsistently implemented and vary widely across institutions.[40] Related to the concept of RCA is ACA, a more limited investigation employed for less severe adverse events. ACAs may be done more quickly and by a broader range of staff members than RCAs, but as with RCAs, their impact is dependent on the quality and rigor with which they are followed up.

Failure modes and effects analysis (FMEA): Originating from engineering, FMEA is, in contrast to RCA, a prospective process that uses five steps to identify potential vulnerabilities in a health care process and to subsequently test the proposed solutions to ensure no new or continued risk to patients.[41] The basic steps for FMEA in health care consist of defining a topic (a process or situation thought to represent a potential safety risk), assembling a multidisciplinary team, graphically describing the process with a flow diagram, conducting a hazard analysis (reviewing any/all ways in which the process in question may fail and compromise patient outcomes), and finally developing actions and outcome measures.[43] The FMEA model has been associated with successful reduction of postanesthesia complications, improved safety in radiology departments, decreased error in chemotherapy orders, and safety gains in many other components of health care delivery.[42-44]

Structured morbidity and mortality reviews: This is a general categorization of a helpful construct—that of approaching traditional "M&M" conferences with a specific structure to better uncover and deconstruct issues underlying serious safety breaches. A growing body of evidence suggests a structured morbidity and mortality conference can be a driver of quality improvement initiatives and practice changes that increase patient safety.[45-47] This objective can be accomplished in many ways; the reader is directed to resources on the specifics of two selected examples, the Learn From Defects Tool and Ishikawa diagrams, for detailed description of these methods and how to implement them.[48-50]

Threat and error management: Edward Hickey has suggested an intriguing new approach to preventable patient harm that draws direct lessons from the safety culture of the airline industry. Aviation experts recognize and accept that error is "ubiquitous, inevitable, and needs to be managed"—trained observers of over 3500 commercial flights have concluded that 80% contain error.[51] This model stands in contrast to the traditional approach of the medical profession to underestimate frequency of errors, to view errors as stemming from personal failure, and to resist making errors and their impacts transparent to the public.[51] The concept of threat and error management is a tactic that therefore encourages medical teams to actively seek error and review all patient cases, rather than focus only on morbidities and mortalities.[51] Hickey's group instituted a model of real-time assessment of every pediatric cardiac surgical patient and included a combination of third-party review of active clinical management, weekly discussion of each patient in an open forum, and preoperative completion of a "flight plan." The flight plan is how the medical team views each patient's hospital course and contains a description of the potential threats for that specific case and the operative intentions and models the patient's projected journey from operating room (OR) to ICU to discharge, similar to an aircraft's intended flight plan.[51] When 524 consecutive patient "flights" were analyzed, 70% had threats; 66% had consequential errors; and 60% of consequential errors led to a chain of further error and progressive deviation from the ideal flight plan.[51] These findings suggest that as in aviation, it is these *chains of events* that lead to progressive loss of safety margins and increasing danger of adverse outcomes. Halting such a chain requires the ability to recognize when one is in such a cycle and active effort to rescue the situation using the principles of *crew resource management*—nontechnical skills that are mandatory for airline pilots and crews but which medicine has yet to embed into training or practice.[51]

Specific Safety Issues for the Pediatric Cardiac Intensive Care Patient: Team Performance, Surgical Handoff, and Nosocomial Infections

Complexity of the Cardiac Intensive Care Unit Environment

The PCICU is particularly vulnerable to adverse safety events, given that the patients are a heterogeneous population with a variety of anatomy, physiology, ages, and management needs, being cared for in a dynamic, complex environment where medical, surgical, nursing, pharmacy, respiratory therapy, and myriad other teams must collaborate seamlessly to provide care in critical scenarios. Information must be transferred accurately between providers, often coordinated between an operating theater or catheterization laboratory and the ICU, and decisions about the plan of action are often required rapidly in the face of emerging clinical information. To minimize the occurrence of events that cause preventable morbidity or mortality, a PCICU must recognize the high-risk state it is continually operating in and mitigate this risk with continuous attention to safety principles throughout the provision of care to every patient. Particular consideration should be devoted to the following three components of care that are especially fraught with risk for unintended patient harm: team dynamics, surgical handoff, and hospital-acquired infections.

Team Training, Teamwork, and Simulation

Poor teamwork and communication are known to contribute to adverse patient events, whereas team training and debriefing have been demonstrated to reduce mortality.[52] Understanding, evaluating, and improving team performance has subsequently emerged as a top priority in institution- or unit-level safety work. Cardiac surgical team performance is particularly critical, given the wide range of providers, equipment, and environments that are called on to assemble quickly and navigate complex cases under severe time constraints.[53] In effective teams a team leader is clearly identified and is proficient in the following skills: prioritizing and delegating tasks, supervising the progress of both patient and team throughout the clinical encounter, formulating the definitive treatment plan (via analysis/synthesis of information presented to the leader from various sources and in coordination with consulting services), and keeping all team members aware of that evolving treatment plan.[54] Work in aviation has demonstrated that teams whose leaders have attributes termed *the right stuff* (active, self-confident, empathetic, possessing interpersonal warmth, seeking challenging tasks, and striving for excellence) perform better than teams led by individuals who are authoritarian, arrogant, impatient, or unassertive, another useful lesson for health care that has yet to be well integrated into routine performance.[55] Strong team performance, however, is driven by much more than simply a good leader. Effective teams are committed to achieving clear and specified goals, are composed of diverse members with complementary skill sets, maintain situational awareness despite dynamic or evolving events, expect the unknown, and demonstrate consistent trust and respect between members.[54]

The importance of the concept of *situational awareness* cannot be overstated. It is defined in health care as a comprehensive and coherent representation of the patient's current status and is continuously updated by way of repetitive reassessment.[54,56] Accurate situational awareness is essential to successful cardiac surgical care, facilitating a shared mental model of a patient's status for all team members to carry through from preoperative evaluation to the OR and into postoperative ICU management.

Evaluating the performance of health care teams is necessary but not without significant challenges. Guided debriefing, review of recorded clinical encounters, simulated scenarios, and the use of trained observers are examples of common approaches, but in general, few well-defined validated metrics are available for assessing team performance in complex tasks such as resuscitation or during unexpected surgical complication.[54] Simulation has long been standard in training for high-risk fields like aviation and the military, and there is growing recognition of its benefits in medicine as well. High-fidelity simulation in particular aims to create realistic clinical scenarios by using sophisticated mannequins that demonstrate a wide range of physiologic responses. Such simulations are designed to induce reactions from the learner that are similar to those that occur during real patient care encounters, and to do so while providing a safe environment and the freedom to fail without endangering live patients.[57,58] There is growing appreciation that both simulation and crew resource management courses can aid surgical teams in acquiring essential skills in the nontechnical domains that underlie a great deal of adverse patient events (adaptability, prioritization of tasks, communication, performance monitoring, situational awareness, conflict resolution), and the implementation of this type of education will likely continue to increase.[54]

Surgical Handoff—Risk and Opportunity

Perhaps no event outside of the surgical procedure itself is as fraught with risk for adverse events as the process of OR-to-PCICU handoff. Three domains—physical equipment, clinical information, and clinical ownership/responsibility—are simultaneously transferred during a time of significant hemodynamic and physiologic vulnerability.[59] Accordingly, much effort has been undertaken to standardize this process and embed into it multiple safeguards against patient harm during this critical event. A standardized method for OR-to-PCICU handoff has been shown to increase patient safety in multiple ways: by improving teamwork, decreasing technical errors, helping to ensure complete transfer of information, and reducing distractions and interruptions during handoff discussions.[59-63]

Although individual hospitals are encouraged to tailor their handoff process to the specifics of their work environment, the Formula 1–style handoff is often cited in discussion about the concept of a standardized OR-to-PCICU transfer of care and provides useful lessons. The pit stop in Formula 1 car racing is an event in which a multidisciplinary team comes together to perform a complex task (change four tires and refuel the car) under intense time pressure (7 seconds) and must do so with minimal error.[60] Similarly, for pediatric cardiac surgery a multidisciplinary group of surgeons, anesthesiologists, and ICU staff meet at the bedside and work as a united team to efficiently and safely transfer equipment, information, and responsibility with minimal error. Catchpole et al.[60] engaged directly with the Formula 1 racing team (Ferrari F1) to watch practice pit stops and visit the team headquarters; conducted detailed discussions with the race director; reviewed safety themes that were common between racing and health care; and identified new practices through subsequent collaborative discussions with anesthetists, surgeons, intensivists, and nurses. This work led to a new conceptualization of four critical phases of patient handover: (1) preparation of monitors, equipment, medications, and fluids before patient arrival in the PCICU and regular updates from the OR team to the receiving PCICU team about the patient's status; (2) physical transfer of patient and equipment from OR systems to the PCICU systems before any verbal transfer of information, minimizing time the patient is unmonitored and off the ventilator; (3) once all team members are ready, verbal transfer of clinical information in a "sterile cockpit" environment—only one person speaks at a time and only patient-specific conversations occur; and (4) questions, clarifications, and concerns are addressed before the receiving team formally accepts responsibility for the care of the patient.[59,60] Rates of both technical errors and communication errors decreased after introduction of Catchpole's Formula 1 framework (depicted in Fig. 8.1) to pediatric cardiac surgical handover, and it is considered foundational to work that strives to improve handover in multiple disciplines.[60]

In addition to the process framework, the use of a formal, structured handoff tool to transition patients from the OR to the PCICU is strongly encouraged. Multiple studies have demonstrated improvement in communication quality and accuracy and in patient outcomes when such a tool is in place.[62-64] See Fig. 8.2 as an example, though these tools can and should be customized to the needs of individual institutions and units.

Nosocomial Infections in Children With Cardiac Disease

Postoperative infection complicates up to 8% of surgical procedures for children with acquired or congenital cardiac disease and is a significant cause of morbidity and mortality.[65,66] Recent single-center work by Turcotte et al.[67] demonstrated that 6% of pediatric cardiac surgical cases had a documented health care–associated infection (HAI) within 90 days of surgery, and the infections were most frequently found to be central line–associated bloodstream infections (CLABSIs), followed by non-CLABSI bacteremia, infective endocarditis, ventilator-associated pneumonia, and surgical site infections (SSIs). HAI in pediatric cardiac surgical patients may increase hospital length of stay and costs, and nosocomial bloodstream infection in particular has been associated with an increase in mortality rate from 2% to 11%.[68,69]

Given that both patient outcomes and use of hospital resources are affected negatively by HAI, a great deal of effort on a national scale has focused on reducing or preventing these infections. Hospitals that participate in the Centers for Medicare and Medicaid

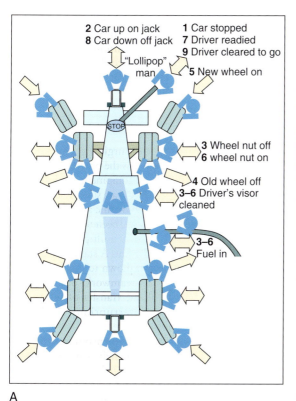

A

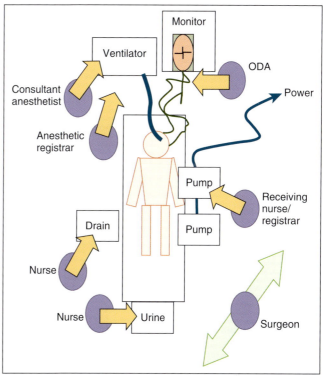

B

• **Figure 8.1** Formula 1 pit stop (A) and its adaptation for postoperative cardiac surgical handoff (B). *ODA,* Operating department assistant. (From Catchpole KR, de Leval MR, McEwan A, et al. Patient handover from surgery to intensive care: using Formula 1 pit-stop and aviation models to improve safety and quality. *Pediatr Anaesth.* 2007;17:470-478.)

<u>OR to CICU sign out</u>   Present (OR team): Surgeon___   Anesthesiology___   Perfusionist ___
                                            Present (CICU): Attending ___   APN___   Nurse___   RT ___
*Sign out time out: Are we ready for sign out: OR team___   ICU med team ___   ICU nursing team ___   Room silence ___

Patient name_____   MR#_____   Age_____   Weight_____kg   Date_____
Diagnosis/problems_____
Surgical repair _____

Pertinent past history
PMHx_____   Pre-op medications _____   Allergies_____
      _____   _____   _____
      _____   _____   _____

Airway/respiratory
Endotracheal tube size_____ depth____cm   Laryngoscope miller / mac___   Airway easy / difficult
Ventilator setting   PIP___   PEEP___   Rate___   FiO2____   NO___ppm
Baseline SpO2 _____   Most recent SpO2____   Most recent ABG pH ____/pCO2____/pO2 ____/HCO3 ____
Precautions/plan:_____

Cardiovascular
Access: PIV_____   Arterial catheter_____ Central venous catheters_____ Thoracic catheters_____
Times: CPB_____mins   Aortle XClamp_____ mins   DHCA_____mins   MUF yes / no
ECG rhythms: Pre-CPB NSR /_____   Post-CPB NSR /_____
Inotropic support: None / milrinone load___meg/kg/milrinone gu___meg/kg/min / Epinephrine___ meg/kg/min/_____
Most recent HR_____   Most recent BP_____   CVP/RAP_____   PAP_____   LAP_____
Precautions/plan:_____

Neurologic
Pain meds given_____   Last dose _____
Precautions/plan:_____

Renal
Urine output_____ml   Most recent chemistries   Na_____   K_____   Glucose_____
Precautions/plan:_____

Hematologic
Most recent Hgb_____ Hct_____
Blood products given RBC / FFP / PLTS / CRYO / cell saver / autologous Available RBC / FFP / PLTS / CRYO / cell saver / autologous
Precautions/plan:_____

ID
Last dose of antibiotic   Ancef_____ mg at ____: ____ / other _____

Additional surgical concerns: Additional anesthesia concerns:

• **Figure 8.2** Example of a postoperative surgical handoff tool. (From Joy BF, Feltes TF. The role of communication and patient handovers in pediatric cardiac care centers. In: Barach PR, Jacobs JP, Lipshultz SE, Laussen PC, eds. *Quality Improvement and Patient Safety.* London: Springer-Verlag; 2015:349-354. *Pediatric and Congenital Cardiac Care;* vol 2.)

TABLE 8.2	Distinguishing Between Community-Acquired Infections, Nosocomial Infections, and Colonization
Community-Acquired Infection	Infection present at time of admission, even if not causing symptoms at admission
Nosocomial Infection	Infection acquired during hospitalization and not present on admission
Colonization	Presence of potentially infectious organisms without causing disease or clinical symptoms

Services funding must report rates of CLABSI, catheter-associated urinary tract infection, nosocomial *Clostridium difficile* infections, and SSI.[70] Financial penalties are incurred from state, federal, and private payers when nosocomial infections occur during hospital admission. Accordingly, dedicated clinical teams or working groups that specifically target preventing and reducing HAI are increasingly common in the inpatient pediatric setting. The reader is encouraged to review the extensive resources on this topic available from organizations like The Joint Commission and the AHRQ. Tables 8.2 to 8.4 and Box 8.3 are an introductory summary of important terms and definitions that the PCICU clinician should understand when considering nosocomial infection as a major contributor to preventable patient harm.[71-75]

Conclusion

Enormous advances have been made in pediatric cardiac care in the last several decades, but preventable harm and adverse events continue to pose a significant threat to patients. Important lessons can be learned from high-reliability organizations that perform safely despite incredibly high risks. Understanding that communication, team dynamics, and standardized best-practice protocols play critical roles in reducing patient harm continues to grow. Medicine must continue to evolve from a culture that tolerates blame and

TABLE 8.3	Definitions of CLABSI, CAUTI, VAP, and SSI	
	Definition	**Notes**
CLABSI (central line–associated bloodstream infection)	A laboratory-confirmed bloodstream infection (LCBI) where central line (CL) or umbilical catheter (UC) was in place for >2 calendar days on the date of event, with day of device placement being day 1, **AND** the line was also in place on the date of event or the day before	LCBI: Patient of any age has a recognized pathogen identified (i.e., an organism that is not on the NHSN common commensal list) from one or more blood specimens by a culture or nonculture based microbiologic testing method **AND** organism(s) identified in blood is not related to an infection at another site
CAUTI (catheter-associated urinary tract infection)	A UTI where an indwelling urinary catheter was in place for >2 calendar days on the date of event, with day of device placement being day 1, **AND** an indwelling urinary catheter was in place on the date of event or the day before	See https://www.cdc.gov/nhsn/PDFs/pscManual/7pscCAUTIcurrent.pdf (for distinguishing symptomatic UTI vs asymptomatic UTI)
VAP (ventilator-associated pneumonia)	A pneumonia where the patient is on mechanical ventilation for >2 calendar days on the date of event, with day of ventilator placement being day 1, **AND** the ventilator was in place on the date of event or the day before	Pneumonia is identified by using a combination of imaging, clinical, and laboratory criteria. For details, see https://www.cdc.gov/nhsn/pdfs/pscmanual/6pscvapcurrent.pdf
SSI (surgical site infection)	Superficial SSI Date of event for infection occurs within 30 days after any NHSN operative procedure (where day 1 is the procedure date) **AND** involves only skin and subcutaneous tissue of the incision **AND** patient has at least *one* of the following: a. Purulent drainage from the superficial incision. b. Organisms identified from an aseptically obtained specimen from the superficial incision or subcutaneous tissue by a culture or non–culture-based microbiologic testing method that is performed for purposes of clinical diagnosis or treatment (e.g., not active surveillance culture/testing [ASC/AST]) c. Superficial incision that is deliberately opened by a surgeon, attending physician, or other designee and culture or non–culture-based testing is not performed **AND** patient has at least one of the following signs or symptoms: pain or tenderness; localized swelling; erythema; or heat d. Diagnosis of a superficial incisional SSI by the surgeon or attending physician or other designee	Deep SSI Date of event for infection occurs within 30 or 90 days after the NHSN operative procedure (where day 1 is the procedure date) **AND** involves deep soft tissues of the incision (e.g., fascial and muscle layers) **AND** patient has at least *one* of the following: a. Purulent drainage from the deep incision. b. A deep incision that spontaneously dehisces or is deliberately opened or aspirated by a surgeon, attending physician, or other designee and organism is identified by a culture or non–culture-based microbiologic testing method that is performed for purposes of clinical diagnosis or treatment (e.g., not ASC/AST) or culture or non–culture-based microbiologic testing method is not performed AND patient has at least *one* of the following signs or symptoms: fever (>38°C); localized pain or tenderness. A culture or non–culture-based test that has a negative finding does not meet this criterion. c. An abscess or other evidence of infection involving the deep incision that is detected on gross anatomic or histopathologic examination or imaging test.

NHSN, National Healthcare Safety Network; *UTI*, urinary tract infection.
Modified from Bloodstream infection event (central line-associated bloodstream infection and non-central line-associated bloodstream infection). https://www.cdc.gov/nhsn/pdfs/pscmanual/4psc_clabscurrent.pdf; Urinary tract infection (catheter-associated urinary tract infection [CAUTI] and non-catheter-associated urinary tract infection [UTI]) and other urinary system infection [USI]) events. https://www.cdc.gov/nhsn/PDFs/pscManual/7pscCAUTIcurrent.pdf; Pneumonia (ventilator-associated [VAP] and non-ventilator-associated pneumonia [PNEU]) event. https://www.cdc.gov/nhsn/pdfs/pscmanual/6pscvapcurrent.pdf; Surgical site infection (SSI) event. https://www.cdc.gov/nhsn/pdfs/pscmanual/9pscssicurrent.pdf.

TABLE 8.4 Practices Associated With Pediatric CLABSI

Practices Associated With Prevention or Reduction of CLABSI	Practices Not Associated With Prevention or Reduction in CLABSI
Preinsertion hand hygiene and aseptic technique throughout insertion	Routine replacement of catheters
Skin preparation with chlorhexidine	Tight glycemic control
Maximal barrier precautions	Avoiding the femoral vein site in pediatric patients
Placement of a transparent, semipermeable dressing, which is replaced regularly per protocol and when damp/soiled/loosened	
Insertion of line with fewest number of required lumens	
Insertion of antibiotic-impregnated or antiseptic-coated catheters	
Implementation of formal insertion and maintenance bundles	
Routine replacement of tubing and infusion sets	

CLABSI, Central line–associated bloodstream infection.
Modified from Custer JW, Siegrist TJ, Straumanis JP. Nosocomial infections in the PICU. In: Nichols DG, Shaffner DH, eds. *Rogers' Textbook of Pediatric Intensive Care.* 5th ed. Philadelphia: Wolters Kluwer; 2016:1503-1523.

• BOX 8.3 General Risk Factors for Nosocomial Infections in Pediatric Intensive Care Unit

Younger age and neonates
    Prematurity
    Use of total parenteral nutrition with high glucose concentrations and lipids
    Compromised immune system such as from chemotherapy, HIV infection, steroid use, etc.
    Increasing severity of illness score
    Increasing length of stay
    Prior antimicrobial therapy
    Blood transfusion
    Device utilization ratios
    Understaffing of the ICU

HIV, Human immunodeficiency virus; ICU, *intensive care unit.*
Modified from Custer JW, Siegrist TJ, Straumanis JP. Nosocomial infections in the PICU. In: Nichols DG, Shaffner DH, eds. Rogers' Textbook of Pediatric Intensive Care. *5th ed. Philadelphia: Wolters Kluwer; 2016:1503-1523.*

views errors as personal failures into a culture of transparency, reliability, justice, and ultimately, of safety.

Selected References

A complete list of references is available at ExpertConsult.com.

1. The Institute of Medicine. Kohn LT, Corrigan JM, Donaldson MS, eds. *To Err Is Human: Building a Safer Health System.* Washington, DC: The National Academies Press; 2000:26.
2. The Institute of Medicine. *Committee on Quality of Health Care in America. Crossing the Quality Chasm: A New Health System for the 21st Century.* Washington DC: National Academy Press; 2001:5.
4. The Joint Commission Center for Transforming Healthcare. *Facts about the safety culture project.* Available at: http://www.centerfortransforminghealthcare.org/assets/4/6/CTH_SC_Fact_Sheet.pdf.
14. Reason J. Human error: models and management. *BMJ.* 2000;320(7237):768–770.
19. Weick KE, Sutcliffe KM. *Managing the Unexpected: Assuring High Performance in an Age of Complexity.* 1st ed. San Francisco: Jossey-Bass; 2001.
38. Patient Safety Primer. *Voluntary Patient Safety Event Reporting (Incident Reporting).* Available at: https://psnet.ahrq.gov/primers/primer/13.
54. Barach PR, Cosman PH. Teams, team training, and the role of simulation. In: Barach PR, Jacobs JP, Lipshultz SE, Laussen PC, eds. *Pediatric and Congenital Cardiac Care Volume 2: Quality Improvement and Patient Safety.* London: Springer-Verlag; 2015:69–90.
59. Joy BF, Feltes TF. The role of communication and patient handovers in pediatric cardiac care centers. In: Barach PR, Jacobs JP, Lipshultz SE, Laussen PC, eds. *Pediatric and Congenital Cardiac Care: Volume 2: Quality Improvement and Patient Safety.* London: Springer-Verlag; 2015:349–354.
60. Catchpole KR, de Leval MR, McEwan A, et al. Patient handover from surgery to intensive care: using Formula 1 pit-stop and aviation models to improve safety and quality. *Paediatr Anaesth.* 2007;17:470–478.
67. Turcotte RF, Brozovich A, Corda R. Health care-associated infections in children after cardiac surgery. *Pediatr Cardiol.* 2014;35:1448–1455.
71. Custer JW, Siegrist Thomas J, Straumanis JP. Nosocomial infections in the PICU. In: Nichols DG, Donald H, Shaffner DH, eds. *Rogers' Textbook of Pediatric Intensive Care.* 5th ed. Philadelphia: Wolters Kluwer; 2016:1503–1523.
72. *Bloodstream Infection Event (Central Line-Associated Bloodstream Infection and non-central line-associated Bloodstream Infection).* Available at: https://www.cdc.gov/nhsn/pdfs/pscmanual/4psc_clabscurrent.pdf.
73. *Urinary Tract Infection (Catheter-Associated Urinary Tract Infection [CAUTI] and Non-Catheter-Associated Urinary Tract Infection [UTI]) and Other Urinary System Infection [USI]) Events.* Available at: https://www.cdc.gov/nhsn/PDFs/pscManual/7pscCAUTIcurrent.pdf.
74. *Pneumonia (Ventilator-associated [VAP] and non-ventilator-associated Pneumonia [PNEU]) Event.* Available at: https://www.cdc.gov/nhsn/pdfs/pscmanual/6pscvapcurrent.pdf.
75. *Surgical Site Infection (SSI) Event.* Available at: https://www.cdc.gov/nhsn/pdfs/pscmanual/9pscssicurrent.pdf. Accessed Mar 7, 2017.

9

Decision Making and Ethics

JOHN R. BROWNLEE, MD; JAMIE DICKEY UNGERLEIDER, MSW, PHD

The thoughts expressed in this chapter are derived from 35 years of working with families, colleagues, and ethics committees and from dedicated study of these issues. The intent is to promote reflection on the process of decision making in the care of patients with congenital heart disease. This includes the context of the parent, their family and friends, and the environment in the neonatal, pediatric, and cardiac intensive care units (which includes the physical setting that is typically alien and imposing to most families and the medical and professional staff, who interject their own experiences, biases, and usually well-intentioned attempts to be helpful).

Ethics

"Ethics is a branch of philosophy which seeks to address issues related to concepts of right and wrong. It is sometimes referred to as moral philosophy and can be divided into different subject areas including, amongst others, meta-ethics (e.g. the role of truth, God, reason and the meanings of various terms used); normative ethics (which focuses on how moral values are determined and what is needed to ensure that they are achieved) and applied ethics (examining controversial issues) (Fieser, 2006)."[1]

Biomedical ethics is a discipline that is taught in most U.S. medical schools and often uses widely accepted principles and guidelines. These four principles are (1) beneficence—the obligation to do good, (2) nonmaleficence—the obligation to avoid harm, (3) autonomy—the principle of self-determination, and (4) justice—"fair distribution of scarce resources (distributive justice), respect for people's rights (rights based justice) and respect for morally acceptable laws (legal justice) (Gillon, 1994)."[2]

Many concerns with the care of children in intensive care areas revolves around autonomy and surrogacy. Autonomy has developed as a concept embraced by our society. Much of the discourse came from enlightenment philosophers.

According to Kantian ethics, autonomy is based on the human capacity to direct one's life according to rational principles. He states,

"Everything in nature works in accordance with laws. Only a rational being has the capacity to act in accordance with the representation of laws, that is, in accordance with principles, or has a will. Since reason is required for the derivation of actions from laws, the will is nothing other than practical reason." (In Korsgaard, 2004)

Rationality, in Kant's view, is the means to autonomy. Autonomous people are considered as being ends in themselves in that they have the capacity to determine their own destiny, and as such must be respected.

For John Stuart Mill, the concept of respect for autonomy involves the capacity to think, decide and act on the basis of such thought and decision freely and independently. Mill advocated the principle of autonomy (or the principle of liberty as he called it) provided that it did not cause harm to others:

"That the only purpose for which power can be rightfully exercised over any member of a civilized community, against his will, is to prevent harm to others. His own good, either physical or moral, is not a sufficient warrant. … Over himself, over his own body and mind, the individual is sovereign" (Mill, 1968, p. 73).

The principle of not causing harm to others (known as Mill's "harm principle") provides the grounds for the moral right of a patient to refuse medical treatment and for a doctor to refrain from intervening against the patient's wishes. Nevertheless, Mill believed that it was acceptable to prevent people from harming themselves provided that their action was not fully informed.

Nowadays, an autonomous decision might be described as one that is made freely/without undue influence, by a competent person, in full knowledge and understanding of the relevant information necessary to make such a decision. It should also be applicable to the current situation or circumstances.[3]

In children or severely debilitated patients, this rationality is lacking, and so surrogate decision makers are given the task of making medical decisions to define what the best choice is for their critically ill dependents. The obligation of a surrogate is "to promote the patient's welfare." If the patient has been able to express preferences in the past and has done so, the surrogate must use the knowledge of these preferences, or at least the known values of the individual, in making the decision. If the patient's own preferences are unknown or unclear, the proxy must consider the "best interests" of the patient. This requires that the surrogate's decision promote the welfare of the individual. Welfare is defined as "the relief of suffering, preservation or restoration of function, extent and quality of life that a reasonable person in similar circumstances is likely to choose."[4]

Challenging Environment of Health Care Decisions

When an infant is born into a family, the family's most typical and natural response is to love, hold, nourish, and protect that infant. Bonding after birth is a key component of care built into modern hospitals with birthing rooms and family attendance and participation in the birth.

When an infant is born with serious congenital heart disease or other birth defects, the process of nurturing and the ability to nurture are interrupted. The health care system moves in and adopts the role of surrogate family and begins a process of control to which the family must often accede. The physicians begin to bombard the family with information regarding the nature of the disease. The nurses, respiratory therapists, and other bedside caregivers control breathing, fluid, and skin care. Daily and continuing care of the infant is removed from the parents, causing a gradual withdrawal because they may feel inadequate or unable to bond with their baby.

Further adding to this confusion is the constant changing of bedside caregivers, who may rotate as often every 8 to 12 hours. It is often unclear to the family who is their infant's primary physician or care provider/decision maker. Different physicians arriving at different times may say things that seem contradictory to the family. Different rounding times of specialty services interfere with clear communication to the family, who may not have timed their visits to this seemingly erratic and unpredictable schedule. The communication about the disease is further complicated when the mother is a teenager. (Approximately 1 in 10 births in the United States are to mothers less than 18 years of age.)

Age and Cognitive Development

In considering how to counsel a teenage mother who has just given birth to a baby with hypoplastic left heart syndrome (HLHS), it might be helpful for the physician to consider some of the following information about adolescent development.

In late adolescence the prefrontal cortex is still developing. Brain imaging studies demonstrate that this process of development continues into the mid-20s. This is significant because the prefrontal cortex is the part of the brain that works with the limbic system to regulate emotions. When an individual's emotions are regulated, he or she is more capable of thinking clearly with concomitant awareness and understanding of his or her own perspectives, as well as consideration of the likely perspectives of others. Wise decision making occurs when the individual is not in the grip of intense fear—characterized by sympathetic system overload (reflected as a flight/fight response and manifested as anger, anxiety, or overly intense emotions) at one end of the spectrum or by a parasympathetic response in which the person shuts down or freezes and is unable to think or act, at the other end of the spectrum. This has been described in the literature as an internalized "window of tolerance" that each of us possesses. When life events or stressors overwhelm us and take us to the edges or outside of our window of tolerance, we become emotionally and cognitively underresourced and less capable of managing the cognitive and emotional demands of our lives. Because the prefrontal cortex and limbic system may not be fully available, due to normative developmental issues, this is a concern for the adolescent who is called upon to make critical decisions. The part of the brain most involved in self-regulation is simply not fully formed.

This limitation in emotional regulation and ability to engage in wise decision making is even more pronounced in adolescents and young adults who have grown up in stressful, dysfunctional, abusive, or neglectful households. Growing up in a single-parent household and/or in poverty are just two adverse childhood events that have the potential to impact the adolescent and young adult's capacity to focus, access working memory, and use cognitive flexibility—all skills important for executive functioning and decision making.

Underdevelopment of the prefrontal cortex is also linked to deficiency in temporal integration, and this is another important factor for the medical team to appreciate when counseling young patients. Temporal integration provides the ability to separate past, present, and future events into a contextual framework that is distinguishable and then link them in a way that allows for reflection on the past, awareness of the present moment, and the capacity to imagine a future that may or may not be like the past or present moment. When a person lacks temporal integration, past, present, and future become merged into a perpetual present experience, and there may be a loss of imagining a future different from the present moment. A young mother might focus only on the emotions of the present situation and be unable to imagine what life would be like raising a child with a chronic disability. Consequently, she would be unable to discern how the meaningful events of her past may not be similar as she moves forward through choice into various future options. Additionally, she may also be in the grip of emotions from previous difficult and overwhelming situations in a way that collapses the present experience into the past experience. The consequence of this may be that she is unable to sort out her present experience as separate from previously emotionally painful experiences, thereby clouding her judgment. Robert Kegan[5] described this by writing that "the future is not the present that hasn't happened yet." The future can change in multiple dimensions related to numerous factors (some internal and some external) that influence experience and context. A person with lack of mature temporal integration might let his or her past intrude on the present moment (e.g., by thinking "I've always made things work in the past," or "things never worked in the past"), impairing the person's ability to project that things might be different in the future. The ability to engage in wise decision making requires the ability to abstract and to integrate events over time. Lack of full development of the temporal cortex impedes this process.

Health care professionals who counsel patients need to have a well-developed sense of self-awareness and self-concept with a capacity to see and know one's own mind and to have empathic awareness of what might be happening in the minds of others. Dan Siegel[6] coined the term *mindsight* to refer to a process in which the individual is able to have insight into his or her own mind and apply this same insight into empathically seeing the differing perspectives in the minds of others and finally have the capacity to link his or her own mind with the minds of others in a way that is harmonious. An individual who has developed this capacity for mindsight has awareness of his or her own sensations, images, feelings, and thoughts, as well as the understanding that others are also having their own personal experiences of sensations, images, feelings, and thoughts that may be very different and for them, very valid. Additionally, people with mindsight are able to link their personal, differentiated processes coherently and harmoniously with another's differentiated process. This means that these individuals have greater awareness and access to their subjective experience and to the subjective experience of others—understanding that both experiences are subjective and uniquely personal. They are also able to attune and regulate their emotional process and from a place of emotional regulation, help to regulate the emotions of others. As the individual self-regulates and relates with curiosity to another person's experience, he or she is also more able to think rationally and objectively. Considering the biologic limitations that young patients bring to this process and the impairment that other patients may bring related to external stressors in their lives, the health care provider needs to develop an educated sense of mindsight and not simply imagine that the patient or family members have experiences or abilities similar to the provider's own.

Whereas Siegel discusses empathy and understanding the mind of another as aspects of mindsight, Kegan, drawing on the research of Piaget, describes abstraction, or the ability to rotate objects, as a necessary developmental milestone for empathy. In other words, in order to understand that another person's subjective experience may be very different from one's own experience, there must be a capacity to rotate objects to see the same issue from multiple perspectives or positions. Because empathy requires an understanding of the perspectives of others or their subjective experience, empathy is not possible until a person has developed the cognitive ability of abstraction. Individuals who have not reached this level of development lack the capacity to perceive another's perspective as being different from one's own. There is a tendency to take things personally and to attribute one's own meanings to another person. Interestingly, according to Kegan, many people well into adulthood have never developed the capacity for abstract thought.

This information about late adolescent development may be helpful for health care professionals when they encounter what might appear to be a limited capacity for understanding the perspectives and complexity that are a part of the decision making required of an adolescent mother with an infant who has a complex congenital heart defect. It may also be helpful for the health care professional because we are all in varying stages of our own emotional and psychologic development. Developmental maturity as described earlier is not age based and for our patients and for the medical team may be advanced or delayed and therefore be a factor in effective decision making. For health care professionals it is helpful to continue to develop mindsight, which simply stated is "unflinching self-awareness with empathic openness to the experiences of others."[7]

When the family and caregivers of patients with congenital heart disease are confronted with the complex physiologic concepts associated with decision making for medical and surgical care, understanding the anatomy and physiology is difficult. Many times the heart disease does not lend itself to an easy description found on the Internet. The bedside nurses, resident physicians, and intensive care physicians are often unsure about the details of the surgeries and long-term outcomes or do not discuss these issues due to the pressing need for interventions or practitioner time constraints.

In this context, who is making informed decisions for this infant? Is the mother informed enough or emotionally developed enough to competently give consent? Does the family act as a team to assist with this decision? Should the family acquiesce to the superior knowledge of the neonatologist, critical care physician, surgeon, or cardiologist? What factors go into these decisions?

Paternalism Versus Autonomy

Parents can usually understand and make surrogate decisions in the simplest cardiac cases, such as patent ductus arteriosus ligation, or in device closures of secundum atrial septal defects. In more complex congenital heart diseases the full extent and ramifications of the disease and consequences of treatment are much harder to grasp, and the parents are often left to trust that the treating medical team is recommending the best decisions for their infant. Although the informed consent documents that the parents sign attest to understanding the risks and benefits of the proposed treatment, the parents often need to turn to other hospital employees or family for support after the cardiologist or surgeon has left the bedside. The document in most instances does not ensure

understanding of the particular procedure or all risks and benefits but instead demonstrates trust in the cardiologists and surgeons.

The fiduciary duty of the physician obtaining consent is not to make the best choice but rather to provide a duty of care, good faith, and competence in guiding the parents/guardians. To accomplish this, most congenital heart centers have multidisciplinary presurgical conferences to discuss treatment/surgical plans. In these sessions the primary cardiologist (or surgeon) acts as a surrogate in representing the agreed-upon best interest of the infant from the perspective of the medical team. They then return to the bedside to explain these plans to the family and gain assent and consent.

Providing Informed Consent for a Patient With Complex Congenital Heart Disease

In American society the medical community has decided it is best for the patient or the patient's surrogate to know what medical treatment is being performed before that treatment begins. This process entails a "discussion" culminating in a signature on every consent form indicating that the family member has an understanding of the risks and benefits of the planned procedure. Ideally, the decision maker signing the document would have a full understanding of the care to which he or she is agreeing.

The problem with doing this for complex congenital heart disease can be best understood with an example: An infant is born with heterotaxy, asplenia, dextrocardia, abnormal pulmonary venous return, unbalanced atrioventricular canal deformity, ventricular inversion, double-outlet right ventricle, and malposition of the great vessels with a right aortic arch. For untrained parents, noncardiac bedside nurses, or even a medical student, an expectation that they can comprehend the anatomy, physiology, and gravity of the problem is unrealistic in the short term. The signed decision of the family more likely reflects whether or not they trust the team who is caring for their baby. If they trust the team, the family may sign the informed consent despite incomplete understanding of the full implications of risks and benefits. If they do not trust the team, then everyone is in for a difficult time.

In an ideal world, full informed consent consists of a long conversation and full understanding of the physiology and anatomy and surgical treatments and short- and long-term risk and benefits associated with these. The medical team should strive for giving full informed consent as the right thing to do, but being able to accomplish this in a thorough manner is difficult.[8]

Barriers to fully informed consent are potentially numerous and can include age of the parents, understanding of pathophysiology, language, level of cognitive development, emotional and psychologic health, intelligence and education, stress from just having given birth, and situational depression from finding out their infant has heart disease and/or other significant diseases/syndromes. Parents and grandparents may be influenced in their trust of the physicians and nurses based on their previous experiences or based on what they have read in the literature or on the Internet. The choices and understanding of young parents are different than those of a 45-year-old mother of a patient with Down syndrome. Instability within the family and social issues such as family dysfunction, sleep deprivation, and poverty with lack of financial or transportation resources may present additional challenges.

Other factors may be affecting family decision making. Occasionally the parents have other children or other family members in a different city who require care, and so arrangements need to be made. Bringing the entire family to the hospital may impose logistic difficulties or constitute a great expense. The usual care of multiple children in a family setting is a full-time job. A suddenly imposed absence from a paying job may mean losing health care benefits and the ability to care for one's family, so an important family figure may be torn between his or her need to show up at work and the desire to be present for these critical family events. Expenses related to staying in the hospital with an ill family member can cost a minimum of $30 to $50 a day with housing assistance such as Ronald McDonald House (personal experience). If the family does not want to eat only fast food and wants to stay at an average hotel for privacy and showering, the cost can easily triple that amount. The length of stay for many infants with critical heart disease is often greater than 2 weeks (creating a living expense cost of $420 to $2300 over and above the normal life expenses for a family). Although there are sometimes ways to provide help and support for families, this added stress (and financial concerns can be an enormous stressor for families who are barely making ends meet) should be appreciated by the health care providers.

Defining the Decision Maker

In legal and practical terms the mother has all the rights as a surrogate for the infant in decision making, even if she is less than 18 years of age. Of course, both parents have equal rights if they are both on the birth certificate and if those rights have not otherwise been reduced by a court. Surrogacy means that the designated guardian (parent) would make a decision considering "the best interest of the patient." This requires that the surrogate's decision promote the welfare of the individual. Welfare is defined as "those choices about relief of suffering, preservation or restoration of function, extent and quality of life sustained that reasonable persons in similar circumstances would be likely to choose."

This life and death responsibility can be a huge burden to a young mother or father. In the case of congenital heart disease the physician does his or her best to explain the complex heart problem and tells the mother and available family members what plan is recommended. Because of the complexity of the diagnosis, the multiple steps and time required to achieve surgical palliations or corrections, the myriad complications to multiple organ systems that can occur, and the expected lifelong disability that accompanies many heart defects, there is often an enormous (virtually unattainable) challenge to the medical team to outline a cogent message that informs the consent for procedures and does not leave families in some confusion. Support staff (e.g., nurses, chaplains, social workers) who listen in on these informed consent conversations commonly describe that after the family has completed the process of signing needed documents after extensive conversations and the physicians have left, the family members frequently turn to the remaining caregivers and then ask for an explanation of their infant's problems and for clarification of the medical/surgical plan. The primary cardiologists and intensive care physicians need to be attentive to this problem and strive for the best care standard of communication. A liaison such as a cardiac nurse—often a highly trained nurse practitioner—who is available daily can help clarify the message or redirect the physicians back to the bedside to help invite further explanation.

It is also important that the care team understand the family's context. Where did this family come from? What are their resources? How many children or other family members are dependents in the family? What is a prolonged absence of the mother, father, or grandparent who is now required to be far from home mean to supporting the other family members left at home? What spiritual resources or experiences affect their decision-making ability? How much of this information that is acquired should go into counseling the family about the procedures and outcomes expected in their baby?

From the physician and caregivers' viewpoint, their information and experience may give them a different view of the infant's peril and outcome. (I [JB] have personally attended several national congenital heart disease conferences during which the audience of surgeons and pediatric cardiologists were polled regarding offering comfort care to a natural death versus having their hypothetical children undergo the multiple surgeries for HLHS. At least half of these professionals favored offering comfort care in this hypothetical situation.) This raises the ethical questions about what constitutes a reasonable quality of life and what constitutes futile treatment. (It also raises the question of how the moral biases of caregivers affect the counsel and actions in treatment of their patients.) None of the long-term outcomes includes a normal physiologic adult from HLHS palliation or, for that matter, for any of the patients with single ventricles. This invites a discussion of what level of survival and functionality constitutes a good outcome. With so many variables, should we allow/encourage acceptance of the natural death option? The resources required for lifetime care are enormous, and the psychologic toll on the family raising a child with chronic and sometimes debilitating disease can be significant. This discussion is offered only to remind the care providers of the difficulty of these decisions and of their long-term implications. There is no "right" answer. Therefore we simply recommend awareness that there are issues around the treatment decisions that extend far beyond our ability to "fix" the anatomic abnormality.

This question often comes up with patients who have trisomy 18 and the usual associated congenital heart disease of a large ventricular septal defect. Some of these patients live to be older than 10 years of age. Most patients die by 1 year of age. The cause of death is usually apnea or seizures. No child with trisomy 18 has an expectation of living an adult life. Given this information, how much palliation should be given to a patient with this burden of disease? If the family member wants the child to have heart surgery, should it be offered? If the family member desires a tracheostomy and ventilation for supportive care of the child, should be offered? This series of questions and concerns are almost universal when an infant is born with this disease. In contrast to the response to choices for HLHS patients, the physicians I have worked with at several institutions encourage minimal treatment and allowing natural death. In my (JB) experience, the bedside care becomes unequal as the treating nurses and physicians try to determine if the infant is in a comfort-care mode or a mode of surviving and going home. In this situation I find it best practice to partner with the family in discussing what treatment goals and outcomes are expected and not prejudge the imminent death of the patient. All patients deserve normative basic care if it does not increase pain and suffering. The concepts of pain and suffering must be discussed with the family of a patient with a terminal illness! The treating physician needs to be brave enough to walk this difficult path with the family. The family's acceptance of quality of life and suffering are often different than that of the care team.

Multidisciplinary Cardiac Conference in Management and Decision Making in Cardiac Care

Throughout the United States multidisciplinary cardiac conferences occur to discuss surgical management and offer case presentation and management discussion for challenging patients. The concept is that more knowledge and experience applied to patients with difficult anatomy and physiology often yields the best treatment plans for these patients. Typically the patient has a history, physical, and information from echocardiography, electrocardiography, catheterization, and other imaging modalities displayed. The question is asked regarding the management, and discussion ensues. Several times a month a challenging patient case comes up who has multiple congenital anomalies in addition to the heart disease. The context of the burden of the other diseases often raises the question of whether treatment should be offered. This discussion then centers on the medical and surgical goal of treatment in these patients. Is the goal to avoid suffering in the patients? Is the goal to give them a normal life and expect them to become productive adults? Is the goal to allow them to be functional in their home, where they can remain in a state of dependency and be loved and cared for? For many practitioners the goal seems to be "let's give this a try and see if we can make it better." As success in cardiac surgery has allowed examination of collateral damage to other organ systems and development of statistics, the behavioral, psychologic, and neurologic sequelae of our actions are becoming apparent and are causing reflection. The community of caregivers for congenital heart disease needs to constantly analyze and be aware of the evolving data regarding life expectancy, neurologic outcomes, and social outcomes for our patients and to present these data to families to inform them of what we know and do not know as we ask them to journey with us in deciphering the natural history of treated congenital heart disease.

It may be fair to have an initial discussion about offering natural death in some cases. The ones who are best informed, the cardiologist and surgeons, should bear the brunt of decision making in some of these cases. In reality we are already deciding treatments for them because the cardiology team often begins care with central lines, prostaglandins, and vasoactive drips to stabilize the baby or keep the baby alive. In some cases in which a prenatal diagnosis has been made, these actions may have been discussed with the family well in advance. However, this is not always the case. As the months of care accumulate, the infant may have had multiple procedures, and the family is often looking to the team of providers to get their infant home. Many infants survive and go home, but others dwindle and succumb to a complication or reach a point where further palliation is not feasible. The burden of end-of-life/do-not-resuscitate (DNR) decisions is higher and more difficult for the family and the treatment team, and neither side is anxious to own the decision.

Spiritual history may be important to understanding how the family views these events. In some cases the family may see this outcome as punishment for indiscretions (use of drugs, illicit sex, or many other types of behavior). Some may see the birth of the abnormal baby as a gift from God because it presents a new challenge with lessons for the entire family. In matters of deciding for withdrawal of care or do-not-resuscitate status the parents or family members may not see this decision as being within their rights as human beings. If they believe "only God can take a life," this often leads to requesting that everything be done. Even those on the medical team are uncomfortable with deciding to stop care and allowing death.

Very often the family also begins to exhibit forms of magical thinking. This often manifests as a prayer request that healing would occur instantaneously or that the medical diagnosis was wrong. This type of thinking is part of the grieving process and can be an impediment to making medical/surgical decisions. The

hospital chaplains can be invaluable in helping to sort these issues out. They frequently spend long hours with the grieving family and come to understand the family's view of the situation in ways that few other members of the health care team can fully assess. Often they are members of the ethics committee with some additional helpful training.

The nurses at the bedside have their own challenges. They may be performing shift work that may or may not be in their primary area of expertise. They may have been working long hours or have been on the same job for years and are starting to experience burnout and fatigue. It is possible that they may be additionally stressed by not having adequate education about their patient's complex congenital heart.

Additional stress is added to the bedside nurse when his or her patients are hospitalized for prolonged periods of time. As the patient languishes in the ICU, the medical goals may become less clear. A sense of futility may occur when original medical goals cannot be achieved.

This problem is further amplified if the patient's status has been declared do not resuscitate. Understanding of the short- and long-term medical goals becomes clouded. The nurse often wonders if certain treatments or medications are still indicated. The care team can be discouraged by a prolonged gradual downhill course that seems to have no conclusion except death. They may feel extra stress by wondering why the treating physicians and parents have not surrendered to the inevitable conclusion of this struggle. Communication with the family may become more strained as the ability to speak of progress is challenged. Prolonged exposure to dying patients in the ICU can also lead to burnout or post-traumatic stress disorder.

After a do-not-resuscitate order is on the chart, there is a change in perception of the patient. Before the patient was someone who needed everything done to preserve life, now the patient is perceived as someone who is dying. Often the bedside nurses and members of the team wonder what constitutes extraordinary care. "Should we order this laboratory test? Should we start this new intravenous infusion? Should we add this vasopressor?" The usually friendly team begins to withdraw from the family. The decision for death often makes most of the team members uncomfortable, and they are at risk for perceiving themselves as "failures."

The decision for withdrawal of care has greater clarity than the order for do not resuscitate. Medical goals shift to avoidance of suffering with subsequent doses of narcotics and benzodiazepines that ease the patient's process of dying. If the care team feels that further care is futile, then that needs to be expressed to the family and permission given for them to withdraw support. Futility is described as something that has less than a 1% chance of success by many publications from ethicists. The patient is described as terminal if he or she is not expected to live 6 more months with the present diagnosis. The order for do not resuscitate refers only to actions not taken when the patient has a cardiopulmonary arrest. The team must understand that the order does not lead to cessation of care and is different than withdrawal of care. Withdrawal of care means that the decision to allow natural death has occurred, and life-supporting/life-sustaining treatments are now being stopped. It is very important to remember the dignity of the dying patient no matter what the age or condition and to respect the deep emotions of the parents and family during this occurrence. When possible, sustaining treatment should be allowed until the family has supporting family members and friends nearby.

When a disagreement occurs within the medical team about the treatment desired (this usually involves withdrawal-of-care decisions), then an ethics consultation is warranted. The ethics consultation clarifies the issues by defining the medical goals and their achievability, the decision makers, the legality of decisions being made, and the contextual issues that influence these decisions. It often allows patients who are chronically ill to have an outside voice step back and speak to the situation. In the state of Texas the decision of the ethics committee is binding if it involves withdrawal of care. If the family disagrees with the ethics committee's decision, they have 10 days to find another facility who will care for their family member. Much has been written concerning the pros and cons of this approach to decision making. Ideally the ethics committee should have a diverse membership and include nonmedical representatives.

Physician Burnout

Physician burnout has been the subject of numerous studies over the past 10 years.[9] *Physician burnout* is a term that is used to describe a condition of emotional exhaustion related to overwhelming and/or chronic stressors present in many physicians' lives. However, burnout has also been found to occur when there is a high level of cynicism and depersonalization, as well as when there is a lack of efficacy or a feeling of being unable to have influence or make a difference. Although it is ultimately people who "burn out," burnout is not a deficiency or a mental illness. Burnout is often created by our systems and the excessive demands placed on us as caregivers—demands to do more than we can humanly do (witness the increase in clerical work now being demanded of caregivers *on top* of demands to provide care to an increasingly sick group of patients). In general, burnout often comprises numerous emotional, cognitive, social, and physical distress experiences, leading to a collection of conditions such as depression, anxiety, depersonalization, fatigue, loss of relationships, impaired decision making, and health impairment.

Physicians treating patients with life-threatening diseases are continuously exposed to patients and families in distress. Our bodies are designed to monitor and respond to both internal and external demands. We can maintain a balanced and healthy response to these demands if we have adequate internal and/or external resources with which to manage them. Some examples of resources contributing to internal or biologic/physiologic support include a healthy diet, exercise/yoga, sleep, meditation, and centering prayer. Examples of external resources leading to healthy psychosocial experiences are work cultures that invite autonomy, mastery, and relatedness, including collaborative colleagues and adequate professional resources to do one's job. Other psychosocial influences include adequate financial resources and living conditions, as well as connected and secure relationships with family and friends. If any of the internal physical demands or external social and contextual demands exceeds an individual's capacity to manage them, then their biologic and social systems begin to break down. This may take the form of illness, impaired cognitive and technical functioning, safety violations at work, and damage to relationships. In addition to the many demands of their professional context, physicians have personal lives, which also have demands that must be supported in order for the physician to be able to be present and fully functioning at work. (To think that physicians are immune to the influences of their lives apart from work would be to imply that they are not human, and depersonalization—lack of acceptance of their humanness—not only is a fast track to burnout, but also is associated with an 11-fold increase in medical errors, as well as unprofessional/immoral acts and lack of empathic connection with

others.) Some factors contributing to an underresourced work environment include the following demands: long work hours, not enough sleep and disrupted sleep patterns, demands of keeping abreast with the latest research for current medical practice, being present to gravely ill and dying patients, interpersonal conflicts, excessive paperwork, and pressure to see increasing numbers of patients in a limited time frame.

In addition to the numerous stressors just mentioned, the medical culture with its demands for perfectionism and its propensity to punish errors, as opposed to understanding them and learning from them, can easily overwhelm a physician's capacity to manage the demands of his or her professional context, leading to burnout and illness. Cultures of perfectionism and blame have been linked to toxic shame and secondary victimization,[10] which interferes with the physician's emotional well-being and also contributes to the increased likelihood of physician error.

One can imagine the inherent difficulties built into a stressful situation when a physician is not adequately resourced and is also in the grip of burnout as the physician tries to engage a teenage mother, who also may not be adequately resourced, to make a meaningful and difficult decision regarding the care of a child with complex congenital heart disease. Both individuals are most likely at the ends of their internalized windows of tolerance, which has the potential to impact their capacities for mindsight, abstract thinking, temporal integration, empathic responsiveness, and ability to engage in wise decision making. Add to this the factors of sleep deprivation, poor nutrition or physical health, and outside stressors (marital discord, issues with their own families, financial stressors), and it compounds the complexity of decision making. The first important step to managing these varying demands is simply becoming aware that they exist. Although that awareness does not abolish them or change them, acceptance of their presence reconnects us with our humanness and invites us to be able to connect with our patients, who have their own extraordinary demands, as humans and not simply as "diseases."

Social and Cognitive Bias and Unconscious Bias

Most people have some awareness that they have biases or preferences for one thing or person over another thing or person. Another way to think about bias is as a form of prejudice, which all individuals experience based on their natural biologic proclivities and their social, educational, and cultural conditioning. Bias and prejudice are commonly considered in respect to race, gender, age, religion, sexual orientation, social class, weight, and physical abilities but can also appear in decision making and diagnosis. When an individual has awareness of his or her biases or prejudices and can notice them with a degree of objectivity, these biases can be more easily managed.

Unconscious bias, on the other hand, operates outside of conscious awareness and prejudices the actual way individuals see and interpret their experiences of people, events, and experiences both within the self and in the world around them. Because unconscious biases operate so secretly, they can encourage the brain to use shortcuts based on previous experiences and aimed at categorizing and reaching quick conclusions. In this manner, unconscious biases cloud judgment, awareness, and choices in ways that are outside of the individual's control. The purpose of the brain using these shortcuts is to save energy for more complex tasks. Unfortunately, the down side of this is that these "shortcuts" place individuals at risk of arriving at inaccurate conclusions based on false and/or inadequate information. Physicians may be particularly susceptible to unconscious bias because they experience an overwhelming workload with great complexity. It would make sense that their brains would be primed to use shortcuts outside of conscious awareness.

Much has been written about stereotype bias in which we tend to attribute certain qualities to individuals based on previously mentioned categories such as race, age, gender, and socioeconomic status. One thing physicians can do to decrease the impact of stereotype threat is to develop internal awareness or mindsight regarding their experience of another person. They can also check out their experiences of a person or event with others or with the person directly. Another tool is to take the Implicit Association Test, which is an online evaluation offered through Harvard that provides individuals with awareness of their own implicit or unconscious biases.

Another form of implicit bias that is similar to stereotype bias is often described as an implicit schemata or mental representation of a person, a relationship, or a group of people (such as physicians in general). This type of schemata can also manifest as an implicit bias against a specific disease process or even interventional/operative procedure. These mental representations and physiologic responses develop from previous familial, social, religious, cultural, and educational conditioning. The experiences we have throughout our lives get internalized as mental representations and also as physiologic responses that seem to bypass the prefrontal cortex. Once we have formed a schema around an experience of a person, place, event, or disease process, we tend to select only information that supports our belief system, and we respond physiologically in previously programmed ways by our experience of similar people, places, events, and diagnoses. We are literally "trapped in our stories" and prior physiologic conditioning, and as a result we are unable to be available to the present moment without the bias of implicit mental models and memories.

A physician engaging with a teenage parent (or really any parent) about his or her child with a congenital heart defect is an encounter that should immediately get the physician's attention for the potential for stereotype threat because it is likely that many unconscious biases are present. There is certainly an age, educational, and developmental difference, as well as possible socioeconomic, religious, or gender differences. If the physician has a child of similar age or is asked to recommend to a family what the physician would do if this were his or her own child, the injection of bias is virtually invited. Awareness of this potential offers the physician an opportunity to take a step back and consider the possibility of one or more of these unconscious biases operating, so that the physician can then bring these implicit biases into his or her own conscious awareness. Siegel describes a process of opening to new situations with COAL,[11] which stands for curiosity, openness, acceptance, and loving-kindness (or nonjudgment). Naming one's experience and treating others and ourselves with COAL allows for more "presence" to the other person with better management of both conscious and unconscious bias.

Improving Informed Consent, Decision Making, and Care of the Health Care Givers

Clear treatment goals are needed for parents, nurses, house staff, and cardiac teams to align vision and action. For infants admitted with congenital heart disease all invested parties benefit from being informed of short-term and long-term goals. Daily rounds can set immediate (hourly to daily) goals of therapy. These goals may include the steps for stabilizing the baby, the need for various diagnostic tests, the timing of interventions (including surgery), conditions required before surgery can be undertaken, the nature and the expected outcomes of the surgery (reparative versus palliative), the length of stay following an individual procedure, and the expectation for the need and timing of future surgeries. All of this information needs to be communicated in a manner that can be understood by the entire team as well as by the parents. A nurse (usually a nurse practitioner or even a physician's assistant) assigned to the cardiac service who rounds daily with the team can be invaluable in helping the family navigate all the various opinions and plans expressed by the many physicians who passed by the bedside. This individual can serve to translate the complex concepts and discussions that occurred during teaching rounds into something more understandable for the family when they have ambiguity or questions, and if needed, this team member can be invaluable in redirecting the physician to the family for further discussion. In addition, this nurse (or physician's assistant) will be able to assist with education and be able to field questions back to the team that will allow the family to have a better understanding and give real informed consent when procedures are needed. Educational materials given to the family need to reflect the infant's immediate condition and expected treatment. Explanation of medications being used is also needed. For the longitudinal medical and surgical goals, the use of life pathways can be a useful map for the family. Figs. 9.1 and 9.2 demonstrate examples of these pathways for tetralogy of Fallot (see Fig. 9.1) and HLHS (see Fig. 9.2). These samples are illustrative of possible means to communicate a more complete picture of the infant's progress over time as the infant is launched on his or her life journey.

Multidisciplinary rounds are needed in which all members feel welcome to give input into the family situation. Chaplains and social workers may give more insight into the family circumstances, needs, and challenges, and this can help the caregivers when asking for consent for procedures. The primary physicians treating the patient (most often the intensivist and cardiologist) should seek to become aware of all these aspects involved in the family dynamics in order to best counsel the family.

In busy intensive care units it is frequently difficult for the providers to remain connected to the human experience that the family is confronting because the contextual needs of providing acute and sometimes life-sustaining care (see Chapter 1 on whole brain leadership) often overwhelm the relational needs of recognizing that the child has a family who have been pushed to the limits of their window of tolerance (or *bandwidth* to manage the cascading demands that are likely new and overwhelming to them). Although emotions often need to be repressed to function efficiently when caring for the patients who are in severe distress or dying, the strategy of keeping emotions suppressed over time leads to depersonalization, burnout, medical errors, and overall suboptimal outcomes (for the patient and the providers). Providers need to find time to care for their own humanity. Exercise, spirituality, meditation, singing, creating art, vacations, or allowing time for family are needed activities to allow the mind to shift gears and regenerate. It is important for physicians or nurses to know themselves and to understand their own limitations. It is important for them to find time for self-healing because wounded healers often have impaired outcomes for their patients. In this regard the addition of professional coaches/counselors into highly stressful units to work with the caregivers, to help them debrief and process the enormity of what transpires in their "everyday" world, and to

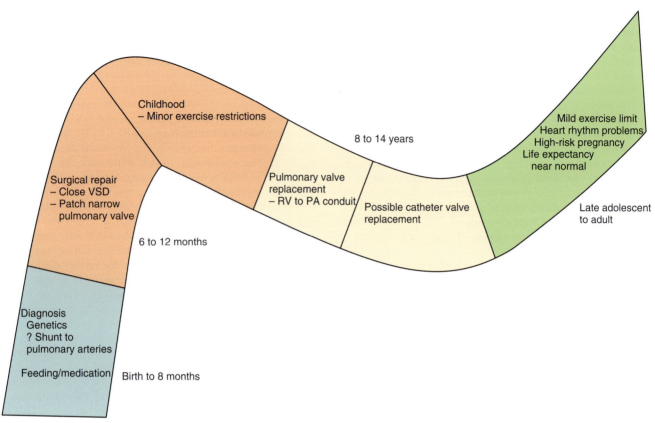

• **Figure 9.1** Life Pathway for Tetralogy of Fallot. An example of a tool to help families understand the timing of surgeries and potential problems from their child's heart disease during the child's lifetime. *PA,* Pulmonary artery; *RV,* right ventricle; *VSD,* ventricular septal defect.

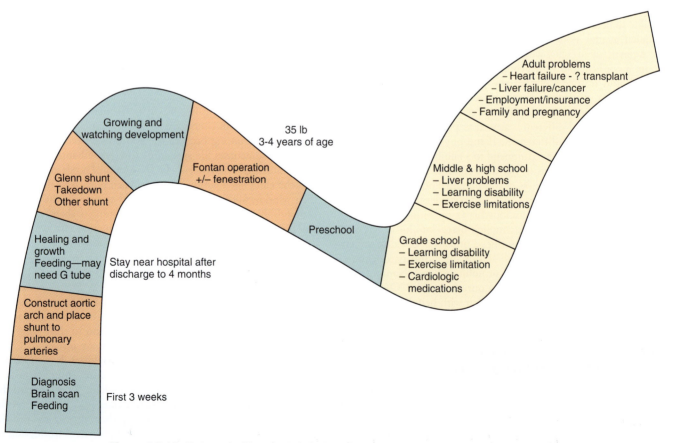

• **Figure 9.2** Life Pathway for Hypoplastic Left Heart Syndrome. An example of a tool to help families understand the timing of surgeries and potential problems from their child's heart disease during the child's lifetime.

simply help them take time to grieve (or celebrate) before they "move on to the next patient" can pay long-term dividends for the caregivers and for those they care for.

Ultimately the relationship between treating physicians, other caregivers, and the family is the primary one. Even though multiple other opinions have been gathered through the cardiology/surgery conference and through the ethics committee and rounds, those who have the power to make decisions, the designated legal guardians, are the ones who get to make the call on what needs to be done. The medical team's duty is to help the patient guardians navigate the complex medical and personal issues that surround the care of the patient with complex heart disease so that an informed best choice can be made for their child and his or her family.

Author's Comment

The preceding discussion represents 35 years of experience working with patients, nurses, cardiologists, and surgeons and personal experience with illness in my family (JB). It also includes 20 years of experience of being a member and clinical consultant to ethics committees in three institutions. Where my expertise lags, others with more knowledge have interjected their thoughts as well. What we do is hard. It is intellectually, technically, and emotionally challenging. As published results become the currency of expectation, struggle and failure have been suppressed to the shadows. The need for perfection (an impossible outcome) breeds shame that often gets manifested as blame (to deflect personal accountability), burnout (escape from stress and ineffectiveness), depression, substance abuse, or disruptive behaviors. Families need the best of us, and the best of us is to simply show up, to understand the complexities of what they are experiencing (as much as we try to understand the complexity of the heart defect itself), and to function as a unified group helping them toward a realistic and shared goal.

References

A complete list of references is available at ExpertConsult.com.

10

Advanced Nursing Practice in Pediatric Cardiac Critical Care

KRISTEN M. BROWN, DNP, CRNP, CPNP-AC; MELISSA B. JONES, MSN, APRN, CPNP-AC; LISA MOORE, RN, MSN, MHA, NEA-BC; CHRISTINE MELIONES, MSN, CPNP-AC/PC, FNP; JENNY A. MONTGOMERY, RN, MSN, CPNP-AC; JUDITH ASCENZI, DNP, APRN-CNS, RN, CCRN

Nurses play a critical role in the lives of children with congenital heart disease (CHD) and their families. This chapter describes the advanced skills and knowledge needed by nurses who care for the child with CHD, discusses the various complex and challenging roles and responsibilities of the pediatric cardiac nurse, explores the psychosocial impact of CHD on children and families, and discusses the nurse's role in assisting family adaptation at each phase of the illness and treatment.

Nursing Roles in Cardiac Critical Care

Bedside Nurse

One of the most crucial members of the multidisciplinary team, caring for a complex cardiac patient is the role of the bedside nurse. Pediatric cardiac critical care nurses are often the first to identify subtle changes in the assessment of the complex cardiac patient. They play an essential role in interdisciplinary rounds, where the continuity of care is centered. Professional nurses link quality care to best practice. They take responsibility for their practice by monitoring sensitive clinical indicators and applying evidence-based initiatives. Bedside nurses collaborate and partner with the multidisciplinary team to deliver the highest quality of care.

Higher levels of nursing education and experience positively impact patient outcomes.[1] Although many bachelor's- and master's-prepared graduate nurses are being hired into intensive care units (ICUs), a vigorous orientation program is necessary for new graduates or those hired with previous experience for successful transition. Orientation should include didactic classes, simulation training, and comprehensive preceptor time. Certification, continuous education, and engagement are important elements in the professional development of a critical care nurse.

Nursing Leadership

The American Nurses Association revised the Scope and Standards for Nurse Administrators in 2013, outlining the professional accountabilities for those nurses serving in leader roles. Certain elements are applicable to nursing administrators of pediatric cardiac critical care environments. Graduate education is necessary to develop expertise in nursing practice, science, innovation, strategic planning, communication, fiscal management, and resource allocation.[2] Nurse administrators must recognize the growing diversity of the workforce and their accountability to consumers. The revised standards also included eight core accountabilities: safety and quality management, health advocacy, care delivery and patient outcomes, healthy work environments, strategic and fiscal management, compliance, partnership and collaboration, and employee advocacy.

Nurse administrators must consider all aspects of the patient care experience, across the continuum. Those who inspire, motivate, and create high-performance teams are considered transformational leaders. Often they possess emotional intelligence and are moral and ethical role models. Transformational leaders challenge themselves, and their teams, to take risks. They learn from their failures, accept responsibility, and hold themselves accountable.[3] These visionary and innovative leaders help to advance the nursing profession for pediatric cardiac critical care nurses.

Advanced Practice Providers

Pediatric Nurse Practitioners. Advanced practice providers (APPs), such as nurse practitioners (NPs) are now the frontline providers in many pediatric cardiac intensive care units (PCICUs). Work-hour limitations of trainees in recent years has compelled units to develop creative care delivery models. Models that combine APPs and physician trainees are now commonplace in the United States.

APPs come into the role with varied educational preparation and clinical experience. The licensure, accreditation, certification, and education (LACE) consensus model was developed by 40 organizations in the United States to standardize NP practice. This model recommends aligning each of the elements (licensure, accreditation, certification, and education) with the desired job description and patient population served.[4] For example, completion of an acute care nursing practitioner curriculum at an accredited program, certification through the pediatric nurse practitioner acute care (PNP-AC) board examination, and licensure by the state board are qualifications of the ideal candidate for a pediatric cardiac critical care NP position. APP orientation programs vary considerably in length and structure; some centers offer a 6- to

8-week program, whereas others offer up to 9-month-long fellow-ships. Many orientation programs combine precepted clinical time, didactic lectures and simulation experiences. An understanding of the individual's background should help shape a strong, customized orientation program.

APPs are consistent direct care providers in the PCICU. Their clinical responsibilities include obtaining comprehensive histories and performing complete physical examinations; ordering and interpreting appropriate laboratory and imaging studies; prescribing and titrating medications; evaluating the effects of interventions; performing invasive procedures, including tracheal intubation, central and arterial line placement, and chest tube insertion; and collaborating with the multidisciplinary team to coordinate care.[5,6] APPs educate families and prepare technology-dependent children for discharge to home. In addition to clinical responsibilities, APPs are well positioned to identify processes in need of improvement in the unit, improve adherence to existing policies and protocols, participate in nursing education, and work with the multidisciplinary team on research and quality improvement projects.

Development of Advanced Pediatric Cardiovascular Curriculum

The care of infants and children with congenital heart disease is complex and challenging. A solid knowledge base facilitates the delivery of quality care by the pediatric critical care nurse. The bedside nurse needs to demonstrate advanced clinical judgment and reasoning skills to provide care for these complex, critically ill children.

A systematic, comprehensive curriculum addressing issues specific to the child with CHD enhances the skills and competency of an experienced ICU nurse. The curriculum is presented in various formats, including lectures, workshops, self-learning activities, one-to-one preceptor opportunities, and simulation. The goals of the program are for the learner to be able to (1) describe common congenital heart defects and surgical interventions, (2) perform a safe admission of a child to the ICU after cardiac surgery, (3) identify potential postoperative complications, and (4) demonstrate appropriate nursing interventions (Box 10.1). Early recognition and prompt treatment of potential complications greatly affect outcome and length of hospital stay.

Nurse's Role in the Pediatric Cardiac Intensive Care Unit

Preoperative Care

In the current health care era, most children receive preoperative evaluations in the outpatient setting. However, neonates with ductal dependent cardiac defects require immediate care in an ICU. As congenital cardiac diagnosis is increasingly made in utero, related to the advent of maternal fetal medicine programs, the delivery of a child with a ductal dependent lesion can be planned before the baby's birth. Arrangements for the infant to be delivered in the hospital where the baby's cardiac care will be provided eliminates potentially dangerous transfers and separation from parents. State-mandated pulse oximetry screening tests have assisted in better detection of infants who have not been diagnosed in utero. This screening has ensured earlier diagnosis after birth, minimizing the delay in transfer to an ICU for further management and diagnostic

---

• BOX 10.1   Advanced Pediatric Cardiac Core Curriculum

Congenital Heart Defects and Associated Surgical Interventions
Atrial septal defect
Ventricular septal defect
Atrioventricular septal defects
Pulmonary stenosis
Aortic stenosis
Coarctation of the aorta
Tetralogy of Fallot
Transposition of the great arteries
Tricuspid atresia
Total anomalous pulmonary venous return
Truncus arteriosus
Hypoplastic left heart syndrome

Cardiopulmonary Bypass
Routine Preoperative and Postoperative Care
Pharmacology
Complications
Low cardiac output
Excessive bleeding/tamponade
Acute renal failure
Electrolyte imbalances
Arrhythmias
Pulmonary hypertension
Other respiratory-pleural effusion
Neurologic deficits
Infection

Advanced Technical Skills
Cardioversion/defibrillation
Open thoracotomy tray
Pacemakers

---

workup.[7,8] Urgent transfer can create a great deal of anxiety for the family and require extensive communication and planning if the mother is hospitalized elsewhere.

Prostaglandin E1–Dependent Neonate (Balancing Q_p:Q_s). The goals for preoperative ICU care consist of maintaining hemodynamic stability and preventing infection and ensuring adequate nutrition.[9,10] Most children needing an ICU as a neonate require prostaglandins to maintain ductal patency before surgery or hemodynamic support in the form of vasoactive infusions, diuretics, and mechanical ventilation due to severe cardiorespiratory compromise. Balancing systemic (Q_s) to pulmonary (Q_p) circulation is a critical step in ensuring ideal preoperative hemodynamics. Goal-directed therapy is aimed at maintaining adequate cardiac output (CO) and balancing adequate oxygenation. Depending on the type of lesion, infants are often managed with diuretics, careful fluid balance, mechanical ventilation, use of vasoactive infusions, and ensuring optimal nutrition.[9,10]

Postoperative Care

Preparation for Admission From the Operating Room. The ICU nurse makes preparations to ensure the delivery of safe, efficient, individualized care to the child and family in the postoperative period. Preparation for admission of a postoperative cardiac surgery patient starts with careful review of all preoperative clinical data, including echocardiographic or cardiac catheterization results, surgical history, current medications and diet, recent physical examination results, and an understanding of the surgical plan. Synthesis of this information is important for the nurse to appropriately anticipate the postoperative care and potential complications. Additionally, the ICU nurse prepares the environment before admission with necessary equipment. The goal of the admission process to the ICU is to ensure safe transfer of care from the operating room (OR) team to the ICU team. An admission protocol is useful to guarantee a safe, efficient admission each time, regardless of individual personnel involved in the process.

Handoff From Operating Room to Intensive Care Unit. The OR team may contact the ICU team to provide information about the course and expected time of admission before arrival at the ICU. The personnel at the bedside during the admission process should be limited to those required for direct patient care responsibilities, including the cardiac anesthesiologist, surgeon, intensive care providers, respiratory therapist, and two ICU nurses. The anesthesiologist is usually responsible for overseeing care during the transition from the OR to the ICU.

Once the patient arrives at the ICU, the team must safely transfer all monitoring equipment and medication infusions. In a hemodynamically stable patient, the information handoff should begin after equipment handoff. Typically a minimum of two nurses is required to admit a cardiac surgery patient to the ICU. Each ICU nurse is assigned a role to ensure a smooth and safe admission to the critical care unit.[11] The nursing team works with the anesthesia team to safely transfer all monitoring equipment and infusions. The first nurse, usually the nurse assigned to care for the patient, performs a baseline physical assessment. The second nurse is responsible for managing drainage tubes and hemodynamic monitors. Respiratory therapists usually work with the anesthesia team and the ICU providers to determine the ventilator settings.

Initial assessment of the intubated patient is focused on confirming correct endotracheal positioning and adequate ventilation. Once adequate ventilation has been established, the primary nurse performs an initial physical examination. Frequent focused cardiac examinations are done until hemodynamic stability is achieved, and then examinations are spaced out.

The second nurse at the bedside transfers monitoring equipment to the ICU monitor. The use of a transport monitor compatible with the ICU monitors simplifies this procedure and eliminates interruption of monitoring vital signs. This nurse also labels intravascular infusion lines and drainage systems, including chest tubes, urinary catheters, and nasogastric tube. This nurse then obtains admission blood work consisting of complete blood count, chemistry panel, arterial blood gas levels, and coagulation panel. Performing these tasks in a sequential fashion promotes order during the admission process and allows completion of these vital tasks in an expeditious fashion.

During the information handoff the anesthesiologist provides information about the airway, vascular access, hemodynamic trends, vasoactive infusions, and external pacing requirements. The surgical team provides information about the procedure, residual defects, cardiopulmonary bypass (CPB), cross-clamp, and circulatory arrest times. Ideally, all members of the team are available for the information handoff and have the opportunity to ask clarifying questions. Once the ICU assumes care of the patient, the ICU providers communicate a plan, specific postoperative concerns, and expected parameters to the bedside nursing team (Table 10.1).

Hemodynamic Monitoring: Evaluation of Oxygen Delivery

Matching oxygen delivery and oxygen demand is the primary goal of the postoperative period. Synthesis of cardiac examination findings, vital sign trends, and laboratory results is essential for the PCICU nurse to determine adequacy of oxygen delivery.

Focused Cardiac Examination

A thorough cardiac examination includes auscultating heart sounds, palpating liver border, measuring urine output, and assessing central and distal pulses, skin color and temperature, and capillary refill time. Evaluation of a heart murmur or rub may identify residual heart disease or the presence of a pericardial effusion. Palpation of the liver edge is especially useful in children with right-sided heart dysfunction or failing single-ventricle physiology. An enlarged liver can indicate worsening function or volume overload. For example, a patient with poor Fontan physiology may develop worsening hepatomegaly in the setting of excessive volume repletion. Trending urine output is often used as a surrogate marker for renal perfusion. Poor urine output may be an indication of inadequate renal perfusion as a result of poor CO. Physical examination findings that focus on the presence and strength of both central and peripheral pulses, skin color and temperature, presence or degree of peripheral edema, and capillary refill time are critically important to evaluating overall perfusion.

Monitoring

Closely monitoring heart rate and rhythm, blood pressure, intracardiac pressures or central venous pressure, oxygen saturation, venous oximetry, near-infrared spectroscopy (NIRS), and end-tidal carbon dioxide ($ETCO_2$) trends is a key nursing responsibility. Twelve-lead electrocardiogram (ECG) is routinely obtained after admission from the OR and obtained as needed thereafter.[5] Atrial wire ECGs may help detect an atrial arrhythmia when the surface lead ECG is difficult to interpret. Tachycardia may be noted in the setting of hypovolemia, fever, or pain or may be a new arrhythmia. Simultaneous monitoring of intracardiac pressures may help delineate the problem. For example, tachycardia associated with elevated atrial pressures may be onset of a new tachyarrhythmia or worsening ventricular function; however, tachycardia associated with low intracardiac pressure is likely the result of hypovolemia. Bradycardia may be noted with sinus node dysfunction, atrioventricular (AV) block, or hypothermia or may be the side effect of analgesia or sedation medications. External pacemaker availability is essential to managing arrhythmias in the postoperative period.

Arterial lines are used for direct and continuous blood pressure monitoring and easy blood gas sampling. Common sites for arterial lines in children include the radial, femoral, and umbilical arteries. Arterial blood pressure measurements are correlated with noninvasive blood pressure monitoring whenever there is a question regarding the accuracy of the arterial line. A poor waveform on the monitor or the inability to withdraw blood from the catheter may give false readings. The ICU nurse troubleshoots the monitoring issues to determine accurate patient data. Nonfunctioning arterial lines are replaced or removed. Depending on ICU protocols, umbilical artery catheters are removed within 7 to 10 days to avoid infection

TABLE 10.1 Interventions for Postoperative Care After Cardiac Surgery

Problem	Patient-Specific Intervention	Problem	Patient-Specific Intervention
Hypoxia	1. Assess respiratory status every 15 min until stable, then every hour 2. Monitor rate and depth of respirations 3. Monitor presence and quality of breath sounds 4. Assess color of mucous membranes and lips 5. Obtain arterial blood gas levels as ordered and as needed with changes in patient's condition 6. Turn every 2 h unless contraindicated by hemodynamic instability	Decreased urine output	1. Record accurate intake and output every hour 2. Obtain electrolytes as ordered 3. Institute peritoneal dialysis or continuous arteriovenous hemofiltration as ordered 4. Daily weights on same scale, with same clothing
Respiratory distress	1. Assess breath sounds before and after suctioning 2. Maintain patency of artificial airway 3. Two-person suctioning for patient with pulmonary hypertension or hemodynamic instability	Pain	1. Pain management per pain service 2. Provide incisional site splinting as necessary 3. Provide diversional activities
Decreased cardiac output	1. Cardiovascular assessment every hour and with changes 2. Vital signs every 15 min until stable 3. Measure four-extremity blood pressure on admission 4. Record accurate intake and output 5. Measure chest tube drainage every hour, replace output as ordered 6. Check external pacemaker settings 7. Six- to 12-lead ECG on admission and every morning 8. Laboratory studies as ordered	Infection	1. Suture line care every day and as needed 2. Invasive site care every day 3. Monitor temperature every hour for 24 h, then every 2 h, if afebrile 4. Get patient out of bed as soon as possible
		Parental stress	1. Encourage parents to express feelings related to child's illness, hospital experience, and current fears 2. Provide information to assist parents in their basic needs 3. Encourage parents to establish their parent role in PICU through participation in child's care 4. Invite participation in parent support group 5. Provide parents with information about stress, adjustment, and parenting roles[a]
Neurologic deficit	1. Assess neurologic status every 4 h and with changes 2. Provide age-appropriate diversional activity as tolerated 3. Plan care to allow uninterrupted periods of rest 4. Minimize noxious effects of PICU environment	Child/parent education	1. Arrange preoperative PICU tour 2. Provide information about child's condition 3. Prepare parent for child's transition from PICU

[a]Visconti KJ, Sandino KJ, Rappaport LA, et al. Influence of parental stress on the behavioral adjustment of children with transposition of the great arteries. *J Dev Behav Pediatr.* 2002;23:314-321.
ECG, Electrocardiogram; *PICU,* pediatric intensive care unit.

and/or thrombosis. Noninvasive pressure monitoring may be adequate once hemodynamic stability is achieved and less vasoactive support is needed.[12]

Central venous and intracardiac pressure monitoring provides valuable information regarding intravascular volume and right ventricular compliance and onset of new arrhythmia.[12] These lines are also useful for blood sampling and medication administration. Common cannulation sites for central venous pressure monitoring include internal and external jugular veins, femoral veins, and umbilical veins. Central venous lines often have multiple lumens that allow for the administration of multiple medications and fluids while monitoring venous pressures. Intracardiac monitoring lines are placed either percutaneously or transthoracically. Left atrial catheters are usually placed at the junction of the left atria and upper pulmonary vein, and pulmonary catheters are placed in the main pulmonary artery.[13] The surgeon places transthoracic lines in the OR based the child's physiology and anticipated postoperative course. Right-sided lines may be used for infusions in the absence of other central lines and any residual right-to-left shunt. Left-sided transthoracic lines are not routinely used to infuse fluids or medications due to increased risk of introducing air or particulate matter emboli into the arterial circulation. Chest tubes

generally remain in place until transthoracic lines are removed, due to potential bleeding after catheter removal.

Careful assembly of the transducers, tubing, and stopcocks is essential to preventing contamination and incomplete priming of the tubing resulting in entrapped air. Air within the closed system will alter the accuracy of the monitoring system and may result in an embolic event. Ensuring that precise information is obtained from the transducers depends on the accuracy of leveling and calibrating the system. The ICU nurse routinely calibrates and levels the transducers at change of shift and after a change in the patient's position.

Oxygen saturation monitoring is a bit more complicated in patients with complex CHD than in patients with normal cardiac anatomy. Oxygen saturation goals depend on the degree of intracardiac shunting. A solid understanding of the anatomy and physiology of each patient is essential to targeting the appropriate saturation goals. For example, patients after a tetralogy of Fallot (TOF) repair with a residual atrial level communication and right ventricular dysfunction may have acceptable oxygen saturation range of 80% to 100% in the immediate postoperative period; however, a TOF patient with an intact atrial septum should have oxygen saturation target of 96% to 100%. Hypoxia in the absence of cyanotic heart disease needs to be addressed and corrected urgently.

ETCO$_2$ monitoring can confirm that the endotracheal tube is in the airway; however, it does not confirm appropriate positioning of the endotracheal tube.[5] Assuming the presence of a pulse in the patient, an abrupt drop in ETCO$_2$ must trigger an immediate evaluation of endotracheal tube placement, including assessment of chest rise, breath sounds, and tube patency and placement.[12] Once ETCO$_2$ is correlated with arterial carbon dioxide levels, the ETCO$_2$ may be trended and spare unnecessary arterial blood gas sampling. Additionally, if airway patency is confirmed, continuous ETCO$_2$ measurement is used as an indicator of CO, and an acute change may prompt the nurse to deterioration in the patient, including worsening perfusion and a diminishing pulse. Also, ETCO$_2$ is used to assess adequacy of chest compressions during resuscitation.

NIRS monitoring is a noninvasive method of evaluating regional tissue oxygenation. NIRS sensors are generally placed over the abdomen or flank region and on the forehead. Trending NIRS values can detect fluctuations in perfusion.[12] Used in conjunction with other monitoring devices, NIRS may be an early warning sign of low CO (LCO).

Early recognition of a deteriorating cardiac examination, vital signs, or laboratory results, anticipation of appropriate treatments, and communication to the provider team expedites time-sensitive interventions. Distilling the pertinent data from the vast amount of information a nurse receives is a high-level, critical thinking skill that distinguishes pediatric cardiac critical care nurses.

Unexpected residual cardiac disease has become rare in the era of intraoperative transesophageal echocardiography (TEE).[14] Intraoperative TEE after the surgical repair gives the surgeon information regarding cardiac function and anatomy before separation from CPB. If significant residual lesions (intracardiac shunts, obstruction to flow, valve regurgitation) exist, the surgeon may correct the remaining problem before leaving the OR.

Inadequate intravascular volume as measured by right atrial pressure, left atrial pressure, and blood pressure can result from hemorrhage, inadequate fluid administration, fluid leaking into the third space, and excessive diuresis. Postoperative bleeding can occur from cannulation sites, suture lines, or postbypass coagulopathy. Long CPB time can lead to platelet dysfunction and diffuse capillary leak. Packed red blood cells, platelets, and fresh frozen plasma should be readily available for replacement due to grossly abnormal coagulation laboratory values or prolonged and excessive bleeding.

Despite ongoing improvements in perfusion techniques, the use of CPB continues to be associated with postoperative morbidity. CPB affects both intravascular volume and cardiac contractility. The use of an external circuit for circulation and oxygenation has been shown to result in the stimulation of an inflammatory response and subsequent capillary leak. This inflammatory response syndrome results in injury to multiple body systems, including the lungs, systemic vasculature, and myocardium. The systemic effects of the CPB inflammatory syndrome may result in substantial increase in intravascular permeability with fluid moving into the tissues, resulting in decreased intravascular volume. Close monitoring of the child's vital signs, perfusion, and urine output is essential to ensuring that fluid shifting into the third space does not result in hypotension and poor end-organ perfusion.

Hypoxemia and acidosis are identified by routine arterial blood gas monitoring. Knowledge of the surgical procedure performed is essential to determining the expected oxygen saturation for a patient. Patients with uncorrected single-ventricle physiology (e.g., those with shunts or Glenn anastomoses) will be hypoxemic because they have mixing lesions, and oxygen saturations in the 80% range may be normal and expected, whereas patients with corrected circulation and normal lungs should be expected to have saturations above 90%. Inadequate CO will result in poor oxygen delivery to tissues and metabolic acidosis. Serial lactic acid measurement provides information regarding the adequacy of perfusion.[15] Persistently elevated lactic acid levels are a marker for poor outcome after cardiac surgery. Mixed venous saturation (SvO$_2$) monitoring also provides information regarding oxygen delivery and utilization. Low mixed venous saturation levels may indicate a residual right-to-left cardiac shunt or decreased CO. Continuous noninvasive monitoring provides trends in the patient's perfusion. Commonly patients have continuous pulse oximetry and NIRS monitoring in the early postoperative period. Analyzing laboratory data and monitoring trends must be done in conjunction with physical examinations.

Postoperative Problems

Low Cardiac Output Syndrome

Low cardiac output (LCO) is a known risk factor after cardiac surgery.[16-20] Several factors influence the likelihood of LCO after surgery, including myocardial ischemia from aortic cross-clamping, activation of inflammatory pathways related to cardiopulmonary bypass, and the residual effects of cardioplegia,[16-18] all of which can negatively impact end organ perfusion. Decreased cardiac output in the postoperative period may be due to the surgical procedure, hypoxemia, acidosis, electrolyte imbalances, prolonged bypass time, or arrhythmias. Treatment options include fluid boluses, vasoactive infusions, temporary pacing, and/or mechanical support. The postoperative management of these patients should be directed at optimizing oxygen delivery to maintain end organ function.[19-22] An understanding of the early signs of impaired cardiac output and implementation of appropriate treatments by the nurse may prevent morbidity and mortality.[16,17] The evaluation of adequate tissue oxygenation is dependent on early and on-going assessments by the bedside nurse, which goes beyond the standard approach of identifying shock.[23-25] Cardiovascular monitoring alone may not be adequate to quickly identify early signs of tissue hypoxia[24,26]; therefore the nurse needs to have an advanced understanding of cardiac output and the effects of preload, afterload, and contractility.[26]

Arrhythmias

Arrhythmias in the immediate postoperative period may have a significant impact on CO due to loss of AV synchrony or inadequate filling time. These arrhythmias may result from electrolyte imbalances, intracardiac monitoring lines, tissue swelling, catecholamine response, or surgical injury to the conduction system. Less commonly, they result from congenital abnormalities of the conduction system associated with channelopathies, structural defects, and myocardial disease secondary to poor postoperative perfusion.[27]

Junctional ectopic tachycardia (JET) is the most common *postoperative* arrhythmia, which typically presents within the first 24 hours of surgery. Several risk factors increase the incidence of JET, including type of repair (i.e., TOF), younger age, lower body weight, longer CPB, aortic cross-clamp time, hypokalemia, hypomagnesemia, acidosis, and high dose of inotropy. Treatment involves mild hypothermia, a reduction of exogenous catecholamines, and sedation.[28] Amiodarone is the preferred first-line agent in supporting hemodynamics in the unstable patient and can significantly reduce the incidence of postoperative JET if given prophylactically.[27]

Postoperative (AV) block may result from inflammation or direct insult to the conduction system in up to 3% of postoperative patients. Complete AV canal and TOF repair are at the highest risk for transient and permanent AV block. Transient AV block is most common with approximately 97% of patients regaining AV conduction by postoperative day 10. Patients require the use of a temporary pacemaker until normal sinus rhythm returns or a permanent pacemaker is placed. The recovery waiting time before proceeding to permanent pacemaker is broadly accepted as 7 to 14 days. Steroids are frequently used to reduce tissue edema and hasten return to normal conduction.[29]

Determining whether the patient is in sinus rhythm versus supraventricular tachycardia may be challenging. Patients with temporary atrial and ventricular pacing wires in place can have an atrial lead study. To perform this, first obtain a 12-lead ECG. Then connect the limb leads to the atrial wires. This can assist in the diagnosis by evaluating the atrial electrogram. Atrial pressure lines can also be useful for diagnosis. Cannon A waves demonstrated on atrial lines will not be present during sinus rhythm.

Hematologic Considerations

After surgery, chest tubes are placed in the pleural and mediastinal spaces. Chest tubes facilitate drainage of blood and serous fluid and are assessed frequently for patency and amount of drainage. The heparin used during CPB is partially reversed with protamine in the OR. The process of returning to a noncoagulopathic state may not be present on arrival to the ICU and can take more than 8 hours in certain patients, such as the neonate with immature liver function, patients who require significant products secondary to bleeding in the OR, and patients with undiagnosed coagulopathy. Excessive drainage should be reported to the surgical team. Drainage from the chest tubes typically changes from bloody to serosanguinous in the first few hours after surgery. Once the chest drainage has diminished, the chest tubes are removed, often 2 to 3 days postoperatively.

A sudden cessation of drainage from previously draining chest tubes coupled with decreasing systemic perfusion and rising right or left atrial pressures is regarded with a high degree of suspicion for cardiac tamponade. Blocked chest tubes prevent adequate drainage of fluid from the pericardial space. CO is impaired due to fluid accumulation around the heart, which interferes with diastolic filling and systolic ejection. Signs of cardiac tamponade include hypotension, tachycardia, narrowing pulse pressure, and elevated right atrial and left atrial filling pressures. Pulsus paradoxus, a fall in systolic blood pressure by 8 to 10 mm Hg during inspiration, is a classic sign in a spontaneously breathing patient but may be difficult to appreciate in a child with tachycardia and hypotension. Other signs may include muffled heart sounds and decreased voltage on the surface ECG. Impending tamponade is a clinical diagnosis as described earlier that can be confirmed by echocardiography, which will demonstrate whether or not there is substantial fluid around the heart and in some cases show compression of cardiac chambers by the fluid. Clearing occluded chest tubes or opening the chest will rapidly restore hemodynamic stability.

Altered Neurologic Status

There is potential for serious neurologic complications after CPB. The ICU nurse performs a comprehensive neurologic examination soon after admission to assess pupillary response and movement of all extremities. As the child emerges from anesthesia, the neurologic examination includes the child's responses. Cerebral protection during CPB has become very sophisticated during the past decade, resulting in few adverse neurologic events.[30] Repair of coarctation of the aorta requires special attention to the movement of the lower extremities due to the risk of interrupted perfusion to the spinal cord subsequent to clamping of the aorta. An extremely small percentage of these patients can have lower extremity paralysis following surgery, and although this cannot be altered by postoperative ICU care, recognition of this possibility (or more often, elimination of this as a possibility by observing movement in the lower extremities as the child recovers) provides important information to the other members of the health care team as well as to anxious family members. Infants and children undergoing surgery that requires circulatory arrest warrant extra attention to monitor their neurologic status. The presence of seizures in the postoperative period following neonatal CPB can be a harbinger of brain injury and should be rapidly investigated and treated with anticonvulsant therapy. The occurrence of major, hemispheric stroke is uncommon following infant cardiac surgery but should be considered if the child demonstrates major focal findings suggestive of this diagnosis. Control of fever in the postoperative cardiac patient is especially important in patients at risk for neurologic injury.

Respiratory Complications

Although some postoperative cardiovascular patients will be extubated, many of the neonates with complicated lesions will remain intubated and mechanically ventilated after surgery. The management of these patients requires an understanding of oxygenation, ventilation, and the effects of cardiopulmonary interactions in CHD. Oxygenation is dependent on adequate delivery of oxygen to the alveolus, presence of shunts, and hemoglobin levels. In postoperative CHD patients, atelectasis, pulmonary edema, mucous plugs, bronchospasm, and collaterals can all impact oxygenation and ventilation. From a nursing perspective, the evaluation requires meticulous assessment of the patient and attention to basic respiratory parameters. Inadequate ventilation is assessed by measuring $PaCO_2$ and end-tidal CO_2 ($ETCO_2$). These parameters can be deranged in conditions such as hypoventilation, abnormalities in lung compliance, increased airways resistance, pleural effusions, and pneumothorax.

Cardiopulmonary interaction plays an important role in the respiratory management of CHD patients. The right ventricle (RV) fills "passively," and any increase in right atrial pressure due to increased intrathoracic pressure can lead to a decrease in RV filling or preload. This can lead to RV dysfunction and decreased CO. On the contrary, an increase in intrathoracic pressure can cause a reduction in left ventricle (LV) afterload, which may decrease the workload of the LV. This may result in an increase LV stroke volume and CO.

Pleural effusions also occur frequently after CHD surgery and may interfere with weaning from ventilator support or necessitate reintubation in the previously extubated child. Small to moderate pleural effusions can be treated with aggressive diuresis; however, large effusions, and especially those that result in hemodynamic changes, require drainage. Children with elevated venous pressures are at higher risk for developing pleural effusions, with some surgeries increasing the risk for chylothorax. Serial respiratory assessments and chest x-ray examinations are needed to monitor the size of pleural effusions and response to therapy. Chylothorax may require adjustment in dietary fat intake, in addition to diuretics. In the usual postoperative course without complication, chest tubes are commonly removed when drainage has significantly decreased, which usually occurs within 24 to 72 hours after surgery.

Infection

Broad-spectrum antibiotics are started intraoperatively to prevent infection. Antibiotics are continued during the immediate ICU recovery phase until central lines and drainage tubes are removed. Early signs of infection, including fever, elevated white blood cell count, thrombocytopenia, elevated C-reactive protein level, and wound drainage, warrant careful monitoring and cultures. Good hand washing and timely removal of central monitoring lines and tubes decrease the incidence of infection.

Electrolyte Imbalance and Acute Renal Failure

Normal levels of sodium, potassium, calcium, and magnesium are essential for excitable membrane function and effective myocardial contraction. A full serum chemistry blood panel, including magnesium, should be obtained with the postoperative admission blood work. Hypokalemia resulting from an increase in intravascular water, treatment of acidosis, and use of diuretic therapy may result in conduction and rhythm disturbances. Hyperkalemia resulting from impaired renal function (acute tubular necrosis) or administering excessive doses of potassium chloride is also detrimental to the cardiac system.

Calcium is essential for adequate cardiac contractility. A decreased ionized calcium level has been demonstrated after CPB. In young infants, hypocalcemia is more likely to develop due to the lack of adequate calcium reserves in the sarcoplasmic reticulum. Calcium stores increase with age and muscle mass, therefore making it less of a postoperative problem in older children. Hypocalcemia may also result from multiple blood transfusions due to citrate used as a blood product preservative.

Hypomagnesia may occur after CPB and intense diuresis. Cardiovascular effects of decreased magnesium levels include depressed myocardial contractility, arrhythmias, and increased sensitivity to digoxin. Low magnesium levels have been shown to be associated with an increased incidence of JET in the immediate postoperative period.[31]

Renal insufficiency after cardiac surgery results in decreased urine output, increased water weight gain, and elevated serum creatinine, blood urea nitrogen, and potassium values. Urine output is closely monitored during the immediate postoperative period, with expected urine output of 1 mL/kg/h. Decreased urine output associated with low filling pressures (left atrial and central venous pressures) is challenged with 5 to 10 mL/kg fluid boluses. Decreased urine output associated with normal or elevated filling pressures is treated with intravenous diuretics. Because excessive fluid overload delays extubation, increases the risk of infection, and prolongs the ICU recovery time, more aggressive diuretic therapy may be indicated. Critically ill newborns and infants undergoing complex surgery may have temporary peritoneal dialysis (PD) catheters placed in the OR during surgery. PD can assist with management of fluid volume overload in patients with hemodynamic instability or who may need considerably higher doses of diuretics to achieve a targeted fluid balance. PD catheters are generally used as short-term management.

Accurate intake and output records are calculated hourly, maintenance fluid goals are carefully considered, and children are weighed daily to assess weight gain or loss compared to their preoperative weight. Length of diuretic therapy is dependent on the patient cardiac lesion, surgical repair (complete repair versus palliative procedure), and postoperative recovery.

Pain Management and Sedation

Pediatric pain teams assist in the management of pain and sedation after surgery. Infants and children who will remain intubated overnight receive intravenous narcotics and sedatives to keep them comfortable. However, the goal is to minimize the use of these agents and facilitate early extubation. Dexmedetomidine (Precedex) is another agent used as an adjust therapy for postoperative ICU sedation. It has fewer side effects related to respiratory depression than other sedative agents and may reduce the risk of arrhythmia and acute kidney injury after surgery. It is generally used as a short-term therapy when early extubation is expected or as adjunctive therapy to facilitate weaning of other sedatives, such as narcotics.[32,33]

Sedation medicines are weaned or withheld before extubation to facilitate wakefulness and adequate respiratory effort. Pain medications are titrated to attain an adequate level of pain management and alertness with acceptable hemodynamic parameters.

It is important to evaluate both pain and the response to therapy closely. Pain evaluation can be accurately assessed and reported by using self-reporting tools or behavioral observational scales.[34,35] Nonopioid agents, such as acetaminophen or ketorolac, should be implemented to aid in pain control and reduce the amount of narcotic administration. It is also important to institute other nonpharmacologic interventions and therapies such as range of motion, massage, and music, art, or physical therapy.

Infants and children who have required extensive use of narcotics and benzodiazepines may experience withdrawal if medications are abruptly discontinued. Signs and symptoms of withdrawal include jitteriness, insomnia, seizures, diarrhea, diaphoresis, agitation, nausea and vomiting, tachycardia, and hypertension. Careful attention should be given to implementing a slow wean approach over 5 to 10 days. The patient's response to therapy during weaning should be carefully monitored and evaluated at regular intervals. Pain management strategies should be addressed daily in multidisciplinary rounds with the ICU team, pharmacist, and pain management service. Delirium screening is also an important tool being increasingly used as part of nursing assessment.

Feeding Intolerance

Early feeding is now the goal in the early postoperative period. Careful consideration should be given when implementing oral and enteral nutrition. Neonatal patients with complex heart disease, a history of feeding intolerance, and failure to thrive are at greater risk for feeding intolerance.[32,34] Hemodynamic stability, need for mechanical ventilation, and use of vasoactive agents, sedation, and narcotics should be taken into consideration. Patients who require prolonged mechanical ventilation may benefit from parental nutrition support until adequate enteral or oral feeds have been well established.

Pediatric dietitians play a key role in evaluating patients and determining appropriate nutrition and feeding goals. Oral and enteral feeds should be initiated when the patient is hemodynamically stable to allow for adequate calories necessary for growth. Oral feeds should be implemented as soon as possible to establish effective oral-motor coordination. Feeds are often established slowly, increasing caloric density (supplemented breast milk or formula) over volume. The establishment of feeding algorithms or protocols has been beneficial in providing a framework for initiating and advancing enteral and oral nutrition in high-risk infants and children.[32,33,35] It is important for the bedside nurse to assess for early signs and symptoms of feeding intolerance because high-risk neonates are at a greater risk for bowel ischemia, which can lead to necrotizing enterocolitis.[34] Patients receiving enteral nutrition should have routine assessment of feeding tube placement and interval abdominal girths until goal feeds have been well established. Abdominal distention, lethargy, vomiting, an increase in gastric residual, or any noted feeding change from baseline should be promptly investigated.

Mechanical Circulatory Support

Extracorporeal Membrane Oxygenation. When a child's cardiac function is inadequate to sustain sufficient CO after surgery, extracorporeal membrane oxygenation (ECMO) or ventricular assist device may be required. If unable to wean from CPB in the OR, the child may be placed on mechanical support for early postoperative cardiac failure. ECMO can be initiated in the ICU for increased pressor and inotropic requirements, metabolic acidosis, and an acute deterioration. ECMO may also be deployed if the postoperative patient remains unstable after cardiac arrest. The bedside ICU nurse plays a crucial role in the early identification and communication of alarming hemodynamic trends.

Ventricular Assist Devices. The number of children on ventricular assist devices has increased over the past decade, which has compelled PCICU nurses not only to learn the technical aspects of the devices, but also how to meet the unique needs of these infants and children.[36] Rehabilitation and normalization of organ function is the goal of long-term support devices. Patients on ventricular assist devices require a multidisciplinary team approach to their care.[37] PCICU nurses are well positioned to promote consistent practice, through protocol development, specifically related to wound care, anticoagulation, and rehabilitation. Ventricular assist devices allow children to be off the ventilator, sedation, and vasoactives, and in some cases, to go home. Meticulous attention to detail is imperative for a patient to be successfully supported. The major risks that the devices present are bleeding, embolic stroke, and infection.[38]

The Berlin Heart is a pulsatile, paracorporeal device that supports infants and children waiting for a heart transplant. Patients on the Berlin Heart have either biventricular support (biventricular assist device [BiVAD]) or isolated left ventricular support (left ventricular assist device [LVAD]) and are kept in the hospital while on the device. Nurses may closely monitor the pump(s) for complete filling and emptying and for any evidence of fibrin or thrombus. Before changing pump settings, the team must target interventions to improve the patient's clinical status. Incomplete filling may be an indication of inadequate preload, or in the case of an LVAD it may represent right ventricular dysfunction. Incomplete emptying may be an indication of high afterload. Fibrin must be monitored closely, and if an organized thrombus is noted, a pump change must be considered. Anticoagulation protocols or teams are often developed to provide a standardized, consistent approach to the complex anticoagulation and antiplatelet management required.

On-time administration of anticoagulation and antiplatelet medications is imperative. Collecting the specific coagulation studies at the appropriate time is also vitally important to managing the balance between bleeding and thrombus formation in the pumps.

Berlin Heart cannula exit sites require careful assessment for signs of infection or loss of skin integrity, including redness, swelling, drainage, pain, or separation of the skin from the cannulas. Nurses often take the lead on the development of a dressing change protocol. Wound care nurses are an important resource for the development of the procedure and interventions to treat areas of concern.

Given that patients on a Berlin Heart are inpatient for the duration of support, the PCICU and inpatient teams must consider not only the immediate medical needs of the patient, but the long-term developmental needs. Child life, physical and occupational therapy, the medical team, and nurses collaborate to deliver care to meet the specific developmental and rehabilitation needs of each patient. Physical rehabilitation, maintenance of a day and night schedule, play therapy, academic tutoring, and time with family are all very important pieces of the long-term care of a patient with a Berlin Heart.[37]

Implantable, continuous-flow devices are another option to support children in decompensated heart failure awaiting transplant. These devices, designed for adults, have been used more frequently in pediatrics over the past 5 years.[39] Unlike the Berlin Heart, patients on a continuous-flow LVAD may be eligible for discharge to home.

Immediate postoperative management of a patient after implantation of a continuous-flow device is focused on right ventricular support and careful management of preload and afterload to the LV. Though the risk of thromboembolism is lower in continuous-flow devices than it is with the Berlin Heart, patients on continuous-flow LVAD require careful anticoagulation management.[40] As with the Berlin Heart, establishing a dressing change procedure and schedule for the driveline exit site is often lead by PCICU nursing and/or the wound care nursing team.

Preparing a patient for discharge home involves teaching the patient and family the process of changing and charging the batteries, emergency procedures, dressing change procedures, and medication administration. The VAD team also needs to perform outreach teaching to the community to ensure a safe transition to home. Nurses play a key role in helping patients and families take ownership of the device and to safely integrate this technology into their lifestyle.

Psychosocial Impact of Congenital Heart Disease in the Child

Initial Presentation and Diagnosis

The diagnosis of CHD imposes significant changes and adjustments to family life.[41] Parental expectations and hopes for a healthy child are altered by the presence of heart disease. The severity of illness, the timing of the diagnosis, the presentation leading to the diagnosis, previous experiences with illness, and individual and family adaptation skills affect the family's responses to the child. The nurse plays an important role in the family's adaptation through each stage of the child's care by providing education, educational material, and support dependent on the family's needs. In fact, some centers have adopted the practice of developing a group of continuity nurses (and physicians) for patients that have extended PCICU stays, as a source of support for both the patient and the family.

Advances in medical technology have increased the prenatal diagnosis of CHD. If a prenatal diagnosis is made describing a critical congenital heart defect, the pregnancy is closely monitored and plans made to deliver at an institution where appropriate support is available for the baby. Maternal anxiety is typically increased when the diagnosis of CHD is made by fetal echocardiography.[42] Support and information provided to the parents is crucial at this point.

If not diagnosed prenatally, serious CHD is usually detected during the first few weeks to months of life. Presentation in the neonatal period varies greatly. Symptoms that may lead to diagnosis include tachypnea with feeding intolerance, a murmur noted on a routine well-baby examination, cyanosis, and/or complete cardiovascular collapse. These differences in symptoms may influence the severity of the child's physiologic state but have little influence on parental reactions to the diagnosis. Three issues typically confront the family of an ill infant: (1) fear of loss and the unknown, (2) grief, and (3) guilt. Each family member individually prepares for what is to come. Frequently parents do not communicate their feelings to each other and may need help acknowledging and communicating their feelings. During the initial workup, denial is the strongest coping mechanism.

The final diagnosis of the child's heart defect presents a new reality and summons the family's previous coping mechanisms. At this time, parents experience grief for the loss of their expected normal child. This mourning is necessary for them to accept the imperfect child. The family will cope only as well as each of its members do. Each family member needs to express individual feelings before the family unit is able to cope. The family's ability to cope at this time is related to other factors, including the severity of illness; the suddenness of diagnosis and treatment; the meaning of the diagnosis to each individual member; the effect of the diagnosis on the family, including financial and lifestyle changes; and the presence and effect of support systems.

After diagnosis, anger is a common parental response. Guilt often accompanies this anger. Interventions by the health care team need to focus on the implications of these feelings. Time spent understanding the parents' perceptions of the child's illness is imperative for proper family functioning. Successful coping is contingent on parents' beliefs about what is wrong and the resultant consequences of their perceived diagnosis. Open, honest communication about the child's condition needs to be repeated to allow absorption and acceptance of facts in the face of stress.

Parent groups can be an additional source of support for families.[43,44] Parents who share similar experiences and solutions are able to help others. These groups allow family members to validate their thoughts and feelings in attempts to adjust to changes resulting from caring for their child with CHD. Parent support groups aid families through individual meetings during particularly stressful times. Parents find these meetings worthwhile at significant times in the child's life. Meetings usually concentrate on life experiences rather than focusing on medical details. Typical discussions concentrate on children playing with other children, starting school, and engaging in sport activities; sibling reactions; and acceptance by family members, teachers, friends, and neighbors. By participating in these groups, parents benefit from receiving guidance and support in addition to the rewards gained by helping others.[45]

If CHD is not detected during early childhood, a preschool or presports physical examination is another period when it is identified. Typically, cardiac lesions diagnosed at this time are usually not life threatening. However, CHD diagnosed at this time needs to be evaluated and treated to maintain good future health. Because the age of the child at the time of elective cardiac surgery or catheter intervention does not influence the course of psychologic distress of parents or the styles of coping used by the parents, nursing interventions should be aimed at education and support of the child and family.[46]

Medical-Surgical Plan

After diagnosis a strategy is proposed by a multidisciplinary group, including pediatric cardiac surgeons, pediatric cardiologists, anesthesiologists, nurses, and social workers, outlining the medical and surgical care plan. The decision to perform surgery presents another crisis point for the child and family. A host of emotions accompany this time, including relief that the decision is made, fear of the unknown, anxiety over the outcome of surgery, and anticipation of changes in family life after surgery. At this time an enormous amount of information is presented to the family. Despite efforts to answer all parental questions, there are topics that parents find difficult to discuss.[47] The staff must be aware of these issues and willing to explore them with family members.

Surgery on a child's heart inflicts fear and apprehension in family members.[48] Parents of a critically ill infant will be absorbed with thoughts of their child's survival,[49] whereas parents of an asymptomatic, healthy child may actually have a more difficult time accepting the diagnosis and surgical plan. Nursing interventions at this time need to focus on each family individually. The team should take cues from the family regarding the timing for preparation and the depth of information given at this time. Honest information about what to expect during and after surgery should be the central theme of interventions.

Developmental Needs of Children

The developmental characteristics of children must be taken into account by staff members as they respond to their physical needs (Table 10.2).[47,50] The essential task during infancy involves the development of a trusting relationship,[50] and the infant and parents must participate in the bonding process. Staff should encourage parents to interact in the care of their infant. Appropriate sensory experiences are fulfilled when familiar toys are placed within the infant's view or reach, musical toys are used, and the child is touched or cuddled. Noxious stimuli should be controlled if possible. Sufficient lighting in the ICU allows adequate observation and assessment of the child; however, glaring lights should be avoided. Nursing care should be planned to provide uninterrupted sleep periods; a day/night sequence is useful to help reduce the development of delirium. Reduction of loud noises as much as possible fosters the short sleep cycles in the ICU.

Toddlers' developmental needs include autonomy, exploration, and security.[47] During times of stress, they demonstrate signs of regression. Their relationship with parents is intense; separation anxiety occurs in their absence. Nursing interventions for toddlers in the ICU include promotion of the parent-child relationship. Parents are encouraged to visit often and participate in the child's care, including bathing, holding, and soothing during and after painful procedures. During the parents' absence, family pictures and tape recordings maintain the child's family contact. Routine care delivered by consistent caregivers adds to the toddler's sense of security. Choices should not be offered if there are none. The child should be encouraged to participate in care activities and allowed to express fear and anger by crying during painful procedures.

TABLE 10.2	Interventions to Care for Developmental Needs of Hospitalized Children		
Age	**Developmental Task**	**Effects of Hospitalization**	**Nursing Interventions**
Infant	Develop sense of trust	Separation from parents is stressful. Hospital's strange environment, including sights, sounds, and smells, produces anxiety. Disruption of routines results in distrust.	Provide consistent caregivers. Decrease separation from parents. Tape family pictures to child's crib. Provide comforting, familiar environment, including blankets and toys from home. Promote uninterrupted periods of rest while avoiding overstimulation by performing all tasks at one time.
Toddler	Develop autonomy	Frightened by strange environment. Perceives illness and hospitalization as punishment for bad behavior.	Minimize separation from parents. Involve family in procedures. Provide consistent caregivers to decrease number of people toddler must adapt to, thereby increasing child's sense of trust. Allow as much movement as possible, using loose restraints only if necessary. Encourage hospital play. Acknowledge child's feelings while providing appropriate means to deal with them. Include familiar toys at bedside. Provide constant reassurance.
Preschool age	Develop initiative and autonomy	Difficulty separating reality from fantasy. Fears unknown. Frightened of bodily injury. Threatened by procedures.	Provide reassurance about healing and getting better. Provide appropriate choices in care. Support family if child engages in regressive behavior. Encourage hospital play for child to act out aggressions; allow child to assume role of nurse or doctor.
School-age	Develop sense of industry and accomplishment	Loss of control produces anxiety. Concerned with privacy and modesty. Fears of bodily mutilation and injury are prevalent.	Tell child what is going to occur. Provide time for explanations about procedures.[a] Repeat explanations frequently. Reduce stimuli. Provide periods of undisturbed sleep. Respect child's privacy. Provide realistic choices that children can make (e.g., do not ask if they want blood drawn, but allow them to choose from which finger or site to have blood drawn).
Adolescent	Develop sense of identity	Fears loss of control. Anxious about loss of identity, separation from peer group. Apprehensive about changes in body image.	Provide privacy to teenager. With teen's approval, facilitate contact with peers. Involve adolescent in decision making. Verify understanding of perceptions of illness, procedures, and hospitalization.[b] Provide time for favorite activities.

[a]Purcell C. Preparation of school-age children and their parents for intensive care following cardiac surgery. *Intensive Crit Care Nurs.* 1996;6:218-225.
[b]Velldtman GR, Matley SL, Kendall L, et al. Illness understanding in children and adolescents with heart disease. *Heart.* 2000;84:395-397.

Preschool children are involved with discovery and initiative.[51] They are egocentric, seeing the world from their viewpoint. The preschool child interprets events in response to good or bad behavior; illness and surgery are therefore seen as punishments.[50] Staff should reassure the child by saying "this is not your fault." Strategies to promote preschoolers' sense of psychologic well-being include preparing them for procedures shortly before carrying them out; explaining who you are, what you are going to do, what the purpose of the procedure is, and what it will feel like, and providing opportunities for them to make choices. Engaging children in therapeutic play allows expressions of aggression and fear.[51] Preschoolers should be given permission to scream or cry during painful procedures and again be assured that what is happening is not their fault.

School-age children are achieving a sense of industry.[47] The socialization process associated with attending school aids in this accomplishment. This is an age when peer approval and acceptance is essential. Interventions guided toward school-age children in the ICU include encouragement of visitors, provision of privacy, and honest explanations regarding procedures, including what will be done, the effects on body parts, and associated pain. The school-age child is inquisitive about the environment and should if possible be protected from scenes involving other patients.

The major developmental task of adolescence is to develop a sense of identity.[52] The importance of body image to the teenager contributes to self-conscious behavior related to appearance and the imperfections imposed by CHD and cardiac surgical repair. Relationships with and acceptance by peers are critical. Privacy is important to the teenager and should be provided in the ICU. Honest communication regarding the physical consequences of surgery, a forum to express fears, and contact with peers during the hospitalization will aid the adolescent patient in recovery after surgery for repair of CHD.

Family-Centered Care

Medical and surgical treatments of CHD are addressed throughout this textbook. The child with CHD must be viewed as an individual, as well as a member of a family unit, whose illness affects all members. Knowledgeable, trusting, calm, and secure parents are the child's best support. Therefore the care of the child must extend to include care of all family members. In addition to delivering high technologic care, the ICU staff must understand and respond to the psychologic needs of the child and family and deliver care to meet those needs.[53] Involving families in the care of children is the underpinning of quality pediatric health care.[54] Parents' participation in the postoperative care of the child in the ICU is an essential part of recovery.

Despite preoperative preparation, the family experiences a wide array of emotions during their first visit to their child in the ICU. This first visit should take place as soon as possible after admission and usually can happen within the first hour after surgery. Ideally, the ICU nurse should greet the family outside the child's room, provide a brief description of the child's appearance, and enter the room with the family. Brief explanations of the use and purpose of each device aid parents' adjustment to the sight of their pale, motionless, seemingly lifeless child surrounded by a maze of monitors, wires, and tubes. The family may be overwhelmed at first by the appearance of their child but should be encouraged and assisted in touching and speaking to the child in an effort to restore their parenting roles. The ICU nurse plays a pivotal role in identifying and alleviating parental fears at this time by encouraging parents to ask questions and express their fears and anxieties. A liberal visiting policy for the parents is crucial.

Parental involvement in the child's care benefits both the child and the parents. The extent of involvement depends on the child's condition. A critically ill child profits from the presence of the family through emotional and physical support. Through touching, holding, talking, and reading, family members provide emotional support. Encouragement by the staff to join in these activities allows the family to take an active role in the child's recovery. Parents may take part in their child's physical care by bathing, dressing, and feeding him or her. Participation in these tasks maintains the parenting role in the ICU setting. Parents' responses to their child's stay in the ICU are influenced by communication with staff members. Honest, current, and accurate communication strengthens the relationship between family and staff. Parental adaptation to their child's ICU admission contributes to the recovery of both child and family.

The impact of CHD on the child and family continues after surgical correction of the lesion. Adjustments must be made to accept the "new" child into the family. A second mourning period often accompanies this change. Families experience grief over the loss of a "perfect" child after the diagnosis of CHD. Difficulties with acceptance of the child after corrective surgery lead to continued overprotection of the child by family members and result in problems of psychologic adjustment and adaptation. Strategies to assist parents during this time include (1) providing information about the child's recovery and restrictions, (2) acknowledgment of the second mourning phase, (3) referral to parent groups, and (4) attention to the family's emotional support.

At first, families may find it difficult to allow the child whom they regarded as ill with cardiac problems before surgical correction

to assume the role of a healthy, normal child. Children are often best able to gauge their own abilities and limitations. Encouraging family members to allow the child to adapt to new or familiar activities is crucial. Most children recover rapidly from heart surgery and are ready to return to active play, day care, or school in just a few weeks. The family's ability to encourage normal activities and to allow the child to participate at his or her own pace will enhance the child's recovery and adjustment after surgical repair of the CHD.

Development of a PCICU Advanced Practice Provider Service

When developing a PCICU advanced practice service, education of the entire PCICU team and hospital leadership should focus on how the addition of these providers can improve patient care delivery and the effect that those improvements have on patient care outcomes and costs. Some studies have shown a decrease in morbidity and mortality, decrease in cost, or decrease in infections associated with the implementation of such a service. Some studies have also demonstrated decreased length of stay with NPs as frontline providers, working in conjunction with physicians.

Beyond the impetus to start such a program, the keys to successful development and implementation of a PCICU APP service are (1) to define the roles of the APPs within the medical team and specific delineation of their responsibilities, (2) to develop clinical practice documents, and (3) to communicate their role and their responsibilities to the entire care team. When developing the clinical practice documents, they should include "role definition, standards of care, educational expectations and career development plans."[6]

Regarding hiring of APPs, the ideal candidate for the PCICU is someone with 3 or more years of prior PCICU nursing experience. It is important to match newly hired providers with a primary advanced practice preceptor and physician mentor for their successful integration into the PCICU. Programs should also include protected off-service time to develop or enhance existing policies and protocols, participate in nursing education, and work with the multidisciplinary team on research and quality improvement projects. Ensuring funding for continuing educational opportunities such as attending, presenting, and ultimately leading academic meetings and/or review courses is important for optimizing patient outcomes and may assist in retention of providers.

A structured educational curriculum is important, both during orientation and for continuing education and refreshers. Use of simulation as an educational tool can increase procedural competency, improve decision-making skills and enhance understanding of important pathophysiology concepts, all while reinforcing teamwork principles.

Conclusion

The addition of APPs to the PCICU team "addresses medical provider shortages while allowing PCICUs to deliver high-quality, cost-effective patient care."[6] Advanced nursing practitioners provide a source of continuity through "consistent clinical presence, effective communication and facilitation of interdisciplinary collaboration."[6] Furthermore, they are important educators of both patient and staff; can facilitate implementation of evidence-based practice, protocols, and quality improvement initiatives; and can perform clinical research in the PCICU, as well as becoming important leaders not only within their institution but also within the nursing community as a whole.

Selected References

A complete list of references is available at ExpertConsult.com.

12. Tucker D, Hazinski MF. The nursing perspective on monitoring hemodynamics and oxygen transport. *Pediatr Crit Care Med.* 2011;12(suppl):S72–S75.

19. Tweddell JS, Hoffman GM. Postoperative management in patients with complex congenital heart disease. *Semin Thorac Cardiovasc Surg Pediatr Card Surg Annu.* 2002;5:187–205.

23. Bronicki RA. Hemodynamic monitoring. *Pediatr Crit Care Med.* 2016;17:S207–S214.

25. Beke DM, Braudis NJ, Lincoln P. Management of the pediatric postoperative cardiac surgery patient. *Crit Care Nurs Clin North Am.* 2005;17(4):405–416.

28. Jones MB, Tucker D. Nursing considerations in pediatric cardiac critical care. *Pediatr Crit Care Med.* 2016;17:S383–S387.

11

Family Needs and Expectations

VALERIE KING, BS; AMY BASKEN, MS; EMILY JOHNSON, MSN, RN, CPNP-PC/AC;
ALISON MILES, DO

When a mother learns that her child has a congenital heart defect, excited anticipation for the promise of the future can transform into fear and uncertainty about how to manage the present. In many cases the mother (as well as the father and other important family members) may move through a cycle of shock, anxiety, fear, anger, worry, blame, and guilt. In our current era, diagnoses are being made earlier in pregnancy and often during the prenatal gestational period. However, there are also numerous times that babies with congenital heart disease (CHD) are born without a prior diagnosis having been made. Regardless, parents can all remember vividly the moment when they were first informed that "something wasn't quite right." They can remember where they were and the time of day when their world spun off its axis.

This chapter is new to this textbook. Two of the contributors are parents of children with CHD, and it is an attempt to help care providers understand the perspectives of the parents of the children they work so hard to care for. As such, it should be stated that we all have enormous respect and love for so many members of the health care units where we have spent some of the most anxious days of our lives. We know that there are dedicated, loving professionals like them all around the world. We simply want to share a little of what we need (in general) and how the members of the cardiac care team might be able to better understand and meet those needs.

Family-Centered Care

In 1999 the Institute of Medicine (IOM) published its now famous monograph *To Err Is Human.* This monograph described the high incidence of medical error leading to death in the United States (predicted to be 100,000 lives lost per year). Some other estimates placed this number (considering errors from omission and not simply from commission) as high as 225,000 lives per year. In their next publication, *Crossing the Quality Chasm,* the IOM suggested six important domains for improved health care, including patient (family)-centered care (in addition to care that is safe, equitable, efficient, timely, and effective). Family-centered care is based on "understanding that the family is the child's primary source of strength and support and that the child's and family's perspectives and information are important in clinical decision making."[1] The family-centered care model is founded on the premise that unlimited presence and involvement of family members in care will optimize outcomes for the child, family, and institution.[2]

According to Ames et al.,[3] parents of children in the intensive care unit (ICU) had three main priorities: "(1) being present and participating in the child's care; (2) forming a partnership of trust with the PICU health care team; and (3) being informed of the child's progress and treatment plan as the person who 'knows' the child best." This can be challenging for numerous reasons, as McDonald et al. demonstrated when they examined the experiences of parents with children admitted to the ICU. The themes that emerged in their study were (1) the transformation from parent and child to visitor and patient, and (2) routines and habits of ICU care that impeded the care a child received from being experienced by the parents as truly family centered. Issues that interfered with care included limitations on visitors allowed, high noise levels, concerns about privacy, and others. These authors concluded that there is a divergence between the priorities of the family members of sick children and those of the staff caring for them, and that this can compromise the delivery of family-centered care.[4]

Effective communication is also essential to building trust with families, and without trust in the medical team, family-centered care cannot exist. A study of pediatric intensive care unit (PICU) parent opinions regarding factors that increased trust identified "good" communication as communication that is honest, inclusive, compassionate, clear, comprehensive, and coordinated.[5] Parents must be incorporated into the health care team as collaborators and advisors, and they prefer a model of open communication and shared decision making.[6]

Intake

Parents who get a prenatal diagnosis of CHD have time to read. Often they have surfed the Internet, and some parents can become well educated about their child's condition. In fact, they may be more familiar (though less educated) with the diagnosis, treatment options, and outcomes than some of the care providers in the ICU. In many cases they have had time to discuss concerns with their cardiologist and surgeon before the baby's birth. Compared to families without a prenatal diagnosis, they are generally better prepared for the hospitalization, except for the fact that all the information and education available is not really a preparation for the reality of the experience. Nothing can prepare a family for that. So, expect that even the most educated, prepared, and intelligent parents will be in shock—a bit numbed, overwhelmed, and scared. That is the best scenario a care provider can hope for when first meeting a family member. For parents who are not prepared by prenatal conversations and for whom the diagnosis of CHD is a surprise, expect to get them early in the cycle of shock. Regardless, it is essential for the cardiac care team to know that in addition to treating a baby with CHD, they will also need to learn how to connect with the family, because no matter how good the care team is, they will need to cultivate a relationship with the family that engenders trust, collaboration, and transparency. This chapter will describe ways that health care professionals, often untrained in these relational matters, can become a better resource and support for families in this regard.

The first thing that the cardiac care team can do is simply connect with the family members. Let them know who the members of the team are, what roles they will play in the child's care, and what the ICU policies are regarding visitation, rounds, and organized family conferences. Although this is often done by the nursing staff, it is valuable for the ICU physician, after the baby has been stabilized, to meet with the family and provide them with an update on their child's condition, as well as a general agenda for what the team sees transpiring over the ensuing 24 to 36 hours.

Our initial advice to the care team members here is to take a breath, slow down, and center themselves so that they can engage with parents in a genuine and connecting manner. Although this comes easier for some than for others, it is very reassuring to families to know that they are in an environment that appreciates that their lives at that moment in time are no longer "normal" and that they have educated and caring "partners" in the experience. Pay attention to the family dynamics, because they are different for all families. As discussed in Chapter 9, try to recognize your own implicit biases and the stories that you might be telling yourself about the family based on unconscious stereotyping. Listening takes an enormous amount of energy, discipline, and attention. But good, careful listening is critical. If you approach the family in the mode of "telling" as opposed to connecting, they are liable to tune out and not take in the full conversation. It is vital to first take in to account the family's own emotional, intellectual/educational, and resourced state. Some families may simply want overarching reassurances without the need (at this time) for a lot of details. Others may want to know as much detailed information as possible. Do not beat families to a pulp with data if they are not in a space to hear it, but be prepared to answer insightful questions with accurate data regarding your own experience, your institution's experience, and the regional/national experience with patients who have similar problems. Do your homework, be prepared, and more importantly, connect. At the initial intake, it may be sufficient to simply connect with families and let them know that you will be a resource to them all along the way.

Health care providers are trained to "fix" things. They are trained to "know" and to "act." There will be numerous opportunities for you to do this during the child's hospital course. However, listening does not require action. It does not require "knowing." It requires that you simply become a "witness," a calm container that the family can simply fill with worry and concern that you will willingly hold for them. That is much more difficult than determining what pharmacologic agent to use to treat hypotension. Pay attention to nonverbal cues—facial expressions, body position, and dynamics between mother and father (and other family members)—to determine how receptive they are to information or to "who's in charge" or whether there are some important tensions that need to be communicated to the rest of the health care team. Most importantly, simply listening to the family, connecting with them in a meaningful way, and acknowledging their fears and anxieties (without having to say or do anything to make those fears go away—because they will not—simply providing compassionate understanding that they exist) goes a long way to establishing trust—and you will need that as the hospitalization continues.

Be aware, too, that the family is likely undergoing stress beyond the diagnosis of the congenital heart defect. They may have financial concerns. Treatment of a congenital heart defect is not planned in most people's budgets. They may have guilt ("What did I do, or not do, to cause this?"). Sometimes, family members overtly blame one another. This is simply a manifestation of great stress and shame. You can simply be a witness to it and let them know that they did not cause this. There may be issues relating to the care of other family members such as siblings who will still need to be cared for at home. There may be stress (and guilt) related to the father needing to still go to work (meaning he will be absent sometimes—and how is this perceived by the mother and/or care team). Mothers may have postpartum issues (and may even not be present for the initial intake—in which case it is very valuable for someone from the team to call them and keep them informed). All family members may have the stress of the situation exacerbated by sleep deprivation or inconsistent eating. Asking a family if they need any water or food is a nice consideration.

Use simple language, and repeat yourself. From our own experiences, families are not totally attentive during the initial meetings. They have so many distractors in their lives, and so much of what is happening is simply new and overwhelming. You may think you have presented a very organized, comprehensive, and accurate explanation of their child's problems and upcoming treatment plans, only to learn that they have hardly "heard" or processed a word you have said. They may simply want reassurance that they are in a good place and they will have skilled people caring for their child.

Families are also trying to process a lot of fears. They have grief from the loss of the dream of having a healthy child. They are now scared that their child might die or be disabled. They know there is nothing you can say to guarantee that this will not be the case. If there were, we would tell you what to say. If you can help reassure them that they are in a safe and caring environment, you can initiate the development of the relationship that you will need to have with each other to cultivate the kind of shared decision making that helps empower the family to be an advocate for their child's care and that will likely contribute to overall best outcomes.

It may be that the patient first comes to the ICU following a surgical procedure, and this is the first time many of the ICU staff have met the family. This underscores how helpful it is, whenever possible (such as during a prenatal visit when there is a prenatal diagnosis), to have the family "tour" the ICU and hopefully briefly meet some of the staff (nurses and physicians). Even when different nurses and physicians are in the ICU when the family tours, the family can establish an initial sense of safety and trust if the ICU staff takes a few moments to engage with them and connect to them. When their child arrives in the ICU following surgery, most of what was described earlier cascades over the family—fear, anxiety, guilt. They see their child with tubes and lines and often looking critically ill, and they have lost all control. They are vulnerable. A pre meeting and tour can be extremely valuable.

Settling In

After the initial intake the child will now be in the ICU getting stabilized, readied for treatment, or recovering from a procedure. This might be the time to begin transforming the family into members of the medical team. If the ICU has an open visitation policy (most ICUs today have open visitation), the family will likely be around and quickly adapting to the ICU culture. They will learn when rounds occur, and they will be developing relationships. It is helpful for the family to have the same nurse as much as possible, and most ICUs try to provide this. From a family perspective, the nurse becomes a valuable, knowledgeable liaison and partner who knows the "language" and who will advocate for them. In today's care models, families are (or should be) invited to participate in formal rounds, meaning it is helpful for rounds to occur at the same time each day or for the family to be informed when this schedule might be altered. It is easy to imagine how overwhelming it can be for parents to be confronted with a large group of medical providers wheeling computers, speaking in medical jargon, and rattling off numbers and phrases they do not understand. For rounds to be useful for family members, it is essential that time is taken to summarize and explain, and that the families leave rounds with a true understanding of the assessment and plan for the day. Additionally, it may not be possible for family members to be present at bedside rounds because these occur during working hours. Parents need clear communication—both the absence of medical jargon and an explanation in layman's terms afterwards—as well as transparency from their providers, even if the information that is to be provided is perceived as bad news. Parents also frequently ask for preparation from the team and for anything they can do to help inform themselves. They expect the team members on rounds to know all of the details about their child and often cite team turnover, with new, less preferred or informed team members, as a frustration. Additionally, families often express that they would like the opportunity to prepare themselves for rounds, with some suggesting consistent daily rounding time and a handout or protocol that defines the purpose of rounds and roles of the participating staff members, as well as the expectations for parent participation.

This means that today's health care professionals need to learn how to round in a way that communicates information and allows for vital information to come forward and to make plans in a way that involves the family and that represents the functionality of the team. In particular, at the end of the rounding process, please ask the family if they have questions. Did they understand what was said? Do they feel that their concerns have been addressed? It is helpful to ask them what they "heard" and what they are expecting to see happen in the next day. It is damaging to trust for the rounding team to rush over to the next patient without connecting with and engaging with the family. If the family's needs are considerable and require more time than the rounding team has, it is reasonable either to leave a team member behind to address these or to tell the family that you will circle back to them within a reasonably short time frame. (And make it a short time frame because what the family is really saying is, "We're anxious and worried or confused and just need to have someone talk with us.") The longer you make them sit with worry, anxiety, and concern or confusion, the more you erode trust in a very vulnerable population.

It is important for the person directing rounds to demonstrate how the team functions with adversity or stress—this is the time to model composure. It is extremely damaging to ask questions of team members that show how little they know and how smart the rounding attending is—this simply creates shame in the person who does not know the answer and consternation for the family that their care providers do not know what they need to in order to care for their child. It is equally damaging to be unprofessional (irrelevant joking—particularly sarcasm, making disparaging comments about other team members/consultants), or to be dismissive of the contributions of other team members. There is a lot written in leadership circles about how to create a resonant environment that engenders a feeling of safety and trust (see Chapter 1), and it is critical for team leaders to adapt to this changing culture. When a team leader needs to say direct things to team members that might not be well perceived by the family, this should be done in a more private setting so as not to diminish or devalue critical personnel in the eyes of the family. If the ICU leader creates a collaborative, inviting, and supportive/productive rounding culture, the family will feel that much more confident that they are in good hands. It is not helpful to anyone, particularly to parents and to other staff, for the physicians to demean each other (such as the surgeons criticizing the intensivists, or the intensivists demeaning the cardiologists).

Rounding is also a time for other important members of the ICU team such as social workers, chaplains, care navigators, or concierges to identify specific needs for their services, and they can use these rounds to seize upon these windows into the family to circle back and provide needed services. Be cognizant not just to what the family says, but also to what they do not say. Be present and mindful.

As the child proceeds through his or her care, a number of issues might present, and these need to be addressed. Families have a huge need for information. Some simply want to know that everything is okay. Others want details. Disruptions in expectations, such as a complication or poor response to therapy, can lead to an increase in anxiety, worry, and fear. This might be manifested in a variety of ways, and it is helpful for the care team to be attuned to this. Often the physicians are informed by the nursing staff that the family has several concerns or desires more communication, and a multidisciplinary care conference is scheduled. The IOM 2001 recommendations regarding shared decision making led to the American College of Critical Care Medicine (2004–2005) task force's recommendation that family conferences occur regularly. An additional recommendation was that family conferences including all pertinent members of the multidisciplinary team happen within 24 to 48 hours of ICU admission and recur "as dictated by the condition of the patient."[7] These conferences are very important to families. This is the time that families will be attentive to information and data, so come to these conferences prepared.

Numerous studies have addressed family conferences in the ICU, although a large proportion has focused on discussions regarding end-of-life decision making. Data on family conferences not exclusively involving end-of-life care are less common. One study found that within 24 hours of the occurrence of a conference during which a treatment was discussed, a treatment decision was made 42% of the time. When discussions involving withholding or withdrawing life-sustaining therapies occurred, a decision was made (again within 24 hours) 58% of the time. Meetings held in conference rooms were more likely to involve both parents and "clinical support members." Disturbingly, though perhaps not unexpectedly given physician turnover (often, attending physicians switch weekly) and the fact that many ICUs follow a shift-work model, the majority of family conferences involved an ICU attending physician who did not have a previously established relationship with the child's parents.[8]

A 2010 study interviewed 122 English-speaking parents of 96 children who were not at risk for imminent death admitted for at least 48 hours to a single, university-based ICU. Overwhelmingly, the parents cited communication as most important in building trust between themselves and health care providers. Honesty, compassion, explanations for care decisions, including parents in decision making, and cohesiveness among the health care team were noted as parental needs in communication from their providers.

When questioned on barriers to communication, parents in this study most often stated that they were fearful of expressing concerns so as not to be perceived negatively by the health care team. Barriers to building trust included lack of continuity of care among providers and lack of understanding of different provider roles.[5]

There is a difference between being "involved" with the child's care and being "engaged" with the family. A family conference helps create the engagement. It not only clarifies communication (for both the medical staff and the family), but it creates the process for shared decision making while honoring the family's culture, needs, hopes, and expectations. Family conferences empower the family to advocate for their child and become members of the health care team. The engagement that emanates provides the family with resources (information, dialogue, a sense of being heard and empowered) to help them collaborate in the process of caring for their child. These conferences also help the health care team learn what resources the family might need, including support for their physical and emotional needs, financial support, theological guidance, social networking, information or research pertinent to their child's convalescence, or even simply a chance to talk. Do not undervalue the need of the family, especially during prolonged hospitalizations, to simply have a chance to talk, vent, or ask questions to a receptive group of multidisciplinary team members. Creating frequent, short, focused meetings is a way to indicate to the family that their concerns matter. Performed artfully, these offer opportunities to teach the family, providing them with information tailored as much as possible to the individual learner. These considerations in teaching need to include race, ethnicity, educational background, stress level (considering the current status of the child), and even learning style. As the team becomes familiar with the family, these meetings can become a wonderful source of information sharing that will help the family better understand what the health care team is trying to accomplish.

Often family conferences are used to convey medical information, make recommendations, and/or make treatment decisions. Generally the medical team members enter these conferences with an agenda that has been shared among the provider participants. It is less common for that agenda to be discussed in advance with the family members attending the conference. There are recommendations in the literature regarding structure and organization of family conferences as well as location (conference room versus bedside) but a paucity of literature regarding families' perceptions and needs.

We advocate for guided participation for families, including joint agendas made in advance. Depending on the circumstance, families may have well-organized thoughts and questions, or they may require assistance in verbalizing their priorities for the conference. In either situation, the medical team, as well as liaisons such as social workers, chaplains, and patient advocates, as appropriate, can help family members formulate a plan and manage expectations, thus promoting a more productive meeting for all involved.[9,10]

Finally, it is incumbent upon the health care team to meet before these conferences so that they can clear up any disagreements and present a unified, agreed-upon message to the family. Disagreements between team members should not be worked out in front of the family—nothing can do more to erode trust and increase anxiety. It is also valuable for the health care team professionals to exhibit humility and compassion as opposed to arrogance and disdain. This includes openness to differences in culture and beliefs, and it is critical that health care team members have the capacity to try and understand and accept the perspectives and beliefs of others, even when they are (especially when they are) different from their own.

Transparency of Information Sharing

From the perspective of families, transparency from the medical field is essential. They want and have a right to know outcomes before selecting a center/physician(s) to provide care for their child. Additionally, families should be made aware of significant differences in opinions among their medical providers, so that they can weigh these opinions when making decisions. Finally, it is imperative that families be made aware of medical errors/adverse events when these occur. What qualifies as appropriate transparency when there are differing opinions between medical providers is a difficult question to address and one not well studied. In addressing this issue, it is important to provide transparency while not overwhelming families with options. When faced with difficult or significantly course-altering decisions, it is advisable to seek consensus, both among the current treatment team members and the wider group. If consensus, or at least a majority opinion, cannot be reached, engaging outside experts for a second opinion may be appropriate. If, despite all efforts to come to consensus, significant differences in opinion remain, this should be honestly presented to the family, with clearly delineated reasons for the differences.

Transparency in reporting adverse events, both to colleagues and the institution as well as to patients and/or families, is a key component of patient safety and family-centered care. Unfortunately, providers may be reticent about making these disclosures, fearing professional or legal ramifications. Numerous studies have shown that adverse events are underreported in the medical field. Considering that 44% of adverse events are potentially preventable, transparency regarding these events is essential to promoting learning and improvement in patient safety.[11]

A 2014 literature review explored barriers to physician reporting of adverse events and, unsurprisingly, found the issue to be complex and multifactorial. The authors categorized the barriers as intrapersonal, interpersonal, institutional, and societal.

Intrapersonal barriers cited include (1) failure of the medical training system to focus on developing good moral character (rather focusing on technical skills), (2) lack of whistle-blowing among physicians secondary to perceptions that it is not an individual's responsibility to report his or her colleagues' mistakes, (3) fear of questioning those in authority about ethical concerns, and (4) fear of personal failure/failing in front of junior colleagues.

Interpersonal barriers included (1) physician-patient communication and (2) peer relations. Although physicians may fear disclosure of adverse events due to concern for litigation, patients are more likely to sue when they perceive the physician to have communicated poorly or covered up an adverse outcome. Additionally, some patients may have unrealistic expectations of their treatment plan, making realistic discussions at the onset of the physician-patient relationship imperative. Further complicating the matter is that physicians are hesitant to report colleagues' errors in the name of preserving friendships and workplace harmony.

Institutional barriers noted were health care culture and policies. In the past, attorneys, insurance companies, and hospital administrators have advised health care providers not to apologize for medical errors because this could be used against them as evidence of malpractice. Research shows that physicians' willingness to report adverse events increases when they believe that this will not lead to punishment or retaliation from supervisors or peers. Additionally, studies have found that physicians are unsure about how to report mistakes, suggesting that clear guidelines would improve transparency.

Societal barriers revolved around the current medicolegal environment. Mandatory error-reporting laws for physicians have been in place in many states since 2007 but have not contributed to a significant improvement in error trends for numerous reasons. More recently, 36 states have also enacted "apology laws," which allow physicians to express to patients their regret for errors, and in some cases admit responsibility, without having these statements later used against them in court. The goal of these laws is to encourage good physician-patient communication around the topic of medical errors while decreasing medical malpractice cases, though research on outcomes is lacking.[12]

A survey-based study published in 2015 examined the attitudes of over 3800 physicians in the United States and Canada regarding transparency in reporting errors to patients, peers, and institutions. Predictors of support for transparency in all three domains included beliefs that reporting errors would decrease the chance of litigation, and that meaningful change would come as a result of error reporting. Support for transparency with patients was increased in physicians who had previous experience with disclosure of a serious error and decreased in those who believed that such disclosure would decrease patient trust. Finally, support for transparency with peers/institution was associated with having been previously educated regarding disclosure of errors.[13]

Overall, these themes indicate that fear is a major contributor to physicians' lack of transparency regarding medical errors. Improvements in physician education starting in medical school and continuing through training and beyond regarding the importance of disclosure, methods by which to do so, as well as nonpunitive systems within institutions are essential to fostering the culture change that is needed.

Anticipatory Guidance

Just as their counterparts with healthy hearts, the needs of children with CHD change as they grow and develop with age. Barring no catastrophic events or genetic syndromes, the intelligence quotient in children with CHD is relatively well preserved; however, the increased risk of socioemotional, cognitive, and academic problems in children and adolescents with CHD is well documented.[14] Variability in outcomes is tremendous across the pediatric years, with subtle to severe concerns. However, school-age children with complex CHD experience more problems with executive functioning than their peers with healthy hearts, with executive functioning being defined as broadly encompassing two main components: behavior regulation (control of emotional and behavioral impulses) and metacognition (planning, organization, self-monitoring, initiation, and follow-through).[15] Clinicians need to assess how these neurodevelopmental comorbidities affect aspects of everyday life. Matching children and families with available support services, such as early intervention, speech/language, tutoring, and other behavioral health programs should be prioritized.

For adolescents and young adults, transitioning to adult care providers is likely one of the most critical steps to occur during this developmental stage.[16-18] Transitioning is a documented stressor for patients, families, and health care providers.[19-21] In adult medicine, young adults are responsible for making their own medical decisions with little consideration for the psychosocial factors that influenced their relationships with their pediatric providers, such as patterns of family decision making, adjustments to their condition, and cognitive and verbal abilities. Moreover, as adolescents transition into adult medicine, the approach to care is even more specialty focused rather than holistic or individualized, thus making symptom management, care coordination, and quality-of-life decision making more difficult.[22]

Professional organizations such as the American Academy of Pediatrics, American Academy of Family Physicians, and American College of Physicians have emphasized the need for greater support for children with chronic health conditions as they transition to adult care providers; however, few strides have been made in this area over the last decade.[23] According to Gurvitz et al. (2013),[24] lapses in care are unfortunately common in the adult CHD population, with percentages as high as 50% to 70% being reported. Mild disease was associated with higher rates of gaps in care; however, over one-fourth of patients surveyed with severe CHD disease experienced a gap of more than 3 years between cardiology appointments.[24] First lapses in care most often occur around 19 years of age, with admissions through the emergency department nearly doubling surrounding this transition.[24,25]

There are currently no published metrics for assessment of transition readiness in this population. For best results, studies suggest starting transition readiness assessments around age 12 years, thus allowing adequate time for information sharing and reassessment; however, the burden of the transitioning experience is not felt until the late adolescent and young adult years.[26,27] Successful transitioning is not solely the responsibility of the individual patient or family; the burden should be shared with the primary care, pediatric cardiology, and other subspecialist teams. To decrease the fragmented care that occurs during the transition to adult medicine, solutions are needed at the patient, family, and health care system levels.

Pediatric palliative care teams are an emerging solution to ease the burden of transitioning on all three levels of care. Although commonly misconceived as applying only to end-of-life care, the primary goal of pediatric palliative care teams is to improve the quality of life for the patient and family through expert management of physical symptoms, care coordination, and psychosocial support throughout the spectrum of disease.[16] Pediatric palliative care teams are experienced in caring for children and young adults with complex medical conditions, and interdisciplinary communication is one of their strengths. Because they routinely facilitate communication between multiple caregivers and different medical teams, pediatric palliative care teams are naturally structured to support patients and families between continuums of care. Involving pediatric palliative care specialists early in the disease trajectory, even at the time of diagnosis, allows for a longitudinal relationship that can follow children with CHD into adulthood and ease the burden of transitioning to adult care.

With the advances in surgical interventions and medical management, children with CHD are living longer; there are now more adults living with CHD than children.[26] With this shift in population demographics, adult patients experience the majority of the mortality associated with CHD. Not all adult cardiologists are equipped to recognize and manage the effects of aging on pediatric-specific physiologies, thus leaving the adult CHD population largely underserved.

Neurodevelopmental challenges continue to affect individuals with CHD throughout their life span, because executive functioning difficulties are also present in adults with CHD. Additionally, a recent study found that visuospatial skills and working memory were worse in adults with CHD compared with the typical population of the same age.[27] Neurologic comorbidities such as stroke and seizure were higher in those with more severe heart disease, and executive functioning was lower in those with neurologic comorbidities. Within the geriatric CDH population, dementia has been reported as the comorbidity affecting older adults with the highest magnitude.[28]

Despite the remarkable advances in management of CHD, 10% of children with CHD die during childhood, and of those who live into adulthood, many die prematurely from advanced myocardial failure.[29] Although the majority of mortality associated with CHD occurs in adult medicine, adult providers struggle with addressing end-of-life needs in this population. One reason is age, because people with end-stage CHD are often younger than people with acquired end-stage heart disease, with the median age of death across all types of CHD remaining under 50 years.[30] Across numerous subspecialties, clinicians find the provision of end-of-life care to be more distressing when caring for younger patients, thus putting this population at risk for receiving overly aggressive treatment at the end of life. Furthermore, as the CHD community lauds significant advances in life-prolonging measures and interventions, it may be difficult to transition to principles of supportive rather than life-prolonging care.[31]

Palliative care specialists are a valuable addition to the care of CHD patients at any age. With standard prenatal ultrasound screenings, CHD allows for earlier involvement with palliative care compared with other specialties, maximizing the opportunity for longitudinal relationships. Many pediatric cardiology programs incorporate palliative care team members as part of their prenatal counseling sessions. Early involvement of palliative care for fetuses or newborns allows palliative care providers to be a source of continuity between the obstetric and pediatric environments, supporting both short- and longer-term decision making. Pediatric palliative care teams can serve as a similar connection between the pediatric and adult environments, allowing for parallel planning in adults with CHD. The absence of palliative care is particularly noticeable in the care of patients with lesions that are traditionally believed to be "cured," like tetralogy of Fallot, in spite of the significant longer-term morbidity and risk of mortality that these patients experience as adults.[31] Because children and adults with CHD frequently encounter clinical scenarios that impact individual and family quality of life, integrating palliative care into standard practice for children and adults with CHD could address some of the unmet needs in this population, including end-of-life planning.

Conclusion

This chapter provides an emphasis for cultivating the relationship with the family as an essential component of the care team for the child with CHD. The processes for engendering trust and for improving communication with families will serve as a mechanism to improve the abilities of most team members to provide outstanding care. Developing courage, a moral compass, compassion (for the self as a learner, as well as for the family as the involuntary recipient of a demanding life event), and willingness to connect to the family while applying knowledge and skill to care for their child, is ultimately the art of the practice of medicine.

References

A complete list of references is available at ExpertConsult.com.

12

Simplified Guide to Understanding the Anatomy of Congenital Heart Disease

KAREN McCARTHY, PHD; RODNEY FRANKLIN, MD; ZDENEK SLAVIK, MD; SIEW YEN HO, PHD

Over 90% of cardiac pathologic conditions in the pediatric population in the developed world are congenital in origin, in that it is present at birth even if undetected until older; in contrast, adult heart disease is largely classified as being acquired. In less developed countries, rheumatic fever is still prevalent. The incidence of congenital heart disease is 6 to 8 per thousand live births (approximately 1 in 130 to 145 live births),[1] whereas at 20 weeks' gestation this figure is 5 to 10 times higher, due to associated lethal chromosomal abnormalities. Approximately 25% of congenital heart lesions can be considered more complex, and one-third will require intervention during infancy. These figures do not include the presence of a bicuspid, nonstenotic aortic valve (2%) or the association of a patent arterial duct in those born prematurely. The incidence of the various lesions is detailed in Table 12.1.

An understanding of the anatomy of congenital cardiovascular malformations is essential for early recognition, diagnosis, and timely management of critically ill pediatric patients. Critical congenital heart defects lead to death in the neonatal period or in early infancy if left untreated. The morphologic characteristics and variations related to these lesions form the basis for understanding the clinical presentation, results of clinical and laboratory assessment, and responses to treatment. Moreover, even relatively simple, well-tolerated, and otherwise benign congenital cardiovascular defects (e.g., muscular ventricular septal defect) may have a profound impact on other organ function and recovery (e.g., the lungs) when an extracardiac organ is adversely affected by another disease (e.g., infection).

Sequential Segmental Approach

Before describing the lesions found within the congenitally malformed heart, it is important to be aware of three fundamental conventions used to describe the components of the normal heart. First, when cardiac chambers are described, the qualifiers *right* and *left* refer only to the morphologic characteristics of the chambers usually designated as being right and left, and not their position in the thorax, as originally proposed by Lev[2] in 1954. If a spatial frame of reference is required, then this first convention mandates that the terms *right-sided, left-sided, anterior,* and *posterior* are used. When dealing with cardiovascular structures other than cardiac chambers, in contrast, *right* and *left* do refer to the spatial position

of these structures within the thorax, and not to their morphologic counterparts. Thus the right superior caval vein (vena cava) refers to the caval vein on the right side of the body.

The second convention, known as the *morphologic method,* states that variable features within the heart should be defined in terms of their own intrinsic morphologic characteristics, and not on the basis of other features that are themselves variable.

The final convention, known as the *segmental approach,* as described by Van Praagh[3] in the early 1970s, is now established as fundamental to imparting the full nature of a cardiac defect, particularly when the malformation is complex and involves multiple cardiac segments. When using this approach, the analyses and descriptions of the malformed heart are made in a logical sequence, permitting the anomalies to be described with precision and in unambiguous fashion. The heart is approached in terms of three major building blocks: the atria, the ventricular mass, and the arterial trunks. There is limited potential for variation in each segment. Segmental analysis therefore depends upon the recognition of the topologic arrangement of the three cardiac segments.

Subsequently, two systems of classification evolved to describe the malformed heart. The sequential segmental variant of the system, emanating from the so-called European School led by Anderson and colleagues in the 1970s,[4,5] combines this morphologic information with the ways in which the segments are joined, or not joined, to each other (Fig. 12.1), and then to their relationships. To avoid ambiguity the system is designed so that each segment can be described according to how it is linked to the subsequent one, while fully describing each segment and the nature of the junctional connections.

The alternative classification system, emanating from the so-called Boston School, uses independent descriptions of three major segments: viscero-atrial situs, ventricular loop and great arterial situs, based originally on embryologic assumptions. Adjacent segments are related to each other by intersegmental alignments, which may not equate to connections.

For the purposes of this chapter, the so-called European approach has been adopted when describing congenital heart malformations. Therefore when describing a malformed heart, particularly when a complex lesion is present, the sequence used begins with the position and orientation of the heart and then follows the flow of blood through the heart in a sequential manner from the great

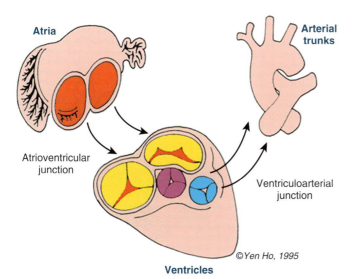

• **Figure 12.1** Diagram showing the three cardiac segments. Sequential segmental analysis requires identification of each of the chambers and great arteries according to morphologic criteria followed by stating how these are connected across the atrioventricular and ventriculoarterial junctions. The location of the heart and its apex are then described, followed by a list of all associated cardiac and vascular defects, such as ventricular septal defect, coarctation, mitral stenosis, or anomalous pulmonary venous connection.

TABLE 12.1	Frequency of Congenital Heart Lesions
Ventricular septal defect	32%
Atrial septal defect	8%
Pulmonary stenosis	7%
Patent arterial duct	7%
Tetralogy of Fallot	5%
Coarctation of the aorta	5%
Transposition of the great arteries	4%
Aortic stenosis	4%
Atrioventricular septal defect	4%
Hypoplastic left heart syndrome	3%
Complex functionally univentricular lesions (double-inlet ventricle, tricuspid or mitral atresia)	3%
Pulmonary atresia with intact ventricular septum	2%
Double-outlet right ventricle	2%
Common arterial trunk	1%
Totally anomalous pulmonary venous connections	1%
Miscellaneous	13%

Data from Hoffman J. Incidence, mortality and natural history. In: Anderson RH, Baker EJ, Macartney FJ, Rigby ML, Shinebourne EA, Tynan M, eds. *Paediatric Cardiology*. Vol 1. 2nd ed. London: Churchill Livingstone; 2005:122-123.

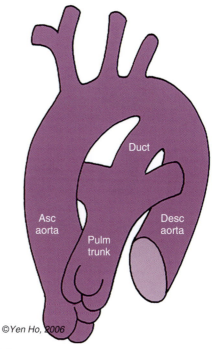

• **Figure 12.2** The arterial duct is the normal fetal channel connecting the bifurcation of the pulmonary *(Pulm)* trunk to the aorta. *Asc,* Ascending; *Desc,* descending.

mediastinal veins to the atria, then ventricles via the atrioventricular (AV) valves, before reaching the arterial trunks via the ventriculoarterial semilunar valves. Additional lesions such as septal defects and arterial obstruction are then described.

From the view of the pediatric cardiac intensivist, this segmental approach allows for structured and reproducible clinical and noninvasive laboratory (x-ray examination, echocardiography, computed tomography, magnetic resonance imaging) assessment of congenital pediatric cardiovascular anomalies. Finding common hemodynamic features and the impact of various anomalies makes their understanding easier and more relevant to the practicing intensivist.

Congenital cardiac lesions can be divided on this basis into:
1. Congenital heart defects with dominant left-to-right shunt, including anomalous pulmonary venous connections
2. Cyanotic congenital heart disease
3. Obstructive congenital heart disease
4. Complex congenital heart disease

Congenital Heart Defects With Dominant Left-to-Right Shunt

Patent Ductus Arteriosus (Patent Arterial Duct)

The ductus arteriosus (arterial duct) joins the pulmonary trunk with the descending aorta. It is part of the normal fetal circulation as it carries most of the blood reaching the pulmonary trunk to the aorta, bypassing the lungs (Fig. 12.2). The direction of blood flow through the patent ductus arteriosus (PDA) reverses postnatally. There is spontaneous ductal closure in most neonates. Patency beyond 1 month of age (3 months in premature infants) is considered abnormal and is common in preterm neonates. The PDA is mostly left sided but right-sided or bilateral PDA can

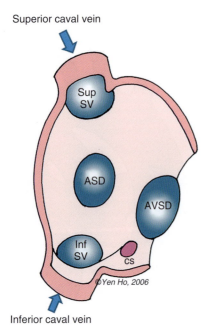

Superior caval vein

Inferior caval vein

• **Figure 12.3** Diagram showing the locations of the various types of interatrial communication. The true atrial septal defect *(ASD)* is at the site of the oval fossa. The superior *(Sup SV)* and inferior sinus venosus *(Inf SV)* defects are at the entrances of the caval veins. The coronary sinus *(cs)* defect is at the site of its orifice. The atrial component of an atrioventricular septal defect *(AVSD)*, also termed *primum ASD*, is classified with other lesions characterized by a coexistent common atrioventricular junction.

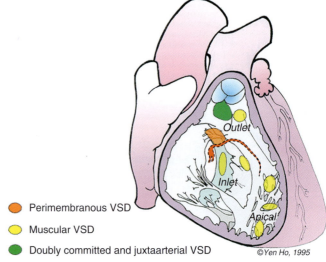

- ● Perimembranous VSD
- ● Muscular VSD
- ● Doubly committed and juxtaarterial VSD

©Yen Ho, 1995

• **Figure 12.4** The normal ventricle has inlet, outlet, and apical trabecular components. The right ventricular surface of the septum is depicted with examples of the morphologic types of ventricular septal defects *(VSDs)* relative to their locations, valves, and the atrioventricular cardiac conduction system *(red shape with broken outline)*.

be present. It is the only source of pulmonary blood supply in some complex congenital heart defects (e.g., pulmonary atresia with intact ventricular septum), but it can be absent in others (e.g., common arterial trunk). The risk of developing pulmonary vascular disease is high if a large PDA is left untreated into childhood.

Interatrial Communications (Including Atrial Septal Defect)

Various parts of the interatrial septum can be affected by defects. Interatrial communications are described according to their developmental locations: *secundum* atrial septal defect (ASD) (within oval fossa and its vicinity), *primum* ASD (part of atrioventricular septal defect [AVSD]; see later discussion), *sinus venosus defect* (superior or inferior adjacent to the orifice of superior or inferior caval vein), or at the coronary sinus (Fig. 12.3). The size of secundum ASDs depends on the extent of deficiency of the fossa valve. Small defects (less than 3 to 4 mm) are often considered part of the spectrum of a patent foramen ovale and often undergo spontaneous closure. Secundum ASDs may be associated with other congenital heart defects (e.g., pulmonary valve stenosis). Transcatheter device closure of larger defects is dependent upon there being sufficient rims for the device to affix to the surround of the defect and size of the defect in relation to size of the patient. A superior sinus venosus defect is commonly associated with partial anomalous pulmonary venous drainage that involves the right upper pulmonary vein joining the superior caval vein (vena cava). The volume of left-to-right shunt depends on the size of the defect and the relative compliance of right and left ventricles. The low kinetic energy of blood reaching the pulmonary arteries makes any increase of

pulmonary vascular resistance associated with isolated ASD in childhood very rare. Large ASDs left untreated until adulthood are associated with risk of atrial dysrhythmias, congestive heart failure (right heart failure), and pulmonary vascular disease and are therefore closed in childhood even in asymptomatic individuals. Paradoxical embolism may occur regardless of ASD size but is rare in children.

Ventricular Septal Defect

The ventricular septal defect (VSD) is the most common congenital heart defect (30%) and can be defined as a hole or pathway between the ventricular chambers. The normal ventricular septum is composed of muscle apart from a very small portion that is a fibrous membrane at the border between the aortic and tricuspid valves. The categorization of VSDs depends on their position relative to this membranous septum and its geographic location with respect to the right ventricular side of the interventricular septum, that is, the ventricular inlet, outlet, or trabecular (apical) portion (Fig. 12.4). *Perimembranous* VSDs have a border that abuts the remnant of the membranous septum, that is, they are situated in a central geographic location and there is atrioventricular valvar and arterial valvar continuity (the aortic and tricuspid valve in the normally connected heart). Of importance is that the conduction system is positioned along the posteroinferior rim of the defect, making it vulnerable to injury during a therapeutic procedure to close such a hole. The VSD in this central perimembranous position may involve the ventricular inlet (perimembranous inlet VSD) or the ventricular outlet (perimembranous outlet) portions of the septum. Perimembranous inlet defects have two independent AV valves and AV junctions and must be distinguished from hearts with a common AV junction and valve with associated AVSD (see later discussion). Perimembranous outlet defects almost invariably are associated with a varying degree of outlet septal malalignment with respect to the trabecular muscular septum, as classically seen in tetralogy of Fallot (TOF), where there is marked anterior septal malalignment and aortic override.

The second group of VSDs is the *muscular defects.* These have exclusively muscular rims around the hole through the ventricular septum and are remote from the major bundles of the cardiac conduction system. They are then further described based on their geographic location within the interventricular septum as opening to the ventricular inlet, outlet, or specific parts of the trabecular portion (midseptal, anterosuperior, posteroinferior, and apical).

When the VSD is in the outlet portion and there is no muscular separation between the aortic and pulmonary valves (absent or purely fibrous outlet septum) such that the valves are in fibrous continuity with each other at the defect's cranial border, this is termed a *doubly committed juxta-arterial* VSD. These may also have perimembranous extension with a fibrous posteroinferior rim, or a muscular posteroinferior rim, which results in some protection to the conduction bundle. Outlet VSDs of all types may have a degree of anterior or posterior malalignment of the outlet septum with respect to the trabecular muscular septum, posterior deviation being associated with aortic arch obstruction, whereas anterior deviation as seen in TOF is associated with right ventricular outlet narrowing or even atresia in extreme cases.

The position of the VSD has implications for spontaneous closure rate (highest in muscular defects) and function of surrounding valves (aortic and pulmonary valvar regurgitation in doubly committed defects, aortic and tricuspid valvar regurgitation associated with perimembranous defects). Multiple defects can be present most often in the muscular part of interventricular septum. The majority of VSDs are small (<3 mm diameter) with a high rate of spontaneous closure, especially in isolated small defects (up to 90% by 6 years of age). The size of the defect is only one factor influencing the volume of left-to-right blood shunting across the defect. The relative right and left ventricular pressure and compliance, and ratio of pulmonary and systemic vascular resistance all play an important role too. The high kinetic energy of blood reaching the pulmonary circulation due to a large left-to-right shunt through the VSD represents a risk for early onset of pulmonary vascular disease, and timely VSD closure (before 2 years of age, or much earlier if associated with other congenital heart lesions such as transposition of the great arteries) is advocated. There is a frequent association with other congenital heart defects (e.g., aortic coarctation), or the defect is an integral part of more complex congenital cardiac malformation (e.g., TOF, functionally univentricular heart). There is a significant risk of infective endocarditis in association with small VSDs.

Atrioventricular Septal Defect (Atrioventricular Canal Defect)

The AVSD is characterized by a common AV junction owing to a lack of division of the embryonic AV canal into separate left and right parts together with a failure of fusion between the downgrowing atrial septum and the up-growing ventricular septum. The valve guarding the common AV junction can have a common valvar orifice guarded by five leaflets, inclusive of superior and inferior bridging leaflets that have commitment to both ventricles, or discrete left and right orifices that are separated by conjoined leaflet tissues (Fig. 12.5). In the latter variant, there are three leaflets in the left-sided valve. AVSDs are usually associated with near equal commitment of each AV valve to each ventricle with equal ventricular sizes (AVSD with balanced ventricles), or there may be ventricular imbalance with relative hypoplasia of either ventricle, which may be so severe as to result in a functionally univentricular circulation.

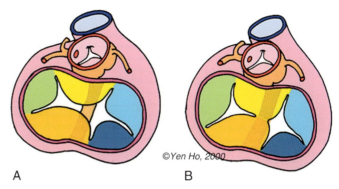

©Yen Ho, 2000

A   B

• **Figure 12.5** In atrioventricular septal defect the common atrioventricular junction is guarded by a five-leaflet valve that has a common orifice (A). Fusion of the opposing inferior *(orange)* and superior *(yellow)* bridging leaflets separates the common orifice into discrete left and right orifices (B). The left atrioventricular valve has three leaflets, the left mural leaflet *(green)* and the two bridging leaflets, whose zone of apposition is often termed the *cleft,* and it is this that is partially closed during surgical repair.

In the *complete form* of AVSD there is deficiency of both the interatrial septum and the interventricular septum resulting in a lack of septal apposition at the AV junction with a common valvar orifice allowing shunts at atrial and unrestrictive flow at ventricular levels (see Fig. 12.5). Associated dysplasia or hypoplasia of leaflets can give rise to valvar regurgitation. The *partial form* affects either the interatrial or the interventricular septum. In cases in which there are separate valvar orifices and the conjoined bridging leaflets are adherent to the crest of the ventricular septum, there is potential for atrial shunting only, in other words, of persistence of the ostium primum (primum ASD). When the conjoined bridging leaflets are adherent to the atrial septum, there is potential for ventricular shunting only (AVSD with isolated ventricular component). A third variant is recognized, particularly in North America, in which there is an interatrial communication immediately above the AV valve and a restrictive interventricular communication immediately below the AV valve (intermediate [or transitional] AVSD).

The complete form of defect is often associated with trisomy 21 in two-thirds of cases (33% of those with trisomy 21 have a complete AVSD), and it can lead to early development of pulmonary vascular disease in these patients. Surgical repair is therefore usually undertaken at 3 to 6 months of age. AVSD is also strongly associated with left and right atrial isomerism (heterotaxy) and may be associated with TOF (also most commonly seen in trisomy 21).

Common Arterial Trunk (Also Known as Persistent Truncus Arteriosus)

The common arterial trunk (CAT) is a solitary arterial trunk that arises from the heart with a single arterial semilunar truncal valve to continue into both the ascending aorta and the pulmonary trunk or separate right and left pulmonary arteries (Fig. 12.6). The truncal valve has a variable number of leaflets that may be dysplastic. It usually overrides a VSD, allowing the CAT to receive blood from both the left and right ventricles. Stenosis and/or regurgitation of the truncal valve is not rare. The origin of the pulmonary arteries from the common trunk varies[6]: the pulmonary trunk arises from the CAT and then divides into the left and right pulmonary arteries (Type I); the left and right pulmonary arteries arise close together from the left-posterior aspect of the CAT (Type II); or the pulmonary arteries are well separated and arise from

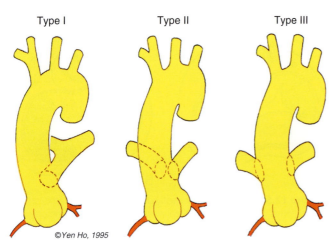

• **Figure 12.6** Three variants of common arterial trunk as explained in the text, based on the classification by Collet and Edwards (1949).[6]

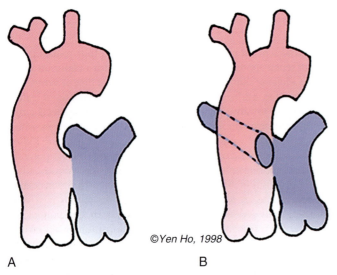

• **Figure 12.7** Aortopulmonary window with normal origin of the right pulmonary artery (A) and a distally situated window with abnormal origin of the right pulmonary artery (B).

the lateral walls of the common trunk (Type III). In addition, CAT may be classified as having aortic dominance, without aortic arch obstruction, or having pulmonary dominance with associated aortic interruption or coarctation (approximately 15%).

The arterial duct is usually absent. The large volume of pulmonary blood flow leads to early-onset congestive heart failure, and the high kinetic energy of blood reaching pulmonary arterioles causes early pulmonary vascular disease in untreated patients. Cyanosis is typically mild but may be more significant in the presence of reduced pulmonary blood flow due to high pulmonary vascular resistance or pulmonary arterial stenoses. There is a strong association of CAT with chromosome 22q11 microdeletion, especially if associated with aortic arch obstruction (e.g., interrupted aortic arch).

Aortopulmonary Window

Direct communication through an opening between the adjoining walls of the ascending aorta and the pulmonary trunk is the hallmark of the aortopulmonary window (Fig. 12.7). Unlike the CAT, there

are separate aortic and pulmonary valves. In most cases the window is large and extends distally to the level of the pulmonary bifurcation with the right pulmonary artery arising from the posterior wall of the aorta. Free transmission of aortic blood pressure into pulmonary arteries represents a high risk of early onset of pulmonary vascular disease.

Partially or Totally Anomalous Pulmonary Venous Connection

The partial variety (partially anomalous pulmonary venous connection [PAPVC]) involves one or more (not all) of the pulmonary veins connecting directly to the right atrium, the superior or inferior caval vein, the coronary sinus, or the brachiocephalic vein, allowing some pulmonary venous blood to drain into the systemic venous system. The partial variety involving the right upper pulmonary vein and the superior caval vein (vena cava) is often associated with a superior sinus venosus defect. PAPVC to the inferior caval vein may also be associated with right (usually) or left lung and bronchial anomalies and dextrocardia, when the combination is known as scimitar syndrome.

In totally anomalous pulmonary venous connection (TAPVC), none of the pulmonary veins connect to the left atrium. Systemic blood flow is dependent upon an interatrial communication (ASD), and the shunt is from *right to left.* The pulmonary veins emerging from the lungs usually merge into a pulmonary venous confluence, which then connects to the right atrium or, more commonly, connects to a systemic venous channel such as the superior or inferior caval vein, brachiocephalic vein, or coronary sinus. Depending on the site of anomalous connection, the TAPVC can be categorized as *supracardiac* (into the brachiocephalic vein or superior caval vein via an ascending vein), *cardiac* (directly into coronary sinus or right atrium), and *infracardiac* (into hepatic or portal veins via a descending vein) (Fig. 12.8). More rarely and most difficult to surgically repair, there may be TAPVC of a mixed type with anomalous connections at more than one level. Narrowing in the pulmonary venous channel is mainly found in the supracardiac, and almost invariably in the infracardiac, form and leads to severe pulmonary hypertension and right ventricular failure presenting soon after birth, requiring urgent surgery with a high risk of postoperative pulmonary hypertensive crises. This latter may be worsened by any residual postoperative defects causing a significant left-to-right shunt due to associated early postoperative reperfusion injury related to myocardial and lung functional impairment.

Unobstructed TAPVC presents with signs and symptoms of mild cyanosis with congestive heart failure due to high pulmonary blood flow, and it is the severity of these symptoms, including failure to thrive and frequent chest infections, that influences the timing of surgery. TAPVC is without exception seen in right atrial isomerism (heterotaxy), and in this setting may also be associated with pulmonary atresia.

Cyanotic Congenital Heart Disease

Tetralogy of Fallot

TOF is the most common cyanotic congenital heart defect. Its four features are a *VSD with overriding aorta, muscular right ventricular outflow tract obstruction,* and *right ventricular hypertrophy* (Fig. 12.9). Malalignment of the outlet septum in a cephalad and anterior direction within the right ventricle is the anatomic substrate

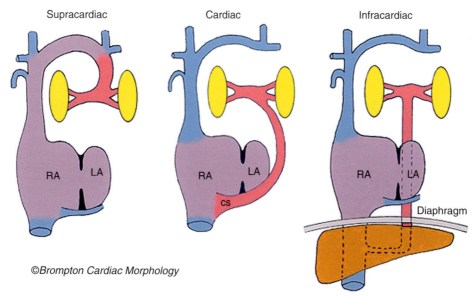

Supracardiac   Cardiac   Infracardiac

RA   LA   RA   LA   RA   LA

CS

Diaphragm

©Brompton Cardiac Morphology

• **Figure 12.8** Examples of the different types of totally anomalous pulmonary venous connections. The pulmonary veins from the lungs (*yellow ovals*) join at a confluence, and the common vein connects anomalously to a systemic vein at three potential levels. *cs,* Coronary sinus; *LA,* left atrium; *RA,* right atrium. (Copyright Brompton Cardiac Morphology.)

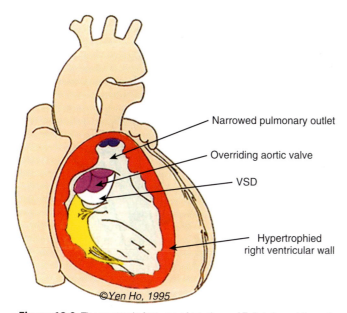

Narrowed pulmonary outlet

Overriding aortic valve

VSD

Hypertrophied right ventricular wall

©Yen Ho, 1995

• **Figure 12.9** The anatomic features of tetralogy of Fallot viewed through an opening into the right ventricle. *VSD,* Ventricular septal defect.

for muscular subvalvar pulmonary stenosis. The VSD is usually large, and right ventricular pressure overload results in hypertrophy of the right ventricular wall. Some degree of pulmonary valvar and arterial hypoplasia may be present. Pulmonary stenosis ranges from the mild form, so-called pink Fallot, to more severe associated with increasingly severe central cyanosis. Its severest form may involve pulmonary atresia with neonatal ductal dependency (left-to-right flow) and variable degrees of central pulmonary arterial hypoplasia or atresia, sometimes with additional systemic-to-pulmonary collateral arteries supplying different segments of the pulmonary circulation. Additional muscular VSD, ASD, AVSD, anomalous origin of the left anterior interventricular (descending)

coronary artery from right coronary artery, and right-sided aortic arch are the most common associated anomalies. TOF may be associated with chromosome 22q11 microdeletion, especially with a right aortic arch.

Another variant is TOF with absent pulmonary valve syndrome, in which the ventriculoarterial junction of the right ventricle with the pulmonary trunk features an atypical valve with absent or rudimentary cusps that do not coapt. In its usual form there is dilation of the pulmonary trunk and central right and left pulmonary arteries, which when extreme, is associated with abnormal arborization of lobar and segmental pulmonary arterial branches, with compression of the trachea and mainstem bronchi, often with tracheobronchomalacia. The physiologic consequence is usually a combination of variable degrees of both stenosis and regurgitation of the pulmonary valve.

It is common to develop significant pulmonary regurgitation, requiring valvar replacement late after surgical repair of TOF in infancy, usually in adolescence or adulthood. A residual VSD is poorly tolerated early postoperatively, contributing to increased right-sided filling pressures, particularly when restrictive right ventricular physiology is present.

Pulmonary Atresia With Intact Ventricular Septum

In pulmonary atresia with intact ventricular septum (PAIVS) there is total occlusion of the right ventricular outflow tract and lack of any interventricular communication. Pulmonary atresia may be due to an imperforate valvar membrane or a blind-ending pulmonary trunk with muscular obliteration of the right ventricular outflow tract. There is a variable degree of right ventricular and tricuspid valvar hypoplasia. A patent arterial duct provides the only source of pulmonary blood flow (Fig. 12.10), coming off the aorta in a reverse angle from usual, corresponding to prenatal flow from aorta into the pulmonary trunk. The pulmonary arteries are usually of normal size. Coronary arterial fistulae connecting with the right

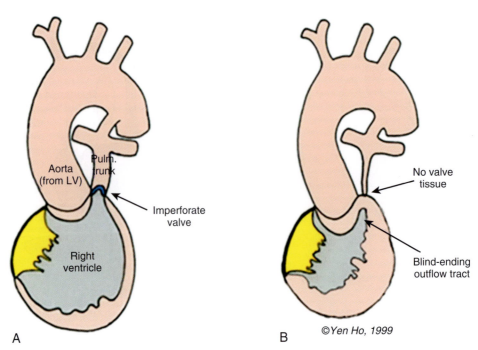

A B

©Yen Ho, 1999

• **Figure 12.10** Variants of pulmonary atresia with intact ventricular septum. The right ventricular outflow tract may be occluded by an imperforate pulmonary valve or by muscle tissue. (A) Valvar or "membranous" atresia. (B) Muscular atresia. *LV,* Left ventricle, *Pulm.,* pulmonary.

ventricular cavity are present in up to one-third of all cases, occurring most commonly in those with a small or diminutive right ventricular cavity. These can be associated with coronary anomalies, including arterial stenoses and a right ventricular dependent coronary circulation such that there is a coronary steal phenomenon and left ventricular myocardial ischemia postnatally. The size of the tricuspid valve, the degree of right ventricular hypoplasia, and the presence of coronary arterial anomalies determine suitability for a biventricular or univentricular repair.

The size of branch pulmonary arteries at birth may influence decision making about the type of initial palliative treatment offered (ductal stenting versus systemic-to-pulmonary arterial shunt). The postoperative course following a postnatal palliative procedure can be complicated by myocardial ischemia in the presence of coronary arterial anomalies. Attention needs to be paid also to the size of the interatrial communication because this may become restrictive with ensuing systemic venous congestion and limitation to systemic cardiac output.

Transposition of Great Arteries

When the atrial chambers are connected to the correct ventricles (concordant AV connections) but the aorta arises from the right ventricle and the pulmonary trunk from the left ventricle (discordant ventriculoarterial connections), there is complete transposition of great arteries (TGA). Consequently, the systemic and pulmonary blood flow are in parallel circuits (Fig. 12.11) instead of the normally configured series circuit. Postnatal survival depends on mixing of blood between the systemic and pulmonary circulations, usually at atrial and arterial ductal level. The size of the native interatrial communication, or that created by a balloon atrial septostomy, does not always correlate with systemic oxygen saturations because the extent of mixing at this level depends on other factors (such as the degree of streaming of venous return across the atrial

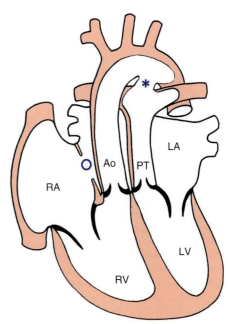

• **Figure 12.11** After birth in transposition of the great arteries, and in the absence of ventricular or atrioventricular septal defects, the systemic and pulmonary blood flows run in parallel circuits. This would be incompatible with life if it were not for an interatrial communication *(circle)* and/or the patency of the arterial duct *(asterisk)*. *Ao,* Aorta; *LA,* left atrium; *LV,* left ventricle; *PT,* pulmonary trunk; *RA,* right atrium; *RV,* right ventricle.

communication; pulmonary vascular resistance—influencing flow to the pulmonary bed; ventricular compliance; and presence of flow from a PDA, to name a few), and oxygen as a pulmonary vasodilator may be helpful. Ventricular septal defect and subvalvar and/or valvar pulmonary stenosis are the most frequently associated cardiac defects. Coronary arterial anatomy varies and is an important consideration for surgical treatment involving the arterial switch and concomitant coronary arterial transfer, particularly if there is a single coronary supplying the whole heart or if there is an intramural proximal coronary arterial course. Coronary arterial anatomy may therefore influence the postoperative course after the arterial switch procedure, leading to a higher risk of myocardial ischemia and myocardial dysfunction.

Obstructive Congenital Heart Defects

Pulmonary Stenosis

The most common cause of pulmonary valvar stenosis is a variable degree of lack of separation of the valvar leaflets. A valve with a dome-shaped "membrane" and central orifice is at the severe end of the spectrum (Fig. 12.12). Thickening of the leaflet edges and dysplasia of the leaflets themselves are less common substrates of stenosis. A bicuspid valve, often associated with TOF, is infrequent in isolation. Mild isolated stenosis rarely progresses. Concomitant presence of right ventricular hypertrophy depends on the hemodynamic significance of stenosis, and severe right ventricular hypertrophy may contribute to subvalvar stenosis. Supravalvar pulmonary stenosis affecting the pulmonary trunk or its branches may occur in isolation or in combination with valvar and subvalvar stenoses, a combination that may be present in TOF (see earlier discussion). Concomitant pulmonary regurgitation is more common in previously treated valves. Pulmonary valvar stenosis, often with pulmonary trunk narrowing, is associated with Noonan syndrome,

which frequently requires surgery because it is resistant to transcatheter pulmonary balloon dilation. Atrial and ventricular septal defects are the most common associated cardiac defects.

Critical neonatal pulmonary stenosis may be associated with hypoplasia of the tricuspid valve and right ventricular cavity, as well as coronary arterial anomalies, in a way similar to pulmonary atresia with intact ventricular septum. These may impact the success of initial treatment intervention (mostly transcatheter balloon dilation) and postprocedural course. Persistent cyanosis following initial intervention is common and may not allow for early discontinuation of prostaglandin treatment due to residual muscular obstruction inside the right ventricular cavity.

Aortic Stenosis

Stenotic aortic valves can be described as unicuspid, bicuspid, or tricuspid depending on the number of functional commissures between the valvar leaflets (Fig. 12.13). Unicuspid valves are usually most severely stenotic. Bicuspid valves, on the other hand, may present without stenosis or regurgitation in childhood and into adult life. Gross dysplasia of valvar cusps has been described in up to 10% of patients with congenital aortic valvar stenosis and are the most difficult to treat effectively either with balloon dilation or surgical repair. Concomitant aortic regurgitation is more common in previously treated valves. Aortic coarctation is the most common associated defect. Any malformed aortic valve is likely to undergo calcification in adulthood.

Congenital supravalvar aortic stenosis is characterized by narrowing of the aorta at the level of the sinotubular junction, which may extend into the ascending aorta. This may be in the form of an hourglass deformity, a fibrous membrane, or a diffuse narrowing of the ascending aorta. It may involve the coronary arterial ostia, along with tethering of the aortic leaflets. It is common in Williams syndrome, when it is often associated with a widespread vasculopathy, including the renal arteries with secondary systemic hypertension.

Congenital subaortic stenosis is associated with narrowing within the outflow tract supporting the aortic valve (left or right ventricular). This may be localized with a fibromuscular ridge extending to the anterior leaflet of the mitral valve or be a diffuse tunnel with circumferential narrowing commencing at annular level and extending downward into the ventricular outflow tract. There are a variety of other causes, including accessory mitral valve tissue with abnormal septal insertion, deviation of the outlet

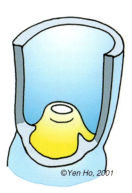

• **Figure 12.12** Diagram of a dome-shaped pulmonary valve.

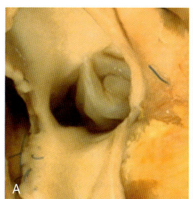
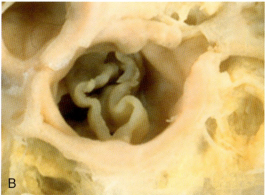
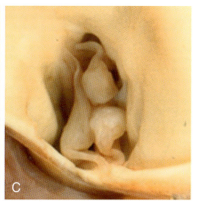

• **Figure 12.13** Variants of aortic valvar morphology. (A) Unicuspid aortic valve with severely stenotic keyhole orifice. (B) Bicuspid aortic valve with redundant leaflets. (C) Tricuspid and stenotic aortic valve with three unequal-sized and thickened leaflets. (Copyright Brompton Cardiac Morphology.)

septum (seen in coarctation of the aorta and interrupted aortic arch), and a restrictive VSD in functionally univentricular hearts with a dominant left ventricle and discordant ventriculoarterial connections.

Critical neonatal aortic stenosis may be associated with hypoplasia of the mitral valve and left ventricular cavity (sometimes forming part of the hypoplastic left heart syndrome spectrum) and endocardial fibroelastosis.

Early postnatal treatment, including initial stabilization and surgical or interventional cardiac catheterization procedures, may be complicated by pulmonary hypertension related to pulmonary arteriolar changes present in the majority of neonates with severe congenital obstructive lesions to the left heart.[7]

Aortic Arch Obstruction: Aortic Coarctation or Interruption

In aortic coarctation the discrete narrowing in the distal part of the aortic arch at the aortic isthmus may be accompanied by a variable degree and extent of aortic arch hypoplasia (Fig. 12.14). The most common site of aortic coarctation is on the aortic wall opposite the orifice of the arterial duct. The discrete coarctation shelf narrowing the aortic lumen may become obvious only when the duct closes after birth, including abnormal ductal tissue encircling the adjacent aorta. Patency of the arterial duct plays an important role in the majority of cases with severe neonatal aortic coarctation, allowing blood flow to reach the lower body (right-to-left shunt). Collateral arteries bridging the narrow aortic segment develop gradually during childhood in untreated patients and are characteristic when presentation occurs in adolescence and beyond, often triggered by the finding of systemic hypertension. Ventricular septal defect, bicuspid aortic valve (25%), and aortic and mitral valve stenoses are the most common associated anomalies, as is Turner syndrome, and there may be associated hypoplastic left heart syndrome. Systemic hypertension due to abnormal arterial wall structure and function and intracranial arterial aneurysms represents a long-term risk, even in successfully treated patients.

In aortic arch interruption a segment of aortic arch is absent or is represented by a fibrous cord. Depending on the location of the missing or atretic aortic arch segment, arch interruption is categorized into type A, interruption distal to the subclavian artery (usually left subclavian); type B (most common), interruption between the common carotid and subclavian arteries; and type C, interruption between the carotid arteries[8] (usually innominate and left carotid), noting that these generic terms take into account the possibility of an aberrant subclavian artery. A PDA with right-to-left shunt is the only source of blood supply for parts of the body distal to the interruption. A VSD is the most common associated heart defect. Typically there is also posterior deviation of the outlet septum into the left ventricle outflow tract, resulting in varying degrees of subaortic stenosis. Chromosome 22q11 microdeletion is strongly linked with type B interruption.

Pulmonary hypertension is present in severe forms of coarctation or aortic arch interruption in most neonates, relating to abnormal pulmonary arteriolar development as found in critical aortic stenosis.

Vascular Rings

The term *vascular ring* refers to a group of congenital vascular anomalies that encircle and compress the esophagus and trachea. The compression may be from a complete anatomic ring (double aortic arch, right aortic arch with pulmonary trunk and left arterial ligamentum, or left aortic arch with pulmonary trunk and right arterial ligament) or from a compressive effect of an aberrant vessel (innominate artery compression syndrome). The final variant is when there is an anomalous origin of left pulmonary artery from right pulmonary artery (pulmonary arterial sling). Esophageal atresia and a degree of tracheobronchial malacia may be present. Classic symptoms are stridor, particularly with chest infections, and occasionally dysphagia.

Complex Congenital Heart Defects

Ebstein Malformation of Tricuspid Valve

This is a tricuspid valve anomaly characterized by apical rotational displacement of the functional annulus, involving the septal and inferior (also called the posterior or mural) leaflets, toward the ventricular apex to variable extents and degrees of severity (Fig. 12.15).

The annular insertion of the anterosuperior leaflet is as normal, at the AV junction, but its distal or free margin is variably malformed, fenestrated, or tethered. All the leaflets of the valve may be larger or smaller than normal, contributing to the failure of all three leaflets to coapt adequately in ventricular systole, which when severe results in bifoliate closure. Consequently, the most frequently encountered hemodynamic abnormality is a variable degree of tricuspid regurgitation. Marked apical displacement of the tricuspid valve orifice limits the size of the right ventricular cavity and may contribute to right ventricular outflow obstruction. An ASD is the most frequently associated anomaly. The wide morphologic and physiologic spectrum of Ebstein malformation influences the clinical presentation, from the asymptomatic child or adolescent presenting with supraventricular tachycardia or mild cyanosis (due to right-to-left interatrial shunt) to the critically ill cyanotic neonate with marked right atrial dilatation affecting development of the right lung and with severe functional or anatomic obstruction to

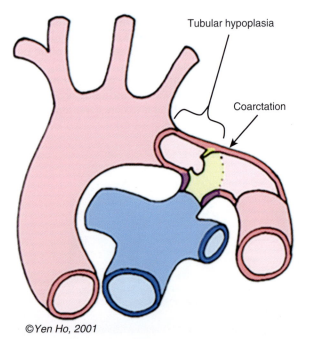

Tubular hypoplasia

Coarctation

©Yen Ho, 2001

• **Figure 12.14** Diagram showing tubular hypoplasia at the isthmus of the aortic arch and a shelf-like discrete coarctation lesion. Ductal tissue is shaded *yellow*.

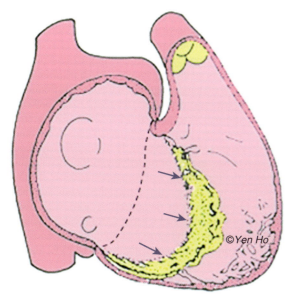

• **Figure 12.15** In Ebstein malformation of the tricuspid valve, the septal and inferior (posterior or mural) leaflets are displaced and rotated *(arrows)* apically and away from their normal level at the atrioventricular junction *(broken line)*.

the RV outflow tract. The association of clinically significant accessory conduction pathways in up to 20% of patients with Ebstein malformation may manifest as supraventricular tachycardia (Wolff-Parkinson-White syndrome) in the fetus, in infancy, or at an older age. Some patients with discordant atrioventricular and ventriculoarterial connections (congenitally corrected transposition) have an Ebstein-like deformity of the left-sided morphologically tricuspid valve.

Functionally Univentricular Hearts

Functionally univentricular hearts refers to a spectrum of congenital cardiac malformations in which the ventricular mass may not readily lend itself to partitioning that would commit one ventricular pump to the systemic circulation and another to the pulmonary circulation. Truly univentricular hearts are very rare. Most often, hearts that are functionally univentricular have one ventricle that is so small (hypoplastic) that the other ventricle, which is considerably larger, has the dominant role in supporting the circulation. Within this group of hearts there is a subgroup that have a *univentricular AV connection* such that both atrial chambers are connected to the dominant ventricle of right, left, or indeterminate morphology (double-inlet AV connection) via two separate, or a common, AV valve(s), or the AV connection on one side is missing (absent right or left AV connection) (Fig. 12.16). There may be a VSD, anomalies of the ventriculoarterial connections and systemic or pulmonary venous connections, and stenosis or atresia of the aortic or pulmonary valve. Right atrial and to lesser extent left atrial isomerism (both atria of the same morphology), also referred to as visceral heterotaxy, are strongly linked with these complex congenital heart defects. Complete intracardiac mixing of pulmonary and systemic venous return leads to a variable degree of cyanosis from birth.

In the other subgroup, each atrium is connected to its own ventricle *(biventricular AV connections)*. A typical example is *hypoplastic left heart syndrome,* in which the left ventricle is hypoplastic and there are variable degrees of associated stenosis, hypoplasia, or atresia of the mitral valve together with stenosis,

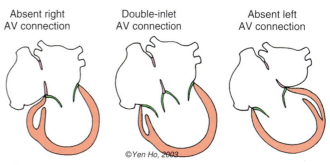

• **Figure 12.16** In hearts with univentricular atrioventricular *(AV)* connection the atrial chambers are connected primarily to one dominant ventricle (double inlet) or there is absence of connection on the right side or the left side, resulting in only one atrium connecting to the dominant ventricle and an absence of connection to the small rudimentary ventricle.

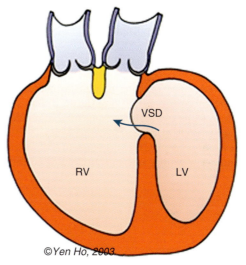

• **Figure 12.17** When both great arteries arise from the right ventricle *(RV)*, the left ventricular outlet is through an interventricular communication (ventricular septal defect *[VSD]*). *LV,* Left ventricle.

hypoplasia, or atresia of the aortic valve. Where the mitral valve is an imperforate membrane (mitral atresia), the circulation is akin to that of absent left AV connection, and the presence of an adequate interatrial communication is vital. The left ventricle is unable to support the systemic circulation postnatally. Systemic arterial blood flow and survival depend on arterial ductal patency (right-to-left shunt). After birth the pulmonary vascular resistance drops, and systemic perfusion (Q_s) decreases due to excessive pulmonary (Q_p) blood flow (increased $Q_p:Q_s$ ratio). The right ventricle sustains both pulmonary and systemic circulation. A severely restrictive interatrial communication at birth is associated with very poor outcome. Associated anatomic anomalies of the central nervous system are common.

Double Outlet Right Ventricle

Double outlet right ventricle (DORV) is a congenital cardiac anomaly in which both the aorta and pulmonary trunk arise from the morphologically right ventricle. Although DORV can exist with any combination of atrial arrangement and AV connection, its most typical form is with usual atrial arrangement and concordant AV connections. The only outlet for the left ventricle is through a VSD (Fig. 12.17), or more correctly termed in this scenario, *interventricular communication.*[9] The relative position of the VSD to the aortic or pulmonary valves determines its classification into four main types, as well as likely associated anomalies and postnatal hemodynamics. A subaortic position of the VSD is more common, and when associated with pulmonary stenosis the hemodynamic situation is similar to TOF and is classified as *Fallot-type DORV.* When the subaortic VSD is not associated with pulmonary stenosis, the physiology is similar to that found in a large perimembranous outlet VSD with pulmonary overcirculation and heart failure; referred to as *VSD-type DORV.* When the VSD is subpulmonary, aortic coarctation is commonly associated, whereas pulmonary stenosis is rare. The physiology in this situation is similar to transposition of the great arteries with VSD, as blood from the left ventricle crosses the VSD into the pulmonary trunk, and the lesion is classified as *transposition-type DORV.* Finally, when the VSD is remote, in the inlet or trabecular muscular septum, this is termed *DORV with noncommitted VSD.* In this scenario, there is no commitment of the VSD to either great artery, and biventricular repair is often not possible.

Conclusion

CHD is the most common congenital malformation, causing up to 10% of infant deaths and 50% of deaths due to a congenital malformation, while extracardiac congenital anomalies are also present in up to 25% of neonates.[10]

Complex and/or severe CHD may present with severe neonatal cyanosis and a low cardiac output state leading to early death if left untreated. The immediate postnatal introduction of a prostaglandin infusion in those neonates with clinical evidence of severe pulmonary or systemic outflow tract or great arterial obstruction is likely to be lifesaving, as well as enabling careful planning of early surgical or transcatheter intervention. Such planning is further facilitated when a prenatal diagnosis is made, as is frequently the case with complex lesions that are relatively easily picked up at routine fetal anomaly screening at 14 to 20 weeks' gestation by obstetric sonographers. However, considerable morbidity and even mortality may follow despite apparently successful early treatment, largely linked to the severity of underlying cardiovascular anatomic or functional malformations and impaired function of other key organ systems, as well as associated extracardiac anomalies. Examples include severe hypoplasia of the ascending aorta with associated coronary artery anomalies and severe tricuspid valve regurgitation in hypoplastic left heart syndrome; and pulmonary venous obstruction with a functionally univentricular heart, TAPVC, and visceral heterotaxy.

A thorough understanding of the complete anatomic substrate related to the patient's specific congenital cardiac lesion and resultant hemodynamic pathophysiology is essential for early recognition, diagnosis, and planning of optimal ICU management of critically ill pediatric patients by the pediatric intensivist, both before and after surgical- and/or catheterization-based interventions

References

A complete list of references is available at ExpertConsult.com.

13

Cardiovascular Physiology for Intensivists

**KARAN R. KUMAR, MD; ROXANNE E. KIRSCH, MD, MBE;
CHRISTOPH P. HORNIK, MD, MPH**

The primary function of the cardiovascular system is to deliver sufficient amounts of oxygen and other nutrients to organs and tissues to meet their metabolic demands. Disruption of this normal cardiovascular function is commonplace in a variety of pediatric critical illnesses, including heart failure, cardiac arrhythmias, congenital heart disease, and shock. To manage these and other disease states, many pharmacologic and surgical interventions are routinely used in the intensive care unit that directly affect the cardiovascular system. A comprehensive understanding of cardiovascular physiology is therefore essential for all practitioners involved in the care of critically ill children.

The purpose of this chapter is to review essential physiologic concepts of the cardiovascular system. It will summarize hemodynamic principles that control circulatory flow, the basic processes that govern the mechanical function of the heart, and the critical determinants of cardiac output. It will also explore vital cardiopulmonary interactions and important crosstalk between the right and left sides of the heart.

Hemodynamic Principles

The foundation of cardiovascular physiology is based on the principles of fluid mechanics and hydrodynamics. These concepts are fundamental in explaining the relationship between blood flow, blood pressure, and the physical properties of the systemic circulation. An understanding of these principles is crucial to the care of critically ill children with cardiovascular disorders.

Flow, Velocity, and Area

The velocity of blood in the circulation is dependent on flow through a vessel and the vascular cross-sectional area of that vessel. Velocity describes the rate of fluid movement in terms of distance per unit time (e.g., cm/s). The flow through the circulation is determined by volume of blood per unit time (e.g., cm^3/s or L/min). In a circulatory system with blood vessels of varying cross-sectional dimensions, velocity of blood is expressed by:

$$v = \frac{Q}{A}$$

where v is velocity (in cm/s), Q is flow (in cm^3/s), and A is the cross-sectional area of the vessel (in cm^2).

For a constant flow the velocity through a blood vessel is inversely proportional to the cross-sectional area of that blood vessel. Accordingly, the highest velocity in the circulatory system occurs in the aorta and the lowest velocity in the capillary bed, which has a very large total cross-sectional area (Fig. 13.1).[1]

Pressure, Flow, and Resistance

Blood flows through a vascular segment in the circulation only when the inflow pressure (P_i) and outflow pressure (P_o) are different, creating a driving pressure (ΔP) between the two ends. However, friction between the vessel walls and the moving fluid creates an intrinsic vascular resistance (R) in the circulatory system. The relationship between flow, driving pressure, and resistance can be described by the *basic flow equation,* a variation of Ohm's law:

$$Q = \frac{(P_i - P_o)}{R}$$

where Q is flow (in cm^3/s), P_i is inflow pressure (in cm H_2O), P_o is outflow pressure (in cm H_2O), and R is resistance (in s/cm^2).

Flow through a vessel is inversely proportional to the vascular resistance and is dependent on the existence of pressure gradients in a vascular segment. This basic equation can be applied to not just a single blood vessel, but also the vascular bed of an organ or the entire systemic circulation.[1]

French physiologist Jean Poiseuille derived one of the most fundamental laws describing the relationship between various physical properties of liquids and fluid flow, which can be extrapolated to the circulatory system. *Poiseuille's law* describes the relationship of the various physical factors to flow as:

$$Q = \frac{(P_i - P_o)\pi r^4}{8\eta L}$$

where Q is flow (in cm^3/s), P_i is inflow pressure (in cm H_2O), P_o is outflow pressure (in cm H_2O), r is radius (in cm), η is viscosity (kg/cm·s), and L is length (in cm).[2]

Even small changes in the diameter of a vessel will result in very large increases in flow. Changes in the contractile state of the vasculature can therefore be significantly altered and play an important regulatory role. Conversely, increases in blood viscosity and vessel length will result in a decrease in blood flow.

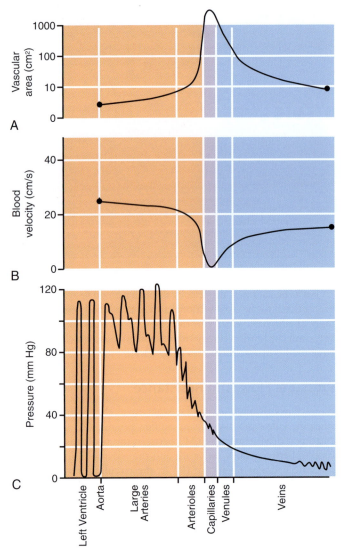

• **Figure 13.1** Relationship between total vascular cross-sectional area, blood velocity, and pressure of the systemic circulation. (A) The largest total vascular cross-sectional area occurs in the small capillary beds. (B) Because blood velocity is inversely proportional to cross-sectional area, the minimal flow rate occurs in the capillary bed. (C) The largest pressure drop occurs across the small arteries and arterioles.

By applying Poiseuille's law to Ohm's law, it can be determined that resistance to flow is affected solely by vessel dimensions (length and radius) and blood viscosity, as explained by the *hydraulic resistance equation*:

$$R = \frac{(P_i - P_o)}{Q} = \frac{8\eta L}{\pi r^4}$$

where *R* is resistance (in s/cm^2), *r* is radius (in cm), η is viscosity (kg/cm·s), and *L* is length (in cm).[2]

Animal studies have confirmed these relationships. Targeted pressure measurements showed a progressive pressure decline from the aorta to the venous circulation, with the largest drop occurring in the arteriole system (see Fig. 13.1).[3] Thus, given constant blood flow through the circulation, resistance must be greatest at the level of the arteriole system because of the smaller radius of the arterioles and the fact that the arteriole system exists in series. The

total resistance of a system (R_{total}) in series is equal to the sum of the individual resistances:

$$R_{total} = R_1 + R_2 + R_3 + \ldots + R_n$$

whereas the reciprocal of the total resistance of a system in parallel is equal to the sum of the reciprocals of the individual resistances:

$$\frac{1}{R_{total}} = \frac{1}{R_1} + \frac{2}{R_2} + \frac{3}{R_3} + \ldots + \frac{4}{R_n}$$

Therefore, although the radius of a capillary is even smaller than an arteriole, the capillary network exists in parallel, and the total resistance is less than the resistance of an individual capillary.

This can be used to explain the physiologic concept of vessel recruitment. As more vessels are recruited to regional capillary beds in parallel—such as in skeletal muscle during active exercise—resistance to flow will decrease.[4-8] Conversely, the loss of vessels in parallel—such as in end-stage pulmonary arterial hypertension—will result in increased pulmonary resistance.[9]

Laminar and Turbulent Flow

Poiseuille's law is most applicable to steady and streamlined flow of Newtonian fluids. Blood normally flows through the circulation in this orderly fashion—called *laminar flow*. In this type of motion, fluid moves as a series of layers with differing velocities. Velocity along the central axis of the vessel is the highest and decreases to zero at the wall of the vessel. The parallel layers of fluid with different velocities move in straight streamlined paths resulting in minimal energy expenditure.[10]

When blood is forced to move at higher velocities through a narrow opening, irregular motions of blood flow develop in a vessel—called *turbulent flow*. In this type of motion there is rapid mixing and much friction. Therefore the vessel's resistance to blood flow is substantially higher, an increased pressure is needed to drive blood flow, and the cardiovascular system must expend more energy to generate the increase pressure.[10]

A dimensionless number in fluid mechanics called the *Reynolds number (R_e)* can predict whether blood flow will conform to a laminar or turbulent flow state. This number represents the ratio of inertial forces to viscous forces within a fluid flowing through a cylindric tube:

$$R_e = \frac{2\rho v r}{\eta}$$

where ρ is the density (in kg/cm^3), *v* is the velocity (in cm/s), *r* is the radius (in cm), and η is the viscosity (in kg/cm·s). At high R_e, turbulent flow occurs due to predominance of inertial forces.[1] At low R_e, laminar flow occurs due to predominance of viscous forces. Therefore less viscous blood that is flowing rapidly through a vessel with a large radius is most susceptible to turbulent blood flow based on the R_e. An R_e of less than 2000 usually results in laminar flow, whereas at an R_e greater than 3000, flow is usually turbulent. This turbulence may result in vibratory patterns that are detected in the circulatory system as an audible murmur. For example, in severe anemia a "flow murmur" is often heard due to a decrease in blood viscosity and increase in cardiac output or blood flow velocity. Various flow conditions may occur in the transition range with R_e between 2000 and 3000.

Vessel Wall Shear Stress

Alterations in the hemodynamic conditions inside blood vessels can lead to the development of stresses near the vessel walls: (1) circumferential stress due to the phasic pressure of blood flow and (2) shear stress on the vascular endothelium of a vessel wall due to the changes in blood flow mechanics. These stresses, in combination with vascular wall compliance and endothelial-induced vasodilation, also help to regulate blood vessel diameter.[11]

Shear stress is the force applied by the blood against a vessel wall and is determined by the following equation:

$$\tau = \dot{\gamma}\eta$$

where τ is shear stress (in kg/cm·s²), η is viscosity (in kg/cm·s), and $\dot{\gamma}$ is shear rate (in s⁻¹).

The determination of shear stress on a surface is based on the fundamental assumption of fluid mechanics that the velocity of fluid on the surface is zero (no-slip condition). This assumption leads to the establishment of a velocity gradient, with the velocity of the fluid particles increasing the further they move away from the vessel wall. The maximum velocity of fluid particles is then reached at the location in the vessel that is furthest removed from the vessel walls. If we consider the blood vessel as a straight cylindric tube with nonelastic walls, then the shear rate, the rate at which neighboring layers of fluid move with respect to each other, can defined as:

$$\dot{\gamma} = du/dr$$

where u is the blood flow velocity (in cm/s) and r is the vessel radius (in cm).[1] Therefore, at a faster rate of blood flow, the shear rate on a vessel wall is greater, which results in more vessel wall shear stress (Fig. 13.2).

Through mathematical derivation the shear stress on the wall can be related to blood flow (Q) by the *Hagen-Poiseuille equation*:

$$\tau = \frac{4\eta Q}{\pi r^3}$$

This states that the shear stress on a vessel wall is directly proportional to the rate of blood flow and inversely exponentially proportional to the radius of the blood vessel.[10] It is important to recognize that applying the Hagen-Poiseuille law in vivo requires the following assumptions: (1) blood is considered a Newtonian fluid (linear relationship between shear rate and shear stress), (2) the blood vessel cross-sectional area is cylindric, (3) the vessel is straight with nonelastic walls, and (4) blood flow is steady and laminar. Under normal conditions, shear stresses are maintained within a range of values that help maintain endothelial integrity against thrombosis, atherosclerosis, leukocyte adhesion, and vascular smooth muscle proliferation.[12] This range varies across the arterial and venous vascular tree, as determined by flow velocity characteristics.[13] However, abnormal vascular anatomy from underlying congenital heart disease or as a result of surgical intervention can dramatically alter shear stress and affect endothelial integrity.[14-17]

Initially, acquired low–shear stress conditions, such as hypertension, induce a decrease in vessel radius and increase in wall thickness by intimal hyperplasia to return shear stress to a normal value.[18] However, despite this compensatory mechanism, low–shear stress conditions are also frequently accompanied by unstable flow conditions such as recirculation and "stagnant" flow and help promote thrombosis, atherogenesis, and stent restenosis.[19-22]

More dramatic alterations in shear stress are frequently seen in the congenital heart disease population, such as the postsurgical physiology after the Fontan operation in patients with single-ventricle physiology. The resulting lack of pulsatile pulmonary blood flow after Fontan surgery diminishes vessel wall shear stress.[23-25] This has been shown to cause an increase in pulmonary vascular resistance (PVR), which is a significant predictor of Fontan failure.[26] In fact, pulsatile blood flow and the resultant shear stress are important in stimulating vasodilatory mechanisms in the pulmonary and systemic endothelium.[27,28] Therefore a lack of pulsatile pulmonary blood flow has been proposed to decrease shear stress, cause endothelial dysfunction, impair vessel recruitment and angiogenesis, and increase PVR.[26,29-31]

As mentioned earlier, shear stress plays an important role in the integrity and function of the vascular endothelium. Recent evidence has shown that vascular endothelial cells respond to shear stress through a mechanosensory complex called *PECAM* (platelet endothelial cell adhesion molecule) located at cell junctions and a luminal endothelial polymeric substance called *glycocalyx*.[32-35] This results in downstream activation of calcium-sensitive ion channels, stretch-sensitive channels, endothelial nitric oxide (eNO)

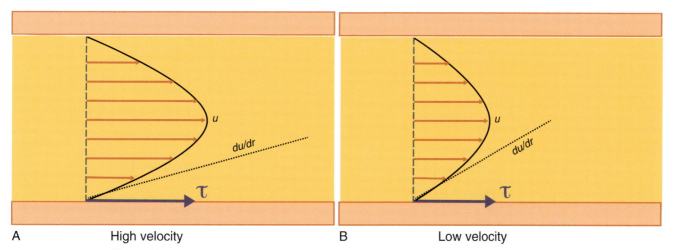

| A | High velocity | B | Low velocity |

• **Figure 13.2** Relationship between vessel wall shear stress and velocity. (A) At higher blood flow velocity *(u)* the shear rate *(du/dr)* is higher, and therefore vessel wall shear stress will increase. (B) At lower blood flow velocity the shear rate will decrease, and vessel wall shear stress will decrease.

production, vessel recruitment, and angiogenesis through activation of a vascular endothelial growth factor (VEGF)–associated gene.[36-44]

Higher shear stress values have been shown to occur in vascular regions that promote turbulent flow or increased flow velocity, such as the aortic arch, arterial bifurcations, and anastomoses.[11,45] Eventually, uncontrolled high shear stress conditions can cause tears in the endothelial lining, resulting in aneurysmal formations and possible rupture or dissection.[11] This is also important in systemic-to-pulmonary artery shunts placed during surgical palliation of congenital heart diseases. It is well known that postoperative thrombosis and occlusion of the modified Blalock-Taussig shunt (mBTS) can be sudden and fatal in the postoperative period.[46] It has been shown that large wall shear stress forces (due to flow channeling and the formation of large "eddies") and low-speed flow areas predominate near the anastomotic site of the mBTS to the pulmonary artery.[47,48] This may stimulate platelet aggregation and subsequent thrombus formation leading to conduit occlusion and significant postoperative complications.

Compliance and Distensibility

The concepts of compliance and distensibility are important in understanding the pressure-volume (P-V) relationships in the cardiovascular system. Compliance is the ability of an organ or blood vessel to distend and increase volume with increasing transmural pressure (P_{tm}) and is determined by the following equation:

$$C = \frac{\Delta V}{\Delta P}$$

where C is the compliance (in mL/cm H_2O), ΔV is the change in volume (in mL), and ΔP is the change in pressure (in cm H_2O).

The distensibility of a specific vessel or organ can be evaluated by dividing compliance by the base volume of the vessel or organ and is defined as the change in volume as a proportion of the initial volume for a given change in pressure:

$$\text{Distensibility} = \frac{\Delta V}{V \cdot \Delta P}$$

where ΔV is the change in volume (in mL), V is the initial volume (in mL), and ΔP is the change in pressure (in cm H_2O). The walls of veins are thinner and less elastic than arterial walls, and veins are therefore much more distensible and approximately 20 to 30 times more compliant. As a result, a majority of the circulating volume is located in the venous system. Therefore, during fluid resuscitation, therapeutic volume expansion has a greater effect on venous blood volume.

Computational Fluid Dynamics

Recent technologic and engineering advances in computational simulations have enabled the creation of accurate patient-specific models of local hemodynamics, blood-flow patterns, and global circulatory physiology in congenital heart disease. This modeling has the potential to have tremendous utility for clinical decision making and the evaluation of existing and novel surgical methods and interventions in a wide range of pediatric heart diseases.[49]

Early computational modeling in congenital heart disease was performed in the mid-to-late 1990s, simulating the hemodynamics of the classic Fontan circulation.[50,51] This pioneering work found reduced energy loss in a novel "offset design" modification between the inferior and superior vena cava at the Fontan junction—leading to changes in surgical practice. Since that time, further advances in modeling have allowed for the creation of image-based models for hemodynamic simulation, fluid-structure and geometric interaction analysis, and scalar models of circulatory physiology in congenital heart disease.[52-54] Work is now being performed on understanding the physiologic interplay between biologic processes and hemodynamic forces such as thrombosis, growth and remodeling, and vascular endothelial changes.[55-57] Creation of these models has the potential to predict postsurgical vascular remodeling, prevent shunt thrombosis, and optimize the formation of collateral vessels and graft hemodynamics.

There now exist multiple reports of patient-specific studies of computational fluid dynamics for surgical care that show good correlation between predictions and clinical follow-up measurements.[58,59] For instance, predictive modeling and virtual surgery for two options for stage 2 palliation (bidirectional Glenn and hemi-Fontan operation) in an infant with single-ventricle physiology has been described (Fig. 13.3).[60] Direct comparison of the outcomes confirmed the reliability of patient-specific simulations and allowed the quantification of the changes between preoperative and postoperative conditions.

Measuring hemodynamics such as blood flow velocity, wall shear stresses, and pressure can be critical in planning treatment of congenital heart disease, where alterations in geometry can lead to physiologic and hemodynamic disturbances.

Cardiac Pump

The heart is a dynamic organ with significant functional capacity. The ability of the heart to perform a large amount of work over the life span of an individual is owed to the interrelated structure and synchronous function of individual cardiac muscle cells.

Contractile Apparatus

The myocardium is a type of striated muscle in the heart composed of a bundle of integrated cardiac muscle fibers grouped into fascicles by a sheath of connective tissue. This sheath consists of a perimysium composed of numerous collagen fibers that connect the epimysium to the endomysium.[61] The neonatal myocardium has many unique structural and anatomic features that distinguish it from the mature myocardium. It is inherently disorganized due to fewer, more rounded, and relatively short cardiac muscle fibers that are not arranged in parallel arrays; a greater percentage of water and cytoplasm; and a lower density of contractile proteins.[62] This contributes to the relatively impaired contractile and relaxation functions of the immature heart.[63]

Each cardiac muscle fiber consists of bundles of cardiomyocytes connected in series by intercalated disks composed of adherens junctions, desmosomes, and gap junctions.[64-66] The cardiomyocyte consists of multiple elements, including the sarcomere, which contains the myofibrillar contractile apparatus and is the basic contractile unit of the cardiomyocyte; the sarcolemma, which contains the excitable cell envelope and its invaginations into the cytoplasm; the mitochondria, which is vital for adenosine triphosphate (ATP) production; the sarcoplasmic reticulum, which stores the intracellular calcium essential for contraction; and numerous proteins, which are important for cardiac muscle structure and function.[67]

The myofibrillar contractile element consists of thick and thin filaments. The filaments are made up of multiple proteins,

Hemi-Fontan (hF) **Bidirectional Glenn (bG)**

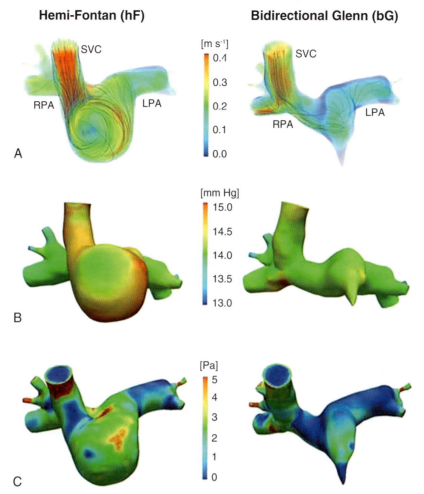

• **Figure 13.3** Comparison of the hemodynamics in the hemi-Fontan (hF) and bidirectional Glenn (bG) models. (A) Time-averaged, volume-rendered flow velocities with color map representing the velocity magnitude and lines representing the velocity streamlines. In the hF the superior vena cava *(SVC)* inflow runs along the side of the cavopulmonary junction, creating a vortex and maintaining a higher velocity (than the bG) before entering the pulmonary artery. In the bG the flow is predominant at the base of the right pulmonary artery *(RPA)* after entering from the SVC and splits into the left and right directions. (B) Wall pressure at peak flow shows larger values at the inlet for the hF compared to the bG. (C) Time-averaged wall shear stress (WSS) magnitude in the hF and bG geometries. Areas of high WSS close to the inlet are present in both due to vessel curvature. The hF model has high WSS throughout most of the surgical junction due to the presence of a swirling vortex. The bG model has a more limited area of high WSS concentrated at the base of the RPA near the SVC inflow junction. *LPA,* Left pulmonary artery. (From Corsini C, Baker C, Kung E, et al. An integrated approach to patient-specific predictive modeling for single ventricle heart palliation. *Comput Methods Biomech Biomed Engin.* 2014;17[14]:1572-1589.)

including actin, tropomyosin, titin filaments, troponin complexes, and myosin filaments. These filaments are organized into a sarcomere, which is located between two transverse Z disks, composed of the proteins that connect adjacent actin and titin filaments (Fig. 13.4).[68,69] On either side of the Z disk is a light zone, which contains the I (isotropic) band. This band includes thin filament couplets of coiled actin protein connected to the Z disk. These paired actin filaments lie in a complex with two long tropomyosin filaments and multiple calcium-sensitive troponin complexes at regularly spaced intervals.[70,71] The overlap of thin filaments with thick myosin filaments occurs at the A band, which encompasses the majority of the sarcomere. Adjacent A bands are separated by a light H band, which contains only thick filaments.[69,71] In the middle of the sarcomere is a dark thin M line. Myosin in the thick filament contains globular heads, which

join to actin-binding sites on parallel thin filaments when the tropomyosin–troponin C complexes are exposed in the setting of calcium flux from the sarcoplasmic reticulum. The large macromolecular titin extends from the Z disk to the M line and supports the actomyosin filaments, contributes to elastic behavior of the cardiomyocyte, and is important for sarcomere length-tension relationships.[72,73]

Mutations or alterations in many of these cytoskeleton filaments and cardiac proteins can contribute to significant myocardial dysfunction.[67,71,74] For example, mutations in beta-myosin S2 and cardiac myosin-binding protein C (cMyBPC), which contribute to thick filament structure, are common causes of familial hypertrophic cardiomyopathy.[75-77] More recently discovered proteins, such as striatin, which controls cardiomyocyte calcium homeostasis and contraction;[78] and novel Z-line proteins, such as

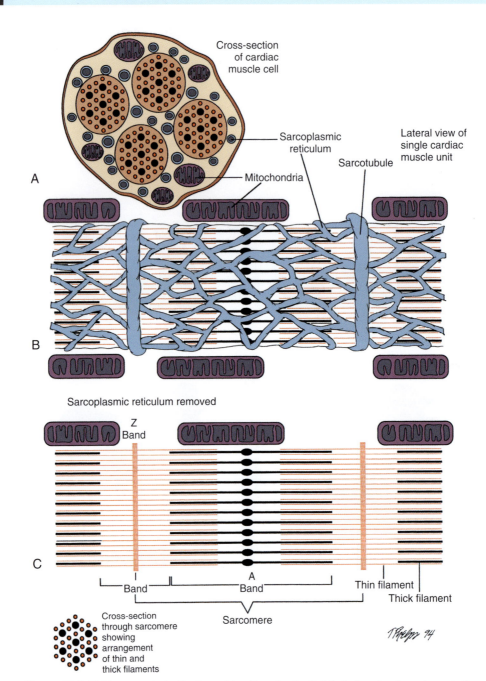

• Figure 13.4 (A) The myocyte (or fiber) consists of bundles (or fibrils) of aligned actin and myosin filaments surrounded by cytoplasm containing mitochondria. (B) The fibrils with sarcoplasmic reticulum and T-tubule systems are responsible for conduction of ionic currents and electrical depolarization, which increases the intracellular calcium around the actin and myosin. (C) Each fibril consists of sarcomeres connected in series, and each sarcomere consists of bundles of actin and myosin connected at the Z plates. The muscle bundles consist of thick filaments (myosin) and thin filaments (actin) and multiple regulatory protein compounds (tropomyosin, troponin C complex). The myosin heads join to their actin-binding sites when the tropomyosin–troponin C complex exposes these binding sites in the presence of increasing calcium concentrations. This is the actual process of contraction.

α-actin, desmin, and filamin C, have been implicated in cardiac arrhythmias and a wide range of cardiomyopathies.[79] Furthermore, new research has shown that oxidative and nitrosative stress can alter the contractile function of cardiomyocytes, contributing to myocardial dysfunction and heart failure.[80-82] Evidence has shown that the targets of these chemical stresses are the contractile and regulatory proteins of the sarcomeres, which can result in altered calcium sensitivity, contractile impairment, and cardiomyocyte dysfunction.[83,84]

Cardiac Muscle Cell Contraction

The contraction of cardiomyocytes is initiated by spreading action potentials through a network of intracellular organelles, resulting

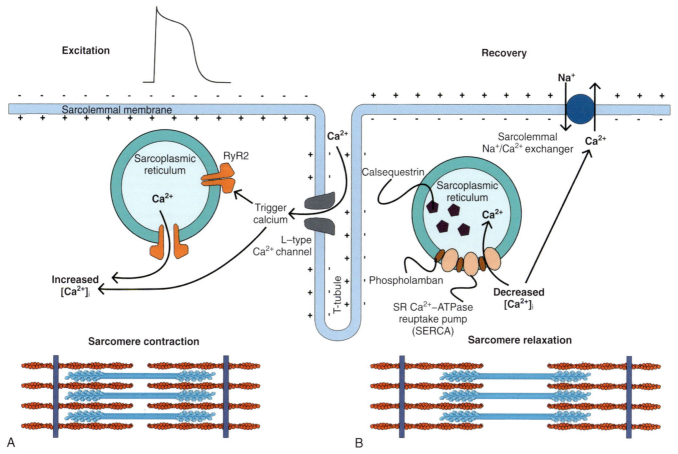

• Figure 13.5 Cardiomyocyte excitation-contraction coupling. (A) Following depolarization of the cardiomyocyte, extracellular calcium enters the cell through dihydropyridine-sensitive L-type calcium channels, triggering the release of calcium in the sarcoplasmic reticulum *(SR)* through the ryanodine receptor *(RyR2)*; this brings about the conformational change in troponin for sarcomere contraction to occur. (B) Cardiomyocyte relaxation occurs from removal of cytoplasmic calcium via the SR Ca²⁺-ATPase pump *(SERCA)* or the sarcolemmal Na⁺/Ca²⁺ exchanger in conjunction with phospholamban and calsequestrin.

in the production of tension or shortening and ultimately contraction.[70] In addition to the sarcomere, cardiomyocytes contain structures and organelles vital to cardiac muscle cell contraction such as the sarcoplasmic reticulum, mitochondria, extracellular matrix, cytoskeleton, and cytoplasm.

The sarcoplasmic reticulum is a complex intracellular membrane system that sequesters calcium during diastole with the assistance of calsequestrin (a calcium-binding storage protein) and SERCA (the sarcoplasmic reticulum Ca²⁺-ATPase).[85] Connected to parts of the sarcoplasmic reticulum is an extensive network of invaginations of the cardiac cell membrane known as *T-tubules*. This tubular system carries the action potential signal to the interior of cardiomyocytes and helps modulate calcium flow through phospholamban.[85] This protein inhibits the binding of calcium to the SERCA pump, preventing calcium entry into the cytoplasm. Phosphorylation of phospholamban reverses this inhibition, resulting in calcium influx and cardiac contractility.[86,87] Perturbations of this interaction are common in heart failure, sepsis, and forms of dilated cardiomyopathy.[88-91]

The cytoplasm contains mitochondria, which provide energy for contraction and relaxation. During development the mitochondria demonstrate increased cristae formation and become larger and plumper. The neonatal cardiomyocyte is relatively deficient

in mitochondria, which accounts for 35% to 40% of the muscle mass by adulthood.[62]

Excitation-Contraction Coupling

The spreading action potential in the myocardium leads to mechanical contraction through a process called excitation-contraction coupling (Fig. 13.5). Once an electrical impulse reaches the myocardium, cardiomyocytes depolarize along their sarcolemma and the T-tubule system, and spread the impulse to adjacent cardiomyocytes through gap junctions. These gap junctions are composed of proteins from the connexin family and are located at the intercalated disks of the cardiomyocyte.[92,93] They play a pivotal role in the speed and safety of action potential propagation from one cell to the next.[94]

High concentrations of extracellular calcium enter the cell through voltage-gated calcium channels at the sarcolemmal membrane and the T-tubules. The increase in cytoplasmic calcium concentration leads to the release of intracellular calcium stores from the sarcoplasmic reticulum (SR) via the ryanodine receptor and a further rise in cytoplasmic calcium content. This process is called *calcium-induced calcium release*.[70,95] It is important to mention that the neonatal myocardium is disproportionately reliant on extracellular calcium because neonatal myocytes are smaller, have a greater area-to-volume ratio, lack T-tubules, and have an underdeveloped sarcoplasmic reticulum. Therefore calcium-induced calcium release is limited, and instead, trans-sarcolemmal movement of extracellular calcium plays a much larger role in excitation-contraction coupling.[96-98]

Free intracellular calcium causes actin-myosin binding, which is the basis of cardiomyocyte contraction. In the resting state, actin and myosin binding is inhibited by troponin and tropomyosin, the filament that overlies actin. Troponin exists as a complex of three subunits: troponin T attaches to the tropomyosin, troponin C is a high-affinity calcium-binding site, and troponin I inhibits the actin-myosin interaction. When intracellular calcium content rises, it binds to the troponin C subunit. This binding antagonizes troponin I and causes a conformational change in tropomyosin and troponin that exposes the myosin-binding sites on the actin filaments.[70,95] These actin-binding sites are then free to bind with the myosin heads forming cross-bridges. As this binding occurs, the actin and myosin filaments slide along each other and draw the cardiomyocyte Z disks closer together, resulting in cardiomyocyte and ultimately myocardial contraction. The force and rapidity of contraction are directly proportional to the amount of free intracellular calcium. The myosin head contains the actin-myosin ATPase that is responsible for the hydrolysis of ATP and the release of energy that allows relaxation of the actin and myosin cross-bridges. The mutual affinity of actin and myosin is so great that energy is required to separate them and allow further cross-bridging, which leads to contraction. The amount of ATP hydrolyzed determines the rapidity of this unbridging and relinking cycle and thus the velocity of fiber shortening.[62,99,100]

Clearly the intracellular calcium content is the crucial determinant of myocardial contraction. Intracellular calcium increases during contraction from 10^{-7} M during diastole to 10^{-5} M during systole.[101] Cyclic adenosine monophosphate (cAMP) plays an important role in regulating contractility by (1) enhancing inward calcium flow, (2) increased sarcoplasmic reticulum calcium release, (3) phosphorylation of troponin I to promote binding of myosin to actin, (4) phosphorylation of sarcoplasmic reticulum to decrease reuptake of calcium, and (5) possibly enhancing mitochondrial release of calcium. Thus agents that stimulate adenylate cyclase will act as inotropes.[102] Most inotropic agents (including catecholamines) increase intracellular calcium, whereas negative inotropes (including calcium channel blockers and beta-antagonists) decrease intracellular calcium. Drugs such as phosphodiesterase inhibitors (amrinone, milrinone) that prevent the breakdown of cAMP to 5′-AMP will also have a positive inotropic effect.

Cardiac Muscle Cell Mechanics

The actin-myosin cross-bridge that forms after cardiomyocyte activation provides the potential energy for muscle contractile force and shortening. External constraints placed on the muscle during the process of contraction determine whether muscle tension, shortening, or both occur.

The *sarcomere length-tension* relationship has been inferred from studies of myocardial muscle strips. Starling's famous demonstration of the length-tension relationship, describing how preload and afterload affect contractility, underlies the concepts that continue to influence patient management in the intensive care unit (Fig. 13.6).[103-107]

Two types of contraction mechanisms exist. In *isometric ("fixed length") contraction,* activation of muscle whose ends are immobile generates muscle tension but impedes muscle shortening. In *isotonic ("fixed tension") contraction,* activation of free muscle causes it to shorten without development of force or tension. Adding additional load ("afterload") to this muscle will decrease the speed and extent of its shortening.

Isotonic and isometric contractions are important to the understanding of ventricular function because cardiomyocytes in the ventricular wall function under different mechanical constraints during different phases of the cardiac cycle.

Isometric Contractions

The association of increasing fixed muscle lengths on the generation of muscle tension during isometric contraction is displayed in Fig. 13.6A. Although muscle strips are initially resting before a contraction stimulus in each of the three muscle lengths, it is important to realize that force is still required to stretch a muscle to different lengths. This is graphically represented as the exponential-like *resting length-tension curve* shown in the bottom graph and is mainly mediated by the cytoskeleton component, titin.[72,108,109] When the fixed muscle strip is activated to contract, it produces additional tension called *active tension.* The *total tension* is the sum of the resting and active tensions as represented by the *peak isometric tension curve.* This is the Starling relationship.[110,111]

The magnitude of active tension that is generated by the cardiac muscle during an isometric contraction is dependent on the muscle length at which the contraction takes place. As shown in the bottom curve, the greatest active tension produced occurs at the intermediate muscle length, whereas little tension is generated at very short or very long muscle lengths.[110,111]

The proposed mechanism for the relationship between muscle length and generated muscle tension is multifaceted. First, the degree of thick and thin filament overlap in the resting sarcomere must be optimal to allow for sufficient actin-myosin cross-bridge formation (see Fig. 13.4). The resting sarcomere Z-Z distance is approximately 1.6 μm. Optimal overlap and peak isometric tension development occurs at approximately 2.2 μm, and distraction occurs at approximately 3.5 μm. At sarcomere lengths shorter than 2.0 μm, the opposing thin filaments buckle, and at long sarcomere lengths the decreased myofilament overlap interferes with cross-bridge generation—hindering active tension generation.[69,100] Second, there exists a length-dependent sensitivity of thick and think filaments to calcium. At short sarcomere lengths, only a small number of cross-bridges are exposed by a measured increase in intracellular calcium concentration. As the sarcomere lengthens, more cross-bridges are activated, and the magnitude of active tension increases.[112,113] It is thought that troponin C acts as the "sensor" responsible for this length-dependent activation of the cardiac muscle.[114,115] Third, it is proposed that stretch-sensitive ion channels in the cardiac cell membrane cause an increase in the amount of calcium released with excitation as the resting length of cardiac muscle increases.[116]

Isotonic and Afterloaded Contractions

The association of muscle length on the generation of tension and muscle shortening during isotonic and afterloaded contractions is displayed in Fig. 13.6B. When a muscle contracts isotonically against a constant load, the muscle will shorten and develop a "threshold" tension needed to lift the fixed weight. As the muscle shortens, its magnitude of potential active tension will also decrease, as shown by the convex slope of the peak isometric tension curve.

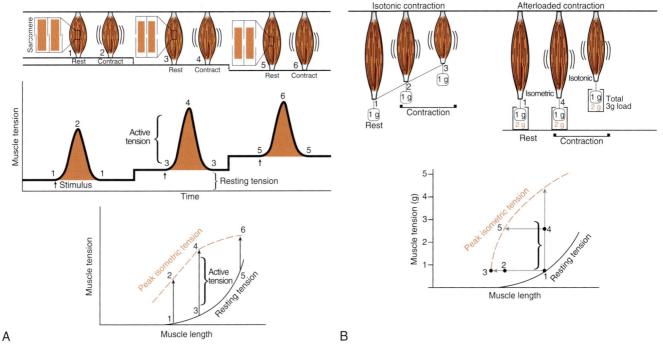

• **Figure 13.6** The classic Starling experiment. (A) Isometric contractions: the top panel shows the experimental setup for measuring muscle force at rest and during contraction of muscle strips at three different lengths; the middle panel shows the muscle tension generated over time during a contraction for each of the three lengths; the bottom panel shows the resting and peak isometric muscle tension as a function of muscle length. (B) The top left panel and bottom graph describe isotonic ("fixed load") contraction; the top right panel and bottom graph describe afterloaded contractions. These are the classic length-tension relationships, which are by analogy extrapolated to our understanding of pressure-volume relationships. (Modified from Mohrman DE, Hiller LJ, eds. *Cardiovascular Physiology*. 8th ed. New York: McGraw-Hill Education; 2014.)

Therefore the peak isometric curve not only indicates how much isometric tension a muscle can generate at different lengths, but also determines the extent of muscle shortening with different loads.

Afterloaded contractions are more clinically relevant because they are more typical of the cardiomyocyte contractions in the heart. In these contractions the *preload* (load on the muscle at rest) and *afterload* (load against which a muscle contracts) determines the *total load* on the muscle during contraction. The afterloaded muscle initially contracts isometrically with a fixed muscle length until it generates sufficient muscle tension to equal the total load. Once this threshold is reached, it will isotonically shorten.

In the clinical setting, preload augmentation is most likely to increase resting fiber length and, if all other conditions remains the same, to increase developed tension, which is associated with increased stroke volume (SV). Clinically, excessive preload does not overdistend the myocyte (although it may overdistend the ventricle and lead to atrioventricular valve regurgitation and increased volume load on the heart) but rather alters myocardial perfusion and energy balance in such a fashion as to decrease contractile function. This system is best represented by a shift of the Starling curve downward to the right: that is, for the same preload, less tension is developed (if afterload is constant). Clinically this is manifested as decreased SV.

Cardiac Cycle

The sequential contraction and relaxation of the atria and ventricles produced by electrical changes, pressures, and mechanical actions constitute the cardiac cycle. Understanding this cycle is important in assessing normal and dysfunctional cardiac function in the critically ill pediatric patient. A single cardiac cycle is defined as one complete sequence of cardiac contraction (systole) and relaxation (diastole). Fig. 13.7 describes the cardiac cycle in terms of pressure, volume, and flow changes.[117]

Atrial Systole

Before the beginning of ventricular systole, the left atrium contracts in response to depolarization initiated by the P wave. This results in a pressure increase within the left atrium, forcing blood to flow across the open mitral valve, leading to rapid blood flow into the left ventricle (LV). Atrial contraction generates a small increase in venous pressure, which is noted as the *a* wave of the left atrial pressure (LAP) tracing. It is important to note that atrial contraction only accounts for one-tenth of left ventricular (LV) filling at rest and in otherwise healthy hearts because most filling occurs passively from the pulmonary veins, through the left atrium, and into the LV. As a result, cardiac output can be perservered in settings of diminished or absent atrial contraction, as seen in atrial fibrillation or even complete heart block. However, as chronotropy increases, the fraction of atrial contraction that contributes to ventricular filling increases because there is less time in the cardiac cycle for passive movement of blood. This active atrial contraction (referred to as the *atrial kick*) is important for contributing a significant volume of blood toward ventricular preload. Consequently, situations with rapid ventricular contraction and absent atrial kick, for example

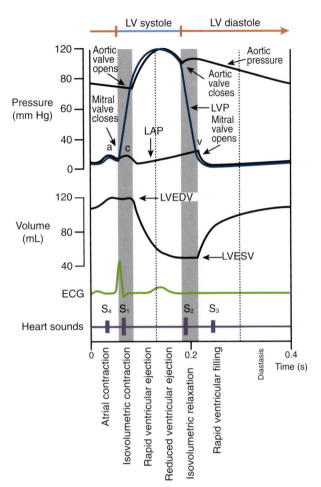

• **Figure 13.7** The cardiac cycle of the left heart. Aortic, left ventricular pressure *(LVP),* and left atrial pressure *(LAP)* tracings as they correspond to the electrocardiogram *(ECG),* mitral and aortic valve opening and closing, and heart sounds. *LV,* Left ventricular; *LVEDV,* left ventricular end-diastolic volume; *LVESV,* left ventricular end-systolic volume.

in the setting of junctional ectopic tachycardia (JET), may result in diminished ventricular filling and cardiac output.

After atrial contraction is complete, the atrial pressure falls and results in a reversal of the pressure gradient across the mitral valve, resulting in inversion of the valve (preposition) before closure. This is the point at which the ventricular volume is at its maximum and is referred to as the *left ventricular end-diastolic volume (LVEDV).* This represents the preload of the LV.

A fourth heart sound (S_4) is sometimes heard during atrial contraction and is caused by vibratory movements of the ventricular wall. It is usually present when there is a significant decrease in ventricular compliance.

Ventricular Systole

Isovolumetric Contraction. This phase of the cardiac cycle marks the beginning of ventricular systole, coincides with the peak of the R wave on the electrocardiogram (ECG), and produces the initial vibration of the first heart sound. The process of excitation-contraction coupling and cardiomyocyte contraction during this phase results in the rapid increase in intraventricular pressure.

The atrioventricular valve closes once the intraventricular pressure exceeds atrial pressure. Following closure of this valve and before opening of the semilunar valve, the ventricular pressure rapidly

increases without a corresponding change in ventricular volume. This brief time period represents isovolumetric contraction.[118] It is important to note, however, that individual cardiomyocyte contractions are not exclusively isometric. Individual cardiac muscle fibers undergo a combination of eccentric (lengthening), isotonic (fixed tension), and isometric (fixed length) contractions, which results in the heart becoming more spheroid in shape in preparation for ventricular ejection. On the atrial pressure tracing a *c* wave is present during isovolumetric contraction. This represents the bulging of the atrioventricular valve back into the atrium, resulting in a small and brief increase in atrial pressure.

Ejection. Ejection of blood from the ventricle begins once the intraventricular pressures exceed the pressures within the corresponding great vessel, resulting in the opening of the semilunar valve. Blood is ejected due to the development of a pressure and energy gradient between the ventricle and the arterial vasculature. This phase of the cardiac cycle can be subdivided into an earlier and shorter phase of rapid ejection and a longer phase of reduced ejection.

The rapid ejection phase can be distinguished from the reduced ejection phase by (1) a large rate of rise in ventricular and aortic pressures, (2) termination at peak ventricular and aortic pressures, (3) faster rate of ventricular blood ejection, and (4) a greater amount of aortic blood flow.

The reduced ejection phase coincides with the culmination of ventricular repolarization, as indicated by the T wave of the ECG. This leads to a drop in ventricular tension, ventricular pressure generation, ventricular ejection rate, and pressure.

During the first third of the ejection period, LV pressure exceeds aortic pressure, and blood flow accelerates. However, during the remaining portion of ventricular ejection, the aortic pressure exceeds the LV pressure. Despite this pressure gradient reversal, there is continued blood flow from the LV into the aorta. This occurs because of the potential energy sorted in stretched arterial walls, which generates a deceleration of blood flow into the aorta.

The exact pattern of ventricular wall shortening and compression of the chamber is complex and is designed to maximize efficiency of the right and left ventricles. Normally during systole, individual cardiac muscle fibers move synergistically with each other to produce torsion and energy-conserving ventricular shape changes necessary for optimal systolic ejection.[119] This has been observed as far back as the late-17th century, when Richard Lower[120] described the large amount of cardiac motion as akin to the wringing out of wet linen cloth to squeeze out the water. Recent studies have demonstrated that these energy-efficient torsion-related shape alterations do not occur effectively in patients with single-ventricle physiology.[121-123] Therefore volume change during ventricular ejection is likely exclusively dependent on cardiomyocyte shortening.

Normally no heart sounds are noted during ventricular ejection because semilunar valve opening is silent in healthy subjects. The presence of systolic murmurs during ventricular ejection can indicate valvular disease or intracardiac shunting.

During the beginning of ventricular ejection, it is important to note that there is an initial downslope in the atrial pressure tracing (*x* descent). This left atrial pressure decrease occurs as the atrial base is pulled downward, resulting in expansion of the left atrial chamber. Following this initial pressure decrease, venous blood continues to flow passively into the left atrium, and the atrial pressure rises until the end of isovolumetric relaxation.

At the end of LV ejection and before the start of isovolumetric relaxation, a volume of blood remains in the ventricular cavity called the *left ventricular end-systolic volume* (LVESV). The difference between the end-diastolic volume and end-systolic volume (ESV) represents the SV.

Ventricular Diastole

Isovolumetric Relaxation. This phase of the cardiac cycle marks the start of ventricular diastole.[124] The closing of the semilunar valves marks the beginning of isovolumetric relaxation and is responsible for the second heart sound (S_2). The closure of the aortic valve is also associated with backflow of blood into the LV and the characteristic incisura or dicrotic notch seen in the descending limb of the aortic pressure tracing. This is followed by a slight rise in the aortic pressure, termed the *dicrotic wave*, followed by a slow decline in pressure throughout diastole. Because the atrioventricular and semilunar valves are closed during this phase, only ventricular pressure decreases, while ventricular volume remains constant.

Ventricular pressure decline is determined by the rate at which individual ventricular muscle fibers relax and is the molecular basis behind the concept of lusitropy. This rate of myocardial relaxation is regulated by resequestration of calcium into the sarcoplasmic reticulum through the sarcoplasmic-endoplasmic reticulum calcium ATPase (SERCA) pump, and extracellular efflux of calcium through the sarcolemmal sodium-calcium exchanger following sarcomere excitation-contraction coupling.[85] The SERCA pump is regulated by the inhibitory protein phospholamban, which once phosphory-lated, allows the calcium reuptake by the SERCA pump.[86,87] Because calcium stored in the sarcoplasmic reticulum is immediately available for the next systolic contraction, failure of the SERCA pump can result in both systolic and diastolic dysfunction.[88-91]

The left atrial pressure continues to increase throughout iso-volumetric relaxation due to passive venous return from the systemic and pulmonary veins and culminates in the *v* wave, which is the peak of the atrial tracing before ventricular diastole.

Rapid Ventricular Filling. The majority of ventricular filling occurs once the ventricular pressure falls below the atrial pressure and coincides with the opening of the atrioventricular valves. The result is passive ventricular filling, called the *rapid filling phase.* Ventricular pressures will continue to fall during the inflow of blood from the atrium due to continued ventricular relaxation.

Although ventricular filling is usually silent, a third heart sound (S_3) is sometimes audible when ventricular filling is rapid. This heart sound is common in pediatric patients but can be pathologic in states of ventricular dilation.

The opening of the atrioventricular valves is following by the rapid *y* descent of the atrial pressure tracing due to flow of blood from the atria into the ventricles.

Diastasis. The rapid filling phase is followed by a period of reduced filling called *diastasis.* During this phase, complete ventricular relaxation has occurred, and LV pressure will gradually rise again. Toward the end of ventricular filling the ventricles become less compliant, and the rate of filling falls even further in late diastole.

Ventricular Pressure-Volume Relationship

The relationship between the cardiac cycle, ventricular pressure, and ventricular volume can be graphically represented by the left P-V loop (Fig. 13.8).[117] This P-V relationship represents a single cardiac cycle and can be divided into four distinct phases: LV filling, isovolumetric contraction, LV ejection, and isovolumetric relaxation. Additionally, each of these phases corresponds to specific length-tension relationships and is the underlying basis for ventricular function.

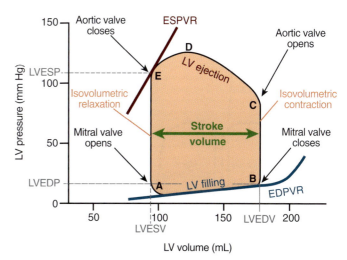

• **Figure 13.8** Left ventricular pressure-volume loop. Demonstrates the events of the cardiac cycle with respect to left ventricular *(LV)* volume and LV pressure, opening and closing of the aortic and mitral valves, end-systolic pressure-volume relationship *(ESPVR)*, and end-diastolic pressure-volume relationship *(EDPVR)*. *LVEDV*, Left ventricular end-diastolic volume; *LVESV*, left ventricular end-systolic volume.

The end of ventricular filling represents the left ventricular end-diastolic pressure (LVEDP) and the left ventricular end-diastolic volume (LVEDV), which corresponds to ventricular preload (point B in Fig. 13.8). The progressively small increase in the ventricular pressure during this phase causes a corresponding increase in muscle tension and passively stretches the resting cardiomyocyte to greater lengths (passive stretch) until it reaches its end-diastolic length.

At the onset of systole the LV undergoes isovolumetric contraction following mitral valve closure. The LV pressure increases as the LV volume remains the same, which results in a vertical line on the P-V loop (B to C). During this phase, ventricular cardiomyocytes develop tension isometrically.

Once the LV pressure exceeds the aortic pressure, the aortic valve opens, and ventricular ejection ensues as a consequence of cardiomyocyte shortening (C). During this phase the LV volume decreases as LV pressure increases to a peak systolic pressure (D) and then decreases as the ventricle begins to relax. The ventricular cardiomyocytes simultaneously generate active tension and shorten during ventricular ejection, which is similar to an afterloaded isotonic contraction. Therefore the amount of LV volume change produced during ejection (SV) is determined by the degree of cardiomyocyte shortening during contraction. The end of LV filling occurs when the aortic valve closes and represents the LV end-systolic pressure (LVESP) and LVESV (E).

This point marks the beginning of diastole and results in the LV undergoing isovolumetric relaxation secondary to a drop in ventricular wall tension (E to A). Cardiac muscle cells undergo isometric relaxation during this phase until the mitral valve opens again (A).

The width of the loop represents the difference between LVEDV and LVESV, which is defined as the stroke volume (SV). The slope of the diastolic ventricular filling curve, also known as the end-diastolic pressure-volume relationship (EDPVR), presents the reciprocal of the LV compliance. The slope at the end of systole defines the end-systolic pressure-volume relationship (ESPVR) and represents the contractility of the LV. The ejection fraction (EF) is the ratio of SV to end-diastolic volume (EDV). The area enclosed within the loop is the external stroke work of the ventricle. The

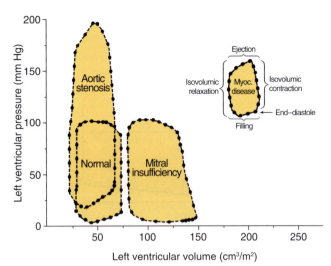

• **Figure 13.9** Pressure-volume loops for children with various congenital heart diseases. Myocardial (Myoc.) disease, volume overload (chronic mitral insufficiency), and pressure overload (aortic stenosis) are demonstrated. (From Graham TP Jr, Jarmakani MM. Evaluation of ventricular function in infants and children. *Pediatr Clin North Am.* 1971;18:1109-1132.)

concepts of elastance and compliance are important to describe the changes in P-V loops when preload, afterload, or contractility of the heart is altered. Elastance is the change in pressure per unit change in volume. Compliance is the change in volume per unit change in pressure (reciprocal of elastance). For a given LVEDV, the LVEDP will depend on the compliance of the ventricle. Thus, for a given LVEDV, cardiac abnormalities such as hypertrophy, ischemia, infarction, or structural anomalies may decrease ventricular compliance and therefore increase the LVEDP.

P-V loops in children with heart disease are shown in Fig. 13.9.[125] In children with mitral insufficiency, as the LV contracts, blood is ejected into the aorta but also backs up into the left atrium. This increases left atrial volume and pressure during ventricular systole. Because blood begins to flow retrograde across the mitral valve and into the left atrium before aortic valve opening, the isovolumetric contraction phase is compromised (loss of vertical line between mitral valve closure and aortic valve opening). In addition, this volume overload state results in larger amount of ventricular filling and larger LVEDV. In chronic mitral insufficiency, children may have some degree of systolic failure, and therefore the LVESV is also increased. In aortic stenosis, LV emptying is impaired because of high aortic outflow resistance. This also results in a large pressure gradient across the aortic valve during ejection, with a greatly increased peak systolic pressure within the ventricle. Increased systolic pressures result in higher ventricular wall stress, a decrease in SV, and an increase in LVESV. Lastly, myocardial disease consists of impairment of ventricular filling (diastolic heart failure) and systolic ejection (systolic heart failure) and is characterized by a marked decrease in SV, elevation in both LVESV and LVEDV, and poor ventricular ejection (decreased LVEDP and peak systolic pressure).

Determinants of Cardiac Output

Cardiac output is determined by heart rate and SV:

$$CO = HR \times SV$$

where *CO* is cardiac output (in L/min), *HR* is heart rate (in beats/min), and *SV* is stroke volume (in L). The heart rate is controlled

by chronotropic influences on the spontaneous electrical activity of the sinoatrial (SA) nodal cells, whereas SV is controlled by three distinct influences on the contractile performance of the heart—preload, afterload, and contractility. Each of these primary determinants of cardiovascular function must be individually understood to comprehend the integrated function of the cardiovascular system.

Heart Rate

Heart rate is an important physiologic regulator of total cardiac output. Through strong influences of the autonomic nervous system, the heart rates in a newborn can range from 70 to 220 beats/min and profoundly impact cardiac output. Coordinated electric activity and automaticity of the conduction system in the newborn heart are essential to maximizing the active phase of ventricular filling. Overall, the relationship between heart rate and total cardiac output is complex.

The most important influences on the automaticity of the SA node come from the sympathetic and parasympathetic divisions of the autonomic nervous system. Fibers from these two divisions alter the intrinsic heart rate by changing the course of spontaneous diastolic depolarization on pacemaker cells in the SA node. Activation of the cardiac sympathetic fibers will increase the heart rate, whereas stimulation of cardiac parasympathetic fibers will decrease the heart rate. These neural influences have immediate effects and can therefore cause very rapid adjustments in cardiac output.

However, the effect of changes in heart rate on cardiac output is complex, and the relationship is not linear. This is because a change in heart rate can alter the three determinants (preload, afterload, and contractility) of SV. A significant increase in heart rate would decrease the duration of diastole and diminish ventricular filling, thereby reducing preload.[126] On the other hand, this rise in heart rate would also increase the net rate of calcium influx into the cardiomyocyte, enhancing contractility. This effect of heart rate on cardiac output has been verified in many types of experimental studies in animals and humans (Fig. 13.10).[127-130]

This characteristic relationship between cardiac output and heart rate is critically important in the postsurgical care of patients with congenital heart disease with excessively slow or fast heart rates. For example, complete heart block from procedures involving the closure of a ventricular septal defect can result in a profound decrease in cardiac output because the compensatory increase in SV is insufficient to offset the very slow heart rate and lack of atrioventricular synchrony.[131] Medication with the potential to slow heart rate should be used cautiously in the postoperative setting to minimize risk of lowering cardiac output. At the other extreme, JET is common postoperatively in infants and requires emergency treatment because cardiac output might be significantly compromised due to decreased diastolic filling time resulting from excessively rapid heart rates and lack of atrioventricular synchrony.[132,133]

Stroke Volume

The SV represents the volume of blood ejected from the ventricle with each heartbeat. It can be calculated as the difference between the volume inside the ventricle at the end of diastole (end-diastolic volume) and the end of systole (end-systolic volume):

$$SV = EDV - ESV$$

where *SV* is stroke volume (in L), *EDV* is end-diastolic volume (in L), and *ESV* is end-systolic volume (in L). Thus SV can be

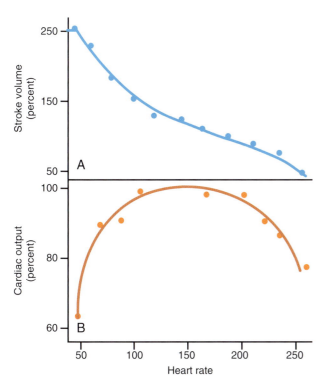

• **Figure 13.10** Effect of heart rate on cardiac output in an anesthetized dog undergoing atrial pacing. (A) There is a progressive decrease in stroke volume as heart rate increases due to shortening of diastolic filling time. (B) The relationship of cardiac output to heart rate is characteristically an inverted U shape with low cardiac output at very low and very high atrial rates.

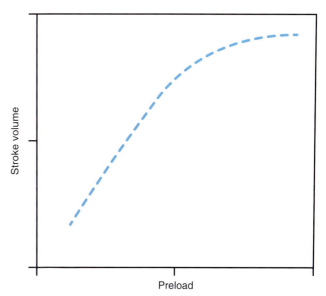

• **Figure 13.11** Frank-Starling curve. Stroke volume of the heart increases in response to an increase in the ventricular filling (preload) when contractility, afterload, and ventricular compliance remain constant.

changed only by alterations in EDV and/or ESV. An increase in ventricular filling (preload) will result in an increase in the EDV and a larger SV. A larger systemic arterial pressure (afterload) will increase the ESV, thereby resulting in a smaller SV. Finally, release of norepinephrine from the sympathetic nervous system (resulting in increased myocardial contractility) will decrease the ESV and result in a larger SV.

Preload

Groundbreaking work in the late 19th century and early 20th century by William Howell, Otto Frank, and E.H. Starling determined that the ventricular ejection volume (SV) of the heart increases in response to increased diastolic filling of the heart (preload).[103,107,134] This observation resulted in a landmark principle of cardiovascular physiology, named the Frank-Starling law (Fig. 13.11). As previously stated, this phenomenon is based on the intrinsic mechanical properties of myocardial muscle fibers. Increased preload is accompanied by longer initial myocardial muscle fiber length, resulting in greater -shortening capacity. Additionally, there is an increase in calcium responsiveness of the cardiac myofilament structure at these longer sarcomere lengths.[112,113,135]

Now consider the changes that occur in the Starling curve and P-V loop with an isolated increase in preload. An infusion of volume will increase preload, resulting in a concomitant rise in SV on the Starling curve (Fig. 13.12A). This is represented as an increase in the end-diastolic volume in the associated P-V loop (see Fig. 13.12B). It is important to note that the contractility (represented as the ESPVR) has not changed, and therefore the end-systolic pressure (ESP) and ESV do not change. This constant

ESP in the face of volume infusion is mediated in part by the baroreceptor reflex, which results in vasodilation and bradycardia in response to increased stretch in the walls of the atria, aorta, and carotid sinus. Note that the EF is also increased. Thus pure preload augmentation may increase EDV, SV, and apparent EF without changing contractility.

The exact relationship between preload and EDV is complex and has important clinical consequences. It is demonstrated by the end-diastolic pressure volume relationship (as shown previously in Fig. 13.8), which is representative of ventricular compliance.[136,137] Although this relationship is curvilinear, especially at very high EDPs, it is mostly linear over the normal operating range of the ventricle. This low slope indicates the substantial compliance of the normal ventricle during diastole. In diastolic heart failure the heart is characterized by a low ventricular compliance, which results in decreased cardiac function as evidence by a depressed Starling curve (see Fig. 13.12A). This results in less filling during diastole, a reduced EDV, and markedly decreased SV (see Fig. 13.12B).

As described previously, it has been demonstrated that the newborn heart responds to increased preload in a fashion similar to the adult heart.[130] Although increased preload increases SV in neonates, there are important developmental differences between newborns and adults. For instance, the newborn heart is stiffer and less compliant and maintains an equivalent volume at a higher EDP. In the neonate, normalized LVEDV is less than in children (42 ± 10 versus 73 ± 11 mL/m^2) even though LVEDP is similar. With less contractile structures per gram of tissue, the ventricles do not tolerate excessive preload as well as later in life.[138] Excessive increases in preload, which readily lead to increased EDP with elevated venous pressures, limit the effectiveness of volume infusion in neonates. Evidence in the fetal lamb indicates that when EDPs are greater than 10 to 12 mm Hg, further preload augmentation does not increase SV. With less compliant ventricles, heart failure may occur earlier in newborns. Therefore, with less tolerance of preload and maximized contractility, the stressed newborn augments cardiac output by increasing heart rate. This mechanism is in part responsible for the heart rate dependence of cardiac output in newborns and infants, as mentioned previously.

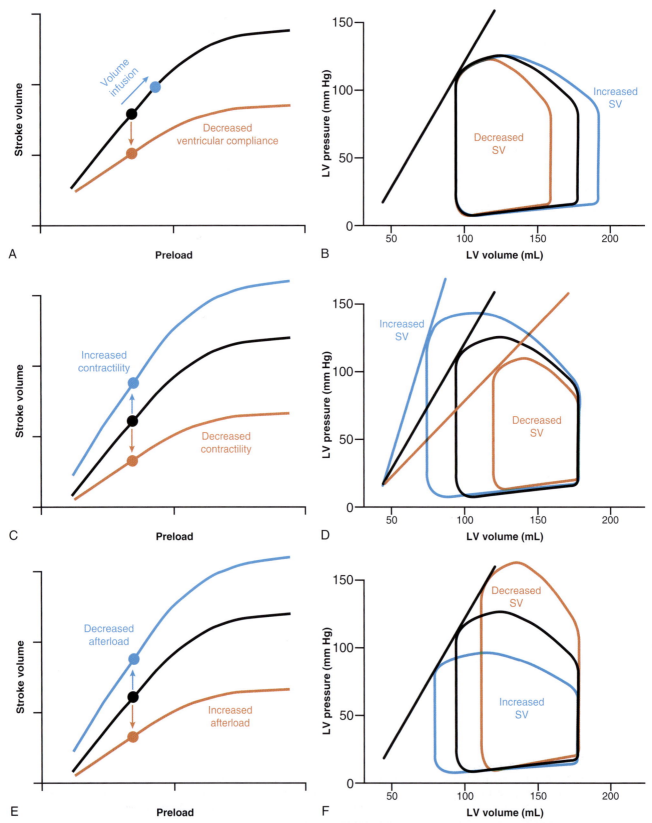

• **Figure 13.12** Effect of volume infusion, decreased ventricular compliance, altered contractility, and altered afterload on the Starling curve and pressure-volume (P-V) loops. (A and B) Volume infusion *(blue)* results in movement to the right in the Starling curve and an augmentation of stroke volume *(SV)* secondary to increased end-diastolic volume (EDV). Decreased myocardial compliance *(red)* results in reducing filling during diastole, decreased EDV, and smaller SV. (C and D) Increased *(blue)* or decreased *(red)* contractility results in enhanced or depressed Starling curves, respectively. Increased contractility results in steeper slope of the end-systolic pressure-volume relationship, decreased end-systolic volume (ESV), and increased SV. Depressed contractility results in decreased slope, increased ESV, and decreased SV. (E and F) Increased afterload results in a depressed Starling curve for a given preload, an increased ESV, and decreased SV *(red)*. Decreased afterload results in an enhanced Starling curve for a given preload, a decrease in ESV, and an increase in SV *(blue)*.

Contractility

Increases in cardiac contractility are produced by the activation of the sympathetic nervous system and result in the release of nor-epinephrine or epinephrine. These substances increase the contractility of individual cardiac muscle cells and are the primary way in which cardiac output is augmented physiologically. This is manifested by an increase in the shortening of a muscle contracting with constant preload and afterload. Therefore this causes an increase in ventricular SV by decreasing ESV, without altering the EDV.

The term *ejection fraction* (EF) is clinically useful to assess cardiac muscle contractility and is defined as the ratio of SV to EDV (fraction of blood in the ventricle at the end of diastole that is ejected during systole). Because an increase in cardiac contractility causes an increase in SV with constant EDV, EF will also increase.

In addition to the change in the extent of muscle shortening, an increase in contractility will also increase the rate of muscle tension development and shortening. This will result in an increase in the rate of isovolumetric pressure development, rate of ejection during systole, peak systolic pressure generation, and magnitude of EDP.

To further understand the relationship between preload and contractility, consider the series of Starling curves and P-V loops related to alterations in myocardial contractility in Fig. 13.12C and Fig. 13.12D. With a change in contractility the heart will be characterized by completely new Starling curves, which reflect the length dependence of cardiac contraction (see Fig. 13.12C). In the corresponding P-V loops, alterations in contractility are reflected by changes in the ESPVR line (see Fig. 13.12D).[139,140] A shift in this line upward to the left (increased slope) indicates increased contractility, where EF and SV are increased for a given EDPVR. A shift in the ESPVR down to the right is consistent with decreased myocardial contractility, where EF and SV are decreased for a given EDPVR.

Afterload

In the Starling muscle strip preparation the afterload is represented as the weight against which a cardiac muscle fiber contracts (see Fig. 13.6B) or the mass that resists contraction. The magnitude of muscle shortening is directly related to the afterload, so that with increasing afterload, shortening is decreased and slowed. Alternatively, a decrease in afterload will result in increased muscle fiber shortening.

However, this concept is deceptively simple, and transferring an in vitro experiment to the intact heart has significant limitations. One reason for this is that it is not the load on the muscle strip that is important, but rather the stress—defined as the load per cross-sectional area. Ventricular stress is a function of both load and geometry, and this concept is important in considering the in vivo determinants of afterload.[141,142] This concept is especially important in certain congenital heart diseases in which the right ventricle (RV) inappropriately acts as the systemic pump. The RV is geometrically well suited for preload changes but is poorly tolerant of acute changes in afterload.[143] The RV is three to four times thinner than the LV, maintains trabeculations that are coarse compared to the finely trabeculated LV, and has a muscular and elongated outflow tract. Therefore the systemic RV has a high propensity to fail due to its inability to accommodate large increases in ventricular stress (see later equation).

It should be remembered that the one-dimensional concept of systemic vascular resistance (SVR) as afterload is only a gross approximation of afterload and has gained use only because it is a measurable parameter of cardiovascular function. The concept of afterload can be generalized as any factor that resists the ejection of blood from the heart. There are several determinants of afterload in the intact heart:

1. *Impedance* of the vasculature, which is related to the elastance of the great vessels and the resistance of the smaller vessels. In children the latter is generally of greater significance.
2. The *ejection pressure* is also important and is in part determined by the vascular resistance. An increase in this resistance decreases fiber-shortening velocity of cardiac myocytes and results in higher peak ventricular ejection pressures. Because the period of time for systolic ejection is finite, an increase in ejection pressure will result in higher ESP and ESV.
3. *Ventricular outflow tract obstruction* significantly affects ventricular afterload, as can be seen with semilunar valve stenosis.
4. *Ventricular wall stress* is also a major determinant of afterload. Laplace's law simply states that the circumferential wall stress is equal to the pressure times the radius divided by twice the wall thickness:

$$T = \frac{(P \times r)}{2t}$$

where T is the circumferential wall stress (in N/cm^2), P is pressure (in N/cm^2), r is radius (in cm), and t is wall thickness (in cm).

In the heart, which is exposed to pressure from the outside (pericardial or intrathoracic pressure) and the inside (intraluminal pressure), the pressure driving wall tension is the transmural pressure or LV_{tm} (in mm Hg):

$$LV_{tm} = LV_{intraluminal} - LV_{extraluminal}$$

As a result, when intrathoracic pressure (ITP) becomes more negative, as with inspiration, then P_{tm}, ventricular wall stress, and afterload will increase. This also partly explains why positive end-expiratory pressure (PEEP), which elevates ITP, may also act as afterload reduction for the heart (see cardiopulmonary interactions discussed later).

Note that wall stress increases with increasing radius, so that volume loading the ventricle (increasing preload) will increases the wall stress. Therefore afterload is preload dependent. Additionally, hypertrophy will cause an increase in wall thickness and therefore a decrease in ventricular wall stress.

5. *Inertia*. Preload not only acts to increase wall stress, but also provides an inertial mass against which the heart must work to eject blood: the greater the mass, the greater the inertia and therefore the greater the afterload.

All of these effects, because they increase afterload, decrease SV for a given contractility and preload. This apparent change in cardiac function with increasing afterload can be understood by analyzing the effects of afterload on the Starling curve and P-V relationship (see Fig. 13.12).

As afterload is increased and the heart ejects against a higher pressure, the Starling relationship for a given preload is diminished, resulting in the movement of the curve downward. On the other hand, a decrease in afterload on the heart results in enhancement of the Starling relationship for a given preload and the movement of the curve upward (see Fig. 13.12E). The P-V loop for an increase in afterload demonstrates that the point for aortic valve opening (at the end of isovolumetric contraction) moves upward along the pressure axis, which results in higher pressures generated throughout ventricular ejection. This causes an increase in both the ESV and

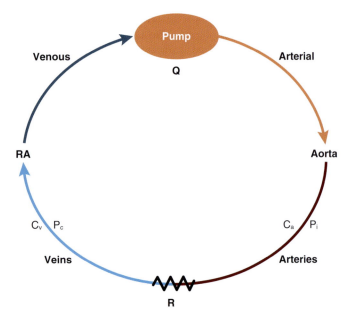

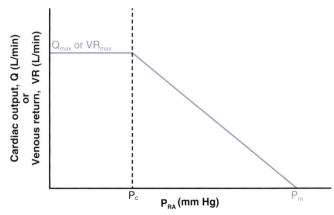

• **Figure 13.14** Venous return curve. As venous return *(VR)* or cardiac output *(Q)* decreases from its maximal point, right atrial pressure *(P_{RA})* increases due to redistribution of blood between the venous and arterial system. The P_c is the critical closing pressure and represents the point at which VR or Q can no longer be increased further. The P_m is the mean circulatory pressure and represents the P_{RA} at a no-flow state (Q or VR equals zero).

• **Figure 13.13** Conceptual model of the cardiovascular circulation to illustrate relationship between venous return, cardiac output, and right atrial pressure. The heart is represented by a mechanical pump, similar to a roller pump in venoarterial extracorporeal support, which drains the right atrium *(RA)* and forces blood into the aorta. Blood then moves through the arterial system, which has a certain capacitance *(C_a)* and inflow pressure *(P_i)*, which is determined by the flow rate *(Q)* and resistance *(R)*. Finally, blood returns via the veins to the right atrium through a venous system with a certain capacitance *(C_v)* and critical closing pressure *(P_c)*.

ESP and ultimately results in decreased SV when preload remain constant. For a decrease in afterload the point for aortic valve opening moves downward along the pressure axis, and therefore ventricular ejection occurs at lower systolic ejection pressures. This results in a decreased ESP and ESV and consequently an increase in SV with constant preload (see Fig. 13.12F).

Venous Return

Normally the heart passively pumps all of the venous return it receives. It has tremendous preload reserve and can increase cardiac output threefold with increasing venous return. Under most conditions, it is venous return that determines cardiac output. Therefore understanding what regulates venous return becomes the key to understanding further regulation of cardiac output.[144]

One model that illustrates this interdependency is shown in Fig. 13.13. It describes the relationship of the intrinsic properties of the systemic vasculature in relationship to cardiac output.[145] In this model the heart acts like a mechanical roller pump and mimics a cardiovascular circulation similar to venoarterial extracorporeal membrane support. As blood moves out of the pump, flow rate (Q or cardiac output) increases, and blood is partitioned into the arterial system at the expense of the venous system. Note that in this closed system model, Q is equal to the venous return. The determinants of this process are arterial capacitance (C_a), venous capacitance (C_v), and flow resistance (R). At maximal levels of Q the P_i and arterial blood volume are both high. Therefore the right atrial (or venous) pressure is low. When this right atrial pressure (P_{RA}) reached the critical closing pressure (P_c), the Q cannot increase further because veins will have the tendency to collapse when the P_{RA} is lower than the P_c. If Q is reduced at the roller pump, the

arterial P_i and arterial blood volume will drop, whereas the P_{RA} will increase, and venous return will drop. As Q approaches zero the P_{RA} approaches an important maximal number, called the mean circulatory pressure (P_m). At this point, venous return therefore approaches zero. This model is important in demonstrating the role of venous return as an independent determinant of cardiac output.[145,146]

This model can also be graphically displaced by the venous return curve (or vascular function curve) in Fig. 13.14. As the flow rate (Q) or venous return is varied, the P_{RA} is altered by the redistribution of blood between the arterial and venous system.[147] VR or Q cannot be increased above a maximum amount because P_{RA} would fall below the P_c of the venous system, resulting in venous collapse. When P_{RA} is high enough, venous return stops, as shown by the intercept point indicated by the P_m.[146] This pressure has also been called the dead pressure (the pressure measured at any point in the circulation when the heart stops), the mean circulatory filling pressure, and the mean systemic pressure (P_{ms}). It is the mean weighted pressure throughout the circulation when the pump (heart) is removed. It represents the capacitance and the relative filling of the entire circulation, both venous and arterial sides.

It is important to realize that the venous return curve is influenced by changes in circulating blood volume and vascular tone, as shown in Fig. 13.15. A blood transfusion (or any increase in intravascular volume) will increase the maximal venous return and cardiac output that can be achieved before the P_{RA} reaches P_c. On the other hand, hemorrhage (or any decrease in intravascular volume) has the opposite effect, resulting in a decrease in maximal venous return or cardiac output. In addition, because veins are more compliant than other blood vessels, changes in circulating blood volume produce larger alterations in the volume of the venous system than any other vascular segment. Therefore a reduction in venous compliance will have a similar effect to increasing blood volume on the venous return curve, and vice versa for an increase in venous compliance. Because transfusion, hemorrhage, and alterations in venous compliance do not directly alter vascular tone, the slope of the venous return curve (which represents resistance to venous return) is not altered. Therefore these

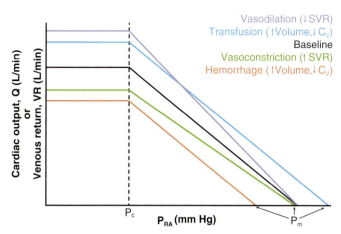

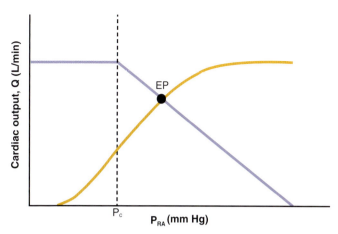

• **Figure 13.15** Effects of changing blood volume and vascular resistance on the venous return curve. Changes in blood volume or venous compliance *(blue and red curves)* are parallel to baseline *(black curve)* but have different mean circulatory pressure (*P_m*) at zero flow. Changes in vascular tone *(purple and green curves)* alter the slope of the venous return curve (venous resistance), resulting in a change in the maximal cardiac output or venous return at the critical closing pressure (*P_c*). *C_v*, Venous capacitance; *P_RA*, right atrial pressure; *SVR*, systemic vascular resistance.

• **Figure 13.16** Superimposition of cardiac function (Starling) and vascular function (venous return) curves. For a certain cardiac and vascular state, these curves intersect at the equilibrium point *(EP)*, which characterizes right atrial pressure (*P_RA*) and cardiac output (*Q*).

interventions alter P_m because they change blood volume or venous compliance.[148]

Changes in vascular tone will alter the maximum venous return (and cardiac output) before venous collapse at the P_c, at any given intravascular volume. However, the P_m at zero flow will remain constant, indicating that P_m is most directly related to volume of blood within the vessels. As shown in Fig. 13.15, a decrease in SVR caused by vasodilation will increase the slope of the venous return curve, whereas an increase in SVR caused by vasoconstriction will decrease the slop of the venous return curve.

Clinically these changes in vascular mechanics rarely occur in isolation. For instance, dilation of arteriolar vessels is usually accompanied by dilation of capacitance vessels, and these have opposite effects on the venous return curve and cardiac output. For example, afterload reduction with nicardipine or milrinone infusions is often accompanied with volume expansion to ensure adequate cardiac output and venous return. In patients with circulatory shock, systemic vasodilation can result in a high or low cardiac output state, depending on changes in vascular mechanics (such as C_v, vascular resistance, vascular volume expansion, and contractile state of the heart).

Veno-Cardiac Coupling

To achieve a combined understanding of contractility, preload, afterload, and venous return on cardiac output, the Starling curve (or cardiac function curve) can be superimposed on the venous return (or vascular function) curve (Fig. 13.16). Cardiac output occurs at the theoretical intersection of these two curves, representing a given state of cardiac function and vascular properties—called the *equilibrium point* (EP).[149]

Fig. 13.17 shows the effect of different cardiovascular changes on this combined curve to provide simultaneous information on the cardiac function, vascular function, and cardiac output. Intravascular volume expansion (point a to b), results in the movement of the venous return curve up to the right with the same

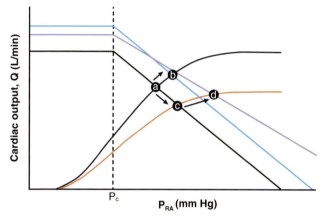

• **Figure 13.17** Veno-cardiac coupling for different cardiovascular states showing superimposition of cardiac function and venous return curves. Baseline curves are shown in black with intersection of two curves at equilibrium *(point a)*. Increasing intravascular volume moves venous return curve up to the right *(point a to b)* on the cardiac function curve, augmenting cardiac output. In systolic heart failure the equilibrium point moves down along the venous return curve to the depressed cardiac function curve *(point a to c)*. Chronic compensation due to fluid retention, decreased venous compliance, and increased systemic vascular resistance results in slight augmentation of cardiac output but at the expense of having higher right atrial pressures *(point c to d)*. *P_c*, Critical closing pressure; *P_RA*, right atrial pressure.

cardiac function curve. Therefore a new equilibrium is established, resulting in a greater cardiac output and slightly higher P_{RA}. Hemorrhage or decrease in intravascular volume will have the opposite effect (not shown).

Now consider the effect of decreased contractility or increased afterload on veno-cardiac coupling. In the case of systolic heart failure the cardiac function curve shifts down to the right along the same venous return curve (point a to c). Therefore P_{RA} is much greater, and cardiac output is decreased. The chronic physiologic adaptation to this heart failure is to increase the P_m by fluid retention, but this also is accompanied by venous constriction (decreased venous compliance) and arterial constriction (increased SVR). Therefore the vascular function curve will shift to the right and have a reduced slope. The new equilibrium point (d) represents this set of vascular and cardiac compensatory mechanisms. Notice that these changes help to partially restore cardiac output (from point c to d) despite the depressed cardiac function curve. This, however, occurs at the expense of further increasing P_{RA} and venous pressures.

Ventriculoarterial Coupling

An analogous situation exists for the systemic arterial circulation, but the forces involved are different. Ohm's law (as described previously) can be used to describe these forces:

$$R_a = \frac{P_p}{Q}$$

where R_a is arterial resistance (in mm Hg·min/L), P_p is perfusion pressure (in mm Hg) and Q is cardiac output (L/min). Therefore an increase in R_a from vasoconstriction will increase P_p. At the same time a significant increase in R_a will raise the afterload to the heart and hence decrease Q, unless compensatory mechanisms increase contractility and heart rate. It is important to realize that this system is much less sensitive than veno-cardiac coupling in regulating cardiac output. On the venous side a pressure change of 1 or 2 mm Hg can alter cardiac output significantly. In fact, Guyton[150] estimates a decrease of 14% in cardiac output for every 1 mm Hg decrease in $P_m - P_{RA}$. On the arterial side, pressure changes of 30 to 40 mm Hg may not alter function significantly, due to the great inotropic reserve of the myocardium when healthy. Conversely, in the impaired myocardium, small increases in afterload may seriously affect cardiac output.

These concepts of venous and arterial coupling to cardiac function can be generalized to the left and right ventricles. Cardiac output and venous return are closely interconnected and must be taken together whenever a therapeutic intervention is considered. Because the vasculature plays a major role in cardiovascular function and the regulation of cardiac output, a detailed discussion of regulation of vascular tone follows.

Cardiopulmonary Interactions

The common location of the cardiac and pulmonary systems within the thoracic cavity subjects them to interdependence. ITP, P_{tm}, systemic venous return, and systemic arterial output are affected by the interplay of this inseparable connection. In the presence of cardiopulmonary disease, understanding the impact of this interaction is of supreme importance in treating the physiologic perturbations of critical illness.

Hydrodynamic Principles

The foundations of understanding cardiopulmonary interactions come from the general laws of hydrodynamics as applied to a compressible structure. The distention or compression of a structure depends on the compliance of the structure itself as well as the pressure exerted across its wall, known as the *transmural pressure* (P_{tm}). A positive P_{tm} would distend the structure, either through increased internal pressure or from decreased external pressure. The opposite is true for a negative P_{tm}. The compliance of the structure dictates the degree of deformation. The more compliant, the more it will be deformed.[151]

Flow (Q) through a compressible tube depends on the P_i, P_o, surrounding pressure (P_s), and the compliance of the tube wall (Fig. 13.18). With a positive P_{tm}, the distended tube is patent, and Q is proportional only to the gradient between P_i and P_o (zone III condition). If P_i and P_o are constant but P_s increases, then P_{tm} will decrease and result in a narrower tube. Therefore the resistance to inflow will increase. In this situation Q is determined by the gradient between P_i and P_s (zone II condition). Should the P_s increase further, the P_{tm} becomes negative, and the tube collapses, resulting in cessation of flow (zone I condition).[151] In this manner hydrodynamic principles affect the compressible structures of the pulmonary bronchial and pulmonary vascular as well as the cardiovascular systems.

Mean Systemic Venous Pressure and Venous Capacitance

In addition to having basic knowledge of the principles of hydrodynamics, it is important to understand the determinants of venous pressure and capacitance to comprehend the effect of preload and afterload on the cardiopulmonary system (Fig. 13.19). The venous system pressure, or P_{ms}, is determined by pressure in veins and venules, which is governed by the interplay between intravascular volume and vascular compliance.[152-154] The major capacitance vessels are located in the splanchnic, splenic and hepatic circulations and are low-pressure venous volume reservoirs, containing approximately 70% of intravascular volume.[149,151,155] The venous system will fill with as much as 25% of the total blood volume without an appreciable change in pressure or distention because the reservoirs recruit a significant amount of volume into the system. Therefore these vascular beds are the biggest contributors to venous compliance, which is approximately 18 times greater than that of systemic arterial resistance vessels.[151] As intravascular volume expands past a certain amount, the P_{ms} will eventually increase in a linear fashion. Furthermore, vasoconstriction of the C_v vessels will increase P_{ms} and reduce of the capacity of the venous reservoirs due to high venomotor tone.[153,156] Therefore the volume in capacitance vessels combined with venomotor tone determines the P_{ms}. Based on the these principles, it is clear that venous return to the heart occurs due to increased volume, decreased venous compliance, decreased resistance to venous return, and decreased P_{RA}.[147,149,154,157]

Systemic arterial pressure is unrelated to venous return because the flow into the arterial circuit only maintains the volume of venous reservoirs. Arterial flow fills the venous reservoirs, and then blood leaves at a rate dependent on resistance to venous return and the overall volume in the venous system.[153,158-160] It is the pressure gradient between the systemic venous reservoirs (upstream pressure or P_{ms}) and the right atrium (downstream pressure) that dictates systemic venous return because the P_{RA} is the major resistor to venous return.[149,154,157] However, P_{RA} is subject to change due to the dynamic alterations of cardiac function, cardiac cycle, and respiration in various physiologic states.[147,151,161-163] Furthermore, although resistance to systemic venous return is constant in most conditions, it can change with differential blood viscosity, development of arterial venous fistulae, and the collapse of vena cava from negative ITP.[164-168] Generally, acute compensatory changes in systemic venous return are mediated by endogenous catecholamines, angiotensin, and vasopressin. Contraction of smooth muscle vessels due to neurosympathetic activation or exogenous catecholamines reduces the C_v and increase P_{ms}.[154,167,169] Alternately, venodilation from pharmacologic agents or inodilators increases capacitance, decreases P_{ms}, and reduces systemic venous return.[151,153] Finally, spontaneous and mechanical ventilation cause changes in ITP and lung volume, which can consequently affect atrial filling,

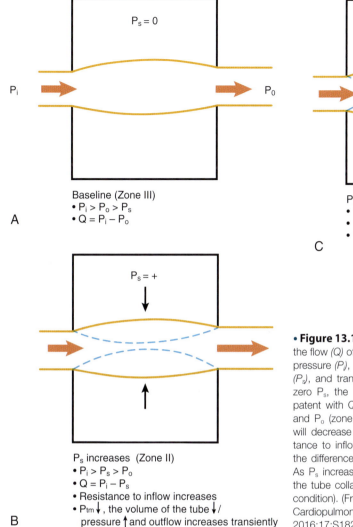

$P_s = 0$

P_i → → P_0

Baseline (Zone III)
- $P_i > P_o > P_s$
- $Q = P_i - P_o$

A

$P_s = ++$

P_s increases further (Zone I)
- $P_s > P_i$
- Resistance to Q increases further
- P_{tm} becomes negative, the tube collapses and flow may cease

C

$P_s = +$

P_s increases (Zone II)
- $P_i > P_s > P_o$
- $Q = P_i - P_s$
- Resistance to inflow increases
- $P_{tm}\downarrow$, the volume of the tube $\downarrow$/ pressure $\uparrow$ and outflow increases transiently

B

• **Figure 13.18** The hydrodynamic principles that govern the flow *(Q)* of fluids through a collapsible tube with inflow pressure *(P_i)*, outflow pressure *(P_o)*, surrounding pressure *(P_s)*, and transmural pressure *(P_{tm})*. (A) At baseline with zero P_s, the P_{tm} is positive, and the distended tube is patent with Q proportional to the difference between P_i and P_o (zone III condition). (B) As P_s increases, the P_{tm} will decrease and result in a narrower tube. The resistance to inflow increases, and Q will be determined by the difference between P_i and P_s (zone II condition). (C) As P_s increases further, the P_{tm} becomes negative, and the tube collapses, resulting in a zero-flow state (zone I condition). (From Bronicki RA, Penny DJ, Anas NG, et al. Cardiopulmonary interactions. *Pediatr Crit Care Med.* 2016;17:S182-S193.)

impedance to ventricular emptying, heart rate, and myocardial contractility.[157]

Intrathoracic Pressure and Right Ventricular Preload

Normal breathing occurs due to the generation of negative ITP. The rib cage expands, and the diaphragm descends to expand the chest cavity. Inspiration creates negative pleural pressure, decreases ITP, and the lungs fill into the created space.[152,157] This negative ITP is transmitted to the right atrium and vena cava, thereby increasing the P_{tm} of the right atrium. This distends the right atrium and reduces the P_{RA}.[151,157,170-173]

As stated earlier, systemic venous return depends on the pressure gradient between extrathoracic veins (driving pressure) and the P_{RA} (back pressure). Spontaneous respiration increases this gradient. As the intraatrial pressure falls, systemic venous return increases, thereby increasing RV preload and SV.[157,174,175] In addition, abdominal pressure is affected by diaphragmatic descent, resulting in an increased P_{tm} of the venous reservoir, decreased capacitance, and a rise in the P_{ms}.[147,151,157,170-173] The end result is a larger pressure gradient between the extrathoracic veins and the right atrium, further augmenting systemic venous return (see Fig. 13.19).[151,152,157]

Venous return will increase as the P_{RA} decreases and then plateau. If the vascular P_{tm} becomes negative at the thoracic inlet, the vena cava will collapse, therefore limiting venous return.[176] Decreasing P_{RA} further creates no additional effect on systemic venous return because flow is now dependent on the difference between P_{ms} and atmospheric pressure (superior vena cava) or abdominal pressure (inferior vena cava).[176]

Finally, increased venous return during inspiration results in a normal physiologic decrease in the systolic blood pressure. As stated earlier, inspiration causes a reduction in the P_{RA} secondary to negative ITP, which consequently increases the filling gradient for the RV. This produces an increase in RV preload with a concomitant decrease in LV compliance, filling, and SV. The end result is a decrease in the systolic blood pressure.[152,178,179]

Positive pressure ventilation (PPV) causes an opposite effect to normal spontaneous respiration. In the 1940s it was demonstrated that RV filling is inversely related to ITP, which leads to decreased cardiac output because of reduced systemic venous return.[157,180,181] Intermittent PPV increases ITP in inspiration above the atmospheric pressure, resulting in increased P_s of the right atrium (thereby decreasing its compliance), decreased right atrial P_{tm}, and therefore increased P_{RA}. If PEEP is added, the ITP is higher than atmospheric for the entire respiratory cycle. In this manner the P_{RA} will be

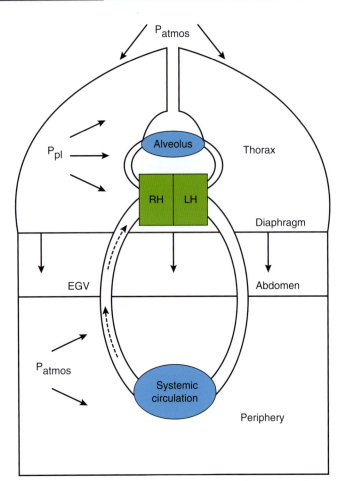

• **Figure 13.19** Model of circulation demonstrating factors that influence venous return. The right heart *(RH)* and intrathoracic veins are subject to pleural pressure *(P$_{pl}$),* which varies during normal respiration. Inspiration results in diaphragmatic descent and increases intraabdominal pressure, which returns to atmospheric pressure *(P$_{atmos}$)* with exhalation. The venous return *(broken arrows)* depends on the pressure gradient between the extrathoracic great veins *(EGV)* and the right atrium. During inspiration, venous return is maximized as the P$_{pl}$ (and right atrial pressure) falls, and the intraabdominal (and EGV) pressure rises. *LH,* Left heart. (From Shekerdemian L, Bohn D. Cardiovascular effects of mechanical ventilation. *Arch Dis Child.* 1999;80[5]:475-480.)

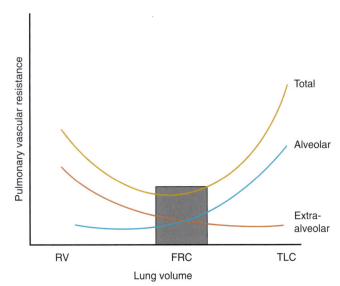

• **Figure 13.20** Relationship between lung volume and pulmonary vascular resistance. As lung volume increases from residual volume *(RV)* to total lung capacity *(TLC),* the alveolar vessels are compressed by overdistention, increasing resistance. As lung volume decreases, extraalveolar vessels become more tortuous secondary to lung atelectasis, resulting in increased resistance. The combined differential effect at various lung volumes produces a typical U-shaped curve as shown with the optimum at functional residual capacity *(FRC).* (From Shekerdemian L, Bohn D. Cardiovascular effects of mechanical ventilation. *Arch Dis Child.* 1999;80[5]:475-480.)

increased, and the gradient of P$_{ms}$ to P$_{RA}$ will be reduced. This will lead to decreased systemic venous return, decreased atrial filling, and ultimately a reduction in RV SV as compared to spontaneous breathing.[a] If the P$_{RA}$ becomes equal to the P$_{ms}$, systemic venous return will cease without compensation by adrenergic stimulation and retention of intravascular volume via the neurohormonal circulatory reflexes.[169,184] Of note, the extent to which systemic venous return is affected by PPV depends on the position of the RV on its pressure-SV curve. In addition to changing RV loading conditions, respiration alters the compliance of the RV by altering ventricular diastolic P$_{tm}$.[185-187]

Intrathoracic Pressure and Right Ventricular Afterload

The impact of ITP on RV afterload depends upon the relationship between pulmonary vascular resistance and lung volume. The

[a]References 149, 151, 157, 180, 182, 183.

resistance of the pulmonary circulation is determined by the effect of differential lung volumes on alveolar, extraalveolar, and parenchymal vessels (Fig. 13.20).[152,157,188,189] The alveolar vessels lie in the septa, and their P$_s$ is alveolar P$_{tm}$. Extraalveolar vessels lie in the interstitium, exposed to intrapleural pressure. Because they are in series, their resistance is additive. Normal tidal volume breathing occurs at functional residual capacity (FRC) lung volume, where PVR is minimal. Due to distention or collapse of the alveoli, PVR is increased at both high and low lung volumes.[151,152,157,188,189] At low lung volumes, atelectatic alveoli compress extraalveolar vessels, whereas at high lung volumes, alveolar overdistention compresses intraalveolar vessels. In both these situations, PVR increases (see Fig. 13.20). Furthermore, atelectasis increases shunting through perfused but nonventilated lung regions and causes hypoxia, whereas overdistention increases dead space ventilation with more ventilated but nonperfused lung regions and causes hypercarbia. Both hypercarbia and hypoxia additionally increase the RV afterload.[151,152]

The degree to which the lung expands with PPV is a function of airway resistance, lung compliance, and chest wall compliance. Regardless, PPV results in a positive interstitial pressure, thereby decreased the P$_{tm}$ for extraalveolar vessels and further increasing PVR. During PPV, alveolar and intrapleural pressures are positive in inspiration and expiration, and resistance is elevated in alveolar and extraalveolar vessels throughout the respiratory cycle.[151,154,157,190]

Finally, the effects of lung volume on PVR also depend on hydrostatic pressures in the pulmonary vasculature, which differ from the dependent zones of the lung to the apical lung fields. In the dependent portion, P$_i$ and P$_o$ are greater than P$_s$, and the P$_{tm}$ of the alveolar vessel is positive throughout (zone III condition). As P$_s$ increases superiorly in the lung, it exceeds the outflow but remains less than the P$_i$ (zone II conditions). If P$_s$ exceeds the P$_i$,

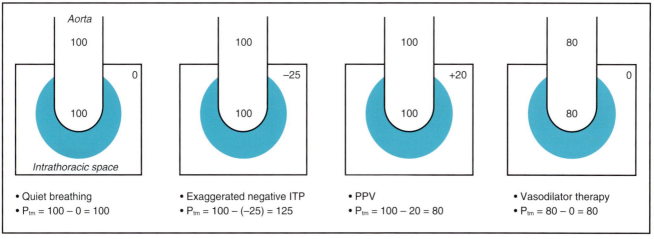

• Figure 13.21 The impact of intrathoracic pressure on left ventricular (LV) transmural pressure (P_{tm}). Changes in the LV P_{tm} are generated by manipulation of the aortic pressure or intrathoracic pressure *(ITP)*. During quiet breathing the LV P_{tm} is equal to the aortic pressure because the ITP is negligible. During exaggerated negative ITP (as occurs in respiratory disease), the P_{tm} of the LV will rise significantly, resulting in increased LV afterload. During positive pressure ventilation *(PPV)*, positive ITP will result in a smaller P_{tm} and therefore offload the LV. Addition of a vasodilator will change only the aortic pressure but have a net effect of decreasing P_{tm} and LV afterload. (From Bronicki RA, Penny DJ, Anas NG, Fuhrman B. Cardiopulmonary interactions. *Pediatr Crit Care Med*. 2016;17:S182-S193.)

the P_{tm} for the alveolar vessel is negative, the vessel collapses, and flow ceases (zone I condition). The zone I condition does not occur without cardiopulmonary disease. PVR is higher in zone I and II conditions, so the use of PPV in those with normal pulmonary venous pressure increases the proportion of lung units under zone I and II conditions, thereby increasing PVR and RV afterload.[151,154,157,190]

Intrathoracic Pressure and Left Ventricular Preload

LV preload is dependent on changes in systemic venous return, RV output, and LV filling. In steady state, cardiac output must equal the blood returning to the heart, determined by circuit function.[149,153,154] The preload to the LV is affected by the alteration of the RV loading conditions and the RV diastolic P_{tm}. Higher ITP reduces systemic venous return and RV output and therefore decreases LV preload. Additionally, the RV is a thinner-walled ventricle and therefore much more sensitive to conditions of increased afterload, such as PPV. Thus RV function might be impeded during PPV, further reducing LV preload.[191] Finally, the RV also affects LV filling due to ventricular systolic and diastolic interdependence.

Intrathoracic Pressure and Left Ventricular Afterload

The degree to which ITP affects LV afterload is determined by the compliance of the LV and the P_{tm} of the thoracic arterial vessels.[192] Peripheral arterial intravascular pressure is measured in relation to atmospheric pressure, but the thoracic aorta, due to its placement in the thorax, is subjected to changes in pleural pressure. Therefore the aorta P_{tm} is the difference between aortic intravascular systolic pressure and pleural pressure.[157,192] In spontaneous respiration the ITP decreases, which increases the P_{tm} of the thoracic arteries and therefore reduces the volume of the thoracic arterial system. The

P_{tm} is increased because the pleural pressure falls to a greater degree than the intravascular aortic pressure. The pressure of the thoracic arterial system is therefore lower relative to the extrathoracic arterial system (Fig. 13.21). This produces higher LV afterload and decreases LV SV.[157,178]

During ventricular systole a decrease in ITP decreases the egress of blood from the thorax. In diastole the decrease in ITP reduces antegrade flow runoff, which increases thoracic arterial blood volume and increases the opposition to ejection after systole. In this manner LV ejection and SV are reduced.[179,193] This produces the decrease in systolic blood pressure in systole with spontaneous inspiration and is the mechanism of the exaggerated systolic drop in pulsus paradoxus.[178] In very negative ITP or with reduced LV function the adverse impact of respiration on LV afterload increases. If this state persists, an increase in catecholamines, SVR, and arterial blood pressure further increase LV afterload.

In contrast, the ITP is increased with PPV, resulting in a reduction of LV afterload and increase in systolic and diastolic pressures.[192,194,195] With increased ITP, the P_{tm} of the thoracic aorta decreases, driving blood into extrathoracic compartments. The LV P_{tm} has decreased because ITP has risen to a greater extent than LV and thoracic arterial pressures (see Fig. 13.21). Therefore patients with LV dysfunction will benefit most favorably by afterload reduction via PPV.[190,196] Additionally, PPV reduces myocardial and respiratory muscle oxygen consumption by unloading the left side of the heart. This improvement in the oxygen supply-demand relationship will dampen the sympathetic nervous system activity and further reduced LV afterload.[177,197]

Special Considerations of Positive Pressure Ventilation in Cardiac Disease

The predominant effects of PPV will be on the RV in diseases in which there is diastolic dysfunction with good LV systolic performance, such as restrictive cardiomyopathy or hypertrophic cardiomyopathy.[198] Additionally, in hypertrophic cardiomyopathy with obstruction to LV outflow, PPV will decrease LV preload and afterload, which can worsen intracavitary obstruction.[199]

In patients with restrictive physiology or normal biventricular function with decreased RV diastolic function (as in postoperative tetralogy of Fallot repair), there is an increase in the SV and cardiac output with negative pressure ventilation.[183,200] Therefore extubating from PPV and allowing resumption of spontaneous breathing improves cardiac output, even in the face of the resultant increase in respiratory muscle oxygen demand.

In the patient with Fontan physiology, systemic venous return is dictated by the gradient between P_{ms} and the pressure downstream at the confluence of the vena cava and pulmonary artery. Flow is passive because there is no subpulmonic pump, and therefore this gradient is the same one driving blood across the pulmonary circulation to the common atrium.[201,202] The venous return downstream resistor is no longer the P_{RA} and instead is the pulmonary circulation. An increase in ITP simultaneously and equally decreases both downstream venous return gradient between P_{ms} and the pulmonary circulation and from pulmonary circulation to the common atrium. Changes in the atrial pressure will not affect systemic venous return, they will only alter pulmonary venous return.[203,204] This means the pulmonary blood flow in Fontan physiology is particularly sensitive to increases in PVR and decreases in systemic ventricular function.[205] These patients also have a marked increase in pulmonary blood flow and cardiac output when they transition from PPV to negative pressure ventilation.[200,206]

Right–Left Heart Interactions

The structural and functional interplay between the LV and RV is essential to the management of the critically ill pediatric cardiac patient. In addition, regulation of RV systolic and diastolic function differs significantly from that of the LV.[207-209] These differences have important therapeutic and surgical implications, especially in congenital heart disease and congestive heart failure.[210]

Comparison of Right and Left Heart Hemodynamics

The hemodynamic mechanisms by which the RV and LV function to generate cardiac output are very different.[207] Although the cardiac output from each ventricle must be essentially equal, the RV performs only 25% of the stroke work (SW) as compared to the LV.[211] This can be depicted graphically using the concepts of the P-V loop introduced in Fig. 13.8. The SW is the area within the PV loop of each respective ventricle. This area represents the external mechanical work done by the ventricle to eject blood and is sometimes used to assess ventricular function. It is essentially the product of the SV and the developed pressure within the ventricle. A comparison of the LV and RV P-V loops shows that the developed pressure and trapezoidal shape of the RV loop results in a significantly decreased amount of SW performed as compared to the LV loop (Fig. 13.22).[208]

Functionally the RV has the ability to eject blood into the pulmonary artery during both systole and diastole; therefore the SW performed by the RV follows a more complex derivation.[211,212] Structurally the RV is a much thinner walled ventricle, and therefore even small changes in preload and afterload can have large alterations in the external mechanical work needed to generate cardiac output of the same magnitude as the LV.[213] Furthermore, the low resistance of the pulmonary vascular bed in normal physiologic states is

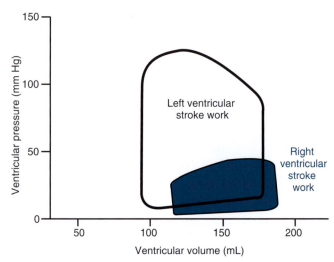

• **Figure 13.22** Schematic representations of left ventricular and right ventricular pressure-volume relationships. The stroke work of the right ventricle is dramatically lower than the stroke work of the left ventricle.

suitably tailored to the trapezoidal shape of the RV P-V relationship.[214] In fact, in healthy individuals the pulmonary vasculature is at maximum vasodilatory capacity, and therefore the amount of work the RV needs to do is much less.[211,215] In comparison, the systemic vasculature is heavily regulated by numerous molecular mediators, physiologic states, and regional circulations. Therefore the amount of work the LV needs to generate to overcome LV afterload is much greater.

Interactions Between the Left Ventricle and Right Ventricle

Classically the function of the LV and the function of the RV have been considered in isolation from one another. However, there has recently been a surge in our understanding and interest in the ways in which both sides of the heart interact with each other.[207,209,216] This is due to the appreciation that both ventricles are contained with a singular pericardial cavity, share an intricate electrical conduction system, have been shown to use common myocardial fibers, and are dependent on each other's cardiac output to function appropriately.[217] Therefore it is clear that the continual communication between the two sides of the heart has profound effects on biventricular function in both the normal and pathologic disease states.

It is known that increased filling of either the LV or RV during diastole results in septal displacement of the opposing ventricle, thereby causing a decrease in the diastolic compliance of the affected ventricle. This effect is further augmented by the fact that the two ventricles share a common pericardium and contiguous myocardium.[218-221] Given that systolic ventricular interactions have the unique potential to affect surgical, therapeutic, and mechanical interventions for cardiac disease, we will primarily focus on the effects of systolic ventricular interdependence.

Effects of the Left Ventricle on the Right Ventricle

In the early 1990s a landmark study established the principle of ventricular interrelatedness by demonstrating the effects of LV performance on RV force generation.[222] This well-designed experimental study examined the mechanical and hemodynamic effects of pacing electrically isolated but mechanically contiguous ventricles. Pacing the electrically isolated RV led to negligible force generation of the LV. However, pacing the electrically isolated LV led to almost normal pressure development of the RV. The authors concluded that dynamic geometric changes occur on the crescentic RV free wall that is contiguous with the LV due to cardiomyocyte shortening during LV contraction.[223] This mechanical effect is independent of the RV free wall function as redemonstrated by a subsequent study in which LV contraction still resulted in significant RV pressure generation after replacement of the RV free wall with a noncontractile patch.[224] These studies suggest that one-third to one-half of the SW performed by the RV is likely a direct effect of LV shortening.

Harnessing this ventricular crosstalk has significant potential for the development of therapeutic modalities to enhance pathologic disease states with significant RV dysfunction. In fact, animal experimental models have shown that an increase in LV afterload by aortic constriction or administration of systemic vasopressors can improve RV dysfunction secondary to acute right heart failure.[225,226] A subsequent experiment demonstrated that chronic LV afterload therapy with long-term aortic constriction not only enhanced biventricular function, but also improved myocardial remodeling in a rabbit model of chronic RV failure.[227]

Effects of the Right Ventricle on the Left Ventricle

In the previous study that demonstrated ventricular interrelatedness in a model of RV free wall replacement, it was also observed that as the size of the artificial RV was augmented, there was a deleterious effect on LV function.[224] As the RV became successively more dilated, there was a consequent drop in LV SW from decreased pressure generation. This experiment was unable to ascertain whether the cause of this decreased LV function was from adverse ventricular cross or reduced LV preload secondary to reduced RV cardiac output. A series of P-V analysis studies were performed in animal models that used isolated RV ischemia to induce right heart dilation.[228] If was found that acute RV dilation resulted in detrimental effects on LV performance, likely secondary to geometric and structural changes influencing LV contraction.[229] It is important to realize that these effects are not entirely due to systolic interactions but likely combined with diastolic interventricular and septal interactions.[230,231] For instance, it is known that ventricular septal

shifts toward the LV in early diastole can reduce early LV filling. This can lead to an increased dependence of LV filling on atrial contraction in certain pathologic conditions, such as pulmonary hypertension.[232]

Conclusion

New insights into the anatomy, physiology, and pharmacology of the developing cardiovascular system and its interaction with other organ systems have provided greater understanding of the action of currently available therapeutic agents and the development of more novel and specific agents. Much more needs to be learned to understand and intervene in the pathology of the cardiovascular system of the child. Congenital cardiovascular defects and their therapy demand a breadth of knowledge of the pathophysiology and available therapies, and an experienced clinician. Through the research of pharmacologists, physiologists, cell and molecular biologists, and clinicians, the development of new therapeutic agents and management strategies to modulate the cardiac vasculature and its interactions with other organs will undoubtedly continue to advance.

Selected References

A complete list of references is available at ExpertConsult.com.

1. Secomb TW. Hemodynamics. *Compr Physiol*. 2016;6(2):975–1003.
60. Corsini C, Baker C, Kung E, et al. An integrated approach to patient-specific predictive modeling for single ventricle heart palliation. *Comput Methods Biomech Biomed Engin*. 2014;17(14):1572–1589.
69. Sonnenblick EH, Spiro D, Spotnitz HM. The ultrastructural basis of Starling's law of the heart. The role of the sarcomere in determining ventricular size and stroke volume. *Am Heart J*. 1964;68:336–346.
121. Fogel MA, Weinberg PM, Fellows KE, et al. A study in ventricular-ventricular interaction. Single right ventricles compared with systemic right ventricles in a dual-chamber circulation. *Circulation*. 1995;92(2):219–230.
151. Bronicki RA, Penny DJ, Anas NG, et al. Cardiopulmonary interactions. *Pediatr Crit Care Med*. 2016;17:S182–S193.
157. Shekerdemian L, Bohn D. Cardiovascular effects of mechanical ventilation. *Arch Dis Child*. 1999;80(5):475–480.
208. Penny DJ, Redington AN. Function of the left and right ventricles and the interactions between them. *Pediatr Crit Care Med*. 2016;17(8 suppl 1):S112–S118.
222. Damiano RJ Jr, La Follette P Jr, Cox JL, et al. Significant left ventricular contribution to right ventricular systolic function. *Am J Physiol*. 1991;261:H1514–H1524.

14

Respiratory Physiology for Intensivists

PLATO ALEXANDER, MD, MBA

Respiratory mechanics and physiology affect the broad spectrum of cardiac physiologies encountered in the cardiovascular intensive care unit (CVICU) in many interconnected and complex ways. Said differently, the patient affected by cardiac disease is often vulnerable to alterations in lung function, and the converse is also true: alterations in cardiac function and anatomy affect respiratory physiology in often dramatic ways. It is therefore imperative for the clinician to be aware of how normal and abnormal respiratory mechanics can create excessive demands on cardiac output, and how they can adversely affect both short- and long-term somatic growth. The mechanisms by which this detriment to cardiac output and somatic growth occurs are multifactorial and truly merit a multivolume textbook dedicated to just this subject. We present to the reader in this chapter an introductory discussion of some of these concepts and mechanisms.

Distribution of Ventilation

Gravity-Dependent Determinants of Ventilation

The lung is a viscoelastic structure that is located inside and is supported by the chest wall. Gravity causes the lung to assume a globular shape with a relatively more negative pressure at the top and a more positive pressure at the base of the lung. The magnitude of the pleural pressure (P_{pl}) gradient depends on the density of the lung. P_{pl} normally increases 7.5 cm H_2O from the top to the bottom of the adult lung.[47]

In normal lungs the pressure of the air in the alveolus (alveolar pressure [P_A]) is equal throughout the lung, and the P_{pl} gradient results in regional differences in transpulmonary pressure ($P_A - P_{pl}$). Where P_{pl} is most positive (i.e., least negative), the transmural pressure differences result in the alveoli being compressed and smaller than the apical alveoli.[65] Thus the small alveoli located in the basal areas of the lung are on the midportion of a normal pressure-volume curve of the lung, and the larger alveoli of the apices of the lung are on the upper portion (Fig. 14.1). Dependent alveoli are relatively more compliant (have a greater volume change for a given change in pressure [i.e., on the steep slope of the pressure-volume curve]), whereas nondependent alveoli are relatively less compliant (on the flatter slope). Therefore the majority of the tidal volume during normal ventilation is preferentially distributed to dependent alveoli because these alveoli expand more per unit pressure change than do nondependent alveoli.

Gravity-Independent Determinants of Ventilation

Muscles of Respiration. In order for gas exchange to occur at the level of the alveoli, inspired air must travel into the lung through the airways. The muscles of respiration, which include the diaphragm and the external intercostal muscles, actively constrict during inspiration to allow air in, whereas quiet expiration occurs passively via elastic recoil of the system. Accessory muscles of inspiration, such as the scalene and sternocleidomastoid muscles, aid respiration during exercise. Expiration also becomes active during exercise with the contraction of muscles of the abdominal wall (i.e., rectus abdominis, internal and external oblique muscles and transversus abdominis), and the internal intercostal muscles.[93]

Lung Volumes and Airway Closure. Functional residual capacity (FRC) is defined as the volume of gas remaining in the normal lungs at the end of an expiration, when P_A equals ambient pressure ($P_{ambient}$). FRC depends on the balance of the lungs' intrinsic elastic properties that favor reduction in volume and the natural tendency of the chest wall to recoil outward. Changes in the elastic properties of either of these components of the respiratory system alter FRC.

Total lung capacity (TLC) is the entire gas volume of the maximally spontaneously inflated pulmonary parenchyma and airways in the thorax. It provides the reference point for all other lung volumes and capacities (Fig. 14.2). Vital capacity defines the volume obtained by maximal expiration from TLC and is the maximum volume possible during spontaneous ventilation. As such, it provides a measure of ventilatory reserve.

A critical relationship occurs between the volume of gas remaining in the normal lungs at the end of expiration (FRC) and the volume of gas in the lung at the point at which conducting airways collapse, which is called the *closing capacity* (CC). Using the inert gas washout technique during maximal inspiratory and expiratory maneuvers, the CC can be identified as the point at which conducting airways in dependent lung regions begin to collapse.[11] If end-expiratory lung volume (EELV) falls below CC, or conversely CC is elevated above EELV, these areas of lung collapse and do not participate in gas exchange.

Compliance. The relationship between the change in volume (ΔV) and change in distending pressure (ΔP) defines compliance.

$$C = \Delta V / \Delta P$$

The elastic properties of the respiratory system and its components, the lungs and chest wall, are graphically defined by their respective

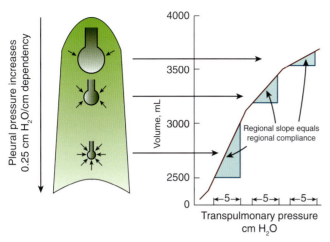

• **Figure 14.1** Pleural pressure increases 0.25 cm H_2O per centimeter down the lung. The increase in pleural pressure causes a fourfold decrease in alveolar volume. The caliber of the air passages also decreases as lung volume decreases. When regional alveolar volume is translated over to a regional transpulmonary pressure–alveolar volume curve, small alveoli are on a steep *(large slope)* portion of the curve, and large alveoli are on a flat *(small slope)* portion of the curve. Because the regional slope equals regional compliance, the dependent small alveoli normally receive the largest share of the tidal volume. Over the normal tidal volume range (lung volume increases by 500 mL from 2500 mL [normal functional residual capacity] to 3000 mL), the pressure-volume relationship is linear. Lung volume values in this diagram relate to the upright position. (From Benumof JL. Respiratory physiology and respiratory function during anesthesia. In: Miller RD, ed. *Anesthesia.* New York: Churchill Livingstone; 1990.)

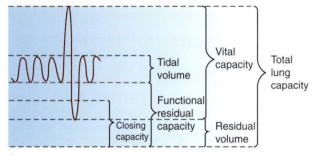

• **Figure 14.2** Functional components of lung volume. (From Scarpelli EM. *Pulmonary Physiology of the Fetus, Newborn, and Child.* Philadelphia: Lea & Febiger; 1975:27.)

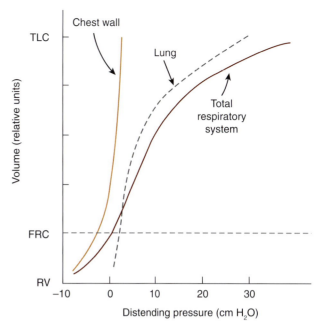

• **Figure 14.3** Pressure-volume relationships (i.e., compliance curves) of the chest wall, lung, and total respiratory system in the normal infant. At FRC the distending pressures of the lung and chest wall are equal and opposite, resulting in the exertion of zero net distending pressure on the total respiratory system. At lung volumes in excess of FRC the chest wall of the infant displays very high compliance characteristics relative to the adult counterpart. In addition, total respiratory system pressure-volume relationships display sigmoid characteristics, with compliance decreasing at either extreme of lung volume. *FRC,* Functional residual capacity; *RV,* residual volume; *TLC,* total lung capacity. (Modified from Kendig EL, Chernick V. *Disorders of the Respiratory Tract in Children.* Philadelphia: WB Saunders; 1977:17.)

volume-pressure relationships (Fig. 14.3). The lung has an *elastic recoil* force due to elastin and collagen fibers that pull the lung toward its deflated state. Lung compliance is determined by ΔV and the *transpulmonary* pressure gradient ($P_A - P_{pl}$, the ΔP for the lung). In contrast, the chest wall has an outward recoil force. The chest wall demonstrates its own compliance, which depends on PV and the *transmural* pressure gradient ($P_{pl} - P_{ambient}$, the PP for the chest wall). FRC occurs at the equilibrium point where these forces are perfectly balanced.[21] The total respiratory system compliance is determined by the compliance of the lungs and chest wall.[68] To determine the total respiratory compliance, PV and the *transthoracic* pressure gradient ($P_A - P_{ambient}$, the ΔP for the lung and chest wall together) must be known.

During certain modes of positive or negative pressure lung inflation, the transthoracic pressure gradient first increases to a peak value and then decreases to a lower plateau value. The peak transthoracic pressure is the pressure required to overcome both elastic and airway resistance (see later). The transthoracic pressure decreases to a plateau value because gas redistributes over time to alveoli with longer time constants. As the gas redistributes into an increased number of alveoli, less pressure is generated by the same volume of gas, and the pressure decreases. Therefore two measures of compliance can be made, dynamic and static. During positive pressure ventilation, *dynamic compliance* can be estimated by calculating the volume change (tidal volume) divided by the *peak* inspiratory pressure minus the end-expiratory pressure (positive end-expiratory pressure [PEEP]). As such, dynamic compliance makes an accounting for the movement of gas through the system. In contrast, *static compliance* can be approximated by measuring the change in volume divided by the *plateau* inspiratory pressure minus the end-expiratory pressure. Plateau pressure falls below peak inspiratory pressure because of gas redistribution; therefore static compliance is greater than dynamic compliance. Static compliance is a better evaluation of the entire respiratory system, because the measurement reflects more of the gas-exchanging alveoli.

The compliance relationship of the chest wall and lung units is sigmoidal. At the extremes of lung volumes, compliance decreases, and a larger increase in peak inspiratory pressure is required to obtain similar changes in volume. Underinflation (atelectasis, hypoventilation, EELV < FRC) and overexpansion (asthma, excessive PEEP, EELV > FRC) should thus be avoided because they require greater peak pressures to change lung volume.

An additional force that contributes to the elastic recoil of the lung is *surface tension.* Surface tension is a force generated by the

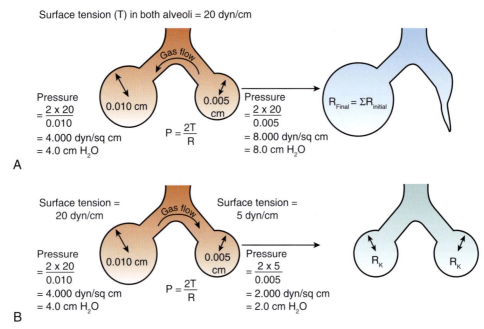

Surface tension (T) in both alveoli = 20 dyn/cm

Gas flow

Pressure
$= \dfrac{2 \times 20}{0.010}$
= 4.000 dyn/sq cm
= 4.0 cm H_2O

0.010 cm   0.005 cm

$P = \dfrac{2T}{R}$

Pressure
$= \dfrac{2 \times 20}{0.005}$
= 8.000 dyn/sq cm
= 8.0 cm H_2O

$R_{Final} = \Sigma R_{initial}$

A

Surface tension =
20 dyn/cm

Gas flow

Surface tension =
5 dyn/cm

Pressure
$= \dfrac{2 \times 20}{0.010}$
= 4.000 dyn/sq cm
= 4.0 cm H_2O

0.010 cm   0.005 cm

$P = \dfrac{2T}{R}$

Pressure
$= \dfrac{2 \times 5}{0.005}$
= 2.000 dyn/sq cm
= 2.0 cm H_2O

R_K R_K

B

• **Figure 14.4** Relationship between surface tension (T), alveolar radius (R), and alveolar transmural pressure (P). A, Pressure relationship in two alveoli of different size but with the same surface tension in their lining fluids. The direction of gas flow will be from the higher-pressure small alveolus to the lower-pressure large alveolus. The net result is one large alveolus ($R_{Final} = \Sigma R_{Initial}$). B, Pressure relationship of two alveoli of different size when allowance is made for the expected changes in surface tension (less tension in smaller alveolus). The direction of gas flow is from the larger alveolus to the smaller alveolus until the two alveoli are of equal size and are volume stable (R_K). K, Constant; ΣR, sum of all individual radii. (From Benumof JL. Respiratory physiology and respiratory function during anesthesia. In: Miller RD, ed. *Anesthesia*. New York: Churchill Livingstone; 1990.)

stronger attraction between adjacent liquid molecules than between molecules of liquid and gas. Because of this force, liquid assumes the shape of a sphere, which provides the smallest possible surface area for a given volume.[93] The liquid that lines the alveolus exerts surface tension and is described by Laplace's law, in which pressure (P) to inflate an alveolus is directly proportional to the surface tension (T) of the fluid lining the alveolus and inversely proportional to the radius (R) of the alveolus:

$$P = 2T/R$$

Using this relationship, the pressure inside small alveoli would be higher than inside large alveoli. Because small alveoli would have greater pressure than large ones, small alveoli would empty into larger ones, until theoretically, one gigantic alveolus would be left (Fig. 14.4A). This phenomenon does not occur in the lung because of the alterations in alveolar surface tension.

In the normal healthy lung, tension is reduced by the presence of surfactant, which is a mixture of phospholipids, neutral lipids, and proteins produced by type II pneumocytes. It greatly reduces surface tension in the alveoli due to the mixed property of its phospholipid molecule being hydrophilic at one end and hydrophobic at the other. By reducing surface tension and therefore the pressure needed to inflate the alveolus, surfactant increases lung compliance. Surfactant also allows stabilization of smaller alveoli, inhibiting them from discharging their contents into large alveoli (see Fig. 14.4B). Pulmonary edema can be exacerbated as surface tension forces draw fluid from the capillaries in the alveoli. By reducing surface tension, surfactant prevents transudation of fluid by reducing the hydrostatic driving force for pulmonary edema.[14]

For preterm infants incapable of producing adequate amounts of endogenous surfactant, exogenous surfactant replacement has been used for many years with great reduction of morbidity and mortality. In addition to bovine- and porcine-derived surfactant, synthetic surfactant has also become available. Newer studies are investigating the effectiveness of minimally invasive surfactant administration techniques, such as nebulization, which would allow administration in nonintubated infants.[71]

Alterations in chest wall and lung compliance are important conditions that require continuous evaluation in critically ill children. Although both an increase and a decrease in compliance can result in a change in lung volume, a reduction in compliance requires prompt identification and intervention. A decrease in intrinsic compliance of the lungs and/or chest wall will result in decreased total compliance and a reduction of lung volume for a given P_A and a decrease in FRC. In many clinical instances this may necessitate the application of additional distending pressure (P_A) in the form of positive pressure ventilation and/or continuous positive airway pressures (continuous positive airway pressure [CPAP]/PEEP) to reestablish normal lung volumes.

Resistance. For gas flow to occur, a pressure gradient must be generated to overcome the nonelastic airway resistance of the lungs. Mathematically, resistance (R) is defined by the pressure gradient (ΔP) required to generate a given flow of gas ($\dot{V}$). Physically, resistance results from the friction during movement of gas molecules within the airways (airway resistance) and friction from motion of the lung and chest wall (tissue viscous resistance). These components make up the total nonelastic resistance of the respiratory system. Normally airway resistance accounts for approximately 75% of total nonelastic resistance.[17] However, in conditions in which respiratory pathophysiology alters tissue viscous resistance, airway resistance may be altered.

The pressure gradient (ΔP) along the airway is dependent upon the caliber of the airway and the rate and pattern of airflow. During laminar flow the pressure drop down the airway is proportional to the flow. When flow exceeds a critical velocity, it becomes turbulent, and the pressure drop down the tube becomes proportional to the square of the flow.[84] As flow becomes more turbulent, pressure increases more than flow, and resistance increases. Increased airway resistance requires a larger pressure gradient between the airway opening and the alveoli to maintain flow. During positive pressure ventilation this requires the generation of higher inspiratory pressures to achieve similar ventilation, whereas during spontaneous breathing a more negative intrapleural and alveolar pressure must be achieved to maintain similar ventilation. In both cases the work required to produce adequate gas flow is increased.

Resistance of the airways is approximated by the diameter of the airway, the velocity of airflow, and the properties of inhaled gases. Resistance is determined by Poiseuille's law, which governs the laminar flow of gas in nonbranching tubes:

$$P = \dot{V}(8L\eta'/\pi r^4)$$

where P is pressure, $\dot{V}$ is flow, L is length, r is radius of the tube, and $\acute{\eta}$ is the viscosity of the gas.[10,29] When flow exceeds critical velocity, its pattern changes from laminar to turbulent. Airway resistance is inversely proportional to the radius of the conducting airways raised to the fourth power during laminar flow and to the fifth power during turbulent flow.

Airway resistance is also dependent on alterations in lung volume. When lung volume is increased above FRC, airway resistance increases by only a small amount.[2,17] In contrast, when lung volume is decreased below FRC, airway resistance increases dramatically. Airway resistance is also dependent on conducting airway patency. During normal negative pressure ventilation, intrathoracic conducting airways have a tendency to narrow on exhalation and open on inspiration. The result is an increase in airway resistance during exhalation. In conditions in which total cross-sectional area is reduced and airway resistance increased, small airways collapse, and flow limitations occur during expiration.

Time Constants. The interaction between compliance and resistance largely determines the distribution of ventilation within the lungs. This relationship is defined as the product of the resistance (R) and compliance (C), which is the time constant (τ), measured in seconds:

$$\tau = R\left(\frac{\text{cm H}_2\text{O}}{\text{L/sec}}\right) \times C\left(\frac{\text{L}}{\text{cm H}_2\text{O}}\right)$$

The time constant defines the time required for each compartment to achieve a change in volume following the application or withdrawal of a constant distending pressure. It also describes the time required for the pressure within alveoli to equilibrate. As an example, a constant distending pressure applied to the airway overcomes airway resistance and expands the lung (elastic forces). The component of the distending pressure overcoming resistance to airflow is maximal initially and declines exponentially as airflow decreases. The component overcoming elastic forces increases in proportion to the change in lung volume. Thus the pressure required to overcome compliance is initially minimal, then increases exponentially with increasing lung volume. Lung volume approaches equilibrium according to an exponential function with the time course of change in these exponential curves being described by

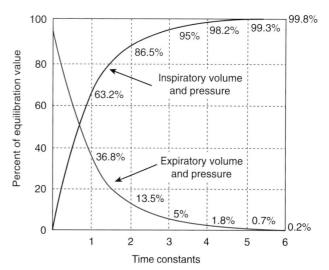

• **Figure 14.5** Exponential rise and fall of lung pressure and lung volume during inspiration and expiration expressed in terms of time constants. (From Chatburn RL. Principles and practice of neonatal and pediatric mechanical ventilation. *Respir Care.* 1991;36:569.)

their time constant. Mathematically, 63% of lung inflation (or deflation) occurs in one time constant (Fig. 14.5).

Most causes of respiratory failure have widespread abnormalities in pulmonary resistance and compliance, resulting in striking inhomogeneity in regional time constants. Consequently, with normal tidal breathing, certain compartments fill and empty rapidly (short time constants) while others fill and empty slowly (long time constants). This inhomogeneity of time constants results in marked irregularities in the distribution of ventilation with abnormal gas exchange.[72,80] Under these conditions, successful positive pressure ventilation may require manipulation of inspiratory and expiratory time to allow more uniform distribution ("homogeneity") of ventilation among lung compartments. This strategy, described elsewhere, frequently improves ventilation/perfusion (V/Q) matching.

Work of Breathing. Work of breathing is defined as the energy necessary to perform tidal ventilation over a set unit of time. The work of breathing is determined by the pressure-volume characteristics (compliance and resistance) of the respiratory system (Fig. 14.6). During breathing, work must be done to overcome the tendency of the lungs to collapse and the chest wall to spring out (see Fig. 14.6, area ADC) and the frictional resistance to gas flow that occurs in the airways (see Fig. 14.6, area ABC). Work of breathing (see Fig. 14.6, area ABCD) is increased by conditions that increase resistance or decrease compliance or when respiratory frequency increases.

If minute volume is constant, the "compliance" component of work is increased when tidal ventilation is large and respiratory rate slow. The "resistance" component of work is increased when the respiratory rate is rapid and tidal ventilation decreased. When the two components are summed and the total work plotted against the respiratory frequency, an optimal respiratory frequency that minimizes the total work of breathing can be obtained (Fig. 14.7). In children with restrictive lung disease (EELV < FRC, low compliance) and short time constants, the optimal respiratory frequency is increased, whereas children with obstructive lung diseases (EELV > FRC, high resistance) with long time constants have a lower optimal respiratory frequency.

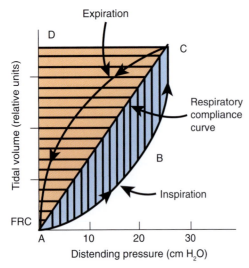

• **Figure 14.6** Inspiratory/expiratory pressure-volume loop recorded during respiratory cycle. The normal respiratory cycle entails the expenditure of work during inspiration to overcome resistive and elastic impedance to allow inflation of the lungs. Total work of breathing (pressure × volume) is defined by the sum of resistive work (area defined by *ABC*) plus elastic work (area defined by *ACD*). Total work of breathing (area defined by *ABCD*) is increased either by an increase in resistive properties of the respiratory system or by a decrease in respiratory compliance (slope of line between *A* and *C*). (From Goldsmith JP, Karotkin EH. *Assisted Ventilation of the Neonate.* Philadelphia: WB Saunders; 1981:29.)

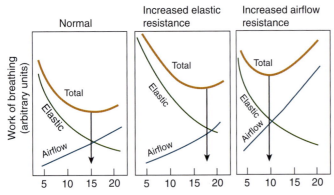

• **Figure 14.7** The work done against elastic and airflow resistance separately and summated to indicate the total work of breathing at different respiratory frequencies in adults. The total work of breathing has a minimum value at approximately 15 breaths/min under normal circumstances. For the same minute volume, minimum work is performed at higher frequencies with stiff (less compliant) lungs and at lower frequencies when the airflow resistance is increased. (From Nunn JF. *Applied Respiratory Physiology.* Boston: Butterworth; 1987:109.)

Distribution of Pulmonary Blood Flow

The pulmonary vasculature can be modeled as having two components: (1) a fixed component that is the primary determinant of regional perfusion and (2) a variable component that acts on top of the fixed structure and is affected by local factors. The fixed structures can best be characterized using fractal geometry, a new mathematical science used to describe "natural objects."[32] The variable component of the vasculature can be influenced by passive and active regional factors such as recruitment and/or distention due to changing hydrostatic or driving pressures. Active factors

such as vasomotion in response to shear stress or hypoxic vasoconstriction will influence regional perfusion. The relative contribution of both the fixed and variable components of the pulmonary circulation to pulmonary perfusion heterogeneity can be quantified.

Passive Pulmonary Blood Flow

Passive alterations in pulmonary vascular resistance (PVR) and blood flow are the primary determinants of the distribution of pulmonary blood flow. In the majority of critically ill patients the primary emphasis in critical care is placed on altering active pulmonary blood flow without a clear appreciation of the importance of passive pulmonary blood flow. Active pulmonary blood flow, however, cannot be fully appreciated without a sound understanding of the passive relationship that occurs between pulmonary artery pressure, P_A, and cardiac output.

Gravity-Dependent Determinants of Blood Flow. For many years it has been held that the primary determinant of the distribution of pulmonary blood flow is gravity. The right ventricle imparts kinetic energy to blood during systole and ejects a stroke volume into the pulmonary artery. The kinetic energy is dissipated in the lungs as blood in the pulmonary artery climbs a vertical column in the gravity-dependent lung. The pulmonary artery pressure therefore decreases by 1 cm H_2O per centimeter vertical distance up the lung (Fig. 14.8). The distribution of pulmonary blood flow to different lung segments is dependent upon the differences between three pressures in the lung: (1) intraalveolar pulmonary artery pressure (P_{pa}) or pulmonary capillary pressure, (2) P_A, and (3) venous pressure (P_{pv}). At some height above the heart the absolute pressure in the pulmonary artery (P_{pa}) becomes less than zero (atmospheric).[92] At that point, P_A exceeds P_{pa} and P_{pv}. In this region the pulmonary vessels are collapsed due to the higher P_A, and blood flow ceases (West zone 1, $P_A > P_{pa} > P_{pv}$). Lung that undergoes ventilation but no perfusion does not contribute to gas exchange and is referred to as physiologic *dead space*. Normally, very few of the lung units function as zone 1. Any factor that alters the P_{pa}/P_A relationship supporting the collapse of pulmonary vessels (i.e., $P_A > P_{pa}$ or $P_{pa}/P_A < 1$) will result in an increase in zone 1 lung. These conditions include an increase in P_A (application of positive pressure to the airways) or a reduction of P_{pa} (decreased cardiac output, shock, pulmonary emboli).

In regions of the lung where P_{pa} exceeds P_A and P_A exceeds P_{pv}, perfusion occurs (West zone 2, $P_{pa} > P_A > P_{pv}$). Pulmonary arterial flow to this region is determined by the mean pulmonary artery versus alveolar pressure difference ($P_{pa} - P_A$).[73] Blood flow is independent of the venous (P_{pv}) or left atrial pressure. Because mean P_{pa} increases down the lung while mean P_A remains constant, the mean driving pressure ($P_{pa} - P_A$) increases, and blood flow in the lower portions of the lung increases. In inferior segments of the lung, P_{pv} exceeds P_A, and blood flow is governed by the pulmonary arteriovenous pressure difference ($P_{pa} - P_{pv}$) (West zone 3, $P_{pa} > P_{pv} > P_A$). The effects of gravity are equal on pulmonary artery and pulmonary venous pressure, and both P_{pa} and P_{pv} increase at the same rate; thus the capillaries are permanently open, and the perfusion pressure ($P_{pa} - P_{pv}$) is constant. However, because the increase in P_{pl} is less than the increase in P_{pa} and P_{pv}, the transmural distending pressure ($P_{pa} - P_{pl}$ and $P_{pv} - P_{pl}$) increases down zone 3. Therefore the resistance is decreased, and for a given driving pressure, flow increases. Thus flow increases at lower lung levels in zone 3. It must be realized that ventilation and pulmonary blood flow are constantly changing forces and any given portion

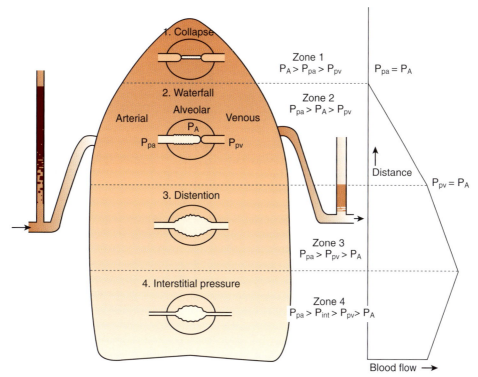

• **Figure 14.8** The four zones of the lung and distribution of blood flow in the upright lung. In zone 1, alveolar pressure (P_A) exceeds pulmonary artery pressure (P_{pa}), and no flow occurs because the intraalveolar vessels are collapsed by the compressing alveolar pressure. In zone 2, arterial pressure exceeds alveolar pressure, but alveolar pressure exceeds venous pressure (P_{pv}). Flow in zone 2 is determined by the arterial-alveolar pressure difference ($P_{pa} - P_A$) and has been likened to an upstream river waterfall over a dam. Because P_{pa} increases down zone 2 and P_A remains constant, the perfusion pressure increases and flow steadily increases down the zone. In zone 3, pulmonary venous pressure exceeds alveolar pressure, and flow is determined by the arterial-venous pressure difference ($P_{pa} - P_{pv}$), which is constant down this portion of the lung. However, the transmural pressure across the wall of the vessel increases down this zone, so that the caliber of the vessels increases (resistance decreases), and therefore flow increases. Finally, in zone 4, pulmonary interstitial pressure (P_{int}) becomes positive and exceeds both pulmonary venous pressure and alveolar pressure. Consequently, flow in zone 4 is determined by the arterial-interstitial pressure difference ($P_{pa} - P_{int}$). (From Benumof JL. Respiratory physiology and respiratory function during anesthesia. In: Miller RD, ed. *Anesthesia*. New York: Churchill Livingstone; 1990; and West JB, Dollery CT, Heard BE. Increased pulmonary vascular resistance in the dependent zone of the isolated dog lung caused by perivascular edema. *Circ Res*. 1965;17:191.)

of the lung may actually move in and out of zone 2 conditions and become either zone 1 or zone 3, depending upon whether the patient is in cardiac systole or diastole, inspiration or expiration, or spontaneous or positive pressure ventilation.

When pulmonary vascular pressures are extremely high, as in volume or pressure loading of the pulmonary arteries, fluid transudate forms in the interstitial space. When fluid flow into the interstitial space exceeds the lymphatic clearance rate, fluid accumulates. This eliminates the normally present negative tension on the extraalveolar vessels. Pulmonary interstitial pressure (P_{int}) eventually becomes positive and exceeds P_{pv} (West zone 4, $P_{pa} > P_{int} > P_{pv} > P_A$).[73] In zone 4, pulmonary blood flow is regulated by the arterial-interstitial pressure difference ($P_{pa} - P_{int}$). The arterial-interstitial pressure difference in zone 4 is less than the zone 3 difference ($P_{pa} - P_{pv}$); therefore zone 4 blood flow is less than zone 3 blood flow.

Alterations of P_{pa} and P_{pv} not only cause changes in regional blood flow but also affect the microcirculation. Three gradual changes take place in the pulmonary circulation when P_{pa} and P_{pv} increase: (1) recruitment or opening of previously nonperfused

vessels, (2) distention or widening of previously perfused vessels (increased cross-sectional area, less resistance), and (3) transudation of fluid at the capillary level.[61] Recruitment occurs when P_{pa} and P_{pv} are increased from low to moderate levels, distension occurs when P_{pa} and P_{pv} are increased from moderate to high levels, and finally, transudation occurs when P_{pa} and P_{pv} are increased from high to very high levels.

Gravity-Independent Determinants of Blood Flow. The first study to demonstrate that the geometry of the vascular bed is an important determinant of pulmonary blood flow distribution was made by Reed and Wood.[75] Later techniques providing high-resolution measurements of pulmonary perfusion have confirmed a large degree of spatial heterogeneity, likely based on the architecture of the vasculature. Neighboring regions of lung have similar magnitudes of flow (i.e., high-flow regions are adjacent to other high-flow regions, and low-flow regions are adjacent to other low-flow regions).[31] This relationship can be quantified using correlation coefficients between flows to pairs of lung regions. The spatial correlation [$\rho(d)$] is the correlation between blood flow to one region at one position and blood flow to a second region displaced by distance d. The correlation can range from 1 (perfect positive correlation) to −1 (perfect negative correlation) with 0 indicating random association between pairs. When the spatial correlation of perfusion is determined for regional pulmonary perfusion, a positive correlation is found for neighboring regions. This spatial correlation is best modeled using fractal methods.[37] When extended to three dimensions, this fractal model is able to explain the high local correlations in blood flow and the decreasing correlation as distance increases.[38] Pulmonary perfusion has also been shown to have temporal variability.[36]

Recent studies using these high-resolution methods[34,35,52] as well as experiments performed in both microgravity[74] and macrogravity[46] settings have demonstrated that pulmonary perfusion is far more heterogeneous than can be explained by gravity alone. Although multiple studies in different species have confirmed gravity-independent perfusion heterogeneity, these observations have not been made in man. Some investigators suggest that gravity is not an important determinant of pulmonary blood flow distribution in quadrupeds (a characteristic common to all species in these studies) because their posture produces smaller lung volumes.[50] Quadrupeds also have a more muscularized vascular system with a smaller proportion of their vascular resistance in the microvascular segments. In an attempt to overcome these potential problems, high-resolution methods were recently used in baboons (a species with pulmonary structures and physiology remarkably similar to man).[33] With the use of multiple-stepwise regression, gravity-dependent perfusion heterogeneity was estimated at 7%, 5%, and 25% in the supine, prone, and upright positions, respectively. Therefore these recent high-resolution experiments continue to suggest that gravity is an important, but not predominant, determinant of pulmonary perfusion heterogeneity.

PVR and blood flow are dependent on a variety of physiologic conditions, including lung volume. As discussed earlier, FRC is the lung volume at the end of an expiration in normal lungs, when P_A equals P_{atm}. Total PVR is increased when lung volume is either increased above or decreased below FRC (Fig. 14.9).[12,81,94] The increase in total PVR at lung volumes above FRC is due to a large increase in vascular resistance contributed by the small intraalveolar vessels, which are extended and compressed by the expanded alveolus and surrounding lung.[6] In contradistinction, the increase in total PVR at lung volumes below FRC is due to hypoxic pulmonary vasoconstriction (HPV), which occurs in collapsed alveoli and the tortuous course of the large extraalveolar vessels at low lung volumes.[4]

FRC can therefore be understood as the lung volume at which PVR is minimized, an observation that should be leveraged when optimizing positive pressure ventilation. It is worth noting that lung compliance and resistance are also optimized at FRC, with compliance being the highest at FRC and resistance being the lowest. Thus in normal lungs EELV is the same as FRC, and the work of ventilation and of perfusion is minimized.

The relationship between lung volume and FRC is obviously variable. Tidal ventilation occurs from EELV (FRC in normal lungs), and thus PVR, airway resistance, and lung compliance cycle dynamically with ventilation. In disease states, EELV can be increased above FRC (obstructive lung disease) or decreased below FRC (restrictive lung disease). This pathologic EELV (i.e., when EELV does not equal FRC) will alter PVR, compliance, and resistance. For these reasons, mechanical ventilation applied during diseased states should be tailored to allow for tidal volume at or near FRC.

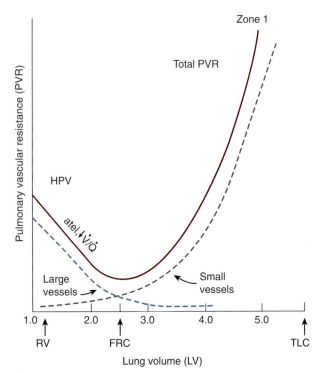

• **Figure 14.9** An asymmetric U-shaped curve relates total pulmonary vascular resistance *(PVR)* to lung volume. The trough of the curve occurs when lung volume equals functional residual capacity *(FRC)*. Total pulmonary resistance is the sum of resistance in small vessels (increased by increasing lung volume) and the resistance in large vessels (increased by decreasing lung volume). The end point for increasing lung volume (toward total lung capacity *[TLC]*) is the creation of zone 1 conditions, and the end point for decreasing lung volume (toward residual volume *[RV]*) is the creation of low $\dot{V}_A/\dot{Q}$ and atelectatic *(atel)* areas that have hypoxic pulmonary vasoconstriction *(HPV)*. (From Benumof JL. Respiratory physiology and respiratory function during anesthesia. In: Miller RD, ed. *Anesthesia*. New York: Churchill Livingstone; 1990.)

Active Pulmonary Blood Flow

Total PVR expresses the relationship between flow and driving pressure (Ohm's law). In the pulmonary circulation the vessels are not rigid tubes but expand as flow increases. Therefore PVR is flow dependent and decreases as flow increases.[25] In addition, previously nonperfused vessels are recruited (opened) as cardiac output increases. Because of these physiologic principles, PVR is not precisely measured in the pulmonary circulation, and the relationship between flow and pressure must be carefully assessed. Two situations, however, can occur in which PVR changes can be accurately measured. One condition is active pulmonary vasoconstriction, which occurs when cardiac output is decreased and P_{pa} remains constant or is increased. Another is active pulmonary vasodilation, which can occur when cardiac output increases and P_{pa} remains constant or decreases.

A variety of physiologic or pharmacologic stimuli may cause alterations of the pulmonary circulation. One of the most frequently encountered is alveolar hypoxia. Alveolar hypoxia of a whole lung, lobe, or lobule of lung causes localized pulmonary vasoconstriction (see Chapter 23), referred to as a *hypoxic pulmonary vasoconstriction* (HPV). HPV is present in all mammalian species.[85] The mechanisms by which alveolar hypoxia causes pulmonary vasoconstriction remain unclear, although two theories have been proposed.[27,89] First, alveolar hypoxia may change the balance between vasoconstrictor substance(s) and vasodilator substance(s) elaborated from multiple potential sources (e.g., endothelium, smooth muscle), with the net result of vasoconstriction. Recent evidence suggests that HPV may in part be a result of a reduction of endothelium-derived nitric oxide. Second, hypoxia may stimulate the metabolic activity of pulmonary vascular smooth muscle, partially depolarizing the cell membrane, influencing excitation coupling, and causing ion fluxes that cause vasoconstriction. Thus HPV appears to be due to hypoxia-induced modulation of vasoactive substances and/or a direct action on the pulmonary vascular smooth muscle. HPV may involve the entire lung or be limited to localized regions of the lung, depending on whether there is global or regional alveolar hypoxia.[60] Regional alveolar hypoxia causes locally increased vascular resistance and shunts blood toward normoxic lung with lower vascular resistance, thereby improving V/Q matching. Global alveolar hypoxia results in an elevated mean P_{pa} and an increased workload for the right ventricle. Regional HPV is therefore a protective mechanism designed to optimize V/Q matching, whereas global HPV is a maladaptive response and can lead to right ventricular dysfunction and failure.

Ventilation/Perfusion Matching. Matching of lung ventilation (V) and perfusion (Q) at the alveolar level is necessary for optimal gas exchange to occur. The ratio of ventilation to perfusion (V/Q) expresses the amount of ventilation relative to perfusion in any given lung region. In the normal healthy lung the idealized lung region has perfectly matched ventilation to perfusion, where V/Q equals 1. Both pulmonary blood flow and ventilation increase with distance down the normal upright lung in a gravity-dependent manner (as discussed previously). However, because blood flow increases more rapidly and from a much lower value than ventilation, V/Q decreases exponentially.

V/Q mismatch alters both arterial oxygen (PaO_2) and carbon dioxide ($PaCO_2$) tensions. Blood flows from underventilated alveoli (with V/Q < 1) tend to have increased $PaCO_2$ and decreased PaO_2. Blood flows from overventilated alveoli (with physiologic dead space and with V/Q > 1) have lower $PaCO_2$ but cannot increase the PaO_2 due to the flat upper portion of the oxygen-hemoglobin dissociation curve. Thus in conditions with V/Q inequalities, carbon dioxide can be eliminated from the overventilated alveoli to compensate for the underventilated alveoli, but large alveolar to arterial oxygen gradients can occur. In fact, V/Q mismatching is the major cause of hypoxemia associated with respiratory diseases. $PaCO_2$ may be normal or even low in response to compensatory hyperventilation for the hypoxemia.[69,90]

V/Q inequality can be altered by a variety of respiratory interventions, which include increasing inspired oxygen or application of positive pressure to the airway. Increasing the concentration of inspired oxygen overcomes the alveolar arterial gradient in poorly ventilated alveoli (i.e., low V/Q lung compartments), resulting in improved oxygen content of the blood.

Physiology of Gas and Fluid Exchange

Gas Properties

The primary function of the respiratory system is to transfer oxygen and carbon dioxide across the alveolar-capillary membrane. This process occurs in the terminal gas exchange unit (alveoli). The transfer of oxygen and carbon dioxide represents the summation of multiple interactions at the level of the alveoli and represents the fundamental process of gas exchange between inspired gases and pulmonary capillary blood. For a more thorough evaluation of these complex interactions, excellent reviews are available.[10,24] The purpose of this section is not to be comprehensive but rather to provide enough background to convey the basic principles of gas exchange.

The behavior of gases and the principles of gas exchange can be expressed by certain laws. The pressure exerted by a gas and its components is observed by Dalton's law. Dalton's gas law states that the pressure exerted by a group of gases is the sum of the partial pressure of these gases. This property defines the pressure exerted by the individual components of a gas mixture. At standard temperature (37°C) and at sea level (atmospheric pressure P_B = 760 mm Hg), air consists of 20.93% oxygen. Therefore the partial pressure exerted by oxygen in air is:

$$P_{air}O_2 = (\% \ O_2 \ in \ air) \times atmospheric \ pressure \ (P_B)$$
$$P_{air}O_2 = 0.2093 \times 760 = 159 \ mm \ Hg$$

The partial pressure of oxygen, however, is altered before gas exchange at the alveolar level. When a gas is inhaled, it is warmed and saturated with water vapor. The partial pressure exerted by water vapor must be accounted for and varies with the temperature of the humidified gas; it is independent of pressure. At 37°C the partial pressure of water vapor is 47 mm Hg. Therefore by the time an inhaled gas has reached the level of the alveoli, the partial pressure of the gas has been reduced to 149 mm Hg (0.2093 × 760 − 47 mm Hg).

At the alveolar level the percentage of carbon dioxide in the alveolus is normally approximately 5.6%, and the partial pressure of alveolar carbon dioxide would be:

$$P_A CO_2 = (\% \ CO_2 \ in \ alveolus) \times (P_B - P_{water \ vapor})$$
$$P_A CO_2 = 0.056 \times (760 - 47 \ mm \ Hg) = 40 \ mm \ Hg$$

Under normal conditions, inspired gas is diluted by gas that remains in the alveoli after expiration. This gas contains water vapor and carbon dioxide. Therefore the partial pressure of oxygen in the alveoli decreases. The sum of the partial pressures must equal the same total pressure, and any increase in partial pressure of a gas must be accomplished with a corresponding decrease in another gas. Under normal conditions the respiratory quotient is 0.8 and the partial pressure of carbon dioxide is 40 mm Hg. Therefore the partial pressure of oxygen at the alveolus is reduced.

$$P_A O_2 = PIO_2 - P_A CO_2/R$$

where *PIO_2* is the partial pressure of inspired oxygen and *R* is the respiratory quotient, or

$$P_A O_2 = 0.2093 \times (P_b - 47 \ mm \ Hg) - 40 \ mm \ Hg/0.8$$
$$= 99 \ mm \ Hg$$

This is known as the alveolar gas equation.

Alveolar Ventilation

When inspiration occurs, gas is drawn into the thorax, and a portion of this gas is distributed to the alveoli. It is this portion of the inspired gas drawn into the alveolus that determines alveolar ventilation. The remaining gas does not contribute to gas exchange and is referred to as *dead space ventilation*. Dead space ventilation can be defined by its location. Gas that does not contribute to gas exchange and is located in the conducting airways is referred to as *anatomic* dead space. This gas is incapable of gas exchange because of the anatomy of the conducting airways. Anatomic dead space as expressed in millimeters approximates the weight of the individual in pounds. The inspired gas that enters the alveolus and does not contribute to gas exchange is referred to as *alveolar* dead space. This distinction is essential because anatomic dead space represents a portion of the gas exchange system that cannot exchange gas and does not change in an individual with a normal airway, whereas alveolar dead space is a portion of the respiratory system that receives gas but is not involved with gas exchange. The amount of this alveolar dead space thus varies with lung perfusion. The total amount of the respiratory system that does not participate in gas exchange is referred to as *physiologic* dead space.

$$V_D \text{ physiologic} = V_D \text{ anatomic} + V_D \text{ alveolar}$$

The tidal volume is distributed between physiologic dead space and those alveoli that provide gas exchange referred to as *alveolar ventilation* (V alveolar).

$$\text{Tidal volume} = V_D \text{ anatomic} + V_D \text{ alveolar} + V \text{ alveolar}$$

Under idealized normal conditions every alveolus participates in gas exchange optimally, and there is no alveolar dead space. Anatomic dead space is thus equal to physiologic dead space. An increase in alveolar dead space occurs in a variety of pathophysiologic conditions, such as acute respiratory distress syndrome. In certain conditions, alveolar dead space may be recruited to exchange gas and therefore, represents a potential area for supplemental gas exchange.

Assessments of alveolar ventilation provide insight into conditions of normal and abnormal cardiorespiratory physiology. The PaO_2 is affected primarily by the presence of right-to-left intracardiac or intrapulmonary shunt and hence is not a good indicator of alveolar ventilation. The $PaCO_2$ is less affected by shunting and is a more accurate assessment of alveolar ventilation than is the PaO_2. The partial pressure of carbon dioxide in pulmonary capillary blood is 46 mm Hg, which differs only slightly from the partial pressure of arterial carbon dioxide ($PaCO_2 = 40$ mm Hg). Therefore a 50% reduction of pulmonary blood flow will result in only a 3 mm Hg increase in the partial pressure of carbon dioxide in arterial blood ($PaCO_2$ from 40 mm Hg to 43 mm Hg). However, a 50% reduction in alveolar ventilation will result in a doubling of the partial pressure of carbon dioxide in arterial blood ($PaCO_2 = 80$ mm Hg). An accurate estimation of alveolar ventilation through measurements of $PaCO_2$ aids in the assessment of the adequacy of respiratory function in patients with hypoxia from right-to-left intracardiac shunting, whereas measurements of PaO_2 may not.

Alveolar-Capillary Membrane

The alveolar-capillary membrane is the gas-exchanging surface that separates alveolar gas and capillary blood.[26] The alveolar side of the alveolar-capillary membrane is bounded by the epithelial cells. Underneath the epithelium is the epithelial basement membrane. The blood side of the alveolar-capillary membrane is the capillary endothelial cells and the endothelial basement membrane. At the alveolar-capillary membrane the basement membrane of the alveolar epithelial cells and the capillary endothelial cells is fused and, in health, watertight. The alveolar-capillary membrane is contiguous with the interstitial space that contains lymphatic channels and connective tissue. There are important differences between the epithelial and endothelial junctions that govern fluid flow. The junctions between the alveolar epithelial cells are tight, whereas the endothelial cell junctions are loose and permit fluid transfer into the interstitium. The tight epithelial junctions help prevent the accumulation of intraalveolar fluid, that is, alveolar pulmonary edema.

Diffusion. Diffusion is defined as the energy-independent (passive) transfer of gas across the alveolar-capillary membrane. The Fick principle of diffusion governs the movements of gases across the alveolar-capillary membrane. Gases move from an area of high partial pressure to an area of lower partial pressure. The amount of gas diffusing across a semipermeable membrane is dependent upon the partial pressure difference of the gas in the two locations ($P_1 - P_2$), the surface area available for diffusion (A) and the diffusion coefficient (K) and is inversely related to the distance of diffusion (d):

$$\text{Amount of gas diffusing}\,(Q/\min) = [(P_1 - P_2) \times A \times K]/d$$

Therefore the propensity of a gas to diffuse across the alveolar-capillary membrane is dependent upon the partial pressure differences of the gas in the two locations and the diffusion coefficient of the gas (K).[70,73] The diffusion coefficient is directly dependent upon the solubility of the gas and inversely proportional to the square root of the molecular weight of the gas. With these formulas it can be demonstrated that carbon dioxide has a much higher solubility than oxygen in water ($24:1$ at $30°C$). Although the partial pressure difference of carbon dioxide between the alveolus and pulmonary capillary is small, carbon dioxide diffuses 20 times faster across the alveolar-capillary membrane than does oxygen because of its high solubility.

Oxygen Diffusion/Transport. As blood enters the pulmonary capillaries, it begins the transfer of gases across the alveolar-capillary membrane. Red blood cells in the pulmonary capillaries are exposed to alveolar gas for approximately 0.75 seconds.[90] The pulmonary capillary transit time depends on the cardiac output and intrapulmonary blood volume. The transport of oxygen across the alveolar-capillary membrane begins immediately upon entry into the alveolar-capillary complex. When capillary blood first enters the alveolar-capillary gas exchange unit, there is a large gradient between the partial pressure of oxygen in the alveolus ($P_AO_2 = 100$ mm Hg) and in the capillary ($P_{capillary}O_2 = 40$ mm Hg). This results in an initial rapid diffusion of oxygen into the capillary. As oxygen diffuses into the capillary, the partial pressure of oxygen in capillary blood increases, and the gradient for diffusion decreases, resulting in a reduction in the diffusion rate over time. Although there is a reduction in oxygen transfer, the transfer of oxygen is not usually limited by diffusion because oxygen transfer is rapid, and the oxygen tension of pulmonary capillary blood approximates the oxygen tension of alveolar gas in the first 0.25 seconds.[91] Under normal conditions little oxygen transfer occurs after the initial 0.25 seconds. This results in a 0.50-second "buffer," which provides extra time for diffusion to occur. Therefore in most pathologic conditions, hypoxia does not occur from impaired diffusion.

In the absence of right-to-left intracardiac shunting, hypoxia most commonly results from V/Q mismatch. This occurs when an alveolus receives inadequate ventilation compared to pulmonary blood flow (V/Q < 1). When individual alveoli receive inadequate quantities of oxygen, P_AO_2 falls. The affected alveolus has less oxygen available for gas exchange, and a reduction in oxygen transfer occurs with resultant hypoxemia. To limit the development of arterial hypoxemia, the respiratory system has intrinsic mechanisms to enhance V/Q matching. In conditions in which alveolar ventilation is inadequate for perfusion, the low alveolar oxygen concentration results in local vasoconstriction and a redistribution of flow to regions with a higher V/Q ratio (hypoxic pulmonary vasoconstriction). In addition, lung regions with a low V/Q ratio have a high alveolar carbon dioxide concentration that dilates the lower airways (but not the local pulmonary vasculature) and increases ventilation to these areas. In regions where the V/Q ratio is high the alveolar carbon dioxide level will be low and promote local airway constriction and a redistribution of airflow to lung units where V/Q ratios approximate unity.

When the transfer of oxygen to the capillaries is complete, oxygen is carried in two forms: (1) oxygen dissolved in plasma and (2) oxygen bound to hemoglobin (Hgb). The amount of oxygen that is carried by the blood is referred to as the *total oxygen content* (CaO$_2$). As will now be shown, only a small portion of oxygen is dissolved in plasma. The majority of oxygen is carried bound to Hgb due to its high affinity for oxygen. One gram of Hgb can carry 1.39 mL of oxygen. For these reasons the oxygen content (CaO$_2$) is critically dependent upon the arterial saturation (SaO$_2$) and Hgb concentration and relatively insensitive to the partial pressure of oxygen.

$$CaO_2 \ (mL \cdot dL^{-1}) = [1.39 \ (mL \cdot g^{-1}) \times Hgb \ (g \cdot dL^{-1}) \times SaO_2] \\ + [0.003 \ (mL \cdot mm \ Hg^{-1} \cdot dL^{-1}) \\ \times PaO_2 \ (mm \ Hg)]$$

It should be noted that in clinical practice it is customary to speak of arterial oxygen content in terms of PaO$_2$, which assumes an implied understanding of where a patient "lives" on his or her oxygen-hemoglobin curve. As such, a normally saturated healthy infant with two ventricles will have a PaO$_2$ of approximately 100 mm Hg, whereas a neonate with "balanced" single-ventricle physiology and equal amounts of pulmonary (Q$_p$) and systemic (Q$_s$) blood flow will generally be said to have a PaO$_2$ of approximately 40 mm Hg. Thus, although helping to convey whether a shunted physiology is properly balanced, this convention of describing oxygen content in terms of the partial pressure of dissolved oxygen can tempt the student of cardiac physiology to underappreciate the profound effect that an adequate red blood cell mass has on the well-being of a cyanotic patient.

As alluded to previously, the amount of oxygen that can be bound to Hgb is related to the partial pressure of oxygen in the blood and the affinity of Hgb for oxygen and is described by the oxygen-hemoglobin dissociation curve. Factors that influence the affinity of Hgb for oxygen include pH, PCO$_2$, temperature, and the amount of 2,3-diphosphoglycerate (DPG) present. Alterations in the oxygen-hemoglobin dissociation curve occur at individual organ levels. At the tissue level a decrease in pH, increase in PCO$_2$, increase in temperature, or increase in DPG results in a shift of the oxygen-hemoglobin dissociation curve to the right. This shift in the oxygen-hemoglobin dissociation curve allows an unloading of oxygen to tissues. At the alveolar level the reverse occurs, and a shift to the left of the oxygen-hemoglobin dissociation curve occurs with increased Hgb affinity for oxygen and increased oxygen uptake by capillary blood.

Maintaining appropriate arterial oxygen content is an important concern in treating infants and children with congenital heart disease (CHD). Patients with intracardiac right-to-left shunting will not significantly increase their arterial saturation and oxygen content with the administration of inspired oxygen. This observation forms the basis in the hyperoxia test classically employed to help discriminate whether a cyanotic neonate has intracardiac shunting

causing the cyanosis. Technically this maneuver involves administering 100% FiO$_2$ to the cyanotic infant and measuring the change in PaO$_2$: absence of a significant rise suggests right-to-left shunting of CHD.

For infants with CHD who are symptomatic from their imbalance of oxygen delivery relative to oxygen consumption, a significant increase in oxygen carrying capacity can be obtained by raising the Hgb concentration. For a given arterial saturation, an increase in Hgb results in an increase in oxygen-carrying capacity and oxygen delivery. Transfusion of red blood cells to a target Hgb of 13 to 15 g/dL may be particularly advantageous in cyanotic infants with relative anemia demonstrating objective evidence of inadequate oxygen delivery to their organs. In practice, even in infants with cyanotic CHD, transfusions are usually avoidable thanks to the presence of fetal Hgb (HbF), a variant of adult Hgb (HbA) that allows for diffusion of oxygen across the placenta from the mother during intrauterine life. Although generally beyond the scope of this text, it is helpful to note that HbF binds the oxygen molecule far more tightly than the HbA found in the red blood cells of adult donors. This means that HbF is generally far more efficient at transporting oxygen in the cyanotic state than HbA, and so neonates with cyanotic CHD often do not demonstrate any untoward physiologic effects of their relative anemia.

Carbon Dioxide Diffusion/Transport. The diffusion of carbon dioxide is similar to the process that occurs with oxygen transfer. As mentioned earlier, carbon dioxide diffusion across the alveolar-capillary membrane is more rapid than oxygen diffusion due to the greater solubility of carbon dioxide. Carbon dioxide transport is dependent upon a variety of interactions in the red blood cell and plasma. The amount of carbon dioxide carried by the blood is dependent on its partial pressure and the presence of oxyhemoglobin. In the presence of oxyhemoglobin there will be a lower carbon dioxide content for a given partial pressure of oxygen. This results in the improved carbon dioxide removal as capillary blood becomes oxygenated. As blood is transported to peripheral tissues, carbon dioxide is taken up from the peripheral tissues and transported to the alveolus for gas exchange.

Fluid Transport. Starling's forces govern the flow of fluid in and out of the capillaries and interstitium.[7,8] The alveolar epithelium is relatively resistant to fluid movement whereas the endothelial membrane is more permeable. The force tending to push fluid out of the capillaries and into the interstitium is the hydrostatic pressure in the capillaries (P$_{cap}$). This is opposed by the hydrostatic pressure in the interstitium (P$_{int}$). The difference between these forces (P$_{cap}$ − P$_{int}$) is the net effect of the hydrostatic forces. Under normal conditions, P$_{cap}$ is greater than P$_{int}$, and the net force promotes fluid movement out of the capillaries into the interstitium. The force tending to promote fluid entry into the capillaries and out of the interstitium is the colloid osmotic pressure difference between the capillaries and interstitium (P$_{cap}$ − P$_{int}$). The balance of these forces is dependent on a number of factors, including the reflection coefficient (K), which delineates the ability of the capillary membrane to prevent the passage of proteins across the capillary membrane. The sum total of these forces defines the flow of fluid into the interstitium and is equal to the filtration rate (Q):

$$Q = K[(P_{cap} - P_{int}) - (\pi_{cap} - \pi_{int})]$$

The phenomena described by the Starling forces help explain the development of cardiogenic pulmonary edema. Under normal conditions the effect of Starling's forces is to promote a small amount of net flux of fluid into the interstitium that is promptly removed by lymphatics. In conditions of left atrial hypertension and/or left ventricular dysfunction (e.g., myocardial ischemia/infarction, cardiomyopathy, pulmonary vein stenosis, mitral stenosis), or increased pulmonary blood flow (as in unrestrictive ventricular septal defect [VSD] physiology) hydrostatic pressure in the pulmonary capillaries may increase dramatically ($P_{cap} \gg P_{int}$), and excessive fluid flows into the interstitium.

As described earlier, the integrity of the alveolar-capillary membrane is essential to regulating the flow of fluid in the interstitium. Disruption of the alveolar-capillary membrane results in an increased permeability to large molecular weight proteins and massive fluid accumulation in the lung. Such disruptions can be expected to occur with some frequency and significance as a result of the generalized inflammatory state that immediately follows bypass surgery. The pulmonary edema that results from this altered membrane integrity and from perturbations in hydrostatic pressures is targeted therapeutically with fluid removal through diuretic therapy or, in extreme cases of renal failure, with mechanical filtration and dialysis.

Developmental Considerations

Significant changes occur in respiratory physiology during the transition from infancy to childhood, with the development of chest wall structures and maturation of the airways and lung parenchyma. These changes are important to recognize in the clinical setting because infants are more vulnerable to many disease states due to higher chest wall compliance, immature control of respiration, and increased airway resistance.

Respiratory Mechanics of the Neonate

In the newborn period the chest wall "system" is composed primarily of cartilage and is therefore more compliant and more easily distortable. Because this allows the lung parenchyma to recoil more easily, FRC occurs at relatively lower lung volumes compared to older children and adults. Another important trait of the neonatal chest is that the orientation of the ribs is more horizontal than that of the older child. This unique orientation causes the intercostal muscles to expand the thorax primarily in an inferior direction, as opposed to lateral and anterior directions, causing them to be less efficient at effectively generating tidal volumes. It should also be noted that the diaphragm and intercostal muscles of infants contain fewer type I intercostal muscles, making them more fatigable. For these reasons, infants typically have smaller reserves of breathing to handle the increased work imposed by disease states of the lung.

It is also important to note that the development of lung parenchyma, or alveolarization, continues well beyond the newborn period into childhood and adolescence. In neonates the area of gas exchange per body surface area is relatively reduced. In addition, during early childhood, collateral pathways of ventilation form (intraalveolar pores of Kohn and canals of Lambert), which make the lung less prone to atelectasis.

Control of Respiration in Neonates

Due to the immature control of respiration in preterm and term neonates, the breathing pattern of the neonate is often irregular, also referred to as *periodic breathing*.[40] In response to hypoxia a neonate may become apneic and bradycardic. For

this reason neonates are often administered bag valve mask ventilation with supplemental oxygen for resuscitation of evolving significant bradycardia. However, in neonates with shunting lesions, extreme vigilance must be maintained so as to expose the pulmonary vasculature to additional FiO_2 for only brief periods of time. Indeed, drops in PVR can be so profound as to cause clinically significant increases in pulmonary blood flow (so-called flooding) that result in even more hemodynamic perturbation.

It should also be noted that prostaglandin infusions, often used to maintain ductal patency in patients waiting for surgical or catheterization intervention, can result in substantial worsening of apnea, culminating in the need for endotracheal intubation. In practice, some clinicians will attempt to titrate down the dose of prostaglandins to mitigate this particular side effect, although this technique both is unproven and requires close clinical monitoring with frequent checks on arterial oxygen content, as well as frequent echocardiographic confirmation of ductal size and/or aortic patency. Additionally, to avoid the pathophysiologic effects of intubation, some clinicians have found that a small subset of neonates may have fewer apneic events from prostaglandins when they are administered humidified room air via high-flow nasal cannula. The authors acknowledge that this technique is unreliable in some patients and remains controversial.

Airway Anatomy and Airway Resistance in Neonates

Another unique but important characteristic of neonatal lung mechanics is the size of their airways, which makes them significantly more prone to high airway resistance if there is minor narrowing. In infants and children, small airways account for approximately 50% of total airway resistance, compared to 20% in adults.[30] Diseases that alter small airways can lead to dramatic alterations in resistance and significant obstruction to gas flow (e.g., bronchiolitis).[19]

It is also important to note that neonates are preferential nose breathers, and therefore obstruction due to mucus or edema of the nasal passages can cause dramatic increases in work of breathing and significant distress. The tongue is relatively larger in this age group as well.

One of the more interesting anatomic considerations unique to the infant is the fact that the epiglottis is omega shaped, and it is longer and less flexible than that of the older child. Meanwhile, the larynx, which marks the entrance to the lower airway, is both smaller and lies higher in the neonate.

The narrowest portion of an infant's airway lies at the cricoid ring, which is the portion of the larynx that is completely surrounded by cartilage. Due to its rigid walls, it is especially prone to increased airway resistance in the presence of mucosal edema or mucous plugging. Lastly, it should be noted that the trachea is proportionally shorter and narrower than that of the older child.[88]

The neonate's smaller nasal passages and lower airway tree, when combined with a lower FRC and less developed muscle mass, places the neonate at increased risk of respiratory failure.[36]

In the neonate, several mechanisms counteract the tendency for the lung to collapse in order to maintain FRC. Laryngeal adduction in expiration increases expiratory airway resistance and functional PEEP. Maintaining inspiratory muscle contraction during expiration makes the chest wall stiffer. Lastly, a higher respiratory rate, which results in starting inspiration before complete expiration, helps maintain lung volumes in infants.[43,49]

Alterations in Respiratory Physiology Secondary to Congenital Heart Disease

Alterations Caused by Airway Compression

The incidence of airway anomalies in patients with CHD is approximately 4%.[19,56] Certain genetic disorders associated with CHD will have some degree of facial dysmorphia, as can be seen in CHARGE syndrome (choanal atresia), Down syndrome (DS) (multiple levels, see later) and Beckwith-Wiedemann syndrome (macroglossia).

Some of the more common examples of upper airway abnormality caused by CHD include laryngomalacia, tracheomalacia, bronchomalacia, or some combination of abnormality involving one more segments of the upper airway (e.g., laryngo-tracheomalacia). These types of "floppy airway" involving abnormalities of the supporting cartilage at different segments of the airway tree can present with symptoms of feeding difficulties and failure to thrive and may be difficult to distinguish clinically from common symptoms of heart failure. Dramatically increased work of breathing, atelectasis, apnea, and occasionally wheezing are other hallmark clinical findings of these conditions. Definitive diagnosis can be accomplished with bronchoscopy during spontaneous ventilation, bronchography, or dynamic computed tomography (CT) evaluation.

Another tracheal lesion to consider is a tracheal bronchus. A tracheal bronchus, defined as a right upper bronchus originating in the trachea, can be occasionally a persistent source of hypoxemia in the ventilated patient with cyanotic heart disease.[33,83]

Cardiovascular causes of airway compression are usually due to abnormal configuration of the tracheobronchial tree in relationship to vasculature structures or due to extrinsic compression of airways from dilated, pulsatile vascular structures.

Compression From Vascular Structures. The incidence of airway compression from cardiovascular causes is 1% to 2% in children with CHD.[63] The most common anomaly associated with airway compression is double aortic arch. Other common causes are included in Box 14.1. Although often symptomatic with dysphagia, respiratory distress, and recurrent respiratory infections early in life, some patients may not manifest symptoms for years. Treatment is surgical correction of the offending vessel or lesion, with patients usually benefiting from immediate relief postoperatively. Often, however, patients will continue to demonstrate symptoms from malacic segments secondary to prolonged extrinsic compression. Although these will usually resolve, surgical intervention on the airway itself may be required.

Airway compression can sometimes occur after repair of interrupted aortic arch. The repair can displace the aorta and cause left main stem bronchus compression between the aorta and left pulmonary artery.

Alterations Caused by Pulmonary Blood Flow

Abnormalities in cardiovascular structure and function can lead to alterations in respiratory mechanics. The alterations in respiratory mechanics that develop in patients with CHD are a direct result of changes in pulmonary blood volume and pulmonary artery pressure. Both of these are dependent on the amount of pulmonary blood flow. Therefore the changes that occur in respiratory mechanics can be classified depending upon the presence of increased or decreased pulmonary blood flow.

> ## • BOX 14.1 Causes of Vascular Compression of the Airway in Children

- Anomalies of the aorta
  - Double aortic arch
  - Interrupted aortic arch (after surgical repair)
  - Right-sided aortic arch
    - With aberrant left subclavian artery
    - With mirror-image branching and right ligamentum arteriosum
  - Left-sided aortic arch
    - With aberrant right subclavian artery and right ligamentum arteriosum
    - Right-sided descending aorta with right ligamentum arteriosum
- Cervical aortic arch
  - Absent pulmonary valve syndrome
  - Aberrant left pulmonary artery ("pulmonary artery sling")
  - Acquired cardiovascular disease
- Dilated cardiomyopathy
- Aneurysm
  - Ascending aorta
    - Ductus arteriosus

From McLaren CA, Elliott MJ, Roebuck DJ. Vascular compression of the airway in children. Paediatr Respir Rev 2008;9:85-94.

Increased Pulmonary Blood Flow

Congenital cardiovascular anomalies associated with increased pulmonary blood flow are due to a left-to-right intracardiac shunt. The respiratory derangements that occur in patients with increased pulmonary blood flow include (1) excessive pulmonary blood volume and (2) excessive pulmonary vascular pressures (Table 14.1).

In patients with excessive pulmonary blood volume, there is an increase in red blood cell mass in the pulmonary circulation. The increased red blood cell mass results in perfusion to alveoli in excess of ventilation and hence V/Q mismatch. When alveolar ventilation is inadequate for pulmonary blood flow, $P_{cap}O_2$ falls. If the V/Q mismatch is significant, hypoxia will ensue. In many patients the left-to-right intrapulmonary shunt is a result of excessive pulmonary blood volume because lung volumes and EELV are not altered.[57,58,87] The alteration in respiratory mechanics may mimic what occurs in patients with atelectasis. The increased pulmonary blood volume can also cause alterations in respiratory mechanics by increasing lung weight. This results in a reduction of compliance and necessitates an increase in airway pressure to generate a given lung volume during positive pressure ventilation.

Excessive pulmonary blood flow can also modify respiratory mechanics by altering pulmonary vascular pressures.[58] Increased pulmonary blood flow results in an increase in pulmonary artery, capillary, and venous pressures, factors that favor the development of extravascular lung water. Extravascular fluid accumulation and alveolar atelectasis cause a loss of lung volume, a reduction of lung compliance, a decrease in tidal volume, and a compensatory increase in respiratory frequency.[48,57] Many of the manifestations of excessive extravascular lung water resolve with surgical correction of the underlying anomaly.[39] The decrease in lung compliance that occurs in patients with increased pulmonary blood flow has been correlated with the estimated blood volume on chest radiography, the ratio of pulmonary artery to aortic diameter determined by echocardiogram, and pulmonary artery pressures.[3,20,39,48]

Both large and small airway obstructions can occur in patients with increased pulmonary blood flow. Small airway obstruction

TABLE 14.1 Effects of Congenital Heart Disease on Respiratory Function

Blood Flow	Abnormality	Pathophysiology	Respiratory Abnormality
↑ Pulmonary blood flow	↑ Pulmonary blood volume	↓ V/Q	Hypoxia
	↑ P_{cap}	R → L shunt	
		↑ Lung weight	↓ Compliance
		↑ Lung fluid accumulation	↓ Compliance
		Interstitial/alveolar edema	↓ Lung volumes
			↑ Airway resistance
	↑ P_{pa}	Large airway obstruction	↑ Airway resistance
	↑ P_{la}	Small airway obstruction	↑ Airway resistance
↓ Pulmonary blood flow	↓ Pulmonary blood volume	↑ Dead space ventilation	Hypoxia
	Airway hypoplasia	↓ Lung weight	↑ Compliance
		Small airway obstruction	↑ Airway resistance

P_{cap}, Hydrostatic capillary pressure; P_{la}, left atrial pressure; P_{pa}, pulmonary artery pressure; R → L shunt, intrapulmonary right-to-left shunt; V/Q, ventilation/perfusion.

results from intrinsic narrowing of the airways due to fluid collecting in the airway lumen or extrinsic compression from interstitial edema or dilation of the pulmonary vasculature.[3] Large airway obstruction occurs when a dilated or high-pressure vascular structure causes external compression of the airway lumen. A classic example of this phenomenon is observed in absent pulmonary valve syndrome, often associated with tetralogy of Fallot (TOF), which results in severe pulmonary regurgitation beginning in fetal life. The end result of this dramatic enlargement of the pulmonary arteries is compression of both bronchi and trachea with resultant severe respiratory distress.[43]

Increased pulmonary blood flow combined with pulmonary artery hypertension causes dilation of the pulmonary arteries and left atrium and predisposes to large airway compression, particularly of the left main bronchus. Large airway obstruction results in a restriction of gas flow, primarily during exhalation. If airway obstruction becomes significant, increased work of breathing, increased respiratory frequency, and abnormalities of gas exchange develop. When the obstruction is severe, inspiration may also be compromised. If dynamic hyperinflation occurs, chest radiographs will demonstrate increased lung volumes, and respiratory mechanics will delineate abnormalities of expiratory flow and increased airway resistance. In patients with large airway disease, application of PEEP may reduce the obstruction and "stent" the airway, pending medical or surgical intervention. Reduction of pulmonary artery volume and pressure reverses these abnormalities, provided tracheomalacia is not present.

Attempts have been made to correlate the alterations in respiratory mechanics with other signs of excessive pulmonary blood flow. Therapy should be directed at reversing the cause of the obstruction because surgical interventions on the airways are frequently unsuccessful. Large airway obstruction can also occur when vascular structures proximal to an area of stenosis become dilated, compress the airways, and present in a similar manner.

Decreased Pulmonary Blood Flow

The effects of a right-to-left shunt and decreased pulmonary blood flow on respiratory mechanics are nearly opposite to those that occur in patients with increased pulmonary blood flow and are due to the reduction of pulmonary blood volume and arterial pressure. The decreased pulmonary blood volume results in a decrease in lung weight, an increase in lung compliance, and alterations in V/Q matching.[3] When decreased pulmonary blood flow is present, ventilation occurs without perfusion, and physiologic dead space increases.[59] The extent of the V/Q mismatch is directly correlated with the severity of hypoxia.[28] The increase in dead space ventilation results in a decrease in ventilatory efficiency, which initiates compensatory mechanisms that include an increase in minute ventilation and a reduction in arterial carbon dioxide.[28,59]

Patients with decreased pulmonary blood flow may also develop hypoplasia of the airways.[94] If the airway hypoplasia is significant, a reduction of the airway lumen and an increase in airway resistance can occur.

Children with uncorrected or palliated cyanotic cardiac defects have chronic hypoxia, which results in a reduced ventilatory response to acute hypoxia. The magnitude of this blunting correlates with the severity of the chronic hypoxemia. These findings explain, in part, the recent observation that cardiac patients with chronic cyanosis have frequent and severe decreases in oxygen saturation during sleep.[45] Other studies demonstrated that these alterations are reversible with correction of the chronic hypoxemia.[9]

In summary, alterations in pulmonary mechanics are expected in nearly every child with CHD. These changes in mechanics can range from subclinical changes to overt respiratory system failure. Clinicians treating patients with CHD must take into account these changes in respiratory mechanics when applying mechanical ventilatory support for this patient population.

Postoperative Effects on Respiratory System

Bypass and Reperfusion

Abnormal pulmonary mechanics after cardiovascular surgery are multifactorial and can be considered secondary either to the effects of cardiopulmonary bypass or to postsurgical physiologic alterations. Cardiopulmonary bypass triggers a systemic inflammatory response that involves the contact system, intrinsic and extrinsic coagulation systems, complement system, platelet activation, endothelial cell activation, and leukocyte activation. Ultimately, there is activation and release of proinflammatory mediators and cytokines. If this response is severe and left unchecked by the antiinflammatory response, the resultant endothelial injury can lead to pulmonary edema and ultimately decreased lung compliance, as described earlier.

In addition to the instigation of the inflammatory cascade, during cardiopulmonary bypass the lungs are excluded from the circulation. The only blood flow received by the lungs during this period is from the bronchial arteries, which normally supply 3% to 5% of pulmonary blood flow, and ischemic injury can result.[49] In coming off bypass, reperfusion injury causes a release of many inflammatory mediators and reactive oxygen species. There is also damage to type II alveolar pneumocytes with reduction in surfactant production and inactivation of surfactant. The result of ischemia-reperfusion is increased microvascular permeability, increased PVR, pulmonary edema, impaired oxygenation, and pulmonary hypertension.[49] The net result of this inflammatory response contributes to fluid accumulation in the interstitial spaces. Clinically, edematous pulmonary tissues demonstrate decreased gas exchange and decreased compliance of the lungs.

Special Postoperative Considerations

Phrenic Nerve Injury. Paralysis or paresis of the diaphragm as a result of injury to the phrenic nerve is a well-known surgical complication and is estimated to occur after 0.28% to 5.6% of congenital heart surgery procedures.[86] It occurs most commonly after bidirectional Glenn, the Fontan procedure, systemic to pulmonary artery shunt placement, VSD repair, TOF repair, and arterial switch procedures. Proposed mechanisms of phrenic nerve injury include thermal injury from cold slush used for myocardial protection, thermal injury from dissection of tissues with an electrocautery device, or direct mechanical trauma during instrumentation.

Patients with this injury can present with an inability to wean from mechanical ventilation, respiratory acidosis, persistent atelectasis, and respiratory distress after extubation. Very young children are more likely to be symptomatic secondary to diaphragmatic paralysis because they are more dependent on the diaphragm while breathing. Single-ventricle patients in particular have substantially longer postoperative recovery if this injury is sustained. Occasionally, although the harm may not result in respiratory failure, it may cause a dramatic increase in work of breathing, thereby inhibiting somatic growth.

Diagnosis can be suspected by elevation of the diaphragm on radiographic studies in patients not on positive pressure ventilation. Confirmation of the diagnosis can be made by ultrasonography or fluoroscopy in the spontaneously breathing child. These studies will show paradoxical motion of the diaphragm.

Management of diaphragm paralysis remains controversial. It is challenging to predict if and when diaphragmatic function returns, and patients may require prolonged intubation to support cardiopulmonary reserve and adequate caloric intake. Plication of the injured diaphragm has been reported to be beneficial in some patients. One study showed that 56.5% of patients experienced return of diaphragm function, and there was no difference in recovery of function in the plicated group versus the nonplicated group.[82]

Recurrent Laryngeal Nerve Injury/Vocal Cord Paralysis. The recurrent laryngeal nerve lies in close proximity to cardiac structures and is therefore subject to inadvertent injury during congenital heart surgery, even in experienced centers. Injury to the nerve occurs most commonly in interventions involving the ductus arteriosus and repairs of the aortic arch. The injury to the nerve can result in unilateral or bilateral vocal cord paresis or paralysis. Paralyzed vocal cords are usually abducted in a paramedian position more often than adducted to a median position. Vocal cord injury can present with a weak or even aphonic cry in infants or as a soft voice or hoarseness in older children. Stridor, occasionally dramatic, can also be present in patients with vocal cord paralysis. If any of these findings are found in the postoperative period, the diagnosis can be quickly confirmed by flexible fiberoptic laryngoscopy at the bedside. Such vocal cord injury can result in respiratory difficulties and feeding difficulties from the inability to protect the airway.

Unaddressed, these difficulties can dramatically increase the work of breathing, hinder adequate caloric intake, and further degrade overall respiratory reserve in the immediate postoperative period. Further evaluation with speech therapy and/or evaluation with a fluoroscopic swallow study may be required to determine the extent of the threat of aspiration with feeds or gastroesophageal reflux. Depending on the severity of insult, the patient may require any number of interventions, including thickening of oral feeds, temporary nasogastric or nasodudodenal tube placement, surgical G-tube placement with or without fundoplication, or laryngeal interventions to attempt to partially correct vocal cord positioning. All of these interventions contribute to the overall intermediate- and long-term morbidity of congenital heart surgery. Fortunately, such injury to the cords is generally thought to be transient, often resolving completely before hospital discharge.

Pleural Effusions and Chylothorax. Pleural effusions occur with some regularity after CHD surgery and are a major reason why chest tube placement represents routine supportive care in the postoperative period. Serous effusions adversely affect both lung compliance and V/Q matching and can substantially contribute to work of breathing. Serous effusions after CHD surgery are gratifyingly responsive to diuretic therapy. Development of a blood-containing effusion (hemothorax) is often associated with clinically significant anemia and may further lower oxygenation already adversely affected by disruptions of respiratory mechanics. A chyle-containing pleural effusion (chylothorax) can develop after 3.8% of CHD surgery.[13] It can occur after Glenn or Fontan surgery, in the presence of elevated central venous pressure, or after direct trauma to the thoracic duct. Treatment of chylothorax may include discontinuation of feeds and implementation of total parental nutrition, conversion to a medium-chain fatty acid formula, ligation of the thoracic duct, pleurodesis, and direct lymphatic embolization.

Trauma of Intubation. Particularly in neonates and small infants, intubation for surgery can result in vocal cord edema and/or subglottic stenosis (SGS) observed at extubation. Vocal cord swelling may reflect the overall edematous state following bypass, or it may be the direct result of even mild impact of the endotracheal tube on the cords during the intubation process. Vocal cord edema can result in significant stridor and increased work of breathing and evolve into respiratory failure reflecting a respiratory and/or metabolic acidosis. SGS can occur after intubation, presenting as mild occasional stridor with minimal respiratory distress, as immediate respiratory failure, or manifesting between these extremes. In one prospective study of 194 children (median age 2.6 months, median duration of intubation 7 days) intubated for any reason in a pediatric intensive care unit (PICU), 84% had acute injury of the larynx, and 10% of all subjects demonstrated SGS of some kind.[79] In another retrospective review of 809 children who underwent CHD surgery at a single institution, the incidence of SGS was 2.3% for children 1 to 12 months and only 1.08% for children less than 18 years. Prolonged intubation and age less than 2 years were found to be risk factors for development of SGS. Treatment may range in intensity from mild (racemic epinephrine, systemic steroids, heliox, or supplemental oxygen) to severe (tracheal dilation, eschar removal, tracheal intubation, tracheal stenting, or tracheal reconstruction).[66]

Transition from invasive ventilation to spontaneous ventilation represents a substantial cardiopulmonary challenge for the postoperative patient, and airway trauma can play a significant role. Indeed, first-time extubation failure is 11% in neonates who underwent CHD surgery.[4] Prolonged mechanical ventilation and postextubation stridor have been shown to affect extubation success rates in the PICU.[16] The same study demonstrated that the addition of pre-extubation steroids increased the odds of extubation success. A study by Kurachek et al. showed that patients who required the use of racemic epinephrine, heliox, and noninvasive positive pressure were at increased risk of extubation failure.[15,55]

Special Cardiopulmonary Considerations Unique to the Cardiovascular Intensive Care Unit

Respiratory Physiology After Cavopulmonary Anastomosis

After total cavopulmonary anastomosis surgery (i.e., the Fontan procedure), patients exhibit several unique physiologic characteristics that must be considered when managing their care. Most important to note in Fontan physiology, blood flows passively from the superior and inferior vena cava into the pulmonary arteries. Pulmonary blood transit is therefore considered to be passive, and any increases in either PVR or intrathoracic pressure are generally considered to be detrimental to optimal blood flow. Early extubation after surgery is therefore considered highly desirable so as to maximize the physiologic benefits of negative pressure ventilation. When positive pressure ventilation is needed, doing so with the lowest possible mean airway pressure is most desirable.[78] Formation of both systemic venous to pulmonary venous collateral vessels and pulmonary arteriovenous malformations are common in certain Fontan patients; either phenomenon can lead to progressive cyanosis independent of V/Q mismatch.[43] When a fenestration is created in the Fontan, right-to-left shunting can occur, which preserves cardiac output at the expense of lower saturation levels. Diagnostic study for loss of fenestration patency (usually with contrast echocardiography) should be considered in such patients demonstrating normal saturation levels. In patients with Fontan physiology that is "failing," plastic bronchitis can develop. In this rare but potentially fatal condition, patients develop bronchial casts that can fill the airways of the lung, which can ultimately lead to complete obstruction. On histologic study, these are typically considered type 2 casts, indicating they contain mostly mucin and fibrin with few or no inflammatory cells. Treatment may include chest percussion therapy, inhaled albuterol, inhaled steroids, inhaled dornase alpha, inhaled hypertonic saline, inhaled tissue plasminogen activator, oral steroids, and/or bronchoscopic extraction. Failing interventional relief of anatomic abnormalities, takedown of the Fontan circuit and/or heart transplant may ultimately be indicated.[23]

Respiratory Physiology in Down Syndrome

Patients born with trisomy 21 often have multiple cardiac and pulmonary abnormalities with consequent interactions that often contribute substantially to their high rates of hospitalization. One of the most significant pulmonary vascular findings in patients with DS is their higher rates and severities of pulmonary hypertension. The proposed reasons behind this are multifactorial but include higher rates of each of the following: CHD with either right-to-left or left-to-right shunting, clinically evident or silent chronic aspiration, obstructive sleep apnea, and primary or secondary lung parenchymal disease.[76] However, it should be noted that patients with DS demonstrate pulmonary arterial hypertension more frequently than patients without DS, even without the presence of lung disease, CHD, or sleep apnea.

The incidence of upper airway abnormalities such as macroglossia and adenotonsillar hypertrophy is known to be increased in patients with DS. Furthermore, a quarter of patients with DS demonstrate lower airway abnormalities, which may include tracheobroncho-malacia, laryngomalacia, SGS, tracheal stenosis, complete tracheal rings, or tracheal bronchus. Respiratory infections also occur at higher rates and with greater severity in patients with DS than in those without, and surgery itself can increase the risk of respiratory infection threefold.[62]

Respiratory Physiology in Primary Ciliary Dyskinesia

Primary ciliary dyskinesia (PCD) is a disorder of ciliary function and structure that is associated clinically with male infertility, otosinopulmonary disease, upper and lower airway disease, and organ laterality (40% to 50% with situs inversus and 12% with situs ambiguous) defects.[54] Respiratory symptoms are typically treated with antibiotics for infection and with bronchodilators. Recent evidence also indicates hypertonic saline nebulization therapy may enhance secretion clearance. PCD can manifest in the neonatal period with tachypnea, increased work of breathing, and prolonged oxygen requirements or at any time throughout childhood. When compared to other patients with heterotaxy, patients with PCD who demonstrate situs ambiguous are at 200-fold increased risk of having structure CHD. It is known that as many as 6% of patients with PCD have cardiac malformations, and 2.6 % have complex CHD. There is a known increase in short- and long-term postoperative morality in patients with CHD and laterality defects in general, compared to those without, and some have speculated that this may be the result of undiagnosed ciliary dysfunction like PCD.[41] Although lung function testing typically demonstrates obstructive lung physiology, these patients also demonstrate higher incidences of scoliosis and pectus excavatum.[54]

Forms of Lung Hypoplasia

Patients with scimitar syndrome, an entity with anomalous pulmonary venous return, often have an associated hypoplastic right lung. The degree of hypoplasia of the lung and the presence of obstruction of pulmonary veins determines the patients' severity of illness.[6,18] Congenital diaphragmatic hernia (CDH), which can present with concomitant congenital heart defects, also predisposes the ipsilateral lung to be smaller. The prevalence of patients with CHD and CDH ranges from 10% to 15%; short-term outcomes of those with both who were treated with extracorporeal membrane oxygenation seem to be similar to those of patients without CHD.[7,23]

Respiratory Infections

Infections of the respiratory tract are a common concern in patients with CHD. Proposed factors that contribute to why patients with CHD have increased incidence of pulmonary infections include underlying parenchymal abnormality, alveolar integrity compromise due to edema, poor nutrition, increased incidence of reflux/aspiration, and increased incidence of immunodeficiency, such as thymic dysplasia and asplenia. Respiratory syncytial virus bronchiolitis is a common cause of hospitalization for patients, as demonstrated in a study by Medrano López.[28,64] Human rhinovirus, although clinically insignificant in most children, causes prolonged intubation times and hospital stay after pediatric cardiac surgery.[5,22] Nosocomial pneumonia estimated at a prevalence of 9.6% to 21.5%, with gram-negative organisms (such as *Klebsiella pneumoniae* and *Pseudomonas aeruginosa*) the most common agents.[10,43] Pulmonary infections can cause significant heterogenous lung disease and desaturation through a combination of V/Q mismatch and alveolar-arterial oxygen gradient. Besides the metabolic demands imposed by an active infection, pneumonia in the patient with CHD can contribute to respiratory failure through these mechanisms.

Long-Term Lung Function in Patients With Congenital Heart Disease

Preoperative lung function is reduced in many patients with CHD. Reduced lung compliance and tidal volumes are present in many patients with left-to-right shunts because of additional extravascular lung water. Agha et al. showed that correction of the shunts in these patients improved pulmonary function test parameters.[1,2] However, the effects of CHD and its interventions on long-term lung function cannot be underestimated. In particular, multiple studies have shown a pattern of restrictive lung function (RLF) in spirometry testing is more common in patients with structural CHD after cardiac intervention than in those with CHD who had not yet undergone intervention. Additionally, some studies have found an increasing prevalence of RLF among patients who have had more surgical interventions and when surgical intervention is performed at an earlier age. Furthermore, in patients who have undergone TOF repair, transposition of great arteries repair or VSD repair, decreases in lung compliance and lung volume have been noted. Mean ventilation at peak exercise is significantly different for patients operated for VSD in early life compared to healthy controls.[11,44] Pulmonary function is better in percutaneously closed atrial septal defect patients than in surgically closed patients, implying that the effects of sternotomy are significant enough to cause a difference.[35,95] Of note, patients with corrected CHD possess lower exercise capacity than their healthy counterparts.[31,77]

In one recent study of 47 adult patients with Fontan physiology, 29.8% demonstrated decreased forced vital capacity on spirometry, whereas only 1 patient demonstrated obstructive lung physiology. Some have speculated that a restrictive thoracic cage is created with the scarring and inflammation caused by sternotomy or thoracotomy, and from bypass itself, and that this contributes substantially to the incidence of RLF findings.[42] Others proposed causes for restrictive lung physiology include higher rates of scoliosis in Fontan patients, diaphragm paralysis, cardiomegaly, pleural adhesions, and hypoplasia and abnormal growth of both pulmonary vasculature and pulmonary parenchyma.[51]

Conclusion

In summary, the principles and complex interactions that govern the relationship between the pulmonary and cardiac systems can tremendously impact the short- and long-term well-being of the child with CHD. These interactions can result in influences that range in intensity from the subtle and perhaps subclinical to the profound and even catastrophic. A thorough appreciation of these concepts is therefore absolutely necessary for the clinician responsible for the care of such patients, and especially when selecting and titrating respiratory support for this population.

References

A complete list of references is available at ExpertConsult.com.

15

Organ System Response to Cardiac Function—Splanchnic

DYLAN STEWART, MD, FACS; DARLA SHORES, MD; SAMUEL M. ALAISH, MD

The term *splanchnic circulation* refers to all blood flow originating from the celiac, superior mesenteric, and inferior mesenteric arteries, which is widely distributed to all abdominal viscera. The splanchnic circulation receives 25% of the cardiac output and therefore holds a similar percentage of the total blood volume under normal conditions. Thus the splanchnic circulation can act as a site of cardiac output regulation and also as a blood reservoir (Fig. 15.1). Multiple regulatory pathways are involved in the distribution of the splanchnic circulation. This chapter will be limited to the intestinal and hepatic circulations because of their functional importance and particularly because they are sites of dysregulation during pathologic conditions and surgical stresses, such as cardiopulmonary bypass (CPB).

Basic Principles of the Splanchnic Circulation

Intestinal Circulation

Anatomy. The named mesenteric arteries branch into multiple serosal arteries, which provide intestinal blood flow. These serosal arteries course from the mesenteric to the antimesenteric surface of the intestine, where they penetrate the muscular layer, giving rise to the submucosal and mucosal vasculature. The terminal arteriolar branches supply blood flow to the intestinal villus. This circulatory arrangement is of particular interest because of the proximity of the arteriole and the venule in the villus, which creates a considerable countercurrent exchange of oxygen. Thus an oxygen gradient is produced between the base and tip of the villus (Fig. 15.2). The potential for arteriovenous shunting and the complex plexus of capillaries contribute to making the distal portions of the villus prone to ischemia. The lability of flow at the villous tip is readily evident in studies examining the progression of mucosal injury to a graded ischemic insult.[1]

Physiology. The balance of systemic constrictor and local dilatory mechanisms regulates intestinal blood flow. Systemic activation of sympathetic nerves results in vasoconstriction of the intestinal vasculature and decreased splanchnic blood flow. Catecholamines and other circulating factors, such as angiotensin II, also contribute to the constrictor response. Substances released from the intrinsic nonadrenergic noncholinergic (NANC) nerves largely mediate the dilatory mechanisms. These include neurotransmitters, adenosine, substance P, and nitric oxide. All of these factors, with the probable exception of substance P, may be released by nonneural tissue.

The constrictor mechanisms act globally on the entire splanchnic circulation, whereas dilators work locally to affect alterations in the distribution of blood flow, particularly between the mucosal and muscular portions of the intestine (see Fig. 15.2). Low concentrations of nitric oxide may also have other potent effects, such as antithrombosis and antiadhesion of leukocytes.[2] Hypothermia, a pertinent factor in patients receiving CPB, may also decrease leukocyte adhesion and help ameliorate ischemia/reperfusion injury.[3]

Unlike the circulating catecholamines and angiotensin II, the constrictor effects of endothelin most likely act in a paracrine fashion. Endothelin-1 and endothelin-3 mediate both vasoconstriction and vasodilation in the intestinal blood vessels and cause contraction of intestinal smooth muscle.[4] Endothelin-A receptors mediate the contractile response, whereas the endothelin-B receptors mediate both contraction and relaxation, the latter via coupling to nitric oxide synthase.[5] Upregulation of the endothelin after CPB may be a factor in decreased intestinal perfusion and villus injury after bypass.[6]

Hepatic Circulation

Anatomy. The terminal portions of the hepatic circulation are arranged in a series of repeating functional units called acini or lobules, depending on whether the portal triad or the central vein is used as the anatomic reference point. The basic unit is approximately 0.5 mm in diameter and consists of a portal venular inflow, a network of sinusoids, and a hepatic venular outflow. Blood flow through these subunits is fairly uniform during normal conditions.

The portal vein provides approximately 75% of the blood supply to the liver. This volume is equal to the total blood flow of the other splanchnic viscera, because it is formed from their venous effluent. Portal vein perfusion pressures are low (approximately 10 mm Hg), and portal blood is relatively oxygen-poor. The low perfusion pressure requires a low vascular resistance to accommodate the relatively high portal venous blood volume. In contrast, the hepatic artery, which supplies the remaining 25% of total hepatic blood flow, is oxygen-rich (mimics the partial pressure in systemic arterial blood) and perfuses the liver at systemic arterial pressure. Because the hepatic artery flow joins the portal venous system in the portal venules or directly in the hepatic sinusoid, arterial resistance must remain high to maintain a sufficient pressure drop to prevent retrograde flow through the portal vein.[7]

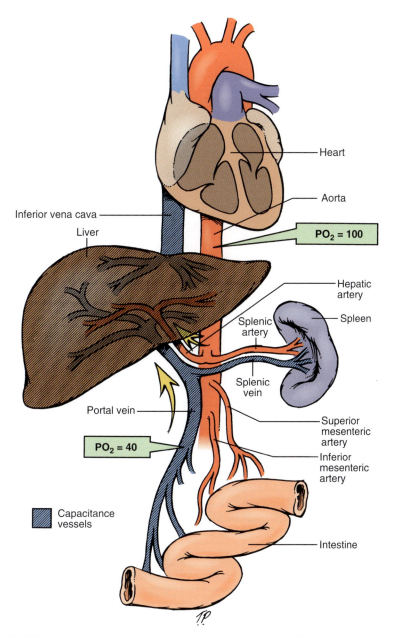

• **Figure 15.1** Schematic representation of the splanchnic circulation. Total flow to the splanchnic viscera is controlled by resistance vessels in the mesenteric and hepatic arterial systems. The venous effluents from the splanchnic viscera converge to form the portal vein, which supplies approximately 75% of the total blood supply to the liver. This portal blood not only is high in substrate concentrations resulting from intestinal absorption but also tends to contain bacteria and endotoxin. Under normal circumstances these are cleared by the resident macrophages of the liver, the Kupffer cells. The venular circulations of the intestines and the liver have a very large blood volume capacity and can thus have a very significant impact on circulating volume and venous return (see text). *PO_2,* Partial pressure of oxygen.

Physiology

Regulation of Hepatic Blood Flow. Blood flow is unidirectional from the portal to the central vein within the sinusoidal beds of the hepatic lobule. Because the oxygen content is low, a significant oxygen gradient is established.[25] This situation results in relative centrilobular hypoxia, even under normal conditions. During conditions of low flow, this gradient becomes greater, and overt ischemia can develop in the centrilobular areas. The tendency toward ischemia may produce *centrilobular necrosis,* the hallmark of low-flow injury in the liver.

The regulation of total portal blood flow lies primarily upstream in the resistance vessels of the intestine during normal conditions. Although intrahepatic or posthepatic diseases have relatively little influence on the total volume of portal blood flow, they can have great significance in the distribution of blood flow and portal pressure. In patients with chronic disease (i.e., cirrhosis), severe disruption of acinar blood flow results in portal hypertension. This leads to the development of extrahepatic shunts. Under these conditions a substantial portion of portal blood can reenter the circulation without first flowing through the liver. Total liver blood

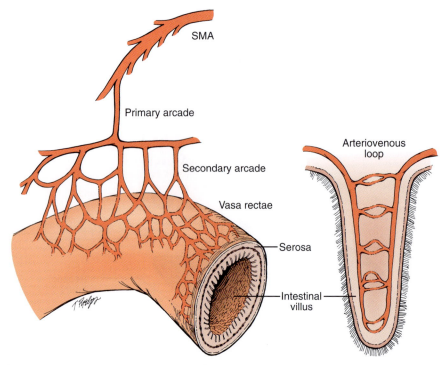

• **Figure 15.2** The superior mesenteric artery *(SMA)* divides into primary and secondary arcades followed by multiple divisions into vasa rectae. The vasa rectae penetrate the serosa, submucosa, and mucosa. Ultimately, the intestinal villus is supplied by an arteriovenous loop. The venous blood supply parallels the arterial system.

flow may not be affected before the development of extrahepatic shunts, which develop over days to weeks. However, heterogeneous distribution of blood flow can exist earlier as a result of intrahepatic shunts, which may impair liver function. In addition to shunting blood, contraction of intrahepatic vessels may cause substantial pooling of blood within the liver and mesenteric veins, resulting in a loss of circulating blood volume.

Systemic Venous Hypertension and Increased Outflow (Downstream) Pressure of the Liver. The portal circulation, with low perfusion pressure, is sensitive to elevation of outflow (downstream) pressures. The site of increased pressure may occur anywhere along the pathway from the sinusoid to the hepatic vein to the right heart. Three cell types line the sinusoid: the endothelial cell, the Kupffer cell, and the hepatic stellate cell. All three cell types are capable of secreting vasoactive substances. Among the various vasoactive substances, endothelin-1 is a prominent vasoconstrictor of endothelial cells and hepatic stellate cells, leading to contraction of the hepatic sinusoid during shock.[8] In addition, sinusoidal contraction resulting in increased portal venous pressures has been associated with CPB. Cytokines, such as interleukin-1 and tumor necrosis factor; arachidonic acid metabolites, including the thromboxanes, leukotrienes, and platelet activation factor; neutrophil products, such as oxygen free radicals and peptidases; and endothelin-1 seem to mediate this process.[9] Sinusoidal perfusion failure is associated with the release of oxygen free radicals, cholestasis, enzyme release from the liver, and hepatocyte necrosis.[10]

Systemic venous pressure elevation represents another cause of increased downstream pressure for the hepatic microcirculation. This increase in systemic venous pressure may arise from a variety of derangements, such as clot in the great veins, right heart failure, tricuspid valve insufficiency, or pulmonary hypertension. A failing Fontan circulation in the patient with a univentricular heart represents a specific cause of systemic venous hypertension. Because the increase in downstream pressure originates in the heart or great vessels, there is a diffuse increase in systemic capillary pressure in addition to the increase in hepatic vein and sinusoidal pressure. Therefore the manifestations are more generalized with hepatomegaly, ascites, pleural effusions, and edema.

Liver dysfunction secondary to high right-sided venous pressure is associated with decreased hepatic blood flow and oxygen delivery. The increased hepatic venous pressure produces pressure atrophy of hepatocytes and perisinusoidal edema. These effects summate to create the classic pathologic picture of centrilobular necrosis.

Hypotension and the Hepatic Artery Buffer Response. Even mild hypotension compromises splanchnic and therefore portal blood flow. However, total liver blood flow and hepatic oxygen delivery are preserved until hypotension becomes severe. Oxygen delivery is maintained as a result of a compensatory increase in hepatic artery flow. This compensation is termed the *hepatic artery buffer response*. Besides hypotension, any condition that results in a decrease in portal blood flow, such as CPB, will invoke a hepatic artery buffer response.[11] Although this arterial buffer response preserves total oxygen delivery, the response does not appear to be regulated by the metabolic needs of the hepatic parenchyma.[7,11] Rather, hepatic arterial resistance is sensitive to changes in the volume of the portal circulation. A vasodilator substance such as adenosine is likely released from hepatocytes at a constant rate. This substance is washed out of the interstitium, so that it does not accumulate, when portal flow is normal or elevated. When portal blood flow decreases, the vasodilator substance accumulates in the vicinity of the hepatic arterial resistance vessels, causing vasodilation and increased flow in the hepatic artery vascular bed. Classic arterial autoregulation can also be explained by this mechanism. Increased hepatic artery blood flow, for example, will cause faster washout of adenosine from the interstitium, with resultant arterial vasoconstriction. Other vasoactive agents such as nitric oxide and angiotensin II may also contribute to regulation of total liver blood flow in this setting.

Effects of Cardiopulmonary Bypass on the Splanchnic Circulation

Overview

A number of factors may play a role in the regulation of hepatic and splanchnic blood flow and organ function during CPB for congenital heart surgery (Box 15.1). A decrease in splanchnic perfusion, detectable via new noninvasive technologies, is associated with early postoperative life-threatening complications.[12] Bypass technique, duration, and mediator release affect splanchnic perfusion.

Physiologic Factors

Bypass flow rate is the major determinant of portal and hepatic arterial blood flow during CPB. Failure to maintain normotension or high flow rates during CPB may jeopardize hepatic blood flow. Normothermic CPB causes a 50% decrease in hepatic blood flow during nonpulsatile bypass in dogs perfused at a lower than normal blood pressure.[13] Under these experimental conditions, hepatic blood flow decreases less than portal venous blood flow. Ostensibly the hepatic artery buffer maintains hepatic flow during low CPB pump flow by increasing the contribution of hepatic arterial blood flow at a time when portal venous flow decreases.[14,15] This is true for any body temperature or perfusion technique. Conversely, portal venous flow improves more consistently by use of a higher flow rate, in keeping with previous studies showing the sensitivity of portal flow during conditions of decreased cardiac output.

The presence of a potent vasoconstrictor, especially in the setting of diminished cardiac output, during or after cardiac surgery may place the splanchnic circulation at risk for ischemia. Vasoactive mediators that may be released during cardiac surgery include angiotensin II,[16] vasopressin,[9] thromboxane A_2 and B_2,[17,18] and catecholamines, including epinephrine and norepinephrine[9] and the endothelins. All these substances may cause vasoconstriction, a potentially catastrophic event in the face of an already diminished oxygen delivery. Clinically the presence of the hepatic buffer to maintain total hepatic flow when portal venous flow falls and the maintenance of portal flow during high-flow CPB may account for the relatively low incidence of gastrointestinal complications after bypass.[13]

The effect of CPB pulsatility on hepatic blood flow depends on the CPB flow rate and temperature. Although some investigators show better preservation of hepatic blood flow by pulsatile bypass perfusion,[13,19] Mathie[19] did not observe any change in hepatic flow as long as the CPB flow rate was maintained at a high level. Pulsatile CPB decreases systemic vascular resistance and increases hepatic blood flow during hypothermia.[20-23] The beneficial effects of pulsatile flow may be apparent only when low-flow CPB is used. Angiotensin II levels increase during and after CPB in dogs[24] and adults, an increase that may be accentuated by nonpulsatile bypass and low perfusion rates.[25] The increase in angiotensin II levels during CPB may depend on the baseline preoperative angiotensin level, because angiotensin II levels actually decreased from very high preoperative levels following CPB in children.[26]

Changes in both PaO_2 and $PaCO_2$ have been shown to affect hepatic blood flow. Hypoxemia causes a mild constriction of the hepatic artery, an effect probably mediated by sympathetic stimulation.[27] Hyperoxia does not appear to alter hepatic blood flow.[28] Acidosis constricts hepatic artery flow but simultaneously dilates portal flow. Total hepatic blood flow will either increase or decrease depending on whether the constrictor or dilator effects predominate.[27,29] Hypocapnia decreases both hepatic artery and portal blood flow in dogs.[30] There are no data on the effect of hypocapnia on hepatic blood flow in infants undergoing congenital heart surgery; however, adults treated with hypocapnia for trauma head injury have been shown to have no decrease in hepatic blood flow.[31]

A general decrease in core temperature unrelated to CPB has little effect on hepatic arterial blood flow but increases intestinal[32] and therefore portal[33,34] blood flow. When flow is kept constant during CPB, the same increase in portal and intestinal blood flow in response to a decrease in core temperature would be expected. Lowering the core temperature from 37°C to 28°C decreases oxygen consumption by 50%.[35] However, hypothermia impairs splanchnic oxygen extraction and may have deleterious effects on splanchnic function during hypothermic CPB.[36,37]

Rewarming after CPB may also affect oxygen delivery. Rewarming is characterized by a decrease in oxygen delivery and an increase in oxygen consumption. This uncoupling of oxygen delivery and consumption may be responsible for the lactic acidosis that occurs after CPB. During rewarming there is a generalized increase in sympathetic nervous system activity, resulting in increased levels of circulating norepinephrine.[38] Selective rewarming of either the spinal cord or the hypothalamus decreases splanchnic oxygen delivery in animal models. Spinal or hypothalamic warming results in increased splanchnic sympathetic nervous system output and thus superior mesenteric artery vasoconstriction.[39] The effects of core rewarming on splanchnic blood flow, mucosal blood flow, and hepatic function have not been fully elucidated.

CPB affects hepatic lactate metabolism. Decreased peripheral oxygen delivery and increased oxygen consumption result in increased lactic acid levels both during and after cardiac bypass. In normal circumstances, hepatic lactate clearance is highly effective,[40] but this clearance capacity is saturated in the presence of very high systemic lactate levels and hepatic blood flow less than 25% of normal.[41] Hepatic venous lactate and pyruvate levels have been shown to increase during the first 30 minutes of CPB.[42] The combination of a rise in both lactate and pyruvate with a relatively constant lactate-pyruvate ratio suggests that there is not only an increase in anaerobic metabolism, but also a possible alteration in the activity of key enzymes such as pyruvate dehydrogenase.[42]

Although prospective data are not available, several retrospective studies reveal that most major gastrointestinal complications occur in CPB patients who experience episodes of hypotension or prolonged shock, particularly when pressor support is required (Box 15.2). Centrilobular hepatocellular necrosis, cholestasis, and intestinal ischemia are perhaps the most common complications, but other disorders such as gastritis, pancreatitis, and intestinal hemorrhage also occur with increased frequency in these critically ill patients.

Clinical Conditions

Congenital Malformations

Certain congenital syndromes combine heart disease and intestinal anomalies. The infant with Down syndrome (see Chapter 75) may have an intracardiac defect combined with duodenal atresia. Bilious vomiting and less commonly abdominal distention suggest the possibility of bowel obstruction, which is confirmed with the classic double bubble sign on abdominal radiograph. The long-term survival rate for duodenal atresia is 86% with virtually all deaths occurring among patients who also had complex cardiac disease.[43]

Heterotaxy syndrome (HS) refers to embryologic abnormalities in the usual left and right asymmetry and results in complex congenital heart disease (CHD) and abnormalities of abdominal organ anatomy. Although intestinal rotational anomalies are the most common finding, gastric volvulus, preduodenal portal vein, esophageal hiatal hernia, and biliary atresia may also occur. The cardiac disease in this population is very complex. Those with asplenia syndrome (right atrial isomerism) demonstrate atrioventricular canal defect, double-outlet right ventricle, transposition of the great arteries, anomalous pulmonary venous return, and pulmonary stenosis or atresia. Bilateral superior vena cavae are usually present. The subgroup with polysplenia syndrome (left atrial isomerism) usually have the combination of ventricular septal defect, atrial septal defect, and pulmonic stenosis. The inferior vena cava is usually interrupted. Instead, a dilated azygous venous system connects the infradiaphragmatic veins with the superior vena cava. The normal visceral asymmetry is absent in this population (particularly in the asplenia group) so that the liver is midline and the stomach is on the side opposite to the cardiac apex. Thus a chest and abdominal radiograph immediately suggest the diagnosis. Given the complexity of the heart disease and the immune deficiency associated with asplenia/polysplenia, the addition of intestinal obstruction leads to a very high (90%) mortality rate.[44]

Much recent interest has focused on the treatment of patients with HS and intestinal rotational anomalies (IRAs). Forty to 90% of HS patients may have some degree of IRA.[45] There is much

debate on whether or not an asymptomatic HS patient should be screened for IRA, or even treated if the condition is discovered. Of note, pediatric surgeons continue to debate this same topic in non-CHD patients as well.[142] Previously mortality rates were reportedly as high as 40%; subsequent advances in pediatric critical care, anesthesia, and cardiac surgical care have vastly improved survival in HS patients. These improved outcomes have lead physicians caring for these children to place more emphasis on treatment of malrotation and to have a desire to avoid the dreaded complication of midgut volvulus. The more interventionist school of thought argues that the known high incidence of malrotation in HS patients warrants screening and prophylactic surgery (the Ladd procedure or intestinal derotation), and that this surgery is much better tolerated in an elective fashion, as opposed to an emergent situation in which volvulus has occurred and bowel ischemia exists. Others have argued that the risk of volvulus is extremely small in HS patients, and that their major morbidities after the Ladd procedure are high.[46,47,47a] The largest review to date suggests that HS patients have a higher morbidity after the Ladd procedure, and a very small percentage of the patients actually had volvulus.[45] However, several single-center retrospective reviews report no difference in the tolerance of the procedure between HS and non-HS populations and advocate an operative approach in asymptomatic patients with HS once the diagnosis of IRA is made.[48] Other studies have suggested the HS patients with predominately right-sided isomerism have a higher risk of narrowed mesentery and therefore catastrophic volvulus than HS patients with left-sided isomerism, further complicating the decision making.[49]

Until a definitive randomized controlled trial is performed, it is reasonable to take an individualized approach to patients with HS and concern for IRA. Patients with abdominal symptoms (feeding intolerance, emesis, signs of obstruction) should be screened with an upper gastrointestinal series, and a decision made regarding surgery should involve cardiology, anesthesia, and the family. Parents should have the opportunity to give fully informed consent to a prophylactic and possibly high-risk surgical procedure, knowing that although the risk of volvulus might be low, it is a catastrophic event. In the case of HS patients with no abdominal symptoms, routine screening does not appear to be mandatory, although increased vigilance in patients with known right-sided isomerism seems warranted. When the decision not to perform prophylactic surgery is made, extensive counseling regarding the signs and symptoms of volvulus, and what to do should those signs and symptoms occur, is extremely important before the patient leaves the hospital setting.

Alagille syndrome (AGS) frequently involves both CHD and liver disease. This is an autosomal dominant disorder with highly variable expressivity characterized not only by liver and heart abnormalities but also by a characteristic facies, butterfly vertebrae, corneal opacities, renal disease, and intracranial bleeding.[50] AGS is associated with two mutations in the Notch signaling pathway, which determines cell fate early in embryogenesis.[51,52] Mutations can occur in the *JAG1* gene, found in approximately 95% of affected individuals, or in the *NOTCH2* gene (1% to 2%). Patients with AGS typically exhibit right heart obstructive lesions ranging from peripheral pulmonic stenosis to tetralogy of Fallot. Cholestasis distinguishes the liver disease in this syndrome, which may progress to liver failure. Liver transplantation may be necessary because of intractable pruritus and failure to thrive. Elevated right heart pressure from peripheral pulmonic stenosis is not a contraindication for liver transplantation.[53]

Splanchnic Complications Associated With Specific Cardiac Operations

Etiology. The multiple etiologic factors that produce splanchnic complications with cardiac surgery or CPB are poorly understood (Box 15.3). The prevailing hypothesis is that ischemia/reperfusion injury plays a major role. This is supported by the clinical observation that most splanchnic complications occur in the setting of hypotension or overt shock. The involvement of other factors such as microemboli, toxins, infectious agents, and vasopressors is suggested by the fact that complications do not develop in all patients who experience hypotension or shock. These splanchnic complications can occur without a previous episode of hypotension. Likewise, there does not appear to be a specific splanchnic target organ, although the liver and the intestinal tract appear to be the most vulnerable. Table 15.1 presents some of the potential complications associated with certain operative procedures.

• BOX 15.3   Congenital Cardiac Anomalies Commonly Associated With Splanchnic Complications

Transposition of the great vessels
  Hypoplastic left heart syndrome
  Tricuspid atresia
  Tetralogy of Fallot
  Pulmonary atresia
  Ventricular septal defect (large left-to-right shunt)
  Coarctation of the aorta

TABLE 15.1   Splanchnic Complications Following Pediatric Cardiac Operations

Cardiac Pathology/Operation	Splanchnic Complication	Risk Factors (Perioperative)	Reference
Cardiopulmonary Bypass Group			
Hypoplastic left heart syndrome/Norwood	Mesenteric ischemia	Hypotension Cardiac arrest within 48 h of mesenteric ischemia	134
Tricuspid atresia/Fontan	Acute hepatic failure	Elevated CVP	126
TOF/repair		Low cardiac output	
AV canal/repair			
Pulmonary atresia/repair and valve			
Single ventricle/modified Fontan	Acute hepatic failure	Low cardiac output	135
Tricuspid atresia/modified Fontan		Low urinary output	
Mitral atresia/modified Fontan			
VSD/repair	Perforated peptic ulcer	Hypotension	136
TOF/repair	UGI bleed	Hypoxia	
ASD/repair			
VSD/repair	UGI bleeding—gastric	None reported	137
ASD/repair	Stress ulceration		
Transposition/Mustard	Protein-losing enteropathy	SVC obstruction	71
Tricuspid atresia/Fontan		SVC/IVC obstruction	
Non–Cardiopulmonary Bypass Group			
Coarctation of aorta	Peptic ulcers	Hemoconcentration	138
Subclavian flap			
Coarctation	Perforated peptic ulcer	None	139
Subclavian flap			
Coarctation/end-to-end anastomosis	Renal failure	Associated cardiac anomalies	140
Nonoperated Group			
Hypoplastic left heart	Mesenteric ischemia	Low birth weight	72,141
PDA + CHF		Major associated anomalies	

ASD, Atrial septal defect; *AV,* atrioventricular; *AVR,* aortic valve replacement; *CHF,* congestive heart failure; *CVP,* central venous pressure; *IVC,* inferior vena cava; *PDA,* patent ductus arteriosus; *SVC,* superior vena cava; *TOF,* tetralogy of Fallot; *UGI,* upper gastrointestinal; *VSD,* ventricular septal defect.

Postcoarctectomy Syndrome. The postcoarctectomy syndrome may develop after repair of coarctation of the aorta.[54,55] It consists of abdominal pain and systemic hypertension sometimes accompanied by vomiting, ileus, and melena. The syndrome appears to be less common if the repair is carried out in infancy. The cause appears to be a necrotizing arteritis, which develops after coarctectomy permits a sudden increase in mesenteric vascular pressures. The syndrome is reversible after bowel rest and control of hypertension.

Protein-Losing Enteropathy. Protein-losing enteropathy (PLE) is the abnormal loss of intestinal protein leading to hypoalbuminemia, diarrhea, edema, ascites, pleural effusions, lymphopenia, immunoglobulin deficiency, and hypercoagulability. It is most commonly seen after the Fontan operation.[56] It may also be a manifestation of right heart failure secondary to congenital or acquired valvular disease,[57] constrictive pericarditis,[58,59] or cardiomyopathy.[60]

The pathogenesis of PLE is unclear. It is believed that a chronically elevated systemic venous pressure is transmitted to the mesenteric veins, resulting in lymphangiectasia and protein loss into the gastrointestinal tract. This explanation appears to apply to many but not all patients with PLE because PLE develops in some Fontan patients who have normal systemic venous pressures.[61] Elevated mesenteric vascular resistance may contribute to the pathogenesis.[62] Other factors that may combine with the Fontan operation to predispose to PLE include having the anatomic right ventricle as the systemic ventricle (e.g., hypoplastic left heart syndrome) and prolonged CPB time (>140 minutes).[63] Because prolonged CPB is known to release inflammatory cytokines and cause reperfusion injury, it is plausible that prolonged CPB combined with elevated systemic venous pressures may lead to a vascular or lymphatic injury of the intestinal tract.

The diagnosis of PLE is often clinical, based on symptoms and laboratory values, but diagnostic evaluation for diarrhea in patients after the Fontan procedure may include endoscopy.[64] On occasion, lymphangiectasias resulting from obstruction to lymphatic drainage may be visualized in the jejunum. Small bowel biopsy reveals dilated lacteals. In the face of a consistent history and physical findings, the diagnosis of PLE is supported by determination of fecal alpha-1 antitrypsin (A1AT). This protein accounts for approximately 4% to 5% of total serum protein and is resistant to both intestinal and bacterial proteolysis. It is excreted intact in the stool and therefore can be quantitated as a marker of protein loss from the bowel.

PLE may develop within weeks to years after a Fontan procedure, occurring 5% to 15% of patients.[65] Changes in stool A1AT may occur in the first few months with hemodynamic disturbances even if full symptoms do not develop.[66,67] PLE is associated with decreased long-term survival. Historically the 5-, 10-, and 20-year survival rates were 46% to 59%, 35%, and 19%.[56,61] Better treatment strategies may be improving survival. A more recent, albeit small, study of patients from 1992 to 2010 had improved outcomes, with a 5-year survival of 88%.[68] Outcomes in patients with PLE who undergo cardiac transplant do not seem to be different than those without PLE.[69]

Various medical and surgical treatment regimens have been used for PLE. Edema may be treated symptomatically with diuretics, 25% albumin infusion, and a diet high in protein and medium-chain triglycerides. Angiotensin-converting enzyme (ACE) inhibitors may reduce systemic afterload and improve ventricular function.[70] High-dose spironolactone (2 to 5 mg/kg/day) has also been found to be clinically efficacious for PLE.[71] Intravenous or subcutaneous heparin (5000 to 7500 IU/m^2/day) has improved PLE over the course of weeks in some cases.[73] Some patients respond to oral prednisone (2 mg/kg/day) with clinical and histologic improvement.[74] Oral budesonide, which has fewer side effects than prednisone due to lower systemic absorption, has also shown efficacy in case series.[75-77] Sildenafil may help treat mesenteric artery resistance and has been used successfully in some cases of PLE.[78,79] Octreotide, which modifies intestinal blood flow and lymphatic pressure and has been used to treat PLE due to lymphangiectasia, has also been used in refractory cardiac cases of PLE.[80] However, long-term improvement with any of these medical modalities alone has been limited; side effects must be weighed, and a multifactorial approach is often employed.[68,81]

Patients with PLE should undergo cardiac catheterization to evaluate overall hemodynamics and correct anatomic lesions such as pulmonary artery stenoses or aortopulmonary collateral vessels. If medical therapy has failed and no correctable anatomic lesions are found, the options include (1) fenestration to create a communication between the lateral tunnel or baffle and the atrium, (2) "Fontan-takedown" to restore the bidirectional Glenn anastomosis, and (3) heart transplantation.

Intestinal Ischemia and Necrotizing Enterocolitis

Children with CHD are prone to the serious gastrointestinal complications of intestinal ischemia and necrotizing enterocolitis (NEC) both before and after cardiac surgery. In the past these two conditions were thought to represent the same disease, but recent advances in the understanding of necrotizing enterocolitis coupled with some clinical discrepancies point to two different diseases. NEC is now thought to develop in the premature baby in the setting of bacterial colonization, particularly after non–breast milk feeds, and disease onset is believed to be due to an increased expression of the bacterial receptor Toll-like receptor 4 (TLR4) leading to an increased reactivity of the premature intestinal mucosa.[82] This leads to mucosal destruction and impaired mesenteric perfusion, which, if left unchecked, can progress to frank necrosis. On the other hand, a term infant with CHD and intestinal ischemia likely has a different pathogenesis.[134] It is more likely that impaired circulation, particularly in infants with left ventricular outflow obstruction and single-ventricle physiology, the stress of cardiac surgery and CPB, and the underlying baseline elevation of serum endotoxin and proinflammatory cytokines all play a role.[83] Unfortunately, these two entities are often lumped together in the literature, thus making any distinction blurry at best. In support of two diseases, infants with CHD and NEC had better short- and long-term outcomes than infants with NEC but without CHD. After controlling for birth weight and gestational age, the CHD group had decreased risk of perforation, need for bowel surgery, strictures, sepsis, and short bowel syndrome compared with the non-CHD group.[84] Another study of neonates with NEC after surgical correction of a congenital heart defect found all patients missing typical radiologic findings of NEC, including pneumatosis.[85] However, the two diseases share a similar clinical presentation because the signs and symptoms are indistinguishable (Table 15.2).[86,87] Moreover, the two both predominantly affect the small intestine.[88]

There is no controversy regarding the increased risk of bowel ischemia, whether it be true NEC or not, in infants with CHD. The increased incidence of NEC (3% to 7%) in the cardiac population clearly points to heart disease as a risk factor.[87,89] It greatly exceeds the incidence of 0.3 per 1000 recorded in the largest

TABLE 15.2	Modified Bell Staging Criteria for Necrotizing Enterocolitis			
Stage	Classification	Systemic Signs	Intestinal Signs	Radiologic Signs
1a	Suspected NEC	Temperature instability, apnea, bradycardia, lethargy	Elevated residuals, emesis, mild abdominal distention, guaiac-positive stool	Normal or intestinal dilation, mild ileus
1b	Suspected NEC	Same as 1a	Bright-red blood from rectum	Same as 1a
2a	Proven NEC—mildly ill	Same as 1b	Same as 1b, plus absent bowel sounds, with or without abdominal tenderness	Intestinal dilation, ileus, pneumatosis intestinalis
2b	Proven NEC—moderately ill	Same as 2a, plus mild metabolic acidosis, mild thrombocytopenia	Same as 2a, plus definite abdominal tenderness, with or without abdominal cellulitis or right lower quadrant mass	Same as 2a, plus portal vein gas with or without ascites
3a	Advanced NEC—severely ill, bowel intact	Same as 2b, plus hypotension, bradycardia, severe apnea, combined respiratory and metabolic acidosis, disseminated intravascular coagulation, and neutropenia	Same as 2b, plus signs of generalized peritonitis, marked tenderness and abdominal distention	Same as 2b, plus definite ascites
3b	Advanced NEC—severely ill, bowel perforated	Same as 3a	Same as 3a	Same as 3a, plus pneumoperitoneum

NEC, Necrotizing enterocolitis.
From McElhinney DB, Hedrick HL, Bush DM, et al. Necrotizing enterocolitis in neonates with congenital heart disease: risk factors and outcomes. *Pediatrics*. 2000;106:1080-1087, with permission.

surveillance study of greater than 500,000 live-birth infants.[90] A database analysis of 11,958 neonates undergoing cardiac procedures found that 194 developed NEC.[91] Nevertheless, premature infants still have the highest incidence of NEC (10% to 17%).[92]

Although cardiac disease in general is a risk factor for NEC, univentricular heart disease and especially the hypoplastic left heart syndrome stand out. In addition, prostaglandin E_1 (PGE_1) administration increases the risk of NEC independent of univentricular heart disease.[93,94] The risk of NEC with PGE_1 administration may be dose dependent and requires doses greater than 0.05 mcg/kg/min.[87] Other anatomic lesions have also been reported in association with NEC, including truncus arteriosus, aortopulmonary window, transposition of the great arteries, and coarctation of the aorta. Severe CHD, including univentricular disease[95] and atrioventricular canal,[96] appears to have the highest risk.[97] In addition, acquired pulmonary vein stenosis had a 50% incidence of NEC in one small study of 20 premature infants.[98] Birth weight less than 1500 g, the need for surgical correction of CHD, and a clinical picture of septicemia were all independently associated with an increased risk of NEC following multivariate analysis of almost 8000 infants.[99]

The pathophysiology of NEC in the infant with cardiac disease presumably entails intestinal hypoperfusion. Diastolic runoff and low diastolic pressures in truncus arteriosus and aortopulmonary window may contribute to intestinal hypoperfusion. Persistent diastolic flow reversal on Doppler study of the abdominal aorta is associated with an increased risk of NEC in term infants with CHD irrespective of gestational age or anatomic type of CHD.[100] Similarly, infants with hypoplastic left heart syndrome and NEC had a lower abdominal aorta pulsatility index compared with those without NEC both on stage 1 preoperative and postoperative echocardiograms despite similar ventricular function and operative

risk.[101] Perioperative shock in the infant with hypoplastic left heart syndrome or critical coarctation might lead to the same result. Finally, the therapeutic interventions with PGE_1, cardiac catheterization, or umbilical artery catheters might compromise gut perfusion.

No matter the cause of the poor perfusion, splanchnic near-infrared spectroscopy (NIRS) is becoming an accepted and frequently used noninvasive means to assess gut perfusion and may be a useful tool for assessing risk of NEC.[102] NIRS devices measure the amount of oxygenated hemoglobin and deoxygenated hemoglobin in a vascular distribution and provide information about regional perfusion. In the splanchnic bed this information is thought to be of extremely high value because in periods of hypoperfusion the gastrointestinal track is often the first to experience ischemia.[103] The gut has been called "the canary of the body" in reference to its potential ability to predict impending worsening of clinical status.[104] Splanchnic circulatory compromise may be the first step to overall hemodynamic collapse. For this reason, routine NIRS monitoring of the splanchnic bed has become standard in many pediatric cardiac critical care units. However, some authors have cast doubt on the reliability of NIRS to accurately predict a low-flow cardiac state.[105,106] As more studies are performed and more clinical experience gained, splanchnic NIRS is likely to find a permanent place in the postoperative monitoring of patients with CHD, with NIRS data simply becoming another important value to assess in the overall clinical picture.

Regardless of the target population (premature versus cardiac), the end result is the same. Bowel ischemia progresses to infarction, bacterial translocation, sepsis, and multiple organ dysfunction syndrome if these conditions are undiagnosed or untreated. The clinical presentation typically includes abdominal distention, absent bowel activity, and lower gastrointestinal bleeding (see Table 15.2).

The diagnosis of NEC is difficult, and delay often results in death of the patient. Clinical findings usually begin with an increased abdominal girth and feeding intolerance, which typically presents with increased aspirates. Occasionally stools are grossly bloody. Fever, persistent tachycardia, and abdominal tenderness may be present. Flank edema, abdominal wall cellulitis, and limb edema are usually seen as late findings. Bowel sounds are absent or hypoactive. Suggestive laboratory data include metabolic acidosis, hyperkalemia, hyponatremia, leukocytosis with a left shift, thrombocytopenia, and hemoconcentration. Fluid resuscitation alone does not resolve these clinical and laboratory disorders. Flat plate and left lateral decubitus radiographs may show distended intestinal loops, pneumatosis intestinalis, portal or biliary air, or pneumoperitoneum. The presence of pneumoperitoneum is an absolute indication for laparotomy. Portal venous gas is a serious relative indication for laparotomy. Some pediatric surgeons even consider it an absolute indication because of its high correlation with intestinal necrosis. Rowe and colleagues[107] reported intestinal necrosis in more than 90% of NEC patients with portal venous gas, including pan-necrosis in 52%. Combinations of hyponatremia despite adequate fluid resuscitation, persistent left shift of the white blood cell count, thrombocytopenia, and metabolic acidosis are relative indications for laparotomy.[108] Erythema of the abdominal wall with a palpable mass is diagnostic of a localized perforation and is an indication for laparotomy. A static loop on serial abdominal radiographs is concerning for necrotic bowel and is a relative indication for surgical exploration as well. Doppler ultrasonography is helpful to identify flow in the aorta and superior mesenteric artery and vein roots.[109] However, because the pathologic condition is nonocclusive ischemia, flow to vessels beyond 3 to 4 cm from the root of the superior mesenteric artery is difficult to image by Doppler techniques. Gastric tonometry with mucosal pH measurement has been assessed in children as a method for diagnosing intestinal ischemia but has met with limited success.[109] Angiography[110] and selective infusion of either papaverine or glucagon have not been evaluated in a large prospective pediatric series.

In the absence of a clear indication for laparotomy, management is generally resuscitative and supportive. Enteral feeding is withheld, and aggressive intravenous volume replacement instituted. A nasal or orogastric tube is mandatory for gastrointestinal decompression. Broad-spectrum antibiotic therapy is instituted. Should the patient develop pneumoperitoneum or fail to improve and meet relative indications for exploration, then a laparotomy is needed.

The operative approach is generally via a right supraumbilical transverse incision. All necrotic bowel is resected, and a diverting stoma and mucous fistula are generally performed. A primary anastomosis can be performed if the infant is hemodynamically stable and the intestinal blood supply adequate; however, this is much less common practice. The high likelihood that the anastomosis has compromised albeit viable bowel increases the complication rate, especially if there is progression of the disease before resolution. If lesions do not appear to be transmural or appear patchy throughout the midgut and no resection is necessary, a second-look laparotomy may be indicated within 24 to 48 hours. Intraoperative evaluation of mesenteric blood supply is feasible using Doppler imaging and fluorescein, but once again the technology has marginal sensitivity and specificity and has not been evaluated in infants by a prospective randomized format.

Prevention strategies have focused on feeding patterns and the use of synbiotics. Many practitioners advocate keeping the infant on nothing by mouth (NPO) status to reduce the incidence of NEC; however, enteral feeding was not associated with an increased odds of NEC in two separate studies.[111,112] In fact, in the latter study, preoperative NPO status was associated with more ventilator-dependent days. The benefits of graduated feeding advancements to avoid NEC remain unproven.[113] Currently, considerable variation exists in feeding patterns for infants with univentricular CHD as shown in a study of 46 centers participating in the National Pediatric Cardiology Quality Improvement Collaborative.[114] This might be another area of medicine in which standardization improves outcomes. One promising additional avenue for prevention may be through the use of synbiotics. In a prospective, blinded, randomized controlled trial of 100 infants, the synbiotic *Bifidobacterium lactis* plus inulin, reduced the NEC incidence from 10% to 0% and the risk of death from 28% to 10%.[115]

Hepatic Complications

Ischemic Hepatitis. Ischemic hepatitis or "shock liver" may occur as a result of decreased total hepatic blood flow secondary to low cardiac output, shock, or cardiac arrest.[116] Serum transaminase levels rise rapidly, generally peaking in 48 to 72 hours (often in the thousands), and are usually accompanied by twofold to fourfold elevations in total serum bilirubin, which may take longer to peak.[117,118] A dramatic rise in lactate dehydrogenase is often seen and can help distinguish ischemic hepatitis from viral or drug-induced hepatitis.[119] Lactate may also be elevated. A mild coagulopathy may occur, usually resolving within 10 days; an international normalized ratio (INR) greater than 1.5 is suggestive of acute liver failure. A liver biopsy is not necessary to confirm the diagnosis; however, histopathologic study typically reveals centrilobular hepatocellular necrosis. In a systematic review of adult patients, ischemic hepatitis was associated with a high mortality rate (up to 50%).[120] Extreme liver injury resulting from prolonged shock or sepsis may produce total infarction of an entire lobe or the entire liver without evidence of vascular occlusion. In contrast to ischemic hepatitis, patients with fulminant hepatic failure may show a rapid decrease in serum transaminase levels, a rising total bilirubin, and a worsening coagulopathy.

Chronic Hepatic Dysfunction and Cirrhosis. Abnormalities in hepatic blood flow associated with cardiac pathologic conditions have previously been described in the chapter, and hepatic dysfunction is more commonly being recognized. The development of hepatic fibrosis is associated with the Fontan operation, with abnormalities seen before and after surgery.[121] Hepatic sinusoidal and portal fibrosis are common pathologic findings on autopsy post Fontan, with more severe fibrosis found in those with heterotaxy or who died early following the Fontan operation.[122] Liver cirrhosis is more commonly being seen in young adults who had Fontan operations.[117,123] Cases of hepatocellular carcinoma have also been reported in cardiac-related cirrhosis.[124] There is limited experience with combined heart and liver transplantation.[125]

Acute Hepatic Failure. Acute hepatic failure develops in less than 1% of children after cardiac surgery.[126] It typically occurs in the setting of multiple organ dysfunction following severe hypotension or shock. The histopathologic pattern consists of progressive centrilobular hepatocellular necrosis.[93,127] In contrast to the periportal hepatocytes, cells in the centrilobular region are particularly sensitive to hypoperfusion because of their position in the hepatic acinus.[128] Chronic passive venous congestion, typically secondary to high right-sided venous pressure, increases the risk of ischemic injury and centrilobular necrosis.

The child with acute hepatic failure exhibits jaundice, obtundation progressing to coma, and a coagulopathy. Biochemical studies reveal hypoglycemia, hyperbilirubinemia, markedly elevated serum transaminase levels (which may return to normal with worsening failure), and an elevated serum ammonia level. Acute renal failure occurs commonly.

Treatment is supportive. The obtunded patient requires airway protection. Hypoglycemia is corrected. Salt and water intake is restricted. Therapies aimed at lowering the serum ammonia level include lactulose, antibiotics, and dietary manipulation (protein restriction of 1 g/kg/day protein). If these measures fail, continuous venovenous hemofiltration may lower ammonia levels, but it has not been shown to alter outcome. Despite the coagulopathy in acute hepatic failure, fresh frozen plasma administration is hazardous, because the attendant protein load may increase serum ammonia levels.

The mortality rate in the setting of acute hepatic failure after congenital heart surgery exceeds 50%, because cardiorespiratory, renal, or neurologic dysfunction is almost always present as well.[129] Survivors regain nearly normal liver function with only mild liver enzyme and coagulation abnormalities.[130] However, most survivors have residual neurologic deficits.

Pancreatitis

Pancreatitis has been reported in adults undergoing cardiac surgery and can also be seen in pediatric patients, particularly those who have Fontan operations.[131] Although the mechanism is not clearly understood, elevated serum amylase level is common after CPB, occurring in up to 34% to 88% of patients.[132,133] Hyperamylasemia may have no association with pancreatic injury; therefore lipase levels should also be measured if there is a strong clinical suspicious of pancreatitis because lipase is a more specific test (more than three times normal is suggestive of pancreatitis). Postoperative pancreatitis in patients with CHD is associated with greater morbidity and carries a significant mortality rate of 21% to 50%.[131,132]

In addition to blood testing, the postoperative diagnosis of pancreatitis in children depends on clinical suspicion (vomiting, abdominal pain) and radiologic studies. Swelling of the pancreas and surrounding tissue is seen on ultrasonography or computed tomography scan. Fluid resuscitation, antacid therapy, and nasogastric decompression are mainstays of therapy in children. Parenteral nutrition and antibiotics are reserved for selected patients whose disease process does not respond to these other supportive measures.

Summary

The splanchnic circulation can act as a site of regulation of distribution of cardiac output and also as a blood reservoir. Multiple regulatory pathways are involved in both intestinal and hepatic blood flow. Bypass flow rate is the major determinant of portal and hepatic arterial blood flow during CPB. Most major gastrointestinal complications occur in CPB patients who experience episodes of hypotension or prolonged shock, particularly when pressor support is required. Centrilobular hepatocellular necrosis, cholestasis, and intestinal ischemia are the most common complications, but gastritis, pancreatitis and intestinal hemorrhage also occur with increased frequency in these critically ill patients.

Selected References

A complete list of references is available at ExpertConsult.com.

54. Ho EC, Moss AJ. The syndrome of "mesenteric arteritis" following surgical repair of aortic coarctation. Report of nine cases and review of the literature. *Pediatrics.* 1972;49(1):40–45.
56. Pundi KN, Johnson JN, Dearani JA, Pundi KN, Li Z, Hinck CA, et al. 40-Year Follow-Up After the Fontan Operation: Long-Term Outcomes of 1,052 Patients. *J Am Coll Cardiol.* 2015;66(15):1700–1710. doi:10.1016/j.jacc.2015.07.065.
82. Nino DF, Sodhi CP, Hackam DJ. Necrotizing enterocolitis: new insights into pathogenesis and mechanisms. *Nat Rev Gastroenterol Hepatol.* 2016;13(10):590–600.
112. Scahill CJ, Graham EM, Atz AM, Bradley SM, Kavarana MN, Zyblewski SC. Preoperative feeding neonates with cardiac disease. *World J Pediatr Congenit Heart Surg.* 2017;8(1):62–68.
115. Dilli D, Avdin B, Zenciroglu A, Ozyazici E, Beken S, Okumus N. Treatment outcomes of infants with cyanotic congenital heart disease treated with synbiotics. *Pediatrics.* 2013;132(4):e932–e938.
117. Ford RM, Book W, Spivey JR. Liver disease related to the heart. *Transplant Rev (Orlando).* 2015;29(1):33–37. doi:10.1016/j.trre.2014.11.003.

16

Organ System Response to Cardiac Function—Renal

DAVID M. KWIATKOWSKI, MD, MS; KATJA M. GIST, DO, MSCS;
STUART L. GOLDSTEIN, MD; CATHERINE D. KRAWCZESKI, MD;
DAVID S. COOPER, MD, MPH

Acute kidney injury (AKI) is one of the most common comorbidities among patients with congenital and acquired heart disease. Patients with AKI after cardiac surgery or with congestive heart failure (CHF) have significantly higher incidence of morbidity and mortality.[1-4] Surgery for congenital heart disease (CHD) is the most common cause of AKI in childhood and the leading risk factor for mortality among patients with renal injury.[5,6] In addition, the heart and kidney are intimately involved in maintaining homeostatic conditions in various disease states. This chapter will focus on normal and pathologic cardiorenal interactions. The diagnosis and significance of AKI in this population will be reviewed. Because there are no validated medication treatments for chronic kidney disease (CKD) or AKI, this chapter will focus on the treatment of fluid overload, the primary sequela of kidney disease. Although diuretic medications are predominantly used as the primary therapy, renal replacement therapy (RRT) has an important and growing role in this population.

Vasomotor Balance in the Kidney

As with all organs, the kidney has the ability to maintain constant perfusion during a period of diminished blood flow through a process known as *autoregulation*. Afferent and efferent arterioles within the nephron dilate or constrict to modify vascular resistance and ensure a constant perfusion pressure in response to changes in cardiac output or metabolic demand. Although modulation of this system is necessary to ensure renal blood flow (RBF), this often has maladaptive effects, which in part explain sequelae such as AKI, fluid overload, and long-term outcomes of chronic cardiac and renal disease.

Renal Vasodilation

The *natriuretic peptides,* including atrial natriuretic peptide (ANP) and brain natriuretic peptide (BNP), produce multiple effects that collectively decrease blood pressure, commonly in response to fluid excess. Natriuretic peptides have properties that directly prevent salt and water retention, inhibit expression of vasoconstrictor peptides, decrease vascular resistance, down-regulate sympathetic activity, and increase vascular endothelial permeability.[7] They also possess central activity to inhibit salt and water appetite[8] and prevent compensatory cardiac hypertrophy.[9] Natriuretic peptides are released in response to an increase in atrial-wall tension, often due to volume expansion, but are also released in response to ventricular stretch and an elevation in plasma levels of angiotensin II and endothelin-1. Renal effects of natriuretic peptides are mediated by direct activity on renal vasodilation and suppression of the renin-angiotensin-aldosterone system (RAAS).[10] Sympathetic tone in the peripheral vasculature is decreased by a suppression of baroreceptors and decrease in catecholamine and sympathetic expression.[11]

Systematic responsiveness to natriuretic peptides depends on patient age and duration of elevation. Animal models suggest the newborn is relatively insensitive to ANP after volume expansion,[12] which may explain the diminished ability of infants to tolerate volume overload. Although natriuretic peptide concentrations are increased in patients with chronic heart failure, receptor downregulation and enzymatic upregulation cause a decrease in the renal responsiveness to ANP, resulting in hypertension and sodium and water retention.

Intrarenal *prostaglandins* such as prostaglandin E_1 (PGE$_1$), E_2, and I_2 are renal cyclooxygenase metabolites that have vasodilatory properties. These molecules are important to balancing the vasoconstrictive effects of angiotensin and vasopressin on RBF to maintain fluid and salt removal. In animal models, prostaglandins have been demonstrated to maintain preservation of RBF during a period of acute reduction in total cardiac output and acute fluid volume depletion.[13,14] In both infant and adult populations the use of medications that inhibit prostaglandin synthesis, such as nonsteroidal antiinflammatory drugs (NSAIDs), has been associated with acute renal failure and progression of CHF.[15,16] Administration of a PGE$_1$ infusion in adults with chronic heart failure in a randomized clinical trial improved RBF and cardiovascular hemodynamics.[17]

Nitric oxide (NO) has potent vasodilatory effects in the kidney and is involved in key pathways to counteract angiotensin's effects.[18] NO has been hypothesized to be involved in normal renal homeostasis, tubuloglomerular feedback response in pathologic processes, and natriuresis.[19] However, in reperfusion/ischemia models, the roles of NO are less clear. Increased production of NO in AKI has been hypothesized to be protective by mediating vasodilation, inhibiting leukocyte adhesion, and reducing platelet aggregation. However, it is also believed that NO reacts with oxygen or superoxide to form injurious metabolites that cause oxidation injury

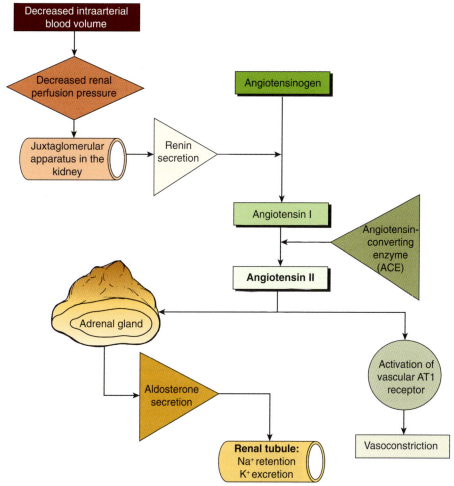

• **Figure 16.1** Feedback loop of the renin-angiotensin-aldosterone system. A reduction in blood volume or renal perfusion pressure leads to a cascade of events, which ultimately restore blood volume and perfusion pressure. Angiotensin II is central to this cascade. *AT1,* Angiotensin II subreceptor type 1.

and further upregulate the maladaptive inflammatory responses associated with AKI.[20]

Bradykinin dilates the renovascular bed and is a key vasodilator targeted by pharmacologic intervention. Blockade of the renin-angiotensin system with angiotensin-converting enzyme (ACE) inhibitors decreases angiotensin II levels but also increases bradykinin levels.[21] The angiotensin II receptor is divided into two subtypes (AT1 and AT2). AT1 blockade, with drugs such as losartan, appears to increase levels of angiotensin II, which is free to bind to the AT2 receptor subtype. The subsequent AT2 activation initiates a vasodilator cascade involving both bradykinin and NO.[22] Animal models have demonstrated that bradykinin may play an important role in ameliorating renal ischemia-reperfusion injury by vascular changes, in addition to reducing DNA damage, apoptosis, and other morphologic renal changes.[23] It may also have important protective roles in chronic renal failure to prevent hypertension, cardiac remodeling, and renal fibrosis.[24]

Adrenomedullin is a peptide that functions as a renal vasodilator and has been posed to be protective in chronic heart failure. Adrenomedullin infusions in CHF patients decreased blood pressure, increased cardiac output, increased urine and sodium excretion, and decreased plasma aldosterone levels.[25] It appears that the ability of adrenomedullin to inhibit oxidative stress production may combat changes induced by AKI and inflammatory pathways.[26]

Renal Vasoconstriction

Physiologic stability of blood pressure, renal vascular tone, cardiac function, and salt and water homeostasis rely heavily upon the RAAS (Fig. 16.1). Likewise, an exaggerated response of this hormonal system is a major driver of renal ischemia and AKI. In response to renal artery hypovolemia or hypotension, the kidney releases renin, which converts angiotensinogen to angiotensin I. This is converted to angiotensin II by ACE. Angiotensin II is a major vasoconstrictor and also stimulates the secretion of aldosterone from the adrenal cortex. Increased aldosterone levels promote sodium and water retention and potassium excretion by the kidney. Animal data suggest that the neonatal RAAS system is necessary for renal development because neonatal rats given ACE inhibitor medications developed persistent irreversible histopathologic renal abnormalities and abnormal renal functioning in adult life.[27] This effect is diminished after the period of nephrogenesis, during the first 2 weeks of life in murine models.[28] The activity of RAAS depends on age. Newborns have a very active RAAS with increased renin gene expression, angiotensin II expression, and plasma renin activity.[29] The greater activity of RAAS in the newborn may explain their increased sensitivity to ACE inhibitors.

In response to hypovolemia and hypotension the endothelium releases various *endothelial vasoconstrictor agents* that are essential to maintaining consistent glomerular filtration rate (GFR). However, this response can cause excess vasoconstriction, which may impede RBF and lead to AKI. Ischemia may cause renal endothelial cell injury and microvascular dysregulation that might not improve when perfusion recovers. Primary pathways include the potent vasoconstrictor *endothelin* and products of the cyclooxygenase pathway, including thromboxane A_2, prostaglandin H_2, and superoxide anions. Animal models of AKI demonstrate increased local and systemic levels of endothelin, which are associated with increased endothelial dysfunction and renovascular constriction.[30] Mouse models of renal artery ischemia demonstrated that blockade of endothelin results in increased RBF, increased GFR, and decreased afferent and efferent arteriolar resistance.[31]

In response to a variety of physiologic stressors, *catecholamines* and *arginine vasopressin (AVP),* also known as antidiuretic hormone (ADH), are released. These endogenous hormones cause renal vascular vasoconstriction, which limits RBF and causes a reduction in GFR. Although commonly elevated in the postoperative setting, these hormones are also increased during states of hypovolemia, hypoxia, acidosis, hypercarbia, hypothermia, and pain.[32] AVP can be administered as a synthetic peptide for maintenance of blood pressure and is commonly used in septic or cardiovascular shock.[33] The renal effects of administration of AVP must be considered when using the medicine for hemodynamic purposes.

Cardiorenal Interactions

Pathophysiology of Salt and Water Retention

Cardiorenal interactions are central in the clinical presentation of CHF, low cardiac output syndrome, and other cardiac pathophysiology. Regardless of the primary cause, the body responds to a decrease in cardiac output via neurohormonal activation of the pathways mentioned earlier to maintain organ perfusion. With an upregulation in stress hormone response and the RAAS system, renal vasoconstriction causes a decrease in RBF and GFR (Fig. 16.2). Increases in angiotensin II causes the release of endogenous vasopressin, and together these lead to increased absorption of sodium and free water from the renal tubule. This protective mechanism to maintain blood volume and blood pressure quickly becomes maladaptive

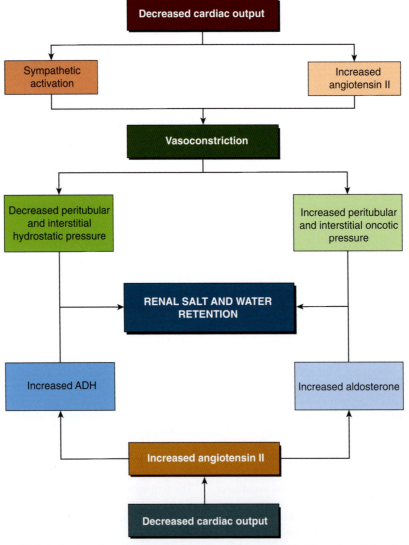

• **Figure 16.2** Pathophysiology of salt and water retention in the child with cardiac dysfunction. Note the combination of physical factors (hydrostatic and oncotic pressure changes) with hormonal stimuli (antidiuretic hormone *[ADH]* and aldosterone).

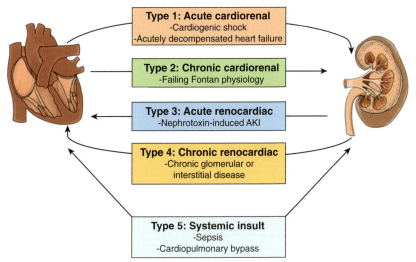

• **Figure 16.3** Cardiorenal syndrome: pathologic interactions of the heart and kidney with examples. Type 1: acute decrease in cardiac output leading to acute kidney injury *(AKI)*. Type 2: chronic heart dysfunction leading to progressive chronic kidney disease. Type 3: acute worsening of renal function causing acute cardiac dysfunction. Type 4: chronic kidney disease that contributes to adverse cardiovascular health. Type 5: systemic condition that causes cardiac and renal dysfunction. (Courtesy Charitha Reddy, MD.)

as the renal tubules face the risk of ischemia, excess fluid is retained, and the struggling heart is forced to work against an increase in afterload.

In healthy patients, homeostasis is maintained because fluid retention causes atrial stretch stimulating the release of natriuretic peptides, which promotes salt and water excretion. However, persistent elevation of natriuretics with CHF causes the development of resistance to the renal effects, particularly in children.[34] Elevation of BNP has been used in adults with CHD to predict mortality and in children with CHF to guide placement of ventricular assist devices (VADs)[35,36] and has been demonstrated to correlate with outcome in the single-ventricle population.[37] However, the BNP level in CHD is better used for monitoring trends because great variation is seen among different cardiac lesions and surgical procedure.[38]

Angiotensin and Aldosterone Effects on the Heart

The effects of the RAAS pathway are more far-reaching than the temporary renal and vascular effects mentioned. Angiotensin acts as a growth factor, promotes fibrosis, and stimulates inflammation.[39-41] Aldosterone has a maladaptive influence on the cardiac extracellular matrix in patients with CHF by stimulating cardiac collagen synthesis and fibroblast proliferation.[42] Chronic elevation of angiotensin, renin, and aldosterone lead to pathologic left ventricular hypertrophy and myocardial fibrosis, independent of hypertension.[43,44] In an effort to blunt these maladaptive interactions, pediatric and adult patients with CHF are treated with ACE inhibitors and spironolactone, an aldosterone receptor antagonist.

Cardiorenal Syndrome

Cardiorenal interactions are abundant in all critically ill patients, particularly those with impaired cardiac output. The pathophysiology of these interactions is best described by Ronco and colleagues,[45] who defined the concept of the cardiorenal syndrome (CRS), a classification system that describes the time frame and origin of organ system dysfunction (Fig. 16.3). Type 1 CRS describes an acute decrease in cardiac output leading to AKI. Type 2 is defined as chronic heart dysfunction leading to progressive CKD. Type 3 describes an acute worsening of renal function causing acute cardiac dysfunction. Type 4 is defined as CKD that contributes to adverse cardiovascular health. Type 5 is defined as a systemic condition such as sepsis, which causes both cardiac and renal dysfunction. Although most of the literature focuses on the effects of cardiopulmonary bypass (CPB) on AKI, a type 5 CRS, type 1 and 2 are frequently encountered. For example, type 1 CRS is seen during viral myocarditis, postoperative low cardiac output syndrome, acute heart transplant rejection, and innumerable other conditions with an acute decrease in cardiac output. Type 2 CRS is seen in patients with cardiomyopathy, failing Fontan physiology, or with graft dysfunction of a transplanted heart.

Defining cardiorenal interactions within this framework helps the clinician understand pathologic processes and appropriate management. For example, if a patient managed for chronic cardiomyopathy has an elevated creatinine level, oliguria, and fluid overload, a type 2 CRS, more diuretic may be detrimental, and some method of cardiac support may be necessary.

Cardiorenal Interactions in Specific Populations

There are specific pediatric cardiac cohorts that are particularly vulnerable to pathologic cardiorenal interactions. AKI after Fontan palliation is frequent in the postoperative period, but CKD remains common years after completion.[46,47] This is likely secondary to multiple renal insults and persistence of a high central venous pressure (CVP). Even with the best Fontan hemodynamics, the renal venous pressure elevates 8 to 10 mm Hg above typical, significantly affecting renal perfusion pressure.[48] Therefore patients with CKD secondary to suboptimal Fontan hemodynamics may see improvement with diuretics, pulmonary vasodilators, a Fontan revision, or improvement in atrioventricular synchrony.

Kidney injury among pediatric patients with CHF is common and associated with a higher rate of transplantation, mechanical support, and mortality.[3,4,49] Among patients with a new diagnosis of dilated cardiomyopathy, one study showed 61% had decreased renal function, and this conferred a 5-year mortality hazard ratio of 2.4.[4] The pathophysiology of cardiorenal interactions is often twofold; left heart failure causes decreased cardiac output and decreased renal perfusion, whereas right heart failure causes venous congestion and an elevation in renal venous pressure. This dichotomous etiology causes some to improve with diuresis and others to improve with vasoactive medications improving cardiac output, although often both are required. The presence of AKI in acute decompensation is especially common among those with an ejection fraction less than 25%.[3] Among patients with CHF and CKD, some centers endorse a strategy of VAD placement to improve end-organ function before listing for transplantation. Unfortunately, adult data show the incidence of AKI remains high after VAD placement and portends a worse outcome.[50] After cardiac transplantation in pediatric patients, AKI is common, affecting up to 73% of patients, and is associated with a worse outcome.[51] This population continues to be at risk for CKD due to diastolic dysfunction of the graft transplant and need for treatment with nephrotoxic immunosuppressants.

An example of a type 3 cardiorenal interaction in children with heart disease is a patient who develops AKI due to nephrotoxic medication, leading to fluid retention. This may cause an increase in left ventricular afterload and depression of systolic cardiac function as the ventricle stretches along its Starling curve, particularly in a patient with impaired baseline cardiac function. Pediatric patients with cardiac disease, especially those with a history of AKI, are at risk for contrast- and medication-induced kidney injury due to the need for ACE inhibitors, NSAIDs, calcineurin inhibitors, or diuretics. Monitoring inpatient use of nephrotoxins with electronic medical records to limit overuse has been associated with decreased AKI incidence.[52] Modifying composition and osmolality of contrast has been studied but not found to be protective.[53] The use of N-acetylcysteine to prevent contrast-associated AKI has also been proposed, but thus far, avoidance of nephrotoxin exposure is the only proven method of decreasing the risk of nephrotoxic AKI.

Although less common, type 4 interactions are present in pediatric populations. Among children on dialysis, mortality has been reported to be as high as 50%,[54] and the incidence of cardiovascular mortality of children on maintenance dialysis is roughly 1000-fold as high as the general population, most commonly due to cardiac arrest or arrhythmia.[55] CKD leads to cardiac morbidity via multiple mechanisms, including chronic uremia, renal osteodystrophy, vitamin D pathophysiology, and fibroblast growth factor–related direct effects on the myocardium and the large vessels.[56] It is hypothesized that younger pediatric patients are more sensitive to uremia because their rate of mortality is highest, despite the fact that they had not yet developed chronic changes of atherosclerosis, left ventricular hypertrophy, and cardiomyopathy.[55]

Acute Kidney Injury

Pathophysiology of Acute Kidney Injury After Cardiac Surgery

The etiology of cardiac surgery associated AKI is multifactorial and incompletely understood, extending beyond low cardiac output and impaired RBF.[57] The primary driving mechanisms include ischemia-reperfusion injury, mechanical blood trauma, oxidative stress, venous congestion, and proinflammatory cytokine activation.[58-62] A reduction in mean arterial pressure and nonpulsatile flow during CPB result in activation of apoptotic and necrotic pathways of tubule and endothelial cell death.[61,63] The kidney is able to tolerate up to 60 minutes of ischemia with only mild structural changes and no loss of function,[64] but with release of vascular clamps, subsequent reperfusion injury results in activation of the oxidative pathways that exacerbate tubular and microvascular injury.[61,63] Red cell hemolysis due to the CPB circuit releases free hemoglobin and iron, which exacerbates oxidant-mediated injury, resulting in release of proinflammatory cytokines from injured tubules and endothelial cells. Contact of the blood with the artificial surfaces of the CPB circuit exacerbates injury via activation of neutrophils, platelets, and proinflammatory cytokines. Perioperative nephrotoxic medication use may increase the severity of existing injury.

Incidence and Risk Factors for Acute Kidney Injury

AKI occurs in approximately 40% of children following cardiac surgery.[65] AKI has consistently been associated with increased morbidity and mortality, including prolonged length of stay, prolonged need for mechanical ventilation, fluid and electrolyte disturbances, and changes in drug metabolism.[65,66] The incidence of AKI is similar among those with CHF and receiving extracorporeal therapies.[3,49,67] Adults with CHD may have other renal comorbidities, including diabetes and hypertension, and are at significant risk for postoperative AKI and CKD.[68,69] In fact, nearly 50% of adults with CHD have some degree of renal dysfunction, and approximately 20% of those patients have moderate CKD.[70] Compared to the general population, the incidence of renal dysfunction has been found to be 18 times higher in acyanotic adult patients, and 35 times higher in cyanotic patients.[70] Renal function also is found to decline at a faster rate than in the general population.[71]

Although perioperative risk factors for the development of AKI have been identified, few of them are modifiable. Younger age, longer CPB duration, higher surgical complexity, and preoperative ventilator support are risk factors for the development of AKI but also correlate with a sick patient substrate.[65,72-74] Intraoperative risk factors include low blood pressure and hemoglobin during CPB, need for emergent intervention, and need for thoracic aortic surgery.[75] After controlling for age and surgical severity; bypass times above 180 minutes had an odds ratio of 7.6 for the development of AKI.[2] Postoperative risk factors include volume overload, preexisting CKD, nephrotoxin use, and use of mechanical circulatory support.[2,57]

In patients with acute heart failure, age, inotrope use, and higher admission creatinine and blood urea nitrogen (BUN) were associated with severe AKI, in-hospital mortality, and need for mechanical circulatory support.[3,49] Lesions with a high postoperative CVP also have high incidence of AKI. This includes lesions with residual right ventricular hypertrophy and diastolic dysfunction, such as tetralogy of Fallot, and lesions with obligate CVP elevation due to surgical palliation, such as the Fontan surgery.[48]

Given the same set of risk factors and a similar renal insult, there will be some patients who develop AKI and others who do not. Although some of this may be due to chance or differences in surgical or bypass techniques, there is growing evidence that there may be gene variations that either predispose patients to or protect them from the development of AKI. Given the common mechanisms of postoperative AKI, polymorphisms associated with renal inflammatory, oxidative stress, or vasoconstrictor responses have been of highest interest.[76,77] A study among adult patients undergoing aortic-coronary surgery found two alleles (interleukin 6–572C and angiotensinogen 842C) associated with AKI in whites.[76] The ability to predict AKI increased fourfold when genetic polymorphism use was added to clinical risk factors.

Acute Kidney Injury Definitions

One of the major limitations for assessing AKI prevalence was lack of consensus definition, and many studies use variable definitions for AKI. A decade ago the Acute Dialysis Quality Initiative Group created the RIFLE criteria due to the lack of a consistent definition of AKI.[78] Since then, several modifications have occurred. The RIFLE (Risk, Injury, Failure, Loss, End Stage) criteria were adapted to include children (pediatric RIFLE [pRIFLE]).[79] This was followed by the Acute Kidney Injury Network (AKIN) criteria that expanded the diagnosis of AKI to include patients with an increase of 0.3 mg/dL or higher in serum creatinine level in a 48-hour period.[80] Most recently the Kidney Disease Improving Global Outcomes (KDIGO) classification system integrated the RIFLE, pRIFLE, and AKIN classifications systems.[81] The different classifications systems are summarized in Fig. 16.4. All three definitions offer advantages: pRIFLE is sensitive, identifying more mild AKI cases; AKIN does not require heights or baseline creatinine; and KDIGO is applicable to both pediatric and adult populations with a less restrictive diagnostic time frame compared to AKIN.

Several adult and pediatric studies have compared incidence and outcomes across all definitions. Most recently Sutherland et al.[82] reported an AKI incidence ranging from 37% to 51% of hospitalized children depending on the definition used. In this study intensive care unit (ICU) mortality increased with each AKI severity stage. Outside the ICU, AKI was not associated with mortality, but length of stay increased with AKI severity stage among all patients.[82] Application of the three definitions with regard to the presence of AKI resulted in only moderate agreement. For AKI staging, AKIN and pRIFLE had 77% agreement, compared to KDIGO and AKIN, which had 93% agreement.[82] These findings are similar to those described by Zappitelli et al.,[83] who found pRIFLE more sensitive than AKIN because it picked up more stage 1 events. Several adult studies have evaluated outcomes across definitions and have found that regardless of the definition used, AKI was associated with higher mortality.[84-87]

Unfortunately, many studies use only creatinine criteria rather than urine output due to difficulties quantifying urine, use of diuretics, and the laborious data collection necessary for analysis. This may underestimate the incidence of AKI, in which urine output is a more sensitive marker of kidney injury.[88] Furthermore, diagnosis is difficult in neonates who are born with an elevated creatinine level and a depressed GFR, which improves over the ensuing months.[89]

Outcomes After Acute Kidney Injury

AKI after CPB is often a self-limited complication, occurring in the first 24 to 48 hours postoperatively. In the Translational Research Investigating Biomarker Endpoints in Acute Kidney Injury (TRIBE-AKI) consortium, almost half of patients met AKI diagnostic criteria

AKIN		pRIFLE		KDIGO	
Stage 1: SCr increase ≥0.3 mg/dL, **or** >1.5 times baseline	UOP <0.5 mL/kg/h for 6 hours	**Risk:** GFR decrease >25% from baseline	UOP <0.5 mL/kg/h for 8 hours	**Stage 1:** SCr increase ≥0.3 mg/dL within 48 hours, **or** >1.5 times baseline within 7 days	UOP <0.5 mL/kg/h for 6 hours
Stage 2: SCr increase >2 times baseline	UOP <0.5 mL/kg/h for 12 hours	**Injury:** GFR decrease >50% from baseline	UOP <0.5 mL/kg/h for 16 hours	**Stage 2:** SCr increase ≥2 times baseline	UOP <0.5 mL/kg/h for 12 hours
Stage 3: SCr increase >3 times baseline, **or** SCr ≥4 mg/dL with an acute increase of at least 0.5 mg/dL, **or** need for RRT	Anuria for ≥12 hours **or** <0.3 mL/kg/h for 24 hours	**Failure:** GFR decrease >75% from baseline **or** <35 mL/min/1.73 m^2	<0.3 mL/kg/h for 24 hours -OR- Anuria for ≥12 hours	**Stage 3:** SCr increase >3 times baseline, **or** SCr ≥4 mg/dL, **or** initiation of renal replacement therapy, **or** GFR <35 mL/min/1.73 m^2 if age <18 years	Anuria for ≥12 hours **or** <0.3 mL/kg/h for 24 hours
		Loss: Complete loss of renal function for greater than four weeks			
		End-stage renal disease: Requirement of RRT for greater than 3 months			

• **Figure 16.4** Common acute kidney injury definitions and staging criteria.[79-81] Note the similarities and differences among the commonly used staging criteria: AKIN (Acute Kidney Injury Network), pRIFLE (pediatric Risk, Injury Failure, Loss, End Stage), and KDIGO (Kidney Disease Improving Global Outcomes). KDIGO criteria are the most recent and most accepted classification criteria. *GFR,* Glomerular filtration rate; *RRT,* renal replacement therapy; *SCr,* serum creatine; *UOP,* urinary output.

for just 1 day and only one of nine patients still met the definition by the fourth postoperative day.[2] For this reason the importance of postoperative AKI has historically been minimized. However, recent research has emphasized the strong association of AKI with worse postoperative and long-term outcomes.

AKI has been shown to be an independent risk factor for prolonged duration of mechanical ventilation, longer ICU and hospital stays, and mortality.[1,2,72] In the TRIBE-AKI consortium 30% of patients with AKI were mechanically ventilated at 48 hours after surgery as opposed to 8% of those without AKI.[2] Blinder and colleagues studied 430 infants after bypass, finding that 52% developed AKI. Stage 2 AKI was associated with a 5-times risk of death, and stage 3 AKI was associated with nearly a 10-times risk. These were stronger predictors of death than having single-ventricle physiology or needing mechanical circulatory support.[1]

Even small increases in creatinine level are important. Compared to those with no change in creatinine level, adults after cardiac surgery with a creatinine level increase of just 0.1 to 0.5 mg/dL had a threefold increase in the rate of mortality, and this association worsened with larger creatinine changes.[90] There are also data among pediatric patients after cardiac surgery that small early changes in creatinine level predict later development of AKI.[74]

It previously was assumed that patients with a single episode of AKI would recover kidney function without long-term consequence. However, during the last decade epidemiologic data from critically ill children and adults suggest that AKI survivors are at considerable risk of developing CKD.[91-93] Coca and colleagues[94] demonstrated that adults who experienced AKI have a ninefold increased risk of developing CKD, a threefold increased risk of developing end-stage kidney disease, and a twofold increased long-term mortality risk as compared to those without AKI. Mammen and colleagues[95] found that 10% of previously critically ill children (including patients following cardiac surgery) had developed CKD 1 to 3 years following AKI, and almost half were considered at risk of CKD development. Wong and colleagues[96] describe the incidence and significance of AKI throughout the three stages of palliation for hypoplastic left heart syndrome and its variants. AKI was common among these high-risk patients, and

the sequelae of severe AKI as a neonate were substantial, predisposing patients to death or need for extracorporeal membrane oxygenation (ECMO) after stage 1 palliation. Despite normalization of creatinine level, risk of severe AKI after stage 2 was elevated in those affected as a neonate. Morgan and colleagues[72] followed a cohort of neonates after cardiac surgery and found that 2 to 4 years later those who developed AKI were at higher risk of growth impairment, cardiac-related hospitalization, and increased health care utilization, even when controlling for gestational age, surgical type, preoperative ventilation, lactate level elevation, and use of mechanical circulatory support. Additionally, although the creatinine level typically normalizes before discharge, there is evidence that those who were affected by AKI have persistent elevation of kidney injury biomarkers up to 7 years postoperatively.[97] These data highlight the importance of following AKI survivors throughout adulthood to understand the long-term implications of AKI.

Acute Kidney Injury Biomarkers

Novel AKI biomarkers in the serum and urine have been developed that offer additive benefit to the traditional approach of measuring serum creatinine level. Many of these biomarkers have been studied in children following cardiac surgery because children lack the comorbidities seen with adults, and the timing of injury is well defined. Biomarkers are rapidly becoming the framework for research investigation and clinical management and are being used to leverage the possibility of detecting kidney injury before obvious functional changes such as a decrease in urine output or increase in serum creatinine level occur (Fig. 16.5).

Several biomarker categories exist: (1) markers of glomerular filtration, (2) markers of tubular injury, (3) markers of cell-cycle arrest, and (4) markers of inflammation. A detailed discussion of each group is beyond the scope of this chapter and can be found elsewhere.[57,98-100] Three biomarkers, cystatin C, neutrophil gelatinase–associated lipocalin (NGAL), and [TIMP-2]*[IGFBP-7] (the product of tissue inhibitor of metalloproteinase-2 [TIMP-2] and insulin-like growth factor–binding protein 7 [IFGBP-7]) are currently being used clinically and are discussed briefly.

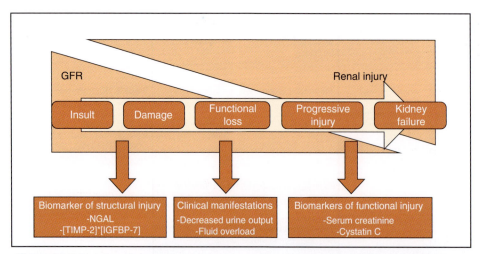

• **Figure 16.5** Evolution of acute kidney injury and corresponding diagnostic modalities. Note that immediately after insult, glomerular filtration rate *(GFR)* is unaffected, and only biomarkers of structural injury will detect acute kidney injury. As injury progresses and GFR decreases, clinical manifestations develop, and eventually biomarkers of functional injury can be used to diagnose kidney injury. *NGAL,* Neutrophil gelatinase–associated lipocalin; *[TIMP-2]*[IGFBP-7],* product of tissue inhibitor of metalloproteinase-2 (TIMP-2) and insulin-like growth factor–binding protein 7 (IGFBP-7).

Cystatin C is a marker of glomerular filtration that is not subject to the inherent limitations seen with creatinine, specifically gender and muscle mass. Measurement is available in many hospitals and laboratories. Two meta-analyses demonstrated that serum cystatin C is superior to creatinine for the diagnosis and risk stratification of AKI severity.[101,102] A prospective multicenter study in children following cardiac surgery showed that early measurement of cystatin C by 6 hours following CPB initiation strongly and independently predicted the later development of serum creatinine–based AKI with an adjusted odds ratio (OR) of 17.2 and an area under the curve (AUC) of 0.89.[103]

NGAL is a marker of tubular injury, and is upregulated very early after injury. Well over 300 publications have reported on NGAL in human AKI, with several systematic reviews and meta-analyses of its diagnostic utility.[104-106] NGAL significantly improved risk prediction over clinical models alone and is predictive of graded AKI severity and duration.[107,108] Clinical trials are beginning to use NGAL as an outcome because it is a more sensitive and earlier indicator of AKI then other methods. Most recently a prospective randomized double-blind controlled trial demonstrated a renoprotective effect of fenoldopam by a dramatic reduction in urine NGAL levels compared to the placebo group in children following cardiac surgery.[109] Although clinical use is becoming more common outside the United States, it is not yet FDA approved. Increased sensitivity above the "gold standard" of creatinine allows discovery of subclinical AKI, in which serum creatinine is negative but NGAL is positive. Subclinical AKI is associated with a twofold to threefold increased risk of death or dialysis in both adults and children.[110,111] NGAL has important limitations, including persistent elevation in CKD. It has also not performed as well in adult cohorts, possibly due to other comorbidities.[112] This test has a fairly large indeterminate zone (100 to 150 ng/mL), which requires the clinician to use other clinical or laboratory corroborators of renal risk.[104,106]

Recently the FDA approved a urine-based test (NephroCheck) that uses the product of two cell-cycle arrest biomarkers, TIMP-2 and IFGBP-7, to risk stratify critically ill adults for developing AKI within 12 hours after testing. These individual biomarkers are inducers of G1 cell-cycle arrest, a mechanism in the progression of AKI. In adults, [TIMP-2]*[IGFBP-7] has been shown to predict AKI as early as 4 hours post bypass and to accurately predict renal recovery.[113] Although not yet validated in pediatric populations, this biomarker combination shows promise of early diagnosis and may be useful particularly in postoperative patients.[114]

It is likely that future diagnostics will be aided by the use of biomarkers. Furthermore, panels of biomarkers that detect different injury pathways, often with different temporality, will maximize the diagnosis of AKI and potentially illustrate the pathophysiology of injury.[107] As a precursor to this concept, Basu and colleagues[115] demonstrated that combining the functional biomarker cystatin C and the tubular injury biomarker NGAL could increase sensitivity and specificity of the diagnosis of AKI in children after CPB superior to creatinine alone.

Fluid Overload

It has been hypothesized that AKI and CKD are markers of poor perioperative condition and hemodynamic instability and that kidney disease itself does not lead to morbidity and mortality, but that continued poor cardiac output is ultimately to blame. In fact, there is an adage, "No acute renal failure patients have ever died because of acute renal failure, but they have died in acute renal failure."[116] This notion has lost favor as research has stressed the independent association of kidney disease with morbidity. The mechanism by which AKI and CKD cause worse outcomes is primarily the development of fluid overload. Renal tubule injury and hypoperfusion lead to a decrease in GFR, which causes retention of free water along with the other retained filtrate. Progressive oliguria or anuria leads to fluid overload. In addition to external swelling, edema of various organs occurs, with ascites, pulmonary edema, pleural effusions, myocardial wall edema, and bowel wall edema. These edematous organs all individually become dysfunctional; pulmonary gas exchange is impaired and lung compliance decreases; bowel walls absorb less nutrition; skin breakdown leads to pressure ulcers and infection at catheter sites; ascites impairs cardiac preload, limits lung excursion, and causes abdominal tamponade of peritoneal organs; and the swollen cardiac myocardium is less contractile and suffers from diastolic dysfunction. Among the other morbid effects, these collectively further impair cardiac output and renal perfusion, which worsens renal dysfunction, leading to progressive fluid overload. Without the ability to break this cycle, AKI and CKD quickly may become major contributors to morbidity and mortality.

A large study from the Prospective Pediatric Continuous Renal Replacement Therapy Registry group showed that patients with multiorgan failure had a 3% higher risk of mortality for every additional 1% of fluid overload, and that a greater than 20% fluid overload conferred an 8.5-times mortality risk.[117] It has been demonstrated that increasing percentage fluid overload is associated with worsening oxygenation index in children.[118] In the pediatric population with cardiac disease, retrospective studies have demonstrated an association between early postoperative fluid overload and worse outcomes, including the duration of ICU stay, inotropic medication use, duration of mechanical ventilation, and oxygenation index.[119-121] In neonates after cardiac surgery, greater than 16% fluid overload was an independent predictor of poor outcome (death, ECMO, or need for dialysis).[122]

In addition to its negative sequelae, fluid overload may also obfuscate the diagnosis of AKI if the excess intravascular volume dilutes the measured creatinine concentration. In a study of postoperative neonates, correcting serum creatinine concentration for the degree of fluid overload unmasked additional cases of AKI.[123] In these patients, previously unrecognized AKI was associated with a worse outcome. Novel biomarkers that are less affected by dilution may help diagnose this "subclinical" AKI. Among patients after cardiac surgery, NGAL elevation, even in the absence of a creatinine rise, is associated with worse outcomes.[110]

Because there are no validated medications to treat AKI, the focus of management often shifts to control of fluid overload. Without a doubt, the most quintessential management for fluid overload is restriction of input, but this is easier said than done. A common postoperative total fluid allowance for an infant after surgery is two-thirds of maintenance. However, the challenge of management can be illustrated in the example of a critically ill 3-kg patient who is restricted to 8 mL per hour. This volume will be exceeded by inotropic infusions, continuous sedation medications, diuretics, necessary electrolyte replacements, and line flushes, even if adequate nutrition is withheld. Furthermore, if the infant is oliguric, they may make 1 mL of urine per hour, and even the most modest fluid inputs will lead to fluid overload.

Pharmacologic interventions intended to improve urine output include diuretics, renal vasodilators, and medications to improve cardiac output. Renal vasodilators and medications to improve cardiac output are theorized to improve glomerular perfusion, therefore improving urine output and potentially mitigating AKI.

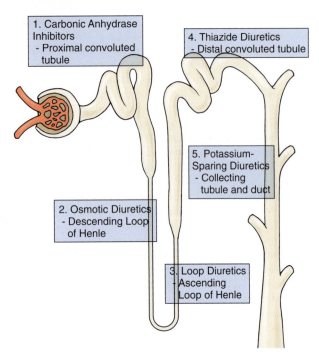

1. Carbonic Anhydrase Inhibitors
   - Proximal convoluted tubule

2. Osmotic Diuretics
   - Descending Loop of Henle

3. Loop Diuretics
   - Ascending Loop of Henle

4. Thiazide Diuretics
   - Distal convoluted tubule

5. Potassium-Sparing Diuretics
   - Collecting tubule and duct

• **Figure 16.6** List of diuretic medications and primary site of action. (Courtesy Charitha Reddy, MD.)

Although retrospective studies of fenoldopam, nesiritide, and aminophylline have suggested an improvement in urine output in neonates after cardiac surgery,[124,125] prospective studies have not shown benefit.[126-128] Diuretic use in critically ill patients with AKI is ubiquitous; however, diuretics are often ineffective and may even be detrimental, associated in some studies with a higher risk of mortality.[129,130]

Renal Pharmacology

Diuretics

Diuretics are the mainstay of fluid removal in critically ill children with heart disease. The location of action of the various diuretic classes can be seen in Fig. 16.6. In the case of tubular immaturity, delivery of diuretics to their site of action is slower, leading to a delayed onset of action and an increased elimination time, which may prolong diuretic effect. Disease states may decrease renal sensitivity to diuretic medications. Specific dosing and monitoring recommendations are beyond the scope of this chapter and can be found in several other excellent sources.[131]

Loop Diuretics. Loop diuretics are the most commonly used diuretic in the management of volume overload in CHF and following cardiac surgery. They may be used alone or in combination with other diuretic classes to achieve a synergistic response. Of all the diuretics classes, they are functionally the most potent and can block up to 25% of sodium reabsorption. They inhibit sodium and chloride reabsorption in the thick ascending loop of Henle via the sodium-potassium-chloride ($Na^+/K^+/2Cl^-$) cotransporter.[132] This receptor is located in the urinary side of the tubular lumen, and thus the loop diuretic must be filtered to be effective. This is critical because if filtrate is not produced due to AKI or inadequate renal perfusion, loop diuretics cannot reach their target. Therefore increasing the dose may be ineffective, and alternative fluid removal strategies may be needed. Common loop diuretics include

furosemide, bumetanide, and ethacrynic acid, and are administered intravenously or orally. To avoid rapid fluid shifts and hemodynamic instability, continuous infusions may be used.

Furosemide. Furosemide is the most common diuretic used. It is a potent bilirubin displacer of the albumin binding sites, and therefore critically ill premature neonates may be at higher risk for hyperbilirubinemia. Furosemide is eliminated by hepatic and renal glucuronidation, with 90% appearing as unchanged drug in the urine.[132]

Bumetanide. This loop diuretic is 40 times more potent that furosemide. Because therapeutic concentrations displace bilirubin from albumin to a lesser extent, it may be safer in neonates with hyperbilirubinemia.[133] There is anecdotal evidence that a bumetanide infusion has increased compatibility with a large group of drugs compared to furosemide.

Ethacrynic Acid. Ethacrynic acid is rapidly absorbed and hepatically metabolized to an active cysteine conjugate. A recent clinical trial compared furosemide and ethacrynic acid in pediatric patients after cardiac surgery and found ethacrynic acid produced more urine output with no differences in renal function.[134]

Side Effects. The most significant effects include electrolyte derangements: hyponatremia, hypocalcemia, hypokalemia, hypochloremia and hypomagnesemia, and a resultant contraction metabolic alkalosis.[135] Transient or permanent ototoxicity may occur with prolonged administration and high doses of all loop diuretics, especially ethacrynic acid, but potentially less likely with bumetanide.[133,136,137] Nephrocalcinosis may also occur with higher doses and increased duration and is more common among premature infants.[135]

Thiazide and Thiazide-like Diuretics. Thiazide diuretics are considered to be of moderate potency and are most often used in combination with loop diuretics to achieve a more potent effect. They function by blocking the thiazide-sensitive Na^+/Cl^- cotransporter in the distal convoluted tubule. Potassium reabsorption is blocked, and carbonic anhydrase is also is inhibited, thereby allowing for the excretion of bicarbonate, sodium, and chloride, along with water.[132,138] Thiazide-like diuretics primarily act upon the distal convoluted tubule and secondarily upon the proximal tubule. In these regions, metolazone inhibits sodium reabsorption, causing increased excretion of sodium and water, as well as potassium and hydrogen ions. When thiazides and thiazide-like diuretics are used in combination with loop diuretics, there is a synergistic diuretic effect created by sequential nephron blockade of the proximal and distal tubule.[139,140] The risk for electrolyte disturbances, renal dysfunction, and hypovolemia is enhanced with drug combinations. Common thiazides include chlorothiazide and hydrochlorothiazide. Metolazone is the most commonly used thiazide-like diuretic but is erratically absorbed, unlike the less commonly used Mykrox formulation, which is 100% bioavailable.[141] Side effects of this class include electrolyte disturbances, hyperuricemia, drug fever, hypersensitivity reaction, cholestasis, dermatitis, and vasculitis. Lipid and carbohydrate metabolism disturbances have been seen in adults with long-term thiazide diuretic use but have not been described in children.[142] Thiazides cause less calcium loss and therefore are sometimes preferred in the premature neonatal population.

Aldosterone Receptor Antagonists/Potassium-Sparing Diuretics. Spironolactone, a synthetic steroid, is an aldosterone receptor antagonist with relatively weak diuretic effects and is most commonly used for its potassium-sparing effects. It is the only diuretic that does not need to reach the tubular lumen to exert its action. Spironolactone competes with aldosterone for the mineralocorticoid receptor, leading to decreased potassium secretion and decreased sodium and chloride reabsorption.[138,142] In conjunction with other diuretics, there is an increased diuretic effect due to sequential nephron blockade. This drug class has antifibrotic effects and promotes reverse remodeling through antagonizing the RAAS. Although no pediatric data exist, adult data showed improved survival when combined with ACE inhibitors and beta-blockers.[143] Potassium levels should be monitored closely, especially when using with other medications that can increase serum potassium (e.g., ACE inhibitors). Gynecomastia is related to dose and duration of therapy and is usually reversible with cessation of spironolactone.

Other Diuretics. Carbonic anhydrase inhibitors (acetazolamide) are weak diuretics, with the main site of action in the proximal tubular lumen and cell. Blockade of carbonic anhydrase leads to decreased bicarbonate and sodium reabsorption via the Na^+/HCO_3^- cotransporter, resulting in reduced water reabsorption. They are most often used for the treatment of a significant metabolic alkalosis. Acetazolamide may promote nephrocalcinosis and nephrolithiasis when combined with loop diuretics. Osmotic diuretics (mannitol) act mainly in the proximal tubule. Mannitol undergoes glomerular filtration and is not reabsorbed along the tubular system. Osmotic diuretics increase osmolality of the tubular fluid and subsequently water and sodium excretion. Mannitol results in a shift of extracellular fluid into the intravascular space in infants with low cardiac output and poor renal perfusion after cardiac surgery. It therefore has the potential to exacerbate CHF and pulmonary edema in patients with myocardial dysfunction.

A common complication of CHF is acute and chronic renal disease with hypervolemic hyponatremia. This can be attributed to venous congestion, decreased renal perfusion, and extended use of diuretics. Although diuretics are necessary, the associated electrolyte abnormalities may exacerbate hyponatremia by limiting the kidney's ability to excrete free water. Tolvaptan is an oral selective vasopressin V_2-receptor antagonist that induces hypotonic diuresis without affecting electrolytes.[144] The efficacy and safety of tolvaptan is established in adult patients.[144-147] A multicenter clinical trial of tolvaptan in children with euvolemic or hypervolemic hyponatremia is currently under way (ClinicalTrials.gov, NCT02012959).

Angiotensin-Converting Enzyme Inhibitors/Angiotensin Receptor Blockers

The primary goal of ACE inhibitors is typically to decrease ventricular afterload via blockade of the RAAS system and vasodilation. However, as mentioned previously, ACE inhibitors also prevent and even reverse pathophysiologic myocardial remodeling and have been demonstrated to decrease mortality and hospitalization in adults with CHF.[148] Several pediatric retrospective cohort and case-control studies have demonstrated improvement in hemodynamics and echocardiographic parameters. A prospective randomized controlled trial in which patients with single ventricle were randomized to receive enalapril or placebo did not result in improved outcomes, and therefore the routine use of ACE inhibitors in this population is not substantiated.[149] It is recommended to start at the lowest dose and titrate to avoid hypotension. ACE inhibitors may cause hyperkalemia, and potassium levels should be monitored closely, particularly in patients also receiving spironolactone or other potassium replacements. Renal function may worsen with ACE inhibitors and should also

be periodically monitored. In adults, angiotensin receptor blockers (ARBs) have similar benefits to ACE inhibitors.[150] There is no evidence in children to suggest that ARBs are superior to ACE inhibitors.

Medications to Prevent Acute Kidney Injury

Several pediatric trials have been conducted evaluating pharmacologic methods to reduce rates of AKI and its associated complications with mixed results. *Fenoldopam* is a short-acting dopamine A1 receptor agonist that promotes renal artery vasodilation and is proposed to be renal protective. Unfortunately, the evidence in both adults and children is equivocal. Adult studies have shown that fenoldopam may reduce AKI but has no effect on survival or need for RRT.[151-153] Retrospective studies in children demonstrated increased urine output in some studies[124,154] but no effect in others.[155] Ricci and colleagues[156] performed a placebo controlled trial of fenoldopam in neonates after CPB and found no difference in renal function, frequency of AKI, fluid balance, duration of ventilation, or hospital length of stay, although in a subsequent trial they found biomarker improvement of AKI and decreased use of diuretics.[109] *Aminophylline* is a phosphodiesterase inhibitor and adenosine receptor blocker, which both result in renal vasodilation. Tamburro and colleagues[157] recently found that administration of aminophylline was associated with an increase in urine output, without a change in creatinine or BUN, but a larger placebo controlled trial by Axelrod and colleagues[126] found no effect of aminophylline to prevent AKI in children after cardiac surgery. Importantly, in this study aminophylline was administered as late as 10 hours after initiation of CPB. At this time, injury may have already occurred, thus mitigating any potential benefit of the drug.[126] *N-acetylcysteine (NAC)* is a derivative of the naturally occurring amino acid L-cysteine and is thought to prevent oxidative stress and scavenge oxygen free radicals, limiting ischemia reperfusion and modulating apoptosis.[158] It has been used prophylactically to prevent renal injury after intravenous contrast for radiology studies. Two studies in patients with CKD found a reduction in mechanical ventilation duration,[159] intensive care length of stay, and mortality.[160] In a placebo controlled trial, neonates receiving perioperative NAC after the arterial switch procedure demonstrated better urine output, shorter time to negative fluid balance, and less creatinine elevation.[161]

Drug Dosing in Acute Kidney Injury and Renal Replacement Therapy

Much of the pediatric drug dosing in patients with depressed GFR or in those receiving RRT is derived from adult data. There are several considerations specific to drug dosing in children. Critical illness can affect the GFR more in neonates than in adults, and GFR does not reach adult levels until 2 years of age.[162,163] The quality and quantity of plasma proteins do not reach adult levels until a year of age, and protein binding may vary. The volume of distribution of water-soluble drugs is larger relative to body weight in pediatric patients than adults. Nephrotoxic medications should be avoided when possible because this is one of the only modifiable AKI risk factors, and review of all medications should be performed in a patient with a creatinine elevation irrespective of AKI diagnosis. In addition, factors that affect creatinine levels, including volume status, muscle mass, and medications, should be accounted for, and use of cystatin C should be considered for a more accurate assessment of GFR.[164-167]

Drug clearance on RRT is dependent on rate of ultrafiltration and several molecular characteristics of the specific medication, including[168]:

1. *Molecular weight*: Smaller molecules are more readily removed. Continuous renal replacement therapy (CRRT) membranes have larger pores than intermittent hemodialysis (HD) and thus cause greater clearance.
2. *Charge*: Drugs with an anionic charge pass through the membrane more easily than cationic drugs, such as aminoglycosides.
3. *Volume of distribution*: Drugs with a greater volume of distribution are less cleared by RRT. However, this property is less important with slow continuous CRRT.
4. *Water solubility:* Drugs that are highly water soluble have a lower volume of distribution, and thus more drug is available for removal by RRT. In contrast, highly fat-soluble drugs are not removed easily.
5. *Protein binding:* Drugs that are highly protein bound are not readily removed. The clinician should consult both pharmacy and nephrology experts for drug dosing on RRT.

Renal Replacement Therapy

Because medical interventions are often ineffective at preventing and treating AKI and fluid overload, RRT may become necessary in pediatric patients with cardiac disease. In critically ill patients it is well established that mortality is significantly lower if dialysis is commenced before significant fluid overload.[117,169] However, it has only recently been demonstrated that children with fluid overload after cardiac surgery who go on to require RRT have improved mortality if dialysis is performed earlier.[170] The indications for RRT in patients with cardiac disease are similar to those in all critically ill children:

1. *Hypervolemia:* volume overload with evidence of organ dysfunction, particularly in the setting of impaired myocardial function
2. *Hyperkalemia:* potassium level greater than 6.5 mEq/L despite conservative measures or greater than 6.0 mEq/L in hypercatabolic (CHF and postoperative) patients
3. *Metabolic acidosis:* persistent metabolic acidosis with a serum HCO_3 level less than 10 mEq/L and arterial pH less than 7.2, with no response to therapy
4. *Azotemia:* elevated BUN level greater than 150 mg/dL, or lower if rapidly increasing or symptomatic (change in mental status, bleeding, pericardial rub)
5. *Neurologic complications:* presence of neurologic symptoms and signs secondary to uremia or electrolyte imbalance
6. *Calcium and phosphorus imbalance:* symptomatic hypocalcemia with tetany or seizures in the presence of high serum phosphate level

Given the decision to dialyze, the ideal modality must be determined. Options include peritoneal dialysis (PD), hemodialysis (HD), and continuous venovenous hemofiltration (CVVH).

Peritoneal Dialysis

PD is the most common form of postoperative RRT. Although the use of PD after pediatric heart surgery is rare and associated with high mortality rates,[171,172] studies suggest that PD may be used too infrequently and too late.[170,173] In addition to preventing the edema associated with multiorgan dysfunction, PD may allow increased administration of fluids to provide adequate nutrition, essential blood products, and beneficial medications. It has also been suggested that PD may help clear maladaptive proinflammatory cytokines.[174]

Reports of the systematic use of PD as an adjunct to postoperative fluid overload were published decades ago, and many studies since have reported safety in this cohort.[170,173-178] The benefit of this invasive procedure to prevent fluid overload in infants with oliguria after cardiac surgery has only recently been established. A case-matched cohort study comparing patients with a PD catheter placed at the time of surgery to infants of similar age and surgical procedure demonstrated that those with a PD catheter were less likely to develop fluid overload, had shorter durations of mechanical ventilation and shorter ICU stay, and did not have an increase in expenditures.[173] A follow-up clinical trial randomized 73 infants with oliguria after cardiac surgery to either standardized doses of furosemide or PD.[179] Patients who received furosemide were three times more likely to develop fluid overload and more likely to have prolonged mechanical ventilation and electrolyte abnormalities than those randomized to early PD.

Principles and Considerations of Peritoneal Dialysis. PD uses the abdominal viscera as a semipermeable membrane to filter excess free water and solute. The peritoneal cavity is a potential space into which dialysis solution is instilled. The movement of solvent is determined predominantly by the osmotic gradients between the dialysate formulation and intravascular solute concentration. In children the higher ratio of the peritoneal surface area to body mass results in very efficient PD. There are very few contraindications to the initiation of acute PD, including infection of the abdominal wall, significant bowel distention, and communication between the chest and abdominal cavity.

Access for Peritoneal Dialysis. Peritoneal catheters can be placed as a bedside procedure using the Seldinger technique or in the operating room at the time of cardiac surgery, either directly through the diaphragm via the sternotomy or through the abdominal wall.[180] Either a cuffed or uncuffed PD catheter can be used. Although use of cuffed catheters may minimize leakage or peritonitis, they require a more complicated placement and removal. Cuffed tubes are mainly used for patients expected to require prolonged dialysis or large volumes of fluid instillation. PD can be performed with a pigtail catheter, but this is often complicated by catheter occlusion. Some centers balance these strengths by using a cuffed tube but leaving the cuff outside the skin.[179]

Equipment and Initiation of Peritoneal Dialysis. After placement, PD can be initiated immediately with several different dialysis systems. Most consist of Y tubing with separate inflow and outflow segments, although a PD cycler can be used in patients requiring chronic dialysis. Commercial dialysis fluid is available and can be modified to match patient needs. Increasing the dextrose concentration of the dialysis fluid (D1.5% to D4.25%) increases the ultrafiltrate removed per cycle (Table 16.1). Commercial dialysate solutions contain a relatively low concentration of sodium and also contain lactate. Lactate may be poorly tolerated in children with impaired liver function or lactic acidosis and can be circumvented by using a bicarbonate-based solution.

Several specific considerations are necessary for pediatric patients with cardiac disease. Unless patient cooling is the objective (e.g., junctional ectopic tachycardia), PD fluid should be warmed to 38°C before instillation. PD should be initiated with small volumes—approximately 10 to 15 mL/kg per dwell over the first several days. This allows the catheter placement site to heal, avoids catheter leaks, and ensures minimal hemodynamic effect. A common initial neonatal prescription is 10 mL/kg D1.5% solution with 2 to 3 mEq/L potassium chloride and 200 units/L unfractionated

TABLE 16.1	Approaches to Optimizing Ultrafiltration and Solute Clearance During Peritoneal Dialysis	
To Improve Ultrafiltration	**To Improve Solute Clearance**	
Increase dextrose concentration	Increase dialysate volume	
Increase frequency of cycles	For potassium and urea: Increase frequency of cycles	
Increase dialysate volume	For phosphorus: Decrease frequency of cycles	

TABLE 16.2	Recommended Dialysis Catheter Sizes	
Patient Size	**Catheter Size**	**Special**
Neonates	7 French	Triple lumen is available for $CaCl_2$ if providing citrate regional anticoagulation.
3-6 kg	7 French	Triple lumen is available for $CaCl_2$ if providing citrate regional anticoagulation.
6-12 kg	8 French	
12-20 kg	9 French	
20-30 kg	10 French	
30+ kg	10 or 11 French	Triple lumen 11.5 French **should always** be used for $CaCl_2$ if providing citrate regional anticoagulation.

heparin; 5-minute fill, 45-minute dwell, 10-minute drain. The final dialysate volume and composition and the cycle frequency will vary based upon need (see Table 16.1).

Instilling fluid in the abdomen has a risk of compression of the inferior vena cava and thoracic cavity and can decrease venous preload or cause lung atelectasis. This risk is particularly high among patients following surgery, neonates, those with depressed cardiac function, and those requiring positive pressure ventilation. However, using a relatively small dwell volume (10 to 15 mL/kg), multiple studies have demonstrated safety in ventilated neonates following surgery.[170,173,174,179] It remains critical to monitor hemodynamics during initiation.

Complications of Peritoneal Dialysis. Although PD is generally considered a safe procedure, complications may occur. Catheters may become occluded by fibrin deposit or omentum, potentially allowing flow into the abdominal cavity but with poor drainage. If this does not resolve with catheter flushing and patient repositioning, the catheter will likely need to be removed, potentially with ligation of adhered omentum. Use of streptokinase or tissue plasminogen activator to clear fibrin deposits has been reported.[181,182]

Bowel injury during placement or due to adhesion formation is possible, although rare. Although infection may occur, it is infrequent. When detected early, peritonitis is often successfully treated with broad-spectrum intraperitoneal antibiotics.[183] Intraoperative placement of PD catheters is associated with a decrease in these complications[173,174,179]

Pleural-peritoneal communication and hydrothorax may occur in patients receiving PD, particularly in smaller neonates, when placing PD catheters through a sternotomy, and in patients after placement of a VAD or pacemakers with thoracic communication. To diagnose this complication, simultaneous measurement of glucose in the chest tube drainage, PD effluent, and serum should be performed. In patients without a chest tube, it may be necessary to perform a diagnostic or therapeutic thoracentesis. If communication is present, the peritoneal catheter should be placed to drain, and dialysis may be attempted again in several days.[179]

Hemodialysis

All dialysis procedures involve three primary processes, diffusion, convection, and ultrafiltration, which occur across a semipermeable membrane between blood and dialysate compartments. In HD and CVVH therapy the membranes are composed of synthetic hollow fibers through which the blood runs countercurrent to a balanced electrolyte solution. Solute clearance, either by diffusion driven by concentration gradients across the membrane or by convection employing solute drag across the membrane, are affected by a number of factors, including solute concentration in blood

and dialysis fluid, surface area and permeability characteristics of the dialyzer, solute size, protein-binding properties, and the blood and dialysis flow rates. Ultrafiltration refers to fluid removal across the membrane. The primary determinant of ultrafiltration is the hydrostatic pressure generated across the membrane. At present, HD technology is fairly advanced, and the hydrostatic pressure differential can be easily manipulated, with predictable and adjustable fluid removal.

The cardiovascular burden of HD—large solute and intravascular fluid shifts, relatively rapid blood flow rates, and significant extracorporeal blood volume—may be poorly tolerated in children with cardiac disease. Additionally, significant hypoxemia may occur during HD, making these patients poor candidates for this aggressive therapy. Caution must be used during the initiation phase of HD to avoid overzealous correction of metabolic and fluid derangements associated with AKI. In the setting of critical illness one must consider if the patient can tolerate the total daily fluid removal goal within the 3- to 4-hour HD treatment time frame.

Hemodialysis Access. HD can be performed in most infants and children because of advances in dual-lumen catheter access. In newborns, although umbilical artery vessels may be used, they generally do not provide adequate flow rates for HD. Even in the smallest infant a 7 Fr dual-lumen catheter may be adequate.[184] Subclavian veins should be avoided, particularly in neonates because resultant subclavian stenosis will preclude use of that limb for permanent access in patients who do not recover kidney function.[185] Catheter size should be matched to patient size to allow for maximal flow and minimal risk of placement (Table 16.2).[186]

Equipment and Initiation of Hemodialysis. There are many available dialysis machines suitable for children that incorporate bicarbonate buffer, variable dialysate sodium concentration, and volumetric technology, all of which have led to improved safety and accuracy of the HD procedure. In addition, application of noninvasive monitoring of hematocrit allows for real-time assessment of intravascular fluid shifts to adjust ultrafiltration rates during the treatment.[187,188]

The circuit and dialyzer chosen for a given patient are predominantly determined by body size. The volume of the extracorporeal circuit (blood tubing and dialyzer) should not exceed 10% of the child's calculated blood volume. If that cannot be achieved, the circuit should be primed with packed red blood cells or albumin.

In this situation the prime volume should not be returned to the patient at the end of the procedure. Tubing size is chosen according to weight: neonatal tubing for any child less than 13 kg, pediatric tubing for a child between 13 and 30 kg, and standard adult tubing for any person greater than 30 kg. During the initiation phase, flow rates as low as 3 mL/kg/min are recommended and may be increased to 5 to 8 mL/kg/min by the third HD run.

HD circuits require anticoagulation to maintain patency, and heparin requirements are difficult to predict for critically ill children. Heparin is typically given as a bolus at the start of the procedure (10 to 20 units/kg) and then continuously throughout (starting at 10 units/kg/h). The activated clotting time (ACT) can be used to guide systemic heparinization, with an ACT goal of 120 to 150 seconds measured hourly throughout the dialysis run. Many children have associated coagulopathies and are relatively anticoagulated and do not receive heparin. Often, acutely ill children receive no heparin through the entire procedure.

Continuous Renal Replacement Therapy

CRRT is particularly attractive in the patient with hemodynamic instability, allowing for slow, continuous, adjustable fluid removal rates throughout the day to account for the fluid volumes associated with provision of nutrition, blood products, and medications. Gradual fluid removal can be achieved with less risk for acute hemodynamic compromise compared to HD.

CRRT initially included both continuous arteriovenous hemofiltration (CAVH) and continuous venovenous hemofiltration (CVVH). However, the development of continuous venovenous machine platforms with precise pump technology and volumetric or gravimetric measurement for fluid removal volumes has led to almost all CRRT being performed more safely in venovenous modes in pediatrics. CRRT clearance can be prescribed as purely convective (CVVH), purely dialytic (continuous venovenous hemodialysis [CVVHD]), or a combination (continuous venovenous hemodialysis filtration [CVVHDF]). Small solute clearance is equivalent between the three modalities, but convective modalities effect relatively greater clearance of molecules larger than 1000 Da. Access considerations are similar to those discussed earlier for HD (see Table 16.2).

Continuous Renal Replacement Therapy Equipment and Prescription. Many different venovenous CRRT platforms are available for pediatric CRRT. Some employ a single integrated set of blood tubing and dialyzer, and others are similar to HD with interchangeable combinations of tubing and dialyzers. The choice of hemofilter is based on the CRRT system used and the size and needs of the patient. As with HD, blood priming should be done for circuits with an extracorporeal volume greater than 10% of the patient's blood volume. Some practitioners opt for circuits with an AN-69 composition because these filters may improve inflammatory cytokine clearance, but care must be taken to avoid a bradykinin release syndrome, and associated hypotension, with these filters, especially when blood priming is needed.[189]

As with HD, continuous anticoagulation is necessary to maintain patency of CRRT systems with similar parameters. Many prefer regional citrate anticoagulation to heparin because some studies demonstrate improved filter life span and decreased patient sequelae.[190,191] This requires a citrate solution to be infused into the blood line coming from the patient and a calcium chloride solution to be infused systemically to the patient. Most protocols aim to keep the circuit ionized calcium level below 0.45 mmol/L and the patient ionized calcium level above 1.0 mmol/L, thereby maintaining anticoagulation in the circuit without systemically anticoagulating the patient.

The dose of CRRT is based on the total effluent volume delivered, which is the sum of the convective clearance achieved with replacement fluid, the diffusive clearance achieved with dialysis fluid, and the additional ultrafiltration volumes prescribed for net patient fluid removal.

Complications of Continuous Renal Replacement Therapy. CRRT is a relatively gentle and accurate form of RRT and as such has no absolute contraindications. Hypotension may occur as a consequence of hypovolemia, so the cardiorespiratory status should be monitored frequently along with assessment of hourly intake, ultrafiltration volume, and urinary output to ensure that significant volume shifts do not occur. Significant electrolyte changes can be observed with correction of acidosis, hyperkalemia, and hyperphosphatemia as the CRRT course progresses. Twice daily monitoring of electrolytes will allow for the ability to alter the composition of the dialysis and replacement fluid accordingly. Hypotension during initiation may be secondary to blood binding of calcium or bradykinin release and is often treated with calcium chloride boluses or low-dose inotropic infusions.

Continuous Renal Replacement Therapy With Extracorporeal Membrane Oxygenation. In patients who require either ultrafiltration or solute clearance while on ECMO, placing a hemofilter within the circuit is simple and efficient due to the large blood flow rates and consistent heparinization.[192] Ultrafiltration is achieved easily with this configuration, and solute clearance can be achieved by running CRRT dialysis fluid countercurrently using an IV pump. However, care must be taken to ensure that the dialysis fluid volume is removed accurately in addition to the desired ultrafiltration volume, and IV pumps are not as accurate as CRRT machines.[193] In addition, the maximal flow rates of IV pumps of 1000 mL/h limit the clearance capabilities significantly. When greater accuracy and clearance are desired, insertion of a CRRT machine parallel to the ECMO circuit, usually in the postpump/premembrane configuration, is commonly used. Usually no additional anticoagulation is needed. The CRRT pump rate should not exceed 10% of the ECMO flow rate.

Conclusion and Future Directions

Management of critically ill pediatric patients with cardiac disease requires a multidisciplinary approach with involvement of specialty services for optimal outcome. Unfortunately, despite meticulous management, AKI and CKD will continue to exist in this population. We expect that innovation will enable improved diagnostic abilities and expand therapeutic options for those with AKI. Validation and clinical utility of novel biomarker and genetic polymorphism testing will help identify patients at risk for kidney disease earlier and with better certainty than current laboratory testing. Earlier recognition of a high-risk cohort will not only augment medical decision making to direct RRT initiation and nephrotoxin avoidance but may also aid in the investigation of potential pharmacologic therapies. Options for RRT in small patients may expand with the introduction of the novel neonatal CRRT device, the **Ca**rdio-**R**enal **Pe**diatric **Di**alysis **E**mergency **M**achine (CARPEDIEM), or by the adaptation of the Aquadex FlexFlow device, a machine developed for ultrafiltration in adults with CHF.[194,195] Although the presence of negative cardiorenal interactions may not be avoidable, diagnostic and therapeutic innovation may help minimize the adverse outcomes associated with cardiorenal disease.

Selected References

A complete list of references is available at ExpertConsult.com.

2. Li S, Krawczeski CD, Zappitelli M, et al. Incidence, risk factors, and outcomes of acute kidney injury after pediatric cardiac surgery–a prospective multicenter study. *Crit Care Med*. 2011;39(6):1493.

45. Ronco C, Haapio M, House AA, Anavekar N, Bellomo R. Cardiorenal syndrome. *J Am Coll Cardiol*. 2008;52(19):1527–1539.

61. Devarajan P. Update on mechanisms of ischemic acute kidney injury. *J Am Soc Nephrol*. 2006;17(6):1503–1520.

81. Kellum JA, Lameire N. Diagnosis, evaluation, and management of acute kidney injury: a KDIGO summary (Part 1). *Crit Care*. 2013;17(1):204.

117. Sutherland SM, Zappitelli M, Alexander SR, et al. Fluid overload and mortality in children receiving continuous renal replacement therapy: the prospective pediatric continuous renal replacement therapy registry. *Am J Kidney Dis*. 2010;55(2):316–325.

179. Kwiatkowski DM. Peritoneal Dialysis is Superior to Furosemide for Preventing Fluid Overload in Infants after Cardiac Surgery: a Randomized Controlled Trial. *JAMA Pediatrics*. 2017.

17

Organ System Response to Cardiac Function—Neurology

ROCKY TSANG, MD; DANIEL J. LICHT, MD; KEN BRADY, MD

Care of the child with congenital heart disease (CHD) has evolved rapidly in the decades since the 1980s, some adaptations driven by evidence, some not. Changes in operative techniques, cardiopulmonary bypass (CPB) strategies, postoperative care, monitoring, interventional cardiac catheterization, and echocardiography are collectively and nonspecifically associated with a dramatic improvement in mortality for patients with CHD.[1-4] With improving survival there has also been a trend to perform more complex surgeries on younger patients with more comorbidities.[5] Despite improvement in mortality, many survivors of CHD suffer high rates of long-term neurodevelopmental abnormalities: limitations of executive functioning, impulse control, language, and cognition, as well as attention deficit.[6-9] The focus of pediatric cardiology and pediatric cardiac surgery has made a pivot from improving survival to improving the quality of life of survivors, including prevention of acquired neurologic injury from CHD.[10,11]

Neonates with critical CHD who require surgery in the first month of life are particularly vulnerable to neurologic injury. In the last two decades, magnetic resonance imaging (MRI) has been methodically applied to neonates who require cardiac surgery with CPB using both preoperative and postoperative scans.[12-18] These studies include different surgical and CPB approaches and different MRI scanners and protocols; however, taken together, they collectively describe the nature of presurgical and perioperatively acquired brain lesions seen in neonates with critical CHD. Twenty percent to 40% of neonates have a brain injury before surgery. It is unknown what percentage of these injuries occur in utero or postpartum.[12,16,17] Postoperative scans show new injury, acquired in the perioperative period in 35% to 75% of newborns who require heart surgery with CPB, and these are most commonly located in the white matter (Fig. 17.1).[12,13,18]

There are two potential susceptibilities seen in preterm infants with similar patterns of white matter injury (WMI) that are invoked to describe the prominent finding of WMI after neonatal cardiac surgery. The white matter is a watershed region in the immature brain, where penetrating arterioles have less overlap than is found in the mature brain. Further, oligodendrocyte precursors in the immature brain have increased susceptibility to hypoxia/ischemia.[19-21] Consistent with that theory is the finding that infants with critical CHD have immature myelination patterns at term birth, and immature myelination is associated with an increased risk of neonatal WMI after cardiac surgery.[16,22]

It is widely assumed that the impaired oxygen delivery contributes to WMI and is caused by cyanosis, inadequate cardiac output, CPB strategies, circulatory arrest, and/or low blood pressure with diastolic runoff to pulmonary shunts. However, there are few evidence-based practices that have been shown to modify the incidence of any brain injury in neonates with CHD.[23] Nonmodifiable factors, such as genetic abnormalities, and socioeconomic factors often have greater significance than modified parameters of care in neurodevelopmental studies of CHD patients.[24] This chapter will review the physiology of cerebral vasculature, vulnerabilities to central nervous system (CNS) pathologic conditions seen in CHD patients, perioperatively acquired neurologic injury and relevant perioperative practices, and the neurodevelopmental sequelae of CHD.

Physiology of the Cerebral Vasculature

The patient with CHD is at risk for impairment of cerebral oxygen delivery from multiple factors in the oxygen delivery equation, including both oxygen content and blood flow. Perioperative management of CHD, more than any other category of pediatric critical illness, requires repetitive assessment and modulation of oxygen delivery to the various organ beds. In these patients, interventions do not necessarily align the goals of maintaining oxygenation, cerebral blood flow, coronary blood flow, and splanchnic/renal blood flow. In other words, interventions to improve perfusion of the brain may come at the expense of visceral perfusion and vice versa. In this section the peculiarity of cerebral vascular homeostasis is described and compared to other systemic vascular behaviors.

Perfusion of the brain is unique when compared with other mammalian organs. The brain has minimal glycemic reserves in the form of glycogen storage, and neurons are not tolerant of anaerobic respiration. The brain has an obligate need for an uninterrupted supply of glucose and oxygen. The maintenance of a constant ratio of cerebral substrate delivery and cerebral metabolic demand is the consequence of an intricate overlay of several known vascular responses that have presumably evolved from the selective pressure of the brain's unique vulnerability. Each of these servomechanisms act on similar targets: modulating cerebral vascular resistance or perfusion pressure to constrain cerebral blood flow. Each of these mechanisms has a different stimulus, regional specificity, and frequency bandwidth (time delay) of operation. With increasing precision the systemic vasoconstrictive response, pressure autoregulation, and neurovascular coupling constitute three principal mechanisms of cerebrovascular control in a dynamic pressure-flow system.

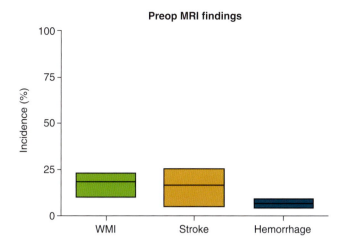

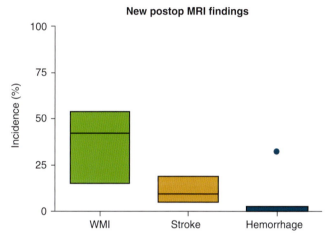

• **Figure 17.1** The incidence of neonatal neurologic injuries before and after cardiopulmonary bypass. Data are compiled from seven published reports, over 400 subjects, across seven centers. Median and range are shown with outlier. White matter injury *(WMI)* is the most common perioperatively acquired brain lesion. *MRI,* Magnetic resonance imaging; *postop,* postoperative; *preop,* preoperative. (Used with permission from Wiley.)

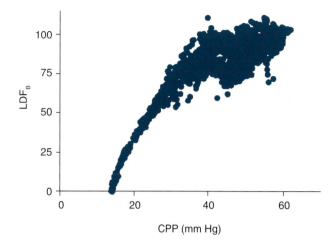

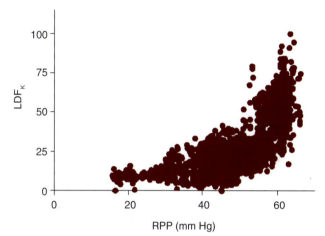

• **Figure 17.2** Comparison of cerebral *(top)* and renal *(bottom)* blood flow responses with progressive low-output shock in a piglet. Hemorrhage was induced from baseline over 4 hours with continuous measurements of cerebral and renal blood flow (y-axes) shown as a function of cerebral perfusion pressure *(CPP)* and renal perfusion pressure *(RPP)* (x-axes). In the initial phase of low-output shock the mean arterial pressure does not change from the baseline mean of 55 to 65 mm Hg due to vasoconstriction. The cerebral blood flow is unaffected by this mild to moderate reduction in cardiac output, but renal blood flow is reduced to 25% of baseline value. Once the systemic vasoconstriction response is exhausted, arterial blood pressure falls, and cerebral blood flow becomes vulnerable. LDF_B, Laser Doppler flux brain; LDF_K, laser Doppler flux kidney. (Modified from Rhee CJ, Kibler KK, Easley RB, et al. Renovascular reactivity measured by near-infrared spectroscopy. *J Appl Physiol [1985].* 2012;113[2]:307-14. Used with permission.)

Systemic Vasoconstrictive Response

A decline in cardiac output triggers vasopressin output, the renin-angiotensin-aldosterone system, and the sympathetic nervous system. Activation of this neurohormonal axis promotes systemic vasoconstriction, but the cerebral vessels are relatively spared due to a paucity of receptors for these vasoconstrictors. The overall result is preservation of the cerebral perfusion at the cost of systemic perfusion.[25-28] The systemic vasoconstrictive response allows the brain to maintain cerebral blood flow across changes in cardiac output and renders cerebral perfusion independent of cardiac output up to a threshold.[29,30] This response is demonstrated in Fig. 17.2, which compares cerebral blood flow with renal blood flow during progressive hemorrhagic shock in a newborn swine. In the early stage of low-output shock in this example the mean arterial pressure is preserved between 55 and 65 mm Hg by systemic vasoconstriction. Cerebral blood flow is unaffected by the increased systemic vascular resistance, but renal blood flow is reduced to 25% of its baseline value.[31]

The effect of the systemic vasoconstrictive response can also be seen during CPB. Michler et al.[32] have shown that independent

of bypass flow rates, if perfusion pressure is adequate, cerebral blood flow is preserved (Fig. 17.3).

Perioperative and CPB strategy for infants in many centers includes alpha-adrenergic inhibition or other vasodilators to maintain systemic perfusion. This strategy is a blockade of the systemic vasoconstrictive response. Splanchnic and renal perfusion are improved, and this strategy is credited with improved survival, especially in the single-ventricle, shunted patient.[33,34] Because this strategy results in low perfusion pressures when output is compromised, it is a potential vulnerability to cerebral perfusion pressure. To some degree the vasodilator strategy places renal protection and survival at odds with cerebral protection (Fig. 17.4).

The contribution of this strategy to the burden of neurologic injury is unknown and is likely modulated by the second-tier vascular response of the brain: pressure autoregulation.

Pressure Autoregulation

When the systemic vasoconstrictive response is exhausted, or pharmacologically ablated, arterial blood pressure falls with reductions in cardiac output. Changes in arterial blood pressure, either up or down, engage the servomechanism of pressure autoregulation in the cerebral vasculature. Pressure autoregulation constrains cerebral blood flow fluctuations caused by perfusion pressure changes.[35] Changes in the transmural pressure gradient of muscular arterioles trigger myogenic responses of constriction and relaxation in a dynamic fashion (Fig. 17.5).

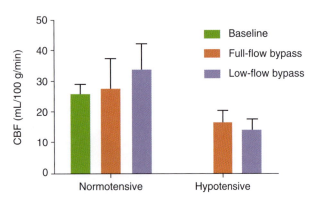

• **Figure 17.3** Cerebral blood flow *(CBF)* in baboons at full- and low-flow cardiopulmonary bypass. When normotensive, regardless of bypass flow rates, cerebral blood flow is at baseline values. When hypotensive, regardless of bypass flow rates, cerebral blood flow is reduced. (Modified with permission from Michler RE, Sandhu AA, Young WL, et al. Low-flow cardiopulmonary bypass: importance of blood pressure in maintaining cerebral blood flow. *Ann Thorac Surg.* 1995;60:S525-S528.)

These vascular changes have been observed to occur rapidly in animal models and between 2 and 10 seconds in pediatric and adult clinical studies, dependent on the magnitude of the transmural pressure change.[36-38] The pressure autoregulation response is fully engaged when changes in arterial blood pressure last longer than 30 to 60 seconds.[39] Thus it allows for passive transmission of perfusion pressure changes at the pulse and respiratory frequencies but acts as a high-pass filter preventing the transmission of sustained perfusion pressure changes into cerebral blood flow changes.

Pressure autoregulation allows for tolerance of mild to moderate hypotension when vasodilators are used, without causing a vulnerability for cerebral ischemia. The limit of this tolerance is the blood pressure at which pressure autoregulation is exhausted, termed the *lower limit of autoregulation,* easily observed in Fig. 17.2 at 40 mm Hg and in Fig. 17.4 at 50 mm Hg. The lower limit of autoregulation was originally estimated in adults to be 50 mm Hg by Lassen and is now understood to have variability between patients and conditions.[40,41] The lower limits of autoregulation are poorly defined, especially for pediatric populations, so absolute safe arterial blood pressures cannot be recommended. Two pediatric studies of CPB suggest a lower limit on average near 40 mm Hg, but the use of a global threshold ignores wide intersubject variability.[42,43] A single threshold for all patients places some at risk of inadequate pressure and some at risk of inadequate vasodilation.

Neurovascular Coupling

Metabolic autoregulation is distinct from pressure autoregulation. Metabolic autoregulation, also known as neurovascular coupling, links neuronal activity to cerebral blood flow, mediated at the level of the neurovascular unit: individual astrocytes linking neuronal synapses and penetrating arterioles.[44] These glial cells release both vasoconstrictors and vasodilators on associated muscular arterioles.[45] In contrast with pressure autoregulation, neurovascular coupling is both rapid and regionally specific. Vascular dilation occurs in specific regions of neuronal activity, causing a match between the

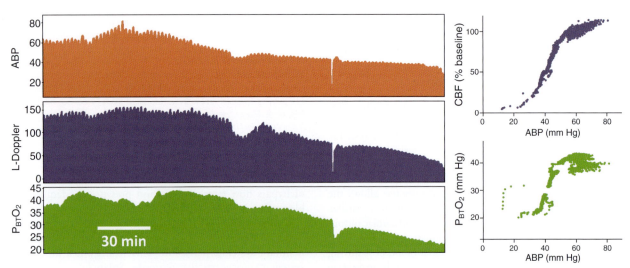

• **Figure 17.4** Arterial blood pressure *(ABP;* mm Hg), cerebral blood flow *(CBF)* (L-Doppler; arbitrary units), and brain tissue oxygen tension in the white matter ($P_{BT}O_2$; mm Hg) measured in a piglet on full-flow cardiopulmonary bypass. ABP, CBF, and $P_{BT}O_2$ all decrease as a function of time with progressive addition of vasodilator (enalaprilat). Top right, CBF (L-Doppler normalized to baseline) as a function of ABP (mm Hg) showing preserved flow to a lower limit of autoregulation between 40 and 50 mm Hg. Bottom right, $P_{BT}O_2$ falls at a similar lower limit of autoregulation between 40 and 50 mm Hg. Even at full flow, ABP greater than the lower limit of autoregulation is required to maintain pressure autoregulation and oxygen delivery.

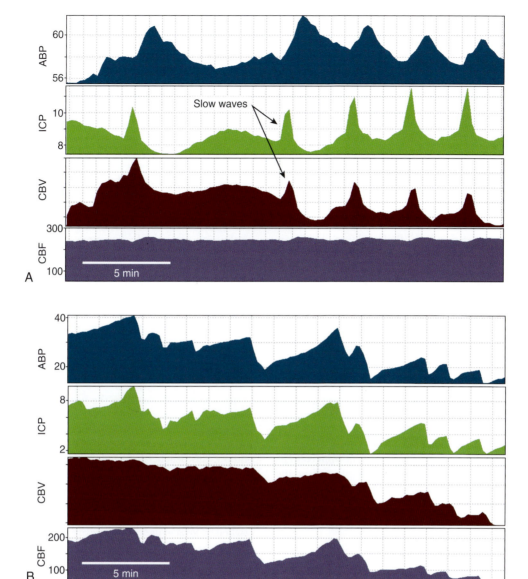

• **Figure 17.5** Intact pressure autoregulation (A) and impaired pressure autoregulation (B). Spontaneous fluctuations in arterial blood pressure (*ABP;* mm Hg) and intracranial pressure (*ICP;* mm Hg) called "slow waves" occur in mammals, shown in this normotensive (A) and hypotensive (B) piglet. During normotension the ABP and ICP waves occur in opposition: increases in ABP render decreases in ICP. This inverse relationship is due to dilation and constriction of blood vessels from pressure autoregulation, shown in the cerebral blood volume (*CBV;* arbitrary units [A.U.]) tracing. With normotension and intact pressure autoregulation, cerebral blood flow (*CBF;* A.U.) is relatively constrained across the changes in ABP. The same animal with hypotension has a passive relationship across ABP, ICP, and CBV because the vasculature is no longer reactive to changes in perfusion pressure. The lack of vascular pressure reactivity results in impaired autoregulation, and CBF becomes fluctuant, also passive to the ABP.

rate of oxygen consumption and oxygen delivery. Factors that reduce neuronal activity and cerebral metabolism cause reductions in cerebral blood flow, cerebral blood volume, and intracranial pressure. Metabolic autoregulation is an important aspect of therapies such as hypothermia and anesthesia for intracranial pressure reduction and neuroprotection of the injured brain.

Carbon Dioxide, Oxygen, and Glucose Reactivity

In addition to the pressure and flow homeostasis described above, the vasculature of the brain is highly responsive to perturbations of the basic chemistry of the cerebrospinal fluid, with mechanisms that can override pressure and metabolic autoregulation. Hypoxia, hypercarbia, and hypoglycemia all cause cerebral vasodilation.

Acute hypercarbia increases cerebral blood flow, and acute hypocarbia decreases cerebral blood flow, with an effect mediated by changes in cerebrospinal fluid pH. Intentional hypoventilation uses arterial carbon dioxide as a drug to increase cerebral blood flow. Single-ventricle patients with large left-to-right shunts have higher pulmonary vascular resistance and higher cerebral blood flow when they are hypercarbic.[46] The combined effect of hypercarbia is to mitigate pulmonary overcirculation and enhance cerebral oxygen delivery.

However, carbon dioxide as a therapy is likely time limited in its effectiveness. Carbon dioxide diffuses freely across the blood-brain barrier, which is not permeable to hydrogen ions. The spinal fluid compartment has an independent pH buffering system from the blood within the choroid plexus. The choroid plexus can produce appropriately buffered spinal fluid much faster than the kidney buffers the pH of blood, in part because of the high rate of production of cerebrospinal fluid. Spinal fluid pH changes (and thus cerebral blood flow changes) induced by hypocarbia or hypercarbia are limited to 3 to 6 hours, and the serum pH is not an accurate reflection of spinal fluid pH over time.[47,48]

The cerebral vasculature is also responsive to changes in oxygen tension when oxygen delivery is below the threshold to meet metabolic oxygen consumption demands.[49,50] Profound vasodilation can occur in the face of arterial oxygen tension of less than 60 mm Hg or anemia. These data come from animal and biventricular subjects, whereas the cerebrovascular effect of chronic exposure to cyanosis in the patient with CHD has not been elucidated.

Causes of Impaired Neurodevelopment in Congenital Heart Disease Outside the Perioperative Period

Identifying modifiable causes of brain injury and neurodevelopmental abnormality for children with CHD is nontrivial. Injuries that occur in an early perioperative period cannot be assessed for impact until years later, when development has occurred. Countless causes of neurodevelopmental abnormality can occur from conception to adulthood, making it difficult to isolate the effect of specific perioperative injuries or care practices. Very few perioperative practices have been shown to associate with long-term developmental outcome, so there has been a proliferation and divergence of practices between centers. This section describes known and potential contributors to impaired neurodevelopment in CHD outside the perioperative period.

Congenital Neurologic Abnormalities

Up to 30% of patients with cardiac defects have genetic abnormalities that affect other organ systems.[51] Aneuploidies such as trisomy 21, 18, and 13; multiple syndromes such as Noonan, Williams, DiGeorge, and CHARGE; and the VACTERL association are all correlated with both CHD and developmental delay.[6,52-54] Cohorts of CHD subjects with these recognizable patterns of malformation have developmental testing results that are below population norms and also below the norms of subjects across a wide range of cardiac lesions other than CHD.[55-57]

Genetic-environmental interactions during illnesses and stressors such as inflammation, hypoxia, and coagulopathy are also postulated to contribute to the neurologic sequelae of CHD.[58,59] Gaynor et al. studied apolipoprotein E (APOE) alleles for association with neurodevelopment in children with CHD. The APOE ε2 allele was associated with worse scores on multiple parameters of the child behavior checklist indices at the fourth and fifth birthdays, whereas the APOE ε4 allele was associated with better scores.[60,61] The APOE lipoprotein is thought to have function in lipid transport and neuronal repair in the CNS.[62,63]

Microcephaly and CNS immaturity are prevalent in patients with complex CHD.[15] The increased incidence of microcephaly at birth persists into childhood and is independently associated with developmental delays.[64-66] Microcephaly is thought to be caused by in utero hemodynamic perturbations associated with specific heart defects. Shillingford et al. found that in patients with hypoplastic left heart syndrome (HLHS) the degree of microcephaly is correlated with ascending aorta diameter. This finding suggests that interruption of the normal streaming of oxygenated blood from the placenta to the brain via the left ventricular outflow tract leads to reduced brain growth in utero.[24,64]

CHD is associated with delayed brain maturation, detectable by MRI as both delayed white matter myelination and cortical folding abnormalities. Brain MRIs of fetuses with CHD show significant differences in brain volume that diverge from the normal trajectory in the third trimester.[67] Licht et al. used a validated scoring system of brain maturity to assess four different parameters: myelination, cortical infolding, presence of germinal matrix tissue, and involution of glial cell migration bands. In a cohort of 29 infants with HLHS and 13 patients with transposition of great arteries (TGA), the preoperative brain MRI showed that term infants with CHD have a total maturation score comparable to a 35-week premature infant without CHD.[68,69] Miller et al.[15] demonstrated similar immaturity patterns using MRI measures of white matter integrity.

Neurologic Injury in Utero

In the normal fetal circulation the eustachian valve and the foramen ovale direct the most highly oxygenated blood to the developing fetal brain via the left ventricular outflow tract. In many complex structural heart defects, especially those with interrupted left-sided outflow, this beneficial streaming is not present, and oxygenated blood flow is directed toward the ductus arteriosus.[70,71] Studies of patients with TGA, for instance, show that fetal blood with the lowest saturation is directed to the brain and blood with the highest saturation is directed inferiorly to the abdominal organs. Relative cerebral hypoxia in utero may contribute to the neurodevelopmental delays seen among these patients.[24,72,73]

Fetal ultrasonography and Doppler ultrasonography of the circle of Willis have demonstrated abnormal responses of the cerebral vasculature in fetuses with systemic outflow obstruction, showing lower than normal cerebral vascular resistance. Donofrio et al. reported this low resistance by measuring the cerebroplacental Doppler ratio (CPR) in a study of fetuses with CHD. CPR is the ratio of the pulsatility index measured in the middle cerebral artery to the pulsatility index measured in the umbilical artery. The pulsatility index is the difference between systolic flow velocity and diastolic flow velocity, divided by the time-averaged flow velocity ($\frac{Sfv - Dfv}{Mfv}$), and is related to downstream vascular resistance (higher pulsatility index is associated with higher downstream vascular resistance). Normal CPR is less than 1, meaning that cerebrovascular resistance is greater than placental vascular resistance. Only 48% of patients with HLHS have a measured CPR greater than 1, whereas 95% of normal fetuses have a measured CPR greater than 1—suggesting lower cerebral vascular resistance in fetuses with HLHS.[74]

By contrast, patients with right-sided obstructive lesions can have high cerebral vascular resistance. Kaltman and colleagues reported low middle cerebral artery pulsatility index in HLHS fetuses, and high middle cerebral artery pulsatility index in fetuses with right-sided obstructive lesions compared with fetuses that have a normal heart (Fig. 17.6).[75,76]

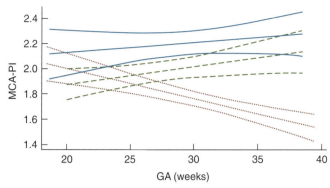

• **Figure 17.6** Pulsatility index *(PI)* with 95% confidence intervals in the middle cerebral artery *(MCA)* of normal fetuses *(green dashed lines)*, fetuses with pulmonary obstruction *(blue solid lines)*, and fetuses with aortic obstruction *(red dotted lines)*. As the fetus with hypoplastic left heart syndrome approaches term, cerebrovascular resistance is falling, whereas it is increasing or stable in normal subjects and in the fetus with right-sided obstructive lesions. *GA,* Gestational age. (Modified from Szwast A, Tian Z, McCann M, et al. Comparative analysis of cerebrovascular resistance in fetuses with single-ventricle congenital heart disease. *Ultrasound Obstet Gynecol.* 2012;40[1]:62-67. Used with permission.)

These observed differences in cerebral vascular resistance are consistent with differences in arterial flow patterns at the aortic arch in utero. Normally, cephalad aortic flow in utero is from the left ventricular outflow tract (streamed oxygenated blood from the placenta across the foramen ovale), and caudad flow in the descending aorta is from the right ventricular outflow tract across the ductus arteriosus. With a left-sided obstruction there is loss of streaming of oxygenated blood to the brain. From the physiologic principles outlined, hypoxia may result in a decrease in cerebral vascular resistance. The effect of this change in cerebral vascular resistance on the developing brain is unknown and is a focus of current study.[24]

Innate Vulnerabilities to Acquired Neurologic Injury in Patients With Congenital Heart Disease

Hypercyanotic Spells. "Tet" spells occur in 10% to 20% of patients with CHD caused by either fixed or dynamic pulmonary outflow tract obstruction.[77] These episodes of cyanosis occur most frequently between the ages of 6 months and 3 years and are associated with sudden drops in arterial oxyhemoglobin saturation. They are caused by marked increases in right ventricular outflow resistance and right-to-left shunting. Unrelenting episodes lead to cerebral hypoxia, loss of consciousness, convulsions, and seizures.[78] Cerebrovascular accidents, hypoxic-ischemic injury, and permeant neurologic sequelae have been reported.[79]

Cerebrovascular Accidents. Arterial ischemic stroke, as manifested by arterial occlusion seen with vasospasm or clot, is less common than WMI in the perioperative period (see Fig. 17.1). However, patients with CHD that involves cyanosis, right-to-left shunting, failing ventricles, or the placement of hardware in the form of valves, conduits, or ventricular assist devices all have an increased risk of cerebrovascular accidents.[80] CHD-related cerebrovascular accidents were more common and more well described in the era preceding surgical repair of CHD. The natural history of unrepaired cyanotic heart disease includes a 75% incidence of cerebrovascular accidents with the majority of these occurring before 2 years of age.[81,82] Berthrong and Sabistion[83] reported that venous occlusion and thrombus occurs with a higher incidence than arterial embolus. Anemia places infants at higher risk of ischemic events that are arterial in origin, and high hemoglobin concentrations associated with cyanosis increase the risk for venous thrombosis.[79] Most arterial thromboembolic events have a single vessel involvement and are characterized by a focal deficit of the affected vascular territory. If multiple arterial territories or both cerebral hemispheres are involved, then an intracardiac thrombus or vegetation should be suspected and investigated. In the case of venous thrombosis, onset of symptoms is more indolent and often preceded by dehydration, which increases blood viscosity and the polycythemic state. Up to 20% of CHD patients with a frank cerebrovascular accident will suffer severe intellectual disability.[81]

In the more modern era, mechanical cardiac support and the ventricular assist device have increased survival to transplant but have become an important risk factor for frank cerebrovascular accidents. In a trial of 48 pediatric patients less than 16 years of age with chronic heart failure, Fraser et al. compared the Excor Pediatric ventricular assist device against extracorporeal membrane oxygenation (ECMO) for survival to heart transplantation. Although survival to transplant was significantly higher in the ventricular assist device group, the rate of adverse events overall was sizable. The incidence of major bleeding—including intracranial bleeding—was reported at 50%, and thromboembolic events were reported at 29%.[80]

Bacterial Endocarditis and Brain Abscess. Patients with palliated single-ventricle anatomy and patients with unrepaired ventricular septal defects (VSDs) have the highest documented risk of developing bacterial endocarditis. Endocarditis associated with rheumatic valve disease has become less common with widespread antibiotic treatment for group A streptococci infections.[84] Endocarditis is more likely to result in brain abscess when intracardiac shunt is present. Endocarditis with brain abscess before 2 years of age is still relatively uncommon in children with CHD in the developed world. However, brain abscess associated with CHD is far more prevalent in developing countries, where children with cyanotic cardiac defects often go unrepaired into school age. In this population, morbidity and mortality from endocarditis are correlated with the degree of hypoxia.[85] Most brain abscesses are identified on neuroimaging with a characteristic ring enhancement associated with surrounding cerebral edema.[86] Although they can be solitary, multiple lesions are found in up to 30% of cases, with the frontal lobe being the common site of infection.[86,87] A study in Taiwan found a relatively low in-hospital mortality rate for brain abscess of 4%.[88] However, another study in Turkey found that more than 50% of survivors had significant neurologic sequelae, including neuromotor deficits, seizures, and hydrocephalus.[89]

Perioperative Neurologic Injury

Perioperative neuroprotection is a field of study with more hypotheses than results, more opinions than facts, and more controversy than standard of practice. Centers of excellence have seen dramatic improvements in outcome with divergent practices that evolve without guiding evidence. Practices that have not been assessed by evidentiary standards are locked in place for fear of disrupting the unidentified elements that caused overall outcome improvement. This section focuses on perioperatively acquired neurologic injury and potentially modifiable aspects of neurodevelopmental outcome for children with CHD. For some of these aspects the quality of data is compelling (e.g., hemodilution and transfusion during CPB).

For some of these aspects the available data are either contradictory or leave room for debate (e.g., the use of deep hypothermic circulatory arrest [DHCA] or selective cerebral perfusion). It is reemphasized here that the primary lesion acquired in the perioperative period for newborns with CHD is WMI, which suggests a deficit of oxygen delivery. The link between WMI and neurodevelopmental delay is inferred, but the studies to assess this association have mixed results.[18,90,91]

Timing of Surgical Intervention

Longer delays to surgical palliation of critical heart disease in the newborn may increase the likelihood of neurologic injury—specifically WMI. Lynch et al. studied 37 neonates with HLHS. Eight patients suffered preoperative WMI, and 28 patients, or 76%, were found to have postoperative WMI. In that study larger volume of new or worsened WMI was associated with a delay greater than 4 days from birth to Norwood palliation.[92]

Petit el al. reported similar findings in patients with TGA. In that study 26 patients with TGA underwent preoperative and postoperative MRI scans. Ten patients were found to have preoperative WMI, and longer time to surgery was associated with presence of WMI on preoperative MRI. The WMI group underwent surgery at 5.6 ± 2.9 days compared to the no-WMI group, who were operated on at 3.9 ± 2.2 days ($P = .028$).[93]

A retrospective analysis of CHD patients undergoing both the arterial switch operation and the stage I repair for HLHS showed that timing of surgery was associated with outcome. For patients with TGA, surgical correction after day of life 3 was associated with increased rates of major morbidity and associated hospital costs.[94] For patients with HLHS, morbidity and hospital costs increases were associated with each day of life that surgery was delayed. The mortality rate in that cohort of 134 neonates with HLHS was 7.4%, and all deaths occurred in subjects operated on after day of life 4, with a median age at operation of 5 days.[95]

Deep Hypothermia and Blood Gas Management

Some degree of hypothermia is applied during CPB at most centers. For surgeries that require periods of time with permissive low-flow or absent-flow states, deep hypothermia is the mainstay of neuroprotection. Hypothermia reduces the metabolic rate of oxygen consumption in the brain. Neurovascular coupling dictates that reduced oxygen consumption concomitantly reduces cerebral blood flow. However, it has been shown that profound hypothermia causes a relative uncoupling of cerebral metabolism and flow, resulting in "luxury perfusion" (Fig. 17.7). In infants and children with CHD, Greeley et al. showed that although cerebral metabolism is reduced exponentially by hypothermia, cerebral blood flow is reduced linearly.[96,97] From these studies it was estimated that an infant in a state of deep hypothermia could tolerate between 39 and 65 minutes of circulatory arrest before developing an oxygen deficit that would lead to ischemic injury.[98]

During profound hypothermia, either pH-stat or alpha-stat blood gas measurements are used to account for the increased solubility and decreased partial pressure of carbon dioxide in blood. Both are used at centers with good outcomes. The alpha-stat approach seeks to adjust the P_aCO_2 to maintain the degree of ionization (alpha) of histidine imidazole groups. The pH-stat method seeks to adjust the P_aCO_2 to maintain pH at the temperature of the patient. Changes in P_aCO_2 solubility with temperature do not

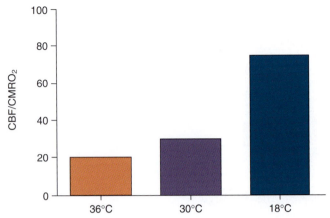

• **Figure 17.7** The ratio of cerebral blood flow (*CBF*) to cerebral oxygen metabolism (*CMRO₂*) increases with decreasing temperature in a state of profound hypothermia. Uncoupling of flow and metabolism during hypothermia results in a relative excess of CBF to metabolic need, termed *luxury perfusion*. (Kern FH, Greeley WJ, Duke RU. The effects of bypass on the developing brain. *Perfusion*. 1993;8[1]:49-54. Used with permission from Sage.)

change ionization of histidine but do change pH due to decreased partial pressure of P_aCO_2. Carbon dioxide diffuses freely across the blood-brain barrier to the cerebrospinal fluid, which has a bicarbonate buffer that is independent of serum buffers (and measurements). In contrast to the alpha-stat strategy, the pH-stat strategy *corrects for blood temperature*, results in *higher P_aCO_2, lower pH,* and *increased cerebral blood flow*.

It has been postulated that the "luxury flow" seen in deep hypothermia may be a consequence of a shift in the oxygen-hemoglobin dissociation curve that impairs oxygen unloading to brain tissue (hypoxic vasodilation).[99] Hypercarbia associated with the pH-stat strategy causes a shift in the oxygen-hemoglobin dissociation curve that facilitates oxygen unloading, in theory counteracting the effect of temperature on the oxygen-hemoglobin dissociation curve.[100] Increased cerebral blood flow with pH-stat management facilitates even cooling in the brain, and in animal models there is improved early metabolic recovery from deep hypothermia when compared with alpha-stat management.[101] A comparison of alpha-stat and pH-stat management in piglets showed improvements in both functional disability scores and histopathology when pH-stat was used.[102]

Studies comparing alpha-stat and pH-stat strategies in adults have shown a trend for improved neurocognitive outcome with alpha-stat management.[103] However, the results are not generalizable to the pediatric population in part due to gross differences in the etiology of neurologic injury: embolic lesions are most common in adults during bypass, and ischemic WMI is most common in pediatric patients. A prospective, randomized trial of alpha-stat versus pH-stat management in 182 infants and neonates under deep hypothermia (with and without circulatory arrest) showed no measurable difference in neurodevelopmental outcome.[104] However, subjects in the pH-stat group had more hemodynamic stability, earlier recovery of electroencephalographic activity, and a trend for fewer seizures, which were rare in both groups.[105] The early benefits seen in both clinical and animal models with the pH-stat strategy have not been shown to provide long-term benefit for neonates who require cardiac surgery.

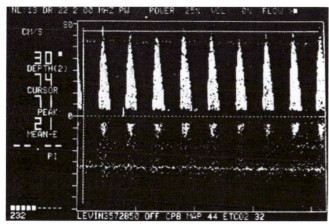

• **Figure 17.8** Flow velocity (FV) in the middle cerebral artery of a newborn after deep hypothermic circulatory arrest for repair of congenital heart disease. The pulsatility index is high ([systolic FV − diastolic FV]/mean FV), and there is no flow during diastole. This pattern is indicative of high cerebrovascular resistance. (From Jonassen AE, Quaegebeur JM, Young WL. Cerebral blood flow velocity in pediatric patients is reduced after cardiopulmonary bypass with profound hypothermia. *J Thorac Cardiovasc Surg.* 1995;110[4 Pt 1]:934-943. Used with permission.)

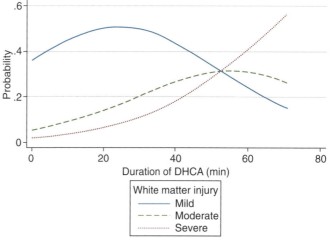

Assuming median values (CPB time of 191 min, brain maturation score 11, and no WMI before surgery)

• **Figure 17.9** The Hearts and Minds Study from Australia and New Zealand showed that longer circulatory arrest times are associated with increased severity of white matter injury in neonates who require cardiopulmonary bypass and cardiac surgery. *CPB,* Cardiopulmonary bypass; *DHCA,* deep hypothermic circulatory arrest; *WMI,* white matter injury. (Modified from Beca J, Gunn JK, Coleman L, et al. New white matter brain injury after infant heart surgery is associated with diagnostic group and the use of circulatory arrest. *Circulation.* 2013;127[9]:971-979. Used with permission.)

Deep Hypothermic Circulatory Arrest or Selective Cerebral Perfusion

When reconstruction of the aortic arch is required for neonatal cardiac surgery, as in the Norwood operation, interrupted arch repair, or arch advancement, optimal visualization cannot be achieved with normal bypass flows and a standard cannulation technique. Traditionally DHCA has been used to maintain a bloodless field and facilitate these surgeries. As described earlier, the reduced metabolism associated with deep hypothermia provides a window of time that is estimated to be between 39 and 65 minutes to perform the operation and reestablish bypass flow before ischemic injury occurs.[98] However, even when DHCA is restricted to 40 minutes, a characteristic pattern of cerebrovascular and metabolic disturbance has been observed in neonates, including (1) lowered cerebral metabolism that fails to return to baseline values after restoration of full flow, (2) decreased cerebral blood flow (with a normal CBF:$CMRO_2$ ratio), and (3) a transcranial Doppler flow pattern showing a high pulsatility index (elevated cerebrovascular resistance) and absent flow velocity in diastole (Fig. 17.8).[106-109] These disturbances may be mitigated by avoiding DHCA and using low-flow bypass, slower rewarming, pH-stat management during cooling, modified ultrafiltration, thromboxane A_2 antagonists, and nitric oxide donors.[107,110-114]

Does DHCA contribute to brain injury and neurodevelopmental abnormality in the neonate with CHD? The Hearts and Minds study conducted in Australia and New Zealand demonstrated that longer periods of DHCA were associated with increased severity of WMI (Fig. 17.9). However, that study of 122 neonates with CHD found no association between WMI and neurodevelopmental testing at 2 years. In a separate study at the Children's Hospital of Philadelphia, neurodevelopmental testing was done at 4 years' follow-up of 238 subjects after neonatal CHD repair. In that cohort there was no association between duration of DHCA and neurodevelopmental performance.[18,115] The Boston Circulatory Arrest Study randomized newborns with TGA to DHCA or low-flow bypass and showed, in 170 enrolled patients, that DHCA was associated with postoperative seizures and worse 12-month and 8-year neurodevelopmental testing. However, in the 139 subjects that were tested at age 16, the use of DHCA was not associated with abnormalities on neuropsychologic testing.[7,9,116,117] This study highlights the problem of measuring cause and effect between neonatal surgery and long-term outcome. At the time of mature neuropsychiatric testing the results are difficult to apply to current methodologies. Practice at the time of the Boston trial included hemodilution and profound anemia, which is now known to contribute to brain injury.

An alternative to DHCA is the use of selective cerebral perfusion, which has been called *antegrade cerebral perfusion* and *regional cerebral perfusion.* Variations in selective cerebral perfusion techniques achieve the end results of supporting normal cerebral blood flow while providing a bloodless surgical field at the aortic arch. At Texas Children's Hospital the technique includes the steps:

1. A polytetrafluoroethylene graft is sewn to the innominate artery (to subsequently become the Blalock-Taussig shunt if indicated) and cannulated for full bypass.
2. Transcranial Doppler measurements are made at deep hypothermia with full perfusion.
3. When selective perfusion is desired, the great vessels are snared at their aortic arch origins (Fig. 17.10).[118]
4. Bypass flow rates are increased from zero until the transcranial Doppler imaging shows the same flow velocities as full-body bypass with full-flow rates.[119]

Pressure monitoring of the right radial arterial line facilitates management of flow rates with selective perfusion cannulation because the right subclavian artery is open to pump flow, while the left subclavian is snared and pressurized across the circle of Willis, basilar artery, and left vertebral artery with retrograde flow.

Three studies have compared DHCA with selective cerebral perfusion. Visconti et al.[120] studied selective perfusion for the Norwood procedure against DHCA in 29 neonates without randomization. Neurodevelopmental scores at 1 year showed no

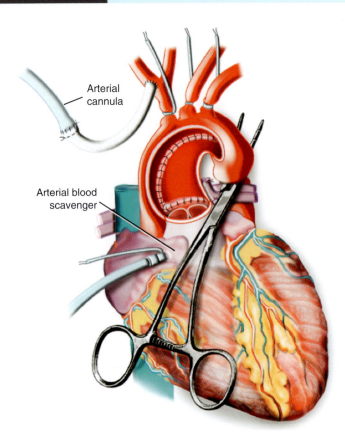

• **Figure 17.10** Selective cerebral perfusion is achieved by cannulation of a graft sewn to the innominate artery and snaring of the great vessels at the aortic arch origins. The aortic arch is in a bloodless field for optimal visualization while the brain can be perfused at normal perfusion pressures and cerebral blood flow rates. (From Pigula FA, Nemoto EM, Griffith BP, et al. Regional low-flow perfusion provides cerebral circulatory support during neonatal aortic arch reconstruction. *J Thorac Cardiovasc Surg.* 2000;119[2]:331-339. Used with permission.)

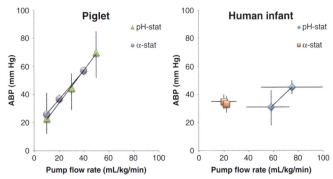

• **Figure 17.11** Arterial blood pressure *(ABP)* and bypass pump flow rates during selective cerebral perfusion. (Data from piglet studies showing similarities between alpha-stat and pH-stat management *[left]* are markedly different when compared to human studies. For the human infant under pH-stat management, a much higher pump flow rate is required to achieve the same cephalad arterial blood pressure.)

difference. Goldberg et al.[121] found the same result in a randomized cohort of 77 subjects. Another randomized trial of 37 neonates requiring arch construction showed a high rate of embolic brain injury ipsilateral to the cannulation site when selective perfusion was used, and more than 70% of new MRI injury in both groups.[122] These studies have both small sample sizes and higher than expected neurologic abnormalities in both groups. By contrast, a 57-subject observational cohort at Texas Children's Hospital, where selective perfusion is universally applied, had a 40% incidence of new injury, mostly WMI, and no evidence of unilateral embolic load.[90] A much larger cohort of 1250 subjects from Shanghai was studied to compare DHCA with selective perfusion.[123] In that study, without imaging or neurodevelopmental testing, gross neurologic abnormalities such as coma, seizure, choreoathetosis, and irritability were recorded and collectively found to be higher in the DHCA group.

There is no consensus among centers of excellence for the use of selective perfusion or DHCA for neonatal arch repair. Further, when selective perfusion is used, there are variations in the pump flow rates used, with published rates ranging from 10 to 100 mL/kg/min.[118,124] It is not known but seems improbable that pressure reactivity and autoregulation is possible in the cerebral vasculature when it is isolated from the rest of the systemic circulation. Regulation of cerebral blood flow requires shunting and stealing flow to and from noncerebral vascular beds when cerebral blood flow is

excessive or inadequate. Discontinuity with the rest of the systemic circulation may markedly narrow the range of tolerated pump flow rates, making choice of perfusion settings paramount.

Three studies have addressed this question with piglet bypass models.[125-127] These studies collectively suggest that pump flow rates between 20 and 30 mL/kg/min provide appropriate cephalad arterial blood pressure and cerebral blood flow without predisposing to hyperperfusion and brain edema. When alpha-stat is used for hypothermic blood gas management, the clinical experience shows similar pressures in newborns for the flow rates used in the piglet studies. However, when pH-stat is used, a much higher flow rate is required to achieve the same cephalad arterial blood pressure.[16,118,128-130] For the piglet studies, alpha-stat and pH-stat management resulted in the same optimization of flow rates (Fig. 17.11). These differences are possibly accounted for by the difference, piglet to human, in the ratio of cerebral to noncerebral tissue that is perfused by selective perfusion. Piglets have a 60-g brain and human neonates have a 450-g brain that vasodilates under pH-stat management. A monitoring-based approach with individual pump flow rates to optimize both flow velocity in the circle of Willis and arterial blood pressure has been advocated.[118]

Hemodilution and Transfusion During Cardiopulmonary Bypass

Historically, permissive anemia was standard of care during CPB to decrease blood viscosity during cooling. However, anemia during CPB is now a known risk of neurologic injury. Sakamoto et al.[131] showed an increased incidence of histologic brain injury in a piglet model of hypothermic circulatory arrest with a goal hematocrit of 20% versus 30%. This finding was further substantiated in a randomized study of 271 infants who had biventricular repair without aortic arch intervention randomized to different hematocrit goals during bypass. Neurodevelopmental testing at 1 year of life showed that the psychomotor development index increased with higher hematocrit up to 23.5%, but a plateau of the psychomotor development index was seen with hematocrit higher than 23.5%. (*P* < .001) There was no association found between the mental development index and hematocrit levels. Lower hematocrit levels were also associated with higher serum lactate levels and higher fluid balance postoperatively.[132] Although the ideal hematocrit for hemodilution is not clear, hematocrit below 24% is associated with abnormal neurodevelopment and should be avoided.

Glucose Management During Cardiopulmonary Bypass

Tight glycemic control has not been found to improve outcome in patients undergoing cardiac surgery.[23,133] Serum glucose level above 200 was not associated with worse neurodevelopmental scores in the Boston Circulatory Arrest Study (BCAS).[9,116] In a prospective trial of 171 neonates undergoing the arterial switch operation, hypoglycemia was associated with increased incidence of electroencephalographic seizures, but the intraoperative glucose level was not associated with worse neurodevelopmental outcomes at 1, 4, and 8 years of age.[134] In another study of postoperative glycemic level and neurodevelopment outcome in 188 patients undergoing cardiac surgery before 6 months of age, Ballweg et al. reported no association between postoperative hyperglycemia and neurodevelopmental outcome at 1 year of life.[135]

Intensive Care Unit Management of Low Cardiac Output Syndrome and Mechanical Ventilation

Numerous hemodynamic disturbances occur in the intensive care unit (ICU) after neonatal cardiac surgery that may cause or exacerbate CNS injury. Bassan et al.[136] has shown that the mechanisms of neurovascular regulation can be impaired after CPB when there are instabilities of arterial blood pressure or arterial blood gas levels. In addition, low cardiac output syndrome (LCOS)— a state of decreased cardiac output, perturbed systemic vascular resistance, and compromised oxygen delivery—is well documented and is predictable in the postoperative period after CPB.[137-139] Survival of LCOS and preservation of renal and visceral blood flow is dependent on reduction of afterload and systemic vascular resistance.[33,34,138] However, if this therapy lowers arterial blood pressure below the lower limit of autoregulation for the brain, then the brain is at risk of ischemic injury (see Figs. 17.2 and 17.4). Although there is limited data for LCOS causing neurologic injury, Galli et al.[13] have reported that profound postoperative hypotension is associated with WMI in postoperative MRI scans. Striking a balance between adequate afterload reduction and adequate arterial blood pressure is a delicate and nuanced aspect of ICU management of the neonate with CHD following surgery.

Evidence also suggests that suboptimal ventilation may contribute to neurologic injury. The mechanism of carbon dioxide reactivity can override metabolic and pressure autoregulation to reduce cerebral blood flow when hypocarbia is present. Samanta et al.[140,141] used computational intelligence techniques to identify prognostic factors for periventricular leukomalacia. In addition to low systolic and low diastolic blood pressure, hypocarbia (P_aCO_2 <34 mm Hg) featured prominently in the statistical model of prediction. Intentional hyperventilation is generally believed harmful in the postoperative setting, so these associative findings are not likely to be tested in randomized trial, but they do underscore the importance of appropriate mechanical ventilation when needed postoperatively.

Sedation and Intensive Care Unit Length of Stay

In the immediate postoperative period the risk of CNS injury may be increased when there is increased cerebral oxygen demand. Hyperthermia can lead to increased cerebral oxygen demand, and it has been found to be associated with neurologic injury after CPB in animal models.[142] When cooling is initiated in a child or infant, some degree of sedation is usually required. The long-term neurodevelopmental sequelae of anesthesia and sedation are a subject of vigorous investigation. Numerous studies have linked neuronal apoptosis with γ-aminobutyric acid receptor inhibition (benzodiazepines, barbiturates, volatile anesthetics, propofol) and N-methyl-D-aspartate glutamate receptor agonists (ketamine) when applied to the developing mammalian brain.[143-147] Because many anesthetic and sedative agents (with the exception of most opioids and dexmedetomidine) act on one of these receptors, there are growing concerns about the use of pediatric anesthesia and sedation. Nondefinitive clinical evidence thus far does not refute the animal studies. Observational and matched-sibling cohort studies in humans have linked anesthesia exposure, especially multiple exposures, and prolonged exposure to sedatives to long-term language and cognitive delays and learning disabilities.[143,148-150] Randomized trials of inhaled anesthetic exposure against regional anesthesia are imminent at this writing, but preliminary analysis has not yet confirmed the observational data that have been amassed.[151] Prolonged sedative exposure, sedation resistance, and sedation dependence contribute to increased ICU length of stay. Studies of long-term neurodevelopmental outcomes in patients with CHD consistently find ICU length of stay to be associated with poor developmental outcome, but it is difficult to account for the underlying instability that necessitates increased length of stay and isolate care patterns such as anesthetic exposure that associate with poor outcome.[7,117,152-154] Newburger et al.[155] showed that protracted length of stay is associated with lower verbal IQ, performance IQ, and math achievement even after controlling for medical factors that would increase length of stay, such as perfusion times, postoperative hypotension, and days of mechanical ventilation. As a counterpoint, the stress response after repair of neonatal congenital heart surgery is known to be mitigated by the appropriate use of analgesia and anesthesia. Anand et al.[156] showed decreased neurohormonal and metabolic responses to stress as well as improved survival in 30 neonates randomized to deep sedation (sufentanil) compared with 15 neonates who received lighter (halothane and morphine) anesthesia. As we await further clarification of the effects of anesthesia and sedation on the newborn brain, the goal of the authors is to strike a balance between adequate pain control and unnecessary oversedation to control the stress response but facilitate rapid transition through the perioperative period.[24]

Long-Term Neurodevelopmental Outcomes in Patients With Congenital Heart Disease

The remainder of the chapter will include a review of the most notable investigations of long-term neurodevelopmental outcomes in survivors of CHD repair. Most of these studies are single-center cohorts with some more recent multicenter trials. Together they provide our current understanding of the risk factors that contribute to low neurodevelopment performance in 30% to 40% of neonates who require newborn repair of CHD.

Boston Circulatory Arrest Study

The original long-term neurodevelopmental study of patients with CHD, the BCAS is a single-center cohort study of 170 neonatal patients with TGA who underwent the arterial switch operation between 1988 and 1992. Patients in the study were randomized to receive low-flow CPB or DHCA intraoperatively. The hematocrit goal was consistent with hemodilution and viscosity theories at that time: 20% while on CPB in the trial, with alpha-stat blood gas management. Repetitive neurodevelopmental testing was conducted at 12 months, 8 years, and 16 years.[7,9,117]

At 12 months of life, 155 patients were tested with Bayley Scales of Infant Development-I (Bayley-I). As a whole, their Mental Development Index (MDI) was 105 ± 15 (normal, 100 ± 15), and their Psychomotor Development Index (PDI) was 95.1 ± 15.5. Subjects who received DHCA had a lower PDI than those who received low-flow bypass ($P = .01$). Furthermore, in the DHCA group the scores on the PDI were inversely related to the duration of circulatory arrest ($P = .02$). There was no association between CPB support strategy and MDI or MRI abnormalities conducted at 12 months of life. However, postoperative seizure was associated with lower PDI on the Bayley scales ($P = .002$) and findings of MRI abnormalities ($P < .001$).[9]

At 8-year follow-up, subjects in the study had scores of 94.9 ± 14.3 on performance IQ, 99.8 ± 16.6 on verbal IQ, and 97.1 ± 15.3 on full-scale IQ. Although their overall academic performance was considered normal, more than one-third required remedial academic services, and approximate 10% had repeated a grade. There was no difference between the two treatment groups (DHCA or low-flow bypass) regarding full-scale or performance IQ scores or academic achievement. However, the DHCA group, specifically those with VSDs, had lower verbal IQ scores ($P = .04$), and this effect was seen for circulatory arrest times greater than 41 minutes (95% lower confidence limit, 32 minutes).[117]

At 16 years, 139 of the enrolled subjects returned for neurodevelopmental testing and brain MRI. More than two-thirds of the subjects had received some form of specialized education or behavioral services. Although most results of academic achievement, executive function, memory, visual-spatial, and social cognition testing did not differ between the two treatment groups, they were all below population norm. Additionally, postoperative seizures were associated with lower scoring across all measures. MRI abnormalities were not associated with test scores, but longer ICU length of stay and need for additional interventions after the arterial switch operation were associated with white matter abnormalities.[7]

The strength of the BCAS lies in its randomized and controlled intervention design, high rate of follow-up spanning 16 years, and a homogenous study population with a single lesion (TGA) absent other genetic abnormalities, requiring a single corrective surgical intervention. However, because the BCAS was initiated in the late 1980s, the results are the product of an earlier era of cardiac surgery, and thoughtful consideration should be given to generalizability to the current CHD population.

Children's Hospital of Philadelphia Study

The Children's Hospital of Philadelphia enrolled 550 neonates between 1998 and 2003 who underwent cardiac surgery before 6 months of life. The patients underwent neurodevelopmental follow-up at 1 and 4 years of age. In the first follow-up at 1 year, 359 infants underwent testing using the Bayley scales version II. Overall, MDI was 90 ± 15, and PDI was 78 ± 18. DHCA was not found to be associated with lower Bayley scores. Low birth weight, preoperative mechanical ventilation, lower hematocrit on CPB, and postoperative length of stay were associated with worse outcome.[51] At 4 years of life, 381 subjects returned for testing. Cardiac diagnosis of HLHS was associated with worse developmental outcome when compared to the diagnoses of TGA, VSD, and tetralogy of Fallot.[157] Gestation less than 39 weeks was associated with worse outcome, and the occurrence of postoperative seizure was associated with poor executive function and impaired social

behaviors.[157-159] Although DHCA was the only support strategy used for single-ventricle patients, over the entire cohort the use of DHCA was again not found to be associated with neurodevelopmental delays at 4 years of age.[115] The presence of a known or "suspected" genetic syndrome was associated with a worse developmental outcome in a graded fashion such that "known" was worse than "suspected," and "suspected" was worse than no syndrome.

Western Canadian Cohort

The Western Canadian Complex Pediatric Therapies Follow-Up Group collected data of neonates and infants who underwent cardiac surgery at less than 6 weeks of age. Two cohorts were included, the first from 1996 to 1999 and the second from 2003 to 2006. The Western Canadian Study included patients with both single and biventricular circulations. HLHS and TGA diagnoses made up one-third of the cohort each. The first reported cohort consisted of 85 subjects, with 67 surviving to Bayley-II testing at 18 to 24 months of age. The study cohort had a MDI of 84 ± 17 and PDI of 80 ± 22. By multivariable analysis, length of preoperative mechanical ventilation, time of CPB and DHCA, highest serum lactate level, acidosis, and chromosomal abnormalities were associated with worse developmental status on Bayley testing. Subjects with genetic abnormalities were included, and their Bayley scores were significantly lower.[160] A separate analysis of the 16 patients with 22q11.2 deletion (DiGeorge syndrome) against 16 matched patients without 22q11.2 deletion found that DiGeorge syndrome was associated with lower MDI and PDI ($P < .001$).[54] Guerra et al. investigated the later cohort for associations between opioid, benzodiazepine, chloral hydrate, ketamine, and volatile anesthetic exposure and neurodevelopmental outcomes at 18 to 24 months; 135 subjects were included with 116 survivors at the time of testing. Approximately 75% of subjects had biventricular repair, and the rest had HLHS. The overall cohort had mental and motor scores below developmental norms, with the majority within 1 standard deviation of normal. No associations were found between cumulative sedation exposure in the first 6 weeks of life and neurodevelopmental delays. However, days of mechanical ventilation, lowest PaO_2 in the first day post surgery, DHCA use, older age at surgery, and less maternal education were all associated with worse outcomes.[161]

Hearts and Minds Study

The Hearts and Minds Study enrolled 122 subjects from Australia and New Zealand. Patients who underwent cardiac surgery at less than 8 weeks of age were enrolled in a prospective longitudinal cohort study. Preoperative and postoperative MRI scans were obtained along with Bayley-III testing at 2 years of age. Approximately half of the cohort were single-ventricle patients, with the rest undergoing biventricular repair. The study investigated associations between WMI, cardiac diagnosis, surgical and CPB management, and neurodevelopmental outcome. Although DHCA and cardiac diagnosis were associated with WMI, the presence of WMI was not associated with worse Bayley-III scores. Brain immaturity and structural abnormalities were associated with worse neurodevelopmental outcomes.[18]

Milwaukee Cohort

Subjects with HLHS undergoing stage I Norwood palliation were monitored perioperatively with regional cerebral oxygen saturation (rSO$_2$) between 2002and 2005 by Hoffman et al.[162] at the Children's Hospital of Wisconsin. Neurodevelopmental testing was conducted at 4 to 5 years of life. Of 51 enrolled subjects, 21 (41%) completed neurodevelopmental testing. Lower rSO$_2$ (63.6 ± 8.1 versus 67.8 ± 8.1, P = .026) in the first 48 hours after cardiac surgery was associated with abnormal visual motor integration. The proposed cutoff for lower visual motor integration score was rSO$_2$ less than 55%.

Texas Children's Hospital Cohort

Andropoulos et al.[17,90,91,163] enrolled 93 neonatal subjects who required cardiac surgery before 30 days of life in two separate prospective studies between 2005 and 2011 at Texas Children's Hospital. Fifty-nine survivors (63%) were tested with the Bayley-III examination at 12 months of age. Overall, cognitive score was 102 ± 13.3, motor score was 89.6 ± 14.1, and language score was 87.8 ± 12.5. Longer duration of selective cerebral perfusion was not associated with lower Bayley scores. However, DHCA use, lower preoperative rSO$_2$, volatile anesthesia exposure, ICU length of stay, and chromosomal abnormalities were associated with lower Bayley-III test scores.

Single Ventricle Reconstruction Trial

The Single Ventricle Reconstruction Trial enrolled subjects with HLHS in a multicenter randomized controlled comparison of two different stage I Norwood palliations. Subjects were randomized to receive either the modified Blaylock-Taussig shunt or the Sano conduit. Neurodevelopmental assessment was conducted at 1 year; 314 patients from the cohort underwent Bayley-II testing. Their score was significantly lower than the population norm with mean MDI of 89 ± 18 and mean PDI of 74 ± 19. Multivariate analysis showed that surgery site, birth weight of less than 2.5 kg, duration of interstage, length of stay, and number of interstage complications were associated with lower PDI scores. Lower MDI scores were associated with genetic abnormalities, lower birth weight, days of mechanical ventilation, and number of interstage complications. The use of DCHA was not associated with worse Bayley scores.[164]

International Cardiac Collaborative on Neurodevelopment Cohort

The International Cardiac Collaborative on Neurodevelopment investigators collected Bayley-II test scores between 1996 and 2009 (some reported earlier in this chapter) from 23 centers for patients with CHD between 6 and 30 months of age. Over 1770 patients were included. Patients were evaluated at a mean age of 14.5 ± 3.7 months. Multivariate analysis found that genetic abnormalities, male gender, cardiac diagnosis, lower birth weight, need for ECMO or ventricular assist device, length of stay, and less maternal education were associated with worse Bayley scores. Another significant finding was that despite impressive improvements in survival, the MDI and PDI scores improved by only 0.4 points per year over the 14 years analyzed in the study.[165,166]

Summary

Survivors of CHD have high rates of neurodevelopmental abnormalities that leave room for the CHD care teams to improve care strategies. The greatest impediment to that effort has been our inability to delineate specific care practices that are (1) modifiable and (2) related to both brain injury and neurodevelopmental outcome. Nonmodifiable, social, and genetic factors dominate the findings of long-term studies in this population.

The most common acquired neonatal brain injury after repair of CHD is WMI, which implies a deficit of perfusion. The principles of cerebral perfusion are well delineated, and the neonate with CHD is fundamentally not aligned for optimization: The mammalian brain requires a minimal arterial pressure to maintain adequate perfusion, but the neonate will be more likely to survive cardiac surgery with afterload reduction. The mammalian brain has obligate requirements for continuous oxygen delivery, but the normal streaming of placental return to the brain is disrupted by left-sided outflow lesions. Persistent cyanosis and low diastolic pressure from shunted circulation are intuitively contributors to failure of cerebrovascular homeostasis, but these physiologic principles have not been clearly seen to contribute to the current state of neurodevelopmental outcome.

Profound divergences of practice exist between centers of excellence, such as the use of DHCA or selective perfusion, blood gas management, and anesthesia/sedation practices. These differences will continue to persist until evidence is available to demonstrate a clear link between practice, MRI-detectable injury, and neurodevelopmental outcome.

Selected References

A complete list of references is available at ExpertConsult.com.

16. Andropoulos DB, Hunter JV, Nelson DP, et al. Brain immaturity is associated with brain injury before and after neonatal cardiac surgery with high-flow bypass and cerebral oxygenation monitoring. *J Thorac Cardiovasc Surg.* 2010;139(3):543–556. doi:10.1016/j.jtcvs.2009.08.022.

23. Hirsch JC, Jacobs ML, Andropoulos D, et al. Protecting the infant brain during cardiac surgery: a systematic review. *Ann Thorac Surg.* 2012;94(4):1365–1373, discussion 1373. doi:10.1016/j.athoracsur.2012.05.135.

39. Fraser CD, Brady KM, Rhee CJ, et al. The frequency response of cerebral autoregulation. *J Appl Physiol.* 2013;115(1):52–56. doi:10.1152/japplphysiol.00068.2013.

95. Anderson BR, Ciarleglio AJ, Salavitabar A, Torres A, Bacha EA. Earlier stage 1 palliation is associated with better clinical outcomes and lower costs for neonates with hypoplastic left heart syndrome. *J Thorac Cardiovasc Surg.* 2015;149(1):205–210.e1. doi:10.1016/j.jtcvs.2014.07.094.

166. International Cardiac Collaborative on Neurodevelopment (ICCON) Investigators. Impact of Operative and Postoperative Factors on Neurodevelopmental Outcomes After Cardiac Operations. *Ann Thorac Surg.* 2016;102(3):843–849. doi:10.1016/j.athoracsur.2016.05.081.

18

Endocrine Function in Critical Heart Disease

ILIAS ILIOPOULOS, MD, FRCPCH, FRCPC, FAAP; CHRISTIN HUFF, MSN, CPNP-AC;
ERIC M. GRAHAM, MD

The role of the endocrine system in regulation of the stress response to cardiac surgery and postoperative recovery has been increasingly recognized over recent years. Evidence associating the magnitude of hormonal stress response to postoperative morbidity have led to efforts to suppress this response. As we will discuss later in this chapter, the results of this strategy have been conflicting. It has become increasingly appreciated that some of the hormonal alterations following cardiac surgery are adaptive and necessary. However, maladaptive responses that are likely to lead to unfavorable outcomes also exist and have been linked to the release of proinflammatory cytokines and activation of chemokine responses that in turn propagate endocrine and metabolic alterations.[1-3] Changes in plasma levels of catecholamine, thyroid-stimulating hormone (TSH), thyroid hormones, cortisol, vasopressin, insulin, growth hormone, and the renin-angiotensin-aldosterone axis have been documented as part of the hypermetabolic stress response to cardiac surgery and critical illness.

The most prominent hormonal response to cardiopulmonary bypass (CPB) in children, especially neonates, is the tremendous increase of endogenous catecholamines.[4] Surgical stress, pain, acidosis, lack of pulsatile flow, and relative ischemia have all been implicated as potential causes. Elevation of plasma epinephrine levels has been described in neonates after sternotomy and before initiation of CPB, after deep hypothermic circulatory arrest, at the end of the operation and 6, 12, and 24 hours postoperatively and has been associated with decreased survival. Norepinephrine levels, in some studies, appear to increase intraoperatively and normalize more quickly.[4] Both contribute to postoperative vasoconstriction and impaired cardiac function. Given that sympathetic activation plays a key role in mediation of the stress response, opioid use to achieve deep level of anesthesia and postoperative analgesia has been shown to attenuate the catecholamine surge and potentially decrease postoperative complications.[5]

Alterations in levels of TSH, thyroid hormones, and cortisol will be discussed later in detail. Briefly, children after cardiac surgery develop a nonthyroidal illness (sick euthyroid) syndrome (NTIS) with low thyroid hormone levels and inappropriately low or normal TSH levels.[6] Cortisol levels, if not confounded by the use of perioperative steroids, are elevated in most patients as a result of hypothalamic-pituitary-adrenal (HPA) axis activation and increased responsiveness of the adrenal cortex.[7] However, a significant minority of children after cardiac surgery have low baseline cortisol levels and an inadequate response relative to severity of illness.[8]

The release of vasopressin is also part of the stress response. Significant elevations of plasma vasopressin levels have been documented in children after CPB. However, recent reports have indicated that a small subgroup of patients have absolute or relative (for the severity of illness) vasopressin deficiency and if hypotensive, exhibit a favorable hemodynamic response to low-dose vasopressin (that will not cause vasoconstriction in healthy subjects).[9]

Similar to adults undergoing cardiac operations, plasma insulin concentration in children usually decreases during the initial stages of CPB and hypothermia, partly related to impaired splanchnic perfusion. Insulin levels frequently then increase at the end of the surgery and remain high for the first 24 postoperative hours.[4,10] However, this is associated with a decreased peripheral response to insulin and elevation of glucagon and growth hormone levels, with the net effect of transient postoperative hyperglycemia in the majority of cases.[4,2,11] Glucagon secretion is also proportional to the magnitude of insult, being markedly elevated after complex surgery. Indeed, it is very likely that the observed postoperative elevation in insulin levels is secondary to perioperative hyperglycemia rather than a primary stress response.[3,12] Notably, the insulin/glucagon molar ratio is decreased after cardiac surgery in children and can be viewed as the primary driver to postoperative hyperglycemia.[4]

Although many pediatric cardiac patients have elevated plasma aldosterone levels preoperatively related to fluid status and heart failure, aldosterone levels have been found to decrease below preoperative levels during the first 24 postoperative hours.[4] Conversely, brain natriuretic peptide (BNP) level commonly peaks 6 to 12 hours postoperatively, but the timing and magnitude of its elevation demonstrates age dependency. Neonates exhibit earlier peak and higher levels than older children. Perioperative BNP levels have been associated with morbidity and postoperative outcomes.[13] Higher BNP levels have been associated with longer ventilation time, duration of intensive care unit (ICU) stay, and higher inotropic needs.[14]

Summarizing, major catabolic stress responses under neuroendocrine axis control have been found in children undergoing cardiac surgery. Neonates are particularly affected due to the enhanced metabolic response to surgical stress and the maturational variation in endocrine function occurring in the first month of life.

Glycemic Control After Pediatric Cardiac Surgery

Transient hyperglycemia in children with previously normal glucose homeostasis is ubiquitous after cardiac surgery. The prevalence of blood glucose levels above 126 mg/dL is reported as high as 90% in some series.[15] Hyperglycemia in an individual patient resolves over time, and the majority of the hyperglycemic patients have normalized blood glucose levels within 24 to 48 hours after cardiac surgery.[10]

The etiology of critical illness–associated hyperglycemia is multifactorial. It involves both increased hepatic production of glucose (glycogenolysis and gluconeogenesis) and decreased peripheral utilization and so is part of the response to the severe physiologic stress of surgery and illness.[2-4,11,12] This response involves activation of the HPA axis, release of stress hormones such as cortisol, epinephrine, norepinephrine, glucagon, and adrenocorticotropic hormone (ACTH) and generation of proinflammatory cytokines (interleukin-6 [IL-6], IL-8, tumor necrosis factor-α) that are implicated in the development of peripheral resistance to insulin.[2,3,16] Furthermore, as indicated by low endogenous C-peptide production, primary beta-cell dysfunction with relative insulin deficiency relative to the degree of hyperglycemia has been documented in children with cardiorespiratory failure and can contribute to the development of hyperglycemia after cardiac surgery.[17]

Several retrospective studies have associated postoperative hyperglycemia after cardiac surgery with adverse clinical outcomes such as higher mortality, lactic acidosis, cardiac arrest, vasopressor use, and longer ventilation and ICU stay.[15,18] However, no evidence exists to date to associate hyperglycemia with adverse neurodevelopmental outcomes in children with cardiac disease.[19,20]

In a large two-center retrospective study of 378 children undergoing complex heart surgery, average (≥143 mg/dL) and peak early postoperative glucose levels (≥250 mg/dL) were independently associated with a composite outcome of morbidity and mortality.[21] In the same study the duration of hyperglycemia in the first 72 hours was associated with prolonged hospital stay. Similarly, low average glucose level (<109 mg/dL) and lower minimum glucose levels were also associated with higher odds of morbidity. The authors concluded that both hyperglycemia and hypoglycemia are associated with adverse outcomes, and the optimal blood glucose level in children after heart surgery might be between 110 and 126 mg/dL. Nevertheless, it appears that hyperglycemia and the odds of adverse outcome have a dose-dependent relationship. Increased duration and severity of hyperglycemia renders more likely an association with inadvertent outcomes.[15]

It is unclear whether hyperglycemia is a marker or a cause of adverse outcomes. In critically ill adult surgical patients, an initial single-center randomized controlled trial showed that tight glycemic control reduced morbidity and mortality, but subsequent trials have not shown benefit.[22,23] In children following cardiac surgery, three randomized clinical trials so far have attempted to investigate these associations and evaluate the effect of targeted glucose management. First, in a single-center trial of 700 critically ill children (75% after cardiac surgery), Vlasselaers et al.[24] showed that tight glycemic control (blood glucose level 50 to 80 mg/dL) led to reduction in inflammation and length of ICU stay. Although the study was not powered to determine differences in mortality, the tight control group had fewer deaths. The second trial to

discuss is the Safe Pediatric Euglycemia After Cardiac Surgery (SPECS) trial, which enrolled 980 children up to 3 years of age after cardiac surgery.[25] No differences existed between the tight glycemic (blood glucose 80 to 100 mg/dL) group and standard care group in the primary outcome (health care–associated infections) or secondary outcomes such as mortality, length of stay, or measures of organ failure. However, a secondary analysis of this trial indicated that tight glycemic control may lower the risk of infection in children older than 2 months at the time of cardiac surgery.[26] Finally, the Control of Hyperglycaemia in Paediatric Intensive Care (CHiP) trial, randomized 1369 critically ill children (60% after cardiac surgery) to tight (blood glucose level 72 to 126 mg/dL) or conventional glycemic control (blood glucose level <216 mg/dL).[27] No difference in mortality or other major clinical outcomes were found. In the noncardiac cohort, tight glycemic control led to decreased length and reduced cost of hospital stay. This benefit was not apparent in the children after cardiac surgery. Although it excluded patients after cardiac surgery, recently the Heart and Lung Failure—Pediatric Insulin Titration (HALF-PINT) trial that randomized children with cardiovascular or respiratory failure and confirmed hyperglycemia to a lower target (80 to 110 mg/dL) versus a higher target (150 to 180 mg/dL) of glycemic control was interrupted early due to lack of benefit and possibility of harm, given the higher incidence of catheter-associated infections and severe hypoglycemia in the lower target group.[28]

When used, the treatment of hyperglycemia in critically ill children is with regular insulin. Insulin acts on liver receptors to inhibit hepatic glucose production and synthesis of fatty acids and on peripheral tissues (muscle and adipose tissue) to stimulate the uptake and metabolism of glucose. It also has an anabolic effect through increased synthesis and decreased breakdown of protein and decreased lipolysis.

Insulin treatment in the pediatric cardiac ICU (CICU) setting is usually in the form of a continuous intravenous infusion at a dose of 0.01 to 0.1 units/kg/h. Subcutaneous intermittent injections are used less frequently due to variable bioavailability depending on preparation used and perfusion of injection site. Regular IV insulin has a half-life of 5 to 15 minutes and will reach a steady state by approximately 45 to 60 minutes. Insulin metabolism takes place mainly in the liver (50%) but also in the kidneys (30%) and peripheral tissues (20%).[29]

The major adverse effect of insulin treatment is hypoglycemia with its associated concerns regarding deleterious effects to brain and neurodevelopment. The study by Vlasselaers et al.[24] had a very high incidence of hypoglycemia (25%) but did not demonstrate a difference in neurodevelopment between the two groups. However, children were followed up at an older age (4 years) with no information regarding early neurodevelopment.[30] In the CHiP trial, severe hypoglycemia occurred in only 1.5% of the conventional treatment group, but its incidence increased to 7.3% in the tight control group.[27] Furthermore, in the subgroup of patients after cardiac surgery, patients who had at least one hypoglycemic episode had a higher rate of mortality compared to those with no hypoglycemia. This is consistent with data from critically ill adults that associate hypoglycemia during intensive glycemic control with mortality.[31] In the SPECS trial the incidence of severe hypoglycemia was 3% in the glycemic control group compared to 1% in the standard care group.[25] This study showed that safe insulin therapy can be achieved with a novel continuous glucose monitoring system and an explicit insulin infusion algorithm. Follow-up of this study indicated that, although tight glycemic control did not offer any measurable neurodevelopmental benefit at 1 year of age, moderate and severe hypoglycemia were associated with worse functioning in the cognitive, language, and motor domains.[32]

Summarizing, the current evidence does not support tight glycemic control in children after cardiac surgery. Given reported benefits in critically ill children without cardiac disease and apparent positive effects in some cardiac studies, it is plausible that tight glycemic control might be beneficial in a subgroup of children after cardiac surgery. Identification of this speculative cohort is currently elusive. Emerging evidence on metabolic, inflammatory, and biomarker profiling that can be used to identify cases in which the perioperative inflammatory and metabolic responses are suggestive of adverse clinical outcomes could be potentially useful to this direction. However, at present, a strategy of tight glycemic control cannot be recommended in children after cardiac surgery.

Thyroid Disease and Thyroid Hormone Therapy After Cardiac Surgery

Thyroid hormone production is regulated by a loop mechanism involving the hypothalamus, hypophysis, and thyroid gland. Hypothalamic thyrotropin-releasing hormone (TRH) stimulates secretion of TSH by the anterior hypophysis, which in turn promotes synthesis of thyroxine (T_4) and triiodothyronine (T_3) by the thyroid gland through iodination of the tyrosine residues into thyroglobulin.[33] Circulating thyroid hormones (plasma free and bound to thyroid-binding globulin, transthyretin, and albumin) exert negative feedback on the release of TSH and TRH.[33] T_3 is secreted directly by the thyroid gland (20%) and also produced in the liver and peripheral tissue (80%) by deiodination of T_4, which can be considered a prohormone for T_3.[33]

Thyroid hormones bind to receptor proteins in the cell nucleus and have a number of physiologic effects, including brain development, bone maturation through influence on calcium and phosphorus metabolism, and increase of basal metabolic rate. T_3 promotes protein synthesis and affects carbohydrate, lipid, and vitamin metabolism. On the cardiovascular system, thyroid hormones increase contractility, chronotropy, and oxygen consumption and decrease systemic vascular resistance.[34] Thyroid hormones also influence calcium transport pathways through the cell membrane and sarcoplasmic reticulum in cardiac myocytes. T_3 is also a nuclear transcription factor and contributes to upregulation and downregulation of genes important for cardiac contractility. The consequent end-organ effects depend on circulating levels of active T_3 and thyroid receptor occupancy.[35]

Children with congenital hypothyroidism have been found to have up to 10-fold higher incidence of congenital heart disease (5.5% to 8%) compared to the general population.[36] Therefore newborns with elevated TSH level on screening should be examined carefully for cardiac malformations in addition to confirmatory thyroid function testing. In the CICU environment, exposure to iodine, such as during cardiac angiography with iodinated contrast or iodine-containing antiseptics, has been implicated in developing hypothyroidism (Wolff-Chiakoff effect).[37] This is characterized by high TSH level and low/normal T_4 level, and it is distinct to the sick euthyroid syndrome induced by CPB, although it may play a contributory role in postoperative thyroid hormone changes. However, other studies have indicated that use of povidone-iodine irrigation in cases of delayed sternal closure is not associated with abnormalities in thyroid function.[38] Data are insufficient at present to advise on the need for thyroid function testing after

cardiac angiography or prolonged exposure to iodine-containing antiseptics.

CPB induces thyroid hormone level alterations that exhibit features similar to sick euthyroid syndrome (or NTIS) seen during critical illness: an initial surge of free thyroid hormones is followed by marked and persistent decrease of circulating T_3 (total and unbound) with an inappropriately normal or low TSH level.[6] This is due to impaired deiodination from T_4 to T_3 in the peripheral tissues, in addition to blood dilution and central inhibition of the HPA axis induced by nonpulsatile flow. An increase in biologically inactive reverse T_3 is also noted. Inflammatory cytokine levels such as IL-6, macrophage inhibitory factor, and IL-8 have been linked to the development of these abnormalities.[39] In severe cases T_4 level is also decreased. Low thyroid-binding globulin levels can further influence the metabolism of T_4. The nadir is seen at 24 to 48 hours, and recovery starts with a rise in TSH level within 1 to 2 weeks, although very sick patients can exhibit slower recovery. Suboptimal nutrition can delay the recovery of thyroid function. The NTIS syndrome changes have been correlated with increased severity of illness. Total and free T_3 levels and, even more, T_3 uptake have been suggested as the best predictors of postoperative clinical course.[40]

Given the association of thyroid hormone deficiencies with unfavorable clinical outcomes, exogenous thyroid hormone administration to correct postoperative deficiencies and restore thyroid hormone homeostasis has been proposed. This strategy has been shown to offer a dose-dependent benefit in cardiac output and improved outcomes in adults undergoing open heart surgery.[41] In children, five randomized controlled trials have attempted to date to investigate the effect of thyroid hormone therapy after cardiac surgery.

First, Portman et al.[42] evaluated a small group of 14 infants after tetralogy of Fallot or ventricular septal defect repair. The treatment group received a bolus of T_3 (0.4 mg/kg) before CPB and at myocardial reperfusion. The treatment group, although found to have similar low T_4 levels to the control group, maintained free and total T_3 levels at prebypass values for 24 hours and higher than the control group for 72 hours. However, there was no difference in inotropic requirements between the groups. Heart rate was transiently elevated and peak pressure-rate product increased after 6 hours in the treatment group. This finding correlated with the peak T_3 levels in the treatment group. The authors concluded that T_3 therapy corrects T_3 deficiencies and implied that it improves myocardial oxygen consumption and possibly enhances cardiac function reserve in infants after CPB.

In a randomized, double-blind, placebo-controlled trial, Bettendorf et al.[43] evaluated 40 children after cardiac surgery with CPB. The treatment group was given a daily infusion of T_3 (2 mg/kg on postoperative day 1 and 1 mg/kg on subsequent days) for 12 days. Both groups were found to have low postoperative plasma concentration of thyrotropin, T_4, free T_4 and T_3, and elevated levels of reverse T_3. Treatment with T_3 raised T_3 plasma concentration without affecting postoperative recovery of thyroid function. Furthermore, patients in the treatment group demonstrated increased cardiac index (as assessed by Doppler echocardiography) and had a lower mean therapeutic intervention score than patients treated with placebo. The improvement in cardiac function was more pronounced in patients who had longer operations and duration of CPB. No adverse effects with respect to heart rhythm or rate were associated with thyroid repletion.

Subsequently, Chowdhury et al.[44] evaluated postoperative serum total T_3 levels in 75 children after cardiac surgery. Patients in their cohort who had T_3 below a prespecified level (<40 ng/dL and <60 ng/dL in neonates) and were mechanically ventilated (n = 28) were randomized to either continuous T_3 infusion or placebo. The continuous T_3 infusion dose (0.05 to 0.15 mcg/kg/h) was titrated to maintain serum levels between 80 and 200 ng/dL. Overall, no differences were found between treatment and control group in inotropic score, mechanical ventilation, or hospital stay. However, in the small subgroup of nine neonates (five treated, four controls) the overall postoperative management requirements (as analyzed by Therapeutic Intervention Scoring System [TISS] score) and inotropic score were lower in the T_3-treated group. Furthermore, in the T_3-treated group of neonates, mixed venous oxygen saturation increased by 17% between 18 and 24 postoperative hours versus only 2% in the nontreated group, albeit this difference did not reach statistical significance. No adverse effects were noted with T_3 treatment on heart rate, blood pressure, or arrhythmias.

Mackie et al.[45] randomized 42 neonates after aortic arch reconstruction (Norwood operation or biventricular repair of interrupted aortic arch and ventricular septal defect) to receive either a continuous infusion of T_3 (0.05 mcg/kg/h) or placebo for 72 hours. Primary outcome was a composite clinical outcome score (based on time to negative fluid balance, sternal closure, and extubation) and cardiac index at 48 hours. No differences were found in cardiac index, time to sternal closure, and extubation, but T_3-treated neonates more rapidly achieved negative fluid balance, obtaining a favorable composite clinical outcome score compared to controls. No serious adverse effects were attributed to T_3 therapy.

Recently the results of Triiodothyronine Supplementation in Infants and Children Undergoing Cardiopulmonary Bypass (TRICC) trial were reported. This was a multicenter, randomized, double-blind, placebo-controlled trial that evaluated 193 children less than 2 years of age after cardiac surgery.[46] There was no difference in the primary outcome (time to extubation) between treatment (T_3 0.4/kg bolus immediately before CPB and on the release of the aortic clamp followed by 0.2/kg bolus at 3, 6, and 9 hours after cross-clamp release) and placebo group. Overall, no difference in time to extubation and inotropic scores between T_3-treated and placebo group was found. Again, treatment with T_3 was considered safe with no difference in adverse events between groups. In a prespecified secondary analysis, response to thyroid treatment was found to be age specific. In particular, patients less than 5 months of age demonstrated a significant shortening in the time to achieve extubation (primary outcome), whereas older patients had a small but statistically significant delay. Furthermore, the younger cohort showed reduced inotropic requirements and improvement in cardiac function as evaluated by echocardiography.

Thyroid replacement therapy in the CICU setting usually takes place in the form of intravenous T_3 therapy.[29] Regimens that have been used include continuous infusion at 0.05 to 0.15 mcg/kg/h to maintain serum levels within 80 to 200 ng/dL or bolus therapy with 0.4 mg/kg at initiation and termination of CPB and followed by 0.2 mg/kg every 3 hours for another three doses (hour 3, 6, and 9 after completion of CPB). The half-life of intravenous T_3 is approximately 7 hours in children but considerably longer (up to 16 hours) in infants.[46] Oral T_3 administered at a dose of 0.5 mcg/kg every 12 hours has been shown to prevent the decline in T_3 levels that typically occurs after pediatric cardiac surgery.[47] The oral form is inexpensive and more widely available, but it remains unclear if normalization of T_3 levels affects clinical outcomes. Furthermore, concerns relating to absorption in cases

of impaired splanchnic perfusion due to low cardiac output or use of vasoactive medications will need to be addressed in future studies.

Summarizing, children after cardiac surgery typically develop a nonthyroidal illness (sick euthyroid) syndrome, which can occasionally be clinically important. It is still unclear if this response is adaptive or maladaptive, contributing to severity of illness and organ dysfunction. Given the unclear benefit of the T_3 supplementation therapy in the aforementioned studies, one can argue that severe illness causes severe NTIS and not vice versa. Although T_3 treatment in this setting appears safe, its clinical efficacy has not been proven in the entire cohort of children after cardiac surgery. Subgroups such as neonates and young infants are more likely to be benefited, but the evidence is not yet conclusive. Therefore data are not currently sufficient to support the routine use of T_3 supplementation in children after cardiac surgery.

Calcium Homeostasis and Hypocalcemia in Cardiac Surgery Patients

Calcium (Ca^{+2}) is an essential element in myocardial contractility.[48] Intracellular calcium concentration determines the tension developed in the plateau phase of contraction and thus is proportional to contractility. The amount of intracellular Ca^{+2} is determined by the amount of calcium released by the sarcoplasmic reticulum and the Ca^{+2} current influx during the plateau phase.

Hypocalcemia is not uncommon in the critical care setting. The cause of hypocalcemia is usually associated with a disturbance in the parathyroid hormone (PTH)–vitamin D response pathway or their end organs—kidneys, intestine, and bones. PTH increases serum calcium level and decreases serum phosphorous level, whereas vitamin D increases both calcium and phosphorous level. Therefore hypocalcemia can be caused by either decreased levels or resistance to PTH and/or vitamin D, inadequate absorption of calcium in the gastrointestinal tract, kidney failure, or changes in bone deposition of ionized calcium. Frequently seen in the ICU environment, causes of hypocalcemia include loop diuretics that enhance kidney calcium excretion and blood transfusion due to calcium chelation by citrate, which is used as a blood preservative.[48] In the neonatal period, causes of hypocalcemia also include intrauterine growth restriction, diabetic mother, and perinatal stress. These conditions can exacerbate the transient "early neonatal hypocalcemia" that occurs in the first 2 to 4 days of life due to physiologic transient deficiency of PTH. Hypomagnesemia frequently occurs with hypocalcemia and must be looked for, especially in cases that are difficult to manage. Magnesium is important for cyclic adenosine monophosphate production in the parathyroid, a second messenger needed for release and end-organ responsiveness to PTH. Ionized calcium is altered based on available albumin as well as plasma acid-base status. Alkalosis increases the affinity of calcium to albumin and therefore decreases ionized calcium levels.[49]

As mentioned, PTH plays an important role in regulation of calcium homeostasis. A decrease in serum ionized calcium concentrations causes secretion of PTH from the parathyroid gland. PTH then causes an increase in serum calcium through increase in bone reabsorption, increase in intestinal absorption, and renal reabsorption of calcium (alongside a decrease in renal phosphate reabsorption). Hypoparathyroidism and hypocalcemia is commonly seen in genetic syndromes associated with chromosomal deletions at the 22q11 locus such as DiGeorge syndrome. DiGeorge syndrome occurs in

1 of every 4000 births and is associated with conotruncal malformations; therefore a high percentage of neonates with DiGeorge syndrome are admitted to CICUs.[50] Neonatal hypocalcemia in the preoperative or postoperative setting can be the first presentation of hypoparathyroidism in patients with 22q11 deletion. Genetic testing for 22q11 should therefore be considered for patients with persistent hypocalcemia.

Hypocalcemia can be defined using total serum calcium (tCa^{+2}) or ionized calcium (iCa^{+2}) level. Given that iCa^{+2} is the biologically active form and total calcium levels have been shown to not be predictive of ionized calcium, current practice in most CICUs is based on maintaining iCa^{+2} levels within normal range.

Signs and symptoms of hypocalcemia in the first week of life include apnea, laryngospasm and stridor, jitteriness, tremors, muscle spasms, tetany, and seizures. Untreated severe hypocalcemia in the critically ill child can lead to hypotension, conduction abnormalities, or life-threatening arrhythmias secondary to QT interval prolongation. Later in life, additional symptoms and signs such as lethargy, feeding intolerance, abdominal distention, and bone demineralization (radiographic evidence of rickets may exist) with fractures and elevated alkaline phosphatase level can be seen. Occasionally hypocalcemia is asymptomatic.

Acute treatment of symptomatic hypocalcemia consists of intravenous administration of a calcium infusion usually as 10% calcium chloride (10 to 20 mg/kg) or 10% calcium gluconate (100 to 200 mg/kg). Calcium chloride is thought to result in a greater and faster increase in ionized calcium level (does not require first-pass metabolism in the liver) and may be preferred in critically ill children, whereas calcium gluconate is less irritating to the vein and a better option if only peripheral venous access is available. Calcium can be administered as a bolus over minutes in emergencies or a slow infusion over 2 to 4 hours. Calcium extravasation is very caustic, resulting in destructive tissue injury; therefore calcium is always given through a central venous line (unless in a life-threatening emergency). Attention should also be given to correction of any coexistent hypomagnesemia and hyperphosphatemia. If the product of total serum calcium (mg/L) and serum phosphorus (mg/dL) levels exceeds 80, there is risk of tissue deposition of calcium. In such cases, correction of hyperphosphatemia with phosphate binders should be considered.

In addition to correcting hypocalcemia, calcium chloride infusions have been used as an inotropic adjunct based on the physiologic importance of calcium homeostasis, especially in the neonatal myocardium.[48] However, literature support for this practice is scarce. Hypocalcemia is associated with hypotension and myocardial dysfunction.[51] Dyke et al.[52] demonstrated that patients with severe hypocalcemia requiring increased calcium supplementation in the postoperative period had increased morbidity and mortality. Recently a retrospective review of pediatric cardiac surgery patients who received calcium chloride infusions postoperatively showed an improvement in arterial–mixed venous oxygen saturation difference and decrease in serum lactate level after initiation of calcium chloride therapy.[53] The neonatal subgroup seemed to benefit the most in this study, presumably for reasons related to the immature nature of the neonatal sarcoplasmic reticulum. An attractive feature of calcium chloride therapy is the presumed hemodynamic benefit in the absence of chronotropic effect that potentially minimizes the metabolic demand associated with traditional inotropes. Nevertheless, further studies are required. Despite the physiologic intuition that may justify calcium infusion in patients with myocardial dysfunction, data are insufficient at present to allow an evidence-based recommendation.

Critical Illness–Related Corticosteroid Insufficiency and Steroid Replacement Therapy

The HPA axis plays an essential role in the human body's maintenance of homeostasis and response to stress. This axis involves a pathway of hormones that are activated in response to a variety of stimuli, including infection, trauma, burns, illness, and surgery.[53] The hypothalamus releases corticotropin-releasing hormone, which leads to the release of ACTH by the pituitary. ACTH leads to the synthesis and release of the primary effector glucocorticoid, cortisol, from the adrenal glands. Cortisol has a myriad of downstream effects important to the response to stress and maintenance of homeostasis, including vascular responsiveness to catecholamines, suppression of inflammatory and immune responses, and gluconeogenesis. Cortisol is roughly 90% bound to corticosteroid-binding globulin, and 5% to albumin, so that only 5% is present in the biologically active form, free cortisol. Both corticotropin-releasing hormone and ACTH are subject to negative feedback control by cortisol and exogenous corticosteroid administration.

Adrenal Insufficiency

Acute adrenal insufficiency is a life-threatening event that manifests when the adrenal cortex fails to produce enough steroids in response to metabolic stress. In the majority of cases it remains challenging to recognize adrenal insufficiency in a patient in the CICU. Important clinical signs are hemodynamic instability despite adequate fluid resuscitation and vasopressor and inotropic support. In primary adrenal insufficiency both glucocorticoid and mineralocorticoid properties are affected due to an intrinsic defect in the adrenal gland. In secondary adrenal insufficiency there is a failure of ACTH release or action resulting in insufficient glucocorticoid production. Mineralocorticoid release from the adrenal gland is primarily driven by the renin-angiotensin-aldosterone system and not ACTH, and therefore mineralocorticoid function is preserved in secondary adrenal insufficiency. Exogenous administration of corticosteroids is a common cause of secondary adrenal insufficiency in the CICU.

Challenges of Defining Adrenal Insufficiency in Critical Illness

Diagnosis of adrenal insufficiency is dependent on the demonstration of an inappropriately low level of cortisol in the blood. Classically this is best demonstrated on a plasma cortisol level measured at 8 a.m., although this is often unrealistic in the CICU given the loss of diurnal rhythm and confounding factors during critical illness. Adrenal responsiveness can be evaluated by the ACTH-stimulation test, which assesses the response of cortisol level to an exogenous dose of ACTH. Challenges for defining adrenal insufficiency in the critical care setting are many.[7] There is variation in the ACTH dose used in ACTH-stimulation tests: the "standard" test uses 125 to 250 mcg, whereas a "low-dose" test uses 1 mcg. There is also disagreement regarding what change in cortisol level from baseline constitutes an appropriate response during critical illness (>9 or >18 mcg/dL) and at what time to measure the response (30 or 60 minutes following ACTH stimulation). Finally, it is unclear whether total cortisol or the biologically active form free cortisol levels more accurately reflect the integrity of the HPA axis. Despite these diagnostic challenges the concept of relative adrenal insufficiency, referred to as *critical illness–related corticosteroid insufficiency* (CIRCI), is used to describe the patient who fails to mount an appropriate glucocorticoid response for the severity of illness.[54] Although the diagnostic criteria remain controversial, the clinical phenotype is characterized by hemodynamic instability despite adequate fluid resuscitation and vasopressor and inotropic support. The challenges of determining adrenal insufficiency are further amplified when cardiac surgery and CPB are confounders. Several studies have demonstrated that levels of cortisol (both total and free) and ACTH decrease significantly after CPB.[55-58] However, these have been confounded by the use of preoperative or intraoperative steroids. In contrast, a previous study examining postoperative cortisol levels with no preoperative steroid exposure found that both cortisol and ACTH increased post CPB.[59] Further uncertainty exists because some investigators have demonstrated that reduced cortisol metabolism contributes to hypercortisolemia and hence ACTH suppression, and therefore exogenous steroid supplementation may not be indicated.[60]

Steroid Therapy in the Cardiac Intensive Care Unit

Over the last 10 years there has been a myriad of studies on the effects of the adrenal axis and steroids in children with congenital heart defects. Several of the studies have been prospective randomized controlled trials[55,61-64] Despite this, the role of perioperative steroids remains anything but clear, in part due to wide variations among the studies. The variations have included the study population (age, complexity), steroid regimen (prophylactic versus targeted), timing of administration (preoperative, anesthesia induction, CPB prime, postoperative), as well as steroid type, dosing, and route. As a consequence, many questions in this area remain unanswered.

Steroid Supplementation for Refractory Hypotension

Evidence to support targeted corticosteroid use in critically ill children with congenital heart disease is limited. Several small retrospective studies have demonstrated that steroid therapy when administered selectively to surgical and nonsurgical patients with catecholamine resistant hypotension improves hemodynamics while reducing inotropic requirements.[65-68] Millar and colleagues[66] undertook a retrospective review of 51 children in their CICU who received steroids for hypotension in an attempt to identify predicators of a hemodynamic response. For the group as a whole, in the 24 hours following initiation of steroid treatment there was a significant increase in mean blood pressure, heart rate decreased, the volume of fluid infused decreased, urine output increased, and inotrope score declined. A hemodynamic response to steroids as defined by an increase in mean blood pressure of greater than 20% without an increase in inotrope score was seen in 41%. However, they were unable to identify any variable predictive of a hemodynamic response, including cortisol level.

Prophylactic Steroid Infusions in the Postoperative Period

Given the challenges of diagnosing adrenal insufficiency in the critically ill child, especially after CPB, and the potential benefits

of exogenous steroids irrespective of the integrity of the HPA axis, some investigators have advocated for prophylactic steroid infusions. Ando et al.[55] randomized 20 neonates undergoing biventricular repair to a postoperative 7-day continuous hydrocortisone infusion or placebo to determine if adrenal insufficiency exists after CPB. As such it was not powered to detect clinical outcomes, but they found steroid treatment was associated with some clinical improvements. It was also noted that the placebo group had low cortisol levels in the first 24 to 72 hours following surgery, although both groups received methylprednisolone at the induction of anesthesia. Robert and colleagues[64] performed a double-blind randomized controlled trial of postoperative hydrocortisone versus placebo in 40 infants undergoing cardiac operations with CPB to determine if prophylactic hydrocortisone could decrease the incidence of low cardiac output syndrome (LCOS). The main findings of the study were that a prophylactic 5-day continuous infusion of hydrocortisone reduced the incidence of LCOS, improved fluid balance and urine output, and attenuated inflammation after CPB compared to placebo. Despite these improvements there was no difference between groups in duration of mechanical ventilation and ICU or hospital stay. As we continue to explore the post-CPB inflammatory cascade and its contribution to alterations in the HPA axis and complicating postoperative recovery, we must remain cognizant of both the risk and benefits of steroids.[69-71] Although some studies demonstrate an improvement in hemodynamic parameters and inflammatory markers with perioperative steroids, these findings are not universal, and no study has demonstrated marked improvements in significantly meaningful outcomes such as length of stay, survival, or neurodevelopmental outcomes.

In summary, although many children in the CICU have evidence of altered adrenal function, no laboratory parameter has consistently been demonstrated to either predict a response to exogenous steroid administration or correlate with clinical outcomes. In patients with postoperative catecholamine-resistant hypotension, selective, targeted steroid therapy can be effective, regardless of cortisol levels. However, a blood test or assay to predict which patients might benefit from prophylactic or targeted steroid supplementation remains elusive.

Conclusion

Children after cardiac surgery exhibit a significant neuroendocrine response, consisting of sympathetic nervous activation, release of proinflammatory cytokines, and hormonal imbalances with potential of metabolic decompensation. Its magnitude has been associated with severity of illness and unfavorable outcomes. Despite initial enthusiasm, attempts to restore normal hormonal homeostasis by exogenous administration of deficient hormones have not been conclusively shown to modify outcomes. It is plausible that response to such therapies is not universal and further efforts are needed to identify the subgroups of patients who are likely to be benefited.

References

A complete list of references is available at ExpertConsult.com.

19

Pharmacology of Cardiovascular Drugs

DAVID E. PROCACCINI, PHARMD; JACLYN E. SAWYER, PHARMD; KEVIN M. WATT, MD, PHD

The triad of preload, afterload, and inotropic state of the heart determines stroke volume, which together with heart rate, determines cardiac output. The parasympathetic and sympathetic nervous systems regulate cardiac inotropy (contractility), chronotropy (heart rate), and lusitropy (myocardial relaxation). An understanding of the anatomy, physiology, and molecular biology of the sympathetic and parasympathetic nervous systems forms the basis of pharmacologic manipulation of the cardiovascular system. This chapter presents basic principles and clinical applications of medicinal therapies used to optimize cardiac output and systemic perfusion. Antiarrhythmic drugs are presented in Chapter 27. Medications for treatment of pulmonary hypertension are presented in Chapter 71.

Autonomic Control of the Cardiovascular System

Sympathetic (Adrenergic) Control

Sympathetic Neuroanatomy. Autonomic control of the cardiovascular system is determined by the sympathetic and parasympathetic inputs. The cell bodies of the preganglionic sympathetic neurons are located in the anterolateral gray matter of the spinal cord from T1 to L3. Preganglionic axons synapse with postganglionic neurons at sympathetic ganglia, which are collected into two paravertebral chains, three abdominal prevertebral ganglia (celiac, superior mesenteric, and inferior mesenteric ganglia), and left and right cervical ganglia (inferior, middle, and superior cervical ganglia) (Fig. 19.1).

The sympathetic nervous system also directly innervates the adrenal gland and controls the release of the catecholamines epinephrine and norepinephrine. Innervation occurs via preganglionic fibers that travel through the sympathetic chain, exit via the splanchnic nerve, pass through the celiac ganglion without synapsing, and directly innervate the adrenal medullary cells. During sympathetic stimulation, acetylcholine is released by the preganglionic fibers, resulting in the opening of calcium-mediated channels on the cell membranes.[1,2] These calcium channels then modulate the exocytosis of granules containing epinephrine and norepinephrine. Epinephrine and norepinephrine then travel through the systemic circulation, where they act on adrenoreceptors throughout the body.

Adrenoreceptors. Endogenous neurohormones (e.g., epinephrine and norepinephrine) and exogenous adrenergic drugs exert their cardiovascular effects by combining with adrenergic receptors in the heart and vasculature. Although genes for at least nine distinct adrenoreceptor subclasses have been identified and cloned,[3-5] the clinical pharmacology of adrenergic drugs is still largely based on the four classic receptor subtypes: alpha₁, alpha₂, beta₁, and beta₂. Norepinephrine and epinephrine are agonists for alpha and beta receptors in the vasculature and the myocardium. Myocardial adrenergic receptors are primarily (80% to 85%) of the beta subclass.[6,7] Stimulation of the myocardial beta receptor leads to increased sinus node firing rate, more rapid atrioventricular conduction, and increased myocardial contractility. Alpha₁ receptors constitute a minority of the total adrenergic receptors in ventricular myocardium. Stimulation of alpha₁ receptors also has a positive inotropic effect. The central cellular mechanism underlying increased myocardial contractility is an increase in intracellular Ca^{2+} concentration in response to stimulation of adrenergic receptors in the sarcolemma. This process is initiated and amplified by a membrane-bound transduction system consisting of adrenergic receptors, guanine nucleotide-binding proteins (G proteins), and the effector enzyme adenyl cyclase.[8]

Vascular smooth muscle contains mainly beta₂ and alpha₁ receptors with beta₂ agonism leading to vasodilation and alpha₁ agonism to vasoconstriction. Norepinephrine has only a small effect on beta₂ receptors but is a potent alpha₁ agonist leading to intense vasoconstriction. Conversely, low concentrations of epinephrine are sufficient to stimulate beta₂ receptors, whereas higher epinephrine concentrations are required for alpha₁ receptor stimulation.

Alpha₂ receptors are found primarily in preganglionic and postganglionic sympathetic nerve terminals to peripheral vasculature and within the central nervous system (CNS).[9] Whereas stimulation of postganglionic alpha₂ receptors leads to vasoconstriction, the overall effect of an alpha₂ agonist such as clonidine is sympathetic inhibition because norepinephrine secretion is inhibited from the preganglionic nerve terminal and/or sympathetic outflow is decreased from the CNS.

Myocardial Beta₁ and Beta₂ Receptors. Myocardial adrenergic receptors in the nonfailing heart are 65% beta₁ and 20% beta₂.[10] Norepinephrine, the dominant endogenous cardiac neurotransmitter, has 30 to 50 times greater affinity for the beta₁ compared with the beta₂ receptor. Thus in the nonfailing heart, beta₁ is the predominant regulator of contractility and heart rate.[11] Activation of myocardial beta₁ and beta₂ receptors results in increased inotropy and chronotropy.[12] The different adrenoreceptor subclasses use different G proteins and second messengers. In the case of the beta receptor the major events in this process consist of a first messenger (e.g., epinephrine) binding to a beta₁ or beta₂ receptor,

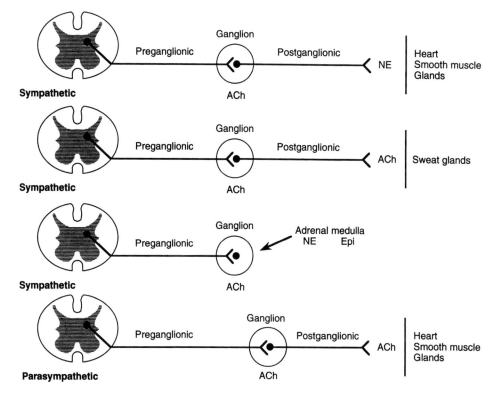

• **Figure 19.1** Neurotransmitters for the sympathetic and parasympathetic nervous system. *ACh,* Acetylcholine; *NE,* norepinephrine; *Epi,* epinephrine. (Modified from Merrin RG. Autonomic nervous system pharmacology. In Miller RD, ed. *Anesthesia.* New York: Churchill Livingstone; 1990; with permission.)

which produces a conformational change in the receptor so that it can activate the stimulatory G protein (Gsα) (Fig. 19.2). The G protein functions as a transducer of the signal by activating the effector enzyme adenyl cyclase. Activation of adenyl cyclase amplifies the signal through the production of the second messenger, cyclic adenosine monophosphate (cAMP). Finally, cAMP activates protein kinase A, leading to phosphorylation of a variety of cAMP-dependent proteins, which ultimately effect excitation-contraction coupling. Because cAMP is broken down by specific phosphodiesterase, inhibition of phosphodiesterase raises cAMP levels and increases myocardial contractility (see section on phosphodiesterase inhibitors).

Among the proteins activated by protein kinase A is the L-type, voltage-sensitive calcium channel in the sarcolemmal membrane. Activation of this calcium channel allows entry of a small amount of extracellular calcium into the cell, which binds to the ryanodine receptor (RyR2) on the sarcoplasmic reticulum. Binding of calcium to the ryanodine receptor triggers the release of micromolar amounts of calcium from sarcoplasmic reticulum into the cytoplasm. This process is known as calcium-induced calcium release, which initiates contraction by binding to the troponin complex, a series of regulatory proteins on the actin molecule. The conformational changes within the troponin complex reverse the inhibition of actin and myosin, thereby allowing contraction to take place. Relaxation of the myocardial fiber becomes possible when reuptake of cytosolic calcium into sarcoplasmic reticulum occurs via energy-dependent sarcoplasmic reticulum/endoplasmic reticulum calcium adenosinetriphosphatase (ATPase) (SERCA) pumps. Any drug that improves myocardial fiber contractility must either increase the concentration of intracellular calcium or increase the sensitivity of the myocardial fiber to calcium.

Vascular Beta₂ Receptors. Beta₂-adrenergic receptors in the vascular smooth muscle mediate dilation and relaxation. Activation of the beta₂ vascular receptor similarly results in increased intracellular cAMP. However, here cAMP inhibits myosin light chain kinase, resulting in vascular smooth muscle relaxation (Fig. 19.3).[13]

Myocardial and Vascular Alpha Receptors. Alpha₁ receptors constitute 13% to 15% of the adrenergic receptors in ventricular myocardium.[10] Once an alpha₁ agonist binds to the alpha₁ receptor, a different G protein (Gαq) is activated and, in turn, activates phospholipase C (see Fig. 19.2). The activated phospholipase C hydrolyzes membrane-bound phospholipids to inositol triphosphate (IP₃) and diacylglycerol (DAG). IP₃ stimulates the release of Ca²⁺ from sarcoplasmic reticulum. DAG activates protein kinase C and subsequent phosphorylation of intracellular proteins, which regulate cell responsiveness.

Adrenoreceptors in Heart Failure. Circulating levels of norepinephrine are raised in heart failure.[14] There is a selective downregulation in the number of myocardial beta₁ receptors without a change in the number of beta₂ or alpha₁ receptors, resulting in an increased percentage of the latter two receptors (47% beta₁, 25% beta₂, and 28% alpha₁).[6,7,15,16] Either increased receptor destruction or decreased receptor synthesis (or both) may cause downregulation. In addition, uncoupling of the beta₂ receptor from the G protein–adenylate cyclase complex prevents effective signal transduction.[10] Another proposed mechanism of beta-receptor desensitization involves sequestration or internalization of the receptor away from the cell surface. In contrast to downregulation, sequestration permits recycling the receptor back to the cell surface once chronic beta agonist exposure has ceased.[17]

Cardiopulmonary bypass (CPB) with aortic cross-clamping is a potent stimulus for release of myocardial norepinephrine.[18] This

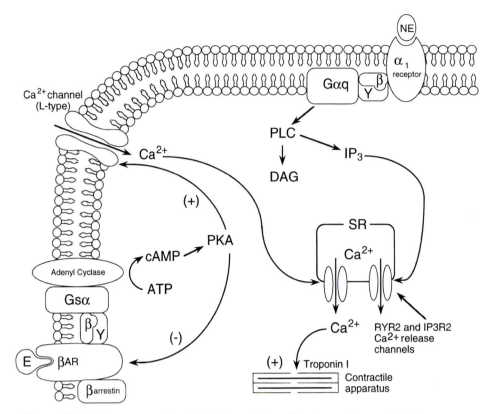

• **Figure 19.2** Major components of signal transduction within the cardiomyocyte. First messenger (epinephrine *[E]*) binds to the beta$_1$ adrenoreceptor *(βAR)*. The resultant conformational change in the stimulatory G protein *(Gsα)* activates the effector enzyme adenyl cyclase, which increases production of the second messenger, cyclic adenosine monophosphate *(cAMP)*. cAMP activates protein kinase A *(PKA)*, which phosphorylates the L-type calcium channel to allow calcium entry into the cytoplasm. Calcium binding to the ryanodine receptor *(RYR2)* on the sarcoplasmic reticulum *(SR)* results in calcium efflux from SR to raise cytoplasmic calcium levels to micromolar levels. Calcium efflux from SR could also be accomplished by norepinephrine *(NE)* binding to the alpha-adrenergic receptor *(α$_1$ receptor)* leading to a conformational change in the Gαq protein, which activates phospholipase C *(PLC)*. PLC breaks down membrane-bound phospholipids to produce inositol triphosphate *(IP$_3$)* and diacylglycerol *(DAG)*. IP$_3$ binds to the IP3R2 calcium release channel on SR (or endoplasmic reticulum), resulting in calcium efflux. The final step to effect muscle fiber contraction requires binding of calcium to troponin I to disinhibit the contractile apparatus. *ATP,* Adenosine triphosphate.

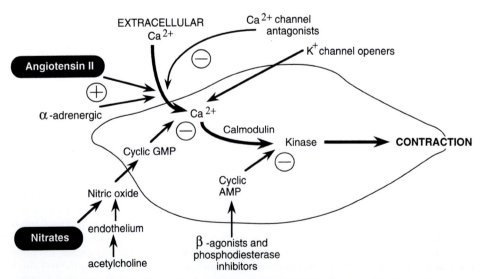

• **Figure 19.3** Cellular mechanisms of actions of vasodilators. *AMP,* Adenosine monophosphate; *GMP,* guanosine monophosphate; *Kinase,* myosin light chain kinase. (Adopted from Opie LH, Kaplan N, Poole-Wilson PA. Angiotension-converting enzyme inhibitors and conventional vasodilators. In: Opie LH, ed. *Drugs for the Heart.* 4th ed. Philadelphia: WB Saunders; 1995.)

could explain myocardial beta-adrenergic desensitization observed in children following CPB with aortic cross-clamping, which is postulated to result from beta-receptor uncoupling.[19]

As a result of beta$_1$ downregulation and beta$_2$ uncoupling, inotropic drugs fail to yield previously attainable levels of hemodynamic support in conditions of heart failure or following CPB with aortic cross-clamp.[17,19,20]

Adrenoreceptors and Exogenous Agonists. Similar to chronic exposure to elevated endogenous norepinephrine levels in heart failure, chronic administration of exogenous agonists induces downregulation of beta receptors.[20] Animal studies indicate that after 7 days of isoproterenol (beta$_1$ and beta$_2$ agonist), beta$_2$ receptors are decreased 60% to 80%, whereas beta$_1$ receptors remain unchanged.[21,22]

Parasympathetic Control

The parasympathetic innervation to the heart is provided by the vagus nerve. The long preganglionic fibers synapse in ganglia within the heart from which very short postganglionic fibers travel to the sinus node, atrioventricular node, and cardiomyocytes. Acetylcholine is the neurotransmitter released by both preganglionic and postganglionic parasympathetic nerve terminals (see Fig. 19.1). Myocardial muscarinic receptors are predominantly of the M2 subtype.[23] Vagal (cholinergic) stimulation depresses cardiac rate and contractile function by limiting the accumulation of intracellular Ca^{2+}. These negative inotropic effects are mediated by activation of inhibitory receptors in the sarcolemma.

Muscarinic receptor density is 2- to 2.5-fold greater in the atria than in the ventricles in contrast to the uniform distribution of beta receptors.[23] Muscarinic receptors are bound to an inhibitory G protein. Activation of this receptor leads to inhibition of adenylate cyclase activity and the subsequent decrease in intracellular cAMP levels.[23] Muscarinic agonists may also stimulate opening of K$^+$ channels in atrial pacemaker cells, leading to K$^+$ influx and hyperpolarization of the cell membrane.[24] The latter mechanism may also be linked to G proteins and account for the bradycardic effect of muscarinic drugs.[25]

Similarly, the transmembrane adenosine A$_1$ receptor is coupled to inhibitory G protein. Activation of the adenosine A$_1$ receptor in the myocardium decreases cardiac oxygen demand by opening sarcolemmal K$^+$ channels, resulting in decreased heart rate and decreased contractility. In addition, activation of adenosine A$_1$ receptors antagonizes beta-adrenergic stimulation by inhibiting the formation of cAMP by adenylate cyclase. Thus the adenosine A$_1$ receptor mediates the negative chronotropic, inotropic, and anti–beta-adrenergic effects of adenosine.[26]

Transplanted Heart

In humans, cardiac beta$_1$ receptors may represent "innervated" receptors and are involved mainly in neuronal control of the heart. Beta$_2$ receptors may represent "hormonal" receptors, responding more to circulatory agonists, and mediate both chronotropic and inotropic responses. In healthy hearts of humans the proportion of beta$_2$ receptors in ventricular myocardium is approximately 20% and between 25% and 40% in atrial tissue. Hemodynamic responses to the endogenous catecholamines, norepinephrine and epinephrine, differ markedly between heart transplant patients and nontransplant patients with mild essential hypertension. Cardiac transplantation results in near complete sympathetic and parasympathetic denervation of the donor heart, which results in an altered hemodynamic

response to beta-receptor stimulation. Beta-adrenergic stimulation of the transplanted heart results in increased heart rate because the denervation removes parasympathetic buffering that would otherwise be activated by the arterial baroreflex. For example, a transplanted heart may respond to exercise via increases in heart rate (as opposed to an inotropic response) that are largely related to increases in circulating endogenous catecholamines, secondary to release from the adrenal medulla. Heart rate responses to isoproterenol have been shown to be enhanced in cardiac transplant recipients compared with healthy subjects but not enhanced or decreased compared with healthy subjects treated with atropine, to exclude potential reflex negative inotropic changes in innervated hearts mediated by the parasympathetic nervous system. In addition to increased responsiveness to isoproterenol,[27] the denervated heart also has increased responsiveness to dobutamine,[28] both of which may reflect upregulation of beta-adrenergic receptors.

Inotropic Drugs

Dopamine

Dopamine is a sympathomimetic amine capable of directly stimulating beta$_1$ and alpha$_1$ receptors and works indirectly as an intermediary in the enzymatic pathway leading to the production of norepinephrine and epinephrine. Dopamine receptors are found in the coronary, renal, mesenteric, and cerebral arteries. Dopaminergic-1 receptors are postsynaptic and result in vasodilation. Dopaminergic-2 receptors are presynaptic and result in vasodilation due to inhibition of release of norepinephrine (Table 19.1).[29]

The pharmacokinetics of dopamine in children is not clearly characterized due to the difficulty in differentiating endogenous versus exogenous concentrations. The pharmacokinetic data that exist suggest high interindividual variability. In a heterogeneous group of pediatric intensive care unit patients, the t$_{1/2}$ α, (distribution half-life) was 1.8 ± 1.1 minutes, and the t$_{1/2}$ β, (elimination half-life) was 26 ± 14 minutes compared with another study of newborns in which the t$_{1/2}$ β was 7 minutes.[30,31] The impact on t$_{1/2}$ by liver or renal dysfunction in unknown because some studies have shown decreased clearance and others no change compared with individuals without hepatic or renal dysfnction.[31-33] Thirty percent of plasma dopamine is protein bound. Dopamine is degraded by two enzyme systems: catechol-O-methyl transferase (COMT) and monoamine oxidase (MAO).

Concomitant administration of dobutamine may affect dopamine clearance. In the presence of dobutamine, dopamine clearance increases linearly as the dopamine infusion rate is raised.[31]

Children younger than 2 years of age clear dopamine twice as fast as those older than 2 years.[32] This may in part explain the fact that infants require a higher dopamine infusion rate to achieve an effect equivalent to that found in older children and adults.

The hemodynamic effects of dopamine are dose dependent, with renal vasodilation evident at low infusion rates of less than 5 mcg/kg/min, increased inotropy at moderate infusion rates of 5 to 10 mcg/kg/min, and increased vascular resistance at higher infusion rates, greater than 10 mcg/kg/min (see Table 19.1). There is little, if any, cardiovascular improvement with lower doses of dopamine (<5 mcg/kg/min), but cardiac index has been shown to increase by 17%, with a concomitant 70% rise in renal plasma flow with doses greater than or equal to 5 mcg/kg/min. The effects of dopamine on heart rate appear to be dose dependent, with tachycardia contributing significantly to the rise in cardiac index at infusion rates greater than 7.5 mcg/kg/min.[34-36] In adults with

TABLE 19.1   Pediatric Adrenergic Cardiovascular Infusions

Drug	Dose	α_1	β_1	β_2	Dopa	Usual Titration[a]	Cautions/Comments
Dobutamine	Usual: 2-20 mcg/kg/min MAX: 30 mcg/kg/min	+	+++	+	0	1-2 mcg/kg/min every 10 min until desired effect is reached	• Increases CO • Higher doses can cause tachyarrhythmias and changes in BP leading to myocardial ischemia
Dopamine	<5 mcg/kg/min	0	++	0	++++	1-5 mcg/kg/min every ≥5 minutes	• Initial dose based on clinical indication and patient status • <5 mcg/kg/min = renal, coronary, mesenteric, and cerebral arterial vasodilation and natriuretic response • 5-10 mcg/kg/min = increased contractility/CO • >10 mcg/kg/min = increased contractility/CO and vasoconstriction/increase in SVR • If >20 mcg/kg/min needed, a more direct-acting pressor should be added (i.e., epinephrine, norepinephrine) • Can induce arrhythmias • Prolonged infusions can deplete endogenous NE resulting in a loss of vasopressor response
	5-10 mcg/kg/min >10 mcg/kg/min	++ ++++	+++ +++	+ +	++ +	1-10 mcg/kg/min every ≥5 min	
Epinephrine	Usual: 0.01-1 mcg/kg/min MAX: 2 mcg/kg/min	++	+++	++	0	0.01-0.1 mcg/kg/min every ≥1 min until desired effect is reached	• Low dose = increased contractility and CO • Escalating doses = increase in SVR and BP • Can induce arrhythmias • Inotropic/chronotropic effects can induce myocardial ischemia
Norepinephrine	Usual: 0.05-1 mcg/kg/min MAX: 2 mcg/kg/min	++++	++	0	0	0.01-0.1 mcg/kg/min every ≥2 min until desired effect is reached	• Increases SVR and BP • Decreases renal perfusion • Can induce tachyarrhythmias and myocardial ischemia • Extravasation can produce ischemic necrosis and sloughing
Phenylephrine	Usual: 0.04-2 mcg/kg/min MAX: 4 mcg/kg/min	++++	0	0	0	0.05-0.3 mcg/kg/min every ≥5 min until desired effect is reached	• Decreases renal perfusion • Pure α-adrenergic agonist with minimal cardiac activity • Rapid increase in SBP and DBP can cause reflex bradycardia • Extravasation can produce ischemic necrosis and sloughing

[a]Titrations may vary based upon clinical indication and patient status.

BP, Blood pressure; *CO,* cardiac output; *DBP,* diastolic blood pressure; *NE,* norepinephrine; *SBP,* systolic blood pressure; *SVR,* systemic vascular resistance.

cardiac dysfunction, dopamine lowers systemic vascular resistance (SVR) in doses up to 10 mcg/kg/min[34,35] and increases SVR with doses greater than or equal to 10 mcg/kg/min.[34] Dopamine increases myocardial oxygen consumption, but it also increases oxygen delivery, leaving the coronary sinus and mixed venous oxygen saturation unchanged.[37]

Clinical correlation of the impact of low-dose dopamine on urine output and creatinine clearance in pediatrics is not well supported.[38] Although case studies support the use of low-dose dopamine to augment urine output, the literature to support its use is insuffient.[38]

Management of the hypotensive premature infant represents a special circumstance in which dopamine infusions have been used.

Systemic hypotension is associated with cerebral injury in very low-birth-weight infants.[39] Although there is no significant difference between dopamine and dobutamine in the incidence of periventricular leukomalacia, grade III to IV intraventricular hemorrhage, or mortality, dopamine is more successful than dobutamine in short-term blood pressure elevation.[40-44] Premature infants seem to require higher doses than children and adults for an equivalent inotropic effect; however, they demonstrate alpha effects at lower doses.[45]

Common scenarios for administration of dopamine include (1) low cardiac output following cardiac surgery, (2) septic shock with low cardiac output and low SVR, and (3) premature infants with hypotension. (See also Chapter 16 on renal function.)

The major complications of dopamine therapy in children are extravasation and arrhythmia. Given the potential for tissue necrosis and gangrene, central administration is the preferred route of administration. Supraventricular tachydysrhythmias have been reported after dopamine infusion in infants and children.[46,47] Risk factors include a preexisting supraventricular rhythm disturbance and high-dose dopamine (10 to 20 mcg/kg/min).[46] Increased frequency of premature ventricular beats occurs at dopamine greater than 5 mcg/kg/min.[34]

Dobutamine

Dobutamine is a synthetic catecholamine that improves the inotropic state of the heart with little effect upon chronotropy. Dobutamine acts primarily on beta$_1$ receptors, with some beta$_2$ and alpha effect. Unlike dopamine, dobutamine does not release norepinephrine. Dobutamine used clinically contains two enantiomeric forms. The ($-$) isomer is a potent alpha agonist, causing an increase in vascular resistance. However, the (+) isomer is a potent beta agonist as well as an alpha antagonist, which blocks the effects of the ($-$) isomer.[48] Dobutamine is metabolized by glucuronidation via COMT.

Most studies indicate that plasma dobutamine concentrations increase proportionally with increasing infusion rate (i.e., linear kinetics). However, other studies showed that higher doses resulted in a smaller increase in concentration (e.g., nonlinear kinetics). Among children in the pediatric intensive care unit, the $t_{1/2}$ α of dobutamine was 1.65 ± 0.2 minutes, and the $t_{1/2}$ β was 25.8 ± 11.5 minutes. Half-lives did not correlate with age, weight, gender, disease state, or duration of dobutamine infusion. The half-lives were shorter when dopamine was coadministered.[49] There seems to be a shift in the dose-response curve in younger (less than 1 year of age) children, leading to younger children needing a higher dose than adults to achieve the same pharmacologic effect.[50]

The myocardial effects of dobutamine are not completely explained by its beta$_1$-adrenergic receptor stimulation. Interestingly, there is an increase in cardiac index that results from an increase in stroke volume index without a significant increase in heart rate.[34,50-52] At low infusion doses (less than 5 mcg/kg/min), children experience a decrease in pulmonary capillary wedge pressure and an increase of cardiac output and blood pressure without an increase in heart rate (see Table 19.1).[51,53,54] At higher doses (greater than 5 mcg/kg/min), there is an associated increase in heart rate (Fig. 19.4; see Table 19.1).[51,54] SVR is either unchanged[51] or decreased[34,50] after dobutamine. There is no effect on pulmonary vascular resistance (PVR).[50,51] The effect of dobutamine may be different following CPB in children. However, data are inconsistent because some studies have shown a more pronounced chronotropic effect without an impact on stroke volume and other studies have shown a significant increase in heart rate with an increase in cardiac index and SVR.[55,56]

Dobutamine may be useful for patients admitted with decompensated systolic heart failure to improve inotropy and augment diuresis and heart failure symptoms or for patients with hemodynamically significant aortic or mitral regurgitation requiring afterload reduction and inotropy. Of note, adult data have shown increased in-hospital mortality, heart failure readmissions, and arrhythmias associated with the use of dobutamine compared to nesiritide for treatment of acute decompensated heart failure.[57,58] Dobutamine causes fewer arrhythmias than epinephrine or isoproterenol.

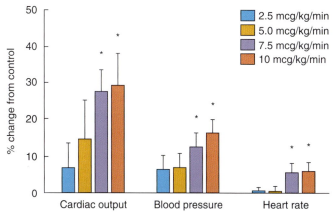

• **Figure 19.4** Effects of dobutamine infusion on cardiac output, blood pressure, and heart rate at different infusion rates in children. Note the increase in cardiac output and blood pressure with dopamine infusion at greater than 5 mcg/kg/min. (From Habib DM, Padbury JF, Anas NG, et al. Dobutamine pharmacokinetics and pharmacodynamics in pediatric intensive care patients. *Crit Care Med.* 1992;20:601-608; with permission.)

Epinephrine

Epinephrine is a mixed beta$_1$ and beta$_2$ agonist at low doses and an alpha agonist at higher doses. Thus it functions as combined inotrope and chronotrope, and at higher doses as a vasoconstrictor.

The pharmacokinetics of epinephrine in critically ill children is variable but correlates with age and body weight. Endogenous production of epinephrine is based upon enzymatic maturation and negligible during epinephrine infusions given the near 50-fold increase in concentration while on an infusion.[59] Epinephrine infusion rates designed to increase myocardial contractility (0.03 to 0.2 mcg/kg/min) yield plasma epinephrine levels of 670 to 9430 pg/mL.[60] Plasma epinephrine concentrations vary linearly with epinephrine infusion rate, suggesting first-order kinetics.[60] The half-life ($t_{1/2}$) of epinephrine is approximately 2 minutes. Epinephrine is degraded via the COMT and MAO systems.

Epinephrine is used frequently in the management of children with septic shock or low cardiac output syndrome (LCOS) after cardiac surgery when other inotropic agents have failed. Early administration of epinephrine was associated with increased survival when compared to dopamine in a single-center double-blind, prospective, randomized controlled trial of patients 1 month to 15 years of age with fluid-refractory septic shock, whereas dopamine was related to an increased risk of death and health care–associated infection.[61]

Epinephrine infusion (3 to 30 mcg/min) improves oxygen delivery by increasing cardiac index without increasing SVR in adults with septic shock unresponsive to fluid resuscitation.[62,63] After open-heart surgery, adult patients demonstrate a marked increase in cardiac output at infusion rates of 0.02 to 0.08 mcg/kg/min.[64]

As epinephrine infusion rates increase, alpha$_1$ agonist effects predominate, and at the highest infusion rates SVR is greatly increased and cardiac index begins to fall. Newborns may be more susceptible than adults to myocardial injury, including sarcolemmal rupture and mitochondrial Ca^{2+} granule deposition after prolonged high-dose epinephrine infusion.

The pulmonary vascular bed contains alpha and beta$_2$ receptors, so that pulmonary vasoconstriction (alpha stimulation) or vasodilation (beta$_2$ stimulation) can be expected depending on a variety of circumstances.[65] At low and medium doses (<0.8 mcg/kg/min), epinephrine decreases PVR and increases pulmonary blood flow. Ventilation/perfusion mismatch may result.[66] Higher doses appear to raise PVR if the preinfusion PVR was normal. Conversely, if the preinfusion PVR was elevated by either hypoxia or sepsis, even high-dose epinephrine administration (1 to 3.5 mcg/kg/min) may yield predominantly beta$_2$-adrenergic stimulation and pulmonary vasodilation.[67]

The effects of epinephrine infusion on regional blood flow have been evaluated primarily in animal studies showing renal vascular resistance increases in a dose-dependent manner with epinephrine infusion in adult sheep. Similarly, newborn piglets demonstrate decreased superior mesenteric artery, hepatic, and renal blood flow with epinephrine (less than 3 mcg/kg/min).[68] Following cardiac surgery in adults, epinephrine administration (0.04 mcg/kg/min) reduces the ratio of renal blood flow to cardiac index, whereas this ratio is not changed with dobutamine (2 to 8 mcg/kg/min) and is improved with dopamine (4 mcg/kg/min).[64]

Epinephrine is still considered the drug of choice in cardiopulmonary resuscitation (CPR) (see Chapter 31). In a witnessed pediatric cardiac arrest the standard initial dose of epinephrine is 10 mcg/kg, and high-dose epinephrine (100 mcg/kg) has been controversial in the past,[35] including a randomized controlled trial indicating that high-dose epinephrine may actually worsen outcomes after cardiac arrest in children.[69] Bolus administration of epinephrine to a compromised myocardium may result in ventricular fibrillation.

Epinephrine can be administered down the endotracheal tube at a dose of 100 mcg/kg, 10 times the recommended intravenous (IV) dose, resulting in rapid absorption and an increase in systolic blood pressure.[70]

Patients with depressed ventricular function, low cardiac output, and systemic hypotension can benefit from epinephrine infusion. It should be avoided in patients at high risk for ventricular arrhythmia.

Hypokalemia and hyperglycemia represent the most common metabolic side effects during epinephrine administration. Hypokalemia results from K$^+$ uptake into skeletal muscle cells after beta$_2$-receptor stimulation. Hyperglycemia results from suppressed insulin release as well as increased glycogenolysis and gluconeogenesis.

Epinephrine may cause extravasation and skin necrosis when administered via non–central venous access. For this reason, epinephrine infusions should be administered through a central venous access device whenever possible.

The most serious side effect of epinephrine is ventricular arrhythmia. Myocarditis, hypokalemia, and hypercapnia, particularly in the presence of inhaled anesthetics such as halothane, predispose patients to ventricular arrhythmia during epinephrine administration.

Norepinephrine

Norepinephrine is an endogenous catecholamine that is the neurotransmitter at sympathetic postganglionic fibers (see Fig. 19.1). It has potent beta$_1$- and alpha-stimulating effects. In contrast to epinephrine, norepinephrine has only minor effects on beta$_2$ receptors.

Variability in norepinephrine pharmacokinetics is related to body weight, age, and severity of illness.[71] Norepinephrine has a short half-life. After secretion of norepinephrine by the nerve endings, most of it is reabsorbed (where MAO can degrade it); the remainder diffuses into the bloodstream, where it remains active for at most minutes. Like epinephrine, norepinephrine is degraded via the COMT and MAO systems

The clinical effects of norepinephrine administration are mainly increased cardiac index and increased vascular (systemic and pulmonary) resistance. Several adult studies have suggested that norepinephrine is useful in increasing SVR in patients with hyperdynamic or vasodilatory septic shock that is not responsive to dopamine or epinephrine.[72,73] Additionally, it can augment coronary blood flow by increasing systemic diastolic pressure, at the expense of increasing afterload.

Given the significant vasoconstrictive properties of norepinephrine, the risk of extravasation and skin necrosis upon administration is quite high, and therefore it should be administered via central venous access.

Isoproterenol

Isoproterenol is a nonspecific beta agonist with no alpha-adrenergic activity and therefore increases inotropy, chronotropy, and systemic and pulmonary vasodilation.

Isoproterenol has a short half-life of 2 to 5 minutes, requiring a continuous infusion. Clearance is mostly in the urine as sulfate conjugates. Postoperative cardiac patients have lower clearance rates and require significantly lower infusion rates than patients with reactive airway disease to achieve clinical effect, potentially due to differences in metabolism, distribution related to plasma protein binding, and cardiac output and related perfusion of the liver and kidneys.[74] The major degradative pathway for isoproterenol is via COMT.

In vitro isoproterenol has greater positive inotropic effects in newborns than in adults.[75] Systolic blood pressure is increased, and diastolic and mean blood pressures are decreased because of systemic vasodilation.[75]

Isoproterenol may increase ventricular escape rate in cases of complete heart block. It is used to maintain heart rate, decrease afterload, and decrease right ventricular pressures immediately following heart transplantation. Isoproterenol may be administered through peripheral IV access.

Arrhythmia, both atrial and ventricular, can occur with isoproterenol. Isoproterenol should be avoided in patients with hypertrophic cardiomyopathy, fixed outflow tract obstruction, or compromised coronary blood flow because it can increase myocardial oxygen consumption and decrease coronary perfusion pressure. When it is used to stabilize complete heart block or effects of beta-blockade, hypotension can occur if the isoproterenol fails to effectively increase the heart rate. Due to potential risk of myocardial ischemia,[76] isoproterenol has been replaced by the more beta$_2$-specific terbutaline in treatment of the child with status asthmaticus.

Milrinone

Milrinone is a bipyridine derivative that inhibits cyclic nucleotide phosphodiesterase (III) resulting in increased cAMP. Increased cAMP causes an increase in intracellular ionic calcium concentration[77] and therefore improved myocardial contractility by increasing calcium transit and myofilament binding.[78] In the systemic vasculature, increased cAMP results in relaxation, decreasing afterload.

Phosphodiesterase III inhibitors may have antiinflammatory effects in septic shock. In vitro cardiac myocytes exposed to tumor necrosis factor-α (TNF-α) have a reduced contractile response to epinephrine compared with controls, whereas myocytes exposed to TNF-α have an augmented contractile response to phosphodiesterase III inhibitor compared with controls.[79]

Milrinone is primarily excreted by the kidneys as an unchanged drug (83%) and a glucuronide metabolite (12%) and must be used with caution in patients with renal impairment.

For infants and children the typical loading dose for milrinone is 50 mcg/kg with an infusion at 0.2 to 1 mcg/kg/min.[80,81]

Milrinone pharmacokinetics in pediatrics has been studied primarily following cardiac surgery. Milrinone does not bind to the bypass circuitry.[82] Milrinone steady state volume of distribution is larger in infants (0.9 L/kg) compared with children (0.7 L/kg) and three times that of adults (0.3 L/kg).[80,82,83] The elimination clearances rates for milrinone following CPB are lower for infants compared with children but twofold to threefold greater than milrinone clearance in adults.[80,82,83] The half-life ($t_{1/2}$) of milrinone is shortest in adults at 1.7 hours compared with children and infants (1.9 hours and 3 hours).

In adults with significant chronic congestive failure, phosphodiesterase inhibitors improve cardiac index, reduce left ventricular filling pressures, and improve the speed of contraction without significant side effects such as tachycardia.[84] After cardiac surgery in adults and neonates, cardiac index increases and heart rate increases, whereas systemic and pulmonary vascular resistance decrease with milrinone[81,85-87] administration (Figs. 19.5 and 19.6). These findings were most pronounced in those individuals with heart failure.[86]

Administration of phosphodiesterase inhibitors to children with left-to-right intracardiac shunts resulted in a more dramatic decrease in PVR in those patients with baseline elevation of their pulmonary artery pressures and PVR compared with those with normal pulmonary artery pressures and PVR.[88]

Barton and colleagues[89] administered milrinone to children with nonhyperdynamic septic shock and demonstrated that milrinone significantly increased cardiac index, increased stroke volume index, and increased oxygen delivery while decreasing systemic and pulmonary vascular resistance and not affecting heart rate.

Milrinone is used following cardiac surgery to augment inotropy and decrease SVR during periods of low cardiac output (Table 19.2). Hoffman and colleagues[90] demonstrated in a double-blind, placebo-controlled multicenter trial in infants and children following corrective heart surgery (n = 227) that milrinone (0.75 mcg/kg/min) significantly decreased the incidence of LCOS compared with placebo (Fig. 19.7). A meta-analysis confirmed the efficacy of prophylactic milrinone in reducing the incidence of LCOS but concluded there is insufficient evidence that prophylactic milrinone reduces mortality.[91] Milrinone is also an excellent agent for dilated cardiomyopathy due to myocarditis, graft rejection, and sepsis-associated cardiac dysfunction and a potential therapy as a bridge to transplantation in patients with advanced heart failure.[92] Additionally, milrinone can be used as adjunct therapy in managing pulmonary hypertension. Milrinone can improve cardiac index and oxygen delivery in children with nonhyperdynamic septic shock.[89] Preliminary data suggest that some phosphodiesterase inhibitors reduce systemic inflammatory response by reducing tumor necrosis factor and interleukin-1.

Hypotension is the most frequent cardiovascular side effect due to the vasodilatory properties noted previously, which may be prevented by alleviating the loading dose, administering a lower dose or administering the loading dose more slowly (over 10 to

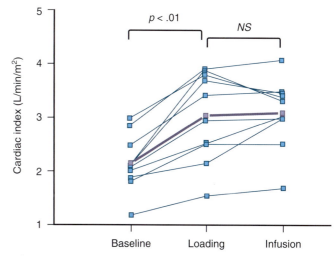

• **Figure 19.5** Cardiac index in neonates following cardiac surgery, with milrinone loading (50 mcg/kg) and infusion (0.5 mcg/kg/min). *NS,* Nonsignificant; *purple squares,* mean values; *blue squares,* individual values. (From Chang AC, Atz AM, Wernovsky GW, et al. Milrinone: systemic and pulmonary hemodynamic effects in neonates after cardiac surgery. *Crit Care Med.* 1995;23:1907-1914; with permission.)

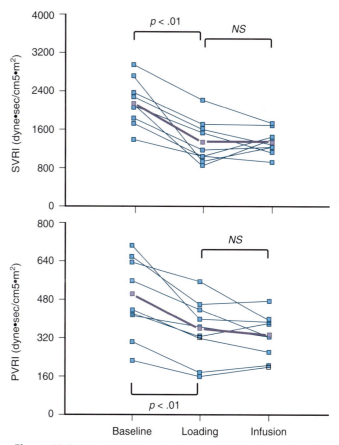

• **Figure 19.6** Systemic *(top)* and pulmonary *(bottom)* vascular resistance indexes in neonates following cardiac surgery, with milrinone loading (50 mcg/kg) and infusion (0.5 mcg/kg/min). *NS,* Nonsignificant; *PVRI,* pulmonary vascular resistance index; *SVRI,* systemic vascular resistance index; *purple squares,* mean values; *blue squares,* individual values. (From Chang AC, Atz AM, Wernovsky GW, et al. Milrinone: systemic and pulmonary hemodynamic effects in neonates after cardiac surgery. *Crit Care Med.* 1995;23:1907-1914; with permission.)

TABLE 19.2   Pediatric Nonadrenergic Cardiovascular Infusions

Drug	Dose	Clinical Effects	Usual Titration[a]	Cautions/Comments
Esmolol	Load: 100-500 mcg/kg infused over 1 min Usual starting: 50-100 mcg/kg/min Usual range: 50-250 mcg/kg/min MAX: 1000 mcg/kg/min	• Competitively blocks β_1 stimulation with little effect on β_2 receptors • (−) chronotropic effect/decrease in HR • Lusitropy	50-100 mcg/kg/min every ≥10 min until desired effect is reached • Smaller titrations may be warranted in patients with asthma/reactive airway disease	• Bradycardia, hypotension, peripheral ischemia • Phlebitis, necrosis after extravasation • Diaphoresis • Caution should be exercised when discontinuing infusions to prevent rebound hypertension
Milrinone	Load: 50-100 mcg/kg Usual starting: 0.5-1 mcg/kg/min Usual range: 0.25-1 mcg/kg/min MAX: 1.5 mcg/kg/min	• Positive inotropic effects/increase in CO • Reduction in SVR/afterload • Lusitropy	0.125-0.25 mcg/kg/min every ≥30 min until desired effect is reached	• Noncatecholamine, phosphodiesterase III inhibitor • Arrhythmias • Duration of effects remain for ≈6 h in patients with normal renal function • Patients in renal failure may respond with lower doses • Long-term use associated with thrombocytopenia
Nitroglycerin	Usual starting: 0.25-0.5 mcg/kg/min Usual range: 0.25-3 mcg/kg/min MAX: 5 mcg/kg/min • Max adult dose exceeded at >80 kg MAX adult dose: 400 mcg/min	• Converted to nitric oxide in vascular smooth muscle leading to vasodilation of venous and arterial smooth muscle • Venous effect greater than arterial	0.5-1 mcg/kg/min every ≥3 min until desired effect is reached	• Headache, flushing, hypotension, pallor, reflex tachycardia • With abrupt withdrawal: severe hypotension, bradycardia, acute coronary vascular insufficiency • Contraindicated in patients with glaucoma, severe anemia, increased ICP, hypotension, uncontrolled hypokalemia, pericardial tamponade, constrictive pericarditis • Use with extreme caution with sildenafil or other PDE-5 inhibitors
Nitroprusside	Usual starting: 0.3-0.5 mcg/kg/min Usual range: 1-3 mcg/kg/min MAX: 10 mcg/kg/min • Max adult dose exceeded at >40 kg MAX adult dose: 400 mcg/min	• Induces release of nitric oxide leading to vasodilation of venous and arterial smooth muscle	0.5 mcg/kg/min every ≥5 min until desired effect is reached	• Hypotension, palpitations • Elevated ICP, headache, restlessness • Nitroprusside is metabolized to cyanide in the bloodstream, then to thiocyanate in the liver, which is then renally eliminated • Risk of thiocyanate or cyanide toxicity is increased in patients with renal or liver dysfunction and at doses ≥1.8 mcg/kg/min
Vasopressin (pressor effect)	Usual starting: 0.05 mU/kg/min Usual range: 0.05-2 mU/kg/min	• Vasoconstriction/increase in SVR and BP	0.05-0.5 mU/kg/min every ≥30 min until desired effect is reached	• May cause hyponatremia

[a]Titrations may vary based upon clinical indication and patient status.

BP, Blood pressure; *CO*, cardiac output; *HR*, heart rate; *ICP*, intracranial pressure; *PDE-5*, phosphodiesterase-5; *SVR*, systemic vascular resistance.

20 minutes), and/or by concomitant volume expansion. Milrinone should be avoided in patients with severe left or right heart outflow tract obstruction because of the risk that fixed outflow tract obstruction in the presence of vasodilation may compromise coronary perfusion.

Thrombocytopenia has been reported with milrinone in patients following cardiac surgery, but there was no nonsurgical control group.[82] Other studies found no effect of milrinone on platelet count or function.[93]

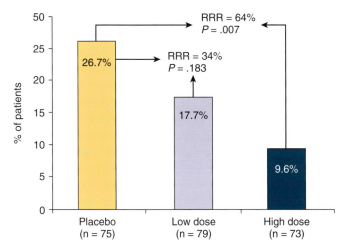

• Figure 19.7 Primary end point: development of low cardiac output syndrome (LCOS)/death in the first 36 hours (preprotocol population, n = 227). Therapy for LCOS was defined as an increase in pharmacologic support (100% over baseline), addition of a new inotropic agent, initiation of extracorporeal life support, or mechanical pacing. High-dose milrinone was 0.75 mcg/kg/min. Low-dose milrinone was 0.25 mcg/kg/min. *RRR*, Relative risk reduction. (From Hoffman TM, Wernovsky G, Atz AM. Efficacy and safety of milrinone in preventing low cardiac output syndrome in infants and children after corrective surgery for congenital heart disease. *Circulation.* 2003;107:996-1002; with permission.)

Calcium

In the past, calcium was routinely administered in situations where improved cardiac function was needed. In newborn lambs with single-ventricle physiology, Reddy and colleagues[94] demonstrated that administration of calcium (10 mg/kg of calcium chloride) significantly increased systolic blood pressure and decreased pulmonary-to-systemic blood flow ratio ($Q_p:Q_s$) prebypass (Table 19.3). The maximal inotropic effect of calcium in the newborn was significantly greater than in adults, perhaps because of a lower intracellular calcium concentration.[75] Calcium is of particular importance in newborns with congenital heart disease (CHD), particularly those with conotruncal abnormalities, for which there is an increased prevalence of 22q11 deletion (DiGeorge syndrome) and associated hypoparathyroidism.

Studies in adults have suggested that calcium is ineffective in the face of refractory asystole,[95] yet of potential benefit in a subset of patients with refractory electromechanical dissociation.[96] Current CPR guidelines discourage use of calcium for treatment of asystole and recommend its use in cases of hyperkalemia, hypermagnesemia, and calcium channel blocker overdose.

Significant hypocalcemia is very common in critically ill children, is associated with poor outcomes,[97] and may be due to relative or absolute hypoparathyroidism. Modestly low calcium levels are not related to impaired cardiac function, but infusions of calcium in this setting can improve mean arterial pressures.[98] In adults following CPB, calcium increases blood pressure without improving cardiac index.[99] However, in infants and children, maintaining ionized calcium levels is important for maintaining blood pressure and cardiac output, perhaps due to relatively diminished intracellular calcium stores or perhaps due to the relative increased volume of transfused citrated blood products. Calcium chloride infusions in pediatric patients with LCOS have been shown in a small retrospective study to improve hemodynamics and end-organ perfusion without an increase in heart rate and without relation to low baseline ionized calcium.[100]

	PAP (mm Hg)	SAP (mm Hg)	Q_p (mL/min/kg body weight)	Q_s (mL/min/kg body weight)	$Q_p:Q_s$	PVR (mm Hg/min/kg)	SVR (mm Hg/ min/kg)
Before Cardiopulmonary Bypass							
Precalcium	31.7 ± 5.4	55.5 ± 11.6	249 ± 30	130 ± 39	2.09 ± 0.80	0.101 ± 0.031	0.41 ± 0.15
Postcalcium	32.0 ± 5.4	59.0 ± 12.5	268 ± 26[b]	150 ± 41[c]	1.90 ± 0.58[d]	0.100 ± 0.025	0.38 ± 0.14[d]
After Cardiopulmonary Bypass							
Precalcium	28.6 ± 4.4	51.7 ± 8.8	238 ± 55	149 ± 49	1.71 ± 0.55	0.101 ± 0.027	0.34 ± 0.14
Postcalcium	28.9 ± 4.0	58.0 ± 7.8[d]	268 ± 62[a]	174 ± 50[c]	1.60 ± 0.44	0.090 ± 0.025[c]	0.32 ± 0.11

TABLE 19.3   Prebypass and Postbypass Hemodynamic Measurements Before and After Administration of Calcium

[a]Neonatal lambs with single-ventricle physiology created in utero (Damus-Kaye-Stansel, main pulmonary artery ligation, and placement of 5-mm aortopulmonary shunt) had direct measurement of systemic and pulmonary blood flow both before and after cardiopulmonary bypass 48 to 72 hours postnatally. Administration of calcium (calcium chloride 10 mg/kg) increased systemic arterial pressure both prebypass and postbypass and decreased $Q_p:Q_s$ prebypass.
[b]$P < .001$
[c]$P < .0001$, relative to preadministration values.
[d]$P < .05$
Data presented are mean values ± SD.
PAP, Pulmonary artery pressure; *PVR,* pulmonary vascular resistance; Q_p, indexed pulmonary blood flow; $Q_p:Q_s$, pulmonary-to-systemic blood flow ratio; Q_s, indexed systemic blood flow; *SAP,* systemic arterial pressure; *SVR,* systemic vascular resistance.
From Reddy VM, Liddicoat JR, McElhinney DB, et al. Hemodynamic effects of epinephrine, bicarbonate and calcium in the early postnatal period in a lamb model of single-ventricle physiology created in utero. *J Am Coll Cardiol.* 1996;28:1877-1883; with permission.

Thyroid Hormone

Thyroid hormone directly affects inotropy and peripheral vascular resistance. Thyroxine (T_4) is synthesized by the thyroid gland and converted by deiodinase enzymes to the active compound triiodothyronine (T_3). T_3 increases synthesis of the fast alpha-myosin heavy chain, increases sarcoplasmic reticulum Ca^{2+} adenosine triphosphatase, and increases intracellular cAMP, resulting in increased inotropy and decreased peripheral vascular resistance.[101]

Thyroid hormone abnormalities, including decreased T_3, normal or decreased T_4 and thyrotropin, and increased reverse T_3, are well documented in children following cardiac surgery[101-104] and in adults following cardiac bypass,[105] post myocardial infarction, and with severe congestive heart failure.[106] In adults with congestive heart failure, a low T3:reverse T_3 index was associated with lower cardiac index, elevated filling pressures, and poorer outcome.[106] *Euthyroid sick syndrome* is a constellation of abnormal thyroid function test results in a clinically euthyroid patient who is suffering from critical illness that appears to involve decreased peripheral conversion of T_4 to T_3, decreased clearance of reverse T_3 generated from T_4, and decreased binding of thyroid hormones to thyroid-binding globulin.

Administration of T_3 to adults following coronary artery bypass surgery and heart failure improved hemodynamic parameters increasing cardiac output and decreased SVR (Fig. 19.8),[107,108] whereas Bennett-Guerrero and colleagues[105] found no significant change in cardiac index or SVR. Currently T_3 seems more beneficial in the setting of congestive heart failure or dilated cardiomyopathy. Bettendorf and colleagues[109] found that T_3 administration to infants

increased cardiac index during the first 24 hours after cardiac surgery, particularly for those with prolonged CPB (>1.8 hours), compared to the placebo group, and by 72 hours both groups had similar cardiac indices and T_3 levels. Chowdhury et al.[110] studied T_3 infusions post CPB with T_3 level of less than 40 ng/dL (or <60 ng/dL for newborns) and found that the T_3 infusion group had significantly lower inotropic requirements. The Transfusion Requirements in Critical Care (TRICC) study was a large multicenter, double-blind, randomized, placebo-controlled trial in pediatric cardiac surgery patients less than 2 years of age that evaluated the use of IV T_3 post CPB. Results of the study were significant in patients less than 5 months of age, resulting in a shortened time to extubation correlating to reduction in inotrope use and improved cardiac function.[111]

Digoxin

Digoxin is a cardiac glycoside that inhibits Na^+-K^+ ATPase in the cardiomyocyte, resulting in increased intracellular Na^+ concentration, thereby increasing intracellular Ca^{2+} through a Na^+-Ca^{2+} exchange mechanism. Contractile force and velocity depend on the concentration of and sensitivity to Ca^{2+} in the contractile apparatus. The ability of digoxin to drive the Na^+-Ca^{2+} exchanger may be limited in the immature heart.[112]

Digoxin undergoes metabolism in the liver and limited enterohepatic circulation. In addition, bacteria in the large intestine may metabolize the drug. Unmetabolized digoxin and metabolites are then excreted in urine and feces.

Absorption of oral digoxin from the gastrointestinal tract is variable from one individual to another and dependent upon

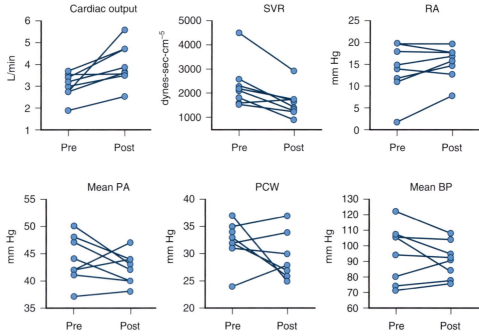

• **Figure 19.8** Hemodynamic parameters at baseline *(pre)* and 2 hours after *(post)* initial triiodothyronine bolus (0.7 mcg/kg) followed by infusion (0.2 mcg/kg/h) in adults with congestive heart failure. There is a significant increase in cardiac output at 2 hours (3 ± 0.6 to 4 ± 1 L/min, P = .03), with a reduction in systemic vascular resistance (2291 ± 1022 to 1664 ± 629 dynes × s × cm^{-5}, P = .02) without change in other parameters. *BP,* Arterial blood pressure; *PA,* pulmonary artery pressure; *PCW,* pulmonary capillary wedge pressure; *RA,* right atrial pressure; *SVR,* systemic vascular resistance. (From Hamilton MA, Stevenson LW, Fonarow GC, et al. Safety and hemodynamic effects of intravenous triiodothyronine in advanced congestive heart failure. *Am J Cardiol.* 81:443-447, 1998; with permission.)

the formulation. The onset of action after an oral dose occurs within 30 to 120 minutes and peaks at approximately 6 to 8 hours. The effects of IV digoxin begin after 5 to 30 minutes. The elimination half-life in adult patients with normal renal function is between 36 and 48 hours and prolonged in renal dysfunction. In preterm neonates and full-term neonates the half-life is 60 to 170 hours and 35 to 45 hours, respectively. In toddlers and younger children the half life is 18 to 35 hours (Table 19.4).

The hemodynamic effects of digoxin include increased contractility, cardiac output, and renal perfusion.[113] These effects may arise from neurohumoral modulation, including decreased plasma renin

activity, attenuated sympathetic drive, and improved baroreceptor sensitivity.[114]

Digoxin may be used to treat children with congestive heart failure or supraventricular tachyarrhythmias. The antiarrhythmic applications of this drug are discussed in Chapter 27. Patients with systolic ventricular dysfunction who have mild to moderate ventricular dysfunction with stable blood pressure and perfusion may benefit from the addition of digoxin. Regarding use in single-ventricle patients following stage I palliation with no history of arrhythmia, use of digoxin at discharge was associated with reduced interstage mortality.[115] There is relative contraindication for the use of digoxin in the presence of atrioventricular block,

TABLE 19.4 Oral Digoxin[a] Total Digitalizing (Loading) Dose and Maintenance Doses in Children With Normal Renal Function

Digoxin Loading/Digitalizing Dose Table (mcg/kg per dose)[a-h]

	ORAL			INTRAVENOUS		
	First Dose	Second Dose	Third Dose	First[t] Dose	Second Dose	Third Dose
Preterm neonate	10-15	5-7.5	5-7.5	7.5-12.5	3.75-6.25	3.75-6.25
Full-term neonate	12.5-17.5	6.25-8.75	6.25-8.75	10-15	5-7.5	5-7.5
1 mo-2 y	17.5-30	8.75-15	8.75-15	15-25	7.5-12.5	7.5-12.5
2-5 y	15-20	7.5-10	7.5-10	12.5-17.5	6.25-8.75	6.25-8.75
5-10 y[i]	10-17.5	5-8.75	5-8.75	7.5-15	3.75-7.5	3.75-7.5
>10 y[i]	5-7.5	2.5-3.75	2.5-3.75	4-6	2-3	2-3
ADULT maximum dose (Do NOT Exceed)	500 mcg (FLAT dose)	250 mcg (FLAT dose)	250 mcg (FLAT dose)	500 mcg (FLAT dose)	250 mcg (FLAT dose)	250 mcg (FLAT dose)

Digoxin Maintenance Dose Table (mcg/kg per dose)

	Oral	Intravenous
Preterm neonate	2.5-3.75 mcg/kg/dose q12h	2-3 mcg/kg/dose q12h
Full-term neonate	3-5 mcg/kg/dose q12h	2.5-4 mcg/kg/dose q12h
1 mo-2 y	5-7.5 mcg/kg/dose q12h	3.75-6 mcg/kg/dose q12h
2-5 y	3.75-5 mcg/kg/dose q12h	3-4.5 mcg/kg/dose q12h
5-10 y[i]	2.5-5 mcg/kg/dose q12h	2-4 mcg/kg/dose q12h
>10 y[i]	2.5-5 mcg/kg/dose once daily	2-3 mcg/kg/dose once daily
Usual ADULT dose (Do NOT Exceed)	125-375 mcg once daily (FLAT dose)	125-375 mcg once daily (FLAT dose)

Digoxin Renal Dose Adjustment Table

Loading/digitalizing dose	Reduce each part of loading dose by 50% in patients with end-stage renal disease.		
Maintenance dose	Administer percentage of dose indicated in lower part of table, based on creatinine clearance determined by the bedside Schwarz equation [0.413*Ht(cm)/Scr (mg/dL)].		
Creatinine clearance	30-50 mL/min/1.73 m^2	10-29 mL/min/1.73 m^2	<10 mL/min/1.73 m^2
Percentage of maintenance dose	Administer 75% of normal dose	Administer 50% of normal dose	Administer 25% of normal dose

[a]IV doses are 80% of the oral doses.
[b]The total loading/digitalizing dose is divided into three doses with first = 50%, second and third = 25% each of total loading dose. Dosing references typically list the TOTAL digitalizing dose. In the chart each INDIVIDUAL dose is precalculated by age in mcg/kg per dose, except the adult maximum, which is NOT weight based.
[c]The adult maximum dose is NOT weight based.
[d]When digoxin is used for tachyarrhythmias, a loading or "digitalizing" dose is administered in three doses at 6- to 12-hour intervals (see Digoxin Loading/Digitalizing Dose Table).
[e]Electrocardiogram should be evaluated before each portion of the loading "digitalizing" dose.
[f]In congestive heart failure, or in tachyarrhythmias after completion of the loading dose, the patient is started on a maintenance dose (see Digoxin Maintenance Dose Table).
[g]Digoxin should be dosed based on lean body weight in obese adolescents.
[h]Digoxin is largely eliminated via the kidneys; patients with reduced or changing renal function must receive lower doses and be closely monitored (see Digoxin Renal Dose Adjustment Table).
[i]Consider rounding dose to nearest tablet size for children ≥10 years of age, if appropriate.

TABLE 19.5	Digoxin Immune Fab Dosing

Dosing for Acute Ingestion/Overdose Based on Amount of Digoxin Ingested in Acute Overdose[a]

Number of Digoxin Tablets or Capsules Ingested	Dose of Digoxin Immune Fab (mg)
5	80
10	160
15	240
25	400
50	800
75	1200
100	1600
150	2400
200	3200

Dosing Based on Steady-State Serum Digoxin Concentration[b]

Patient Weight (kg)	SERUM DIGOXIN CONCENTRATION (ng/mL)						
	1	2	4	8	12	16	20
≤1	1 mg	1 mg	1.5 mg	3 mg	5 mg	6.5 mg	8 mg
>1 to 3	1 mg	2.5 mg	5 mg	10 mg	14 mg	19 mg	24 mg
>3 to 5	2 mg	4 mg	8 mg	16 mg	24 mg	32 mg	40 mg
>5 to 10	4 mg	8 mg	16 mg	32 mg	48 mg	64 mg	80 mg
>10 to 20	8 mg	16 mg	32 mg	64 mg	96 mg	128 mg	160 mg
>20 to 40	20 mg	40 mg	80 mg	120 mg	200 mg	280 mg	320 mg
>40 to 60	20 mg	40 mg	120 mg	200 mg	280 mg	400 mg	480 mg
>60 to 70	40 mg	80 mg	120 mg	240 mg	360 mg	440 mg	560 mg
>70 to 80	40 mg	80 mg	120 mg	280 mg	400 mg	520 mg	640 mg
>80 to 100	40 mg	80 mg	160 mg	320 mg	480 mg	640 mg	800 mg

[a]For every 250-mcg tablet (80% bioavailability) or 200-mcg capsule (100% bioavailability) ingested, administer 16 mg of dioxin immune Fab (see table for estimated doses).
[b]Estimated doses correlate with measured serum digoxin concentration.

sinus bradycardia, ventricular tachycardia, Wolff-Parkinson-White syndrome, hypokalemia, hypercalcemia, hypomagnesemia, or renal insufficiency and should be used with caution in hypertrophic cardiomyopathy due to the known association with accessory pathways.

Dysrhythmias constitute the most serious manifestation of digitalis toxicity, and adults may exhibit nausea and vomiting as the first sign of digitalis toxicity, whereas children usually present with dysrhythmia as the first sign of toxicity. The most common precipitating factors are hypokalemia or various drug interactions. Serum digoxin concentrations of 0.8 to 2 ng/mL represent the therapeutic range. Table 19.5 illustrates the treatment algorithm for digitalis intoxication.

Beta-Blockade

Esmolol

Esmolol is a relatively specific beta$_1$ antagonist. It undergoes rapid hydrolysis in the blood by red cell esterases. Pharmacokinetic data

in children indicate a faster elimination ($t_{1/2}$ of 2.7 to 4.5 minutes) than reported in adults (9 minutes).[116-118]

Esmolol can be administered as a loading dose (100 to 500 mcg/kg) followed by an infusion (100 to 1000 mcg/kg/min) titrated to response.[116,117] The antiarrhythmic properties of esmolol are described elsewhere (see Chapter 27).

Esmolol has been shown to control hypertension in children following coarctation repair.[118-120] Persistent hypertension, or paradoxical hypertension, occurs in 63% to 100% of patients during the postoperative period following surgical coarctation repair.[121-123]

Esmolol can increase ventricular filling time and augment cardiac output in patients with heart failure without cardiogenic shock or cardiomyopathy. Similarly, it can improve antegrade blood flow in infants following balloon dilation of critical or severe pulmonary stenosis, with significant right-to-left atrial shunting. Esmolol can help treat hypercyanotic spells in tetralogy of Fallot.[124] Esmolol can be used for pheochromocytoma after effective alpha-blockade has been established to prevent unopposed alpha-adrenergic stimulation and severe hypertension.

Extravasation can cause tissue necrosis. Esmolol can induce bronchospasm or hypoglycemia.

Carvedilol

Carvedilol is an oral nonselective beta-receptor and alpha$_1$-receptor antagonist with strong antioxidant properties. It is 98% protein bound with a t$_{1/2}$ of 7 to 10 hours in adults.[125]

Carvedilol has been shown to be effective therapy for chronic heart failure. Carvedilol attenuates the upregulated beta-adrenergic activity associated with heart failure, and as an alpha$_1$-blocker, it reduces ventricular afterload by lowering blood pressure and may play a role in cardiac remodeling and reducing hypertrophy.

A large (n = 1094) double-blind, placebo-controlled trial comparing placebo to carvedilol in adults with chronic heart failure concurrently treated with digoxin, diuretic, and angiotensin-converting enzyme inhibitor showed a significant reduction in mortality (7.8% versus 3.2%) and in cardiovascular-related hospitalizations (27% reduction).[125-134]

Use of beta-blockers in children is derived from adult experience and limited based on heart failure cause and ventricular morphology (Table 19.6). In children with dilated cardiomyopathy and biventricular CHD with a systemic left or right ventricle there is evidence showing improvements in ventricular function and heart failure symptoms, but evidence showing reduced mortality is lacking. A few studies in biventricular CHD heart failure did not show improvements in ventricular function or symptoms.[135-139] A small study in CHD single-ventricle patients showed improvements in ventricular function and symptoms.[140] Side effects, including dizziness (19%), hypotension (14%), and headache (14%), occur in approximately 54% of pediatric patients with heart failure.[125]

Vasodilation

Basic Principles

The work that the heart must perform is proportional to the pressure (ΔP) against which it must pump multiplied by the volume (V) that it pumps.

$$\text{Work} = \Delta P \times V$$

Decreasing the pressure against which the heart pumps decreases the work of the heart. The pressure against which the heart pumps is best understood as vascular resistance, which is proportional to afterload. In normal cardiac physiology, the afterload in the right ventricle is proportional to the PVR, and the afterload in the left ventricle is proportional to SVR. A more elaborate model accounts for the fact that the systemic ventricle must raise the potential energy of the blood from the level at which it exists in the thorax to one that exists in the descending aorta. Therefore the change

TABLE 19.6	Oral Beta-Blockers in Pediatric Patients With Heart Disease					
Oral Beta-Blocker	Pediatric Use	Dosing	Receptor Selectivity	Partial Agonist Activity	Adverse Effects	
Atenolol	• HTN • Arrhythmia	0.5-1 mg/kg/d given one or two times/d (Max: 2 mg/kg/d or 100 mg/d)	• β$_1$	No	Bradycardia, hypotension, hypoglycemia	
Carvedilol	• CHF	0.08-0.3 mg/kg/dose twice daily (Max: 0.75 mg/kg/dose twice daily or 25 mg/dose twice daily)	• β$_1$ • β$_2$ • α$_1$	No	Bradycardia, hypotension, hypoglycemia	
Labetalol	• HTN	1-3 mg/kg/d divided twice daily (Max: 12 mg/kg/d or 1200 mg/d)	• β$_1$ • β$_2$ • α$_1$	Yes	Bradycardia, hypotension, hypoglycemia	
Metoprolol	• HTN • Arrhythmia • CHF	Children 1-17 y: 1-2 mg/kg/d given twice daily (Max: 6 mg/kg/d or 200 mg/d)	• β$_1$	No	Bradycardia, hypotension, hypoglycemia	
Nadolol	• Arrhythmia	Infants, children, adolescents: 0.5-1 mg/kg/day once daily (Max: 2.5 mg/kg/d or 320 mg/d)	• β$_1$ • β$_2$	No	Bradycardia, hypotension, hypoglycemia, AV block, peripheral vascular insufficiency (Raynaud phenomenon)	
Propranolol	• HTN • Arrhythmia	Neonates: 0.25 mg/kg/dose every 6 h (Max: 5 mg/kg/d) Infants and children: 0.5-1 mg/kg/d in divided doses every 6-8 h (Max: 60 mg/d)	• β$_1$ • β$_2$	No	Bradycardia, hypotension, hypoglycemia	
Sotalol	• Arrhythmia	Children ≤2 y: 30 mg/m^2/dose every 8 h adjusted per age nomogram (Fig. 19.9) OR 2 mg/kg/d divided every 8 h OR 80-200 mg/m^2/d divided every 8 h Children >2 y: 80-200 mg/m^2/dose divided every 8 h	• β$_1$ • β$_2$	No	Bradycardia, hypotension, hypoglycemia, TdP • ECG monitoring for QT prolongation necessary • Females at greater risk for TdP than males	

AV, Atrioventricular; *CHF*, congestive heart failure; *ECG*, electrocardiogram; *HTN*, hypertension; *TdP*, torsades de pointes.

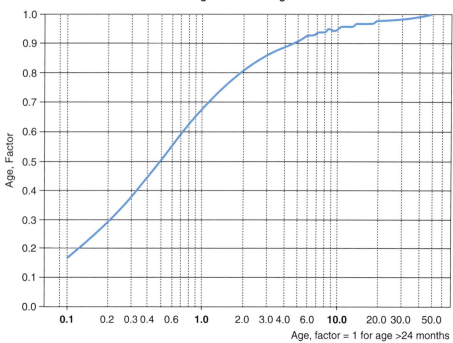

Age Factor Nomogram

Age, factor = 1 for age >24 months

Age, months

• **Figure 19.9** Age nomogram for patients ≤2 years of age. See Table 19.6. (From https://www.access-data.fda.gov/drugsatfda_docs/label/2011/021151s010lbl.pdf.)

TABLE 19.7	Ductal Dependent Lesions Requiring Stabilization With Prostaglandin E₁ Infusion		
Parameter	Ductal Dependent Pulmonary Blood Flow	Ductal Dependent Systemic Blood Flow	Inadequate Mixing
Presenting Symptoms	Cyanosis	Shock	Cyanosis
Lesions	Severe tetralogy of Fallot Pulmonary atresia with intact ventricular septum Critical pulmonary stenosis Severe Ebstein anomaly Single ventricle with severe pulmonary stenosis or atresia	Hypoplastic left heart syndrome Critical aortic stenosis Interrupted aortic arch Critical coarctation Single ventricle with severe aortic stenosis or atresia	Transposition of the great arteries Taussig-Bing double-outlet right ventricle

in pressure will be proportional to the mean arterial pressure in the descending aorta subtracted from the intrathoracic pressure (ΔP). Thus positive pressure ventilation (which increases intrathoracic pressure) decreases the work that the heart must perform to bring blood to the descending aorta. Pharmacologic reduction of afterload can be attained by administration of an arterial vasodilator.

Alprostadil (Prostaglandin E₁)

Alprostadil, or prostaglandin E₁ (PGE₁), is a potent vasodilator and specifically maintains patency of the ductus arteriosus in the fetus and newborn. The introduction of PGE₁ into clinical practice in 1976 allowed stabilization and recovery of newborns with nearly all ductal dependent cardiac lesions before repair or palliation of complex congenital heart lesions.[141] Although the mechanism resulting in the vasodilatory effect of PGE₁ has not been fully described, a dose-related increase in nitric oxide and nitric oxide synthase has been seen in other tissues. PGE₁ also has

inhibitory effects on platelet aggregation and can increase the risk of bleeding.

PGE₁ is nearly completely metabolized on first pass through the pulmonary circulation to the active metabolite 13,14-dihydro-15-keto-PGE₁.

The usual starting dose is 0.05 mcg/kg/min, which can be increased every 15 to 30 minutes up to 0.4 mcg/kg/min, with the maximum response occurring 15 minutes to 4 hours after start of the infusion.[141] Once the duct is open, patency should be maintained at the lowest effective dose, which is generally 0.01 to 0.03 mcg/kg/min. Newborns up to a month of age may still respond to PGE₁ infusion as long as ductal closure is not complete.[141,142]

The major indication for PGE₁ is maintaining patency of the ductus arteriosus in infants with CHD. Ductal dependent CHD includes lesions with inadequate pulmonary blood flow, inadequate systemic blood flow, and inadequate mixing (Table 19.7). Newborns with right-sided obstructive lesions may have ductal dependent pulmonary blood flow and present with cyanosis and paucity of pulmonary blood flow, which will improve with initiation of PGE$_1$.[143] PGE$_1$ also causes pulmonary vasodilation at a dose as low as 0.05 to 0.1 mcg/kg/min with an increase in pulmonary blood flow in patients with pulmonary hypertension.[144] Additionally, infants with left-sided obstructive lesions may have ductal dependent systemic blood flow and present with systemic hypoperfusion and shock. PGE$_1$ administration usually results in resolution of acidosis and increased pulses.[143]

Newborns with transposition of the great arteries (TGA), with or without a ventricular septal defect (VSD), will have ductal dependent mixing if the intracardiac shunting is inadequate. A subset of these patients with nearly intact atrial septum will present with early shock; however, a majority of infants with TGA present with isolated cyanosis. Initiation of PGE$_1$ will help stabilize these patients until a balloon atrial septostomy can be performed.

A few cardiac lesions cannot be stabilized by PGE$_1$ therapy alone, and infants with these lesions will rapidly progress to shock. Total anomalous pulmonary venous return with obstruction requires urgent surgical repair or stabilization on venoarterial extracorporeal membrane oxygenator. Administration of PGE$_1$ to these patients can worsen symptoms.[145] Hypoplastic left heart syndrome with intact atrial septum requires opening of the atrial septum in the catheterization laboratory or operating room. TGA with inadequate intracardiac shunting requires emergent balloon atrial septostomy.

Side effects of PGE$_1$ include primarily hypotension, fever, edema, and hypoventilation.[146] These complications were more common with intraaortic administration, which is a less common route of administration than IV administration. Respiratory depression, including apnea, occurred in 12% of children and was most common in infants with a birth weight less than 2 kg.[146] Thus premature infants, those requiring high-dose PGE$_1$, or those with inadequate observation time on PGE$_1$ may benefit from a secure airway for transportation.

Nitroprusside

In vitro data suggest that nitroprusside causes release of nitric oxide, which then reacts with a variety of thiols to produce unstable S-nitrosothiols, which are potent activators of guanylate cyclase. This, in turn, causes a rise in intracellular cyclic guanosine monophosphate (cGMP), which activates cGMP-dependent protein kinases and ultimately leads to smooth muscle relaxation and vasodilation.

Nitroprusside combines with hemoglobin to produce cyanide and cyanmethemoglobin. Cyanide detoxification mainly occurs in the liver via rhodanase-mediated conversion of cyanide to thiocyanate (Fig. 19.10). Thiocyanate is then renally excreted. A cofactor in this reaction is vitamin B$_{12}$.[147]

Nitroprusside has a rapid onset of less than 2 minutes and a t$_{1/2}$ of less than 5 minutes. Thiocyanate has a half-life of approximately 3 days; however, it can be prolonged in patients with renal insufficiency. Nitroprusside is light sensitive and can be administered through peripheral IV access.

Nitroprusside is a mixed vasodilator that results in preload reduction (venous vasodilation) and afterload reduction (arterial vasodilation). It has no direct cardiac effects (Table 19.8) but indirectly can enhance cardiac output. General dosing is 0.3 to 3 mcg/kg/min and may be titrated every 5 minutes or longer until the desired effect is reached (maximum of 10 mcg/kg/min or 400 mcg/min).[148,149] Nitroprusside has been found to be efficacious in maintaining mean arterial blood pressure within the

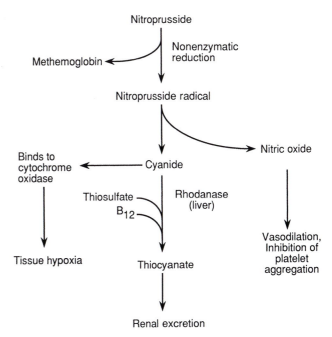

• **Figure 19.10** Metabolic pathway for the degradation of nitroprusside.

TABLE 19.8	Nitroprusside Pharmacology
Dose (mcg/kg/min)	0.5-10
Mechanism	Direct smooth muscle relaxation
Major effects	Venous and arteriolar vasodilation Decreases SVR, PVR Decreases preload
Indications	Hypertensive emergencies Deliberate hypotension technique during major surgery Blood pressure control after coarctation repair Afterload reduction after cardiac surgery
Major complications	Severe hypotension Tachycardia Compromised cardiac output in preload-dependent physiology Hypertension after weaning nitroprusside Ventilation/perfusion mismatch Increased Q$_p$:Q$_s$ in infants with large left-to-right shunt Cyanide and thiocyanate intoxication

PVR, Pulmonary vascular resistance; *Q$_p$:Q$_s$*, pulmonary-to-systemic blood flow ratio; *SVR*, systemic vascular resistance.

recommended dosing range, following a 12-hour infusion, without the development of tolerance.

Indications. *Ventricular dysfunction* has been evaluated as a potential indication for nitroprusside administration, specifically in patients with diastolic abnormalities.[150] This is secondary to reduction in systemic afterload with concomitant optimization of preload. Similarly, children with mitral regurgitation benefit from nitroprusside administration[151] with reduced SVR and enhanced forward cardiac output.[152]

Low cardiac output syndrome (LCOS) after open-heart surgery is an indication for nitroprusside, most often in conjunction with inotropic agents. The addition of epinephrine to nitroprusside further augments the cardiac index without increasing SVR.[153] The combination of these may necessitate the need for volume expansion to maintain adequate preload. Nitroprusside, supplemented by blood transfusion to maintain filling pressure, significantly increases cardiac index in children with low output syndrome following cardiac surgery.[153,154]

Hypertensive emergencies have been managed safely using nitroprusside in the pediatric population.[155] Nitroprusside infusion avoids neurologic complications associated with bolus administration of vasodilators such as diazoxide and hydralazine. Progressive increases in cardiac index in children with hypertensive crisis receiving nitroprusside may simulate nitroprusside tachyphylaxis because higher nitroprusside doses are generally required to achieve equivalent blood pressure control.[156] In addition, nitroprusside can be used alone or in conjunction with beta-blockers for systemic hypertension following coarctation repairs.

The major side effects of nitroprusside are predictable from its hemodynamic and metabolic properties. Profound systemic hypotension can occur with boluses or high-dose infusions, for which invasive arterial pressure monitoring is beneficial. Patients should have large-bore IV access established so that intravascular volume can be expanded rapidly if needed. If necessary, children can be placed in the Trendelenburg position, which shifts blood volume to the central circulation and restores adequate blood pressure. Discontinuation of nitroprusside may produce rebound hypertension, which may be aggravated by increased SVR, hypervolemia, or tachycardia.

Nitroprusside can worsen ventilation/perfusion mismatch resulting in hypoxemia, particularly in patients with pulmonary edema or lung disease.

Cyanide (CN^-) and, to a lesser extent, thiocyanate toxicities are the most feared metabolic complications. Inadequate levels of thiosulfate and rhodanase in conjunction with high nitroprusside infusion doses may lead to accumulation of free CN^-, which will inhibit oxidative phosphorylation and may lead to tissue hypoxia. Patients with cyanide toxicity exhibit a metabolic acidosis in spite of adequate oxygen delivery and increased mixed venous saturation. Thiocyanate is normally excreted in the urine, but when this compound accumulates, psychosis and convulsions can ensue. Although thiocyanate toxicity is unusual in children with normal hepatic and renal function,[157] doses of 1.8 mcg/kg/min or higher are associated with increased cyanide concentration in pediatric patients following cardiac surgery. Treatment of cyanide toxicity in adults includes administration of sodium nitrite and sodium thiosulfate.[158] Pediatric dosages depend on the child's hemoglobin concentration (Table 19.9). Coadministration of thiosulfate with nitroprusside may also decrease the risk of cyanide toxicity in adults and children. Hydroxocobalamin has been shown to prevent accumulation of cyanide and acidosis.[159] Pediatric dosing is 70 mg/kg (maximum 5 g) administered over 30 minutes, with optional repeated doses of 35 mg/kg depending on severity.

Nitroglycerin

Nitroglycerin induces the release of nitric oxide in vascular smooth muscle via aldehyde dehydrogenase. In contrast to nitroprusside, the major effect of nitroglycerin is dilation of the venous capacitance vessels and coronary arteries, with lesser effects on systemic arterioles. This results in reduction of both right and left atrial pressures and also pulmonary and systemic arterial pressures. Nitroglycerin

TABLE 19.9	Sodium Nitrite and Sodium Thiosulfate Doses for Treatment of Cyanide Poisoning From Nitroprusside Toxicity	
Hemoglobin (g/dL)	Initial Dose of 3% Sodium Nitrite[a] (mL/kg IV)	Initial Dose of 25% Sodium Thiosulfate[b] (mL/kg IV)
8	0.22	1.10
10	0.27	1.35
12	0.33	1.65
14	0.39	1.95

[a]Maximum initial dose is 10 mL.
[b]Maximum initial dose is 50 mL.
IV, Intravenously.

is not as effective as nitroprusside in lowering blood pressure in healthy children undergoing major surgery[160]; however, it is favorable in regard to coronary vasodilation. In adult patients nitroglycerin has been shown to improve myocardial ischemia, presumably due to improvement in the ratio of myocardial oxygen supply and demand.[161] Likewise, in adults after coronary artery bypass surgery, nitroglycerin can be as effective as nitroprusside in treating postoperative hypertension. Endothelin-1, which is elevated following cardiac surgery in infants and children, results in coronary vasoconstriction that is reversed by nitroglycerin.[162] The coronary vasodilatory effects may be suppressed in patients with aneurysms. Patients with persistent or regressed aneurysms following Kawasaki syndrome demonstrate decreased coronary vasodilation to nitroglycerin both at the site of the regressed aneurysm[163] and at angiographically normal coronary segments. The diminished reactivity to nitroglycerin suggests fixed stenosis or ongoing vasculitis with endothelial dysfunction in some patients who appear to have recovered from the acute phase of Kawasaki syndrome.

Nitroglycerin has been used for treatment of LCOS in children who had undergone cardiac surgery and had low cardiac indexes (less than 2.5 L/min/m²) with left atrial pressures of 10 to 14 mm Hg.[164] Administration of nitroglycerin resulted in a significant improvement of cardiac index without significant hemodynamic changes or need for inotropic support in those with adequate intravascular volume (Fig. 19.11). These outcomes may be due to improvements in myocardial oxygen supply (via coronary vasodilation and improved myocardial regional blood flow), use of blood transfusion (made possible by the vasodilation), decreased myocardial oxygen demand (by reduction of afterload), or a combination of all.[164]

Nitroglycerin has been used as a pulmonary vasodilator in children with variable success depending on the cause and duration of pulmonary hypertension. Successful pulmonary vasodilation has been achieved after the arterial switch procedure for TGA and after closure of intracardiac left-to-right shunts.[165] Although the nitroglycerin dose has ranged from 2 to 10 mcg/kg/min, significant lowering of pulmonary pressure has required infusion rates of 5 mcg/kg/min or greater. Conversely, nitroglycerin was not effective in lowering pulmonary artery pressure and resistance in a neonatal sepsis model. Taken together, these data suggest that nitroglycerin at higher doses may be useful for some cases of reactive pulmonary hypertension; however, fixed pulmonary

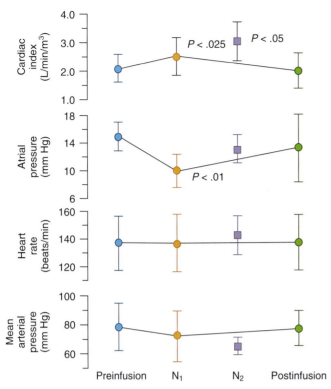

• **Figure 19.11** Hemodynamic effects of nitroglycerin infusion in children after cardiac surgery. There is a significant increase in cardiac index and a fall in atrial pressures during nitroglycerin infusion (N_1). A further increase in cardiac index is noted in four patients during nitroglycerin infusion and preloading (N_2). (From Benson LN, Bohn D, Edmonds JF, et al. Nitroglycerin therapy in children with low cardiac index after heart surgery. *Cardiovasc Med.* 1979;4:207-215; with permission.)

vascular disease, sepsis, and chronic lung disease do not respond. Regarding effect on gas exchange, nitroglycerin increases the alveolar-arterial O_2 gradient ($AaDO_2$) only modestly, whereas nitroprusside administration was associated with a significant rise in $AaDO_2$.

Nicardipine

Nicardipine is a calcium channel blocker belonging to the smooth muscle–selective class known as dihydropyridines. Prevention of movement of calcium ions into vascular and myocardial smooth muscles results in peripheral arterial vasodilation. Because of their high vascular selectivity, these drugs are primarily used to reduce SVR and arterial pressure and therefore are used to treat hypertension in pediatric patients.[166] Nicardipine is metabolized via cytochrome P-450 isoenzyme CYP3A4, resulting in risk of several drug interactions and decreased clearance in hepatic dysfunction. Nicardipine has a rapid onset of action within minutes and can be quickly titrated. The half-life is dose dependent with an alpha half-life of 2 to 3 minutes and a terminal half-life of 14 hours with prolonged infusions resulting in a 50% decrease of effect at 30 minutes after the cessation of an infusion and reduction of antihypertensive effects over 50 hours. Central administration is preferred due to risk of venous irritation with peripheral administration. The recommended initial dose of continuous infusion nicardipine is 0.5 to 1 mcg/kg/min with titration every 15 to 30 minutes up to 5 mcg/kg/min. Nicardipine is used for

pediatric hypertension and hypertensive emergencies.[80] In the CHD population, nicardipine is often used to manage postoperative hypertension, particularly postcoarctectomy to prevent risk of stroke and adverse outcomes. Calcium channel blockers had been generally avoided in children less than 6 months given concerns for myocardial depression, although there are data that support the safety and efficacy of nicardipine in this age-group without undesired myocardial effects.[167-172] The systemic vasodilating effects can lead to reflex tachycardia, which can offset the beneficial effects of afterload reduction on myocardial oxygen demand.

Angiotensin-Converting Enzyme Inhibitors

Angiotensin-converting enzyme (ACE) converts angiotensin I to angiotensin II, which is a potent systemic vasoconstrictor and induces sodium and water retention via aldosterone activation. Hence administration of ACE inhibitor lowers SVR and increases venous capacitance. Blood pressure does not change significantly if cardiac output can increase to compensate for the fall in SVR.

Enalaprilat is an IV form of ACE inhibitor. In adults with congestive heart failure secondary to ischemic heart disease, enalaprilat administered either as a bolus or continuous infusion improves hemodynamics and oxygen delivery, with no impact on cardiac index.[173]

With the exception of treatment of acute hypertension/hypertensive crisis, the reported use of enalaprilat in children is limited. Extrapolation of the indications for enalaprilat can be made from the oral ACE inhibitors and provides an option for patients acutely unable to tolerate oral medications.

ACE inhibitors are used predominantly in three populations: congestive heart failure in dilated cardiomyopathy, congestive heart failure in large left-to-right shunts, and systemic hypertension. A hyperreninemic state and consequently increased angiotensin levels characterize all of these conditions (Table 19.10). Infants with large left-to-right shunts (e.g., VSD) and congestive heart failure may have a favorable response to ACE inhibitors.[174-176] The hemodynamic response depends on the baseline SVR; thus infants with increased SVR (greater than 20 U/m²) as well as increased Q_p:Q_s and pulmonary artery pressure are most likely to achieve a reduction in Q_p:Q_s after captopril.[176]

There are few significant complications from ACE inhibitors. Hypotension is the major hemodynamic complication. It is more common at high doses and in young infants and in the setting of hyponatremia. Blood pressure should be monitored closely at the start of ACE inhibitor therapy, and dosages are increased gradually. Hyperkalemia may also result due to a decrease in aldosterone, which is normally responsible for potassium excretion. Renal insufficiency has been reported with use, secondary to reduction in efferent arteriolar tone and therefore glomerular filtration[29]; however this effect rarely occurs.[176]

Angiotensin Receptor Blockers

Angiotensin receptor blockers (ARBs) have very similar effects to ACE inhibitors and are used for the same indications. Their mechanism of action, however, is very different from that of ACE inhibitors, in that ARBs are receptor antagonists that block angiotensin II receptors on blood vessels and other tissues such as the heart. These receptors are coupled to the $G\alpha^q$-protein and IP_3 signal transduction pathway that stimulates vascular smooth muscle contraction (see Fig. 19.2). ARBs also have transforming growth factor-beta blocking properties, which have been shown to slow

TABLE 19.10 Oral Angiotensin-Converting Enzyme Inhibitor and Angiotensin Receptor Blocker Dosing in Pediatric Patients With Heart Disease

Oral Agents		Dosing	Adverse Effects
ACE inhibitors	Captopril[a]	Initial: 0.2-0.4 mg/kg/d divided q6-8h Max: 6 mg/kg/d (Max: 450 mg/d) divided q6-8h	• Hyperkalemia • Hyponatremia • Increased SCr • Anemia • Cough • Thrombocytopenia
	Enalapril[a]	Initial: 0.04-0.1 mg/kg/day (Max 5 mg/d) divided every day to twice daily Max: 0.8 mg/kg/d (Max: 40 mg/d) divided every day to twice a day	
	Lisinopril[a]	Initial: 0.07 mg/kg (Max: 5 mg) orally every day Max: 0.6 mg/kg (Max: 40 mg) orally every day	
ARBs	Candesartan	Initial: 0.2 mg/kg/d (Max: 8 mg) divided every day to twice a day Max: 0.4 mg/kg/d (Max: 32 mg/d) divided every day to twice a day	• Hyperkalemia • Hyponatremia • Increased SCr • Anemia • Thrombocytopenia
	Losartan	Initial: 0.7 mg/kg/d (Max: 50 mg/d) divided every day to twice a day Max: 1.4 mg/kg/d (Max: 100 mg/d) divided every day to twice a day	
	Irbesartan	6 to <13 y: Initial: 75 mg/d orally divided every day to twice a day Max: 150 mg orally every day ≥13 y: Initial: 150 mg/d orally divided every day to twice a day Max: 300 mg orally every day	
	Valsartan[246]	1 to <6 y and ≥8 kg: Initial: 0.4-1 mg/kg orally every day Max: 8-18 kg: 3.4 mg/kg (Max: 40 mg) ≥18 kg: 3.4 mg/kg (Max: 80 mg) ≥6 y: Initial: 1.3 mg/kg (Max: 40 mg) orally every day Max: 2.7 mg/kg (Max: 160 mg) orally every day	

[a]Requires dose adjustments in renal impairment.
ACE, Angiotensin-converting enzyme; *ARB,* angiotensin receptor blocker; *SCr,* serum creatinine.

progression of aneurysm formation in some connective tissue diseases, such as Marfan syndrome and Loeys-Dietz syndrome.[177] Because ARBs do not inhibit ACE, they do not cause an increase in bradykinin, which contributes to side effects of ACE inhibitors (cough and angioedema). Hyperkalemia may also be seen with ARB use.

In 2015 the Food and Drug Administration approved an angiotensin receptor–neprilysin inhibitor (sacubitril/valsartan [Entresto]) following a clinical trial of more than 8000 adults in which this drug was shown to reduce the rate of cardiovascular death and hospitalizations related to heart failure when compared with enalapril.[178] There was also less kidney injury with Entresto than with enalapril. Sacubitril is a neprilysin inhibitor, and administration results in increased natriuresis, increased urine cGMP levels, and decreased plasma levels of N-terminal pro-brain natriuretic peptide (NT-proBNP). Valsartan is an angiotensin II receptor type I inhibitor. The safety and efficacy of Entresto has not been established in pediatric patients.

All of the drugs in this section can promote reverse ventricular remodeling, resulting in improved ventricular mechanics and function.

Vasoconstrictors

Phenylephrine

Phenylephrine is an alpha$_1$ agonist with very little beta effect. Its major action is systemic and pulmonary arterial vasoconstriction, increasing SVR and systemic arterial pressure (systolic, diastolic,

and mean). Reflex bradycardia can occur. The increase in pulmonary artery pressure is less pronounced than the increase in aortic pressure.

Phenylephrine has been used in a variety of settings. Bolus (10 mcg/kg) and/or continuous (2 to 5 mcg/kg/min) IV phenylephrine have been used to reverse and treat the hypercyanotic spells of tetralogy of Fallot. By increasing the SVR in excess of the PVR, this alpha$_1$ agonist lessens right-to-left ventricular shunting and improves arterial oxygenation.[179,180]

Septic shock with low SVR has been considered an indication for phenylephrine in adults. In a small series of patients, oxygen delivery, oxygen consumption, stroke volume index, and urine output all increased after phenylephrine infusion.[181] Phenylephrine is rarely used in pediatric septic shock.

The use of phenylephrine after CPB is more controversial. In a low-cardiac-output state, phenylephrine may improve hemodynamics and right ventricular coronary driving pressure but at the cost of increasing myocardial oxygen demand.[182-184] These studies are limited to adults and animal models.

Arginine Vasopressin

Arginine vasopressin (or antidiuretic hormone) is a neuropeptide secreted by the posterior pituitary gland in response to increases in serum osmolality or decreases in plasma volume. At low concentrations, vasopressin causes free water retention by the kidney. At higher concentrations, vasoconstriction occurs.[185]

Adults with vasodilatory septic shock have been shown to have low vasopressin plasma levels.[186] Vasopressin (0.04 U/min) improves arterial blood pressure by increasing SVR without affecting cardiac index in adults with vasodilatory septic shock.[185] Similarly, adults with vasodilatory shock following cardiac surgery have inappropriately low serum vasopressin concentrations and demonstrate increased mean arterial pressure with vasopressin (0.09 ± 0.05 U/min).[187] Vasopressin has also been shown to improve systemic blood pressure without affecting cardiac index in patients with milrinone-induced vasodilation and hypotension following cardiac surgery.[188]

In children, plasma levels of vasopressin following congenital cardiac surgery appear to be elevated compared with preoperative levels.[189] However, infants and children with acceptable cardiac function but vasodilatory shock following cardiac surgery that is refractory to inotropes and vasopressors demonstrate a significant increase in systemic blood pressure with vasopressin infusion (0.0001 to 0.002 U/kg/min).[122,190] Vasopressin should be considered in the patient with adequate cardiac function but severe vasodilatory shock that is not responsive to dopamine or epinephrine.

In addition to the role of vasopressin as a pressor, studies in animals suggest that vasopressin can decrease capillary leak and the resultant edema.[81] Decreased capillary leak may also decrease the volume of chest tube output in children following the Fontan procedure, thereby decreasing hospital length of stay.[191]

Please refer to Tables 19.1 and 19.2 for additional dosing and monitoring information for use of adrenergic and nonadrenergic infusions in pediatric patients.

Diuretics

Loop Diuretics

Loop diuretics work by inhibiting the sodium-potassium-chloride ($Na^+/K^+/2\ Cl$) cotransporter in the thick ascending loop of Henle, which inhibits reabsorption of sodium and chloride in this part of the nephron, thereby causing excretion of water and sodium, chloride, calcium, magnesium, potassium, and hydrogen ions.

Commonly used loop diuretics are furosemide and bumetanide. The bioavailability of oral furosemide is approximately 50%.[192] If a switch is made from IV to oral administration, doubling the dose should be considered to maintain equivalency. Bumetanide bioavailability can be as high as 90%, so the IV to oral dose conversion is 1 : 1.[193-197]

Comparison studies of continuous infusion versus intermittent infusion of furosemide have shown that diuresis is more controlled with fewer hemodynamic and electrolytic variations during continuous infusion. Infusion rates of furosemide range from 0.05 to 0.4 mg/kg/h. Bumetanide is approximately 40 times more potent than furosemide. Bumetanide intermittent IV doses range from 0.005 to 0.1 mg/kg every 24 hours and continuous infusion rates from 0.01 to 0.05 mg/kg/h, although higher doses have been reported.[198]

Unlike the other loop diuretics, ethacrynic acid is not a sulfonamide, and thus its use is not contraindicated in those with sulfa allergies. It can be administered by oral or IV route.

Thiazide and Other Drugs With Diuretic Effect

Thiazide and thiazide-like diuretics (chlorothiazide, hydrochlorothiazide, metolazone) inhibit reabsorption of sodium in distal tubules, causing increased excretion of sodium and water, as well as potassium and hydrogen ions. Hydrochlorothiazide and metolazone are available only in oral dosage forms. Chlorothiazide is available for intermittent IV or oral dosing. It has a bioavailability that ranges from 50% to 75%; however, this is reduced in patients with congestive heart failure or when administered with food.[199]

Aminophylline also has diuretic effect, acting on the renal vasculature by adenosine receptor blockade or type IV phosphodiesterase inhibition. However, reports on use of aminophylline in diuretic-dependent children are limited to a few studies. Administration of aminophylline at low doses (3 mg/kg) before administration of furosemide has been shown to promote increased urine output.[200,201]

Nesiritide is the recombinant human form of brain natriuretic peptide (BNP). BNP is a hormone that is released from ventricular myocytes subjected to increased volume stretch. BNP leads to a vascular smooth muscle (vasodilation), natriuresis, and diuresis. In addition, BNP decreases the synthesis of a variety of hormones associated with congestive heart failure, including norepinephrine, endothelin-1, angiotensin, and aldosterone. BNP does not have inotropic or chronotropic effects. Initial enthusiasm for its use declined with results from adult studies revealing worsening renal function and increased mortality.[202,203] However, a recent systematic review of these trials revealed no adverse effect on survival, and use was not associated with worsening renal function.[204,205] Although there are no pediatric trials of nesiritide to date, there have been retrospective studies in pediatric patients with critical congenital cardiac disease in which nesiritide had a favorable impact on hemodynamics and urine output in children with no worsening of renal function. Adult studies have used a loading dose of 1-2 mcg/kg IV bolus followed by an infusion at 0.005 to 0.01 mcg/kg/min, titrated to a maximum of 0.03 mcg/kg/min.[206-211]

Pharmacology in Children on Extracorporeal Support

Children with CHD may require extracorporeal life support (ECLS). Although ECLS is often lifesaving, these devices can affect drug exposure. Drug exposure can be impacted in three primary ways: (1) drug extraction by the circuit; (2) ECLS-associated organ dysfunction; and (3) for drugs whose distribution is limited to the blood, hemodilution due to the volume of exogenous blood required to prime the circuit.

Drug Extraction by the Circuit

Multiple ex vivo experiments have shown that certain drugs are directly extracted by the ECLS circuit.[212-221] Drug extraction is likely due to nonspecific adsorption by the various materials that constitute the circuit (e.g., tubing, oxygenator).[214,222-225] Whether or not a drug is extracted depends on the interaction between the circuit material and the physicochemical properties of the drug. For example, fentanyl was highly extracted (>99% loss over 180 minutes) in an extracorporeal membrane oxygenation (ECMO) circuit with a silicone membrane oxygenator but showed only 66% loss over the same time frame in a circuit with a microporous, hollow-fiber polypropylene oxygenator. Other studies of fentanyl showed that the vast majority of extraction can be attributed to tubing, and the extent of extraction is impacted by the type of tubing coating.[223,224] Although ex vivo studies have generally demonstrated increased extraction of highly lipophilic and protein-bound drugs, this relationship is not entirely predictable and likely depends on other factors such as the degree of drug ionization driven by blood pH and the negative logarithm of the ionization constant of an acid (pKa) of the drug.[214,219,220,226] Knowing how much extraction occurs can help clinicians decide whether higher doses might be necessary. However, determining an exact dose with ex vivo data has been problematic. Further, many questions remain about whether drug adsorption is saturable and reversible.[213,221] Efforts are under way to study these topics in systematic fashion.[227]

Extracorporeal Life Support–Related Organ Dysfunction

ECLS-related organ dysfunction can cause alterations in both volume of distribution and clearance. Exposure to the ECMO circuit results in an inflammatory response, resulting in capillary leak and increased volume of distribution.[228-232] In addition, altered blood pH can affect the ionization of a drug and distribution into tissues. Renal dysfunction is common in patients on ECMO, occurring in more than 30% of ECMO patients.[233] Reasons for the renal dysfunction are not entirely clear but appear to be multifactorial.[233,234] Altered renal function can substantially increase exposure of renally cleared drugs and places children at risk for toxicity. It is postulated that altered liver blood flow and inflammation could decrease metabolism for some drugs.[231,235-240] However, this has not been demonstrated in children supported with ECLS. There are no data describing the impact of ECLS on drug transporters. Because transporter function can be impacted by inflammation, it is possible that ECLS could also impact exposure of drugs that rely on transporters.

Hemodilution

Hemodilution is common, especially in ECMO, and occurs due to the large volume of exogenous blood required to prime the circuit, frequent transfusions of blood products, and administration of crystalloid to maintain circuit flows. Hemodilution has the largest effect on drugs whose distribution is primarily confined to the bloodstream. The impact of hemodilution is less for drugs with a large volume of distribution because drug diluted in the bloodstream may be replaced by drug stored in the tissue. Further, the impact of hemodilution is inversely related to age. For a 3-kg infant the circuit prime volume (250 to 400 mL) might exceed the infant's native blood volume (≈250 mL), whereas in a 70-kg adolescent, the prime volume is approximately 8% of the child's blood volume (≈5 L).

Most of the work studying the impact of ECLS on drug dosing has focused on ECMO, but studies are now being done in ventricular assist devices. Among the cardiovascular drugs discussed in the chapter, only esmolol and PGE$_1$ have been described in children, and both are limited to case reports.[241,242] Epinephrine and dopamine were evaluated in an isolated ECMO circuit. After spontaneous degradation is accounted for, epinephrine and dopamine lost less than 10% of their original concentration due to interaction with the circuit. Due to the limited data available, no definitive dosing recommendations can be made for the drugs in this chapter. For drugs such as inotropes that can be titrated to effect, standard dosing should be used, though the upper limit of safe dosing is unknown. Dosing recommendations for other classes of drugs commonly used on ECMO are published but in many cases are based on limited data.[243-245] Given the differences reported in drug extraction between older components (e.g., silicone membrane oxygenators) and newer technology (e.g., polymethylpentene-fiber oxygenators), it is unknown whether dosing recommendations derived from trials using the older technology can be extrapolated to children supported with modern ECLS circuits.

Conclusion

The interplay between clinical trial and molecular biology has been particularly fruitful in the understanding, design, and clinical application of cardiovascular drugs. In the future, cardiovascular therapy will become more specific and safer as further insights into basic mechanisms are developed.

References

A complete list of references is available at ExpertConsult.com.

20

Anesthesia and Sedation for Pediatric Heart Disease

EULECHE ALANMANOU, MD, FAAP; NINA DEUTSCH, MD; VYAS M. KARTHA, MD, FAAP;
JAMIE MCELRATH SCHWARTZ, MD

Pediatric cardiac anesthesiology is a dynamic field with its unique impact and challenges. Our field has grown from skilled anesthesiologists with an interest in cardiac patients, to the development in 2005 of the Congenital Cardiac Anesthesia Society, which eventually led to a proposal for formal training pathways in 2010.[1] Our practice spans anesthesia and sedation for neonatal critical cardiac disease, palliation for children with cardiac disease with and without cardiopulmonary bypass (CPB), cardiac and lung transplantation, interventional cardiology, advanced imaging, patients with cardiac disease for noncardiac surgery, electrophysiology, and adult congenital heart disease. As outcomes from congenital cardiac surgery improve, over a million children and adults are living with corrected or palliated congenital heart disease; these patients with sometimes significantly altered physiology present challenges to the anesthesia community. Pediatric cardiac anesthesiologists are key members of the multidisciplinary team that cares for these patients.

Anesthesia Risk for Children With Congenital Heart Disease

Children with cardiac disease are at substantially increased risk when undergoing anesthesia when compared with children without cardiac disease. Specifically, infants with single-ventricle physiology, left ventricular outflow tract obstruction (LVOTO), cardiomyopathy, and pulmonary hypertension are at greatest risk.[2-7]

A critical role of the cardiac anesthesiologist is to know and integrate these risk factors with the patient's specific information to provide risk stratification and consultation. In many centers the number of needed procedures on patients with cardiac disease is greater than the availability of anesthesiologists who specialize in cardiac anesthesia, and therefore anesthesia for some lower-risk patients or procedures can be successfully performed by noncardiac anesthesiologists in consultation with cardiac anesthesiologists. Additionally, because anesthesia has significant risk for patients with cardiac disease, cardiac anesthesiologists often serve in the role of perioperative care coordinator, combining procedures to minimize anesthetics and improve care efficiency for our patients.

Preoperative Management

The cardiac anesthesiologist is part of the team that makes critical cardiac surgical planning decisions. Most centers have a surgical planning multidisciplinary conference to discuss upcoming surgeries and patients who may need repair. Patient history, physical examination, comorbidities, imaging, and preoperative testing results are reviewed and discussed. These data add to the anesthesiologist's understanding of preoperative condition and physiology. The anesthesiologist's attendance at this conference is essential for both obtaining information about upcoming cases and providing input for patient optimization before surgery.

Immediate standard anesthetic preoperative assessment includes a review of preoperative history, including symptoms, medications, allergies, and imaging studies. Additionally, the patient/family should be queried about anesthesia-associated issues, including recent infection, malignant hyperthermia, difficult airway, and nothing by mouth (NPO) timing.

Physical examination before cardiac anesthesia focuses on areas that may cause intraoperative challenges, as well as areas that may be modified before surgery. Head and neck examination looks for dysmorphism and possible difficult airway risk. Indeed, the incidence of difficult airway is higher in children with congenital cardiac disease, and difficult airway can complicate an already complex anesthesia for this patient population.[8] Loose teeth should be noted and discussed with parents. Excessively loose primary teeth are often removed under anesthesia to prevent accidental dislodgement and aspiration. Nares should be examined for signs of acute viral infection, and chest examination should look for signs of respiratory compromise. Excessive pulmonary blood flow lesions put children at increased risk for reactive airways disease and infection; these pathologic conditions should be addressed and optimized before surgery. Acute viral infection is common in children, especially in winter months, and it may increase perioperative risk of pulmonary complications.[9] Risk of pulmonary complications from viral infections should be weighed against the urgency of surgery. Although cardiac examination often confirms the findings associated with recent imaging studies, it should not be minimized. Abdominal examination can reveal distention, ascites associated with high venous pressure, and organomegaly from elevated right heart pressures or left-to-right (L-R) shunt. Pulses and perfusion are useful to assess before induction because children with compromised ventricular function are at risk for cardiovascular instability during induction and before placement of invasive lines. Palpation of the arterial pulse can provide real-time information about blood pressure when noninvasive cuff cycling is slower than the fluctuating clinical situation.

Because many of these patients have had many anesthetics, parents are often knowledgeable about anesthetic issues. They may have preferences about induction or information about previous positive or negative anesthetic experiences. Many centers include anesthetic evaluation and consultation during the preoperative visit performed in the days before surgery. This approach allows for a more deliberate assessment and communication than the immediate preoperative period. It provides time for anesthetic fine-tuning optimization, including shortened NPO times for patients with fluid-sensitive physiology or holding on the day of surgery of medications that may impact the anesthetic or hemodynamics.

There is a trend toward less preoperative laboratory study. In the relatively healthy outpatient, few laboratory values will impact preoperative planning. A hemoglobin test is needed before initiation of CPB to calculate hemodilution hemoglobin value. Because arterial blood gas level is typically obtained after induction and placement of invasive monitoring lines, hemoglobin value can be obtained at that time. Electrolytes, coagulation assays or tests to examine end-organ function are typically not indicated for outpatients unless there is high suspicion of abnormalities that will prompt preoperative changes in care or operative plan. Two required laboratory values are pregnancy test in menstruating females and preoperative type and screen for CPB cases. Because type and screen testing can take hours, it may need to be performed before

the day of surgery to avoid unacceptable delays and length of anesthetic. For inpatients, as well as patients who have end-organ dysfunction, the appropriate additional laboratory tests are ordered after surgical and anesthetic review.

Intraoperative Management

General Principles

The principles underlying anesthetic management of children with congenital heart disease are based on an understanding of each disease process, pathophysiology, and a working knowledge of anesthetic effects and other pharmacologic interventions on a specific patient's condition. Cardiac and great vessel structural abnormalities may result in shunt, outflow obstruction, regurgitation, common mixing, or a combination of lesions. Interactions between those lesions determine the clinical presentation and anesthetic considerations. Anesthesia and surgery will impact patient physiology, setting the stage for potential cardiovascular instability. Without being overly simplistic, once the defect characteristics, predominant physiology, and impact of surgery and anesthesia are understood, anesthesia for cardiac and noncardiac operations can be competently performed using a physiologic approach (Table 20.1).

Critical to understanding congenital cardiac physiology and anesthesia is the concept of shunting. A shunt is defined as an abnormal connection between two chambers or vessels that allows passage of blood. The direction and magnitude of shunting depends on defect size and pressure gradient between the chambers connected to that defect. Shunting is typically fixed in a restrictive defect, whereas it varies with the relative vascular resistances of the connected structures in a nonrestrictive defect.

TABLE 20.1 Intraoperative Hemodynamic Goals					
Condition	**HR**	**Contractility**	**Preload**	**Pulmonary Vascular Resistance**	**Systemic Vascular Resistance**
Shunts					
L → R (all types)	Normal	Normal	↑	↑	↓
Ventricular septal defect R → L	Normal	Normal	Normal	↓	↑
Obstructive					
Aortic stenosis	↓*	Normal-↑	↑	Normal	↑
Aortic coarctation	Normal	Normal	↑	Normal	↓
Mitral stenosis	↓	Normal-↑	↑	Normal-↓	Normal
Pulmonary stenosis	↓	↑	↑	↓	Normal
Dynamic subaortic obstruction	↓*	↓*	↑	Normal	Normal-↑
Dynamic subpulmonic obstruction	↓	↓*	↑	↓	Normal
Regurgitant					
Aortic insufficiency	Normal-↓	Normal-↓	↑	Normal	Normal-↓
Mitral regurgitation	Normal	Normal-↓	↑	Normal-↓	↓
Pulmonary insufficiency	Normal-↓	Normal	↑	↓	Normal
Tricuspid regurgitation	Normal	Normal	↑	↓	Normal

Many congenital heart defects include several of the above lesions; for dynamic outflow obstruction, an asterisk (*) marks the most important consideration.
HR, Heart rate; *L*, left; *R*, right.
Modified from Steven JM, Nicolson SC. Congenital heart disease. In: Greeley WJ, ed. *Pediatric Anesthesia*. New York: Harcourt Pub Ltd; 1999. *Atlas of Anesthesia*; vol. 7.

TABLE 20.2 Factors Affecting PVR/SVR			
Factors Increasing PVR	**Factors Decreasing PVR**	**Factors Increasing SVR**	**Factors Decreasing SVR**

• PEEP
• High airway pressure
• Atelectasis
• Low FiO_2
• Acidosis and hypercapnia
• Increased hematocrit
• Sympathetic stimulation
• Pain and agitation
• Epinephrine, dopamine
• Direct surgical manipulation
	• No PEEP
	• Low airway pressure
	• Normal FRC
	• High FiO_2
	• Alkalosis and hypocapnia
	• Low hematocrit
	• Blunted stress response
	• Nitric oxide
	• Vasodilators (milrinone)
		• Sympathetic stimulation
		  • Pain and agitation
		  • Epinephrine, dopamine
		  • Norepinephrine
		  • Ketamine
		• Vasopressin
		• Negative intrathoracic pressure
		• Hypothermia
			• Adequate sedation and analgesia
			• Vasodilators
			  • Milrinone, dobutamine
			  • Nitroprusside
			  • ACE inhibitors
			• Positive pressure ventilation
			• Fever, sepsis

ACE, Angiotensin-converting enzyme; *FiO₂*, fraction of inspired oxygen; *FRC*, functional residual capacity; *PEEP*, positive end-expiratory pressure; *PVR*, pulmonary vascular resistance; *SVR*, systemic vascular resistance.
Modified from Chan D, Schure A. Congenital heart disease. In: Vacanti C, Sikka P, Urman R, eds. *Essential Clinical Anesthesia.* New York: Cambridge University Press; 2011.

Cyanotic patients with right-to-left (R-L) shunt have too little pulmonary blood flow. This makes them less tolerant of airway obstruction or apnea during sedation or anesthesia. Systemic vasodilation may worsen a R-L shunt and cyanosis. R-L shunts slow the rate of inhalation induction by delaying the equilibration of partial pressure of alveolar-to-inspired anesthetic. This delay is more pronounced with the less soluble inhalation agents.[10]

Depending on the type and size of defect, lesions with L-R shunt are generally better tolerated under anesthesia. Nevertheless, depending on location of shunt, increasing L-R shunt by maneuvers that decrease pulmonary vascular resistance (PVR) may lead to some degree of systemic hypotension with reduction of coronary perfusion. Uncorrected L-R shunting and pulmonary overcirculation over the long term may produce changes that increase pulmonary vasculature reactivity, especially when weaning from bypass. The onset of intravenous (IV) anesthetic is slower in L-R shunting, whereas inhalational anesthetic pharmacokinetics remain unchanged.

Right heart obstructive lesions are either dynamic or fixed and may create R-L shunt where pulmonary to systemic defect is present. The degree of cyanosis will depend on the degree of right-sided obstruction, PVR, and systemic vascular resistance (SVR). It is advantageous to avoid systemic vasodilation. Reducing dynamic obstruction (by decreasing contractility) is helpful by reducing R-L shunting and improving cyanosis during anesthesia.

Patients with left heart obstructive lesions have decreased cardiac output and systemic perfusion. Consequently, they can rapidly decompensate with anesthesia and surgical manipulation. For the ductile-dependent left heart obstructive lesions, maintenance of prostaglandin infusion is necessary. An increase in the fraction of inspired oxygen (FiO_2) with concomitant decrease in PVR leads to steal from systemic circulation, which could be detrimental.

Management of regurgitant lesions (e.g., atrial-ventricular canal, Ebstein anomaly) includes reduction of regurgitant fraction by decreasing afterload (PVR for right-sided lesions, SVR for left-sided lesions), improvement in ventricular contractility, and heart rate increase.

Mixing lesions (e.g., single ventricle, total anomalous pulmonary venous return, tricuspid atresia, truncus arteriosus) are characterized by complete mixing of deoxygenated systemic venous blood and fully oxygenated pulmonary venous blood. Balance between systemic and pulmonary vascular resistances determines arterial blood desaturation. In a patient with single-ventricle physiology, PVR and SVR are the key determinants of hemodynamic stability. The desirable ratio of pulmonary blood flow to systemic perfusion (Q_p:Q_s) of approximately 1 (balanced) leads to an oxygen saturation as measured by pulse oximetry (SpO_2) of approximately 80%.[11] This delicate balance of PVR/SVR will place a patient with single-ventricle physiology at a higher risk of myocardial ischemia during induction of anesthesia and surgical manipulation.[12] Factors affecting the balance of PVR/SVR are listed in Table 20.2.[13]

The anesthesiologist will work toward hemodynamic goals by manipulating factors affecting cardiac output, systemic and pulmonary flow, and oxygen delivery with consideration of the specific anatomy and physiology as well as factors affecting the arterial O_2 content, especially the hemoglobin level (see Table 20.1). Specific anesthetic strategies will be further discussed later in the chapter.

Physiologic Monitoring

Noninvasive monitors are placed before anesthesia induction. They include a five-lead electrocardiography system (one lead for each extremity and one precordial lead in V_5 position), two pulse oximetry probes (preductal and postductal), and an appropriately sized blood pressure cuff. A nasopharyngeal temperature probe is inserted after intubation and is most closely reflective of brain temperature. Depending on the child's condition and planned procedure, additional monitoring is necessary: an indwelling arterial catheter, a central line, and a urinary catheter. A second temperature monitor is added (often rectal to reflect core temperature) when planning to go on bypass.

SpO_2 and capnography (end-tidal carbon dioxide [$ETCO_2$]) provide instantaneous feedback concerning adequacy of oxygenation and ventilation. Capnography is of great value and remains the gold standard to confirm tracheal intubation. SpO_2 and $ETCO_2$ direct ventilatory and hemodynamic adjustments to optimize Q_p:Q_s in patients with shunts and pulmonary artery bands. Differences in preductal and postductal SpO_2 values indicate shunting through a patent ductus arteriosus (PDA). SpO_2 and $ETCO_2$ can also be used to assess the adequacy of cardiac output.[14] Low systemic arterial saturation or inability of the oximeter probe to register a pulse wave may be a sign of a very low cardiac output and high systemic resistances.[15] SpO_2 values less than 80% often overestimate arterial oxygen saturation,[16] which make other means of tissue oxygenation measurement necessary.

Near-infrared spectroscopy (NIRS) measures regional oxygen saturation. Whereas the oxygen saturation displayed by the

TABLE 20.3	Factors Affecting NIRS
Factors Raising Cerebral NIRS	Factors Reducing Cerebral NIRS
↑ Hemoglobin	↑ Oxygen consumption
↑ PaO$_2$	↑ ICP (brain edema, decrease venous drainage)
↑ CPB flow or cardiac output	↑ Sweep rate/ hyperventilation
↑ Mean arterial pressure (↑ cerebral perfusion pressure)	
↓ Sweep rate (↑ CO$_2$)	

CPB, Cardiopulmonary bypass; *ICP,* intracranial pressure; *NIRS,* near-infrared spectroscopy.

pulse oximeter represents only the pulsatile component of light transmitted to tissues, signal received by the NIRS represents the nonpulsatile blood (75%) as well as pulsatile blood (20%).[17,18] Normal range of regional cerebral oxygen saturation (cerebral rSO$_2$) for a noncyanotic patient is 60% to 85%. The somatic rSO$_2$ is generally 10% higher than the cerebral. Any fall of rSO$_2$ 20% or more below the baseline obtained before induction warrants interventions aimed at improving oxygen delivery and/or decreasing oxygen consumption to restore rSO$_2$ (Table 20.3). Numerous studies have indicated good correlation between rSO$_2$ and central venous oxygen saturation (SvO$_2$).[18-21]

Continuous monitoring of arterial pressure is possible only through an indwelling intraarterial catheter. Previous procedures or currently planned procedure, such as radial artery cut-down, Blalock-Taussig shunt, or a subclavian flap for coarctation of the aorta repair, can impact the arterial pressure monitoring site. Other sites available for cannulation include ulnar, femoral, axillary, or umbilical arteries. Posterior tibial or the dorsalis pedis arterial catheters function poorly after CPB and do not reflect central aortic pressure when the temperature of the distal extremities remains low.[22] The optimal position of the umbilical artery catheter tip is just above the aortic bifurcation between L3 and L4 or preferably, high above the diaphragm between T6 and T9. To decrease the risk of thrombosis of the renal and mesenteric arteries, the tip should not be left in the area of T12 to L2.[23]

Major cardiovascular surgeries require some type of central venous pressure (CVP) monitoring. The CVP catheter is also used for administration of fluid, drugs, and blood products. Alternatively, directly placed transthoracic atrial lines may be used to deliver medications and to evaluate filling pressures during the separation from CPB and the postoperative period. Most often the right internal jugular is accessed. The left internal jugular is avoided in case of persistent left superior vena cava. Other percutaneous options include cannulation of subclavian, femoral, external jugular, or axillary veins. The use of real-time ultrasound guidance reduces the time and number of needle insertions required for successful venous cannulation and decreases the rate of complication compared to the use of anatomic landmarks. The greatest benefit was found for internal jugular cannulation.[24] In case of preexisting peripherally inserted central catheters anesthesiologists should ascertain that the catheter is at least 3 French for rapid fluid and blood infusion, and that the tip is positioned centrally for infusion of vasoactive agents. For patients with single-ventricle physiology, superior vena

cava thrombosis could be catastrophic, and femoral or atrial lines are sometimes the preferred options.

Another reliable source of central venous access is the umbilical vein. It is cannulated within the first week after birth. To use it as a central line, the optimal position of the tip should be in the right atrium or high in the inferior vena cava.

The utility of intraoperative echocardiographic assessment with Doppler color flow imaging in predicting outcome after repair of congenital heart defect was first demonstrated in 1989 by Ungerleider and associates,[25] using an epicardial echocardiography probe. Since then, many authors have published strong evidence supporting transesophageal echocardiography (TEE) use for all cardiac defects requiring repair under CPB.[26-29] Advances in probe technology make multiplane TEE use routine to confirm or revise the initial diagnosis and assess the heart function during the prebypass period, even in small neonates. In the postbypass period, TEE assesses repair adequacy, presence of residual defects, and ventricular filling and function. Bettex et al.,[30] in a series of 865 intraoperative TEE examinations for congenital heart defect surgeries, found that alteration in surgical management occurred in 12.7% of cases, including 7.3% repeat bypass run; alteration in medical management occurred in 19.4% of cases. The occurrence of airway compression or hemodynamic instability after insertion should prompt the removal of the TEE probe; using an intraoperative epicardial probe should be considered instead.

Preoperative Medication

For infants less than 6 month of age, no premedication is necessary. Children older than 9 months may require a dose of midazolam given orally 0.3 to 0.7 mg/kg to a maximum of 20 mg, 10 to 20 minutes before induction, to provide effective anxiolysis. If an IV access is available, then midazolam 0.05 mg/kg up to 4 mg may be given a few minutes before operating room transfer. On occasion, a child or adult with developmental delay and without IV access is given ketamine 4 to 5 mg/kg with glycopyrrolate 20 mcg/kg and midazolam 0.1 mg/kg via the intramuscular route; oral ketamine (5 mg/kg) and midazolam (0.5 mg/kg) is also an option for an older child with developmental delay or a patient who requires denser preoperative sedation.

Induction and Maintenance of Anesthesia

Although it is important to comprehend the complexities of shunt and vascular resistance changes, airway and ventilation effects on the cardiovascular system are of equal importance during induction and maintenance of anesthesia. Selection of an induction technique depends on the cardiac defect, the degree of cardiac dysfunction, and the level of preinduction sedation. Anesthetic agent titration is more important than specific anesthetic technique in patients with reasonable cardiac reserve. Successful and safe induction is possible with volatile agents such as sevoflurane and nitrous oxide or IV agents such as etomidate, fentanyl, midazolam, and ketamine.

Induction method choices include IV (when an IV catheter is present) and inhalational. Skillful airway management and adequacy of ventilation are essential during induction no matter what induction method is used.

The use of inhalation induction should be reserved for children with reasonable cardiac reserve. Sevoflurane is currently the only halogenated anesthetic used for induction in the United States. Sevoflurane may be combined with up to 50% of nitrous oxide during initial induction to speed induction and decrease patient response to pungent Sevoflurane odor. Sevoflurane increases the heart rate slightly, mildly depresses myocardial contractility, and lowers SVR and PVR. Depression of myocardial contractility and blood pressure with volatile agent use is more pronounced in neonates compared to older children and adults due to the effect of volatile agents on calcium channels in the immature cardiovascular system.[31,32] Pronounced bradycardia is frequent during sevoflurane induction of patients with trisomy 21 with and without heart defects.[33] Inhalation induction is generally well tolerated by most children, including some with cyanotic defects such as tetralogy of Fallot (TOF).

In situations in which a higher minimum alveolar concentration (MAC) is used during prolonged sevoflurane induction, cardiovascular compromise or collapse can occur, in particular when positive pressure ventilation is applied indiscriminately with excessive depth of anesthesia. Careful titration of anesthetic agent and depth is required.

After anesthetic induction, IV access is established or augmented as appropriate. A nondepolarizing muscle relaxant is usually administered, and an IV opioid and/or inhalation agent is chosen for maintenance of anesthesia. The child is preoxygenated before intubation, and a nasal or oral endotracheal tube is carefully positioned. Some degree of alveolar preoxygenation is recommended, even in an infant whose systemic perfusion might be jeopardized by PVR decrease. This maneuver delays desaturation during intubation. If the child arrives in the operating room with an endotracheal tube in place, it should be changed if the benefit of a new tube outweighs the reintubation risk.

Intravenous induction is preferable when a child arrives with a well-functioning preexisting IV catheter. For neonates and sick children, IV opioid plus relaxant induction is most prevalent. In patients with limited cardiac reserve, inhalation agents are less well tolerated as a primary anesthetic, especially after a CPB. Titrated doses of fentanyl or sufentanil are excellent induction and maintenance anesthetics for this group of patients because these opioids generally have a low impact on hemodynamics. After repair of a congenital heart defect, the hemodynamic effects of fentanyl at a dose of 25 mcg/kg with pancuronium given to infants in the postoperative period show no change in left atrial pressure, PVR, and cardiac index. There is only a small decrease in SVR and mean arterial pressure (MAP).[34] Higher doses of fentanyl at 50 to 75 mcg/kg with pancuronium result in a slightly greater fall in arterial pressure and heart rate.[35] Fentanyl has also been shown to block stimulus-induced pulmonary vasoconstriction and contributes to pulmonary circulation stability in neonatal congenital diaphragmatic hernia repair.[36] Thus fentanyl use may be extrapolated post CPB in newborns with pulmonary vascular responsiveness. The ultra–short-acting opioid remifentanil has not shown any significant advantage over fentanyl.[37,38] It is often possible to titrate low-dose inhalational agents with opioids and maintain hemodynamic stability. The combination of fentanyl/midazolam as an alternative to fentanyl/low-dose volatile agents is frequently used for maintenance of anesthesia. But this results in lower cardiac output due to a decrease in heart rate.[39,40] Despite a widespread safety margin exhibited by opioids, it should be noted that patients with marginally compensated hemodynamic function sustained by endogenous catecholamines may decompensate with higher-dose opioids.

Isoflurane or sevoflurane may be used for maintenance of anesthesia. Inhalation agents can provide both anesthesia and vasodilation when a vaporizer is connected to the circuit during CPB. Some studies have found volatile agents to be neuroprotectors on CPB.[41,42] Isoflurane and sevoflurane maintain the ratio $Q_p{:}Q_s$ when the controlled ventilation is adequate.[43]

Dexmedetomidine is a highly selective alpha-2 adrenergic receptor agonist that produces sedation. It is useful as an adjunct to a volatile agent or narcotic-based anesthetic to decrease surgical stress response. The reduction in central sympathetic outflow can lead to bradycardia and hypotension.[44,45] Dexmedetomidine bolus of 0.5 mcg/kg over 10 minutes, followed by an infusion of 0.5 mcg/kg/h attenuates hemodynamic and neuroendocrine response to surgery and CPB.[45] Dexmedetomidine is associated with a reduction in the incidence of postbypass ventricular and supraventricular tachyarrythmias.[46] Because of its antiarrhythmic effects, it is not an ideal sedative for electrophysiologic studies.

Ketamine used to be popular for anesthetic induction in patients with cyanotic conditions because it increases SVR and diminishes the magnitude of R-L shunting. Administration of ketamine can be IV or intramuscular. Ketamine also increases salivation. It exerts a central nervous system–mediated sympathetic activation and catecholamine release, which makes ketamine an attractive anesthetic for patients with decreased function. However, it is a direct myocardial depressant and should be used with caution in very sick patients with exhausted sympathetic responses.[47,48]

Another option for induction in hemodynamically unstable patients is etomidate. This imidazole derivative does not change the hemodynamic parameters at clinical doses.[49,50] Etomidate has the undesirable effect of possible adrenal suppression, particularly when repeated doses are used.

Cardiopulmonary Bypass

For cardiac anesthesiologists, CPB is not a passive time. It can test the quality of interteam communication, even during a routine case. This is especially true when monitors or laboratory test results show anomalies (e.g., decreased cerebral and/or somatic NIRS, abnormal arterial blood gas values, worsening of lactic acidosis, elevated central venous pressure) and when problems occur as a result of poor myocardial protection or residual defects. Good communication is essential during separation from CPB and the decision-making process regarding mechanical circulatory support when things do not go according to plan (e.g., native cardiac output not sufficient to terminate CPB, difficult to control arrhythmia).

The major advances in pediatric CPB are improved circuitry, technology, and management strategies to reduce systemic inflammatory response and improve organ protection. Oxygenators specifically designed for neonates were developed and combined with an integrated arterial filter. There has been a wider adoption of mast-mounted pumps that are closer to the patient to shorten the length of the tubing line. These improvements provided significant reduction in prime volume and foreign surface area.[51]

Hemodilution

Hemodilution to a hematocrit value of 24% or higher is associated with reduced lactate levels and better neurologic outcomes.[52] Hemodilution to a hematocrit value of 25% versus a value of 35% during hypothermic CPB in infant surgery for two-ventricle repair shows no difference in hemodynamics during the procedure.[53]

Temperature

The three ranges of hypothermia used are mild (30°C to 35°C), moderate (22°C to 30°C), and deep (<22°C). No proven benefit has been associated with normothermic CPB.[54,55] Hypothermic CPB is used to preserve organ function during cardiac surgery. The scientific rationale for the use of hypothermia rests primarily on temperature-mediated reduction of metabolism. Whole body oxygen consumption metabolic rate, including cerebral, decreases by a factor of 2 to 2.5 for every 10°C reduction.[56] Hypothermia significantly decreases excitatory amino acids release, suggesting an additional mechanism for protective effect.[57]

Deep hypothermia is generally reserved for neonates, infants, and children requiring complex cardiac repair. Deep hypothermic circulatory arrest (DHCA) allows removal of atrial and/or aortic cannula. Using this technique increases precision and ease of surgical repair through a bloodless and cannula-free operative field. Duration of DHCA should be under 41 minutes to reduce permanent neurologic damage, according to the Boston Circulatory Arrest Trial.[58] During DHCA it is recommended to cool evenly and slowly over at least 20 minutes to reduce risk of neurologic injury.[59] The head must be covered with ice packs to avoid brain rewarming during DHCA.

Antegrade Cerebral Perfusion

Also known as regional cerebral perfusion, antegrade cerebral perfusion (ACP) may be used in lieu of DHCA. An arterial cannula flows into the innominate artery after direct insertion or via a prosthetic graft. Only the brain is actively perfused. To prevent the risk of cerebral hypoperfusion and hypoxemia, an ACP flow rate of at least 40 mL/kg/min is necessary for adequate flow to reach the left hemisphere via the circle of Willis.[60] Furthermore, ACP times are frequently longer than DHCA, so adequate cerebral flow, deep hypothermia, and monitoring of NIRS are essential for brain protection.[60,61]

pH-Stat Strategy

pH-stat blood gas management is preferred for deep hypothermic CPB, particularly during cooling. Hypothermia-induced alkalosis is corrected by adding CO_2 to the circuit or by reducing CO_2 removal. This strategy provides cerebral vasodilation and a more even cerebral cooling. Review of published data suggests better neurodevelopmental outcomes for pH-stat compared to alpha-stat management in pediatric cardiac surgery and possibly a reduction in intensive care unit (ICU) stay.[62-64]

Perfusion Flow

Full bypass perfusion flow rate for a 2- to 7-kg patient is 120 to 200 mL/kg/min. For patients above 20 kg, it is 50 to 75 mL/kg/min.[65] Monitors of adequate CPB flow include MAP, SVO_2, NIRS, lactate, and acid-base status.[66] Vasodilators such as phentolamine, nitroprusside, or nitroglycerine may be used during hypothermic bypass to promote even organ perfusion, prevent hypertension on bypass, improve oxygen delivery, minimize acidosis, and improve patient outcome.[66-69] During separation from bypass, excessive vasodilation may be reversed with low-dose vasopressin infusion if necessary.

Discontinuation of Cardiopulmonary Bypass

When weaning from CPB, blood volume is assessed by direct cardiac visualization sand monitoring right and/or left atrial filling pressures. When filling pressures are adequate, patient fully warm,

acid-base status normalized, and heart rate adequate and in sinus rhythm, CPB venous drainage is decreased, and the patient is weaned from bypass. The arterial cannula is temporarily left in place so that infusion of residual pump blood can be used to optimize filling pressures.[70] Myocardial function is assessed by direct cardiac visualization, left and/or right atrial pressures, percutaneous jugular venous pressure, or echocardiography. After complex congenital heart defect repair the anesthesiologist and surgeon may have difficulty separating a patient from CPB. Under these circumstances the differential diagnosis may include an inadequate surgical result with a residual defect, pulmonary artery hypertension, right or left ventricular dysfunction, arrhythmia, bleeding, or any of these combined. TEE may be used to provide an intraoperative image of structural or functional abnormalities and to assist in the evaluation of the postoperative cardiac repair.[71,72] Strategies will involve identification and correction of reason for failure to wean, including consideration of return to hypothermia and repair of residual defect. Leaving the operating room with a significant residual structural defect adversely affects survival and increases patient morbidity.[71,72]

If the patient is unable to come off bypass due to early postoperative cardiac failure and has severe metabolic acidosis and high inotropic and/or pressor requirement, postoperative mechanical support with extracorporeal membrane oxygenation (ECMO) may be considered.[73] Typically the same aortic and right atrial cannulae are used for conversion from bypass to ECMO.

Ultrafiltration

Conventional ultrafiltration or modified ultrafiltration (MUF) is used to remove excess total body water and reduce proinflammatory factors in almost all pediatric cardiac surgical centers in the United States. Conventional ultrafiltration is performed during bypass, whereas MUF is performed for 10 to 15 minutes after the discontinuation of bypass (Figs. 20.1 and 20.2). MUF filters the patient's blood volume and improves hemodynamic and pulmonary performance.[74,75] After the patient is weaned from CPB, blood is removed from the patient via aortic cannula, fed through an ultrafilter, and then returned via venous cannula to the right atrium. A constant left or right atrial pressure is maintained for hemodynamic stability. Ultrafiltration is carried out with end points being either time of 15 to 20 minutes or hematocrit value of approximately 40%.[76]

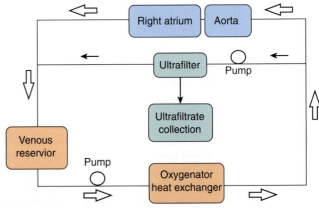

• **Figure 20.1** Conventional ultrafiltration throughout cardiopulmonary bypass.

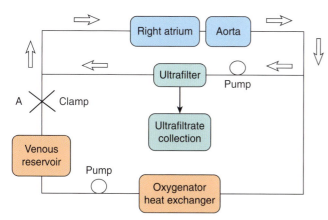

• **Figure 20.2** After the patient is weaned from bypass, the circuit tubing is clamped at *A* to perform arteriovenous modified ultrafiltration. Blood from the venous reservoir can undergo ultrafiltration and be transfused as needed.

Anticoagulation and Hemostasis

CPB is a significant thrombogenic stimulus, requiring anticoagulation with heparin. The effect of heparin is followed by activated clotting time (ACT) monitoring. The effect of heparin is primarily due to antithrombin III coupling; because there are age-related and quantitative differences in procoagulants and inhibitors, heparin dosing may be variable. Maintaining an ACT above 400 seconds is recommended. Heparin is neutralized by protamine after CPB and MUF, but protamine excess may actually contribute to postoperative bleeding.[77]

Bleeding after CPB is not an unusual occurrence. Neonates and young infants with congenital heart disease have low circulating levels of procoagulants and inhibitors. Thrombogenic and dilutional effects of CPB further contribute to hemostatic abnormalities. Furthermore, DHCA causes increased clotting and fibrinolytic activities. There are pharmacologic interventions aimed at reducing bleeding after CPB. Desmopressin acetate[78,79] and antifibrinolytics aminocaproic acid or tranexamic acid have been tried with variable success. However, the most impressive results have been demonstrated with the use of aprotinin.[80] It is a proteinase inhibitor with antifibrinolytic properties at low concentrations and a kallikrein inhibitor at higher levels. Aprotinin is not available in the United States at the time of this writing due to studies associating it with renal failure in adults.

When postoperative bleeding occurs, the surgeon should first attempt to identify any source of surgical bleeding. Next, adequate protamine reversal of heparin is assessed by ACT and laboratory evaluation. In general, standard coagulation tests show prolongation of prothrombin time, partial thromboplastin time, hypofibrinogenemia, and dilution of other procoagulants, as well as prolonged bleeding time in patients with and without bleeding. The most common reason for persistent bleeding is platelet dysfunction.[81,82] Administration of platelets is warranted in those bleeding situations. Routine administration of blood products to correct laboratory coagulation abnormalities in the absence of bleeding is not indicated. If bleeding persists after platelets have been given, reassessment and a repeat of platelet infusion or cryoprecipitate administration may be beneficial, whereas fresh frozen plasma has not been found to be effective.[83] When facing persistent bleeding despite repeated previously described interventions, recombinant activated factor VII may be used as a last resort.[84]

Patient Transport and Handover to Intensive Care Unit

After surgery, when the patient is deemed stable for transport, report should be given to the ICU staff before departing from the operating room. All transport equipment is checked beforehand to confirm proper functioning. The patient is carefully transferred to the transport bed. The trip to the ICU requires full, continuous monitoring without any interruption of vasoactive medication infusion. The patient is manually ventilated at the appropriate FiO_2. If there is pulmonary hypertension that requires the use of nitric oxide post bypass, nitric oxide should not be interrupted during transport.

The complex nature of pediatric cardiac defects and procedures necessitates a structured and efficient handover process to ensure patient safety and continuity of care[85,86] (Box 20.1, Fig. 20.3). A systematic review by Segall et al.[87] offers the following recommendations: "(1) standardize processes (e.g., using checklists and protocols); (2) complete urgent clinical tasks before information transfer; (3) allow only patient-specific discussions during verbal handovers; (4) require that all relevant team members be present; and (5) provide training in team skills and communication." It is imperative that each institution develops a handover process tailored to its setting. The sequence of events during a routine cardiac surgery done under CPB is listed in Box 20.2.

Specific Anesthetic Considerations

According to the Society of Thoracic Surgeons Congenital Heart Surgery Database, nine congenital heart operations constitute approximately 50% of reported cases. It is beyond the scope of

Patient Label

Driscoll CHILDREN'S HOSPITAL

Pediatric Heart Center Handoff Tool

Present: Anesthesia ☐ CV Surgeon ☐ IC/EP Attending ☐ Perfusion ☐ CRNA ☐ ICU Attending ☐ APP ☐ Nursing ☐ Respiratory Therapy

Time Out: Completed ☐

PMH/PSH _____

Diagnosis/Surgical Repair _____

_____

Airway

Pox _____ Supplemental Oxygen _____ ETT Size _____ Difficult Intubation: No/Yes, Ventilation Concerns _____

Cardiovascular

CPB_____ Cross clamp_____

Access: PIV ☐ Arterial Line ☐ CVL ☐ Intracardiac Line ☐ UAC ☐ UVC ☐ PICC (SL/DL) ☐ Broviac **Chest Open**: (yes/no)

Drains: ☐ MCT ☐ Right Pleural ☐ Left Pleural **CV Gts**: Epi @ _____ Milrinone @ _____ Dopamine@ _____ VP @ _____

Rhythm Concerns (yes/no) _____ Defibrillated: Y __ N___ Cardioverted: Y __N___ (rhythm) Paced (yes/no)_____ (mode) BP_____

Recent Lactate _____

Diagnostic Cath_____ Ballooned _____ Stent(s) _____ Location _____ Size _____

ASD Closure _____ Device _____ Size _____ Coil _____ Location(s) _____

PDA Closure _____ Device _____ Size _____ Melody Valve____ Size _____ Septostomy _____

Cath Site: Arterial: L / R   Venous: L / R   Location: Groin_____ L __ R ___ Neck: _____

Neurological:

NIRS/Somatic Range Intra-Op _____

Recent Narcotics/Sedation/Neuromuscular blockade given _____

Renal:

Urine Output: _____ mL/kg/hour

Hematology/Blood Products/Volume Expanders:

Cellsaver _____ (mL) PRBC _____(mL/units) Platelets ___(mL/unit) FFP ___ (mL/units) Cryo _____(mL/units) Crystalloids _____ (mL)

ID/Skin:

Last Dose of ABX _____   MRSA Status: +/–/unknown

This Handoff information is in addition to the report given utilizing SBAR in EPIC and not part of the medical record

Children's Heart Center of South Texas ❤️

• **Figure 20.3** Pediatric Heart Center Handoff Tool. (Courtesy Jenny Montgomery, RN MSN CPNP-AC, Driscoll Children's Hospital, Corpus Christi, TX.)

this chapter to address anesthetic approach to all surgical procedures performed on children with congenital heart defects. Instead, we will concentrate on most of these nine defects with principles applicable to the vast majority of procedures.

Anesthesia for Simple Open-Heart Procedures

"Simple" open-heart procedures include those defects that involve relatively straightforward surgical repair, uncomplicated hemodynamics, minimal to moderate postoperative intensive care, and mechanical ventilation or no mechanical ventilation. *Simple* is a relative term. A case that may be classified as simple may unexpectedly become more complicated (Table 20.4, Box 20.3). Examples of simple open-heart procedures include repairs of atrial septal defect (ASD), ventricular septal defect (VSD), TOF, and atrioventricular (AV) canal defect in otherwise healthy children with good cardiopulmonary reserve. ASD closure is often performed in the

cardiac catheterization laboratory, so it is less often repaired surgically. Patients may present with a range of symptoms from no medical management, minimal management with afterload reduction or diuretic, to congestive heart failure with minimal reserve. The latter will require a different level of care, despite the relatively simple surgical procedure.

Every center has a team of nurses, cardiologists, anesthesiologists, perfusionists, congenital cardiac surgeons, and cardiac intensivists whose familiarity establishes a well-scripted synergism in caring for children with congenital heart defects. Within each center exists different management styles and strategies in caring for patients coming for open-heart surgical procedures. In general, designing an anesthetic plan will take into consideration numerous variables and goals.

Specific anesthetic considerations for patients undergoing simple procedures, in addition to the general guidelines previously discussed, are predicated on clinical state; surgical plan, including

TABLE 20.4	Risk Stratification for Patients With Congenital Heart Disease		
Cardiac Lesion	**Low Risk**	**Moderate Risk**	**High Risk**
Structural lesions	• Repaired atrial or ventricular septal defect (ASD, VSD) • Mild valvular stenosis or regurgitation	• Simple unrepaired lesions such as ASD or VSD • Fully repaired complex cardiac lesions • Single ventricle with Glenn or Fontan palliation	• Unrepaired complex cardiac lesions • Systemic arterial to pulmonary arterial shunts • Severe valvular disease
Pulmonary hypertension		• New York Heart Association functional class I • Normal cardiac index	• New York Heart Association functional class III or IV • Pulmonary artery pressures equal or higher than systemic pressures • Decreased cardiac index
Miscellaneous		• Post heart transplant	• Severe heart failure • Ventricular assist devices • Williams syndrome • Hypertrophic obstructive cardiomyopathy

Modified from Saettele AK, Christensen JL, Chilson KL, et al. Children with heart disease: risk stratification for non-cardiac surgery. *J Clin Anesth*. 2016;35:479-484.

• BOX 20.2 Sequence of Events During Routine Cardiovascular Procedures With Cardiopulmonary Bypass

- Standard monitors
- NIRS cerebral + somatic
- Induction/IV/intubation
- Maintenance of anesthesia
- IV augmentation + antibiotic if not already administered
- Arterial line
- Baseline laboratory values (ABG, ACT, TEG)
- Aminocaproic acid/tranexamic acid
- Central venous line
- Gastric suction, then TEE
- Median sternotomy
- Heparin + ACT
- Aortic cannulation
- Venous cannulation
- CPB initiation + cooling
- Aortic cross-clamp + cardioplegia
- Surgical repair ± additional cardioplegia
- Cross-clamp release
- Ionotrope ± vasodilator
- Rewarming, pacing wires, atrial lines
- TEE
- End CPB (hemodynamically stable, warm, adequate laboratory values)
- MUF
- Protamine, then ACT
- Hemostasis + chest closure
- Transport to ICU and handover

ABG, *Arterial blood gas;* ACT, *activated clotting time;* CPB, *cardiopulmonary bypass;* ICU, *intensive care unit;* IV, *intravenous;* MUF, *modified ultrafiltration;* NIRS, *near-infrared spectroscopy;* TEG, *thromboelastography;* TEE, *transesophageal echocardiography.*

• BOX 20.3 Criteria for Cardiac Anesthesia or Equivalent Care

1. Unrepaired congenital heart disease
   - *Excluding* straightforward physiology (e.g., ASD, VSD, PDA)
2. Repaired or palliated congenital heart disease with abnormal residual physiology
   - Significant systemic valvular regurgitation or outflow tract obstruction (i.e., mitral or aortic valvular disease or obstruction)
   - Symptomatic patient (CHF, short of breath, respiratory failure, need for inotropes)
   - Patient palliated with Blalock-Taussig shunt
3. Significant ventricular dysfunction
   - Right or left or both
   - Echocardiographic shortening fraction < 25% (or qualitative diagnosis by cardiologist as dysfunction moderate to severe)
   - Symptomatic patient (CHF, short of breath, respiratory failure, need for inotropes)
   - Listed for transplant
4. Pulmonary HTN
   - RV or pulmonary pressures > 3/4 systemic (outside the physiologic neonatal period)
   - Treated with vasoactive infusions (i.e., epoprostenol [Flolan]; prostacyclin)
   - Treated with inhaled nitric oxide
5. Any patient undergoing procedure with planned ECMO backup

ASD, *Atrial septal defect;* CHF, *congestive heart failure;* ECMO, *extracorporeal membrane oxygenation;* HTN, *hypertension;* PDA, *patent ductus arteriosus;* RV, *right ventricular;* VSD, *ventricular septal defect.*

CPB and/or aortic cross-clamping or cardiac arrest; degree of cooling; and specific physiologic goals associated with these defects (see Table 20.1). Additionally, the anesthetic plan is guided in part by postoperative management and is based on input from the cardiothoracic surgeon and cardiac intensivist. In general, anesthetic management can be divided into three phases: precorrection, immediate postcorrection, and postoperative. During the precorrection phase, plans for premedication, induction and maintenance of anesthesia, and selection of monitors are based on the patient's pathophysiology and plans for postoperative care.

Premedication maybe selected for patients depending on the level of anxiety. Most patients with a "simple procedure" will tolerate an oral or IV sedative. Depending on the physiology (e.g., TOF), premedication may be warranted if one is trying to avoid unexpected catecholamine surge during the preinduction and induction period. Intravenous or inhalation induction is usually well tolerated. Patients with high right ventricular (RV) outflow tract obstruction benefit from particular vigilance to adequate airway and ventilation to prevent pulmonary hypertension, impaired pulmonary blood flow, and diminished left-side filling. These lesions benefit from preinduction IV access, so once IV is established, additional anesthesia can be provided even before intubation. Aside from necessary preparation for airway management, agents to maintain SVR (phenylephrine) and reduce PVR (oxygen, opioid) should be readily available throughout the precorrection period, particularly during induction.

The level of monitoring also reflects the nature of the procedure. Adequate IV access is established for fluid or blood transfusion in anticipation of the potential for bleeding. Additionally, invasive central venous pressure monitoring is established in preparation for CPB, or transthoracic atrial lines are placed before discontinuing CPB. Although simple patent foramen ovale/secundum ASD closures do not typically require central catheters, some still advocate central venous access in case an untoward event occurs in the immediate postoperative period.

ASDs and VSDs require the use of CPB to facilitate access to the surgical site. Right atriotomy allows visualization of most ASDs. The technique for ASD closure may be associated with atrial arrhythmia and conduction delay. VSD repair is done through the tricuspid valve or a ventriculotomy. Consequences of ventricular incision include AV node dysfunction with various degrees of heart block and ventricular myocardial dysfunction.

For patients with TOF, the precorrection time period can be challenging. Hypercyanotic spells can plague transition to CPB, and its management may depend on the time of desaturation and hemodynamic compromise. Before incision or sternotomy, hypercyanosis can be managed with a bolus of fluid (10 to 15 mL/kg) and/or a bolus dose of phenylephrine (0.5 to 1.0 mcg/kg IV).[88] Alternatively, if the sternum is open and the surgeon has aortic access, a gentle squeeze on the aorta by the surgeon can reverse acute R-L shunting. Typically a repair of TOF requires both CPB and aortic cross-clamping to address the VSD.

Of the diagnostic criteria for TOF (malaligned VSD, overriding aorta, RV hypertrophy, and RV outflow obstruction), the RV outflow obstruction is the most variable in both degree and location. The spectrum ranges from dynamic subpulmonic obstruction with normal anatomy distally to small pulmonary valve to absent pulmonary valve and arteries. In the latter cases, pulmonary blood flow occurs either through a PDA or by aortopulmonary collateral circulation. These complex cases of TOF require more extensive surgical interventions and are discussed in a later section.

Cyanosis and compensatory polycythemia are frequent findings in these patients. In addition, 5% to 6% of patients have abnormal coronary anatomy, with the anterior descending artery originating from the right coronary artery and traversing the RV outflow tract. This necessitates a careful preoperative evaluation before the RV outflow tract incision is planned.[89] Depending on the size and inflow source of the pulmonary circulation, surgical options range from augmentation of small pulmonary arteries to reimplantation of aortopulmonary collaterals onto an RV–pulmonary artery conduit. Although these plans theoretically provide pulmonary blood flow, small vessel caliber can result in high PVR. The decision to close the VSD may also impact postcorrection myocardial function. However, most seem to close the VSD in the modern era. Mechanisms to minimize PVR through a reconstructed pulmonary circulation include mild hypocapnia, high inspired oxygen concentration, adequate anesthesia/analgesia, and other pharmacologic therapy. Although the ASD and VSD repairs share many of the same potential postoperative complications, such as bleeding, ventricular dysfunction, and arrhythmias, each type of case raises its own set of anesthetic issues.

With these relatively straightforward repairs, separation from CPB is achieved with minimal to no inotropic support. Dopamine may be administered to assist recovery from mild ventricular dysfunction. The potential for conduction disturbances, particularly after ventriculotomy, supports temporary epicardial pacing wire placement. Other immediate postcorrection issues include residual shunt. Postoperative care depends on the level of mechanical ventilation and inotropic support and the presence of comorbidity or complication. Tables 20.5 and 20.6 list common postoperative issues by surgical site and procedure, and Table 20.7 presents the anesthetic considerations for complex versus simple repairs.

TABLE 20.5	Postoperative Complications by Procedure	
Procedure	**Extubation Time Frame**	**Postoperative Issues, Potential Problems**
Percutaneous device closure (ASD, PDA)	Early	Residual shunt flow
Thoracoscopy	Early	Mild pain; atelectasis; pneumothorax, chylothorax, hemothorax; pleural effusion; inadvertent ligation of thoracic duct; injury to vagus/recurrent laryngeal nerve; sequelae of lateral decubitus position
Thoracotomy	Early-intermediate	Significant pain (impaired pulmonary mechanics if unresolved), atelectasis; other issues same as thoracoscopy; lung contusion from direct retraction
Median sternotomy	Early-late	Pericardial, pleural effusion; brachial plexus injury; phrenic nerve paresis (impaired diaphragmatic function); pain
Ventriculotomy	Intermediate-late	Ventricular arrhythmias, conduction delay, ventricular dysfunction
Atriotomy	Early-late	Atrial arrhythmias, conduction delay, sinoatrial and atrioventricular node dysfunction
Cardiopulmonary bypass	Early-late	Activation of inflammatory cascade; platelet dysfunction; bleeding; transfusion requirement; short- and long-term neurologic sequelae
Deep hypothermic circulatory arrest	Intermediate-late	Same as for cardiopulmonary bypass; higher incidence of short- and long-term neurologic sequelae

ASD, Atrial septal defect; *PDA,* patent ductus arteriosus.

TABLE 20.6 Postoperative Complications by Surgical Site

Specific Procedure	Postoperative Complication
Percutaneous device closure (ASD, PDA)	Residual shunt, delayed detection of cardiac perforation
Coarctation repair	Neurologic dysfunction from thoracic aortic cross-clamp
Arterial switch, anomalous coronary repair	Coronary insufficiency/myocardial ischemia
Atrial switch (Mustard, Senning)	Loss of sinus rhythm, venous baffle obstruction
Stage I for HLHS	Inadequate shunt (pulmonary) blood flow, aortic arch obstruction/coarctation
Stage II, III for HLHS	Arrhythmias, baffle or venous pathway obstruction, ventricular dysfunction
AV canal repair	AV valve dysfunction (stenosis/regurgitation) conduction disturbance
Truncus arteriosus repair	Semilunar valve dysfunction
Tetralogy of Fallot repair	Heart block, RV dysfunction, pulmonic regurgitation, residual RVOT obstruction
Resection subaortic membrane	Recurrence of subaortic obstruction

ASD, Atrial septal defect; *AV*, atrioventricular; *HLHS*, hypoplastic left heart syndrome; *PDA*, patent ductus arteriosus; *RV*, right ventricular; *RVOT*, right ventricular outflow tract.

TABLE 20.7 "Simple" Versus "Complex" Congenital Open-Heart Procedures: Anesthetic Considerations

Consideration	Simple Open Procedure	Complex Open Procedure
Preoperative evaluation	Growth history/symptoms, medications, CBC, ECG, echocardiogram	Growth history/symptoms, medications/inotropes, ventilatory support, CBC count, electrolytes ECG, echocardiogram, cardiac catheterization data, MRI
Premedication (>6 mo of age)	Midazolam 0.5-0.75 mg/kg with or without acetaminophen	Midazolam 0.5-0.75 mg/kg or diazepam 0.05-0.1 mg/kg PO
Induction	Inhalation (if no IV)	Inhalation or intravenous
Maintenance	Fentanyl 10-40 mcg/kg[a] + rocuronium 0.6-1.0 mg/kg[a] + inhalation agent if needed	Fentanyl 40-75 mcg/kg[a] + rocuronium 0.6-1.0 mg/kg[a]
Antibiotics	Cefazolin 25 mg/kg IV **or** vancomycin 10 mg/kg IV (if PCN allergy)	Cefazolin 25 mg/kg IV **or** vancomycin 10 mg/kg IV (if PCN allergy)
Special monitors	Arterial line Two temperature sensors (central, peripheral) Urinary catheter ± Atrial lines ± TEE	Arterial line Two temperature sensors (central, peripheral) Urinary catheter Atrial lines ± TEE
Special techniques	CPB, selective cerebral perfusion, occasional DHCA	CPB, selective cerebral perfusion or DHCA
Fluids	Pre-CPB: limited crystalloid Post-CPB: crystalloid, FWB or PRBCs[b]	Pre-CPB: limited crystalloid Post-CPB: FWB or PRBCs[b]
Inotropic/hemodynamic support	Dopamine 3 mcg/kg/min (not always needed)	Almost always: Dobutamine, dopamine, or epinephrine titrated to effect Epinephrine 0.05-0.2 mcg/kg/min Milrinone (bolus ± infusion) Inhaled nitric oxide nitroprusside 0.5-5 mcg/kg/min
Postoperative mechanical ventilation	0-6 h, sometimes longer	6-24+ h

[a]Total dose.
[b]Choice of FWB or PRBCs determined by hematocrit and amount of bleeding.
CBC, Complete blood cell; *CPB*, cardiopulmonary bypass; *DHCA*, deep hypothermic circulatory arrest; *ECG*, electrocardiogram; *FWB*, fresh whole blood; *IV*, intravenous; *MRI*, magnetic resonance imaging; *PCN*, penicillin; *PO*, by mouth; *PRBCs*, packed red blood cells; *TEE*, transesophageal echocardiogram.

Early extubation has emerged over the last 10 to 15 years for simple procedures and has proven to be beneficial for both the patient and the economics of congenital heart surgery. A fast-track strategy, defined as extubation within 6 hours of arriving in the ICU or extubating in the operating room, has proven successful. Extubation in the operating room after surgery was first reported in 1980; in 197 patients less than 3 years of age, including neonates, 61% of patients were successfully extubated in the operating room.[90] A fast-track strategy has the advantages of decreasing ventilator days, length of hospital stays, and cost.[91,92] Appropriate patient selection and anesthetic planning is required for safe fast-track extubation. Studies suggest that patients with Risk Adjustment for Congenital Heart Surgery (RACHS) scores of 1 to 3 are best suited for this strategy.[93]

A 7% incidence of reintubation in patients following TOF repair has been reported.[94] Risk factors contributing to extubation failure include lung disease, cardiac dysfunction, airway edema, diaphragmatic paralysis, and vocal cord paralysis. Some studies have suggested that patients with spontaneous ventilation have better hemodynamics and improved cerebral oxygenation.[95,96] Early extubation after TOF repair has been associated with shorter hospital length of stay.[91] On-the-table extubations of acyanotic patients has been reported.[97]

Anesthesia for Complex Open-Heart Procedures

More extensive surgeries are required for complex TOF with abnormal pulmonary vasculature, univentricular hearts, truncus arteriosus, and transposition of the great arteries (TGA). Surgery for univentricular heart is typically staged over time to allow pulmonary vasculature development and to maintain ventricular function. Following stage I palliation, the parallel arrangement of systemic and pulmonary circulations is maintained. The operation for truncus arteriosus, by contrast, achieves repair in one encounter and results in circulation separation into normal serial arrangement. In the neonatal period, precorrection pulmonary vascular reactivity is useful in achieving a balanced circulation (i.e., $Q_p:Q_s$ of 1). In patients with unpalliated univentricular hearts and truncus arteriosus, pulmonary overcirculation implies systemic hypoperfusion; this state may eventually result in diminished end-organ perfusion and acidosis. As previously noted, hypercapnia and low inspired oxygen concentration promote increases in PVR; these factors can be regulated by altering inspired gas mixtures with the addition of CO_2 or N_2.[98] NIRS monitoring continues on both the forehead and flank, and this provides noninvasive assessment of regional perfusion and oxygen delivery. Improvements in noninvasive imaging such as cardiac magnetic resonance imaging (CMRI) have provided valuable information to the surgical team regarding the approach to palliation. In some instances CMRI can provide a better estimate of left ventricular (LV) volume.[98] In the operating room, CO_2 is added to achieve SpO_2 near 85%. Metabolic acidosis is treated by attempting to improve systemic flow and on occasion with IV sodium bicarbonate. Many patients are on prostaglandin E_1 (PGE_1) and may require balloon atrial septostomy before surgery.

The infant with univentricular heart undergoing initial palliation (the first stage in the series of operations leading to Fontan physiology) requires special considerations to provide pulmonary blood flow. Planned use of an arterial-to-pulmonary artery shunt impacts the site of arterial cannulation. For a planned right modified Blalock-Taussig shunt, the right upper extremity is avoided for blood pressure cuff monitoring or arterial line insertion. The diminutive size of the ascending aorta in hypoplastic left heart syndrome (HLHS) often precludes its cannulation and use for initiating bypass; an alternative strategy employs pulmonary artery cannulation, with subsequent snaring of the branch pulmonary arteries to allow systemic flow through the ductus arteriosus. Traditionally, surgical repair reconfigures the pulmonary trunk into the neo–ascending aorta, and this site can be recannulated after DHCA for reinitiating CPB. More centers are using the distal end of the Blalock-Taussig shunt to provide selective cerebral perfusion to avoid or limit circulatory arrest time. Depending on the native aorta size, homograft or prosthetic material is used for augmentation. An arterial-to-pulmonary artery shunt, either from the right subclavian or right carotid artery, or right innominate artery (modified Blalock-Taussig shunt), will supply the pulmonary circulation. Alternatively, the Sano modification is performed to allow pulmonary blood flow. Occasionally a centrally located shunt between the ascending aorta and the pulmonary artery may be used.

Balancing the circulation can be challenging while providing adequate anesthesia.[99] PGE_1 is continued from the ICU to maintain ductal patency before institution of CPB. Targeting PaO_2 to 40 to 45 mm Hg with SaO_2 70% to 80% is associated with adequate oxygen delivery confirmed by NIRS monitoring. The goal is to provide adequate coronary circulation, cardiac output, and oxygen delivery to systemic organs and reach CPB with preserved ventricular function and end-organ perfusion.

After surgical palliation is performed, separation from bypass is achieved once inotropic support is started, ventilation is initiated, and shunt flow is established. Issues that complicate postcorrection management in the operating room and the ICU include hypoxemia and metabolic acidosis. Hypoxemia following a stage I palliation results from several factors, including inadequate ventilation, impaired shunt flow, and high PVR. Ventilation can be assessed visually by looking at the field to see if the lungs are moving with inspiration. Impaired shunt flow can result from shunt thrombus or kinking, excessive length, or inadequate diameter. Manipulation of PVR by using ventilation, inspired oxygen concentrations, and pulmonary vasodilators may provide some improvement in oxygen saturation. Compression of vascular structures following chest closure occasionally diminishes pulmonary blood flow and may require leaving the sternum open for 24 to 48 hours. Although some metabolic acidosis is anticipated following separation from CPB, its persistence suggests impaired systemic perfusion, either from aortic arch obstruction, ventricular dysfunction, or severe AV valve regurgitation. Echocardiography assists in diagnosing these problems. Inotropic support and afterload reduction may improve systemic flow. Mild arch obstruction may allow balloon dilatation in the cardiac catheterization laboratory at a later date. Severe arch obstruction necessitates surgical revision.

The hybrid procedure is another option for managing HLHS. This strategy employs pulmonary artery banding and a PDA stent. Interventional cardiologists often need to perform balloon atrial septectomy to allow atrial level mixing of blood from systemic and pulmonary circulations. The hybrid procedure strategy avoids the risks associated with neonatal CPB and the challenges that follow. These procedures are performed with the patient under general anesthesia with the expectation of extubation shortly after the procedure. A comprehensive stage 2 procedure (construction of neoaorta, Glenn shunt, possible atrial septectomy, takedown of pulmonary artery bands, and PDA ligation) that follows a hybrid approach to stage 1 is much more challenging.

Patients with TGA usually present at birth or within a few days. The surgical correction of TGA has evolved, allowing nearly 90% of these patients to reach normal adulthood.[100] TGA with intact ventricular septum has a more favorable outcome than a TGA with a VSD. Approximately 10% to 13% of TGA with a VSD have an associated hypoplastic aortic arch, interrupted aortic arch, or coarctation of the aorta.[101,102]

Patients will present for surgery in a variety of clinical states. Some infants have inadequate effective pulmonary or systemic blood flow, requiring balloon atrial septostomy rather urgently after birth or a continuation of PGE_1. Many will arrive on room air, with relatively stable hemodynamics. Saturations in the low 90s to upper 80s may represent adequate mixing. Noninvasive monitoring such as NIRS can assess for oxygen delivery and perfusion. Uterine vein and artery lines are often present and are used for access and to obtain blood gases levels. Preoperative cMRI or echocardiography can delineate the coronary anatomy and aortic arch patency. Depending on the diagnosis, a complete repair with arterial switch operation (ASO) may involve a Rastelli or Nikaidoh procedure, or even a two-stage procedure if LVOTO is present. IV induction includes ketamine or etomidate, usually combined with an opioid. Some advocate high-dose narcotic techniques (fentanyl or sufentanil) along with a paralytic and intermittent benzodiazepines for amnesia.[99] Nasal intubation is an option if a lengthy postoperative ventilation is anticipated. For patients with inadequate mixing, a manipulation of PVR along with inotropic support may be necessary. Reactive pulmonary vasculature is common in neonates.

After separation from CPB, difficulties in management may result from myocardial ischemia due to compromised coronary perfusion, decreased myocardial function, bleeding from extensive suture lines, or pressurized suture lines. Coagulopathy after neonatal CPB exacerbates bleeding. Intraoperative echocardiography can help delineate myocardial function and detect air in the left chambers that may embolize in coronaries. Kinking of reimplanted coronaries may lead to ischemia. Ionotropic support and vasodilator therapy help with separation from CPB. Neonatal ASOs have a 97% 10-year survival.[100] Early extubation or fast tracking is increasingly advocated.

Recent studies have examined immediate extubation (IE; in the operating room) versus non-IE[92] in patients having ASO. IE was associated with shorter postoperative ICU length of stay. Gestational age was a predictor of IE. However, coronary anatomy showed no significant difference in IE, perhaps due to the low number of patients with unusual coronary anatomy. The presence of a VSD played no part in IE versus non-IE. Temperature on CPB did play a role in IE with higher temperature having better success for IE. However, controversy exists regarding temperature management on CPB for ASO procedures.

Truncus arteriosus, or common arterial trunk defect, is another complex mixing lesion. Precorrection ventilator maneuvers or surgical strictures of the pulmonary arteries help balance the circulation. Anesthetic management depends on the degree of congestive heart failure, and patients may be on inotropes preoperatively.[103] Moderate- to high-dose opioid anesthetic technique is typically employed. Truncal valve insufficiency or stenosis, as well as interrupted aortic arch and VSD can accompany common arterial trunk defect, increasing the risk for mortality significantly. Postoperative issues involve bleeding due to extensive suture lines and pulmonary hypertension from uncontrolled precorrection pulmonary blood flow. These patients will return for further surgical intervention owing to the pulmonary artery conduit or homograft's natural history.

Anesthesia for Closed-Heart Procedures

Early corrective repair in infancy has significantly reduced the number of noncorrective, palliative closed-heart operations. Corrective closed-heart procedures include PDA ligation and repair of coarctation of the aorta. Noncorrective closed-heart operations include pulmonary artery banding and extracardiac shunts such as the Blalock-Taussig shunt. All these procedures are performed without CPB. Therefore venous access and intraarterial monitoring are important in evaluating and supporting these patients.

PDA ligation is typically performed through a left thoracotomy, although video-assisted thoracoscopic techniques are increasingly prevalent.[104,105] Physiologic management is that of a L-R shunt producing volume overload. Patients with a large PDA and low PVR generally present with excessive pulmonary blood flow and congestive heart failure. Neonates and premature infants also run the risk of having substantial diastolic runoff to the pulmonary artery, potentially impairing coronary perfusion, and other end organs. Thus patients range from an asymptomatic healthy young child to the sick ventilator-dependent premature infant on inotropic support. The former patient allows for a variety of anesthetic techniques culminating in operating room extubation. The latter patient requires a carefully controlled anesthetic and fluid management plan. Generally a trial of medical management with indomethacin and fluid restriction is attempted in the premature infant before surgical correction. Indomethacin is avoided in very low-birth-weight (VLBW) premature infants at risk for cerebral intraventricular bleeds. In the premature infant, transport to the operating room can be difficult and potentially hazardous, requiring great vigilance to avoid extubation, excessive patient cooling, or venous access disruption. For these reasons, many centers have been performing ligation in the neonatal ICU. Intraoperatively, retractors may interfere with cardiac filling and ventilatory management, leading to hypotension, hypoxemia, and hypercarbia. To counter this, brief periods of high FiO_2 is employed with little sequelae. Some controversies remain regarding the ideal oxygen saturation for VLBW. It is clear that very high oxygen administration is implicated in retinopathy of prematurity.[106] Complications of PDA ligation include inadvertent ligation of the left pulmonary artery or descending aorta, recurrent laryngeal nerve damage, and excessive bleeding due to inadvertent PDA disruption. After ductal ligation in premature infants, worsening pulmonary compliance can precipitate a need for increased ventilatory support. Manifestations of an acute increase in LV afterload should be anticipated, especially if LV dysfunction has developed preoperatively. More recently, PDA ligation has been performed in infants and children using thoracoscopic surgical techniques. This approach has the advantages of limited incisions at thoracoscopic sites, promoting less postoperative pain and discharge from the hospital the same day of surgery. In some institutions, surgical approaches to PDA ligation have disappeared and have become limited to the neonatal ICU (NICU) and premature infants (VLBW). Anesthetic approach to NICU cases tends toward a high-dose narcotic technique along with paralytics. Fentanyl 10 to 25 mcg/kg followed by infusion seems to provide adequate hemodynamics intraoperatively and postoperatively.[106] Glucose level needs to be monitored and addressed because VLBW infants are at higher risk for hypoglycemia. Some anesthesiologists employ NIRS monitoring for regional perfusion or oxygenation. Anesthetic conducted as an outpatient generally consists of inhalational agents and muscle relaxants, with postoperative narcotics for pain management. These patients do well, and if the procedure is done thoracoscopically, they may go home the same day.

Coarctation of the aorta is a narrowing of the descending aorta near the ductus arteriosus insertion. Aortic flow obstruction may range from severe obstruction with compromised distal systemic perfusion to mild upper extremity hypertension as the only manifestation. Associated anomalies of both the mitral and aortic valves can occur. In the neonate with severe coarctation, systemic perfusion is dependent on R-L shunting across the PDA. In these circumstances, LV dysfunction is very common, and PGE_1 is necessary to preserve sufficient systemic perfusion. Generally a peripheral IV line and an indwelling arterial catheter, preferably in the right upper extremity, are recommended for intraoperative and postoperative management. In patients with LV dysfunction a central venous catheter may be desirable for pressure monitoring and inotropic support; however, this is rare. The surgical approach is through a left thoracotomy, whereby the aorta is cross-clamped and the coarctation is repaired with an on-lay prosthetic patch, a subclavian artery flap, or resection of the coarctation with an end-to-end anastomosis. During cross-clamp, we usually allow significant proximal hypertension (20% to 25% increase over baseline), based on evidence that vasodilator therapy may jeopardize distal perfusion and promote spinal cord ischemia.[107] Intravascular volume loading with 10 to 20 mL/kg of crystalloid is given just before removal of the clamp. The anesthetic concentration is decreased, and additional blood volume support is given until the blood pressure increases. Postrepair rebound hypertension due to heightened baroreceptor reactivity is common and often requires medical therapy. After cross-clamp, aortic wall stress due to systemic hypertension is most effectively lowered by use of beta-blockade with esmolol or alpha/beta-blockade with labetolol.[108] Propranolol is useful in older patients but can cause severe bradycardia in infants and young children. Although it actually increases calculated aortic wall stress in the absence of beta-blockade by accelerating dP/dt, the addition of sodium nitroprusside may become necessary to control refractory hypertension. In these instances, central venous lines are not necessary because these medications can be administered safely through peripheral lines. Captopril or an alternative antihypertensive regimen is begun in the convalescent stage of recovery in those patients with persistent hypertension.

The management of infants undergoing placement of extracardiac shunts without CPB centers around similar goals as other shunt lesions: balancing pulmonary and systemic blood flow by altering $PaCO_2$, PaO_2, and ventilatory dynamics. Central shunts are usually performed through a median sternotomy, whereas Blalock-Taussig shunts may be performed through a thoracotomy or sternotomy. In patients in whom pulmonary blood flow is critically low, partial cross-clamping of the pulmonary artery that is required for the distal anastomosis may cause further reduction of pulmonary blood flow and desaturation, necessitating meticulous monitoring of pulse oximetry and NIRS. Careful application of the cross-clamp to avoid pulmonary artery distortion will help maintain pulmonary blood flow. When severe desaturation and bradycardia occur with cross-clamping, CPB is required to proceed. Intraoperative complications include bleeding and severe systemic oxygen desaturation during chest closure, usually indicating a change in the relationship of the intrathoracic contents that results in distortion of the pulmonary arteries or shunt kink.

Pulmonary edema may develop in the early postoperative period in response to the acute volume overload that accompanies the creation of a large surgical shunt. Measures to increase PVR, such as lowering inspired O_2 to room air, allowing the $PaCO_2$ to rise,

and adding positive end-expiratory pressure (PEEP), are helpful maneuvers to decrease pulmonary blood flow until the pulmonary circulation can adjust. Intraoperative lines include usual IV access, arterial line, and possibly central line if CVP monitoring and/or inotropes are anticipated. Diuretics may alleviate the manifestations of congestive heart failure. Continuous narcotic infusions are often used for postoperative pain management.

Given the physiologic vulnerability of neonates, particularly in those with congenital heart disease, early extubation is a risk. However, early extubation has been successfully achieved using paravertebral blocks for pain control. Under ultrasound guidance, paravertebral blocks have been administered using 0.5 mL/kg of 0.25% bupivacaine with epinephrine 1:200,000 at the T5-T6 level. The use of blocks and a regimen of acetaminophen has measurable opioid-sparing effect and facilitates extubation.[109]

Pulmonary artery banding is used to restrict pulmonary blood flow in infants who are poor candidates for immediate correction, either for anatomic or physiologic reasons. These patients are often in congestive heart failure with reduced systemic perfusion and excessive pulmonary blood flow. The surgeon places a restrictive band around the main pulmonary artery to reduce pulmonary blood flow. Band placement is imprecise and requires careful assistance from the anesthesia team to be accomplished successfully. Many approaches have been suggested. One approach is to place the patient on 21% inspired oxygen concentration and maintain the $PaCO_2$ at 40 mm Hg to simulate the postoperative state. Alternatively, the band may be adjusted to achieve hemodynamic (e.g., distal pulmonary artery pressure at 25% to 50% of the systemic pressure) and/or physiologic goals. The band is loosened to correct any unacceptable hypoxemia.

Blalock-Hanlon atrial septectomy is no longer a common procedure for enlarging an intraatrial connection. This procedure is done by occluding caval flow and creating an intraatrial communication through the atrial septum. In patients with HLHS with an intact atrial septum, this procedure is lifesaving and must be performed within hours of birth. Improved safety of CPB and less invasive catheter-based interventions have led to virtual elimination of such intracardiac procedures using inflow occlusion.

Balloon atrial septostomy (Rashkind procedure) and blade septectomy performed in the cardiac catheterization laboratory or at the bedside have replaced surgical intervention, except when the left atrial size is very small or the atrial septum is thickened. Because surgical septectomies are currently confined to the most difficult subset of cases, they are rarely performed without the benefit of CPB.

Anesthesia for Heart and Lung Transplantation

Although perioperative management for thoracic organ transplantation is discussed elsewhere in this text, the application of these procedures to children brings specific concerns, including candidate characteristics, preparation, anesthetic considerations, surgical considerations, postbypass management, and outcome.

Recently heart transplants have seen a reduction in the number of cases. Nearly 10% of all heart transplants are in pediatric patients. Survival has continued to improve; nearly 60% have a 10-year survival. Even though some advocate for ABO-incompatible heart transplants, there continues to be a limited number of donors, forcing palliation or correction strategies in these candidates. In HLHS, for example, 5-year survival for standard three stage palliation and heart transplant, including deaths while waiting, is the same.[99] From 1988 to 1995, 78% of pediatric transplants were in children less than 1 year of age with congenital heart disease and 16% in children with myocarditis. However, between 1996 and 2009, nearly 65% were in children with congenital heart disease and 30% for cardiomyopathies and myocarditis. In the past several years 4% to 6% were retransplants, a population ushering numerous ethical issues. The overwhelming majority of infants undergo transplant for congenital heart malformations for which reconstructive options either have failed or are not believed to exist.[110]

Among defects considered for heart transplants are failed HLHS palliation and HLHS with coronary fistulae. Although hybrid palliation may sustain the latter, many centers prefer heart transplants for these patients.[111] Other candidates for heart transplant are patients with pulmonary atresia with intact ventricular septum, particularly with coronary sinusoids and RV-dependent coronary circulation. Some advocate for transplant in univentricular heart physiology, unbalanced AV canal, or double-outlet RV with inseparable ventricles. Dilated cardiomyopathy is also an indication for heart transplant. Patients with hypertrophic cardiomyopathy can become candidates for heart transplantation. However, surgical intervention or pacemakers/cardiodefibrillators have extended the life span of these patients without transplant. Extracorporeal life support with venoarterial ECMO or ventricular assist devices and total artificial hearts have been used in many centers as the bridge to transplant.

Children considered for heart transplantation are more likely to have pulmonary hypertension than adults. Most adult transplant programs will not offer heart transplant therapy to patients with PVR over 6 Wood units $\times$ m^2.[112] The exclusion threshold in infants and children remains controversial. Some programs accept patients with PVR as high as 12 Wood units $\times$ m^2, particularly if the pulmonary vasculature responds to vasodilators such as oxygen, NO, calcium channel blockers, or prostacyclin.[113] RV dysfunction or critical pulmonary hypertension after transplantation is unlikely in pediatric patients with PVR less than 6 Wood units $\times$ m^2.[114] Neonates are generally assumed to have elevated PVR, but outcome data from some programs suggest that the impact of this factor on postoperative outcome is substantially less in the first year of life, perhaps because the infant donor hearts, having recently undergone transitional circulation, are better prepared to cope with the RV pressure load that elevated PVR imposes.[115]

The anesthetic plan for pediatric heart transplantation must accommodate a wide spectrum of pathophysiologies. Recipients with congenital heart malformations benefit from the same analysis of loading conditions and optimizing hemodynamics previously discussed. Although a few of these patients undergo heart transplant because the natural history of reconstructive heart surgery poses greater risk despite reasonable ventricular function, most candidates exhibit manifestations of impaired ventricular performance. As such, they require careful titration of anesthetic agents with minimal myocardial depressant characteristics to avoid cardiovascular collapse. In this fragile population even modest doses of opioids can be associated with marked deterioration in systemic hemodynamics, presumably by reducing endogenous catecholamine release. A combination of narcotics, low-dose inhalation agents, and paralysis is an anesthetic mainstay. As with most patients with congenital heart disease, skilled airway management and ventilation represent crucial elements in a satisfactory induction, particularly with elevated PVR. No matter how elegant the anesthetic plan is in conception and implementation, a certain proportion of these children will decompensate upon induction, necessitating resuscitative therapy.

Although orthotopic heart transplantation poses some technical challenges in neonates and young infants, the replacement of an anatomically normal heart is less complex than several reconstructive heart procedures commonly performed at this age. However, the need to adapt this procedure to incorporate repair of major concurrent cardiovascular malformations requires the consummate skill and creativity that remains the province of the few exemplary congenital heart surgeons.[116,117] Having withstood extended ischemic periods, heart grafts are extraordinarily intolerant to superimposed residual hemodynamic loads that might accompany imperfect vascular reconstruction. The extensive vascular repair, particularly in older children with long-standing hypoxemia, and the propensity to coagulopathy together elevate hemorrhage to a major cause of morbidity and even mortality in pediatric heart transplantation. Nevertheless, once successfully implanted, these grafts will respond to physiologic factors that stimulate growth and adaptation in the developing infant and child.[118]

Management considerations during separation from CPB and the early postoperative period are primarily focused on three pathophysiologic conditions: myocardial preservation, denervation, and PVR. Even expeditious transplant surgery usually forces the heart to endure ischemic periods that exceed those encountered for reconstructive surgery. Although some centers believe the infant heart is more tolerant of extended ischemia,[115] these hearts will demonstrate a period of reperfusion injury, and virtually all require pharmacologic and, in some cases, mechanical support. In addition, endogenous adaptive responses and exogenous pharmacologic agents that act via myocardial sympathetic activation are ineffective in the denervated graft. Because the majority of children presenting for heart transplantation exhibit some element of elevated PVR, even with isolated end-stage cardiomyopathy, the right ventricle of a newly implanted heart is particularly vulnerable to failure.

As such, ventilatory and pharmacologic interventions are usually configured to exert a favorable impact on PVR and provide inotropic and chronotropic support. Once the lungs are fully expanded, we ventilate to PaCO$_2$ values in the low 30s using a FiO$_2$ of 1. Centers use different ionotropic regimens to achieve the same end. Dopamine (3 to 5 mcg/kg/min) and isoproterenol (0.02 to 0.05 mcg/kg/min) promote inotropy, chronotropy, and lower PVR. If these do not provide sufficient inotropy in significant postischemic dysfunction, additional agents are added (e.g., milrinone, epinephrine). Most transplant centers have a specific regimen for perioperative immunosuppression, some of which may be initiated in the operating room before bypass or following removal of cross clamp, including high-dose steroids and/or tacrolimus.

Lung and heart-lung transplantation have achieved respectable operative survival in children.[119,120] They remain the only viable surgical therapy for infants and children with severe pulmonary vascular disease and selected progressive pulmonary diseases. In 2009 more than 2000 pediatric lung transplants had been performed.[121] Pediatric lung transplants have plateaued since the late 1990s. Wait times have increased and may be as long as 2 years. Organ donation number and variability continue to be the limitation. Around 2005 lung transplant wait times changed to a survival model that attempts to estimate the waitlist survival. It is unclear if this has impacted pediatric lung transplantation candidates. The majority of children are older with cystic fibrosis, pulmonary hypertension, and pulmonary fibrosis. As experience has been gained, lung transplantation in young children has grown to 10% to 20% of recipients being children younger than 2 or 3 years of age.[99] These procedures remain uncommon in pediatrics. Lung transplantation carries the additional morbidity of obliterative bronchiolitis, a debilitating small airway disease that results in gradual deterioration in flow-related pulmonary functions over time. Despite operative mortality that is currently less than 20%, the 3-year survival is only 50% to 60%.[110,120] Double lung transplants are more frequent than single lung transplants in pediatric patients. The compromised lung function can make administering an anesthetic challenging.

Most centers initiate the lung transplantation process in patients with cystic fibrosis when the forced expiratory volume at 1.0 second (FEV_1) falls below 30% to 40% of predicted value, and quality of life is unacceptable. This is a significantly compromised patient at the time of actual transplantation.[122] For those with pulmonary hypertension, lung transplantation survival is inversely related to right atrial and pulmonary artery pressures, as well as the product of right atrial pressure and PVR.[123] Often these patients are hypercarbic and/or hypoxic on supplemental oxygen, which makes preoperative sedation difficult. If given, midazolam can be administered in small incremental doses preferably while being monitored or in the operating room. Monitoring includes arterial line, central venous line, and possibly a pulmonary artery catheter to assess response to pulmonary artery cross-clamping. Intraoperative and postoperative bleeding can be an issue. This may be exacerbated by previous thoracotomies and adhesions, so large-bore IV access is necessary. Epidural catheters at the thoracic level are helpful for management of postoperative pain. However, coagulation status should be assessed before placement because some of these patients may be coagulopathic. Induction is performed with most IV agents or by inhalational techniques. One-lung ventilation can be used for single-lung transplant if CPB is not used. Depending on the disease process leading to lung transplantation, excessive sedation and low oxygenation are problematic. Different issues present for bilateral or sequential lung transplant without CPB versus with CPB. After transplantation there is a "honeymoon" period of excellent gas exchange, which is short lived. Gas exchange worsens with reperfusion injury and pulmonary edema and reduced compliance. Pulmonary hypertension may also result from reperfusion triggered by the ischemic-reperfusion injury. Patients with "septic lungs" occasionally develop sepsis or a syndrome similar to septic shock, likely from bacteremia or release of inflammatory mediators during removal of the native lung. The postoperative period of a transplanted lung is marked by acute dysfunction, infections, hemorrhage, and transplant failure. Acute rejection usual presents after a few months to a year.

Anesthesia for Cases Other Than Open and Closed Cardiac Procedures

Anesthesia for Diagnostic and Interventional Cardiac Catheterization Procedures

Significant advances in both diagnostic and therapeutic capabilities that are achievable in the cardiac catheterization laboratory (CCL) have revolutionized the management of patients with congenital heart disease. Improvements in equipment and imaging have introduced many nonsurgical options and at times have postponed or replaced more invasive interventions.[124] However, these advances in therapy do not come without risk, with the latest Pediatric Perioperative Cardiac Arrest (POCA) Registry demonstrating a significant number of arrests occurred in the CCL.[125] Odegard et al.,[126] in a retrospective review of over 7200 pediatric catheterizations found an arrest risk of 0.96%, with highest risk seen in children under the age of 1 year and in those children undergoing interventional procedures. Several other studies have also verified

these findings,[127-130] and attempts are now being made to stratify risk among pediatric patients undergoing catheterization.[131] In light of these findings, an anesthesiologist who understands the unique environment of the CCL, the physiology of these complex patients, and the implications of the planned intervention should be administering these anesthetics.[12]

There are numerous anesthetic and sedation options for patients undergoing catheterization. To date, no specific combination of anesthetic agents and ventilation technique has been proven superior.[132] Importantly, the choice of anesthetic must be tailored to the specific patient, taking into account the underlying pathophysiology as well as how the anesthetic will impact his or her blood pressure, heart rate, and respirations. Often, a combination of a volatile agent, an opioid, and a supplementary agent such as a benzodiazepine or dexmedetomidine allows for adequate anesthesia while limiting the undesirable side effects of higher doses of any one agent alone. Prolonged NPO times also need to be accounted for, with appropriate fluid resuscitation provided before hemodynamic measurements are taken.[12]

For the diagnostic portion of catheterization the goal is to replicate the patient's normal physiology to determine if further interventions are necessary. To mimic normal conditions in the CCL, hemodynamic measurements are taken on room air with a physiologic $PaCO_2$ and pH. Although spontaneous ventilation is ideal, causing minimal impact on venous return compared to positive pressure ventilation, more commonly, general anesthesia with an artificial airway is being used.[133] Presumably this allows for controlled ventilation to better prevent hypoventilation, respiratory acidosis, and increased pulmonary pressures.[12] Importantly, high peak airway pressures and PEEP should be avoided during the data acquisition period.[124]

During the catheter-based intervention the potential to cause significant alterations in the patient's hemodynamics must be anticipated. For instance, balloon dilation of a valve will disrupt forward flow and potentially cause an acute increase in the pressure load on the heart, resulting in a decrease in cardiac output. These changes may then necessitate initiation of inotropes or further fluid resuscitation. Complications such as bleeding or vascular rupture are also possible, and cross-matched blood should be available in the room for emergency use.

At the end of the procedure a second set of hemodynamic measurements, including blood pressure, mixed venous oxygen saturation, ventricular end-diastolic pressure, and cardiac output, are used to assess the effect of the intervention. The new physiology produced will potentially have significant impact and will determine postprocedural disposition and recovery. The acuity of the patient and the need to remain intubated in light of these changes should be determined to decide if recovery in the postanesthesia care unit (PACU) or the ICU is appropriate. Once the catheters are removed, the operator will often need to hold pressure at the insertion sites for 20 minutes or longer to achieve hemostasis. Ideally the patient should lie flat for a minimum of 2 to 6 hours to prevent rebleeding, but this is often difficult for young children. Therefore, depending on patient age and ability to cooperate, the anesthesiologist will often tailor the anesthetic to allow for some anxiolysis or mild sedation in the recovery period. This can be achieved with benzodiazepines, low-dose opioids, or dexmedetomidine until the critical period for rebleeding has passed.

For certain patients a hybrid procedure is an appropriate option. In this scenario both the interventional and surgical procedures are combined and performed at the same time. One such example is the hybrid for patients with stage I HLHS, in which bilateral pulmonary artery bands are surgically placed and a ductus arteriosus stent is deployed.[134] Intracardiac hemodynamic monitoring helps guide the surgeons in determining how tight to cinch the bands. This complex procedure allows for avoidance of neonatal bypass, often in patients who have comorbidities that prevent them from undergoing a Norwood procedure. However, it requires significant coordination of resources and experienced subspecialists who are well trained to care for these vulnerable patients.[124]

Anesthesia for Magnetic Resonance Imaging and Computed Tomography Diagnostic Procedures

Although cardiac catheterization remains the gold standard for diagnosis and management of many forms of congenital heart disease, it requires exposure to ionizing radiation. In 2009 the American Heart Association published a science advisory that concluded an interventional catheterization could be similar to the exposure of up to 4000 x-ray examinations.[135] In children, exposure is thought to be even greater due to fluoroscopy times being 5 to 10 times longer than adult procedures. Furthermore, children are thought to have a three to four times greater sensitivity to radiation because they have more rapidly dividing cells and most likely will live longer to experience radiation toxicity.[136] Even low-level exposure to ionizing radiation is thought to contribute to the long-term risk of malignancy,[137] and chromosomal damage has been seen in children exposed to catheterization-related radiation.[138,139] Therefore there has been a concerted effort within the medical community to decrease radiation exposure as much as possible.

Magnetic resonance imaging (MRI) has emerged as a useful diagnostic tool in the pediatric cardiac population. Muthurangu et al.[140] demonstrated that phase-contrast MRI accurately quantifies PVR, even in patients with high pulmonary blood flow and with varying amounts of oxygen and nitric oxide therapy. MRI offers the further benefit of improved structural imaging in any plane when compared to conventional catheterization, whereas MR angiography highlights cardiac abnormalities and allows for detailed soft tissue imaging. Importantly, this imaging is all done radiation-free, thereby decreasing the risk of ionizing radiation to the patient and medical staff.

Working in the MRI environment poses many challenges that necessitate the use of special equipment. Anesthetic equipment and monitoring devices all must be ferrous-free and deemed MRI-safe in order to be used in the MRI area. This requires particular vigilance on the part of each member of the care team to guard against inadvertent taking of nonsafe materials into the scanner. Furthermore, scanning sequences can take several minutes, requiring a still patient. Although older, cooperative patients can follow the MRI technologist's instructions and remain still during the scans, younger patients often require sedation at a minimum and general anesthesia and intubation if breath holds are needed.

For MRI scans in which free breathing is appropriate for imaging, deep sedation with IV medications and nasal cannula oxygen is often used. The patient's baseline physiology and functional status should determine the choice of agent. Various medications have been used with success, including propofol, dexmedetomidine, ketamine, and benzodiazepines either alone or in combination.[141-144] Importantly, appropriate MRI-safe monitoring, including pulse oximetry, blood pressure, electrocardiography, and end-tidal CO_2 is mandatory throughout the test.

When breath holds are needed, general endotracheal anesthesia is most often used. Anesthesia induction and intubation occur in an area outside the MRI zone 4, and the patient is then transferred to the MRI scanner. An MRI-safe anesthetic machine can be used to deliver volatile agents. If a standard ventilator is used, total IV anesthesia is required. In both instances, breathing circuit extension tubing will be needed to reach the patient in the MRI bore. The anesthesiologist can then coordinate breath holds with the MRI technologist to provide optimal conditions for imaging while preventing the patient from risk associated with intermittent ventilation. Once scanning is complete, the patient is then transferred to an appropriate area for emergence and extubation.

Several studies have looked at the incidence of complications related to anesthesia for MRI. Most commonly, hypothermia, desaturation, and bradycardia occurred, more commonly in those that undergo general anesthesia compared to deep sedation.[145] However, serious adverse events have occurred in higher numbers, especially in patients with single-ventricle physiology.[146] Based on these findings, particular attention must be paid to temperature maintenance and minimizing NPO times.

In some centers the use of MRI assistance for right heart catheterization is gaining ground. In x-ray magnetic resonance fusion, a three-dimensional MRI image is overlaid on a fluoroscopy image to enable road mapping and thereby decrease radiation exposure.[147,148] In MRI-guided right heart catheterization (MRI-RHC) the radiation-free imaging of MRI is used to guide the interventional cardiologist as he or she performs diagnostic catheterization in the MRI scanner itself.[149]

After induction and intubation of the patient in the CCL the cardiologist places the cardiac catheters, and then the patient is moved to the MRI suite for scanning of the heart and development of the appropriate images. For MRI-RHC the cardiologist performs the right heart catheterization and obtains hemodynamic measurements. Subsequent interventions are then performed in the CCL. As in a regular MRI scan, the same precautions exist regarding the unique environment in which everyone is working. With the additional scanning required, these procedures tend to be longer than traditional catheterization.[132]

Computed tomography (CT) is another diagnostic tool for pediatric patients with congenital heart disease. In contrast to MRI, CT scans take a shorter amount of time to complete, yet they expose the patient to significantly greater amounts of radiation than a standard x-ray examination. Due to the brief time frame of the study, patients often only need to be immobile for less than a minute for the scan itself. Therefore they can typically be sedated with a short-acting agent such as propofol or ketamine if appropriate for the patient's physiology. Coordination of the injection of IV contrast, patient immobility, and scanning is key to producing the best images.

Anesthesia for Noncardiac Procedures

With improvements in the care of children with congenital heart disease, the size of this patient population continues to grow, necessitating an increasing number of these patients to have anesthesia for noncardiac surgery and diagnostic tests. Multiple studies have demonstrated that these patients are at increased risk of anesthetic complications.[125,150] Based on this data, several centers have stratified patients into risk categories based on age and/or complexity of disease to help standardize preoperative evaluation and determine whether subspecialized cardiac anesthesiologists are needed to care for the patients in the perioperative period.[151-153]

Although specific criteria may vary between centers, some stratification should be developed based on the comfort level and training of each group's anesthesiologists.

Compared to children with low RACHS scores, those in higher categories 4 to 6 are more likely to have general, dental, orthopedic, and thoracic surgeries.[154] Patients with single-ventricle physiology, in particular, undergo various types of noncardiac surgery, most commonly placement of peripheral or central venous lines, insertion of gastrocutaneous tubes (percutaneous or laparoscopic), and airway procedures.[155] In this subset of patients, anesthesia-related complications typically range between 11% and 15% but are as high as 31% in older Fontan patients.[155-157]

It is imperative that the anesthesiologist understand the underlying cardiac physiology of these patients to best care for them. This includes a thorough review of the patient's past medical and surgical history and any other comorbidities. Medications, including anticoagulants that the patient may be taking, should also be discussed with the primary cardiologist and surgeon to determine how best to manage them in the perioperative period. The latest echocardiogram and any catheterization or cMRI data available will also need to be obtained. Cardiac function, the presence of shunts, and the relative pulmonary to systemic blood flow described in these reports should correlate with the patient's overall clinical picture. Once all preoperative data are reviewed, risk stratification should be attempted to determine whether a cardiac subspecialty anesthesiologist is better suited to care for a patient.

In addition to the underlying patient physiology, the effects of a prolonged NPO time need to be considered. NPO times have been liberalized in the latest American Society of Anesthesiologists (ASA) NPO guidelines, with clear liquids allowed up to 2 hours before surgery (ASA Guidelines, 2017; https://www.asahq.org/... guidelines/practice-guidelines-for-preoperative-fasting.pdf). Patients in the higher-risk groups (single ventricle, pulmonary hypertension, LVOTO) should be encouraged to drink clear liquids if they are able or should have IV fluids to prevent significant dehydration. Intraoperatively, any fluid deficits should be corrected, and maintenance fluids then initiated. In younger age-groups, maintenance fluids should include dextrose at an appropriate concentration for the patient's age.

Beyond the standard ASA monitors the need for additional invasive monitoring such as an arterial line or central venous catheter will depend on the patient's underlying cardiac disease, the patient's functional status, and the nature of the surgery. In many shorter and less invasive procedures, no additional monitors are needed if there is a well-functioning noninvasive blood pressure cuff and accurate pulse oximeter. However, if there is a high likelihood of needing inotropes intraoperatively or postoperatively, most practitioners will elect to place additional monitors preemptively.

As with any anesthetic, the choice of medications and type of anesthesia will be guided by the underlying cardiac disease and the proposed surgery. Agents such as etomidate, opioids, and ketamine have a favorable hemodynamic profile that allows for smoother IV inductions of patients with even the most complex congenital heart disease. Volatile agents can then be used at lower MAC values (0.5 to 1) for maintenance of anesthesia. Although intubation with positive pressure ventilation is often undesirable in second- and third-stage single-ventricle physiology, many surgeries require intraoperative paralysis for best conditions to be present. If so, limiting the peak inspiratory pressures and PEEP so that venous return is not impeded is key. Finally, the decision to extubate the patient is multifactorial and depends on the length of the surgery, the amount of fluids administered, intraoperative hemodynamic stability, and postoperative pain management.

Because abdominal surgery is one of the most common noncardiac procedures done in this patient population, the question of whether laparoscopic surgery is safe has been investigated extensively. With insufflation, changes in SVR and decreases in venous return have the potential to cause hemodynamic instability, especially in the patients with single-ventricle physiology. Gillory et al. performed a 10-year retrospective review of 121 laparoscopic versus 50 open procedures in children with congenital heart disease. They found no difference between groups with respect to instability.[158] Other studies have also demonstrated safety with laparoscopy in patients with a single ventricle, noting that insufflation pressures should be kept between 8 and 12 mm Hg and low flow.[159,160]

Finally, postoperative disposition needs to be considered. Most first-stage single-ventricle patients should recover in an ICU due to the potential for hemodynamic instability, potential for the need for postoperative ventilation, and closer evaluation of shunt patency. In other populations, disposition will depend on their baseline functional status, the extent of the surgery, and the transition back to baseline medications. Even in patients who are deemed appropriate for the PACU, longer observation times are often recommended before discharge.

How to Interpret an Anesthetic Record

The anesthetic record serves as the official data recording of the perioperative anesthetic course, as a source of information for later anesthetics, and as a legal document. It will contain all pertinent preoperative information, including patient medical history, significant laboratory values, time of last food or liquid intake, vital signs, and a focused physical examination. All anesthesia providers involved care should be listed for reference.

A full description of induction and intubation is recorded, including the drugs given, vocal cord grade view and ease of tube placement, size of the endotracheal tube, whether cuffed or uncuffed, and verification of proper tube air leak. If additional airway devices are needed to secure the airway, this is also recorded. Any anesthetic procedures, such as arterial and central venous lines are also recorded. Gas flow rates, maintenance concentrations and doses of anesthetic and adjuvant drugs, blood pressure, pulse, respiratory rate, temperature, oxygen saturation readings, and end-tidal CO_2 are entered at frequent intervals.

With advances in technology, automated anesthetic record systems are now more widely used. Preoperative data can be obtained from multiple electronic data resources to facilitate more complete evaluations. Intraoperatively, multiple devices can interface with the electronic record to facilitate real-time capture of information. This includes physiologic monitors to record pulse oximetry, blood pressure, and heart rate; gas analyzers; and anesthesia machines to record ventilation parameters.[161] This automation also allows for intraoperative medications and fluids to be fed into the patient's chart to prevent accidental redosing of medications and allow for more accurate accounting of intake and output.

Postoperative handoff to other care providers can be documented appropriately. Automated billing, regulatory compliance, and data capture for research purposes are also aided.[161,162] As automated records continue to evolve, their utility in providing safe and efficient care will only continue to grow.

Conclusion

Anesthesia for children with congenital and acquired cardiac disease is a dynamic field with significant complexity and risk. The congenital cardiac anesthesiologist is a critical part of the multidisciplinary team committed to this patient population. He or she will use a thorough understanding of cardiac anatomy, pathophysiology, and surgical and anesthetic procedures and concerns to provide meticulous perioperative care.

Selected References

A complete list of references is available at ExpertConsult.com.

1. DiNardo JA, Andropoulos DB, Baum VC. A proposal for training in pediatric cardiac anesthesia. *Anesth Analg*. 2010;100:1121–1125.
6. Matisoff AJ, Olivieri L, Schwartz JM, Deutsch N. Risk assessment and anesthetic management of patients with Williams syndrome: a comprehensive review. *Paediatr Anaesth*. 2015;25:1207–1215.
12. Odegard K, Vincent R, Baijal R, et al. SCAI/CCAS/SPA Expert Consensus Statement for Anesthesia and Sedation Practice: Recommendations for Patients Undergoing Diagnostic and Therapeutic Procedures in the Pediatric and Congenital Cardiac Catheterization Laboratory. *Anesth Analg*. 2016;123:1201–1209.
85. Fabila T, Hee H, Sultana R, et al. Improving postoperative handover from anaesthetists to non-anaesthetists in a children's intensive care unit: the receiver's perception. *Singapore Med J*. 2016;57(5):242–253.
91. Mahle WT, Jacobs JP, et al. Early Extubation After Repair of Tetralogy of Fallot and the Fontan Procedure: An Analysis of the Society of Thoracic Surgeons Congenital Heart Surgery Database. *Ann Thorac Surg*. 2016;102(3):850–858.
130. Vincent RN, Moore J, Beekman RH, et al. Procedural characteristics and adverse events in diagnostic and interventional catheterisations in paediatric and adult CHD: initial report from the IMPACT Registry. *Cardiol Young*. 2016;26:70–78.

21

Sedation, Sleep, Delirium, and Rehabilitation

SAPNA R. KUDCHADKAR, MD, PHD; HEIDI A.B. SMITH, MD, FAAP, MSCI;
CHANI TRAUBE, MD, FAAP, FCCM

Advances in cardiac surgery over the last three decades have translated to a shift in the epidemiology of congenital heart disease mortality from childhood to adulthood. As a result, patient and family–centered care with therapies designed to improve neurodevelopmental, functional, and quality-of-life outcomes in children with heart disease are crucial. There is no question that sedation, analgesia, and mechanical ventilation (MV) will always be central aspects of care for children with critical heart disease. However, minimizing the risks associated with these therapies while optimizing patient safety and both short- and long-term outcomes is a practical and achievable goal for all providers caring for these children. There is a strong interplay between sedation, sleep, delirium, and rehabilitation—a child who is heavily sedated and restrained is at high risk for sleep disturbance and delirium and is unable to participate in rehabilitation therapies. Conversely, a child who is awake during the day and engages in rehabilitation in the acute phase of his or her recovery will be more likely to maintain a normal circadian rhythm and less likely to transition to delirium due to decreased administration of sedative medications. When immobilization with sedation is medically necessary (generally only for the most severely ill children) goal-directed and titrated-sedation approaches are needed to optimize outcomes. In the following sections we provide an overview of sedation, analgesia, delirium, sleep, and rehabilitation as they relate to the pediatric cardiac patient.

Pain and Sedation Management in the Cardiac Intensive Care Unit

Pediatric patients with cardiac disease often experience pain and anxiety. Despite substantial advances in perioperative, surgical, and critical care, they remain at high risk for adverse events such as multiorgan dysfunction, need for extracorporeal membrane oxygenation and cardiac arrest.[1,2] Low cardiac output syndrome (LCOS), a period of inadequate oxygen delivery, can occur and usually peaks 8 to 12 hours postoperatively and is associated with increased morbidity and mortality.[3,4] In attempts to circumvent the severity of LCOS, sedation and analgesia have been effectively used to decrease metabolic demand, myocardial oxygen requirement, and the stress response.[5] However, this practice has become skewed over time, resulting in many patients who are either deeply sedated or comatose for prolonged periods of time.

Prolonged MV and intensive care unit (ICU) stay, along with the development of tolerance, withdrawal, posttraumatic stress syndrome, and delirium, have been reported in critically ill children with longer duration of and higher exposure to sedatives.[6-11] Moreover, the US Food and Drug Administration (FDA) recently issued an FDA Drug Safety Communication (https://www.fda.gov/Drugs/DrugSafety/ucm532356.htm) reporting that prolonged (>3 hours) or repetitive exposure to certain groups of drugs (anesthetics and sedatives) in children less than 3 years of age "may affect the development of children's brains." Due to this the labeling of 11 common anesthetics and sedatives, including volatile agents (sevoflurane) and intravenous (IV) agents (barbiturates, benzodiazepines, propofol, and ketamine), have been modified to include this neurodevelopmental warning. The basis for this warning is largely dependent on evidence from animal and in vitro studies, with the available clinical evidence admittedly difficult to interpret. As such, this warning concludes that "additional high quality research is needed to investigate the effects of repeated and prolonged anesthesia exposures in children, including vulnerable populations."[12]

As the care provided in the cardiac intensive care unit (CICU) continues to evolve, using evidence-based medicine, different aspects of the patient assessment, presentation of patient data, and development of patient care plans will be challenged. The foundation to begin this discussion is based on the following conclusions:
- The routine assessment of both pain and sedation level is recommended by the Pediatric Cardiac Intensive Care Society.[13]
- Pain, sedation, and delirium assessments, along with the current disease state and patient-specific psychosocial goals, should be integrated and discussed on medical rounds daily using an interdisciplinary approach.[11,14-17]
- Thoughtful decisions regarding sedation and analgesia should be made, including drug choice and titration, providing a personalized patient approach, recognizing the risks of associated delirium, withdrawal, and possible long-term cognitive outcomes.[10,18]

Pain Assessment

Pain is "an unpleasant sensory and emotional experience associated with actual or potential tissue damage," that is largely *subjective* in the assessed intensity or importance to each patient.[19] Unfortunately, the course of critical illness in the CICU involves numerous sources of pain via necessary therapies such as placement of invasive lines, chest tubes, or Foley catheters; requirement of an endotracheal tube, mask, or nasal cannula; frequent repositioning; and wound care. Due to variation in psychosocial maturity, the emotional component of pain can be greatly magnified in pediatric patients and confused with symptoms of agitation. This emotional component is not restricted to the patient and may extend to the family, thereby changing perceptions of satisfaction with the ICU experience. Moreover, the routine assessment of pain or sedation level in pediatric patients can be complex given variations in cognitive, verbal, and motor skill development, and even regression of previously learned skills. Clinical signs such as restlessness, agitation, grimace, or increased muscle tone in nonverbal pediatric patients may indicate undersedation, pain, fear, or even separation anxiety. Though purely objective assessment tools are preferred, the pain and sedation level evaluation commonly employs observational components based on age and development.

There are two general approaches for pain assessment, using either self-report or observational scales. Self-reporting pain scales are by nature more objective, but their usefulness can be limited by age and development. These tools use a linear display of "no pain" to "worst pain" using phrases and numbers or pictures, like the numeric rating scale (NRS), verbal numeric scale, and visual analogue scale, or the Wong-Baker "faces" pain scales,[20-22] and can be altered for ethnicity and age (Oucher Scale).[23,24] Though a preferred tool for assessment of pain, the NRS cannot be consistently used in children less than 4 years of age. Observer-rated pain tools include the FLACC (acronym for face, legs, activity, crying, and consolability) and COMFORT-B scales.[25-29] The FLACC is a pain assessment tool used in infants and children whereby five variables are observed or assessed and scored, with a maximum score of 10 points (associated with discomfort).[28] The COMFORT-B scale combines assessment of both pain *and* sedation level using two physiologic and seven behavioral variables for estimation of pain and agitation among infants and children.[30,31] Although it may be difficult to differentiate pain from agitation and vice versa in the very young using the COMFORT-B scale, targeting levels[32] and using a treatment algorithm has been associated with decreased ICU length of stay, decreased duration of MV, less withdrawal, and lower sedative exposure in ventilated pediatric patients.[33]

Sedation Assessment

The term *sedation* often is used to encompass components of anxiolysis, amnesia, and analgesia.[34,35] Sedation assessment scales measure arousal or the level of consciousness (LOC).[36] Historically these assessments have been largely subjective with descriptors such as "unresponsive," "lethargic," "obtunded," "calm," "restless," "distressed," "agitated," or "combative." Monitoring LOC in the CICU provides early recognition of worsening neurologic status related to the critical illness, oversedation, or delirium. Routine monitoring also encourages targeted sedation whereby patients are maintained at the most appropriate LOC based on needs and disease state, the goal being a patient who is comfortable and either calm or slightly sedated. This level of sedation allows for more accurate clinical assessment, caregiver interaction, and possibly quicker liberation from MV. Pediatric tools using both objective and observational components to assess LOC have become the cornerstone of CICU care. The Richmond Agitation-Sedation Scale (RASS) has 10 possible levels of arousal (−5 to +4) defined by three clearly defined steps of patient interaction to elicit a response (*look* or *observe* the patient, *talk* to the patient, *touch* the

patient).[34,37] Patients are scored as being alert and calm (RASS 0), agitated (+1 to +4), responsive to voice (RASS −1 to −3), responsive to touch (RASS −4), or comatose (RASS −5). The RASS has been successfully employed in the pediatric cardiac and medical ICUs for routine monitoring, sedation targeting, and delirium monitoring.[18,38,39] The State Behavioral Scale (SBS) is similar to the RASS but has six levels of arousal (−3 to +2).[40] The SBS score is determined by patient observations for respiratory drive, cough, response to stimulation, attentiveness, tolerance to care, consolability, movement after comforting, and pain assessment using the NRS. The SBS has also been successfully used in the ICU setting associated with nurse-driven sedation protocols and delirium.[41]

Nonpharmacologic Management

A major strength of recent pediatric sedation regimens is the importance placed on a patient's baseline psychologic health to include recognition of disorders such as anxiety, depression, or traumatic stress before the critical illness. Another strength is the reliance on comfort measures provided by caregivers through touch and verbal reassurance in conjunction with optimal analgesia when appropriate. The CICU can quickly overwhelm children, challenging them to use often immature coping mechanisms to deal with pain and anxiety from both surgery and necessary procedures.[17] Family presence during procedures has been shown to not only preserve quality of care but also provide enhanced comfort to the patient and decrease pharmacologic needs.[42] The environment of the CICU can either be part of the solution or remain part of the problem for our fragile patients. Moving forward, we may find just how important a regular routine, sleep hygiene, and family presence are to not only the general well-being of our patients, but also how they experience or interpret their circumstances, modulating their responses to pain and anxiety.

Pharmacologic Management (Table 21.1)

Management of pain and anxiety is of the utmost importance to the medical team and the family. Finding the right balance of nonpharmacologic and pharmacologic therapies will be an ongoing challenge in the ICU setting. CICU clinicians must manage (1) targeted sedation, (2) increasing patient wakefulness and attention, (3) early extubation following surgical interventions, (4) early mobility, and (5) greater parental involvement. Understanding the associated pharmacokinetic changes during critical illness when using analgesics and sedatives is extremely important. Many patients in the CICU depend on continuous infusions for sedation and analgesia, for which awareness of the context-sensitive half-time will need to be considered. The *context-sensitive half-time or half-life* is the time required for the plasma drug concentration to decrease by 50% following discontinuation of the infusion.[43] The context-sensitive half-time depends on drug distribution and therefore cannot reliably be predicted by the elimination half-life alone.[13] Some drugs that usually have a short context-sensitive half-time (in which the drug concentration and clinical effect quickly resolve) will demonstrate noncharacteristic action when infusions are continued for long periods due to saturation of both central (blood) and peripheral (adipose tissue) compartments.

Analgesia

Nonopioid analgesics include acetaminophen and nonsteroidal antiinflammatory drugs (NSAIDs). Regimens that combine

TABLE 21.1 Commonly Used Sedative and Analgesic Medications in the Cardiac Intensive Care Unit

Drug Name	Bolus Dose	Infusion Dose	Cardiovascular Effects	Properties
Nonopioid Analgesics: COX-1 and COX-2 Inhibitors → _Analgesia, Antiinflammation_				
Acetaminophen	15 mg/kg PO/PR/IV q6h 7.5 mg/kg IV (<10 kg)	NA	None	↑Analgesia, ↑antipyretic, ↓↓antiinflammatory Overdose: ↑NAPQI requiring _N_-acetylcysteine
Nonsteroidal Antiinflammatory Drugs (NSAIDs): Nonselective COX Inhibitors → _Analgesia, Antiinflammation_				
Ketorolac	2-16 y: 0.5 mg/kg IV q6h × 5 d (maximum single dose 30 mg) <2 y: 0.25 mg/kg IV q6h × 3 d	NA	None	NSAID ↑Analgesia, ↑antipyretic, ↑antiinflammatory Overdose/↑duration: renal insufficiency
Opioid: μ-, κ-, δ- Receptor Agonists → _Analgesia_				
Fentanyl	1-2 mcg/kg IV	1-20 mcg/kg/h	Bradycardia	≈100× potency of morphine Rigid chest
Hydromorphone	5-10 mcg/kg IV	3-4 mcg/kg/h	Minimal when used as single agent	≈10× potency of morphine Faster onset (5 min) than morphine
Methadone	0.05-0.15 mg/kg PO/IV q4-8h	NA	Bradycardia Dysrhythmia (prolonged QT)	Equipotent to morphine
Morphine	0.05-0.2 mg/kg IV/IM/SC	0.01-0.03 mg/kg/h	++Histamine ↓SVR, ↓MAP	Active metabolite, adjust in ARI Pruritus, hallucinations
Remifentanil	1-3 mcg/kg	0.4-1 mcg/kg/min	Bradycardia	Equipotent to fentanyl Constant context-sensitive half-time
Tramadol	1-2 mg/kg/dose PO q4-6h (maximum single dose 100 mg)	NA	None	FDA recommend use in patients at over 12 y of age ≈1/10 potency of morphine Minimal respiratory depression
GABA$_A$ Receptor Agonist → _Sedation_				
Barbiturate				
Pentobarbital	1-2 mg/kg/dose q3-5 min to desired effect (maximum total dose 100 mg/dose)	0.5-5 mg/kg/h	Significant CV depressant	Deep sedation, ↓ICP, antiepileptic
Thiopental	4-6 mg/kg IV	5-10 mg/kg/h	Significant CV depressant	Deep sedation, ↓ICP, antiepileptic
Benzodiazepine				
Midazolam	0.025-0.1 mg/kg IV/IM 0.5-1 mg/kg PO/IN	0.05-0.3 mg/kg/h	Minimal	Active metabolite, adjust in ARI
Lorazepam	0.02-0.1 mg/kg q4-8h	NA	Minimal	Contains propylene glycol
Phenol → Directly Potentiates GABA$_A$ Activity Leading to _Hypnosis, Amnesia, and Sedation_				
Propofol	0.5-2 mg/kg IV	25-350 mcg/kg/min	↓SVR, ↓MAP ↓Contractility	Minimal respiratory depression PRIS (↑dose, ↑duration) Antiemetic, antipruritic, antiepileptic FDA approval: infusion for <48 h
Alpha (α)-adrenergic Receptor Agonist → _Analgesia, Sedation_				
Dexmedetomidine (α₂)	0.1-1 mcg/kg IV over 10-20 minutes	0.2-1.5 mcg/kg/h *Doses as high as 2.5 mcg/kg/h have been reported	SE > bolus and high doses Bradycardia	Minimal respiratory depression Decreased clearance (age <1 y) FDA approval: infusion for <24 h
Clonidine (α₁ , α₂)	1-5 mcg/kg/dose PO q6h - 8h (max dose: 200 mcg/ dose)		Bradycardia	Rebound hypertension IV bolus/continuous sedation under study, few clinical reports.
N-methyl-D-aspartate (NMDA) Receptor Antagonist → _Analgesia, Dissociative Sedation_				
Ketamine	0.5-2 mg/kg IV 3-7 mg/kg IM 5-10 mg/kg PO	0.5-2 mg/kg/h	↑HR, stable MAP Lose CV + effects w/ ↓catecholamine	Minimal respiratory depression Active metabolite (weak) Bronchodilation

ARI, Acute renal insufficiency; _COX_, cyclooxygenase; _CV_, cardiovascular; _FDA_, Food and Drug Administration; _GABA$_A$_, type A γ-aminobutyric acid; _HR_, heart rate; _ICP_, intracranial pressure; _IM_, intramuscular; _IN_, intranasal; _IV_, intravenous; _MAP_, mean arterial pressure; _NA_, not applicable; _NAPQI_, N-acetyl-p-benzoquinone imine; _PO_, by mouth; _PR_, by rectum; _PRIS_, propofol infusion syndrome; _SC_, subcutaneous; _SE_, side effects; _SVR_, systemic vascular resistance.

nonopioid and opioid analgesia are clearly associated with improved pain scores and less total opioid requirement.[44,45] Nonopioid analgesics should be administered early and scheduled as baseline therapy, using opioids for more severe or breakthrough pain. In the CICU, where we are already challenged with oversedation, the use of these adjuncts cannot be emphasized enough.[17]

Pain, fever, and inflammation are mediated through the cyclo-oxygenase (COX) pathway via prostaglandin production and action. There are two forms of the COX enzymes (COX-1 and COX-2), of which analgesia is greatest via COX-2 inhibition, whereas COX-1 inhibition may alter platelet aggregation and protection of the gastric lining. Many NSAIDs are nonselective COX inhibitors, whereas acetaminophen is COX-2 specific. Acetaminophen (paracetamol) is the most widely used analgesic and antipyretic worldwide, though with minimal antiinflammatory properties.[46,47] With the availability of IV formulations of both acetaminophen and ketorolac (an NSAID), the use of nonopioid agents in the ICU is no longer limited by the severity of illness or intolerance of enteral intake.[13,48,49] Recent studies have supported the use of ketorolac to provide rapid and effective analgesia among pediatric cardiac patients, with low reported risk of associated side effects such as clinically significant hemorrhage.[50-55] Changes in routine administration of acetaminophen may increase risk of overdose, requiring early detection because high levels of the metabolite N-acetyl-p-benzoquinone imine (NAPQI) are treated by N-acetylcysteine therapy.[56]

Opioids are potent analgesics that stimulate the μ, κ, and δ opioid receptors in both the peripheral and central nervous systems. Most analgesic properties are mediated via the μ_1-receptor, with less potent analgesia via the μ_2-receptor and naturally occurring dynorphin/encephalin-stimulated κ- and δ-receptors.[57] The majority of opioid-associated respiratory depression, bradycardia, and physical dependence occur via the μ_2-receptor activity. Most opioids undergo hepatic metabolism and renal elimination.

Morphine is considered the archetypal opioid. Morphine is highly water soluble, subject to extensive first-pass metabolism, and undergoes glucuronide conjugation to morphine-6 glucuronide, an active and potent metabolite dependent on renal elimination. Cardiac patients with low cardiac output and requiring inotropic support are at risk for decreased metabolism and up to a threefold decrease in clearance among patients with hemodynamic instability.[58,59] Although normovolemic patients tolerate morphine administration without hemodynamic effects, patients with low cardiac output may have an exaggerated histamine effect, causing impaired compensatory sympathetic reflexes, increased venous capacitance, and decreased perfusion.[10]

Fentanyl is a synthetic opioid that is highly lipid soluble, with a rapid clinical onset, and is converted primarily to inactive metabolites. Fentanyl is routinely used in the perioperative period, providing safe and effective analgesia and sedation to cardiac patients.[47,49,60,61] In the CICU prolonged use of fentanyl infusions for analgesia and sedation may lead to tachyphylaxis and require transition to other opioids.[62] Studies have demonstrated a positive safety profile and clinical benefit of the associated blunted sympathetic stress response in infants and children with LCOS, pulmonary hypertension, and critically balanced systemic/pulmonary circulations.[58,63]

Hydromorphone (Dilaudid) is a semisynthetic opioid, with greater potency and quicker onset (5 to 10 minutes) compared to morphine.[64-67] Metabolism occurs via conjugation and forms two nonactive metabolites that undergo renal elimination.[68] The absence

of significant associated hemodynamic side effects makes its use an advantageous option for analgesia in the CICU.

Methadone is a long-acting opioid analgesic,[69] most commonly used in the ICU setting for opioid withdrawal. Though the long half-life of methadone prevents its use in critically ill patients with a rapidly changing clinical course, methadone can be as a useful adjunct when a regimen is required for prolonged MV, gradual weaning, or a stable level of analgesia.[70,71] Potential adverse effects include prolongation of QTc and hypotension.

Remifentanil is a pure μ-receptor agonist with equipotency to fentanyl, an ultrashort onset of action, and a constant context-sensitive half-time regardless of duration of infusion. These properties make remifentanil an important option for intraoperative and procedural anesthesia. The associated bradycardia common with higher doses and hyperalgesic component following prolonged exposure make its usefulness in the CICU for analgesia less apparent.[60,69]

Tramadol is a synthetic 4-phenyl-piperidine analogue of codeine with a dual mechanism of action; it is a μ-, δ-, and κ-opioid receptor agonist. Though less potent, its lack of respiratory depression and low risk of dependence lead to its role as an adjunct for breakthrough pain and opioid-sparing effects.[72-74]

Sedation

Benzodiazepines bind to the postsynaptic type A γ-aminobutyric acid (GABA_A) receptor, which increases the affinity of the receptor to GABA. GABA-ergic activity leads to inhibition of the central nervous system (CNS), resulting in sedation, hypnosis, amnesia, anxiolysis, and anticonvulsant effects.[75,76] In general, metabolism of benzodiazepines is hepatic mediated and elimination is renal mediated.

Midazolam is the most commonly used sedative in the CICU with its rapid onset and ease of titration as a continuous infusion. Midazolam may lead to respiratory depression, especially with coadministration of an opioid. However, it can provide safe sedation/induction for some patients with cardiac disease, usually at lower doses. Although many patients may tolerate benzodiazepine use, administration can result in hypotension, particularly in patients with decreased cardiac function or in conjunction with additional sedative therapies. Midazolam has a short context-sensitive half-time; however, these properties are lost following infusions lasting multiple days, leading to longer duration of action and delayed elimination.[69] The free (active) fraction of midazolam can be increased in critically ill children who are malnourished, have hepatic dysfunction, or are receiving other protein-bound drugs. Midazolam is metabolized via cytochrome P-450 to an equipotent metabolite, of which approximately 80% of conjugated 1-OH-midazolam is renally eliminated; therefore the risk of prolonged sedation should be considered in the setting of renal dysfunction.[77-79] Due to the reliance on midazolam for continuous sedation, associated tolerance, dependence, and withdrawal is common.[57,75] The clinical benefit of dose titration occurs at lower doses, with only marginal clinical improvement at higher levels. With the heavy reliance on benzodiazepines in the CICU, including high exposure and prolonged administration, association with delirium, prolonged ICU stay, and MV, and recent concerns regarding neurodevelopment, clinicians must seriously consider the appropriate role of this drug class in ICU sedation regimens.

Lorazepam is a long-acting benzodiazepine used for intermittent sedation and treatment for withdrawal following long-term midazolam infusions. It undergoes metabolism via hepatic-mediated phase II reactions that are not as sensitive to low cardiac output or hepatic dysfunction.[47,69] Lorazepam infusions are frequently used in the adult ICU but are not used in the pediatric setting due to its long context-sensitive half-time and risk of propylene glycol (an additive in lorazepam) toxicity. Propylene glycol toxicity presents as an osmolar-gap metabolic acidosis and can be fatal if not recognized in a timely manner.[47]

Alpha-2 adrenergic receptor agonists inhibit adenylyl cyclase via the alpha-2-adrenergic receptor located in both the peripheral and central nervous system. The greatest density of receptor activity occurs in the locus coeruleus (pons) and is responsible for mediating the sympathetic responses to stress, reducing brainstem vasomotor center–mediated CNS activation, in addition to treating pain, agitation, and withdrawal.[80] The quality and characteristics of sedation differ based on drug choice. Sedation produced by alpha-2 agonists occurs by decreasing sympathetic neurotransmission, with a clinical picture of a calm-appearing yet easily aroused and attentive patient.[81] (This is in contrast to GABA-ergic agents [benzodiazepines], which suppress arousal, producing an alteration of consciousness and even paradoxical agitation, with negative effects on cognition and behavior. Opioids too have inhibitory effects on the locus coeruleus; therefore when consumption is discontinued, abrupt increases in adrenergic neurotransmission from the locus coeruleus produce significant symptoms of withdrawal). The alpha-2 adrenoceptor activity of both dexmedetomidine (selective alpha-2 adrenergic receptor agonist) and clonidine (nonselective alpha-adrenergic receptor agonist) counteract these withdrawal effects.[80] Due to their broad activity and favorable safety profiles, the roles of the alpha-2 adrenergic receptor agonists in the CICU continues to increase.

Dexmedetomidine is a selective alpha-2 adrenergic receptor agonist that demonstrates both sedative and analgesic properties.[82] Dexmedetomidine is currently approved for procedural sedation of nonintubated patients, though off-label use for prolonged continuous sedation (>24 hours) in the ICU setting among adults, infants, and children is becoming commonplace.[83,84] To that end, successful use of dexmedetomidine has been demonstrated in multiple studies of critically ill pediatric patients, including those with cardiac disease, for surgical anesthesia, postoperative sedation, and procedural sedation.[85-88] Similar to ketamine and propofol, dexmedetomidine has opioid- and benzodiazepine-sparing effects when continuous sedation is required. Due to its large volume of distribution, a loading dose is required before starting an infusion for acute sedative/analgesic effects. In infants and younger children the terminal half-life is longer, and therefore a lower maintenance dose is required.[82] Because its properties are favorable for continuous sedation, the longer context-sensitive half-time requires thoughtful titration in advance when weaning is desired. Dexmedetomidine is metabolized via the hepatic-mediated cytochrome P-450 pathway but does not depend on renal elimination and is therefore safe in patients with renal insufficiency.[89] The safety profile of dexmedetomidine has been promising in the critically ill population, though bradycardia and hypotension have been reported regardless of the mode of administration (bolus versus infusion).[83,85] Uniquely, the electrophysiologic effects of dexmedetomidine may be advantageous in some patients, with fewer episodes of perioperative junctional ectopic tachycardia and supraventricular tachycardia reported.[90-92] As the routine use of dexmedetomidine increases, the risks of dependence and significance of symptoms, such as agitation and hypertension, will need to be further studied.[93]

Clonidine is a nonselective alpha-adrenergic receptor agonist with greater alpha-2 activity. Historically used for the treatment of hypertension, clonidine is increasingly being tapped for sedation, analgesia, and opioid/benzodiazepine withdrawal.[94,95] Though the most effective dosing regimen of clonidine in the pediatric intensive care unit (PICU) has not been determined, available evidence supports both infusion and bolus dosing.[96] In a recent report, infusion dosing as high as 3 mcg/kg/h was reported to have excellent analgesic and sedative properties while maintaining stable hemodynamics in patients less than 2 years of age following repair of congenital heart disease.[95] In combination with NSAIDs, local anesthetics, opioids, or ketamine, clonidine been shown to be a successful adjunct for analgesia.[97]

Ketamine is a phencyclidine compound that antagonizes the N-methyl-D-aspartate (NMDA) receptor and has some opioid, nicotinic, and monoamine oxidase action as well. The dissociation created between the thalamocortical and limbic systems leads to a cataleptic-like state of unresponsiveness (sedation), intense analgesia, and amnesia. Despite the significant degree of anesthesia, with appropriate titration both airway reflexes and spontaneous respiration can remain intact.[98] Ketamine is metabolized via N-methylation to form norketamine, a less-potent active metabolite, which undergoes conjugation and renal-mediated elimination. Ketamine undergoes rapid redistribution due to its lipophilicity. Ketamine causes both release of and reuptake inhibition of endogenous catecholamines that increase/maintain vascular tone and increase heart rate and contractility. Patients with severe uncompensated cardiomyopathy often have depleted catecholamine stores; hence the direct myocardial depressant properties of ketamine may be unmasked and lead to hypotension during bolus administration.[57] Psychedelic effects, including emergence delirium, and the risk of tolerance with prolonged use require consideration.[99,100]

In the perioperative setting, oral ketamine provides excellent sedation for IV access in patients with cardiac disease who cannot tolerate the hemodynamic effects associated with a volatile induction. Intramuscular ketamine provides safe, emergent anesthesia for intubation of uncooperative or critically ill patients who do not have IV access. Ketamine has been successfully used intraoperatively as continuous IV anesthesia for cardiac catheterizations and repair of congenital heart lesions on cardiopulmonary bypass,[101-103] without significant dose-related elevations in heart rate.[104,105] With a short context-sensitive half-time, ketamine is ideal for CICU sedation because titration is predictable. Low-dose (<2 mg/kg/h) ketamine infusions provide effective analgesia and decrease the total opioid and benzodiazepine exposure, without clinically significant hypertension, tachycardia, increased intracranial pressure, or hallucinations.[106]

Propofol is an IV-administered sedative-hypnotic commonly used for procedural sedation, intubation, and anesthetic induction and maintenance in pediatric patients. As a lipophilic phenol, propofol potentiates and directly facilitates the action of the $GABA_A$ receptor, causing hypnosis, amnesia, and sedation, without analgesia. Propofol has several unique actions, including antiemetic, antipruritic, and anticonvulsant properties. It is metabolized rapidly by the liver with no active metabolites.[107] In the CICU population, propofol has been advantageous as an adjunct for continuous sedation with opioid/benzodiazepine-sparing effects and a short context-sensitive half-time for infusions of short duration (<10 hours) due to its large volume of distribution and increased clearance in pediatric patients.[108,109] Though low-dose continuous infusions may be tolerated, induction bolus doses (1 to 3 mg/kg) can lead to profound decreases in systemic vascular resistance, myocardial depression, and bradycardia in settings of significant myocardial depression, shunt-dependent pulmonary/systemic flow, or hypovolemia.[110,111] Propofol has not been associated with withdrawal syndrome and may be advantageous during rapid titration of opioids and benzodiazepines. The use of propofol in the pediatric population must be weighed against the risk of developing propofol infusion syndrome (PRIS). Key risk factors associated with PRIS include high infusion rates (>4 mg/kg/h), infusion duration longer than 48 hours, critical illness, young age, concurrent catecholamine infusion, and steroid use. PRIS results in impaired oxidative phosphorylation, leading to a life-threatening metabolic acidosis, myocardial failure, rhabdomyolysis, and renal failure. The FDA provided recommendations in 2001 against prolonged propofol infusion sedation regimens in critically ill children, and therefore it is usually employed for less than 48 hours or during early extubation in most pediatric ICUs if at all.[10]

Barbiturates are global CNS depressants that provide sedation, amnesia, and anticonvulsant activity. Barbiturates are not routinely used in the CICU because even lower doses can have profound effects on cardiac output and vasomotor tone, leading to poor oxygen delivery. The duration of action is determined by the rate of redistribution from the CNS to other tissue compartments. As these compartments become saturated due to high exposure or prolonged administration, patients are at risk for protracted sedative effects.

Tolerance and Dependence

Prolonged sedation in the ICU setting can lead to iatrogenic withdrawal syndrome (IWS). The most predictive risk factors for IWS are duration and cumulative exposure, with other associated factors, including age, drug class, bolus versus continuous administration, and use of weaning protocols.[8] Prolonged exposure to opioids and sedatives can produce tolerance and dependence. Tolerance results in less clinical effect for a given dose, and therefore higher doses are required to achieve therapeutic effect. Dependence occurs when ongoing drug administration is required to prevent symptoms of abstinence syndrome. Abstinence syndrome can develop within 24 hours following cessation of chronic medications and is characterized by symptoms such as restlessness, insomnia, diaphoresis, tachycardia, hypertension, movement disorders, abdominal cramps, vomiting, diarrhea, delirium, and seizures.[112] Amigoni and colleagues[113] recently reported the extremely high prevalence (>60%) of IWS among survivors of critical illness. Both methadone and lorazepam are commonly required to treat IWS. The hope is that with optimization of targeted sedation and analgesia regimens, IWS will decrease over time.

Implementation of Sedation and Analgesia Regimens

To optimize sedation and analgesia in the CICU, a change in culture is required. It is necessary to routinely monitor pain and sedation scores, consider both pharmacologic and nonpharmacologic interventions, and recognize the physiologic implications of both inadequate treatment and overtreatment. For every patient, every day, three questions should be asked: (1) Where is my patient now? (pain, sedation, and delirium assessments); (2) Where is my patient going? (incorporation of the current physiologic/disease state and establishment of patient goals for the day); and (3) How do I get the patient there? (setting new sedation targets and planning for titration). In a systematic review by Vet and colleagues[114] it is reported that daily sedation targets are achieved only approximately 60% of the time, with oversedation common. In fact, when sedation scores were below the target (oversedation), clinicians seemed to tolerate the more undesirable LOC because weaning of sedating medications rarely occurred. With recent recognition of the dangers of oversedation, clinicians are beginning to tolerate patients' being more awake to benefit from touch, family present, and early mobilization (EM). In addition, interdisciplinary and multimodal approach, incorporating active waiting, and consideration of intermittent dosing rather than continuous infusions may benefit children in the CICU. [114]

Delirium in the Cardiac Intensive Care Unit

Children are at high risk for developing delirium in the CICU.[115,116] Delirium is defined as an acute and fluctuating state of neurologic dysfunction, manifested by altered awareness and cognition.[116] It develops as a direct result of the underlying illness or as an unwanted side effect of hospital treatment. This is a medical diagnosis (rather than a psychiatric one) and can be conceptualized as a hospital-acquired complication. Delirium is a reversible process, and duration can be shortened with early detection and appropriate intervention.[117-119]

Three subtypes of pediatric delirium are described: hyperactive, hypoactive, and mixed. Hyperactive delirium is easily recognized, with refractory agitation impeding caregivers' attempts to administer necessary treatment. Hypoactive delirium, characterized by age-inappropriate lethargy, apathy, and withdrawal, is often overlooked. In mixed delirium, children vacillate between the motoric subtypes over the course of a 24-hour period. In children, disrupted sleep is a hallmark of all delirium subtypes.[117,120-123] It is estimated that without routine screening, most cases of delirium remain undiagnosed.[124]

Etiology of Delirium

The pathophysiology leading to delirium is complex and multifactorial.[125] Hypoxia, inflammation, and altered neurotransmission all play key roles in delirium development. The neuroinflammatory hypothesis suggests that inflammation or oxygen deprivation leads to cytokine release with subsequent modification of the blood-brain barrier (BBB). Alteration in BBB permeability, in addition to dysregulation of the hypothalamic-pituitary-adrenal axis, lead to disruption of second messengers and neurotransmitters.[126] All neurotransmitters are involved to some extent, with acetylcholine playing a prominent role.[127] Neurons may also be directly injured due to oxidative stress, with possible exacerbation by the neuro-humoral response, with research suggesting that endogenous glucocorticoids contribute to neuronal injury, particularly in the hippocampus.[125,128] Delirium is also more likely to occur in those with less physiologic reserve, where serious illness unmasks those brains with the least resilience.[129,130] Regardless of cause, most researchers agree that delirium represents acute whole brain dysfunction, with interruption of brain network connections and alteration in neurotransmission leading to the cognitive and behavioral changes that we recognize as delirium.[125]

Clinically it is useful to think of pediatric delirium as a consequence of three interrelated factors: the underlying medical illness, unwanted side effects of treatment, and the unnatural and stressful environment in the ICU.[17,117,120] Accordingly, children with congenital heart disease are at particular risk. As an example, consider a 4-month-old infant with trisomy 21 and an atrioventricular canal defect. She is admitted with congestive heart failure and undergoes surgical repair. After general anesthesia and bypass surgery the infant is admitted to the CICU. In the postoperative period she is mechanically ventilated, with multiple indwelling lines and tubes, pharmacologically sedated with narcotics and benzodiazepines, and restrained in her ICU bed. There she is immobilized while being exposed to noise and lights 24 hours a day. This child will likely become delirious early in her CICU stay.

Epidemiology of Delirium

The prevalence of pediatric delirium reported in the literature ranges from 13% to 65%, depending on the population studied.[11,18,115,120,131-133] A large multinational study (n = 835 subjects) showed an overall frequency of 25%. In this mixed population, factors independently associated with increased delirium risk included need for MV or inotropes, receipt of benzodiazepines and narcotics, and age less than 2 years. For children in the ICU for 6 or more days, delirium frequency increased to 38%.[11] Children with critical cardiac disease have many (if not all) of these risk factors, suggesting that our patients are at particular risk for developing delirium during their hospital stay.

Other single-institution studies have identified an extremely high delirium prevalence in children less than 5 years of age. In two separate studies, delirium rates were 56% and 65% in patients younger than 2 years, and 35% and 40% in patients 2 to 5 years of age.[18,115,120] Children with preexisting neurodevelopmental delay are more likely to become delirious when compared to children with typical development.[120] Severity of illness is also independently associated with delirium.[134,135]

Postcardiotomy delirium is a specific delirium subtype described in adults after cardiac bypass surgery, which can affect up to 70% of patients in a CICU.[136-138] This high prevalence is attributed to perioperative insults (including hypoperfusion, hypoxia, and cerebral microinfarcts) in an already vulnerable population.[139,140] Until recently, little was known about delirium in children after bypass surgery.

A single-center prospective observational study followed 194 children after cardiac bypass surgery.[115] These children were screened for delirium daily, and 49% were diagnosed with delirium during their ICU stay. In most children, delirium developed within the first 3 days after surgery, with a median duration of 2 days. Consistent with other pediatric delirium literature, the youngest children (less than 2 years of age) were most likely to develop delirium, as were children with the highest severity of illness, and those with baseline cognitive impairment. Cardiac-specific risk factors that were identified were presence of cyanotic heart disease and duration of bypass. Data suggest that poor nutritional status preoperatively increased the chance for development of postoperative delirium. As a marker of good nutritional status, children with a preoperative albumin level of more than 3 mg/dL had a lower odds of delirium development (odds ratio [OR] for delirium diagnosis 0.2; $P = .028$).[115] Close attention should be paid to vulnerable children with these risk factors because they are most likely to become delirious during their hospital stay.

Importantly, there are hospital-related factors that contribute to delirium development in at-risk children. These include use of restraints and benzodiazepines. A large multicenter study showed an independent association between the use of physical restraints and delirium (OR 4.0), after adjusting for MV, sedating medication, and other potential confounders.[11] A recent single center study has shown that the use of benzodiazepines confers a fivefold risk of delirium in children, even after controlling for age, developmental delay, severity of illness, MV, and use of other narcotics and sedatives.[135] In adults, dexmedetomidine has been associated with

decreased delirium, when compared to benzodiazepine-based sedation.[141-144] It is likely that sleep deprivation and immobilization both play a role in the evolution of pediatric delirium.[145-147]

Outcomes Related to Delirium

Not only is delirium highly prevalent, it also is associated with short-term distress and long-term harm. Delirium has been tightly linked to increased time on MV and longer hospitalization.[135,148] A 2016 study demonstrated a 60% increase in CICU length of stay in children diagnosed with delirium, after controlling for relevant confounders.[115] Even early-onset delirium of only 1 to 2 days' duration was associated with poor short-term outcomes.[115,132] Delirium during hospitalization has also been linked to delusional memories and posttraumatic stress symptoms in PICU survivors.[6] From an economic perspective, pediatric delirium is associated with a dramatic increase in hospital costs, estimated at more than $560 million annually in the United States.[149]

Most significantly, delirium has been shown to be an independent predictor of pediatric in-hospital mortality, with a quadrupling of mortality rates beyond that predicted by severity of illness on admission (adjusted OR 4.39; CI 1.96-9.99; $P < .001$).[135]

Delirium Assessment

Clinical guidelines recommend routine monitoring of all critically ill children for delirium at least once every shift.[150] The gold standard for delirium diagnosis is a psychiatric evaluation using the *Diagnostic and Statistical Manual of Mental Disorders,* fifth edition (DSM-5) criteria.[151] This is time-consuming and clearly not feasible for twice-daily use in every patient in the CICU. Recognizing the need for delirium diagnosis by nonpsychiatrists, experts have developed appropriate tools for use at the bedside.[152] There are two validated instruments suitable for use in children.

The Pediatric Confusion Assessment Method for the ICU (pCAM-ICU) is an interactive bedside tool for use in children 5 years of age and older (Fig. 21.1A). The medical provider assesses for alteration from baseline mental status, then evaluates attention by asking the child to squeeze the provider's hand in response to the letter *A* (or as an alternative, using memory pictures if appropriate). If altered LOC is also present, then the pCAM-ICU is positive. Occasionally, when the child is alert and calm, an additional step to assess cognition (yes/no questions and hand gestures) may be required.[133] There is a preschool version, the Preschool Confusion Assessment Method for the ICU (psCAM-ICU) available for use in children between 6 months and 5 years of age (see Fig. 21.1B).[18] The pCAM-ICU and psCAM-ICU provide point-in-time assessments for delirium and can be completed in a short amount of time.

The Cornell Assessment of Pediatric Delirium (CAPD) is an observational tool scored by the bedside nurse (Fig. 21.2) and is validated for children of all ages. After a period of observation of the child (generally toward the end of the nurse's shift), the nurse scores a Likert type of scale, consisting of eight questions (evaluating the child's eye contact, purposefulness, awareness, communication, restlessness, consolability, activity, and response to interactions). A score of nine or higher is consistent with a diagnosis of delirium. This provides a longitudinal assessment for delirium because the CAPD score can be trended in the individual child over time to assess delirium trajectory and treatment response.[131]

Both the pCAM-ICU and CAPD have been shown to be quick to complete, are reliable for use in seriously ill children, and can detect all delirium subtypes. Neither can be used in children who

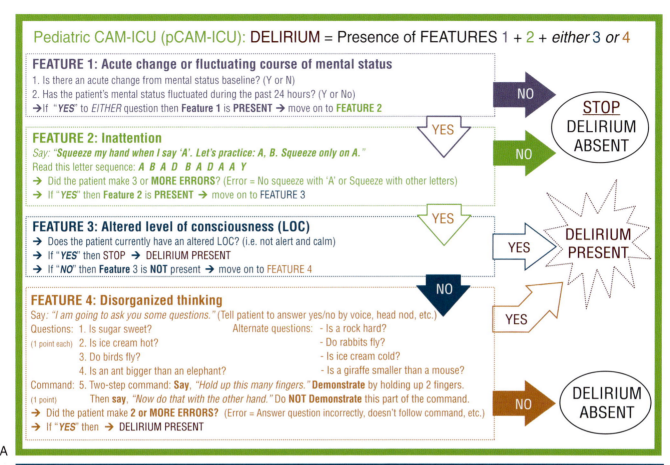

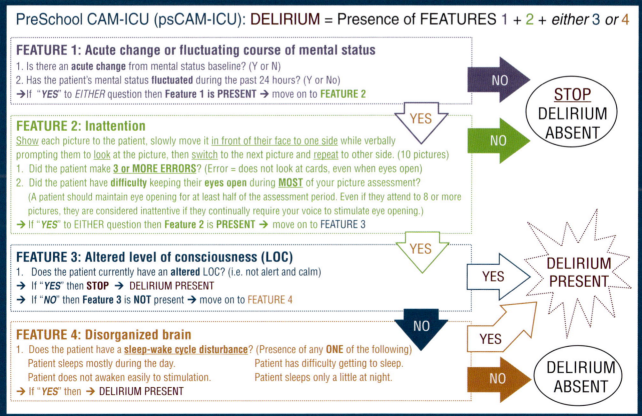

• **Figure 21.1** (A) Pediatric Confusion Assessment Method for the ICU (pCAM-ICU). (B) Preschool Confusion Assessment Method for the ICU (psCAM-ICU). The pCAM-ICU and psCAM-ICU are interactive cognitively oriented tools validated in children from 6 months to 18 years of age. ([A] From Smith HAB, Boyd J, Fuchs DC, et al. Diagnosing delirium in critically ill children: validity and reliability of the Pediatric Confusion Assessment Method for the Intensive Care Unit. *Crit Care Med.* 2011;39[1]:150-157. [B] From Smith HA, Gangopadhyay M, Goben CM, et al. The Preschool Confusion Assessment Method for the ICU: valid and reliable delirium monitoring for critically ill infants and children. *Crit Care Med.* 2016;44[3]:592-600.)

CORNELL ASSESSMENT OF PEDIATRIC DELIRIUM

Please answer these questions based on your interactions with the patient over the course of your shift:

	Never 4	Rarely 3	Sometimes 2	Often 1	Always 0	Score
1. Does the child make eye contact with the caregiver?						
2. Are the child's actions purposeful?						
3. Is the child aware of his/her surroundings?						
4. Does the child communicate needs and wants?						
	Never 0	Rarely 1	Sometimes 2	Often 3	Always 4	
5. Is the child restless?						
6. Is the child inconsolable?						
7. Is the child underactive—very little movement while awake?						
8. Does it take the child a long time to respond to interactions?						
					TOTAL	

• **Figure 21.2** Cornell Assessment of Pediatric Delirium (CAPD). The CAPD is an observational longitudinal tool validated in children from birth to 18 years of age.

are deeply sedated (i.e., unarousable to verbal stimulation) because their depressed LOC precludes a clinical determination of delirium.[150]

Children with cognitive disabilities are challenging to assess for delirium because there is a need to establish an alteration from neurologic baseline. However, these children with developmental delay are at significant risk for delirium, with multivariable analyses showing a more than threefold increase in delirium frequency as compared to children with typical development.[120] They also represent a substantial minority (greater than 15%) of children admitted to the cardiac ICU, so it is imperative that they be included in routine delirium screening.[115]

Treatment of Delirium

Just as the etiology of delirium is multifactorial, the approach to treatment should be multilayered as well (Fig. 21.3). First, the clinician should investigate for an underlying medical cause that may have precipitated the delirious episode; then, minimize iatrogenic causes; and finally, optimize the ICU environment.[153,154] If this is not enough, and the child remains delirious, then pharmacologic therapy for the delirium may be considered.

Underlying Illness. With delirium diagnosis a focused physical and neurologic examination is required. On occasion this will dictate the need for further laboratory or radiologic studies. Delirium is associated with hypoxia, hypotension, anemia, and infection. In particular, occult urinary tract infections and peritonitis have been associated with delirium. A new neurologic process (such as

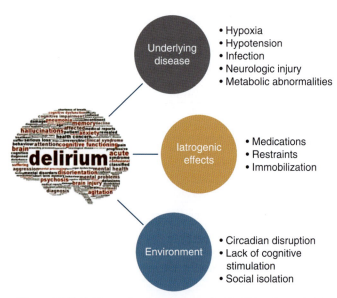

• **Figure 21.3** Delirium: a treatment approach. Identifying the underlying cause of the delirious episode is often the key to successful treatment.

a cerebrovascular accident) may need to be excluded if there are any focal signs on the neurologic examination. Attention should be paid to electrolyte abnormalities and anemia.[120,139,155-157]

Iatrogenic Factors. When a child is diagnosed with delirium, review of the medication list is warranted. Any nonessential drugs (particularly benzodiazepines and anticholinergics) should be eliminated.[158] Pain control should be optimized and sedation minimized. Restraints should be removed if safety allows.[11,156] If concern exists that the child may remove necessary medical devices, consider a one-to-one companion at the bedside to monitor and redirect the child, rather than physical restraints. Immobilization may be a potent precipitator of delirium in young children. With minimization of sedation, early and progressive mobilization will be facilitated.[145,159,160]

Environmental Modifications. The child's environment can be optimized with fairly modest changes. A schedule can be implemented, with lights on and cognitive stimulation during the day, and lights off with minimization of noise and interruptions at night. Familiar items from home (pajamas, blanket, security objects) can be brought to the bedside. Bedtime routines can be implemented. Family involvement should be encouraged, with parents physically interacting with their child (holding, touching) as much as feasible.[154,161,162]

Pharmacologic Therapy. With respect to pharmacotherapy for delirium, there is a scarcity of data within pediatrics. Most experts recommend an atypical antipsychotic as first-line therapy when a nonpharmacologic approach to delirium is inadequate.[156,163,164] With fewer side effects than typical antipsychotics, these procognitive drugs have been used effectively in children of all ages.[165-167] Monitoring the QTc is recommended because children in the cardiac unit are often on multiple medications that can prolong the QT interval. A retrospective study evaluated the short-term safety of quetiapine (an atypical antipsychotic with a favorable side-effect profile) for treatment of delirium in critically ill children. The study included 50 consecutive PICU patients ranging in age from 2 months to 20 years, and there were no serious adverse events.[168] It is important to note that this is an off-label use of neuroleptics (both with respect to indication and population) because the FDA has not approved these drugs for treatment of pediatric delirium. Antipsychotics should be considered to treat delirium when the risk/benefit ratio is favorable.

Prevention of Delirium

With a change in CICU culture, it may be possible to decrease the frequency of delirium. The Society of Critical Care Medicine has embraced a holistic approach to culture change, termed *ICU liberation.* The initiative incorporates six bundles of care that seek to optimize pain control, minimize sedation, encourage ventilator weaning, screen for delirium, and promote EM and family involvement.[169] Increasingly ICUs are embracing "analgo-sedation," using an analgesic-based approach to sedation, with sedatives added only if necessary.[156] With adequate pain control, need for sedatives is decreased (and sometimes eliminated entirely). When patients are less sedated, they are better able to communicate pain, which then further optimizes pain control. With less pharmacologic sedation, this happy cycle also leads to a decrease in delirium incidence and duration.[170]

Sleep Promotion and Acute Rehabilitation in the Cardiac Intensive Care Unit

Balancing goal-directed pain and sedation management with close attention to delirium prevention and treatment is critical to optimizing outcomes in critically ill children with cardiac disease. A multicomponent approach integrating sleep promotion and acute rehabilitation into the routine care of each child will help create a healing environment and foster recovery. Traditional paradigms of heavy sedation, restraints, and immobility during a child's most acute phase of illness or postoperative recovery are shifting to promotion of natural circadian rhythms with good sleep hygiene and incorporation of EM activities soon after ICU admission.[145,160,169,171-177] The following sections discuss the current evidence supporting sleep promotion and acute rehabilitation for the child in the CICU, with practical approaches for implementation.

Sleep

Sleep continues to be one of the most mysterious aspects of physiologic function. Although sleep is traditionally thought of as a time of passivity and rest, the human brain is very active during sleep. Sleep is integral to homeostasis of multiple organ systems, and the trajectory of sleep behavior during infancy, childhood, and adolescence demonstrates the importance of sleep in healthy neurodevelopment.[178] Differences in sleep with age include change not only in total sleep time, but also in sleep architecture (or stages) of sleep. Each sleep stage is characterized by distinct electroencephalographic (EEG) patterns and representative changes in eye movement, muscle tone, and muscle activity. During sleep humans cycle from wakefulness through three stages of non-REM (NREM) sleep before completing each cycle with a rapid eye movement (REM) period and starting the next cycle. Whereas adults spend approximately 20% of their sleep time in REM sleep, 50% of infant sleep is spent in this active phase, which is considered to be integral to promotion of cortical plasticity in the developing brain.[179] Insufficient sleep in childhood is associated with negative cognitive, behavioral, and mental health outcomes.[180]

The majority of sleep research has focused on duration of sleep in healthy children in the home environment. Emerging data demonstrate that children in the PICU have severe disruption of natural circadian rhythmicity, with decreased NREM sleep and severe sleep fragmentation.[171,181-183] In children admitted to the ICU after cardiac surgery, significant sleep fragmentation is evident, as demonstrated by long-term actigraphic monitoring, and persists through discharge from the hospital.[172] Although total sleep time is not significantly changed, approximately 40% of these patients have no discernible difference in daytime versus nighttime activity, suggesting that sleep is occurring in short fragments throughout a 24-hour period.

As a rule the hospital environment brings a host of challenges to optimizing sleep hygiene for patients, and hospital routines are not conducive to consolidated sleep at night due to constant noise, artificial light, and frequent interventions. Admission to the ICU is stressful for children and their families, and the chaotic environment compounds the anxiety a child experiences. Despite World Health Organization recommendations to maintain noise levels below 30 dB, the vast majority of ICUs far exceed these levels on average, often peaking to 100 dB.[184-186] In a 2012 international survey sample of pediatric intensivists, less than a quarter of all respondents were aware of any protocols in place for either noise reduction or lighting optimization. The child admitted to the CICU is often exposed to the highest levels of noise and light due to high acuity and intensive monitoring in the immediate postoperative period. Lights often remain on at full intensity at night due to concerns of missing key physical examination changes that may occur with acute decompensation. Noise from staff voices and technology augment the risk of severe sleep disruption.

In addition to environmental risk factors for sleep disruption, cardiac patients are exposed to a multitude of pharmacologic agents that contribute to poor sleep. The cardiac surgery patient is subjected to prolonged duration of general anesthesia, and the most commonly used sedative-analgesic medications in the postoperative period are benzodiazepines and opioids, which both negatively impact sleep quality.[145] Dexmedetomidine and clonidine, both alpha-agonists, are the only commonly used sedatives that do not share this same impact, demonstrating an EEG pattern most consistent with natural sleep.[187] Of special relevance to the CICU patient, inotropic medications are known to have deleterious effects on sleep.[178]

Often clinicians add other medications in an attempt to promote sleep, but this may further exacerbate sleep disruption. For example, diphenhydramine is sometimes prescribed for insomnia. However, diphenhydramine is known to be deliriogenic, and although it improves sleep latency (time to sleep onset) and increases sleep duration, the quality of sleep is severely diminished.[188] Benzodiazepines are also commonly added to help children "sleep"; however, this practice is beginning to change with education and awareness among PICU physicians and staff. Clinicians sometimes prescribed melatonin, a naturally occurring hormone produced by the pineal gland, which plays a key role in maintenance of the circadian rhythm and regulation of other hormones. However, melatonin levels in critically ill pediatric patients can be elevated or depressed.[189] Atypical antipsychotics have also been prescribed to improve sleep in the PICU; however, there is no current evidence to support this practice.

Early Mobilization and Acute Rehabilitation

As mortality rates decrease, the impact of functional impairments on children and their families' quality of life is drawing increased attention in the pediatric critical care community. Historically, cardiac surgery patients have been prescribed bed rest in the immediate postoperative period to reduce cardiac load.[190,191] A culture of immobility in the pediatric ICU setting to promote recovery and ensure safety is being scrutinized thanks to a strong foundation of adult studies demonstrating that ICU-acquired weakness (ICU-AW) affects greater than 50% of all patients.[192,193] ICU-AW refers to the presence of clinically detectable muscle weakness in critically ill patients in the absence of weakness caused by factors other than the critical illness itself.[194,195] ICU-AW is characterized as critical illness polyneuropathy (CIP), critical illness myopathy (CIM), or both, and is independently associated with post-ICU mortality in adults.[196] CIP has a pathogenetic basis with an increase in glucose level preceding reactive oxygen generation and bioenergetics failure, leading to toxic peripheral nerve outcomes. CIM is a result of muscle inactivity due to dysfunction of the excitation-contraction calcium ion channels, leading to ICU-AW.[197] In adult patients after cardiac surgery there is evidence to suggest that acute muscle loss occurs due to an imbalance of mediators of muscle hypertrophy (insulin-like growth factor-1) and atrophy (myostatin).[198] Immobility also impairs oxygen transport in lung and tissue and increases the risk of deep vein thrombosis and thromboembolism.[199] Although children in the ICU are exposed to all of the same risk factors for immobility-related complications as critically ill adults, research is just now emerging in the pediatric population.[200,201]

EM, or progressive mobility, is defined as initiation of rehabilitation activities early in the ICU stay, generally in the first 48 hours. In adults, EM has a low reported rate of adverse events, and expert consensus is that EM and rehabilitation is safe in intubated patients with careful planning and close monitoring during and after the process.[194,202] Data from clinical trials in adult medical ICU

patients investigating the effects of EM interventions demonstrate significant variability in results, with accompanying heterogeneity in inclusion criteria, methodology, and interventions. However, several studies have demonstrated benefit with outcomes including reduced duration of MV and ICU and hospital length of stay and improved functional independence at discharge.[194,203-206] A systematic review of randomized controlled trials investigating EM in cardiac surgery patients identified nine studies for inclusion, with varying interventions and timing of EM.[190] Only two studies provided a clear definition of EM, and interventions included body positioning, sitting at the edge of bed, passive range of motion, virtual reality exercises, breathing exercises, and ambulation. For trials comparing EM to no treatment, EM was found to be beneficial for length of hospital stay, functional capacity, and incidence of postoperative complications.

The impact of EM on outcomes in the pediatric population has not yet been systematically evaluated. However, there is a growing base of evidence to support the safety and feasibility of EM for children in the ICU.[173] A systematic review of EM studies in critically ill children identified six studies for inclusion and concluded that EM is likely safe and feasible in the PICU. One study focused on pediatric cardiac patients to determine the safety and feasibility of an inpatient acute rehabilitation program using standardized patient and family–centered care pathways after ventricular assist device placement.[207] Among 14 patients ranging from 6 months to 14 years of age, structured rehabilitation resulted in no adverse events, and predefined goals were achievable. A subsequent single-center quality improvement study demonstrated the safety and feasibility of a tiered, multicomponent approach to EM in the PICU; 14% of the patients evaluated were children admitted to the PICU after cardiac surgery.[208] The most common barriers to EM for pediatric patients across studies were lack of appropriate equipment for heterogeneous patient sizes and weights, staffing availability, and the need for physical and occupational therapy consultation to be ordered by the physician staff.[174,175,208]

Promoting Sleep Hygiene and Acute Rehabilitation in the Cardiac Intensive Care Unit

Integration of sleep hygiene and acute rehabilitation with EM plays a key role in decreasing exposure of the developing brain to sedative-analgesic medications and prevention of delirium. Silo-based approaches to tackling each issue separately are rarely successful due to the intricate connectivity and dependence of each issue on another. Therefore a team-based approach to maintaining healthy sleep/wake patterns and facilitating EM must take into account the pediatric CICU's current practices surrounding sedation, analgesia, and delirium assessment/prevention, with a focus on potential nonpharmacologic interventions. Additionally, the perioperative nature of the management of the cardiac patient necessitates close collaboration with surgeons and anesthesiologists to optimize preoperative discussions and intraoperative care for streamlined transition to the CICU.

The first step in culture change to create a healing environment for children in the CICU is to engage collaborative, multidisciplinary teams to initiate the process.[209] All stakeholders in sedation, delirium assessment and prevention, sleep promotion, and early rehabilitation must be involved from the very beginning to ensure that all potential barriers to and facilitators of creating change have been considered during the evaluation process.[208] In the CICU these team members will likely include champions representing each of the disciplines listed in Box 21.1. Seeking input from *all* stakeholders increases

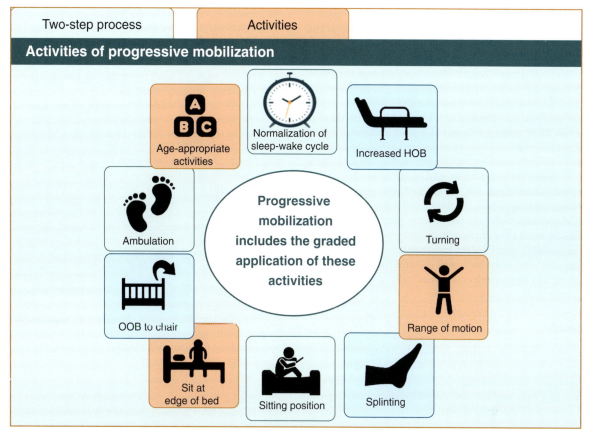

• **Figure 21.4** Activities of progressive mobilization. *HOB*, Head of bed; *OOB*, out of bed.

the chance of identifying a comprehensive list of local barriers and facilitators.[209]

Interventions to promote mobility and sleep hygiene range from simple, inexpensive, and noninvasive approaches (e.g., earplugs, eye masks) to complex and resource-intensive interventions (ambulating an intubated patient). Specifically for sleep promotion, a logical first step is to create unit-wide protocols for lighting optimization with exposure to sunlight during the day and noise reduction during nighttime hours. Nurses are the cornerstone of these protocols, given their presence at the bedside 24 hours a day. In fact, exposure to natural light and reducing noise has a positive impact on nursing work satisfaction, in addition to benefits for patients.[162] There are a variety of approaches to bedside sleep promotion interventions that are reviewed extensively in the pediatric and adult literature.[171,210,211] CICU architectural design is also an important consideration because private rooms with adjustable window shades and sliding doors can be beneficial for sleep promotion. However, although private room design may decrease exposure to outside noise, conversations at the bedside are still a common issue described by nursing staff.[162]

Although sleep promotion interventions are commonly perceived as low risk and feasible, EM often raises concerns from ICU staff due to fear of adverse events and heavy resource utilization. Indeed, despite growing evidence in adult ICUs, mobilization activities for critically ill adults are still uncommon internationally.[212,213] In the pediatric CICU, immediate attention is on resuscitation and stabilization in the postoperative period. Unfortunately, discussions about EM and acute rehabilitation are often deferred until the patient has reached a point of stability. In most ICUs a physician order is required for consultation of physical and occupational therapy (PT/OT), which can lead to significant delays in initial evaluation by rehabilitation experts. Even when PT/OT consultations are made, it is not uncommon for therapists to be sent away by PICU staff (nurses, physicians) due to a perception that the patient is "too sick" for mobility. Therefore education about the wide spectrum of EM activities (Fig. 21.4) is crucial for initial culture change to promote mobility.[160]

Pediatric PT and OT staff are well versed in the assessment and treatment of critically ill children and can provide an outstanding resource for educating staff on not only the range of EM activities but also techniques that can be performed at the bedside by nursing staff when therapy staff are not physically present. PTs and OTs with specific cardiac focus are exceptional educational resources in the CICU and benefit from continuity of care with their patients after CICU discharge to the floor and home settings. Therefore probably the single most effective intervention is implementation of uniform consultation of PT and OT within the first 48 hours of CICU admission. PTs and OTs work collaboratively—therefore consulting both services does not automatically translate to requirement of both services. The consult enables the rehabilitation team to make an assessment and determine the child's immediate and future needs. In the single-center experience at Johns Hopkins, creating a basic leveling criteria based on patient acuity for EM activities with "rest and reassess" guidelines provided a shared mental model for therapy staff and nursing when collaborating on a child's care.[160] Sleep hygiene, sedation assessment, and delirium screening were built into the criteria to ensure that all members of the multidisciplinary medical team incorporate these issues into their management plan.

Conclusion

CICU paradigms nationwide have begun the transition from a culture of deep sedation to one of mobility. With increased awareness as to the importance of optimal analgesia, minimal sedation, routine delirium screening, early mobility, and sleep hygiene, we can improve outcomes in pediatric cardiac patients.

Selected References

A complete list of references is available at ExpertConsult.com.

6. Colville G, Kerry S, Pierce C. Children's factual and delusional memories of intensive care. *Am J Respir Crit Care Med.* 2008;177(9):976–982.

11. Traube C, Silver G, Reeder RW, et al. Delirium in Critically Ill Children: An International Point Prevalence Study. *Crit Care Med.* 2017;45(4):584–590.

18. Smith HA, Gangopadhyay M, Goben CM, et al. The Preschool Confusion Assessment Method for the ICU: Valid and Reliable Delirium Monitoring for Critically Ill Infants and Children. *Crit Care Med.* 2016;44(3):592–600.

38. Smith HA, Boyd J, Fuchs DC, et al. Diagnosing delirium in critically ill children: Validity and reliability of the Pediatric Confusion Assessment Method for the Intensive Care Unit. *Crit Care Med.* 2011;39(1):150–157.

41. Curley MA, Wypij D, Watson RS, et al. Protocolized sedation vs usual care in pediatric patients mechanically ventilated for acute respiratory failure: a randomized clinical trial. *JAMA.* 2015;313(4):379–389.

115. Patel AK, Biagas KV, Clarke EC, et al. Delirium in Children After Cardiac Bypass Surgery. *Pediatr Crit Care Med.* 2017;18(2):165–171.

131. Traube C, Silver G, Kearney J, et al. Cornell Assessment of Pediatric Delirium: a valid, rapid, observational tool for screening delirium in the PICU. *Crit Care Med.* 2014;42(3):656–663.

135. Traube C, Silver G, Gerber L, et al. Delirium and Mortality in Critically Ill Children: Epidemiology and Outcomes of Pediatric Delirium. *Crit Care Med.* 2017.

145. Kudchadkar SR, Yaster M, Punjabi NM. Sedation, Sleep Promotion, and Delirium Screening Practices in the Care of Mechanically Ventilated Children: A Wake-Up Call for the Pediatric Critical Care Community. *Crit Care Med.* 2014;42(7):1592–1600.

160. Wieczorek B, Ascenzi J, Kim Y, et al. PICU Up!: Impact of a Quality Improvement Intervention to Promote Early Mobilization in Critically Ill Children. *Pediatr Crit Care Med.* 2016;17(12):e559–e566.

175. Hopkins RO, Choong K, Zebuhr CA, Kudchadkar SR. Transforming PICU Culture to Facilitate Early Rehabilitation. *J Pediatr Intensive Care.* 2015;4(4):204–211.

22

Monitoring Systems

NANCY S. GHANAYEM, MD; MUBBASHEER AHMED, MD; MARC M. ANDERS, MD;
SEBASTIAN C. TUME, MD; ERIC L. VU, MD; GEORGE M. HOFFMAN, MD

Critically ill patients are vulnerable to organ injury and circulatory failure due to cellular hypoxia. Monitoring for perturbations in circulatory well-being, early recognition of tissue hypoxia, and prevention of organ injury via preservation of adequate oxygen delivery are at the core of critical care medicine. Oxygen must make the journey from the atmosphere to the intracellular environment to take part in the oxidative energy generation process. To sustain cellular obligatory and facultative functions, cells must consume adenosine triphosphate (ATP) generated from oxygen. If oxygen delivery (DO_2) is limited, loss of facultative function occurs first and is then followed by loss of obligatory functions. Thus insufficient oxygen delivery creates a hypoxic tissue environment culminating in organ malfunction and followed by eventual organ death.

This chapter provides a broad overview of the noninvasive and invasive monitoring modalities and biochemical markers commonly employed to assess the circulatory status and organ function in critically ill infants and children with acquired and congenital heart disease. Although each system is described in isolation, simultaneous use of multiple modalities in critical illness is necessary to quantify adequacy of oxygen delivery and to guide management during physiologic volatility. In fact, technologic innovation is dependent upon synchronized, concurrent integration of multiple systems and the electronic medical record for the development of advanced monitoring systems, real-time analytics, and risk-prediction.

Noninvasive Monitoring

Electrocardiographic Monitoring

The electrocardiogram (ECG) is the graphic representation of the electrical activity of the heart, a necessary but insufficient component of myocardial function.

Since the introduction of continuous ECG monitoring more than 60 years ago,[1] the goals of ECG monitoring in the cardiac intensive care unit (ICU) have expanded beyond simple heart rate and basic rhythm determination and currently encompass detection of complex arrhythmias, myocardial ischemia, conduction defects, and electrolyte abnormalities. Recent advances in rhythm monitoring systems expand beyond computerized arrhythmia analysis into advanced ST-segment ischemia analysis[2,3] and predictive modeling.[4] ECG algorithms are often limited by false alarms due to the need for high sensitivity at the expense of specificity. Hence human interpretation and oversight of ECG systems are still necessary.

With these challenges in mind, it is essential that providers have a complete understanding of ECG monitoring systems, including their benefits and pitfalls.

The ECG is recorded by placing an array of monitoring electrodes in specific locations on the body surface to capture various axes of electrical vectors. The most commonly recognized ECG setup consists of a 12-lead system. Standard 12-lead ECG requires placement of electrodes on both the limbs and precordial position. Because this is difficult to achieve in a patient following cardiac surgery, simplified configurations are often used. They allow for limb lead placement on the torso to reduce muscle artifacts during limb movement and avoid lead cable tethering.

The basic ECG monitoring setup involves a three-electrode lead monitoring system (Fig. 22.1A). The potential difference between two electrodes is recorded and allows for monitoring of three leads (leads I, II, and III). The three leads record positive P and T waves as well as major portions of QRS complex. Bipolar lead monitoring provides a single-lead display and is often used for portable monitor-defibrillators because the system allows for evaluation of the heart rate and time relation between different waves of the cardiac cycle, detection of R waves for synchronized cardioversion, and detection of ventricular fibrillation. This type of monitoring is inadequate for the sophisticated arrhythmia and ST-segment monitoring required in the cardiac ICU because it lacks the anterior lead necessary to delineate arrhythmia origin.

The five-electrode lead system remains the most commonly used setup in the ICU and enables seven-lead monitoring (see Fig. 22.1B). The leads from the extremities act as common ground (negative electrode) for the precordial unipolar lead (positive electrode), enabling display of leads I, II, III, aVR, aVL, aVF, and a single precordial lead (V_1 to V_6). The advantages of seven-lead monitoring are the ability to detect ischemic events utilizing ST-segment trending and to define the mechanism of arrhythmias as well as supraventricular tachycardia (SVT). It should be noted that although the V_1 lead location is excellent for diagnosis of wide QRS complex arrhythmias (bundle branch block, wide QRS tachycardia, and pacemaker rhythms), it is poorly sensitive in detection of myocardial ischemia. Leads III and V_5 appear to be the most sensitive pair for recognition of myocardial ischemia in the postoperative setting.[5,6] More advanced 12-lead ECG systems are less frequently used in children compared with adults due to body surface limitation. If advanced arrhythmia or ischemia workup is required, the standard portable 12-lead ECG system should be employed.

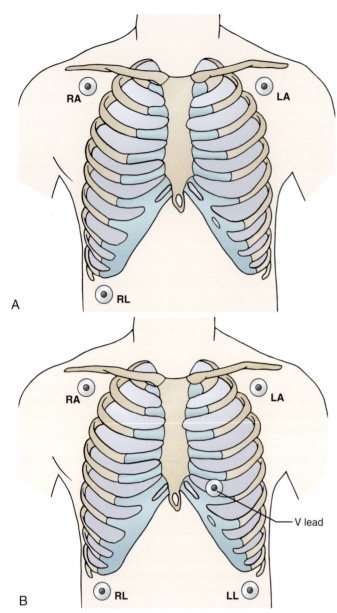

• **Figure 22.1** (A) Three-lead electrode placement. (B) Five-lead electrode placement.

All patients admitted to the ICU should be continuously monitored using a central telemetry system that records and stores ECG information, allowing for retrospective analysis. The standard for ECG recording is a 1-mV deflection equaling 10 mm on the strip chart recorder and with the paper speed set to 25 mm/s.

Arrhythmias are commonly encountered in the cardiac critical care unit with prevalence reported at 15% to 29%.[7,8] The incidence of arrhythmias in the postoperative period for cardiac congenital repairs can be as high as 48%.[7,9] Because postoperative arrhythmias are associated with significant morbidity and higher mortality,[10,11] prompt diagnosis and appropriate management are crucial. Postoperative arrhythmias occur due to a variety of factors such as mechanical irritation of the conduction system, postoperative metabolic derangements, electrolyte disturbances, increased adrenergic tone from surgical stress, and use of inotropic medications. Surgical repairs involving ventriculotomies and coronary reimplantations predispose these children to transient ventricular dysrhythmias. Ventricular arrhythmias that occur in the setting of myocardial

ischemia are associated with mortality as high as 61%.[12] More common postoperative arrhythmias in children include junctional ectopic tachycardia (JET), SVT, and atrioventricular (AV) block,[9,11] which might be difficult to diagnose using surface ECG.

Transcutaneous epicardial atrial leads (Fig. 22.2), which record electrical activity directly from the atria and allow for pacing of atria and/or ventricles, can aid in diagnosis and management of complex rhythm and conduction disorders following open-heart surgery.[13,14] P waves on the surface ECG may be buried in the QRS complex or T wave, complicating diagnosis of supraventricular arrhythmias such as JET. Atrial ECGs provide the ability to clearly identify atrial activity and localize P waves.

Myocardial ischemia in children in the postoperative setting can be the result of intraoperative hypoxia or mechanical stress of the coronary arteries due to prolonged cardiac surgery.[15] Other described causes include acute myocarditis,[16] postoperative pericarditis, acute graft rejection, transplant-related coronary artery disease,[17] and cardiotoxicity from pharmacologic therapies and chest trauma. The ability to detect these complications via advanced ST-segment monitoring is uncertain. The ST amplitude is normally measured at a fixed interval of approximately 60 milliseconds after the J point. The steep slope of these ST segments cause ST amplitude to vary with heart rate triggering ST segment, resulting in frequent false ST alarms. For example, the presence of bundle branch block results in ST-T waves that markedly deviate in a positive or negative direction depending on the lead being monitored. Any questionable ECG changes especially those complemented by change in clinical status should always be evaluated with 12 lead ECG and additional diagnostic workup.

Software used for ST segment monitoring has undergone modifications to include trend analysis and noise reduction. This allows for improved ECG signal processing and measurement of ST-segment changes; however, little information is available regarding optimal lead systems for ischemia detection in children. When compared with Holter monitoring for ischemia in adults, the sensitivity and specificity of ST-trend monitors are described at 74% and 73%, respectively.[2] The normal ST segment in a child is isoelectric with baseline elevations of the ST segment ±1 mm in the limb leads and up to ±2 mm in the precordial leads, but ST-segment elevations greater than 2 mm might be valuable in making the diagnosis of ischemia in children.[12]

Pulse Oximetry

Pulse oximetry is a noninvasive spectroscopic technique that estimates arterial oxygen saturation. Since 1986 the American Society of Anesthesiologists has included in its "Standards for Basic Anesthetic Monitoring" that "during all anesthetics, a quantitative method of assessing oxygenation such as pulse oximetry shall be employed."[18] The American Academy of Pediatrics mandates the use of pulse oximetry for sedation in children.[19] The widespread adoption of pulse oximetry as a safety monitor is intuitive, but evidence for such efficacy is surprisingly lacking. The widespread adoption of pulse oximetry to evaluate and monitor sick children has virtually eliminated unrecognized arterial hypoxia as a cause for patient harm, and it allows continuous assessment of right-to-left shunting in children with congenital heart disease.

Most modern pulse oximeters merge two physical principles: spectrophotometry and optical plethysmography. The spectrophotometry component of pulse oximetry operates on the theory that oxygenated hemoglobin (O_2Hb) and deoxygenated hemoglobin (HHb) show different absorption in red (660 nm) and infrared

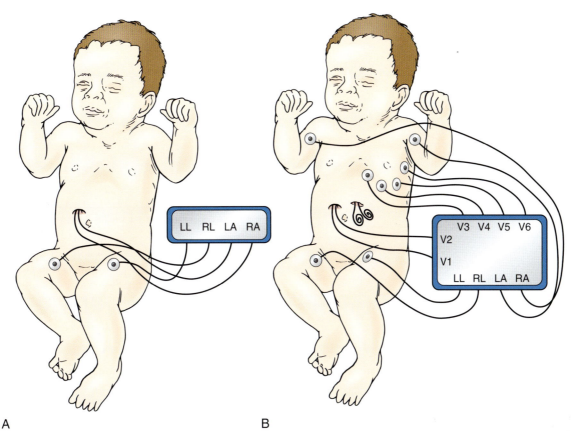

A

B

• **Figure 22.2** Lead placement for atrial electrocardiogram. (A) Method for recording a bipolar atrial electrocardiogram using temporary pacing wires by connecting the atrial leads to the right arm *(RA)* and left arm *(LA)* leads. The atrial impulse will be very prominent in lead aVF and observable in other leads but less prominent. (B) Method for recording a unipolar atrial electrocardiogram from temporary pacing wires. This setup requires attachment of all limb leads and precordial leads V_3 to V_5. The atrial wires are connected to V_1 and V_2, giving two unipolar atrial electrocardiograms with large-amplitude ventricular electrograms displayed in leads V_1 and V_2.

light (940 nm). O_2Hb absorbs more infrared light, whereas HHb absorbs more red light. The Beer-Lambert Law (Eqs. 22.1a and 22.1b) defines the attenuation of light through the material traveled:

$$T = I/I_O \qquad \text{Eq. 22.1a}$$

$$A = -\log(T) = -\log(I/I_0) = \varepsilon * b * c \qquad \text{Eq. 22.1b}$$

where T is transmittance, A is the measured absorbance, I_0 is the initial light intensity, I is the light intensity after it passes through a sample, ε is the molar absorptivity wavelength dependent, b is the path length, and c is the concentration of the analyte.

During the cardiac cycle the proportion of the light that strikes fat, connective tissue, skin, bone, and venous blood remains relatively constant (direct current). During systole a small increase in arterial blood volume increases light absorption (alternating current). Hence the total absorption (A_{total}) is time dependent (dt) during the cardiac cycle (Eq. 22.2) with more absorption during arterial dilation ($A_{arterial}$)—systole—and less during arterial constriction (A_{venous})—diastole (Fig. 22.3).

$$d(A_{total})/dt = d(A_{arterial})/dt + d(A_{venous})/dt$$
$$= d(\varepsilon_{arterial} * b_{arterial} * c_{arterial})/dt + d(\varepsilon_{venous} * b_{venous} * c_{venous})/dt$$

Eq. 22.2

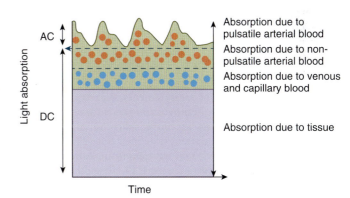

• **Figure 22.3** Light absorption through living tissue. Note that the AC signal is due to the pulsatile component of arterial blood, whereas the DC signal is composed of all the nonpulsatile absorbers in the tissue: nonpulsatile arterial blood, venous and capillary blood, and all other tissues. (From *Ohmeda Pulse Oximeter Model 3700 Service Manual.* Ohmeda, Boulder 1986.)[20]

Under the assumption that arterial pulsation is much more than venous pulsation during the cardiac cycle (b_{venous} is constant), the total absorption over time is almost exclusively dependent on the arterial absorption.

$$d(A_{total})/dt = d(A_{arterial})/dt = \Delta A_{total} = \Delta A_{arterial} \qquad \text{Eq. 22.3}$$

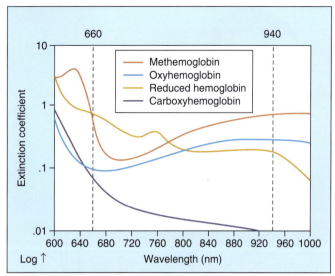

• **Figure 22.4** Hemoglobin extinction curves. Transmitted light absorption spectra of four hemoglobin species: oxyhemoglobin, reduced hemoglobin, carboxyhemoglobin, and methemoglobin. (From Tremper KK, Barker SJ. Pulse oximetry. *Anesthesiology.* 1989;70[1]:98-108.)

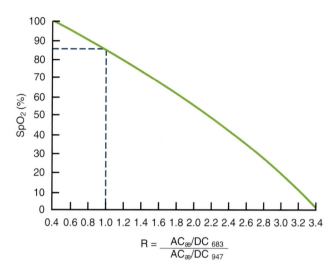

$$R = \frac{AC_{\text{æ}}/DC_{683}}{AC_{\text{æ}}/DC_{947}}$$

• **Figure 22.5** Pulse oximeter calibration curve. Pulseoximetric arterial oxygen saturation (SpO$_2$) estimate is determined by the ratio (R) of the pulse-added red absorbance at 660 nm to pulse-added red absorbance at 940 nm. (Data from Tremper KK, Barker SJ. Pulse oximetry. *Anesthesiology.* 1989;70[1]:98-108.)

By comparing the peak absorption during arterial pulsation (alternating current) to a baseline, through absorption (direct current), only the arterial pulsation remains relevant (Eq. 22.4)[20]:

$$A = AC/DC \qquad \textbf{Eq. 22.4}$$

where AC is alternating current and DC is direct current.

The combination of the ratios of absorbances at two distinct wavelengths (660 nm and 940 nm) with distinct absorbance characteristics for O$_2$Hb and HHb (Fig. 22.4) leads to a ratio of ratios (Eq. 22.5):

$$R = A_{660nm}/A_{940nm} = (AC_{660nm}/DC_{660nm})/(AC_{940nm}/DC_{940nm})$$

$$\textbf{Eq. 22.5}$$

where R is the ratio of ratios, A_{660nm} / A_{940nm} absorbance at 660 nm / 940 nm, AC_{660nm} / AC_{940nm} is the alternating current at 660 nm and 940 nm, and DC_{660nm} / DC_{940nm} is the direct current at 660 nm / 940 nm.

Averaged over a series of measurements, R is expressed on a calibration curve based on healthy volunteers with alterations of their saturations from 70% to 100%, where an almost linear relationship from R to saturations is defined (Fig. 22.5).[20]

The pulse oximeter with two wavelength measurements can distinguish a maximum of two substances: O$_2$Hb and HHb. Hence pulse oximeter measurements are referred as *functional saturations,* defined as the ratio of O$_2$Hb compared to total hemoglobin (Eq. 22.6):

$$\text{Functional SpO}_2 = O_2Hb/(O_2Hb + HHb) \qquad \textbf{Eq. 22.6}$$

Pulse oximeters are empirically calibrated on normal, healthy volunteers during desaturation studies. The Food and Drug Administration and US Department of Health and Human Services mandates an accuracy between oxygen saturation as measured by pulse oximetry (SpO$_2$) and measured arterial oxygenation by A$_{rms}$ ≤ 3.5% under normal conditions with SpO$_2$ ranging from 70% to 100%. A$_{rms}$ is defined as the root mean square, which reports accuracy as a function of bias and precision. All modern pulse oximeters meet those requirements under normal conditions;

however, there are significant limitations in bias and precision of pulse oximeter readings in various settings (Table 22.1).

The application of the pulse oximeter reaches far beyond its initial application for measurement of functional saturation and heart rate. During systole AC increases and more light is absorbed, whereas in diastole only DC contributes to the light absorption. The alteration of AC and DC during the cardiac cycle is a mirror image of an arterial blood pressure waveform, which is often displayed as a plethysmographic waveform. Further parameters can be derived as displayed in Table 22.2.

Pulse oximetry is one of the standard tools for patient monitoring during anesthesia, the critical care setting, and even the acute care setting. Aside from the original application of the pulse oximeter for noninvasive arterial saturation and heart rate monitoring, recent improvements enable the use of the pulse oximeter in more challenging situations with low perfusion or hypoxemia, and analysis of the plethysmographic waveform may lead to more clinical information in the future.

Near-Infrared Spectroscopy

Optimal oxygen delivery to tissue beds occurs through not only global, but regional circulatory mechanisms. Regional perfusion is determined by perfusion pressure and regional vascular resistance, affected by local, humoral, and neural mechanisms that have complex inputs. Near-infrared spectroscopy (NIRS) provides a continuous, noninvasive estimate of regional tissue oxygen saturation that is highly venous weighted and thus can be conceptualized as an estimate of regional venous oxygen saturation, indicating changes in regional oxygen economy that occur both in normal circulatory adaptations and in more serious circulatory disturbances, including developing shock states. NIRS assists in the characterization of regional and global circulatory function directly and by facilitation of continuous, noninvasive application of the Fick principle.[21]

NIRS utilizes a modified Beer-Lambert principle to provide a continuous noninvasive assessment of tissue oxygenation through quantitative assessment of the color of hemoglobin in blood in the optical field beneath the probe. Because approximately two-thirds

TABLE 22.1	Limitations in Bias and Precision of Pulse Oximeter Readings
Hypoxia and congenital heart disease	Pulsoximetric measured saturations below 70% show an increased bias and decreased precision. Multiple studies confirmed that the assessment of hypoxic states is unreliable and should be reconfirmed by cooximetric assessment.[176-180]
Hyperoxia	Hyperoxia (cooximetric measured saturations >100 mm Hg or >150 mm Hg) may lead to increased mortality in critical care patients. SpO_2 measurements are not reliable to detect hyperoxic states.[181-183]
Increased carboxyhemoglobin (COHb)	Significant COHb poisoning increases false high readings of SpO_2; recent advances in pulse oximeters use multiple wavelengths to quantify COHb and MetHb.[184]
Increased methemoglobin (MetHb)	MetHb absorbs light at almost similar wavelengths (660 nm/940 nm) as conventional pulse oximeter readings; hence in the presence of MetHb, SpO_2 readings are commonly between 82% and 86%; recent advances in pulse oximeters use multiple wavelengths to quantify COHb and MetHb.[184]
Hemoglobinopathies[a]	Hemoglobin Sydney and hemoglobin Southampton lead to falsely low SpO_2.[185]
Body temperature	Increased body temperature causes more venous pulsation, which results in lower SpO_2 readings.
Cardiac arrhythmia	See reference 176.
Poor perfusion	See reference 186.
Excessive ambient light	See reference 187.
Motion artifacts	See reference 187.
Probe miscalibration	
Probe misplacement	
Nail polish	Although traditional pulse oximeters may have been susceptible to nail polish decreasing SpO_2 reliability, newer models yield almost no difference in healthy volunteers.

[a]The absorbance of red and infrared light by fetal hemoglobin (HbF) is essentially the same as adult hemoglobin (HbA), and thus SpO_2 measurement is as reliable in newborns as in adults.

SpO_2, Oxygen saturation as measured by pulse oximetry.

TABLE 22.2	Derivation of Select Circulatory Indices With Pulse Oximetry	
Perfusion Index (PI)	PI = AC/DC * 100%	PI reflects the peripheral vasomotor tone. Low PI suggests peripheral vasoconstriction (or severe hypovolemia), and high PI suggests vasodilation.[188]
Pleth Variability Index (PVI)	PVI = (PImax − PImin) / PImax * 100%	PVI quantifies the variability due to respiration and is thought to be a surrogate measure of intravascular volume.[189-191]

of the total blood volume resides in the venous circulation, the optical field coverage is predominantly a venous-weighted tissue hemoglobin-oxygen saturation (rSO$_2$) and thus provides an estimation of the regional oxygen supply-demand relationship. Continuous, real-time changes in rSO$_2$ reflect changes either in metabolic demand or supply: as an approximation of regional venous oxygen saturation (SvO$_2$), rSO$_2$ = SaO$_2$ − VO$_2$/DO$_2$ (where SaO$_2$ is arterial oxygen saturation and VO$_2$ is oxygen consumption) and is thus a function of systemic cardiac output (CO), arterial oxygen content, and total or regional resistance. Clinical studies have initially focused on cerebral NIRS and have validated cerebral rSO$_2$ with jugular bulb venous saturation (SjvO$_2$) measurements.[22-25] The strongest correlation between rSO$_2$ and SjvO$_2$ has been observed in infants less than 10 kg (r = 0.83).[25]

Several studies have reported the relationship between cerebral rSO$_2$, somatic rSO$_2$, and venous saturation from the superior vena cava (SvO$_2$).[26-31] Because the mixed venous saturation is the flow-weighted average of regional venous saturations, attempts to show a univariate correlation between single-site rSO$_2$ and a mixed venous measure should be viewed as oversimplified. A global, quasi-mixed SvO$_2$ can be reasonably approximated by NIRS models that include multiple sites (Fig. 22.6).[32]

The relationship between rSO$_2$ and organ injury has been established in animal models of cerebral injury. Cerebral hypoxia below a normothermic rSO$_2$ threshold of 45% has been associated with progressively increased lactate production, intracellular anaerobic metabolism, depletion of ATP, and electroencephalographic slowing and silence.[33] Specific "thresholds" for cerebral injury in adults have been established in prospective observational studies of adults undergoing cardiac surgery. Absolute cerebral rSO$_2$ less than 50% or a 20% decline from baseline is associated with a higher likelihood of cognitive decline, frontal lobe injury, increased incidence of stroke, electroencephalographic silence, prolonged mechanical ventilation, and prolonged hospitalization.[34-37] In a randomized, prospective study of adults having coronary artery bypass grafting, prolonged cerebral desaturation was associated with greater incidence of organ dysfunction.[36] A higher likelihood of adverse neurologic outcomes has been associated with lower intraoperative cerebral rSO$_2$ saturation in children.[38]

Application of NIRS technology relies on knowledge of normal rSO$_2$ values in healthy patients as well as knowledge of baseline versus abnormal values in patients with vulnerable physiology. Healthy children and those with acyanotic heart disease have baseline cerebral rSO$_2$ values similar to adults with an arterial saturation (SaO$_2$) and cerebral rSO$_2$ difference of approximately 30%.[39] Resting and postprandial cerebral and somatic rSO$_2$ values in healthy neonates demonstrated cerebral rSO$_2$ of 78% with a somatic rSO$_2$ of 88%, consistent with higher oxygen extraction across the cerebral bed. In sick patients with cyanotic heart disease before surgical palliation, cerebral rSO$_2$ values were 46% to 57% with a wider

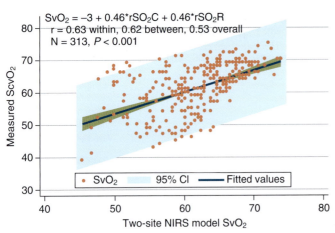

• **Figure 22.6** Estimation of SvO_2 from cerebral and somatic NIRS in 10 patients with hypoplastic left heart syndrome after stage I palliation, with an average of 31 measures per patient in the first 48 postoperative hours. $ScvO_2$ was measured by an oximetric catheter (Abbott Oxycath) in the superior vena cava. Cerebral and somatic rSO_2 were measured by Somanetics Invos 4100A with probes in the midline frontal and right T12 through L2 flank region. The best linear model was fit as $SvO_2 = -3 + 0.46*rSO_2C + 0.46*rSO_2R$. This can be transformed as $SvO_2 = 0.92*$ (average of cerebral and somatic rSO_2) -3. *CI*, Confidence interval; *NIRS*, near-infrared spectroscopy; *rSO₂*, regional oxygen saturation; *rSO₂C*, cerebral oxygen saturation; *rSO₂R*, renal oxygen saturation; *ScvO₂*, central venous saturation; *SvO₂*, venous oxygen saturation. (Modified from Hoffman GM, Ghanayem NS, Tweddell JS. Noninvasive assessment of cardiac output. *Semin Thorac Cardiovasc Surg Pediatr Card Surg Annu.* 2005:12-21.)

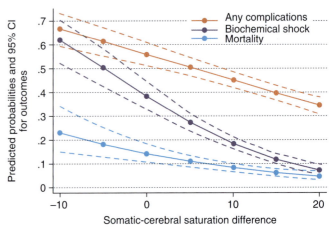

• **Figure 22.7** Predicted probability of complications, biochemical shock, and mortality in 79 neonates with hypoplastic left heart syndrome. A somatic-cerebral rSO_2 difference of less than 10 during the first 48 postoperative hours after stage I palliation is associated with an increased risk of biochemical shock and postoperative complications. A somatic-cerebral rSO_2 difference of zero or less is associated with an increased risk of mortality. *CI*, Confidence interval; *RR*, relative risk; *rSO₂*, regional oxygen saturation. (From Ghanayem NS, Hoffman GM. Near infrared spectroscopy as a hemodynamic monitor in critical illness. *Pediatr Crit Care Med.* 2016;17[8 Suppl 1]:S201-S206.)

SaO_2-rSO_2 difference.[39] Pediatric patients with clinical evidence of left-to-right shunts with or without cyanosis had lower baseline cerebral rSO_2 compared with those without left-to-right shunts regardless of arterial saturation.[40]

Prospective observational studies of infants and children with congenital heart disease requiring surgery have evaluated the relationship of multisite NIRS and SvO_2 or indicators of anaerobic metabolism.[21,28,29,32,41,42] Dorsal lateral flank and anterior abdominal rSO_2 exhibited strong correlation with SvO_2 and/or lactate within 48 hours of surgery.[27,41] Actual cerebral and somatic rSO_2 are loosely related with SvO_2 but are more closely related when considering both cerebral and somatic rSO_2 in a linear relationship. Cerebral and somatic rSO_2 differences of less than 10% predicted anaerobic metabolism.[42] In a series of patients who underwent Norwood palliation for hypoplastic left heart syndrome (HLHS), somatic rSO_2 less than 60% and progressive somatic ischemia indicated by a cerebral-somatic rSO_2 difference approaching zero, predicted biochemical shock, an increased number of complications, and a longer ICU length of stay (Fig. 22.7).[21] A larger series of 329 patients with comprehensive postoperative monitoring identified that two-site rSO_2 can predict mortality and need for postoperative extracorporeal membrane oxygenation (ECMO) use after Norwood palliation. Furthermore, a bivariate analysis of mean arterial blood pressure and somatic rSO_2 allowed identification of low CO and mortality risk (Fig. 22.8).[43]

Prolonged cerebral desaturation in the perioperative period has been shown to be associated with early childhood developmental delay.[44-46] Cerebral rSO_2 desaturation within the first 48-hour postoperative period following Norwood palliation was more predictive of low neurodevelopmental performance in children at preschool age.[44] A prospective observational assessment of infants

with congenital heart disease following cardiac surgery correlated new or worsened postoperative magnetic resonance imaging (MRI) lesions with prolonged cerebral rSO_2 declines (rSO_2 <45% for more than 180 minutes).[47] Lower psychomotor development index (Bayley scale) scores have been found to be associated with lower rSO_2 60 minutes following separation from cardiopulmonary bypass (CPB) following biventricular repair without arch obstruction in infancy.[48]

Finally, NIRS can be used to trend conditions noninvasively in less acute environments or before invasive or laboratory measures can be obtained.[49,50] Specifically, in infants with single-ventricle disease and parallel circulation, optimization of the pulmonary-to-systemic flow ratio can be critical to avoiding end-organ injury. Consequently, changes in pulmonary and systemic flows can be approximated by trending systemic and pulmonary arteriovenous differences with SvO_2 or noninvasively with NIRS.[51,52] More generally, the combination of arterial and two-site NIRS (venous) oximetry can provide a continuous real-time noninvasive "virtual cardiac catheterization" by exploiting the Fick principle.

Temperature

Heat loss occurs through radiation, conduction, convection, and evaporation. Radiation and convection contribute to most of the heat loss in the critical care setting. Hypothermia can result from a combination of anesthetic-impaired thermoregulation and exposure to a cold operating room environment. Thermoregulatory vasoconstriction is comparably impaired in infants and children exposed to anesthetic gases[53,54] and can be further affected by factors like sedation, pain, and vasoactive agents. Cutaneous vasoconstriction is the most important mechanism used by the body to reduce heat loss. Thus body heat is distributed with the peripheral temperature 2°C to 4°C cooler than the core. Sustained shivering, another compensatory mechanism, has been shown to increase heat production by 50% to 100% in adults. Newborn infants lack this

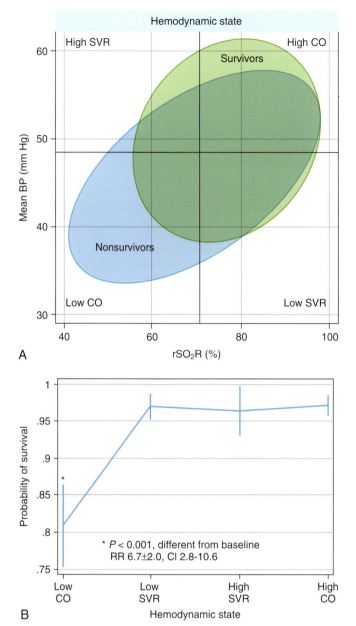

A

B

• **Figure 22.8** (A) Bivariate plot of mean arterial pressure *(BP)* versus somatic regional oxygen saturation *(rSO₂R)* with cut points dividing regions of high cardiac output *(CO)*, high systemic vascular resistance *(SVR)*, low SVR, and low CO. Ellipses show the 95% confidence interval of measures for survivo**r**s *(green)* and nonsurvivors *(blue)*. Nonsurvivors were overrepresented in the low cardiac output region. (B) Predicted survival by bivariate circulatory characterization over the first 6 hours. (From Hoffman GM, Ghanayem NS, Scott JP, et al. Postoperative cerebral and somatic near-infrared spectroscopy saturations and outcome in hypoplastic left heart syndrome. *Ann Thorac Surg.* 2017;103[5]:1527-1535.)

mechanism, which does not become fully effective until several years of age.[55] However, nonshivering thermogenesis in neonates and infants can increase oxygen consumption by 300% through activation of futile cycling in brown adipose tissue, and maintenance of a neutral thermal environment by monitoring both skin and core temperature is critical.

Thermoregulatory vasodilation and rapid rewarming following hypothermic circulatory arrest can lead to core-to-peripheral redistribution of body heat with resultant redistribution of

circulating intravascular volume and hemodynamic compromise.[56] Although core to peripheral temperature difference has been shown to be a poor marker of hemodynamic status in children,[57,58] careful monitoring of temperature changes may be of help in predicting hemodynamic alterations. Skin surface temperatures are considerably lower than core temperatures and should not be used alone in the operative or critical care setting.[59]

Temperatures are not uniform within the body compartments. Thus the location and value of temperature measurements have different physiologic significance. The core compartment is composed of highly perfused tissues whose temperature is uniform and higher compared with the peripheral compartment. Common core sites used for monitoring in the operating room include tympanic membrane, nasopharynx, esophagus, rectal, or pulmonary artery (PA) catheter.[60] In the event of CPB or ECMO, the temperature is monitored and regulated using the heat exchanger on the arterial line of the circuit.

Various adult studies have shown that even mild hypothermia increases incidence of myocardial damage, surgical wound infections, bleeding, and need for blood transfusions and prolongs postoperative recovery and hospitalization.[61-65] Pediatric data are lacking; however, a clear understanding of the thermoregulation mechanisms and careful temperature monitoring and control may help prevent temperature-related complications in the perioperative period. Therapeutic induction of mild to moderate hypothermia to reduce oxygen demand, control dysrhythmia, and ameliorate hypoxic-ischemic insult requires not only continuous temperature monitoring of core and gradient temperatures but also a thorough understanding of the concepts discussed earlier.

Invasive Monitoring

The heart and vasculature are coupled to provide efficient distribution of substrate to sustain organs. Hemodynamic monitoring allows measurement of the functional characteristics of the cardiac and circulatory systems in an effort to understand factors impacting tissue oxygen delivery.[66] Cardiac output (CO) measurement has been an integral component of advanced hemodynamic monitoring and diagnostics. Accurate measurement of CO, however, continues to present a challenge, and although its relationship to outcome is intuitive, evidence for this relationship is weak. Clinical parameters such as the comprehensive physical examination, pulse amplitude, capillary refill, blood pressure, and urine output are routinely used to provide a qualitative assessment of "cardiac output," but these assessments show low concordance with true CO measurements.[67]

The Fick method is most frequently used for measurement of either pulmonary or systemic blood flow and hence CO. According to the Fick principle, CO is equal to oxygen consumption divided by the arterial-venous oxygen content difference:

$$VO_2 = CO \times CaO_2 - CvO_2 \text{ and } CO = VO_2/CaO_2 - CvO_2$$

Eq. 22.7 (Fick equation)

where VO_2 is oxygen consumption, CaO_2 is arterial oxygen content, and CvO_2 is venous oxygen content.

The Fick principle can further be used to determine the ratio of systemic and pulmonary flow in parallel circuits. For assessment of pulmonary blood flow (Q_p), the rate of oxygen uptake by the red blood cells in the pulmonary bed is divided by the difference between the pulmonary venous and pulmonary arterial oxygen content. Systemic blood flow (Q_s) is calculated using systemic oxygen consumption divided by the difference between the arterial and mixed venous oxygen content. It is important to note that true mixed venous oxygen content should be sampled from the PA to represent global tissue oxygen utilization. Understanding this relationship enables one to determine the degree of intracardiac shunt Q_p/Q_s:

$$Q_p/Q_s = SaO_2(Ao) - SaO_2(PA)/SaO_2(PV) - SaO_2(PA)$$

Eq. 22.8

Limitations of the Fick method include a high risk of cumulative errors of measurements. Measurement of VO_2 is frequently extracted from nomogram charts that provide derived VO_2 from healthy subjects. Directly measured VO_2 through indirect calorimetry requires certain obligatory conditions to be met such as the use of low fraction of inspired oxygen (FiO_2). Finally, it is important to understand that the Fick method measures CO at one point in time and thus is not able to represent CO variability.

Pulmonary Artery Catheter Thermodilution Method

The thermodilution method using the PA catheter has been one of the most commonly used tools to measure CO and is considered the gold standard. The introduction of the PA catheter in 1970 revolutionized the clinical management of critically ill patients.[68] The early PA catheters allowed for assessment of hemodynamic conditions through direct monitoring of pressures in the right atrium, right ventricle (RV), and PA, as well as assessment of left heart pressures using the pulmonary wedge technique (Fig. 22.9).[174] Since then these catheters underwent significant technological advancements incorporating thermodilution, continuous assessment of CO and mixed venous saturations (MvO_2), and pacing capabilities.

Thermal energy can be used as an indicator in the form of cold saline or dextrose. The PA catheter contains a proximal injection port located in the right atrium and a thermistor at the distal end of the catheter positioned in the PA. During a thermodilution measurement a specified volume of cold or room temperature injectate is introduced into the circulation at the proximal port, and the resultant change downstream in the PA temperature is recorded by the thermistor at the catheter tip, producing a thermodilution curve (Fig. 22.10). A modified Stewart-Hamilton

equation is then used to calculate the CO, incorporating difference between the blood and indicator temperature, the specific gravity and volume of the solution injected, and the area under the thermodilution curve.

$$CO = \frac{(T_b - T_i) \times V_i \times K}{\Delta T_b \times dt}$$

Eq. 22.9

where T_b is blood temperature, T_i is injectate temperature, V_i is volume of the injectate, K is computational constant, $\int \Delta T_b(t)dt$ is change in temperature as a function of time.

PA catheter use in children is limited by size because its insertion is difficult in patients weighing less than 10 kg.[69] Also, potential sources of error should be considered, especially in structural heart disease. Left-to-right shunt causes recirculation of the injectate, resulting in underestimated measured CO. Right-to-left shunt allows for injectate to bypass the thermistor, resulting in overestimation of CO. Tricuspid or pulmonic valve regurgitation leads to prolonged decay time and unreliable measurement that depends on severity of regurgitation and typically underestimates CO.[70]

The use of PA catheters remains controversial because numerous adult studies show increased hospitalization costs, longer length of stay, and lack of positive effect on mortality.[71-73] A combination of risk factors associated with use of the catheter (PA rupture, pulmonary embolism, or arrhythmia), use of potentially harmful therapies based on incorrect interpretation of data, and poor patient selection are thought to be contributors to high morbidity associated with the device.[71]

Transpulmonary Thermodilution and Pulse Contour Analysis

Transpulmonary thermodilution (TPTD) is gaining popularity in the pediatric population due to its limited invasive nature. A TPTD measurement involves an ice-cold saline injectate that is introduced using any central venous line. The change in temperature is measured distally via an arterial line catheter equipped with a thermistor. Like PA thermodilution, a modified Stewart-Hamilton equation is used to calculate flow. The accuracy of this technique depends on the assumption that the injectate is introduced at a constant blood flow, distributed throughout the central circulation with minimal loss of the injectate, completely mixed with blood, and has a single pass through the circulation as it travels from the venous to the arterial system.[74] Due to the longer travel distance

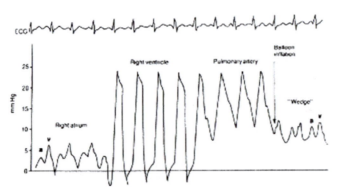

• **Figure 22.9** Pressure waveform tracing with advancement of pulmonary artery catheter from right atrium to pulmonary capillary occlusion. The terminal tracing represents pressures transmitted from the left atrium. (From Matthay MA. Invasive hemodynamic monitoring in critically ill patients. *Clin Chest Med.* 1983;4[2]:233-249).

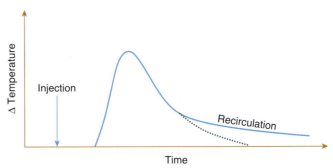

• **Figure 22.10** Thermodilution response curve. During a measurement a specified volume of cold or room temperature injectate is introduced into the circulation at the proximal port, and the resultant change downstream in the pulmonary artery temperature is recorded by the thermistor at the catheter tip, producing a thermodilution curve.

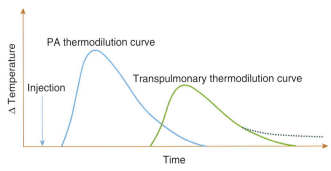

• **Figure 22.11** Comparison of pulmonary artery *(PA)* catheter thermodilution and transpulmonary thermodilution temperature curves. Note the delayed response and lower amplitude of the transpulmonary thermodilution curve.

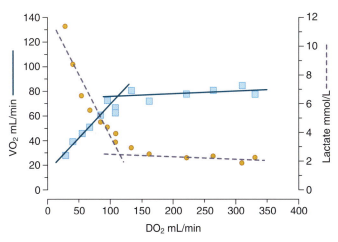

• **Figure 22.12** Relationship between oxygen consumption *(VO₂)*, oxygen delivery *(DO₂)*, and anaerobic metabolism when DO₂ is acutely reduced by tamponade or hemorrhage in anesthetized animals (data pooled from several studies). (From Vincent JL, De Backer D: Oxygen transport—the oxygen delivery controversy. *Intensive Care Med.* 2004; 30[11]: 1990-1996.)

of the indicator, the temperature-time curves obtained during TPTD measurements are broader and lower in magnitude, making them more prone to errors caused by baseline drift and indicator microcirculation (Fig. 22.11).

As with PA thermodilution, TPTD measurements can be affected by intracardiac shunts, valvular insufficiencies, and unaccounted loss of thermal indicator due to pericardial or pleural effusions. The accuracy of the transpulmonary technique has been investigated and found to have a high degree of correlation when compared with PA thermodilution[75] and the Fick method[67,76] in critically ill children.

Pulse contour analysis (PCA) has emerged as another method for measurement of CO. Its minimally invasive nature and continuous display of CO makes the technology attractive. Cardiac output measurement using PCA is based on using the area under the systolic portion of the arterial pressure waveform divided by aortic impedance. The algorithm can compute the left ventricular (LV) stroke volume which when multiplied by heart rate gives CO.

$$CO = \frac{HR \times A_{sys}}{Z_{ao}} \qquad Z_{ao} = \frac{SV_{pc}}{SV_{td}} \qquad \textbf{Eqs. 22.10a and 22.10b}$$

where A_{sys} is the area under the systolic pressure waveform, Z_{ao} is aortic impedance, SV_{pc} is uncalibrated stroke volume based on pulse contour, and SV_{td} is stroke volume measured by thermodilution.

PCA is most accurate when calibrated using the TPTD method to compensate for changes in arterial compliance. When CO is necessary for interpretation of a hemodynamic state, a calibration of the system should be performed to achieve better accuracy. This technology has been validated in adults and children and shown to have satisfactory accuracy in stable hemodynamic conditions[77,78] with potential loss of precision when faced with rapidly changing hemodynamics.[77-81]

Hemodynamic parameters can be measured using a combination of PCA and TPTD technique found in PiCCO (Pulsion Medical Systems, Munich, Germany) or VolumeView (Edwards Lifesciences, Irvine, CA) monitoring systems. Preload and intravascular volume can be calculated using TPTD with specific measures of global end-diastolic volume index (volume of all cardiac chambers at the end of diastole), intrathoracic blood volume index, and extravascular lung water index (fluid that accumulates in the interstitial and alveolar spaces). Dynamic markers of cardiac preload such as pulse pressure variation and stroke volume variation are used for guidance of fluid therapy and are calculated from beat-to-beat analysis of the arterial pressure waveform. Because these parameters represent cardiopulmonary interactions in patients on positive pressure ventilation, their validity has been studied only in intubated patients with controlled ventilation.[82]

Venous Oximetry

When oxygen supply decreases below a critical threshold, cellular oxygen consumption is reduced because cellular function is now supply dependent.[83] This leads to tissue hypoxia and lactate production as anaerobic metabolism ensues (Fig. 22.12). Tissue hypoxia may escape detection by conventional hemodynamic measures and by bedside physical examination because these do not provide knowledge of oxygen supply-demand economics (see Fig. 22.12).[84-87] The oxygen supply-demand relationship can be mathematically expressed by the Fick principle:

$$VO_2 = CO \times davO_2 \qquad \textbf{Eq. 22.11}$$

where VO_2 is O_2 consumption, CO is cardiac output, and $davO_2$ is arterial-venous content difference.

Manipulation and simplification of this equation leads to:

$$SaO_2 - SvO_2 \approx VO_2/DO_2 \qquad \textbf{Eq. 22.12}$$

Mixed venous saturation (SvO_2) reflects the oxygen supply and demand relationship and provides a global measure of whole-body oxygen utilization. This global oxygen utilization can be quantified as a proportion via calculation of the oxygen extraction ratio (OER). OER is approximately 25% in a state of health, and generally an OER of 60% marks supply-dependent consumption (i.e., critical DO₂, anaerobic threshold). In neonates this anaerobic threshold occurs at an SvO_2 of 30% to 40%.[88]

$$OER = (SaO_2 - SvO_2)/SaO_2 \qquad \textbf{Eq. 22.13}$$

Venous oximetry has shown to be prognostic of outcomes and has served as a therapeutic goal in various disease states. As a target for goal-directed treatments, evidence is better for SvO_2 than for CO or oxygen delivery. In patients with major trauma with traumatic brain injury, central venous saturation ($ScvO_2$) of 65% or less in the first 24 hours heralded higher mortality and longer hospitalization.[89] Rivers et al.[90] showed a significant reduction in mortality and organ dysfunction when employing early goal-directed therapy targeting specified hemodynamic parameters and $ScvO_2$ greater than or equal to 70% in adult patients with severe sepsis and septic shock. Significant improvement in survival and reduction in organ injury was noted in patients with single-ventricle disease following stage I palliation when postoperative management was based on goal-directed therapy targeting $ScvO_2$.[90]

Completely mixed SvO_2 can be obtained only from a PA blood sample. Modern PA catheters allow for continuous SvO_2 measurements, but there is an inherent risk and an additional cost associated with placement of these catheters. Moreover, it is not feasible to establish SvO_2 in patients with congenital heart disease who have parallel circulations or left-to-right shunts. Due to the routine use of central venous catheters, central venous saturation ($ScvO_2$) has been proposed as an alternative measure based on the notion of functional equivalence.[84] $ScvO_2$ is measured at the superior vena cava and right atrial junction and represents the oxygen balance of the upper body. Generally, the upper body extracts more oxygen than the lower body, and in infants the upper body receives a greater portion of the CO. Although $ScvO_2$ normally closely approximates SvO_2 and generally moves in parallel with SvO_2 with alterations in O_2 supply and demand, deviations from this relationship may occur in various low-flow or high-flow states.

Use of venous oximetry and understanding its limitations requires a thorough grasp of the cellular O_2 consumption and O_2 delivery relationship and pathophysiologic alterations during periods of stress. Low venous saturations clearly mark cardiocirculatory insufficiency and require further investigation, but normal or high venous saturations can mask underlying tissue hypoxia. For example, an elevation of $ScvO_2$ may occur in patients with septic shock secondary to arteriovenous shunting, mitochondrial dysfunction, or inability to extract O_2, producing tissue hypoxia while $ScvO_2$ may remain elevated. Blood flow to areas with cellular death or inhibition of mitochondrial function (cyanide toxicity) essentially creates arteriovenous shunt conditions and can elevate venous O_2 levels. Because the oxygen saturation in any venous blood sample reflects the flow-weighted average of the heterogeneous circulatory beds from which it derives, the high-flow regions will be over-represented in the sample, thus masking the detection of lower-flow desaturated regions.

Invasive Pressure Monitoring

Invasive pressure monitoring systems are composed of a catheter in the compartment of interest, fluid-filled tubing to transmit the pressure signal, a transducer to convert the pressure signal to an electronic signal, an amplifier within the monitor, and a visualization and storage scheme.[91,92] The whole monitoring system is designed to produce an accurate reproduction of pressure waveforms, as well as to characterize dynamic responses. Dynamic response characteristics include natural frequency (oscillations after stimulus) and dampening coefficient (absorption of oscillatory energy) and are generated from elasticity, mass, and friction of the system. The combined monitoring system and biologic system characteristics generate the numeric and graphic representation on the display module, and thus interpretation of invasive pressures necessitates an understanding of both systems. Setup of the system requires referencing pressures to atmospheric pressure ("zeroing") and then horizontally aligning with a phlebostatic axis ("leveling"), most commonly the right atrium.[92,93]

Arterial Blood Pressure. The arterial circulatory system serves dual functions: first as a conduit for transfer of metabolites to tissues and organs, and second to convert pulsatile flow to continuous flow at the arteriolar and capillary level to ensure metabolic exchange (i.e., cushioning function).[94] Arterial blood pressure is a measure of the force responsible for the work of the circulatory system to achieve its dual purpose.[86] Invasive arterial blood pressure monitoring is the recognized standard for blood pressure measurement in critically ill patients for diagnostic purposes, titration of vasoactive medications, and when blood pressure cannot be reliably measured via noninvasive methods.[66,86,93]

The arterial waveform represents a cyclic pressure oscillating wave around a mean pressure, where the peak and trough represent the systolic and diastolic pressures.[94,95] The arterial waveform contour is developed from a summation of a series of waves that are multiples of the fundamental frequency (i.e., heart rate).[93] Clinically the arterial waveform contour and pressure is derived from a combination of phasic CO and systemic vascular resistance and to a lesser extent viscoelastic properties of the arterial tree and viscosity of blood.[95,96] Numeric values and waveform shape are impacted by the site of catheter position. Due to reflected wave augmentation, peripheral arterial waves have a higher and steeper systolic peak and a more defined diastolic component compared with more central arterial measurements (Fig. 22.13).[93,95] The waveform contour relays the phases of the cardiac cycle: rapid upstroke and initial downslope aligns with systolic ejection, the dicrotic notch with closure of the aortic valve, and a tailed runoff indicating diastole.[95] A steeper upstroke thus reflects better contractility. The position of the dicrotic notch may assist in determination of peripheral vascular resistance. In infants the dicrotic notch is normally in the upper half of the descending pressure waveform, but with a low peripheral resistance state, such as with runoff through a patent

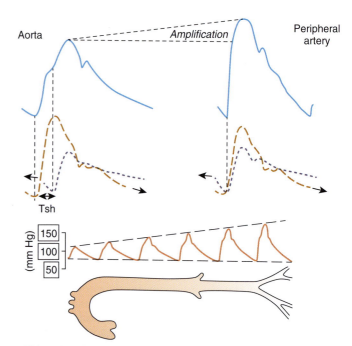

• **Figure 22.13** Schematic representation of arterial waveform amplification. Reflected waves are not in phase with forward wave in the aorta, and thus systolic pressures are lower than in periphery. In the periphery the phase reflected wave is in phase and summed with the forward wave, augmenting the systolic pressure.[95]

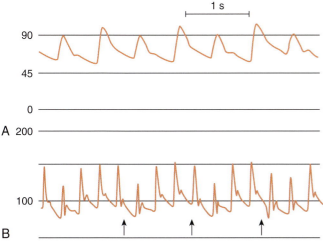

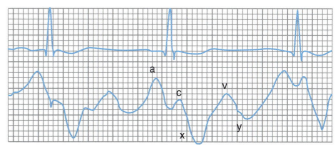

• **Figure 22.15** Central venous pressure and relation to electrocardiogram. Systolic phase (*c* wave, *x* descent, *v* wave) and two diastolic phases (*y* descent, *a* wave). (From Pittman JA, Ping JS, Mark JB. Arterial and central venous pressure monitoring. *Int Anesthesiol Clin.* 2004;42[1]:13-30.)

• **Figure 22.14** Arterial pressure waveform morphologies. (A) Pulsus alternans. Amplitude change with each pulse. (B) Pulsus paradoxus. Decline in systolic pressure with spontaneous inspiration *(arrows)*. (From Schroeder R, Barbeito A, Bar-Yosef S, et al. *Miller's Anesthesia.* Philadelphia: Elsevier; 2015.)

ductus arteriosus, the dicrotic notch will be lower on descending limb of the waveform.

Aside from absolute numeric pressure values displayed, the contour and variation in arterial waveform can convey clinical information to the bedside provider.[66,93] Multiple physiologic derangements show characteristic arterial tracings: pulsus alternans with LV systolic failure, pulsus paradoxus with cardiac tamponade, and pulsus bisferiens with aortic insufficiency (Fig. 22.14).[93,175] Variations in pulse pressure, systolic pressure, and stroke volume (based on waveform analysis) due to intrathoracic pressure changes with cyclic respiratory phases have shown to be a clinically useful marker for detecting a state of volume responsiveness, indicating that an increase in CO will likely result from preload augmentation.[92,97,98] More esoteric techniques, such as application of enhanced mathematic methodologies to deconstruct arterial waveforms, allow for a clearer understanding of the interactions between cardiac and circulatory systems.[96] Additionally, values derived from arterial wave contour analysis (pulse wave velocity) permit elucidation of arterial tree features (i.e., elastance, resistance).[95] Total arterial compliance can be estimated from measuring the area under the curve for systolic and diastolic portions of an aortic pressure wave.[99] Although the clinical effectiveness of these nuanced derivatives awaits broader demonstration, they can be diagnostic and provide guidance for intervention in specific circumstances.

Central Venous Pressure. Adequate functioning of the cardiovascular system requires effective intravascular volume, myocardial performance (rate and contractility), vascular tone, and optimal cardiac rhythm. The venous system is integral in regulation of the circulatory system given CO is strongly determined by the venous pressure resulting from volume returned to the heart (i.e., venous return).[100] A predominant feature of the venous system is its ability to shift blood from a physiologically inert state (unstressed volume) to a hemodynamically active state (stressed volume).[100] Central venous pressure (CVP) or right atrial pressure is directly coupled to both cardiac and venous vascular functions and has been primarily monitored as a surrogate for intravascular volume status, AV synchrony, and right heart function.

CVP reflects the right atrial pressure, and when there is no tricuspid stenosis, it reflects the end-diastolic RV pressure.[93] The transduced CVP is referenced to ambient atmospheric pressure, but it is the transmural pressure (CVP minus extramural pressure) that determines wall stretch, ventricular filling, CO, and venous flow.[93]

The normal CVP waveform contour aligns with the cardiac cycle and consists of three waves (*a, c, v*) and two descents (*x, y*). The *a* and *c* waves represent atrial and ventricular contractions, respectively, and the *v* wave represents atrial filling (Fig. 22.15). The *x* descent occurs with downward displacement of the AV valve with ventricular contraction, and the *y* descent is correlated with the AV valve opening. Clinically the waveform can be divided into systolic components (*c* wave, *x* descent, *v* wave) and diastolic components (*y* descent, *a* wave).

The morphology of the CVP waveform components provides insight into intracardiac blood flow and cardiac conduction. Atrial contraction against a closed or stenotic AV valve produces a tall *a* wave ("cannon *a* wave"), such as in the setting of tricuspid stenosis and junctional rhythm. An elevated *a* wave may also occur with RV diastolic dysfunction. Merging of *c* and *v* waves is characteristically seen with AV valve regurgitation due to loss of the *x* descent. During these conditions, changes in the CVP waveform morphology still allow a transduced pressure but may not be reliable indicators of RV end-diastolic pressures.[93] In states of extramural restriction (constrictive pericardial disease and tamponade) the transduced CVP will read higher due to elevated *v* and *a* waves.[93]

The use of CVP to guide fluid resuscitation is widespread, but evidence supporting CVP for fluid-responsive increase in CO is poor.[101,102] Marik et al. performed a meta-analysis of adult patient studies reporting an area under receiver operating characteristic curve (AUC) between the CVP and change in cardiac performance following an intervention that altered preload. The summary AUC for the population was 0.56 (95% CI, 0.52-0.60), and the correlation coefficient was 0.18 (95% CI, 0.1-0.25).[101] CVP cannot be equated with end-diastolic volume due to continually changing venous tone, ventricular compliance (LV and RV), ventricular loading conditions, and intrathoracic pressure in the critical illness period.[101,103] Further, RV end-diastolic volume in itself is a poor measure of fluid responsiveness because volume alone does not indicate where one lies on the Frank-Starling curve.[101,103]

Central venous line (CVL) access can be attained in a multitude of veins, including axillary, internal jugular, subclavian, femoral, and inferior vena cava, or CVLs can be placed directly into the atria. The complications of venous access include pneumothorax (<1%), arterial puncture (<2%), thrombosis (≈3.7%), and bloodstream infections (≈8.7%).[104,105]

Left Atrial Pressure. Left atrial pressure (LAP) monitoring is performed to obtain hemodynamic insight into left-sided cardiac structures. LAP may provide value when there is concern for LV function (systolic and diastolic), left atrial hypertension, or concern for LV preload (acute right heart failure, pulmonary hypertension). Access to left atrial pressures can be acquired via the transthoracic route or via the transseptal route.[71,106] LAP monitoring can impact management in patients when apprehension exists in regard to LV function, such as when separating from CPB, following heart transplantation, and in neonates with arterial switch procedures. Left atrial hypertension is a typical concern in patients with diminutive left-sided structures following a two-ventricle repair, mitral valve repair, and acutely following LV assist device placement. Patients at risk for right heart failure or vulnerable to pulmonary hypertensive crisis may benefit from LAP monitoring because an acute decrease in LAP can signify loss of LV preload.

Given the risk of introducing thromboemboli to the systemic circulation, the risk of bleeding, and the potential for catheter retention at the time of removal, caution has been taken in limiting routine placement of these catheters and emphasis directed to early removal. A review of 5815 transthoracic left atrial catheter implants over a 7-year period found the overall bleeding requiring transfusion or mediastinal reexploration to be less than 0.24%, whereas Gold et al. found the bleeding risk to be 0.13%.[107,107a]

Capnometry

CO_2 is the end product of cellular metabolism delivered to the lungs via systemic and pulmonary circulation. Hence exhaled CO_2 is not only a marker of ventilation, but also of cellular metabolism and systemic and pulmonary blood flow. Capnometry refers to the measurement and numeric display of carbon dioxide (CO_2) during the respiratory cycle. *Capnography* or *capnogram* refers to the graphic display of the concentration of exhaled and inhaled CO_2 over time. CO_2 measurements are expressed in partial pressure PCO_2 (mm Hg, kilopascals, torr, bar, or atmosphere), or FCO_2 (fraction of CO_2 in gas mixture in %). A normal capnogram displays exhaled CO_2 over time during the respiratory cycle[108] (Fig. 22.16 and Table 22.3). Variations of the capnogram in clinical conditions are represented in Fig. 22.17.

Time-based capnograms can give important information about exhaled and end-tidal CO_2, respiratory frequency, and inspiratory CO_2 (if present), and the visual analysis of the waveform can give further important clinical information (Fig. 22.18). However, time-based capnograms are correct only when no significant rebreathing occurs because every inspiratory effort leads to transition from phase III to phase 0; and during the beginning of expiration, anatomic dead space already contributes to a small rise in exhaled CO_2 (phase I). Those potential drawbacks have led to the development of volumetric capnograms.

The simultaneous measurement of flow and/or volume during the respiratory cycle and of exhaled CO_2 is defined as volumetric capnography.[109] Although newer ventilators have integrated mainstream volumetric CO_2 analyzers, only volumetric capnographs enable breath-to-breath analysis of volumetric CO_2 waveforms. The phases in volumetric capnography are synonymous with the phases in time-based capnography. However, when CO_2 is plotted versus volume, more detailed information about the anatomic source of CO_2, mixed expired CO_2, CO_2 elimination (VCO_2), and calculation of anatomic, physiologic, and alveolar dead space can be obtained.

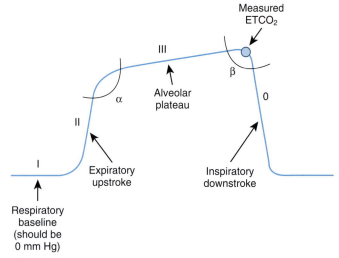

• **Figure 22.16** Capnometry. A normal capnogram displays exhaled CO_2 over time during the respiratory cycle. *ETCO$_2$,* End-tidal carbon dioxide.

TABLE 22.3	**Physiologic Components of Time Capnogram**	
Phase I	No/minimal CO_2	Physiologic (upper airway and alveolar) and artificial (ventilation circuit) dead space
Phase II	Increasing CO_2	Transition from alveolar dead space to alveolar ventilation
α angle	Between Phase II and III	Indirect parameter for ventilation/perfusion
Phase III	Plateau	Exhaled CO_2 represents alveolar gas exchange
β angle	Between Phase III and IV	
Phase IV	Terminal upswing of CO_2	While slow alveoli exhale constant CO_2 during expiration, fast alveoli exhale initially fast, but close earlier
ETCO$_2$	End-tidal, end-expiratory CO_2	End of expiration
Phase 0	Decreasing/no CO_2	Inspiration

CO_2, Exhaled carbon dioxide.

Measurement of exhaled CO_2 is a noninvasive technique to estimate the arterial CO_2 partial pressure ($PaCO_2$). Although in healthy subjects the relation of end-tidal CO_2 is close to $PaCO_2$, this relationship is more discrepant in patients with pulmonary disease or increased alveolar dead space,[110-114] alteration of positive end-expiratory pressure,[115] or decreased CO[111] or changes in arterial and venous CO_2. The accuracy of capnography can be challenging in neonates and infants because of leaks with uncuffed endotracheal tubes, lower lung compliance, and higher respiratory rate with shorter exhalation times, and apparatus size may distort the alveolar plateau.[114] Despite these limitations, exhaled CO_2 monitoring improves patients' safety and provides essential for an array of monitoring indications, including ventilation and circulation.

The arterial-alveolar (end-tidal) CO_2 difference has contributions both from alveolar dead space (alveolar-capillary difference) and from

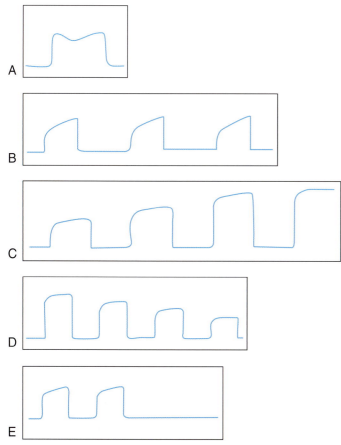

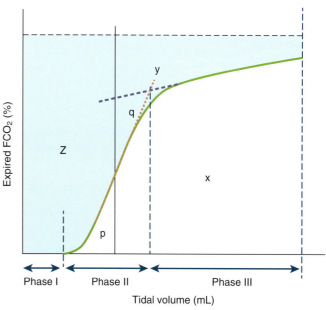

• **Figure 22.18** Time capnogram. Expiratory segment (divided into phases I, II, III). Angle between phase II and phase III; angle between phase III and descending limb of phase 0 (inspiration); FCO_2, fractional concentration of carbon dioxide. Airway deadspace as illustrated by triangles p and q are of equal area. Area X is the volume of CO_2 in the expired breath while area Z and y are from airway and deadspace ventilation. Because they do not contribute to CO_2 elimination, this is wasted ventilation. (Fletcher R. *The Single Breath Test for Carbon Dioxide.* Lund, Sweden, Berlings, Arlov, 1986.)

• **Figure 22.17** Clinical capnograms. (A) Rebreathing. (B) Obstruction of endotracheal tube or airway obstruction. (C) Gradual increase of end-tidal carbon dioxide ($ETCO_2$) in hypoventilation, fever, sepsis, increase in cardiac output ([C] illustrates changes in malignant hyperthermia). (D) Gradual decline in $ETCO_2$ in hyperventilation, hypothermia, decrease in cardiac output. (E) Sudden decrease in $ETCO_2$ in extubation, loss of cardiac output, pulmonary embolism.

venoarterial admixture (capillary-arterial difference).[116,117] Thus the arterial-to-end-tidal PCO_2 difference will be progressively larger as the arterial saturation falls from increasing right-to-left shunt, without any intrinsic lung disease. Recognition of this principle allows for proper interpretation of capnometry in patients with cyanotic heart disease. The combination of pulse oximetry and capnometry can aid in diagnosis of alterations of pulmonary blood flow.

Echocardiography

Comprehensive echocardiography is a fundamental tool in the cardiac ICU and provides detailed information, including morphology, systolic and diastolic function, pressure gradients, coronary anatomy, and postsurgical assessment. Performing and interpreting the comprehensive examination requires lengthy training and can be time consuming. With development of portable ultrasonography and growing comfort with its use, a simplified focused cardiac ultrasound (FoCUS) platform has been developed to answer limited time-sensitive queries in critical scenarios.[118] With its ability to rapidly provide diagnostic information in acute settings, FoCUS has become a vital part of bedside assessment, allowing providers to diagnose and to monitor the effect of interventions. FoCUS has gained traction in the both cardiac and general pediatric intensive care settings, emergency medicine, and anesthesiology. Specialists

have taken to incorporating FoCUS training into their respective training curriculum.[119,120]

The abbreviated transthoracic ultrasound examination is structured to evaluate (1) systolic LV function, (2) the severity of valvular stenosis or regurgitation, (3) PA systolic pressure, (4) presence of a pericardial effusion, and (5) intravascular volume status. Typically the examination is performed to answer dichotomous clinical questions (e.g., "Does the patient have depressed systolic function?"). Additional uses of bedside echocardiography include assessment during cardiopulmonary resuscitation. There is agreement from both the International Evidence-Based Recommendations for Focused Cardiac Ultrasound and the 2010 international pediatric advanced life support recommendations to consider FoCUS in cardiac arrest to evaluate for potentially treatable causes of a cardiac arrest while weighing the risk of known deleterious consequences of interrupting chest compressions.[118]

Biochemical Assessment

Acid-Base Status

Three major methods to describe alterations of acid-base balance are as follows:

1. The physiologic approach by Henderson-Hasselbalch assesses acid-base disorders on the relation of bicarbonate (HCO_3^-) and partial pressure of carbon dioxide (PCO_2). Henderson defined the equation relating the concentration of [H^+] to the base pair [CO_2] / [HCO_3^-]:

$$pH = pKa + \log([HCO_3^-]/[H_2CO_3])$$ **Eq. 22.14**

where pKa is the acid dissociation constant for carbonic acid (6.1).

2. In the approach by Van Slyke, base excess is defined as the amount of acid or base needed to restore a normal pH in vitro while PCO_2 (40 mm Hg) and temperature (37°C) are held constant:

$$BE = \{HCO_3^- - 24.4 + (2.3 \times [Hb] + 7.7)\} \times (1 - 0.023 \times Hb)$$

Eq. 22.15

To improve measurements in vivo, base excess was standardized to the effect of Hb on CO_2 titration, the standard base excess (SBE):

$$SBE = 0.9287 \times ([HCO_3^-] - 24.4 + 14.83) \times (pH - 7.40)$$

Eq. 22.16

3. The physicochemical approach by Stewart uncovers acid-base disturbances by evaluating electrolyte distribution and dissolved CO_2 in the extracellular space and deriving the strong ion difference (SID):

$$SID = [Na^+] + [K^+] + [Ca^{2+}] + [Mg^{2+}] - [Cl^-] - [A^-]$$
$$= 40 - 44 \text{ mEq} \approx [HCO_3^-] + [A^-]$$

Eq. 22.17

Practical Approach to Assess Acid-Base Disturbances. An acid-base disorder is described as primary respiratory when it is caused primarily by abnormality of the respiratory function (changes in PCO_2) and primary metabolic when it is caused primarily by changes in the HCO_3^- concentration as with the Henderson-Hasselbalch equation or in SID with Stewart's approach (Table 22.4). The most common analytic tools to further investigate metabolic disturbances are based on the principle of electrical neutrality and the sum of charges of extracellular ions, known as the *anion gap*.[121,122]

$$\text{Anion Gap} = Na^+ + K^+ - Cl^- - HCO_3^- = 10 \text{ to } 12 \text{ mEq/L}$$

Eq. 22.18

In the setting of acidemia a widening anion gap (AG) represents measurement of unmeasured anions (for example, uremia, ketones, lactate, hyperosmolar hyperglycemic nonketotic coma, toxicity due to salicylates, methanol, ethylene glycol, paraldehyde), whereas an acidosis with normal AG represents that anions are measured

(for example, gastrointestinal bicarbonate loss, drugs [acidifying agents and carbonic anhydrase inhibitors], dilutional acidosis with hyperchloremia, renal tubular acidosis). The urine AG ($Na_{urine}^+ + K_{urine}^+ - Cl_{urine}^- = 3$-$11$ mEq/L) can further discriminate renal (high urine AG) or gastrointestinal losses (normal urine AG) in metabolic acidosis. The original approach for AG lacked the implication of albumin or phosphate as weak acids, hence Figge modified the original equation[123]:

$$\text{Albumin corrected } AG = AG + 2.5 \, (\text{normal albumin in g/L}$$
$$- \text{measured albumin in g/L})$$

Eq. 22.19

An alternative approach to the calculation of AG,[121] is the calculation of strong ion gap (SIG), based on the Stewart and Fencl concept of SID, which explores the small differences of apparent SID ($[Na^+] + [K^+] + [Ca^{2+}] + [Mg^{2+}] - [Cl^-]$) and effective SID, the sum of bicarbonate and nonbicarbonate buffers ($HCO_3^- + [Albumin_{charge}] + [Phosphate_{charge}]$).[124] This difference of apparent and effective SID is a marker for the presence of abnormal anions (SIG). Theoretically the SIG maybe superior to the conventional calculation of AG, and calculation of unmeasured anions using the Fencl-Stewart concept is superior to lactate in identification of patients at high risk of death.[125]

Cardiac Biomarkers

In monitoring cardiac health concurrent with physical measures, emphasis is given to quantifying biochemical changes as a consequence of myocyte injury, myocyte stress, and neurohormonal responses to inadequate cardiac function.[126] Cardiomyocyte injury due to ischemia, trauma, or necrosis is routinely evaluated by measurement of released cardiac troponins. The troponin complex is composed of three proteins (troponin C, I, T) that regulate contraction by governing the actin-myosin interaction. Cardiac troponin I (cTnI) and cardiac troponin T (cTnT) are specific to the cardiomyocyte.[127] The rate of rise and clearance from peripheral circulation depends on the extent of injured tissue, the blood flow and lymphatic drainage in the area of the injury, and the rate of elimination of the marker from the blood.[128] The typical pattern for a distinct non-reoccurring injury is a rise during the first 24 hours, followed by a plateau for 12 to 24 hours, then a steady fall thereafter.

TABLE 22.4	Practical Approach to Acid-Base Disturbances		
Primary	**Acidemia**		**Alkalemia**
Respiratory	Increase in PCO_2		Decrease in PCO_2
Metabolic			
• By Henderson-Hasselbalch	Decrease in HCO_3^-		Increase in HCO_3^-
• By Stewart			
• Abnormal SID	Decrease in SID	Extracellular water dilution Increase in lactate and ketoacid	Increase in SID	Extracellular water depletion Decrease in chloride
• Abnormal total weak acids	Increase in albumin		Decrease in albumin
	Increase in phosphate		Decrease in phosphate

HCO_3^-, Bicarbonate; *PCO_2*, partial pressure of carbon dioxide; *SID*, strong ion difference

According to the American College of Cardiology/American Heart Association, cardiac troponin levels are the mainstay of diagnosing acute coronary ischemia and highly sensitive and specific for myocardial necrosis.[129] A negative troponin confers a greater than 99% negative predictive value for myocardial infarctions when using a high-sensitivity assay. Following ischemic injury, a rise in troponin levels should be detectable in 3 to 4 hours.

Inflammation of the myocardium (myocarditis) due to infections, toxins, hypersensitivity reactions, or autoimmune processes can cause necrosis of the cardiomyocyte. Studies are inconclusive as to the sensitivity and specificity of troponin levels in diagnosing myocarditis.[130] Following pediatric heart transplant, cTnI concentrations have been found to be significantly higher in rejection versus nonrejection samples. With a cTnI cutoff of 15 ng/L, sensitivity was 94%, specificity 60%, positive predictive value was 18%, and negative predictive value was 99%.[131]

Cardiac troponin levels appear to have a prognostic role in pediatric heart surgery. A retrospective review of 1001 children having heart surgery found cTnT levels greater than 5.9 µg/L on the first postoperative day to be independent risk for 30-day mortality.[132] Additionally, peak cTnI levels have been correlated with increased inotropic support and ICU stay in neonates undergoing arterial switch operations.[133] A prospective study found cTnI level greater than 14 ng/mL 2 hours after CPB to be an independent predictor of low CO syndrome.[134]

Cardiomyocyte stress due to distention of the myocardium from volume load is primarily quantified by natriuretic peptides.[126] Use of natriuretic peptide levels for establishing the presence of heart disease and its severity has been recommended by the AHA.[135] B-type natriuretic peptide (BNP) and N-terminal pro-BNP (NTproBNP) are considered gold standard biomarkers for diagnosis, management, and prognostication in heart failure patients.[136] BNP production is predominantly stimulated by myocardial stretch of the LV but can be induced via inflammation, sympathetic activity, and myocardial ischemia. Transcription of the BNP gene leads to proBNP protein, which is cleaved into the inactive N-terminal BNP and the active form BNP, and then these products are released into the bloodstream.[137] BNP has both paracrine and endocrine functions and balances the autonomic neurohormonal effects of heart failure and thus promotes diuresis, natriuresis, and vasodilation and inhibits myocardial remodeling.[137] BNP reaches the circulation within minutes of production, is cleared by receptor-mediated processes and enzymatic breakdown with a small portion requiring renal filtration, and generally exhibits a circulating half-life of 20 minutes.[136]

BNP has been well established in the pediatric population with heart failure as a marker that correlates with severity of clinical heart failure and with severity of ventricular dysfunction.[138] In patients without structural heart disease and heart failure, NTproBNP levels are higher compared with healthy children, negatively correlated with ejection fraction, and positively correlated with clinical heart failure scores.[138] NTproBNP and BNP levels have correlated with modified Ross heart failure classification.[139] BNP levels of 300 pg/mL or higher have been forecasted to predict the 90-day composite end point of death, hospitalization, or listing for cardiac transplantation in heart failure patients.[140]

Urine Output and Biomarkers of Renal Perfusion

Generous urine output is commonly considered as a marker of optimal CO and renal perfusion pressures. Although oliguria may reflect a reduction in glomerular filtration rate (GFR), the rate of urine formation is more strongly determined by tubular and collecting system function, and the activation of the stress response increases levels of antidiuretic hormone and renin-angiotensin-aldosterone so that "hormonal" oliguria is commonly observed without a reduction in GFR. Moreover, urine formation can be a lagging indicator of renal perfusion. Thus oliguria is a sensitive but very nonspecific indicator of reduction in GFR and of renal ischemia.

The kidneys are one of the most highly perfused organs in the body, receiving almost 25% of CO.[141] Perfusion of renal parenchyma, however, is not uniform. Significant regional differences in blood flow and high metabolic demand paradoxically make areas like the renal medulla extremely vulnerable to ischemic injury because the tissue oxygen tension is extremely low in a setting of very high extraction. Even a mild reduction in total and cortical renal blood flow in the medulla may induce ischemic and hypoxic injury.

Monitoring tools for traditional renal failure are typically insensitive until more than 60% of nephrons are injured.[142] This small margin of remaining renal function before symptoms of irreversible injury ensue leaves little opportunity for the early treatment of acute kidney injury (AKI).[143] GFR is considered the best indicator of renal function but is challenging to accurately measure in clinical practice. Thus urine output continues to remain a clinical indicator of renal function at the bedside. Perioperative oliguria in children is defined as a urine flow rate of less than 0.5 mL/kg/h. It is often interpreted as a sign of renal dysfunction, but in the perioperative period oliguria is common and might represent an appropriate prerenal response to intravascular hypovolemia or a manifestation of the physiologic response to CPB or surgical stress. When arterial blood pressure and intravascular volume are restored to normal levels and surgical stress resolves, urinary flow should return to normal.

The range of perfusion pressure over which the kidney can autoregulate may be limited in certain conditions, including extracellular fluid depletion, renal ischemia, or renal vascular disease. Constriction of the afferent arteriole may be stimulated by increased sympathetic nervous system activity and increased levels of endogenous or exogenous circulating catecholamines.[144] Reduction in CO and effective intravascular volume can further increase activity of the sympathetic nervous system, vasopressin levels, and the renin-angiotensin-aldosterone system, stimulating increased reabsorption of sodium and water to help restore CO and intravascular volume. Fluid overload on the other hand is countered by a series of vasodilating, salt-excreting neuropeptides.

Intravascular volume monitoring in the perioperative setting is essential to identifying physiologic conditions that influence renal perfusion. Monitoring of central venous pressure can help to assess preload or elevated venous pressures. Direct measurements of left atrial pressure offers some insight into the kidney pressure-flow relationship because left atrial hypotension is a known stimulus for renal vasoconstriction.[145] Somatic NIRS is commonly used after congenital heart surgery and allows for monitoring of regional renal circulation. Its use for predictability of renal injury is still not clearly delineated, but some studies show promise for detection of conditions indicative of renal ischemia.[146-148]

Serum chemistry values and urinary indices such as GFR, creatinine clearance, or fractional secretion of sodium may enable the assessment of CO distribution but function poorly as predictors of early renal failure.[149,150] Limited progress in early diagnosis of AKI has stimulated interest in investigation of other biomarkers of renal injury. These biomarkers attempt to expose three early signs of renal damage during AKI, including tubular cell damage, cell dysfunction, and renal adaptive stress response. Some of the extensively investigated renal biomarkers include cystatin C[151] and neutrophil gelatinase–associated lipocalin (NGAL).[152] Others in early stages of clinical investigation include urinary interleukin-18, kidney injury molecule 1 (KIM1),[153] and liver-type fatty acid binding protein (L-FABP).[154] Cystatin C remains the most extensively studied in the pediatric population as a filtration-based marker. Like creatinine, it accumulates in the circulation in the setting of renal impairment and thus is used as a marker of glomerular filtration. Cystatin C is thought to have potential advantage over creatinine as an indicator of mild chronic kidney disease and its sequelae, although studies remain conflicting.[155-157] NGAL is one of the most promising markers of renal injury. Its levels rise before creatinine elevation is seen[157a,157b] and show promising specificity for predicting AKI.[158]

Advanced Monitoring Systems

With the development of modern-day ICU monitors, computational processors, and methods of information storage, we have entered an era of data-driven health care. The increasingly complex medical system is burdened with an estimated 180,000 to 440,000 preventable medical errors leading to patient mortality.[159,160] Additionally, the burden of alarm fatigue is a real and significant challenge in the critical care setting. In a pediatric ICU study 68% of alarms were false, and 94% of alarms were likely to be clinically unimportant.[161] Present monitoring systems are limited in predicting adverse events, and the opportunity for the development of improved and more intelligent monitoring systems is real.

Adoption of electronic health and medical records has increased the accessibility of patient information. However, to truly advance the monitoring of the patient in the cardiac ICU, the basic recording and viewing of single-patient data points are no longer sufficient. Historical and real-time physiologic patient data can now be synthesized to create an integrated representation of the patient's overall state of health. In the future, relevant medical information, including sensitive and specific alarm conditions, risk-index scores, and potential suggestions for care, may be presented on a single screen.[162] There is a substantial benefit in the creation of such a display that not only integrates the sizable amount of ICU data in a meaningful way, but also provides the medical team with a hypothesis-driven display so that a patient's clinical trajectory may be followed over time.

The velocity and volume of patient data generated on a day-to-day basis has led to the concepts of big data, data mining, and statistical learning, particularly in the ICU.[163,164] The growing ubiquity and collection of this patient data allows for the intersection of technology and intensive care medicine in a way in which data mining, predictive analytics, and artificial intelligence can flourish. The pursuit of real-time analytics methods and risk prediction is an evolving field with the goal of improving patient outcomes through early diagnosis. At the University of Michigan, complex network infrastructures capture physiologic data from both patient monitors and electronic health record data to Structured Query Language (SQL) databases, which are then being utilized to create patient risk scores and more intelligent alarms in the ICU setting.[162]

High-resolution physiologic data allow for the development of metrics that may be more specific and sensitive to a patient's condition than current pediatric acuity scores; these metrics include the Pediatric Risk of Mortality, third version (PRISM III), and the Pediatric Index of Mortality, second version (PIM2).[37,165-167] Advanced analytics, such as probabilistic network models, neural networks, classification trees, logistic regression, and random forest algorithms can be used to create complex models of disease.[168,169] Using the information from the publicly available Physionet database, artificial neural networks have been developed to detect patients at high risk of clinical deterioration with better performance than traditional acuity scores.[170,171] Cardiopulmonary monitoring systems have also been developed using neural networks to diagnose arrhythmic cardiac arrest, tension pneumothorax, pericardial tamponade, venous air embolism, and exsanguination in the adult ICU setting.[172] In a multicenter study using electronic health record information, Churpek et al.[173] have applied machine learning methods to predict cardiac arrest, ICU transfer, and death in an adult hospital ward. In the pediatric cardiovascular ICU setting, Rusin et al. have used continuous, high-resolution, physiologic recordings to develop a model that predicts cardiorespiratory deterioration 1 to 2 hours before the event in the patient with single-ventricle disease.[3,4] For all cases, early recognition of impending deterioration would allow the medical team time to intervene in hopes of improving patient outcomes.

Though many advanced monitoring systems are still in their infancy, they will likely continue to evolve. As patient databases continue to grow in scope and size, so will the medical system's contextual knowledge base and ability to develop intelligent monitoring through advanced computational techniques.

Selected References

A complete list of references is available at ExpertConsult.com.

20. Tremper KK, Barker SJ. Pulse oximetry. *Anesthesiology.* 1989;70(1): 98–108.
43. Hoffman GM, Ghanayem NS, Scott JP, Tweddell JS, Mitchell ME, Mussatto KA. Postoperative cerebral and somatic near-infrared spectroscopy saturations and outcome in hypoplastic left heart syndrome. *Ann Thorac Surg.* 2017;103(5):1527–1535.
44. Hoffman GM, Brosig CL, Mussatto KA, Tweddell JS, Ghanayem NS. Perioperative cerebral oxygen saturation in neonates with hypoplastic left heart syndrome and childhood neurodevelopmental outcome. *J Thorac Cardiovasc Surg.* 2013;146(5):1153–1164.
66. Dorfman MV, Schenkman KA. Principles of invasive monitoring. In: Fuhrman BP, ed. *Pediatric Critical Care.* 5th ed. Philadelphia, PA: Elsevier; 2017:279–291.
67. Tibby SM, Hatherill M, Marsh MJ, Murdoch IA. Clinicians' abilities to estimate cardiac index in ventilated children and infants. *Arch Dis Child.* 1997;77(6):516–518.
68. Swan HJ, Ganz W, Forrester J, Marcus H, Diamond G, Chonette D. Catheterization of the heart in man with use of a flow-directed balloon-tipped catheter. *N Engl J Med.* 1970;283(9):447–451.
73. Sandham JD, Hull RD, Brant RF, et al. A randomized, controlled trial of the use of pulmonary-artery catheters in high-risk surgical patients. *N Engl J Med.* 2003;348(1):5–14.
88. Hoffman GM, Ghanayem NS, Kampine JM, et al. Venous saturation and the anaerobic threshold in neonates after the Norwood procedure for hypoplastic left heart syndrome. *Ann Thorac Surg.* 2000;70(5):1515–1520, discussion 1521.
90. Rivers E, Nguyen B, Havstad S, et al. Early goal-directed therapy in the treatment of severe sepsis and septic shock. *N Engl J Med.* 2001;345(19):1368–1377.
124. Stewart PA. Modern quantitative acid-base chemistry. *Can J Physiol Pharmacol.* 1983;61(12):1444–1461.

23

Ventilators and Ventilator Strategies

KONSTANTINOS BOUKAS, MD; IRA M. CHEIFETZ, MD; JON N. MELIONES, MD, MS

Respiratory Support

Classification of Positive Pressure Ventilators

A mechanical ventilator is designed to replace or support lung function by altering, transmitting, and directly applying energy in a predetermined way to perform the work of the thorax and lungs. Nomenclature to classify the essential features of positive pressure ventilators has been described by many authors and continues to be an area of confusion for practitioners not closely involved in the design and development of ventilators.[1-3]

A classification system provides a common knowledge base of terms and concepts to facilitate the understanding, interpretation, and assessment of ventilator operating systems and performance characteristics. The classification system must be clinically relevant and accurately reflect the pattern of respiratory support a patient receives. This section will present a classification system as it supports the clinical practice of ventilatory care.

Power Input/Transmission. Ventilator power input is either electrical or pneumatic (compressed gas). The transmission of input power is a function of the drive and control mechanisms of the ventilator. Ventilator classification focuses on the control variables, output parameters, and alarm systems as applied to their clinical utility. More specifically, clinicians focus on how each tidal volume (VT) is delivered to describe the type of respiratory support a patient receives.

Control Schemes and Control Variables. Ventilator control variables address the physical qualities adjusted, measured, and/or used to manipulate the various phases of the ventilatory cycle. The four general control variables are inspiratory flow pattern, limit, trigger, and cycle. Classifying ventilators with this system may seem cumbersome and challenging to practitioners; however, this system is designed to address advances in ventilator operation, is based on the physiology of the ventilatory strategies, and provides a platform for new technology without confounding terminology.

Typically the control variables remain constant despite changes in ventilatory load. Therefore the ventilator sacrifices other preset variables (i.e., dependent variables) to keep the control variables constant despite changes in the patient's compliance and resistance.[4] The dependent variables depend on the controlled variable(s) as well as changes in compliance and resistance of the patient's respiratory system. Although each manufacturer develops and refines its control scheme for the manipulation of these variables, commonalities exist between ventilators, which allow clinicians to describe the resultant respiratory patterns with common terminology.

Inspiratory Flow. The inspiratory flow pattern sets the characteristics of gas flow during a positive pressure breath and affects the distribution of that breath within the patient's respiratory system. Clinicians must consider several factors when selecting an inspiratory flow pattern for an individual patient. Airway pressures are dependent on the mechanical properties of the lungs and movement of gas into the lungs. The airway pressures generated during inspiration increase as flow enters the respiratory system and encounters the resistance of the airways. The gas volume must also overcome the elastic recoil of the lung. Therefore peak pressure = (flow)(R_{aw}) + (VT)(elastance), where R_{aw} is the airway resistance and VT is the tidal volume. The shape of the inspiratory flow pattern as it delivers the positive pressure breath determines the shape of the pressure curve and the peak pressure generated.[5] This can be predicted given knowledge of the characteristics of the various flow patterns and the pneumatic characteristics of the patient's lungs, as subsequently described. As derived from the equation, the selection of an appropriate inspiratory flow pattern based on a patient's pulmonary pathophysiology will improve the effectiveness of ventilation, reduce peak inspiratory pressure, and optimize mean airway pressure, while promoting patient-ventilator synchrony.[6]

Fig. 23.1 illustrates typical inspiratory flow patterns available with positive pressure ventilators.[7] Four inspiratory flow patterns exist, although only the first two are generally available on current ventilators. A square-wave pattern is produced by a constant flow of gas throughout inspiration. Variable decelerating flow is a waveform characterized by peak flow early in inspiration and then a decrease in flow until end-inspiration. This decrease in flow is generally curvilinear but may vary based on the specific programming of the ventilator. Ascending, accelerated flow patterns produce a ramp pattern with low flow at beginning inspiration and a linear increase in flow throughout inspiration with peak flow delivered at end-inspiration. A sine wave pattern is generated by a variable flow with a rapid increase during the early phase of inspiration, a peak at midinspiration, then a decrease in flow until end-inspiration.

The functional performance of the various inspiratory flow patterns remains constant across manufacturers but may be produced by dramatically different control schema. The flow pattern characteristics of a specific mechanical ventilator significantly influence the airway pressures generated. Clinicians should monitor inspiratory/expiratory (I:E) ratios when selecting flow patterns during volume-limited ventilation and adjust the peak flow to maintain an appropriate inspiratory time.

Gas flow always follows the path of least resistance. Alterations in inspiratory flow pattern affect the distribution of gas flow based

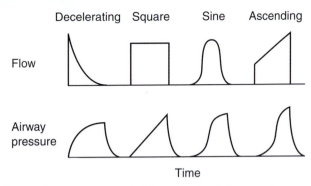

Decelerating   Square   Sine   Ascending

Flow

Airway
pressure

Time

• **Figure 23.1** Tracings typical of the various inspiratory waveforms available with mechanical ventilators. Pressure control ventilation uses a descending waveform that results in lower peak and higher mean airway pressures. Volume control uses a square waveform. (Modified from Pontoppidan H, Geffin B, Lowenstein E. Acute respiratory failure in the adult. 3. *N Engl J Med.* 1972;287:799–806.)

on the underlying pathophysiology and anatomic considerations of the respiratory system. Ascending (accelerating) flow patterns deliver the highest flow at end-inspiration when the effects of resistance and elastance are increased. Ascending flow patterns produce higher peak pressures compared to other flow patterns and are generally no longer in clinical use. A decelerating flow pattern has several advantages over an ascending pattern. Decelerating flow patterns deliver the highest flow at the beginning of inspiration when volume and elastance are low. Inspiratory flow then decreases during inspiration as delivered volume increases. Therefore peak airway pressure is lower, but mean airway pressure is higher. In general, as the maximum flow moves from the beginning to the end of the inspiratory cycle, peak pressure increases and mean airway pressure decreases.

Inspiratory flow patterns should be matched to each patient's clinical condition. In situations in which the patient has high airway resistance (e.g., asthma, bronchiolitis, large airway obstruction), peak airway pressures may be reduced by avoiding a flow pattern with high peak inspiratory flow rates. In these patients a square-wave, constant flow pattern may generate a lower peak pressure than a descending flow pattern as a result of the decrease in peak flow. The actual effects in individual patients may vary widely with those patients who have a strong inspiratory demand being more comfortable with the generally high flow rate of a variable, decelerating pattern. In contrast, respiratory pathology characterized by a low compliance may benefit from a descending flow pattern in which the peak pressure is reduced but the mean airway pressure is increased. Variable flow ventilation (e.g., pressure control ventilation [PCV]) uses a decelerating flow pattern, which can significantly decrease the peak inspiratory pressure and increase the mean airway pressure to recruit collapsed alveoli and potentially improve oxygenation.[8-10]

Trigger. The inspiratory phase of a breath can be initiated by (1) patient effort, as determined by a change in either pressure or flow in the ventilator circuit, or (2) time. Therefore mechanical breaths may be pressure, flow, or time triggered.[11,12] Flow triggering increases the sensitivity of the ventilator to the patient's spontaneous demands and can decrease the response time of VT delivery. The ventilator "sensitivity" determines the degree of inspiratory effort a patient must exert to trigger the ventilator to deliver a VT. Ideally, this should be adjusted to 0.1 to 3.0 L/min of flow or −0.5 to −1.5 cm H_2O to minimize the patient's imposed work of breathing.

Cycle. The cycle variable determines when inspiration ends. This variable is used as a feedback signal to terminate gas flow and allow the patient to passively exhale. Time is the most common cycle variable for mechanical breaths (time cycled). Certain spontaneous breaths (e.g., pressure supported breaths) can be flow cycled. In a flow-cycled breath the expiratory valve opens when inspiratory flow decreases to a preset percentage of peak inspiratory flow. This algorithm is generally preset, not adjustable, and varies among ventilators.

Limit. During inspiration, pressure, volume, and flow increase above the end-expiratory values. Limit variables allow the clinician to control the upper limits of pressure and/or volume of the mechanical breath a patient receives, hence the description "pressure limited" and "volume limited."

Ventilatory Modes

Using the terminology described earlier, a system can be developed that describes the ventilatory modes and specific breathing patterns used during positive pressure ventilation (PPV). Ventilatory modes may include mechanical breaths, spontaneous breaths, or a combination of both.

Mechanical Breaths. Assist control mode delivers a patient-triggered ventilator VT with each spontaneous effort. In an assist control mode the ventilatory rate is determined by the patient and therefore may be in excess of the preset control rate. When there is no spontaneous respiratory effort, the minimum ventilatory rate is that which is set by the clinician. Assist control modes should be contrasted with support modes of ventilation. In both modes a predetermined level of support is adjusted by the clinician. In assisted modes the inspiratory time is determined by the clinician. In contrast, in supported modes the inspiratory time is determined by the patient. Assist control breaths may be limited by either volume or pressure. A patient may receive volume control ventilation (VCV), in which a predetermined minimum breath rate is delivered and breaths are volume limited, or PCV, in which a preset minimum breath rate is delivered along with a preset pressure limit.

In previous modes of ventilation the decelerating flow pattern was available only on the PCV mode. Now several vendors have combined the attributes of a decelerating flow pattern with a volume guarantee. In these modes, the ventilator guarantees a preset minute ventilation. In one such mode, pressure-regulated volume control (PRVC), the ventilator monitors the airway resistance and compliance of the lungs and adjusts the inspiratory pressure level via a predetermined algorithm to deliver a preset volume limit. PRVC provides the benefit of a stable minute ventilation while providing the opportunity to use a decelerating inspiratory flow pattern.

Spontaneous Breaths. Spontaneous breathing may be supported with continuous positive airway pressure (CPAP), a mode in which the ventilator maintains a constant airway pressure throughout inspiration and expiration. A preset expiratory pressure limit prevents the patient from exhaling down to atmospheric pressure at end-expiration. Continuous or demand flow during inspiration maintains airway pressure above atmospheric pressure. Raising the expiratory pressure above atmospheric pressure increases end-expiratory lung volume (EELV) proportionate to the pressure applied and total respiratory compliance. The CPAP mode can be used alone or in conjunction with mechanical breaths. Of note, when used in combination with mechanical breaths, the term *positive end-expiratory pressure (PEEP)* is used instead of CPAP.

Pressure support ventilation (PSV) is a spontaneous breathing mode that can be used alone or in combination with other modes

TABLE 23.1 Classification of Modes of Positive Pressure Ventilation Used for Cardiac Patients

Mode	MECHANICAL BREATH VARIABLES			SPONTANEOUS BREATH VARIABLES		
	Trigger	Cycle	Limit	Trigger	Cycle	Limit
Control ventilation	Time Flow Pressure	Time	Volume Pressure	—	—	—
Synchronized intermittent mandatory ventilation	Time Flow Pressure	Time	Volume Pressure	Flow Pressure	Flow	Pressure
Supported ventilation (PSV or VS)	—	—	—	Flow Pressure	Flow	Pressure Volume

PSV, Pressure support ventilation; *VS*, volume support.

(synchronized intermittent mandatory ventilation [SIMV], CPAP). A preset level of inspiratory pressure is delivered above the baseline end-expiratory pressure with each spontaneous respiratory effort. PSV is initiated when pressure or flow decreases to the preset threshold level during inspiration. When this trigger is sensed by the ventilator, flow accelerates into the breathing circuit and increases proximal airway pressure to the preset pressure level. The pressure support breath is usually terminated when flow decreases to 25% of peak flow.[13] The VT delivered in this mode will vary with changes in lung compliance, airway resistance, pressure support level, and inspiratory time.

Volume support (VS) combines the benefits of PSV with a volume guarantee during spontaneous breathing. The ventilator monitors airway resistance and pulmonary compliance and adjusts the pressure support level using a predetermined algorithm to deliver a preset minute ventilation. In this mode the pressure used to deliver the VT is automatically adjusted (a dependent variable).

Combined Breaths. SIMV modes combine mechanical breaths with spontaneous breaths. Flow for spontaneous breathing may be provided by a continuous flow of gas through the breathing circuit, a demand valve, or a combination of both. If PEEP is applied with continuous and demand flow, the spontaneous breaths become CPAP breaths. Pressure support is often administered in conjunction with SIMV.

Neonatal and Pediatric Ventilators

In this classification system the mechanical breaths produced by most traditional neonatal ventilators would be considered constant flow, time-triggered, time-cycled, and pressure-limited breaths. The advances in neonatal ventilator design have enabled most modes that are available on pediatric and adult ventilators.[14] Improvements in calibration and the measurement of smaller volumes have facilitated volume-limited mechanical SIMV breaths with CPAP or pressure support.[15,16] Mechanical breaths can be pressure or flow triggered, time cycled, and volume or pressure limited. Spontaneous breaths are constant flow, CPAP, or variable flow, pressure-supported breaths.[17]

The primary difference between neonatal and pediatric/adult ventilators is the range of flows and volumes the ventilator can deliver. Neonatal ventilators are able to deliver lower flows and volumes at faster rates and deliver breaths with a shorter response time to patient-triggered effort. Pediatric ventilators are essentially the same ventilators used in adults, only at lower ranges of flow and volume.

As technology has advanced, ventilator manufacturers have developed ventilators that are capable of ventilating patients ranging from small neonates to large adults. Table 23.1 contains the common classifications of mechanical ventilator breaths by mode of ventilation.

Output Waveform Analysis

Ventilators provide continuous monitoring of respiratory mechanics, including displays of gas flow, volume delivery, and airway pressure. Output waveforms are a useful tool for understanding the characteristics of ventilator operation and provide a graphic display of the various modes of ventilation.[18] Waveform analysis can be used to optimize mechanical ventilatory support and analyze ventilator incidents and alarm conditions. Using this technology, it is possible to tailor the form of ventilatory support, improve patient-ventilator synchrony, reduce patient work of breathing, and calculate a variety of physiologic parameters related to respiratory mechanics.

The most useful waveforms are flow, pressure, and volume graphed over time (termed *scalars*). Convention dictates that positive values correspond to inspiration and negative values to expiration; horizontal axes represent time in seconds, and vertical axes represent the measured variable in its common unit of measurement. Optimal measurements are obtained when the pressure and flow monitoring device is positioned between the endotracheal tube (ETT) and the ventilator circuit.[18,19] Measurements may also be obtained from the inspiratory or expiratory limbs of the ventilatory circuit. Integration of intrapleural pressure from an esophageal balloon further enhances graphic data and enables assessment of the patient's work of breathing. During spontaneous breathing, patient effort, work of breathing, and the level of intrinsic PEEP are best evaluated using esophageal pressure measurements.[20]

In addition to plotting flow, pressure, and volume versus time, each of these parameters can be plotted against each other. Pressure-volume and flow-volume loops can be particularly helpful in assessing alterations in resistance or compliance, work of breathing, overdistention of the lung, and intrinsic PEEP.

Flow Graphics. Flow sensors should be capable of measuring a wide range of flows (−300 to +150 L/min) and be resistant to motion artifact, moisture, and respiratory secretions.[5] The flow graphic has two distinct parts: inspiratory flow and expiratory flow. The inspiratory flow graphic displays the magnitude, duration,

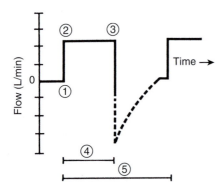

• **Figure 23.2** Inspiratory flow graphic of a square-wave mechanical breath. Positive deflections indicate flow from the ventilator to the patient. *1*, Initiation of flow from the ventilator; *2*, peak inspiratory flow; *3*, end-inspiration; *4*, inspiratory time; *5*, total cycle time. (Modified from MacIntyre NR, Ho L. Weaning mechanical ventilatory support. *Anesth Report.* 1990;3:211–215.)

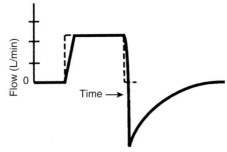

• **Figure 23.3** Constant inspiratory flow graphic of a mechanical breath, modified by ventilator response time. Note the phase shift and alteration in shape of the flow curve during inspiration. (Modified from MacIntyre NR, Ho L. Weaning mechanical ventilatory support. *Anesth Report.* 1990;3:211–215.)

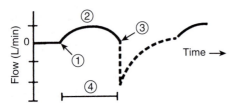

• **Figure 23.4** Inspiratory flow graphic of a spontaneous breath. Inspiratory flow from the patient to the ventilator by convention is represented as a positive deflection. *1*, Start of inspiration; *2*, peak inspiratory flow; *3*, end-inspiration; *4*, inspiratory time. (Modified from MacIntyre NR, Ho L. Weaning mechanical ventilatory support. *Anesth Report.* 1990;3:211–215.)

and flow pattern of the positive pressure breath or spontaneous breath. Fig. 23.2 is a theoretical inspiratory flow pattern of a continuous flow mechanical breath. In actual application, flow delivery mechanisms have response times that alter the shape of the flow graphic. These response times result in a positive slope at the start of inspiration and a negative slope at end-inspiration (Fig. 23.3).

The flow graphic of a spontaneous breath is demonstrated in Fig. 23.4. The characteristic of the flow graphic is determined by the characteristics of the patient's inspiratory demand and the ventilatory support provided to the spontaneous breath (i.e., continuous flow CPAP, demand flow CPAP, and/or pressure support).

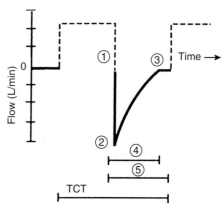

• **Figure 23.5** Representation of a normal expiratory flow graphic. Expiratory flow from the patient to the ventilator by convention is represented as a negative deflection. *1*, Start of expiration; *2*, peak expiratory flow; *3*, end expiratory flow; *4*, duration of expiratory flow; *5*, expiratory time; *TCT*, total cycle times. (Modified from MacIntyre NR, Ho L. Weaning mechanical ventilatory support. *Anesth Report.* 1990;3:211–215.)

The expiratory flow of gas is generally passive for mechanical and spontaneous breaths, although patients may forcibly exhale to assist exhalation. The magnitude, duration, and pattern of the expiratory graphic are determined by the resistance of the patient's respiratory system and ventilator circuit. Important features of the ventilator circuit that affect the flow graphic include the size and length of the ETT, internal diameter and length of the ventilator circuit, resistance of the expiratory valve, and distensibility of the circuit itself. Fig. 23.5 represents a typical expiratory flow graphic for a positive pressure breath. The expiratory flow, by convention, is shown below the zero baseline. Because the characteristics of the patient circuit that affect the expiratory flow pattern are generally fixed, dramatic changes in the expiratory flow curve may be attributable to changes in the patient's resistance, compliance, or activity. For example, an increase in airway resistance due to obstructive disease or secretions may result in decreased peak expiratory flow, increased duration of flow, or failure of flow to return to baseline (Fig. 23.6).

Pressure Graphics. Although resistance of the ETT is a component of the pressure graphic, pressures measured are generally considered to reflect airway pressure. In a typical pressure-triggered breath from a demand-flow valve, there is a slight pressure drop at the beginning of inspiration, and the magnitude of the drop is proportionate to the patient's peak inspiratory flow rate, sensitivity of the demand valve, and response of the flow delivery system. Of note, this pressure drop usually is not seen in a flow-triggered breath. During a mechanically supported breath the peak inspiratory pressure is determined by the patient and circuit compliance, resistance, delivered VT, and inspiratory flow (Fig. 23.7). Baseline pressure reflects the expiratory pressure in the circuit (i.e., PEEP or CPAP). The pressure-time graphic is useful for evaluating the stability of PEEP in the presence of an air leak.

Volume Graphics. Volume is generally measured by integrating the flow signal with inspiratory time (Fig. 23.8). The upsweep of the graphic represents the volume delivered to the patient and/or circuit. The "downsweep" of the graphic represents the total expiratory volume. Typically, inspiratory and expiratory volumes should be equal. Nevertheless, it is not uncommon in infants and children with uncuffed ETTs for the expiratory volume to be less than the inspiratory volume. An actual percentage leak can be calculated and may aid in the decision to change the ETT size.

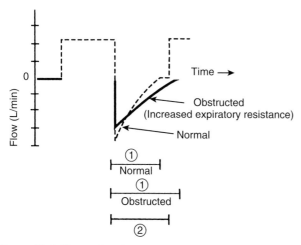

• **Figure 23.6** Abnormal expiratory flow graphic in a patient with airway obstruction. The expiratory flow exceeds the available expiratory time, and exhalation is not complete. If expiratory time is short (as occurs in the expiratory waveform marked *obstructed*), premature termination of exhalation will occur with resultant gas trapping and increased dead space/tidal volume ratio. Normal time *(1)* equals normal patient expiratory time. Obstructed time *(1)* is prolonged patient expiratory time secondary to obstruction. *2,* Mechanical time for expiration. (Modified from MacIntyre NR, Ho L. Weaning mechanical ventilatory support. *Anesth Report.* 1990;3:211–215.)

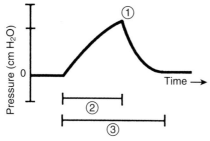

• **Figure 23.7** Pressure graphic of a valved-control mechanical breath. *1,* Peak inspiratory pressure; *2,* inspiratory time; *3,* duration of positive pressure. (Modified from MacIntyre NR, Ho L. Weaning mechanical ventilatory support. *Anesth Report.* 1990;3:211–215.)

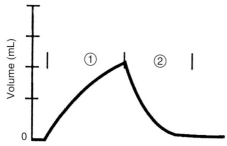

• **Figure 23.8** Volume graphic of a volume control mechanical breath. The volume that is delivered to the patient during inspiration is the delivered inspiratory volume. The volume that returns during expiration is the expiratory volume. *1,* Time for inspiration; *2,* expiratory time. (Modified from MacIntyre NR, Ho L. Weaning mechanical ventilatory support. *Anesth Report.* 1990;3:211–215.)

Patient-Ventilator Synchrony. The timing sequence of various respiratory events can be determined by displaying volume, flow, and pressure over time (Figs. 23.9 and 23.10). Comparisons of all three graphics simultaneously facilitate analysis of ventilator-patient interactions. Ventilator dyssynchrony becomes evident when the timing and magnitude of flow, pressure, and volume are disproportionate or delayed.

Ventilator Parameters and Alarm Systems

Parameters. Spontaneous VT and respiratory rate are a reflection of circuit characteristics, respiratory system compliance and resistance, and respiratory muscle function. Assessment of mechanical VT and preset rate ensures delivery of the prescribed alveolar ventilation and facilitates detection of endotracheal or ventilator circuit leaks. Inspiratory time is selected by the clinician to facilitate patient comfort and synchronous breathing during PPV. The patient's age and respiratory pattern are major considerations in the selection of inspiratory time. Recommended inspiratory times by age-group are as follows:

Newborns: 0.3 to 0.5 seconds
Toddlers: 0.5 to 0.75 seconds
Children: 0.75 to 1.0 seconds
Adults: 0.75 to 1.5 seconds

Total cycle time is the time allotted for one complete inspiratory (I) and expiratory (E) cycle. I:E ratio is an expression of the set inspiratory time and the remaining expiratory cycle time. Recommended I:E ratios vary greatly with ventilator rate. Ratios of 1:2 or 1:3 are most desirable but should be no lower than 1:1 in assisted ventilation to allow adequate time for exhalation. Peak flow should be titrated to the spontaneous demands of the patient.

Peak inspiratory pressures during volume-limited ventilation are a reflection of volume, flow, inspiratory time, airway resistance, and respiratory system compliance. Peak inspiratory pressures vary with alterations in the patient's respiratory physiology. The presence of airway secretions, bronchospasm, tubing kinks, pneumothorax, agitation, and decreased lung compliance all may increase peak inspiratory pressures. Decreased peak pressures reflect an air leak around the ETT, a leak in the ventilator circuit, or an improvement in the child's lung mechanics. Peak pressure is not an indicator of changes in patient condition with time-cycled, pressure-limited ventilation.

Mean airway pressure closely reflects alveolar pressure and is an important indicator of the degree of PPV required to achieve adequate oxygenation. Mean airway pressure is principally a function of inspiratory time and PEEP; however, VT, peak inspiratory pressure, inspiratory flow pattern, and ventilator rate also play a role.

Plateau pressure is obtained by recording the pressure following an inspiratory hold maneuver. Plateau pressure reflects the compliance of the lung without gas flow and eliminates the airway resistance component. A plateau pressure must be obtained with a constant inspiratory flow pattern and cannot be measured in the presence of an air leak.

PEEP is produced by closure of the ventilator expiratory valve. The volume of gas remaining in the lung is proportionate to the end-expiratory pressure and the patient's compliance. Increasing the volume of gas increases EELV.

Alarms. Ventilator alarm systems have improved dramatically with microprocessor technology.[21] Input power alarms notify clinicians of changes in electrical or pneumatic supplies. Control circuit

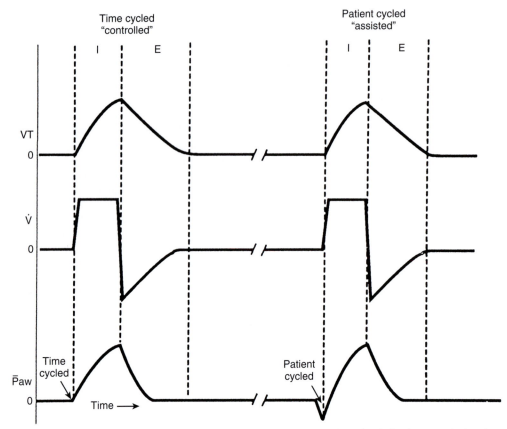

• **Figure 23.9** Graphic orientation of volume, flow, and pressure of mechanical volume control and volume assist breaths. *E,* Expiratory; *I,* inspiration; *P̄aw,* airway pressure; *V̇,* flow; *VT,* tidal volume. (Modified from MacIntyre NR, Ho L. Weaning mechanical ventilatory support. *Anesth Report.* 1990;3:211–215.)

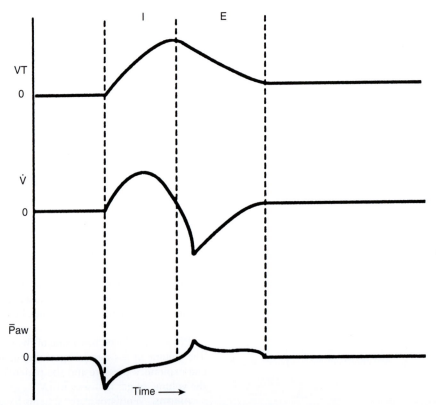

• **Figure 23.10** Graphic orientation of volume, flow, and pressure of a spontaneous breath. *E,* Expiratory; *I,* inspiration; *P̄aw,* airway pressure; *V̇,* flow; *VT,* tidal volume. (Modified from MacIntyre NR, Ho L. Weaning mechanical ventilatory support. *Anesth Report.* 1900;3:211–215.)

alarms notify the clinician of incompatible parameters or that the ventilator self-test has failed. Output alarms indicate unacceptable levels of ventilator output, including peak airway pressure, end-expiratory pressure, volume, flow, minute ventilation, respiratory rate, and inspired gas concentration. The fraction of inspired oxygen (FiO_2) should be analyzed continuously with high and low alarm limits set to prevent inadvertent hyperoxemia or hypoxemia.

Nonconventional Modes of Ventilation

High-Frequency Ventilation. High-frequency ventilation (HFV) refers to a variety of technologies that use VTs smaller than the patient's anatomic dead space and high ventilatory frequencies to minimize the effects of increased peak pressure. HFV consists of a variety of ventilatory strategies, including high-frequency oscillatory ventilation (HFOV) and high-frequency jet ventilation (HFJV).

High-Frequency Oscillatory Ventilation. HFOV uses an electrically powered piston diaphragm oscillator to alternate positive and negative pressures in the airway. With use of this diaphragm, VTs between 1 and 3 mL/kg are generated with cycles ranging from 300 to 900 beats/min (5 to 15 Hz). During HFOV, inspiration and expiration are both active and occur above and below the mean airway pressure baseline. HFOV has been used successfully in neonates with respiratory distress syndrome and children with acute respiratory distress syndrome (ARDS).[22-25] HFOV has also been used successfully in air leak syndrome in both neonates and children. Recently in a large pediatric observational study, HFOV was shown to increase length of ventilation and possibly increase mortality. The HFOV should be used with caution because the data have not shown improvements in outcomes.[26]

The exact mechanisms of gas exchange during HFOV remain controversial. The potential mechanisms include convective gas transport, coaxial flow, Taylor dispersion, molecular diffusion, and the pendelluft effect.[27-34] Conventional bulk flow is responsible for gas delivery to the larger airways and potentially to the alveoli close to these larger airways. Coaxial flow is the bidirectional flow of gas in the airways at the same time. A net flow of gas can occur in one direction through the center of the airway and in the other direction in the area closer to the airway wall. Taylor dispersion describes gas flow along the front of a high-velocity gas flow. Gas transport occurs as a result of gas dispersion beyond the bulk flow front. Molecular diffusion is known to occur at the alveolar level during conventional ventilation, and enhanced diffusion may play a role during HFV. The pendelluft effect is the phenomenon of intraunit gas mixing due to the impedance difference among lung units.

Any strategy that results in increased mean airway pressure may result in rapid transmission of the increased intrathoracic pressure to the cardiovascular structures and subsequently to cardiovascular compromise. HFOV should be used with caution in patients with congenital heart disease (CHD) associated with passive pulmonary blood flow and/or right ventricular (RV) dysfunction and in those with hemodynamic instability because these patients may be sensitive to the resulting higher mean airway pressures. Also, HFOV should be used with caution in those with severe asthma given the less efficient active expiratory flow.

High-Frequency Jet Ventilation. Most HFJV systems use a high-pressure, air-oxygen gas source that generates gas flow. A rapid solenoid valve allows for flow interruption, which regulates the frequency of ventilation.[35] A reducing valve is present that allows adjustments of inspiratory driving pressure from 10 to 50 psi.

The current US Food and Drug Administration–approved HFJV system (Bunnell LifePulse Ventilator, Bunnell Inc., Salt Lake City, UT) requires a second ventilator in tandem.

During HFJV, peak inspiratory pressures can be controlled from 8 to 50 cm H_2O, inspiratory time from 20 to 40 milliseconds, and respiratory rate from 150 to 600 insufflations per minute. The PEEP and sigh breaths are regulated by the tandem ventilator. Previously a specific ETT was necessary for HFJV, which required reintubation. This is no longer required because specific jet adapters are now used.

Effect on Gas Exchange. Although the mechanism of gas exchange during HFJV has not been well defined, convection streaming and enhanced molecular diffusion are known to occur.[35] Simply defined, convection streaming is the flow of gas in a bulk flow manner to the level of the alveoli. Gas is injected into the airway at high speed during HFJV. The gas molecules located in the center of the inspired gas travel faster than those at the edges (asymmetric velocity profiles). Exhalation is passive and promoted by an extremely short inhalation time (20 to 40 milliseconds) and long exhalation times. The exhaled gas travels at a slower velocity than the inspired gas. When exhaled gas encounters the rapidly moving inspired gas, it is extruded along the tracheal walls. The net result is continuous exhalation of gas around the inspired gas. Molecular diffusion is the rapid kinetic motion of molecules and occurs in the terminal bronchioles and alveoli. A variety of other theories have been proposed to explain the ability of HFJV to provide adequate ventilation at VTs below dead space.[35]

Carbon Dioxide Elimination. During PPV, manipulations in minute ventilation, ventilatory rate, and VT allow alterations in CO_2 elimination. During HFJV, CO_2 elimination is governed by the relationship $(VT)^a \times f^b$, where VT = tidal volume, f = frequency.[36] In this relationship a ranges from 1.5 to 2.5 and b from 0.5 to 1.0. Because $a > b$, alveolar ventilation during HFJV has a greater dependency on alterations in VT than frequency.

The primary method of eliminating CO_2 during HFJV is by increasing the delivered VT. Increasing the delivered VT can be accomplished by increasing the inspiratory pressures during HFJV. This increases alveolar ventilation and may improve ventilation/perfusion matching. If atelectasis develops, increasing the PEEP (i.e., mean airway pressure) may help recruit lung volume. PEEP is adjusted during HFJV on the tandem ventilator. The tandem ventilator is usually set to administer 0 to 10 sigh breaths per minute. The sigh breath should be set at a peak pressure less than that set on the HFJV (HFJV breaths are not interrupted) and should not exceed 30 cm H_2O. In patients, sigh breaths are designed to prevent atelectasis and allow for appropriate recruitment of lung volume. Alternatively, EELV may be maintained without any sigh breaths if the PEEP (i.e., mean airway pressure) is titrated upward. When the $PaCO_2$ becomes elevated, increasing the HFJV peak pressure (i.e., VT) may be necessary to increase alveolar ventilation.

During HFJV, VT is dependent on the respiratory frequency, which also affects CO_2 elimination. When the respiratory frequency is increased, a reduction of VT may occur, resulting in decreased tidal alveolar ventilation.[36] Therefore under certain conditions, increasing the respiratory frequency may result in a reduction in alveolar ventilation. For these reasons, manipulations of VT remain the most important determinant of alveolar ventilation during HFJV.

In premature infants, HFJV is initiated at frequencies of 360 to 480 insufflations per minute. This can be accomplished because the premature lung has a short time constant, and b approximates

1.0. In premature infants, increasing the respiratory frequency results in improved alveolar ventilation. In older patients and those with compliant lungs the lung has a longer time constant, and *b* approaches 0.5. In comparison with premature patients, increasing the respiratory frequency in older patients and patients with normal compliance results in a reduction of the delivered VT and an overall reduction of alveolar ventilation. For these reasons HFJV is usually begun at a frequency of 240 to 300 insufflations per minute in children with respiratory or cardiovascular dysfunction.

Lung Volumes. During HFJV, lung volumes do not vary dramatically because peak pressures are low, inspiratory time is short, and mean airway pressure is constant. Mean lung volume is determined by the mean airway pressure. Therefore lung volumes remain relatively static around the mean lung volume. During HFJV, oxygenation is primarily dependent upon mean airway pressures, and increasing mean airway pressures will increase lung volume and improve ventilation/perfusion ($\dot{V}/\dot{Q}$) matching. Mean airway pressure is most affected by increasing the PEEP on the tandem ventilator. Peak inspiratory pressure of the jet ventilator and the VT and rate of the sigh breaths play a lesser role.

Effect on Cardiovascular Parameters. The primary physiologic effect of HFJV is improved ventilation at equivalent mean airway pressures developed during conventional mechanical ventilation. Therefore during HFJV the mean airway pressures can be reduced while maintaining alveolar ventilation and CO_2 clearance, thus limiting the potential adverse effects of positive intrathoracic pressure on cardiovascular performance.[35,37,38]

Negative Pressure Ventilation. Negative pressure ventilation (NPV) can be used in patients after surgery for CHD and in pediatric patients with respiratory dysfunction.[39-41] Currently NPV is usually performed using a chest cuirass that covers the patient's chest and abdomen. Negative pressure is generated within this cuirass. Such cuirass devices avoid the limitations of body tank devices (iron lung type of devices), which are rarely used today. The advantage of NPV is that intubation is avoided, sedation requirements may be decreased, and systemic venous return may be improved. However, the disadvantage of NPV is that left ventricular (LV) afterload may be increased. The regulation of respiratory parameters during NPV, including I:E ratios, can be difficult. NPV is not routinely used in patients with CHD; however, it may be an effective technique in patients with passive pulmonary blood flow such as following Glenn shunt and Fontan procedures.[40,41]

Cardiorespiratory Interactions

Providing adequate gas exchange with mechanical ventilation requires a clear understanding of how the cardiorespiratory system functions as a unit and how alterations in the respiratory system lead to changes in cardiovascular function.

Alterations in intrathoracic pressures are transmitted to cardiac structures and can dramatically alter cardiovascular performance, especially in those with CHD. Alterations in cardiovascular performance may be more dramatic in neonates and children than adults. First, ventricular dysfunction can be particularly severe in infants and children after cardiac surgery. In infants the myocardium is immature and intrinsically noncompliant, and surgical interventions frequently require transmyocardial incisions and intracardiac repair. Also, congenital cardiac surgery may require the placement of prosthetic material into the heart, which can disrupt normal myocardial architecture and function, resulting in myocardial injury, myocardial edema, and abnormal ventricular function. These factors

cause the neonatal myocardium to be more sensitive to alterations in preload and afterload after cardiac surgery.

A second factor is myocardial wall tension. The myocardium of neonates and young children generates a low pressure. Therefore small changes in intrathoracic pressure can lead to relatively large changes in transmural pressure ($P_{transmural} = P_{intracardiac} - P_{pleural}$). In contrast, the adult myocardium generates a higher intraventricular pressure, resulting in only minimal changes in the transmural pressure for a given change in intrathoracic pressure. Transmural pressure affects cardiovascular performance because it contributes to myocardial wall tension.[42-44] Because changes in intrathoracic pressure result in a more dramatic change in myocardial wall tension, PPV has a more dramatic effect on ventricular function in infants and children compared to adults.

Finally, the pulmonary and systemic circulations of neonates and children are highly reactive to alterations in intrathoracic pressures. Minor changes in intrathoracic pressure and lung volume can alter the afterload imparted on the right and left ventricle, resulting in altered ventricular wall stress and performance.

In the following sections the effects of a variety of respiratory interventions on cardiac function will be enumerated. These sections are not designed to be all-inclusive but rather to present cardiorespiratory interactions that are clinically relevant to physicians caring for infants and children with CHD. Interested readers are encouraged to review the references provided for a more in-depth review of this topic.[42,45-47]

Effect of Oxygen Administration

A primary goal of the cardiorespiratory system is to deliver oxygen to the tissues. One method to improve oxygen delivery (DO_2) is to increase the oxygen content of the blood by increasing the concentration of inspired oxygen. Oxygen administration results in an increase in both alveolar and arterial oxygen content. Alterations in alveolar and arterial oxygen content independently result in a reduction of pulmonary vascular resistance (PVR). Neonates are more sensitive to alterations in P_AO_2 and PaO_2 than adults. In conditions of increased afterload a reduction of PVR will decrease RV afterload and may improve RV function. These beneficial cardiorespiratory interactions may be used in the perioperative period in an attempt to assist patients with RV dysfunction.

It should be noted that a reduction of PVR may or may not be beneficial. An increase in the inspired oxygen concentration can reduce PVR and subsequently increase pulmonary blood flow in the presence of a systemic-to-pulmonary shunt. In conditions of decreased pulmonary flow, this may improve DO_2 by increasing arterial oxygen content. In those patients with increased pulmonary flow (e.g., ventricular septal defect, large patent ductus arteriosus, hypoplastic left heart syndrome), the increase in pulmonary blood flow can occur at the expense of systemic flow, and thus a reduction in systemic DO_2 may result.

Effect of Nitric Oxide Administration

A complete discussion of nitric oxide is beyond the scope of this chapter and is contained elsewhere. However, nitric oxide, a powerful pulmonary vasodilator, has been shown to reduce low cardiac output syndrome in selected patients.[48] The data on the use of nitric oxide are variable. Despite this, the selective use of nitric oxide appears to be justified in patients in whom pulmonary artery hypertension and/or RV dysfunction is present.

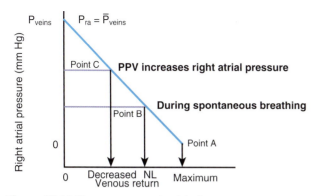

• **Figure 23.11** Venous return to the right heart occurs passively and is dependent on a pressure gradient from the systemic veins to the right atrium. When right atrial pressure (P_{ra}) is zero, there is no impedance to flow back to the right heart, and venous return is maximum *(Point A)*. As right atrial pressure is increased, and mean systemic pressure (P_{veins}) is held constant, there is a progressive reduction in venous return. When right atrial pressure exceeds mean systemic venous pressure, venous return ceases. During spontaneous breathing, right atrial pressure is low, and systemic venous return is high *(Point B)*. During positive pressure ventilation, intrathoracic pressure and right atrial pressure increase, resulting in a reduction of venous return *(Point C)*. *PPV*, Positive pressure ventilation; P_{veins}, venous pressure; $\bar{P}_{veins}$, mean venous pressure. (Modified from Pontoppidan H, Geffin B, Lowenstein E. Acute respiratory failure in the adult. 1. *N Engl J Med.* 1972;287:690–698.)

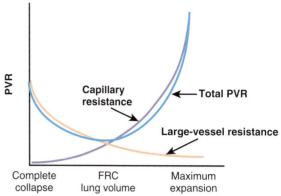

• **Figure 23.12** Pulmonary vascular resistance *(PVR)* is dependent on lung volume and the sum of the resistance contributed by the large- to medium-sized pulmonary vessels and pulmonary capillaries. At lung volumes less than functional residual capacity *(FRC)*, pulmonary vascular resistance is high due to hypoxic pulmonary vasoconstriction and the increased resistance contributed by the tortuous large- and medium-sized vessels. As lung volume increases, pulmonary vascular resistance falls. High lung volumes are associated with an increase in pulmonary vascular resistance due to increased resistance contributed by compression of the pulmonary capillaries. (Modified from West JB, Dolbry CT, Naimark A. Distribution of blood flow in isolated lung: relation to vascular and alveolar pressures. *J Appl Physiol.* 1964;19:713.)

Effect of Ventilatory Manipulations on Right Ventricular Function

Important differences exist between the physiologic response of the right and left ventricles to alterations in intrathoracic pressures and lung volumes.[47] The RV is extremely sensitive to alterations in intrathoracic pressure for a variety of reasons. Systemic venous return to the right atrium (RA) is passive and occurs as a result of a pressure gradient. When the RA pressure is 0 mm Hg or negative, the pressure gradient for venous return is greatest (Fig. 23.11). As RA pressure increases, there is a decreased pressure gradient for venous return, and RV preload falls. During spontaneous breathing, RA pressure and impedance to blood flow to the right heart are low, and thus venous return is high. Positive pressure ventilation alters RV preload by increasing intrathoracic pressure. During PPV the increase in intrathoracic pressure is transmitted to the right heart, resulting in an increase in RA pressure. The increase in RA pressure causes a decreased pressure gradient for venous return, and RV preload decreases. Therefore PPV can reduce RV output by decreasing RV preload. The magnitude of the effect on RV output is dependent upon the mean airway pressure associated with PPV and the intravascular volume status of the patient.

A determinant of ventricular contractility is myocardial oxygen delivery. In the nonhypertensive RV, coronary flow occurs primarily in systole and is dependent on the systolic pressure difference between the aorta and RV.[49] Because PPV results in increased RV pressure, the pressure difference between the aorta and RV is decreased, and RV coronary flow falls during inspiration. As a result, RV contractility, cardiac output (CO), and DO_2 may decrease, especially when the RV end-diastolic pressure is also elevated. Myocardial blood flow is determined by the myocardial perfusion pressure, which depends on intrathoracic, aortic, and RV pressures. An increase in intrathoracic or RV systolic pressure or a reduction in aortic pressure will cause a reduction in RV myocardial blood

flow. In the majority of clinical conditions the pressure difference is such that aortic pressure far exceeds RV and intrathoracic pressures, and RV myocardial blood flow is relatively unaffected by PPV. In certain pathophysiologic conditions, including low aortic pressure, RV dysfunction, and increased intrathoracic pressure, these interactions can become clinically important. When these conditions are present, the adequacy of RV blood flow should be addressed and interventions taken to optimize RV perfusion. Interventions consist of minimizing peak and mean intrathoracic pressures, as possible, and increasing aortic pressure.

The RV has been shown to be exquisitely sensitive to changes in intrathoracic pressure that alters PVR. Neonates and infants are more sensitive to these changes than adults. Modification of RV afterload through respiratory intervention, as described in a later section, is an important therapeutic option for infants and children with RV dysfunction.

RV afterload is influenced by a variety of intrathoracic processes. One modulator of RV afterload is lung volume (Fig. 23.12). Functional residual capacity (FRC) is the lung volume from which normal tidal ventilation occurs. In restrictive lung disease (e.g., ARDS, pneumonia, and musculoskeletal abnormalities), EELV is less than FRC (i.e., normal EELV). At lung volumes above or below FRC, PVR can be increased. When EELV is below FRC, PVR is increased by hypoxic pulmonary vasoconstriction and the tortuous course of large- to medium-sized blood vessels that supply the lung.[50,51] As lung volume increases, the large vessels become more linear, their capacitance increases, hypoxia subsides, and vascular resistance decreases. As lung volumes continue to increase well above FRC, hyperexpansion of alveoli and compression of the surrounding pulmonary capillaries occur and cause vascular resistance to increase.[52] Thus total PVR is the sum of these forces. PVR is elevated at low or high lung volumes and is lowest when EELV approximates FRC. Positive pressure ventilation can promote a reduction of RV afterload in patients with low lung volumes by expansion of collapsed lung units and reducing vascular resistance. Alternatively, PPV can result in increased RV afterload due to excessive alveolar expansion and compression of capillaries.[52] In the normal lung, EELV is maintained near FRC to minimize pulmonary vascular (and airway) resistance, as well as to optimize lung compliance. Thus at FRC the work of matching ventilation and perfusion is minimized. A primary goal of mechanical ventilation is to maintain EELV at or near FRC.

Effect of Ventilatory Manipulations on Left Ventricular Function

Three physiologic principles have been proposed to explain why LV preload is decreased during PPV. First, the LV can eject only the quantity of blood it receives from the RV.[53] When RV output is decreased during PPV, the LV receives a decreased quantity of blood, and LV preload falls. Second, when RV afterload and RV systolic pressure increase during PPV,[42] the increase in RV pressure results in conformational changes in the intraventricular septum and a decrease in LV compliance and preload. Finally, direct compression of the LV from increased intrathoracic pressure may further reduce preload. Under various circumstances one or all of these mechanisms may reduce LV preload during PPV. LV intrinsic contractility is generally not altered by ventilatory interventions. When contractility is reduced during ventilatory manipulations, it is secondary to high airway pressures. Increased airway pressures reduce preload and alter afterload, resulting in a reduction in CO, myocardial DO_2, and contractility.

LV afterload is altered by ventilator manipulations. One determinant of LV afterload is LV transmural pressure (LVTM).[45] LVTM can be approximated by the difference between the LV systolic pressure and intrathoracic pressure (LVTM = P_{LV} − $P_{intrathoracic}$).[45,46] LVTM can be reduced by either decreasing aortic pressure and therefore LV pressure or increasing intrathoracic pressure. During PPV the increase in intrathoracic pressure is rapidly transmitted to the intrathoracic arterial system. LV wall tension remains the same because both the LV pressure and intrathoracic pressure generated are equal. For example, if LVTM = P_{LV} (100 mm Hg) − $P_{intrathoracic}$ (10 mm Hg) = 90 mm Hg, an increase in intrathoracic pressure by 30 mm Hg causes no net change in LV wall tension because P_{LV} (130 mm Hg) − $P_{intrathoracic}$ (40 mm Hg) = 90 mm Hg. The extrathoracic arterial system also develops an increase in arterial pressure due to propagation of the increased arterial pressure. When the increase in intrathoracic pressure results in a significant increase in arterial pressure, aortic pressure will be autoregulated due to baroreceptor stimulation.[45,46] This results in a reflex decrease in aortic pressure and a compensatory reduction of LV pressure. When aortic pressure returns to baseline due to this reflex action, the LV systolic pressure and the transmural pressure gradient fall. Using the previous example, if LVTM = P_{LV} (100 mm Hg) − $P_{intrathoracic}$ (10 mm Hg) = 90 mm Hg, with an increase in intrathoracic pressure by 30 mm Hg and a return of aortic pressure to 100 mm Hg, LV wall tension = P_{LV} (100 mm Hg) − $P_{intrathoracic}$ (40 mm Hg) = 60 mm Hg. Therefore the end result of a persistent increase in intrathoracic pressure is a decrease in LVTM (decreased afterload), as a consequence of aortic pressure autoregulation. Thus increased intrathoracic pressure decreases LV afterload.

Under usual clinical conditions, intrathoracic pressure is low compared to LV pressure, and inspiration occurs over only one to two cardiac cycles. This results in only minor phasic changes in LV afterload, and hence autoregulation may not occur. If intrathoracic pressure is high and the increased intrathoracic pressure

occurs over multiple cardiac cycles, LV afterload can be reduced. Clinicians should be aware of these interactions, especially in neonates with LV dysfunction and concomitant respiratory dysfunction. Clinical signs that suggest a patient may be experiencing these important cardiorespiratory interactions include a wide fluctuation in arterial tracing during inspiration. If this is observed and improvements in LV performance are the goal, the clinician should consider respiratory strategies that optimize intrathoracic pressure to augment LV performance.

Effect of Ventilatory Manipulations on Heart Rate

The institution of PPV has been shown to cause minor changes in heart rate. A significant increase in lung volume can result in a reflex bradycardia; however, this change is modest at the VTs generally employed in clinical practice. Excessive VT ventilation will, however, result in a reflex bradycardia that could become clinically significant.

Respiratory Support for Children With Heart Disease: a Systematic Approach

The application of respiratory support for children with CHD requires balancing the effects of each respiratory intervention on the cardiovascular and respiratory systems. Because of the cardiorespiratory interactions that occur and the diversity of the conditions treated, a single, standardized approach is not possible. Respiratory strategies therefore should be designed to address the specific pathophysiologic condition of each patient. This section defines respiratory management strategies using the principles outlined previously. First, the initial respiratory support settings will be presented, then a systematic approach will be outlined for pathophysiologic respiratory and cardiovascular conditions.

Goals of Respiratory Support

When the goals of the respiratory system are not met by spontaneous breathing, mechanical respiratory support is required.[54] Despite a wide variety of options, all types of respiratory support have two common goals: (1) optimize DO_2 by improving the oxygen content of blood (i.e., increase systemic arterial saturation) while decreasing the oxygen needs of the respiratory muscles (i.e., decrease work of breathing), and (2) improve CO_2 elimination. Respiratory support should meet these goals while minimizing the deleterious effects of these interventions on other organ systems.

The initial ventilatory strategy for all patients should be one that is simple, meets the needs of the patient, provides the greatest benefit with the lowest risk for complications, and represents an approach that is familiar to the multidisciplinary critical care team. The criteria for initiating PPV vary according to the intended goals and needs of each child.

Perioperative Management

Respiratory support should be initiated when arterial hypoxemia (SaO_2 <90% to 92% in the absence of right-to-left intracardiac shunt) and/or alveolar hypoventilation with resultant hypercapnia (generally defined as $PaCO_2$ >60 torr in neonates and $PaCO_2$ >55 torr in children) exists despite pharmacologic therapy and oxygen administration. An additional indication exists when DO_2 is

INITIAL VENTILATOR SETTINGS

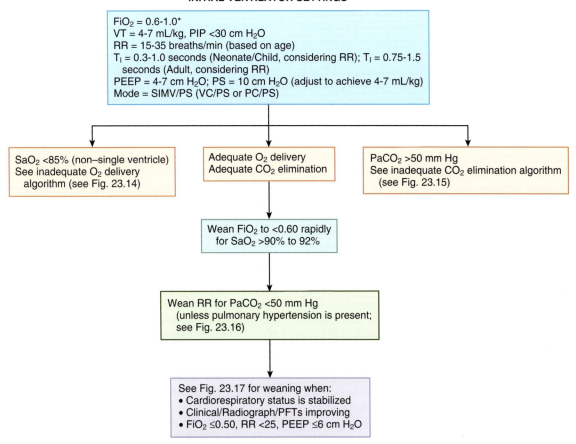

FiO$_2$ = 0.6-1.0*
VT = 4-7 mL/kg, PIP <30 cm H$_2$O
RR = 15-35 breaths/min (based on age)
T$_I$ = 0.3-1.0 seconds (Neonate/Child, considering RR); T$_I$ = 0.75-1.5 seconds (Adult, considering RR)
PEEP = 4-7 cm H$_2$O; PS = 10 cm H$_2$O (adjust to achieve 4-7 mL/kg)
Mode = SIMV/PS (VC/PS or PC/PS)

SaO$_2$ <85% (non–single ventricle)
See inadequate O$_2$ delivery algorithm (see Fig. 23.14)

Adequate O$_2$ delivery
Adequate CO$_2$ elimination

PaCO$_2$ >50 mm Hg
See inadequate CO$_2$ elimination algorithm (see Fig. 23.15)

Wean FiO$_2$ to <0.60 rapidly for SaO$_2$ >90% to 92%

Wean RR for PaCO$_2$ <50 mm Hg (unless pulmonary hypertension is present; see Fig. 23.16)

See Fig. 23.17 for weaning when:
• Cardiorespiratory status is stabilized
• Clinical/Radiograph/PFTs improving
• FiO$_2$ ≤0.50, RR <25, PEEP ≤6 cm H$_2$O

*For infants with single-ventricle physiology, increased pulmonary blood flow, and decreased systemic blood flow, a lower FiO$_2$ may be indicated. (See text for more details.)

• **Figure 23.13** Decision-making algorithm designed for the initiation of positive pressure ventilation in patients with two ventricles after uncomplicated cardiac surgery. Initial ventilatory settings are described, and reduction of ventilatory settings is dependent upon resolution of cardiorespiratory dysfunction. *FiO$_2$,* Fraction of inspired oxygen; *PC,* pressure control; *PEEP,* positive end-expiratory pressure; *PFT,* pulmonary function test; *PIP,* peak inspiratory pressure; *PS,* pressure support; *RR,* respiratory rate (frequency); *SaO$_2$,* arterial oxygen saturation; *SIMV,* synchronized intermittent mandatory ventilation; *T$_I$,* inspiratory time; *VC,* volume control; *VT,* tidal volume.

inadequate to meet tissue/organ oxygen demand. Mechanical ventilation has been shown to be useful in these conditions by reducing work of breathing, which subsequently decreases respiratory muscle oxygen consumption and improves the oxygen supply/demand relationship. The beneficial effects of PPV are especially dramatic in patients who have abnormal pulmonary mechanics and in whom an average reduction of oxygen consumption of 25% can be achieved.[55,56]

PPV reduced lactic acid production in animals with circulatory shock, resulting in the redirection of circulation from respiratory muscles to vital organs.[57,58] The oxygen needs of the respiratory system are high in the newborn period, especially with acute respiratory failure. The withdrawal of either positive or negative pressure ventilatory support in neonatal animals with respiratory failure is associated with a marked alteration in CO attributable to increased work of breathing.[59] For these reasons it is not unusual for neonates with heart disease to require temporary ventilatory support until medical management can be optimized and the patient can adjust to the physiologic changes in the cardiorespiratory system that occur after birth.

Respiratory support in the postoperative period is an extension of the support initiated in the operating room (Fig. 23.13). Communication between the cardiovascular anesthesiologist, cardiac surgeon, and intensive care team is essential. On the patient's arrival in the intensive care unit (ICU), communication is directed at determining the surgical procedure, integrity of the repair, pathophysiology observed after surgery, and potential for cardiovascular or respiratory dysfunction (see Chapter 20 for anesthesia handoff checklist). Next, a complete physical examination should be performed with particular attention to the adequacy of the cardiorespiratory system, including clinical assessments of CO and respiratory function.

Patients who are extubated in the operating room or shortly after admission to the ICU should be monitored for the development of hypoxemia, hypercapnia, and/or increased work of breathing. After a period of time, if hypoxemia and/or hypercapnia is progressive and refractory to conservative therapy (e.g., supplemental nasal/mask oxygen, chest physiotherapy, noninvasive respiratory support), reintubation and the initiation of PPV may be required.

The development of postoperative metabolic acidosis refractory to medical therapy and noninvasive support may require reintubation to optimize the oxygen supply/demand relationship. One should be cautious in attempting to create a compensatory respiratory alkalosis using PPV because such an approach alone does not address the underlying pathophysiologic disturbance(s) and may reduce cerebral blood flow in an already compromised patient.[60] If arterial oxygen content is high and respiratory muscle oxygen consumption low, management should be directed at augmenting DO_2 by improving CO, thereby directly treating the underlying cause of the metabolic acidosis. Mechanical ventilation can decrease oxygen consumption, increase oxygen content, and increase CO, thus favorably altering the supply/demand relationship.

Inspired Oxygen Concentration. Most postoperative patients transferred to the ICU on PPV are initially ventilated with an oxygen concentration (FiO_2) of 0.60 to 1.0, unless there is a small alveolar-arterial gradient. An important exception is a patient with single-ventricle physiology, especially those with signs of increased pulmonary blood flow and decreased systemic blood flow, in which case a "lower" FiO_2 is indicated. In these patients, oxygen should generally be supplemented to maintain an SaO_2 of 75% to 85%.

During transport, fluid shifts and changes in lung volume with resultant alveolar hypoventilation may occur. The initiation of elevated FiO_2 provides a buffer against the development of hypoxia in patients at risk for ventilation/perfusion mismatch. Once transfer has been completed and stable hemodynamics achieved, weaning of the FiO_2 should begin. In general, inspired oxygen is reduced when SaO_2 is above 92%, in the absence of a right-to-left intracardiac shunt. Certain conditions (e.g., pulmonary hypertension) may require prolonged administration of "high" concentrations of inspired oxygen. In the majority of patients, however, a rapid reduction of FiO_2 to nontoxic levels (<0.50) while maintaining SaO_2 above 92% can be accomplished over the initial 6 to 12 hours.

The benefits of oxygen administration should be continually balanced against the potential risks. Arterial hypoxemia in a patient with a two-ventricle repair without intracardiac shunts should not be tolerated, and hypoxic patients should receive the appropriate oxygen necessary to reverse hypoxemia. If the patient does not tolerate a reduction of the FiO_2 to a nontoxic level (<0.50), a comprehensive investigation into the cause of the hypoxemia should be performed. Weaning of inspired oxygen below 0.50 will be discussed in the section on weaning from PPV.

Tidal Volume. In postoperative cardiac patients, careful attention should be paid to the delivered VT because the VT set on the ventilator may be significantly higher than the VT the patient actually receives (referred to as the *delivered or effective* VT).[18,19] This is a result of the distensibility of the ventilator circuit, air leak, and circuit dead space.[19,61-64] This problem is magnified in neonates, in whom a small change in VT leads to a large percentage change in effective VT.[19] For these reasons the delivered VT should be set on the ventilator using a pneumotachometer placed at the ETT (generally, spontaneous breath VT = 4 to 7 mL/kg, mechanical breath delivered VT = 4 to 7 mL/kg). The VT can then be titrated to provide adequate chest excursion and appropriate gas entry as determined by physical examination. The corroboration of adequate gas exchange can then be obtained by blood gas analysis.

Ventilator Frequency. The ventilator frequency should be set based on the physiologic norms based on patient age. Adjustments should then be made based on noninvasive (e.g., pulse oximetry, end-tidal CO_2 monitoring) and invasive (e.g., blood gas analysis) monitoring as clinically indicated. Treatment for alveolar hypoventilation is outlined in the text that follows. Increases in ventilatory frequency above 35 breaths/min may be associated with inadvertent inverse ratio ventilation (depending on the inspiratory time) and subsequently increased EELV and pulmonary overdistention. These higher ventilatory rates should be used cautiously due to the potential detrimental effects of increased lung volume and intrinsic PEEP on gas exchange and cardiorespiratory performance.

Inspiratory Time. The inspiratory time is generally set between 0.3 and 1.0 seconds in infants and children and between 0.75 and 1.5 seconds in adults. A reduction of the inspiratory time below 0.3 seconds does not allow adequate time for the distribution of gas to alveolar units. Prolongation of the inspiratory time in infants may result in an excessively high I:E ratio and inadequate ventilation due to inadequate expiratory time. An excessive prolongation of inspiratory time can also result in significant elevations in mean airway pressure, decreased venous return, and decreased CO.[65]

Prolongation of the inspiratory time with an increased or reversed I:E ratio was historically advocated as a means of increasing mean airway pressure and recruiting low ventilation/perfusion compartments in diseases involving decreased pulmonary compliance.[66] As oxygenation improves with elevation of mean airway pressure, regardless of the phasic pattern of airway pressure,[67] the application of PEEP (see the following section) elevates mean airway pressure with less risk of barotrauma and circulatory depression and is the preferred approach.[68] The precise relationship between inspiratory and expiratory times during PPV should be tailored to address the patient's underlying pathophysiology. As a general guideline, deviation from normal physiologic respiratory patterns with regard to rate and inspiratory time should be avoided.

Positive End-Expiratory Pressure. The application of PEEP is an essential step in providing respiratory support for postoperative patients.[69-72] PEEP opens atelectatic regions of lung, increases EELV, improves ventilation/perfusion matching, and reduces right-to-left intrapulmonary shunting. The net effect of PEEP is generally improved oxygenation.[73-75] In postoperative patients, PEEP is initiated at 4 to 7 cm H_2O to recruit lung volume and prevent alveolar atelectasis. Increased PEEP should be used in specific conditions, including severe reductions in lung compliance (e.g., ARDS). Except in those with severe ARDS, high levels of PEEP (>10 cm H_2O) may result in overexpansion of normal lung units, reduced compliance, increased PVR, increased dead space ventilation, and ventilation/perfusion mismatch due to shunting of blood away from normal yet overexpanded alveoli to abnormal alveoli.[76-81] High PEEP should therefore be avoided unless specifically required for ARDS and must be appropriately monitored. In general, in the absence of intrinsic lung disease, children following cardiac surgery do not require PEEP greater than approximately 8 cm H_2O.

Attempts have been made to physiologically define "optimal PEEP" in terms of total DO_2. However, defining the optimal PEEP level strictly in terms of DO_2 has been criticized because decreased DO_2 secondary to a fall in CO with high levels of PEEP can often be reversed by intravascular volume expansion and/or inotropes. Thus a further enhancement of DO_2 may be achieved by higher levels of PEEP if CO is otherwise maintained.[80,82-84] The level of PEEP associated with maximal DO_2 generally coincides best with the achievement of ideal lung volume and maximum total respiratory compliance.[80]

Ventilator Mode. No data exist to definitely support one mode of ventilation over another for patients with CHD. Thus no recommendations can be made for specific modes. The mode chosen

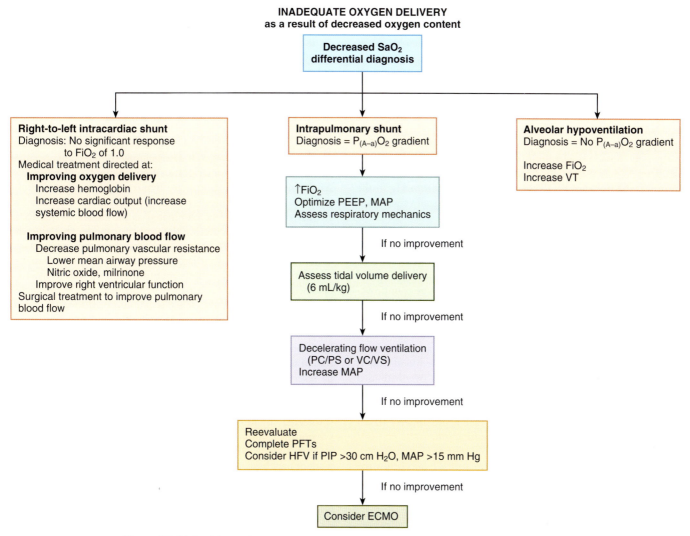

INADEQUATE OXYGEN DELIVERY
as a result of decreased oxygen content

Decreased SaO_2
differential diagnosis

Right-to-left intracardiac shunt
Diagnosis: No significant response
to FiO_2 of 1.0
Medical treatment directed at:
 Improving oxygen delivery
  Increase hemoglobin
  Increase cardiac output (increase
   systemic blood flow)

 Improving pulmonary blood flow
  Decrease pulmonary vascular resistance
   Lower mean airway pressure
   Nitric oxide, milrinone
  Improve right ventricular function
Surgical treatment to improve pulmonary
blood flow

Intrapulmonary shunt
Diagnosis = $P_{(A-a)}O_2$ gradient

↑FiO_2
Optimize PEEP, MAP
Assess respiratory mechanics

If no improvement

Assess tidal volume delivery
(6 mL/kg)

If no improvement

Decelerating flow ventilation
(PC/PS or VC/VS)
Increase MAP

If no improvement

Reevaluate
Complete PFTs
Consider HFV if PIP >30 cm H_2O, MAP >15 mm Hg

If no improvement

Consider ECMO

Alveolar hypoventilation
Diagnosis = No $P_{(A-a)}O_2$ gradient

Increase FiO_2
Increase VT

• **Figure 23.14** Decision-making algorithm for postoperative patients who develop decreased DO_2 during positive pressure ventilation. Identification of the cause for the decreased DO_2 is the initial step in managing this pathophysiology. Causes of decreased SaO_2 include right-to-left intracardiac shunt or ventilation/perfusion mismatch. *DO_2,* Oxygen delivery; *ECMO,* extracorporeal membrane oxygenation; *FiO_2,* fraction of inspired oxygen; *HFOV,* high-frequency oscillatory ventilation; *HFV,* high-frequency ventilation; *MAP,* mean arterial pressure; *P_{(A-a)}O_2,* alveolar-arterial oxygen tension gradient; *PC,* pressure control; *PEEP,* positive end-expiratory pressure; *PFT,* pulmonary function test; *PIP,* peak inspiratory pressure; *PS,* pressure support; *SaO_2,* arterial oxygen saturation; *VC,* volume control; *VS,* volume support.

should be based on the general practices of the ICU with consideration of the pathophysiology of the individual patient. A detailed discussion of the various modes of ventilation is beyond the scope of this chapter. However, it is our general practice to provide a mode with a volume guarantee. That way the $PaCO_2$ and pH will not vary as much as with a pressure control mode. This is important because wide swings in either $PaCO_2$ or pH may affect myocardial performance and vascular resistance.

Physiologic Conditions Requiring Alterations in Support

Inadequate Oxygen Delivery. When DO_2 is inadequate to meet tissue needs, metabolic acidosis develops. In the postoperative period, inadequate DO_2 is usually related to decreased CO from myocardial dysfunction and/or intravascular depletion.

If inadequate DO_2 results from an intracardiac right-to-left shunt, respiratory interventions play a minor role and are directed at decreasing PVR and/or improving RV function. If the primary cause of the decreased DO_2 is a decreased arterial oxygen content, respiratory support is the primary intervention (Fig. 23.14). Alterations in oxygenation are most commonly a result of hypoventilation or ventilation/perfusion mismatch.

The transfer of oxygen from inhaled gas to the pulmonary capillaries is dependent on inspired gas reaching the alveoli, pulmonary blood flow perfusing ventilated alveolar units, presence of an adequate alveolar-to-capillary oxygen gradient, and diffusion of oxygen across the alveolar-capillary membrane. Alterations in oxygen transfer occur when the P_AO_2 in perfused alveolar units falls. This can occur as a result of alveolar hypoventilation (reduction of P_AO_2 in normally functioning alveolar units), low ventilation/perfusion ratio (P_AO_2 falls because of an inability of inspired gas to reach perfused injured alveoli), or high ventilation/perfusion ratio (inability of pulmonary blood to reach ventilated alveoli).

In the postoperative period the cause for arterial hypoxemia is often ventilation/perfusion mismatch. Chest radiography generally demonstrates a reduction in lung volumes with evidence of atelectasis. Respiratory mechanics can help to confirm a reduction in lung volumes by demonstrating a decrease in pulmonary compliance and a prolonged recruitment phase in the inspiratory limb of the pressure-volume curve. The diagnosis of a significant intrapulmonary shunt and hypoxemia from ventilation/perfusion mismatch is made by determining the alveolar-to-arterial oxygen gradient. When the patient breathes 100% oxygen for 15 to 30 minutes, the presence of a PaO_2 of less than 250 mm Hg in the absence of intracardiac shunting indicates a clinically significant intrapulmonary shunt.

The systematic approach outlined for conditions with a low ventilation/perfusion ratio is directed at decreasing intrapulmonary shunt by increasing lung volumes. Initially this is accomplished by increasing PEEP to restore collapsed alveolar units and improve pulmonary compliance. PEEP is increased until there is improvement in arterial hypoxemia or toxicity occurs.[80,85] Excessive PEEP may reduce CO, especially in conditions of hypovolemia and/or myocardial dysfunction. Such a situation can lead to a significant reduction in DO_2.[76,78,80] A worsening of oxygenation has been reported with excessive PEEP, presumably because blood flow is shunted to poorly ventilated alveolar units from overdistended regions of the lung due to a local increase in PVR.[81] These potentially adverse cardiorespiratory effects of PEEP require clinicians to be cautious in applying PEEP levels greater than approximately 10 cm H_2O in children with cardiovascular dysfunction.

During PEEP titration, close attention to respiratory parameters, including VT and compliance, is warranted. If VT falls below the level that provides adequate chest excursion, an increase in VT may be required. If the patient demonstrates hypoxemia despite alterations in PEEP, the VT should be increased to provide adequate VT by examination and respiratory mechanics. If the peak airway pressure exceeds 30 cm H_2O during constant inspiratory flow ventilation (e.g., SIMV, volume control), a decelerating inspiratory flow pattern should be considered. The use of a decelerating flow pattern will usually result in a lower peak airway pressure, a higher mean airway pressure, and improved oxygenation when compared to VCV (square wave, constant inspiratory flow). PCV provides a consistent peak pressure but varying VT depending on lung compliance. Changes in compliance in either direction during PCV can result in swings in oxygenation and ventilation, which may be detrimental. Another approach is to use a mode of ventilation that guarantees minute ventilation/VT while providing a decelerating flow pattern (e.g., PRVC).

If arterial hypoxemia persists, careful reevaluation of the patient is required. The need for FiO_2 above 0.60, PEEP above 6 to 10 cm H_2O, peak airway pressure above 30 cm H_2O, and/or mean airway pressures above 15 cm H_2O likely indicates the presence of respiratory failure and may be associated with a worse prognosis in postoperative CHD patients.[86]

Physical examination, noninvasive testing, and invasive testing should be directed at reevaluating the possibility of a residual or previously undiagnosed right-to-left intracardiac shunt, inadequate pulmonary blood flow, or left heart abnormalities. If severe respiratory failure continues to be the cause of the hypoxia, increasing the PEEP, increasing the inspiratory time, or changing to HFV should be considered. One must assess the effects of these maneuvers on CO, which can generally be done with echocardiography, measurements of lactic acid and mixed venous saturation, and, if indicated, cardiac catherization.[87,88]

Increased Oxygen Consumption. Patient-ventilator dyssynchrony defines a condition in which spontaneous inspiratory efforts are out of phase with positive pressure breaths, resulting in the patient "fighting" the ventilator. During patient-ventilator dyssynchrony, work of breathing is increased, oxygen consumption of the respiratory muscles may be high, and a reduction in effective VT may result. In addition, barotrauma may occur, and cardiac afterload may be adversely affected. The clinical diagnosis is made with the assistance of airway graphics. If dyssynchrony continues, oxygenation and ventilation may deteriorate. When patient-ventilator dyssynchrony is significant, primary hypoxemia due to ventilation/perfusion mismatch, mucous plugging, pneumothorax, and reactive airways disease should be eliminated as the causes. When these causes are eliminated, altering the ventilator mode, changing the inspiratory flow pattern, improving the ventilator trigger sensitivity, or increasing overall ventilator support may improve patient-ventilator synchrony. When manipulation in the ventilator parameters does not improve patient-ventilator synchrony, increased sedation can be attempted. When sedation is instituted/increased, spontaneous ventilation may reduce or cease, and thus ventilatory support should be increased to ensure appropriate gas exchange. Persistence of dyssynchrony after these maneuvers may prompt a trial of neuromuscular blockade. This is rarely required and should be reserved for patients with uncontrollable dyssynchrony and elevated peak airway pressures.

Following cardiac surgery the impaired myocardium can be "protected" by judicious management of mechanical ventilation. Obviously, if respiratory function is completely furnished by the ventilator, there will be no respiratory muscle effort. Subsequently work of breathing, and the associated cardiac work, will be reduced. Using the ventilator to maintain EELV near FRC will minimize the work of $\dot{V}/\dot{Q}$ matching. Preventing patient-ventilator dyssynchrony prevents increased RV afterload and decreased preload while minimizing barotrauma and limiting excessive oxygen consumption. Finally, alleviation of LV afterload by eliminating negative intrathoracic pressure may also be beneficial.

Inadequate Carbon Dioxide Elimination. Another goal of the respiratory system is to remove CO_2 generated from the body's metabolic processes. When CO_2 elimination is inadequate, hypercapnia develops. Although hypoxemia is the most frequently observed abnormality in the immediate postoperative period, hypercapnia more often occurs in the weaning phase. Hypercapnia can have profound effects on a variety of organ systems, including alterations in PVR, myocardial performance, and catecholamine release. Inadequate CO_2 elimination is a result of inadequate minute ventilation or increased alveolar dead space.

Hypercapnia occurs if total minute ventilation is decreased or if dead space ventilation (VD) is increased. The latter is more common in children with heart disease. Because dead space is ventilated but not perfused lung, alterations in CO and pulmonary perfusion can alter dead space. In low cardiac output states, lung perfusion is low, and hypercapnia in the face of normal total minute ventilation indicates increased VD. If pulmonary perfusion can be increased in this setting, $PaCO_2$ should decrease (all other factors being the same). Because the lung is perfused primarily during expiration, an adequate expiratory time is critical. Therefore increasing PPV may actually increase VD and worsen hypercapnia if expiratory time is shortened. Collapsed alveoli require a higher transpulmonary pressure to increase their diameter in comparison to open alveolar units. Therefore a given volume of inspired gas is distributed primarily to open alveoli, and overdistention may occur. Overdistention compresses capillaries, decreases perfusion, and results in increased VD. The volume of inspired gas that results in overdistention does not contribute to gas exchange and results in increased VD and potentially increased volutrauma. As a result of these abnormalities, alveolar minute ventilation (volume of gas involved in gas exchange per unit time) falls.

In all patients with hypercapnia, before the initiation of respiratory interventions a comprehensive examination of the respiratory system is required. Patients with inadequate ventilation or obstruction of medium to large airways have a decreased gas entry to alveoli. The clinical manifestations will be dominated by decreased alveolar ventilation. Tachypnea and tachycardia will be present in the majority of patients with significant hypercapnia. Because patients with inadequate alveolar ventilation and hypercapnia increase work of breathing, they may also demonstrate patient-ventilator dyssynchrony. These patients attempt to compensate for an inadequate alveolar ventilation by increasing the spontaneous rate and may "fight" the ventilator. The presence of hypercapnia can lead to systemic arterial hypertension and occasionally ventricular ectopy secondary to endogenous catecholamine release. Systemic hypertension in this clinical scenario should not be misinterpreted as patient agitation, and administration of sedatives should be avoided until arterial blood gas analysis, clinical assessment, and radiographic assessment are performed. If sedatives are administered to hypercapnic patients, a further reduction in alveolar ventilation may develop, and a worsening of hypercapnia can be precipitated.

The examination of the respiratory system in patients with airway obstruction may demonstrate decreased chest excursion and expiratory wheezing. With inefficient ventilation, symmetric decreased breath sounds will be present. This is in contrast to patients with mechanical obstruction who may demonstrate asymmetric breath sounds. Chest radiographs in patients with inadequate effective alveolar minute ventilation demonstrate decreased lung volumes throughout all lung fields and may show diffuse atelectasis. If mechanical obstruction of the large to medium airways is the cause, larger areas of hypoaeration will be present adjacent to areas of normal aeration. In extreme cases of large airway obstruction, total lobes of the lung can collapse.

The pathophysiology of small airway obstruction caused by bronchospasm differs from the previous causes of airway obstruction. When small airway obstruction from bronchospasm occurs, there is an inability of alveolar gas to be expelled from the lungs. This results in increased lung volumes, development of intrinsic PEEP, and increased VD. On physical examination these patients have evidence of increased lung volume. A markedly prolonged expiratory phase and expiratory wheezing will generally be present on auscultation. Chest radiography demonstrates hyperlucent areas of the lung and increased lung volumes. Respiratory mechanics are diagnostic and will show an increase in expiratory resistance with EELV greater than FRC.

In postoperative patients, hypercapnia generally results from inadequate effective alveolar ventilation secondary to collapsed alveoli and small airways. When this occurs, an appropriate increase in VT and/or PEEP may be required. Airway pressures should be monitored to ensure that they are not in the toxic range. If the measured VT is appropriate, an increase in the respiratory frequency should be attempted, while monitoring the I:E ratio. Continued hypercapnia may require an increase in sedation or neuromuscular blockade if patient-ventilator dyssynchrony is present.[62,74,89,90] In the presence of continued hypercapnia, VT could be increased

until hypercapnia resolves or until a peak airway pressure of approximately 30 cm H_2O is reached. If hypercapnia continues, one could consider conversion to an alternative mode of ventilation to provide improved effective minute ventilation at a lower peak airway pressure (Fig. 23.15).

Patients with small airway disease require therapy directed at reversing bronchospasm, promoting the ability of retained alveolar gas to be exchanged with inspired gas, and increasing alveolar ventilation. The initial approach should be to increase the expiratory time by reducing the respiratory rate while maintaining the inspiratory time in the appropriate physiologic range. When the respiratory rate is reduced, the VT may be increased to provide an adequate alveolar ventilation. If this does not allow adequate emptying of the alveoli, a reduction of inspiratory time can be attempted. Bronchodilator therapy should be considered early in the management of patients with CHD and small airway obstruction. In these patients, alveolar hyperexpansion and hypercapnia can result in dramatic alterations in cardiovascular function, and aggressive respiratory interventions are required to prevent the development of severe cardiorespiratory failure. Respiratory mechanics are recommended in all patients with significant gas trapping because a variety of management approaches may be necessary.

Therapy for Specific Pathophysiologic Conditions

Left Ventricular Dysfunction. In postoperative patients with LV dysfunction, cardiorespiratory interactions should be evaluated and directed at optimizing LV function.[37,91-93] Because PPV decreases venous return and LV afterload (which have contrasting effects on CO), careful attention to hemodynamic function is required when ventilating children with LV dysfunction. Maintaining EELV near FRC while minimizing airway pressure will optimize LV function.

If patients with LV dysfunction develop pulmonary edema and decreased systemic oxygen saturation, oxygen content may fall, and DO_2 will be further compromised. In these instances an increased FiO_2 may be needed, PEEP should be titrated to improve oxygenation, and packed red blood cell transfusion may be considered to augment oxygen-carrying capacity.

Right Ventricular Dysfunction. Patients with RV dysfunction will benefit from manipulations of cardiorespiratory interactions to optimize RV preload and minimize RV afterload. In patients with RV dysfunction, PPV is initiated with settings as previously described. RV afterload can be reduced by hyperoxygenation and alkalization if pulmonary hypertension is present. Inhaled nitric oxide may also be considered. Because the majority of pulmonary blood flow occurs during expiration, inspiratory time should be short compared to expiratory times. PEEP should be set to maintain EELV near FRC to minimize PVR as described earlier. Patients with RV dysfunction are particularly sensitive to changes in intrathoracic pressure because CO is preload dependent. These patients may benefit from ventilation strategies that reduce intrathoracic pressure and increase preload, such as reducing the mean airway pressure. This can be accomplished by minimizing end-expiratory pressure, decreasing inspiratory time, and using the mode of ventilation with the lowest intrathoracic pressure. The RV response to ventilatory manipulations is more dramatic in patients with concomitant hypovolemia because RV preload is already reduced. Therefore strict attention to intravascular volume status is required in patients with RV dysfunction and elevated intrathoracic pressures. HFJV may be considered in patients with

INADEQUATE CARBON DIOXIDE ELIMINATION
INADEQUATE ALVEOLAR VENTILATION

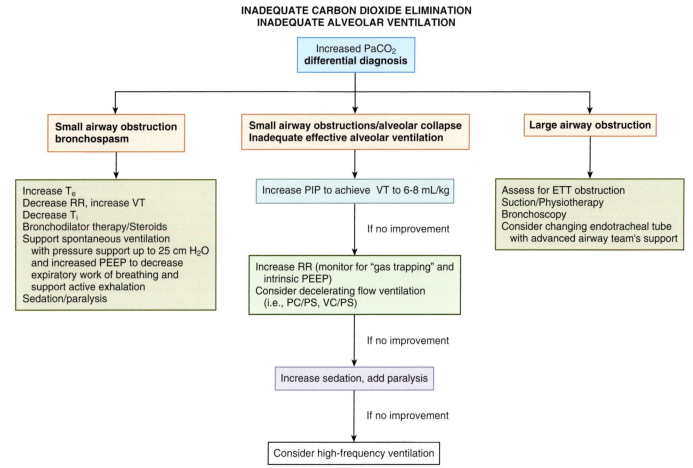

• **Figure 23.15** Decision-making algorithm designed for postoperative patients who develop increased $PaCO_2$. Elevated $PaCO_2$ is a result of inadequate alveolar ventilation. This can be categorized into patho-logic conditions that result in small or large airway obstruction or alveolar collapse. Strategies are then dependent upon the underlying pathophysiology. All approaches require an increase in effective alveolar ventilation. *ETT*, Endotracheal tube; *PC*, pressure control; *PEEP*, positive end-expiratory pressure; *PIP*, peak inspiratory pressure; *PS*, pressure support; *RR*, respiratory rate; T_e, expiratory time; T_i, inspiratory time; *VC*, volume control; *VT*, tidal volume.

RV dysfunction who require mean airway pressures greater than 12 cm H_2O. HFJV may allow a reduction of mean airway pressure, improved RV preload, and increased RV output.[37]

Pulmonary Artery Hypertension. Therapy for pulmonary artery hypertension is directed at lowering pulmonary artery pressures and improving RV function by optimizing preload and contractility (Fig. 23.16).[94-96] Patients with elevated PVR are sensitive to changes in RV preload. Because of the increased afterload, the RV will require increased RV preload to maximize RV stroke volume. Therefore these patients often require higher than usual filling pressures. As afterload increases, the end-systolic volume of the RV increases. An increase in RV diastolic and systolic volume can result in conformational changes of the intraventricular septum, which can cause a reduction of LV preload and thus stroke volume.[53] Patients with pulmonary hypertension frequently require inotropic agents to increase RV output. However, the use of inotropic agents in patients with pulmonary artery hypertension has had limited success. This may be related to the relative insensitivity of the RV to inotropes. Agents such as dopamine, epinephrine, and dobu-tamine have limited utility in treating patients with pulmonary hypertensive crisis, and these patients are more successfully treated by decreasing the RV afterload. Maintaining RV coronary perfusion

pressure through inotropic support may be helpful because RV perfusion occurs primarily during systole as previously described.[97]

Therapy directed at reducing pulmonary hypertension consists of increasing pH, decreasing $PaCO_2$, increasing PaO_2 and P_AO_2, and optimizing intrathoracic pressures.[94-96,98,99] (Inhaled nitric oxide can also be administered and is discussed in detail in Chapter 13). When treating pulmonary hypertension with decreasing $PaCO_2$, the potential adverse physiologic effects on the cerebral vasculature must be considered. Both an increase in pH and a reduction in $PaCO_2$ could independently result in a reduction in RV afterload. Studies have shown that an increase in both alveolar oxygen (P_AO_2) and arterial oxygen (PaO_2) by increasing inspired oxygen concentra-tion reduces PVR.[94,96] Increasing inspired oxygen in patients with intracardiac shunts may result in little change in PaO_2; however, a reduction in PVR may occur. This effect is related to an increase in P_AO_2 and demonstrates that an increase in both alveolar and arterial oxygen content can alter PVR. In animal studies, increasing inspired oxygen concentration has been shown to be a more potent pulmonary vasodilator in neonates compared with adults.[96] The use of inspired oxygen to reduce PVR has been useful in the ICU and is a frequent mode of interrogating pulmonary vascular responsiveness in the cardiac catheterization laboratory.[96]

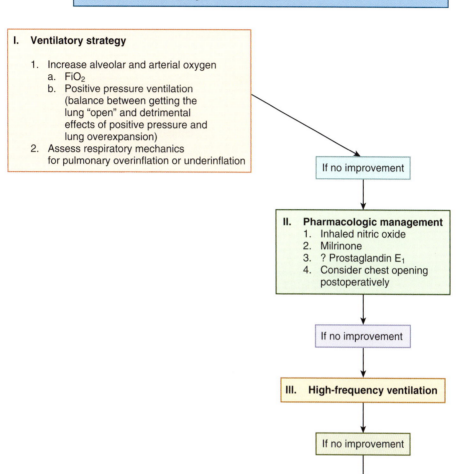

PULMONARY ARTERY HYPERTENSION

Diagnosis: Decreased oxygen delivery as a result of pulmonary hypertension, decreased right ventricular output, and decreased pulmonary blood flow
Treatment: Decrease right ventricular afterload

I. **Ventilatory strategy**

1. Increase alveolar and arterial oxygen
   a. FiO_2
   b. Positive pressure ventilation (balance between getting the lung "open" and detrimental effects of positive pressure and lung overexpansion)
2. Assess respiratory mechanics for pulmonary overinflation or underinflation

If no improvement

II. **Pharmacologic management**
1. Inhaled nitric oxide
2. Milrinone
3. ? Prostaglandin E_1
4. Consider chest opening postoperatively

If no improvement

III. **High-frequency ventilation**

If no improvement

IV. **ECMO**

• **Figure 23.16** Decision-making algorithm for postoperative patients with pulmonary artery hypertension. Manipulations of pH, FiO_2, and ventilatory mechanics are the most crucial. *ECMO,* Extracorporeal membrane oxygenation; *FiO_2,* fraction of inspired oxygen.

PPV is often required in patients with pulmonary artery hypertension. The effects of different types of ventilation on PVR are not well established. A reduction in mean airway pressure has been shown to reduce PVR.[37] Patients with pulmonary artery hypertension may benefit from hyperventilation, but because of the detrimental effects of elevated mean airway pressure on PVR and RV filling, mean airway pressure should be limited.[100,101] PEEP must be used judiciously in these patients. High PEEP (>10 cm H_2O) / high mean airway pressure may result in alveolar overdistention and compression of the pulmonary capillaries with a resultant increase in PVR.[15] Therefore the overall approach to these patients should be directed at providing the necessary amount of PEEP to maintain the lungs at FRC (see Fig. 23.12).

Several differences in lung physiology in infants lead to EELV less than FRC, increased closing capacity, and increased airway collapse during normal tidal breathing.[102-105] This process results in a ventilation/perfusion mismatch with segments of lung demonstrating perfusion without ventilation.[106] As these nonventilated lung segments become hypoxic, a secondary hypoxic response can develop, and PVR increases. Respiratory mechanics can be used to optimize VT delivery and PEEP in these patients.

Weaning From Positive Pressure Ventilation

When PPV is required for a longer time than expected for the surgical procedure performed, a thorough investigation for the presence of residual cardiac disease or intercurrent illness is necessary. Weaning from PPV requires the patient to gradually assume the entire work of breathing. Understanding respiratory muscle performance in infants and children is necessary to transition from PPV to unassisted ventilation.[107]

As a patient assumes an increase in respiratory muscle work, inadequate gas exchange with resultant hypoxemia and hypercapnia

WEANING

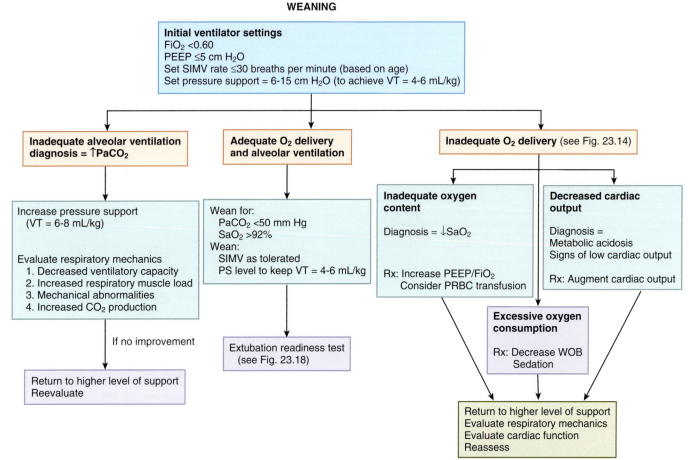

• **Figure 23.17** Decision-making algorithm designed to promote weaning. The SIMV rate and pressure support levels are reduced as respiratory mechanics improve. Weaning is terminated when inadequate DO_2 or inadequate alveolar ventilation (increased $PaCO_2$) occurs. When this occurs, the strategy is directed at treating reversible causes and supporting the cardiorespiratory system until resolution of cardiorespiratory dysfunction has occurred. *DO_2*, Oxygen delivery; *FiO_2*, fraction of inspired oxygen; *PEEP*, positive end-expiratory pressure; *PIP*, peak inspiratory pressure; *PRBC*, packed red blood cells; *PS*, pressure support; *Rx*, treatment plan; *SaO_2*, arterial oxygen saturation; *SIMV*, synchronized intermittent mandatory ventilation; *VT*, tidal volume; *WOB*, work of breathing.

and inadequate DO_2 will occur if the cardiorespiratory system is unable to achieve its goals (Fig. 23.17).

Oxygenation. Hypoxia during weaning from PPV usually results from ventilation/perfusion mismatch (intrapulmonary shunt). As PEEP and peak airway pressures are reduced, atelectasis may develop with resultant loss of lung volume and increased intrapulmonary shunt. Impaired gas exchange from right-to-left intrapulmonary shunting can be identified by the presence of an elevated alveolar-arterial oxygen tension gradient, $P_{(A-a)}O_2$. When hypoxemia is encountered, an increased FiO_2 may be necessary. If the hypoxemia persists, the cause of the hypoxemia must be investigated and corrected. If loss of lung volume is the cause of the ventilation/perfusion mismatch, an increase in PEEP may be necessary and weaning suspended until improvements in pulmonary compliance are seen.

Oxygen Delivery. Abnormalities of respiratory mechanics lead to increased work of breathing. When the patient is sedated and receiving high levels of cardiorespiratory support, respiratory muscle oxygen consumption may be minimal. In contrast, in critically ill patients, 50% of total oxygen consumption may be used by the respiratory muscles in response to the increased workload.[56]

Therefore significant resolution of cardiorespiratory dysfunction should occur before weaning from PPV is performed. If marginal DO_2 and abnormal respiratory mechanics are present, weaning may result in an imbalance between oxygen supply and demand, anaerobic metabolism, and metabolic acidosis.[58] The development of a metabolic acidosis during the weaning phase requires reinstitution of previous ventilatory support and an aggressive evaluation for the underlying pathophysiologic disturbance.

Carbon Dioxide Elimination. In infants and children the most common cause of failure to wean from PPV is inadequate alveolar ventilation due to respiratory muscle pump failure. The etiology of respiratory muscle pump failure can be categorized into two causes: decreased ventilatory capacity and increased respiratory muscle load (Box 23.1). Respiratory muscle failure can be caused by a variety of events, including shock, hypoxemia, and hypercapnia. These conditions diminish the contraction of the diaphragm and may cause a decrease in VT via impairment of excitation-contraction coupling by intracellular acidosis.[108-110] When the respiratory muscles cannot provide adequate alveolar ventilation, respiratory acidosis results from an inadequate effective VT. The patient will attempt to compensate for the reduced VT by increasing the respiratory

Decreased Ventilatory Capacity

Neurologic
- Decreased respiratory center output
- Cervical spinal cord surgery
- Phrenic nerve dysfunction

Respiratory muscle
- Hyperinflation
- Malnutrition
- Metabolic derangements
- Decreased oxygen supply
- Disuse atrophy
- Fatigue
- Abdominal wall defects

Increased Respiratory Muscle Load

Increased ventilatory requirements
- Increased CO2 production
- Increased dead space ventilation
- Inappropriately elevated ventilatory drive

Increased work of breathing

Decreased efficiency of breathing
- Increased chest wall compliance
- Respiratory pattern

Data from Martin LD, Rafferty JF, Walker LK, et al. Principles of respiratory support and mechanical ventilation. In: Rogers MC, ed. Textbook of Pediatric Intensive Care. *Baltimore: Williams & Wilkins; 1992:135-203.*

frequency. The presence of hypercapnia despite a significant increase in respiratory frequency necessitates termination of weaning. Patients who require diuretic support may develop a metabolic alkalosis and a mild-to-moderate compensatory respiratory acidosis. These patients will have an increased $PaCO_2$ and normal (or possibly increased) pH, and weaning should continue provided the increased pH does not significantly reduce the respiratory drive.

Failure to wean from PPV can also occur from a variety of conditions that reduce ventilatory performance. Airway obstruction with lung hyperinflation from diseases such as bronchomalacia, bronchopulmonary dysplasia, airway compression by vascular structures, or chronic lung disease may occur.[111] Hyperinflation of the lungs leads to a flattened diaphragm and shortened fiber length, which results in a decreased transdiaphragmatic pressure generation. Additionally, tidal breathing occurs at the upper, less compliant portion of the pressure-volume curve of the lung.[112] Malnutrition[113,114] and metabolic derangements such as hypomagnesemia, hypophosphatemia, hypocalcemia, and hypokalemia may impair respiratory muscle performance and present as an inability to wean from ventilatory support.[115-117]

Disuse atrophy of the respiratory musculature may complicate weaning attempts.[118] Infants lack fatigue-resistant type I fibers and may be more susceptible to fatigue.[119] Phrenic nerve dysfunction or, less commonly, neurologic causes such as inadequate respiratory center output can cause failure to wean from PPV. Residual respiratory depressant drugs, such as opioids and benzodiazepines, may complicate weaning attempts. These patients hypoventilate but do not demonstrate increased work of breathing. Finally, the highly compliant chest wall and the rapid, shallow respiratory pattern of the neonate significantly decrease ventilatory efficiency, increase work of breathing, and may result in weaning failure.

Increased Ventilatory Requirements. Rarely, failure to wean from PPV can occur when there are increased ventilatory requirements without adequate compensation. Increased ventilatory requirements may be a result of increased tissue CO_2 production necessitating increased alveolar ventilation to preserve normocapnia. Excessive carbohydrate calories during enteral and parenteral nutrition can cause hypercapnia due to excessive CO_2 production. In addition, CO_2 production increases with fevers (10% increase for each degree centigrade) and excessive muscle activity (e.g., seizures, shivering, rigor). Conditions that increase the ratio of physiologic dead space to tidal volume (VD/VT) such as reduced CO, airway obstruction, or excessive positive airway pressure require an increase in minute ventilation to maintain effective ventilation and normocapnia. Increased dead space is common postoperatively, and virtually all children require minute ventilation greater than normal following surgery. Increased ventilatory requirements can also occur from other pathophysiologic conditions. Excessive respiratory drive from psychologic stress, neurologic lesions, or pulmonary irritant receptor stimulation may lead to inappropriate hyperventilation and increased respiratory muscle load.

Techniques for Weaning. Following uncomplicated closed-heart or simple bypass procedures such as atrial septal closure or correction of aortic or pulmonary obstruction, extubation can occur shortly after surgery when the patient is awake and fully recovered from anesthesia.[120] This may occur in the pediatric ICU or the operating room. Other children may require more prolonged ventilation. Risk factors predicting the potential need for prolonged PPV include younger age (<10 months), lower weight, greater STAT* (Society of Thoracic Surgeons–European Association for Cardio-Thoracic Surgery) Congenital Heart Surgery Mortality Categories, and longer length of stay.[121,122] Preexisting pulmonary disease and severe systemic disease complicated by malnutrition may also prolong the need for ventilatory support.

During weaning the patient assumes the work of breathing, which includes both patient demands and the demands imposed by the artificial respiratory support. The mechanically imposed work of breathing is a function of the ETT size, circuit size, inspiratory gas flow rate, and ventilator type. The work of breathing imposed by these factors can be quite substantial, especially in the neonate who requires a small ETT. Any method of weaning ventilatory support must take these considerations into account. There are no well-controlled clinical trials that demonstrate a clear superiority for any one approach over another.[123]

The appearance of respiratory distress, hypoxemia, or CO_2 retention at any point should temporarily halt further weaning efforts.

Criteria for Extubation. Predicting successful extubation in infants and children presents unique challenges to the pediatric intensive care physician. Currently there are no widely accepted criteria for predicting successful extubation in children. Methods used to predict extubation in adults, such as respiratory frequency to VT ratio,[124,125] CROP index (compliance, rate, oxygenation, and pressure),[125] T-piece trials, and negative inspiratory effort measurements,[126] are either unreliable or not easily performed in children. Recently, a pediatric clinical study by Khan and colleagues[127] characterized multiple predictors of extubation failure. Unfortunately, these authors were unable to identify a single parameter or formula for predicting extubation in children and concluded that a combination of factors should influence any extubation decision.

The use of extubation readiness testing (ERT) has received increased interest. Several studies have shown that this reduces the length of ventilation and reintubation rates. The criteria for a methodology for ERT are outlined in Fig. 23.18.

Extubation Readiness Testing (ERT)

- Indications
  - Spontaneous respiratory drive
  - PEEP setting between 5 and 8 cm H_2O
  - FiO_2 requirement less than 0.50
  - Hemodynamically stable

- ERT

  - Set FiO_2 to <0.5
  - Set PEEP to 5 cm H_2O
  - Set PSV mode as follows:

ETT	PSV
3.0-3.5	10
4.0-4.5	8
≥5.0	6

- Monitor patient SpO_2, VT, RR, work of breathing for 60-90 minutes (RN documents BP)

  - Exhaled VT should be at least 5 mL/kg
  - RR

Age	RR
<6 mo	20-60
6 mo–2 y	15-45
2 y–5 y	15-40
>5 y	10-35

  - SpO_2 must maintain within the prescribed range for the duration of the test on FiO_2 <0.5.

Extubation Guideline*

- Patient passes an ERT
- PIP ≤25 cm H_2O
- PEEP ≤5 cm H_2O
- Set respiratory rate ≤10 breaths/min
- Pressure support adequate to overcome resistance of ETT
- Blood gas analysis results at clinical goals

• **Figure 23.18** Extubation Readiness Testing Indications and Process. *BP,* Blood pressure; *ERT,* extubation readiness testing; *ETT,* endotracheal tube; *FiO₂,* fraction of inspired oxygen; *PEEP,* positive end-expiratory pressure; *PIP,* peak inspiratory pressure; *PSV,* pressure support ventilation; *RN,* registered nurse; *RR,* respiratory rate; *SpO₂,* oxygen saturation as measured by pulse oximetry, *VT,* tidal volume.

Several studies have attempted to define criteria for extubation in children.[128-131] Hubble and colleagues[129] demonstrated that the V_D/V_T ratio may be a useful, objective determinant of the readiness for extubation in infants and children. Shoults and colleagues[132] were unable to find a correlation between maximum negative inspiratory airway pressure and successful removal of PPV in a group of neonates. In a group of older infants receiving postoperative PPV the combination of a crying vital capacity above 15 mL/kg and a maximum negative inspiratory airway pressure greater than 45 cm H_2O accurately predicted successful discontinuation of ventilatory support. Failure to meet these criteria was associated with a failure to tolerate withdrawal of PPV and extubation.[132] In a separate study, DiCarlo and colleagues[128] demonstrated a reduced mean lung compliance during the acute phase of ventilation. However, the primary determinants of the inability to extubate were an elevated airway resistance during the weaning phase and postoperative weight gain. In neonates weight gain may be an important determinant of the ability to extubate. Weaning should

be considered when there has been adequate resolution of cardiovascular dysfunction and respiratory mechanics have improved such that the work of breathing is not excessive.

Extubation of the trachea should be considered in the presence of normal arterial oxygenation and CO_2 elimination ($PaCO_2$ <45 torr) on minimal ventilatory support (PEEP 5 cm H_2O, pressure support 6 to 10 cm H_2O, and inspired oxygen < −0.50). Monitoring of the patient includes oxygen saturation as measured by pulse oximetry (SpO_2), VT, respiratory rate, work of breathing, and blood pressure for 60 to 90 minutes with an arterial blood gas analysis to help determine success. Exhaled VT should be at least 5 mL/kg. Taken together with the previously mentioned indices of respiratory reserve, these criteria indicate the ability to tolerate independent ventilation with acceptable requirements for supplemental oxygen.

Noninvasive ventilation use is prevalent in patients with CHD. In a study by Romans and colleagues, nearly 4000 patients in the Pediatric Cardiac Critical Care Consortium clinical registry were begun on high-flow nasal cannula and positive airway pressure support during a 2-year period. These data underscore the important role of noninvasive support for these patients. They noted that neonates, extracardiac anomalies, single ventricle, procedure complexity, preoperative respiratory support, mechanical ventilation duration, and postoperative disease severity were associated with noninvasive ventilation therapy ($P < .001$ for all). There was also a wide range of use from 32% to 65%, and adjusted mean noninvasive ventilation duration ranged from 1 to 4 days.[133]

The method of noninvasive ventilation varies as well. High-flow nasal cannula (HFNC) and CPAP have advantages and disadvantages. HFNC has the advantage of being "less invasive" because it does not require a device that encompasses the face. In studies on HFNC the delivered PEEP is variable. In a recent study the effects of HFNC showed a nonlinear increase in PEEP in closed-mouth modes, but in open-mouth modes, a disadvantage of HFNC, there was an actual decrease in PEEP. Although HFNC improved expiratory CO_2 elimination, there is a maximum flow at which this benefit ceases to occur, which was 4 L/min in the preterm infant and 10 L/min in the small child.[134]

Positive airway pressure support is usually provided as CPAP either nasally or by mask. Nasal CPAP has been studied in patients with bronchiolitis and has shown some evidence for a benefit versus HFNC. CPAP does have significant compliance issues, which may limit its use.[135]

Our approach: We typically start with HFNC. If there is failure of this therapy (defined as increased work or breathing, increased respiratory rate, desaturation or destabilization of cardiovascular status, or alterations in ABG levels), CPAP is instituted. The CPAP is initially begun as nasal CPAP. Again, if there is failure as defined earlier, then mask CPAP is begun. Each institution must develop a protocol that is standardized and that the institution is comfortable with.[136]

Conclusion

Respiratory support for infants and children with CHD requires a thorough understanding of cardiorespiratory performance. With use of the principles of cardiac function, respiratory physiology, and cardiorespiratory interactions, a management strategy can be developed that is matched to the pathophysiology of the patient. This strategy will vary depending upon the pathophysiology of the patient. The principles outlined in this chapter will allow clinicians the opportunity to maximize patient care and improve outcome variables.

Selected References

A complete list of references is available at ExpertConsult.com.

26. Bateman ST, Borasino S, Asaro LA, et al. Early High Frequency Oscillatory Ventilation in Pediatric Acute Respiratory Failure: A Propensity Score Analysis. *Am J Respir Crit Care Med.* 2015 Oct 22.

48. Millar JC, Horton J, Brizard C. Nitric oxide administration during paediatric cardiopulmonary bypass: a randomised controlled trial. *Intensive Care Med.* 2016;42(11):1744–1752.

60. Mott AR, Alomrani A, Tortoriello TA, et al. Changes in cerebral saturation profile in response to mechanical ventilation alterations in infants with bidirectional superior cavopulmonary connection. *Pediatr Crit Care Med.* 2006;7(4):346–350.

86. Gupta P, Rettiganti M, Gossett JM, et al. Risk factors for mechanical ventilation and reintubation after pediatric heart surgery. *J Thorac Cardiovasc Surg.* 2015 Sep 28. pii: S0022-5223(15)01789-4).

122. Winch PD, Staudt AM, Sebastian R, et al. Learning From Experience: Improving Early Tracheal Extubation Success After Congenital Cardiac Surgery. *Pediatr Crit Care Med.* 2016;17(7):630–637.

133. Romans RA, Schwartz SM, Costello RA, et al. Epidemiology of Noninvasive Ventilation in Pediatric Cardiac ICUs. *Pediatr Crit Care Med.* 2017;18(10):949–957.

134. Nielsen KR, Ellington LE, Gray AJ. Effect of High-Flow Nasal Cannula on Expiratory Pressure and Ventilation in Infant, Pediatric, and Adult Models. *Resp Care.* 2017 Oct 24.

135. Milesi C, Essouri S, Pouyau R, et al. High flow nasal cannula (HFNC) versus nasal continuous positive airway pressure (nCPAP) for the initial respiratory management of acute viral bronchiolitis in young infants: a multicenter randomized controlled trial (TRAMONTANE study). *Intensive Care Med.* 2017;43(2):209–216.

24

Coagulation Disorders in Congenital Heart Disease

KRISTEN NELSON MCMILLAN, MD; JENNIFER KRAMER, MD; CLIFF M. TAKEMOTO, MD; CAROLINE P. OZMENT, MD

In 1950 Bahnson and Ziegler first observed a hemorrhagic diathesis in patients with congenital heart disease (CHD). In fact, hemorrhage was the fourth leading cause of mortality in the first group of patients to undergo the Blalock-Taussig shunt.[1] In his classic article, "A Hemorrhagic Disorder Occurring in Patients With Cyanotic Congenital Heart Disease," Hartmann[2] noted that 18 patients bled to death after this surgery. He noted that these patients had thrombocytopenia, abnormal clot retraction, low fibrinogen levels, and prolonged bleeding times and observed an association between the degree of polycythemia and the hemorrhagic diathesis.

Over 60 years of progress in hematology and CHD have confirmed Hartmann's observations. Despite significant advances in the characterization of hemostatic abnormalities in CHD, the precise nature of the defect remains incompletely understood due to its multifactorial nature and individual variation. Preoperative hematologic screening has improved, yet perioperative hemorrhage still complicates approximately 5% of pediatric open-heart surgery, and thrombosis is now recognized as a significant problem often long after the recovery from surgery is complete.[3,4]

This chapter will review the process of normal coagulation in infants and children, examine the various tests of the clotting mechanism, review the alterations of hemostasis in CHD, consider the impact of cardiopulmonary bypass (CPB) and other mechanical circulatory support devices on hemostasis, and develop strategies for the diagnosis and management of bleeding and thrombosis after pediatric cardiac surgery.

Hemostasis: Cell-Based Coagulation

The classic coagulation cascade model, proposed in 1964 by Macfarlane[5] and Davie and Ratnoff,[6] was accepted for almost 50 years, and although it tremendously improved the understanding of coagulation, we now know this model has some limitations and cannot satisfactorily explain all phenomena related to in vivo hemostasis. The conventional cascade model proposed that coagulation occurs through sequential proteolytic activation of proenzymes by plasma proteases, resulting in the formation of thrombin, which then breaks up fibrinogen to fibrin. This model divided coagulation in an extrinsic pathway (involving components that are usually not found in the intravascular space) and an intrinsic pathway (started by components that exist in the intravascular space), which converge to a common pathway with the activation of factor X.

The current cell-based model, on the other hand, proposes that hemostasis requires activated procoagulant substances that remain at the site of the injury and are involved in the formation of platelet and fibrin plugs.[7-10] The process for clotting is initiated by contact of tissue factor (TF) to the bloodstream. TF is a transmembrane protein that acts as a receptor and cofactor for factor VII (FVII). TF is not constitutively expressed in endothelial cells but is present in the membranes of cells around blood vessels, such as in smooth muscle cells and fibroblasts. Thus TF is exposed to the bloodstream due to damage to the endothelium and surrounding cells or by the activation of endothelial cells or monocytes.[11,12] As we begin this discussion of the complex process of coagulation, it is important to understand the concept of a cofactor. Cofactors are necessary for the appropriate subsequent reactions to occur, such as TF serving as cofactor for FVII to initiate the clotting process. Calcium is also necessary for this reaction, serves as a cofactor for several other reactions in clotting, and has been referred to as factor IV. Reactions involving cofactors generally require phospholipid surfaces, which become exposed due to injury. This requirement ensures that clot forms only at sites of vascular injury.

The model of cell-based coagulation has been described to have four phases[7-10]: (1) initiation of coagulation on TF-bearing cells, (2) amplification of the procoagulant signal by thrombin generated on the TF-bearing cell, (3) propagation of thrombin generation on the platelet surface, and (4) termination to prevent pathologic thrombosis. Given the complexity of the coagulation system, it is recommended that you refer to Figs. 24.1 and 24.2 as you read through the phases of coagulation and the role of anticoagulants in this chapter.

Initiation Phase

The initiation phase of coagulation occurs when cells or cellular fragments that express TF on their surface are exposed to blood components at the site of injury.[7-10] Injury encompasses a number of conditions, including surgery, trauma, and infection. Inflammation releases cytokines, which can also induce cells to express TF in the absence of overt vessel injury, which is why inflammatory conditions are often considered procoagulant states. Regardless of how TF is expressed, once TF is bound to FVII in blood, it quickly activates FVIIa, forming the FVIIa/TF complex, which is responsible for the subsequent activation of small amounts of FIX and FX. The FVIIa/TF complex appears to be essential for initiation of in

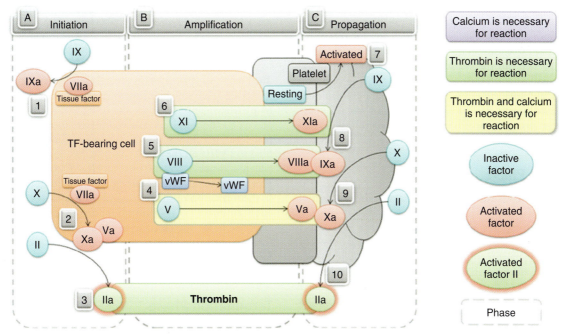

• **Figure 24.1** Cell-based model of blood coagulation. Initiation phase *(A)*. *(1)* On the TF-bearing cell, TF-FVIIa complex converts FIX to FIXa and *(2)* converts FX to FXa. *(3)* FXa combines with FVa to convert II to IIa (thrombin). Amplification phase *(B)* (involves TF-bearing cells and platelets). *(4)* Thrombin converts FV to FVa in the presence of calcium. *(5)* Thrombin assists cleavage of FVIII-vWF to FVIII and free vWF. *(6)* Factor XI is converted to XIa through actions of thrombin. Propagation phase *(C)*. *(7)* Resting platelet is activated. *(8)* FIX is converted to IXa through actions of FXIa. *(9)* FIXa combines with FVIIIa to convert FX to FXa. *(10)* FXa combines with FVa to convert II to IIa (thrombin). *a,* Activated; *TF,* tissue factor; *vWF,* von Willebrand factor. (From Swanepoel AC, Nielsen VG, Pretorius E. Viscoelasticity and ultrastructure in coagulation and inflammation: two diverse techniques, one conclusion. *Inflammation.* 2015;38[4]:1707-1726.)

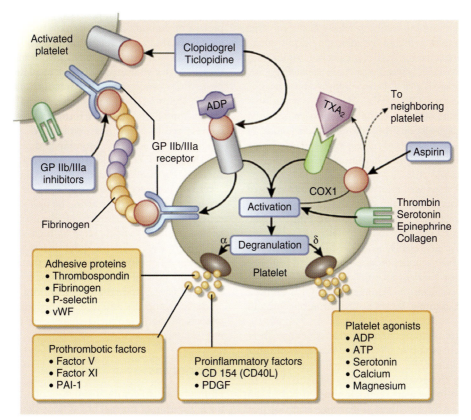

• **Figure 24.2** Mechanisms of platelet activation. *ADP,* Adenosine diphosphate; *ATP,* adenosine triphosphate; *CD,* cluster of differentiation; *COX1,* cyclooxygenase-1; *GP,* glycoprotein; *PAI-1,* plasminogen activator inhibitor type 1; *PDGF,* platelet-derived growth factor; *TXA₂,* thromboxane A₂; *vWF,* von Willebrand factor. (From Daugirdas JT, Bernardo AA. Hemodialysis effect on platelet count and function and hemodialysis-associated thrombocytopenia. *Kidney Int.* 2012;82[2]:147-157.)

vivo clotting. FXa can activate factor V (FVa), which is a cofactor for FXa, and together they form a complex called prothrombinase on the surface of cells that express TF. This complex transforms small amounts of prothrombin (factor II) to thrombin (Fig. 24.1). It has been suggested that the initiation phase remains continuously active, with small quantities of activated factors being produced at baseline. Thus small amounts of thrombin are continuously produced outside the vascular space, independent of vascular injury. The coagulation process proceeds to the amplification phase only when there is vascular damage.

Amplification Phase

The amplification phase involves the process of thrombin activation of platelets and cofactors V, VIII, and IX on the surface of platelets. FVIII is actually composed of two parts: (1) factor VIII, which helps IXa activate factor X, and (2) von Willebrand factor (vWF), which binds to a platelet membrane protein (glycoprotein Ib) and promotes platelet adhesion. Due to their large sizes, platelets and FVIII/vWF can pass to the extravascular space only when there is vascular injury. Furthermore, the intact endothelium produces the platelet-inhibiting substances nitric oxide and prostacyclin. When a vessel is injured, platelets leave the vessel and bind to collagen and other components of the extracellular matrix at the site of injury, where they are partially activated and form a platelet plug responsible for primary hemostasis. Small amounts of thrombin produced by cells that express TF as described earlier can then interact with platelets and the FVIII/vWF complex. The FVIII/vWF complex then dissociates, allowing vWF to mediate platelet adhesion and aggregation at the site of injury. This begins the hemostatic process that culminates in the formation of stable fibrin, referred to as secondary hemostasis, which consolidates the initial platelet plug.[7-15]

Platelet activation by thrombin results in release of the contents of their cytoplasmic granules, including adenosine diphosphate (ADP), serotonin, platelet factor 4 (PF_4), catecholamines, and thromboxane A_2. Upon platelet activation by these released agonists a signalling process is initiated, giving rise to conformational changes within the platelet receptor GPIIb/IIIa. These conformational changes increase the affinity of this receptor for fibrinogen, resulting in platelet bridging and aggregation. Thromboxane A_2 also produces vasoconstriction and causes platelets to further aggregate, recruiting circulating platelets into the primary hemostatic plug formed at the site of vascular injury.[16]

When there is blood vessel wall injury, factor XII is also exposed to collagen or connective tissue in the subendothelium, resulting in its activation. FXIIa catalyzes the conversion of FXI to FXIa. Thrombin also activates FXI (FXIa) on the platelet surface during this phase. FXIa in turn cleaves FIX to FIXa. FIXa then cleaves FX into FXa. However, FIXa requires the cofactor FVIII to complete the reaction.[7,8,10,12] Factor XIIa triggers not only coagulation, but also fibrinolysis, the dissolution of clot. Therefore CPB-induced stimulation of XIIa, for example, causes both a thrombogenic and fibrinolytic response.

Although deficiencies of components of this system, such as FVIII and FIX, in patients result in bleeding, deficiencies of other factors, such as FXII, do not. Ex vivo this system is activated by contact with negatively charged surfaces. Hence factors XI, XII, prekallikrein, and high-molecular-weight kininogen have been termed *contact activation* factors. There is growing evidence that activation of this system plays a major role in catheter-related thrombi. In addition to activation of thrombin, this system will result in activation of the bradykinin system and thus also participates in vasoregulation.

Propagation Phase

The goal of the propagation phase is to produce large amounts of thrombin and allow bleeding to cease. This phase is characterized by platelet migration to the site of injury and by the production of tenase and prothrombinase complexes on the surface of activated platelets. First, FIX activated during the initiation phase can now bind to FVIIIa on the platelet surface, forming the tenase complex, which activates large amounts of FXa. FXa then associates with FVa bound to the platelet during the amplification phase, resulting in the formation of the prothrombinase complex, which converts large amounts of prothrombin into thrombin. Thrombin is responsible for the cleavage of fibrinogen into fibrin monomers that, in turn, polymerize to consolidate the platelet plug. The formation of insoluble fibrin polymers that are cross-linked by peptide bonds occurs under the influence of factor XIIIa.[7-10]

Termination Phase

Once a stable fibrin clot is formed at the site of injury, the clotting process must be limited to the injury site to prevent pathologic thrombosis and occlusion of the vessel. Four natural anticoagulants are involved to control the spread of coagulation activation: tissue factor pathway inhibitor (TFPI), protein C, protein S, and antithrombin (AT).

TFPI is a protein secreted by the endothelial cells and platelets that forms a quaternary complex, TF/FVIIa/FXa/TFPI, which inactivates activated factors to limit coagulation. Protein C is a vitamin K–dependent plasma glycoprotein that circulates in an inactive form. However, upon exposure to the endothelial-derived protein thrombomodulin and in the presence of thrombin, protein C is converted to its active form. Once activated, it participates with its cofactor, protein S, to inactivate cofactors V and VIII. Protein S is a vitamin K–dependent plasma protein that enables protein C to more efficiently inhibit binding of Xa to V and to inhibit factor VIII. As a reminder, factor VIII is necessary for the conversion of X to its active form, and FV is necessary to help Xa convert prothrombin to thrombin. AT is a plasma protein that binds to and inactivates thrombin and other serine proteases such as FIXa, FXa, FXIa, and FXIIa, as well as kallikrein and plasmin. Biologic heparan sulphate and medicinal heparin bind to and accelerate the reaction between thrombin and AT, with medicinal heparin accelerating the reaction by up to 10,000-fold. Endothelial cells also produce a variety of glycosaminoglycans (including heparan sulfate), which serve as high-affinity binding sites for AT, which are crucial for quick inactivation of thrombin.[12,17,18] There are other physiologic controls that limit the spread of clot. The rapid flow of blood dilutes the effective concentration of activated factors and removes them from sites of injury. Once the activated factors are removed, the hepatic and reticuloendothelial systems promptly and preferentially clear the activated factors from the circulation.

Fibrinolysis

Fibrinolysis involves the dissolution of a stable fibrin clot to allow for restoration of normal blood flow. Once a stable fibrin clot has formed and injured tissues have been repaired, fibrinolysis is initiated through the attraction of plasminogen and tissue plasminogen activator (t-PA) to the lysine residues of fibrin. Plasminogen activators are a heterogeneous group of proteases that are located both within the circulation and in organs such as the lungs, heart, adrenal glands, and ovaries. When it is time to limit the spread of clot, t-PA catalyzes the conversion of plasminogen to plasmin. Plasmin then digests the fibrin clot, which yields fibrin degradation products. Once clot lysis is complete, plasmin enters the circulation, where it is rapidly inactivated by antiplasmin, a serum protein that forms an enzyme-inhibitor complex with plasmin. Thus four reactions counteract fibrinolysis by promoting fibrin stability: (1) factor XIIIa results in cross-linking of fibrin, (2) thrombin-activatable fibrinolysis inhibitor removes lysine residues from fibrin, (3) plasminogen activator inhibitor type 1 (PAI-1) inactivates t-PA and urokinase plasminogen activator (u-PA), and (4) α2-antiplasmin inactivates plasmin.[12,13,19,20]

Two forms of fibrinolysis are worth noting. Primary fibrinolysis is associated with rapid breakdown of clot and is usually due to excess circulating t-PA, as discussed earlier. Secondary fibrinolysis, on the other hand, is a result of hypercoagulability (increased breakdown of clots due to increased formation of clots). Because the causes of primary and secondary fibrinolysis are different, the treatments are also different. In the case of primary fibrinolysis the goal is to treat excessive plasmin activity, which is the consequence of excess circulating t-PA. Administration of an antifibrinolytic agent, with specific or nonspecific antiplasmin activity, is commonly the treatment of choice (see the cardiopulmonary bypass section later) for primary fibrinolysis, whereas anticoagulant therapy is the common treatment for secondary fibrinolysis.[19]

Developmental Changes in Hemostasis

Healthy neonates and infants maintain a balance of procoagulant and anticoagulant states, despite dramatically different levels of the involved factors when compared with older children and adults. Children under 6 months of age have decreased levels of coagulation factors (II, VII, IX, X, XI, and XII) but also decreased levels of other molecules within the antithrombotic pathway (protein C, protein S, and AT).[2,21-26] The fibrinolysis pathway also shows age-related changes with diminished plasminogen and tissue plasminogen activator (t-PA) but increased PAI-1.[19-21] Traditional tests of coagulation function show results consistent with these principles. Studies have shown an inverse relationship between age and prolongation of prothrombin time (PT) and partial thromboplastin time (PTT), with neonates having the greatest prolongation of both tests. Coagulation factor levels typically reach adult values by 6 months to 1 year of age.[24-28] The presence of low factor levels that might predispose to bleeding is balanced by low levels of circulating inhibitors of coagulation. As a result, infants and young children without heart disease in general are not felt to have an increased propensity toward thrombosis due to the continued balance of procoagulant and anticoagulant factors, which may not be accurately measured by common coagulation studies. However, the delicate balance can easily be disrupted by any number of medical interventions needed in the care of children with cardiac disease, especially in the postintervention period or if the need for mechanical circulatory support arises.

Tests of Coagulation

With the traditional intrinsic and extrinsic coagulation pathways, it made sense that the PT was reflective of the extrinsic pathway (which reflected coagulation outside of the vessel), with the activated

partial thromboplastin time (aPTT) reflective of the intrinsic pathway (which reflected coagulation inside the vessel). Given what we now know regarding the interplay between these pathways and other substances leading to the cell-based model, how do we explain what these tests reflect? The PT assesses the levels of procoagulant involved in the initiation phase of coagulation, whereas the aPTT assesses the levels of procoagulant generated during the propagation phase, which are involved in the production of a large amount of thrombin on the surface of activated platelets.[12,29] No currently available test is able to provide a complete and reliable profile of the hemostatic function.

The normal aPTT is 25 to 35 seconds. The aPTT test will be prolonged when there is less than 30% activity of factors I, II, V, VIII, IX, X, XI, or XII.

The normal PT is 10 to 12 seconds but varies among laboratories. Prolonged PTs are seen when there is less than 30% activity of factors II, V, VII, or X or when there is dysfibrinogenemia or hypofibrinogenemia (factor I). Note that three (factors II, VII, X) of the four vitamin K–dependent clotting factors are evaluated in this test.

What is the significance of vitamin K? The majority of the coagulation factors are synthesized in the liver. Factors II, VII, IX, and X undergo enzymatic transformation in the hepatocyte after synthesis. This transformation involves the addition of a carboxyl (COOH) moiety. Carboxylation is possible only with the help of vitamin K. The COOH addition allows for these factors to bind via a Ca^{2+} bridge to phospholipid. Vitamin K–deficient patients produce these factors, but they are nonfunctional. Vitamin K antagonists (VKAs), such as warfarin, exert their anticoagulant effect by inhibiting the carboxylation step in the hepatocyte. Remember that the anticoagulant proteins C and S are also vitamin K dependent.

The international normalized ratio (INR) has been adopted in an attempt to standardize the results of the PT test. INR guides the use of the oral anticoagulant warfarin, which is required in patients at high risk for thrombosis. Typically warfarin is initiated while the patient is still receiving heparin because warfarin will initially decrease protein C levels before achieving therapeutic INR, such that patients may be prothrombotic in the initial stage of warfarin use. Infants require higher doses and take longer to achieve the targeted INR range than older children, such that many choose to use other options for anticoagulation for infants (such as low-molecular-weight heparin [LMWH]). Fontan patients and patients with liver disease require lower Coumadin doses (when it is used), and it is often difficult to determine ideal anticoagulation for such patients.

The activated clotting time (ACT) is a modification of the whole blood clotting time. It is a global measure of anticoagulation and is quickly accomplished at the bedside. The normal range is 80 to 140 seconds. The ACT is performed by automated equipment, and results are provided almost instantaneously. It is used in the operating room as a measure of heparin effect. Heparin activates AT and inhibits FIIa, FIXa, FXa, and FXIa and thus will prolong the ACT. ACT is, however, also affected by hypothermia, thrombocytopenia, and disseminated intravascular coagulation (DIC), to name a few examples in which the result may be prolonged and not be reflective of heparin effect alone.

Tests of Platelet Function

Platelet count is a quantitative measure only, telling us nothing about platelet function. Normal values are 150,000 to

400,000/mm³. Platelet counts less than 20,000/mm³ are usually associated with spontaneous bleeding. Surgical bleeding may occur at counts of 40,000 to 70,000/mm³.

Other tests of platelet function available now include the PFA-100, platelet aggregation testing, and thromboelastography (TEG).[30] (Platelet pathways and common antiplatelet therapies are depicted in Fig. 24.2). The PFA-100 (platelet function assay) will provide a closure time (CT), which signifies time to formation of a platelet plug. If there is platelet dysfunction, the CT will be increased with epinephrine and/or ADP depending on the disease. For example, PFA-100 may be used to screen for aspirin nonresponsiveness, with CT increased with epinephrine but not ADP. If PFA-100 results are unexpectedly abnormal, formal platelet aggregation testing is then performed in most circumstances.[30,31]

Light transmission aggregometry (LTA) testing can be used to assess response to different platelet agonists such as thrombin, collagen, arachidonic acid, ADP, epinephrine, and ristocetin cofactor. Born's PLA is the most widely employed methodology for detecting platelet function disorders and monitoring antiplatelet therapies. It is often the first step in the evaluation of hemorrhagic patients with inherited or acquired platelet dysfunction. The antibiotic ristocetin is another agent used as an agonist in the assessment of platelet function. It facilitates the binding of vWF to the glycoprotein Ib/IX/V complex. For a normal result, both functional vWF and normal glycoprotein Ib/IX/V complex must be present. Hence ristocetin-induced platelet aggregation is considered a test that can detect both von Willebrand disease and platelet dysfunctions.[30] Monitoring antiplatelet therapies (e.g., aspirin) by using LTA has permitted the prediction of major adverse cardiovascular events in adult cardiovascular patients at high risk. Identifying pediatric patients who are nonresponders to antiplatelet agents and are at high risk for thrombosis appears to be important as well because studies have reported 10% to 25% of pediatric cardiac surgical patients are nonresponders to aspirin and aspirin is often the sole anticoagulant used for the Blalock-Taussig shunt and Fontan prophylaxis, for example.[32] In fact, the highest incidence of nonresponsiveness has been reported in patients weighing less than 5 kg given 20.25 mg/d of aspirin.[33]

The VerifyNow system (ITC, Edison, NJ) is a point-of-care test that assesses platelet aggregation in whole blood based on the capacity of activated platelets to bind to fibrinogen. This initial VerifyNow test was used to verify the inhibitory effect of platelet GPIIb/IIIa antagonists (abciximab or eptifibatide) in adult cardiovascular patients undergoing percutaneous coronary intervention and reported as platelet aggregation units (PAUs). Now two more assays, each sensitive to targeted drugs, are available: Aspirin Test with arachidonic acid as agonist, whose results are expressed as aspirin reaction units (ARUs), and PRUTest (sensitive to thienopyridines, such as clopidogrel), whose results are expressed as P2Y12 reaction units (PRUs), by using ADP as agonist.[34-37]

TEG can also be used to evaluate platelet function with measurement of the maximal amplitude and platelet mapping (see section on TEG later).

Tests of Fibrinolysis

A useful screening test for fibrinolysis is a fibrinogen level combined with D dimer level. If the D dimer level is elevated, fibrinolysis is likely, meaning that the fibrinolytic system is trying to break up a cross-linked clot. D dimer is a specific fibrin degradation product, competing with thrombin to slow down additional clot formation by preventing conversion of fibrinogen to fibrin. Several more specific tests of fibrinolysis are available, including TEG and euglobulin clot lysis time (ECLT). The ECLT is a confirmatory test for fibrinolysis. The euglobulin fraction of plasma is free of inhibitors of fibrinolysis and contains plasminogen, plasminogen activators (primarily t-PA) and fibrinogen. This fraction of plasma is mixed with thrombin, and the time to clot lysis is measured. Normally the ECLT ranges from 90 to 240 minutes. If the ECLT is less than 90 minutes, hyperfibrinolysis is likely. If ECLT is abnormal, it may be useful to undertake specific assays of the components of the fibrinolytic pathway or to perform TEG. TEG often serves to monitor fibrinolysis and is a considerably more rapid test to perform than the ECLT.[19,38]

Thromboelastography and Thromboelastometry

There has been renewed interest in the use of TEG, first described in 1948, to rapidly assess global in vivo hemostatic function. TEG provides a real-time assessment of viscoelastic clot strength in whole blood. Rotational thromboelastometry (ROTEM) evolved from TEG technology, and both devices generate results of the changes in the viscoelastic strength of a small sample of clotting blood (usually 2 to 3 mL for the test) to which a constant rotational force is applied. These devices allow visual assessment of blood coagulation from clot formation, propagation, stabilization, and clot dissolution (Figs. 24.3 and 24.4).[38,39] Activation of clot formation can be initiated with both intrinsic (kaolin, ellagic acid) and extrinsic (TF) activators. The two tests use different nomenclature to describe the same parameters. CT (clotting time) for ROTEM and reaction rate (R) for TEG are both defined as the time in minutes it takes for the trace to reach an amplitude of 2 mm. Clot formation time (CFT) and kinetics time (K) are defined as the time necessary for clot amplitude to increase from 2 to 20 mm. Angle (a) is determined by creating a tangent line from the point of clot initiation (CT or R) to the slope of the developing curve. Maximum clot firmness (MCF) for ROTEM and maximum amplitude (MA) for TEG are the peak amplitudes (strength) of the clot. For TEG, Lysis 30 and Lysis 60 (LY30 and LY60) are

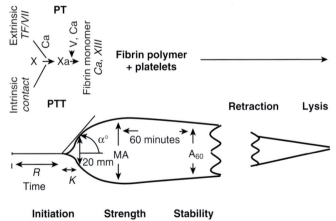

• **Figure 24.3** Thromboelastography and standard coagulation tests. *K,* Kinetics time; *MA,* maximum amplitude; *PT,* prothrombin time; *PTT,* partial thromboplastin time; *R,* reaction rate; *TF,* tissue factor. (From Whiting D, DiNardo J. TEG and ROTEM: technology and clinical applications. *Am J Hematol.* 2014;89[2]:228-232.)

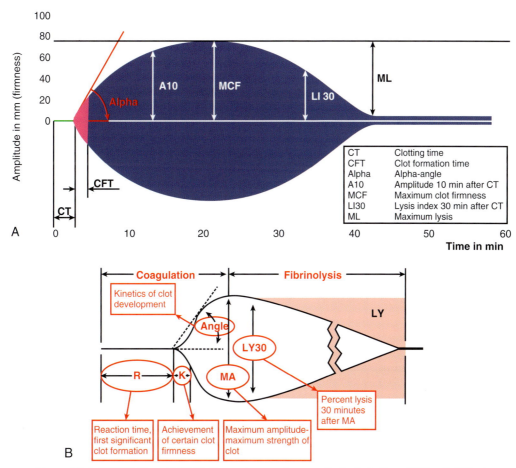

• **Figure 24.4** ROTEM (A) and TEG (B). Parameters are discussed in the text. (From Whiting D, DiNardo J. TEG and ROTEM: technology and clinical applications. *Am J Hematol.* 2014;89[2]:228-232.)

the percent reductions in the area under the TEG curve, assuming MA remains constant, that occur 30 and 60 minutes after MA is reached. For ROTEM, Lysis Index 30 (LI30) is the percent reduction in MCF that exists when amplitude is measured 30 minutes after CT is detected (see Fig. 24.3).[39] Respectively, these parameters measure fibrin formation (R and CT), fibrinogen turnover (K and CFT), speed of clot formation (α-angle), platelet-fibrin interactions (MA and MCF), and fibrinolysis (LY30, LY60, and LI30). Thus R and CT times will be prolonged in the presence of coagulopathy (i.e., factor deficiencies) and shortened in hypercoagulability. The TEG K and α-angle represent cross-linking of fibrin and thus reflect the levels of circulating fibrinogen available for this process to occur. Platelet aggregation is represented in the MA or MCF, with lower values being representative of a potential platelet dysfunction or deficiency with possible fibrinogen deficiency or dysfunction to a lesser degree because fibrinogen is an activator of platelets. The whole blood Thromboelastograph (TEG) Platelet Mapping assay provides a more specific way of detecting the reduction in platelet function, presented as percentage inhibition, by both aspirin and clopidogrel.

TEG and ROTEM may be incorporated into algorithms to diagnose and treat bleeding in high-risk populations such as those undergoing cardiac surgery or suffering from blunt trauma (Fig. 24.5). Some evidence suggests that these algorithms appear to reduce the overall transfusion of erythrocyte and nonerythrocyte

blood products compared with empiric therapy, but further study is needed to assess patient outcomes. Additional curves obtained from these tests, such as thrombin generation, may help give insight into thrombus formation, but more work is also needed in this area to determine specific application.[38]

Hemostasis and Coagulation in Congenital Heart Disease

The incidence of abnormalities on preoperative screening tests in CHD patients varies from 20% to 60%.[40-43] In addition, genetic conditions predisposing to thrombosis (i.e., factor V Leiden, prothrombin gene mutation 20120, and methylene tetrahydrofolate reductase [MTHFR]) have a disproportionally higher prevalence within the CHD population.[44-47] In general, children with cyanotic heart disease or whose hematocrit values are greater than 60% are most likely to have clinically relevant hemostatic abnormalities. However, acyanotic patients with CHD also manifest dysfunctional coagulation. There is no consistent pattern of abnormality among CHD patients. This wide range and variable presentation are likely due to the heterogeneous population that children with CHD represent. In clinical practice, basic preoperative laboratory assessment includes a hemoglobin and hematocrit determination along with a quantitative platelet count, a PT, and an aPTT. Some centers

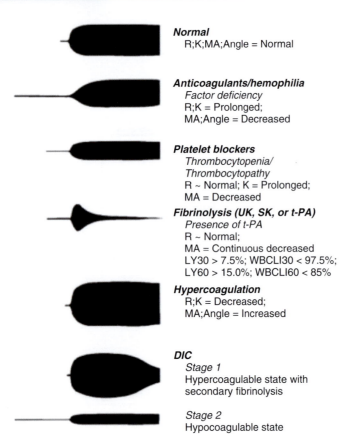

Normal
R;K;MA;Angle = Normal

Anticoagulants/hemophilia
Factor deficiency
R;K = Prolonged;
MA;Angle = Decreased

Platelet blockers
Thrombocytopenia/
Thrombocytopathy
R ~ Normal; K = Prolonged;
MA = Decreased

Fibrinolysis (UK, SK, or t-PA)
Presence of t-PA
R ~ Normal;
MA = Continuous decreased
LY30 > 7.5%; WBCLI30 < 97.5%;
LY60 > 15.0%; WBCLI60 < 85%

Hypercoagulation
R;K = Decreased;
MA;Angle = Increased

DIC
Stage 1
Hypercoagulable state with
secondary fibrinolysis

Stage 2
Hypocoagulable state

• **Figure 24.5** Thromboelastography examples. *DIC*, Disseminated intra-vascular coagulation; *K*, kinetics time; *LY*, lysis; *MA*, maximum amplitude; *R*, reaction rate; *SK*, streptokinase; *t-PA*, tissue plasminogen activator; *UK*, urokinase; *WBCLI*, whole blood clot lysis index. (From Whiting D, DiNardo J. TEG and ROTEM: technology and clinical applications. *Am J Hematol.* 2014;89[2]:228-232.)

are beginning to include additional testing, including TEG/ROTEM, factor activity levels, and AT activity in their initial preoperative evaluation for high-risk patients.

Coagulation Factors

Several studies have demonstrated prolongation of the PT and aPTT in CHD. Low levels of factors I (fibrinogen), II, V, VII, VIII, IX, and X have been observed, with elevated levels of factor VIII also being reported, which may be reflective of its role as an acute phase reactant. Quantitative abnormalities are even more pronounced in neonates. Factor levels are approximately 30% to 40% lower in newborns with CHD than in those neonates without structural cardiac abnormalities. One postulated cause for these low levels is impaired hepatic synthesis secondary to liver hypoperfusion, such as following CPB or in hypoplastic left heart syndrome patients with an imbalance of pulmonary-to-systemic blood flow ratio ($Q_p:Q_s$) with inadequate systemic cardiac output as examples. Other proposed mechanisms for decreased production included low cardiac output for a variety of conditions, genetic predisposition, or hepatic synthetic abnormalities, although the latter has not been demonstrated in current studies. Children with cyanotic CHD also often demonstrate delayed maturation of their coagulation system, whereas those with acyanotic heart disease will often demonstrate normal levels by 5 years of age.[40-43]

The single-ventricle patients are at particularly increased risk of coagulation factor abnormalities. Up to 33% of patients following a Fontan procedure demonstrated thrombotic events, which was initially thought to be multifactorial but in part due to acquired hypercoagulable state from decreased levels of protein C, S, and AT3. However, more recent studies have demonstrated abnormal levels of coagulation factors predating the Fontan surgery. Studies have also demonstrated elevated factor VIII levels in Fontan patients who develop thromboses, which may serve as a predictive tool in the future. Elevated factor VIII levels in adults have been predictive of recurrent deep venous thrombosis (DVT), for example.[48-51]

Anticoagulant factor abnormalities are also seen with CHD patients, again with increased prevalence among cyanotic children. In cyanotic CHD, hyperviscosity can be the limiting factor in oxygen delivery to tissues because it further decreases flow in small capillaries. This hyperviscosity can occur as a result of increased red cell production and can be further exacerbated by iron deficiency anemia by altering the shape of red cells. Furthermore, AT activity is often significantly lower than in age-matched controls. The utility of replacement in children with documented deficiency remains controversial, but careful repletion may improve coagulation balance or anticoagulation effectiveness. Protein C and S levels are often decreased in CHD patients with a similar exaggeration of the deficiency in both newborns and cyanotic heart disease.[40-43]

Whatever the exact mechanisms, children at highest risk of coagulation factor abnormalities and thrombosis are those with hematocrit values above 60%, cyanotic defects, left-sided obstructive lesions, and poor cardiac output. Younger age appears to have a variable effect. There are limited data on coagulopathy in adults with CHD, but these patients appear to be at an increased risk compared with their peers. Potential mechanisms include continued abnormal levels of coagulation factors, endothelial dysfunction, mechanical factors, and additive risk from protein-losing enteropathy, pregnancy, or oral contraceptives.

Anatomic considerations include increased blood viscosity within small vessels or shunts. In addition, alterations in blood flow may occur secondary to nonpulsatile flow (such as after bidirectional cavopulmonary anastomosis or Fontan or with mechanical circulatory support) or to vessel or chamber dilation (such as with dilated cardiomyopathy). As a result, children with CHD with extreme alterations in blood flow (stenotic or static) may be at increased risk of thrombosis. However, increased bleeding risk may also occur secondary to increased shear stress, with resultant acquired vWF deficiency[52] (discussed in more detail in ventricular assist device section later).

Platelets

Children with cyanotic CHD demonstrate both quantitative and qualitative platelet defects. Thrombocytopenia occurs in approximately one-third of the children. Even if the absolute platelet count is normal, many of these patients have prolongation of the bleeding time. These findings suggest defects in platelet adhesion and aggregation. Quantitative functional platelet assays have demonstrated elevated levels of beta-thromboglobulin and PF_4 in CHD patients compared with controls. This observation suggests that in CHD, platelets are chronically activated and thus depleted of their vesicle contents. They exist in a functionally refractory state, unable to mount a normal response by aggregating and adhering at sites of vascular injury.[40-43,53]

Children with noncyanotic CHD also demonstrate platelet abnormalities. These abnormalities include the loss of the vWF portion of the factor VIII complex. The absence of a portion of vWF leads to bleeding that can be clinically significant. This abnormality is likely due to aberrant flow patterns or altered hemodynamics associated with the specific cardiac lesion, such as in patients with aortic stenosis and in patients with continuous-flow ventricular assist devices (VADs), leading to acquired vWF deficiency. In most affected children studied, the vWF abnormality corrects when the cardiac defect is repaired or the device is removed (see later in VAD section).[54]

Newborns with ductal dependent pulmonary or systemic blood flow receive prostaglandin E infusions preoperatively to maintain ductal patency. These infusions affect platelet function by preventing activation.

Sometimes children receive heparin preoperatively. Heparin-induced thrombocytopenia (HIT) is a rare complication of heparin therapy, occurring with an incidence of 0.5% to 5% in adult patients. The incidence in pediatric patients is presumably less. HIT is an idiosyncratic, antibody-mediated reaction that occurs within 6 to 12 days of heparin administration. The clinical features of HIT are thrombocytopenia (platelet counts typically are around 50,000/mm^3; however, values as low as 10,000/mm^3 have been reported) and thrombosis with an increasing heparin requirement. (See HIT section later for additional detail.)[55-61]

Fibrinolysis

Fibrinolysis may be a contributing factor in the coagulopathy of CHD. Perioperative inhibition of primary fibrinolysis may decrease blood loss during palliative or corrective surgery for CHD through the use of aminocaproic acid or tranexamic acid (discussed in more detail under pharmacologic strategies to treat bleeding).

Anticoagulation Medications

Anticoagulation is frequently used for patients with heart disease, both congenital and acquired, as noted earlier, for prevention or treatment of thrombosis and thromboembolism. Unfractionated heparin (UFH), LMWH, or warfarin is often the anticoagulant of choice in the pediatric population for prevention and treatment of thrombosis. If UFH and LMWH cannot be used due to HIT and if warfarin is not an option due to the lack of oral access or concern for difficulty achieving consistent therapeutic INR, other alternatives such as bivalirudin, argatroban, and fondaparinux can be used. Published literature exists supporting the use of these three latter anticoagulants in pediatric patients.

Unfractionated Heparin and Low-Molecular-Weight Heparin

UFH has been used for the prevention and treatment of thrombosis for several decades. Heparin is mainly obtained from porcine intestine. UFH is a mixture of sulphated glycosaminoglycans of variable lengths and molecular weights and is administered parenterally. Anticoagulant effects and pharmacologic properties vary with the size of the molecules. UFH inactivates several coagulation enzymes, including FIIa (thrombin), IXa, Xa, XIa, and XIIa, by binding to the cofactor AT. Several studies have also shown that heparin possesses various antiinflammatory and immunomodulatory properties. Binding of heparin to different mediators involved in the immune system response (cytokines and chemokines), acute phase proteins, and complement complex proteins may contribute to the antiinflammatory activity of heparin. Use of heparin-treated

surfaces in CPB circuits, for example, has been shown to decrease activation of leukocytes and the complement cascades.[62,63]

LMWHs are derived from UFH by depolymerization. Each LMWH product has a specific molecular weight distribution that determines its anticoagulant activity and duration of action, so one product cannot always be substituted for another. LMWHs in current use globally include enoxaparin, dalteparin, and tinzaparin as examples, with enoxaparin being most commonly used in the United States. They are administered subcutaneously for venous thromboembolism (VTE) prevention and treatment. Like UFH, LMWHs inactivate several coagulation enzymes by binding to AT but have a lower affinity for binding to proteins other than AT and are therefore associated with a predictable dose response and have fewer nonhemorrhagic side effects in patients with normal renal function and without significant inflammation. If these conditions do not exist, LMWHs have improved bioavailability mainly due to reduced reactivity with PF$_4$, a release product of activated platelets acting as an antiheparin and as such inhibiting a certain, variable amount of circulating heparin.[55,64-66]

Anti-FXa levels are used to measure the effect of UFH and LMWH. Recommended anti-FXa levels in children have been extrapolated from adult studies. In neonates and young infants the PTT may not correspond to anti-FXa levels because of developmental hemostasis. In children or adults with high FVIII or fibrinogen levels (nonspecific acute phase reactants) or in the presence of an antiphospholipid antibody or nonspecific inhibitor, the PTT is not a good reflection of heparin effect. LMWH is a short-chain heparin that does not influence the PTT; therefore the anti-FXa level is the only measure of the effect of LMWH therapy.

Parenteral Direct Thrombin Inhibitors

The most common parenteral direct thrombin inhibitors (DTIs) include argatroban and bivalirudin.[67-71] Bivalirudin is cleared by proteolytic mechanisms (80%) and to a lesser degree via renal mechanisms (20%), with argatroban cleared mostly by hepatic mechanisms. DTIs are a useful alternative to heparin for anticoagulation in infants and children. They have been found to be effective for treatment of thrombosis and for anticoagulation during CPB and extracorporeal membrane oxygenation (ECMO) or with VADs.[67,68] Although they have traditionally been used in patients who were unresponsive to heparin or who developed HIT, they are now being studied as first-line agents. Bivalirudin, unlike heparin, does not require AT to be effective, having the potential to provide more consistent anticoagulation, especially during critical illness. Available literature reports equivalent or lower rates of bleeding or thromboembolic complications. It is more expensive than heparin, but the cost may be offset by reductions in costs associated with heparin use, including anti-factor Xa testing and the need for administration of AT. Studies prospectively evaluating bivalirudin efficacy and safety in the pediatric population are under way.

Warfarin

Warfarin is a vitamin K antagonist (VKA). It is completely absorbed orally and 98% bound to plasma proteins. Warfarin therapy in neonates and infants is associated with significant challenges because of developmental hemostasis with decreased levels of vitamin K–dependent factors in newborns, increased variability in nutritional intake, higher dose requirements, increased incidence of viral infections, and less time in therapeutic range (as high as 50%

in some studies). In general, warfarin therapy is not recommended in infants less than 1 year of age unless they have a mechanical valve. A number of drugs are known to interact with warfarin, affecting anticoagulant effect, with some drugs being highly likely to inhibit warfarin, such as carbamazepine, phenobarbital, and rifampin, whereas others increase the risk of bleeding, such as cephalosporins, macrolide antibiotics, acetaminophen, and nonsteroidal antiinflammatory drugs (including aspirin). The mechanism of interference of acetaminophen with warfarin metabolism appears to be through cytochrome P450. If acetaminophen use is necessary, it is recommended to use as low a dose as possible for short duration. Although concomitant use of warfarin and aspirin generally should be avoided, studies in patients at high risk for thromboembolic events (i.e., patients with mechanical heart valves, combination of tissue valves and atrial fibrillation, and VADs) have demonstrated that the increased risk of bleeding with combined warfarin and aspirin therapy is outweighed by the benefit in decreased thromboembolic events.[72-76]

Genetic polymorphisms may also impact warfarin metabolism. In 2007 the Food and Drug Administration (FDA) approved the Nanosphere Verigene Warfarin Metabolism Nucleic Acid Test capable of detecting variations in the metabolism of two genes, *CYP2C9* and *VKORC1*. The frequency of these abnormalities varies among individuals and among people of different races and nationalities.[77-80]

Although there are no well-designed studies evaluating the safety and efficacy of warfarin after the Fontan procedure in children, it may be used for thromboprophylaxis, with typical target INR of 2.0 to 3.0. Lower doses of warfarin are usually needed for Fontan patients, with a typical starting dose of 0.1 mg/kg.[75,76]

Antiplatelet Medications

Antiplatelet drugs are commonly used in children for both prophylaxis and treatment of thrombosis (see Fig. 24.2). Agents that irreversibly inhibit platelet function include aspirin and the thienopyridines clopidogrel, ticlopidine, and prasugrel. Ticagrelor is a direct-acting, reversibly binding, oral $P2Y_{12}$ receptor antagonist that exhibits a rapid onset and offset of antiplatelet effect. Other reversible antiplatelet drugs include dipyridamole and cilostazol, and the nonsteroidal antiinflammatory agents also have a transient antiplatelet effect.[55,65,81]

Direct Xa Inhibitor

Fondaparinux is an AT-dependent, selective anti-Xa inhibitor with a half-life of 17 to 21 hours in patients with normal renal function, longer if renal impairment exists. In the FondaKIDS trial, dosing of fondaparinux at 0.1 mg/kg subcutaneously once daily in children resulted in pharmacokinetic (PK) profiles comparable to those in adults receiving standard dosing. This study and a subsequent follow-up suggests that fondaparinux can be considered an attractive alternative to LMWH given its once-daily dosing, acceptable safety data, and other favorable properties.[82,83]

Direct Oral Anticoagulants

Direct oral anticoagulants (DOACs), also known as novel oral anticoagulants (NOACs), are in wide use for adult patients requiring both short- and long-term anticoagulation with increased interest in pediatric use now as well. The increased implementation of DOACs has been due to ease of use, favorable pharmacokinetics

with typically short half-lives, decreased drug-drug interactions, and lack of monitoring requirements. Although routine laboratory monitoring is not recommended, it is possible for the DOACs and will be specified later for each drug. Management of patients on DOACs in the perioperative period involves an assessment of thromboembolic event risk while off anticoagulation compared to the relative risk of bleeding if such drug is continued. Based on current adult literature, DOACs are used for treatment and prevention of DVT and PE and for prevention of stroke and embolism in patients with nonvalvular atrial fibrillation and should be avoided in patients who are pregnant and those with mechanical heart valves, rheumatic mitral stenosis, and/or stage V chronic kidney disease. Limited data exist on the use of DOACs in pediatric patients, and none of them currently have FDA-approved pediatric labeling. Off-label use of these DOACs in pediatrics is largely extrapolated from adult dosing guidelines. We will briefly discuss currently available DOACs because we expect their use will increase in the coming years as more data become available for pediatric patients.[84-87]

Dabigatran etexilate mesylate, known by the brand name Pradaxa, is a DOAC that directly binds to thrombin's active site, competitively inhibiting both free and clot-bound thrombin, and is therefore an oral DTI. In October 2015 an antidote for dabigatran known as idarucizumab (Praxbind) was approved by the FDA. This is the only DOAC for which there is currently a reversal agent available. PTT or thrombin time will be prolonged with therapeutic dosing. Rivaroxaban (Xarelto) is a DOAC that directly inhibits factor Xa, which is a part of the prothrombinase complex. The most accurate means of measuring rivaroxaban levels in the blood is to perform a calibrated specific anti-Xa assay. Apixaban (Eliquis) is a DOAC that directly and selectively inhibits factor Xa, like rivaroxaban, and therapeutic levels can also be assessed through a specific anti-Xa assay. Edoxaban (Savaysa) also directly inhibits factor Xa, much like rivaroxaban and apixaban. Edoxaban can prolong PTT and the anti-Xa assay, which have both been shown to accurately indicate drug levels within the plasma. Rivaroxaban, apixaban, and edoxaban do not have a drug-specific reversal agent currently available. Current management options for reversal include use of four-factor prothrombin complex concentrate or fresh frozen plasma. There are also reversal agents in development for oral direct anti-Xa inhibitors.[84-87]

Due to the lack of published clinical trials, it is too early to recommend one of the DOACs as an initial alternative for thrombosis treatment or prevention. More data are needed to determine the appropriate dosing of these agents in different age-groups. To date the available evidence for use of rivaroxaban in this population is from four completed studies, the results of which suggested that in children less than 40 kg of body weight there are significantly reduced serum concentrations, suggesting the need for higher doses. Pharmacokinetic and pharmacodynamic results of apixaban and edoxaban may increase their use in children with study results suggesting different dosing regimens for pediatric patients varying by age, as one would expect.[87]

Thrombosis in Pediatric Cardiac Disease and Use of Anticoagulation

Thromboembolic disorders in pediatric patients have historically been reported to be relatively rare compared with adults. However, during the past 10 years there has been an increase in the incidence of VTE in children.[88-97] In fact, it was reported that the annual rate of VTE increased by 70% from 2001 to 2007 for pediatric patients, including neonates, infants, children, and adolescents.[98] In the congenital and acquired heart disease population, thrombosis has long been recognized as a potentially life-threatening complication. The American Heart Association (AHA) released a scientific statement, "Prevention and Treatment of Thrombosis in Pediatric and Congenital Heart Disease," in 2013, citing the prevalence in high-risk groups, including patients with shunt-dependent single ventricles (shunt thrombosis, 8% to 12%; 4% risk of death resulting from shunt failure), postoperative central lines (13% thrombosis in central venous lines [CVLs]), Fontan circulation (17% to 33% incidence of thrombosis after Fontan with 2% to 12% of stroke), arrhythmias, Kawasaki disease with coronary aneurysms, and cardiomyopathy/myocarditis.[3] For most of these conditions there remain a wide variety of preventive and management strategies.[3,55,65]

In one study, children with stroke and heart disease had an increased prevalence of one or more prothrombotic abnormalities, including the presence of lipoprotein(a), anticardiolipin antibodies, and protein C deficiency.[3,99] Thus for evaluation of thrombosis or thromboembolism in pediatric patients, according to the AHA guidelines, it is reasonable to evaluate the following in an initial assessment: levels of protein C, protein S, AT, lipoprotein(a), homocysteine, anticardiolipin antibodies, and lupus anticoagulant; mutations of factor V Leiden; and prothrombin genes.[3,88,89] As noted earlier, the incidence of CVL-associated venous thromboembolic events was 13% as documented by venogram in infants and children (158 evaluable patients, all >3 months of age) in patients in the multicenter Prophylaxis of Thromboembolism in Kids Trial (PROTEKT).[3,100] It is also reported in various studies that in published series, approximately 90% of neonates and 50% of children with venous thrombosis had a CVL with one prospective cohort study demonstrating an incidence of 25%.[3,101-103] More specifically, in symptomatic and asymptomatic neonates and children with CHD a prospective cohort study demonstrated an incidence of thrombosis of 25% resulting from CVLs.[103] There is also growing evidence that activation of contact activation factors plays a major role in catheter-related thrombi.[92-97]

Use of Anticoagulation in Pediatric Heart Disease (Table 24.1)

A variety of anticoagulation prophylaxis and treatment regimens exist for a number of cardiac conditions, although there is often a lack of uniformity across institutions, likely related to the lack of prospective pediatric studies. Manlhiot et al.[104] evaluated risk factors associated with significantly increased odds of thrombosis following pediatric cardiac surgery: age greater than 31 days, baseline oxygen saturation less than 85%, previous thrombosis, heart transplantation, use of deep hypothermic circulatory arrest, longer cumulative time with CVLs, and postoperative use of extracorporeal support. Regarding CVL risk in particular, radiographically confirmed asymptomatic CVL-related thromboses (1) may be associated with increased CVL-related sepsis, (2) are the most common source of pulmonary embolism (PE),[105,106] (3) may result in loss of crucial (and often limited) vascular access, and (4) may have the potential to result in embolic stroke in patients with right-to-left intracardiac shunts.[3,96,97,101-103,107-109] Due to these risks the AHA guidelines state that in infants or children with a CVL who will ultimately require a palliative Fontan procedure or in those with concomitant bacteremia or a hypercoagulable risk factor (increased hematocrit, history of thrombosis, confirmed thrombophilic abnormality),

low-dose intravenous heparin may be reasonable until the CVL is removed.[3]

PE is discussed in more detail in Chapter 74, but we will briefly mention management here based on AHA guidelines. Infants and children with PE and heart disease who are clinically stable should be treated with anticoagulation according to the guidelines for deep venous thrombosis. In infants and children with PE and heart disease who have life-threatening cardiorespiratory compromise and positive radiographic findings for PE, rapid removal of pulmonary thrombi by thrombolytic therapy, pulmonary embolectomy, or stent placement can be beneficial.[3,55]

Regarding shunt prophylaxis, low-dose aspirin (1 to 5 mg/kg) is recommended for prevention of long-term polytetrafluoroethylene systemic to pulmonary shunt thrombosis in infants and children. According to AHA guidelines, anti-platelet therapy for long-term antithrombotic therapy is "reasonable" after cavopulmonary anastomosis and "probably indicated" after Fontan procedure, although long-term therapy with warfarin may be indicated after the Fontan procedure for higher-risk patients, such as those with arrhythmias, ventricular dysfunction, and prolonged immobilization.[3] Shunt thrombosis management can be life-threatening and should include immediate systemic anticoagulation with a bolus of intravenous heparin (50 to 100 U/kg) and ongoing heparin infusion, as well as maneuvers to increase Q_p with lowering of pulmonary vascular resistance (PVR) and increasing systemic vascular resistance, such as increasing systemic blood pressure (e.g., intravenous phenylephrine or epinephrine) in an effort to improve blood flow through the shunt, and intubation, mechanical ventilation, and neuromuscular blockade to maximize oxygen delivery and to minimize oxygen consumption with consideration of inhaled pulmonary vasodilators to lower PVR. Cardiac catheterization with directed t-PA, surgical exploration, and/or ECMO may be required.[3,55,110-116]

After superior cavopulmonary anastomosis or Fontan palliation, patients are at increased risk of developing pleural effusions, with chylous effusions likely the most concerning.[3,75,76,107] Chylothoraces are associated with an increased risk of thrombosis, as they are associated with the loss of natural anticoagulant proteins, including proteins C and S and AT, the deficiency of which can limit the effectiveness of heparin.[3,107,117] Serious thrombotic complications can include pulmonary artery and cerebral sinovenous thrombosis, the latter of which can be associated with stroke. According to the AHA guidelines, anti-platelet therapy for long-term antithrombotic therapy is "reasonable" after cavopulmonary anastomosis and "probably indicated" after Fontan procedure, although long-term therapy with warfarin may be indicated after the Fontan procedure for higher-risk patients, such as those with arrhythmias, ventricular dysfunction, and prolonged immobilization.[3] Given that there is some evidence that the first 3 to 12 months after Fontan procedure may be a higher-risk period, warfarin or LMWH may be indicated, particularly for patients at increased thrombotic risk. Likewise, given that older patients may be at higher risk, escalation or initiation of antithrombotic therapy may be indicated in adolescence or adulthood.[3,55,75,107]

Refractory intraatrial reentrant tachycardia, atrial flutter, and atrial fibrillation are less common in pediatric patients than in adults, but when present may be associated with left atrial thrombus. When a thrombus has been found, the recommendation for adult patients is anticoagulation with a VKA for 4 weeks before cardioversion with a repeat transesophageal echocardiography to confirm resolution of thrombus. In adults, anticoagulation is also recommended for a minimum of 4 weeks after cardioversion. Although

TABLE 24.1	Anticoagulation/Antithrombotic Prophylaxis for Pediatric Cardiac Conditions	
Condition	**Anticoagulant/Antithrombotic Prophylaxis**	**Comments**
Patients with CVL who will ultimately require a Fontan OR those with concomitant bacteremia OR a hypercoagulable risk factor[a]	Consider low-dose heparin infusion until CVL removed	Typically initiated once postoperative bleeding controlled or at time of diagnosis of other risk factors
Shunts: BT or central shunt, Sano shunt	Low-dose heparin infusion if no hypercoagulable risk factors	Typically initiated once postoperative bleeding controlled or at time of diagnosis of other risk factors
With risk factors[a]	Consider systemic heparin or DTI if suspected or confirmed infection, known CVL-associated thrombus, stented shunt, or hypercoagulable state (including persistently draining pleural effusions or chylothorax); aspirin as long-term therapy	Consider additional antiplatelet therapy in patients with coronary artery disease or prior stent/shunt thrombus
Glenn shunt With risk factors[a]	Aspirin Consider long-term therapy with warfarin or LMWH may be indicated for higher-risk patients (i.e., arrhythmias, ventricular dysfunction, and prolonged immobilization)	Usually started within 48 h postoperatively
Fontan shunt With risk factors[a]	Aspirin Consider long-term therapy with warfarin or LMWH may be indicated for higher-risk patients	Usually started within 48 h postoperatively Consider warfarin for first 3-12 months in high-risk patients Consider addition of warfarin to adolescents/adults
Conduits: RV-PA valved conduits • Homograft (cadaveric pericardium) • Xenograft (Contegra bovine jugular vein; Hancock Dacron tube with porcine valve) • PTFE/Gore-Tex	Consider aspirin	Usually started within 48 h postoperatively
Cardiomyopathy with any risk factor[a] (including shortening fraction ≤10% or ejection fraction ≤25%)	Systemic anticoagulation initially with heparin or DTI or LMWH; transition to warfarin once therapeutic for older patients Consider addition of aspirin	Usually started at diagnosis if no imminent procedures planned and bleeding risk is low
Patients presenting with shortening fraction ≤20% or ejection fraction ≤45%	Systemic anticoagulation initially with heparin or DTI or LMWH; transition to warfarin once therapeutic for older patients if degree of heart failure persists Consider addition of aspirin	
Noncoronary endovascular **stents** (including stented shunts) With risk factors[a]	Low-dose aspirin for 6 mo Consider LMWH or warfarin plus aspirin or clopidogrel	
Stents for higher thrombotic-risk lesions (nonpulsatile flow, previous complete occlusion, thrombophilic abnormality)	Warfarin or LMWH with or without antiplatelet therapy for 3-6 mo after implantation and then continue antiplatelet therapy alone	Consider additional antiplatelet therapy in patients with coronary artery disease or prior stent/shunt thrombus
Transcatheter ASD closure	Low-dose aspirin for 6 mo Additional anticoagulant may be added for 3-6 mo in older children and adults	
Transcatheter VSD closure	Low-dose aspirin for at least 6 mo	
Transcatheter PDA closure	Low-dose aspirin for 6 mo	
Aortic and/or Mitral Valves		
Mechanical aortic valve (e.g., St. Jude, Medtronic, Carbomedics)		Heparin use started 48-72 hrs post-op
With no additional thrombotic risk factors	Systemic heparin or DTI until therapeutic warfarin plus aspirin	Goal INR 2-3
With risk factors[b] (plus atrial fibrillation, older-generation mechanical aortic valves)	Systemic heparin or DTI until therapeutic warfarin plus aspirin	Goal INR 2.5-3.5
Mechanical aortic valve (On-X)	Systemic heparin or DTI until therapeutic warfarin plus aspirin	Heparin use started 48-72 hrs post-op Goal INR 2-3 for 3 mo, then 1.5-2

TABLE 24.1	Anticoagulation/Antithrombotic Prophylaxis for Pediatric Cardiac Conditions—cont'd	
Condition	**Anticoagulant/Antithrombotic Prophylaxis**	**Comments**
Mechanical mitral valve (e.g., St. Jude, Medtronic, Carbometrics)	Systemic heparin or DTI until therapeutic warfarin plus aspirin	Goal INR 3 (2.5-3.5)
Mechanical mitral valve (On-X)	Systemic heparin or DTI until therapeutic warfarin plus aspirin	Goal INR 2.5-3.5 for 3 mo, then 2-2.5
Bioprosthetic aortic or mitral valve (use rare in children)	Low-dose aspirin; Consider warfarin for 3 mo	Goal INR 2-3
If risk factors present[b]	Systemic heparin or DTI until therapeutic warfarin plus aspirin	Goal INR 2-3
Pulmonary and/or Tricuspid Valves		
Bioprosthetic pulmonary valve	Consider aspirin for 3-6 mo	
Bioprosthetic tricuspid valve	Consider life-long aspirin; consider warfarin for 3-6 mo	Goal INR 2-3
If risk factors present[b]	Systemic heparin or DTI until therapeutic warfarin plus aspirin	Goal INR 2-3

[a]Potential risk factors include (1) atriopulmonary type of Fontan connection, (2) bilateral bidirectional cavopulmonary anastomoses, (3) hypoplastic cardiac chambers with flow stasis, (4) presence of a blind-ended pulmonary artery stump, (5) history of previous thrombosis, (6) protein-losing enteropathy, (7) prolonged pleural effusions/chylothoraces, (8) prolonged immobilization, (9) ventricular dysfunction, (10) arrhythmia, (11) presence of thrombogenic foreign material, (12) atrial-level fenestration, (13) Kawashima connection, (14) polycythemia, and (15) an abnormal thrombophilia profile.
[b]Potential risk factors for valve replacement: (1) previous thromboembolism, (2) systemic ventricular dysfunction, and (3) hypercoagulable condition.
ASD, Atrial septal defect; *BT*, Blalock-Taussig; *CVL*, central venous line; *DTI*, direct thrombin inhibitor; *INR*, international normalized ratio; *LMWH*, low-molecular-weight heparin; *PDA*, patent ductus arteriosus; *PTFE*, polytetrafluoroethylene; *RV-PA*, right ventricle–pulmonary artery; *VSD*, ventricular septal defect.

there are currently no data in the pediatric age-group on the timing or need for anticoagulation after cardioversion of refractory atrial arrhythmias, it is common pediatric practice to continue postcardioversion anticoagulation.

To prevent coronary thrombosis in coronary aneurysms, such as in patients with Kawasaki disease, aspirin is used, with a second antiplatelet agent added for moderate-size aneurysms (4 to 6 mm).[3] Most commonly, patients with giant aneurysms (≥8 mm), with or without stenoses, are treated with low-dose aspirin, together with warfarin, maintaining an INR of 2.0 to 3.0 or therapeutic LMWH.[3,118,119] In patients with giant aneurysms with a recent history of coronary thrombosis, triple therapy may be considered (two antiplatelet agents and LMWH or warfarin).[3,119]

For cardiomyopathy patients with arrhythmias, previous thrombosis or thromboembolism, thrombophilic conditions, or shortening fraction of 10% or less or ejection fraction of 25% or less, it is "reasonable" to use systemic anticoagulation according to the AHA guidelines.[3] Furthermore, for patients presenting with shortening fraction of 20% or less or ejection fraction of 45% or less, systemic anticoagulation (warfarin or heparin therapy with or without aspirin) for the first three months may also be "reasonable."[3] Assessment for thrombophilia abnormalities may be undertaken for those patients with thrombus or if VAD use is necessary.[3,55,119,120]

For children undergoing placement of endovascular stents for non-coronary lesions, low-dose aspirin should be used for at least 6 months after implantation according to AHA guidelines.[3] In children undergoing stent implantation for higher thrombotic-risk lesions, such as nonpulsatile flow, previous complete occlusion or thrombophilic abnormality, it is "reasonable" to use warfarin or LMWH with or without antiplatelet therapy for 3 to 6 months after implantation and then continue antiplatelet therapy alone according to these same guidelines.[3,55,121]

According to the AHA guidelines, for transcatheter atrial septal defect device closure in children, low-dose aspirin should be used for 6 months following implantation, with an additional anticoagulant potentially added to aspirin therapy for 3 to 6 months in older children, while for transcatheter ventricular septal defect closure, low-dose aspirin may be used for at least 6 months after implantation.[3,55]

Anticoagulation in the first few months after surgical valve replacement has traditionally been used to protect against thrombotic complications, presumably related to suture material and to a device that does not yet have biofilm and endothelialization (a process that usually takes 3 to 6 months).[3,55,122]

Based on adult data, the addition of aspirin to VKA therapy in patients with mechanical valves leads to reduction in risk of thromboembolism and mortality when compared to VKA therapy alone (65% observed risk reduction in major systemic embolism or death in the aspirin plus VKA group). The addition of at least 50 to 100 mg/d of aspirin is therefore recommended in the current American College of Cardiology (ACC)/AHA and American College of Chest Physicians guidelines for all patients with mechanical valves, though consideration must be given to an individual patient's bleeding risk. The ACC/AHA "Guideline for the Management of Patients With Valvular Heart Disease" recommends VKA therapy with a target INR of 2.5 for patients with mechanical aortic valves if no additional risk factors are present (see Table 24.1). Additional risk factors are defined as atrial fibrillation, prior thromboembolism, left ventricular dysfunction, or hypercoagulable state. For patients with mechanical mitral valves, older-generation mechanical aortic valves, or risk factors in addition to any type of mechanical aortic valve, a target INR of 3.0 is recommended.[3,55,123-137]

Based on the 2017 focused update on management of patients with valvular heart disease, the AHA/ACC recommends use of a VKA after bioprosthetic valve replacement for aortic and/or mitral bioprosthesis for 3 to 6 months after surgery in patients at low risk for bleeding. In children, however, tissue valves, particularly xenografts, deteriorate rapidly when used in the aortic or systemic atrioventricular (mitral) valve position, such that mechanical valves are usually used in these positions. A lower INR target of 1.5 to

2.0 for patients with an On-X bileaflet mechanical aortic valve and no additional thromboembolism risks can also be considered. Aspirin is recommended in patients regardless of whether additional anticoagulation is employed. There are no specific recommendations offered in regard to duration of aspirin therapy in this population.[125-131] Tissue valves are generally considered to be more durable when placed on the right side for replacement of the pulmonary and tricuspid valves. For bioprosthetic pulmonary valves, which may be commonly used for pulmonary valve replacement in patients following tetralogy of Fallot (TOF) repair, for example, some centers use aspirin for 3 to 6 months postoperatively. Tricuspid valve replacement is less common, being used most commonly for Ebstein anomaly, followed by pulmonary atresia and TOF. For bioprosthetic tricuspid valves, it is reasonable to use warfarin to achieve an INR goal of 2.0 to 3.0, particularly if there is decreased ventricular function. Long-term aspirin is also a reasonable antithrombotic regimen for bioprosthetic tricuspid valves, often used in conjunction with warfarin.[3,55,123,124]

Heparin-Induced Thrombocytopenia

HIT occurs in approximately 2% of adult patients and less than 1% of pediatric patients who are exposed to heparin. HIT is a hypercoagulable state resulting in the formation of immunoglobulin G antibodies produced against the complex of PF_4 on the surface of activated platelets and heparin, resulting in thrombocytopenia and significant platelet activation. Both clinical and laboratory tests are used to diagnose HIT. The clinical signs include thrombocytopenia (platelet drop of 50% within 24 hours) 5 to 8 days after the first heparin exposure (or sooner if heparin exposure has occurred in the past few weeks or months because HIT antibodies are transient). Two laboratory assays are available to detect HIT antibodies: platelet serotonin-release assay (SRA) and PF_4-dependent enzyme immunoassays (EIAs). The SRA is the gold standard test because it has high sensitivity and specificity. The anti-PF_4/heparin EIA is the laboratory test most commonly carried out, and it has the same high sensitivity as the SRA; however, a lower specificity results in a high false-positive rate (approximately 50% of patients clinically suspected to have HIT and a positive EIA actually have HIT type 2).[56-61,138,139] In one study a positive EIA of more than 2.0 optical density (OD) units had approximately 90% predictivity for the presence of platelet-activating antibodies and a positive SRA. With an EIA of 1.4 OD units or higher, there was a 50% probability of the presence of platelet-activating antibodies.[60,140]

Perioperative Discontinuation of Anticoagulants

If and when anticoagulation is discontinued before surgery depends on a number of factors, including the type of anticoagulant and type of surgery (Table 24.2). The effect of most antiplatelet agents lasts for the duration of the life of a platelet, which is typically 7 to 10 days. Aspirin is often not stopped before surgery but may be stopped 5 to 7 days before in some cases. Clopidogrel (Plavix) is often stopped 5 to 7 days preoperatively, whereas Prasugrel (Effient) is discontinued 7 days before surgery. Dipyridamole is not typically stopped preoperatively, but when other antiplatelet agents are continued preoperatively, dipyridamole is usually discontinued 24 hours preoperatively. Warfarin is often stopped 5 days preoperatively, with LMWH initiated 3 days preoperatively as a bridge if the patient is high risk for being off anticoagulation

completely. LMWH is then discontinued 12 to 24 hours before surgery. Fondaparinux is discontinued typically 5 days preoperatively. In patients undergoing procedures with moderate to high bleeding risk, it is recommended to stop a DOAC based on the creatinine clearance, which is unique for each DOAC subclass, but often 3 to 5 days preoperatively. Given the short half-life of DOACs, no bridging heparin is usually necessary for these patients.[3,55,84,85,123,124,141]

Hemostatic Alterations Caused by Cardiopulmonary Bypass

Surgical repair of pediatric cardiac lesions often requires the use of CPB for both definitive repairs and for palliative procedures. CPB is associated with significant alterations in coagulation homeostasis. The foreign surface of the bypass circuit is highly thrombogenic, making systemic anticoagulation with heparin necessary. Heparin exerts its effect as previously stated by irreversibly binding to and potentiating the effects of the endogenous anticoagulant, AT, by up to 10,000-fold. Unfortunately, anticoagulation does not totally mitigate the risk of clotting and places the patient at risk for paradoxical life-threatening hemorrhage. Additional factors such as surgical trauma, hypothermia, and underlying critical illness further contribute to the coagulation disturbances seen in pediatric and neonatal CPB patients.[142] Recent advances in circuit technology such as smaller surface area oxygenators and heparin-coated tubing, as well as the addition of fresh frozen plasma (FFP) to the circuit prime, have helped reduce some coagulation complications; however, a significant number of CPB patients still experience postoperative bleeding requiring significant transfusion and/or reexploration. Risks for severe bleeding with CPB include young age, low weight, deep hypothermia, high preoperative hematocrit, and complex surgery.[143-145] The need for surgical reexploration for postoperative bleeding is associated with significantly increased mortality and morbidity, including prolonged mechanical ventilation, increased infections, and increased transfusions.[146-148] The etiology of CPB-associated coagulopathy is multifactorial and can be broken down into five categories that occur simultaneously and include activation of the coagulation system, inflammation, hemodilution, platelet dysfunction, fibrinolysis, and heparin effect.

Activation of Coagulation

Activation of the coagulation process occurs immediately in CPB due to exposure of vascular endothelium during surgical incisions, as well as exposure of blood to the foreign surface of the CPB circuit. Exposure of the vascular endothelium initiates the normal, appropriate cell-based process of hemostasis seen in nonbypass patients. When blood is exposed to the foreign circuit surface, circulating proteins such as fibrin, fibrinogen, and vWF immediately bind these surfaces and attract platelets, leukocytes, red blood cells (RBCs), and other circulating coagulation factors. What follows is a complex, intertwined process that culminates in continuous clot formation on the circuit surface. Circulating thrombin binds to circuit-bound fibrin and fibrinogen and participates in a positive feedback loop of further thrombin production and platelet activation. It is important to note that once thrombin is bound it is no longer susceptible to the inhibitory effect of the heparin-AT complex, so this process can continue unchecked until bound thrombin is degraded and circulating thrombin is neutralized. Initial platelet aggregation leads to activation, further aggregation, release of procoagulant proteins (vWF, fibrinogen, and factors V and XIII)

TABLE 24.2   Perioperative Management of Anticoagulants

Drug	Mode of Action	Half-Life	Preoperative Management	Agents Currently Used to Reverse Bleeding
Warfarin	Vitamin K antagonist, factors II, VII, IX, X, protein C and S	40 h (duration of effect 2-5 d)	Stop 2-5 d	Prothrombin complex concentrate
Unfractionated heparin	Thrombin and factor Xa	60-90 min	Variable practice—often not stopped before surgery	Protamine sulphate
Low-molecular-weight heparin	Factor Xa and Thrombin	3-5 h	Stop 12-24 h before surgery	None
Dabigatran	DTI	14-18 h[a]	Stop 3-5 d[b]	Hemodialysis
Rivaroxaban	Factor Xa	8-10 h[a]	Stop 3-4 d[b]	Prothrombin complex concentrate
Apixaban	Xa	7-18 h[a]	Stop 3-4 d[b]	
Enemol (Argatroban)	DTI	50 min	Stop 4 h before surgery	None
Bivalirudin	DTI	30 min		None
Aspirin	Antiplatelet—cyclooxygenase inhibitor	Effect present for life of platelet	Variable practice—thought to have limited impact on postoperative bleeding and often not stopped	Platelet transfusion
Clopidogrel	Antiplatelet—ADP receptor antagonist	Effect present for life of platelet	Stop 5-7 d before surgery. Some patients have normal platelet function at day 3 and approximately 30% do not respond to treatment	Platelet transfusion
Prasugrel	Antiplatelet—ADP receptor antagonist	Effect present for life of platelet	Stop 7 d before surgery	Platelet transfusion
Ticagrelor	Antiplatelet—ADP receptor antagonist	7-8.5 h, metabolite 12 h Reversible binding to ADP receptor	Stop 24-72 h before surgery	Platelet transfusion

[a]Half-life varies depending upon renal impairment.
[b]Cessation of drug will vary depending on degree of renal impairment.
ADP, Adenosine diphosphate; *DTI,* direct thrombin inhibitor.
From Davidson S. State of the art: how I manage coagulopathy in cardiac surgery patients. *Br J Haematol.* 2014;164:779-789.

from alpha granules and perpetuation of the clotting process. The negatively charged phospholipid surface of the activated platelet acts as a platform for prothrombinase (factor Xa and Va complex) formation, which then further activates circulating thrombin, and the process continues. Bound monocytes express TF, the most potent stimulator of coagulation initiation. TF binds circulating factor VIIa, leading to activation of both factors X and IX and further propagation of the coagulation process.

Inflammation

CPB causes systemic inflammatory response syndrome via a variety of paths.[147,148] Blood exposure to the circuit and surgical disruption of the vascular endothelium both lead to activation of the alternative complement pathway via C3. Activated C3 (C3a) causes a variety of changes that impact coagulation, including increases in TF-bearing cells, procoagulant alterations in vascular endothelium, and further platelet activation.[149] Interestingly, the classic complement pathway is also activated in CPB patients by the heparin-protamine complex during heparin reversal, contributing to further

inflammation. Increases in classic complement proteins, C2 and C4, major players in this pathway, are not seen in nonbypass cardiac surgery.[150] Endotoxin and other inflammatory mediators such as tumor necrosis factor-α, interleukin-6 (IL-6), and IL-8 are all increased in CPB patients and are potent stimulators of TF production.[151-154] Nuclear factor-κB (NF-κB), a transcription factor responsible for the transcription of many proinflammatory genes, also appears to play a role in CPB-induced inflammation and coagulopathy.[155,156] Inhibition of NF-κB in CPB leads to decreases in TF expression, thrombin generation, and clot formation.[157,158] Tissue injury leads to the migration of activated neutrophils to injured tissues, upregulation of cytokine expression, and degranulation with the release of proinflammatory molecules such as free radicals, histamine, leukotrienes, and platelet-activating factor. This leads to further TF expression by monocytes, and the cycle continues.[156] Finally, blood salvaged from the pericardial space and thoracic cavity and returned to the patient after being in contact with extravascular TF-expressing cells leads to further inflammatory insult and activation of coagulation.[159] Patients who do not have blood salvage have lower levels of clot breakdown products such as thrombin-AT complex, t-PA antigen, and fibrin degradation products.[160,161]

Hemodilution

The initiation of CPB is associated with a reduction in the plasma concentrations of coagulation factors (Fig. 24.6). The younger the patient, the more pronounced the effect, because the circuit to blood volume ratio may be quite high. In neonates undergoing deep hypothermic CPB, Kern and colleagues[162] demonstrated a 50% reduction in circulating coagulation factors (Table 24.3). Priming the CPB pump with FFP as well as RBCs helps mitigate this, but thrombocytopenia and factor depletion are common in pediatric and neonatal CPB patients and likely contribute to increased risk of bleeding. Intraoperative transfusion may be required.

Recognition of the importance of supplying coagulation factors to smaller infants is reflected in the practice at some centers of priming the pump with whole blood or FFP and having whole blood available for transfusion after separation from CPB. Whole blood contains RBCs, platelets, and coagulation factors and is a balanced product. There are potential advantages to this approach: (1) the transfused blood product is from a single donor and (2) the use of a balanced product avoids depletion of red cells, which can occur with component therapy. The availability of whole blood frequently requires close cooperation with local transfusion therapy services and may limit its use.[163-165]

Platelet Dysfunction

Many consider platelet dysfunction to be the primary cause of excessive bleeding in CPB patients, and results of tests of function such as bleeding time and thromboelastograms are altered after CPB.[166] Platelet dysfunction is a combination of qualitative and quantitative defects with qualitative being the most important.[167-172] Qualitative defects result from activation and degranulation of platelets due to stimulation by circulating inflammatory mediators, vascular injury, and contact with the non–prostacyclin-producing circuit surface. Serum thromboxane concentration increases

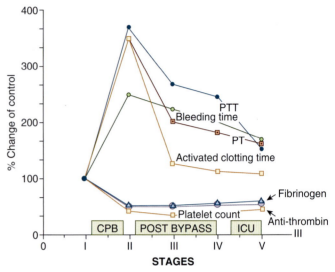

• **Figure 24.6** Plot of blood coagulation profile changes before, during, and after cardiopulmonary bypass (CPB) in 25 children. Clotting times and coagulant factors are shown as percentage change from control. Stage I, baseline, before CPB; stage II, post-CPB, before protamine reversal of heparin; stage III, after protamine; stage IV, just before leaving the operating room; stage V, after 3 hours in the intensive care unit (ICU). *PTT*, Partial thromboplastin time; *PT*, prothrombin time. (From Greeley WJ, Bushman GA, Kong DL, et al. Effects of cardiopulmonary bypass on eicosanoid metabolism during pediatric cardiovascular surgery. *J Thorac Cardiovasc Surg.* 1988;95:842-849.)

TABLE 24.3	Coagulation Factor Activity and Functional Tests of Coagulation in 30 Neonates					
Assay	Before CPB	1 Min on CPB	Cold CPB	Warm CPB	After Protamine	ICU
Fibrinogen (% activity)	210 ± 52	91 ± 15[a]	92 ± 19[a]	105 ± 22[a]	159 ± 58[a]	183 ± 33
Factor II (% activity)	56 ± 14	28 ± 8[a]	29 ± 9[a]	32 ± 10[a]	56 ± 14	64 ± 13[b]
Factor V (% activity)	70 ± 21	ND	ND	ND	40 ± 11[a]	48 ± 14[a]
Factor VII (% activity)	55 ± 13	26 ± 6[a]	27 ± 7[a]	29 ± 8[a]	50 ± 14[c]	63 ± 24[b]
Factor VIII (% activity)	58 ± 26	ND	ND	ND	36 ± 26[d]	73 ± 40[b]
Factor IX (% activity)	39 ± 19	24 ± 10[d]	22 ± 7[d]	33 ± 13[b]	39 ± 23	51 ± 20[b]
Factor X (% activity)	53 ± 13	31 ± 9[a]	30 ± 8[a]	33 ± 10[a]	53 ± 16	55 ± 17
Platelets (× 10⁹/L)	219 ± 57	64 ± 26[a]	65 ± 24[a]	93 ± 31[a]	161 ± 65[b]	
Antithrombin III (% activity)	50 ± 17	29 ± 11[a]	28 ± 12[a]	31 ± 12[a]	51 ± 17	64 ± 21[b]
Heparin (U)	0.05 ± 0.09	0.36 ± 0.11[a]	0.39 ± 0.10[a]	0.39 ± 0.11[a]	0.08 ± 0.14	0.08 ± 0.09
ACT (sec)	167 ± 20	>700[a]	>700[a]	700[a]	148 ± 22[b]	
PT (sec)	13.4 ± 2.4	25.1 ± 3.1[a]	25.0 ± 7.1[a]	22.2 ± 5.3[a]	15.2 ± 1.6[b]	13.9 ± 1.7
PTT (sec)	58.2 ± 16.7	>90[a]	>90[a]	>90[a]	72 ± 18.8[d]	53.7 ± 14.1

[a-d]Significance versus before CPB: [a]$P < .0001$, [b]$P < .05$, [c]$P < .01$, [d]$P < .002$.

ACT, Activated clotting time; *CPB*, cardiopulmonary bypass; *ICU*, intensive care unit; *ND*, not detected; *PT*, prothrombin time; *PTT*, partial thromboplastin time.

From Kern FH, Morana NJ, Sears JJ, et al. Coagulation defects in neonates during cardiopulmonary bypass. *Ann Thorac Surg.* 54:541-546, 1992; with permission.

significantly after the initiation of CPB in infants and children compared with control patients not undergoing extracorporeal circulation.[173] Thromboxane A_2 is a potent mediator of platelet microaggregation during CPB. Also during CPB, serum levels of PF_4 and beta-thromboglobulin are elevated. These peptides are found in the alpha granule and are secreted by activated platelets. Once activated, platelets lose both the ability for further degranulation and important surface receptors (i.e., GPIb and GPIIb/IIIa) involved in coagulation, leaving them functionally spent.[174-177] Heparin also induces platelet activation and qualitative dysfunction. Bleeding times are prolonged and microaggregation impaired after heparin administration even before the initiation of CPB. These effects appear to be independent of dose, although high-dose heparin may protect against excessive platelet activation by inhibiting thrombin formation.[178-180] Finally, increased fibrinolysis may play a role in platelet dysfunction. Plasmin and t-PA inhibit platelets by breaking down vWF and GPIb and GPIIb/IIIa receptors on the cell surface. This platelet effect may be one of the reasons t-PA is effective in the treatment of coronary artery occlusion. CPB patients receiving the antifibrinolytic aprotinin, for example, have higher levels of GPIb receptors, better platelet function, and less bleeding than those who do not receive aprotinin.[181-184]

Fibrinolysis

Upregulation of fibrinolysis may also play a role in altered hemostasis in neonatal and pediatric CPB patients. Products of fibrinolysis are elevated in bypass patients over levels seen in patients receiving cardiovascular surgery without bypass.[185,186] Fibrin formation stimulates t-PA and u-PA synthesis and release. These two serine proteases, in conjunction with factor XIIa, formed in response to blood contact with the foreign circuit, convert plasminogen to plasmin. Plasmin is the workhorse of fibrinolysis and is responsible for the breakdown of fibrin and fibrinogen into inactive fragments such as D-dimer. Levels of plasminogen, t-PA, u-PA, and D-dimer are elevated in patients undergoing CPB over levels seen in patients undergoing nonbypass cardiac surgery.[187,188] Inflammatory mediators such as cytokines and endotoxin also stimulate plasminogen synthesis and further the process of fibrinolysis.[189-191]

The exact role of fibrinolysis in the pathogenesis of post-CPB bleeding awaits further clarification. Nonetheless, inhibitors of fibrinolysis such as aprotinin, epsilon-aminocaproic acid (EACA), and tranexamic acid are routinely used after open-heart surgery to decrease bleeding.[192,193] Aprotinin, a serine protease inhibitor that functions at many points in the coagulation cascade, including the inhibition of fibrinolysis, produces laboratory evidence of inhibition of fibrinolysis and decreased blood loss.[194] However, aprotinin is no longer in use in the United States (see later).

Hypothermia

Hypothermia impairs clotting ability by inhibiting platelet activation and aggregation as well as clotting factor activity. Some of these effects appear to be dependent on the level of hypothermia, with platelet function being impacted at higher temperatures than coagulation factors.[195] The progression of coagulopathy can be seen with decreasing temperatures ($37°C$ to $25°C$) via whole blood thromboelastogram with prolongation of clotting time, CFT, alpha angle, and maximum clot firmness.[196] Hypothermia inhibits the activity of both the TF/FVIIa and FXa/Va complexes, which in turn inhibit thrombin formation.[197-199] Acidosis in conjunction with hypothermia further worsens coagulation deficits.[200]

Heparin Effect

Heparin exerts its effect by potentiating the inhibitory activity of AT, as previously discussed. Monitoring of heparin effect is imprecise, and point-of-care tests such as ACTs have proven less than perfect in predicting bleeding and clotting outcomes. Further, the effect of heparin on the CPB patient is complex. Excessive heparin dosing may lead to bleeding or may more effectively inhibit thrombin formation, leading to decreased factor consumption and platelet activation, as well as decreased fibrinolysis. Less bleeding may occur with lower doses of heparin, but insufficient dosing may lead to thrombin formation, further factor consumption and platelet activation, and increased fibrinolysis. In both situations inappropriate bleeding or clotting may occur.

Hematologic Management During Cardiopulmonary Bypass in Children

Heparinization

Heparin quickly and effectively blocks the generation of fibrin, is rapidly titratable, and is easily reversible. Unfortunately, heparin is effective against only circulating thrombin and does not affect thrombin already bound to the CPB circuit. It is also highly protein bound and has variable metabolism and clearance, especially in the pediatric population, making optimal dosing and monitoring challenging.

Neonates are thought to have a significantly altered response to heparin for several reasons. The levels of most of the coagulation factors are altered in infants for the first several months to years of life.[201-203] This is evidenced in the prolongations seen in the clot-based monitoring tests such as the activated PTT and the PT. These differences are even more pronounced in children with CHD and, in particular, those with single-ventricle physiology.[204-206] Of special importance, average AT activity levels at birth are only 40% and increase to 100% by around 6 months of age. Pediatric patients also have increased heparin clearance and a lower dose response to heparin than adult patients, making them relatively heparin resistant.[207,208]

At many institutions the initial intravenous heparin bolus dose of 300 to 400 U/kg is empiric. It is administered before cannulation of the great vessels either by direct injection into the right atrium or through a functioning central line to ensure that heparin enters the central circulation. Heparin is also added to the CPB circuit prime in a concentration equal to 2 U/mL. The most common manner of assessing the biologic effect of heparin in the operating room is measurement of the ACT, which is a measure of contact activation of the coagulation system and is prolonged with systemic heparinization. The advantage of the ACT is that it provides rapid results at the bedside. An ACT of greater than 400 seconds is generally felt to prevent fibrin deposition in the extracorporeal circuit and provide adequate anticoagulation for the institution of CPB. However, the ACT is neither a sensitive nor a specific test of heparin concentration or effect. Further, multiple studies have shown that ACT is a poor predictor of heparin effect in pediatric patients.[209-211] Hypothermia, hemodilution, and platelet abnormalities can also prolong the ACT. Finally, ACT also does not provide direct information on the level of thrombin suppression, the primary goal in systemic anticoagulation during CPB.

A more individualized approach to heparin management has been proposed in recent years. The premise for this approach comes from data indicating that heparin concentration, which varies greatly based on individual patient factors and variable clinical scenarios, better estimates thrombin suppression.[212,213] Traditionally heparin concentration has been measured using the plasma-based anti–factor Xa assay, which is time consuming and not readily available for point-of-care testing. A comparable bedside method uses a combination of a heparin dose response (HDR) curve and a heparin protamine titration (HPT). In the HDR, samples of the patient's blood are added to increasing known amounts of heparin, and an ACT is calculated for each dose. From this, an individualized initial heparin bolus dose is calculated to achieve the desired ACT. During CPB an HPT can be used to maintain the desired concentration of heparin. In this assay, known amounts of the patient's whole blood are added to increasing doses of protamine sulfate. Protamine neutralizes heparin in a 1 : 1 ratio so that the vial with the protamine dose closest to the heparin dose will clot the fastest, providing the clinician with an estimate of the patient's blood heparin concentration. The HPT is also used to determine the ideal protamine dose for heparin reversal at the conclusion of CPB. Accurate protamine dosing is important because excess protamine contributes to platelet inhibition and bleeding risk. The HMS Plus Hemostasis Management System (Medtronic, Minneapolis, MN) is a commercially available method that uses HDR, HPT, and ACT technology to guide intraoperative heparin management during CPB. It correlates well with laboratory-based methods of plasma heparin concentration (anti-Xa assay). Individualized heparin and protamine management has been associated with higher intraoperative heparin doses, lower protamine doses, and decreased platelet and factor consumption, postoperative bleeding, and transfusion requirements.[213,214]

Heparin resistance refers to the clinical situation in which standard heparin doses fail to produce an effect on the ACT. AT deficiency is suspected when the ACT fails to prolong beyond 300 seconds despite the administration of more than 600 U/kg heparin.[215] Low levels of AT appear to be a major culprit in heparin resistance and inadequate thrombin suppression, especially in neonates and infants. Normal neonatal prebypass levels of AT are approximately 40%. When combined with the hemodilution from the circuit prime, even if the prime includes FFP, AT levels after the initiation of bypass may be even lower. FFP has been the traditional method of treatment for heparin resistance. However, 1 mL of plasma provides only 1 unit of AT; therefore replacement volumes to achieve significant increases in AT activity may be prohibitively high. For this reason some centers supplement with AT concentrates instead.[216-218] Antithrombin concentrates contain between 50 and 175 U/mL of AT, depending on the formulation (pooled human or recombinant). Replacement goals vary by institution. Normal AT activity (100%) is based on adult norms. Goals for replacement in pediatric bypass often range between 80% and 100%, and required dosing to achieve these goal levels varies by baseline patient AT level and product concentration. Antithrombin supplementation in adult CPB patients has shown promise in reducing heparin resistance.[219,220] The safety and efficacy of AT supplementation in neonatal and pediatric CPB patients remains unknown at this time. Other factors may also contribute to heparin resistance, including ongoing active coagulation, previous heparin therapy, and drug interaction. The prospective identification of patients with heparin resistance is vital so that thrombin generation can be sufficiently suppressed during CPB.

Alternatives to heparin use in pediatric patients (due to HIT or heparin resistance) undergoing operations with CPB include danaparoid (synthetic heparinoid not available in the United States) and the DTIs argatroban and bivalirudin. There are limited data on the use for CPB of these agents, but they have been used successfully.[68-71]

Heparin Neutralization

Protamine is used to neutralize heparin and restore clotting activity after CPB. Protamine is a polycationic alkaline molecule that combines with the negatively charged sulfated mucopolysaccharide heparin to produce a dense precipitate that is biologically inactive.

Analogous to the situation with heparin dosing, the dosing of protamine is often empiric. Usually 1 to 1.5 mg of protamine is administered for each 100 U of heparin given during bypass. Alternately, protamine dosage may be based on weight or on protamine titration as noted earlier. Protamine dosing based on heparin dose or weight typically results in an intentional protamine excess. This surfeit of protamine is felt to minimize the possibility of residual heparin causing postoperative hemorrhage.

Protamine dose requirements are higher in neonates younger than 1 month compared with older infants and children. This is presumably due to the fact that heparin effect is more pronounced in neonates because of their reduced metabolic capability and their exposure to hypothermia.

Protamine frequently produces systemic hypotension in adults. Hypotension after protamine in infants and children does occur but appears to be less of a problem. It is unclear why pediatric patients are spared many of the complications of protamine therapy. When hypotension occurs, it is transient and felt to be due to histamine release. Injecting the drug over 5 to 10 minutes and adequate volume replacement usually avert the fall in blood pressure in patients with a marginal cardiac output. More worrisome are anaphylactic or anaphylactoid reactions to protamine. These reactions can manifest as cutaneous flushing or protracted systemic hypotension associated with noncardiogenic pulmonary edema. A more ominous event, catastrophic pulmonary vasoconstriction (CPVC), has been reported to occur in adults at rates anywhere from 0.2% to 4% following protamine administration. CPVC reactions appear to be complement mediated. Previous sensitization to protamine may play a role, and populations deemed by some experts to be at risk include insulin-dependent diabetic patients who receive protamine-containing insulin preparations and patients with cross-reacting antigens such as those with fish allergies and vasectomized men. Whatever the mechanism of these adverse reactions to protamine, the reactions appear to be relatively rare in infants and children.[221-225]

The end point for protamine administration is an ACT value within 10% of the baseline value obtained before heparinization. There are further limitations of titrating protamine effect to the ACT: thrombocytopenia, hypothermia, and hemodilution, a triumvirate frequently present after CPB, all adversely affect the ACT. Bleeding after heparin reversal is a common and difficult problem in neonates and infants.

Diagnosis and Management of Bleeding After Cardiopulmonary Bypass in Infants and Children

At the conclusion of CPB, many patients exhibit a multifactorial coagulopathy with relatively severe quantitative and qualitative factor and platelet deficits. This effect is exaggerated in neonates and smaller children. The incidence of excessive bleeding after surgical repair of congenital heart defects is approximately 5% to 10%. Blood loss in excess of 10% of the child's circulating blood volume in any hour or blood loss greater than 5% of the patient's blood volume per hour for more than 3 consecutive hours often mandates surgical reexploration.

Continued blood loss following heparin neutralization is common and must be treated with transfusion of whole blood or RBCs, platelets, and/or coagulation factors depending on the likely defect. Large-volume blood loss should be replaced in a manner similar to massive hemorrhage seen in trauma patients with extra focus on platelet replacement because qualitative abnormalities may be significant even in the face of sufficient quantity. It is reasonable to replace in a 1 : 1 : 1 ratio in this scenario. Manno and colleagues[163] have shown that the administration of fresh whole blood (less than 48 hours old) after CPB is associated with significantly less bleeding compared with component therapy. The group treated with whole blood demonstrated improved platelet function as well. The potential additional advantage of whole blood is that it may minimize donor exposure when compared to component therapy. However, fresh whole blood is often not readily available in hospital blood banks and may require coordination with the local blood banks.

Coagulation factors are replenished with FFP or cryoprecipitate. FFP contains normal plasma levels of most procoagulant and anticoagulant proteins. Cryoprecipitate provides a higher concentration of fibrinogen than FFP, as well as some vWF, factor VIII, and factor XIII. Cryoprecipitate is used as the first-line replacement for isolated hypofibrinogenemia or when volume is of concern because it is a more concentrated product. In clinical practice, 1 unit of cryoprecipitate per 5 kg of patient weight will increase fibrinogen by approximately 100 mg/dL. Another method of determining the number of units of cryoprecipitate needed is to multiply 0.2 times the weight (in kilograms) to provide approximately 100 mg/dL fibrinogen.

Some centers use bedside TEG to guide transfusion therapy; for example, a low angle in a bleeding patient may suggest a need for cryoprecipitate. Treatment should not be delayed by pending laboratory results, or the clinician is likely to be significantly behind in replacement therapy. The use of rapid TEG, however, may allow for results within approximately 10 minutes to allow potential real-time decision making regarding blood product repletion.

Surgical bleeding should be considered a cause for significant bleeding that does not respond to factor and platelet replacement, and reexploration should be considered. However, differentiation between medical and surgical bleeding can be difficult. Although cyanotic, polycythemic children have the highest incidence of coagulation abnormalities on preoperative screening tests of coagulation, it is impossible to prospectively identify a population at risk for postoperative hemorrhage. Severely polycythemic children are also seen with decreasing frequency in the current era of congenital heart surgery. Furthermore, advances in anesthetic and surgical techniques have resulted in a shift from palliative procedures to total correction in the neonatal period. Early total correction avoids hypoxia and the hemostatic alterations due to polycythemia and cyanosis. In place of these alterations are substituted the new hemostatic challenges of the neonate and young infant undergoing extensive surgical repairs using CPB, hypothermia, and total circulatory arrest.

There are no data on the optimal hematocrit after weaning from CPB. Decisions regarding hematocrit level are individualized based on the patient's postrepair function and anatomy to optimize oxygen delivery. Newer data indicate that previously unrecognized complications related to transfusion may counteract the benefit of transfusion in some instances. Transfusion of RBCs has been associated with increased length of mechanical ventilation, nosocomial infection, and increased hospital length of stay in pediatric cardiac surgery patients.[219,220] A more restrictive transfusion strategy is likely to be beneficial in both cyanotic and noncyanotic CHD.[226-228] In a recent study by Cholette et al. there was no benefit to a liberal transfusion strategy (goal hemoglobin of 13.9 g/dL) over a more restrictive transfusion strategy (11 g/dL) in single-ventricle patients undergoing cavopulmonary anastomosis. Further, patients in the restrictive transfusion cohort received significantly fewer transfusions and donor exposures.[229] Children who have moderate to severe myocardial dysfunction may still benefit from the improved oxygen-carrying capacity provided by hematocrit levels of 40%, but a lower hematocrit (30% to 35%) may be well tolerated in some cyanotic and noncyanotic postoperative patients with mild to moderate myocardial dysfunction. Hematocrit levels of 21% to 25% are usually acceptable in patients with a physiologic two-ventricle correction and excellent myocardial function.

Pharmacologic Methods to Reduce Bleeding

Many centers use pharmacologic agents to reduce bleeding and restore hemostasis after congenital heart surgery. Because platelet activation appears to be the predominant hemostatic derangement associated with CPB, the pharmacologic prevention of activation with synthetic prostaglandins has been proposed as one strategy to decrease blood loss. In animal studies PGI_2 decreases blood loss and prevents platelet activation.[230] In humans there is no conclusive evidence for benefit with this approach. A problem associated with prostaglandin administration is side effects because these drugs are potent vasodilators, and life-threatening hypotension may accompany their use.

Desmopressin acetate, a synthetic vasopressin analogue whose mechanism of action, although not well understood, appears to involve VIII:vWF, has not demonstrated any benefit in decreasing blood loss during pediatric cardiovascular surgery.[3,231] The authors do not recommend its routine use in children with CHD with post-CPB bleeding, but it could be considered with ongoing nonsurgical bleeding.

In children undergoing CPB, inhibition of fibrinolysis can be achieved with lysine analogues, which bear structural similarity to lysine. These lysine analogues competitively bind to plasmin and plasminogen and prevent breakdown of fibrin or fibrinogen and are known as antifibrinolytic agents. As previously discussed, EACA is one such drug and has been shown to produce a significant reduction in blood loss compared with placebo-treated controls.[192] The dose of EACA often used is 100 to 150 mg/kg load followed by an infusion of 15 to 30 mg/kg/h. The use of tranexamic acid (TXA) (100 mg/kg bolus followed by infusion of 10 mg/kg/h), another antifibrinolytic agent, has also significantly decreased blood loss compared to placebo-treated control patients.[193,232] Aprotinin was another antifibrinolytic previously available but now removed from the market in the United States due to reports of renal and cardiovascular toxicity. A Society of Thoracic Surgeons Congenital Heart Surgery Database study suggested relatively equivalent results between aprotinin and EACA in pediatric patients but improved outcome with TXA in terms of lower mortality and bleeding overall, and this benefit extended into the neonatal age range.[233]

Human-derived medium-purity FVIII concentrates complexed to vWF (Humate-P) are approved for pediatric patients with von Willebrand disease for the prevention of excessive bleeding during and after surgery. This applies to patients with severe von Willebrand disease and patients with mild to moderate von Willebrand disease in whom the use of desmopressin is known or suspected to be inadequate.[234] Reports of the use of vWF in pediatric patients undergoing cardiac surgery are limited to case reports. Activated factor VII (FVIIa) has been used off-label to treat severe bleeding in a variety of conditions, with dosing ranging from 20 to 180 mcg/kg. Among postcardiotomy patients with life-threatening hemorrhage despite every effort at surgical hemostasis and unabated by blood product transfusion, the use of recombinant FVIIa may be considered, weighing the risk of thrombosis.[235-243]

Surgical causes of bleeding must always be considered, especially in complex repairs with lengthy suture lines such as the arterial switch operation for transposition of the great arteries. If bleeding through the chest tube exceeds 10 mL/kg in the first postoperative hour and 5 mL/kg/h thereafter, or if blood loss is greater than 10% of the circulating blood volume per hour despite adequate heparin neutralization and correction of hemostatic defects with the appropriate blood products, emergent surgical reexploration may be indicated.

Hematologic Alterations on Extracorporeal Membrane Oxygenation

Patients on ECMO have many of the alterations in hemostasis seen in CPB with several important differences. First, the duration of CPB is much shorter than that of ECMO: hours versus days to sometimes weeks or months for ECMO patients. Depending on their recent operative history, ECMO patients may or may not have the disruptions in hemostasis caused by surgical trauma, hypothermia, and/or circulatory arrest. Those patients who fail to separate from bypass and are converted to ECMO immediately postoperatively will experience all of these derangements. This is in contrast to the patient with severe cardiomyopathy and poor function placed on ECMO before any operative procedure. However, the initial inflammatory reaction and hemodilution is similar to that seen in CPB.[228,229,244,245] ECMO patients also require systemic anticoagulation, most commonly with heparin, and therefore experience the effects related to this need. Further, successful anticoagulation, the balance between bleeding and clotting, must be achieved for much longer periods. Over time, coagulation factors, platelets, and RBCs are continuously consumed and must be replaced as needed on a regular basis.

Anticoagulation on ECMO

ECMO is similar to CPB in that it uses an extracorporeal circuit made up of thrombogenic foreign substances that dictate the use of systemic anticoagulation. ECMO is different from CPB in that patients are often maintained on this extracorporeal support for days to weeks instead of hours. Despite improvements in the ECMO circuit technology over the past several decades, bleeding and clotting complications continue to account for the majority of ECMO-related complications. Based on a recent analysis from the Extracorporeal Life Support Organization (ELSO) registry, bleeding occurs at a rate of approximately 38%, and thrombosis is nearly as commonly reported at 31%.[246] Bleeding and thrombosis are associated with increased mortality, and pediatric patients with heart disease are particularly vulnerable to both.[247-249] Within this group the highest incidence of bleeding occurs in postoperative patients (57%). Mediastinal exploration, high pre-ECMO surgical

complexity, longer CPB time, and early postoperative cannulation all increase risk of hemorrhage in this patient population.[248] The most dreaded bleeding complication, intracranial hemorrhage, occurs in up to 5% to 20% of pediatric cardiac ECMO patients. Other sites for bleeding include the pericardial space, pleural site, cannula site, and surgical site(s) and occur with an incidence of between 3% and 30%.[246,249] Reed and Rutledge[247] reported that thrombosis was noted in two-thirds of ECMO nonsurvivors on autopsy. Further, clotting in the circuit and oxygenator occurs in an estimated 15% and 12% of pediatric ECMO patients, respectively.[246] Careful systemic anticoagulation is therefore essential to balancing circuit clotting and patient bleeding.

In a recent survey of ELSO centers, all reported using a continuous infusion of UFH for ECMO anticoagulation. Despite the universal use of heparin, ECMO anticoagulation management varies widely among centers, and there are very few data points on which to base standardization of management.[250] In 2014, ELSO published a recommended framework for ECMO anticoagulation.[251] These recommendations are described in the following discussion.

Patients who require ECMO support are almost always critically ill and may have underlying coagulation disturbances related to recent surgery, DIC, inflammation, infection, and/or liver disease. Every attempt should be made to correct preexisting coagulopathy before initiation of ECMO. This may include administration of FFP, cryoprecipitate, vitamin K, and/or platelets. The ECMO circuit should be primed with RBCs and FFP when possible with 50 to 100 units of UFH per unit of RBCs to decrease hemodilution. When blood priming is not possible due to the urgency of the clinical situation (i.e., extracorporeal cardiopulmonary resuscitation or ECPR), then the pump may be saline primed, although emergency release blood may be preferable, especially in neonates and smaller children.

Systemic anticoagulation includes an empiric initial bolus dose of UFH (usually 50-100 U/kg body weight) just before cannulation for systemic anticoagulation followed by an UFH infusion. If patients are immediately postoperative and bleeding is a concern, it may be reasonable to decrease the bolus dose, delay initiation of UFH infusion, or use smaller starting doses. Dosing of the UFH infusion varies depending on individual patient factors such as platelet count and renal function, but the recommended starting range is 7.5 to 20 U/kg/h. Larger patients will require smaller starting doses. Neonates have a relative heparin resistance due to baseline differences in coagulation factors (including AT), underdeveloped kidneys, altered metabolism, and a different volume of distribution than older patients and usually require higher starting UFH doses.

The ideal heparin monitoring strategy for ECMO patients is a subject of great debate in recent years. For many years, management using ACTs via adaptations of CPB practices was the standard of care in ECMO. Recent studies suggest that ACT measurements are highly variable and often inaccurate measurements of heparin effect in both CPB and ECMO patients.[252-254] The reasons for this include variability between the point-of-care test devices and individual patient factors such as factor consumption, hemodilution, hypothermia, thrombocytopenia, and acidosis. Despite these issues, in a 2013 survey of ELSO centers done by Bembea et al., 97% still reported using ACTs to guide heparin management. The most common goal ACT range for heparin therapy on ECMO was reported to be 180 to 220 seconds.[250] It is important to note that ECMO patients have varying degrees of coagulation factor and platelet consumption at all times during their prolonged course;

therefore a multipronged approach to anticoagulation monitoring and management is likely to be beneficial. Patients may be at high risk of bleeding due to underlying factor deficiency or platelet dysfunction while experiencing subtherapeutic heparin effect. Insufficient heparin effect may lead to excess thrombin formation and exacerbation of factor and platelet consumption. A comprehensive approach that includes measurements of individual patient coagulation status such as aPTT, PT, TEG, and AT activity level combined with a measurement heparin effect (anti–factor Xa assay) may prove to provide superior information for safe and effective heparin management of ECMO patients. The use of additional assays is becoming more common, with 76% of respondents reporting the use of aPTT at least every 12 hours, and 51%, 40%, and 12% of respondents reporting the routine use of AT activity levels, anti–actor Xa levels, and TEG, respectively.[250]

Successful anticoagulation with heparin depends on adequate AT levels. Neonatal patients have lower baseline AT levels ($\approx$40%) until approximately 6 months of age, and ECMO patients of any age may experience AT deficiency due to consumption, liver disease, or hemodilution. Low levels of AT may lead to the need for escalating doses of heparin to achieve appropriate anticoagulation. This heparin resistance may be treated by supplementing AT, using either recombinant or pooled human AT. The exact AT levels needed to successfully anticoagulate pediatric and neonatal ECMO patients is unknown and likely variable depending on the underlying clinical situation, but many centers advocate replacement of AT when levels are low and/or heparin dose needs are high. The safety and efficacy of such practices remain unknown.

Bleeding may complicate ECMO, with every effort made to correct coagulation deficiencies, including maintaining the hemoglobin level above 10 mg/dL, platelet count above 100,000/mm^3, and fibrinogen level above 200 mg/dL. EACA or TXA may be considered if bleeding remains excessive.

There is a growing interest in anticoagulation of ECMO patients using a newer class of anticoagulants, the DTIs (argatroban and bivalirudin). These drugs directly bind and inhibit factor Xa and are not dependent on the presence of AT, making them appealing when AT levels are unpredictable. In addition, unlike UFH, they are able to inhibit both bound and circulating thrombin and do not cause immune-mediated reactions like HIT. Routine use of DTIs has been limited by expense and the lack of a reversal agent. There is increasing use of DTIs, and we expect there will be additional literature available on outcomes in the coming years.

Ventricular Assist Device–Associated Coagulation Abnormalities

When a VAD is implanted, the interaction between the device material and blood affects the delicate balance of hemostasis. Major complications of VAD therapy include both thrombosis and bleeding.

Thrombotic complications can occur in all VADs, but studies of the pulsatile extracorporeal devices such as the Berlin Heart EXCOR report approximately 30% neurologic complications. Bleeding complications with VADs also occur at a higher rate than would be expected based on use of systemic anticoagulation alone. Factors implicated in an increased risk of bleeding with VADs include acquired von Willebrand syndrome, impairment in platelet aggregation, and lack of pulsatility.[255-260] Acquired von Willebrand disease can be responsible for significant bleeding, with gastrointestinal (GI) bleeding most common, and appears to be related

to loss of large vWF multimers in continuous flow (CF) VADs[256] (see Chapter 40 on VADs). A similar pathologic bleeding condition resulting in a high incidence of GI bleeding was discovered in 1958 in patients with aortic stenosis (Heyde syndrome). Warkentin et al.[259] subsequently found that a severely stenotic aortic valve predisposes patients to the development of acquired von Willebrand syndrome (type 2A) characterized by the loss of large vWF multimers. This is thought to be the mechanism of high bleeding rates from GI angiodysplasia in patients with aortic stenosis. vWF abnormalities are directly related to the severity of aortic valve disease and are improved by valve replacement. A loss of large, high-molecular-weight vWF multimers similar to that described in patients with critical aortic stenosis has been observed in patients with implanted CF-LVADs.[255,256] In a series of 101 patients, Crow and colleagues[256] reported that GI bleeding was higher in patients with CF-LVADs than in those with pulsatile devices. This hemostatic abnormality is a contributor to excessive, typically mucosal bleeding in patients with CF-LVADs. Narrow pulse pressure has been hypothesized to dilate mucosal veins, increase smooth muscle relaxation, and cause arteriovenous dilation, also leading to arteriovenous malformation and bleeding. LVAD-associated vWF degradation alters angiogenesis in the bowel mucosa, which proliferates continuously, thus promoting GI angiodysplasia and predisposing LVAD patients to bleed. Shear force activates hemostasis by a few mechanisms, including microparticle production from endothelium, leukocytes, and platelets and alteration of von Willebrand multimers. Anticoagulation for VADs is discussed in Chapter 40.

Summary

Postoperative bleeding and thrombosis continue to be a problem for patients with heart disease, despite years of progress in pediatric cardiac surgery, intensive care, anesthesiology, and hematology. This chapter has addressed normal coagulation from a developmental perspective, discussed ways of investigating both bleeding and thrombosis risk in these high-risk cardiac patients, highlighted preexisting coagulation abnormalities in CHD, discussed common use of anticoagulant regimens in the cardiac population, and examined the relationship of those abnormalities to the hematologic derangement of CPB, ECMO, and VADs. Pediatric cardiac disease involves many hematologic considerations that continue to provide challenges and opportunities for ongoing clinical investigation.

Selected References

A complete list of references is available at ExpertConsult.com.

3. Giglia TM, Massicotte MP, Tweddell JS, Barst RJ, Bauman M, Erickson CC, et al; American Heart Association Congenital Heart Defects Committee of the Council on Cardiovascular Disease in the Young, Council on Cardiovascular and Stroke Nursing, Council on Epidemiology and Prevention, and Stroke Council. Prevention and treatment of thrombosis in pediatric and congenital heart disease: a scientific statement from the American Heart Association. *Circulation.* 2013;128(24):2622–2703.

7. Hoffman M, Monroe DM 3rd. A cell-based model of hemostasis. *Thromb Haemost.* 2001;85:958–965.

41. Zabala LM, Guzzetta NA. Cyanotic congenital heart disease (CCHD): focus on hypoxemia, secondary erythrocytosis, and coagulation alterations. *Paediatr Anaesth.* 2015;25(10):981–989. doi:10.1111/pan.12705. [Epub 2015 Jul 17]. Review. PubMed PMID: 26184479.

55. Monagle P, Chan AKC, Goldenberg NA, Ichord RN, Journeycake JM, Nowak-Göttl U, et al; American College of Chest Physicians. Antithrombotic therapy in neonates and children: antithrombotic therapy and prevention of thrombosis, 9th ed: American College of Chest Physicians evidence-based clinical practice guidelines. *Chest.* 2012;141(suppl):e737S–e801S.

120. Giglia TM, Witmer C, Procaccini DE, Byrnes JW. Pediatric Cardiac Intensive Care Society 2014 consensus statement: pharmacotherapies in cardiac critical care anticoagulation and thrombolysis. *Pediatr Crit Care Med.* 2016;17(3 suppl 1):S77–S88. doi:10.1097/PCC.0000000000000623. Review. PubMed PMID: 26945332.

123. Nishimura RA, Otto CM, Bonow RO, Carabello BA, Erwin JP 3rd, Guyton RA, et al; ACC/AHA Task Force Members. 2014 AHA/ACC guideline for the management of patients with valvular heart disease: a report of the American College of Cardiology/American Heart Association Task Force on Practice Guidelines. *Circulation.* 2014;129(23):e521–e643. doi:10.1161/CIR.0000000000000031. [Epub 2014 Mar 3].

124. Nishimura RA, Otto CM, Bonow RO, et al. 2017 AHA/ACC focused update of the 2014 AHA/ACC guideline for the management of patients with valvular heart disease: a report of the American College of Cardiology/American Heart Association Task Force on Clinical Practice Guidelines. *J Am Coll Cardiol.* 2017;70(2):252–289.

169. Besser MW, Klein AA. The coagulopathy of cardiopulmonary bypass. *Crit Rev Clin Lab Sci.* 2010;47(5–6):197–212. doi:10.3109/10408363.2010.549291. Review. PubMed PMID: 21391830.

202. Monagle P, et al. Developmental haemostasis. Impact for clinical haemostasis laboratories. *Thromb Haemost.* 2006;95(2):362–372.

208. Yee DL, O'Brien SH, Young G. Pharmacokinetics and pharmacodynamics of anticoagulants in paediatric patients. *Clin Pharmacokinet.* 2013;52(11):967–980.

218. Finley A, Greenberg C. Review article: heparin sensitivity and resistance: management during cardiopulmonary bypass. *Anesth Analg.* 2013;116(6):1210–1222. doi:10.1213/ANE.0b013e31827e4e62. [Epub 2013 Feb 13]. Review. PubMed PMID: 23408671.

246. Dalton HJ, et al. Factors associated with bleeding and thrombosis in children receiving Extracorporeal Membrane Oxygenation (ECMO). *Am J Respir Crit Care Med.* 2017;196(6):762–771.

251. Lequier L, Al-Ibrahim O, Bembea M, Brodie D, Brogan T, Buckvold S, et al. *ELSO Anticoagulation Guidelines.* 2014.

256. Crow S, Chen D, Milano C, Thomas W, Joyce L, Piacentino V 3rd, et al. Acquired von Willebrand syndrome in continuous-flow ventricular assist device recipients. *Ann Thorac Surg.* 2010;90(4):1263–1269, discussion 1269.

25

Blood Utilization and Conservation

JILL MARIE CHOLETTE, MD; BRANDEN ENGORN, MD; DHEERAJ GOSWAMI, MD

The use of blood products is common in patients who have surgery for congenital heart disease (CHD). Ninety-eight percent of these patients receive at least one red cell transfusion, and greater than 50% receive fresh frozen plasma (FFP) or platelets.[1] Transfusions are given to improve oxygen delivery and to prevent or improve coagulation abnormalities. Pediatric cardiac surgical patients have varying physiologies, and oxygen delivery needs can be different for neonates compared to teenagers and for cyanotic patients compared to acyanotic patients. This variation can complicate a provider's decision making on when, what, and how much to transfuse.

Transfusions also are not without risks. Immunologic reactions may occur, and the risk of infectious transmission remains despite thorough screening. Blood transfusions also lead to increased risk of infection, ICU and hospital length of stay (LOS), duration of mechanical ventilation, and mortality.[2-4] The benefits of transfusing a critically ill child and the potential harms must be carefully balanced.

The concepts of blood utilization and blood conservation originated in attempt to optimize the balance of benefit and harm from transfusion. These concepts are similar but focus on two slightly separate components when trying to minimize transfusions. Blood utilization focuses on how and what is transfused; blood conservation attempts to minimize the likelihood or potential need for transfusion. In this chapter we will discuss both concepts throughout the entire perioperative period.

Preoperative

The preoperative period offers the provider a unique opportunity to engage the patient in strategies for blood conservation and utilization that will last throughout the perioperative course. Many of these strategies have been studied and proven in adults, whereas the pediatric literature relies more on institutional experience and case reports. The preoperative strategies can be divided into the following: general strategies, iron replacement for iron deficiency anemia, recombinant human erythropoietin, preoperative autologous donation, and optimization of other blood components

General Strategies

First, it is important to recognize that cell counts are individual to the patient and rely on other factors, including age of the patient, medications, syndromes, and comorbidities. Although it is imperative to obtain a complete blood cell count (CBC) before surgery, attention should be paid to being judicious and thoughtful about preoperative phlebotomy and making sure blood draws are limited to those tests that are absolutely necessary. Furthermore, hemodilution via volume administration should be avoided for any patient admitted preoperatively.

Patients with CHD are often on numerous medications, including those that may affect bleeding. Acetylsalicylic acid (aspirin) is commonly prescribed, and adult literature shows it can have an effect on postoperative bleeding.[5] An analysis of the risks and benefits of continuing aspirin, other nonsteroidal antiinflammatory medications that may affect platelet function, and other anticoagulant and antiplatelet agents should be made with the patient's surgeon and cardiologist and in consideration of the patient's comorbidities.

As with the general preoperative evaluation of the pediatric cardiac surgery patient, it is necessary to maximize nutrition in an effort to maintain levels of hemoglobin (Hgb), albumin, and other plasma proteins. Furthermore, although there is concern for increased morbidity with blood transfusion, the clinician must balance this risk with concerns that preoperative anemia may have adverse effects. It is independently associated with adverse outcomes after cardiac surgery in adults[6] and a risk factor for postoperative mortality in both neonates and children undergoing noncardiac surgery.[7,8] Although the risk of preoperative anemia in pediatric cardiac surgical patients not been studied, it is important to consider that the strategies discussed in the following sections could both conserve blood and treat a potentially modifiable preoperative risk factor.

Iron Replacement

As mentioned previously, nutrition is an important aspect of the preoperative evaluation, particularly with a goal of blood conservation. One modifiable nutritional risk factor that is of particular benefit is iron deficiency anemia (IDA). IDA is a very common pediatric condition that most often affects toddlers and adolescent girls.

The prevalence of IDA is 3% to 7% and is increased in patients with prematurity, Hispanic ethnicity, obesity, and low socioeconomic status.[9,10] Laboratory workup shows a decreased Hgb, decreased mean corpuscular volume, increased red cell distribution width, decreased serum iron concentration, increased total iron-binding capacity, and decreased transferrin saturation. One can often see low ferritin levels as a surrogate of iron stores. However, in the setting of acute inflammation, ferritin level may be elevated because it is an acute phase reactant. If IDA is suspected, the child can be given enteral iron (premature infant: 2 to 4 mg elemental iron/kg/24 h divided twice a day; child: 3 to 6 mg elemental iron/

kg/24 h divided twice a day; adult: 60 to 100 mg elemental iron twice daily), and Hgb values can be reassessed in 4 to 6 weeks.[11]

Recombinant Erythropoietin

Erythropoietin (EPO) is an endogenous hormone that is produced by the kidney and allows for differentiation and proliferation of erythroid precursor cells resulting in increased hemoglobin. Recombinant human EPO (rHuEpo) has been used in pediatrics for anemia related to many conditions such as chronic renal failure, oncologic disease, human immunodeficiency virus, and anemia of prematurity with an established safety profile and dosing.[12] It is important to provide concomitant iron supplementation unless iron stores are already in excess, and the peak effect is seen in 2 to 3 weeks. Perioperatively there has been success in pediatric critical care and pediatric anesthesia in other procedures that have a high risk for bleeding and need for blood transfusion, including patients who are Jehovah's Witnesses and craniosynostosis repair.[13-14] In pediatric cardiac surgery there have been reports of the successful use of EPO in the preoperative period, and the dose recommendation is 300 U/kg of EPO 7 days before surgery supplemented with iron.[12,15] EPO has been proven to be safe, and, although it may increase hematocrit in the pediatric cardiac patient, the effect on outcome and blood utilization in the perioperative period is still questioned. Given the variable response and rare usage in pediatrics, consultation with a pediatric hematologist may be beneficial in select patients.

Autologous Blood Donation

Preoperative autologous blood donation (PAD) has been shown to be safe and efficacious in adult cardiac surgery.[16] It should be noted that differences in adult and pediatric physiology should be taken into consideration when planning for PAD. Adults after PAD are able to benefit from enteral rehydration to replenish the reduction in intravascular volume and increase stroke volume. Older children may have a similar physiologic response; however, pediatric patients less than 4 years of age cannot compensate with increased stroke volume due to differences in myocardial muscle fibers and may be unable to rehydrate with oral fluids and require intravenous fluid replacement.[17] Furthermore, infants and young children, often require sedation or anesthesia during procedures. The strategy of PAD has been shown to safely and effectively minimize homologous blood transfusion in the perioperative period in pediatric cardiac surgery patients older than 5 years.[18] Various protocols have been studied for PAD in smaller children. Masuda et al. showed that autologous donation can be performed in children weighing less than 20 kg through collection of volumes 5 to 10 mL/kg over six PAD sessions in the 50 days before surgery. In this study the patients received no homologous blood donations; however, many of the children did not cooperate with the PAD procedure.[19] Fukahara et al.[20] showed that the lack of cooperation with the donation procedure could be overcome with PAD at the time of preoperative cardiac catheterization. Hibino et al. studied children 6 months to 5 years of age undergoing primary cardiac surgery who underwent PAD via two donations of 5 to 10 mL/kg collected via the femoral vein under general anesthesia at 2 and 3 weeks preoperatively. They found a significant decrease in homologous transfusion with no difference in intraoperative or postoperative Hgb levels.[21] Although there are no randomized trials for PAD, careful patient selection could allow this strategy to be employed for pediatric patients undergoing cardiac surgery.

However, one must remember that through PAD the patient will often become anemic and therefore may benefit from adjunctive preoperative EPO and iron.[16] PAD is not without cost to the patient and medical system, and because preoperative autologous blood units are often wasted if not needed in the perioperative period, patient selection is crucial. The blood bank can store the preoperative autologous blood for 3 weeks with citrate phosphate dextrose adenine solution or 6 weeks with cryopreservation.[22]

Other Blood Components

It is important to recognize that perioperative bleeding can be multifactorial, and it is important in the preoperative, intraoperative, and postoperative periods to maximize other factors in the coagulation cascade. Cardiopulmonary bypass–associated platelet dysfunction can contribute to postoperative bleeding. Some studies have suggested that platelet dysfunction diagnosed by thromboelastography (TEG) indicating an increased time to platelet plug formation are at increased risk for intraoperative red blood cells and FFP transfusions.[23] Most pediatric anesthesiologists would agree that for both cardiac and noncardiac surgery platelets should be transfused preoperatively if the platelet count is less than $50,000/\mu L$.[24] Because there are few well-defined preoperative laboratory values that require preoperative transfusion, it is important to have a personalized approach to each patient's history and comorbidities, which can allow further evaluation with platelet counts, coagulation studies, fibrinogen, bleeding times, and TEG.

Intraoperative

Intraoperative blood conservation and utilization are important components of blood management for a child undergoing cardiac surgery. The focus is on minimizing the amount of blood loss and using various methods of returning the patient's blood back to the intravascular space while optimizing the benefits when transfusing. Both these methods can be made more complicated by patient factors and variations in physiology during the intraoperative period.

This period of physiologic variability can begin with the transition from negative pressure ventilation to positive pressure ventilation that occurs with intubation. There is also the hemodynamic transition that occurs coming on and off cardiopulmonary bypass (CPB), as well as the physiologic change that occurs with the repair. These transitions can alter oxygen delivery and utilization for each patient and potentially the transfusion thresholds for the practitioner. Furthermore, just the initiation of CPB can involve the use of blood products and/or significant hemodilution. The CPB circuit has numerous deleterious effects on the coagulation cascade and blood product function, as does the process of cooling and rewarming that is required in many pediatric cardiac surgeries. These factors, along with the surgery itself, can make it difficult to know how to treat any bleeding that occurs. A thorough understanding of these transitions, the patient's physiology, and the surgical repair will better allow one to make an educated decision on transfusion practices during the intraoperative time course.

Blood Conservation

General Strategies. Minimizing blood loss is not just a component of surgical technique. Laboratory draws, waste, and line insertion are small but not insignificant causes of blood loss especially in children. New technology has allowed for a minimal volume of blood, less than 0.1 mL in the newest blood gas machines, to be drawn and still provide the same information as the older machines.[25] These machines are often used as a point-of-care service, which could potentially increase their overall utilization. Judicious use of blood draws and laboratory tests will minimize blood loss directly and also by reducing the waste that occurs each time that blood is obtained.

Invasive lines are placed in many patients undergoing cardiac surgery. The placement of invasive lines can be difficult due to the size of the vessels, cannulation sites, and the number of previous cannulation attempts. Techniques to minimize blood loss should be used, including holding pressure at the line site, optimizing positioning for line placement, and occluding infusion sites once the line is in the vessel. Some blood loss is inevitable with both line placement and blood draws, but a focus on the details will make this minimal even in the smallest of children.

Acute Normovolemic Hemodilution. Acute normovolemic hemodilution (ANH) is an excellent method of minimizing actual hemoglobin loss during surgery. Blood is removed from the patient in the operating room, replaced with an equal volume of crystalloid, and stored at room temperature until transfusion is required. The hemoglobin is diluted, and thus hemoglobin loss from the surgery is decreased. Transfusion of whole blood containing all the coagulation factors and platelets may minimize further transfusions. ANH can be difficult in neonates and small children. The amount of blood that must be removed is likely to cause a large drop in hemoglobin and potentially affect oxygen delivery for the patient. There are only small studies of ANH in pediatric patients, and none are in patients with congenital cardiac disease.[26,27] These studies showed no effect on transfusion requirements, but the theoretical benefits exist and could manifest with larger studies. A recent meta-analysis did find that ANH reduced red blood cell transfusions in adults undergoing cardiac surgery.[28] This may be the best evidence for its use in large children, teenagers, or adults with CHD, though the need for surgery is quite different between the populations.

Cell Salvage/Pump Blood. There can be a large amount of blood loss during cardiac surgery. The easiest way to minimize the effect of this blood loss is to return it to the patient in some form. Generally this can be done via "pump blood" or cell salvage devices. The majority of blood loss during CPB is returned to the pump via drains or the pump sucker (dedicated suction line that returns to the bypass circuit). Blood that is lost post bypass is collected via a dedicated suction line and then stored via a cell salvage device. This stored blood will be washed and filtered and will contain only red cells. The pump blood, on the other hand, is whole blood and will contain factors, platelets, and residual amounts of heparin. Therefore new or persistent bleeding should likely be addressed differently depending on which of these two was used for blood return.

There are multiple cell salvage systems, but the most common use saline to wash the salvaged blood and centrifuge off the supernatant and heparin, creating a hemoconcentrated product for reinfusion. The efficiency of the system is based on the ratio of blood suctioned to red cells salvaged. This ratio is not 1:1 due to red cell injury or loss at separate aspects of the system. The first and likely most damage is at the suction tip. There is also clotting and damage through the suction tubing and injury of the red cells during the washing method.[29]

The literature regarding cell salvage in adults is robust and relatively consistent in its benefits in decreasing transfusion needs.[30] The pediatric literature shows similar efficacy, although the number

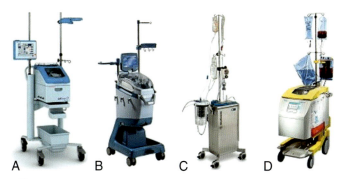

• **Figure 25.1** Popular cell salvage devices. A, Cell Saver Elite (Haemonetics Corporation, Braintree, MA). B, Sorin XTRA autotransfusion system (LivaNova, London, UK). C, autoLog autotransfusion system (Medtronic, Minneapolis, MN). D, C.A.T.S *plus* Continuous Autotransfusion System (Fresenius Kabi, Bad Homburg, Germany).

of studies is much less robust.[31-33] The only study in the pediatric cardiac population included 106 patients weighing less than 20 kg, but investigators stored the cell-salvaged blood for up to 24 hours following its collection, which is not consistent throughout pediatric cardiac institutions, which generally limit reinfusion for 4 to 6 hours following collection. The study demonstrated significantly fewer autologous RBC transfusions, coagulant product transfusions, and donor exposures early in the hospital course, but there was only a trend toward significance by the end of the hospital stay, likely due to heterogeneity in subjects and procedures. This study is discussed further in the postoperative portion of the chapter.[33]

Cell salvage efficiency has been one of the limitations in its use in pediatrics. The older devices often required more than 300 mL of volume to be able to adequately wash and filter the blood for reinfusion. New technology has improved this process significantly, and now there are devices that require between 40 and 60 mL (Fig. 25.1).[34] Further studies are needed to evaluate the efficacy of the superefficient cell salvage devices in the pediatric population.

Mechanisms to Minimize Surgical Blood Loss

Antifibrinolytics. There are two primary antifibrinolytics currently used in pediatric surgery, tranexamic acid (TXA) and epsilon-aminocaproic acid (EACA). These medications are similar and work primarily by inhibiting plasmin, but TXA is more potent and generally more expensive.[35] Their efficacy in both adult and pediatric cases are similar in many surgical situations. There are two prospective comparison studies in newborns undergoing cardiac surgery that show similar efficacy.[36,37] Generally both medications are thought to decrease blood loss and potentially decrease transfusion requirements. The choice of which antifibrinolytic to use is based on institutional preference.

There have been a number of pharmacokinetic studies completed in an attempt to determine the optimal dosing parameters for both TXA and EACA. There was single study in neonates undergoing CPB with EACA in which a loading dose of 40 mg/kg, an infusion of 30 mg/kg/h, and a pump prime concentration of 100 mg/L maintained an optimal concentration in the majority of the patients.[38] Dosing for other age-groups is usually a load of 100 mg/kg with an infusion range between 30 and 50 mg/kg/h.[39] A similar study in patients with TXA showed that an optimal dosing strategy was based on the age and weight of the patient.[40] In 2007 approximately 50% of all patients undergoing cardiac surgery in the Society of Thoracic Surgery database received antifibrinolytics.[41] The current percentage is likely significantly higher with more widespread use at pediatric cardiac institutions and the removal of aprotinin from the US market in 2007. Certain institutions are selective with their use of antifibrinolytics, with the Fontan surgery and other single-ventricle repairs being common exceptions.

Surgical Technique. Surgical technique is the most important component of blood conservation in pediatric cardiac surgery. Excellent surgical hemostasis can make much of intraoperative blood conservation moot. The same can be said of poor surgical hemostasis because surgical bleeding will persist until the cause is found and repaired. A combination of excellent surgical technique and a blood conservation plan is the most optimal for the patient. Significant blood loss often is expected in many pediatric cardiac cases, and some amount of blood use is inevitable. Approximately 90% of all pediatric cardiac surgical patients are transfused with some component of blood products during the entire perioperative period.[42] Therefore the question for the practitioner is often what, when, and how much to transfuse rather than if transfusion should occur.

Blood Utilization

Packed Red Blood Cells. The purpose of transfusing packed red blood cells (PRBCs) is to attempt to optimize systemic oxygen delivery. Anemia has been found to be a risk factor in some studies for infections, acute kidney injury, and mortality in pediatric patients undergoing cardiac surgery.[43-45] The same adverse outcomes are present in patients who are transfused more than others.[45-47] The balance between oxygen delivery via transfusion and minimizing the risks of transfusion is the goal of optimal PRBC utilization.

The oxygen delivery in healthy individuals at rest is thought to be at least twice the amount required.[48] However, patients with congenital cardiac disease have variable physiologies (e.g., mixing lesions, differential pulmonary to systemic blood flow) that can significantly alter expected oxygen requirements. Cyanosis further alters oxygen content, thereby increasing the need for circulating red blood cells as an adaptive response. Multiple studies have attempted to find the optimal transfusion trigger intraoperatively. The most in-depth study looked at psychomotor development scores at nonlinearly increasing hematocrit levels. This study found developmental delays at hematocrit levels less than 24%.[49] The generalizability of this study can be questioned due to the fact that it was completed only in infants, none of whom were patients with single-ventricle physiology or had aortic arch reconstruction. It was also completed on infants who underwent low-flow bypass for a period of time. The study gives a basic framework on which future investigations may be based, though adjustment for cardiac lesion, age, and bypass technique needs to be considered. Though there have been other transfusion threshold studies, only one has been initiated in the operating room. The study was in noncyanotic patients with CHD between 6 weeks and 6 years of age and had a liberal threshold of 10.8 g/dL and a conservative threshold of 8 g/dL for hemoglobin. Outcome differences were shown in LOS and amount of PRBCs transfused benefiting the conservative group.[50]

Fresh Frozen Plasma. Approximately 50% of pediatric patients undergoing cardiac surgery receive a transfusion of FFP in the operating room.[42] The primary purpose of FFP use is to minimize alterations in the coagulation cascade during CPB. Generally FFP is used in pump priming for infants and neonates despite limited evidence for its use. A single study of only 20 patients showed a decrease in blood product and cryoprecipitate use but not platelets, FFP, or PRBCs.[51] Two other studies, including the largest on this topic (80 patients), showed no clinical benefit of priming with FPP.[52,53] Once again, the variability in the pediatric cardiac population makes it difficult to accurately generalize any of the studies. There were no patients undergoing reoperations included in the studies, and some did not include higher-complexity operations.

Platelets. Intraoperative platelet use is variable, with only approximately 30% of all pediatric patients undergoing cardiac surgery receiving them. The percentage is higher for neonates and infants compared with older patients and is associated with longer duration of surgery.[42] Platelet-associated bleeding on bypass is likely multifactorial. Platelet destruction occurs when blood flows through the oxygenator and CPB tubing.[54] The functional abnormalities are widespread, including increased activation, alteration of platelet surface adhesion receptors, and platelet signaling.[55-57] Indications for platelet transfusion differ across institutions. Many transfuse platelets to all neonates, whereas some transfuse platelets according to CPB duration or specific surgical procedure. The timing of platelet administration is more uniform because they are given after CPB once protamine has been completed. Further platelet administration is often considered if the site of persistent bleeding is thought to be the microvasculature.[58]

Cryoprecipitate. Although cryoprecipitate initially was used to treat hemophilia A, its use has been expanded to acquired causes of hypofibrinogenemia, including that which occurs with CPB. The likely mechanism of hypofibrinogenemia in CPB is a consumptive process that occurs with a large amount of blood loss and as a result of the effects of blood flowing through the bypass circuit.[59] It is the least likely blood product to be transfused in patients with CHD undergoing cardiac surgery.[42] The potential benefits are the small volume compared to the amount of fibrinogen contained when compared to FFP. There are no studies evaluating its use, but it may be beneficial in infants and neonates who may not tolerate large volumes of FFP or who have isolated hypofibrinogenemia.

Transfusion Algorithms/Coagulation Studies. The overwhelming evidence of the harm of transfusions has forced pediatric cardiac centers to alter their transfusion practices. Many centers have started to use laboratory data in an attempt to decrease the amount of blood products used.[60-66] Laboratory data may help identify underlying causes of bleeding and address the appropriate causes. Some studies have shown the efficacy of using laboratory data and demonstrated a decreased use of overall blood products.[60,61,63,66]

A variety of laboratory studies may be considered from basic coagulation studies, such as international normalized ratio, prothrombin time, partial thromboplastin time, platelet count, and fibrinogen, to functional studies (Fig. 25.2) like TEG (TEG; Haemonetics Corporation, Braintree, MA), thromboelastometry (TEM) and rotational thromboelastography (ROTEM) (Pentapharm GmbH, Basel, Switzerland). Please refer to Chapter 24 for additional explanation of these laboratory studies. There are some concerns that the routine use of these studies could potentially increase blood product utilization in attempt to make laboratory study results normal without the abnormality showing any clinical effect. Therefore an important component for some of these algorithms is the presence of "abnormal" bleeding. This is a subjective evaluation

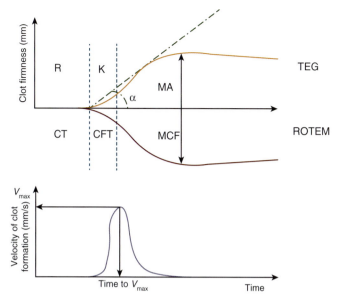

• **Figure 25.2** Sample tracing from a viscoelastic clotting analyzer. *α*, Angle formed by a tangential line to the curve starting from the split point; *CFT*, clot formation time; *CT*, clotting time; *K*, time from an amplitude of 2 mm to 20 mm; *MA*, maximal amplitude; *MCF*, maximal clot firmness; *R*, reaction time; *Vmax*, maximum velocity of clot formation. (Hans GA, Besser MW. The place of viscoelastic testing in clinical practice. *Br J Haematol.* 2016;173:37-48.)

by the surgeon and impacts the potential accuracy and generalizability of the algorithms.[62,67] For these reasons some experts advocate the use of coagulation studies only in high-risk bleeding patients (e.g., redo sternotomies, neonates, and patients undergoing deep hypothermic circulatory arrests).[68]

Factor Concentrates. Please refer to Chapter 24 for a full discussion of factor depletion and potential mechanisms for bleeding.

The primary factors in coagulation are present in FFP. Factor concentrates give a concentrated dose of specific factors and are primarily used in patients with hemophilia who lack specific coagulation factor(s). There has been an increase both in the number of factor concentrates available in recent years and in their use in pediatric cardiac surgery. There is little high-quality evidence for the use factor concentrates, and much of the literature is limited to case reports or relatively small case series.[69-71] Factor concentrates have been used predominantly as a rescue therapy for patients with persistent medical bleeding during the perioperative period (Table 25.1). The lack of empiric data along with the expense, and risks, of these products has led many institutions to create strict protocols for their use. Further studies are needed to establish the role of factor concentrates in blood conservation and utilization.

Ultrafiltration. Ultrafiltration is a method of removal of fluid and high-molecular-weight solutes and inflammatory mediators across a semipermeable membrane after or during CPB. There are numerous types of ultrafiltration, but the most common in pediatrics is modified ultrafiltration. This process occurs immediately after bypass and was first described in the early 1990s. Conventional ultrafiltration is still used at some centers, and fluid removal occurs while on CPB. Ultrafiltration has beneficial effects on blood conservation and utilization, including increasing hematocrit, platelets, and coagulation factors and decreasing postoperative transfusions.[72-75]

Special Considerations

Fresh Whole Blood

The use of fresh whole blood (FWB) in pediatric cardiac surgery is still a topic of debate. The proponents believe that giving blood with all its procoagulant and anticoagulant factors allows for a better balance between clot formation and destruction, which may minimize the amount of blood required during the surgery. There may also be benefits with minimizing the number of donor products in decreasing the overall risk with transfusion and the associated inflammatory response. The contrary view is that whole blood can be difficult to obtain at many centers, and there is a potential waste of products by not partitioning out each component. Most centers that use FWB primarily use it in neonates and infants, who have a higher rate of overall blood utilization. The evidence for FWB use in priming the circuit and for continued resuscitation is not completely clear. The studies have primarily been completed in single centers with differing methods. Three prospective studies have shown a benefit to the use of whole blood. Two of these studies used FWB not only in the prime but also for continued resuscitation. These studies were consistent in showing that FWB decreased postoperative blood loss.[76,77] The more recent study also showed a decrease in LOS, inotropic scores, and ventilation times with FWB. This blood was also reconstituted from separate components from the same donor.[77] Priming with FWB alone has two conflicting studies; Mou et al. showed no benefit and at worse, possible harm, whereas Valleley et al. demonstrated a benefit in donor exposure and postoperative bleeding.[78,79] Complicating this further is that the study by Mou et al. compared a reconstituted blood prime (PRBCs and FFP) to whole blood, whereas the study by Valleley et al. had a CPB prime containing only PRBCs. The conflicting data, the difficulty in obtaining FWB, and the potential waste of products have kept it from being consistently used in neonates and infants throughout the United States.

Blood Utilization and Blood Conservation—Postoperative Management

Iatrogenic anemia is common in infants and children following cardiac surgical procedures secondary to hemodilution and hemolysis related to CPB strategies, crystalloid and albumin boluses/infusions postoperatively, and frequent sampling.[80,81] Ongoing blood loss through mediastinal and chest tubes is commonplace, particularly in the first 48 hours after surgery, and can be significant when compounded by inadequate surgical hemostasis or exacerbated by hypothermia, coagulopathy, hypofibrinogenemia, platelet dysfunction, and thrombocytopenia.[82] Efforts to maintain hemodynamic stability and ensure adequate oxygen delivery include PRBC transfusion for volume expansion and improved oxygen-carrying capacity and plasma products to correct coagulopathy and replace fibrinogen and platelets and control/resolve bleeding.[83,84]

Complicating postoperative management is the prevalence of decreased myocardial performance and systemic vasodilation/systemic inflammatory response syndrome that occurs following CPB, which may impair the patient's ability to increase cardiac output and maintain oxygen delivery in response to anemia.[85-87] Unique factors related to CHD impact blood conservation and utilization. First, morphologic/structural changes (single-ventricle physiology and/or intracardiac or great-vessel-level shunting) may increase the volume and/or pressure load on either the systemic and/or pulmonary ventricle(s) and may limit the patient's ability

TABLE 25.1	Common Factor Products Available in the United States	
Drug Name	**Accepted Clinical Use**	**Dosing**
Antithrombin III (Thrombate III)	Hereditary antithrombin deficiency Possible clinical use: low antithrombin III in the setting of ECMO or CPB	Prophylaxis: 25-40 units/kg Treatment: (Desired − Measured AT III level) × wt in kg/1.4
Factor VIIa (NovoSeven)	Hemophilia A/B, factor VII deficiency, Glanzmann thrombasthenia Uncontrolled bleeding despite adequate FFP, cryoprecipitate, platelets Intrabronchial administration for pulmonary hemorrhage	Dosing dependent on diagnosis: For bleeding post cardiac surgery: 60 mcg/kg
Factor VIII (Advate)	Hemophilia A	Prophylaxis: 20-40 units kg Treatment: (Desired VIII − Baseline VIII level) × (weight in kg)/2
Factor VIII (Recombinant)	Hemophilia A	Treatment: (Desired FVIII increase [%]) × (weight in kg)/2
Factor IX (BeneFix)	Hemophilia B	Prophylaxis: 25-40 units/kg twice weekly Treatment, children: (Desired IX − Baseline IX level) × (weight in kg) × 1.4 Treatment, adult: (Desired IX − Baseline IX level) × (weight in kg) × 1.2
FEIBA (aPCC antiinhibitor)	Bleeding in the setting of oral anticoagulants Hemophilia A and B with inhibitors	50-75 units/kg
Fibrinogen concentrate (RiaSTAP)	Congenital fibrinogen deficiency	Prophylaxis: 20-30 mg/kg weekly Treatment: 70 mg/kg
Prothrombin complex concentrate (Kcentra)	Reversal of vitamin K antagonists (Warfarin)	Dependent on INR: 25-50 units/kg for children
von Willebrand factor (Humate-P)	von Willebrand disease	Type I: Loading dose: 50-75 IU Maintenance: 40-60 IU every 6-25 h (target VWF concentration of > 50) Type II/III: Loading dose: 60-80 IU Maintenance dose: 40-60 IU

aPCC, Activated prothrombin complex concentrate; *AT III*, antithrombin III; *CPB*, cardiopulmonary bypass; *ECMO*, extracorporeal membrane oxygenation; *FEIBA*, factor eight inhibitor bypass activity; *FFP*, fresh frozen plasma; *INR*, international normalized ratio; *VWF*, von Willebrand factor.

to augment cardiac output by increasing ventricular stroke volume (hypertrophy and/or diastolic dysfunction) and overcome increased afterload (systolic dysfunction). Additionally, in cases of single-ventricle physiology and/or intracardiac or great-vessel-level shunting, changes in downstream pulmonary and/or systemic vascular resistance threaten the adequacy of blood flow to the other vascular bed (pulmonary or systemic). For these reasons, patient status post palliation or repair for CHD is uniquely vulnerable to anemia, bleeding, and alterations in hemodynamics, oxygenation, and ventilation. Red cell and coagulant product transfusions are important components of the medical management of these patients (see Table 25.1).

It is impossible to control for all the confounding factors that affect anemia, severity of illness, PRBC transfusion, and outcomes, which is why use of prospective randomized controlled trials (RCTs) is paramount (Fig. 25.3). There are now a few RCTs examining transfusion strategies in postoperative pediatric cardiac surgery, but it must be emphasized that the results of such trials should be interpreted with caution because each pediatric patient undergoing cardiac surgery has unique cardiac morphology and physiology that may change over time and may differ depending on the clinical situation, which may also change. For example, even when grouped according to cardiac diagnoses, developmental differences (gestational age, postnatal age, weight), and the presence of additional congenital

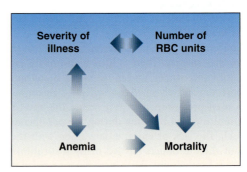

• **Figure 25.3** The number of RBC transfusions received by severely ill cardiac patients during their stay in an ICU is associated with short-term mortality. Anemia and severity of illness are also associated with mortality in these patients. What makes things even more complex is that RBC transfusions, anemia, and severity of illness are closely interconnected to one another. No multivariate analysis can deconstruct such confounding by indication; only a randomized clinical trial can disentangle these interactions. *RBC,* Red blood cell. (From Lacroix J. RBC transfusion: risk marker or risk factor? *Pediatr Crit Care Med.* 2013;14[3]:330-331.)

extracardiac defects and/or chromosomal abnormalities or genetic syndromes, prevent the generalization of transfusion management of these children. Great differences in physiology exist even in those who carry the same cardiac diagnosis. For example, patients with tetralogy of Fallot have varying degrees of right ventricular outflow tract obstruction and may have supravalvar, valvar, or subvalvar pulmonary stenosis, resulting in different degrees of right ventricular hypertrophy and varied atrial level shunting These anatomic differences lead to variation in oxygen saturations, preload dependence, and cardiac function and make generalization of anemia tolerance, even with this specific structural diagnosis, impossible. CPB and surgical techniques vary greatly among surgeons and across institutions. Differences in anesthesia, perfusion, and critical care management strategies also impact anemia tolerance and complicate generalization of transfusion strategies in the literature to the specific patient.

The bedside practitioner must have a good understanding of the pathophysiology of the cardiac lesion and the physiology resulting from the surgery performed, in the context of the postoperative alterations across all organ systems, in order to judge the risks and benefits of transfusion in these fragile patients (Table 25.2).

Red Blood Cell Transfusions—Restrictive Transfusion Practices.

The majority of the literature regarding postoperative transfusions in pediatric cardiac surgery is focused on transfusion of PRBCs, which is not surprising given the large number of PRBCs transfused in this population.[88,89] Children with CHD are routinely transfused and maintained at higher hemoglobin levels even when they are not anemic.[90-92] Observational studies demonstrate an association between RBC transfusion and worse clinical outcomes in pediatric cardiac surgery, including pediatric heart transplant and those on extracorporeal membrane oxygenation.[93-96]

The use of restrictive transfusion practices in critically ill patients was first presented by Hebert et al. in the landmark Transfusion Requirements in Critical Care (TRICC) trial and followed by similar studies across various patient populations and disease states, including critically ill adults with coronary artery disease.[97-101] Adults undergoing cardiac surgery also appear to tolerate restrictive transfusion practices, and perhaps more importantly, patients receiving the largest number of transfusions demonstrate the worst clinical outcomes.[102]

The landmark 2007 pediatric transfusion trial, the Transfusion Requirements in Pediatric Intensive Care Units (TRIPICU) study, concluded that hemodynamically stable critically ill children demonstrated no increase in new or progressive multiorgan failure when managed with a restrictive transfusion strategy.[103] Subgroup analysis of children with CHD from the TRIPICU trial found similar results.[104] However, authors of both studies cautioned that their work was not definitive. Indeed, TRIPICU study patients could be enrolled within 7 days of ICU admission, and inclusion criteria required that they be hemodynamically stable, defined as no increase in vasopressor agents and stable mean systemic pressures for 2 hours preceding enrollment. Unfortunately, these criteria prevent generalization of the results to the patients most likely to have PRBC transfusion entertained—those earliest in their postoperative course and those who are hemodynamically unstable. Furthermore, the subgroup analysis of children with CHD excluded those less than 28 days of age, those with cyanotic heart disease, and those undergoing palliative procedures for single-ventricle physiology, excluding the more complex children in whom RBC transfusion may provide the greatest potential benefit (and possible risk).

The second prospective RCT of blood utilization in pediatric cardiac patients was performed by Cholette et al.[105] and was the first to examine transfusion strategies in children with single-ventricle physiology and those undergoing cavopulmonary connection with bidirectional Glenn and Fontan procedures. Sixty patients were managed with either a restrictive or liberal transfusion strategy from time of pediatric cardiac intensive care unit (PCICU) admission to 48 hours post surgery. The primary outcome was peak and

TABLE 25.2	Variables Impacting Oxygen Delivery in the Pediatric Patient Following Cardiac Surgery		
Anemia	**Bleeding**	**Decreased Cardiac Output**	**Hypoxia/Desaturation**
Dilutional	Poor surgical hemostasis	Tachycardia leading to decreased cardiac filling time and increased myocardial oxygen demand	Intracardiac mixing • Cyanotic lesions
Blood loss	Thrombocytopenia	Arrhythmias AV dissociation • Heart block • Junctional rhythm	Elevated pulmonary vascular resistance
Active bleeding	Decreased platelet function	Post-CPB diastolic dysfunction	V/Q mismatch • Parenchymal lung disease • Effusion • Atelectasis
Iatrogenic anemia • Frequent blood tests • Blood "waste"	Hypofibrinogenemia	Inadequate preload	Fluid overload • Pulmonary edema
	Fibrinolysis Coagulopathy/factor deficiency	Decreased contractility Univentricular physiology • Single ventricle provides systemic and pulmonary circulations	

AV, Atrioventricular; *CPB*, cardiopulmonary bypass; *V/Q*, ventilation/perfusion.

mean arterial lactate levels and arteriovenous and arteriocerebral oxygen content differences as measures of oxygen utilization. No between-group differences were found, and those in the restrictive group received significantly fewer numbers of PRBC transfusions. This study is not without limitations as a small, single-center study, and its generalizability across centers has not been tested. The study was not powered for clinical outcomes, but no statistically significant clinical differences were seen. Despite its limitations, this study provides the first evidence that transfusion based on Hgb values to maintain higher Hgb levels is not required in this population as a matter of "routine"; the subjects did not appear disadvantaged by the lower Hgb levels and received significantly fewer PRBC transfusions. Of particular significance is that the study intervention included the highest-risk period when patients are most vulnerable to altered hemodynamics and blood loss.

The third prospective RCT, performed by de Gast-Bakker et al.,[50] included children 6 weeks to 6 years of age from time of anesthesia initiation to hospital discharge, randomized to a restrictive versus liberal transfusion strategy with transfusion thresholds of 8.0 and 10.8 g/dL, respectively. The authors excluded children with cyanotic defects and those with peripheral oxygen saturations below 95%. Of the 107 subjects, those managed with a restrictive strategy received significantly decreased PRBC transfusion volume and had significantly shorter hospital LOS, which resulted in significant cost savings. This study provides additional evidence that acyanotic children undergoing biventricular repairs can also tolerate lower Hgb levels and further encourage bedside clinicians to base their decisions to transfuse on clinical parameters.

A 2014 Cochrane review sought to determine the impact of PRBC transfusions on morbidity and mortality in neonatal and pediatric patients with CHD undergoing cardiac surgery.[106] Eleven trials with 862 cumulative patients were included, covering restrictive versus liberal transfusion trials (two trials), leukoreduction versus nonleukoreduction (two trials), and standard versus nonstandard CPB prime (seven trials). Unfortunately, wide heterogeneity in subjects, degree of cyanosis, and intervention precluded ability to pool data for meta-analysis. The authors concluded that additional studies that control for presence or absence of cyanosis are warranted.

In 2016 Cholette et al.[107] performed another prospective RCT that included neonates and infants weighing less than 10 kg, who traditionally receive the greatest number of transfusions from time of PCICU admission to 28 days post surgery. Children who required extracorporeal membrane oxygenation to wean from CPB were excluded. This study was unique in that it included neonates and infants undergoing palliative procedures and did not have any exclusion parameters regarding hemodynamic stability or oxygenation. Conservative transfusion strategy was PRBC transfusion for a Hgb less than 7.0 g/dL for biventricular repairs or less than 9.0 g/dL for palliative procedures plus a clinical indication. Liberal group strategy was PRBC transfusion for Hgb less than 9.5 g/dL for biventricular repairs or less than 12 g/dL for palliative procedures regardless of clinical indication. One hundred sixty-two infants were studied, 82 conservative (53 biventricular, 29 palliated) and 80 liberal (52 biventricular, 28 palliative), including 12 patients following Norwood procedure (6 conservative, 6 liberal). There was 100% protocol compliance in biventricular subjects managed with a restrictive transfusion strategy with no difference in outcomes. There was 80% protocol compliance in the palliated restrictive group, with only 6 patients receiving transfusions above their threshold. The authors concluded that neonates and infants could be managed with a conservative transfusion strategy with few protocol deviations and receive significantly fewer number and volume of PRBC transfusions even in the immediate postoperative period. Daily Hgb concentrations were significantly lower in the conservative group by postoperative day 1 and remained lower for more than 10 days after surgery. Despite maintenance of lower Hgb levels within the conservative group, arterial lactate level, arteriovenous oxygen difference, and clinical outcomes were similar between groups. This study's findings support the conclusion that clinical indications should guide PRBC transfusions, even in this uniquely vulnerable population, and provide further evidence for conservative transfusion practices in the neonate and infant undergoing complete biventricular repair. Whether these results can be replicated in a large, multicenter trial with clinical outcome differences would be of great interest, with particular focus on the highest-risk group, those undergoing palliative procedures (Table 25.3).

Red Blood Cell Storage Age and Modification

Further complicating matters is that practices differ across institutions in regard to PRBC storage duration of units utilized or reserved for pediatric cardiac surgery and other potential

TABLE 25.3	Red Blood Cell Transfusion Threshold Trials in Pediatric Cardiac Surgery					
Study	**Population**	**Patients (n)**	**Inclusion Criteria**	**Hb Thresholds**	**Outcomes**
Willems et al.[104] (2010)	Biventricular Noncyanotic	125	>28 d to <14 y	7 vs. 9.5 g/dL	New/progressive MODS
Cholette et al.[105] (2011)	Univentricular Cyanotic	60	Stage 2 or 3 Cavopulmonary connection	9 vs. 13 g/dL	Mean/peak lactate avDO$_2$ and acDO$_2$
de Gast-Bakker et al.[50] (2013)	Biventricular Noncyanotic	103	>6 wk to <6 y	8 vs. 10.8 g/dL	Hospital LOS Cost
Cholette et al.[107] (2017)	Univentricular and biventricular Cyanotic and noncyanotic	162	≤10 kg	(C) 9 vs. 12 g/dL + clinical (NC) 7 vs. 9.5 g/dL	Hb level, RBC transfusions, mean/peak and lactate clearance avDO$_2$

acDO$_2$, Arteriocerebral oxygen difference; *avDO$_2$,* arteriovenous oxygen difference; *C,* cyanotic; *Hb,* hemoglobin; *LOS,* length of stay; *MODS,* multiorgan dysfunction; *NC,* noncyanotic; *RBC,* red blood cell.

modifications (e.g., saline washing). The storage age of PRBCs may be of relevance, because the "storage lesion" that occurs as blood cells mature changes the structure and function of the cells, producing microparticles and mediators, and impairs red cell rheology and oxygen off-loading.[108-110] Despite the results from observational studies that found an independent association between longer storage age and multiple organ dysfunction in critically ill children,[111,112] two follow-up large, prospective RCTs failed to identify in-hospital mortality differences between hospitalized adults receiving either the freshest available (mean storage 13 days) or oldest available (mean storage 23.6 days) RBCs or 90-day mortality in critically ill adults.[113,114]

The patient undergoing CPB may be particularly affected by PRBC transfusions because of the already heightened inflammatory and immune response to CPB. Neonates and small infants are even more susceptible due to the large volume of PRBCs relative to blood volume they require. To determine whether patients undergoing cardiac surgery with CPB are vulnerable to differences in PRBC storage duration, a large, prospective RCT of 1098 subjects above 12 years of age undergoing complex cardiac surgery across multiple sites randomized to PRBCs of 10 or less versus 21 or more days of storage was performed.[115] Median age in each group was 73 and 72 years, respectively, and 98% to 99% of cases were coronary artery bypass grafts with or without valve repairs and not congenital cardiac surgery. The authors found no significant difference in multiple organ dysfunction scores between groups.

Retrospective pediatric studies of PRBC storage age have demonstrated varied results. An observational study of children following cardiac surgery did not find maximal or mean storage age to be associated with serious adverse events, although number of donors was.[116] Ranucci et al.[117] found that the storage of the PRBCs composing the blood prime for the CPB circuit was associated with a "major complication" (derived from a composite score). However, this association was not found for patients receiving PRBC after CPB. For example, Manlhiot and colleagues found in their retrospective review of 1225 pediatric cardiac surgeries that in patients receiving "high PRBC transfusion volumes" (>150 mL/kg), longer storage duration was associated with bleeding complications, renal insufficiency, higher inotrope score, longer chest tube drainage, longer hospitalization, and increased in-hospital mortality, with these associations strongest for storage duration above 14 days. This led the authors to conclude that the freshest available units should be used in pediatric cardiac surgery in which large-volume transfusions are anticipated, with no units above 14 days used as possible.[118] The study is confounded by the fact that the "high PRBC transfusion" group also received higher amounts of platelets, FFP, cryoprecipitate, albumin, and recombinant factor VII and underwent more complex surgeries.

Data from a prospective RCT examining washed versus standard transfusions were evaluated for an association of PRBC storage age and clinical outcomes.[1,119] Longer storage duration was significantly associated with increased postoperative nosocomial infections. A strength of the study was that the dose of PRBCs per kilogram in the study was large and mainly came from a single donor unit. Almost none of the patients received platelets or plasma, and the patient sample was recruited prospectively and consecutively as part of a controlled clinical trial.

Of the available pediatric cardiac surgical literature, differences in study design, confounders, and the varied "age" of stored blood has limited making strong conclusions about the impact of the storage age on clinical outcomes. It appears that the number of donors, as well as total transfused number and volume, adversely

impacts the recipient. Whether the storage age of the PRBCs transfused is independently associated with poor clinical outcomes is yet to be confirmed by larger multicenter trials.

Cholette et al. sought to answer whether the impact of the storage lesion could be ameliorated by modification of blood cell products by saline washing. The authors performed a prospective RCT in 162 children undergoing cardiac surgery with CPB to either an unwashed or washed transfusion protocol for PRBC and platelets during the operation and following the operation.[120] The primary outcome was use of the interleukin (IL)-6 to IL-10 ratio as a biomarker of altered balance of the proinflammatory and antiinflammatory response. Storage duration was similar between groups. The washed group had an improved inflammatory profile with significantly lower IL ratios, which suggests an improved balance of proinflammatory and antiinflammatory mediators. The study was not powered for clinical outcomes; however, the washed group demonstrated a nonsignificant trend toward reduced mortality. A larger study powered for clinical outcomes is needed to examine whether the storage lesion can be mitigated by washing blood cell products before their transfusion.

Blood Cell Conservation—Reinfusion of Cell Saver Blood. Reinfusion of autologous blood collected during cardiac, orthopedic, and vascular surgeries, commonly termed *cell salvage,* has proven effective in reducing need for subsequent allogeneic PRBC transfusions according to a 2010 Cochrane meta-analysis.[121] In pediatric cardiac surgery there is concern that reinfusing "pump salvage" may increase postoperative bleeding due to its heparin content and inflammation due to circulating mediators in the supernatant, and technical difficulties with small-volume collection have limited its use. These concerns have been ameliorated by technologic advances that make small-volume collection possible and remove heparin and the supernatant of the pump salvage, providing a heparin-free, hemoconcentrated product termed *cell saver.* A 2016 systematic review and meta-analysis of 46 prospective randomized trials (21 in cardiac surgery) supported the findings of the previous meta-analysis. Not only did reinfusion of washed cell salvage significantly reduce allogeneic PRBC exposure, but it also was associated with a reduction in the rate of infection by 28% and in-hospital LOS by 2.31 days.[122]

This meta-analysis included two pediatric studies, one in cardiac surgery.[33] That trial in 106 neonates and infants demonstrated significantly fewer allogeneic RBC transfusions, donor exposures, and coagulant product transfusions in the first 48 hours after surgery in the cell saver group. These differences persisted over the first postoperative week but did not reach statistical significance. The methodology of the trial was unique; cell saver was maintained at the bedside in a temperature-controlled cooler with strict quality assurance procedures for up to 24 hours after collection for immediate reinfusion in small sterile aliquots. Although it was not powered to detect difference in clinical outcomes, postoperative complications and mortality were similar between groups. Results of this trial led the authors to implement a cell saver protocol as standard of care, which allowed for review of an additional 110 children receiving cell saver blood for up to 24 hours.[123] No differences in postoperative infection rates were found when compared to historical controls, and fewer allogeneic red cell transfusions were given. A multicenter trial examining this practice would be of great interest and would potentially expand cell saver utilization and blood conservation practices. Expansion of cell saver use will decrease PRBC transfusions and donor exposures, will likely improve clinical outcomes, and will decrease hospital costs and conserve limited resources.

Pediatric Cardiac Intensive Care Unit Conservation Strategies. The great number of blood tests performed daily in a pediatric intensive care setting is well documented and is independently associated with subsequent PRBC transfusion.[124] Efforts to limit "routine" bloodwork are ongoing.[125,126] In addition to reducing the number of blood tests performed, limiting the blood volume drawn as "waste" may also decrease iatrogenic blood loss.[127] Use of pediatric tubes and in-line arterial systems also decreases iatrogenic blood loss and anemia due to blood sampling.[128,129] Most large centers have created multidisciplinary adult patient blood management (PBM) programs designed to increase education, implement blood conservation practices, and decrease the number of transfusions provided by an institution.[130] Adoption of blood conservation programs reduces PRBC and coagulant product transfusions, renal failure, hospital LOS, and costs in adult and pediatric cardiac surgery.[131,132] However, adult PBM standards do not apply to neonates and children, and development of pediatric-specific blood management programs is important not only to assist investigators but to support clinicians in the care of their patients.[133] Multidisciplinary efforts must include anesthesia, perfusion, congenital cardiac surgery, and critical care, in addition to nursing, transfusion medicine, and blood bank specialists.

Coagulant Products

Coagulant products often are required in the PCICU following pediatric cardiac surgery to control bleeding. Not surprisingly, neonates undergoing the longest and most complex procedures and those undergoing "redo" operations receive the largest number of PRBC and coagulant product transfusions.[134] Bleeding and transfusion of coagulant products following open-heart surgery are also associated with increased morbidity and mortality.[135,136]

Viscoelastic whole blood hemostasis analyzers TEG, TEM, and ROTEM are able to provide data on the patient's hemostatic function (even in the setting of heparin) and separate out coagulation factors, platelet function, and subsequent fibrinolysis (see Fig. 25.2). Use of these point-of-care devices allows for targeted, goal-directed coagulant product therapy, helps discern surgical bleeding from true aberrant hemostasis, and has been found to decrease postoperative transfusions in pediatric cardiac surgery.[65,137]

Children undergoing cardiac surgery with CPB complicated by significant bleeding have different TEG results than those children without, and bleeding can be controlled when TEG results are used to drive interventions.[138,139] In pediatric cardiac surgery, perioperative TEG has been found to decrease blood product transfusions and limit exposure to unnecessary coagulant product transfusions with similar hospital LOS, mechanical ventilation,

mortality, and thrombotic events.[65,140] Indiscriminant coagulant product transfusions should be avoided, and blood product transfusions should be goal directed. These tests of hemostasis should not be limited to the operating room and should be available to direct postoperative blood product management.

Conclusion

Optimal blood conservation and utilization in a patient with congenital cardiac disease can be difficult to achieve. The literature seems to support limiting and having a lower threshold for transfusions. This is complicated in the perioperative period by changes in physiologic state and coagulation and volume status in a patient who is attempting to recover from a surgical insult. The sickest of these patients often have the most hemodynamic variability, but the preconceived notion that they need more blood and blood products must come to an end. Many of the recent studies discussed in this chapter have helped the PICU community care for these patients. However, there is still much uncertainty on how to manage these patients; what is clear is the need for further studies on how to optimize transfusion and coagulation.

Selected References

A complete list of references is available at ExpertConsult.com.

6. Karkouti K, Wijeysundera DN, Beattie WS, et al. Risk associated with preoperative anemia in cardiac surgery: a multicenter cohort study. *Circulation.* 2008;117(4):478–484.
63. Nakayama Y, Nakajima Y, Tanaka KA, et al. Thromboelastometry-guided intraoperative hemostatic management reduces bleeding and red cell transfusion after pediatric cardiac surgery. *Br J Anaesth.* 2015;114(1):91–102.
103. Lacroix J, Hebert PC, Hutchison JS, et al. The TRIPICU Investigators, the Canadian Critical Care Trials Group, and the Pediatric Acute Lung Injury and Sepsis Investigators Network. *N Engl J Med.* 2007;356(16):1609–1619.
106. Wilkinson KL, Brunskill SJ, Doree C, Trivella M, Gill R, Murphy MF. Red cell transfusion management for patients undergoing cardiac surgery for congenital heart disease. *Cochrane Database Syst Rev.* 2014;(2):Art No.: CD009752.
107. Cholette JM, Swartz MF, Rubenstein J, et al. Outcomes Using a Conservative Versus Liberal Red Blood Cell Transfusion Strategy in Infants Requiring Cardiac Operation. *Ann Thorac Surg.* 2017;103:206–215.
132. Karimi M, Forentino-Pineda I, Weatherred T, Qadeer A, Rosenberg CA, Hudacko A, et al. Blood Conservation Operations in Pediatric Cardiac Patients: A Paradigm Shift of Blood Use. *Ann Thorac Surg.* 2013;95:962–967.

26

Nutrition and Metabolism in the Critically Ill Child With Cardiac Disease

DARLA SHORES, MD; LEAH SIMPSON, RD; SAMUEL M. ALAISH, MD

Nutrition is a vital consideration in children with critical heart disease for several reasons: (1) nutritional deficiency may cause heart disease; (2) congenital heart disease (CHD) may cause malnutrition and poor growth, which can delay or complicate corrective surgery[1,2]; and (3) congenital heart surgery may be associated with complications that lead to life-threatening metabolic and nutritional derangements.

Nutritional Deficiency as a Cause of Heart Disease

Malnutrition (Protein-Energy Deficiency)

Protein-energy malnutrition (PEM) is the inappropriate loss of body cell mass secondary to reduced intake or inadequate use of substrate. Children, especially neonates, are particularly prone to developing PEM because they have minimal metabolic reserve to combat illness. PEM may arise from reduced intake or inadequate absorption leading to caloric deprivation or may be a result of a hypermetabolic inflammatory process that triggers inadequate use of protein substrate while nonprotein caloric intake remains relatively unaffected. The prevalence of PEM in hospitalized children was previously reported as 36% to 54%, but in 2010 the estimates were 1.3% to 28%.[3-5] This lower prevalence may be related to inconsistencies in documentation and coding of malnutrition, which have changed in recent years. Other pediatric studies in intensive care units continue to find deficiencies in meeting caloric and micronutrient needs.[6,7] Children with malnutrition continue to have worse outcomes compared with nourished children. The distinction between starvation and hypermetabolism is important and will affect the choice of nutritional therapy to prevent the detrimental complications of underfeeding or overfeeding.[8] Because PEM contributes greatly to morbidity in heart disease, it is important to understand this entity.

Metabolic Adaptations in Starvation. Glucose is the principal energy substrate in the body and vital for the central nervous system and red blood cells, so the body adapts to preserve glucose homeostasis during starvation (Fig. 26.1). Hepatic glycogenolysis provides the first defense for glucose homeostasis during starvation. However, the hepatic glycogen supply is depleted after 24 hours in adults and sooner in infants. A fall in serum glucose concentration results in a release of the counterregulatory hormones epinephrine, cortisol, and glucagon. These hormones stimulate proteolysis to provide amino acids for gluconeogenesis. Increased counterregulatory hormones combined with decreased levels of insulin stimulate lipolysis and accelerate the production of ketone bodies and fatty acids, which serve as alternative fuel sources in the brain, heart, and muscle. After several days the brain adapts to the use of ketones, and the rate of muscle proteolysis declines.

Specific Micronutrient Deficiency Syndromes and Heart Disease

Iron Deficiency. Iron deficiency is a common and potentially life-threatening problem in children with cyanotic CHD. It is associated with hypercyanotic attacks ("tet spells"), cerebral thromboses, metabolic acidosis, and infection especially in the younger child.[9] Because the adequacy of tissue oxygen delivery is dependent on the hemoglobin concentration, and thus indirectly on iron stores, maintenance of iron sufficiency is paramount.

The iron-deficient cyanotic patient may exhibit an elevated red blood cell count with relatively normal hemoglobin concentration. Another clue to the presence of iron deficiency in this population comes from the fact that the hematocrit is usually greater than three times the hemoglobin level, in contrast to the usual 3 : 1 ratio in the iron-sufficient patient. The mean corpuscular volume may also be low, reflecting the presence of a hypochromic microcytic anemia. The child with critical heart disease and iron deficiency should receive iron therapy. The supplemental iron administration is usually required for over a month until the hematocrit increases. Serial hematocrits during this period are essential, because some patients will experience rapid increases in hematocrit after iron therapy and develop polycythemia (hematocrit >60%). Polycythemia increases blood viscosity and also increases the risk of cerebral thromboses.

L-Carnitine Deficiency and Fatty Acid Oxidation Defects. Recurrent exacerbations of systemic carnitine deficiency or a fatty acid oxidation defect are heralded by vomiting, diarrhea, and mental status changes associated with nonketotic hypoglycemia, hyperammonemia, elevated liver transaminases, lactic acidosis, and coagulopathy.[10] The cardiac manifestations include right or biventricular hypertrophy and cardiomegaly with decreased contractility. This presentation is reminiscent of Reye syndrome with encephalopathy, shock, and weakness.

L-Carnitine is an essential cofactor in fatty acid oxidation and energy production for myocardial contraction. This dependence on fatty acid metabolism as a source of energy is especially

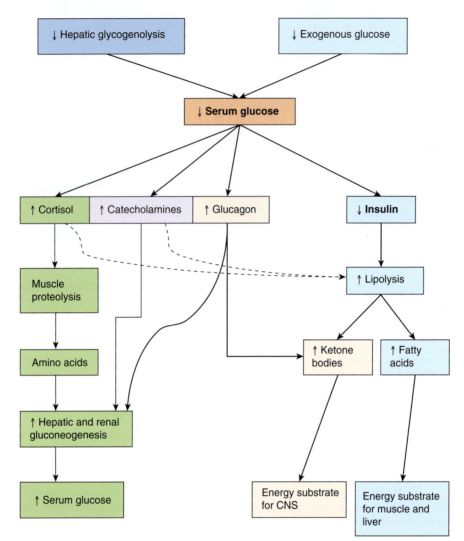

• **Figure 26.1** Metabolic and hormonal adaptation to starvation and hypoglycemia. The increased levels of counterregulatory hormones (cortisol, catecholamines, and glucagon) generate the amino acid substrate for gluconeogenesis by promoting muscle proteolysis. The decreased insulin levels, aided by counterregulatory hormones, generate ketones bodies and fatty acids as alternative fuels for the central nervous system *(CNS)*, muscle, and liver, thus sparing glucose utilization.

acute during periods of fasting, when the glucose supply is inadequate.

Primary carnitine deficiency results in low plasma and tissue carnitine levels and generally presents with varying combinations of cardiomyopathy, skeletal muscle weakness, and encephalopathy. Laboratory examination usually reveals hypoketotic hypoglycemia. The specific carnitine enzyme defects associated with critical heart disease are given in Table 26.1.

Secondary carnitine deficiencies are the result of excessive carnitine losses or inadequate carnitine intake or production. Inadequate carnitine production in the liver may arise in cirrhosis, in malnutrition, or after valproate therapy. Carnitine intake may be deficient with chronic parenteral nutrition (PN) or certain vegetarian diets. Excess carnitine losses may occur with diuresis, diarrhea, or hemodialysis.[11]

Fatty acid oxidation defects include very long chain acyl-coenzyme A (CoA) dehydrogenase (VLCAD) deficiency, long-chain acyl-CoA, long-chain L-3-hydroxyacyl-CoA dehydrogenase (LCHAD) deficiency, or medium-chain acyl-CoA dehydrogenase (MCAD) deficiency, and glutaric acidemia type II. Patients with

these enzymopathies typically have low plasma and tissue carnitine levels and an associated cardiomyopathy. The specific diagnosis is made based on the serum acylcarnitine profile and elevated urinary dicarboxylic acids. Table 26.2 lists the specific clinical findings in fatty acid oxidation defects.

Glucose supplementation during periods of stress is the most important therapy for patients with any of the fatty acid oxidation defects. However, some patients have been successfully treated with carnitine supplementation. An inverse correlation between survival and plasma carnitine levels has been demonstrated in cardiomyopathic patients.[12] L-Carnitine supplementation in these circumstances normalizes mitochondrial function and myocardial performance.[13] Critically ill children with carnitine deficiencies should receive adequate dietary carnitine supplementation and have their serum glucose levels monitored frequently to avoid potentially catastrophic hypoglycemia. Carnitine supplementation has been successfully used in children with cardiomyopathy.[14,15]

Medium-chain triglyceride (MCT) administration may alleviate the cardiac manifestations of secondary carnitine deficiency. MCTs are transported across the mitochondrial membrane independently of carnitine and are mainly oxidized. Consequently, MCTs provide a greater energy substrate than long-chain triglycerides (LCTs) and may minimize the consequences of a secondary carnitine deficiency.

Thiamine Deficiency. Beriberi is caused by a dietary deficiency of thiamine. Thiamine pyrophosphate, vitamin B_1, acts as a cofactor for pyruvate dehydrogenase and other enzymes involved in the pentose and tricarboxylic acid pathways needed to metabolize pyruvate and lactate in the Krebs cycle. In developed nations thiamine deficiency occurs in alcoholics and in selective diets. Childhood beriberi is seen in patients receiving unsupplemented PN and in infants breast-fed by thiamine-deficient mothers.[16] Thiamine deficiency may occur in critically ill children; 12.5% of children receiving care in a pediatric intensive care unit (PICU) for more than 2 weeks and 18% of children admitted for surgical correction of complex congenital heart defects were thiamine deficient.[17] Clinicians should have a low threshold for suspecting and treating thiamine deficiency in critically ill children given the severe neurologic consequences.[18] Long-term treatment of heart failure with furosemide may also predispose patients to thiamine deficiency.[19,20]

There are three forms of beriberi heart disease. Shoshin beriberi is acute fulminant myocardial depression, on the verge of acute cardiovascular collapse. These patients are dyspneic, cyanotic, and display restlessness with an increasing metabolic acidosis. Physical examination reveals severe tachycardia, massive cardiomegaly, jugular venous distention, and hepatomegaly in the absence of peripheral edema. Although thiamine supplementation rapidly restores peripheral vascular resistance, improvement in contractility is often delayed. Acute infantile beriberi presents between the ages of 1 and 4 months in children breast-fed by thiamine-deficient mothers. Infants are pale, irritable, edematous, and often hoarse. Trivial infections can precipitate acute, life-threatening Shoshin beriberi. In the chronic form, wet beriberi, patients appear diaphoretic and edematous with sinus tachycardia, a widened pulse pressure, and a diminished arteriovenous extraction of oxygen. Skeletal muscle blood flow is increased at the expense of cerebral, hepatic, and renal perfusion.[21]

Vitamin D and Calcium Deficiency. Vitamin D deficiency may both contribute to and be a result of pediatric cardiac dysfunction. Vitamin D is a pleotropic hormone that is not only important to bone health but also impacts cardiac function and immunomodulation. Vitamin D deficiency is associated with cardiomyopathy, organ dysfunction, and prolonged PICU stay.[22]

Many infants with CHD have vitamin D deficiency. Although infants are often deficient preoperatively, Vitamin D levels drop intraoperatively during initiation of cardiac bypass and with the administration of catecholamines.[23] It is still unknown if this is a modifiable risk factor that affects outcome. In the outpatient setting, vitamin D supplementation has been associated with improved cardiac function.[24-26]

Hypocalcemia, as a manifestation of hypoparathyroidism, is seen in the 22q11 deletion syndromes, DiGeorge syndrome or

TABLE 26.1 Carnitine Deficiency and Fatty Acid Oxidation Defects Presenting With Critical Heart Disease

Enzyme Defects Associated With Carnitine Deficiency	Features
Carnitine-acylcarnitine translocase deficiency	Life-threatening episodes in the neonatal period Cardiac arrhythmia Generalized weakness Hyperammonemia Variable hypoglycemia
Carnitine palmitoyltransferase II deficiency (hepatocardiomuscular form)	Infants or children Cardiomegaly Cardiac arrhythmia Liver disease Encephalopathy Fasting hypoketotic hypoglycemia Mild myopathy Sudden death
Primary systemic carnitine deficiency (carnitine membrane transporter deficiency) (defect on chromosome 5q)	Dilated cardiomyopathy ECG: peaked T waves Endomyocardial biopsy: massive lipid storage and low carnitine concentration Poor response to inotropes and diuretics Dramatic response to carnitine supplementation Acute encephalopathy Hypoketotic hypoglycemia Hepatomegaly with liver steatosis Myopathy

ECG, Electrocardiogram.

TABLE 26.2 Clinical and Laboratory Characteristics in Various Fatty Acid Oxidation Defects

Defects	CLINICAL FINDINGS						LABORATORY FINDINGS					
	CM	AR	SD	RM	HM	EC	↓Glu	↓Ket	Met Acid	↓Car	↑LFTs	↑NH₃
VLCAD	✓	✓	✓	✓	±✓	✓	✓	✓	✓	✓	✓	✓
MCAD			✓		✓	✓	✓	✓		✓		✓
LCHAD	✓			✓ child	✓						✓	
GA II	✓	✓					✓	✓	✓			✓

AR, Arrhythmia; *Car,* carnitine; *CM,* cardiomyopathy; *EC,* encephalopathy (coma, seizures); *GA II,* glutaric acidemia type II; *Glu,* glucose; *HM,* hepatomegaly; *Ket,* ketones; *LCHAD,* long-chain L-3-hydroxyacyl-CoA dehydrogenase deficiency; *LFT,* liver function test; *MCAD,* medium-chain acyl-CoA dehydrogenase deficiency; *Met Acid,* metabolic acidosis; *NH₃,* ammonia; *RM,* rhabdomyolysis; *SD,* sudden death; *VLCAD,* very long-chain acyl-CoA dehydrogenase deficiency.

velocardiofacial syndrome. Ten percent to 20% of these will present with hypocalcemia in the first 3 months of life; 10% of these babies will present with hypocalcemic seizures.[27,28]

Other factors that affect calcium, vitamin D, and bone mineralization may be more specific to the surgery itself. Following the Fontan operation, children and young adults are more prone to skeletal muscle deficits and vitamin D deficiency compared with their peers.[25,26] Additionally, decreased bone density has been seen in children who have undergone Fontan palliation compared with other forms of CHD, despite normal vitamin D levels.[29] Hyperparathyroidism has also been described in children following Fontan palliation.[26]

Refeeding Syndrome With Hypophosphatemia. Children with PEM are at risk for developing refeeding syndrome, which manifests as hypophosphatemia and other electrolyte derangements if caloric intake is advanced too quickly. Patients may have normal serum phosphorus concentrations, but their total body phosphorus is depleted. During nutritional intervention, anabolic processes increase cellular uptake of serum phosphate, usually between the second and fifth day, but this can occur as late as 7 to 10 days after initiating feeding.[30,31] If serum phosphate levels fall below 1 mg/dL, encephalopathy, diaphragmatic failure, dysrhythmias, acute renal failure, or hepatocellular injury may result.[32] Refeeding syndrome can be prevented by gradually increasing caloric supplementation, although aggressive nutritional support and vigilant phosphate monitoring and replenishment may be just as effective.[33]

Multifactorial Nutritional Syndromes in Children With Critical Heart Disease

Overview

Undernutrition and growth retardation are common complications of CHD. The magnitude of growth failure can be astounding and continues to be a significant problem.[34] Over 70% of children with cardiac disease are below the 50th percentile for height and weight, 50% are below the 16th percentile for height and weight, and over 35% are below the 3rd percentile for both height and weight.[1] Prolonged nutritional deficits and growth failure related to congestive heart failure may result in heightened surgical risks, particularly in infants with single-ventricle defects.[35,36] The etiology of undernutrition seen in children with CHD is multifactorial. Contributing factors include age at surgery, the increased energy expenditure of frequent infections and congestive heart failure, as well as inadequate intake due to dysphagia and frequent feeding interruptions, feeding intolerance, and intestinal malabsorption.[37,38]

Hypermetabolism in Uncorrected Congenital Heart Disease

A meta-analysis comparing 65 infants with CHD and 124 healthy controls found that total daily energy expenditure in infants with CHD is 35% more than that of healthy controls.[39] Presumably the elevated catecholamine levels increase oxygen consumption significantly. This increase in basal metabolic rate (BMR) reduces the calories that usually supply growth during infancy and childhood. Even if a normal caloric intake could be ensured, this would be insufficient to replenish the deficit. Often a caloric intake of 150% of normal values for age is necessary to support normal growth in this population.

Insulin and Glucose Homeostasis in Congenital Heart Disease

In children with CHD, alterations in insulin secretion and glucose homeostasis can occur. Children with symptomatic ventricular septal defects have normal fasting glucose levels and glucose tolerance test results but lower insulin levels and surprisingly higher rates of insulin secretion, as demonstrated by higher plasma concentrations of C-peptide.[40] The higher rates of insulin secretion seen in children with CHD are a consequence of high levels of sympathetic activity, resulting in increased glucose release.[41] Conversely, children with cyanotic heart disease have *lower* fasting glucose levels, normal glucose tolerance, and insulin levels with higher rates of insulin secretion.[42] If the cyanotic infant has inadequate glucose stores, *hypoglycemia* may be the net result of the high insulin secretion rate.[43] Conversely, increases in pulmonary circulation increase *insulin clearance*, which may minimize the risk of hypoglycemia in CHD. Following cardiac surgery, infants are likely to experience transient hyperglycemia, which is often associated with intraoperative glucocorticoid administration.[44]

Growth Hormone Insensitivity

Children with CHD and malnutrition may be insensitive to growth hormone (GH), which may partially explain growth failure in this population. Normally GH affects metabolism in diverse ways. Its effect on protein metabolism is anabolic and leads to positive nitrogen balance. Conversely, GH has catabolic effects on fat metabolism by increasing lipolysis. The resultant increase in free fatty acids accounts for the ketogenic effect of GH. GH has an antiinsulin effect and raises serum glucose levels by increasing hepatic glucose output and decreasing glucose uptake into muscle.

GH promotes growth through its effects on cartilage and protein metabolism, which require the interaction between GH and somatomedins, such as insulin-like growth factors (IGFs) 1 and 2. GH stimulates local IGF secretion in various tissues, including liver, cartilage, and heart. Local and circulating IGFs stimulate growth. Insulin-like growth factor–binding protein 3 (IGFBP-3), also synthesized under GH control, is the most important carrier of circulating IGF-1.[45] The GH:IGF-1:IGFBP-3 axis plays an important role in the preservation of anabolism following stress.[46]

This axis is altered in critical heart disease. Malnourished children with CHD have elevated levels of circulating GH but markedly decreased levels of IGF-1 and IGFBP-3, suggesting GH insensitivity.[47,48] Children undergoing cardiac surgery for complex CHD exhibit this GH resistance preoperatively. In the initial postoperative week the discrepancy between elevated GH levels and depressed IGF-1 and IGFBP-3 worsens. These GH:IGF-1: IGFBP-3 abnormalities resolve within 6 months after corrective surgery.[48] GH also regulates ventricular size and myocyte contractility.[49] Both Turner syndrome and Noonan syndrome are associated with congenital cardiac anomalies and short stature and frequently require GH replacement.[50,51]

Heart Failure

Heart failure may result in poor appetite, tachypnea, vomiting, or dysphagia. Others have emphasized the importance of anorexia and early satiety in the development of this malnutrition state.[52] When heart failure is mild, the hungry infant overfeeds, resulting in fluid overload and impaired cardiorespiratory function. Increased patient fatigability during oral feeding then limits feeding volumes, resulting in underfeeding, as well as prolonged feeding times.[53] Persistent vomiting, thought to be a manifestation of left-to-right intracardiac shunts, which resolves following surgical correction, may be an additional contributor to inadequate intake. Underweight children with CHD have inadequate diets compared with their normal-weight cohorts. With nutritional counseling these children demonstrate a 10% weight gain from baseline over a 6-month period.[54]

Intestinal Malabsorption and Nutrient Loss (Protein-Losing Enteropathy, Chylothorax)

Children with CHD may accrue nutritional deficits through intestinal malabsorption or leakage of nutrients into the intestinal lumen or the pleural space. In some settings the nutrient leakage follows the malabsorption syndrome. Intestinal malabsorption may result from heart failure and is thought to be a form of intestinal lymphangiectasia. As right heart failure increases, lymphatic drainage from the gut is impeded, and a functional lymphatic obstruction develops. Consequently, intestinal absorption and digestion of protein and fats are altered. Carbohydrate absorption is generally normal.[55] Fat malabsorption may occur in some patients with symptomatic congestive heart failure regardless of the underlying cardiac anomaly, but not if the heart failure has been treated effectively with diuretics.[37,56]

Absorption of protein can be impaired in children with heart disease, particularly in patients with a single ventricle who have undergone the Fontan operation. This *protein-losing enteropathy* (PLE) is thought to be due, in part, to increased systemic venous and mesenteric lymphatic pressure resulting in the leakage of protein in the lumen of the gut (see Chapter 15 on splanchnic function for a full discussion of PLE, including dietary and therapeutic options).[37]

Chylothorax, a well-recognized complication of thoracic procedures, has an incidence of 0.25% to 1.9% after surgery for CHD. These chylothoraces are thought to be the result of intraoperative damage to the thoracic duct and accessory lymphatic channels.[57,58] Systemic venous hypertension can also result in chylothorax formation by impeding lymphatic duct emptying. Chylothorax should be suspected whenever a pleural effusion develops after a thoracic procedure, including both median sternotomies and thoracotomies. Chylothorax following thoracotomy was noted to present later in the postoperative period when compared with median sternotomy.[59] Additional risk factors for chylothorax after congenital heart surgery include the Fontan procedure itself and central line insertion in either the subclavian or internal jugular vein.[60,61] Chylothorax is a significant complication because large chylous effusions result in immune, nutritional, and cardiovascular derangements secondary to the loss of T lymphocytes, chylomicrons, and electrolyte-containing fluid.

If the patient has been receiving enteral nutrition, including long-chain fatty acids, chyle has a creamy appearance because it contains chylomicrons and LCTs. The diagnosis of a chylothorax is confirmed by the presence of a pleural fluid triglyceride level of more than 1.2 mmol/L and a total cell number of greater than 1000 cells/μL, consisting predominantly of lymphocytes.[62] However, in the typical postoperative case of chylothorax, the child has been fasting. Therefore the chylous effusion may appear serosanguinous without an elevated triglyceride content. Although an elevated lymphocyte count in the pleural effusion may suggest the diagnosis

of chylothorax, the laboratory analysis is often nondiagnostic. The diagnosis is then made retrospectively after therapy directed at chylothorax results in resolution of the effusion.[57] The initial management consists of tube thoracostomy for large effusions and dietary modification (Fig. 26.2).

Nutritional management of chylothorax traditionally includes a regimen that is very low in LCTs and high in MCTs and contains sufficient protein and electrolytes to replace nutrient losses in chyle. The use of MCT-enriched diets is based on the understanding that enterocytes directly absorb medium-chain fatty acids into portal circulation, reducing lymphatic flow and enabling healing of the damaged lymphatic vessels.[63] Commercially prepared infant formulas containing at least 80% of fat as MCT oil can be used to meet the nutrient needs of infants with chylothorax.[64] Application of a MCT diet alone was effective in resolving the chylothorax in 71% of patients in one study.[65] The use of fat-free human milk may be an important dietary approach to consider in infants with chylothorax due to its immunologic qualities.[66] Through the process of cold centrifugation, human milk can be separated into a solidified-fat top layer and a lower fat-free liquid portion. Because removal of the fat portion causes the human milk to become deficient in energy, essential fatty acids, and fat-soluble vitamins, the fat-free human milk must be supplemented with MCT oil, vitamins, carbohydrate modulars, and/or high-MCT infant formula. If the use of fat-free human milk is prolonged (greater than 2 to 4 weeks), supplementation with 2% to 4% of total energy in the form of essential fatty acids may be necessary to prevent essential fatty acid deficiency. This is illustrated in a recent report demonstrating no difference in the resolution of chylothoraces with fat-modified breast milk versus MCT infant formula; however, the fat-modified breast milk group experienced a decline in mean weight and height.[67] If clinical symptoms of chylothorax persist (no decrease in chylous chest tube output) on a low LCT/high MCT diet, complete enteric rest and PN may be required. This approach is successful in a majority of cases. Clinical improvement is defined as a decrease in effusion drainage to less than 10 mL/kg/d.[68] More than a third of patients receiving fat-free formulas will experience resolution of their chylothoraces within 2 weeks.[69] Nutritional management of chylothoraces is typically continued for up to 6 weeks.

Symptomatic venous thrombosis is commonly associated with chylothorax and may contribute to its severity and duration. Of 1396 children who underwent cardiac surgery, 54 developed chylothorax and 28 (52%) had venous thromboembolism confirmed by ultrasonography.[70] Indeed, elevated central venous pressures are associated with more refractory chylothoraces.[58,71] These chylothoraces resolve slowly because of the time it takes to reach a sufficiently high intralymphatic pressure to cause lymphatic rupture.[58] Such patients require a careful hemodynamic evaluation to identify the cause of the systemic venous hypertension. Potential causes in the surgical patient include the aforementioned systemic venous thrombosis, which requires anticoagulation, or pulmonary artery stenosis, which may require stent placement or surgical plasty. Recently balloon angioplasty for the treatment of left innominate vein obstruction in the face of chylothorax led to improvement if not full resolution of the chylothorax.[72] Chylothorax associated with postoperative pulmonary hypertension can be treated with a trial of nitric oxide (NO), which decreases right ventricular afterload and associated tricuspid regurgitation and/or augments forward flow through the pulmonary circulation.[73,74]

Somatostatin and its synthetic analogue, octreotide, have been used successfully to treat chylothorax.[75] There is a subset of patients who seem to respond to octreotide; they have lower chest tube

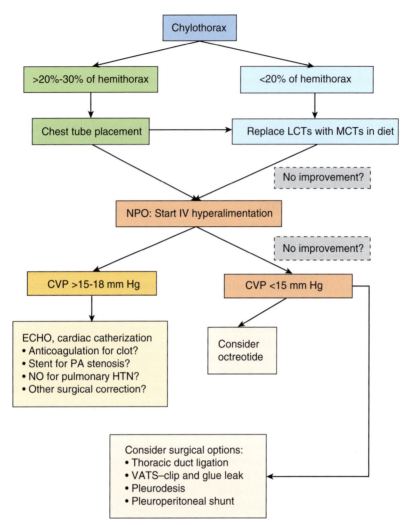

• **Figure 26.2** Management algorithm for persistent chylothorax. *CVP,* Central venous pressure; *ECHO,* echocardiography; *HTN,* hypertension; *IV,* intravenous; *LCT,* long-chain triglyceride; *MCT,* medium-chain triglyceride; *NO,* nitric oxide; *NPO,* nothing by mouth; *PA,* pulmonary artery; *VATS,* video-assisted thoracoscopic surgery.

output, and a higher proportion are patients with single-ventricle anatomy.[76] By acting directly on splanchnic vascular receptors, octreotide reduces chylomicron synthesis and transport into the lymphatic duct, thus decreasing lymphatic flow rate and limiting triglyceride loss into the pleural fluid.[77,78] Octreotide has been used both as a continuous infusion and in divided subcutaneous doses.[79] It is initiated at 10 mcg/kg/d in three divided subcutaneous doses and increased in a stepwise fashion of 5 to 10 mcg/kg/d every 3 days until chyle output decreases to minimal levels for 3 consecutive days. At this point the octreotide is weaned over the next 3 to 6 days. The dose of octreotide required to achieve total suppression of chylous effusion was reported as 20 to 40 mcg/kg/d.[80]

Although as many as nearly 80% of patients respond to dietary and medical management to resolve their chylothoraces, the remainder do not and require surgical interventions.[81,82] Such surgical techniques include pleurodesis with talc/tetracycline or fibrin glue, video-assisted thoracoscopic surgical (VATS) identification and clipping of the site of duct leakage or thoracic duct ligation, or pleuroperitoneal shunting.[71,83] The operations are preceded by consumption of a meal of cream mixed with Sudan black 1 hour before the procedure to identify the leak site. In four

of six adults with a chylothorax the site was successfully identified using a VATS technique, then sealed with fibrin glue and sutures or clips. The remaining two underwent pleurodesis with fibrin glue. All of these chylothoraces resolved completely by the fifth postoperative day.[84] Despite these impressive results, a right-sided thoracic duct ligation, done using either a VATS or open approach, remains the standard procedure for a refractory chylothorax.[81,85] When this fails, consideration should be given to a left-sided approach with left periaortic mass ligation due to the anatomic variation in pediatric CHD patients, especially those with dextrocardia.[86]

In two small series of children with persistent chylothorax, implantation of double-valved pleuroperitoneal shunts resulted in successful resolution of their symptoms, without complications.[87,88] These shunts are removed an average of 1 to 2 months post placement. An advantage of a pleuroperitoneal shunt is to minimize the loss of chyle by facilitating its absorption by the peritoneum and allowing the formation of new lymphatic thoracic channels. The use of these shunts is limited by high right atrial pressure (>25 mm Hg) or by inferior vena cava obstruction.[68,89]

Nutritional Assessment

Anthropometrics

Growth is the primary outcome measure of nutritional status in children and should be monitored at regular intervals from infancy through adolescence and at every preventive, acute, or chronic care encounter. In children less than 36 months of age, growth parameters should include weight-for-age, length-for-age, head circumference-for-age, and weight-for-length. In children 2 to 20 years of age, growth parameters include weight-for-age, standing height-for-age, and body mass index (BMI)-for-age.

The best indicator of growth failure is the change in growth rate over time. Longitudinal growth is preserved during acute short-term nutritional deprivation. Therefore a low weight-for-length percentile in children less than 2 years of age and a low BMI percentile in children greater than 2 years of age suggest an acute energy imbalance, whereas a low length-for-age or height-for-age percentile indicates long-standing deficits. Many children presenting with cardiac disease weigh significantly less than normal for age in the face of appropriate height.[54]

Anthropometric measurements provide the best estimates of muscle and fat content of the body in the clinical setting. In the absence of edema, measuring triceps and subscapular skinfold thickness assesses adipose tissue but is most accurate when serial measurements are taken by the same trained clinician. Skeletal muscle mass can be estimated by measurements of the arm muscle circumference and is useful in assessing the depletion of lean body mass. Mid-upper arm circumference (MUAC) can be used an independent marker in determining malnutrition in children 6 to 59 months of age. MUAC measurements are particularly important in those whose weights alone are unreliable due to fluid status, such as those with lower extremity edema or ascites or those receiving steroids. MUAC has been indicated as a more sensitive prognostic indicator for mortality than weight-for-length or BMI in malnourished pediatric patients.[90] The Academy of Nutrition and Dietetics and the American Society for Parenteral and Enteral Nutrition (ASPEN) have developed standardized guidelines for identifying and documenting pediatric malnutrition (Tables 26.3 and 26.4).

Biochemical Measurements

Nitrogen balance reflects the equilibrium between protein intake and losses. Stress produces nitrogen losses, driven by the catabolic actions of cortisol and epinephrine. Skeletal muscle breakdown provides substrate for gluconeogenesis and also releases nonessential amino acids that are excreted in the urine as urea. All patients with PEM have a negative nitrogen balance. The magnitude of the negative balance is useful in determining the process leading to the patient's malnourished state. In hypermetabolism, tissue is being catabolized for gluconeogenesis and wound repair. Acute negative nitrogen balance is the rule. Chronic starvation leads to a modestly negative nitrogen balance.[91] Drainage of proteinaceous fluids from other body cavities will further increase nitrogen loss.

Although serum protein concentrations (particularly albumin and transferrin) have been used as biochemical markers of nutritional status, these tests are neither sensitive nor specific. Hypermetabolism is associated with negative nitrogen balance, but hypoalbuminemia requires prolonged hypermetabolism because of the long half-life of albumin (20 days) (Table 26.5). Hypoalbuminemia in the face of a hypermetabolic state is associated with increased risk of death. The shorter half-life proteins such as retinol-binding protein and prealbumin correlate better with acute changes in critically ill patients. However, prealbumin levels can be affected by several factors. Lower levels may be seen in liver disease, or they may be

TABLE 26.3	Primary Indicators for Pediatric Malnutrition When Single Data Point Is Available		
	Mild Malnutrition	Moderate Malnutrition	Severe Malnutrition
Weight-for-length z-score	−1 to −1.9	−2 to −2.9	≥ −3
BMI for age z-score	−1 to −1.9	−2 to −2.9	≥ −3
Length/height for age z-score	No data	No data	≥ −3
Mid-upper arm circumference z-score	≥ −1 to −1.9	≥ −2 to −2.9	≥ −3

From Becker PJ, Carney LN, Corkins MR, et al. Consensus statement of the Academy of Nutrition and Dietetics/American Society for Parenteral and Enteral Nutrition: indicators recommended for the identification and documentation of pediatric malnutrition (undernutrition). *J Acad Nutr Diet.* 2014;114(12):1988-2000.

TABLE 26.4	Primary Indicators for Pediatric Malnutrition When Two or More Data Points Are Available		
	Mild Malnutrition	Moderate Malnutrition	Severe Malnutrition
Weight gain velocity (<2 years)	<75% of the norm for expected weight gain	<50% of the norm for expected weight gain	<25% of the norm for expected weight gain
Weight loss (2-20 years of age)	5% usual body weight	7.5% usual body weight	10% usual body weight
Deceleration in weight-for-length or BMI z-score	Decline of 1 z-score	Decline of 2 z-scores	Decline of 3 z-scores
Inadequate nutrient intake	51%-75% estimated energy/protein needs	26%-50% of estimated energy/protein needs	≤25% estimated energy/protein needs

From Becker PJ, Carney LN, Corkins MR, et al. Consensus statement of the Academy of Nutrition and Dietetics/American Society for Parenteral and Enteral Nutrition: indicators recommended for the identification and documentation of pediatric malnutrition (undernutrition). *J Acad Nutr Diet.* 2014 114(12):1988-2000.

TABLE 26.5 Plasma Proteins Used for Nutritional Assessment and Their Half-Lives

Plasma Protein	$t_{1/2}$
Transferrin	8 d
Albumin	20 d
Prealbumin	2 d
Retinol-binding protein	10 h

TABLE 26.6 World Health Organization Equations to Calculate Resting Energy Expenditure

Age	Male	Female
0-3 years	$60.9W - 54$	$61W - 51$
3-10 years	$22.7W + 495$	$22.5W + 499$
10-18 years	$17.5W + 651$	$12.2W + 746$

W, Weight (kg).
Modified from *Energy and Protein Requirements*. Report of a Joint FAO/WHO/UNU Expert Consultation. Technical Report Series 724. Geneva: World Health Organization; 1985.

TABLE 26.7 Schofield Equations to Calculate Basal Metabolic Rate

Age	Male	Female
0-3 years	$0.167W + 15.174H - 617.6$	$16.252W + 10.232H - 413.5$
3-10 years	$19.59W + 1.303H + 414.9$	$16.969W + 1.618H + 371.2$
10-18 years	$16.25W + 1.372H + 515.5$	$8.365W + 4.65H + 200.0$

H, Length/height (cm); W, weight (kg).
Modified from Schofield WN. Predicting basal metabolic rate, new standards and review of previous work. *Hum Nutr Clin Nutr*. 1985;39(Suppl 1):5-41.

falsely elevated in renal failure and steroid use. Visceral proteins such as albumin and prealbumin do not accurately reflect nutritional status and response to nutritional intervention during inflammation. During periods of inflammation the liver reprioritizes synthesis of acute-phase proteins such as C-reactive protein (CRP) over transport proteins such as prealbumin. Therefore levels of serum prealbumin and CRP are inversely related. For the postoperative infant, decreases in serum CRP level to less than 2 mg/dL have been associated with the return of anabolic metabolism and are followed by increases in serum prealbumin levels.[92]

Predictive Methods of Energy Expenditure

An infant's caloric requirement depends on his or her BMR, the rate of growth, and activity. Because adipose tissue is not as metabolically active as other tissue, an undernourished infant with little or no subcutaneous fat has a higher than expected level of metabolism relative to body weight. The caloric requirements of recovering undernourished children are also increased because of active reparative anabolic processes. Fever significantly increases total energy requirements. Each degree Celsius elevation in body temperature increases caloric needs by 12%.[93]

The nutritional needs of patients in intensive care rarely conform to tabular norms because these patients are not in a basal state. The term *resting energy expenditure* (REE) is used for adults when they are supine and quiet or asleep and have not eaten for at least 3 hours.[94] REE is a function of gender, age, height, and weight. However, studies of critically ill children on mechanical ventilation in whom energy expenditures were measured by indirect calorimetry reported wide differences between measured and predicted values, even after stress factors were applied.[95]

Consistent with the ASPEN guidelines, indirect calorimetry to measure REE provides the best estimate of energy requirements in critically ill pediatric patients.[93] Several studies comparing indirect calorimetry versus predictive equations in estimating energy requirements in the critically ill child following cardiac surgery found that predictive equations are unreliable and do not take into account the unpredictable metabolic changes that occur in these patients.[96,97] Because the metabolic response is difficult to estimate and changes throughout the acute and recovery phases, individualized nutrition prescriptions using indirect calorimetry every second day should be the new standard in this population.[98]

If indirect calorimetry is unavailable, basing REE on standard equations without additional stress factors during the acute phase response can help prevent overfeeding and its potential consequences. The end of the acute/catabolic stress response may be estimated through serial monitoring of CRP levels (CRP <2 mg/dL suggests a return to anabolic state). The most commonly used equations

for critically ill patients are the World Health Organization (WHO) equations to calculate REE and the Schofield equations to calculate BMR (Tables 26.6 and 26.7).

Nutritional Management of the Cardiac Surgical Patient

The challenges in the nutritional management of the child with critical heart disease include (1) determining the extent of coexisting undernutrition; (2) defining the metabolic stage of development; (3) estimating the caloric requirements during critical illness; (4) appreciating the extent of exposure to catabolic, hormonal, and immunologic risks that can be modulated through nutritional support; and (5) deciding the appropriate method of providing nutritional support during the critical care period. In a study of over 90 children undergoing cardiac surgery, approximately half were malnourished at the time of surgery, and by 1 week postoperatively, most children were receiving only two-thirds of their recommended calorie and protein requirements.[99] A multidisciplinary team approach to planning nutritional support throughout the course of treatment can improve nutritional delivery and growth.[100]

Preoperative Nutritional Management

A nutritional evaluation should be included for all children with CHD. In children with severe undernutrition the timing of a palliative or corrective procedure should be carefully considered. Although total correction of a long-standing nutritional deficit is unrealistic in the short term, provision of an intensive nutritional program, including the use of continuous nasogastric feeds for a period of 1 to 2 weeks, may restore anabolic balance. For children in whom full enteral feeding is unrealistic, PN augmented with trophic enteral feeds may achieve many of these same salutary effects. A prospective study at two sites found worse clinical outcomes among those children with preoperative acute and chronic malnutrition, as well as an inverse relationship between declining markers of nutrition status and a concomitant rise in B-type natriuretic peptide levels and need for inotropic support.[101] These findings suggest that malnourishment is associated with a decrease in myocardial function.

There is little agreement regarding the safety or risks of early enteral feeding in infants with ductal dependent cardiac lesions who require prostaglandin therapy. However, this practice is becoming more common and is widely used in Europe.[102,103] Reluctance to feed preoperatively is often attributed to the presumed risk of necrotizing enterocolitis. In one hundred thirty consecutive infants who required cardiac surgery, preoperative feeding did not increase the prevalence of necrotizing enterocolitis.[104] Despite variations in clinical practice, the current evidence suggests it is reasonable to attempt enteral feeding in the preoperative cardiac infant as long as the infant is not requiring high-dose vasopressors. A survey of 56 centers participating in the National Pediatric Cardiology Quality Improvement Collaborative found that 65% fed infants with hypoplastic left hearts preoperatively.[105] In one retrospective study of 34 infants with prostaglandin-dependent cardiac defects, 33 infants were successfully enterally fed while awaiting surgical repair. The type of cardiac defect, ductal-flow pattern, and the use of umbilical venous or arterial catheters did not appear to affect feeding tolerance.[106] In another retrospective study of neonates with CHD who underwent surgical repair at less than 1 month of age, enteral feeds were initiated in 50 of 52 infants requiring prostaglandin therapy. Enteral volumes up to 100 mL/kg/d were achieved in 39 (75%) of these infants, and full feeds were achieved by 15 infants (28.8%).[103] Benefits to preoperative feeding may include improved clinical outcomes such as decreased fluid overload, shorter duration of mechanical ventilation, and earlier achievement of full enteral and oral feeds.[107]

There are several strategies available for estimating energy needs in children with CHD. Regardless of the method used, growth parameters must be consistently monitored and adjusted based on individual needs. For infants, starting with 120 kcal/kg/d as a baseline caloric requirement and adjusting based on weight gain is a practical approach. Of note, some infants may require as high as 150 to 175 kcal/kg/d for optimal growth. Fortifying breast milk and increasing the caloric density of infant formulas (typically 22 to 30 kcal/oz), as well as providing supplemental tube feedings, are common strategies to help meet the higher energy needs of this population.

Feeding volumes and solute composition will be dictated by heart failure and intestinal malabsorption. General guidelines for calorie and protein requirements for infants and children are outlined in Table 26.8. Although there is no recommended daily allowance for fat, it is an excellent source of calories and also provides essential fatty acids for growth. Sodium restriction to 2 to 3 mEq/kg/d should avoid exacerbation of congestive heart failure. The osmolality of enteral feeds should be less than 600 mOsm/L to avoid the complications of vomiting, abdominal pain, and diarrhea.

MCTs are frequently used to supplement the caloric content of enteral feeds. These fatty acids provide a high–caloric density, low-osmolality additive that can be absorbed and hydrolyzed directly by the intestinal mucosa independent of pancreatic lipases, bile acid solubilization, and chylomicron formation. A large proportion of administered MCTs is absorbed directly into the portal circulation, bypassing the lymphatic channels that may be congested in heart failure. MCTs are totally saturated, are devoid of the essential fatty acids, and can produce a cathartic effect.

TABLE 26.8	Daily Calorie and Protein Requirements in Infants and Children	
Age	**Calories (kcal/kg/d)**	**Protein (g/kg/d)**
Infants		
0-6 mo	108	2.2
7-12 mo	98	1.6
Children		
1-3 yr	102	1.2
4-6 yr	90	1.1
7-10 yr	70	1.0
Males		
11-14 yr	55	1.0
15-18 yr	45	0.9
Females		
11-14 yr	47	1.0
15-18 yr	40	0.8

From National Research Council Subcommittee on the Tenth Edition of the Recommended Dietary Allowances. *Recommended Dietary Allowances.* 10th ed. Washington, DC.: National Academies Press; 1989.

Postoperative Nutritional Management

Energy Requirements. Nutritional requirements after cardiac surgery vary with age and the nature of the stress response to surgery and cardiopulmonary bypass. The initial goals of nutrition support include minimizing the loss of lean body mass and supporting vital organ function.[108] Despite the well-documented growth failure in infants with CHD, growth is not a critical priority during the immediate postoperative phase. Limited data in infants and children following cardiac surgery suggest that their measured energy expenditure is lower than in adults.[109] In fact, Gebara and colleagues[110] showed that the REE (mean of 55 kcal/kg/d) of children after heart surgery is less than the predicted BMR for normal children in the immediate postoperative phase. Another group of investigators using indirect calorimetry to compare postoperative energy expenditure in 14 cyanotic (mean age: 3.2 months) and 15 acyanotic (mean age: 12.3 months) infants with CHD found that both groups had similar REE measurements following surgery (average REE was 59 ± 10 and 62 ± 10 kcal/kg/d in the cyanotic and acyanotic groups, respectively).[96]

The reasons for the lower than predicted energy requirement are many. The infant subjected to stress responds by first decreasing tissue synthesis. Many of the children are malnourished, causing a similar reduction in growth and overall reduction in their BMR. Postoperatively children are frequently paralyzed, sedated, mechanically ventilated, and receiving PN in a thermoneutral environment.

Of those children not paralyzed and sedated, most postoperative infants are at rest 80% to 90% of the time. Finally, metabolic measurements may not be appropriately timed to reflect the peak metabolism of the stress response.

Although energy requirements during the immediate postoperative period are highly variable, research suggests that they normalize to an anabolic state by approximately 1 week following surgery.[98] Following the immediate postoperative period, energy needs for infants increase to 90 to 100 kcal/kg/d parenterally and 100 to 110 kcal/kg/d enterally (10% increase from parenteral requirements due to the thermic effect of food).[100,108] Although it is well documented that total energy expenditure (TEE) in infants with unrepaired CHD is elevated compared to healthy infants of similar age, studies suggest that energy requirements for infants with CHD following surgical intervention decrease to those of healthy infants. An observational study comparing TEE in infants with CHD who required surgical intervention within the first 30 days of life and healthy infants found that TEE was similar at 3 and 12 months of age between the two groups.[111]

Protein Requirements. Because the catabolism of skeletal muscle protein to generate glucose and inflammatory response proteins is limited in infants and children who have less endogenous protein stores, the provision of adequate dietary protein required to maximize protein synthesis, facilitate wound healing and the inflammatory response, and preserve lean body mass is the single most important nutritional intervention in critically ill and postoperative children. Infants demonstrate 25% higher protein degradation after surgery.[93] Estimated protein requirements are 3 to 3.5 g/kg/d in term neonates with weights appropriate for gestational age and 3 to 4 g/kg/d in low-birth-weight neonates.[108] After the neonatal period, protein requirements are 2 to 3 g/kg/d for infants and children up to 2 years of age, 1.5 to 2 g/kg/d for children aged 2 to 13 years, and 1.5 g/kg/d for children aged 13 to 18 years.[93]

Nutritional Support Techniques

Enteral Nutrition

Enteral nutrition is the preferred method of providing nutrition.[93] It is less costly and has fewer complications than PN.[112,113] Early institution of enteral feedings has been associated with lower infection rates and shorter hospital stays, compared with delayed enteral feeds, in a population of surgical ICU patients.[114] Enteral nutrients are necessary for optimal gastrointestinal function. Fasting studies in young animals show that despite maintenance of a positive nitrogen balance, PN results in atrophy of the pancreas and small bowel mucosa, as well as decreased mucosal height, DNA content, intestinal brush border enzyme activity, and intestinal absorptive capacity.[115] There is an associated increase in bacterial translocation.[115] Enteral feeding reverses these responses.[116] The mechanisms behind the reparative response to feeding include direct intraluminal enterocyte nutrition, decreases in intestinal vascular resistance promoting enhanced intestinal perfusion, as well as the hormonal effects of feeding. Specific intraluminal substances, such as glutamine, may play a very important role in this process.[117]

Hormonal Response to Enteral Nutrition

Enteral nutrition is associated with the secretion of various intestinal hormones that augment the secretion of insulin. Insulin is an important element in the growth of the infant. Infants receiving hypocaloric enteral feeds have less glucose intolerance than do those receiving PN. Compared with PN, enteral feeds produce higher levels of gastric inhibitory polypeptide, insulin, and insulin/glucose ratios.[118] The gastrointestinal tract of the newborn is particularly vulnerable to enteral nutrient deprivation, even with adequate parenteral caloric supplementation.

The composition and route of feeding have major influences on the level of circulating gastrointestinal hormones and regulatory peptides. Even very small amounts of milk induce surges of gut hormones.[119] Enteroglucagon is a trophic hormone for the small intestinal mucosa. Gastrin stimulates the growth of the gastric mucosa and exocrine pancreas, accelerates gastric acid secretion, and promotes glucose-induced insulin release.[120]

Intestinal motility increases after enteral feeding. The peptides gastrin, neurotensin, and motilin modulate intestinal motor activity. Intragastric feeds result in rapidly increasing plasma levels of gastrin and motilin. Infants maintained solely on PN do not have similar rises in plasma levels. Similar changes in plasma gastrin are seen during nasojejunal feeds.[121]

Immunologic Benefits of Enteral Nutrition

A healthy mucosa reduces the risk of bacterial translocation and modulates immune response. Immunoglobulin A (IgA) secretion and the regional lymphoid tissue provide the secondary defense to collect and destroy any bacteria that successfully complete a transepithelial migration. Factors that weaken this multifaceted defense include physical disruption of the mucosal barrier, alteration of the local microflora, and impaired immune defenses.[122] Clinically, shock with reduced splanchnic blood flow, PN, lack of enteral nutrition, intestinal epithelial damage, and antibiotic therapy predispose the critically ill to bacterial translocation.

The endogenous microflora, unique in each section of the intestine, plays a critical role in preventing colonization with exogenous pathogenic organisms. The stomach and the proximal small intestine are relatively sterile, whereas large populations of organisms safely reside in the colon.[123] Antibiotic therapy and PN are well recognized to disrupt this normal flora. Critical illness is often associated with proximal gut overgrowth of enteric gram-negative organisms. It is these organisms that are frequently responsible for nosocomial infections.[124] The institution of enteral feedings alone can produce dramatic improvements in immune function.

Breast milk may provide even further immunomodulatory effects. The protective components in breast milk include not only maternal secretory IgA and the cellular elements (macrophages, lymphocytes, and neutrophils) but also oligosaccharides, iron-binding lactoferrin, and bacterial growth factors.[125] The oligosaccharide fractions of breast milk glycolipids inhibit certain bacteria from adhering to epithelial cells.[126] By binding iron, an important growth factor for many gram-negative organisms, lactoferrin is able to decrease colonization by pathogenic gram-negative bacteria in the colon. Unique to humans, breast milk contains a factor that selectively promotes the growth of *Bifidobacterium bifidum*.[127] The net result is a colonic ecosystem that favors the selective growth of nonpathogenic organisms.[9] Breast milk confers protection against the development of necrotizing enterocolitis.[128,129]

Even if breast milk feeds are not available, some amount of enteral formula feeds are preferable to nothing by mouth and PN. The use of PN has been shown to be one of the most significant predictors for nosocomial infections in pediatric patients after cardiac surgery and other critically ill children.[130,131]

Feeding Protocols

Infants with single-ventricle physiology have worse outcomes if nutrition is suboptimal, particularly between stage 1 (Norwood) and stage 2 (Glenn) palliation.[37,132,133] Through a national quality improvement collaborative, significant work has been aimed at improving outcomes between stage 1 and stage 2 palliation by focusing on improving nutrition.[134,135] Multiple institutions have seen decreased variability in feeding practices and improved outcomes with the implementation of feeding guidelines or protocols, which are also expanding to include infants with multiple causes of CHD.[136-140] However, even with feeding protocols, many infants still fall short of enteral goals frequently due to interruptions in feeding for procedures or intolerance.[141] Others have also reported not meeting goal calories due to fluid restrictions that affect delivery of both enteral and parenteral nutrition.[142]

Route of Enteral Nutrition

The bedside decision of which type of enteral feeding to employ depends on the clinical circumstances. The awake child with intact airway protective reflexes, normal swallowing function, and normal respiratory rate should be allowed to suck or drink. This scenario applies to most cardiac surgical patients within 24 hours after extubation and removal of mediastinal tubes and transthoracic monitoring catheters. If oral feedings fail or are contraindicated, then the physician must choose between intragastric and transpyloric feedings. The absolute contraindications for any form of enteral feeding are intestinal obstruction, necrotizing enterocolitis, severe gastrointestinal bleeding, and intractable diarrhea.

Intragastric feedings via a nasogastric tube generally represent the next step if oral feedings have failed, because nasogastric tubes are somewhat easier to position and maintain. Although the data are conflicting, transpyloric feeding does not appear to have a clear-cut advantage over intragastric feeding in the prevention of aspiration or nosocomial pneumonia.[143,144]

Patients requiring prolonged tube feeds often will require a feeding gastrostomy tube to avoid the complications of long-term nasogastric feeds such as sinusitis, otitis media, hypopharyngeal irritation, and tube dislocation.[145] Under most circumstances a pediatric gastroenterologist or pediatric surgeon can place a percutaneous endoscopic gastrostomy (PEG) tube.[146] The contraindications to a PEG in which a child would require an open or laparoscopic gastrostomy tube include esophageal stricture, previous abdominal surgery, massive ascites, peritoneal dialysis, portal hypertension, severe coagulopathy, and abdominal wall infection. Congenital anomalies of the gastrointestinal tract may be a relative contraindication to PEG placement. A similar caution regarding PEG and laparoscopy exists in patients with a single ventricle and shunt-dependent pulmonary circulation because either the gastric inflation required for PEG or the abdominal insufflation required for laparoscopy may decrease lung volume and increase pulmonary vascular resistance. A number of studies have shown that an antireflux procedure is unnecessary for the majority of patients requiring a feeding gastrostomy who have a negative gastroesophageal reflux (GER) evaluation preoperatively.[147,148]

Transpyloric feedings are superior to intragastric feedings in the patient with delayed gastric emptying. Small intestinal motility and absorptive function remain intact under a variety of pathologic conditions, making transpyloric feedings a viable option for the majority of critically ill patients. Continuous transpyloric feeding in infancy affords a higher average cumulative weight gain than intermittent nasogastric feeds in some centers.[149] If bedside placement fails, transpyloric tubes can be positioned under fluoroscopic guidance.

The placement of a transpyloric feeding tube does not ensure safe, successful enteral nutrition.[150] Nasogastric aspirates have been found to double once transpyloric enteral feeding begins. These aspirates are not refluxed feeds but represent an increase in gastric output, which may be the result of an enteral hormonal response to the presence of feeds in the small intestine.[151] This may explain, in part, the equivalent incidence of aspiration pneumonias in transpylorically fed patients and those fed intragastrically. Transpyloric feeds are associated with accelerated small bowel transit time, more rapid gallbladder contractions, and higher levels of cholecystokinin secretion than are intragastric feeds.[152] Approximately 10% of patients fed transpylorically will experience significant complications such as abdominal cramps, distention, or diarrhea, which force cessation of feeding.[153]

Maintenance of Tube Feedings

Once placed, maintaining a feeding tube in its desired position can be challenging. Patients must be continuously evaluated for feeding intolerance, GER, and microaspiration. Because large-bore nasogastric tubes are associated with a higher risk of GER and prolonged duration of acid in the esophagus, it is advantageous to use as small a bore tube (10 French) as is practical.[154] If long-term transpyloric feedings are required, placement of a PEG tube with wire-guided advancement under fluoroscopy into the jejunum is an excellent option.[155]

Despite the benefits of providing nutrition, many families of infants with CHD report stress and anxiety centered around feeding concerns, especially if feeding tubes are needed.[156]

Parenteral Nutrition

Critical illness often precludes the enteral delivery of complete caloric requirements. PN is an alternative to enteral feeding when gut absorptive capacity or motility is severely disturbed. PN solutions contain hypertonic dextrose, amino acids, vitamins, and trace elements. A lipid emulsion is often administered separately. PN is generally administered by central vein in children, because the solution's hypertonicity causes phlebitis. Long-term PN in critically ill patients is associated with a variety of complications, including excess CO_2 production and difficulty in weaning from mechanical ventilation, hepatic dysfunction, hyperglycemia in stressed patients with a decreased insulin/glucagon ratio, and nosocomial infection. In fact, PN remains one of the most significant risk factors for developing a nosocomial infection in PICUs.[130]

PN in the postoperative cardiac surgery infant is often limited by the total fluid restriction. When cardiopulmonary bypass is used during cardiac surgery, postoperative fluid goals are often restricted to 50% to 80% of maintenance fluid needs. Medication infusions needed to support cardiac function, sedation, and pain control; carrier fluids; and flushes are all included in the total fluid provision, leaving a very small volume allotted for PN. Typically PN is not initiated until more than 30 mL/kg/d of fluid is available. Until sufficient volume is available, intravenous fluids with concentrated dextrose solutions can be provided.

Monitoring of PN in the critically ill patient is based on measurements of nutrient levels in the circulation. Serum glucose levels should be monitored every time a change in glucose delivery rate takes place, when the clinical status of the patient changes significantly, or when the patient receives medications or undergoes procedures presumed to affect glucose metabolism. Sodium, potassium, magnesium, and calcium should be measured every time the rate of infusion is modified or when required by clinical assessment. A particularly hazardous situation may arise in the cardiac patient when a reduction in diuretic dose leads to reduced urine output but potassium concentration in the PN is not adjusted concomitantly. Plasma triglycerides should be measured on a weekly basis unless the rate of intralipid infusion has been changed.

The manifestations of PN-associated liver disease (PNALD) differ by age. Cholestasis is more common in infants, in whom PNALD is defined as a persistent direct bilirubin level greater than 2 mg/dL for more than 1 week in the presence of PN.[157] Biliary sludge and elevated levels of transaminases are more common in older children.[158] Levels of serum transaminases, bilirubin, and alkaline phosphatase should be measured once a week to monitor for PN-induced complications. Children who are unable to tolerate enteral feeds are more likely to develop PNALD. Partial enteral feeding appears to be able to attenuate many of these deleterious processes and is associated with a much lower incidence of PNALD.[159] If PNALD does occur, feeding advancement and reducing the soy lipid dose to 1 g/kg/d can be helpful.[160]

Oral Feeding, Swallowing, and Dysphagia in the Child With Congenital Heart Disease

Etiology of Dysphagia in Children With Congenital Heart Disease

Children with CHD are at risk of developing feeding problems for a variety of reasons related to the underlying pathophysiology of their disease as well as acquired risk factors related to their care, such as cardiac surgery, prolonged hospitalization, or intubation.[161,162] Pharyngoesophageal dysmotility has been reported in infants with CHD, especially those who underwent surgery.[163] Among infants who have undergone a Norwood procedure, recurrent laryngeal nerve dysfunction occurs in 3% to 45% of infants, vocal cord dysfunction occurs in 10% to 45% of infants, and up to 50% of infants have an abnormal modified barium swallow, with 25% showing signs of aspiration.[39] Another study of hospitalized infants less than 7 months of age in a PICU with CHD found dysphagia in 84%. These infants displayed abnormalities in oral motor skills, such as arrhythmic sucking, and had low scores on a feeding readiness evaluation, similar to preterm infants.[164] An absent, poor, or weak suck has been described as a major problem in 7% to 43% of infants with CHD.[165,166] Fatigue and increased respiratory rate may further exacerbate an infant's ability to coordinate the suck-breath-swallow process, especially if they are also preterm.[167] Problems with feeding are often a significant source of stress for parents and in some instances can even outweigh parents' cardiac concerns.[168]

Vocal fold paralysis due to laryngeal nerve injury has been reported in infants having open heart surgery (2% to 9% of patients), particularly with Norwood procedures, and may not resolve over time.[162,169] Common symptoms of vocal fold dysfunction are stridor, breathiness, a hoarse or weak cry, and choking with feeding.[170,171] Silent aspiration, aspiration without coughing, is a twofold problem. The airway's primary defense mechanism does not clear aspirated material, and the presence of swallowing dysfunction is masked. Silent aspiration occurs in 40% to 97% of patients with neurogenic dysphagia.[172,173] Infants who have had open-heart surgery, particularly aortic arch surgery, are also prone to silent aspiration, so a high index of suspicion is needed in high-risk patients.[174]

Prolonged endotracheal intubation with or without subsequent tracheostomy is also associated with pharyngeal phase dysphagia in adults and may be in children as well.[175] In the absence of neurologic injury, most postextubation dysphagia resolves within 96 hours of extubation, concurrent with the healing of mucosal lesions.[176]

Tachypnea alone can impair airway protection. As the respiratory rate increases, the breathing pause that usually occurs during the pharyngeal phase of swallowing is violated, and aspiration becomes more likely.[177]

Evaluation of Dysfunctional Swallowing

A multidisciplinary approach to the child with dysfunctional swallowing provides the best opportunity to define the pathologic process. In high-risk children, such as those undergoing a Norwood procedure, a qualified feeding therapist should perform a bedside feeding evaluation and determine if further imaging is needed.

The child should be alert, interested in feeding, able to tolerate positioning for feeding, and able to handle bolus delivery to the stomach. If these conditions are not met, the child should not be considered ready for oral feeds. The presence of a nonnutritive suck (NNS) is another important feeding prerequisite for infants. Concerted efforts should be made to preserve the NNS through oral-motor stimulation whenever oral feeds are interrupted for prolonged periods of time. Some infants have trouble sustaining sucking because of endurance problems. Others with a disorganized NNS may benefit from oral-motor intervention. Findings of poor oral motor skills in children with CHD and hypotonia should prompt examiners to evaluate the possibility of central nervous system problems.[165]

Imaging studies focus on specific aspects of the swallowing process that cannot be viewed directly during bedside assessment. The most common radiologic procedures used to assess pediatric dysphagia are the barium swallow and the videofluoroscopic swallow study (VFSS). The VFSS is the gold standard for assessing the presence of oropharyngeal dysphagia and concomitant aspiration.[178,179] The VFSS is an appropriate procedure when a child is suspected of having pharyngeal phase dysphagia and the child is ready, willing, and able to participate in the protocol.[178] Although the VFSS provides the most comprehensive information about swallowing function and the risk of aspiration, its findings, even when normal, cannot completely exclude the possibility of aspiration.

Management of Dysfunctional Swallowing

The management goals for children with impaired swallowing are to reduce factors contributing to airway compromise, maintain adequate nutrition, maximize the child's potential for growth and development, and facilitate positive interactions with caregivers.[180] When possible, oral feeding is the desired route of nutrition because swallowing is the best therapy for swallowing dysfunction. Oral-motor and swallowing therapies promote the child's compensatory patterns (e.g., changing position or altering the consistency of foods or liquids) and strengthen the movement patterns of the swallowing structures. Children with dysphagia tend to have less difficulty handling thicker liquids, particularly those children with vocal fold paralysis or neurogenic dysphagia.[171,172] However, some infants with oral-motor dysfunction or poor endurance may fatigue while drinking thicker liquids. The feeding and swallowing evaluation, including the VFSS results, should help guide therapy. Some children with CHD may be unable to handle any risk of aspiration because of an extremely fragile medical status or pending surgical or medical interventions. Limited oral feeding or nonnutritive "tastes" if tolerated may still be beneficial for improving oral motor function.

Management of Gastroesophageal Reflux Disease

The clinical manifestations of gastroesophageal reflux disease (GERD) may include vomiting, poor weight gain, dysphagia, abdominal or substernal pain, esophagitis, feeding intolerance, wheezing, recurrent stridor, chronic cough, recurrent pneumonia, and aspiration. GERD is typically a clinical diagnosis, but pH/impedance monitoring can be used to confirm the diagnosis.

Treatment for the child with GERD includes changes in formula composition, feeding positioning, acid suppression therapy, prokinetic therapy, and surgical interventions. The response to empiric therapy should be prompt, usually within 2 weeks.[181] A 1- to 2-week trial of a hypoallergenic formula may be efficacious in infants suspected of having milk protein intolerance. Milk thickening may decrease the number of episodes of vomiting.[30]

Pharmacologic therapy for GERD has been directed toward (1) acid suppression and (2) accelerating gastric emptying. Gastric acid suppression can be achieved with the use of histamine-2 receptor antagonists and proton pump inhibitors. The available prokinetic agents include erythromycin, metoclopramide, and bethanechol.

Although many infants with CHD require feeding access, relatively few need a fundoplication. In one series of 111 patients who underwent an open gastrostomy, only 3 went on to need a subsequent fundoplication.[182] Therefore fundoplication should be considered only when medical therapy has failed to control GERD symptoms or when severe airway complications occur during treatment. When indications are met, fundoplication has been shown to enable patients to improve perioperative weight gain.[183,184] In a study of 24 consecutive infants with trisomy 21 and atrioventricular septal defect who had GER early after repair of their cardiac anomaly, 14 underwent a Nissen fundoplication, whereas 10 were managed medically. The medical group had significantly longer hospitalization and rehospitalization days over 24 to 56 months' follow-up than the surgical group.[185] Two randomized controlled trials and one meta-analysis found that laparoscopic fundoplication in children appears to have similar results and complication rates as compared with the open procedure.[186-188] Fewer retching episodes after laparoscopy were noted in one trial,[188] whereas longer surgical time and higher operating room costs were associated with laparoscopic Nissen fundoplication in the other trial.[186] Some centers limit the CO_2 insufflation pressure during laparoscopy in pediatric cardiac patients to approximately 10 to 12 mm Hg. At this time we can conclude only that laparoscopic fundoplication is an acceptable option when compared with the traditional open approach. One notable advantage of the open approach is that the gastrostomy has a purse-string suture around the tube, and the stomach is sutured to the anterior abdominal wall, thus making it more secure with less potential for leakage than the laparoscopically created gastrostomy.

Conclusion

Children with CHD frequently are malnourished before surgical intervention. The extent of undernutrition has a significant impact on the timing of surgical interventions, as well as the perioperative outcome. Postoperative nutritional support should be instituted early and aggressively. Enteral feedings should be employed whenever possible. Children with CHD may require a multidisciplinary swallowing evaluation before resumption of oral feeds. GER, PLE, and persistent chylothorax are significant postoperative complications with important nutritional complications in children with CHD. A staged therapeutic approach consisting of dietary changes, medical interventions, and then invasive interventions, if needed, is successful in mitigating the nutritional complications of each of these conditions in a majority of cases.

References

A complete list of references is available at ExpertConsult.com.

27

Arrhythmias and Pacing

ZEBULON Z. SPECTOR, MD; CHRISTINE MELIONES, CPNP, FNP; SALIM F. IDRISS, MD, PHD

The rapid recognition, diagnosis, and management of cardiac arrhythmias are essential skills in the intensive care unit (ICU). Outcomes can hinge on the timely initiation of arrhythmia therapy. The aim of this chapter is to serve as a useful, practical resource by (1) describing the basic physiology of the normal cardiac rhythm followed by the common mechanisms causing rhythm disturbances, (2) describing common tools used to diagnose rhythm, (3) describing specific pediatric arrhythmias, causes, and treatments, and (4) providing a practical guide to pacemakers and pacing in the ICU setting.

Normal Cardiac Rhythm

The normal cardiac rhythm is initiated in the sinoatrial (SA) node, which is a crescent-shaped collection of cells situated in the lateral terminal groove of the right atrium (RA) at its junction with the superior vena cava (SVC). SA nodal cells are specialized myocardial cells that depolarize automatically (Fig. 27.1) and trigger a wave of electrical activation that conducts across the atria. The basal rate of spontaneous SA nodal depolarization, and thus heart rate, is modulated by autonomic nervous system input. Increased parasympathetic tone will slow SA node discharge rate, and increased sympathetic tone will correspondingly increase the rate. The myocardial cells in the remainder of the atrium can also spontaneously depolarize but do so at a slower rate than the SA node. Therefore spontaneous beats from other "ectopic" atrial sites may occur if their rate of depolarization increases or if there is significant slowing of the SA nodal discharge rate caused by damage or other factors.

The atrioventricular (AV) node is located within the muscular atrial septum at the AV junction near the midseptal portion of the tricuspid valve annulus. Its position is approximated, classically, as being at the superior apex of the triangle of Koch. Conduction through the AV node is slow and is modulated by the autonomic nervous system. Increases in vagal tone that slow heart rate will also result in conduction slowing through the AV node and prolongation of the PR interval on the electrocardiogram (ECG). Increases in sympathetic tone that result in higher heart rates will do the opposite and accelerate AV nodal conduction and shorten the PR interval. The delay between atrial and ventricular electrical activation, imposed by the AV node, provides a hemodynamic benefit by allowing time for atrial contraction to contribute to diastolic filling of the ventricles.

Electrical activation conducted through the AV node is routed to the ventricles via the His bundle at the membranous septum. The atria and ventricles are otherwise electrically insulated from one another by fibrofatty tissue planes. Within the ventricular septum the His bundle divides into left and right bundle branches. The right bundle branch runs in the deep subendocardium of the interventricular septum until it emerges in the moderator band. The left bundle branch fans out broadly shortly after emerging on the left ventricular endocardial surface. These large conduction fibers remain insulated from surrounding myocardium by sheaths of fibrous tissue until they have further divided into the Purkinje network of smaller fibers that conduct the wave of depolarization rapidly throughout the ventricular myocardium.

Mechanisms of Arrhythmia

The normal heart rhythm is the product of an elegant system with multiple layers of control at the molecular, cellular, and whole organ levels. However, despite this robust underpinning of rhythm control, an abnormality at any level can result in an arrhythmia. There are multiple factors that cause primary arrhythmias in children and lead to the need for ICU care, but there are also many factors that secondarily cause arrhythmias in the critically ill child. Despite the presence of a primary or secondary rhythm problem, the mechanisms most often responsible for arrhythmias are similar. These include (1) failure of impulse formation, (2) conduction block, (3) reentry, (4) enhanced automaticity, and (5) triggered activity.[1] Reentry and block can be considered abnormalities of impulse conduction. Failure of impulse formation, enhanced automaticity, and triggered activity are abnormalities of impulse generation. One or more of these mechanisms underlie the specific cardiac arrhythmias.

Failure of impulse formation occurs when normal pacemaking tissue (i.e., the SA node) does not reach activation threshold, either at all *(sinus arrest)* or at a rate needed to meet physiologic requirements. This may occur during moments of extreme vagotonia, such as when a newborn receives nasopharyngeal stimulation, or may occur as part of *sick sinus syndrome* chronically following atrial surgery.

Conduction block refers to the failure of an electrical impulse to propagate in its normal direction and sequentially depolarize the myocardium. Conduction block may occur in the atrial or ventricular myocardium itself or in portions of the normal conduction system such as the AV node, His bundle, bundle branches, or Purkinje fibers. Block may occur due to an intrinsic abnormality that prevents depolarization of adjacent cells, such as metabolic derangements (e.g., ischemia), or anatomic barriers such as fibrosis or scar. Extreme vagal tone can cause conduction block within the AV node. Conduction block may also occur physiologically in

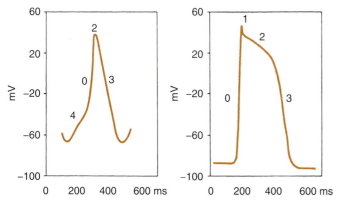

• **Figure 27.1** Cardiac action potentials from a sinus node cell *(left)* and a ventricular myocyte *(right)*. The phases of the action potential are numbered. During phase 0 there is rapid depolarization, mediated by inward calcium flux in sinus node cells and the opening of sodium channels in myocytes. The early rapid repolarization (phase 1) seen in ventricular cells is the result of sodium channel inactivation and a transient outward potassium current. The plateau (phase 2) results from the balance of currents that depolarize the cell membrane, such as the inward calcium current, and currents that repolarize the membrane, principally outward potassium currents. The membrane repolarizes (phase 3) as potassium currents increase and drive the potential more negative. Unique to cells with automaticity, such as the sinus node, is a steady diastolic depolarization during phase 4. Once this depolarization reaches a threshold level, inward calcium currents are activated, and phase 0 is initiated.

response to premature impulses or extremely rapid activation. For example, conduction block within the AV node may occur in response to a premature atrial contraction or depolarization that occurs at a time when the AV node is in its refractory period. Rapid atrial activation, such as during atrial flutter or fibrillation, results in dynamic variability of AV nodal conduction such that impulses are conducted to the ventricle in a regular or irregular periodic pattern.

Reentry is the most common cause of tachyarrhythmias. Reentry is a mechanism for the self-propagation of a wavefront that repetitively travels the same conduction circuit. The conditions necessary to initiate and sustain reentrant arrhythmias include unidirectional block in one limb of the path (e.g., long refractory period at the site of block), sufficiently slow conduction around the other limb of the circuit such that the site of unidirectional block is recovered from refractoriness when the impulse returns, and capacity for retrograde conduction through the area of original block (Fig. 27.2). The path may encircle inexcitable tissue such as surgical injury or scar from previous myocardial infarction or tissue fibrosis, or it may include normally excitable tissues with discrepant conduction properties such as occurs in AV nodal reentry or accessory pathway (AP)–mediated tachycardias. In most cases the initiation of reentry results from unidirectional conduction block created following a premature stimulus encountering refractory tissue (see earlier discussion). This same property can also lead to termination of reentry through timed placement of a prematurely paced beat, which creates refractoriness and blocks ongoing conduction in the reentrant circuit (see "Treatment of Tachyarrhythmias With the Pacemaker" later).

Automaticity is a normal property of several different types of cardiac cells and consists of a gradual depolarization of resting membrane potential during diastole (phase 4) (see Fig. 27.1). Once activation threshold is attained, the rate of depolarization increases steeply (phase 0), and a full action potential ensues. Cells capable

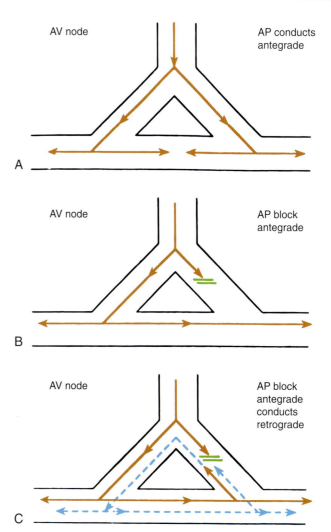

• **Figure 27.2** Mechanism of reentry arrhythmias. (A) Reentry requires two conduction pathways that may be anatomically or physiologically distinct, such as an atrioventricular (AV) node and an accessory pathway *(AP)*. (B) Conduction block may occur in one pathway, such as an AP, with slow conduction over the other pathway, the AV node. (C) If this slowly conducted impulse travels retrograde over the previously blocked pathway, it will reenter the circuit and then initiate a regular tachycardia by repetitively circling the path. As an example of AP-mediated tachycardia, the circuit would be antegrade unidirectional block in the AP with slow antegrade conduction over the AV node to the ventricle and return to the atrium due to retrograde conduction over the AP.

of automaticity include those in the sinus node, specialized regions of the atria, the AV node, and the His-Purkinje system. The cells with the most rapid diastolic depolarization, usually in the SA node, determine the heart rate. *Abnormal automaticity* may develop in cells that are not normally automatic, such as atrial and ventricular myocytes. Conditions that increase the likelihood of enhanced abnormal automaticity include ischemia, electrolyte imbalance, catecholamine excess, and certain drug toxicities. An abnormal automatic rhythm often exhibits a gradual increase in rate, or "warm-up," before becoming a regular tachycardia and a gradual deceleration before termination.[2] Automatic rhythms can usually be transiently interrupted *(overdrive suppressed)* by overdrive pacing, but they cannot be reliably initiated or terminated by these methods.

Triggered activity develops in the setting of low-amplitude secondary depolarizations (afterdepolarizations) of the membrane potential during (phase 3) or after (phase 4) normal repolarization. If an afterdepolarization reaches the activation threshold potential, another action potential is triggered that is coupled closely to the first. If this second action potential is accompanied by another afterdepolarization, the process can be repetitive and give rise to a sustained arrhythmia. Early afterdepolarizations (EADs) are present during repolarization (phase 3) and arise as a result of enhanced calcium or sodium entry through sarcolemmal ion channels.[3,4] Conditions associated with EADs are often present in postoperative patients and include acidosis, hypoxia, hypokalemia, and a variety of antiarrhythmic agents. The development of sustained EAD-triggered ventricular arrhythmias is bradycardia dependent, with an increased frequency of EADs observed at slow rates or following pauses in the cardiac rhythm. Delayed afterdepolarizations (DADs) develop after the membrane potential has fully repolarized (phase 4) and are caused by intracellular calcium overload and a subsequent oscillatory uptake and release of calcium from the sarcoplasmic reticulum.[3] The prototypic arrhythmia associated with DADs is digitalis intoxication. DAD–triggered ventricular arrhythmias may also be associated with catecholamine excess and can be initiated by rapid pacing.

Electrocardiographic Monitoring in the Intensive Care Unit

The Electrocardiogram

Electrocardiography is the measurement of body surface, time-varying voltages generated by electrical activation of the heart. The ECG is a "map" of the body surface voltages based on a standardized set of recording positions. Proper interpretation of the ECG is rooted in a fundamental understanding of how it is generated, and assumptions are made as to how it has been recorded. Simple pattern reading, although potentially accurate in adults with normal cardiac structure and position, will lead to a flawed diagnosis in children with and without congenital heart disease (CHD) given the wide range of variables, including body size, cardiac position, cardiac structure, and nonstandard ECG lead positioning (especially in an ICU setting).

The standard 12-lead ECG is recorded using electrodes placed on each limb and across the chest in a reproducible pattern. Because interpretation of the ECG is usually performed by a provider who did not perform the measurement, adherence to standardized methods and correct electrode placement is critical. The standard limb leads, labeled I, II, and III, are measured from the surface potentials recorded between electrodes placed on the distal extremities: lead I left arm(+)/right arm(−); lead II right arm (+)/left leg(−); lead III left arm (+)/left leg (−). A right leg electrode acts as a ground to reduce noise and stabilize the recording baseline. The precordial leads are placed in standardized positions relative to the chest wall: V_1—fourth intercostal space at the right sternal border; V_2—fourth intercostal space at the left sternal border; V_3—the midpoint between electrodes V_2 and V_4; V_4—fifth intracostal space aligned at the midclavicular line; V_5—horizontally in line with V_4 but at the anterior axillary line (or midway between V_4 and V_6); V_6—horizontally in line with V_4 but at the midaxillary line. In the ICU setting it is common to place leads in nonstandard positions for bedside monitoring or with ambulatory monitors due to limitations on access to the thorax. The ECGs obtained from leads in nonstandard positions are helpful for rhythm interpretation. However, other diagnostic conclusions, such as the

TABLE 27.1	Normal Electrocardiographic Intervals in Children (Defined as the 2nd Through 98th Percentile Values)		
Age	PR (ms, in Lead II)	QRS (ms, in Lead V_5)[a]	QT (ms, in lead V_5)
0-1 d	79-161	21-76	210-370
1-3 d	81-139	22-67	223-346
3-7 d	74-135	21-68	220-327
7-30 d	72-138	22-79	220-301
1-3 mo	72-130	23-75	222-317
3-6 mo	73-146	22-79	221-305
6-12 mo	73-157	25-76	218-324
1-3 y	82-148	27-76	248-335
3-5 y	84-161	31-72	264-354
5-8 y	90-163	32-79	278-374
8-12 y	87-171	32-85	281-390
12-16 y	92-175	34-88	292-390

[a]The QRS duration was measured only in lead V_5 because the onset of the QRS is most sharply defined there. This measurement in a single lead underestimates the full QRS duration because in some cases the beginning or end of the QRS in lead V_5 may not deviate from the baseline and will not be detected.

presence of hypertrophy, should not be made. Final diagnosis should always be made using the standardized electrode positions and lead sets.

Atrial electrical activation is manifest on the surface ECG as the P wave. The shape, duration, and orientation of the P wave is influenced by the site of origin of the activating stimulus, the size of the atria, and the rate of conduction of the electrical impulses through the atria. The PR interval, being the time elapsed from P wave onset to Q wave onset, reflects conduction time from the initial site of atrial activation summed with AV nodal and His-Purkinje conduction times. Depolarization of the ventricles produces the QRS complex on the surface ECG. QRS morphology is influenced by the origin of ventricular activation, the presence of conduction block or delay in the bundle branches, and the rate of electrical conduction within the ventricles. Repolarization of the ventricular myocardium is reflected by the ST segment and T wave. Normal ranges for the PR, QRS, and QT intervals by age are shown in Table 27.1.[5]

Bedside Telemetry

Continuous bedside electrocardiographic monitoring is performed in critically ill children in the ICU. In addition to real-time ECG monitoring from one or more leads for immediate analysis at bedside, ICU telemetry systems provide continuous archiving of data for review. An important skill in the management of postoperative cardiac patients and those requiring intensive care is the review of these recordings. In general, providers should review a patient's telemetry at least daily and with any concern for arrhythmia or change in condition. Important events and useful diagnostic information tend to be found at *inflection points, peaks,* and *troughs* of the heart rate trend graph. Thus in most modern telemetry systems, this graph should serve as the starting point for telemetry review. A straightforward approach to telemetry review is as follows:

1. Review the heart rate trend graph. This graph can typically be set to display 12 or 24 hours of heart rate at a time, although shorter time intervals can usually be set for more detailed review. Attention should be focused on *overall heart rate trend*—has the heart rate been increasing or decreasing? Is there mainly bradycardia or tachycardia? Is there normal heart rate variability? Most patients after orthotopic heart transplant will lack normal heart rate variability due to poor innervation of the graft. Patients after the Fontan procedure or after more extensive atrial surgery, such Mustard or Senning atrial switch procedure, will often have bradycardia and/or a diminished ability to raise heart rate (chronotropic incompetence) due to sinus node dysfunction. Heart rate trend can be a good indication of patient recovery or response to therapy.

2. Heart rate *peaks and troughs* should be identified and rhythm at these points examined in greater detail, looking at the telemetry strips at those times. Is the patient in sinus rhythm? If not, is the rhythm an expected response to change in heart rate, such as junctional escape rhythm in the setting of sinus bradycardia? Is apparent bradycardia caused by frequent ectopy that is either not conducted (blocked premature atrial complexes [PACs]) or followed by a compensatory pause? Is the telemetry indicative of a tachyarrhythmia such as supraventricular tachycardia or junctional ectopic tachycardia?

3. *Inflection points* should be examined in detail. A finding of abrupt or rapid increase in heart rate on the graphic trend followed by a new heart rate plateau can be suggestive of tachyarrhythmia, especially when the heart rate plateaus or varies slightly around a supranormal heart rate. Dysrhythmias often terminate abruptly, but gradual offset can be seen in the setting of automatic rhythms or due to sympathetic stimulation–related sinus tachycardia at termination of tachyarrhythmia.

4. If an arrhythmia is identified, the provider should especially examine the *onset, termination,* and any points of *change or interruption* during the arrhythmia. As described in the section on tachyarrhythmias in this chapter, the mode of onset and termination, the relationship of atrial to ventricular signals, and the effect of PACs, premature ventricular complexes (PVCs), or changes in atrio-ventricular/ventriculo-atrial (A-V/V-A) conduction are important in the identification of type and mechanism of arrhythmia. *Widening* or *narrowing of the QRS complex* (e.g., loss of ventricular preexcitation at the initiation of orthodromic AV reciprocating tachycardia [AVRT] in a patient with Wolff-Parkinson-White [WPW] syndrome, change in the pattern of conduction delay at the onset of ventricular tachycardia [VT] in a patient with tetralogy of Fallot, widening of QRS at the onset of VT or supraventricular tachycardia [SVT] with aberrant conduction in a patient with baseline normal QRS complex), can often be helpful in identifying type of arrhythmia. Proper identification allows targeting of therapy for termination and prevention of the arrhythmia.

5. *Review alarms.* Although much superfluous information will be provided by automatically generated alarm strips, careful review can help focus the provider's attention on areas of telemetry that might otherwise be overlooked.

6. *Distinguish true signals from artifact.* Abnormal telemetry signals can be caused by lead interference, patient movement, or artifacts such as those caused by respiratory care/chest physiotherapy. It is important to distinguish true abnormal rhythms from artifact. Correlation of heart rhythm with other monitoring

signals (which can usually be displayed simultaneously with heart rhythm on telemetry), such as arterial line tracing or pulse oximetry tracing, can be helpful. Also, even in the setting of significant artifact, an R or S wave can often be found that marches out with the QRS complexes preceding and following the period of possible artifact, with some slight leeway given for normal heart rate variation. Examination of the relationship of the abnormal signals in question to P waves or QRS complexes (does the signal appear to be driving the QRS complexes or is there no clear relationship between the two signals) can also help in distinguishing artifact from dysrhythmia.

Atrial and Ventricular Electrograms

In the postoperative patient, bipolar recordings from each pair of epicardial wires may be attached to standard ECG recording devices or to ICU monitors as follows: attach one electrode connecting wire (or use alligator clamps if necessary) to the monitor's cable corresponding to "right arm" and the other electrode to the monitor's cable corresponding to "left arm." Be certain that the monitor's leg cables are appropriately attached to the patient (Fig. 27.3A). Lead I will represent a bipolar electrogram from the chamber in continuity with the epicardial pair of wires. If the chamber being viewed is atrial, there may be minimal ventricular signal, making a simultaneous surface lead desirable; the surface QRS can serve as a ventricular reference. If the lead I, II, III montage is available, leads II and III will represent electrical fusion between the atrial electrogram and QRS, which will serve the same purpose. Alternatively, either or each of the epicardial wires can be connected to a precordial "V" lead input to obtain unipolar recordings of atrial or ventricular activation. Useful activation timing information will be obtained from either of these methods. In addition, there are other methods of obtaining discrete cardiac electrograms using temporary pacing systems (Fig. 27.3B). Examples of bipolar and unipolar atrial electrograms with simultaneous ventricular references appear in Fig. 27.4. These methods are invaluable for discriminating postoperative junctional ectopic tachycardia (JET) from sinus tachycardia or SVT, sinus bradycardia from nonconducted atrial bigeminy, and atrial flutter with 2:1 AV conduction from sinus tachycardia, to name a few. Simultaneous use of pharmacologic agents, such as adenosine, makes this technique even more powerful.

Common Intensive Care Unit Rhythm Issues and Their Management

Using the mechanistic approach described earlier, the most common cardiac arrhythmias encountered in the ICU are listed in Table 27.2. This categorization allows for a more rational approach to the selection of pharmacologic or interventional therapies. This section addresses these heart rhythm issues, focusing on the clinical setting in which the rhythm issue is encountered, diagnosis of the arrhythmia, and treatment options. Before discussing individual clinical entities, a brief review of available medications and other techniques for the management of cardiac rhythm issues is touched upon.

Pharmacology

Pharmacologic Treatment of Tachyarrhythmias

The Vaughan-Williams classification is a widely used antiarrhythmic medication schema based on common actions of different agents

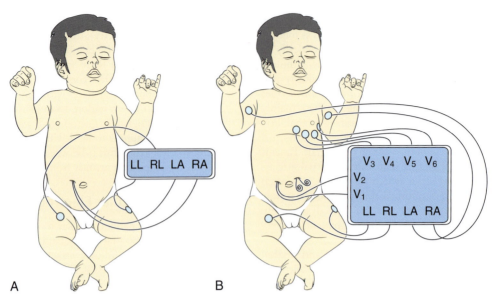

• **Figure 27.3** (A) A method for recording a bipolar atrial electrogram involves connecting the atrial electrodes (or wires) to the right arm *(RA)* and left arm *(LA)* leads and leaving the leg leads connected to the right leg *(RL)* and left leg *(LL)*. The atrial electrogram is very prominent in lead I and observable, but less prominent, in the other limb leads. (B) An alternate method for recording a unipolar atrial electrogram from temporary epicardial wires. This setup requires normal attachment of limb leads to establish a central Wilson terminus (plus V_3). One atrial wire is connected to V_1, the other to V_2, and a V_1-V_2-V_3 montage is recorded. Two unipolar atrial electrograms with large amplitude (far-field) ventricular electrograms will appear as V_1 and V_2. Compare this method with that described in the text.

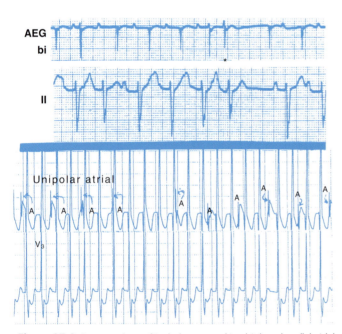

• **Figure 27.4** A comparison of techniques used to obtain epicardial atrial electrograms. *Top,* As described in the text and illustrated in Fig. 27.3A, bipolar *(bi)* atrial electrograms *(AEGs)* are much larger than the ventricular and must be compared with a surface lead *(II)* to identify the QRS. This technique readily identifies a nonconducted premature atrial beat *(*)*. *Bottom,* The technique shown in Fig. 27.3B illustrates the easy identification of the QRS and atrial *(A)* electrograms in one lead, but the atrial signal may be dwarfed by the large ventricular one. This V_1-V_3 montage demonstrates postoperative junctional ectopic tachycardia.

TABLE 27.2	Arrhythmia Types According to Mechanism
Bradycardias	*Failure of impulse formation*
	Sinus bradycardia
	Sinus node arrest
	Conduction block
	Sinus node exit block
	AV node block
	Bundle branch block
Tachycardias	*Reentry*
	Atrial flutter (macroreentry)
	Atrial fibrillation
	Sinus node reentry tachycardia
	AV node reentry tachycardia
	AV reciprocating tachycardia (including permanent form of junctional reciprocating tachycardia)
	Some ventricular tachycardia (including torsades de pointes)
	Enhanced automaticity
	Some atrial ectopic tachycardias
	Junctional ectopic tachycardia
	Accelerated junctional rhythm
	Accelerated idioventricular rhythm
	Some ventricular tachycardias
	Triggered activity
	Some atrial ectopic tachycardias
	Digitalis toxicity
	Initiating beat of torsades de pointes
	Some ventricular tachycardias
	Other mechanisms causing premature beats
	Supernormal conduction
	Parasystole

AV, Atrioventricular.

Class	Subclass	Drug	Pharmacologic Effect
I		Moricizine	Depression of rate of increase of action potential
	IA	Quinidine	Increased action potential duration, and increased atrial and ventricular ERP; increased JT interval; vagolytic action
		Procainamide	
		Disopyramide	
	IB	Lidocaine, mexiletine, tocainide	Decreased action potential duration but increased ventricular ERP; unchanged QRS complex; unchanged JT interval
	IC	Propafenone flecainide (encainide)	Depressed rate of increase of action potential, causing widening of QRS complex; unchanged action potential duration, but increased atrial and ventricular ERP; unchanged JT interval
II		Beta-blockers	Inhibition of beta-adrenergic receptors
III		Amiodarone	Increased action potential duration
		Sotalol	Increased JT interval
		Bretylium	
IV		Verapamil, diltiazem	Blockade of Ca^{++} channels

TABLE 27.3 Classification of Antiarrhythmic Agents

ERP, End resting potential.

(Table 27.3). These medications predominantly affect ion currents responsible for various phases of the cardiac action potential (see Fig. 27.1). Some have their effect on the sympathetic and parasympathetic balance contributing to the persistence of cardiac arrhythmias. Several medications are effective through multiple mechanisms. The same mechanisms responsible for the antiarrhythmic effects may also be responsible for the side effects seen with antiarrhythmic medications.

Class I drugs inhibit inward depolarizing sodium channels, resulting in a slowed upstroke of the cardiac action potential and secondary alteration of action potential duration and refractoriness of excitable tissues. Class II agents block beta-adrenergic receptors altering the sympathetic influence on electrophysiologic properties of cardiac cells. Class III medications predominantly block potassium channels, resulting in prolonged phase 3 repolarization of the cardiac action potential. Class IV antiarrhythmics block calcium channels, which are the depolarizing channels in the sinoatrial and AV nodes.

Class IA Antiarrhythmic Medications (Quinidine, Procainamide, and Disopyramide). Procainamide is the Class IA agent most often used in the ICU setting in the United States due to its availability in parenteral form. The primary action of procainamide is to block the inward sodium channel, with lesser repolarizing potassium channel blockade and vagolytic effects. It can be expected to prolong the cardiac action potential and refractory period of atrial, ventricular, and His-Purkinje cells. Conduction velocity is slowed, and automaticity is decreased. The major effect of these agents on the ECG is prolongation of the corrected QT interval (QTc). The PR interval will prolong in the presence of preexisting His-Purkinje system disease. Likewise, procainamide slows the heart rate in the presence of sinus node dysfunction. Class IA drugs are most useful in treating all reentrant supraventricular tachycardias and some VTs.

The major noncardiac side effects limiting use of procainamide in the acute setting are nausea, vomiting, and central nervous system symptoms. These agents all have negative inotropic properties, especially disopyramide, and due to slight alpha-adrenergic blocking effects, they may also cause hypotension. Due to its vagolytic property, procainamide used in the setting of atrial fibrillation or rapid atrial tachycardia will accelerate AV nodal

conduction, resulting in a rapid ventricular response. In those instances a beta-blocker or calcium channel blocking drug is also necessary. Prolongation of the QTc may predispose patients with an unstable ventricular myocardium to develop torsades de pointes (TdP).

Class IB Antiarrhythmic Medications (Mexiletine, Lidocaine). Lidocaine is a Class IB agent that is available in intravenous form in the United States and had classically been part of Advanced Cardiac Life Support treatment algorithms for VT and ventricular fibrillation (VF). Its primary effects are to slow ventricular conduction and to raise the threshold for VF.[6] It has little effect on atrial and nodal tissue. Lidocaine particularly depresses conductivity in injured or hypoxic myocardium, accounting for its efficacy immediately following myocardial infarction. It has mild negative inotropic effects. Heart block and decreased myocardial function are potential complications of lidocaine therapy in the postoperative period, although it is generally well tolerated. Central nervous system toxicity in the form of seizures, disorientation, drowsiness, agitation, and paresthesias can be expected at supratherapeutic blood levels, especially at levels in excess of 10 to 15 mcg/mL.

Mexiletine is an orally active agent effective at suppressing PVCs and ventricular arrhythmias, especially in patients who have undergone ventriculotomy for repair of congenital heart defects and are having abnormal hemodynamics (e.g., tetralogy of Fallot).[7,8] Mexiletine is increasingly used in patients with long QT syndrome type 3 (LQTS3). It does not depress ventricular function.

Class IC Antiarrhythmic Medications (Flecainide, Propafenone). Flecainide and propafenone are Class IC agents,[8-10] which decrease the phase 0 slope and slow conduction velocities throughout the myocardium. They are available only in oral form in the United States. They are efficacious in treating sustained and resistant ventricular tachyarrhythmias and refractory reentrant SVT. Propafenone also has calcium channel and beta-blocking activity.[11] It has been reported to be useful in treating JET.[8,12] These drugs can increase the PR interval and QRS duration. They have been associated with malignant proarrhythmia, so caution is required when using them, especially in children with impaired left ventricular function or previous cardiac surgery. Proarrhythmia may take the form of worsening of the index VT or SVT[13] or induction of an incessant, difficult-to-terminate VT. Proarrhythmia is usually related to higher doses, and careful monitoring of the rhythm and QRS duration is warranted. Patients initiated on flecainide are typically monitored for at least 72 hours in hospital.

Class II Antiarrhythmic Medications (Beta-Blockers). Class II agents are direct antagonists of beta-adrenergic receptors.[14] They decrease the slope of phase 4 of pacemaking tissues, thus reducing automaticity and lowering heart rates.[8,10] Beta-blockers increase the refractory period of the AV node and are used as chronic therapy to prevent the SVTs that use the AV node as a part of the tachycardia circuit. They are also used chronically to limit the ventricular rate response to atrial flutter and atrial fibrillation,[14] and intravenous preparations are used for immediate reduction in ventricular rate. They may also be useful in suppressing PVCs and VT in persons having no other heart disease.

Propranolol is the prototypic drug in this class, having both beta$_1$ and beta$_2$ receptor–blocking effects. Atenolol and nadolol are also in common use, with nadolol the most efficacious beta-blocker in treatment of long QT syndrome (LQTS). Esmolol, an intravenous agent that is ultra–short acting, has a plasma half-life of 8 minutes and is an excellent alternative when initiating beta-blockade therapy in postoperative or cardiomyopathic patients. It can be delivered in small IV boluses or as a rapidly accelerating IV infusion. When using these drugs in the acute care setting, side effects include depression of ventricular function, vasodilation and hypotension, and bradycardia. Extreme caution should also be used in patients with SA node dysfunction or advanced AV nodal disease. In patients with asthma, beta-blockers may precipitate small airway bronchospasm, and beta$_1$-specific blocking agents such as metoprolol are preferred.

Class III Antiarrhythmic Medications (Amiodarone, Sotalol). The Class III antiarrhythmic agents act principally by potassium channel blockade. Thus they prolong repolarization and refractoriness of most cardiac tissues. Amiodarone and sotalol have additional beta-adrenergic blocking effects,[9,15,16] and amiodarone has lesser sodium and calcium channel blocking effects. The ECG effects of these drugs are to increase the PR and QT intervals without affecting the QRS duration. Oral sotalol and amiodarone are useful agents for chronic prevention of otherwise medically resistant VT and most SVT. They have unique efficacy in treating automatic tachycardias, such as atrial ectopic tachycardia (AET).

Intravenous amiodarone load is administered as 1 mg/kg over 12 minutes or 5 mg/kg over 60 minutes and may be repeated to achieve the desired effect to a maximum of 20 mg/kg/day. An infusion is needed to maintain the effect. Although there are no direct negative inotropic effects of amiodarone, alpha-adrenergic blocking properties and resultant hypotension may occur. Intravenous volume expansion or calcium chloride is used to treat secondary hypotension. Significant prolongation of the QTc may occur, resulting in the development of TdP, and patients should be evaluated with serial ECGs. Additionally, amiodarone decreases conductivity of nodal tissue and may produce significant sinus bradycardia, sinus arrest, or variable AV block. Long-term systemic side effects of amiodarone include phototoxicity, corneal deposits, altered thyroid function, and depressed liver function. Pulmonary interstitial fibrosis rarely occurs with prolonged chronic use, but shock lung may rarely occur in the acute setting. Treatment for these side effects consists of discontinuing the antiarrhythmic medication and supportive therapy. Unfortunately, amiodarone is very lipophilic and has an extremely long elimination half-life, making treatment of chronic side effects a problem.

Sotalol has combined beta-adrenergic and potassium channel blockade, making it a useful agent in the therapy of supraventricular and ventricular arrhythmias. Sotalol is an oral drug (available in IV form in some centers) with similar electrophysiologic effects as amiodarone without the systemic toxicities. Sotalol causes QT prolongation in a dose-related manner, increasing the risk of TdP to a greater extent than amiodarone. In addition, sinus bradycardia, sinus arrest, or AV block may occur. The beta-blocking effects are responsible for other side effects such as decreased ventricular function, fatigue, dizziness, and syncope.

Class IV Antiarrhythmic Medications (Calcium Channel Blockers). The Class IV drugs are calcium channel inhibitors.[8] Verapamil is the most frequently used drug of this class in children, although it has more negative inotropic properties than other subclasses of calcium channel blockers, such as nifedipine and diltiazem.[17] These agents slow conduction in calcium channel–rich tissues such as the SA and AV nodes.

Before the availability of adenosine, intravenous verapamil was widely used to terminate AV nodal reentrant tachycardia (AVNRT) and AVRT. However, due to reports of hypotension, bradycardia, and cardiac arrest in infants, the use of IV verapamil is to be avoided in infants younger than 1 year of age.[18] Although all calcium channel blockers cause some degree of negative inotropy and peripheral vasodilation, diltiazem appears to be safer than verapamil and still provides an excellent negative dromotropic effect. Both agents are excellent choices to slow the ventricular response in the presence of atrial fibrillation or flutter. The exception is in patients with WPW syndrome—the ventricular response during atrial fibrillation may actually be enhanced via the AP, due to *relative* block in the AV node, and therefore it is not indicated in this setting. As discussed later, verapamil is the drug of choice in fascicular VT. Complications of calcium antagonists in the ICU setting are peripheral vasodilation, decreased myocardial contractility, sinus bradycardia, and AV block, any of which may lead to hypotension and shock. The half-life of IV verapamil is extremely short (minutes).

Other Antiarrhythmic Medications

Adenosine. Adenosine is an endogenous nucleoside that in high doses produces sinus bradycardia and transient conduction block in the AV node.[19,20] This effect is mediated through specific membrane A$_1$ adenosine receptors coupled to adenylate cyclase and specific sarcolemmal potassium channels.[8] The transient effects are due to its rapid uptake and deamination by red blood cells, which results in a very short half-life (less than 10 seconds). The effects of adenosine are dose dependent and time dependent. AV block usually develops within 10 to 30 seconds after an IV bolus injection. In general, AP conduction is not influenced by adenosine.

Clinically, IV adenosine will abruptly terminate approximately 90% of cases of reentrant tachycardias that involve the AV node,[21] including AVRT and AVNRT. Adenosine may also be useful for determining the mechanism of unknown arrhythmias.[19] Transient AV block by adenosine may reveal atrial flutter or other atrial tachycardias by blocking the ventricular response,[22] without affecting the primary arrhythmia mechanism. The failure of adenosine to terminate a wide-complex tachycardia suggests that the arrhythmia is VT or a preexcited atrial tachycardia rather than an aberrantly conducted SVT. Some forms of right ventricular outflow tract VT in the otherwise normal heart are also terminated by adenosine.

Adenosine is initially administered as a 100 mcg/kg (to a maximum of 6 mg) rapid bolus into a large peripheral vein.

Failing the initial dose, increasing doses up to 300 mcg/kg (to a maximum of 12 mg) may be administered every 1 to 2 minutes as needed. Following tachycardia conversion, the initial escape rhythm may include PVCs, marked sinus bradycardia, AV block, and, rarely, atrial fibrillation. This drug should not be administered unless an external defibrillator is available. Systemic side effects are common but usually mild and short-lived; they include dyspnea, flushing, chest discomfort, bronchospasm, coughing, headache, and hypotension. In children with impaired contractility and uncertain volume status, cautious monitoring of blood pressure is necessary. Adenosine should be used with caution in patients with asthma. Adenosine is avoided when possible in patients post orthotopic heart transplant because its effect can be prolonged.

Digoxin. The use of digitalis glycosides is time honored.[8] Its primary action is inhibition of membrane-bound Na^+-K^+ ATPase, with resultant intracellular calcium loading. Its primary cardiac electrophysiologic effect is AV conduction delay, related to its effect on calcium traffic, and by enhancing vagal influences. The glycosidic portion of the digoxin molecule enhances carotid sinus baroreceptor reactivity, which leads to increased vagal tone and decreased sympathetic tone. In addition, it appears to have a central parasympathetic influence. In ventricular muscle, digoxin shortens the action potential and decreases the VF threshold, thus explaining the tendency for digoxin to induce ventricular tachyarrhythmias. Digoxin slows the normal sinus rate, increases the PR interval, and causes visible alteration (coving) of the ST segments, even in the absence of toxicity. QRS interval duration is unaffected, even at toxic doses. The QT interval may be shortened as a result of hastened ventricular repolarization.

Similar to calcium channel blockers, the major applications of digoxin are for treatment and prevention of reentrant supraventricular tachyarrhythmias that involve the sinoatrial or AV node, and ventricular rate control in the presence of atrial flutter or fibrillation. Unlike verapamil, however, its AV node–blocking effects are countered by physiologic periods of vagolysis or enhanced adrenergic states, as may occur during exercise. Systemic loading, even when administered parenterally, requires at least 12 to 16 hours; thus its use in the ICU setting may be limited. Digoxin also may shorten AP refractoriness in a patient with WPW, and thus digoxin is considered contraindicated in this setting.

Systemic signs of toxicity include visual disturbances, disorientation, anxiety, drowsiness, abdominal pain, hyperkalemia, nausea, and vomiting. Cardiac signs of toxicity are exclusively proarrhythmias: advanced SA and AV block in younger patients and a variety of ventricular or atrial tachyarrhythmias. An SVT with AV conduction blockade is the classic sign of digoxin toxicity, and failure to recognize this and administration of additional doses of digoxin may be catastrophic. Neonates may have artificially elevated levels due to maternal digoxin-like substances. Furthermore, the pharmacokinetics of digoxin are altered by multiple agents, including phenytoin, lidocaine, quinidine, and amiodarone,[8] and the dose of digoxin should be decreased in patients concomitantly receiving verapamil or amiodarone.

Recognizing digoxin toxicity is important because the emergent use of digoxin-specific Fab fragments (Digibind) may be lifesaving. Indications for the use of Digibind include hyperkalemia, the new occurrence or worsening of bradycardia, or the occurrence of a tachyarrhythmia in a patient in whom digoxin ingestion is known or strongly suspected. Serum concentrations may be misleading and should not be considered steady state unless the ingestion occurred at least 6 hours previously. Especially if there is a delay in Digibind administration, arrhythmias should be aggressively treated. AV block should be treated with atropine or a temporary pacing catheter, and VT with intravenous phenytoin or lidocaine. Hyperkalemia should be treated by standard means, potentially excluding intravenous calcium. The exclusion of calcium in this circumstance was historically due to concern for the development of "stone heart," which is an irreversible noncontractile state due to impaired diastolic relaxation from calcium–troponin C binding. This concern has not been consistently reproduced in the literature. Further concern for calcium repletion in this circumstance may be due to development of calcium excess with repletion, which may predispose to dysrhythmia by causing delayed afterdepolarizations. The dose of Digibind is calculated based on total body load of digoxin. If the amount of digoxin received is known, then 1 vial (40 mg) per 0.5 mg digoxin is given intravenously over 15 to 30 minutes. If a steady-state serum concentration is known, then dosing is based on total body load as calculated from serum concentration. If digoxin toxicity is highly suspected and dose or level of digoxin is unknown, then 10 vials (400 mg) should be administered. A bolus injection may be given should cardiac arrest be imminent. Cardioversion may be necessary should the patient be unstable, although there is additional risk because digoxin lowers the VF threshold. Prophylactic administration of lidocaine is advisable in those cases.

Magnesium. Intravenous magnesium may be helpful to treat TdP and ventricular arrhythmias associated with LQTS. Side effects of magnesium include hypotension and hypotonia, which may lead to respiratory complications. This drug should be considered for patients with ventricular arrhythmias and prolonged QT syndrome.

Pharmacologic Agents for Treatment of Bradyarrhythmias

A wide array of pharmacologic and device treatment options exist for bradycardia encountered in the intensive care setting (see also "Pacing in the Cardiac ICU" later). It must be remembered that in infants and all patients with diminished systolic function, chronotropic support is particularly important due to relatively reduced capacity for inotropic recruitment during periods of hemodynamic stress.

Pharmacologic augmentation of heart rate is accomplished though the use of either vagolytic or beta-adrenergic agents. Atropine is a vagolytic agent that substantially increases sinoatrial rate and improves AV conduction in most patients. However, impaired AV conduction due to surgical trauma or edema of the AV node may not be as responsive to atropine. Also, atropine is not expected to be effective treatment for impaired AV conduction caused by pathology below the level of the AV node (i.e., the bundle of His and bundle branches). Immediately following cardiac transplant, bradycardia may not be responsive to atropine, because the heart has been at least temporarily denervated.

Of the adrenergic agents, isoproterenol is the most widely used for pure heart rate augmentation, although epinephrine and norepinephrine also cause varying degrees of beta-receptor stimulation. Isoproterenol is a nonselective, pure beta-adrenergic agonist. As such, it increases both the chronotropic and the inotropic state of the heart. It also lowers systemic vascular resistance and diastolic blood pressure and, in certain settings of pulmonary arteriolar hypertension, may reduce pulmonary vascular resistance. Its major drawbacks include increase of myocardial and total body oxygen consumption, hyperglycemia, tachyarrhythmias, and increase of metabolic requirements by the injured myocardium.

TABLE 27.4	Physical Maneuvers for Terminating Atrioventricular Node–Dependent Supraventricular Tachycardias
Enhancement of vagal tone to the AV node	Exposure of upper half of face to ice water or ice in washcloth
	Finger in throat (gag maneuver)
	Right carotid sinus massage
Sudden volume/pressure changes to the right heart	Valsalva maneuver (has vagal component)
	Bearing down
	Squatting
	Gentle pressure to abdomen in an infant until he or she resists
	Turning patient upside down

AV, Atrioventricular.

Treatment of Tachyarrhythmias Using Vagal Maneuvers

An abrupt increase in parasympathetic tone generated by a variety of vagal maneuvers can result in transient AV block that will terminate AVRT and AVNRT and rare other tachycardias. The maneuvers in Table 27.4 are most effective when used soon after the onset of symptoms, before sympathetic tone rises to a high level.[23] Failing these maneuvers, pharmacologic intervention often becomes necessary.

Cardioversion and Defibrillation

For unstable patients with hypotension or altered mental status due to atrial or ventricular tachyarrhythmias, prompt cardioversion or defibrillation is indicated. Electrical energy is applied between two paddles or adhesive electrode patches placed on the chest or on the chest and back. The success of this procedure depends on its ability to fully depolarize the heart, thereby terminating most reentrant tachyarrhythmias and allowing sinus rhythm to be restored. Automatic tachyarrhythmias persist despite cardioversion and may actually accelerate due to the release of endogenous catecholamines.

Cardioversion refers to a shock, usually in the range of 0.25 to 4 J/kg, that is delivered synchronously with the QRS complex of the surface ECG. Energy delivery synchronous with the QRS complex reduces the risk of conversion of the tachycardia to VF. The lower energy range is generally used for atrial arrhythmias, and the upper energy range for ventricular arrhythmias. Defibrillation is a high-energy shock, usually 2 to 4 J/kg, delivered asynchronously for the treatment of VF.

Electrophysiology Study

The electrophysiology (EP) study is the most provocative means of tachyarrhythmia induction and analysis.[24] Typically the study involves the placement of either a single esophageal catheter or several multipolar catheters into the right heart from the femoral and/or internal jugular and subclavian veins.[25] In the intracardiac EP study, catheters are placed with electrodes in the high right atrium, right ventricular (RV) apex, coronary sinus (to record left atrial and left ventricular electrograms), and adjacent to the His

bundle. They are used to both record signals and pace the heart to evaluate the conduction system and determine the mechanism of any provoked arrhythmias. An additional steerable catheter can be added to map the arrhythmia substrate and potentially burn (radiofrequency ablation) or freeze (cryoablation) the mapped target.

Ectopy

Premature Atrial Complexes

PACs are common in the intensive care setting, especially in acutely ill patients or following cardiac surgery. A PAC typically originates because of abnormal automaticity or triggered activity outside the sinus node. A PAC can conduct normally, demonstrating the same QRS morphology as in sinus rhythm, though P wave and PR interval may be different than for a normal sinus beat. If the PAC occurs at a short interval after a normal beat (short *coupling interval*), a portion of the conduction system may be in its refractory period from the prior activating beat. In this situation the PAC may demonstrate *aberrant conduction,* resulting in a wide QRS complex. It is important to carefully assess for the premature P wave in the ST segment or T wave of the preceding beat to help differentiate the wide QRS complex as aberrant, rather than being generated by the ventricular myocardium itself (PVC, see later). If the coupling interval is short enough, the AV node or more distal conduction system may be completely refractory when the premature impulse reaches it, and the PAC will be blocked (there will be an abnormal P wave, often within the preceding ST segment, but no QRS following it). A blocked PAC can still reset atrial timing, so a compensatory pause will be noted after the PAC occurs. Frequent blocked PACs can result in ventricular bradycardia, especially if occurring in a pattern of bigeminy, in which every other atrial impulse does not conduct to the ventricle. In this situation, if the P wave of the PAC is not discovered, the ECG may be misinterpreted as marked sinus bradycardia. Therefore careful inspection of the ECG in all bradycardia is warranted to make the proper diagnosis and initiate appropriate treatment as necessary.

PACs are generally benign and well tolerated but can reflect an underlying metabolic derangement. If PACs are frequent, attention should be paid to electrolyte imbalance, choice of medications, hypoxia, and body temperature. Mechanical stretching of the atrial wall, such as from the tip of a central venous catheter, can induce local injury and automaticity resulting in PACs or runs of atrial tachycardia. In these cases a chest radiograph may be diagnostic, and withdrawing the line slightly can be therapeutic.

Premature Ventricular Complexes

PVCs are also common in the intensive care setting. Like PACs, they are generally caused by abnormal automaticity or triggered activity. PVCs can occur in the setting of metabolic derangement, hypoxia, strain, as a result of medications, as a response to catecholamines, or by direct stimulation due to a catheter or a device touching the myocardium. Following aborted cardiac arrest, PVCs may be a harbinger of underlying pathology, such as catecholaminergic polymorphic ventricular tachycardia (CPVT) (increasing PVCs with increasing heart rate), arrhythmogenic right ventricular cardiomyopathy (ARVC) (multiform or polymorphic PVCs with left bundle branch block [LBBB] morphology), or myocarditis (see "Clinical Entities Frequently Associated With Arrhythmias" later). Electrolyte levels should be evaluated, in particular potassium, ionized calcium, and magnesium. In the period following cardiac surgery if no other reversible cause is found for frequent PVCs, an echocardiogram should be performed to assess cardiac function and the integrity of the surgical repair and for the presence of a pericardial effusion.

PVCs can occur as singles, couplets (two PVCs strung together), or triplets and runs. PVCs can be monomorphic (single morphology) or polymorphic (also known as multiform), suggesting multiple abnormal foci or multiple exit points from a reentrant circuit. Up to 2% of normal children have PVCs on routine ECG.[26]

Bradyarrhythmias

Sinus Bradycardia

Normal heart rate range in children is age dependent. In the ICU, sinus bradycardia is commonly observed and has multiple potential causes, including increased vagal tone, medication side effects, and sinus node dysfunction due to surgical injury or scar. Sinus node dysfunction can occur acutely or develop later after complex atrial surgical procedures, including atrial switch (Mustard or Senning operation) and Fontan palliation. Medications are a common cause for sinus bradycardia, especially antiarrhythmics such as beta-blockers, amiodarone, and sedatives such as dexmedetomidine. In sinus bradycardia, P-wave morphology should be normal (upright in ECG leads I, II, and aVF) or reflect a rhythm from low in the sinus node (upright in I, negative in II and aVF). Note that the recording axis of limb lead III tends to be nearly perpendicular to the direction of atrial activation for sinus rhythm, and small deviations in the location of sinus node output could result in a negative P wave in this lead during normal sinus rhythm or sinus bradycardia. If there is significant sinus bradycardia, a junctional escape rhythm may be observed. In general, sinus bradycardia does not require treatment; however, symptomatic sinus node dysfunction may require pacing. Further, following heart transplant, often the new heart cannot mount a sufficient heart rate response for the chronotropic needs of the early posttransplant period. Isoproterenol infusion or temporary atrial pacing may be required to give adequate chronotropy for effective cardiac output.

Sinus Arrest

Sinus arrest results from failure of impulse generation in the sinus node. It is manifested as a pause in the rhythm for a duration that is not a multiple of the sinus cycle length. If sinus arrest is prolonged, another automatic focus in the atria, AV node, or ventricles may become active and generate an escape rhythm that continues until sinus node function recovers. Pauses greater than 3 seconds warrant careful assessment and in some cases manifest as an indication for permanent pacemaker implantation.[27]

Junctional Escape Rhythm

When the sinus rate is significantly slow or abruptly decreases, an ectopic rhythm from a site distal in the conduction system may take over. Junctional escape beats or a junctional escape rhythm should emerge, with the same QRS morphology and duration as in sinus rhythm but without a preceding P wave. If there is intact retrograde conduction during this rhythm, a retrograde P wave may be observed within or immediately following the QRS complex. If there is no retrograde conduction, the rhythm may appear somewhat irregular because sinus impulses occasionally conduct as a sinus capture beat. If a sinus capture beat is closely coupled to the preceding junctional complex, the sinus beat can conduct with aberrant conduction (much like a closely coupled PAC) and generate a wide QRS complex. A sustained junctional rhythm should never be misconstrued as JET given that JET may require aggressive treatment as a clinically significant arrhythmia.

Atrioventricular Block

AV block describes various degrees of slowing or failure of conduction within the AV node or His bundle. First-degree AV block manifests as a prolonged PR interval for age and is generally benign and well tolerated. It can occur in rare disease states such as Lyme disease or acute rheumatic fever but is also seen as a normal variant in conditioned athletes.[28] First-degree AV block can also be seen with high vagal tone and generally resolves with exercise or increased sympathetic tone.

Second-degree AV block describes intermittent failure of an impulse to conduct to the ventricles. Type I second-degree AV block (Wenckebach) is common and manifests as gradual prolongation of the PR interval before a dropped QRS complex. Careful examination for sinus slowing should be performed, in which case the nonconducted beat may be secondary to a vagal response rather than progressive conduction slowing across the AV node. Sometimes prolongation of the PR interval is clearly seen only in the first to second beat of the Wenckebach sequence. The Wenckebach phenomenon is commonly seen during sleep on Holter monitors in healthy children and is generally benign and not considered evidence of conduction system disease.

Type II second-degree AV block is considered *high grade,* tends to occur more distal in the AV node or within the His bundle, and is considered evidence of potentially significant conduction system disease (Fig. 27.5). A stable PR interval is present before

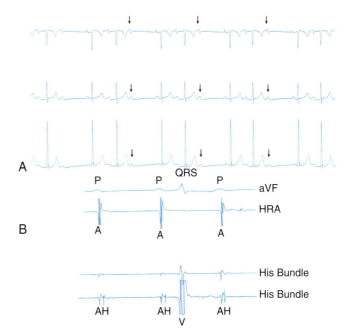

• **Figure 27.5** Second-degree atrioventricular (AV) block. (A) Type I AV block is manifested by a gradual prolongation of the PR interval until an atrial beat is not conducted *(arrow)* to the ventricles. (B) Infranodal second-degree AV block demonstrated by intracardiac electrogram recordings (paper speed 100 mm/s). The *top tracing* is surface lead aVF. The *middle tracing* is an intracardiac electrogram from a catheter placed in the high right atrium *(HRA)* that shows regular atrial activity. The *bottom two tracings* are recorded from a catheter placed across the tricuspid valve in the region of the His bundle. This catheter shows atrial activation (A), the His bundle potential (H) but no ventricular activation (V) for the first and third beats. The second beat demonstrates normal AV conduction, although the H-V interval is prolonged.

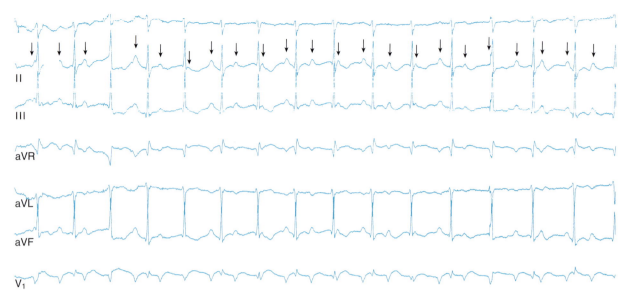

• **Figure 27.6** Complete heart block with atrioventricular dissociation. The atrial rate is 150 beats/min, indicated by *arrows,* which mark the P waves. The ventricular rate (88 beats/min) is completely regular and unrelated to the atrial rhythm.

the dropped QRS in the absence of sinus slowing. Type II second-degree AV block may be a sign of progression to complete heart block (CHB) and may be an indication for permanent pacing. Patients who have recurrent or persistent type II AV block and a low ventricular escape rate for longer than 7 to 10 days postoperatively may require permanent pacemaker implantation.[27] Note that when 2:1 AV block is observed, the cause may be either type I or type II. Therefore the clinical circumstances are included in determining the correct diagnosis because type I 2:1 AV block may be benign, whereas type II may warrant further treatment.

Third-degree or CHB describes dissociation of atrial from ventricular activity (Fig. 27.6). Atrial impulses are not conducted to the ventricles. Retrograde conduction can remain intact in the absence of intact anterograde conduction, allowing junctional or ventricular impulses to be conducted to the atrium. CHB can be congenital (present at birth), associated with certain congenital heart lesions (congenitally corrected transposition of the great arteries, in which it can be present at birth, intermittent, or emerge later in life), or acquired from cardiac surgical damage to the conduction system. Cardiac conduction may recover despite apparent CHB in the immediate postoperative period, and therefore it is customary to wait at least 7 to 10 days postoperatively before implantation of a permanent pacemaker. Congenital heart block is present in approximately 1 of every 20,000 live births.[29] In most patients without structural heart disease, there is an association with maternal anti-Ro (SS-A) or anti-La (SS-B) autoantibodies.[30,31] In congenital heart block, need for a pacemaker is related to age, escape rate, width of escape complexes (junctional versus ventricular), ectopy, QT interval, and perfusion/symptoms. Some patients with congenital heart block can go many years without requiring a pacemaker.[27]

Surgical heart block can be treated with temporary pacing as needed while evaluating for return of intact conduction. In the neonate with congenital heart block with inadequate escape rate and hypoperfusion, isoproterenol infusion is often the first intervention with temporary pacing (transcutaneous pacing can be performed if the patient is sedated, or via a temporary transvenous pacing catheter) as second-line therapy. Note that transesophageal pacing is not indicated for CHB given that only atrial pacing is possible with this modality.

Tachyarrhythmias

Supraventricular Tachycardia

Sinus Tachycardia. Sinus tachycardia is a regular tachycardia with sinus P waves. Table 27.5 presents age-specific ranges of normal heart rates. In infants and children, sinus tachycardia generally does not exceed 230 beats/min. Sinus tachycardia may indicate fever, hypovolemia, hypoxia, pain, hypercarbia, or myocardial failure. Treatment of sinus tachycardia involves treating the underlying cause.

Atrioventricular Reciprocating Tachycardia. AVRT is the most common form of pathologic tachycardia in infants and young children. It is a *reentrant* tachycardia that employs both the AV node and an AP, though atrial and ventricular myocardium are also essential parts of the reentrant circuit. Block in any of these portions of the circuit will terminate AVRT. If the AP is capable of conducting impulses in the anterograde direction during sinus rhythm, the surface ECG may demonstrate ventricular preexcitation, and the AP is considered *manifest* (see "Wolff-Parkinson-White [Ventricular Preexcitation] Syndrome" later under "Clinical Entities Frequently Associated With Arrhythmias"). If the AP does not support anterograde conduction, then the pathway is considered to be *concealed.*

The most common form of AVRT is called orthodromic reciprocating tachycardia (ORT) (Fig. 27.7B) with anterograde conduction over the AV node and retrograde conduction over the AP. Orthodromic AVRT is paroxysmal in onset and is initiated by a PAC or PVC. Because the ventricles are depolarized by normal conduction down the AV node, the QRS complexes are usually narrow, and a delta wave will not be present. The exception would be rate-dependent bundle branch block, in which the QRS is wide and must be differentiated from VT. AVRT is a *short R-P* tachycardia.

Age	Heart Rate (bpm)
0-1 d	94-155
1-3 d	92-158
3-7 d	90-166
7-30 d	107-182
1-3 mo	120-179
3-6 mo	106-186
6-12 mo	108-168
1-3 yr	90-152
3-5 yr	73-137
5-8 yr	64-133
8-12 yr	63-130
12-16 yr	61-120

TABLE 27.5 Age-Specific Range of Normal Heart Rates in Children (Defined as the 2nd Through 98th Percentile Values)

bpm, Beats per minute.
From Davignon A, Rautaharju P, Boisselle E, et al.: Normal ECG standards for infants and children. *Pediatr Cardiol.* 1979;1:123-152.

Antidromic AVRT (*antidromic reciprocating* tachycardia) is rare and occurs when the atrial impulse is conducted to the ventricles via a manifest AP and retrograde to the atria via the AV node. Because the ventricular activation is via the AP rather than the normal AV conduction system, the QRS during tachycardia is wide complex (see Fig. 27.7C) and appears maximally preexcited. In patients with WPW there may be a similar ECG appearance during tachycardias that originate in the atria such as atrial flutter or fibrillation. The latter should always be suspected when there is an irregular, wide-complex tachycardia.

For acute termination of orthodromic AVRT with stable hemodynamics, vagal maneuvers are the first line of therapy. Adenosine is the next line when vagal maneuvers fail to terminate AVRT. If adenosine is ineffective despite escalating doses, intravenous esmolol is generally infused followed by repeat vagal maneuvers/adenosine once a steady state is reached. Esmolol dose range is typically 50 to 250 mcg/kg/min. Amiodarone or procainamide may be alternatively selected in patients with ventricular dysfunction. Chronic medical therapy is aimed at impairing conduction in the AV node and/or AP and suppressing ectopy, which initiates tachycardia. Beta-blockers or digoxin are generally first-line treatments,[32] with flecainide or sotalol second line in refractory cases. Flecainide and sotalol are dosed in most cases by body surface area, and *a nomogram exists to adjust sotalol dosing in infants.* Catheter ablation of the AP is also highly effective and may be chosen as first-line therapy in patients of adequate size.

Atrioventricular Nodal Reentrant Tachycardia. AVNRT is the most common form of SVT in adults and is not uncommon in children over 5 to 10 years of age. It usually occurs in the absence of other cardiac abnormalities. Whereas the substrate for AVRT is present at birth, AVNRT appears to develop later in most patients. It is mediated by functionally discrepant zones of conduction within the region of the AV node. One of these pathways,

the fast pathway, conducts impulses rapidly and has a relatively long refractory period. The other, or slow pathway, has slower conduction velocity but a shorter refractory period. AVNRT is usually initiated by a PAC that blocks in the fast pathway but conducts over the slow pathway. If conduction down the slow pathway is sufficiently delayed, the fast pathway recovers and is able to conduct the impulse in the retrograde direction. At the atrial end of the fast pathway, the impulse can return down the slow pathway, and thus a cycle between these pathways is established that sustains the arrhythmia. The retrograde P wave usually occurs simultaneously with ventricular depolarization and may not be seen on the surface ECG or may be recognized as a *pseudo-r'* or small deflection at the terminal portion of the QRS in V_1. Hence AVNRT is one of the *short R-P* tachycardias. If atrial wires have been placed surgically or an esophageal lead is used, the recording of an atrial electrogram simultaneous with the surface QRS will help to diagnose this rhythm.

Atypical AVNRT develops in a small percentage of patients and is mediated by anterograde conduction along the fast pathway and retrograde conduction via the slow pathway.[33] Because retrograde conduction (from ventricles to atria) in atypical AVNRT is slow, the R-P interval is long and P waves are readily apparent. They are negative in the inferior leads (II, III, aVF).

When the patient is in the emergency department or ICU, this tachycardia will respond to vagal maneuvers or intravenous adenosine. Chronic medical therapy is directed at slowing conduction in the AV node, and therefore digoxin, beta-blockers, and calcium channel agents are often effective. As with AVRT, esmolol can be used in recalcitrant cases, and flecainide and sotalol are considered second-line therapies. In many centers, catheter modification of the slow pathway at EP study is considered first-line therapy. This approach eliminates a critical element of the reentry circuit and is curative.[34]

Atrial Ectopic Tachycardia. AET is a regular narrow QRS complex tachycardia with an abnormal P-wave morphology. As in sinus tachycardia, the P wave is usually temporally nearer to the succeeding (not the preceding) QRS, making this a *long R-P tachycardia.* The majority of cases are due to abnormal automaticity.[35,36] A presumed microreentrant mechanism can be the cause in a smaller proportion of these tachycardias. In those cases the rhythm is typically named a *focal* atrial tachycardia. Diagnosis of this arrhythmia is important because chronic AET at rates greater than 125 beats/min may lead to ventricular dysfunction (tachycardia-induced cardiomyopathy). Although AET may resolve spontaneously, the majority of patients require therapy, especially if a cardiomyopathy has resulted.[37] Pharmacologic suppression with beta-blockers, digoxin, or type IA antiarrhythmic agents is frequently ineffective, prompting the use of type IC or III agents.[38] Calcium channel blockers can be effective in rhythm control, and esmolol will often slow or suppress AET. Cardioversion, atrial overdrive pacing, and adenosine will not terminate these tachycardias if the mechanism is enhanced automaticity (approximately 90% versus 10% triggered activity). Radiofrequency catheter ablation has been demonstrated to be a safe and effective alternative.[39]

Atrial Flutter. Atrial flutter is a rapid, regular macroreentrant atrial tachycardia with atrial rates ranging from 200 to 500 beats/min in children (Fig. 27.8). Less than 10% of children with atrial flutter have a structurally normal heart.[40] Most have repaired or unoperated CHD or a cardiomyopathy.[41] The exception is healthy neonates with a structurally normal heart who may or may not have had a history of atrial flutter as a fetus. In these patients,

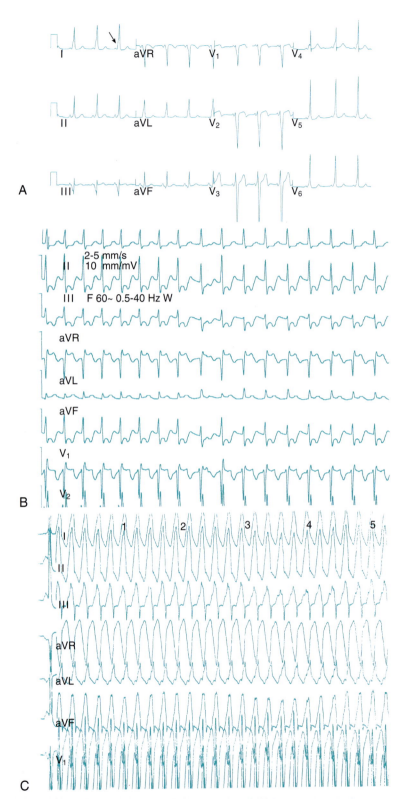

• **Figure 27.7** Electrocardiograms from a patient with the Wolff-Parkinson-White syndrome. During sinus rhythm (A), there is antegrade conduction over both the atrioventricular (AV) node and the accessory pathway, resulting in ventricular preexcitation (*arrow* indicates delta wave). During orthodromic reciprocating tachycardia (B), there is antegrade AV node conduction resulting in a normal QRS complex with retrograde conduction from the ventricle to atria completing the reentry circuit. During antidromic reciprocating tachycardia (C) there is maximal preexcitation with antegrade conduction via the accessory pathway and retrograde conduction over the AV node.

once terminated, atrial flutter tends not to recur and therefore does not need long-term therapy. Different types of atrial flutter have been characterized based on flutter wave morphology and anatomic substrate.[12] Electrophysiologic mapping studies have demonstrated that the slow zone of conduction of the reentry circuit in typical atrial flutter passes between the tricuspid valve annulus and the ostium of the inferior vena cava.[42] In the setting of structural or surgical heart disease involving the atria, critical isthmuses of slow conduction are often related to surgical incisions and adjacent areas of myocardium.[43] In these cases it is referred to as *intraatrial reentrant tachycardia*. AV conduction in the setting of atrial flutter can be variable and dependent on atrial rate, often 2:1. Typically electrical cardioversion or pacing is required to terminate the arrhythmia.

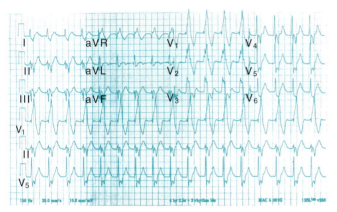

• **Figure 27.8** Atrial flutter in a patient with congenital heart disease. The presence of an unexplained tachycardia with no visible P waves is a common presentation of atrial flutter in these patients. The atrial rate is 204 beats/min with 2:1 atrioventricular block.

Atrial Fibrillation. Atrial fibrillation is a rapid, irregularly irregular rhythm with atrial rates ranging from 350 to 600 beats/min. This rhythm appears to be mediated by multiple microreentry circuits scattered throughout the atria.[12] It may be paroxysmal or persistent. The ventricular response is irregular and is significantly slower than the atrial rate, due to slowed conduction through the AV node. Atrial fibrillation is an increasingly common problem in teenagers and adults with CHD, especially those forms that cause left atrial dilation. In the absence of CHD in older children and teenagers, atrial fibrillation may occur as a result of sudden hypervagotonia, degeneration of SVT, in association with WPW, or rarely, as an isolated, familial disorder. Electrical cardioversion is often necessary for termination of atrial fibrillation. However, a single dose of flecainide or propafenone can be successful in restoring sinus rhythm in carefully monitored patients.[44] Careful consideration of anticoagulation must be given, and patients in atrial fibrillation for more than 24 to 48 hours, for an unknown period of time, or many with CHD require transesophageal echocardiography to examine for atrial thrombus before cardioversion.

Permanent Junctional Reciprocating Tachycardia. Permanent junctional reciprocating tachycardia (PJRT) is a narrow-complex often incessant tachycardia with rates from 120 to 250 beats/min, characterized by sudden onset and termination, negative P waves in leads II, III, and aVF, and a long R-P interval (Fig. 27.9).[45] It must be discriminated from atypical AVNRT and AET, which also have long R-P intervals. This arrhythmia is an unusual variant of orthodromic AVRT. It is the most common form of *incessant* tachycardia in children but is uncommon in neonates and adults. It may lead to tachycardia-induced cardiomyopathy, often necessitating catheter ablation. The underlying mechanism is reentry with retrograde conduction over a slowly conducting AP most commonly located in proximity to the ostium of the coronary sinus. Digoxin, beta-blockers, and type IA antiarrhythmics are generally ineffective in terminating PJRT. Type IC agents and type

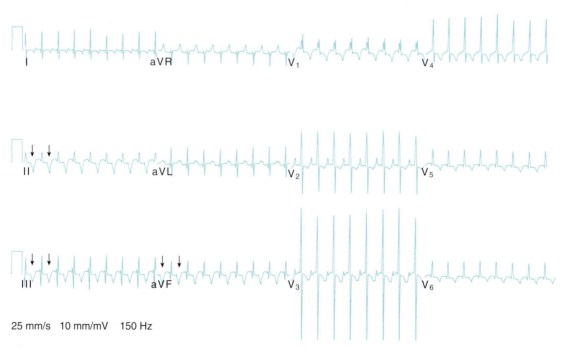

25 mm/s   10 mm/mV   150 Hz

• **Figure 27.9** Permanent form of junctional reciprocating tachycardia with characteristic deeply inverted P waves *(arrows)* in the inferior leads (II, III, aVF).

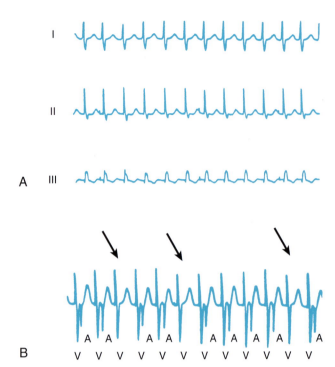

TABLE 27.6	**Causes of Ventricular Ectopy and Ventricular Tachycardia**

Metabolic/electrolyte derangements	Hypoxia/ischemia Hypercarbia Hypothermia Acidosis Hypokalemia, hyperkalemia
Drug/toxin exposure	Any Class I or III antiarrhythmic agent Sympathomimetic agents (e.g., cocaine) Digitalis toxicity Drugs that prolong the QT interval (see Table 27.7)
Myocardial abnormalities	Myocardial infarction Congenital heart disease Cardiomyopathy: dilated, hypertrophic, or restrictive Certain inborn errors of metabolism Certain neuromuscular disorders Myocarditis Myocardial tumors Idiopathic

• **Figure 27.10** Junctional ectopic tachycardia (JET). (A) Electrocardiogram (ECG) leads I, II, and III obtained 2 days following closure of an atrial and ventricular septal defect. The ventricular rate is 180 beats/min, with no apparent P waves. This ECG in the postoperative patient suggests JET. (B) Combined surface ECG and atrial electrogram recording during tachycardia. The ventriculo-atrial (V-A) relationship is irregular, with intermittent V-A block *(arrows)*. This confirms that the origin of the tachycardia is below the common atrioventricular node and that the atrium is not an essential component to sustaining the tachycardia.

III agents can provide partial but frequently incomplete suppression of tachycardia. Catheter ablation offers the potential for a definitive cure with a low risk of inadvertent high-grade AV block.[46]

Junctional Ectopic Tachycardia. Junctional ectopic tachycardia (JET) is an uncommon tachycardia that results from abnormal automaticity within the AV node or His bundle[47,48] and therefore will not respond to cardioversion. JET occurs in a rare congenital form in children younger than 6 months of age or more commonly following surgery for CHD (e.g., ventricular septal defect [VSD], atrioventricular septal defect, transposition of the great arteries with VSD, and tetralogy of Fallot). This rhythm is usually incessant and characterized by a narrow QRS complex, often with AV dissociation and more QRS complexes than P waves (Fig. 27.10). The onset (warm-up) and termination are gradual. The associated symptoms are dependent on the rate and duration of the tachycardia. JET is a serious postoperative rhythm disturbance and at times is associated with impaired hemodynamic performance and poor outcome following cardiac surgery. Initial treatment should include reduction of adrenergic drugs, normalization of electrolyte levels, and atrial pacing at rates slightly faster than the JET rate (if possible) to restore AV synchrony and optimize cardiac output.[49] In refractory cases, infusion of amiodarone or procainamide may be effective in slowing the rhythm, with or without cooling of the patient.[50] Postoperative JET tends to be a transient rhythm that seldom persists longer than 48 to 72 hours. Hence support of hemodynamics and cardiac rhythm during this interval is the primary strategy.

Ventricular Tachyarrhythmias

Ventricular Tachycardia. VT is a potentially life-threatening arrhythmia defined as three or more consecutive beats arising from the ventricles at a rate exceeding 10% above the prevailing sinus rate. The QRS complex is usually widened except in infants and small children, in whom the QRS morphology may be narrow but distinct from the morphology seen during sinus rhythm. If the morphology of the QRS complex is uniform, the VT is considered monomorphic. If the QRS complexes vary, the VT is polymorphic. If VT lasts longer than 30 seconds, it is considered to be sustained; otherwise it is nonsustained.

Sustained VT in children most often develops in association with metabolic/electrolyte derangements, drug/toxin exposure, or myocardial abnormalities (Table 27.6). VT may be the first manifestation of a cardiomyopathy.[51] In children under the age of 3 years, sustained VT is rare, but when present, VT is often incessant (i.e., in VT for greater than 10% of the day) and associated with myocardial tumors.[52]

There are two types of VT that occur in otherwise normal hearts, usually during exercise.[53] The most common is idiopathic outflow tract VT and demonstrates an LBBB QRS morphology and inferior QRS axis (dominant R wave in II, III, and aVF). Origin in the RV outflow tract is most common, but VT originating in the coronary cusps or left ventricular outflow tract can have a similar ECG appearance.[54] The underlying mechanism in approximately 90% of cases is triggered activity with the remainder caused by abnormal automaticity, and therefore this VT tends to be adenosine sensitive, with the initial treatment for these children either calcium channel blockers or beta-blockers.[55] The other form is *fascicular VT* (also known as verapamil-sensitive VT or Belhassen VT) and has a right bundle branch block (RBBB) QRS morphology and superior axis (dominant S wave in II, III, and aVF). It is caused by reentry involving the fascicles of the left bundle branch and is usually sensitive to verapamil. These forms of VT can be targets for catheter ablation.

The diagnostic evaluation of VT begins with the appreciation that not all wide-complex tachycardias are VT. SVT with aberrant conduction or with a bystander AP also has a wide QRS complex.[56] The diagnosis of VT is proven by the finding of AV dissociation in the setting of wide-complex tachycardia or the presence of fusion or capture beats. Careful differentiation of these possibilities is necessary before providing therapy. In patients with VT without clear reversible cause, further workup, including echocardiography, exercise treadmill testing, and cardiac magnetic resonance imaging (MRI), is often pursued to evaluate for underlying scar or cardiomyopathy or ion channelopathy such as CPVT.

Therapeutic management of VT is determined by the cause, hemodynamic stability, and age of the patient. Hemodynamically unstable arrhythmias should be treated by immediate electrical cardioversion. Reversible causes of VT, such as hypoxia or hyperkalemia, must be treated promptly. Pharmacologic therapy with Class I or III antiarrhythmic agents alone or in combination can be employed for acute termination of VT and for chronic arrhythmia suppression.[57] Esmolol is indicated to suppress arrhythmia in CPVT, and isoproterenol or epinephrine in Brugada syndrome. Catheter ablation is often useful in the absence of channelopathy or cardiomyopathy. Tachycardia originating in the right ventricular outflow tract can be cured by radiofrequency catheter ablation in greater than 90% of cases.[58]

Torsades de Pointes. TdP is a form of polymorphic VT that often develops in the setting of prolonged QT interval.[59] A partial list of the causes of QT prolongation, including both acquired and congenital forms, is provided in Table 27.7. TdP is characterized by the following features: (1) in a single ECG lead the polarity of the QRS complexes repetitively twists around an isoelectric baseline, (2) the tachycardia frequently terminates spontaneously, and (3) infrequently the tachycardia sustains and/or degenerates into VF.

TdP may occur in the setting of sinus pauses, especially in the presence of hypokalemia, or by sudden increases in sympathetic tone. The pause-dependent arrhythmias are often associated with a short cycle–long cycle–short cycle sequence of beats, as shown in Fig. 27.11. The QRS complex following the long cycle (i.e.,

TABLE 27.7	Causes of QT Interval Prolongation
Congenital	Long QT syndrome
Medications/toxins	Anesthetic agents: enflurane, isoflurane, halothane
	Antiarrhythmic agents: Class IA (esp. quinidine) and Class III (esp. sotalol)
	Antibiotics/antifungals: erythromycin, trimethoprim-sulfamethoxazole, pentamidine, ketoconazole
	Psychiatric: phenothiazines, tricyclics, tetracyclics
	Antihistamines: terfenadine, astemizole
	Organophosphate insecticides
Metabolic abnormalities	Hypokalemia
	Hypomagnesemia
	Hypocalcemia
	Hypothyroidism
	Hypothermia
	Liquid protein diets
Severe bradycardia	Marked sinus bradycardia or sinus arrest
	High-grade atrioventricular block
Myocardial diseases	Ischemia/infarction
	Myocarditis
	Cardiomyopathy
	HIV disease
Central nervous system	Subarachnoid hemorrhage
	Intracranial trauma
	CNS tumor
	CNS infection
	Cerebrovascular occlusion

CNS, Central nervous system; *esp.,* especially; *HIV,* human immunodeficiency virus.

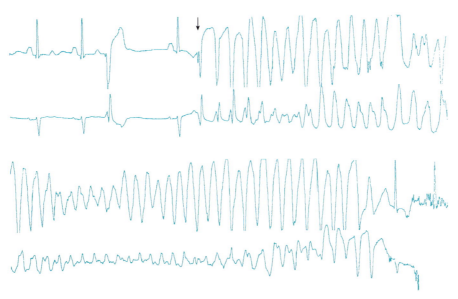

• **Figure 27.11** Torsades de pointes in a patient with the long QT syndrome. Two simultaneous electrocardiogram leads from a Holter monitor are shown (the strip is continuous). Following a long-short sequence that begins after a premature ventricular complex (PVC) (third beat), the T-wave morphology changes markedly *(arrow),* and another PVC results in the initiation of polymorphic ventricular tachycardia.

the pause) usually has a markedly prolonged QT interval and/or bizarre T-wave morphology. In patients with adrenergic-dependent TdP the catecholamine surge may be produced by exertion, fright, or startling noises, or it may exist as part of the stress response to cardiac surgery.

Prolonged TdP is always poorly tolerated hemodynamically and, if it does not spontaneously convert to sinus rhythm, will ultimately degenerate into VF. Therefore prompt direct current cardioversion should be performed. For frequently repeating episodes, initial treatment includes the correction of electrolyte abnormalities and elimination of medications that may have contributed to the QT prolongation (see Table 27.7). In the pause-dependent form, intravenous isoproterenol or cardiac pacing increases the heart rate and thereby shortens the QT interval, suppressing recurrent episodes of TdP. Intravenous magnesium has also proven effective in both terminating and suppressing TdP.[46] For the adrenergic form, chronic beta-blockade therapy represents initial management.

Ventricular Fibrillation. VF is an extremely rapid and irregular ventricular arrhythmia with low-amplitude QRS complexes. It may arise de novo (primary VF) or, more commonly, result from degeneration of hemodynamically unstable supraventricular or ventricular tachycardias. The majority of children who develop VF have experienced a severe metabolic or toxic event, have a structurally abnormal or severely injured heart, have WPW syndrome, or have a channelopathy.[60] Initial treatment includes cardiopulmonary resuscitation and electrical defibrillation. Potential causes should then be identified and treated.

Other Arrhythmias

Sinus Arrhythmia. Sinus arrhythmia describes normal variability in PP intervals with the respiratory cycle (the rate increases with inspiration and decreases with expiration). Generally, sinus arrhythmia is at most mildly symptomatic (e.g., palpitations) and warrants no specific treatment.

Wandering Atrial Pacemaker. Wandering atrial pacemaker is produced by the competing activity of three or more atrial pacemakers, one of which is usually the sinus node. It is an irregular rhythm characterized by variable P-wave morphology and PR intervals. As in sinus arrhythmia, the symptoms are mild, and treatment is not indicated unless long pauses are present.

Accelerated Idioventricular Rhythm. Accelerated idioventricular rhythm (AIVR) is a rhythm originating within the ventricles that has a rate 10% or less faster than the prevailing sinus rate. It is generally well tolerated in children. AIVR may be seen in normal children or in the setting of myocardial ischemia in adults. Specific therapy is usually not needed unless the patient is hemodynamically unstable. AIVR generally terminates when the excitable focus in the ventricle becomes less active or the sinus rate accelerates.

Clinical Entities Frequently Associated With Arrhythmias

This section discusses a variety of entities in which cardiac arrhythmias may play a prominent role in children and teenagers and which may come to the attention of the intensivist.

Syncope

Syncope is common in children with up to 40% reporting at least one episode by adulthood. Neurocardiogenic syncope is the most common cause. In neurocardiogenic syncope, common triggers include postural changes or sympathetic surges. The decrease in systemic vascular resistance and/or cardiac output coupled with an increase in parasympathetic tone mediated by the vagus nerve results primarily in hypotension, with or without bradycardia. These changes lead to cerebral hypoperfusion responsible for the loss of consciousness.[61] The diagnosis is suggested by a careful history that reveals a clear triggering event. Routine laboratory test results after neurocardiogenic syncope are usually normal. However, a 12-lead ECG should be performed to exclude the less than 2% more serious causes of syncope, such as hypertrophic cardiomyopathy, WPW, and LQTS. Red flags suggesting a more serious underlying cause include lack of typical prodrome, syncope with exertion, with palpitations, or family history of sudden cardiac death or related condition.[62] In the presence of congenital heart or other structural heart disease, syncope at rest or with exertion is a red flag that warrants more extensive evaluation to rule out potential life-threatening bradyarrhythmias and tachyarrhythmias.

Sudden Cardiac Arrest

Although the true incidence is unknown due to lack of mandatory reporting, sudden cardiac arrest (SCA) in pediatric patients in the United States has an estimated incidence of 0.6 to 6.2 per 100,000 patient years with approximately 2,000+ sudden deaths annually in the United States. Of those pediatric patients who die, 61% have no known cardiac disease, 45% had prior symptoms (most commonly seizures, dyspnea, or syncope), and only 26% had symptoms immediately before the event. SCA in the pediatric population can be subdivided into four subsets of patients: (1) sudden infant deaths, (2) primary cardiac electrical abnormalities, (3) structural cardiac defects, and (4) acquired (e.g., drug exposure, *commotio cordis*).[63]

Sudden Infant Death Syndrome

The cause of sudden infant death syndrome (SIDS) remains unclear, and research suggests it is probably multifactorial. Cardiac arrhythmias, central nervous system abnormalities, inborn errors of metabolism, central control of breathing, and pulmonary abnormalities have all been proposed. Despite extensive research, objective parameters predicting the likelihood of SIDS are lacking. However, given that ion channel diseases, such as LQTS, are a known cause of SIDS, postmortem evaluation, including genetic testing, is essential to diagnosing a potential inherited condition, thus enabling the possibility of cascade testing and diagnosis of other family members.

Wolff-Parkinson-White (Ventricular Preexcitation) Syndrome

APs are embryonic remnants of direct atrial and ventricular continuity present early in cardiogenesis.[64] APs potentially provide a substrate for tachycardias. They are generally sporadic, but rarely APs are inherited as an autosomal dominant trait (PRKAG2 mutation).[65] When anterograde conduction down an AP results in preexcitation of the ventricles, the patient meets the diagnosis of WPW. This manifests on ECG as a slurred upstroke of the QRS complex (delta wave) and a shortening of the PR interval. On the 12-lead ECG, WPW may be confused with right/left bundle branch block, right or left ventricular hypertrophy, or myocardial infarction. Algorithms have been developed to estimate the location of the AP from the morphology of the delta wave on 12-lead ECG.[66,67]

In addition to AVRT, children with WPW are at risk of developing atrial fibrillation. Unlike the AV node the AP may permit a very rapid ventricular rate response, predisposing to degeneration to VF and sudden death. Digoxin may increase this risk due to its unpredictable effects on AP conduction. In any young person presenting with an irregular, wide-complex tachycardia, the first rhythm a clinician should consider is *preexcited atrial fibrillation*. Furthermore, any patient having a history of syncope and an ECG demonstrating WPW pattern deserves urgent evaluation by an electrophysiologist. Patients with WPW who are asymptomatic also deserve evaluation by an electrophysiologist given the need for sudden death risk stratification and potential catheter ablation of the AP.[68]

Long QT Syndrome

LQTS is a heritable disorder of cardiac potassium or sodium channels. It is one of a group of *channelopathies* that clinically presents as recurrent syncope, seizures, or sudden death.[59,69] Cardiac arrhythmias are typically provoked by physical or emotional stress, although LQTS3 may result in sudden death during sleep. Historically, two clinical variants of LQTS had been identified: an autosomal dominant form with normal hearing (Romano-Ward syndrome) and an autosomal recessive form with congenital deafness (the Jervell and Lange-Nielsen syndrome). However, advances in molecular genetics have led to greater understanding of this group of disorders, with at least 16 forms of LQTS thus far identified. By far the most common causes of LQTS are mutations in the genes KCNQ1 (LQTS1), KCNH2 (LQTS2), and SCN5A (LQTS3).[70] Certain medications or metabolic derangements can also prolong the QT interval (see Table 27.7). The pathogenesis of TdP in most patients having LQTS may be related to exaggerated dispersion of ventricular refractoriness and pause- or catecholamine-induced EADs, which then initiates a malignant, rapid, reentrant VT.

LQTS should be suspected in any child with exertional or emotional syncope, especially if it is associated with a seizure and without a typical prodrome. The surface ECG is often diagnostic in demonstrating a markedly prolonged QT interval, and typical T-wave morphologies—broad and flat (LQTS1), notched (LQTS2), or normal but delayed in onset (LQTS3). *The QT interval should be measured from the onset of the QRS complex to the point where a line tangent to the steepest downslope of the T wave crosses baseline (as defined by the T-P interval).* U waves should not be included in the measurement unless merged with the T wave and greater than one-half the amplitude of the T wave. The QT interval is generally corrected for heart rate using Bazett's formula, defined as the QT interval divided by the square root of the preceding RR interval. Other correction formulas are also used.[71] Patients with LQTS, especially type 1, may have failure of the QT to appropriately shorten with tachycardia. Because of the difficulty in defining the LQTS on the sole basis of the QT interval, additional diagnostic criteria have been proposed (Table 27.8).[72]

A 2014 retrospective multicenter study, including six high-volume pediatric centers in the United States, described the clinical features of patients diagnosed with LQTS. There were 239 patients included who were 21 years of age and younger (median age at presentation is 9.1 years).[73] Five percent of patients presented with SCA, and 22% had LQTS-associated symptoms before diagnosis. A positive family history for a long QT interval was present in 52%. Of the 239 patients, 88% had phenotype-positive LQTS with a prolonged QT interval on ECG. There were 12% with genotype-positive/phenotype-negative LQTS; all were asymptomatic and referred due to family history of LQTS.

TABLE 27.8	LQTS Diagnostic Criteria of 1993 to 2011	Points
Electrocardiographic findings*		
A	QTc,† ms	
	≥480	3
	460–479	2
	450–459 (men)	1
B	QTc† 4th minute of recovery from exercise stress test ≥480 ms	1
C	Torsades-de-Pointes‡	2
D	T-wave alternans	1
E	Notched T wave in 3 leads	1
F	Low heart rate for age§	0.5
Clinical history		
A	Syncope‡	
	With stress	2
	Without stress	1
B	Congenital deafness	0.5
Family history		
A	Family members with definite LQTS‖	1
B	Unexplained sudden cardiac death younger than age 30 among immediate family members‖	0.5

LQTS indicates long-QT syndrome.
*In absence of medications or disorders known to affect these electrocardiographic features.
†QTc calculated by Bazett formula where QTc=QT/√RR.
‡Mutually exclusive.
§Resting heart rate below the second percentile for age.
‖The same family member cannot be counted in A and B.
Score: ≤1 point: low probability of LQTS; 1.5–3 points: intermediate probability of LQTS; ≥5 points: high probability.
From Schwartz PJ, Crotti L, Insolia R. Long-QT syndrome: from genetics to management. *Circ Arrhythm Electrophysiol.* 2012;5(4):868-877.

Beta-blockers are indicated in nearly all patients with LQTS. For patients with continued symptoms on beta-blockers, nonpharmacologic therapies are considered, including pacemaker implantation to prevent excessive bradycardia, left cardiac sympathetic denervation to alter autonomic input to the heart, and defibrillator implantation to treat dangerous arrhythmias.

Catecholaminergic Polymorphic Ventricular Tachycardia

CPVT is a channelopathy caused most commonly by a mutation in the genes encoding the ryanodine receptor in the sarcoplasmic reticulum and affecting calcium trafficking. Ventricular arrhythmias in CPVT are caused by adrenaline-dependent triggered activity. Patients will generally have a structurally normal heart and normal ECG and rhythm at baseline. With exertion/agitation/emotion, first frequent PVCs will develop, followed by runs of VT at faster heart rates. If unabated, VT can degenerate into VF and cause cardiac arrest. A particular form of VT known as *bidirectional VT* is nearly pathognomonic for CPVT. In bidirectional VT, the QRS axis alternates from beat to beat, giving the characteristic pattern. Bidirectional VT can also rarely be seen in digoxin toxicity and in a rare form of LQTS called the Andersen-Tawil syndrome, although in the latter there are generally characteristic facies, frequent PVCs at baseline, and periodic paralysis.

VT in CPVT is treated with beta-blockade and in the outpatient setting, patients are managed with beta-blockers such as nadolol, sometimes with the addition of flecainide. Implantable cardioverter-defibrillator (ICD) implantation in asymptomatic CPVT is considered only infrequently given the potential for ICD shock–induced electrical storm. However, following aborted cardiac arrest, ICD implantation may be necessary.[74]

Brugada Syndrome

Brugada syndrome is caused by a loss-of-function mutation in the sodium channel SCN5A (a gain-of-function mutation in the same gene causes LQTS3). It is frequently associated with a characteristic ECG pattern in the right precordial leads, characterized by an elevated takeoff of the ST segment, with a downsloping ST segment into a negatively deflected T wave. In patients with suspected Brugada syndrome but without the characteristic pattern on ECG, the pattern can often be provoked with infusion of the sodium channel blocker procainamide (or classically ajmaline—no longer available in the United States).[75] Ventricular arrhythmias in Brugada syndrome are often triggered by fever or sleep and are not clearly associated with exercise. VT or arrhythmic storm in Brugada syndrome is treated with beta-agonists, including isoproterenol or epinephrine. Prevention can be affected by use of the drug quinidine.[76] ICD implantation can be indicated.

Congenital Heart Disease

Children with CHD are predisposed to atrial and ventricular arrhythmias both before and after surgical repair.[20,77,78] In general, atrial surgery increases the likelihood of sinus node dysfunction and atrial arrhythmias, and ventricular surgery is associated with ventricular tachyarrhythmias. Rhythm disturbances have a tendency to increase in frequency with time after cardiac surgery and in the presence of new or progressive hemodynamic deterioration. Late sudden death after cardiac surgery appears to be related to surgical scar in the ventricle and the complexity of the congenital lesion.[79] Sudden death occurs in less than 0.1% of patients after pulmonary valvotomy, up to 4% after VSD repair,[80] 3% to 15% after atrial switch operation for d-transposition of the great arteries (Mustard or Senning operations),[81-84] up to 5% after aortic valve surgery,[80] 1.5% to 6% after tetralogy of Fallot repair,[58,85-88] and 18% after repair of truncus arteriosus with a single pulmonary artery.[89] Identifying criteria for risk stratification of these high-risk patients and for selecting which patients to treat with antiarrhythmic drugs or implantable defibrillators is an important problem. Specific criteria for identifying high-risk patients with repaired tetralogy of Fallot have been published.[90] Ambulatory rhythm monitoring, exercise testing, and invasive EP studies have all been used in an effort to determine such risk.[91] Children with corrected CHD who present with cardiac arrest, syncope, or presyncope should be referred to an electrophysiologist skilled in the treatment of patients with CHD.

Of interest to the intensivist are arrhythmias encountered in the immediate postoperative period following surgery for CHD (see earlier discussion of JET). Sinus or junctional bradycardia is not uncommon after any right heart surgery in which there is a period of elevated right atrial pressure or other right atrial distortion. Accordingly, we often encounter this following surgery for AV septal/canal defects and during extracorporeal membrane oxygenation (ECMO) management even in the absence of CHD. Bradycardia may present in the absence of abnormal hemodynamics when damage to the sinus node or its blood supply occurs. This should be considered in patients having just undergone repair of complex anomalous pulmonary venous return, the hemi-Fontan operation, or the Fontan operation. Ventricular arrhythmias, on the other hand, are uncommon immediately postoperatively and may represent ongoing metabolic disturbance, occult oxygen myocardial supply/demand imbalance, or hemodynamic problems, such as a patch or valve leaflet dehiscence or bacterial endocarditis.

Ebstein anomaly is worthy of special comment. It is associated with WPW syndrome and right-sided APs in 10% of patients.[92] WPW should be suspected in patients with Ebstein anomaly who do not manifest RBBB on ECG. Most children requiring right heart surgery for this condition now undergo EP study with potential catheter ablation before surgery to reduce the postoperative arrhythmia risk. Nevertheless, other atrial and ventricular arrhythmias are common perioperatively in these complex patients.

Hypertrophic Cardiomyopathy

Hypertrophic cardiomyopathy (HCM) is a primary disorder of the contractile proteins of the myofibril. Grossly it is characterized by marked thickening of the ventricular myocardium and some combination of hyperdynamic systolic function, left ventricular outflow tract obstruction, and diastolic dysfunction with pulmonary venous congestion. Microvascular changes can be detected early by cardiac MRI, with later development of scar predisposing to ventricular arrhythmia. Over 50% of cases of HCM are inherited (usually autosomal dominant pattern with variable penetrance). Young patients present with a range of symptoms, including fatigue, exercise intolerance, chest pain, shortness of breath, syncope, and sudden death. Sudden death appears to be most common in children and young adults aged 10 to 35 years and not infrequently occurs before the disease is recognized.[93] Approximately 40% of the deaths happen during or just after vigorous physical activities; in the remaining cases, patients were sedentary or engaged in light activities. HCM appears to be the most common cause of sudden death in young athletes (confirmed or suspected HCM accounted for approximately 50% of deaths in the study by Maron et al.[94]). Risk factors for sudden death include a family history of sudden death, a history of syncope, VT on Holter monitor, and—in children—excessive ventricular hypertrophy.[95] The cause of syncope or cardiac arrest in children and young adults appears to be myocardial ischemia and secondary ventricular arrhythmias.[96]

Dilated Cardiomyopathy

Dilated cardiomyopathy (DCM) is a heterogeneous group of conditions having in common diminished left ventricular systolic function. As many as 50% of affected individuals are now thought to have a heritable disorder of a myocyte protein, with dystrophin abnormality as the original protein identified. Of the remainder, many are thought to have sequelae of a prior viral myocarditis that resulted in fibrosis. However, it has been shown that even such patients may have a genetic predisposition for development of cardiomyopathy. One study revealed that 12% of children with acute myocarditis were found to be homozygous for cardiomyopathy mutations, in that previously silent recessive defects of the myocardium may predispose to acute heart failure presenting as acute myocarditis, notably after common viral infections in children.

Patients with DCM present with fatigue, orthopnea, dyspnea on exertion, syncope, and sudden death. Both atrial (especially atrial fibrillation) and ventricular arrhythmias are commonly seen in children with DCM. Amiodarone is the safest antiarrhythmic drug for outpatient management in this patient group because oral dosing in particular does not have appreciable myocardial depressant properties. Those having the most severe left ventricular dysfunction appear to be at greatest risk for sudden death. A left ventricular ejection fraction less than 20% carries a 5-year survival rate of 50%[97] and justifies consideration of ICD implantation as a bridge to cardiac transplantation.

ICU management of these patients requires an aggressive approach to any ventricular ectopy. Normalization of hypoglycemia, hypoxia, and plasma electrolyte concentrations, including magnesium, is paramount. Progression of ectopy to runs of VT may require intravenous amiodarone and consideration of cardiovascular support with an ECMO circuit as an emergency bridge to transplant. Although often necessary, all manner of pressor support is problematic due to proarrhythmic tendency.

Arrhythmogenic Right Ventricular Cardiomyopathy

ARVC is clinically characterized by ventricular arrhythmias, progressive loss/thinning of RV myocardium, and replacement with fibrofatty tissue. As the disease progresses, the ultimate phenotype resembles that of dilated biventricular cardiomyopathy. Gene mutations are reported in up to 60% of patients, commonly within desmosomal proteins.[98] Estimated prevalence of ARVC is approximately 1 in 5000. Some European countries have a much greater incidence (approximately 1 in 2000).[98,99] ARVC may be a more frequent cause of sudden death in young athletes than had been appreciated and should be considered in all children and teenagers with VT having a LBBB morphology, especially if concomitant RV dilation or dysfunction is present.[100]

Patients usually present between the second and fourth decades with palpitations, light-headedness, VT (generally LBBB QRS morphology with superior greater than inferior QRS axis), syncope, or sudden death. Compared with adults, pediatric patients are more likely to present with SCA, which can occur during early stages of the disease. Arrhythmias are thought to be provoked by exercise, and endurance sports especially are thought to hasten the progression of disease. The resting ECG may show right atrial abnormalities, RBBB, and T-wave inversions in the precordial leads. Signal-averaged ECG can reveal epsilon waves. Criteria for the diagnosis of ARVC in probands and first-degree relatives were first published in 1994 and updated in 2010.[101,102] Due to the poor efficacy of echocardiography for imaging the right ventricle, cardiac MRI is an important component in the evaluation of these patients.[103]

International consensus guidelines for the treatment of ARVC have been published.[104] Beta-blockers are indicated in all patients if tolerated. Right ventricular ejection fraction of less than 35% by MRI and sustained VT are considered class I indications for ICD implantation. Standard heart failure management should be considered in those patients with clinical heart failure. Although ARVC has a tendency to progress to clinical heart failure in its later stages, death is more often related to arrhythmia.

Myocarditis

Inflammation of the heart, or myocarditis, is caused by infectious agents, radiation, chemicals, pharmacologic agents/chemotherapy, cocaine, and metabolic disorders. The most common cause is viral infection, especially coxsackievirus A and B, echovirus, influenza A_2, varicella, poliomyelitis, hepatitis B, and human immunodeficiency virus. The pathophysiology appears to involve virus-mediated triggering of an immune response targeting myocytes in the weeks after the initial infection.

The clinical expression of myocarditis ranges from no symptoms to fulminant heart failure. In many patients, transient ECG abnormalities (sinus tachycardia, diminished voltages, and ST-segment and T-wave changes) accompany systemic viral infection, but other cardiac symptoms are absent. With more significant myocardial involvement, patients may report dyspnea, fatigue, palpitations, and chest discomfort. In some patients the first manifestation of myocarditis is a fatal ventricular arrhythmia; 5% to 10% of children with sudden death have active myocarditis on postmortem examination.[105] Up to 10% of children with VT may have occult myocarditis.[106] Myocarditis that extends to the conduction system may produce AV block that is usually transient but may require temporary pacing. The diagnosis is established by an endomyocardial biopsy that demonstrates an interstitial inflammatory infiltrate and myocyte necrosis or by cardiac MRI, especially by late gadolinium enhancement caused by failure of the contrast agent to efficiently wash out of damaged/scarred myocardium. Potentially effective treatment for viral myocarditis includes immunosuppressive therapy to modify the immune response. Circulatory support by ECMO may be necessary during the acute phase.

Pacing in the Cardiac Intensive Care Unit

In the care of cardiac patients in the ICU, knowledge of pacing is essential for optimal outcome. Given the need at times for urgent pacing or modification of pacing parameters following cardiac surgery, caregivers in the ICU must have hands-on familiarity with both permanent internal and temporary external pacemakers.

Classification of Modes

A five-letter code, the NBG code, describing the programming and capabilities of pacemakers was developed by the North American Society of Pacing and Electrophysiology and British Pacing and Electrophysiology Group (NASPE/BPEG). In temporary pacemakers only the first three letters of the code are used, with the fourth letter in common use to denote presence or absence of rate responsiveness in permanent pacemakers. The fifth letter of the code is not commonly used except in cardiac resynchronization therapy (CRT) devices, wherein leads stimulate the myocardium of both the right and left ventricles. The letters can be more easily remembered in thinking of historical context—pacemakers first *paced*, then *sensing* functions were added, and finally different *responses to sensing*.

1. The first letter of the code denotes what chamber(s) are paced:
   A—atrium only.
   V—ventricle only.
   D—dual-chamber pacing/both atrium and ventricle.
   O—pacing function off. The O function is rarely used, except if the indication for pacing is no longer present, in the setting of device malfunction while the patient is in a monitored setting, or at the time of death. In cases of patient death, however, metabolic derangement/acidosis will often rapidly cause loss of capture, rendering the O function unnecessary.

2. The second letter of the code denotes what chamber(s) are sensed:
   A—atrium only.
   V—ventricle only.
   D—dual-chamber sensing/both atrium and ventricle.
   O—sensing function off/asynchronous mode. The device will only pace, ignoring intrinsic heart rhythm. This mode is most frequently used in the operating room to prevent signal interference from electrocautery devices from being mistaken for intrinsic heart rhythm and thereby causing inhibition of pacing by the device in pacemaker-dependent patients.

3. The third letter of the code describes the pacemaker's response to a sensed electrical event:
   I—inhibited. The pacemaker will not pace if it senses an intrinsic event before the programmed amount of time passes.
   T—triggered. The pacemaker will pace in response to a sensed event.
   D—dual response/inhibited and triggered. This function is available only in dual-chamber devices.
   O—No response to sensed events. This function is generally programmed along with O in the second position as part of asynchronous mode.

4. The fourth letter in the code denotes the presence or absence of rate responsiveness[107]:
   R—rate responsiveness. The rate increases in response to sensor-dependent physical or physiologic changes. The rate and degree of response can be programmed.
   Blank or O—rate responsiveness off or unavailable.

5. The fifth letter in the code describes the cardiac chamber with multisite pacing if present, most commonly biventricular pacing in CRT devices with an epicardial lead on the systemic ventricle or systemic ventricular pacing via a transvenous coronary sinus lead. The letter *V* would denote biventricular pacing. The fifth position would otherwise be left blank.

The commonly used modes for programming of temporary pacemakers and those most commonly programmed in permanently implanted pacemakers are as follows:

1. AOO—The atrial lead paces at the programmed *lower rate limit* (LRL) if expressed in beats/min or *lower rate interval* (LRI) if expressed as cycle length/time elapsed in milliseconds (ms), denoting the longest time interval allowed to pass without an event. Sensing is turned off. All intrinsic cardiac activity is ignored. AOO is an example of an asynchronous mode.

2. AAI—The atrial lead is programmed to sense intrinsic electrical activity. If an event is sensed before the LRI elapses, pacing is inhibited, and the LRI clock is reset. If the LRI clock elapses before an intrinsic event is sensed, the atrial lead paces, and the LRI clock is reset. This sequence then repeats.

3. AAIR—Programming is identical to AAI mode, except that the LRL increases/LRI decreases in response to activity or physiologic changes.

4. VOO—The ventricular lead paces at the programmed LRI. Sensing is turned off. All intrinsic cardiac activity is ignored. VOO is an example of an asynchronous mode. It may be used in the operating room in a patient with CHB undergoing electrocautery. The patient should be paced at a rate that will suppress intrinsic ventricular activity to prevent an R on T phenomenon, in which the pacemaker paces the ventricle coincident with a native T wave, potentially inducing a dangerous ventricular arrhythmia.

5. VVI—The ventricular lead is programmed to sense intrinsic electrical activity. If an event is sensed before the LRI elapses, pacing is inhibited, and the LRI clock is reset. If the LRI clock elapses before an intrinsic event is sensed, the ventricular lead paces, and the LRI clock is reset. This sequence then repeats.

6. VVIR—Programming is identical to VVI mode, except that the LRL increases/LRI decreases in response to activity or physiologic changes.

7. DDD—Programming of dual-chamber pacemakers is somewhat more complex than single-chamber devices. In DDD mode, whether timing is determined by atrial activity or ventricular activity will vary among devices. In general, after the last sensed event the atrial lead will check for intrinsic activity. If an event is sensed before the LRI elapses, atrial pacing is inhibited. If the LRI clock elapses before an intrinsic event is sensed, then the atrial lead paces. Once either an intrinsic atrial event occurs or the atrial lead paces, the *atrioventricular interval* (AVI) begins. This programmable setting, similar to the PR interval, determines how long the pacemaker will wait for an intrinsic ventricular event before the ventricular lead paces. On some pacemakers, different AVI can be programmed to follow an intrinsic atrial event versus a paced atrial event. If the ventricular lead senses an event before the AVI clock elapses, then ventricular pacing is inhibited, and the whole sequence repeats. If no ventricular event is sensed before the AVI clock elapses, the ventricular lead paces, and the whole sequence repeats. In some devices, *ventricular safety pacing* is present. If the pacemaker detects an intrinsic ventricular event early after pacing the atrium, a ventricular pace is delivered in case the sensed ventricular event was actually noise from atrial pacing.

8. DDDR—Programming is identical to DDD mode, except that the LRL increases/LRI decreases in response to activity or physiologic changes.

Temporary Pacing

Methods of Temporary Pacing

The most common method of temporary pacing encountered in the cardiac ICU is via postoperative epicardial wires. After most cardiac surgeries a pair of wires is affixed to the atrial epicardium and a second pair to the ventricular epicardium. One wire from each pair serves as a cathode and one from each pair as an anode, allowing bipolar sensing and pacing of either or both chambers. The other end of each pair of wires exits the skin and is capped if not needed, or else attached to a temporary pacing box at the bedside.

Temporary pacing can also be accomplished through several other methods. In sedated patients an esophageal pacing catheter can be positioned behind the left atrium, allowing sensing of atrial and ventricular signals and pacing of atrial tissue (rarely the ventricle can be captured at high outputs). In infants, atrial pacing can be accomplished without undo discomfort with only mild sedation such as a small dose of midazolam, making esophageal pacing an excellent choice for pace termination of atrial flutter, thus avoiding electrical cardioversion. Safe, proper placement of an esophageal pacing catheter requires either fluoroscopic guidance or a means of recording signals detected by the catheter. Thus the EP laboratory is the preferred setting for the placement and use of an esophageal catheter, except where a mobile EP stimulator is available. Transcutaneous pacing can also be accomplished in emergency situations; however, significant sedation is often required due to the discomfort caused by this method of pacing.

In patients without temporary epicardial wires who are in need of continuous pacing, a temporary transvenous pacing wire can be placed. Placement of such a wire requires central access and carries the risk of bacteremia/infection. Appropriate placement should be guided by fluoroscopy, echocardiography, or recording of appropriate electrograms from the catheter. Placement is generally followed by confirmation of position by plain film of the chest.

Setting the Temporary Pacemaker

1. Turn on the temporary pacing box. Note that, at device power-up, default pacing parameters will be present. These parameters may not be applicable to the situation (e.g., too slow for an infant). Therefore power on and setup of the pacemaker should be performed before connecting to the patient's leads.
2. Unlock the box to allow changes to settings.
3. Select a pacing mode based on those described previously. Note that temporary postoperative pacemakers will not have rate responsiveness. Mode will be selected based on the indication for pacing.
   a. *Sinus bradycardia with intact AV conduction:* AAI mode would be appropriate to ensure a specified minimum heart rate. This situation might also include patients with sick sinus syndrome or heart transplant patients whose atrial rates will not rise appropriately due to poor innervation. In the latter case the atrium might be paced at a slightly tachycardic rate to allow more chronotropy.
   b. *Sinus rhythm with high grade or CHB:* VVI or DDD mode would be selected depending on sensing and pacing thresholds of the temporary pacing wires. Although VVI mode would not allow AV synchrony, in the short term in stable patients it would suffice to maintain a minimum ventricular rate while awaiting return of spontaneous conduction or placement of a permanent pacemaker. DDD mode would allow AV synchrony and generally would pace the ventricle at the patient's intrinsic atrial rate.
   c. *Sinus rhythm with intermittent heart block:* VVI or DDD mode would be appropriate in this situation. If all that is desired is a back-up rate below which the patient's heart rate will not drop, then VVI is an appropriate choice. Intrinsic atrial activity will be ignored, and pacing should occur only in the setting of heart block with an escape rate less than the programmed LRL. DDD would not be considered a backup mode. In the setting of a normal sinus/atrial rate, when heart block develops, even if the ventricular escape rate is greater than the LRL, the atrium will be sensed and tracked by the pacemaker and the ventricle paced at the same rate as the intrinsic atrial activity.
   d. *Accelerated junctional rhythm/JET:* To maintain AV synchrony in the setting of a junctional dysrhythmia, the heart is paced at a rate slightly faster than the junctional rate. Anterograde

AV conduction is usually still intact in the setting of JET, and therefore AAI pacing is an appropriate first mode in an attempt to overdrive pace the tachycardia. For example, if the junctional rate is 170 beats/min, pacing the atrium at 175 to 180 beats/min is usually sufficient to restore AV synchrony. As the junctional rhythm accelerates, it may start competing with atrial pacing, with the atrial rate needing to be adjusted upwards. The LRL can occasionally be turned down to check the underlying rhythm, with the LRL turned down or overdrive pacing turned off as allowable.

4. Program the rate at which you would like to pace or below which you would not like the patient's heart rate to drop. In AAI and VVI mode the pacemaker should not pace above this rate. In DDD mode the pacemaker will track the intrinsic atrial activity at rates above the LRL and pace the ventricle accordingly. In DDD mode, if the intrinsic rate is below the LRL, the atrium will be paced at the LRL, and depending on AV conduction, the ventricle may be paced as well.
5. Plug in the atrial and/or ventricular leads. Note that with the pacemaker set to DDD mode, unplugging the atrial leads will effectively give you VVI pacing with the option of rapid switch back to DDD mode by plugging these leads back in. The same can be done with the ventricular leads, resulting in effective AAI pacing.
6. Turn up atrial and ventricular output (in milliamperes [mA]) until capture occurs. Note that bedside monitors with pacing sensing enabled will display a tick mark on the ECG screen tracing when detecting a pacing artifact. However, this does not indicate pacing capture of the myocardium. Capture should be verified by a paced P wave, paced QRS, or appropriate paced heart rate being present. The pacing threshold is the energy output below which the pacemaker fails to capture the heart. Output is usually set at approximately twice the capture threshold to provide a safety margin in case of deterioration of lead function or increase in intrinsic pacing thresholds. Pacemaker output is actually composed of both an amplitude (as in earlier discussion) and a pulse width. Temporary pacing boxes do not allow adjustment of the pulse width.
7. Adjust sensitivity in each chamber as needed so that the pacemaker does not *oversense* (see "Troubleshooting" later) or *undersense.*
8. If using DDD mode, set AVI and *postventricular atrial refractory period* (PVARP). The AVI will determine how long the pacemaker waits after an atrial event to pace the ventricle. In the setting of CHB the AV delay can affect ventricular filling time. PVARP is the period of time in milliseconds following a sensed or paced ventricular event during which any sensed atrial activity/P waves will not be acted upon by the pacemaker. PVARP was designed mainly to prevent the tracking of retrograde P waves following ventricular paced events in the setting of intact *retrograde* conduction (see later discussion of *pacemaker mediated tachycardia* [PMT]), which can occur if the PVARP is too short. With too long a PVARP, *pacemaker Wenckebach* (see later under "Troubleshooting") can occur. The *total atrial refractory period* is not set but is the sum of the AVI and PVARP. The *upper rate interval* is the shortest time in milliseconds allowed between ventricular events (fastest rate at which the atrium will be tracked).

Maintenance and Safety

A few steps should be performed regularly to ensure proper function of the temporary pacing system. Pacing thresholds should be checked at least daily. The atrial lead threshold can be tested in AAI mode in a patient with intact AV conduction or adequate ventricular escape rate but should be tested in DDD mode in patients with heart block who are pacemaker dependent. Set the LRL to 10 to 20 beats/min above the intrinsic atrial rate or to the minimum safe heart rate, whichever is higher. Then slowly turn down atrial output in milliamperes until capture is lost. This loss of capture will likely be most apparent by a sudden slowing of the heart rate despite continued attempts by the pacemaker to pace. Especially with small P waves, it may be difficult to discern whether a P wave follows a pacing spike. Also, as noted earlier, when using bedside monitors as a guide for threshold testing, it should be understood that pacing spikes on the monitor are interpolated by the computer system and do not necessarily mean that pacemaker attempted to pace at that time. The output should then be expediently turned back up to where it captures and ultimately set to an output of about twice the capture threshold to allow an adequate safety margin.

Ventricular lead threshold is most easily tested in VVI mode. Care should be taken in pacemaker-dependent patients to recognize loss of capture immediately and turn ventricular lead output back up before the patient becomes symptomatic. LRL should be set to 10 to 20 beats/min above intrinsic ventricular rate or to the minimum safe heart rate, whichever is higher. Ventricular lead output should then be slowly turned down until there is loss of capture, then immediately turned back up to a capturing output. Loss of capture is generally apparent in ventricular lead testing due to an abrupt drop in heart rate, failure of a QRS to inscribe following a pacing spike, and narrowing of QRS in most patients as the escape rhythm comes through. In patients with frequent PVCs, care must be taken to distinguish true loss of capture from *physiologic noncapture*. In physiologic noncapture, a PVC occurs before a paced ventricular event, and for a period of time following the PVC, ventricular tissue is refractory and will not depolarize even if paced above capture threshold. If unclear, ventricular threshold testing should be repeated. A similar phenomenon can occur with a PAC during atrial threshold testing. Ventricular output is generally set at approximately twice capture threshold to allow an adequate safety margin.

Underlying rhythm should be checked at least daily in most instances as well. Although unplugging the leads from the temporary pacemaker will generally accomplish this aim, it is not ideal for several reasons. First, an abrupt change in heart rate, especially in a postoperative patient may not be well tolerated symptomatically. Second, pacing can suppress intrinsic cardiac activity, and so a true evaluation of underlying rhythm may not be accomplished by briefly unplugging leads. Instead, underlying rhythm should be watched for several minutes if tolerated because often heart rate in the previously paced chamber(s) will gradually increase over this period. Also, if there is intermittent conduction, this phenomenon is more likely to be appreciated with more prolonged observation. In patients with heart block but normal atrial rate, AV conduction can be tested in DDD mode by gradually prolonging the AVI. Alternatively, and to check ventricular escape rhythm/rate in heart block, VVI mode can be used. Ventricular rate is then gradually turned down until intrinsic rhythm emerges or else minimum safe ventricular rate is reached. If minimum safe rate is reached before intrinsic rhythm emerges, then ventricular rate is generally left unchanged for several minutes to see if the intrinsic rate overtakes the low paced rate. Once testing is done, prior pacing settings are resumed, or adjustments made if underlying rhythm is improved.

In terms of mechanical maintenance, batteries should be changed approximately every 2 days, or the temporary pacemaker swapped for another pacemaker with fresh batteries. Temporary epicardial leads tend to last a couple of weeks, but pacing threshold can increase over this time. It is thus important to test threshold on a regular basis. If high thresholds are necessary to capture, preventing an adequate safety margin, or if the pacemaker does not allow capture, polarity of the lead in question can be reversed (switching the wire from the bipolar lead which is the cathode to the one that is the anode). This often will allow for improved thresholds. If atrial leads cease to function, in most patients it is safe to exclusively pace the ventricle for several days. Most modern temporary pacemakers will not allow pacing above 20 mA of amplitude. However, many centers still have on hand older pacing boxes (e.g., those originally designed to pace infants out of atrial flutter using esophageal catheters). These pacemakers may allow adjustment of pulse width and amplitude to greater than 20 mA, or else they may have a switch that multiplies the amplitude of output, effecting greater output. These pacemakers can help short term in an emergency, although they are not designed for continuous pacing, and so batteries will drain rapidly.

Troubleshooting

Oversensing and *undersensing* are problems with *sensitivity* that can affect proper pacemaker function. These problems can usually be diagnosed by telemetry or ECG. *Sensitivity* can be adjusted on temporary pacemakers and determines how large a signal will be detected as an event by the pacemaker. High sensitivity means that the pacemaker will detect lower-amplitude signals as electrical events. Sensitivity is measured in millivolts (mV). It may be counterintuitive, but the smaller the number in millivolts is programmed, the higher the sensitivity. The larger the number in millivolts, the lower the sensitivity, so that only high-amplitude signals will be detected as electrical events. For the atrial lead the sensitivity must be high enough that intrinsic P waves will be detected but not baseline noise. For the ventricular lead, sensitivity must be high enough that QRS complexes are detected as ventricular events, but not far-field P waves or T waves.

Oversensing is a problem with too high a sensitivity (low programmed number in millivolts), wherein the atrial lead is detecting baseline noise or far-field signals as atrial events/P waves, or the ventricular lead is detecting noise, far-field atrial signals, or T waves as ventricular events/QRS complexes. Oversensing generally manifests as inappropriately long pauses in pacing without intrinsic signals visible on telemetry or ECG. Sometimes it is clear what is being oversensed, though at other times this cannot be determined. Oversensing in the ventricular lead in pacemaker-dependent patients can be dangerous and will often lead to symptoms due to bradycardia or prolonged pauses in rhythm. Making the pacemaker less sensitive (increasing the programmed number in millivolts) for the affected lead will usually solve this problem, although sensitivity should not be made so low that intrinsic QRS complexes are no longer detected.

Undersensing is a problem related to too low a sensitivity (high programmed number in millivolts), wherein intrinsic P waves are ignored (not detected) by the atrial lead, or intrinsic QRS complexes are not detected by the ventricular lead. Undersensing manifests as too-frequent pacing in the chamber of concern, or in the case of pacing impulses delivered when the paced chamber is refractory (during or shortly following an intrinsic event), as physiologic noncapture or else a pacing spike buried in the P wave or QRS complex. Occasionally an intrinsic event may occur shortly after a paced or detected event, in an *absolute refractory period,* in which the pacemaker is blinded to any signals that occur for a brief period of time—such a phenomenon does not reflect undersensing by the pacemaker. Undersensing can be corrected by making sensitivity in the affected lead higher (decreasing the programmed number in millivolts).

Failure to capture means that the pacemaker attempts to deliver an electrical impulse but does not succeed in pacing the heart. This can occur with a mechanical problem such as lead fracture or lead dislodgment (which can usually be diagnosed by plain film) or a break in lead insulation but often is caused by insufficient output by the pacemaker such that it is unable to overcome capture threshold. Failure to capture can be consistent or intermittent. In some situations it can appear similar to oversensing, except either pacing spikes will be visible without associated P wave or QRS complex, or else the pacing indicator on the temporary pacemaker will indicate that it is attempting to pace despite no effect on heart rhythm. In a previously functional lead, in addition to mechanical problems as listed earlier, failure to capture may result from the following causes:

1. Insufficient safety margin between capture threshold and programmed amplitude of output. In this situation, slight changes in capture threshold may cause failure to capture.
2. Normal deterioration in lead function. It is therefore important to check capture threshold of temporary pacing leads at least daily.
3. Electrolyte abnormality. Pacing threshold is sensitive to changes in serum electrolyte levels.
4. Temporary pacing box changed without changing from default programmed parameters. When electively switching the temporary pacing box, program appropriate parameters before changing out the box.

Pacemaker Wenckebach is a phenomenon that can take place in DDD mode with sensed atrial activity and paced ventricular activity. Pacemaker Wenckebach is considered a form of upper rate behavior. It occurs when intrinsic atrial activity is occurring around or above the programmed upper rate limit. The pacemaker will not allow the ventricle to track the atrium at a rate higher than the upper rate limit, and therefore the AVI will be extended following sensed atrial activity until the following P wave falls within the PVARP, and the atrial event is not tracked (no ventricular paced event following the P wave). The sequence then resets. If poorly tolerated, pacemaker Wenckebach can be addressed by the following:

1. Address the reason for tachycardia above the programmed upper rate limit.
2. Increase the upper rate limit.
3. Shorten the PVARP. Note that shortening the AVI will not likely have an effect on the pacemaker Wenckebach because the pacemaker is automatically extending the AVI so as not to pace above the upper rate interval.

Pacemaker-mediated tachycardia (PMT) can occur in the setting of anterograde heart block with intact retrograde conduction (conduction from ventricle to atrium), either retrograde via the AV node or via an AV accessory pathway. It is generally triggered by a PVC or transient AV dyssynchrony. The ventricular event conducts retrograde to the atrium. The retrograde P wave is sensed by the pacemaker and tracked by pacing the ventricle, and the cycle repeats. PMT can often be recognized by pacing at or near the upper rate limit. It can be terminated (the cycle broken) by temporarily inhibiting pacing, placing a magnet over a permanent pacemaker, switching to a nontracking mode (e.g., VVI, VOO), or extending the PVARP so that retrograde P waves will fall within

a period in which they will not be tracked. Once terminated, the best way to address PMT is to lengthen the PVARP. Some permanent pacemakers have PMT algorithms designed to recognize and terminate PMT. A mode switch can also be programmed on some permanent pacemakers so that when the atrial rate rises above a certain level, the pacemaker switches to a nontracking mode.

Treatment of Tachyarrhythmias With the Pacemaker

Pacemakers can be used as interventional tools in the case of some tachyarrhythmias. These functions in permanent pacemakers should generally be reserved for use by trained electrophysiologists, and therefore this chapter addresses only temporary pacemakers. Regardless, the use of these specialized pacing functions should be performed by or under the direct guidance of an experienced provider given the potential for inducing potentially harmful arrhythmias. (For JET, see earlier discussion.)

Pacemakers are most useful in the termination of reentrant arrhythmias, because automatic arrhythmias will usually be unaffected or only transiently suppressed. In rare cases seemingly automatic tachycardias that are in fact caused by the mechanism of triggered activity can be initiated and terminated by pacing. The two most common maneuvers for pace termination of arrhythmias are *burst pacing* and *ramp pacing*. In burst pacing, pacing is delivered at a cycle length 10% to 20% faster than the tachycardia cycle length (in 2 : 1 tachycardias, remember to use the atrial cycle length rather than the ventricular cycle length) until the tachycardia is noted to accelerate to the rate of pacing. Pacing is then continued for several seconds then terminated. Sinus rhythm will often resume at this point. In ramp pacing, pacing is delivered at a cycle length near or slightly faster than the tachycardia cycle length then rapidly increased before ceasing pacing. Rapid pacing is generally a special function on a temporary pacemaker selected from the submenus at the bottom of the box. Many include a dial that allows the operator to change the rate of pacing while holding down a button to deliver pacing.

1. *AVRT:* This reentrant tachycardia can generally be pace-terminated by temporarily pacing at a cycle length slightly faster than the cycle length of the tachycardia. It is generally safest to rapidly pace from the atrium, but because the ventricle is involved in the circuit, pace termination from the ventricle would also be expected to be effective. Burst or ramp pacing can be effective.
2. *AVNRT:* This reentrant tachycardia can usually be pace-terminated through ramp or burst pacing. Atrial pacing will usually be more effective, but ventricular pacing can sometimes access the circuit and terminate AVNRT as well.
3. *Atrial flutter:* Flutter is a reentrant tachycardia with the reentrant circuit contained completely within the atrium. In neonates who present in atrial flutter, once the arrhythmia is terminated, often the infant will not suffer a recurrence. Esophageal or rapid atrial pacing is necessary to terminate atrial flutter because the ventricle is distant from the circuit. Either burst or ramp atrial pacing can be effective in terminating atrial flutter. If very rapid pacing is required, atrial flutter may degenerate into atrial fibrillation, which will usually self-terminate after a period, especially in children with normal hearts.
4. *AET:* AET is predominantly caused by the mechanism of abnormal automaticity. Arrhythmias caused by this mechanism usually will be unaffected or only transiently suppressed by atrial pacing. A small percentage of AET is caused by triggered activity, and this subset is often susceptible to pace termination. Ventricular pacing is unlikely to affect AET.

5. *Ventricular tachycardia:* Care must be used when rapidly pacing the ventricle because a more chaotic ventricular arrhythmia may be induced such as VF. Defibrillation pads should be attached to the patient or a resuscitation cart immediately available. Much like with atrial arrhythmias, the effect of pacing on ventricular arrhythmia is determined mainly by mechanism. Ventricular arrhythmias caused by abnormal automaticity will usually be unaffected or transiently suppressed by ventricular pacing. Idiopathic outflow tract VT (VT with LBBB morphology and inferior axis) is predominantly caused by triggered activity and therefore commonly susceptible to pace termination. VT in patients with CHD, especially those with a ventriculotomy who are remote from surgery, is often caused by a reentry circuit around areas of scar tissue. The classic example of this phenomenon is in tetralogy of Fallot. Fascicular VT is caused by a reentrant circuit involving the fascicles of the left bundle branch and should be susceptible to pace termination. Classically, fascicular VT can be pace initiated and terminated from both the ventricle and the atrium. In cases of slower reentrant VT, if only atrial wires are available, in the setting of good AV nodal conduction, overdrive pacing from the atrium may be sufficient to terminate VT caused by reentry or triggered activity.

Care of the Patient With a Pacemaker or Implantable Cardioverter-Defibrillator in the Operating Room

Electrocautery as part of a surgical procedure can interfere with appropriate pacemaker function. Most commonly, the interference generates noise that can be mistaken by the pacemaker for intrinsic cardiac activity. In the pacemaker-dependent patient this can lead to inhibition of pacing and prolonged asystole. In the setting of an ICD the noise may be mistaken for rapid ventricular rhythm and may generate an inappropriate shock. These concerns can be addressed either by placing a magnet over the device or by switching the pacemaker to an asynchronous mode before the case. Application of the magnet will switch a pacemaker into an asynchronous mode as long as the magnet remains over the device. In ICDs, application of the magnet will inhibit delivery of therapies for tachyarrhythmias. In an asynchronous mode any noise or intrinsic electrical activity will be ignored and pacing delivered at a predetermined rate. Guidelines exist for the perioperative evaluation and programming of pacemakers.[108]

Permanent Implantable Defibrillators

For patients with a history of aborted cardiac arrest and those at high risk for lethal ventricular arrhythmias, and especially for those who have failed or are intolerant of antiarrhythmic agents, the ICD is recommended therapy. The basic components of these systems are (1) a lead for sensing the ventricular rate, (2) a lead for delivering energy to the heart, and (3) the generator housing the battery, capacitors, and electronic circuitry. The rate-sensing lead is either a bipolar endocardial lead placed in the right ventricular apex or an epicardial pair of sensing leads attached to a ventricle. The shocking leads include one or more coils, mesh patches, or metal arrays that may be epicardial (patches), intravascular (coils), or subcutaneous (arrays). Most contemporary systems involve a rate-sensing lead and shocking coil(s) that are incorporated into a single transvenous device, and the current is delivered between the coil(s) and the ICD generator. This approach has the added benefit of not requiring a thoracotomy to place defibrillation patches. These systems can be implanted in children down to approximately 25 kg, although the ICD itself may have to be implanted in the abdominal wall and the lead tunneled down to it in smaller patients.

ICDs deliver energy as a biphasic shock, and most can be programmed to deliver up to 40 J for internal defibrillators and up to 80 J in the subcutaneous ICD (SICD), which does not have leads attached to the heart. The current implantable devices are multifunctional and can deliver not only high-energy shocks for defibrillation, but also low-energy shocks for synchronized cardioversion or overdrive pacing (with the exception of SICDs) for termination of sustained VT. ICDs are capable of dual-chamber bradycardia pacing and can discriminate SVTs from VTs using a variety of recognition algorithms. These devices are fully programmable by means of telemetry and are capable of storing data that recall the device status, detected tachyarrhythmias, and delivered therapy.

Selected References

A complete list of references is available at ExpertConsult.com.

1. Hoffman BF, Rosen MR. Cellular mechanisms for cardiac arrhythmias. *Circ Res.* 1981;49:1–15.
5. Davignon A, Rautaharju P, Boisselle E, et al. Normal ECG standards for infants and children. *Pediatr Cardiol.* 1979;1:123–152.
27. Epstein AE, DiMarco JP, Ellenbogen KA, et al. 2012 ACCF/AHA/HRS focused update incorporated into the ACCF/AHA/HRS 2008 guidelines for device-based therapy of cardiac rhythm abnormalities: a report of the American College of Cardiology Foundation/American Heart Association Task Force on Practice Guidelines and the Heart Rhythm Society. *Circulation.* 2013;127(3):e283–e352.
28. Drezner JA, Ackerman MJ, Anderson J, et al. Electrocardiographic interpretation in athletes: the "Seattle Criteria." *Br J Sports Med.* 2013;47:122–124.
31. Reed BR, Lee LA, Harmon C, et al. Autoantibodies to SS-A/Ro in infants with congenital heart block. *J Pediatr.* 1983;103:889–891.
33. Silka MJ, Kron J, Halperin BD, McAnulty JH. Mechanisms of AV node reentrant tachycardia in young patients with and without dual AV node physiology. *Pacing Clin Electrophysiol.* 1994;17:2129–2133.
47. Perry JC, Knilans TK, Marlow D, et al. Intravenous amiodarone for life-threatening tachyarrhythmias in children and young adults. *J Am Coll Cardiol.* 1993;22:95–98.
68. Cohen MI, Triedman JK, Cannon BC, et al. PACES/HRS expert consensus statement on the management of the asymptomatic young patient with a Wolff-Parkinson-White (WPW, ventricular preexcitation) electrocardiographic pattern: developed in partnership between the Pediatric and Congenital Electrophysiology Society (PACES) and the Heart Rhythm Society (HRS). Endorsed by the governing bodies of PACES, HRS, the American College of Cardiology Foundation (ACCF), the American Heart Association (AHA), the American Academy of Pediatrics (AAP), and the Canadian Heart Rhythm Society (CHRS). *Heart Rhythm.* 2012;9(6):1006–1024.
72. Schwartz PJ, Crotti L, Insolia R. Long-QT syndrome: from genetics to management. *Circ Arrhythm Electrophysiol.* 2012;5(4):868–877.
74. Priori SG, Wilde AA, Horie M, et al. HRS/EHRA/APHRS expert consensus statement on the diagnosis and management of patients with inherited primary arrhythmia syndromes: document endorsed by HRS, EHRA, and APHRS in May 2013 and by ACCF, AHA, PACES, and AEPC in June 2013. *Heart Rhythm.* 2013;10(12):1932–1963.
93. Maron BJ, Fananapazir L. Sudden cardiac death in hypertrophic cardiomyopathy. *Circulation.* 1992;85:I57–I63.
102. Marcus FI, McKenna WJ, Sherrill D, et al. Diagnosis of arrhythmogenic right ventricular cardiomyopathy/dysplasia: proposed modification of the Task Force Criteria. *Eur Heart J.* 2010;31(7):806–814.
104. Corrado D, Wichter T, Link MS, et al. Treatment of arrhythmogenic right ventricular cardiomyopathy/dysplasia: an international task force consensus statement. *Circulation.* 2015;132:441–453.

28

Inflammatory Heart Disease: Pericardial Effusion and Tamponade, Pericarditis, and Myocarditis

STEVEN S. MOU, MD; MICHAEL C. MCCRORY, MD

Inflammatory Heart Disease—Pericardial Effusion/Tamponade

Normal Pericardium: Anatomy and Physiology

Anatomy. The pericardium is a dual-layered structure enveloping the heart and proximal great vessels. It consists of an inner visceral pericardium (also called the epicardium when in contact with the myocardium), and an outer parietal pericardium, composed of layers of collagen fibrils and elastin fibers.[1] The pericardium normally contains approximately 10 to 50 mL of fluid, an ultrafiltrate of plasma (the pericardial reserve volume). Pericardial fluid may contain cytokines, prostaglandins, atrial natriuretic peptide (particularly in congestive heart failure [HF]), endothelin, and growth factors that may locally influence myocytes and vascular tissue, as well as albumin and other plasma proteins.[2-4] Drainage of pericardial fluid occurs via lymphatics on the surface of the heart and parietal pericardium.[5]

The pericardium is tethered by its reflection around the great vessels and fibrous connection with the vertebral column, sternum, and diaphragm. The outer surface of the pericardium is in direct contact with the pleura. The lungs constitute a space that envelops the heart and pericardium termed the *cardiac fossa*. Sensory innervation to the pericardium is supplied by the phrenic nerve.[5]

Physiology. Various functions have been attributed to the pericardium, including (1) maintenance of the heart in a fixed position in the chest, (2) protection of the heart from infection, inflammation, or contiguous spread of malignancy from surrounding structures, (3) minimizing friction associated with cardiac motion, and (4) influencing cardiac dynamics by exerting external constraining forces over the heart.[6,7] The pericardium appears to influence cardiac dynamics by maintaining an optimal shape of the heart, enhancing interactions between chambers to balance right and left ventricular output, and attenuating acute changes in preload and afterload.[5,8-11] However, the pericardium is not essential for cardiovascular function as evidenced by the fact that both congenital and acquired deficiency states are compatible with long-term survival.[5,12,13]

Pericardial Effusion and Tamponade

Overview. Pericardial effusion occurs in a variety of clinical settings when excess pericardial fluid accumulates beyond the usual pericardial reserve volume. Pericardial effusion may consist of transudate due to obstruction of fluid drainage and/or low plasma oncotic pressure (e.g., HF), exudate due to inflammatory/infectious processes (e.g., purulent pericarditis), blood (e.g., chest trauma), air (e.g., pneumopericardium), chyle (idiopathic or postoperative chylopericardium), or even intravenous (IV) crystalloid solution (e.g., perforation of the right atrium or intrapericardial cava by a central venous catheter). Causes of pericardial effusion, with indication of presence of inflammation of the pericardium (pericarditis) versus noninflammatory causes, are listed in Box 28.1.

Etiology. The etiology of pericardial effusion varies widely by population studied; however, purulent pericarditis appears to have become less common in the era of antibiotics and routine vaccination against previously common bacterial pathogens. In a 20-year review of children with pericardial effusion from a tertiary care center in the United States, bacterial infections were found in only 3% of patients, with *Haemophilus influenzae*, *Staphylococcus aureus*, and *Neisseria meningitidis* each reported. In this study 39% of patients with pericardial effusion had associated neoplastic disease, 9% collagen vascular disease, 8% renal disease, 5% other diagnoses (human immunodeficiency virus [HIV], viral sepsis, hypothyroidism, anorexia nervosa), and 37% were classified as idiopathic.[14] By contrast, a study of children with pericardial effusion from a tertiary center in India demonstrated tuberculosis in 52%, other bacteria in 23% (including *S. aureus* and *Pseudomonas aeruginosa*), viral causes in 12%, idiopathic effusion in 8%, and only 4% with neoplastic disease.[15] Similar findings have been reported in adult studies of pericardial effusion, with 7% to 50% idiopathic, 10% to 37% neoplastic, 2% to 20% infectious, 4% to 20% uremic, 5% to 15% collagen vascular, 0% to 20% iatrogenic, 0% to 8% post myocardial infarction, and as high as 50% to 70% tuberculous in some areas of the world.[16-18]

Pericardial effusion may occur after surgery for congenital heart disease and is usually transudative but may be chylous. Increased venous pressure is thought to be a principal factor in the pathogenesis. Various conditions, including septal defect repairs, cavopulmonary anastamoses, and repair of lesions with right ventricular (RV) outflow tract obstruction, have been associated with postoperative pericardial effusions, with variable clinical significance and typical detection a mean of 11 days after surgery.[19,20] Prolonged drainage may indicate hemodynamic problems within the

• BOX 28.1 Causes of Pericarditis and Pericardial Effusion

Infectious Pericarditis

Viral
See Box 28.2

Bacterial/Tuberculous
Staphylococcus aureus, Haemophilus influenzae, Neisseria meningitidis, Streptococcus pneumoniae β-hemolytic streptococci, *Mycoplasma pneumoniae, Mycobacterium tuberculosis, Enterobacter cloacae, Corynebacterium diphtheriae*

Fungal
Candida, Aspergillus, Histoplasma, coccidiomycosis

Noninfectious Pericarditis

Cardiac Injury
Postpericardiotomy syndrome, post myocardial infarction

Systemic Inflammatory Disease
Rheumatic fever, juvenile rheumatoid arthritis, systemic lupus erythematosus, inflammatory bowel disease, Kawasaki disease, rheumatic fever, tumor necrosis factor receptor–associated periodic syndrome (TRAPS), familial Mediterranean fever

Neoplasms
Leukemia, lymphoma, metastatic tumor, radiation pericarditis

Renal
End-stage renal disease (uremia), dialysis

Miscellaneous
Hypersensitivity to drugs/toxins (e.g., procainamide, hydralazine, penicillins, cromolyn, dantrolene, anthracyclines), amyloidosis, radiation

Additional Causes of Pericardial Effusion ± Pericarditis

Traumatic and Postoperative
Blunt chest trauma, central line malposition, catheterization/biopsy, rupture of coronary aneurysm (such as with Kawasaki disease), early postoperative hemorrhage

Elevated Central Venous Pressure/Low Plasma Oncotic Pressure
Superior vena cava syndrome, chylous effusion, primary pulmonary hypertension and right ventricular failure, decompensated congestive heart failure, liver failure, anorexia nervosa
    Bone marrow transplant/graft versus host disease
    Hyperthyroidism/Hypothyroidism

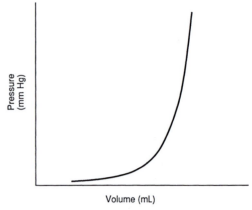

• **Figure 28.1** A schematic illustration showing a typical pressure-volume relationship of the whole pericardium obtained in animal experiments.

repair and should prompt consideration.[21] Postoperative effusions may also occur in patients after heart transplantation,[22] possibly due to the smaller donor heart within the chronically stretched recipient pericardium. Persistence of pericardial effusions after transplant has been correlated with both higher incidence and more severe histology of rejection.[23] Postpericardotomy syndrome following heart surgery is associated with pericardial effusion, with symptoms largely related to pericarditis as discussed later.

Signs and Symptoms. Small pericardial effusions may be asymptomatic or associated with only slightly muffled heart sounds on examination and may be discovered incidentally by widened cardiac silhouette on chest radiograph or on an echocardiogram performed in the context of a workup for an associated systemic illness. Dyspnea or chest discomfort may be present, especially if there is accompanying pericarditis. A classification system has been proposed based on size (large >20 mm in size on imaging, moderate 10 to 20 mm, small <10 mm), distribution (circumferential versus loculated), and duration (acute if <1 week, subacute 1 week to

<3 months, or chronic if >3 months)[5,16,24]; however, clinical manifestations in children are multifactorial and do not necessarily correlate with these features.

Cardiac Tamponade. Cardiac tamponade is a life-threatening clinical condition that occurs when accumulation of material (such as fluid, blood, or air) in the pericardium causes hemodynamic compromise. The classic presentation described by Beck[25] in 1935 includes (1) hypotension, (2) rising central venous pressure, and (3) a small, quiet heart. As pericardial volume increases, intrapericardial pressure undergoes a slow ascent until reaching the limits of extensibility, at which point a rapid rise in pressure occurs associated with cardiac chamber compression (Fig. 28.1). The rate of fluid accumulation, effectiveness of compensatory mechanisms, and stiffness of the pericardium affect the inflection point of the intrapericardial pressure curve and thus the severity and timing of clinical manifestations.[26] Therefore a slowly developing pericardial effusion (such as in a systemic inflammatory state) may result in large volumes of fluid before significant cardiovascular effect, whereas a rapidly accumulating process such as a traumatic intrapericardial hemorrhage may quickly cause hemodynamic collapse.

Progression of hemodynamic changes in tamponade proceeds in a well-described fashion. Increased pericardial pressure leads to increased cardiac diastolic pressure, reduced myocardial transmural pressure, smaller cardiac chambers with decreased compliance, and decreased preload and cardiac output. A compensatory sympathetic response results in tachycardia, increased venous tone, and baroreflex-induced systemic arteriolar vasoconstriction to compensate for the hypotension.[27] Jugular venous distention, hepatomegaly, and elevated central venous pressures may be evident. *Pulsus paradoxus,* defined as an exaggerated decrement in the arterial systolic pressure (>10 mm Hg) during inspiration, occurs in tamponade primarily due to bulging of the interventricular septum into the left ventricle (LV) as the right heart fills and the RV free wall is inhibited from expanding anteriorly due to pericardial constraint. Exceptions to this occur when abnormal communications exist between cardiac chambers (atrial septal defect; patent foramen ovale), when there is alteration of normal ventricular pressure-volume relations (hypertrophic cardiomyopathy, severe aortic stenosis, aortic insufficiency),[28-30] or when there is decreased intravascular volume (low-pressure tamponade).[31] Characteristic echocardiographic findings in pericardial effusion and tamponade are depicted in Fig. 28.2.

Other characteristic findings in pericardial effusion and tamponade include low-voltage QRS complexes on electrocardiogram

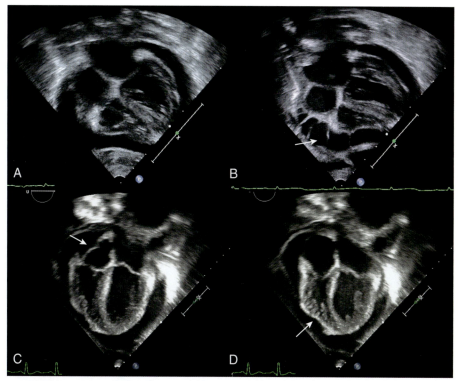

• **Figure 28.2** Echocardiographic findings in pericardial effusion and tamponade. (A) Simple circumferential effusion; (B) Complex effusion with septations *(arrow)* from purulent pericarditis. Blood cultures grew *Staphylococcus aureus*. Right atrial collapse *(arrow;* C) and right ventricular collapse *(arrow;* D) in a patient with tamponade physiology, occurring due to increased pericardial pressure relative to right atrial and right ventricular diastolic pressure, respectively. Other echocardiographic findings in tamponade may include exaggerated respiratory variation in mitral and tricuspid inflow velocity (may be absent in positive pressure ventilation), respiratory variation in aortic outflow velocity (echocardiographic pulsus paradoxus), and inferior vena cava plethora.

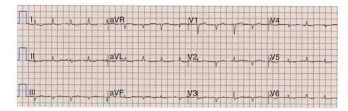

• **Figure 28.3** Electrical alternans. Beat-to-beat variation occurs in both the amplitude and axis of the QRS complex as the heart swings inside of a large pericardial effusion (particularly evident in leads II, V_2, V_3). (From Jehangir W, Osman M. Images in Clinical Medicine. Electrical alternans with pericardial tamponade. *N Engl J Med.* 2015;373:e10, with permission.)

and electrical alternans, which is beat-to-beat alteration of the QRS complex amplitude and axis due to the swinging motion of the heart within a large pericardial effusion (Fig. 28.3).[26] Electrical alternans is considered specific but not sensitive for tamponade. The central venous pressure waveform in tamponade classically shows an exaggerated *x* descent in ventricular systole with a diminished or absent *y* descent in ventricular diastole (Fig. 28.4). This is because in tamponade the intraluminal atrial or ventricular diastolic pressures (i.e., the downstream pressures for venous return) are effectively determined by the pericardial pressure. Ejection of blood in ventricular systole causes a decrease in total intrapericardial volume and subsequent antegrade venous flow, whereas pericardial and atrial pressures remain elevated and unchanged in ventricular

diastole as intrapericardial volume transfer occurs through the atrioventricular (AV) valves.[32]

Management. Management of pericardial effusion consists of treating the underlying disease, with drainage performed when needed for diagnostic purposes or if progression to tamponade appears imminent. Management of tamponade consists of immediate drainage of pericardial fluid via percutaneous catheter pericardiocentesis or surgical pericardotomy/pericardectomy. Volume loading with crystalloid or colloid solution may be considered as a temporizing measure to augment preload, but definitive therapy should not be delayed. Diuretics may worsen the patient's condition by further reducing preload. Inotropic agents may be considered but may have limited effect in the setting of an already brisk endogenous sympathetic response. Endotracheal intubation and mechanical ventilation should be approached with extreme caution because further cardiovascular compromise can occur with increased intrathoracic pressure due to increased lung volumes, further reducing systemic venous return and increasing total external constraint of the heart.[33]

Pericardiocentesis should be performed in an intensive care unit (ICU), operating room, or catheterization laboratory with experienced personnel and resuscitation supplies present and echocardiographic guidance if possible. An illustration of the technique of pericardiocentesis using the Seldinger technique and a pigtail catheter is depicted in Fig. 28.5. The patient should be positioned in the semiupright position. Local anesthesia with 1% or 2% lidocaine may be used to facilitate puncture; systemic

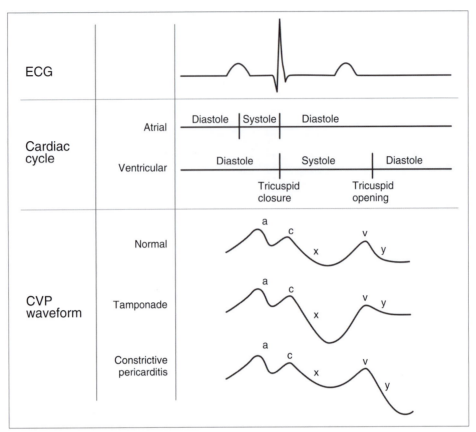

• **Figure 28.4** Central venous pressure *(CVP)* waveform in normal, tamponade, and constrictive pericardial physiology. The *a* (atrial contraction), *c* (closure of the tricuspid valve is followed by bulging into the right atrium in early ventricular systole), and *v* (end of ventricular systole before tricuspid opening, with rapid filling of the atrium) waves are shown corresponding to their position in the cardiac cycle. In tamponade there is a prominent *x* descent as the majority of venous filling occurs during ventricular systole, with an attenuated or absent *y* descent. In constrictive pericarditis the *y* descent is more prominent. *ECG,* Electrocardiogram.

sedation/anesthesia should be used judiciously due to risk of cardiovascular collapse even with administration of agents such as fentanyl or ketamine. An 18-gauge needle long enough to reach the effusion (often 6 cm) is used, with the best site of puncture and angulation determined echocardiographically as the point at which the largest fluid accumulation is closest to the body surface. In an emergency the subxiphoid approach may be used with approximately 15-degree angulation off the skin directed toward the left shoulder.[14] In a retrospective series of 94 procedures in 73 pediatric patients, the optimal site of puncture by echocardiographic guidance was determined to be para-apical (68.1%), subxiphoid (17%), left axillary (5.3%), left parasternal (3.2%), right parasternal (2.1%), posterolateral (1.1%), or unspecified (3.2%).[34]

Continuous suction is held until fluid is aspirated, at which point a 0.035- or 0.038-inch guide wire is advanced, followed by dilation and insertion of a 7 Fr or 8 Fr pigtail catheter, typically left in place for ongoing drainage until the underlying cause is resolved (see Fig. 28.5).[21,34] Fluid may be sent to the laboratory for cell count with differential, determination of glucose, protein, and lactate dehydrogenase levels, and bacterial/fungal culture if further characterization is needed. A cardiac surgeon should be immediately available during the procedure because complications of pericardiocentesis can include laceration/perforation of the myocardium or coronary vessels with hemopericardium; however,

intrapericardial fluid may often be bloody even without cardiac puncture (56% of cases in one study).[34] Bloody pericardial fluid is nonclotting; additionally, bloody pericardial fluid usually sinks to the bottom of a gauze sponge, whereas blood forms clots on the surface of the gauze.[35] Approximately 2 to 5 mL of agitated saline may be instilled under echocardiographic guidance to confirm placement. Other complications of pericardiocentesis include air embolism, pneumothorax, pulmonary edema, arrhythmias (most commonly vasovagal bradycardia), or puncture of the peritoneal cavity.[36]

After placement the pericardial catheter may then be flushed with saline to prevent catheter plugging, and intermittent drainage (frequency dependent on reaccumulation rate and hemodynamics; usual minimum, every 2 hours) is followed by sterile saline catheter flush to maintain catheter patency. This is preferred over continuous drainage for maintenance of catheter patency. Balloon pericardiotomy has been used in adults, and there is some experience in children.[37,38] Pericardial effusions also may be drained surgically via a subxiphoid approach or laparoscopy.[39,40] A pericardial window is a communication created surgically, typically between the pericardial and pleural space. This allows ongoing drainage of effusion and may be used for recurrent effusions (such as in malignancy) or to prevent tamponade after cardiac surgery.[16,41]

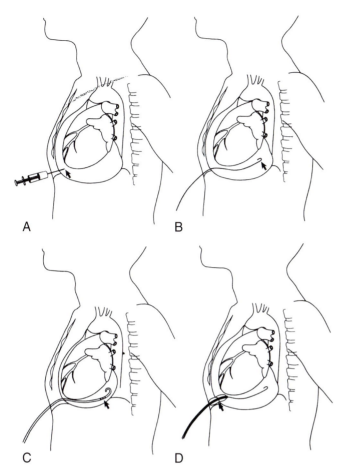

• **Figure 28.5** Schematic of pericardiocentesis technique. (A) Introduction of needle *(arrow)*. (B) Passage of guide wire *(arrow)*. (C) Pigtail catheter in pericardial space *(arrow)*. (D) Balloon inflation to create pericardial-pleural space window *(arrow)*. (From Lang P: Other catheterization laboratory techniques and interventions: atrial septal defect creation, transseptal puncture, pericardial drainage, foreign body retrieval, exercise and drug testing. In: Lock JE, Keane JF, Perry SF, eds. *Diagnostic and Interventional Catheterization in Congenital Heart Disease.* 2nd ed. Boston: Kluwer Academic Publishers; 2000:256-258, with permission.)

Inflammatory Heart Disease—Pericarditis

Overview

Pericarditis is inflammation of the pericardium, which may be acute, incessant (lasting for ≥4 weeks to <3 months without remission), recurrent (symptoms after a documented first episode and a symptom-free period of ≥4 weeks), or chronic (>3 months).[16,42] Acute pericarditis is an infrequent cause of chest pain among pediatric emergency department visits (<0.2%)[43] and among pediatric cardiology consultations for chest pain at a tertiary center (≈5%)[44] and may come to the attention of an intensivist only when associated with a severe systemic disease, a postoperative state, and/or a significant pericardial effusion. Proposed diagnostic criteria for pericarditis include two or more of the following: (1) chest pain, classically pleuritic and relieved by sitting up and leaning forward, (2) pericardial friction rub, (3) new widespread ST elevation or PR depression on electrocardiogram (ECG) (60% or more),[45] and (4) new or worsening pericardial effusion (approximately 80%).[16,42,45] Additional supporting features include elevated markers of inflammation (white blood cell count, C-reactive protein [CRP],

erythrocyte sedimentation rate [ESR]) and evidence of pericardial inflammation on imaging tests such as computed tomography (CT) or cardiac magnetic resonance imaging (MRI), if performed. Assessment of markers of myocardial injury (creatine kinase [CK]-MB, troponin) as well as transthoracic echocardiography is important when pericarditis is strongly suspected in critically ill patients due to the risk of concurrent coronary syndrome and/or myocarditis. Chest x-ray examination results are generally normal in isolated pericarditis but may show an enlarged cardiac silhouette (water bottle sign) if a significant (generally >300 mL in an adolescent/adult) pericardial effusion is present.[16]

Etiology

Pericarditis may be infectious (including bacterial, viral, mycobacterial, or fungal) or noninfectious (see Box 28.1). Viral causes (especially coxsackievirus or echovirus) remain commonly implicated in acute pericarditis in otherwise healthy children, although the true incidence is difficult to determine due to incomplete detection. Purulent pericarditis may be associated with other infections such as septic arthritis, osteomyelitis, pneumonia, and pyelonephritis,[46] with organisms discussed previously in discussion of purulent pericardial effusion. Tuberculosis is a common cause of pericarditis worldwide, especially in patients who also have HIV.[16] A large proportion of patients with pericarditis are labeled idiopathic in multiple series (40% to 90% of all cases of pericarditis)[5,45,47-50]; however, in one multicenter database study of hospitalized children with pericarditis and pericardial effusion, only 5% were classified as idiopathic after an inpatient workup.[51] In this study, cardiac causes (such as post cardiac surgery) were most commonly identified (54%), followed by neoplastic and renal causes (each 13%), contiguous infection or trauma (6%), and rheumatologic disease (5%). Antiheart, antiintercalated disk, antimyolemmal, antifibrillary, and antinuclear antibodies have been detected in patients with idiopathic recurrent pericarditis and/or chronic pericardial effusion,[52-55,55a] suggesting that autoimmune responses develop in predisposed individuals following exogenous triggers.[53,56] Recurrent pericarditis, especially in the context of a family history of inflammatory disorders, is being increasingly recognized as a prominent feature of tumor necrosis factor receptor–associated periodic syndrome (TRAPS) and familial Mediterranean fever.[57,58]

The postpericardiotomy syndrome is an important cause of noninfectious pericarditis and pericardial effusion in the ICU that may occur after any open-heart procedure that involves opening of the pericardium. Features include signs and symptoms of pericarditis (chest pain, pericardial friction rub, patient irritability), pericardial effusion, and fever occurring more than 72 hours postoperatively. In a single-center retrospective study of children following atrial septal defect repair, 28% were diagnosed with postpericardiotomy syndrome within the first year, with a median time of diagnosis 8 days postoperatively.[59] Adult studies describe an incidence of postpericardiotomy syndrome of 9% to 24% after cardiac surgery,[60-62] with more than 50% of cases occurring within 2 weeks postoperatively and more than 80% to 90% within 3 months. Pleural incision is described as a risk factor for postpericardiotomy syndrome, and pleural effusion is also commonly present.[62] Pathophysiology of the postpericardiotomy syndrome is hypothesized to involve an autoimmune inflammatory response to pleuropericardial antigens, with perioperative viral infections also having a potential role.[62-64] Treatment is similar to that for other patients with pericarditis and pericardial effusion, with additional attention to any postoperative concerns regarding the surgical repair or cardiac function. Corticosteroids[65] and aspirin[66] have been shown to be ineffective as prophylaxis for postpericardiotomy syndrome in children, whereas colchicine has shown a preventative effect in adults.[60]

Management

Among critically ill patients, immediate management of pericarditis is directed at draining symptomatic pericardial effusions and treating associated systemic disease. For idiopathic, immune-mediated, or viral pericarditis, the classic first-line therapy has been nonsteroidal antiinflammatory medication (such as aspirin or ibuprofen) for 1 to 2 weeks or until symptom resolution.[16] Colchicine and anti–interleukin-1 therapy with anakinra may be considered in recurrent or refractory cases.[16,60,67] Corticosteroids are not recommended unless indicated for a concurrent disease process such as an autoimmune disorder, due to concerns for adverse effects, prolonged disease course, and increased risk of recurrence.[16,60,68] Azathioprine or IV immunoglobulin (IVIG) have also been used; however, data are limited regarding these therapies.[55]

Outcome

Pericarditis often resolves with treatment of the initial insult or underlying condition; however, recurrence may occur in approximately 15% to 30% of cases in adults.[16] In one multicenter series of 110 children with recurrent pericarditis, median age was 13 years, and the most common symptoms at recurrence were chest pain (94%) and fever (76%).[68] The initial cause of pericarditis in this series was most often idiopathic or viral (89%) or postpericardiotomy (9%).

In some patients, pericardial inflammation may progress to fibrosis, resulting in constrictive pericarditis. In a large prospective cohort of adults after acute pericarditis, 1.8% developed constrictive pericarditis over a median 6-year follow-up, with less than 0.5% of patients with viral or idiopathic pericarditis progressing to constrictive pericarditis and 8.3% of patients with other causes, with the highest risk for those with bacterial or tuberculous pericardial disease.[69] In limited data in children, bacterial pericarditis also appears to be the most common cause of constrictive pericarditis.[70] Constrictive pericarditis may be similar to pericardial effusion clinically with signs and symptoms of systemic venous hypertension (such as jugular venous distention, hepatomegaly, ascites, protein-losing enteropathy); however, cardiomegaly is not seen on radiograph, and pulmonary edema or pulsus paradoxus typically does not occur. The central venous pressure waveform in constrictive pericarditis exhibits a prominent y descent (see Fig. 28.4) with filling in early ventricular diastole, in contrast to the filling primarily in ventricular systole (prominent x descent) in tamponade. This difference is thought to be related to the complex physiology caused by the fibrotic pericardium forming a tight sac around the heart, which causes more "uncoupled" constraint of local pericardial surface pressures rather than the more uniform or "coupled" pericardial surface pressure across chambers that occur in tamponade.[71]

The combination of echocardiography and CT scan or magnetic resonance imaging (MRI) may help establish the diagnosis of constrictive pericarditis. Pericardial biopsy is sometimes needed. Pericardiectomy is the only effective therapy and should be undertaken early before the fibrotic process also has affected the myocardium. The patient's rate of recovery will depend on the extent of comorbid disease and especially the degree of coexistent myocardial fibrosis.

Inflammatory Heart Disease—Myocarditis

Overview

Myocarditis is defined clinically as inflammation of the heart muscle that most often results from common viral infections and postviral immune-mediated responses. There is no clear universally accepted clinical definition of acute myocarditis, and often the diagnosis is presumed upon clinical presentation and noninvasive diagnostic tests such as cardiac echocardiography or cardiac MRI. Endomyocardial biopsy (EMB) remains the gold standard for in vivo diagnosis of myocarditis, but its application in pediatrics is inconsistent because there is concern due to the perceived potential associated complications in such vulnerable patients.[72] The Dallas criteria established in 1986[73] serve to define active myocarditis based upon histopathologic criteria, the presence of infiltrating lymphocytes, and myocytolysis; however, these criteria have been criticized as underestimating the incidence of myocarditis due to large interobserver variability.[74] Nonetheless, the diagnostic and prognostic benefits of EMB results have been demonstrated.[75-77] The development of new molecular techniques such as micro-RNA (miRNA) profiling, nested polymerase chain reaction (PCR), and in situ hybridization has improved the accuracy of diagnosis and prognostic value of EMB sampling, allowing for improved definitions of myocarditis, including the less prevalent subtypes such as eosinophilic and giant cell myocarditis.[78] Despite the value of EMB in adult studies we are seeing a trend away from its use in pediatrics[79] with an increased reliance upon cardiac MRI.[79]

The clinical manifestations of myocarditis are heterogeneous, ranging from virtually asymptomatic cases with vague signs and symptoms to severe myocardial destruction by virus and immune cells with New York Heart Association (NYHA) class IV symptoms to cardiogenic shock and arrhythmia with reports of mechanical support in as much as 23% and mortality as high as 7.2%.[74] Manifestations include flu-like symptoms with LV systolic dysfunction associated with signs of inflammation such as leukocytosis, elevated ESR, and increased levels of cardiac troponin and creatine kinase.

A study using International Classification of Diseases (ninth revision) codes estimated the global prevalence of myocarditis to be approximately 22 of 100,000 patients annually.[80] The potential of myocarditis to be an insidious disease with lack of symptoms makes it difficult to ascertain its true epidemiology. Myocarditis is a major cause of sudden unexpected death[81-83]; the American Heart Association (AHA) and the American College of Cardiology (ACC) rank myocarditis as the third leading cause of sudden cardiac death in competitive athletes.[84] Approximately 1% to 9% of routine postmortem examinations demonstrate evidence of myocarditis.[85-87] A significant discrepancy exists between myocarditis diagnosed in autopsy studies and myocarditis noted clinically because many cases are subclinical and never manifest symptoms severe enough to warrant medical care.

Neonates and children exhibit a more fulminant myocarditis and are typically more susceptible to virus-induced pathogenesis than adults.[88,89] Many studies report a greater prevalence and severity in men, speculated to be caused by a protective effect of natural hormonal influences on immune responses in women when compared to men.[90,91] In a retrospective study that reviewed 5 years of data from the Pediatric Health Information System database, there was a bimodal age distribution for acute myocarditis, with a peak in infancy and a similar peak in mid–teenage years.[79]

The outcome of myocarditis can be predicted based upon initial clinical presentation. Patients with acute myocarditis and preserved

LV ejection fraction have a good prognosis and a high rate of spontaneous improvement without sequelae.[92] Patients with fulminant viral myocarditis as defined by severe hemodynamic compromise requiring inotropic support or mechanical support also have an excellent long-term prognosis and are more likely to experience complete recovery[93] if aggressive management is initiated in a timely manner. Nonfulminant myocarditis may be acute or chronic and so may progress in a more insidious manner with a less predictable long-term outcome with potential for complete resolution or progression to dilated cardiomyopathy (DCM), for which a subset may require transplantation. Virus has been isolated from the hearts of both adults and infants with acute cardiac disease.[94-96] With the identification of the enterovirus genome in the myocardium of patients with myocarditis and DCM,[97,98] a causal link between viral myocarditis and DCM has been widely accepted. It is estimated that roughly 10% to 15% of cases of DCM are due to biopsy-proven myocarditis.[99] It is presumed that it is the adaptive and maladaptive response to such myocardial inflammation that determines the fate of those with myocarditis as to whether resolution occurs or a chronic ongoing immune response commits the patient to chronic HF. This is also the area where more recent attention has been focused toward the application of antiviral therapies to eradicate persistent viral states with immunosuppression that may potentially lead to treatment of such patients with chronic HF. Understanding the cellular and molecular processes responsible for such responses may provide further insight into developing such therapeutic algorithms.

Etiology

The spectrum of possible infectious and noninfectious causes of myocarditis is similar to that of pericarditis (Box 28.2). Infectious agents may produce cardiac damage by direct invasion of myocardial cells, an abnormal immunologic response of the host, or in rare cases, toxin production by the invading organism (e.g., *Corynebacterium diphtheriae*). Despite refinements in identification and viral-isolation techniques and the increased use of PCR, many cases of myocarditis remain idiopathic with no identifiable infectious agent isolated.

Viral Myocarditis

In cases in which the cause can be established, the majority of cases of myocarditis in North America have a viral cause. Although

several viral agents have been implicated as possible causes of myocarditis (Table 28.1), enteroviruses (members of the Picornaviridae family) have been the most frequently identified.[100] Of these agents, coxsackievirus B is the culprit in more than half of the cases.[101] Other enteroviruses associated with myocarditis include enteric cytopathic human orphan (ECHO) E6, E9, E11, and E22 serotypes. As more techniques have been developed, such as PCR and in situ hybridization, we have seen a shift in the typically identified enterovirus and adenovirus[102,103] to mainly parvovirus B19 and human herpesvirus 6.[104,105] Our understanding of the molecular mechanisms of myocarditis, however, largely come from animal and tissue cell culture studies of coxsackievirus B-3 (CVB3).[106] Using CVB3 as a model system, we will discuss our current understanding of disease progression.

Pathogenesis. The pathogenesis of viral myocarditis is both caused by direct injury mediated by viral infection and secondary to the immune response of the host.[107] At the cellular and tissue levels the pathologic progression of viral myocarditis can be divided into three stages. The acute viremic stage, which typically occurs over the first 4 days of disease, is characterized by viral entry and replication with consequential activation of the innate immune response. The subacute phase is characterized by the adaptive immune response with inflammatory cell infiltration over days 4 to 14, with cardiac remodeling being the major feature of the chronic phase, which may lead to DCM in some patients.[108]

The acute viremic stage is characterized by early cardiomyocyte damage associated with prominent viral replication. Viral invasion first begins when the circulating virion enters the myocyte via receptor-mediated endocytosis (Fig. 28.6). The first step in this process is the attachment of the virus to a myocyte cell-surface adhesion molecule. The prototype adhesion molecule in myocarditis is the coxsackie adenovirus receptor (CAR). The predominance of coxsackievirus B group and adenovirus as etiologic agents for myocarditis probably results from the fact that they share a common myocardial cell-surface receptor.[109] After the virus gains entry into the myocyte (see Fig. 28.6), viral genome replication occurs, producing a negative-strand viral RNA intermediate that serves as a template for transcription of progeny genomes.[110] The release of progeny

---

• BOX 28.2   Viruses Implicated in Myocarditis/Pericarditis

RNA Viruses
Coxsackievirus A, B
Echovirus
Hepatitis A
Influenza A, B
Lymphocytic choriomeningitis virus
Measles
Mumps
Poliovirus
Respiratory syncytial virus
Rhabdovirus
Rhinovirus
Rubella

DNA Viruses
Adenovirus
Cytomegalovirus
Epstein-Barr
Hepatitis B
Herpesviruses
Parvovirus
Varicella
Variola

Retroviruses
Human immunodeficiency virus

TABLE 28.1   Etiology of Myocarditis

Infectious Agents	Noninfectious Causes
Viruses	**Toxins**
See Box 28.2	Cocaine
	Toluene
Bacteria	Chemotherapy
Streptococcus	Interleukin-2
Corynebacterium diphtheriae	Ethanol
Neisseria meningitidis	Cobalt
Mycoplasma pneumoniae	Drug hypersensitivity
Chlamydia psittaci	
Staphylococcus aureus	**Autoimmune Diseases**
Shigella sonnei	Systemic lupus erythematosus
Enterococcus	Juvenile rheumatoid arthritis
Borrelia burgdorferi	Giant cell arteritis
	Takayasu arteritis
Parasitic Diseases	Sarcoidosis
Toxoplasmosis	Kawasaki disease
Trypanosoma cruzi	Transplant rejection
Trichinella spiralis	Peripartum
Echinococcosis	

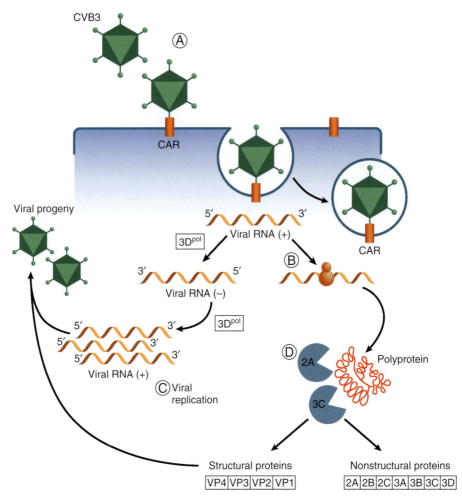

• **Figure 28.6** Viral infection of the cardiomyocyte. A, Viral attachment to coxsackie-adenoviral receptor *(CAR)* and internalization of viral genome via endocytosis. Viral RNA-dependent RNA polymerase 3Dpol synthesizes negative strand viral RNA intermediate that serves as a template for transcription of progeny genomes, *C; B,* The positive strand RNA directs synthesis of a single polyprotein; *D,* This single polyprotein is then cleaved into structural and nonstructural proteins by virus-encoded specific proteinases 2A and 3. *CVB3,* Coxsackievirus B-3.

virion requires that cell destruction be orchestrated, which the virus achieves by disrupting cell integrity and architecture[111,112] and taking control of cellular apoptosis (Fig. 28.7).[113-116]

The immune response to viral infection is crucial in the pathogenesis of myocarditis. Several observations support this theory, including the demonstration of immune complexes in the myocardium,[117] the occurrence of myocarditis in autoimmune diseases such as systemic lupus erythematosus (SLE), and the clinical response of some patients to immunosuppressive and other immune-modulating therapies. The details of the immune response to myocardial enteroviral infection have emerged from numerous experiments using murine models.[98,118]

The initial phase of acute myocarditis that occurs within the first 4 days of viral infection is characterized by viremia and the activation of the innate immune response.[107]

Cell-mediated immunity affects the host response during the subacute phase of myocarditis (days 4 to 14) (Fig. 28.8).[107] Whereas cell-mediated immunity is necessary for viral clearance, persistent T-cell activation may aggravate myocardial damage and lead to chronic myocarditis or DCM.[119]

Clinical Manifestations. Manifestations of myocarditis range from an asymptomatic patient to obvious signs of congestive HF. Infants with HF may present with history of poor feeding, respiratory distress, listlessness, poor weight gain, or irritability. Common adult symptoms such as paroxysmal nocturnal dyspnea and orthopnea are uncommon in pediatric patients. Most older children are somewhere in between these two extremes, with an acute febrile illness and a minor degree of cardiovascular involvement, such as tachycardia or isolated ECG changes. Abdominal pain, anorexia, nausea, and vomiting are often observed and are likely due to liver capsule distention from hepatomegaly and/or intestinal venous congestion. The most common cardiovascular symptom is chest pain, which may be the sole complaint in some patients.[120,121] Other presentations include isolated ventricular ectopy without obvious signs of cardiac failure. Syncope may result from ventricular tachycardia or less frequently from high-grade AV block. The ECG may be normal in between spells, making it more difficult to establish the diagnosis. Sudden death is the most severe presentation, and in such cases the diagnosis of myocarditis is made only at autopsy.[122] Myocarditis and cardiomyopathy also can be causes of sudden death during general anesthesia and surgery among patients not previously suspected of having heart disease.[123]

In most cases the multisystem effects and symptoms of the underlying viral illness outweigh the symptoms related to the

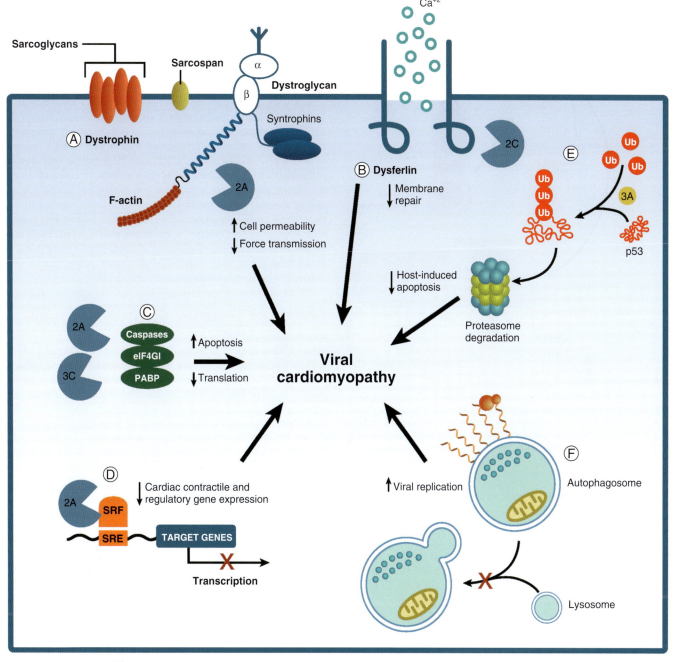

• **Figure 28.7** Direct myocardial injury induced by viral infection. (A) Dystrophin links the cytoskeleton to the extracellular matrix and protects muscle cells from contraction-induced damage. CVB3-encoded proteinase 2A cleaves dystrophin, contributing to myocardial dysfunction by increasing cell permeability and decreasing force transmission. (B) Dysferlin is a transmembrane protein that plays a role in calcium-dependent membrane repair of cardiomyocytes. Proteolytic processing by proteinase 2A contributes to impaired myocardial function by disrupting membrane repair function. (C) Virus-encoded proteinase 2A and 3C can produce direct cytotoxicity by inducing apoptosis through the direct cleavage of caspases and inhibiting host translation through the processing of eukaryotic translation initiation factor 4γ *(eIF4GI)* and poly-A binding protein *(PABP)*. (D) Serum response factor *(SRF)* is a transcription factor that is highly expressed in cardiac muscle that controls the expression of target genes through the binding of serum response element *(SRE)* located on gene promoter regions. SRF is cleaved by CVB3 proteinase 2A, which leads to impaired cardiac function by eliminating SRF-mediated gene expression. (E) The ubiquitin-proteasome system *(UPS)* functions to catalyze the degradation of abnormal proteins and short-lived regulatory proteins by targeting them through the process of ubiquitination. The virus fosters the ubiquitin-dependent proteolysis degradation of p53 via the action of protease 3A to prevent host-induced apoptosis. (F) CVB3 uses autophagosomes as a site for replication machinery. CVB3 prevents autophagosome-lysosome fusion to increase availability of autophagosomes to promote viral replication. *CVB3,* Coxsackievirus B-3.

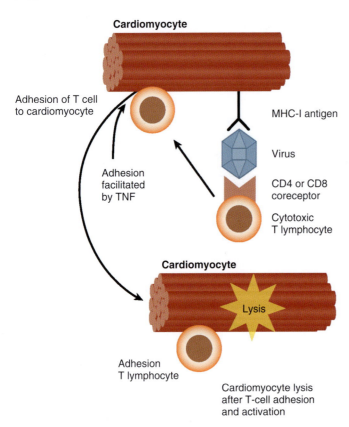

Adhesion of T cell to cardiomyocyte

Adhesion facilitated by TNF

Cardiomyocyte

MHC-I antigen

Virus

CD4 or CD8 coreceptor

Cytotoxic T lymphocyte

Cardiomyocyte

Lysis

Adhesion T lymphocyte

Cardiomyocyte lysis after T-cell adhesion and activation

• **Figure 28.8** Effects of cell-mediated immunity during subacute phase of myocarditis (days 4 to 14). Major histocompatibility complex *(MHC)* class I antigen on myocyte presents virus to CD4 or CD8 receptor on T lymphocyte. Tumor necrosis factor *(TNF)* facilitates T-cell adhesion to cardiomyocyte. Cardiomyocyte lysis occurs after T-cell activation.

cardiovascular system. However, signs and symptoms related to cardiac involvement may be seen. A tachycardia out of proportion to the fever may be present. Signs of cardiac failure such as cardiomegaly, pulsus alternans, hepatomegaly, and third or fourth heart sounds may be present. Decreased exercise tolerance, dyspnea, and easy fatigability may be the only complaints in some children. Associated symptoms such as myalgias, pneumonitis, exanthems, or lymphadenopathy may be suggestive of a viral cause.

On physical examination the child may appear anxious, and sinus tachycardia is usually present. Sweating is common in infants. Pallor and cool extremities may be present and are often associated with poor peripheral pulses and prolonged capillary refill. Resting tachypnea and retractions are common. Crackles are exceedingly rare in infants and young children with HF, unlike adults, even when pulmonary edema is present. Wheezing is more likely to be present, and periorbital edema is more common in children than peripheral edema.

The presentation in infants stands out because it is often very acute and life threatening. Irritability and poor feeding give way after a few hours to signs of overwhelming shock and HF. Respiratory distress, cyanosis, thready pulses, and gallop rhythm all suggest an infant in extremis. Because of the similarity of this presentation to ductal-dependent left-sided obstructive lesions such as coarctation, prostaglandin E_1 is sometimes given before the diagnosis of myocarditis in very young infants.

Laboratory and Electrocardiographic Findings. The majority of laboratory and ECG findings of myocarditis are nonspecific.

Elevations of creatine phosphokinase and lactate dehydrogenase are present in 50% to 75% of cases with ST-segment abnormalities.[124] CK has been previously considered a preferred biomarker to screen for myocarditis; however, its sensitivity in late diagnosis is poor because studies show that CK decreases steadily to basal levels by 36 hours.[125,126] Nonspecific serologic markers of inflammation, including leukocyte count and CRP, may be elevated in suspected myocarditis. The complete blood count reveals a leukocytosis in 50% of patients.[127] The presence of eosinophilia should prompt the search for a parasitic cause of the myocarditis. Another nonspecific indicator of an inflammatory process is an elevated ESR.[128] Nonelevated levels of leukocytes, CRP, and ESR fail to rule out an inflammatory response within the myocardium.[129] Levels of B-type natriuretic peptide and N-terminal pro-B-type natriuretic peptide can be elevated in myocarditis, and elevated levels may aid in distinguishing cardiac from noncardiac reasons for children who present with respiratory symptoms.[130] Cardiac troponin I (cTnI) levels now are the most sensitive diagnostic test for biopsy-proven myocarditis.[131] In addition, cTnI levels may be of prognostic value because they correlate with ejection fraction and clinical HF.[132]

ECG changes in myocarditis also are nonspecific and only support the diagnosis. The ECG most commonly reveals nonspecific ST-T-wave abnormalities. ECGs provide a convenient tool for risk stratification and initial screening, but provide little in diagnostic value. Ukena et al.[133] investigated the prognostic value of ECG in patients suspected of having myocarditis and reported that a prolonged QRS duration may be an independent predictor for cardiac death or heart transplantation. Other abnormalities include ventricular and atrial ectopy, conduction defects, sinus tachycardia, and T-wave inversion. The presence of ventricular ectopy in a febrile, irritable infant represents myocarditis until proven otherwise and should prompt immediate admission to an ICU. In infants with an ECG pattern consistent with acute myocardial infarction, anomalous origin of the left coronary artery from the pulmonary artery should be considered and excluded. Occasionally the ECG may point toward an alternate diagnosis. For example, Pompe disease has a characteristic ECG pattern of a short PR interval with very large precordial voltages. Similarly, the presence of ventricular preexcitation (Wolff-Parkinson-White syndrome) may raise the question of unrecognized sustained tachyarrhythmias as a cause of ventricular dysfunction.

Diagnostic Approach. Because of the wide clinical spectrum in presentation and the diversity of etiologic agents, the diagnostic approach to the patient with myocarditis must include a strategy that attempts to include several etiologic possibilities. A thorough history is imperative and should focus on the possibility of toxic ingestion (including illicit and over-the-counter medications), trauma, and possible exposure to infectious agents (including a complete travel history). Past history should include immunization status, because several infectious diseases of childhood (diphtheria, polio virus) are included in the differential diagnosis. Additionally, the history may reveal signs or symptoms of previously undiagnosed collagen vascular disorder or inflammatory bowel disease.

Echocardiography is a useful measurement tool in the diagnostic assessment of suspected myocarditis and aids in the process of ruling out other causes of HF, such as structural heart disease. Echocardiography may even contribute to the assessment of prognostication in such patients through two-dimensional speckle tracking that evaluates myocardial strain and strain rate.[134] Echocardiography investigates cardiac chamber size, wall thickness, and systolic and diastolic function, but it cannot provide direct evidence to confirm myocarditis. Patients with acute myocarditis often show only a poorly functioning LV with minimal dilation with or without regional wall motion abnormalities. There may be ventricular thickening secondary to myocardial edema, and left atrial enlargement may not be prominent, even when mitral valve regurgitation is present, suggesting an acute disease process.

The diagnosis of viral myocarditis is generally based on circumstantial evidence such as a recent viral infection and the sudden onset of cardiac dysfunction while ruling out other diagnostic possibilities. Although viral cultures (pharyngeal, rectal) should be obtained, the "window of opportunity" for viral isolation is narrow, and therefore isolation of the virus is often not possible. Use of PCR may allow identification of the viral genome even when cultures are negative. Supportive evidence for a viral cause can be obtained by a fourfold or greater increase in antibody titer between acute and convalescent sera. In addition to these titers, the presence of Epstein-Barr virus infection should be investigated with serologic study. Routine bacterial and fungal cultures of blood should be obtained in addition to serologic examination to rule out treponemal infection (Venereal Disease Research Laboratory or rapid plasma regimen).

Pathologic confirmation of myocardial inflammation continues to be required for definitive diagnosis of myocarditis.[135] Edwards and associates[136] suggested a criterion for myocarditis that includes five or more lymphocytes per 20 high-power fields during histologic examination of the endomyocardial specimen. Several biopsy specimens (5 to 10) may be needed because the inflammatory process is focal. These criteria were subsequently refined with the introduction of the Dallas criteria, which state that active myocarditis is present when routine light-microscopy examination of the biopsy specimen reveals lymphocytic infiltration and myocytolysis.[73] Borderline or ongoing myocarditis exists in the presence of lymphocytic infiltration alone without myocytolysis. The specimen is considered negative if both lymphocytic infiltration and myocytolysis are absent. Although the Dallas criteria remain in widespread use, most clinicians believe that they underestimate the true incidence of myocarditis, probably because of the patchy nature of myocardial inflammation and the high degree of interobserver variability.[74]

EMB provides relatively high diagnostic and prognostic value in suspected myocarditis patients[75,77] with reported complication rates of less than 1% among adults.[137,138] Furthermore, it has demonstrated benefits in aiding in clinical decision making[72,76] and in ruling out disorders important in the differential, such as endocardial fibroelastosis, Pompe disease, and eosinophilic and giant cell myocarditis.[78] Additional testing applied to the histologic sample such as RNA/DNA hybridization[139] and PCR[102] allow for more sensitive means to detect the offending virus. Despite these benefits, there has been a trend away from the use of EMB in pediatrics. The major concerns leading to its decrease in use are about its safety and potential for adverse events in a very vulnerable patient. Pediatric patients who are considered for EMB are typically younger, have more impaired hemodynamics, and typically require ICU-level support.[72] In a retrospective multi-institutional study looking at safety and efficacy of EMB among pediatric patients undergoing cardiac catheterization for suspected myocarditis, cardiomyopathy, and new-onset HF found a threefold increase in adverse events versus a posttransplant comparison group with a high-severity adverse event rate as high as 5%.[72] A major concern for EMB is cardiac perforation, which has been reported to be as high as 4% in children less than 1 year of age with primary risk factors of weight less than 8 kg and age less than 6 months.[140]

A report analyzing the Pediatric Health Information System database shows a statistical trend toward fewer EMBs and more

cardiac MRI scans in children with myocarditis in recent years.[79] In a survey of centers assessing the practice of EMB, less than 33% of patients with suspected myocarditis were referred for EMB, with a post hoc survey that reflected such a trend in practice in favor of a greater tendency to use cardiac MRI.[72] The 2007 AHA/ACC/ European Society of Cardiology (ESC) scientific statement also does not support the routine use of EMB for the diagnosis of myocarditis.[78] So despite literature that demonstrates a role for and benefit from the use of EMB, neither is it recommended nor is there evidence that it is commonly performed in pediatric patients.

Cardiac MRI has evolved as a valuable noninvasive clinical tool for the diagnosis of myocarditis.[141] MRI gained acceptance as it demonstrated reliability in tissue characterization of cardiac allograft rejection,[142,143] which histologically appears identical to acute myocarditis.[144] It is the myocardial inflammation that presents itself as an attractive target for cardiac MRI-based imaging. Contrast enhancement (CE) is a more sensitive technique of cardiac MRI and can detect areas of myocardial damage in myocarditis. The International Consensus Group on CMR Diagnosis of Myocarditis published recommendations on the indication, implementation, and analysis of appropriate cardiac MRI techniques for noninvasive diagnosis of myocarditis (Lake Louise criteria). The combined use of three different cardiac MRI techniques is suggested.[145,146] The T2-weighted edema imaging is a tool for evaluating the presence of acute myocardial edema (Fig. 28.9).[145,147] Further evaluation is performed looking at hyperemia and muscular inflammation using ECG-triggered T1-weighted images obtained within the first few minutes after gadolinium-diethylenetriaminepentaacetate (Gd-DTPA) infusion, deemed "myocardial early gadolinium enhancement."[146] This

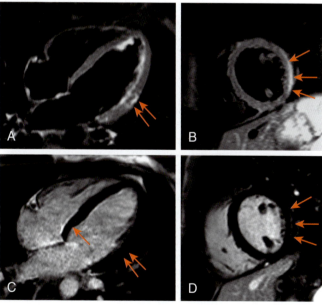

• **Figure 28.9** Magnetic resonance imaging (MRI) findings in patients with myocarditis. Cardiac MRI images of a patient presenting with acute chest pain due to acute myocarditis. Long-axis (A) and short axis (B) T2-weighted edema images demonstrating focal myocardial edema in the subepicardium of the left midventricular lateral wall (red arrows). Corresponding long axis (C) and short axis (D) T1-weighted late gadolinium enhancement images demonstrate presence of typical late gadolinium enhancement in the subepicardium of the left midventricular lateral wall and the basal septum (red arrows). (From Kindermann I, Barth C, Mahfoud F, et al. Update on myocarditis. J Am Coll Cardiol. 2012;59:779-792, with permission.)

sequence has been prone to artifactual interference that decreases specificity.[145] Lastly, a method known as *late gadolinium enhancement (LGE) imaging* looks at evidence of irreversible myocardial injury (i.e., necrosis and fibrosis) by a T1-weight segmented inversion-recovery gradient-echo sequence.[148] LGE images reveal two common patterns of myocardial damage: either an intraluminal rim-like pattern in the septal wall or a subepicardial (patchy) distribution in the free LV lateral wall (see Fig. 28.9).[149] In patients with acute myocarditis, areas of CE are often located in the lateral wall originating from the epicardial quartile, even if the pattern of myocardial injury is influenced by viral infection.[150] It has been suggested that because of the ability of CE to identify areas of myocardial inflammation it can serve as a guide for EMB sampling when necessary,[141] thus enhancing the diagnostic accuracy of biopsy specimens. LGE imaging does not allow differentiation between acute and chronic inflammation; it only represents damaged myocardium, making interpretation dependent upon clinical context.

The limitation associated with cardiac MRI is that it lacks the ability to determine the magnitude of myocardial inflammation and so depends heavily upon clinical context for interpretation. Furthermore, the superior sensitivity is relevant only among patients with acute myocarditis because the clinical features of chronic myocarditis resolve after several weeks to a month. Additionally, cardiac MRI diagnostic criteria have yet to be shown to correlate with EMB samples, which is considered the gold-standard, and so the prognostic value of cardiac MRI remains unclear because criteria have yet to be defined in predicting functional recovery.[146]

Management

Pharmacologic and General Supportive Care. The cornerstones of treatment for myocarditis, regardless of the cause, include removal of any offending agent/toxin and supportive care. Once the diagnosis is established, continuous monitoring in an ICU is recommended because of the risks of ventricular ectopy and hemodynamic deterioration. Offending factors such as toxins, pharmacologic agents, or excessive catecholamines should be eliminated. Limitation of activity or bed rest is recommended because clinical experience suggests that early ambulation and activity may favor viral replication and ongoing myocardial damage. Supportive care is directed at maintaining adequate cardiac output and systemic oxygen delivery. The use of invasive hemodynamic monitoring is based on the patient's clinical status. Although routine use of a pulmonary artery catheter is not recommended, invasive hemodynamic monitoring may be required for the appropriate monitoring of intravascular status and response to inotropic medications. However, the benefits of such monitoring should be weighed against the risks of ventricular ectopy during insertion. Additionally, proper placement may be difficult, requiring fluoroscopic guidance, in the child with a dilated, poorly contractile heart.

The use of inotropic agents may be indicated in patients with signs of poor cardiac output. Because of the irritable state of the myocardium, arrhythmias may be seen with catecholamine administration. In a retrospective database review of the Pediatric Health Information System Database, milrinone was used the majority of the time with the second most-common inotrope choice being epinephrine.[79] Our preference is to use milrinone initially because it has less arrhythmogenicity and can be run more safely through a peripheral IV line. Milrinone is a phosphodiesterase inhibitor and thereby increases the intracellular concentration of cyclic adenosine monophosphate, providing a positive inotropic effect with peripheral vasodilation. In addition, milrinone has lusitropic effects, improving the diastolic function of the myocardium, which may result in improved ventricular relaxation and increased filling volumes during diastole. More aggressive inotropic intervention, such as the combination of inotropic agents and vasodilators, would necessitate stable central access and an arterial blood pressure monitor for continuous hemodynamic monitoring and laboratory surveillance.

Although cardiac failure from myocarditis responds to inotropic agents in the majority of patients,[79] patients who do not respond (patients who have elevated blood lactate levels, who demonstrate evidence of end-organ dysfunction, or in whom the need for excessive inotropic support is associated with worsening ventricular or supraventricular arrhythmias) should be considered for mechanical support. Fulminant myocarditis has a good prognosis with a 61% to 80% survival to discharge after extracorporeal membrane oxygenation (ECMO) with a majority of survivors experiencing recovery of native ventricular function,[151-155] and rescue with mechanical support should be a serious consideration in the failing patient. Furthermore, in a retrospective review of the Extracorporeal Life Support Organization (ELSO) registry, 80% of patients with myocarditis who died on ECMO or were withdrawn from ECMO suffered multiple organ failure,[153] underscoring the importance of expeditious deployment in cases in which there is evidence that standard therapy is insufficient in supporting the patient. In general a low threshold toward early institution of mechanical circulatory support should be maintained because patients with fulminant myocarditis by nature are unpredictable and can often suffer rapid deterioration.

The most commonly used mechanical support is ECMO; it is used in approximately 20% of US children hospitalized with myocarditis.[79] The choice between ECMO and a ventricular assist device (VAD), among centers that can offer both, depends on the size of the patient and the anticipated duration of mechanical support. ECMO can be used in the smallest patients, but the duration of support is usually limited to approximately 3 weeks, during which continuous anticoagulation is required. Patients who undergo ECMO may develop a stunned LV, which may require decompression of the LV in as many as 30% to avoid pulmonary venous hypertension and pulmonary hemorrhage. In those who are cannulated through the chest, a LV vent via the sternotomy is commonly used. In those who are cannulated peripherally, creating an interatrial communication in the catheterization laboratory may be necessary.[151,154] Other disadvantages include platelet and red cell destruction by the pump, necessitating frequent transfusions. Despite these limitations, ECMO has been a very useful tool to support the myocarditis patient because a significant portion will recover sufficient myocardial function to allow weaning from ECMO in 2 to 3 weeks.[151-153,155] Survival, however, drops to below 50% in myocarditis patients who require more than 2 weeks of mechanical support as reported in the ELSO registry.[153] Predictors of mortality include persistent arrhythmia, need for dialysis, and ongoing evidence of end-organ hypoperfusion.[153]

The VAD has revolutionized care in adults with advanced HF, allowing cardiac support for months, even years, without the need for continuous anticoagulation. Continuous-flow VADs used in adults are limited to older children and adolescents.[156] Currently the primary VAD for support in children is the pulsatile Berlin Heart EXCOR, which is a miniaturized, pneumatically driven, pediatric biventricular assist device with a chamber volume as low as 12 mL, which has allowed support in infants as small as 3.5 kg. The US Food and Drug Administration (FDA) approval was obtained for its use in 2011 after an FDA-sanctioned trial demonstrated superior survival and safety compared with a propensity-match cohort of patients supported with ECMO from the ELSO registry.[157] The primary use of the Berlin Heart has been as a bridge to transplant.[158] Mortality has been reported to be as low as 8% with close to 90% receiving transplants.[157] Lower weight, elevated bilirubin level, reduced glomerular filtration rate, and need for biventricular assist device was associated with mortality. Major risk includes a high rate of neurologic adverse events, including thromboembolic stroke, major bleeding, and infection.

Arrhythmias constitute the second life-threatening complication of myocarditis. High-degree AV block may occur in viral myocarditis, but it is especially characteristic of lupus carditis and Lyme carditis. Although patients may respond to isoproterenol administration, such chronotropic drugs entail the risk of inducing ventricular tachycardia, particularly in viral myocarditis. The risk of developing ventricular tachyarrhythmias after chronotropic therapy is perhaps less pronounced in other, nonviral forms of myocarditis. Therefore cardiac pacing is the preferred therapy for life-threatening bradyarrhythmias. Transcutaneous pacing can be placed rapidly and is effective during the resuscitation phase. A temporary transvenous pacemaker can be substituted after the resuscitation is complete. If heart block persists for more than 2 to 3 weeks, the physician should consider replacing the temporary pacemaker with an implanted permanent pacemaker.

Aside from AV block, ventricular ectopy and even sudden death from ventricular fibrillation may occur in myocarditis.[122] Whereas lidocaine has historically been considered standard therapy for ventricular ectopy, no controlled studies support its efficacy in myocarditis. Both clinical experience and studies in other populations, such as cardiac arrest or myocardial infarction, have failed to support its efficacy in ventricular tachyarrhythmias.[159] Conversely, amiodarone may improve survival after cardiac arrest due to ventricular tachyarrhythmias.[160] The AHA now recommends amiodarone as the first-line antiarrhythmic therapy in pulseless ventricular tachycardia or ventricular fibrillation after defibrillation has been attempted.[161] Lidocaine has become a second-tier choice. Antiarrhythmic agents other than lidocaine and amiodarone have a high likelihood of worsening ventricular function and thus are problematic in patients with myocarditis. Aside from pharmacologic therapy, correction of electrolyte imbalances such as hypokalemia and hypomagnesemia may be particularly effective in the treatment of ventricular ectopy. The occurrence of such electrolyte disturbances should be evaluated both initially and periodically during therapy, because diuretic therapy can cause excessive urinary losses of both of these cations.

Supraventricular tachyarrhythmias (SVTs) based on a reentrant mechanism (AV nodal reentrant tachycardia or AV reentrant tachycardia) are treated initially with adenosine if the patient is hemodynamically stable. Intraatrial reentry tachycardia (atrial flutter) often is not responsive to adenosine. In such cases and in patients with frequent reinitiation of SVT, amiodarone is usually the drug of choice. Electrical cardioversion is the treatment of choice in the unstable patient but is of no value in patients with termination and immediate reinitiation of their tachycardia. In the past, digoxin has been used to treat SVT in myocarditis. However, experimental and clinical evidence suggests caution with this approach during the acute phase of myocarditis because digoxin was found to increase myocardial cytokine production.[162] The intracellular calcium loading caused by digoxin may induce or worsen ventricular arrhythmias.

Once the patient's cardiovascular status is stabilized, a gradual switch to more prolonged, oral therapy is indicated. In adults in recent-onset DCM in the Intervention in Myocarditis and Acute Cardiomyopathy 2 (IMAC-2) study, routine use of angiotensin-converting enzyme (ACE) inhibitors and beta-blockers led to a transplantation-free survival of 88% and a survival free of HF hospitalization of 78%.[163] These agents also may be the first-line therapy in patients with a minimal to moderate degree of myocardial dysfunction. Subsequent treatment of HF and LV dysfunction should proceed according to established guidelines of the AHA, ACC, ESC, and Heart Failure Society of America.[164-166] These guidelines suggest ACE inhibition for asymptomatic LV dysfunction, a combination of ACE inhibition and beta-blockade with selective use of aldosterone antagonists in symptomatic HF. Further discussion about the chronic management of HF is beyond the scope of this chapter.

Immunosuppressive Therapy. Although direct viral damage to myocardial cells may be responsible for the cardiac dysfunction in myocarditis, clinical and laboratory evidence also points to immune dysfunction and altered cellular immunity as playing the primary role in many cases.[167] These findings are the foundation on which many have surmised that immunosuppressive therapy may be efficacious in the treatment of viral myocarditis.[168] However, the possible beneficial effects must be weighed against the risks of promoting viral replication during the administration of immunosuppressive agents. Both dramatic improvement and fatal progression of myocarditis have been described after immunosuppressive therapy.[169-171] Once myocarditis is confirmed, the decision to administer such therapy must take into account the morbidity and mortality associated with the use of such agents versus that associated with myocarditis. It also has been recommended that the decision to administer immunosuppressive therapy may be based on the histologic findings, for which immunosuppression is directed toward those with lymphocytic infiltration.

Several reports have described the implementation of immunotherapies in the early treatment of acute myocarditis. These treatments have included the use of IVIG and other immunosuppressant agents such as prednisone, methylprednisolone, azathioprine, and OKT3 at the time of presentation and during the early phase of cardiomyopathy. IVIG has been speculated to be most efficacious during the acute phase of disease with potential benefit in enhancing viral clearance, as well as quenching the inflammatory response triggered by inflammatory cytokines. Other immunosuppressive therapies are felt to aid in suppressing cell-mediated inflammatory and autoimmune reactions, which are more characteristic of the subacute and chronic phase of disease.

Drucker and colleagues[170] noted improved ventricular function and a trend toward improved survival at 12 months for children who received IVIG, 2 gm/kg, as a single dose to treat biopsy-proven myocarditis compared with recent historical controls. To date no randomized controlled trial of immunoglobulin therapy has been conducted in pediatric viral myocarditis. A prospective randomized placebo-controlled study was conducted in adults by McNamara et al.[172] in the IMAC trial that showed a high but not statistically significant different rate of improvement in left ventricular ejection fraction (LVEF) associated with IVIG treatment. Despite this lack of supportive evidence IVIG continues to be used in the acute management of myocarditis. In a study looking at data from the Pediatric Health Information System database, 70% reported use of IVIG in the care of patients with acute myocarditis.[173]

Immunosuppressive therapy is recommended in the management of granulomatous, giant cell,[174,175] and eosinophilic myocarditis[176,177] and lymphocytic myocarditis associated with connective tissue diseases or with heart transplant rejection. Randomized controlled trials of prednisone alone or prednisone plus cyclosporine in adults with acute viral myocarditis have shown either small or no treatment effect.[178,179] In pediatrics there are a number of small case series, retrospective reviews, and mostly uncontrolled studies that have been published on the use of various immunosuppression regimens, including steroids, azathioprine, cyclosporine, and OKT3, in pediatric myocarditis.[88,168,180-184] These studies are small and inadequately powered, so the routine use of immunosuppressive therapy in acute myocarditis cannot be recommended based on current evidence. Despite this lack of evidence, prednisone is currently used in up to 30% of cases of acute myocarditis in the United States.[79]

Immunosuppressive therapy may have a role in the treatment of myocarditis that has progressed to DCM. A study in which patients with evidence of ongoing myocardial injury due to an inflammatory autoimmune process without viral persistence by EMB, termed *inflammatory dilated cardiomyopathy*, were studied in the Tailored Immunosuppression in Inflammatory Cardiomyopathy (TIMIC) trial.[185] This study demonstrated improvement in LVEF and improvement in NYHA class among adults treated with prednisone and azathioprine with concurrent conventional therapy for chronic DCM. A similar study was performed in children also with chronic DCM with evidence of active myocarditis on EMB. Children who were treated with prednisone and azathioprine demonstrated improvements compared to controls. Presence of virus was not a significant predictor of response to treatment in this trial.[186]

Antiviral Therapy. Effective antiviral therapy might have its greatest impact in the very early stages of myocarditis. Most patients with acute myocarditis are diagnosed weeks after viral infection, making it questionable whether therapy during the acute phase could be given early enough to be beneficial. Therapy against the common causes of viral myocarditis has been under investigation over 30 years, during which very few effective agents have been developed. Agents include pharmacologic active low-molecular-weight substances that inhibit the invasion and replication of coxsackievirus, such as pleconaril and ribavirin. Another group includes interferons, which have antiviral and immunomodulating activity, and finally, biologic and cellular therapeutics that interfere with viral invasion by affecting replication and translation at the level of the viral or host RNA. Agents included in this group have their effect through RNA interference and include small interfering RNAs, short hairpin RNAs, and antisense oligonucleotides. These targeted strategies show promise among animal and cell culture studies, but there is presently no evidence in human trials.[187]

Pleconaril represents a class of drugs that specifically targets picornaviruses, including the enteroviruses.[188] This agent integrates into the capsid of the picornavirus and thereby prevents viral attachment to myocyte receptors. Isolated reports have been made showing benefit among children with life-threatening viral infections[189,190]; however, there have been no clinical trials demonstrating the efficacy in patients with myocarditis. Ribavirin is a nucleoside analogue that functions to induce lethal mutations when incorporated into viral RNA. This agent also lacks clinical evidence to support its application.

Treatment with interferon (IFN)-beta has demonstrated potential clinical benefit in patients with long-term LV cardiac dysfunction with clearance of myocardial enteroviral or adenoviral genome and an improvement in LV function.[191] In the double-blind placebo-controlled randomized phase II trial BICC (Betaferon in patients with chronic viral cardiomyopathy) study,[192] 143 patients with inflammatory DCM and confirmed viral genome persistence were treated with Betaferon (IFN-beta-1b). Treatment with Betaferon reduced viral load significantly in the myocardium with a significant improvement in NYHA functional class and patient global assessment. Similar effects on viral clearance have been observed with IFN-alpha in small case series.[193] Natural agents such as astragaloside IV have been shown to decrease CVB3 titers by upregulating IFN-gamma.[173]

Outcome and Natural History. Various factors affect the eventual outcome and natural history of myocarditis, including the cause, the patient's general state of health before the onset of the illness, and the extent of myocardial inflammation. Although mortality early in the course is rare, death may occur related to ventricular arrhythmias, progressive cardiac failure, or conduction disturbances. Early mortality is especially high in infants and young children, approaching 10% to 15%.[93,194] McCarthy and colleagues[93] suggest that adolescent and adult patients may have a better long-term prognosis after fulminant myocarditis, with up to 93% transplant-free survival after 11 years. This has also been observed among pediatric patients, with a 61% to 80% survival to discharge after ECMO with a majority of survivors experiencing recovery of native ventricular function,[151-155] lending to speculation that a more robust inflammatory response as manifested in fulminant disease may be more effective in eradicating viral invasion and thereby ultimately improving recovery and long-term outcomes. Patients with acute myocarditis (nonfulminant) who manifest a less robust immune response during the acute phase of illness demonstrate worse outcomes, with only 45% long-term, transplant-free survival. Data suggest that such chronic patients have evidence of viral persistence on EMB and that antiviral therapies may have a role in this phase of disease. Treatment with immunosuppressants such as steroids, azathioprine,[185,186] and Betaferon[191,192] have demonstrated clearance of viral genome and potential improvement in myocardial function.

Summary

Myocarditis is a descriptive term based on histologic findings showing an inflammatory process of the heart with isolated areas of myocardial cell necrosis. The primary consequences of the inflammatory process are alterations in myocardial function or the potential for arrhythmias or both. Various causes include infectious agents, autoimmune diseases, and drugs/toxins. Autoimmune phenomena may be part of the primary disease process, as with cardiac involvement in SLE or an aberrant immunologic reaction directed at the myocardium such as a postviral myocarditis or the carditis associated with rheumatic fever. With improvements in viral isolation techniques such as PCR, fewer cases are now considered idiopathic. Treatment includes treatment of primary infectious causes, removal of the offending toxin/drug, control of the underlying autoimmune process, and provision of pharmacologic support of the failing myocardium. With the adoption of an aggressive approach toward hemodynamic support, which includes judicious and expeditious deployment of mechanical support, clinical outcomes have been very good with excellent long-term outcomes. Furthermore, with revelation of the association of DCM and myocarditis with viral persistence, we are gaining better insight as to means to help treat such patients. Application of antiviral therapies to eradicate chronic viral myocardial persistence may have a place in future therapeutic algorithms in patients with DCM. Furthermore, investigations into the mechanisms of viral invasion have led to insight toward novel biologic and cellular therapeutics such as RNA interference that will potentially open the door to a completely new armamentarium to treat disease.

References

A complete list of references is available at ExpertConsult.com.

29

Fetus With Critical Heart Disease— Bridging to Birth

RYAN LOFTIN, MD; MIGUEL DELEON, MD

The care of newborns with congenital heart disease (CHD) has changed dramatically in the last 20 years, leading to the improvement of both survival rates and patient outcomes. Prenatal care and prenatal assessment, along with the availability of technology and quality initiatives that have become standard of care, are major contributing factors. With these changes providers are able to conduct a more comprehensive prenatal assessment and better understand the physiologic changes that occur in utero. Advanced technology has made it possible to diagnose CHD and other associated abnormalities during fetal life. The provider is able to have a better understanding about the physiology of complex heart defects and those factors that would indicate deterioration of the cardiac condition. Based on these findings, the provider can decide to either manage certain conditions in utero or refer the patient to a tertiary center that is better prepared and equipped to manage complications. The information also helps both the provider and the family to better prepare for the time of delivery. When families are informed, they are able to make better choices about potential outcomes. When there is limited or no prenatal care, the provider is unable to adequately screen the baby for possible cardiac complications, putting both the provider and the baby at risk. Families are not able to make choices, and providers are not able to adequately plan for the time or place of delivery.

Ultrasound Screening for Congenital Cardiac Defects

Ultrasound screening for anatomic abnormalities is routine in most areas of the United States. The specialties of providers performing the examinations are often regionally varied, with radiology performing examinations in some areas, general obstetrician gynecologists in others, and in a few areas, maternal fetal medicine (MFM) providers perform the screening ultrasound services. The quality of ultrasound equipment has improved dramatically over the past decades. However, the interpreting providers must be competent in the reading of imaging and know when further evaluation is needed. There are organizations that provide certification of prenatal imaging laboratories, such as the American Institute for Ultrasound in Medicine. Part of the certification processes is to ensure that ultrasound technologists are adequately trained and able to acquire appropriate images,

as well as the need for continuing education in ultrasonography for physicians. The certification process may not be feasible for all practices but does provide a means of assessing competency verification.

As part of the general screening of all fetuses, we advocated for acquiring a four-chamber view, outflow tracts, arches, and a three-vessel trachea view. When a cardiac abnormality is suspected or the risk is sufficiently high based on maternal risks, fetal genetics, or family history, a detailed fetal cardiac examination is warranted. This is typically performed by either MFM providers or pediatric cardiologists with a specific interest and training in prenatal cardiac imaging. Fetal echocardiography will provide additional cardiac structural views and functional assessments, with the goal of optimizing diagnosis as much as possible before delivery.

When a fetal cardiac defect is found, the pregnant patient and her family will need additional follow-up and support. In our organization, if the defect is seen initially by MFM, we refer the patient to the fetal cardiology department for the next available appointment. We have a multidisciplinary team consisting of MFM, pediatric cardiology, neonatology, genetics, and pediatric cardiovascular surgery that is available to counsel patients. It is not uncommon for the initial shock of the diagnosis to create a barrier to processing information. Thus parents are often brought back to discuss findings again in a few days or a week later.

After confirming as well as possible the prenatal diagnosis, the team counsels the patient regarding expectations in the early neonatal period and longer-term outcomes. We have a fetal coordinator who is a registered nurse and takes patients through the neonatal intensive care nursery (NICU)/pediatric intensive care nursery (PICU) as appropriate to familiarize the family with the location. As much as possible, we attempt to make plans and contingencies that will be followed known to the patient and her family so that the element of surprise is reduced after delivery. Close contact with the primary obstetric provider is important to continue to support the family and as a means of following up with patients who may withdraw upon receiving bad news.

Our multidisciplinary team meets regularly to go over upcoming patients and to help determine the immediate neonatal plan. As pregnancy progresses, the plans may need to be updated as the condition or diagnosis evolves. The plan is relayed to the obstetric providers, neonatal providers, and facilities where delivery is anticipated.

Care of the Fetus/Neonate With Critical Cardiac Defects

In rare cases, such as fetuses with suspected hypoplastic left heart and restricted atrial septum or transposition of the great arteries with intact septum, an early septostomy may be needed. In these cases delivery in a facility that can provide this emergent procedure may be lifesaving for the child. In these cases abdominal delivery to provide logistic support may be considered as part of the management of the fetus. For example, in some centers, delivery may be performed in the children's hospital or regional maternity hospital with the pediatric catheterization laboratory held open to receive the newborn. The coordination of the resources needed for these deliveries is often intense. Facilities that choose to perform these procedures should have active ongoing training programs and case review for improvement in process. If uncertain whether the child will need immediate intervention, it is better to transfer to a facility for delivery that can handle the emergent procedure if necessary.

Neonatal Resuscitation Program and the Critical Congenital Heart Defect Screen

Although changes in prenatal assessment and technologies can help to improve care and outcomes for babies with CHD, they can pose several challenges at many different levels for providers of both maternal care and newborn care. Providers are responsible for making sure that the necessary technologies and training are made available to support both maternal and newborn care. Two important initiatives are the Neonatal Resuscitation Program (NRP) and the Critical Congenital Heart Defect Screen.

The NRP, sponsored by the American Academy of Pediatrics (AAP), is an evidence-based approach focusing on resuscitation skills for the newborn. The NRP provides a basic algorithm for neonatal resuscitation, offering effective team-based care for health care providers caring for newborns at birth in the delivery room or nursery. It is essential that health care providers caring for newborns obtain and maintain NRP training.

The Critical Congenital Heart Defect Screen is a tool for early detection of critical congenital heart defect (CCHD). Eighteen out of every 10,000 babies are born with CCHD, which requires early intervention. Because CCHD may not be detected prenatally or upon examination, there is a risk that infants with CCHD may quickly decompensate when discharged from the nursery to home. CCHD screening has been found to be an effective way to detect serious health issues in what appears to be a well newborn. The AAP recommends screening after 24 hours of age or right before discharge if the baby is less than 24 hours of age. All babies at risk for undetected CCHD should be screened, which would be any baby that is not known to have CCHD.

Levels of Newborn Care

There are four levels of care for newborn infants: level I, well-newborn nursery; level II, special care nursery; level III, NICU; and level IV, regional NICU. The majority of babies are born in a lower level of neonatal care, so it is necessary to have a basic line of service to manage a potential congenital heart defect and to be prepared for an emergency. This service would include having NRP-certified personnel present at all deliveries and the ability to do CCHD screening. Essentially there are two scenarios for the

birth of a baby with a complex cardiac defect. One scenario is the unknown and undiagnosed cardiac defect with or without cardiovascular compromise that may or may not initially be obvious to the clinician and is asymptomatic at birth. The second scenario is the birth of a baby with a known diagnosed complex cardiac defect.

Unknown Cardiac Defect Preparation

The more frequent scenarios are those in which there has been limited or no prenatal screening and a baby is born with an unidentified cardiac defect. These babies can develop a rapidly deteriorating cardiovascular compromise with or without cyanosis. In this case it is critical to have several processes in place: rapid access to cardiac consultation, preferably in person with a pediatric cardiologist or a consult via telemedicine; access within 60 minutes to an echocardiogram; and a provider who is competent in managing basic airway support and intravenous (IV) access. Additionally, it is important to have available lifesaving medications such as prostaglandin and personnel that are trained to prepare and administer the drug. Personnel should also be familiar with code medications that are routinely used when providing NRP. In addition to providing emergent treatment, it is important to have an established referral agreement with other units that can provide a higher level of care and availability of a transport system that can expedite and facilitate transporting the infant to a tertiary center.

Known Cardiac Defect Preparation

When a pregnancy has been diagnosed with a complex heart defect, it is imperative to discuss the findings, the potential outcomes, and the medical options with the family. There may be a case in which the mother-baby dyad needs to be comanaged with a MFM specialist group that is specialized in obstetric care and competent, certified, and experienced in the care of fetal complications. Special attention should be given to the option of a planned delivery in which multidisciplinary care can be provided for both the mother and baby. This field is rapidly changing, and it is now becoming a common practice for MFMs, along with pediatric cardiologists and neonatologists, to manage fetal congestive heart failure and arrhythmias that otherwise would either affect the outcome of the baby or end up in a premature delivery. It is also important to have access to interventional cardiologists, pediatric cardiovascular anesthesiologists, pediatric cardiovascular surgeons, pediatric cardiac intensivists, and ECMO. Other important ancillary services include genetics, a chaplain, and a dedicated PICU and NICU specialized in congenital heart defects. When the mother is referred to a tertiary center, it is important to have the support of social services and case workers who can assist with relocation, housing needs, care for other siblings, and financial assistance. Ideally, these patients are triaged before birth so that bonding (yes/no), emergent lines (yes/no), PGE dependence, and admitting unit (PCICU/NICU) are all determined before delivery. This ensures that appropriate triage is performed before delivery.

Support for Lower Levels of Newborn Care—Undiagnosed Cardiac Defects

Tertiary care centers can support their referral areas by providing NRP courses and offering cardiac education to assess for clinical signs of a heart defect. In addition to education, tertiary centers can provide to their referral areas algorithms on how to stabilize the baby with a cardiac defect as soon as feasible. Prostaglandin is an essential medication for the treatment of cyanotic heart defects and should be readily available for the appropriate patients. Providing education on mixing and dosing the medication, along with instruction for indication and administration, would be beneficial in care of the baby with a cyanotic heart defect.

Fetal Arrhythmias

Fetal arrhythmias occur frequently, and, although there has been great progress in the interpretation of fetal heart tones associated with fetal compromise, it may be difficult to identify the differences, making it difficult to make medical decisions or to conduct a proper assessment. This can lead to an untimely premature delivery. There is not a clear correlation of fetal heart tones being directly associated with a specific heart defect.

Basic differentiation needs to be established for the clinician. The presence of fetal bradycardia, which may be persistent or intermittent, should be differentiated from the bradycardia caused by fetal distress, fetal hypoxemia, acidosis, or maternal medications or related to heart block with or without structural cardiac anomalies. Fetal tachycardia may typically be associated with maternal fever or chorioamnionitis; however, in situations in which the heart rate is over 220 beats/min careful consideration needs to be given to one of the tachyarrhythmias that poses a high risk for fetal compromise. Therefore establishing a careful differentiation is crucial. In the most complex scenario of significant persistent tachycardia, it is urgent to have proper diagnosis and treatment because it can significantly compromise the cardiovascular fetal system, leading to fetal death or hydrops. Timely consultation either by a pediatric cardiologist or an MFM specialist is imperative to determine the cause and risk. If an MFM specialist is unavailable, the transfer of the mother to a tertiary center for further care is necessary and would be recommended before delivery. Delivery can generally be delayed or the dysrhythmia managed.

As we better understand these complications, it is becoming crucial to establish a network of tertiary services to assist remote areas or low-volume obstetric systems that lack local consultative services.

Monitoring

The fetal cardiovascular profile score provides standard parameters for heart size and cardiac function, presence of hydrops, and arterial Doppler and venous Doppler ultrasonography. The score can be used in the surveillance of fetal hydrops to predict the presence of congestive heart failure and fetal outcome.

Continuous fetal monitoring of patients during labor is important, but the benefits in long-term outcomes have not been proven. There is a correlation with higher incidences of having an emergency cesarean section. Fetal dysrhythmias may also make electronic fetal monitoring in labor impossible. Presently there is no evidence of improved outcomes when choosing an elective cesarean section, but a planned delivery at a center prepared for neonatal complications may offer better access to timely intervention.

Level IV Tertiary Care Centers—Known Cardiac Defects

For patients who have been prenatally diagnosed and delivered in a tertiary center, intense scrutiny should be offered to optimize outcomes. Care needs to be individualized and multidisciplinary.

For a pregnancy with a known complex heart defect the immediate care should be more predictable. Proper counseling should be done in advance by both the neonatologist and pediatric cardiologist. The outcomes should be discussed and the medical options explained. In the case of a lethal condition in which the outcome is poor, compassionate care should be offered, emotional and spiritual support should be made available, and informational literature provided to the families to help them to make decisions that are mutually agreeable in advance. Also a second opinion should be offered.

In the event of a fetus with a complex heart defect that may require invasive management after delivery, advance notice should be given to the ECMO rapid response team and the emergency interventional catheterization team. A skilled and experienced neonatologist should be present at the delivery. In some cases a cesarean section may be considered for logistic reasons to have all the teams ready for delivery.

It is also important to consider some fetal interventions that may improve the outcomes. Fetal septostomy is being used in some tertiary centers in cases that may benefit. This is a technology that is in progress, and the outcomes are being studied to evaluate the benefits. Tertiary centers more commonly perform complex procedures like placement of drainage catheters in case of Hydrops Fetalis for decompression of pleural or abdominal effusions. This consequently can improve pregnancy outcomes.

When decisions are made for a fetal intervention, the risks should be discussed, and families should be prepared for a suboptimal outcome that can be compounded by a preterm birth. This may limit the surgical postnatal options.

Cardiac Defects

The most serious conditions that require immediate care and are at risk for rapid decompensation are uncontrolled arrhythmias, complete heart block, Ebstein anomaly with hydrops, total anomalous venous return, hypoplastic left heart syndrome with restrictive patent foramen ovale, d-transposition of great vessels with intact septum, and tetralogy of Fallot with pulmonary valve atresia (PVA).

In cases of serious arrhythmias a pediatric cardiologist with experience in electrophysiology should assist in the management. The medical team should work together in concert with the obstetrician and the neonatologist to expedite care. Preparation should be done to establish airway and intravenous access. Monitoring electrocardiographic disturbances and making the right diagnosis promptly should optimize the best antiarrhythmic options when needed. Also, cardioversion equipment should be made available and managed by experienced users. All of these actions should be done in a controlled environment in a cardiac intensive care unit (ICU).

The care of these babies is complex and needs to be done by a team of experienced cardiologists and intensivists. The timing of delivery, the preparation, and the execution should provide the best outcomes. The physical location should be a consideration because all these interventions may be needed rapidly. The consequences may be fatal if treatment is delayed, or at best the long-term outcomes may be compromised. Close proximity to the cardiac ICU is important when expecting the birth of a very unstable compromised baby. Preparation for multidisciplinary care may include a tertiary care obstetrician, fetal intervention, immediate care at delivery, heart catheterization, ECMO, and ultimately the arrangement for cardiac surgery. All these disciplines should be part of the care of a newborn with complex congenital heart defect.

For babies that may develop catastrophic cardiovascular collapse a differential diagnosis should be established, managed properly, and transferred to a tertiary care when indicated.

Babies with fulminant sepsis, pulmonary hypertension, and cyanotic heart defects share a lot of the same clinical signs, and, although some of the management choices may be similar, an early proper diagnosis is important to decide further management. When a baby has a ductal dependent lesion, careful use of oxygen is important, and prostaglandin should be readily available. Also it is important to simultaneously make arrangements to transfer to a tertiary center.

Summary

In summary there are two groups of babies that need to be subdivided and managed according to circumstances: the unknown, undiagnosed congenital heart defect and the known fetal cardiac complications. For the unknown defects there are three distinct groups to be identified: (1) association of lethal anomalies so compromised that no viable care would allow time for proper diagnosis and treatment; (2) rapid clinical deterioration with either significant cyanosis or global cardiovascular decompensation requiring rapid intervention, stabilization, specialized cardiology evaluation, and transfer if necessary to a tertiary level institution; and (3) elective evaluation to include stable cyanosis, nondecompensated arrhythmias, heart murmurs, or perhaps failure of the cyanosis CHD test.

For the unknown, undiagnosed cardiac complications, local resources should be considered either in person or via telemedicine in order to perform a full cardiac evaluation. Care should be coordinated based on the availability of local resources, the level of care nursery, and diagnosis. In cases in which a higher-level NICU and a pediatric cardiologist are available, it may be appropriate to monitor and manage as indicated. In case of malignant arrhythmias, proper electrophysiologic management should be arranged to provide the best care either in person or via telemedicine.

For the known fetal cardiac complications the time and the place of delivery should be planned with the expectation of the medical and surgical needs. A neonatologist and a pediatric

TABLE 29.1 Type of Congenital Heart Disease and Delivery Recommendations

Definition	Example CHD	Delivery Recommendations	DR Recommendations
CHD in which palliative care is planned	CHD with severe/fatal chromosome abnormality or multisystem disease	Arrange for family support/palliative care service Normal delivery at local hospital	—
CHD without predicted risk of hemodynamic instability in the DR or first days of life	VSD, ASD, mild TOF	Arrange cardiology consultation or outpatient evaluation Normal delivery at local hospital	Routine DR care Neonatal evaluation
CHD with minimal risk of hemodynamic instability in DR requiring postnatal catheterization/surgery	Ductal dependent lesions, including HLHS, critical coarctation, severe AS, IAA, PA/IVS, severe TOF	Consider planned induction, usually near term Delivery at hospital with neonatologist and accessible cardiology consultation	Neonatologist in DR Routine DR care, initiate PGE if indicated Transport for catheterization/surgery
CHD with likely hemodynamic instability in DR requiring immediate specialty care for stabilization	d-TGA with concerning atrial septum primum (it is reasonable to consider all d-TGA fetuses without an ASD at risk) Uncontrolled arrhythmias CHB with heart failure	Planned induction at 38-39 wk; consider CS if necessary to coordinate services Delivery at hospital that can execute rapid care, including necessary stabilizing/lifesaving procedures	Neonatologist and cardiac specialist in DR, including all necessary equipment Plan for intervention as indicated by diagnosis Plan for urgent transport if indicated
CHD with expected hemodynamic instability with placental separation requiring immediate catheterization/surgery in DR to improve chance of survival	HLHS/severely RFO or IAS d-TGA/severely RFO or IAS and abnormal DA Obstructed TAPVR Ebstein anomaly with hydrops TOF with APV and severe airway obstruction Uncontrolled arrhythmias with hydrops CHB with low ventricular rate, EFE, and/or hydrops	CS in cardiac facility with necessary specialists in the DR usually at 38-39 wk	Specialized cardiac care team in DR Plan for intervention as indicated by diagnosis; may include catheterization, surgery, or ECMO

APV, Absent pulmonary valve; *AS,* aortic stenosis; *ASD,* atrial septal defect; *CHB,* complete heart block; *CHD,* congenital heart disease; *CS,* cesarean section; *DA,* ductus arteriosus; *DR,* delivery room; *d-TGA,* d-transposition of the great arteries; *ECMO,* extracorporeal membrane oxygenation; *EFE,* endocardial fibroelastosis; *HLHS,* hypoplastic left heart syndrome; *IAA,* interrupted aortic arch; *IAS,* intact atrial septum; *PA/IVS,* pulmonary atresia/intact ventricular septum; *PGE,* prostaglandin; *RFO,* restrictive foramen ovale; *TAPVR,* total anomalous pulmonary venous return; *TOF,* tetralogy of Fallot; *VSD,* ventricular septal defect.

Modified from Donofrio MT, Levy RJ, Schuette JJ, et al. Specialized delivery room planning for fetuses with critical congenital heart disease. *Am J Cardiol.* 2012;111:737–747.

TABLE 29.2 Current Recommendations for Fetal Predictors for Delivery Planning

CHD	Fetal Echocardiographic Finding	Delivery Recommendation

Ductal dependent lesions	Ductal dependent pulmonary circulation:
	  Aorta to pulmonary flow in the DA
	  Reversed orientation of the DA
	Ductal dependent systemic circulation:
	  Left-to-right atrial flow across the foramen ovale
		No specialized care in the DR
		Initiation of prostaglandin E_1

HLHS with RFO or IAS	Ratio of pulmonary vein forward to reverse velocity-time integral <3 Maternal hyperoxygenation in third trimester with no change in fetal branch pulmonary artery pulsatility index	Plan for possible urgent intervention to decompress left atrium (catheterization balloon or stent; surgery)

d-TGA	Reported FO findings predictive of restriction:
	  Angle of septum primum <30 degrees to the atrial septum
	  Bowing of septum primum into the left atrium >50%
	  Lack of normal swinging motion of septum primum
	  Hypermobile septum primum (all fetuses with d-TGA and concerning septum primum should be considered at risk)
	Abnormal DA findings:
	  Small (low z score)
	  Accelerated forward, bidirectional, or reversed diastolic flow
		Plan for urgent balloon atrial septostomy, on site if possible in the DR or ICU
		Initiation of prostaglandin E1
		Consider therapy for pulmonary hypertension with abnormal DA flow

TOF with APV	Lung finding suggestive of lobar emphysema (fluid trapping) on MRI	Specialized ventilation Consider ECMO
Ebstein anomaly	Hydrops fetalis Uncontrolled arrhythmia	Consider early delivery with measures to decrease pulmonary resistance, treat arrhythmias, and support cardiac output
TAPVR, obstructed	Decompressing vein below the diaphragm Accelerated flow in decompressing vein	Consider ECMO
Tachyarrhythmias	Rapid heart rate Decreased heart function Pericardial effusion/hydrops fetalis	Consider early delivery if appropriate gestational age Urgent cardioversion or medical therapy in DR if possible
CHB	Decreasing CVP score (to <7) Very low ventricular rate Decreased heart function/EFE Hydrops fetalis	Consider early delivery Consider medical chronotrope or temporary pacing in DR if possible

CHB, Complete heart block; CHD, congenital heart disease; CVP, cardiovascular profile; DA, ductus arteriosus; DR, delivery room; d-TGA, transposition of the great arteries; ECMO, extracorporeal membrane oxygenation; EFE, endocardial fibroelastosis; FO, foramen ovale; HLHS, hypoplastic left heart syndrome; IAS, intact atrial septum; ICU, intensive care unit; MRI, magnetic resonance imaging; RFO, restrictive foramen ovale; TAPVR, total anomalous pulmonary venous return; TOF with APV, tetralogy of Fallot with absent pulmonary valve.
Reprinted with permission Circulation. 2014;129:2183-2242. Copyright 2014 American Heart Association, Inc.

cardiologist should be part of the team planning the delivery. In an unexpected emergency both services should be readily available. Close proximity to a cardiac ICU with experienced staff is important. If a planned cardiac intervention is foreseen, plans should be coordinated with an interventional cardiologist. A pediatric cardiac surgeon should participate in the plan of care. As with all congenital defects, the family should be as informed as possible before delivery and understand the most likely outcome and alternative scenarios. The psychosocial care of the pregnant patient and her family should not be neglected.

A NICU team competent in airway management and experienced with managing critical newborns should be present at delivery. In view of the multilateral complexity, ancillary services are very important, including advanced practice staff, cardiac nurses, chaplains, social workers, and case managers. If indicated, a transport team should be timely informed and prepared in advance. They should be competent in the management and stabilization of critical newborns.

At delivery the team should be prepared to stabilize airway, provide IV access, manage cardiac support, have available antiarrhythmic medications, be prepared for cardioversion, and be prepared for pleural evacuation. A rapid-response ECMO team should be in place when indicated. All of these preparations for the most part would provide the best chance for an optimum transition to newborn circulation in order to make an adequate evaluation and as a team decide the best treatment choices.

Selected Readings

American Academy of Pediatrics and American Heart Association. Textbook of Neonatal Resuscitation, 7th ed.

Altman CA, Identifying newborns with critical congenital heart disease. UpToDate Website. www.uptodate.comPublished 2017. Accessed February 19, 2017.

Hofstaetter C, Hansmann M, Eik-Nes SH, Huhta JC, Luther SL. A cardiovascular profile score in the surveillance of fetal hydrops.

J Matern Fetal Neonatal Med. 2006;407–413. doi:10.1080/14767050600682446.

Simpson JM. Impact of fetal echocardiography. *Ann Pediatr Cardiol.* 2009;2(1):41–50. doi:10.4103/0974-2069.52806.

Sanapo L, Moon-Grady AJ, Donofrio MT. Perinatal and delivery management of infants with congenital heart disease. *Clin Perinatol.* 2016;43:55–71.

Cannobbio MM, Warness CA. American Heart Association Council on Cardiovascular Disease and Stroke, Nursing. *Circulation.* 2017;135(8):e50–e87. Review.

Peterson AL, Quartermain MD, Andes A, et al. Impact of mode of delivery on markers of perinatal hemodynamics in infants of hypoplastic left heart syndrome. *J Pediatrics.* 2011;159:64–69.

Park, Myung K, Parks. The Pediatric Cardiology Handbook, Dosages of drugs used in Pediatric Cardiology (458-89).

Donofrio MT, Levy RJ, Schuette JJ, Skurow-Todd K, Sten MB, Stallings C, et al. Specialized delivery room planning for fetuses with critical congenital heart disease. *Am J Cardiology.* 2013;111(5):737–747.

30

Low Birth Weight and Other High-Risk Conditions

MATTHEW H.L. LIAVA'A, FRACS; GANGA KRISHNAMURTHY, MBBS;
PAUL J. CHAI, MD

The prevalence of congenital heart disease (CHD) ranges from 6 to 10 per 1000 live births, and CHD is the most common birth defect.[1,2] Nearly 40,000 infants are born with CHD each year in the United States, and over 1 million babies are born every year worldwide.[3] Many of these infants will require surgery to correct or palliate their heart defect during their lifetime, and some require surgery in the newborn period.

In North America between 2007 and 2010 the age distribution of the approximately 80,000 patients undergoing cardiac surgery for CHD across 96 centers is shown in Fig. 30.1.[4] Although neonates constituted only 25% of the total surgical volume, they accounted for more than 50% of all the deaths (Fig. 30.2). Continual advances in surgical and cardiopulmonary bypass (CPB) techniques, as well as improved preoperative and postoperative management, have resulted in a general decline in operative mortality across all age-groups.[5] However, neonates have the highest mortality risk.[4] Multiple factors contribute to a mortality rate of approximately 10% after neonatal cardiac surgery.[4]

Lesions requiring surgery in the neonatal period are often quite complex. Technical challenges include tissue fragility, cannulation, and maintenance of adequate CPB. The performance of intricate procedures in tiny hearts requires superior technical skill and years of experience for mastery.[6]

Abnormal preoperative circulation and the effects of CPB on immature organ systems are additional factors that place neonates at greater risk for death after surgery. Premature birth and low birth weight (LBW) add substantial risk.[7,8] Neonates born before 37 completed weeks of gestation are at greater risk of death after cardiac surgery than those born after 37 weeks.[6] However, the risk of death after 37 weeks is not uniformly equivalent. Population and single-center studies have revealed this phenomenon both in babies born with CHD and in those without.[9] There is an incremental decline in death rate from 37 to 40 weeks, with the nadir at 39 to 40 weeks.[6] Death rates increase again if delivery is delayed beyond 41 weeks. Most babies with CHD are born before 39 to 40 weeks of gestation; this is often to allow better coordination of delivery, catheter intervention if necessary, and to avoid in utero demise. Extending pregnancy from 37 to 38 weeks to 39 to 40 weeks provides a significant survival benefit and reduces the risk of complications.[8] Therefore elective delivery of babies before 39 completed weeks of gestation, absent any obstetric or fetal risk, should be discouraged.

Term gestation is actually delineated by statistical probability and ranges from 37 weeks to 42 weeks. Thirty-seven weeks is an entirely arbitrary beginning for term gestation, and the period between the two limits represents a continuum during which organ maturity continues. Therefore babies born in the "early term" period are physiologically less mature than babies born in "late term." The exact physiologic immaturity that places early-term neonates at greater risk of mortality likely represents incomplete development of several organ systems. Even at birth, organ maturation is unlikely to be complete but is a gradual process that continues for several months and years after birth. Neonates are disadvantaged in comparison to infants and older children because of this multiorgan immaturity.

Immature Organ Systems

Cardiovascular

Postnatal Increase in Left Ventricular Output. At birth the ratio of metabolic rate to oxygen consumption increases several-fold because of the additional demands imposed by heat conservation mechanisms and respiratory activity.[10-12] Oxygen delivery increases in a similar proportion to maintain normal oxygen reserve capacity. Much of the increase in oxygen delivery is attributed to a substantial increase in left ventricular output after birth. Enhanced left ventricular output is caused by an increase in heart rate, an increase in left ventricular preload, and greater inotropic state.[13-15] The exact mechanisms causing this postnatal increase in cardiac output are not completely known, but thyroid hormone is believed to play a role.[16] Fetal lambs in which the thyroid gland was removed 2 weeks before delivery demonstrated low plasma levels of triiodothyronine (T_3) and failed to show the expected postnatal increase in T_3 levels and cardiac output.[16] These same lambs had fewer beta-adrenergic receptors on the myocardial surface and exhibited a blunted response to beta-adrenergic stimulation.[16] Elevation in cortisol levels, a catecholamine surge, and relief from ventricular constraint at delivery also contribute to the postnatal elevation in cardiac output.[17-19]

Developmental Differences in Myocardial Structure and Excitation-Contraction Coupling. Generation of myocardial contractile force increases with maturation.[20-22] Developmental differences in contractility are mostly caused by age-related differences in myocardial structure (Fig. 30.3).

The immature myocyte is smaller and has greater intracellular spatial disorganization than its mature counterpart.[22] Also, a large proportion of the immature myocyte is inhabited by noncontractile

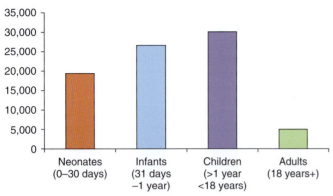

Figure 30.1 Age distribution of patients who underwent cardiac surgery for congenital heart disease between 2007 and 2010 in 96 centers in North America.

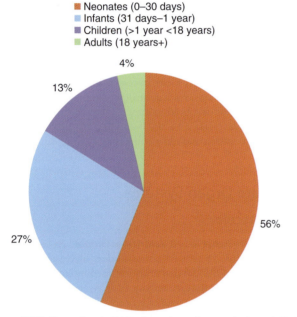

Figure 30.2 Proportional distribution of cardiac surgical mortality by age-group between 2007 and 2010 in 96 centers in North America.

Neonatal myocyte

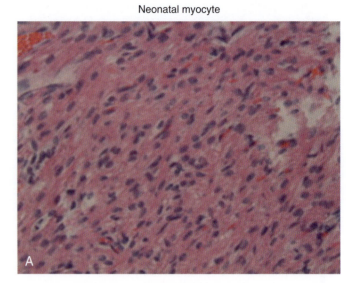

Adult myocyte

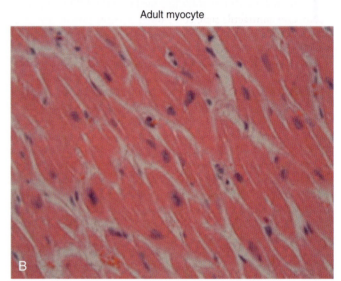

Figure 30.3 Sections of neonatal and adult human myocardium. Hematoxin and eosin stain.

organelles that do not contribute to force generation. The small, spherical structure of the immature myocyte and the central location of noncontractile elements impose a biophysical disadvantage to shortening.[22]

Immature myofibrils assume a random arrangement rather than the parallel arrangement seen in adult myocytes.[21-23] There are also far fewer myofilaments—the fundamental units of cross-bridge formation.[23] An increased number of myofilaments correlates with an increase in myocardial force generation.[24] Isoform switching of myofibrillar proteins with development also contributes to improved contractile efficiency with age.[25,26]

The calcium-handling mechanism in the neonate is both underdeveloped and inefficient.[23] The cytosolic calcium concentration is primarily dependent on transsarcolemmal flux of calcium because T-tubules and sarcoplasmic reticulum are scarce and intracellular calcium regulatory proteins are functionally immature.[27-30] Neonatal myocardium is more sensitive to changes in extracellular ionized calcium and relies more on glucose

metabolism. Thus there is a greater risk for myocardial dysfunction given the neonates' decreased stores of calcium, inadequate glycogen stores, and impaired gluconeogenesis.[31]

Adult myocardium is densely innervated by a plexus of sympathetic nerves.[32] However, sympathetic innervation in neonatal myocardium is incomplete.[24,32] Parasympathetic tone predominates, and hypotensive episodes are easily evoked.[33]

Cardiac stores of norepinephrine, a reflection of sympathetic innervation, is lowest in late-term fetuses but approaches adult levels by 4 weeks of age.[34] This is despite no significant quantitative difference between neonatal and adult beta-adrenergic receptors on the myocardial cell surface.[35,36] Functional uncoupling of beta-receptor–G protein–adenylate cyclase complex in the newborn limits the effectiveness of catecholamine-modulated contractility in this age-group.[37]

Neonatal Ventricular Performance. Circulatory adaptation at birth is vital to meeting the increased metabolic demands of extrauterine life. An acute increase in heart rate, pulmonary venous

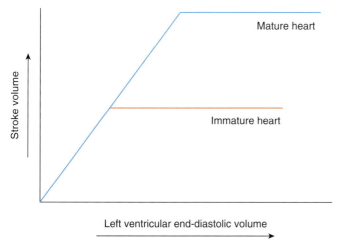

Figure 30.4 Relationship of left ventricular end-diastolic volume and stroke volume in immature and mature hearts.

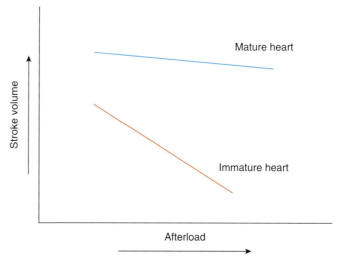

Figure 30.5 Relationship of afterload and stroke volume in mature and immature hearts.

return, and contractile state contributes to the postnatal enhancement in cardiac output.[13,15] High resting inotropism limits contractile reserve in newborns, and immature hearts exhibit a blunted response to exogenous catecholamines compared with mature hearts.[38] Rate-dependent mechanisms to improve cardiac output are thus favored in neonates.

The immature heart has less recruitable preload reserve and demonstrates only a modest Frank-Starling relationship compared to the adult mature heart[39-41] (Fig. 30.4).

This limited response to volume loading is partly due to the decreased compliance of immature hearts. With age, maturational changes in cytoskeleton and extracellular matrix improve myocardial compliance.[42,43]

Volume or pressure loading of one ventricle can impact filling of the contralateral ventricle to a greater extent in immature hearts than in more mature ones.[44] This restrictive effect is particularly evident in neonates who have endured an unfavorable postnatal transition and exhibit persistent fetal circulation. The pressure-loaded right ventricle (RV) alters septal dynamics and limits left ventricular filling and left ventricular stroke volume.

Increases in afterload profoundly diminish ventricular performance in the fetus and neonate.[24] When exposed to similar afterloads, the immature myocyte shortens to a lesser extent and more slowly than a mature myocyte. Developmental changes in myocyte architecture permit the adult heart to counteract afterload stressors more effectively[23] (Fig. 30.5).

Congenital Heart Disease and Postnatal Circulation. Most babies with structural heart disease experience an unremarkable transition to postpartum conditions. In neonates with ductal dependent circulations, symptoms will emerge with constriction of the ductus arteriosus. However, abnormal circulatory patterns in some forms of CHD may impose hemodynamic challenges immediately at birth:

- Babies with hypoplastic left heart syndrome with a restrictive atrial communication
- d-Transposition of the great vessels with intact ventricular septum and restrictive foramen ovale

In some forms of CHD the inherent limitations of the neonatal myocardial mechanics are also exposed:

- Severe aortic stenosis
  - There is limited ability to increase myocardial performance in the face of increased afterload.

- Lesions with left-to-right shunts
  - Recruitment of the Frank-Starling mechanism and increasing the inotropic state accomplish much of the increased stroke work required to maintain adequate systemic flow. However, large shunts may overwhelm the limited preload and contractile reserve of the newborn heart. Babies with hypoplastic left heart syndrome are particularly vulnerable. In these neonates, excessive pulmonary blood flow can limit systemic flow. Right ventricular output must increase several-fold to maintain systemic flow, and the right ventricular functional reserves may be insufficient to maintain systemic flow.

Other Immature Organ Systems

Other organ systems may also be incompletely developed, especially in premature and LBW babies, but even in the infant born at term. A brief summation of critical systems is provided.

Respiratory

Fetal lungs achieve drastic maturation at the end of gestation.[45] In preterm neonates this last surge of lung maturity is absent, resulting in significantly impaired alveolarization and dysmorphic vasculogenesis.[46] As a result, functional residual capacity is reduced and has an adverse impact on respiratory function.[47] Surfactant deficiency is common and leads to respiratory distress syndrome if untreated.[48]

Chest wall structure and limited diaphragmatic apposition introduces mechanical inefficiencies in ventilation. The neonatal lung and chest wall possess variable compliances—the lungs are less compliant, whereas the chest wall is extremely compliant.[49] This uncoupling predisposes the chest wall to deformational forces, and much of the respiratory energy is expended in counteracting these forces.[49] Compensation is with a higher resting respiratory rate than that seen in older children and adults.

Renal and Gastrointestinal

Nephrogenesis is completed at 35 weeks of gestation; however, structural and functional growth of the kidney continues for several months after birth.[50] The biggest limitation in renal function in the neonate is the rate of glomerular filtration, which, in the first few days of life, is one-third that seen in adults.[51] Tubular and medullary renal function limit the maximal urine-concentrating ability of the newborn infant to half that of an adult.[52] These functional limitations make the neonate more vulnerable to fluid overload or depletion.

Premature infants are at increased risk for necrotizing enterocolitis. The main risk factors are poor systemic perfusion (particularly if the cardiac anomaly causes substantial aortic runoff to the lungs) and higher dosage of prostaglandins.[53] Jaundice is more severe, particularly in LBW or very LBW infants because of reduced blood cell survival and liver immaturity.[54]

Temperature Regulation

Newborn infants, particularly those born prematurely, are susceptible to hypothermia.[55] Their large surface area in relation to body weight permits greater heat loss than in older children. Neonates have only a modest ability to conserve heat in the presence of cold stressors.[55,56] Shivering thermogenesis is limited in the first few weeks to months of life. Nonshivering mechanisms such as brown fat metabolism are recruited for heat production in neonates, but this increases oxygen consumption.[55,56] Therefore neonates benefit from care in a thermoneutral environment—the temperature at which normal core temperature is maintained with minimal energy expenditure.

Immune System

Neonatal skin and mucosa are ineffective barriers, and thus they are susceptible to infections. Immature cellular and humoral systems limit their ability to mount an effective immune response.[57] Particularly at risk are premature infants with long-standing indwelling venous catheters.

Low Birth Weight, Very Low Birth Weight, and Prematurity

LBW related to prematurity or small for gestational age is present in 8% to 18% of infants born with CHD.[58] Among LBW (<2.5 kg) and very LBW (<1.5 kg) neonates, CHD accounts for approximately a quarter of all deaths.[59] Approximately one-third of LBW neonates with CHD will have an associated noncardiac abnormality.[60] LBW and prematurity are two separate variables; however, they are intimately related, and we will consider them together rather than apart.

Clinical manifestations of immature organs in LBW and premature neonates requiring cardiac surgery are typically seen in the respiratory, gastrointestinal, and neurologic systems.

Respiratory

Premature lungs are immature in structure and function.[61] A deficiency in surfactant may require exogenous surfactant replacement, oxygen supplementation, and, in severe cases, mechanical ventilation.[62,63] A variety of lung insults result in bronchopulmonary dysplasia, dependency on mechanical ventilation can cause significant barotrauma and interstitial emphysema, and long-standing intubation can cause airway stenosis. Any parenchymal lung disease, fluid, or air accumulation in the pleural space quickly exposes the diminished respiratory reserves of the neonate.[64,65]

Gastrointestinal

Premature neonates have high insensible water losses and are prone to dehydration and electrolyte abnormalities. Gut immaturity often prevents establishment of enteral feedings, and parenteral nutrition is required for prolonged periods. Postnatal closure of the ductus arteriosus is unusual in extremely LBW infants.[66] Wide patency not only causes congestive cardiac failure but also can lead to renal failure and necrotizing enterocolitis.[64,65]

Neurologic

Premature babies have abnormally developed areas of the brain, such as the immature germinal matrix, which are susceptible to injury. These abnormalities are also found in full-term gestation neonates with CHD, probably caused by abnormal cerebral circulation in utero.[67] Extremely premature babies are especially prone to intraventricular hemorrhage because of fragile cerebral vessels.[68] Brain maturation is also considerably delayed in neonates with congenital heart defects and more so if associated with prematurity.

Preterm infants face multiple challenges that are compounded in the presence of CHD and require special attention in perioperative management.

Treatment Options in Low-Birth-Weight or Very Low-Birth-Weight Neonates With Congenital Heart Disease

The three main physiologic issues in neonates with CHD are volume overload, pressure overload, and cyanosis—from reduced blood flow or poor mixing. The goal of neonatal heart surgery is to either correct or palliate these conditions. It is essential to weigh the balance between the risks of waiting and the risk of surgery to achieve the best possible results.

Medical Therapy

Prostaglandin E_1 is used to keep the ductus arteriosus patent and maintain fetal circulation when required for certain types of CHD. However, the use of prostaglandins can be complicated by hypotension, apnea, fever, intraventricular hemorrhage, electrolyte disturbances, and increased fragility in ductal tissue.[69] In LBW babies, duration of preoperative hospitalization significantly correlated with preoperative complication rates, and a longer waiting period caused worse complications, which impacts mortality and morbidity after cardiac surgery.[70]

Effects of Cardiopulmonary Bypass on Neonates

The adverse effects of CPB, including hemodilution, systemic inflammation, and bleeding, are more pronounced in neonates than in older children and adults.[71] The priming volume of the extracorporeal circuit may be as high as two or three times the circulating blood volume of the term neonate (approximately 80 mL/kg).[72] This disparity between the circulating blood volume and bypass circuit size results in marked hemodilution, anemia, hypoproteinemia, and a reduction in coagulation factors. Significant hypoproteinemia leads to greater movement of fluid from the intravascular compartment into the extracellular space.

Surgical trauma and extracorporeal circulation trigger an extensive systemic inflammatory response involving neutrophil, contact, and complement activation; cytokine release; platelet aggregation; and coagulation cascade activation. Systemic inflammatory mediators can cause cellular and organ dysfunction. Release of C3a increases vascular permeability, tumor necrosis factor-α (TNF-α) and interleukin-1-β depress myocardial contractile function, and TNF-α increases vascular permeability and lung water content and decreases glomerular filtration.[73] These adverse effects of global inflammation are more pronounced on the immature organ systems of neonates.

Palliative Surgery

Because of the insult of CPB during corrective cardiac surgery and the limitations of medical therapy, surgeries have been designed to palliate CHD and allow patient growth and organ system maturation before complete corrective repair. These surgeries include systemic-to-pulmonary shunts for patients with decreased pulmonary blood flow, pulmonary artery banding for patients with increased pulmonary blood flow, and surgical septectomy or catheter balloon septostomy for patients requiring mixing to maintain saturations.

These procedures can be performed without the use of CPB and are technically relatively simple; however, postoperative management is complex because it is very difficult to regulate the appropriate amount of pulmonary blood flow because neonatal pulmonary vascular resistance is very mercurial.

Difficulty in managing this abnormal physiology means there is a consistent amount of early postoperative morbidity, which in some institutions may be equivalent to the morbidity from early corrective surgery.[74]

The palliated state also has implications for other organ systems, and palliative surgeries can also create adhesions and distort native tissue, such as the pulmonary artery, which may then require reconstruction at the time of complete repair.

When to Delay Surgery

The rate of complications is clearly related to length of time before corrective surgery.[74] The strategy of "letting the child get bigger" on his or her own is not a good enough reason to delay surgery. One should aim to perform corrective surgery before the development of complications unless there are specific reasons not to operate. Conditions that generally preclude surgery include sepsis, specifically necrotizing enterocolitis, bacteremia, and bronchiolitis; end-organ dysfunction, predominantly respiratory, renal, and liver failure; active bleeding or bleeding tendency; and cerebral hemorrhage or stroke. These conditions should be corrected before surgery.

Some malformations do not impose a severe physiologic impact on the neonate and allow the neonate to grow appropriately, without mechanical ventilation or medication. Small atrial septal defects (ASDs) and ventricular septal defects (VSDs), transposition of the great arteries with VSD and pulmonary stenosis, tetralogy of Fallot without severe cyanosis, double-outlet RV with balanced circulation, and unobstructed total anomalous pulmonary venous return fit into this category. Traditionally, single-ventricle palliation, especially the Norwood procedure for hypoplastic left heart syndrome, has shown high mortality in LBW neonates, and management usually involved delayed surgery if stable hemodynamics can be maintained

on prostaglandins; however, recent data from our own unit showed univentricular palliation was not a risk factor for mortality in the LBW group of patients.[75,76] Technical limitations relate not only to surgical care but also anesthetic and intensive care management. Surgical limitations usually relate to cardiac size and tissue fragility, which predominantly affects those defects requiring intracardiac repair. The deleterious effects of prolonged CPB and myocardial ischemia on immature myocardium should also be taken into consideration before embarking on a prolonged procedure.

Although accurate surgery is requisite, perioperative management by neonatologists, anesthetists, and intensive care physicians is often more difficult. There is an inverse association between pediatric cardiac surgical volume and mortality that becomes increasingly important as case complexity increases.[77] Although volume is not associated with mortality for low-complexity cases, high-volume programs outperform smaller programs as case complexity increases. This reflects not only surgical technique but experienced perioperative care from all treating teams.

Cardiac Surgery at Low Birth Weight and Very Low Birth Weight

The functional limitations of the premature baby must be recognized in the operating room and intensive care unit. Exposure to CPB may result in surfactant dysfunction, hemodilution, inflammation, and postoperative capillary leak syndrome. Ventilator strategies favorable to premature lungs and chest wall should be used. High peak inspiratory pressure and tidal volumes are particularly injurious to immature lungs. Positive end-expiratory pressure stabilizes the highly compliant chest wall and maintains functional residual capacity. The myocardial structural and functional limitations detailed earlier can be managed with inotropes; however, there are no clear data favoring one inotrope over another, and choice is usually driven by institutional practices.

The Society of Thoracic Surgeons database study from 2008 provides a modern data set to guide prognostication.[7] Outcomes for 3000 patients (of which 517 were <2.5 kg) are described. Compared with infants weighing 2.5 to 4 kg, infants weighing less than 2.5 kg had a significantly higher mortality for the following operations: repair of coarctation of the aorta, repair of total anomalous pulmonary venous connection, arterial switch procedure, systemic-to-pulmonary-artery shunt, and the Norwood procedure. Lower infant weight remained strongly associated with mortality risk after stratifying the population by Risk Adjustment for Congenital Heart Surgery-1 levels 2 through 6 and Aristotle Basic Complexity levels 2 through 4.

Our own analysis of cardiac surgery in LBW babies also revealed a significantly higher mortality rate compared to babies weighing more than 2.5 kg (10.9% versus 4.8%; $P = .0069$).[76] We also found that lower gestational age at birth was an independent risk factor for early mortality in neonates or infants weighing less than 2.5 kg at surgery. The rate of early unplanned reintervention was not significantly different between patients weighing less than 2.5 kg and more than 2.5 kg, suggesting that technical surgical factors that might occur in tiny neonates can be overcome and were not the primary cause of the greater mortality seen in the patients weighing less than 2.5 kg. Factors such as the STS–European Association for Cardio-Thoracic Surgery (EACTS) Congenital Heart Surgery (STAT) risk categories, surgeon, and bypass time were also not related to mortality or early reintervention. Several technically complex procedures, such as the arterial switch operation, interrupted aortic arch repair, or truncus arteriosus repair, were performed with no hospital mortality in the patients weighing less than 2.5 kg. The expertise of the surgical and perfusion teams in the management of CPB in low-weight neonates, with significant emphasis on fluid restriction such as priming volume reduction and a lack of postoperative bleeding to avoid blood product transfusion and the lack of a need for permanent pacemaker implantation, should not be underestimated.

Our analysis of "usual" versus "delayed" timing of surgery did not show greater risk for any of the outcomes in the low-weight population. This finding is consistent with a study from Toronto that showed that for neonates weighing less than 2.0 kg, imposed delays in intervention neither compromised nor improved survival. The risk of medical complications from delayed surgery and higher mortality risk in nondelayed surgery seem to be in balance.[74]

Other High-Risk Conditions

Congenital Diaphragmatic Hernia

Congenital diaphragmatic hernia (CDH) is estimated to occur in 1 per 2500 to 1 per 5000 newborn infants.[78] It results from a developmental anomaly of the pleuroperitoneal fold.[79] Lungs in infants with CDH are hypoplastic on both sides, although the lung on the side of the hernia is more severely affected. More importantly, the total cross-sectional area of the pulmonary vascular bed is decreased, and pulmonary arterioles are abnormally and extensively muscularized, which increases pulmonary vascular resistance. There are several subtypes of CDH based upon location of the diaphragmatic defect. The most common type is the Bochdalek hernia, which occurs in more than 90% of cases and results from a posterolateral defect. Left-sided CDH is by far the commonest form (85%), with right-sided CDH occurring in 13% and bilateral CDH occurring very infrequently.[80]

CHD is the most frequent association and is noted in approximately 15% of all infants with CDH.[78,81] Isolated VSD is the most common defect (42%), followed by aortic arch obstruction (15%), univentricular anatomy (14%), and tetralogy of Fallot (11%). Importantly, in infants with a left-sided CDH with otherwise normal heart anatomy, left heart structures can be smaller than gestational-age matched controls.[82]

Left heart hypoplasia is likely related to mechanical compression of left heart structures by herniated abdominal contents and to decreased blood flow to the left heart due to the resultant cardiac malposition. Both of these factors may diminish left atrial and ventricular filling and negatively influence left ventricular size and output.[82]

Prenatal Diagnosis and Prognostic Factors. Prenatal indicators of poor outcome include early diagnosis in pregnancy, intrathoracic liver, and polyhydramnios. The degree of pulmonary hypoplasia and pulmonary hypertension ultimately determines survivability in isolated CDH. Despite inherent limitations the most reliable determinant of lung size and predictor of postnatal outcome is the lung-to-head ratio.[83]

Delivery and Postnatal Management. Delivery of newborns with CDH is recommended at tertiary centers with experienced multidisciplinary teams. No specific mode of delivery confers a significant survival advantage, and no gestational age at delivery offers a clear survival benefit.[84,85]

Infants with CDH are usually symptomatic at birth and present with respiratory distress in the first few minutes. Chest radiographs typically show gas-filled loops within the thorax and mediastinal shift away from the side of the hernia. Bag and mask ventilation should be avoided, and infants should be intubated immediately after birth to avoid gaseous distention of the stomach and intestine, which can worsen overall respiratory compliance. A large-bore Replogle tube connected to continuous low wall suction is useful to evacuate air from the stomach and decompresses the bowel.

Mechanical Ventilation. Until the mid-1980s, standard medical therapy to reduce pulmonary hypertension and reverse atrial and ductal level shunting employed aggressive ventilator strategies to induce hyperventilation and respiratory alkalosis. One of the most significant contributions to improved survival of infants with CDH has been the concept of gentle ventilation, initially proposed in 1985.[86] Minimal inspiratory pressures are used, muscle relaxation and sedation are avoided, and relative hypercapnia and postductal hypoxemia are tolerated.[86,87] One of the main goals of this therapy is to preserve the potential for future lung growth by minimizing ventilator-induced lung injury. Although oxygenation and ventilation targets vary at different institutions, preductal arterial oxygen saturation of greater than 85% and PCO_2 of less than 65 mm Hg are generally accepted goals. The employment of gentle ventilation strategies in single-center experiences results in a significant reduction in mortality.[88]

Pulmonary Vasodilators. Severity of pulmonary hypertension ultimately determines outcome in patients with CDH.[89] Inhaled nitric oxide (iNO) is not as effective in CDH as in pulmonary hypertension associated with other causes.[90] This is most likely related to a disproportionately greater amount of pulmonary vascular resistance resulting from fixed, structural abnormalities rather than reactive mechanisms. Use of iNO in infants with CDH has neither reduced the need for extracorporeal membrane oxygenation (ECMO) nor shown a survival benefit in controlled trials.[90] Most centers, however, continue to use iNO despite evidence of limited benefit due to lack of superior alternatives.[91]

Extracorporeal Membrane Oxygenation. Before clinicians offer ECMO to neonates with CDH, the neonates must satisfy the usual criteria for ECMO eligibility and show evidence of adequacy of lung tissue available for gas exchange. Nonrandomized studies suggest a significant reduction in short- and long-term mortality with the use of ECMO, particularly in those with severe CDH.[92] However, randomized controlled trials show only a short-term survival benefit with ECMO but are limited by small sample sizes.[92] Survival after ECMO in patients with CDH ranges from 53% to 61%; risk factors for mortality include a birth weight of less than 3 kg, birth before 38 weeks' gestation, and severe associated cardiac anomalies.[93] Both venovenous and venoarterial ECMO can be used with similar survival rates.[94] ECMO support for longer than 2 to 3 weeks suggests severe pulmonary hypertension and has a low probability of survival.[93,95]

Surgical Repair of Congenital Diaphragmatic Hernia. In general, when CDH is associated with a cardiac anomaly requiring surgery in the neonatal period, CDH repair is performed first. Timing of surgery is determined by the clinical status of the infant. Infants undergo CDH repair when ventilatory support and supplemental oxygen have been weaned to a minimum and pulmonary hypertension has largely resolved. The notion that CDH might not be a surgical emergency was first proposed in the late 1980s and then more firmly established by Wung and colleagues.[86,87] No trials have adequately addressed the question of urgent versus delayed CDH repair, but current practice has evolved toward allowing some period of stabilization before repair.[96]

If feasible, primary repair of the diaphragm is performed, otherwise in 50% to 70% of cases a prosthetic patch is placed. If there is loss of abdominal domain or concerns of elevated intra-abdominal pressure with risk of compartment syndrome, the abdomen is temporarily closed with a prosthetic patch. This is commonly done for infants who are repaired while on ECMO.

Outcomes. In a recent multicenter cohort, overall hospital survival was 76%. Factors associated with increased risk of mortality include severe pulmonary hypertension, need for ECMO, patch repair, and larger defect size.[97] Several studies report significantly lower survival in infants with CDH and CHD compared to infants with an isolated CDH.[97,98] Survival rates range from 41% to 68% in infants with CDH and CHD; however, survival is significantly worse in infants with CDH and a major cardiac anomaly, with only one-third of patients surviving to discharge and no substantial improvement in survival over the past 20 years.[97,98]

Survivors of CDH with CHD are at high risk for nutritional, gastrointestinal, respiratory, and neurodevelopmental morbidities. Problems include need for supplemental oxygen after discharge, recurrent hernias, gastroesophageal reflux, tube feedings, and failure to thrive. More recently, neurocognitive and learning disabilities and behavioral disorders have been identified in survivors.[99]

Esophageal Atresia and Tracheoesophageal Fistula

Esophageal atresia (EA) is a developmental anomaly characterized by discontinuity between the upper and lower esophagus. A fistulous communication between the proximal and/or distal esophageal pouch and trachea usually exists but is absent in approximately 5% of cases.[100] EA with tracheoesophageal fistula (TEF) occurs with an approximate frequency of 1 per 3500 to 1 per 4000 live births.[100] Approximately 50% of infants with EA/TEF have other associated anomalies.[101,102] Ten percent to 25% of infants have a cluster of anomalies that fall within the VACTERL (vertebral, anal atresia, cardiac, tracheoesophageal, renal, limb) spectrum, 10% are associated with genetic syndromes (trisomies 13, 18, and 21), and 30% have cardiovascular anomalies with VSD being the most common.[101,102]

Preoperative Management. A Replogle catheter should be placed in the proximal esophageal pouch for continuous drainage of oral secretions because episodes of respiratory distress can be caused by inadequate evacuation of saliva from the proximal esophageal pouch. Patient positioning should be upright and side-lying with elevation of the head to minimize reflux of gastric contents through a distal fistula into the lungs. A large distal TEF or associated duodenal or anal atresia can cause progressive gastric distention, in which case an urgent gastrostomy is required.[103]

Occasionally an infant with EA and distal TEF may require mechanical ventilation. Because the fistula is usually near the carina, exclusive ventilation of the lungs may be difficult, and intubation of the fistula sometimes occurs. Adequate tidal volumes may be difficult to generate if lung compliance is diminished, and the distal fistula and gastrostomy tube offer the least resistance to gas flow.[104] Emergent ligation of the fistula or of the gastroesophageal junction may be indicated.[104] A repeat surgery for division of the fistula and repair of the esophagus is accomplished after respiratory stability has been achieved. In stable infants, timing and which defect to repair first is often a point of contention and debate among cardiac and general surgeons. Most general surgeons prefer the cardiac defect to be repaired first.

Outcomes. Overall long-term survival for infants with EA is excellent, but associated cardiac malformations increase mortality approximately threefold.[101,102,105] Early complications include anastomotic leak, anastomotic stricture, and recurrent TEF. Late complications include gastroesophageal reflux disease (GERD), tracheomalacia, respiratory disease, and esophageal dysfunction.[105]

Omphalocele

An omphalocele constitutes herniation of organs (generally intestine and liver) from the abdominal cavity through a midline abdominal wall defect (AWD) into the umbilical cord. The protruding organs are encased in a protective sac and therefore usually uninjured. Omphalocele results from only partial folding of lateral body wall folds and failure of return of physiologically herniated intestinal loops into the abdominal cavity at the end of the first trimester. Chromosomal abnormalities (almost 50%) and other anomalies (80%) are frequent in omphalocele and ultimately determine survival.[106] Cardiac anomalies are seen in almost 30% of infants with omphalocele and most commonly include ASD, VSD, patent ductus arteriosus, dextrocardia, and tetralogy of Fallot.[106]

Delivery and Postnatal Management. Infants with AWDs are usually delivered at term. The optimal mode of delivery of a giant omphalocele is unclear; some groups advocate primary cesarean section to avoid hepatic injury, whereas others favor vaginal deliveries irrespective of size of omphalocele.[107] After birth the protective sac with eviscerated abdominal organs within it must be handled with extreme care to prevent injury, contamination, and sac rupture. Warm saline-soaked dressing is applied over the omphalocele for protection, and continuous gastrointestinal decompression with a Replogle tube is provided. Infants with an omphalocele may encounter respiratory difficulty due to abnormal chest and abdominal wall mechanics and pulmonary hypoplasia.

Cardiac or omphalocele repair should ideally be deferred until a full genetic evaluation is completed. If cardiac surgery is required in the neonatal period, then a conservative approach for the management of a large omphalocele is preferable. Attempts to reduce abdominal contents when the abdominal domain is limited will worsen respiratory compliance and adversely impact gas exchange.

Surgical Management. The size of the omphalocele, respiratory compromise, and associated anomalies, particularly cardiac, determine the course of definitive treatment. A small omphalocele (<4 cm) is easily reduced, and surgical closure is simple. A large omphalocele usually contains stomach, small and large intestine, as well as liver, spleen, urinary bladder, or gonads, and management can be challenging. There are three broad categories of options for surgical management of an omphalocele: primary closure, staged closure with or without mesh or patch, and nonoperative management with delayed closure. A large omphalocele often requires gradual reduction of the organs into the abdominal cavity due to lack of domain. The fascia and/or skin can then be closed primarily with a mesh or a patch. If skin closure is not feasible, either a preformed Silastic (Dow Corning, Midland, MI) silo bag can be placed over the viscera for gradual reduction over a week, or a Silastic sheet can be sutured to the fascia to serve the same purpose. Nonoperative management with delayed closure is used for a large omphalocele in infants with associated comorbidities who cannot tolerate surgery because of prematurity, lung hypoplasia, respiratory insufficiency, or CHD. Commonly, silver sulfadiazine and a covering dressing is applied to the omphalocele sac daily until the sac granulates and eventually epithelializes. The residual large ventral hernia is then repaired later.

Outcomes. The prognosis of the child with omphalocele is determined by the size of the defect and presence of associated anomalies, such as chromosomal abnormalities, CHD, and pulmonary hypoplasia, with an overall mortality rate of approximately 20%.[108] Most infants who do not have other severe anomalies do well, and approximately 90% of survivors have no significant long-term problems. Long-term complications may include GERD, feeding issues, and adhesive bowel obstructions.[109]

Conclusion

The management of LBW and VLBW neonates with CHD should take into account the inherent risks of waiting, the complexity of surgery, and the expertise of the teams providing care. The majority of LBW and VLBW neonates can be operated on early with better results compared with medical management or palliation in experienced centers. Surgery can be delayed in certain patients and situations to improve outcomes; however, patients with single-ventricle physiology remain a difficult group to treat regardless of the strategy, and management should be individualized.

Selected References

A complete list of references is available at ExpertConsult.com.

4. Jacobs JP, Jacobs ML, Mavroudis C, et al. *Executive summary: the Society of Thoracic Surgeons Congenital Heart Surgery Database - Fourteenth Harvest – (January 1, 2007–December 31, 2010).* The Society of Thoracic Surgeons (STS) and Duke Clinical Research Institute (DCRI), Duke University Medical Center, Durham, NC, USA, Spring 2011 Harvest; 2011.
7. Curzon CL, Milford-Beland S, Li JS, O'Brien SM, Jacobs JP, Jacobs ML, et al. Cardiac surgery in infants with low birth weight is associated with increased mortality: analysis of the Society of Thoracic Surgeons Congenital Heart Database. *J Thorac Cardiovasc Surg.* 2008;135(3):546–551.
74. Hickey EJ, Nosikova Y, Zhang H, Caldarone CA, Benson L, Redington A, et al. Very low-birth-weight infants with congenital cardiac lesions: is there merit in delaying intervention to permit growth and maturation? *J Thorac Cardiovasc Surg.* 2012;143(1):126–136, 36.e1.
76. Kalfa D, Krishnamurthy G, Duchon J, Najjar M, Levasseur S, Chai P, et al. Outcomes of cardiac surgery in patients weighing <2.5 kg: affect of patient-dependent and -independent variables. *J Thorac Cardiovasc Surg.* 2014;148(6):2499–2506.e1.

31

Cardiopulmonary Resuscitation (CPR) in Children With Heart Disease

ELIZABETH A. HUNT, MD, MPH, PHD; TIA T. RAYMOND, MD;
KIMBERLY WARD JACKSON, MD; BRADLEY S. MARINO, MD, MPP, MSCE;
DONALD H. SHAFFNER, MD

Cardiac arrest is a relatively rare phenomenon in children. Although the overall incidence is rare, cardiac arrest represents a clinically important event often resulting in death or poor neurologic outcome. Out-of-hospital cardiac arrest (OHCA) is estimated to occur approximately 16,000 times per year (8 to 20 per 100,000 children annually) in the United States.[1] In-hospital cardiac arrest (IHCA) has been variably estimated to occur in 5000 to 10,000 children per year, or in 0.77 per 1000 admissions (or 77 per 100,000 children). Thus IHCA occurs at least four times more frequently than OHCA.[2-5] Higher survival to discharge after in-hospital[6-12] compared with out-of-hospital[13] arrest rates have been attributed to differences in cause of arrest and more rapid recognition and treatment by skilled caregivers in the in-hospital setting.[14] Among hospitalized children, cardiac arrest is reported in 2% to 4% of all children admitted to a pediatric intensive care unit (ICU)[6,15,16] and in approximately 3% to 6% of children admitted to a cardiac ICU.[16,17] Cardiopulmonary resuscitation (CPR) is performed in 7 per 1000 hospitalizations of children with acquired and congenital cardiovascular disease, a rate greater than 10-fold that observed among hospitalized children without cardiovascular disease.[5] Recently published data from the Pediatric Cardiac Critical Care Consortium (PC[4]) demonstrated a cardiac arrest rate of 3.1% among 15,908 cardiac ICU encounters (6498 medical and 9410 surgical) in 23 centers. Observed (unadjusted) cardiac ICU cardiac arrest prevalence varied from 1% to 5.5% with wide variation in cardiac arrest rates per 1000 cardiac ICU days among the 23 centers (1.1 to 10.4).[17]

Survival from IHCA in infants and children has significantly improved over the past four decades, from approximately 9% in the 1980s to at least 14.3% in 2000, and most recent data reports overall survival has increased nearly threefold during the past decade to 43%.[6-12,18] This significant improvement in survival is despite an increase in cardiac arrests resulting from nonshockable rhythms. These improvements have been facilitated by improvements in systems and processes to prevent cardiac arrest and improvements in CPR quality, resulting in higher rates of survival during the acute resuscitation period.[19-21] Notably, these improved survival rates were not accompanied by increased rates of significant neurologic disability among survivors.[18] A number of factors have likely played an important role in achieving these trends. First, clinical practice guidelines over the past decade have emphasized several aspects of the acute resuscitation chain of survival.[22] These include greater vigilance and closer monitoring, which may have resulted in shorter response times. In addition, recent pediatric in-hospital publications have demonstrated a higher proportion of patients located in a monitored unit or an ICU at the time of cardiac arrest, which may have allowed earlier recognition of cardiopulmonary compromise and prompt initiation of resuscitation efforts.[18,23]

Additionally, patients located in an ICU may have patient management/interventions in place at the time of the arrest (e.g., central venous and arterial access, improved cardiac monitoring) and/or the presence of team members experienced with resuscitation of the cardiac patient, which may contribute to improved survival after cardiac arrest. Additionally, specialized cardiac arrest processes, including easier access to extracorporeal life support during resuscitation (extracorporeal CPR [ECPR]), may improve survival after cardiac arrest when it occurs in the ICU.[24] Increased participation in hospital-specific quality improvement efforts like the American Heart Association's (AHA's) Get With the Guidelines—Resuscitation (GWTG-R) registry may also have led to improved survival over time. Improved patient outcomes have also been shown with the use of routine mock codes in pediatric hospitals, audiovisual feedback during resuscitation, and postevent debriefing.[25-27] Additional resuscitation strategies that may have improved outcomes include earlier recognition and management of at-risk patients, better adherence to resuscitation algorithms, improved coordination between code team members, greater emphasis on quality of resuscitation (e.g., high-quality chest compressions with minimal interruptions), and postresuscitation care (e.g., multidisciplinary care).[8,15,16,28,29]

Risk Factors

The cardiac diseases associated with sudden cardiac death can be divided into previously recognized or unrecognized diseases (Table 31.1).[30] Children with repaired congenital heart disease (CHD) constitute the largest group among the patients with previously recognized heart disease. The group with previously unrecognized heart disease is more challenging because cardiac arrest may be the presenting sign of the abnormality. Children with unrecognized heart disease may have underlying structural heart disease such as

TABLE 31.1	Underlying Cardiac Diagnoses in Children Presenting With Sudden Cardiac Death *Patients at Risk for Out-of-Hospital Cardiac Arrest From Cardiovascular Disease (Sudden Cardiac Death)*			
WITH PREVIOUSLY RECOGNIZED HEART DISEASE		**WITH PREVIOUSLY UNRECOGNIZED HEART DISEASE**	
Congenital	Acquired	Structural Heart Disease	No Structural Heart Disease
Tetralogy of Fallot	Kawasaki syndrome	Hypertrophic cardiomyopathy	Long QT syndrome
Hypoplastic left heart syndrome	Dilated cardiomyopathy	Congenital coronary artery abnormalities	Wolff-Parkinson-White syndrome
Transposition of the great arteries	Myocarditis	Arrhythmogenic right ventricular dysplasia	Primary ventricular tachycardia and ventricular fibrillation
Aortic stenosis		Myocarditis	Commotio cordis
Single-ventricle palliative procedures—Fontan, Glenn, hemi-Fontan			Primary pulmonary hypertension
Marfan syndrome			
Eisenmenger syndrome			
Congenital (or postoperative) heart block			

Modified from Berger S, Dhala A, Friedberg DZ. Sudden cardiac death in infants, children, and adolescents. *Pediatr Clin North Am.* 1990;46:221-234.

hypertrophic cardiomyopathy, coronary anomalies, or arrhythmogenic right ventricular dysplasia, or nonstructural heart disease with conduction system abnormalities such as long QT syndrome, Wolff-Parkinson-White syndrome, primary ventricular tachycardia/fibrillation, or commotio cordis. Commotio cordis is an underappreciated syndrome in which low-energy impact to the chest wall leads to ventricular fibrillation because of impact during the vulnerable period just before the peak of the T wave.[31] Many of the entities in the group with previously unrecognized heart disease have an underlying genetic predisposition.

Retrospective analysis of pediatric IHCAs entered into the administrative Kids' Inpatient Database (KID) revealed survival after cardiac arrest was higher among pediatric surgical cardiac patients (52%) than among pediatric medical cardiac patients (43%); however, children with single-ventricle disease had a lower survival rate (35%) than did children with other forms of cardiovascular disease (45%).[5] Variables associated with an increased risk of cardiac arrest on multivariate analysis in the KID inpatient database included age less than 1 year, heart failure, myocarditis, single-ventricle physiology, and coronary artery pathology, whereas patients undergoing cardiac surgery had decreased risk of cardiac arrest.[5] Single-ventricle patients demonstrated a fivefold increased odds of arrest over CHD patients with a biventricular circulation, and they were the only group with increased odds of death after CPR, even after adjusting for age, hospital characteristics, and comorbidities.[5]

More recent data on the epidemiology of cardiac arrest in cardiac ICUs were explored by the PC[4] registry, which analyzed 15,908 medical and surgical encounters from 23 North American centers. Medical encounters had a 50% higher rate of cardiac arrest compared with surgical encounters. On multivariable analysis, prematurity, neonatal age, any Society of Thoracic Surgeons preoperative risk factor, and Society of Thoracic Surgeons–European Association for Cardio-Thoracic Surgery mortality category 4 or 5 had the strongest association with surgical encounter cardiac arrest. In medical encounters, independent cardiac arrest risk factors were acute heart failure, prematurity, lactic acidosis greater than 3 mmol/

dL, and invasive ventilation 1 hour after admission. Return of spontaneous circulation occurred in 64.5%, and ECPR was used in 27.2% of cardiac arrest events. Unadjusted survival was 53.2% in encounters with cardiac arrest versus 98.2% without cardiac arrest. Medical encounters had lower survival after cardiac arrest (37.7%) versus surgical encounters (62.5%), with the Norwood surgical population noted to have less than half the survival after cardiac arrest (35.6%) compared with all others.[17]

The AHA's GWTG-R multicenter registry found significantly improved hospital survival after resuscitation from an IHCA in children who have undergone cardiac surgery compared with children without cardiovascular disease. Among the cardiac patients the survival to hospital discharge in those with surgical cardiac disease (37%) was significantly higher compared with patients with medical cardiac disease (28%) (adjusted odds ratio, 1.8; 95% confidence interval [CI], 1.3-2.5; *P* < .001), and non–cardiac disease (23%) (adjusted odds ratio, 1.8; 95% CI, 1.4-2.4; *P* < .001).[32] Additionally, a report from GWTG-R found that children with cardiac disease were more likely to survive to hospital discharge compared with children without cardiac disease when ECPR was used.[33]

The most recent multi-institutional data from the Society of Thoracic Surgeons Congenital Heart Surgery Database (STS-CHSD) suggests a 2.6% cardiac arrest rate for postoperative patients and a mortality rate of 49.4% among those having cardiac arrest.[34] This publication and previous literature have identified younger age, prematurity, genetic syndromes, preoperative comorbid conditions, and increased surgical complexity as risk factors for cardiac arrest in patients following cardiac surgery.[16,34-36] As hospitals increasingly develop dedicated cardiac ICUs to optimize the care of this complex patient population, practitioners must understand the unique cardiac arrest incidence and outcome data of this population to improve quality of care and clinical outcomes. Specific causes of arrest, the availability of specialized invasive monitoring, and access to interventions and management subsequent to the arrest may explain the differences in survival in these three large retrospective studies.

Overview of Guidelines for Cardiopulmonary Resuscitation

When managing a cardiac arrest patient in the cardiac ICU, it is important for all team members to have a shared mental model of the goals of the resuscitation. The most common approach to defining the goals of the resuscitation would be to use regionally published, evidence-based resuscitation guidelines such as the AHA, European Resuscitation Council, or Australian and New Zealand Committee on Resuscitation guidelines for basic life support (BLS) and pediatric advanced life support (PALS). These guidelines should be used as the default, and then the team can consider alterations to personalize the resuscitation based on specific aspects of the size of the individual patient, disease population, or situation not yet covered in the standard guidelines, such as how to approach arresting ICU patients with an open chest, presence of hemodynamic monitoring information from central venous lines, arterial lines, near-infrared spectroscopy (NIRS), and special considerations based on a patient's anatomy (e.g., single ventricle).

Until 2015 the AHA updated their CPR guidelines every 5 years for both BLS and PALS; it has now shifted to a rolling approach (i.e., with the intent to perform updated reviews as new literature is published). In 2010 the guidelines most notably changed the traditional sequence of basic CPR from A-B-C (airway, breathing, circulation) to C-A-B (circulation, airway, breathing) to decrease time to chest compressions and reduce decreased perfusion time.[37] Differences in time to return of spontaneous circulation (ROSC) and clinical outcomes with this change are yet to be determined; however, time to chest compressions and to starting ventilation strategies have both been shown to be decreased with the C-A-B sequence.[38]

New to the 2015 AHA pediatric BLS guidelines is the idea of compression-only CPR—particularly in the setting of a witnessed cardiac arrest that is presumably nonasphyxial in nature or when a provider is unable or unwilling to perform assisted breaths and most likely in the out-of-hospital setting. When a witnessed sudden cardiac death event occurs, there should be high suspicion for unrecognized heart disease as the cause (see Table 31.1). In these patients, compression-only CPR has been shown to have better outcomes than no CPR at all. However, in all cases, compression-only CPR has been shown to have worse survival compared with conventional CPR for children.[39] The AHA pediatric BLS guidelines recommend conventional CPR for all pediatric cardiac arrests (regardless of cause) when bystanders are able and willing. In 2017 the first updated, rolling review of this topic reviewed the most recent evidence supporting this but again stated if rescuers were not willing or able to provide mouth to mouth, to perform compression-only CPR rather than not performing CPR.[40]

The parameter goals for the AHA 2015 pediatric BLS guidelines can be seen in Table 31.2.[19,41-44] The AHA 2015 updated PALS CPR algorithm can be seen Fig. 31.1.[41]

A focus of the guidelines is to standardize and optimize CPR quality, specifically adequate compression rate and depth. For all ages the recommended compression rate is 100 to 120 per minute (same as for adults). For infants and children (up to onset of puberty), adequate depth of compressions is at least one-third of anterior-posterior chest diameter (typically 4 to 5 cm in children) with full recoil of the chest between compressions. The compressor should rotate every 2 minutes to limit provider fatigue, and interruptions in chest compressions should be minimized in an attempt

TABLE 31.2	The 2013 and 2015 American Heart Association Recommendations for Metrics of CPR Performance by the Provider Team		
Parameter	**Infants**	**Children**	**Adults**
Chest compression rate	100-120 compressions per min[a,b]		
Chest compression depth	≥⅓ AP diameter or ≈38 mm[a,b]	≥⅓ AP diameter or ≈50 mm[a,b]	≥50 mm, <60 mm[a,b]
Chest compression fraction	Minimize interruptions[b], >80%[a]		
Chest compression release	Allow full recoil[a,b]		
Ventilation rate	10[a], <12 breaths per minute[b]		
Ventilation volume	Minimal chest rise[a]		
Epinephrine interval	3-5 min[a,b]		
Perishock pauses	Minimize number and length of preshock and postshock pauses, <10 s each[b]		

[a]Recommendation from 2013 AHA consensus statement.[19]
[b]Recommendation from the 2015 AHA resuscitation guidelines.[41]
AP, Anteroposterior.
Supporting references 19, 30, 41, 43, and 44.

to maximize perfusion to vital organs and to maintain coronary perfusion pressure (CoPP).[37]

Recent literature has shown that early placement of an advanced airway during CPR does not improve survival or neurologic outcome.[45,46] Because of the lack of definitive evidence, the current PALS algorithm suggests one consider advanced airway placement (either a laryngeal mask airway or endotracheal intubation) during resuscitation if an experienced health care provider is present, with focus on minimizing interruptions in chest compressions. When an advanced airway is present, a ventilation rate of one breath approximately every 6 seconds (10 breaths/min) is recommended with adequate, but not excessive, chest rise.[41] Hyperventilation and overdistention of the lungs should be avoided because this could impede venous return to the thoracic cavity. Presence of an advanced airway also allows continuous end-tidal carbon dioxide ($ETCO_2$) monitoring, which can assist in guiding quality chest compressions, though specific values to guide therapy have not been established in children. This is discussed in detail later in the chapter. If no advanced airway is present, effective bag-mask ventilation should be performed at a rate of 2 breaths per 15 chest compressions (or 2 breaths for every 30 compressions in the setting of one health care provider) with focus on adequate, but not excessive, chest rise.[37]

Drug Therapy

Vasopressors

Theoretically, vasopressors are indicated in cardiac arrest to cause systemic vasoconstriction (increase blood pressure) to increase coronary blood flow, providing perfusion to the myocardium,

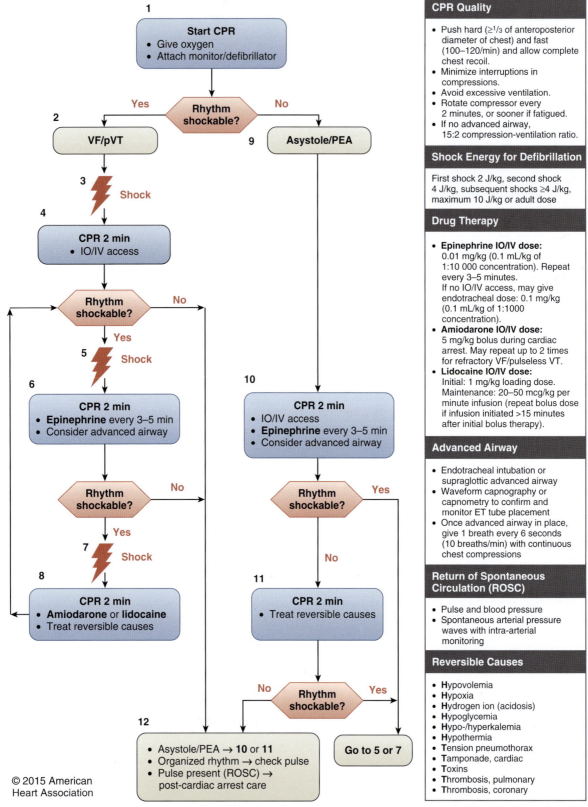

CPR Quality

- Push hard (≥1/3 of anteroposterior diameter of chest) and fast (100–120/min) and allow complete chest recoil.
- Minimize interruptions in compressions.
- Avoid excessive ventilation.
- Rotate compressor every 2 minutes, or sooner if fatigued.
- If no advanced airway, 15:2 compression-ventilation ratio.

Shock Energy for Defibrillation

First shock 2 J/kg, second shock 4 J/kg, subsequent shocks ≥4 J/kg, maximum 10 J/kg or adult dose

Drug Therapy

- **Epinephrine IO/IV dose:** 0.01 mg/kg (0.1 mL/kg of 1:10 000 concentration). Repeat every 3–5 minutes. If no IO/IV access, may give endotracheal dose: 0.1 mg/kg (0.1 mL/kg of 1:1000 concentration).
- **Amiodarone IO/IV dose:** 5 mg/kg bolus during cardiac arrest. May repeat up to 2 times for refractory VF/pulseless VT.
- **Lidocaine IO/IV dose:** Initial: 1 mg/kg loading dose. Maintenance: 20–50 mcg/kg per minute infusion (repeat bolus dose if infusion initiated >15 minutes after initial bolus therapy).

Advanced Airway

- Endotracheal intubation or supraglottic advanced airway
- Waveform capnography or capnometry to confirm and monitor ET tube placement
- Once advanced airway in place, give 1 breath every 6 seconds (10 breaths/min) with continuous chest compressions

Return of Spontaneous Circulation (ROSC)

- Pulse and blood pressure
- Spontaneous arterial pressure waves with intra-arterial monitoring

Reversible Causes

- **H**ypovolemia
- **H**ypoxia
- **H**ydrogen ion (acidosis)
- **H**ypoglycemia
- **H**ypo-/hyperkalemia
- **H**ypothermia
- **T**ension pneumothorax
- **T**amponade, cardiac
- **T**oxins
- **T**hrombosis, pulmonary
- **T**hrombosis, coronary

© 2015 American Heart Association

• **Figure 31.1** Pediatric advanced life support cardiac arrest algorithm as updated in the American Heart Association 2015 guidelines. (Reprinted with permission. *Circulation.* 2015;132:S526-S542. Copyright 2015 American Heart Association, Inc.)

and increase myocardial contractility of the stunned myocardium. Despite the fact that epinephrine is the key drug used during the management of pediatric cardiac arrest, and the first drug listed in every PALS algorithm, there is little human evidence that vasopressors are effective in helping to achieve return of circulation or impact clinical outcomes. One adult study did show that epinephrine administration was associated with increased return of circulation in OHCAs,[47] but no such pediatric data are available. Currently the only recommended vasopressor in pediatric cardiac arrest is epinephrine (0.01 mg/kg intraosseous [IO]/intravenously [IV] or 0.1 mg/kg per endotracheal tube [ETT]) every 3 to 5 minutes.[41]

Antiarrhythmic Therapy

When a patient experiences pulseless ventricular tachycardia or ventricular fibrillation, CPR and defibrillation (2 to 4 J/kg) should be initiated per the PALS algorithm (see Fig. 31.1). If defibrillation is not successful in converting to a perfusing rhythm, amiodarone (5 mg/kg IO/IV bolus) or lidocaine (1 mg/kg IO/IV bolus, 2 mg/kg per ETT) may be given in addition to repeat defibrillation attempts.[41] In a recent systematic review, lidocaine and amiodarone were found to be comparable, so either is acceptable in this setting.[48]

Sodium Bicarbonate

In the past the use of sodium bicarbonate during CPR had been a common practice in an attempt to buffer the metabolic acidosis associated with poor perfusion because acidemia impairs myocardial contraction and cardiac output. In recent years its use has become controversial because some studies have associated its use with worsened outcomes.[49] The administration of sodium bicarbonate during CPR is now recommended only during resuscitation for cardiac arrest specifically related to severe metabolic acidosis, hyperkalemia, and tricyclic antidepressant overdose.

Calcium

Routine calcium administration is not recommended during resuscitation unless there is documented hypocalcemia, calcium channel blocker overdose, hypermagnesemia, or hyperkalemia. Calcium chloride or calcium gluconate may be used; however, calcium chloride should be given through central venous access when possible (i.e., to avoid infiltrates).[41] However, in a true cardiac arrest situation, risk-benefit analysis would suggest the risk of infiltrate should not outweigh rapid administration if clinically indicated.

For a full description of initial dosing of drugs commonly used in the treatment of low cardiac output syndrome in an attempt to avoid a cardiac arrest and during treatment of a cardiac arrest see the Pharmacology: Typical Doses and Indications table in the AHA scientific statement on CPR in infants and children with cardiovascular disease.[50]

Special Considerations for Cardiopulmonary Resuscitation in Patients With Underlying Cardiac Disease

Single-Ventricle Resuscitation

The resuscitation of the child with single-ventricle anatomy is dependent on anatomic factors and cardiopulmonary interaction.

Resuscitation profiles for the structurally normal heart and the single-ventricle palliated states are delineated in Table 31.3,[50] in which the pathway of each circulation and the impact of chest compressions, chest recoil, and positive-pressure ventilation are shown.

Risk Factors for Cardiac Arrest and Death

Anatomic, hemodynamic, and other comorbid factors that contribute to hemodynamic compromise and early death in the infant with single-ventricle physiology include (1) the presence of hypoplastic left heart syndrome (HLHS), pulmonary atresia with intact ventricular septum with right ventricle–dependent coronary circulation, and total anomalous pulmonary venous connection; (2) reduced cardiac function and hemodynamically significant atrioventricular and/or semilunar valve regurgitation; and (3) prematurity and the presence of a genetic disorder or syndrome.[51-54] Neonates with a univentricular physiology are at higher risk of cardiopulmonary arrest secondary to (1) increased cardiac work from volume overload, (2) unbalanced systemic and pulmonary blood flow (i.e., elevated pulmonary-to-systemic blood flow ratio [Q_p:Q_s]), and (3) shunt thrombosis.[55-57] The risk of cardiac arrest remains high until the superior cavopulmonary anastomosis is completed.[58-60] The incidence of IHCA in patients with HLHS after stage I Norwood palliation is higher after modified Blalock-Taussig shunt (MBTS) than after right ventricle to pulmonary artery shunt (RVPAS).[59-61] However, there is no difference in hospital mortality based on shunt type.[53,62,63] The Single Ventricle Reconstruction Trial revealed that one-third of infants after stage I Norwood for HLHS died or underwent heart transplantation at 12-month follow-up,[59] with a nontrivial incidence of cardiac arrest and mortality occurring between 30 days after the stage I palliation and the time of the superior cavopulmonary anastomosis (CPA) procedure (interstage period). Thus the interstage period is considered a prearrest state that warrants active monitoring and intervention to improve survival.[56]

Resuscitation in the Patient With Patent Ductus Arteriosus or Shunted Single-Ventricle Physiology

The prearrest state usually includes some combination of lactic acidosis, intestinal hypoperfusion and feeding intolerance, renal insufficiency, or ST wave changes on ECG indicative of coronary ischemia.[56,57] Q_p:Q_s is increased in patients with large shunt size relative to body weight. In the neonate with significantly elevated Q_p:Q_s, increases in systemic vascular resistance (SVR) may result in rapid deterioration with extreme pulmonary overcirculation and shock ("SVR crisis").[64-66] Hemodynamic compromise in a shunt-dependent physiology can typically be reversed with inotropic support, preload modification, mechanical ventilation and sedation/analgesia, manipulation of SVR and pulmonary vascular resistance (PVR), and anticoagulation if shunt obstruction is suspected.

Recognition and Management of Shunt Obstruction. Decreased systemic arterial oxygen saturation after the Stage I Norwood palliation may result from insufficient pulmonary blood flow, intrapulmonary shunting and pulmonary venous desaturation, and/or diminished mixed venous saturation (SvO_2). Insufficient pulmonary blood flow may result from mechanical obstruction of the shunt, elevated PVR, inadequate shunt perfusion pressure, or from pulmonary vein stenosis or restrictive atrial communication.[62,67]

TABLE 31.3	Resuscitation Profiles for the Structurally Normal Heart and Those That Have Undergone Single-Ventricle Palliation				
Physiology	Circulation Description	Circulation of Blood	Chest Compressions	Chest Recoil	Positive Pressure Ventilation
Structurally normal heart	Two-ventricle series circulation without heart disease	Systemic veins—lungs—Pulmonary veins—body	1. RV compression results in PBF 2. LV compression results in SBF	Increases the transthoracic gradient from the systemic veins to the RA increasing RV filling	Decreases the transthoracic gradient from the systemic veins to the RA decreasing RV filling
Stage I Norwood or shunted physiology	Single-ventricle parallel circulation with shunt-dependent PBF	Systemic veins—single V — Lungs (via shunt) or body	Single-ventricle compression results in PBF (shunt ± PVR) and SBF (SVR)	Increases filling to the preload-dependent single ventricle	Decreases filling to the preload-dependent single ventricle
Bidirectional Glenn and hemi-Fontan	Single-ventricle parallel circulation with PBF dependent on multiple arteriolar vascular beds	IVC—single V—body/brain— SVC—lungs—pulmonary veins—body	Single-ventricle compression results in SBF	1. Predominantly fills the RA from the IVC 2. SVC flow dependent on cerebral vascular resistance and PVR	Decreases filling to the single ventricle by impeding SVC flow and IVC filling
Fontan	Single-ventricle series circulation	Systemic veins—lungs—Pulmonary veins—body	Single-ventricle compression results in SBF	1. Predominantly fills the PAs with IVC blood flow (PVR) 2. SVC flow dependent on cerebral vascular resistance and PVR	Decreases filling to the single ventricle by impeding both SVC and IVC flow

IVC, Inferior vena cava; *LV,* left ventricle; *PA,* pulmonary artery; *PBF,* pulmonary blood flow; *PVR,* pulmonary vascular resistance; *RA,* right atrium; *RV,* right ventricle; *SBF,* systemic blood flow; *SVC,* superior vena cava; *SVR,* systemic vascular resistance; *V,* ventricle.

From Marino BS, Tabbutt S, MacLaren G, et al. Cardiopulmonary resuscitation in infants and children with cardiac disease: a scientific statement from the American Heart Association. *Circulation.* 2018;137(22):e691-e782.

Systemic desaturation with normal systemic blood flow and unchanged arteriovenous oxygen saturation difference (initially) is consistent with shunt obstruction. One clinical sign of shunt obstruction in patients who are intubated and mechanically ventilated, and thus have $ETCO_2$ continuously monitored, is a sudden decline in $ETCO_2$ with an increase arterial $PaCO_2$.[68-72] The risk of shunt thrombosis is higher in those patients after stage I Norwood palliation with a MBTS than with an RVPAS during the interstage period.[62,73,74]

Strategies for prophylactic anticoagulation include heparin therapy in the early postoperative period after shunt placement, followed by enteral aspirin once feeds are initiated.[55] Aspirin may reduce the risk of shunt thrombosis and cardiac arrest during the first year after placement.[73]

Acute shunt obstruction may be treated by (1) oxygen to maximize alveolar oxygenation, (2) bolus dose heparin (50 to 100 U/kg) for rapid anticoagulation,[55,57] (3) systemic vasoconstricting medications to maximize shunt perfusion pressure (e.g., phenylephrine, norepinephrine, epinephrine), (4) cardiac catheterization or surgical intervention to open shunt, and (5) use of extracorporeal life support (ECLS) to support circulation. Therapies that decrease PVR (e.g., oxygen, hyperventilation, inhaled nitric oxide) will provide little benefit if there is complete shunt occlusion. When shunt obstruction occurs with reduced oxygenation, sedation, and neuromuscular blockade, the placement of an advanced airway and mechanical ventilation at low mean airway pressure will reduce oxygen consumption and may maintain oxygen saturation while the patient is waiting for

definitive therapy to open the shunt.[71] If shunt obstruction results in prolonged and severe arterial desaturation, cardiac function will be impaired quickly. In infants with acute shunt obstruction, ECPR may be beneficial if used promptly to support the myocardium during the acute obstruction and/or afterwards during myocardial recovery.[62,75-79]

Unique Challenges in Cardiopulmonary Resuscitation in the Patient With Patent Ductus Arteriosus or Shunted Single-Ventricle Physiology. Cumulative data from the STS-CHSD from 2007 to 2012 revealed a 13% incidence of cardiac arrest in those patients who have undergone stage I Norwood palliation.[36] When the infant with a shunted single-ventricle physiology has cardiac arrest, it is difficult to obtain ROSC. The mortality rate for infants after stage I Norwood palliation who develop cardiac arrest is five times higher than for those infants who do not suffer cardiac arrest.[36] When cardiac arrest develops, providers should begin conventional high-quality CPR.

It is difficult to obtain effective pulmonary blood flow during resuscitation in the infant with shunted single-ventricle physiology because pulmonary blood flow is shunt dependent and is impacted by PVR and aortic diastolic pressure (for MBTS) and SVR (for MBTS and the RVPAS). Compressions generate only one-third of normal blood flow to the heart and brain during CPR in patients with normal cardiac anatomy.[19] In patients with single-ventricle shunted physiology, systemic blood flow during CPR is very likely to be even lower secondary to the loss of some systemic cardiac output to the pulmonary circulation due to the parallel circulation (see Table 31.3). In the neonate with shunted physiology in cardiac

TABLE 31.4 Effect of Respiratory Manipulations on Circulatory Parameters at Different Stages of Palliation of Children With Univentricular Physiology

Stage	Respiratory Strategy (Alveolar Gas)	SaO_2	SvO_2	Q_p/Q_s	TPG	ΔAVO_2	VO_2	Lactate	CBF	rSO_2C	rSO_2S
0	Hypocapnic										
	Hyperoxic										
	Hypercapnic[81,83]	↑	↑	↓↓		↓				↑	
	Hypoxic[81,83]	↓	↓			↔				↔	
1	Hypocapnic[89]	↔	↔			↔					
	Hyperoxic[89]	↑	↑			↔					
	Hypercapnic[86,87]	↔	↔↑	↔		↓	↓	↓	↑	↑	↓
	Hypoxic										
2	Hypocapnic[82]	↓				↔				↓	
	Hyperoxic[86]	↑									
	Hypercapnic[7,20,82,85,86]	↑↑		↔	↑	↓	↓	↓	↑	↑	
	Hypoxic										

Measured parameters in multiple studies are shown.
See references for details.

Stage 0: Uncorrected/unpalliated ductal dependent parallel pulmonary and systemic circulations. Maintenance of ductal patency is necessary for systemic perfusion and prostaglandin E_1 is indicated. No human experimental data exist for measures such as hyperoxic or hypocapnic alveolar gas strategies that tend to reduce pulmonary vascular resistance, and such strategies should generally be avoided without significant monitoring of systemic oxygen delivery. The greatest improvement in systemic oxygenation occurs with induction of hypercapnic ventilation.

Stage 1: Post surgical palliation of parallel circulation with relief of arch obstruction and limitation of pulmonary blood flow with a systemic-to-pulmonary artery shunt. Hypercapnia can improve cerebral more than systemic oxygen delivery.

Stage 2: Post superior cavopulmonary anastomosis. The cerebral and pulmonary circulations are in series, and hypercapnia can improve systemic arterial oxygen saturation and systemic oxygen delivery by increasing cerebral blood flow, SVC flow, and therefore pulmonary blood flow.

Stage 3: Post superior and inferior cavopulmonary anastomoses (post-Fontan). No systematic data exist for alveolar gas manipulation.

AVO_2D, Arteriovenous oxygen saturation difference; *CBF,* cerebral blood flow; *NIRS,* near-infrared spectroscopy; *Lactate,* lactate or metabolic acid change; *Q_p/Q_s,* pulmonary-to-systemic blood flow ratio; *rSO_2C,* cerebral oxygen saturation by NIRS; *rSO_2S,* somatic oxygen saturation by NIRS; *SaO_2,* arterial oxygen saturation; *SvO_2,* systemic venous (SVC) saturation; *TPG,* transpulmonary pressure gradient; *VO_2,* oxygen consumption.
Data from references 7, 20, and 81-90.

arrest the systemic blood flow (SBF) often has low oxygen content and in the presence of reduced coronary perfusion will result in coronary ischemia. As a result, the neonate with shunt-dependent single-ventricle physiology who undergoes a cardiac arrest with prolonged CPR is at particularly high risk for significant end-organ injury, including neurologic injury.

Due to the limitations of conventional CPR in the infant with shunt-dependent physiology, it is important to consider other resuscitation measures early in the resuscitation, including use of a pacer for bradycardia (particularly if pacing wires are already available), treatment of arrhythmias, treatment of possible shunt thrombosis, urgent opening of the sternum (in the immediate postoperative period), and early activation of ECLS, if available in the institution. In the infant with shunted single-ventricle physiology, prolonged in-hospital resuscitative efforts that include ECPR may be successful, whereas out-of-hospital resuscitation efforts are typically not successful.[76,80]

Superior Cavopulmonary Anastomosis and Fontan

In the child with a superior CPA circulation with low cardiac output or respiratory insufficiency or failure, strategies to improve venous return to the superior CPA will increase pulmonary blood flow and improve systemic saturation and systemic oxygen delivery. Ventilatory strategies that promote relative hypoventilation to increase cerebral blood flow and minimize intrathoracic pressure have been shown to be most useful. Although spontaneous breathing

is preferable to augment the extrathoracic to intrathoracic pressure gradient and increase pulmonary blood flow and stroke volume in the superior CPA or Fontan physiology, judicious mechanical ventilation is typically well tolerated in circumstances of respiratory insufficiency or failure or low cardiac output. Positive pressure ventilation lowers systemic afterload and wall stress to the systemic ventricle for the child with poor ventricular function or atrioventricular valve regurgitation; however, positive pressure ventilation will decrease pulmonary blood flow and ventricular preload. Modulation of inotropic support, afterload reduction, and positive pressure ventilation is complex and must be individualized for each child in an effort to avoid cardiac arrest. Table 31.4 delineates the effect of respiratory manipulations on circulatory parameters at different stages of palliation of children with univentricular physiology.[50]

Unique Challenges in Cardiopulmonary Resuscitation in Patients With a Superior Cavopulmonary Anastomosis or Fontan. Only 1% of patients undergoing a Fontan procedure will develop postoperative cardiac arrest, but 40% of those who arrest will not survive.[36] When cardiac arrest develops in patients who have had either of these surgeries, providers should begin conventional high-quality CPR.

There are important physiologic differences between single-ventricle patients with a superior CPA and a Fontan that impact resuscitation (see Table 31.3).[50] In these populations, chest compressions create systemic blood flow; however, pulmonary blood flow can be minimal, resulting in reduced oxygenation and preload to the systemic ventricle, creating a vicious cycle that limits cardiac output. Full recoil in these populations is particularly important (i.e., chest recoil can result in blood flow through the superior CPA and lungs, as well as from the inferior vena cava [IVC] into the systemic venous atrium, providing important preload to the single ventricle for the next compression). In contrast, chest recoil in Fontan physiology results in filling of the total cavopulmonary connection from the superior vena cava (SVC) and IVC. During CPR, cardiac output in patients with a superior CPA may be further reduced when there is hemodynamically significant insufficiency of the atrioventricular or semilunar valves. A further concern in patients with a superior CPA is the reduction in cerebral blood flow and risk of neurologic injury during chest compressions secondary to the elevation in SVC and cerebral venous pressure, minimizing the necessary gradient to perfuse the brain.[91]

Standard Versus Open Chest Cardiopulmonary Resuscitation

There are no data to support changing the AHA-recommended CPR technique in children with CHD, although the effectiveness of chest compressions may be compromised if the patient has an open chest. In addition, there are no data to support changing the techniques for cardioversion and defibrillation in children with CHD.[22]

In defibrillators with pads that contain an accelerometer to measure quality of chest compressions, mattress deflection can confound the measurement of chest compression depth. Thus, when possible, the recommendation would be to use anterior-posterior positioning of these pads such that more accurate measurement of chest compression depth can be made between the pads. These pads can be placed over a sternal dressing to measure quality of chest compressions but will not be able to defibrillate. If the child has dextrocardia, defibrillator pads should be placed over the right side of the chest to keep the heart between the defibrillation pads. If the child's chest is small, placing the pads in the anterior-posterior position will prevent overlap. This can even be done with paddles for very small infants (i.e., turn the infant on his or her side and place paddles on the chest and back to avoid paddles touching each other). For patients with an open sternum or sternal dressing that require defibrillation, paddle and pad positions may need to be modified, or internal paddles can be used under sterile conditions. In the setting of an open sternum and internal paddles, the dose for defibrillation is 10 to 20 J in adults[92,93] and 0.6 to 0.7 J/kg in children.

Monitoring Effectiveness of Resuscitation During Cardiac Arrest

Cardiac arrest is a no-flow or low-flow (during CPR) state that risks ischemic injury to critical organs if perfusion is not promptly restored. CPR is the providers' attempt to restore perfusion and prevent ischemic injury. The prevention of ischemic injury to critical organs depends on early recognition of inadequate perfusion, early institution of resuscitation efforts, the effectiveness of the resuscitation efforts, and the ability to restore adequate spontaneous (or extracorporeal) circulation. Patients with serious cardiovascular disease at risk for cardiac arrest are usually monitored in intensive care, where early recognition and intervention for cardiac arrest are possible. After the early recognition and intervention for cardiac arrest, the intensivist needs to be able to monitor the effectiveness of resuscitation so that efforts can be maximized while attempting to achieve ROSC or initiate ECPR. Monitoring the effectiveness of resuscitation efforts is a rapidly developing field that focuses on maximizing the provider's performance and optimizing the patient's response.

Maximizing the Provider's Performance— Human Feedback and Human Factors

There is increasing recognition of the cognitive load involved in managing a cardiac arrest. It is nearly impossible to ensure exquisite CPR while simultaneously following the rhythm-specific PALS algorithm, identifying and treating reversible causes, and activating ECPR. This is particularly true in the cardiac ICU setting, where teams can be large (including nurses, respiratory therapists, pharmacists, intensivists, and surgeons), there are many streams of information relevant to the cardiac arrest (human voices, bedside monitor with multiple physiologic parameters, NIRS monitor, $ETCO_2$ monitor, defibrillator feedback), and the anatomic and physiologic considerations of the cardiac arrest may be complex. To address this, Hunt et al. developed a model that explicitly distributes the workload of a resuscitation and intentionally cognitively unloads the team leader. Hunt introduced the role of the "quality CPR coach," who is responsible for coaching the team members performing CPR (i.e., compressions and ventilations) to perform within the AHA guidelines (see Table 31.2) or other physiologic goals such as diastolic blood pressure, CoPP, or $ETCO_2$ defined by the team leader and to periodically update the team leader. The goal is for the team leader to be able to focus on *advanced* life support (identifying the cardiac rhythm and following the appropriate PALS algorithm and considering and treating possible reversible causes) while another team member can focus on ensuring very high-quality *basic* life support. Another approach that can decrease the cognitive load of the leader and the team is to optimize and standardize the ergonomics of the room. Potential benefits include (1) optimizing sight lines (i.e., enable compressors to see the arterial line diastolic blood pressure or the depth of compressions reflected on the defibrillator directly in front of them), (2) improved communication, and (3) a shared mental model of how the room should be organized and a decrease in the amount of effort to "figure it out" during an emergency, for example, to enable the team to know ahead of time how to set up the room for ECPR. This entire approach is similar to a pit crew in auto racing or a dance team that creates choreography and practices with each other before important events.

Maximizing the Provider's Performance— Mechanical Feedback

Monitoring the effectiveness of the provider's performance involves feedback on the quality of the resuscitation efforts. This "mechanical" feedback can be used by the providers to meet recommendations for CPR quality. The AHA identifies the five components of high-quality CPR as providing chest compressions of adequate rate, ensuring chest compressions of adequate depth, allowing full chest recoil between compressions, minimizing interruptions in chest compressions (i.e., maximize "compression fraction"), and avoiding excessive ventilation.[44] The recommendations from the AHA for metrics of CPR performance are listed in Table 31.2. Performing high-quality CPR improves the outcome from cardiac arrest.[19]

Providing resuscitation efforts without having a system of ongoing training, practice, feedback, and debriefing often fails to promote

TABLE 31.5 Studies That Examine the Effect of Audiovisual Feedback During Cardiopulmonary Resuscitation on Quality Metrics and on Patient Outcome

Study	CCR (/min) NFB vs. FB	CCD (mm) NFB vs. FB	CCF (%) NFB vs. FB	CCL (%) NFB vs. FB	ROSC (%) NFB vs. FB	STD (%) NFB vs. FB	GNO (%) NFB vs. FB
Kramer-Johansen et al.,[94] 2006	121 vs. 109	34 vs. 38	52 vs. 56	0 vs. 0	17 vs. 23	3 vs. 4	NR
N = 358, OH	P .001	P .001	P .08	P .08	P .3	P .7	
Abella et al.,[25] 2007	104 vs. 100	42 vs. 44	77 vs. 80	NR	40 vs. 44	9 vs. 9	NR
N = 156, IH	P .16	P .47	P .26		P .58	P .97	
Hostler et al.,[95] 2011	108 vs. 103	38 vs. 40	64 vs. 66	15 vs. 10	45 vs. 44	12 vs. 11	10 vs. 10
N = 1586, OH	P .001	P .005	P .02	P .001	P .96	P .21	P .85
Bobrow et al.,[96] 2013	128 vs. 106	45 vs. 55	66 vs. 84	Not %	25 vs. 22	9 vs. 14	7 vs. 11
N = 484, OH					NS	OR 2.7 (1.2-6.4)	OR 2.7 (1.0-6.9)
Couper et al.,[97] 2015	121 vs. 114	45 vs. 53	78 vs. 84	18 vs. 14	35 vs. 50	16 vs. 17	16 vs. 14
N = 249, IH	P .02	P .001	P .002	P .75	P .26	P .28	P .60
Couper et al.,[97] 2015	126 vs. 116	50 vs. 49	78 vs. 82	14 vs. 12	39 vs. 42	17 vs. 13	15 vs. 11
N = 400, IH	P .001	P .38	P .003	P .91	P .60	P .83	P .86
Couper et al.,[97] 2015	120 vs. 116	46 vs. 54	80 vs. 84	14 vs. 12	52 vs. 56	19 vs. 20	18 vs. 18
N = 746, IH	P .08	P .001	P .001	P .87	P .66	P .73	P .80
Couper et al.,[97] 2015	122 vs. 115	46 vs. 54	79 vs. 83	15 vs. 12	45 vs. 51	18 vs. 18	17 vs. 16
N = 1395, IH	P .005	P .009	P .002	P .98	P .03	P .35	P .85

Note that the AHA guidelines increased the CCD from ≥38 mm to ≥50 mm in the 2010 recommendations.

CCD, Chest compression depth; *CCF*, chest compression force; *CCL*, chest compression leaning; *CCR*, chest compression rate; *FB*, feedback; *GNO*, good neurologic outcome; *IH*, in hospital; *NFB*, no feedback; *NR*, not reported; *NS*, not significant; *OR*, odds ratio; *OH*, out of hospital; *ROSC*, return of spontaneous circulation; *STD*, survival to discharge.

Data from references 25 and 94-97.

and ensure quality CPR. The inclusion of real-time audiovisual feedback about the quality (mechanics) of CPR has been effective in improving most CPR metrics in simulation (manikin) and actual clinical scenarios. Audiovisual feedback about CPR mechanics has been used to improve the quality of resuscitation efforts. Studies that have investigated CPR quality in actual clinical scenarios with and without audiovisual feedback are presented in Table 31.5.[25,94-97] Several of the studies show improvements in chest compression rate, depth, fraction, and leaning after audiovisual feedback is enabled. One shows that these metrics improved without feedback over the same time frame.[97] Most of these studies fail to show any improvement in outcome (ROSC, survival to discharge [STD], or neurologic function) despite the addition of audiovisual feedback and improvement in quality, though they were not designed with adequate power to do so (see Table 31.5).

Because it appears that real-time monitoring of the performance metrics of CPR has the potential to improve the quality of resuscitative efforts, it is important for us to consider how to optimize the use of these tools. It is important for caretakers in cardiac intensive care to focus on delivering chest compressions at the rate, depth, and release outlined in Table 31.2 and with minimal interruptions. Real-time feedback about performance metrics can be delivered by audio or visual output from resuscitation aids and/or from quality CPR coaches. It is important that providers be familiar with and not overwhelmed or distracted by the audiovisual input provided as they focus on the quality of their chest compression delivery.

Optimizing the Patient's Response— Physiologic Feedback

The use of real-time physiologic feedback during CPR involves monitoring the patient's response to the resuscitation efforts and has the potential to improve outcome. Using physiologic feedback has important differences from using mechanical feedback. Mechanical feedback is based on recommendations that are meant to be generally applicable to any cardiac arrest and other than slight alterations in the guidelines related to the patient's age, do not include guidance on how to individualize or optimize efforts based on the patient's underlying anatomy or physiologic response. The use of real-time physiologic feedback during CPR allows changes to resuscitation technique to be studied for effects on physiologic metrics.

The 2013 AHA consensus statement on CPR quality and improving resuscitation outcomes recommends the use of physiologic monitoring during CPR. The metrics include coronary perfusion pressure (CoPP), diastolic blood pressure (DBP), and ETCO2 level monitoring.[19] The CoPP is estimated at the bedside by the following parameters (CoPP = diastolic blood pressure − central venous pressure), please see further discussion below on more advanced and accurate calculations.

Studies involving physiologic feedback have focused on prognostication and provide little evidence or guidance about how to use this feedback to optimize resuscitative efforts. There are some animal data to support the timing of vasopressor administration to improve myocardial perfusion during CPR (see hemodynamic-directed CPR). The most commonly studied methods of physiologic monitoring include hemodynamic, $ETCO_2$, cerebral regional oxygen saturation ($rScO_2$), electrocardiogram amplitude spectral analysis, blood gas and blood lactate levels, and cardiac and vascular ultrasonography. These physiologic monitoring methods differ by whether they involve invasive techniques, are continuous or intermittent, are real-time or delayed, and whether they interfere with resuscitative efforts. These methods also differ by whether they represent myocardial, cerebral, or systemic perfusion and whether they can be used for prognostication, to determine futility, to detect ROSC, or to adjust resuscitative efforts. The study of the use of these methods during CPR is complicated by variations in measurement and reporting of clinical targets based on initial, average, 20-minute, peak, final, or trending values. Average values may be useful in research but are the most difficult to use in real time. Peak, 20-minute, and final values tend to be most useful when used for futility determinations. Trends in the values may ultimately be the most important clinically but are rarely reported in studies and deserve further attention. Explanations of these physiologic feedback techniques and the available information about their use are provided in the following sections.

Hemodynamic Monitoring During Cardiopulmonary Resuscitation. Hemodynamic monitoring during CPR involves the use of arterial and/or central venous pressure (CVP) catheters to measure the systolic blood pressure (SBP), DBP, SvO_2) and derived CoPP. Calculation of the CoPP requires both arterial and central venous access and uses the formula CoPP = DBP – the venous relaxation (diastolic) pressure. The CoPP is considered the most useful surrogate for myocardial blood flow during CPR. The next most useful surrogate for myocardial blood flow during CPR is the DBP, which requires arterial access. The SBP also requires arterial access and is a less well-described metric of systemic perfusion. Measurement of the SvO_2 requires central venous access and is a surrogate of systemic perfusion.

All four parameters used for hemodynamic monitoring during CPR require invasive monitoring and may be applicable to children in the cardiac ICU. It is not recommended to interrupt chest compression delivery to place invasive lines for the sole purpose of determining these measurements during CPR. However, if an arterial line can be placed during a cardiac arrest without compromising CPR, the real-time values may be very helpful in directing high-quality compressions. If the lines are already in place, these measurements may be used for optimal direction of high-quality compressions. This is important because it allows the team to maximize coronary perfusion while avoiding overzealous compressions with depths that increase risk of unintended consequences. The CoPP, DBP, and SBP can be measured continuously and in real time. The SvO_2 is measured intermittently unless an oximetric catheter is in place. The calculation of the CoPP during CPR requires both the DBP from the arterial line and the diastolic venous pressure from the central venous line. Because most bedside monitors display the CVP only as a mean value (i.e., does not report the CVP systolic and diastolic values), renaming the "CVP" within the bedside monitoring parameter menu as the "pulmonary artery" on the monitor allows the display of diastolic venous values to be available for CoPP calculation. For any of these four parameters the initial value may indicate the severity of the injury before starting CPR. Initial values that are low may indicate a worse preresuscitation status, whereas high initial values represent a less severe and potentially more recoverable status. Late values that are high or increasing represent a good response, whereas late values

---

TABLE 31.6 Parameters Used for Physiologic Feedback During Cardiopulmonary Resuscitation and Approximate Targets

Perfusion Area	Parameter	Target
Coronary	Arterial relaxation pressure	>25 mm Hg
	Myocardial perfusion pressure	>20 mm Hg
	Amplitude spectral area	>13 mV Hz
Cerebral	Cerebral regional oxygen saturation	>30%
Systemic	End-tidal carbon dioxide	>20-25 mm Hg
	Mixed venous saturation	>30%
	Blood lactate levels	<9-12 mmol/L

---

that remain low or are decreasing may represent a poor response to CPR and lower likelihood of ROSC and thus support strong consideration of ECPR.

Prognostication. In an early study of adults with OHCA a maximal CoPP of greater than 15 mm Hg predicts 50% survival.[98] No data are available for CoPP and survival in children. In a query of the AHA GWTG-R registry the use of DBP to monitor CPR quality was associated with improved ROSC in adults.[99]

Futility. The early study of adults with OHCA also found that a maximal CoPP of less than 15 mm Hg was associated with no survival.[98]

Detection of Return of Spontaneous Circulation. Rapid increase in arterial blood pressures may represent that ROSC has occurred, but no specific values have been suggested for holding chest compression delivery to determine if ROSC is present.

Direction of Resuscitative Efforts. A series of preclinical studies have led to the recommendation to use CoPP, DBP, SBP, and SvO_2 to monitor and optimize chest compression quality and titrating vasopressor therapy. Precise numeric targets have not been established, but approximate values are listed in Table 31.6. Specific target values for blood pressure have not been established in children. Rescuers in advanced care settings with access to invasive arterial blood pressure monitoring can use targets based on expert consensus.[19,41] In swine with ventricular fibrillation (VF)-induced cardiac arrest the adjustment of chest compression depth to obtain a CoPP above 30 mm Hg increased the rate of ROSC and postresuscitation myocardial function.[100] In an adult OHCA study the intraarrest placement of femoral catheters into the aorta and inferior vena cava allowed adjustment of the chest compression rate and depth and administration of intraaortic epinephrine to improve the CoPP from 8 to 25 mm Hg.[101] In a series of studies in 10- to 30-kg swine the use of hemodynamic-directed CPR (HD-CPR) has been compared with standard CPR in both VF and asphyxial arrest models of 7 minutes' duration.[102-108] The HD-CPR group received chest compressions adjusted to a depth to produce a SBP above 100 mm Hg, and epinephrine and vasopressin were titrated to produce a CoPP above 20 mm Hg. The standard CPR group received a chest compression depth consistent with current guidelines, and epinephrine was dosed at 4-minute intervals. The HD-CPR group consistently used a shallower chest compression depth than the standard group yet had an increased DBP, CoPP, rate of ROSC, and survival at 24 hours and improved neurologic outcome. The improvements in these parameters occurred in both VF and asphyxial arrest. In a retrospective review of 3 years of their group's animal experiments, Morgan et al. determined that a DBP less than 34 mm Hg was a threshold that was highly associated with nonsurvival.[107] The evolving data in this field are intriguing because they suggest that compression depth may not be as important as vasopressor administration in achieving target blood pressure goals and that there are potential benefits of individualized resuscitation. It is possible that in children who have hearts or vascular tone that are very responsive to chest compressions or vasopressors, the team might be able to minimize the compression depth needed and/or the amount of vasopressor needed. Alternatively, when the patient is less responsive, it is possible that by using more vasopressor the team may be able to minimize the depth of compressions needed and thus has the potential to decrease complications.

In cardiac intensive care, hemodynamic monitoring during CPR, when the appropriate vascular catheters are in place, may provide real-time information about the effectiveness of resuscitative efforts, myocardial perfusion, and the likelihood of ROSC. Adjusting resuscitative efforts, especially vasopressor administration, holds promise for improving these measurements, myocardial perfusion, and clinical outcomes. However, there are few human data and no current guidelines to clearly outline which physiologic parameters are the most important, what the goals for each parameter should be, and if the goals should vary by age, size, or anatomy. Thus this is a high-priority area of future research.

End-Tidal Carbon Dioxide Monitoring During Cardiopulmonary Resuscitation.

$ETCO_2$ monitoring during CPR involves the measurement of the carbon dioxide level at the end of expiration. The $ETCO_2$ level during CPR is a measure of pulmonary blood flow in low-flow states and has been shown to correlate with cardiac output (systemic perfusion). Capnography during CPR has been used to confirm endotracheal tube placement and maintenance, to monitor for ROSC, and to assess the effectiveness of CPR.

Capnography is preferred to capnometry because visualization of the waveform helps verify the integrity of the values. $ETCO_2$ measurements can be made continuously and in real time. As described in the following discussion, $ETCO_2$ levels during CPR are highly correlated with pulmonary and systemic perfusion. The use of $ETCO_2$ monitoring during CPR has traditionally been described in regard to use with an endotracheal tube. Although little information is available about the reliability of $ETCO_2$ measurements to assess the effectiveness of CPR with mask ventilation, we would still recommend placement of quantitative $ETCO_2$ capnography in line with face mask and bag until an advanced airway is placed. At a minimum, presence of an $ETCO_2$ waveform and numeric values with bag-mask ventilation confirm the airway is open and can confirm both some degree of ventilation and cardiac output are taking place.

Studies report different $ETCO_2$ measurements (initial, average, final, and 20 minute) in relation to a cardiac arrest. The initial value is important for early prognostication and evaluation of efforts. Definition of initial measurement varies by study (the first value after intubation, the value 1 minute after intubation, and the value six breaths after intubation are some of the variations in study design). The average value during an arrest is difficult to use clinically. A 20-minute value may be useful for termination of efforts. The final value may be problematic to interpret because of difficulty separating when ROSC occurred, and so the final value may be falsely elevated. In 30 adults with OHCA and $ETCO_2$ level above 20 mm Hg, between 5 and 10 minutes of CPR had the strongest correlation with ROSC.[109] A systematic review showed that the slope of the $ETCO_2$ trend line and the cumulative

maxETCO₂ were the most consistently significant differences between patients with and without ROSC.[110]

Several factors have an influence on $ETCO_2$ levels during CPR. The cause of the cardiac arrest may influence early $ETCO_2$ levels. Hypercarbia produced during asphyxia may take some time to wash out during CPR before the $ETCO_2$ level represents the effectiveness of resuscitation. In adults with asphyxial arrest the $ETCO_2$ levels after 5 minutes of CPR were useful.[111] In animals with asphyxia the $ETCO_2$ level normalized after five breaths[112] or 1 minute of CPR.[113] Bicarbonate and epinephrine administration during CPR may also influence the $ETCO_2$ level. Bicarbonate administration is associated with a transient increase in the $ETCO_2$ level. Epinephrine administration has been variably reported to transiently increase, decrease, or not affect the $ETCO_2$ level during CPR.

Prognostication. Two studies that evaluated the frequency of use of $ETCO_2$ monitoring in adults with cardiac arrest found an association between the use of $ETCO_2$ monitoring during CPR and ROSC.[107,114] A 2013 systematic review concluded that there was a strong correlation between $ETCO_2$ levels during CPR and outcome. They found that 15 of 18 studies confirmed association of $ETCO_2$ level with ROSC and 5 confirmed association of $ETCO_2$ level with STD.[110] A 2015 systematic review of 27 studies found that the mean $ETCO_2$ level in patients with ROSC was 26 mm Hg and without ROSC was 13 mm Hg. They suggest that developing a target $ETCO_2$ level during CPR has the potential to improve the rate of ROSC or decrease ischemic organ injury and that the potential target for prognostication may be higher than previously believed.[115] In adults with IHCA an initial $ETCO_2$ level (after six manual ventilations) above 25.5 mm Hg was predictive of sustained ROSC and STD but not of favorable neurologic outcome.[116]

Futility. An $ETCO_2$ level during CPR of less than 10 mm Hg immediately after intubation or after 20 minutes of CPR has been associated with extremely poor chances of ROSC.[110] Although proposed cutoff values for $ETCO_2$ have been considered to assist in predicting outcome, this is complicated because the value may be affected by confounders.[117] A confounder that is common clinically is the presence of pulmonary edema fluid in the endotracheal tube, which leads to a falsely low $ETCO_2$ level. There are other potential causes of low $ETCO_2$ levels that can be potential confounders (i.e., still have potential for recovery if the underlying issue is addressed). For example, an infant with a clotting BT shunt will likely have a low $ETCO_2$ level due to hypoperfusion to the lungs and associated poor cardiac output or cardiac arrest that may be reversible with medical management, including a high-dose heparin bolus and ECPR. A similar presentation can occur for a large pulmonary embolism as the cause for cardiac arrest in older children and adults. Finally, profound hypovolemia can also be associated with low $ETCO_2$ levels that may be the reversible cause of a cardiac arrest.[118-120] Recommendations for the use of $ETCO_2$ level in assessing futility apply only to intubated patients, and although an $ETCO_2$ level of less than 10 mm Hg is strongly associated with mortality, $ETCO_2$ values should not be used as a mortality predictor in isolation.[41] If the $ETCO_2$ level is much lower than expected despite optimizing quality of CPR, it is important to consider these potentially treatable alternate causes before considering futility.

Detection of Return of Spontaneous Circulation. An abrupt increase in $ETCO_2$ level during CPR can be the first sign of return of native circulation when CPR efforts are ongoing and may be an indication to stop chest compressions and check the rhythm and presence of a pulse. The size of the increase that indicates ROSC is not known, but author experience suggests a jump from the 20s to the 40s is highly suggestive of ROSC and warrants a coordinated pause to assess for a spontaneous pulse. Alternatively, when the ETCO$_2$ is consistently staying at a value below 25 with no other signs of improved cardiac output (i.e., no improvement in color, no spontaneous movement, no jump in arterial blood pressures,) the authors would avoid stopping chest compressions for pulse checks as very low yield, in order to minimize no-flow time.

Direction of Resuscitative Efforts. When the ETCO$_2$ level during CPR is consistently less than 15 mm Hg, efforts should focus on improving CPR quality (quality of chest compressions and avoiding overventilation).[20] In adults with IHCA and OHCA the ETCO$_2$ values during CPR were significantly associated with chest compression depth but not rate.[121] The use of the ETCO$_2$ level (in isolation from other feedback) to optimize chest compression depth and rate in a neonatal swine was as effective as standard CPR with chest compressions optimized by marker, video, and verbal feedback after a short arrest interval.[122] In a long arrest interval ETCO$_2$-guided CPR provided increased ROSC compared with standard CPR in the same preclinical mode.[122]

In cardiac intensive care, ETCO$_2$ level monitoring during CPR is widely available for intubated patients and should be used to continuously confirm airway access and to reflect and guide quality of CPR. For hospitals in limited-resource areas that do not have ETCO$_2$ monitoring available for every intubated patient, we advise owning even a single portable ETCO$_2$ device to be taken and used in the event of any cardiac arrest in the hospital. This has been a successful strategy as a first step or long-term strategy for cardiac arrest response teams. As an indicator of systemic perfusion, it is recommended as the second choice for monitoring the effectiveness of CPR behind hemodynamic monitoring.[19]

Cerebral Regional Oxygen Saturation Monitoring During Cardiopulmonary Resuscitation.
Cerebral regional oxygen saturation monitoring during CPR involves the use of a NIRS emitter and sensor applied to the patient's forehead. NIRS is not dependent on pulsatile flow and can be used in low-flow states. The measured values represent the saturation in primarily venous (70% venous) blood and are a surrogate for regional brain perfusion.

Cerebral regional oxygen saturation is noninvasive and can be used continuously and in real time. This monitoring may already be in place after a cardiac surgical procedure because cerebral NIRS monitoring is often used intraoperatively and continued postoperatively. Monitoring rScO$_2$ during CPR may provide a surrogate for regional brain perfusion during CPR. In a 2016 systematic review of 19 studies examining the initial, mean, and highest levels of rScO$_2$ during CPR the highest levels were too heterogeneous a subgroup for meta-analysis. The initial level was associated with STD and favorable neurologic outcome, a combination of mean and initial levels was associated with STD and favorable neurologic outcome, but the mean level alone was not associated with STD or neurologic outcome.[123] The mean levels were more likely to be associated with ROSC than initial levels. NIRS is mainly a trend monitoring technique, and trends during CPR may offer the most important prognostic value.[124]

Prognostication. In adults in cardiac arrest, survival has been associated with mean rScO$_2$ levels,[125] an increase in rScO$_2$ level of more than 20% during CPR,[126] an increase from baseline, and percentage of time with rScO$_2$ level above 40%.[127] In adults with IHCA, maintaining the rScO$_2$ level above 50% improved survival with a favorable neurologic outcome, and peak rScO$_2$ (>65%) was associated with ROSC.[128] A 2015 systematic review of nine studies

of adults with OHCA and IHCA found that higher initial and averaged NIRS levels were associated with ROSC.[124] In adults with OHCA going onto ECPR, no change in rScO$_2$ level after initiation of ECPR was a better prognosis for neurologic outcome than if the level improved on ECPR.[129]

Futility. In adults with IHCA or OHCA a persistently low (<25% to 30%) rScO$_2$ may predict futility.[123,125,130]

Detection of Return of Spontaneous Circulation. In adults with OHCA without endotracheal intubation with standard chest compressions, the use of NIRS in the emergency department was associated with ROSC.[131]

Direction of Resuscitative Efforts. In adult IHCA, during four separate episodes of low-quality CPR, no increase in NIRS was observed despite efforts to improve the quality of CPR.[132] In cardiac intensive care, monitoring rScO$_2$ levels during CPR may be useful when available and is easy to apply if not already applied. It may be useful to predict outcome or futility and to detect ROSC. The usefulness of rScO$_2$ to direct resuscitative efforts is still not clear.

Blood Gas and Lactate Level Monitoring During Cardiopulmonary Resuscitation. Blood gas and lactate level monitoring involves the determination of pH, pO$_2$, or pCO$_2$ and lactate levels by blood sampling during CPR. Low pH or lactate levels may be associated with long periods of no or low flow. Trends in any of these values during CPR may reflect systemic perfusion produced by resuscitative efforts. Blood gas and lactate level monitoring during CPR is invasive and requires a vascular catheter or IO access. Continuous and real-time analysis using these methods are not available.

Prognostication. In adults with OHCA an intraarrest pCO$_2$ level of less than 75 mm Hg (either arterial or venous) on arrival to the emergency department was associated with sustained ROSC.[133] Other blood gas variables and the lactate level were not predictive of ROSC. The use of blood gas and ETCO$_2$ measurements to calculate the arterial-alveolar (PaCO$_2$-ETCO$_2$) CO$_2$ difference was inversely associated with survival to hospital admission.[134,135] In adults with IHCA an intraarrest serum lactate level of less than 9 mmol/L measured during first 10 minutes of CPR was associated with STD and favorable neurologic outcome.[136] No study was found that used blood gas or lactate levels during CPR to predict futility, detect ROSC, or direct resuscitation efforts.

In cardiac intensive care, many patients often have catheters that would allow frequent sampling of these parameters during CPR. The contribution of these parameters to the management of children in arrest is unknown but likely similar to the observations from adults. The data could be additive to that from other methodologies when assessing the effectiveness of prolonged CPR efforts.

Ultrasound Monitoring During Cardiopulmonary Resuscitation.
Ultrasound monitoring during CPR involves the use of echocardiography to determine reversible causes of cardiac arrest, mechanical activity versus standstill, or blood flow during resuscitative efforts. Echocardiography, although noninvasive, may interfere with chest compression performance.[137] It is real time but usually not continuous. Intermittent application is used to reduce interference with resuscitative efforts. Ultrasound monitoring during cardiac arrest can demonstrate cardiac mechanical activity and detect carotid blood flow or be used to rule out reversible causes of cardiac arrest.

Prognostication. Mechanical activity on initial ultrasound examination during cardiac arrest is associated with ROSC (84%) versus its absence (14%).[138] Echocardiography use during the 10-second intervals when compressors changed was evaluated to determine reversible causes of pulseless electrical activity (PEA). It detected hypovolemia and trivial effusion but not pneumothorax or tamponade. Treatment based on findings did not improve survival. True PEA did not result in survival.[139]

Futility. Serial ultrasound examinations during the 10-second intervals every 2 minutes for pulse check and compressor change showed that no adult with an OHCA and cardiac standstill at the 10-minute or greater examination had ROSC.[140]

Detection of Return of Spontaneous Circulation. No study was found that used ultrasound measurement during CPR specifically to detect ROSC. Many studies use ultrasonography during CPR to detect mechanical activity when pulses are not present. The distinction between inadequate and adequate mechanical activity is usually made based on hemodynamics.

Direction of Resuscitative Efforts. The feasibility of collection of 5 minutes of common carotid blood flow measurements during chest compressions has been shown in adults with OHCA. The relevance of this technique to the performance of CPR is not known.[141]

Diagnosis of the Cause of Cardiac Arrest. The finding of right ventricle dilation by echocardiography during CPR in a preclinical study was not useful to determining pulmonary embolus.[142] Reversible causes, including hypovolemia, tension pneumothorax, tamponade, pulmonary embolism, and myocardial activity, can be detected using ultrasonography in 10-second intervals during compressor change.[139,143]

In cardiac intensive care, ultrasonography or echocardiography is often available and may be considered during CPR but risks potential harm from interruption of chest compressions. Suspicion of an ultrasound-detectable cause is recommended before use because of the lack of evidence that it changes outcome. Tamponade, hypovolemia, and hemothorax or pneumothorax may be more common in cardiac intensive care and increase the usefulness of intraarrest ultrasonography.

Mechanical Support—Extracorporeal Life Support and Extracorporeal Cardiopulmonary Resuscitation

Since Bartlett and others started using extracorporeal membrane oxygenation (ECMO) to support children with CHD in the 1970s, ECMO has evolved from an extraordinary, last resort, lifesaving intervention to a standard of care in many pediatric centers with thousands of patients supported to date.[130,144,145] Indications for ECMO now include not only cardiovascular and/or respiratory failure but also sustained cardiac arrest. Extracorporeal CPR (ECPR or rescue ECMO) is the initiation of ECMO support while active chest compressions are taking place. ECPR was first described in 1992, and since then its use has increased significantly.[146,147] Improvement in outcomes following in-hospital pediatric cardiac arrest has been attributed in part to the impact of ECMO as a rescue strategy when prolonged conventional CPR cannot restore spontaneous circulation.[33,148-150] Pediatric patients who receive ECPR for refractory cardiac arrest have survival to hospital discharge rates ranging from 33% to 42% in general ICU patients[151-154] and from 23% to 55% in cardiac ICU patients.[153-155] The AHA has recognized a role for ECPR in the 2015 pediatric advanced life support guidelines for CPR and emergency cardiovascular care. These guidelines recommend that ECPR may be considered for pediatric patients with cardiac diagnoses who have IHCA in settings with existing ECMO protocols, expertise, and equipment.[41] The recent AHA scientific statement "Cardiopulmonary Resuscitation in Infants and Children With Cardiac Disease" outlines cannulation strategies (Table 31.7) for ECPR and mechanical circulatory support device strategy in rapidly deteriorating children with heart disease (Fig. 31.2).[50]

TABLE 31.7 Cannulation Strategies for Extracorporeal Cardiopulmonary Resuscitation

General Principles for Efficient Use of ECLS to Support CPR

1. Venoarterial ECLS should be utilized in all cases.
2. Knowledge of venous anatomy and previously occluded vessels is critical for successful and timely deployment of ECLS.
3. Central (transthoracic) cannulation may be considered in patients who have undergone a recent sternotomy.
4. Peripheral (percutaneous) cannulation may be preferred for patients without recent sternotomy.
5. ECLS cannulas should be large enough to provide complete cardiac output (CI greater than 2.5 L/min/ m²). If ECMO flow is limited by inadequate venous drainage, secondary drainage sites should be considered.

| Physiology | PERIPHERAL CANNULATION | | CENTRAL CANNULATION | | Comments |
	Venous	Arterial	Venous	Arterial	
Biventricular circulation	Internal jugular or femoral	Common carotid or femoral	Systemic venous atrium	Aorta	Left atrial decompression may be required.
Single ventricle or shunted physiology	Internal jugular	Common carotid	Systemic venous or common atrium	Aorta	Shunt restriction may be required. For carotid cannulation with a MBTS, cannula position may result in shunt overcirculation or occlusion.
Superior cavopulmonary anastomosis	Internal jugular and/or femoral	Common carotid	SVC and/or systemic venous or common atrium	Aorta	Additional venous cannula may be required.
Fontan	Internal jugular and/or femoral	Common carotid or femoral	Fontan baffle	Aorta	Additional venous cannula may be required. Pulmonary venous atrial drainage may be required.

CI, Cardiac index; *ECLS,* extracorporeal life support; *ECMO,* extracorporeal membrane oxygenation; *MBTS,* modified Blalock-Taussig shunt; *SVC,* superior vena cava.
Modified from Marino BS, Tabbutt S, MacLaren G, et al. Cardiopulmonary resuscitation in infants and children with cardiac disease: a scientific statement from the American Heart Association. *Circulation.* 2018;137(22):e691-e782.

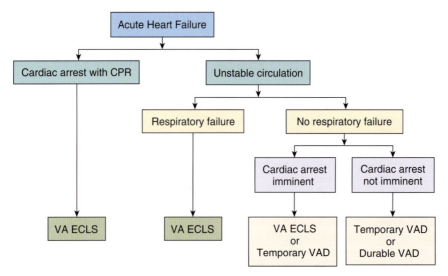

1. Choice of VAD depends on patient size and need for LV or biventricular support.
2. Examples of temporary VAD: centrifugal pump ECLS without oxygenator, Impella, and TandemHeart.
3. Examples of durable VADs: Berlin Heart EXCOR, Thoratec PVAD, HeartMate, HeartWare, and TAH/Syncardia.

• **Figure 31.2** Mechanical circulatory support device strategy in rapidly deteriorating children with heart disease. *CPR,* Cardiopulmonary resuscitation; *ECLS,* extracorporeal life support; *LV,* left ventricular; *TAH,* total artificial heart; *VA,* venoarterial; *VAD,* ventricular assist device. (Data from references 186 through 208.)

Evidence from four observational studies of pediatric IHCA has shown no overall benefit to the use of ECPR compared to conventional CPR.[12,156-158] More recently, however, data from the GWTG-R registry have shown that among pediatric patients treated with at least 10 minutes of in-hospital CPR, those receiving ECPR had greater odds of STD than patients who received continued CPR. Importantly, ECPR patients also had a greater survival with favorable neurologic outcome.[24] Similar improved outcomes have been shown when ECPR is used for children with underlying cardiac disease compared to those with noncardiac disease,[33] with the population of surgical cardiac diagnoses having the greatest likelihood for survival to hospital discharge.[32]

Historically, pediatric CPR was considered futile beyond 20 minutes' duration or more than two doses of epinephrine.[159,160] A recent report from the AHA's GWTG-R analyzed the relationship between CPR duration and survival to hospital discharge after pediatric IHCA.[161] Survival rates fell linearly over the first 15 minutes of CPR, yet patients who received ECPR had no difference in survival across CPR durations. Survival for patients receiving more than 35 minutes of conventional CPR was only 15.9% (survival for patients receiving conventional CPR for <15 minutes was 44.1%). For children with underlying cardiac disease, when ECPR is initiated in a critical care setting, long-term survival has been reported even after more than 50 minutes of conventional CPR.[151] In a report from the Extracorporeal Life Support Organization (ELSO) database on 492 patients with cardiac disease who underwent ECPR,[162] survival to hospital discharge was 42%, with mortality associated with single-ventricle physiology, the stage I Norwood procedure, extreme acidosis before ECMO, renal injury, neurologic injury, and duration of ECMO support. Right carotid artery cannulation was associated with decreased mortality risk and is most likely secondary to the ability to perform high-quality CPR without interruption with neck cannulation, compared to transthoracic cannulation.

Long-term neurologic outcome data are lacking in survivors of ECPR. In the ELSO database, acute neurologic injury was reported in 22% of the 682 patients who had ECPR.[163] Acute neurologic injury was defined in the ELSO database as brain death, cerebral infarction, or intracranial hemorrhage determined by ultrasonography or computerized tomography imaging of the head; 11% had brain death, 7% cerebral infarction, and 7% intracranial hemorrhage, with an in-hospital mortality for patients with acute neurologic injury of 89%. However, this manuscript did not report any medium-term (at hospital discharge) or long-term (following index hospitalization) neurologic outcome data as functional outcome at discharge, and long-term follow-up after index hospitalization was not collected by ELSO. Although recent papers have reported high percentages of children with good neurologic outcome at the time of discharge,[33,152,162] this most likely does not represent true long-term neurologic injury because the majority of survivors are young infants. A small cohort study of 51 pediatric cardiac patients is the only study reporting detailed neurocognitive outcomes of ECPR survivors and found that global intelligence, vocabulary, and adaptation skills were significantly lower than the population mean with 24% having intellectual disability.[164] These results highlight the need for further studies to identify improved ECPR protocols and techniques, as well as early intervention programs for these children to optimize their long-term outcomes. It is also important to consider that ECPR is usually provided to those patients with refractory cardiac arrest, and these children were likely to die if this support was not provided.

Post Cardiac Arrest

In past decades, efforts to resuscitate a child would cease when the child either had ROSC, the team determined it was futile to continue, or the parents asked for the resuscitation to stop. In the era of ECPR there is a fourth option: the team may have achieved "circulation," albeit via the ECMO circuit, but no spontaneous pulse. This is now commonly referred to as return of circulation (ROC), rather than ROSC. If a child was hemodynamically unstable or in a coma, then critical care would continue, but there was not an organized framework for "post–cardiac arrest care" (PCAC). This period has become increasingly complex and nuanced, and efforts to improve processes of care during the post–cardiac arrest period are having an important impact on optimizing neurologically intact survival. The science in this area continues to evolve, but it is clear there are two distinct issues to address regardless of whether the child is resuscitated. The first is postevent debriefing, and the second is performing organized PCAC.

Post–Cardiac Arrest Debriefing

The literature continues to accumulate that debriefing teams on their performance after a cardiac arrest has a positive impact on subsequent resuscitation performance and may impact survival as well.[165-167] There is also evidence to suggest that combining real-time feedback during the cardiac arrest with postevent debriefing is synergistic with a stronger impact than either element alone.[166] A common element to debriefings associated with improved performance is the use of objective performance data. This allows the discussion to move beyond a reflection of the team's subjective experience to a discussion framed around any performance gaps and/or exploring things that went exceptionally well. Despite these data, a survey of a nationally representative sample of US hospitals published in 2014 revealed that only 34% of hospitals report conducting post–cardiac arrest debriefings.[168]

Research is being conducted as to how to optimize debriefing (i.e., hot debriefings [immediately after the event], cold debriefings [separated in time from the event once data have been accumulated and reviewed—e.g., 1 week later], or a combination of the two). Although there is less evidence on the role of the hot debriefing, the authors' experience is that it can be important for several reasons. Traditionally teams have focused on the fact that it can be used to diffuse the situation emotionally and help the team get back to work knowing there will be time for further discussion about what went well and what needs further discussion at a subsequent cold debriefing. The time can be used to create the agenda for that follow-up meeting. In addition, a hot debriefing can be used to make sure that any broken equipment or used-up medication is replaced or restocked before any subsequent events, as well as to clarify and refine the plan for any subsequent cardiac arrests that the child may have. For example, should the child receive ECMO immediately to avoid a second arrest; in the event of ECPR, can the room be optimized for ergonomics (i.e., move the child so the surgeon has easy access to perform the cannulation); have all reversible causes been addressed, or should the parents be approached about limiting further resuscitation efforts? Finally, the postevent hot debriefing is an excellent time to discuss the PCAC goals as defined in the next section.

Post–Cardiac Arrest Care

Ongoing clinical instability in the postresuscitation period often occurs, necessitating continuous cardiopulmonary monitoring and careful management to allow recovery time, optimize systemic perfusion to preserve end-organ function, and optimize outcomes. Precipitating causes of the arrest should be identified and treated promptly to avoid further deterioration and recurrent arrest. Placement of arterial access is helpful for blood gas sampling and blood pressure monitoring. If IO access was placed for resuscitation, more stable venous access is warranted with subsequent removal of the IO as soon as possible. An indwelling urinary catheter is helpful to follow urine output closely as both a surrogate marker to adequate cardiac output and possible renal injury. Laboratory values, including renal function, electrolytes, complete blood count, coagulation studies, venous and arterial blood gases, and lactate, may help guide postresuscitation care, particularly when abnormal values are identified that may have contributed to the cardiac arrest. A chest x-ray should be obtained to assess appropriate ETT placement and to assess for cardiopulmonary pathology (including heart size, parenchymal lung disease, pneumothorax, and/or pleural effusions.)

Myocardial dysfunction and vascular instability are common after arrest, and inotropic support is often required. An echocardiogram to assess for inadequate ventricular filling, myocardial function, and cardiac tamponade can guide therapy for fluid resuscitation, inotropic support, or need for pericardiocentesis, respectively. Hypotension (less than fifth percentile for age) should be avoided in the postresuscitation period because hypotension has been associated with lower likelihood of survival with favorable neurologic outcome.[169] There are no data currently to recommend specific vasoactive medications for blood pressure support, and such infusions should be tailored to patient-specific physiology and cause of cardiac arrest.

Typically 100% oxygen is administered during CPR, especially in the hospital setting. After return of circulation, monitoring of oxygen saturations and PaO_2 is prudent because both hyperoxemia and hypoxemia after cardiac arrest have been associated with worse outcomes.[170,171] Postischemic hyperoxemia contributes to oxidative stress and cellular injury, decreased cardiac output, and decreased oxygen delivery to the cerebral and coronary vascular beds.[172-174] Hypoxemia limits oxygen delivery to tissues that have just experienced ischemic time. The AHA currently recommends targeting normoxemia (defined as a PaO_2 level between 60 and 300 mm Hg) and avoidance of hyperoxemia and hypoxemia. In the absence of arterial blood gas information, one should wean supplemental oxygen as tolerated for a pulse oximetry saturation of 94% to 100% (or patient-specific goal saturations) to avoid hyperoxemia.[41]

Few data exist to support a specific $PaCO_2$ range in the postarrest period. Given that $PaCO_2$ plays an important role in the regulation of cerebral flow, it is sensible to avoid hyperventilation and hypocapnia because this may decrease cerebral blood flow and potentiate neuronal ischemia. In one observational pediatric study, both hypocapnia and hypercapnia post arrest were associated with higher mortality.[171] At this time the AHA recommends targeting $PaCO_2$ for the specific patient's condition and limiting significant hypocapnia or hypercapnia.[41]

Glucose level should be measured during and after resuscitation, particularly in infants because they have a higher glucose requirement and lower glycogen stores. The authors have experienced patients who have been hyperglycemic at the beginning of the arrest with progression to "unmeasurably low values" during prolonged arrests. Thus we would recommend checking the glucose level every 20 to 30 minutes during a prolonged resuscitation attempt (i.e., ECPR). Hypoglycemia should be treated promptly. Hyperglycemia is common in the postarrest period, but with few data to support tight glycemic control, the AHA does not currently have a target glucose range recommendation.

Current AHA guidelines recommend continuous temperature monitoring following cardiac arrest with the primary focus on avoiding fever (>38°C) because fever has been associated with poor outcomes.[41,175] Therapeutic hypothermia following arrest in attempt to prevent neurologic injury has been a controversial topic. Though therapeutic hypothermia has been shown to improve neurologic outcomes in neonates with asphyxia[176] and adults after OHCA with an initial rhythm of ventricular fibrillation,[177] there are conflicting data in infants and children. One study showed improved survival in infants and children after cardiac arrest,[178] whereas others have shown worsened mortality and functional outcome.[179] A recent large multicenter randomized controlled trial evaluating the effects of therapeutic hypothermia (target temperature 33°C) versus therapeutic normothermia (target temperature 36.8°C) for 120 hours post–cardiac arrest showed no difference in survival with a favorable neurologic outcome at 1 year for both the in- and out-of-hospital populations.[180,181] Thus for patients who remain comatose after cardiac arrest, it is not clear whether hypothermia improves outcomes, but clearly fever should be avoided. Thus it is currently recommended to maintain 5 days of normothermia (36°C to 37.5°C) or 2 days of hypothermia (32°C to 34°C) followed by 3 days of normothermia.[41]

Prognostication Post Arrest

Practitioners must consider multiple factors when trying to predict outcome because no sole criterion for prognostication of neurologic outcome and survival after cardiac arrest exists. Many factors have been associated with poor neurologic outcomes and/or increased mortality after pediatric cardiac arrest, including age greater than 1 year, longer duration of CPR,[182] persistent hypotension after resuscitation,[169] persistent lactate level elevation after 12 hours,[183] high and persistently elevated levels of serum neuronal biomarkers (neuron-specific enolase and S100B),[184] poor pupillary response at 12 to 24 hours,[182] and discontinuous or isoelectric tracing on electrocardiogram within 7 days of arrest.[185]

Conclusion

In conclusion, over the past two decades survival from pediatric cardiac arrest has improved dramatically, particularly in the in-hospital setting, from 15% to nearly 50%. The reasons for this are multifactorial, and include but are likely not limited to the use of ECPR, personalizing the care delivered to that child's age and also the child's underlying cardiac anatomy and physiology, and applying a multitude of approaches to improving the quality of care we deliver. Teams are now systematically addressing the quality of CPR delivered during the event with real-time feedback with bedside devices and quality CPR coaches, postevent debriefing, and meticulously managing the PCAC period. Unfortunately, there is evidence of great variability between hospitals, suggesting there are still lives to be saved. In the upcoming decades we need to continue to explore physiologic targets to optimize coronary and cerebral perfusion while minimizing harm from compressions, use human factors to improve team dynamics and room ergonomics, refine approaches to PCAC, and improve our ability to prognosticate on outcomes. Although avoiding a cardiac arrest is always best, we now know that many lives can be saved with exquisite CPR, and we must continue to focus on optimizing outcomes for these most vulnerable of patients.

References

A complete list of references is available at ExpertConsult.com.

32

Pediatric General Surgeon and Critically Ill Cardiac Patient

ALLISON L. SPEER, MD; BETH A. RYMESKI, DO; JOHN K. PETTY, MD

Although congenital heart disease (CHD) most commonly occurs as an isolated condition, approximately one in four newborns with CHD will have other congenital anomalies.[1,2] These noncardiac anomalies may pose a threat to life or function and require the skills of a pediatric surgeon. Specifically, newborns with esophageal atresia (EA), duodenal atresia, malrotation, Hirschsprung disease (HD), and anorectal malformations may also have CHD and thus require multidisciplinary care from the pediatric surgical team and the congenital heart team. In addition to caring for noncardiac congenital anomalies, the pediatric surgeon may care for nonstructural conditions such as necrotizing enterocolitis (NEC), dysfunctional feeding, pathologic gastroesophageal reflux, and difficult vascular access in children with CHD. In all cases a spirit of true collaboration between the surgical and nonsurgical specialists is paramount to achieving the best possible outcome for the child. A comprehensive review of these myriad conditions would exceed the scope of this project. Rather, the following discussion focuses on the bedside evaluation and clinical management of major pediatric surgical conditions in the child with CHD.

Esophageal Atresia and Tracheoesophageal Fistula

EA with tracheoesophageal fistula (TEF) is an uncommon anomaly, occurring in approximately 1 per 3500 to 1 per 4000 live births.[3-5] Several configurations of EA/TEF are recognized, with the most common being proximal EA with distal TEF type C, which occurs in 80% to 85% of cases. At least 50% of newborns with EA/TEF have other associated anomalies.[5,6] Cardiovascular anomalies occur in approximately 30% of these patients, most commonly ventricular septal defect.[5,6] EA/TEF may occur alongside cardiovascular anomalies as part of a recognized association of anomalies. The VACTERL association includes vertebral anomalies, atresia (anus, duodenum), cardiovascular anomalies, TEF, renal anomalies, and limb anomalies. EA/TEF may occur as part of the CHARGE association, which includes coloboma, heart defects, atresia choanae, retardation (developmental delay), genitourinary anomalies, and ear deformities. Severe cardiac anomalies are associated with mortality in newborns with EA/TEF, as is low birth weight. Historically infants with EA/TEF, major CHD, and birth weight less than 1500 g have had mortality as high as 78%, compared with 3% mortality in EA/TEF patients without major CHD or low birth weight.[7] Although mortality has decreased with improvements

in neonatal and cardiovascular care, it serves as an important reminder of the complex nature of these patients.

The congenital heart surgery team and the pediatric surgery team collaborate in two main arenas regarding infants with combined EA/TEF and CHD: preoperative care and intraoperative care. Preoperatively both teams should discuss which anomalies are most life threatening and whether temporizing treatment or definitive treatment should be pursued initially. Newborns with EA/TEF may develop respiratory distress related to several factors. If the TEF is large, they may lose significant tidal volume through the fistula into the GI tract. This can create progressive abdominal distention, which can impair diaphragmatic excursion. In addition, gastric distention may lead to regurgitation of gastric fluid directly into the airways through the fistula. Such patients with progressive respiratory distress may be temporized by an urgent surgical gastrostomy. This approach may get the patient through a period of critical illness, whether from prematurity or physiologically significant CHD. Infants with a decompressive gastrostomy are not safe to feed enterally until they have definitive correction of their TEF.

Intraoperative collaboration between pediatric surgery and congenital heart surgery for EA/TEF typically pertains to aberrant thoracic anatomy. Newborns with EA/TEF should receive an echocardiogram soon after birth to assess the sidedness of the aortic arch. Patients with a left-sided aortic arch have exposure and repair of their esophagus through a right thoracotomy. Patients who have a right-sided aortic arch or a double aortic arch should have preoperative consultation with a congenital heart surgeon. Traditionally patients with a right-sided aortic arch should have a left thoracotomy to repair their EA/TEF. On occasion, preoperative echocardiography will fail to recognize a right-sided aortic arch, and the pediatric surgeon will identify a right-sided arch through a standard right thoracotomy for anticipated repair of EA/TEF. If the length of the upper esophageal pouch is sufficient, it is reasonable to proceed with mobilization of the upper pouch and repair of the EA/TEF without dividing the right-sided aortic arch. If the upper esophageal pouch is short, or if it cannot be adequately mobilized without dividing the right-sided aortic arch, it is advisable to obtain intraoperative consultation with a congenital heart surgeon. The aortic arch should not be divided without a complete understanding of the patient's thoracic vascular anatomy. This knowledge may be obtained by stopping the operation and obtaining a high-resolution computed tomography (CT) angiogram of the chest or by closing the right thoracotomy and performing a left

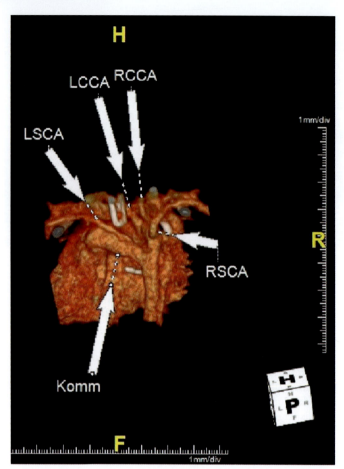

• **Figure 32.1** Computed tomography angiogram reconstruction of a patient with esophageal atresia, tracheoesophageal fistula, and a vascular ring (posterior view). The tube at the center represents the oroesophageal tube, terminating in the proximal esophageal pouch. The vascular ring includes a right-sided aortic arch with a patent ductus arteriosus to a large diverticulum of Kommerell *(Komm)*. This patient has an aberrant left sub-clavian artery *(LSCA)*. *LCCA,* Left common carotid artery; *RCCA,* right common carotid artery; *RSCA,* right subclavian artery.

thoracotomy for vascular exploration (Fig. 32.1). Surgeons who are facile with minimally invasive techniques may consider the use of thoracoscopy in this setting. Once the patient's thoracic vascular anatomy is determined, it is appropriate to proceed with esophageal and vascular repairs at the same operation. Collaboration between the congenital heart surgeon and the pediatric surgeon is paramount in complex newborns such as these.

Malrotation

Intestinal rotation abnormalities (IRAs) manifest across a range of anatomic arrangements and symptomatic presentations. Fundamentally these relate to disruptions in the normal 270-degree counterclockwise rotation of the midgut and retroperitoneal fixation of the duodenum and the right colon during the 4th to 12th weeks of gestation. If the patient's IRA results in a narrow mesentery, the patient is at risk for developing midgut volvulus. True malrotation occurs when the duodenal-jejunal junction is located in the right upper quadrant of the abdomen, the third and fourth portions of the duodenum are intraperitoneal rather than retroperitoneal, and the cecum is nonfixed or poorly fixed to the right upper

quadrant. True malrotation creates a narrow mesentery and risk for midgut volvulus. Nonrotation occurs when the midgut rotates less than 180 degrees, such that the small bowel comes to lie on the right side of the abdomen and the colon on the left side of the abdomen. Patients with nonrotation typically do not have a narrow mesentery and are at lower risk for midgut volvulus. IRAs less than 270 degrees may be considered incomplete rotation. These terms can be confusing and are often incorrectly used interchangeably. It is critical to remember that it is the risk of midgut volvulus that drives the concern for IRAs.

IRAs may present with a wide variety of symptoms, ranging from completely normal gastrointestinal function up to complete midgut necrosis with perforation and sepsis. Other symptoms may be due to intermittent or incomplete volvulus, including feeding intolerance, gastroesophageal reflux disease, abdominal pain, abdominal distention, chylous ascites, protein-losing enteropathy, gastrointestinal bleeding, NEC, or intestinal obstruction. These symptoms can result from other causes as well. In the absence of a clear-cut episode of volvulus on upper gastrointestinal (UGI) contrast study or operative exploration, it is difficult to know the contribution of the IRA to a patient's symptoms (Fig. 32.2).

Infants with CHD, particularly heterotaxy syndrome (HS), have an incidence of malrotation as high as 40% to 90%.[8] Two recent systematic reviews evaluated the published literature regarding malrotation in patients with severe CHD and HS.[8,9] The authors recommend against screening asymptomatic patients for malrotation. GI symptoms are very common in patients with severe CHD. If an UGI contrast study is performed to evaluate these symptoms, and malrotation is discovered, a decision about performing a Ladd procedure must be placed in the context of the CHD. Only 1.2% of patients with HS had the feared presentation of midgut volvulus. A Ladd procedure can result in significant morbidity in this population. Postoperative complications occur in 14% of patients, including a 10% incidence of small bowel obstruction. Overall mortality following a Ladd procedure in these patients is 21%, including a 3% mortality perioperatively. The vast majority of this mortality is from their cardiovascular disease, rather than their GI disease. Accordingly, patients with severe CHD who have malrotation and minor symptoms should be observed until their CHD is palliated. At that point a Ladd procedure may be considered, though it may also be reasonable to continue to observe these patients. Patients with severe GI symptoms or acute volvulus before CHD palliation should undergo a Ladd procedure with the acknowledgment that this is a high-risk intervention. Finally, during the period of observation, health care providers and family members should be aware of the possibility of the patient's developing acute midgut volvulus and the accompanying symptoms that would signal this event. The pediatric surgeon should be consulted to help with these discussions and to be aware of the patient if an acute surgical need should arise. A decision algorithm for the treatment of malrotation in the patient with CHD is illustrated in Fig. 32.3.

Other Congenital Pediatric Surgical Conditions

Because organogenesis of the cardiovascular system occurs simultaneously with organogenesis in the GI system, defects in one system may occur with defects in the other. Although a full review of the interplay between congenital cardiac and GI defects is beyond the scope of the current discussion, several important clinical points

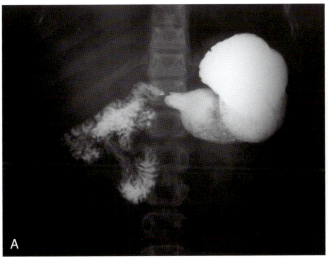
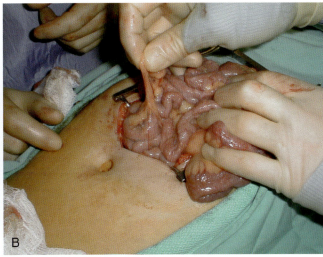

• **Figure 32.2** An 8-year-old girl with a history of "nonspecific" intermittent crampy abdominal pain was involved in a motor vehicle crash. (A) Computed tomography scan for her trauma evaluation suggested malrotation, which was confirmed by upper gastrointestinal series. (B) Operative findings included peritoneal bands across the proximal small bowel.

of pediatric surgical care bear mentioning for the provider whose area of expertise is congenital cardiovascular care.

HD involves the absence of ganglion cells in the hindgut and a variable amount of distal bowel. Neural crest cells form the enteric ganglion cells and are also involved with development of the cardiac outflow tract and aortopulmonary septum. Approximately 5% to 8% of patients with HD will also have CHD, with the majority of these defects being cardiac septation defects.[10] Patients with Down syndrome account for two-thirds of patients with both HD and CHD, followed by patients with Mowat-Wilson syndrome.[10] The cardiovascular physician team should be aware that the pediatric surgeon may have more than one option for initial management of these complex patients. These patients present with varying degrees of intestinal obstruction. It is the rare neonate who presents with overwhelming enterocolitis and requires an emergency colostomy. Most patients can be managed in the initial phase with rectal irrigations to manage their obstruction or enterocolitis symptoms. The key clinical point is that most patients with HD can be managed nonoperatively in the early phase, allowing for evaluation of the anatomy and severity of their CHD and potentially allowing for safe delay of their colorectal operation for HD if their CHD is a higher physiologic priority.

Neonates with anorectal malformations manifest a wide spectrum of severity and may have concurrent CHD in 12% to 22 % of cases.[11] CHD is more likely to occur in newborns with more severe ("high") anorectal malformations. Tetralogy of Fallot and ventricular septal defect are the most common cardiac lesions in these patients. The association between CHD and anorectal malformations presents several points of clinical importance. For the newborn in the delivery room the imperforate anus may be the only abnormal finding on initial physical examination by delivery room providers. Yet if the imperforate anus is diagnosed, this could potentially facilitate early transfer, diagnosis, and treatment for the potentially occult CHD associated with the anorectal malformation. Management of anorectal malformations requires operative treatment under general anesthesia in most cases. Failure to diagnose a neonate's CHD could result in unexpected physiologic derangements under conditions of general anesthesia in the operating room. Similarly, although the GI obstruction of an anorectal malformation may appear to

be an emergency, neonates without a rectal fistula apparent on physical examination are typically observed for 1 to 2 days to determine if a rectal fistula will become apparent. This allows for a neonatal cardiac evaluation to ascertain if the patient has a true emergency of ductus dependent CHD.

Necrotizing Enterocolitis

NEC is the most common gastrointestinal emergency of infancy and occurs primarily in preterm infants (>90%).[12] Birth weight is inversely related to the incidence of NEC with very low-birth-weight (VLBW; <1500 g) infants experiencing an incidence of 6%, whereas extremely low-birth-weight (ELBW; <1000 g) infants have an approximately 8% to 15% incidence.[13,14] Although the incidence of NEC is lower in full-term infants (<10%), it is disproportionately higher (10 to 100 times) in term neonates with CHD.[15] NEC is most common in CHD patients with cyanotic heart disease and is highest among patients with hypoplastic left heart syndrome.[15] As neonatal intensive care has improved over the years, so has survival of infants with ELBW and with complex CHD, and therefore the already high incidence of NEC in these populations continues to rise. It is imperative for those caring for neonates with CHD to have a high index of suspicion for NEC because early diagnosis and prompt treatment is paramount for the best outcomes.

Risk factors for NEC include initiation of enteral nutrition, prematurity, bacterial infection, maternal cocaine use, hypoxia, and CHD, predominantly single-ventricle physiology and left ventricular outflow tract lesions.[12] Although CHD and NEC are distinct diseases, they are undoubtedly related. The increased risk of NEC in infants with CHD may be due to circulatory perturbations that lead to gut hypoperfusion such as diastolic flow reversal in the abdominal aorta, a baseline elevation of circulating proinflammatory mediators, and the stress of cardiac surgery and cardiopulmonary bypass.[16] Prostaglandin administration in CHD infants, especially at higher infusions rates (>0.05 mcg/kg/min), may be a NEC risk factor as well, although its effects are controversial in the literature.[15] Protective strategies to prevent NEC include the use of human breast milk instead of formula, cautious feeding

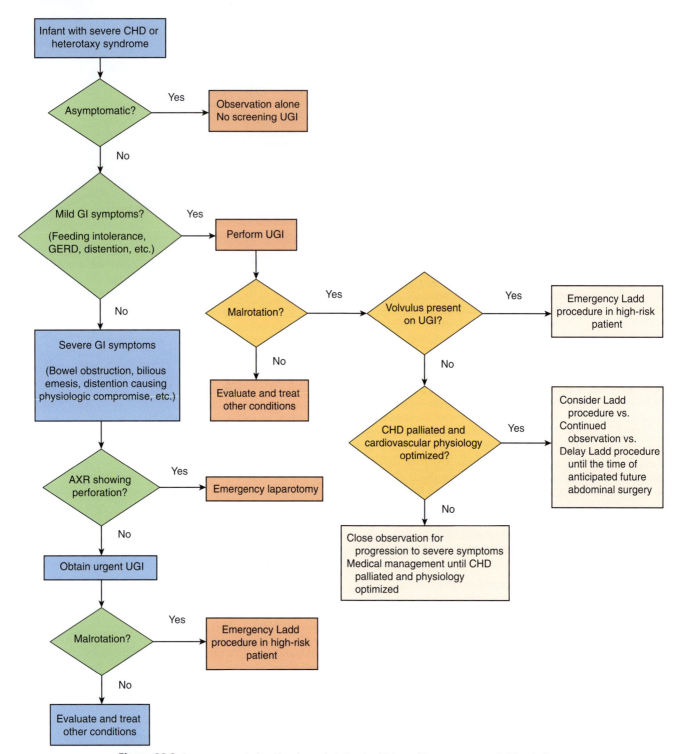

• **Figure 32.3** A management algorithm for malrotation in children with severe congenital heart disease (*CHD*) or heterotaxy syndrome. *AXR,* Abdominal x-ray examination; *GERD,* gastroesophageal reflux disease; *GI,* gastrointestinal; *UGI,* upper gastrointestinal x-ray examination series.

regimens, and probiotics; however, none of these strategies has proven 100% effective.[12,16] Further studies are needed to investigate the pathogenesis of NEC in an effort to develop novel treatments and improve the efficacy of potential preventative therapies. Although the pathogenesis of NEC remains unclear, the contemporary hypothesis is that an ischemic or hypoxic insult occurs in the intestine that damages epithelial mucosal integrity. This allows indigenous pathogenic bacteria from the intestinal lumen to invade the intestinal epithelial barrier and stimulate a release of proinflammatory cytokines that then further aggravate the original epithelial injury. Thus bacterial colonization is required for the development of NEC.[12]

Although the pathogenesis of NEC remains uncertain, the signs and symptoms of NEC are well described. The age of onset is

TABLE 32.1	Evaluation and Treatment of Necrotizing Enterocolitis			
Stage	**Systemic Signs**	**Abdominal Signs**	**Radiographic Signs**	**Management**
IA Suspected	Temperature instability, apnea, bradycardia, lethargy	Mild abdominal distention, emesis, high gastric residuals, fecal occult blood	Normal, nonspecific mild intestinal dilation, mild ileus	Bowel rest (NPO + OGT) Antibiotics (4-7 days) Serial exams + labs AXR q12-24h
IB Suspected	Same as IA	Same as IA + gross fecal blood	Same as IA + intestinal dilation	Same as IA
IIA Definite Mildly ill	Same as IA	Same as IB + absent bowel sounds, ± abdominal tenderness	Same as IB + pneumatosis intestinalis	Bowel rest (NPO + OGT) Antibiotics (7-10 days) Serial exams + labs AXR q8-12h Supportive treatment for sepsis
IIB Definite Moderately ill	Same as IA + mild metabolic acidosis and thrombocytopenia	Same as IIA + abdominal tenderness, ± abdominal cellulitis, ± RLQ mass	Same as IIA + portal venous gas, ± ascites	Bowel rest (NPO + OGT) Antibiotics (14 days) Serial exams + labs AXR q6-8h Supportive treatment for sepsis Consider surgery based on relative indications and clinical judgment
IIIA Advanced Severely ill Bowel intact	Same as IIB + combined metabolic and respiratory acidosis, DIC, severe apnea, bradycardia, hypotension, and neutropenia	Same as IIB + marked abdominal tenderness and distention, peritonitis	Same as IIB + ascites	Bowel rest (NPO + OGT) Antibiotics (14 days) Serial exams + labs AXR q6-8h Supportive treatment for septic shock Consider surgery based on relative indications and clinical judgment
IIIB Advanced Severely ill Bowel perforated	Same as IIIA	Same as IIIA	Same as IIIA + pneumoperitoneum	Same as IIIA + surgery

AXR, Abdominal x-ray examination; *DIC*, disseminated intravascular coagulopathy; *NPO*, nil per os; *OGT*, orogastric tube; *RLQ*, right lower quadrant.
Modified from Castle SL, Speer AL, Grikscheit TC, et al. Necrotizing enterocolitis. In Ziegler MM, Azizkhan RG, Von Allmen D, et al., eds. *Operative Pediatric Surgery.* 2nd ed. New York: McGraw-Hill Education; 2014:597-608.

usually in the first 2 weeks of life after bacterial colonization of the gastrointestinal tract but may occur earlier in neonates with CHD (7 days).[12,16] The Bell staging system was first established in 1978, and a modified version continues to be used today (Table 32.1).[17] This classification system defines three stages of NEC based on systemic, abdominal, and radiographic signs. The Bell staging system is valuable both at the bedside for clinical management decisions and for research in the field because it promotes uniform language. Although some signs and symptoms are more suggestive of NEC, such as peritonitis and pneumoperitoneum, others are nonspecific and overlap with other diagnoses such as sepsis, bacterial or viral enterocolitis, or ileus. These nonspecific signs may be subtle in neonates with complex CHD. Therefore it is important for the intensivist to have a high index of suspicion for NEC and to consult early with a pediatric general surgeon. In an infant with suspected NEC, the following laboratory studies should be checked: complete blood cell count with differential to look for leukocytosis, leukopenia, neutropenia, anemia, and/or thrombocytopenia; electrolyte and blood gas levels to evaluate for metabolic acidosis, as well as hypoxia and hypercapnia; prothrombin time and partial thromboplastin time to assess for coagulopathy; and blood cultures to rule out bacteremia. Notably, bacteremia is confirmed in almost 50% of patients. Patients with severe

thrombocytopenia ($<100 \times 10^9$/L) experience poorer outcomes.[17] Radiographic imaging is critical and should include two-view abdominal radiographs: a supine anteroposterior view and either a left lateral decubitus or cross-table lateral view. Radiographs can identify dilated air-filled loops (a nonspecific finding), a "fixed loop" (a segment of bowel that remains unchanged over serial abdominal radiographs and may be associated with bowel obstruction or transmural necrosis), pneumatosis intestinalis (intramural gas pathognomonic for NEC), portal venous gas (intramural gas absorbed by the venous system), and pneumoperitoneum (free intraperitoneal air from intestinal perforation). Abdominal ultrasonography is a supplementary imaging modality that may identify intraabdominal fluid collections, bowel wall thickness, and intestinal peristalsis with greater sensitivity than radiographs but unlike radiographs is user and experience dependent. Therefore its findings may not have the same clinical significance, and it should be used with caution.

Currently treatment for NEC depends on the stage of disease (see Table 32.1). All infants with any stage of NEC should be placed on immediate bowel rest and an orogastric tube placed to low intermittent suction. Parenteral nutrition should be given while infants are on bowel rest. Additionally, sepsis should be treated promptly and appropriately: intravenous fluid resuscitation should be initiated along with appropriate blood product replacement if anemic, thrombocytopenic, or coagulopathic; vasopressors should be administered if septic shock is present to maintain adequate perfusion pressure; and, finally, proper mechanical ventilation should be initiated in infants with respiratory distress. Broad-spectrum intravenous antibiotics should be administered after blood cultures are drawn. No single organism is responsible for NEC, but bacteria previously isolated include gram-positive cocci such as *Staphylococcus* species, gram-negative rods such as *Escherichia coli, Klebsiella* species, *Enterobacter,* and anaerobes such as *Clostridia.*[12] Common antibiotic regimens include ampicillin or vancomycin for gram-positive coverage, gentamicin or a third- or fourth-generation cephalosporin for gram-negative coverage, and Flagyl or clindamycin for anaerobic coverage. Some institutions will use piperacillin-tazobactam to cover both gram-negative and anaerobic organisms. The institutional nomogram should direct therapy. Antifungals such as fluconazole or amphotericin B may be added if blood cultures or intraoperative cultures indicate the presence of a fungal infection, although this is rare.[17] The duration of antibiotic therapy is often related to disease severity but is highly variable both in the literature and in clinical practice. Stage I may require only 4 to 7 days, whereas Stage III may require 14 days. If the patient has Stage I or II disease, serial examinations, laboratory tests, and imaging should ensue to identify progression of disease as early as possible. The only absolute indication for surgery is pneumoperitoneum. Relative indications for surgery include failure of maximal medical therapy, such as persistent metabolic acidosis and thrombocytopenia; portal venous gas on abdominal radiograph; fixed intestinal loop on serial abdominal radiographs; and abdominal wall cellulitis or a palpable right lower quadrant mass. Approximately 50% of all patients with NEC will require surgical intervention (Fig. 32.4).

Surgical treatment is potentially lifesaving for patients with advanced-stage NEC. The overall goals of surgery are to obtain source control and preserve bowel length. The indications for primary peritoneal drainage (PD) versus laparotomy are still debated today, especially in ELBW infants. Two multicenter randomized controlled trials in VLBW and ELBW infants have found no significant difference in mortality between the two approaches.[14,18] Interestingly, it was noted in the trials that 38% to 74% of patients randomized to PD eventually required a laparotomy.[14,18] The Necrotizing Enterocolitis Surgery Trial (NEST) aims to address this controversy. NEST is a multicenter randomized trial of PD versus laparotomy in ELBW infants with NEC or isolated intestinal perforation with the primary objective of determining survival without neurodevelopmental impairment at 18 to 22 months adjusted age. NEST results are expected in April 2019.[19]

Specific surgical techniques during laparotomy depend on the extent of disease: focal, multisegmental, or panintestinal. Focal disease is most often treated with a simple resection of the necrotic or perforated intestine and a proximal diverting ostomy with or without a distal mucous fistula, depending on the location of the disease. Multisegmental disease involves multiple segments of intestine, but more than 50% remains viable. It may require the use of several techniques, including: a single proximal stoma versus multiple stomas; multiple resections; patch, drain, and wait; or clip and drop. Panintestinal involvement, or NEC totalis, is defined as less than 25% viable intestine. It is the most fulminant form of NEC and occurs in approximately 19% of patients. Surgical options include multiple resections with a proximal stoma or multiple stomas; silo placement followed by reexploration after resuscitation to reassess questionably viable bowel for improvement

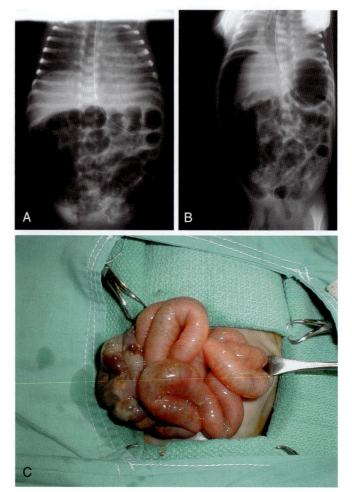

• **Figure 32.4** This patient developed necrotizing enterocolitis. (A) His anteroposterior x-ray image shows pneumatosis intestinalis predominantly in the right lower quadrant. (B) The left lateral decubitus x-ray image shows free intraperitoneal air over the liver. (C) Findings at operation revealed necrotizing enterocolitis in the ileum, including a perforated segment of bowel.

before definitive resection; or, in some patients, foregoing surgical intervention entirely because treatment may be futile and a natural death should be allowed with family at the bedside. NEC totalis mandates a frank discussion with the family not only about survival but also regarding quality of life because essentially all of these children are left with short bowel syndrome. Pediatric intestinal failure leaves them dependent on parenteral nutrition, which has its own morbidities such as central venous catheter (CVC) complications like infection and thrombosis and occasionally liver failure requiring liver or combined liver-intestinal transplant. Mortality for patients with NEC totalis is near 100%, especially in ELBW infants and those with CHD.[17]

The morbidity and mortality of NEC is considerable. Overall mortality ranges from 10% to 50% and is worse in patients requiring surgery (30%), those with CHD (39% to 71%), and those with NEC totalis (near 100%).[12,20] Although the mortality rate of CHD has decreased due to advances in critical care, as well as surgical reparative procedures, morbidities such as NEC remain a major problem for survivors. Long-term complications from surgical NEC include bowel obstruction from adhesions or strictures, pediatric intestinal failure from loss of intestinal length, and neurodevelopmental impairment (NDI) in 15% to 43%.[17] Infants with complex CHD already have an increased risk of NDI with 70% of patients experiencing speech, motor, behavior, or learning disabilities.[21] Thus CHD survivors who develop NEC may have an even more impaired quality of life.

As medical and surgical neonatal care continues to advance, and more preterm ELBW infants with complex CHD continue to survive, it will be crucial for the intensivist to have a comprehensive understanding of the diagnosis and treatment for NEC. Additionally, future studies are necessary to determine the etiology of NEC in neonates with CHD to develop targeted preventive therapies in an effort to lower the significant morbidity and mortality of these two interrelated diseases.

Vascular Access

Patients with CHD frequently require vascular access for treatment. Several catheter types provide meaningful options for patients, depending on the patient's immediate and long-term needs. There is no one ideal location or device for venous access that is appropriate for all patients. Indeed, the best choice for venous access may change even in the same patient over time, with changes in physiology and size.

Several key principles guide decision making regarding venous access in the patient with CHD. First, the anticipated duration of catheter need should be considered. Perioperative patients with CHD and patients in the pediatric intensive care unit require vascular access beyond the peripheral intravenous catheter. A "temporary" CVC that is not cuffed and not tunneled may provide reliable vascular access for up to 2 weeks. A peripherally inserted central catheter typically will last for a month, sometimes more. A cuffed and tunneled CVC generally will last for months if needed. When considering duration of anticipated catheter need, it is important to remember that regardless of the device, every day with a CVC in place presents an incremental risk of infection or thrombosis.

Second, the size of the catheter should be considered. Resistance to flow varies inversely with radius to the fourth power, and it varies directly with catheter length. Smaller, longer catheters are poorly suited to high-volume infusions of blood products or fluids, and they are more prone to occlusion. Larger-diameter catheters occupy more of the venous lumen and increase the risk of venous thrombosis. In children less than 1 year of age, catheters larger than 6 Fr are associated with a higher rate of complications than catheters smaller than 6 Fr.[22]

Finally, the location of catheter placement should be considered in light of often competing factors. As a matter of principle, placement of a catheter peripherally preserves more central sites for future vascular access in the event that the peripheral vein becomes occluded or stenotic. A thrombosed vein tends to resume flow at the site of its next patent venous tributary. This allows a surgeon to potentially access the same vein more proximally for subsequent access if it becomes thrombosed peripherally. Venous stenosis is increased with longer duration of catheter use, left subclavian vein location, or placement on the left side of the neck.[23] Venous thrombosis can be particularly hazardous in infants with CHD. Regardless of anatomy, any infant is at risk for pulmonary embolism or superior vena cava syndrome associated with a venous thrombosis event. Such infants can also develop chylothorax associated with the rise in central venous pressure. Additionally, patients with cavopulmonary anastomoses are at risk for thrombosis of their pulmonary circulation in the setting of a venous thrombus.

Although the causes of thrombosis in patients with CHD are multifactorial, almost one in six vascular thromboses is associated with a catheter in the vessel.[24] For this reason CVC placement is generally avoided in the internal jugular veins and superior vena cava in patients for whom a Fontan type of reconstruction is anticipated. For a short duration of time, such as the perioperative period, it may be safe to place CVCs in the internal jugular or subclavian locations. A recent series of 235 patients with univentricular hearts who underwent intraoperative upper body CVC placement during cardiac surgical procedures had no episodes of venous thrombosis or stenosis. These CVCs were in place for only a median of 4 days.[25]

Lower extremity vascular access may be obtained through the femoral veins or through the greater saphenous vein. Traditional landmark-based and cutdown approaches continue to have clinical relevance, though increasingly ultrasound guidance facilitates access, even in small patients.[26] Whereas in adult critical care medicine femoral lines are associated with a higher rate of infection and thrombosis, in neonates the rates of infection and thrombosis are equivalent if not better with long-term femoral lines than with neck lines.[27,28] In children with CHD, lower extremity access presents a risk of femoral vein thrombosis and thus potential loss of future access for cardiac catheterization from that site. This risk should be weighed against the risk of upper body central venous thrombosis in patients with anticipated Fontan type of reconstruction. In general, lower extremity central venous catheters provide good long-term vascular access for infants with CHD.

Nontraditional approaches may allow additional vascular access for children with CHD who have had multiple CVCs throughout their life but have lost typical sites of venous access. Most neonates begin with an umbilical venous catheter (UVC). Continuing with a UVC rather than immediate placement of a nontunneled femoral CVC is associated with a lower incidence of catheter thrombosis and iliofemoral venous occlusion, with no difference in catheter infection, central venous thrombus, or need for transhepatic access.[29] In one series of patients with single-ventricle physiology, UVCs were left in place for a median of 18 days, and in a randomized trial of premature infants, UVCs that were left in place up to 28 days did not have a significant difference in catheter infection or thrombosis.[29,30] Although the Centers for Disease Control and Prevention recommends that UVC use be limited to 14 days, mounting evidence suggests that it may be reasonable to extend the duration of UVC use in certain patients. In CHD patients with prohibitive upper body venous access and loss of lower extremity venous access, transhepatic central venous access provides an important option. Catheter placement is performed by a cardiologist or interventional radiologist, often in conjunction with a pediatric surgeon. The liver is accessed percutaneously, and a hepatic vein is entered under fluoroscopy, allowing tract dilation and placement of a cuffed and tunneled catheter with its tip at the junction of the right atrium. Transhepatic placement presents a small risk of liver hematoma or intraperitoneal hemorrhage. However, because of the percutaneous approach, transhepatic CVC placement is preferable to the invasiveness of a thoracotomy and direct placement of a CVC into the vena cava or the right atrium.[31,32] Direct atrial placement is the final option for CVC placement, and such morbidity should be considered carefully in high-risk patients.

Although mechanical and positional complications can accompany long-term CVCs, the two most vexing complications of long-term vascular access are infection and thrombosis. Both infection and thrombosis are a function of the amount of time that a CVC remains in place. Prevention of both of these complications is more important than treatment. Accordingly, a patient's need for ongoing central venous access should be reconsidered on a daily basis. Regarding infection, using a series of best practices ("bundle") can reduce the risk of central line–associated bloodstream infection (CLABSI). Key components of such a bundle include hand hygiene, maximum sterile barrier precautions for insertion, chlorhexidine skin preparation, appropriate catheter and site selection, daily review of CVC necessity, and prompt removal of unnecessary CVCs. Temporary catheters that are impregnated with heparin and antibiotics may have a lower incidence of infection. Use of ethanol or vancomycin to lock the catheter when it is not in use may also lower the incidence of CLABSI. Management of CLABSI in a patient with an ongoing need for an indwelling CVC can be challenging. Decisions about removal or continuation of the indwelling catheter are driven by the patient's need for the catheter, the nature of the infecting organism, and the physiologic status of the patient. An approach to management of this problem is illustrated in Fig. 32.5.

Thrombosis of a CVC can cause loss of catheter function, but, more significantly, deep venous thrombosis (DVT) can create distal venous hypertension, pulmonary embolism, loss of the vein for future vascular access, and loss of the vein for possible cardiovascular reconstruction. The incidence of DVT in children with CVCs is estimated at 20%, though not all of these thromboses are symptomatic.[33] This rate of thrombosis was similar for upper body, lower body, and umbilical sites. A number of interventions have been tried to prevent DVT, including unfractionated heparin, low-molecular-weight heparin warfarin, antithrombin concentrate, nitroglycerin, and heparin bonding of the catheter.[33] None of these have been demonstrated to lower the rate of CVC-associated DVT, and thus no intervention can be recommended to decrease CVC-associated DVT other than removal of unneeded CVCs. Many patients with CHD receive anticoagulant or antiplatelet therapy. Such patients should receive therapy on the basis of their cardiac surgical anatomy and not on the basis of having a CVC. Decisions regarding patients with an indwelling CVC and a venous thrombosis can be complicated, particularly if a catheter is still needed and the options for replacement of the catheter are limited. An algorithm for management of CVC-associated DVT is illustrated in Fig. 32.6. Patients who have asymptomatic DVT may be considered either for therapeutic anticoagulation or for close surveillance with physical examination and ultrasonography, based on the clinician's assessment of patient risks and benefits associated with anticoagulation. Children with symptomatic CVC-associated DVT should receive therapeutic anticoagulation for 3 months, though longer courses of treatment may be considered for patients with underlying conditions that predispose to DVT beyond just the presence of a CVC. Management of the CVC in the setting of DVT is influenced by additional factors. Immediate removal of the CVC is not recommended until after the patient has started receiving anticoagulation. Once anticoagulation has been started, a nonfunctional or unneeded CVC may be removed. If a patient has a functioning CVC in place and that patient has an ongoing need for a CVC, it is reasonable to treat with anticoagulation and leave the CVC in place. This option should be considered in patients with limited alternative venous access sites. In patients with multiple access options, treating with anticoagulation and replacing the CVC may be preferable.

Other issues related to vascular access are the complications associated with attempts to gain access in the cardiac catheterization laboratory for diagnostic catheterization or therapeutic intervention.

These complications can include loss of pulse (usually in the femoral artery), disruption of an arterial vessel (most commonly the iliac artery from a "high" inguinal puncture), bleeding around indwelling catheters, or venous thrombosis with peripheral extremity manifestations. Often a pediatric surgeon or vascular surgeon (in many institutions these are the same person for the pediatric service) is called in for consultation, along with the cardiac surgical team. The most serious of these complications is the unrecognized injury to the iliac artery. Even when an inguinal puncture is made below the inguinal ligament, advancement of the needle above the inguinal ligament and penetration of the iliac artery in the retroperitoneum can occur. When the catheters are withdrawn following the procedure, retroperitoneal bleeding can occur, and, because of the difficulty recognizing this or controlling it with pressure in the femoral area, life-threatening hemorrhage can occur. Infants who have interventions with large-bore catheters or who have difficult femoral access may be more at risk for this complication and likely should be followed after their catheterization with serial determinations of hemoglobin level. If the hemoglobin level is found to fall by more than 3 g in the first 6 hours following a high-risk catheterization, investigation for potential sources of bleeding should be undertaken in addition to blood replacement therapy. Abdominal distention or hemodynamic instability without an obvious external source of blood loss can be an indicator that retroperitoneal bleeding might be occurring and require surgical exploration and repair of the iliac artery.

Because large catheters are often left in place following a catheterization procedure, consideration for removing them, particularly if there are signs of vascular compromise to the lower extremity (dusky appearance from venous occlusion or loss of pulses from arterial compromise), should be pursued as soon as the patient's hemodynamics allow. Catheters can be removed or changed over wires (sterilely) to small sizes if vascular access is still necessary. Long-term consideration to preserving vessels is critical in infants with CHD because they may need numerous procedures (both in the catheterization laboratory and in the operating room) in the future. Loss of peripheral vessels can be a significant morbidity for these complex patients. Patients with loss of femoral pulses following an arterial catheterization can be treated with heparin, although the long-term benefit of this for restoring arterial patency is not clear. Although it is difficult to restore lost femoral pulses, extremity loss following a catheterization should be a rare occurrence. There are some studies that suggest that maintenance of arterial patency in infants is likely more associated with need for fewer attempts at access and use of smaller catheter sizes—which is why prolonged attempts in the catheterization laboratory for access or the use of larger catheters (for insertion of stents or balloons) should be communicated to the intensive care unit staff so that they can be more vigilant for these kind of potential access compromises. When there are concerns following an attempt at vascular access, it is reasonable to obtain a consultation from both cardiac and pediatric/vascular surgery to discuss potential options. Obviously, if the patient presents with hemoperitoneum (from iliac artery injury), urgent general surgery consultation is critical.

Feeding Dysfunction

For many infants with CHD, feeding and growth can be areas of incredible challenge. Neonatal growth and nutrition are critical to long-term survival and neurodevelopmental outcomes, but how to safely and successfully meet these goals is not always clear. The

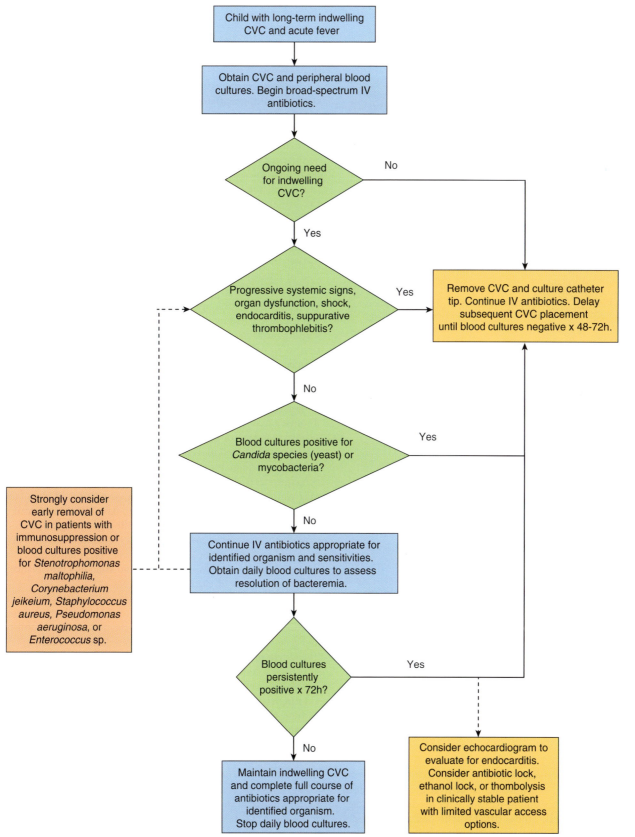

• **Figure 32.5** A management algorithm for central line–associated bloodstream infection in a child with a long-term indwelling central venous catheter *(CVC)*. *IV,* Intravenous. (Modified from Zeller KA, Petty JK. Vascular access procedures. In Ziegler MM, Azizkhan RG, Von Allmen D, et al., eds. *Operative Pediatric Surgery.* 2nd ed. New York: McGraw-Hill Education; 2014:137-149.)

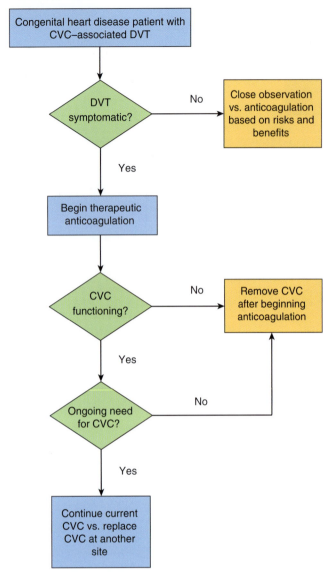

• Figure 32.6 A management algorithm for treatment of a central venous catheter *(CVC)*–associated deep venous thrombosis *(DVT)* in children with congenital heart disease.

showed that timing of gastrostomy (with or without fundoplication) yielded similar morbidity and mortality, regardless of which stage it was performed after, but that patients who required gastric access surgery had overall worse outcomes than patients who did not.[35]

The more controversial issue probably is which type of operation is the most appropriate—gastrostomy alone versus gastrostomy with fundoplication versus gastrojejunostomy tube placement—and the role of laparoscopy in this population. Unfortunately, data to drive this decision are mostly retrospective and often support conflicting conclusions. No prospective randomized trials have been performed. There appears to be strong institutional bias as to the best procedure for infants with CHD. A recent review of the pediatric National Surgical Quality Improvement Program (NSQIP) identified increased odds of morbidity or mortality with fundoplication in 2346 infants with CHD. When compared with gastrostomy alone, gastrostomy performed with fundoplication carried an odds ratio of 1.82 for morbidity and mortality.[36] The role of laparoscopy is debated, but recent reports from several centers have failed to show significant morbidity or mortality related to the use of laparoscopy in these infants.[37,38] It is probably safe and reasonable to attempt to perform the operation laparoscopically, keeping intraabdominal pressure at 12 mm Hg or less, with conversion to an open approach if the infant is experiencing cardiopulmonary effects that cannot be easily managed or corrected by the anesthesiologist. Certainly a primary open operation would also be acceptable.

For the infant who is able to tolerate gastric bolus feedings through a nasogastric feeding tube and who needs long-term feeding access, a gastrostomy alone is the appropriate surgical choice. Gastroesophageal reflux is normal in infancy, and it is not pathologic unless its frequency or severity is accompanied by physiologic consequences to the patient. Esophageal pH and impedance testing may clarify the severity and symptom correlation of an infant's gastroesophageal reflux. In patients who have significant reflux or who are unable to tolerate gastric feeding, the surgical decision making becomes more complex. In this population the cardiology team and pediatric surgical team must work together to determine the best course forward for the patient, understanding the advantages and disadvantages of each of the choices.

In deciding between fundoplication with gastrostomy tube (GT) versus gastrojejunostomy (GJ) tube, several factors should be considered, including the weight of the patient, family abilities and geographic concerns, and long-term implications of each option. The weight of the patient is an important factor in the consideration of placing a conventional GJ tube because increased complications have been seen in smaller infants undergoing this procedure.[39-41] Commercially available GJ tubes are larger devices (14 or 16 Fr) with relatively stiff tubing that passes through the pylorus and into the small bowel. Use of these tubes in small infants with thin bowel walls has resulted in an increased perforation rate as compared with older and larger children. Recommendations based on these small series have been to use caution in GJ tube placement in infants under 10 kg, with one of the studies recommending 6 kg or less than 6 months of age as the highest risk group for perforation.[41] Another technique of GJ feeding is to place a standard gastrostomy button device and to thread a small-caliber feeding tube through this into the jejunum for feedings. A study of this technique specifically in the cardiac population has shown a low complication rate and no mortality attributed to the surgery or its anesthetic.[42] Not reported in this paper is the incidence of dislodgment or clogging of the jejunal feeding tube extension because dislodgment or clogging of this tube

two questions that seem to come up most frequently in infants with CHD who require long-term enteral access for feeding are when to proceed with surgical feeding access and what the best operation is to provide this access. The answers to each of these questions are driven by a number of factors that may differ between individual patients.

Timing of surgical placement of feeding access is an important consideration. The majority of patients with single-ventricle physiology will require some form of tube feeding during the course of their infancy, with a smaller percentage going on to need more long-term access. Among patients who needed three-stage palliation for their CHD, those patients who had a gastrostomy within 90 days of their stage 1 operation have been compared to those who received a gastrostomy more than 90 days after their stage 1 operation. There were no major differences in outcome between the two groups, other than a slightly shorter hospital length of stay in the group that had the gastrostomy within the first 90 days of their stage 1 operation.[34] Another study similarly

would result in additional procedures to replace the feeding tube portion.

In addition to the size of the child, the ability of the family to return the child to a pediatric center for tube maintenance needs to be considered. Unlike a standard GT device that parents and caregivers can be taught to replace at home with minimal training, a GJ tube will always require radiologic or endoscopic guidance to replace the tube. So, if the tube becomes dislodged or clogged and the family lives a long distance from a facility capable of replacement, then additional burden may be placed on the family to maintain this type of tube.

Disadvantages of fundoplication include that it is a permanent alteration of anatomy that cannot easily be undone in the future, whereas a GJ tube can always be changed back to a standard GT. Fundoplication is also reported to cause retching and gagging. It may affect swallowing in patients with baseline poor esophageal motility. It carries a risk of wrap failure with recurrent symptoms or herniation of the stomach through the hiatus. In the absence of clear superiority data the care team should discuss the advantages and disadvantages of each option for a particular patient to arrive at a patient-centered consensus decision.

Summary

Infants and children with CHD often need collaborative care from a pediatric surgeon. For many of these gastrointestinal and vascular access conditions, more than one good treatment option may be possible. Decisions for surgical care should be made with open communication between the pediatric surgical team and the congenital heart team to optimize care for the patient.

Selected References

A complete list of references is available at ExpertConsult.com.

2. Krishnamurthy G, Ratner V, Bacha E, et al. Comorbid conditions in neonates with congenital heart disease. *Pediatr Crit Care Med*. 2016;17:S367–S376.
9. Landisch R, Abdel-Hafeez A, Massoumi R, et al. Observation versus prophylactic Ladd procedure for asymptomatic intestinal rotational abnormalities in heterotaxy syndrome: A systematic review. *J Pediatr Surg*. 2015;50:1971–1974.
12. Petrosyan M, Guner YS, Williams M, et al. Current concepts regarding the pathogenesis of necrotizing enterocolitis. *Pediatr Surg Int*. 2009;25:309–318.
16. Giannone PJ, Luce WA, Nankervis CA, et al. Necrotizing enterocolitis in neonates with congenital heart disease. *Life Sci*. 2008;82:341–347.
25. Miller JW, Vu DN, Chai PJ, et al. Upper body central venous catheters in pediatric cardiac surgery. *Pediatr Anesth*. 2013;23:980–988.

33

Management of Common Postoperative Complications and Conditions

JAVIER J. LASA, MD, FAAP; PAUL A. CHECCHIA, MD, FCCM, FACC;
RONALD A. BRONICKI, MD, FCCM, FACC

The critical care of neonates, infants, children, and adults with acquired heart disease and/or congenital heart disease (CHD) recovering from cardiac surgery has evolved over the last 40 years, paralleling improvements in pediatric cardiac surgical techniques, pediatric cardiac anesthesia, pediatric cardiac nursing, and cardiology. Although the complexity and heterogeneous nature of CHD have not changed, our understanding of the physiologic derangements that occur in the postoperative period has grown along with the subspecialization of pediatric cardiac critical care practitioners.[1] Identifying risk factors for postoperative complications continues to remain a focus among cardiac critical care practitioners, cardiothoracic surgeons, cardiologists, anesthesiologists, and cardiac nurses. Yet translating our understanding of risk factors into effective and efficient management strategies remains the next frontier for the practice of pediatric cardiac critical care.

The recovery period after cardiac surgery represents one of the highest-risk periods for patients with CHD requiring palliative or corrective surgery. Successful congenital heart surgery requires a comprehensive, well-coordinated team-based care delivery model that incorporates several key elements of postoperative care: a broad knowledge base of the patient's preoperative condition; precise anatomic diagnosis of the congenital heart defect; pathophysiologic impact of the defect(s) on cardiopulmonary and other organ system function; noncardiac medical and surgical history; anesthetic agents used in the operating room; details of the operative procedure and cardiopulmonary bypass (CPB) strategy; intraoperative complications, including dysrhythmias and bleeding; real-time interpretation of vital signs, hemodynamic data, and physical examination results; pharmacology of drugs effecting cardiovascular homeostasis; management of respiratory support devices; and indications for advanced procedures such as pacing and mechanical circulatory support.

Anticipating postoperative complications is as much an art form as it is a science. Pattern recognition and the complex incorporation of bedside physiologic data with limited evidence-based practice strategies constantly challenge the practitioner. This chapter aims to inform cardiac critical care clinicians with an informative appraisal of the current state of postoperative care for the patient with acquired heart disease and CHD, with a focus on the management of postoperative complications and conditions.

Cardiopulmonary Bypass in Neonates, Infants, and Children—Impact on Postoperative Care

CPB stimulates complement activation and the release of endothelial, parenchymal, and inflammatory cell-derived mediators, leading to a proinflammatory cascade. This was termed the *systemic inflammatory response syndrome* (SIRS) by the American College of Chest Physicians and Society of Critical Care Medicine in 1992; we now know that noninfectious triggers such as exposure of blood elements to the nonendothelial lining of the CPB circuit stimulate a SIRS state.[2] The hallmark of SIRS is an increase in microvascular permeability and the development of interstitial edema. In addition to SIRS, ischemia-reperfusion injury (IRI) contributes substantially to the overall inflammatory state, as well as to the injury of the organ(s) that undergo reperfusion. In an additive fashion SIRS and IRI induce myocardial injury, causing ventricular systolic and diastolic dysfunction and parenchymal lung injury, causing pulmonary edema and impairing respiratory mechanics and gas exchange. In addition, IRI injures the pulmonary endothelium, contributing to a state of heightened vascular reactivity. The SIRS response also impacts other organ functions, contributing to central nervous system (CNS), kidney, mesenteric, and endocrine injury and dysfunction.[3-10]

Postoperative Cardiac Dysfunction—Pathophysiology

The interplay of the inflammatory response to CPB, IRI, cardiac surgery, and age and developmental status place the patient at risk for developing a low cardiac output syndrome (LCOS) following surgery. LCOS is a historical term that seeks to encapsulate the transient myocardial injury and dysfunction resulting from the effects of CPB, direct myocardial trauma, and the lingering impact of preoperative ventricular volume and pressure loads. This transient depression in cardiac function and cardiac output (CO) generally improves after the first 24 hours.[11,12] Table 33.1 highlights the hemodynamic profile of conditions that can lead to cardiovascular instability in the postoperative period.

TABLE 33.1	Hemodynamic Profile of Conditions That Lead to Cardiovascular Instability in the Postoperative Period					
	HR	CVP	Pulse Pressure	MAP	Urine Output	Capillary Refill Time
Hypovolemia	↑	↓	Normal to narrowed	↓	↓	↑
Tamponade	↑	↑	Narrowed	↓	↓	↑
LCOS	↑	↓/↑	Narrowed	↓	↓	↑

CVP, Central venous pressure; *HR*, heart rate; *LCOS*, low cardiac output syndrome; *MAP*, mean arterial blood pressure.

Contributing factors to the development of postoperative LCOS include intravascular volume depletion secondary to excessive ultrafiltration, hemorrhage, excessive diuresis or inadequate fluid administration, and excessive capillary leak post CPB. Complicated surgical procedures associated with long CPB times may result in myocardial swelling and/or excess bleeding. Both sequelae may prohibit immediate sternal closure. Hemodynamic instability or ongoing bleeding can be managed more efficiently with delayed sternal closure, although mechanical ventilatory strategies must reflect the changes in functional residual capacity (FRC) and respiratory compliance that occur with sternal closure. Delayed sternal closure can be associated with transient respiratory deterioration and a similar decrease in cardiac output, often requiring a temporary escalation of ventilatory and vasoactive support and increase in intravascular volume.[13]

Despite several working definitions for LCOS, a lack of consensus and variability in diagnostic criteria have limited scientific query into its epidemiology. Current definitions place emphasis on therapeutic interventions (e.g., inotrope dosing), yet efforts to refocus diagnostic criteria on patient-specific markers of impaired oxygen delivery have also gained traction,[14,15] suggesting LCOS could be rephrased as "post–cardiac surgery shock" or "CPB-induced shock."

Hemodynamic Monitoring in the Postoperative Period

The transition of care from the cardiac operating room to intensive care unit (ICU) occurs at a time of significant hemodynamic vulnerability, often accompanied by a complex interplay of cardiopulmonary pathophysiology and pharmacologic manipulation(s). At its core the goal of postoperative care is to optimize oxygen and substrate delivery to the myocardium and key organs while minimizing oxygen demands and other acquired comorbidities. This overarching principle of postoperative care is translated into intense vigilance and focus on invasive and noninvasive markers of cardiac function, CO, systemic oxygen delivery, and tissue oxygenation. Qualitative and quantitative determination of these parameters can be accomplished by routine physical examination aided by the interpretation of hemodynamic data, including transthoracic echocardiography, and indicators of tissue oxygenation such as serum lactate levels, near-infrared spectroscopy (NIRS), and venous oximetry. Additional parameters that are essential to determining the hemodynamic profile include the central venous pressure (CVP)/right atrial pressure (RAP), heart rate, blood pressure, and in some patients a left atrial pressure. The monitoring of urine output also provides some indication of CO and renal perfusion.

Several studies have demonstrated the limitations of the standard assessment of cardiac function, CO, and tissue oxygenation, which relies on conventional "hemodynamic" monitoring (CVP, heart rate, blood pressure, and urine output) and the physical examination.[16,17] Several investigations have demonstrated discordant values between estimations and measurements of the aforementioned parameters, which occur irrespective of training and level of experience. The clinician should have a low threshold for using adjunctive monitoring modalities, including NIRS and venous oximetry, serial lactate levels, and transthoracic echocardiography. Several studies in adults and children have demonstrated the utility of venous oximetry in assessing the adequacy of tissue oxygenation. It should be appreciated that oxygen extraction increases well before serum lactate production exceeds clearance and levels begin to rise.[18-20] NIRS has been studied extensively in animals and clinical studies validating regional cerebral oxyhemoglobin saturation with jugular and superior vena cava saturations.[21,22] In some cases the use of transpulmonary or pulmonary artery thermodilution may be indicated, providing a measurement of CO as well as enabling the derivation of pulmonary vascular resistance (PVR) and systemic vascular resistance (SVR). The pulmonary artery catheter also enables the clinician to determine the left ventricular filling (LV) pressure and, if pulmonary hypertension (PH) is present, differentiate between pulmonary venous hypertension and/or pulmonary arteriolar disease. Please refer to Chapter 22 for further in-depth discussion of monitoring systems in the cardiac ICU (CICU).

Postoperative Cardiac Dysfunction— Medical Management

Several pharmacologic agents are available to aid in the manipulation and optimization of ventricular loading conditions and, if necessary, to provide inotropic support. The mechanisms of action and side-effect profile of each vasoactive agent should be weighed on an individual basis for each lesion and/or condition in the postoperative period (Table 33.2). Catecholamines include dopamine, dobutamine, norepinephrine, epinephrine, and isoproterenol, all of which increase heart rate, inotropic state, and myocardial oxygen consumption. Atrial and ventricular dysrhythmias can be seen with higher frequency when using these agents. Moderate to high doses of dopamine, epinephrine, and norepinephrine vasoconstrict venous capacitance vessels (increasing systemic venous return and ventricular end-diastolic pressure) and arterial resistance vessels, which will decrease stroke volume if systolic function is impaired. Phosphodiesterase type 3 inhibitors (e.g., milrinone) and dobutamine provide inotropic support while vasodilating venous capacitance and arterial resistance vessels. Milrinone has less chronotropic effect than catecholamines and is immune to adrenergic receptor desensitization. If systolic function is severely impaired, epinephrine may be indicated because it provides unparalleled inotropic support without increasing SVR at low to moderate doses (<0.03 to 0.20 µg/kg/min).[23] Another consideration is the use of calcium chloride as a continuous infusion, especially in neonates, who are sensitive to exogenous calcium due to an immature sarcoplasmic reticulum. Calcium offers the benefit of increased contractility without chronotropy. Although not approved by the US Food and Drug Administration, levosimendan is a calcium sensitizer with inotropic

TABLE 33.2 Inotropic and Vasopressor Classification, Standard Dose Range, Receptor Binding (Catecholamines), and Major Clinical Side Effects

Drug	Dose Range	α1	β1	β2	DA	Major Side Effects
Dopamine	2-20 μg/kg/min	+++	+++	++	++++	Hypertension, ventricular arrhythmias, cardiac ischemia, tissue necrosis with extravasation
Dobutamine	2-20 μg/kg/min	+	++++	+++	N/A	Tachycardia, hypertension, ventricular arrhythmias, cardiac ischemia, hypotension
Norepinephrine	0.01-1.0 μg/kg/min	++++	+++	++	N/A	Arrhythmias, bradycardia, peripheral ischemia, hypertension
Epinephrine	0.01-0.2 μg/kg/min; 1 mg IV Q 3-5 min (max 0.2 mg/kg)	+++	++++	+++	N/A	Ventricular arrhythmias, severe hypertension, cardiac ischemia, cerebrovascular hemorrhage
Isoproterenol	0.01-1.0 μg/kg/min		++++	++++	N/A	Ventricular arrhythmias, cardiac ischemia, hypertension, hypotension
Phenylephrine	0.01-1.0 μg/kg/min	++++			N/A	Reflex bradycardia, hypertension, severe peripheral and visceral vasoconstriction, tissue necrosis with extravasation

DA, Dopamine; *IV,* intravenously; *N/A,* not applicable.

properties used in international centers. Levosimendan provides an alternative pharmacologic approach for patients experiencing postoperative cardiovascular dysfunction/shock and/or heart failure. The effects of pure vasodilating agents such as nitroprusside and nitroglycerin are limited to altering ventricular loading conditions. Both agents vasodilate venous capacitance and arterial resistance vessels, with nitroglycerin having a significant impact on SVR at moderate to high doses (>3 μg/kg/min).

Management of the Shunt-Dependent Single-Ventricle Patient

Patients with single-ventricle physiology undergoing shunt placement and/or first-stage palliation for hypoplastic left heart syndrome (HLHS) are at significant risk for developing postoperative cardiovascular dysfunction and shock. The limitations of the neonatal myocardium, cardiac surgery, the adverse effects of CPB and IRI on the myocardium, and the inefficiencies of a parallel circulation present an enormous challenge to the critical care clinician in the management of these patients.

The immediate postoperative period following the Norwood procedure involves dynamic changes in circulatory function, with risks for pulmonary overcirculation at the expense of systemic oxygen delivery. This tenuous balance between the systemic and pulmonary circulations is often expressed as a ratio of pulmonary perfusion (Q_p) to systemic perfusion (Q_s), or $Q_p{:}Q_s$, with the partitioning of total CO into Q_p and Q_s determined by the relative resistance in each circulation. As SVR rises, the Q_p/Q_s ratio increases, which may result in inadequate Q_s. It is particularly important to make a timely and accurate assessment of Q_s in these patients because as Q_s wanes, neurohormonal activation increases, driving further increases in the Q_p/Q_s ratio and decreases in Q_s. The use of NIRS and venous oximetry as discussed previously is useful for assessing the adequacy of Q_s; it is also imperative to understand that the arterial oxygen saturation (SaO_2) and blood pressure provide little if any indication of the adequacy of Q_s. Using nonselective vasodilators reduces SVR and PVR, increasing stroke volume and simultaneously increasing Q_s and Q_p (increasing arterial oxygen

content), with the net effect being a marked increase in systemic oxygen delivery.[12,24] In cases of impaired ventricular systolic function, inotropic support in the form of epinephrine may be required, although doses higher than 0.3 μg/kg/min should be avoided due to unwanted vasoconstriction of arterial resistance vessels.[23] If Q_s remains inadequate despite the manipulation of vasoactive therapy, then mechanical support in the form of extracorporeal membrane oxygenation (ECMO) may be necessary. Please refer to Chapter 39 for further in-depth discussion of ECMO in the CICU.

Shunt Malfunction

The surveillance of aortopulmonary shunt function in the postoperative period requires an understanding of the causes of arterial hypoxemia: parenchymal lung disease leading to pulmonary venous desaturation, inadequate Q_p, and/or low mixed venous saturation due to limited Q_s (in the presence of intracardiac and/or pulmonary shunt). Partial aortopulmonary shunt obstruction leads to hypoxemia and impaired carbon dioxide (CO_2) elimination due to wasted ventilation, the latter of which is reflected in an arterial to end-tidal CO_2 gradient. Auscultation may be effective in ruling out a complete occlusion, but more advanced imaging is required to accurately confirm the diagnosis. Echocardiography with color Doppler assessment lacks adequate sensitivity to detect shunt malfunction. The definitive assessment of shunt function requires angiography.

Shunt obstruction that occurs immediately after surgery most likely requires reoperation, although some cases that involve narrowing at the proximal/distal anastomotic site may be treated with percutaneous balloon angioplasty. Medical interventions to temporize the patient with acute shunt malfunction include pharmacologic manipulation of SVR to increase the perfusion gradient across the shunt (epinephrine/phenylephrine), increasing the partial pressure of alveolar oxygen (supplemental O_2), immediate systemic anticoagulation (50 to 100 U/kg heparin), and the rapid reduction in O_2 demand/consumption (sedation, muscle relaxation, and mechanical ventilation). Surgical and/or catheter based intervention is the ultimate goal although a subset of shunt-dependent patients may require ECMO for immediate rescue after cardiac arrest.[25]

Cardiopulmonary Interactions in the Postoperative Period

Optimizing the care of critically ill children with congenital and/or acquired heart disease requires an understanding of the physiologic principles that govern the interactions between the cardiovascular and respiratory systems. Respiratory mechanics and cardiovascular function are linked primarily through changes in lung volumes and intrathoracic pressure (ITP).

Positive pressure ventilation (PPV) increases ITP, decreasing the transmural pressure of the right atrium, which causes the RAP to increase and the pressure gradient for systemic venous return to decrease.[26] Subjects with low CO due to inadequate ventricular filling (diastolic dysfunction), may benefit from spontaneous respiration or minimizing ITP during PPV.[27] Right ventricular (RV) afterload is also affected by respiration. In addition to blood pH and alveolar oxygen tension, changes in lung volume and ITP also impact RV afterload. As lung volume rises above FRC, PVR increases due to compression of interalveolar vessels and the creation of zone I conditions. This is particularly important to consider in patients with elevated PVR and/or RV dysfunction. Respiration also effects LV afterload through changes in ITP. As ITP rises, the transmural pressure for the thoracic arterial system decreases, the volume within these structures decreases, and as a result the pressure within rises relative to the extrathoracic arterial system, creating a waterfall-like effect, enhancing the egress of blood from the intrathoracic to extrathoracic compartment. The benefits of PPV in patients with systolic heart failure cannot be overstated. The benefits are greatest in those patients with exaggerated negative ITP due to impaired airway/lung mechanics or elevated minute ventilation (as seen in patients compensating for a metabolic acidosis) and/or in patients with impaired systolic function of the systemic ventricle. An additional so-called cardiopulmonary interaction occurs when blood flow is redistributed from the respiratory muscles to other vital organs with the initiation of mechanical ventilation in a limited CO state. Under normal conditions, respiratory muscle oxygen consumption is minimal. However, when the respiratory load is increased (as described earlier), respiratory muscle (pump) metabolic demand rises, requiring a commensurate increase in respiratory pump perfusion. Mechanical ventilation unloads the respiratory pump, decreasing respiratory muscle oxygen demand, allowing for a redistribution of a limited CO to other vital organs.[28]

Extubation Failure

Respiratory failure due to diaphragmatic paresis or paralysis may manifest as extubation failure in neonates and infants because they rely on diaphragmatic contraction for chest wall expansion more than older children. Intraoperative injury to the phrenic nerve (usually left-sided) is most commonly caused by direct trauma, although thermal injuries have also been reported.[29] The diagnosis is confirmed by fluoroscopy or by bedside ultrasonography, demonstrating paradoxical or paretic motion of a raised hemidiaphragm in conjunction with paradoxical abdominal wall motion.[30] In such cases, diaphragmatic plication is recommended should the patient demonstrate increased work of breathing and/or failure to wean from mechanical ventilation.

An infrequent complication from open-heart surgery that parallels injury to the phrenic nerve is trauma to the recurrent laryngeal nerve, which results in unilateral vocal cord paralysis and leads to

---

a hoarse voice or weak cry. Because airway protection is potentially compromised, previously normal feeding neonates can demonstrate signs of aspiration (coughing, gagging, respiratory distress, and hypoxemia) when bottle-fed. Vocal cord dysfunction is transient in the majority of patients, yet consultation with an otorhinolaryngologist or speech-language therapist may help determine if the child will require thickened oral feeds or will be completely dependent on nasogastric (NG) feeds.

Although many postoperative CHD patients remain intubated and mechanically ventilated after surgery, specific patient populations may benefit from early extubation. Older children and those with less complex lesions requiring shorter CPB times have been shown to be successfully extubated in the operating room or within hours of arrival to the ICU.[31] Several criteria should be evaluated to minimize the incidence of respiratory failure following extubation in the postoperative patient (Box 33.1). The patient's hemodynamic status should be evaluated with the goal of maintaining adequate perfusion at an acceptable heart rate; the patient should demonstrate adequate gas exchange with normal respiratory effort; hemostasis should have been achieved; and the patient's neurologic status should be evaluated, titrating sedation and analgesia accordingly.

Pleural and Pericardial Diseases

Pleural effusions may also complicate the postoperative course. Severe cases can compromise cardiopulmonary function and may lengthen the CICU and/or hospital stay. The majority of filtered fluid is reabsorbed by the microvasculature (90%), with the remaining fluid captured by the lymphatic system, which drains into the central venous system via the thoracic duct. An elevated central venous pressure, commonly observed after repair of tetralogy of Fallot and the Fontan procedure, decreases lymphatic clearance and may lead to a transudative pleural effusion. Conversely, exudative pleural effusions are caused by increased microvascular permeability related to nonspecific inflammation. Chylothorax is a variant of pleural effusion that must be considered in the postoperative period, especially in patients with high-risk comorbidities (age <1 year, single-ventricle physiology, extracardiac anomalies, longer CPB time, and thrombosis associated with an upper-extremity central venous line).[32] Causes of chylothorax in the postoperative period include traumatic disruption of the thoracic duct and thoracic duct occlusion due to venous thrombus and/or external compression, leading to elevated central venous pressures with subsequent rupture of thoracic duct. Chylous drainage causes a significant loss of plasma proteins, lymphocytes, and lipids, leading to lymphopenia and impaired immunologic function, coagulation abnormalities, and malnutrition, all of which requires an integrative and intensive multidisciplinary approach to management.

Pneumothorax is an equally serious complication that results from air entry into the pleural space(s), often resulting from surgical trauma or PPV-induced alveolar rupture. Prophylactic percutaneous insertion of catheters in the pleural space is often performed after cardiothoracic surgical procedures in which pleural spaces have been opened. Applying continuous negative-pressure suction (15 to 20 cm H_2O) to these tubes minimizes potential cardiorespiratory compromise. Tension pneumothorax is a life-threatening form of pneumothorax that requires emergent intervention due to hemo-dynamic compromise related to the rapid increases in intrathoracic pressure and subsequent limitation of systemic venous return. Needle decompression followed by thoracostomy tube insertion allows for emergent stabilization of cardiopulmonary function.

Pericardial effusions may cause hemodynamic compromise in the early and late postoperative period. Acute and rapid accumulation of fluid in a noncompliant pericardial space in the early postoperative period will lead to a significant decrease in the right atrial transmural pressure, causing the right atrium to collapse and the central venous pressure to rise. Early clinical manifestations include tachycardia with evolution to exaggerated respiratory variation in systolic blood pressure (pulsus paradoxus) with or without associated fever, chest pain/discomfort, irritability, nausea, poor appetite, and intolerance of feeds in the infant. The physical examination reveals a pleural or pericardial rub, and chest radiography confirms a widened mediastinum with occasional accompanying pleural effusions. Mild cases require observation with serial examinations and echocardiograms. However, moderate effusions with symptoms usually require treatment with nonsteroidal antiinflammatory agents and close follow-up. Larger pericardial effusions may require pericardiocentesis to prevent cardiac tamponade, and chronic effusions may require a surgically created pericardial window.

Pulmonary Hypertension

Pulmonary hypertension (PH) presenting in the postoperative period contributes substantial morbidity and mortality to the CHD population.[33] Acute pulmonary hypertensive crises are life-threatening emergencies requiring immediate aggressive treatments to avoid circulatory collapse.

The mainstay of therapy for acute PH involves optimizing RV loading conditions, augmentation of RV contractility, and avoiding triggers that may precipitate and/or contribute to a PH crisis. Caution must be taken when considering volume loading because increases in RV diastolic volume and pressure may reduce LV compliance and filling via encroachment of the interventricular septum on the LV during diastole. In some situations, acute diuresis and/or phlebotomy may be necessary. Table 33.3 lists several pharmacologic treatment options for the management of acute PH in the CICU.[34] Inhaled nitric oxide (iNO) is a specific pulmonary vascular smooth muscle relaxant that can lower pulmonary artery pressure in a number of diseases without the unwanted

TABLE 33.3	Medications Used for Treatment of Pulmonary Hypertension in the Cardiac Intensive Care Unit	
Drug	**Dose**	**Comment**
Epoprostenol *intravenous*	Start with 1-2 ng/kg/min, increase gradually to 60 ng/kg/min IV	Caution: systemic arterial hypotension Need to change drug vial/delivery system every 12-24 h
Iloprost *inhaled, IV*	0.25 µg/kg inhaled, max. 10 µg; 6×/day or 1-5 ng/kg/min IV	Caution: systemic arterial hypotension
iNO	2-40 ppm inhaled	
Sildenafil *intravenous*	0.4 mg/kg bolus over 3 h (optional), then 1.6-2.4 mg/kg/day continuous infusion	Do not exceed 30 mg/d. Higher sildenafil doses up to 7.2 mg/kg/day IV have been used in newborn infants with PPHN associated with congenital diaphragmatic hernia
oral	Weight 8-20 kg: 10 mg TID Weight >20 kg: 20 mg TID	In children weighing <8 kg, dosage of 1 mg/kg TID[a]
Epinephrine	0.01-1 µg/kg/min IV	Inotropy. Increases myocardial oxygen consumption. Dose-dependent effects on SVR
Norepinephrine	0.01-1 µg/kg/min IV	Increases SVR
Vasopressin	0.0003-0.002 IU/kg/min IV	Probably does not increase PVR (advantage vs. norepinephrine)
Dobutamine	5-20 µg/kg/min IV	Increases myocardial oxygen consumption, tachycardia
Isoproterenol	0.05-2 µg/kg/min IV	Caution: dose-dependent vasodilation may occur due to unopposed beta₂-agonism
Milrinone	0.375-1.0 µg/kg/min IV	Caution: systemic arterial hypotension Lowers PVR
Levosimendan	0.1 µg/kg/min IV	Caution: systemic arterial hypotension Lowers PVR

[a]https://www.fda.gov/Drugs/DrugSafety/ucm317123.htm.
iNO, Inhaled nitric oxide; *IV*, intravenous; *PPHN*, persistent pulmonary hypertension of the newborn; *PVR*, pulmonary vascular resistance; *SVR*, systemic vascular resistance; *TID*, three times daily.
Modified with permission from Kaestner M, Schranz D, Warnecke G, et al. Pulmonary hypertension in the intensive care unit. Expert consensus statement on the diagnosis and treatment of paediatric pulmonary hypertension. The European Paediatric Pulmonary Vascular Disease Network, endorsed by ISHLT and DGPK. *Heart.* 2016;102(suppl 2):ii57-ii66. doi:10.1136/heartjnl-2015-307774.

effect of systemic hypotension. Abrupt withdrawal of iNO can lead to rebound PH, thus requiring a slow wean from support. An additional therapy that may attenuate or prevent a withdrawal phenomenon after weaning iNO includes the use of sildenafil, a phosphodiesterase type 5 inhibitor.[35] Pretreatment with sildenafil, which is well tolerated and available as an oral preparation, produces acute and relatively selective pulmonary vasodilation while acting synergistically with iNO. Hyperventilation was previously proposed as a strategy for the management of PH but is no longer used because it causes a compensatory increase in SVR, decrease in cardiac output, and reduction of cerebral blood flow. However, adequate ventilation and avoidance of hypercapnia remains important. In addition to avoiding known triggers, analgesia and sedation in the ICU play a large role in avoiding or treating postoperative PH crises. Please refer to Chapter 71 for further in-depth discussion of PH in the CICU.

Arrhythmias

Arrhythmias are one of the most commonly reported complications in the cardiac critical care setting, affecting between 15% and 49% of patients after cardiac surgery.[36-38] This wide distribution of arrhythmia frequencies can be accounted for by the heterogeneity of the patient population and types of arrhythmias described. Most arrhythmias occur within the first 48 hours and include both bradyarrhythmias (sinus bradycardia, varying degrees of atrioventricular [AV] block) and tachyarrhythmias (atrial ectopic tachycardia, reentrant supraventricular tachycardias, atrial flutter, atrial fibrillation, junctional ectopic tachycardia [JET], and ventricular tachycardia). These dysrhythmias may impact the patient's hemodynamic stability due to loss of AV synchrony, inadequate ventricular loading, and/or inadequate ventricular output.

Ultimately, significant morbidity may occur, including prolongation of mechanical ventilation and duration of ICU and hospital length of stay. In addition, arrhythmias are independently associated with increased risk of mortality and therefore require an in-depth understanding of arrhythmia diagnoses and therapeutic options to mitigate their impact on outcomes.[39-41]

Postoperative arrhythmias often have multiple causes, combining to alter the underlying electrophysiologic substrate, both iatrogenic (postoperative, mechanical, ischemic, metabolic/electrolyte) and noniatrogenic (genetic, metabolic, ischemic/scar-related, infectious). Specific risk factors to consider in the postoperative patient include myocardial IRI, multiple intracardiac suture lines near the conduction tissue, electrolyte imbalances, irritation of the endocardium from intracardiac monitoring lines, long-standing volume overload, and direct surgical trauma to the conduction system. Rhythm duration may provide clues to the underlying mechanism (paroxysmal, recurrent, or permanent) because gradual changes in cycle length during tachycardia are most commonly encountered in disorders of automaticity (impulse generation). In contrast, tachyarrhythmias caused by reentrant mechanisms (impulse conduction) tend to start and terminate abruptly and demonstrate a relatively constant cycle length.

For life-threatening acute tachyarrhythmias, electrical cardioversion may take precedence over pharmacotherapy. JET is common after pediatric cardiac surgery, especially after repair of tetralogy of Fallot in young infants and after repair of ventricular septal defects and atrioventricular septal defects. The diagnosis of JET is made in the presence of a narrow complex tachycardia and accompanying AV dissociation. Often, retrograde P waves can be seen immediately after the QRS complex, suggesting retrograde conduction via the AV node (Fig. 33.1). Effective treatment strategies for this automatic tachycardia include adequate sedation and

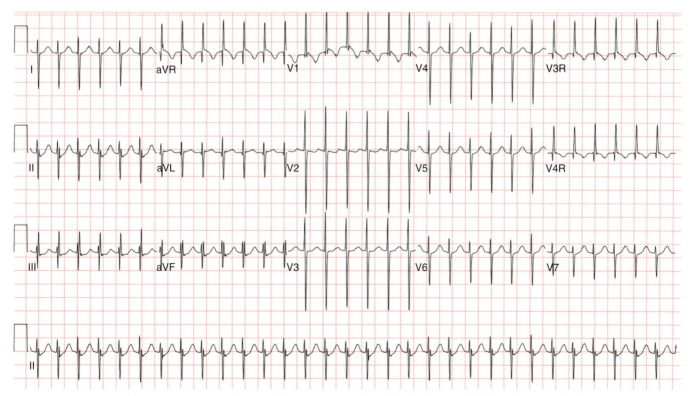

• **Figure 33.1** Fifteen-lead surface electrocardiogram demonstrating junctional ectopic tachycardia with retrograde P waves in a 3-month-old infant after undergoing congenital heart surgery.

analgesia, minimizing exposure to catecholamines, correction of electrolyte derangements, and avoidance of hyperthermia through the use of antipyretics or institution of mild hypothermia (35°C). Temporary overdrive atrial pacing may also be instituted once the JET rate has been reduced by medical therapies. Antiarrhythmic medications such as amiodarone (class 3) are particularly effective in treatment of hemodynamically significant JET, as well as other automatic and ventricular arrhythmias in the postoperative period. Amiodarone exerts a negative inotropic effect and decreases conductivity of nodal tissues, potentially producing significant sinus bradycardia, sinus arrest, or variable AV block, especially if preexisting disease is present. The medical team should therefore be prepared to initiate temporary pacing when administering amiodarone in the early postoperative period. Permanent pacing may also be needed. Coexisting medications must also be considered when treating cardiac arrhythmias, especially adrenergic agents, digoxin (dose adjustment is required when given with amiodarone), and drugs known to alter electrolyte levels.

Up to 3% of postoperative cardiac surgical neonates and infants will experience surgically induced permanent complete AV block. The majority of patients require transient pacing via temporary pacing wires that are placed and tested in the operating room. Consensus recommendations for postoperative advanced second- or third-degree AV block in the pediatric population suggest permanent pacemaker implantation if heart block is not expected to resolve or persists for more than 7 to 10 days after cardiac surgery[42] (Fig. 33.2). Please refer to Chapter 27 for further in-depth discussion of arrhythmias and pacing in the CICU.

Central Nervous System Injuries

The CNS may be particularly susceptible to injury following CPB and may be exacerbated during periods of low CO and/or IRI associated with deep hypothermic circulatory arrest (DHCA). Many efforts have been focused on the operating room as the site of primary CNS injury, yet events in the CICU may also contribute to CNS morbidity, including CNS ischemic insults from low CO, severe hypoxemia and/or severe anemia, and unmatched metabolic demands resulting from pain, agitation, or hyperthermia. Preoperative morbidity, complicated postoperative hospitalizations, in addition to intraoperative perfusion strategies, likely coalesce in a multifactorial fashion to impair normal neurocognitive development in varying degrees as yet to be determined. Additional considerations during the postoperative period include the use of invasive monitoring lines, which may increase the risk of paradoxical embolus, as well as complications from prolonged hospital course such as fever, infections, hyperglycemia and hypoglycemia and perhaps the use of sedatives and analgesics.[43]

Although usually transient, clinically detectable seizures have been reported in 5% to 20% of neonates in the immediate postoperative period and should be investigated rapidly and treated with anticonvulsant therapy.[44] The potential deleterious effects of prolonged circulatory arrest with profound hypothermia may contribute to adverse neurologic outcomes. Conversely, bypass strategies that avoid prolonged DHCA, use antegrade cerebral perfusion strategies for aortic arch reconstruction, and avoid low-flow CPB have been demonstrated to significantly reduce the incidence of postoperative seizures and improve neurologic outcomes.[45,46] Risk factors for seizures include younger age at the time of surgery, longer periods of DHCA, and the presence of coexisting CNS abnormalities. Perioperative seizures are a marker for early CNS injury and have been reported to be associated with worse scores on developmental testing of children several years after undergoing CPB and complex congenital heart surgery.[47] Due to the lack of generalizability of prior studies of seizure incidence and outcomes, no consensus exits to recommend routine postoperative

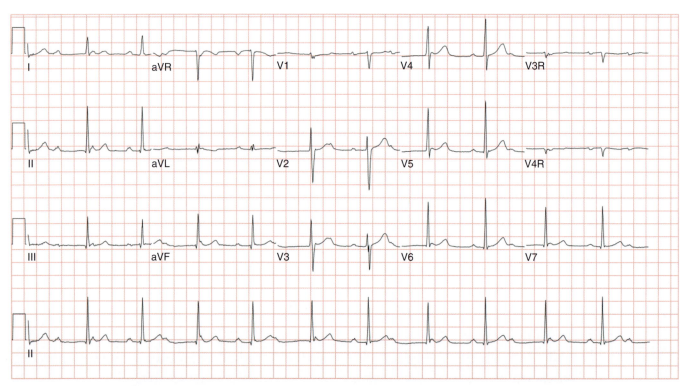

• **Figure 33.2** Fifteen-lead surface electrocardiogram demonstrating complete atrioventricular block.

electroencephalography in neonates and infants undergoing CPB and/or DHCA.

Children with congenital and acquired heart disease are known to be at greater risk for arterial ischemic stroke than the general population.[48] Yet the true incidence, risk factors, and outcomes in children experiencing thrombotic complications after undergoing cardiac surgery for CHD is unknown due to a paucity of data and challenging epidemiology during the acute postoperative period. CNS thrombotic complications further narrow the population after excluding peripheral and/or central venous thromboses in the total frequency. Stroke syndromes related to thromboembolic disease represent only one aspect of the spectrum of cerebral abnormalities, which includes cerebral dysmaturity, periventricular leukomalacia, ischemic and hemorrhagic stroke, and disturbed cerebrovascular physiology.[49] Ventricular assist device recipients are also at risk for ischemic and hemorrhagic stroke(s) and require a high degree of suspicion when neurologic deficits are manifested. Although the prevalence of strokes is consistently low throughout the first 2 months after continuous-flow device implantation, the risk of stroke in pulsatile devices is highest in the first 30 days.[50,51]

Patients undergoing the Fontan procedure are an additional subgroup of patients at increased risk for postoperative stroke. Although not confined to the acute postoperative period, strokes may occur in a variety of settings and require cardiac critical care providers to be aware of the consequences of thrombosis in patients with Fontan physiology. Thromboembolic events within Fontan venous pathways have historically been associated with early morbidity and mortality, with reported incidences of stroke from 3% to 19%.[52]

In the acute phase of an arterial ischemic stroke, general supportive interventions should be considered, regardless of cause. These include ensuring adequate systemic oxygen delivery, maintenance of euglycemia, correction of anemia, avoidance of hyperthermia, and treatment of clinically evident seizures with anticonvulsants. The safety and efficacy of thrombolysis for acute ischemic stroke in children have not been established, yet formal recommendations for "children with a cardiac embolism unrelated to a patent foramen ovale who are judged to have a high risk of recurrent embolism, it is reasonable to initially introduce UFH (unfractionated heparin) or LMWH (low molecular weight heparin) while warfarin therapy is initiated and adjusted (Class IIa, Level of Evidence B)."[53] Please refer to Chapter 17 for an in-depth review of neurologic system responses to cardiac function.

Acute Kidney Injury and Fluid Management

Acute kidney injury (AKI) is a term that encompasses all forms of insults to the kidney, ranging from a minimal rise in serum creatinine (SCr) to anuric renal failure and need for renal replacement therapies (RRTs). Epidemiologic studies have demonstrated an incidence of AKI of 30% to 40% in adult and pediatric patients after CPB, with neonates, younger infants, and adults with comorbidities especially vulnerable to the period of planned renal ischemia. The recognition of this in-hospital complication has revealed striking independent associations with longer lengths of stay, hemodynamic monitoring, need for RRT, hospital costs, lower long-term quality of life, and mortality.[54,55] Despite novel improvements in recognition (biomarkers) and technical treatment options, mortality and morbidity associated with AKI remain high.

CPB-induced SIRS, renal IRI in those undergoing DHCA, low CO, and nephrotoxins all contribute to the development and progression of AKI. Volume overload, although independently associated with adverse outcomes in children recovering from cardiac surgery, may not always accompany AKI in the clinical setting. Increases in microvascular permeability may contribute to total body fluid overload despite having intact renal function. Although less common in the pediatric population after CHD surgery, severe renal failure with anuria, life-threatening hyperkalemia, intractable metabolic acidosis, and fluid overload that compromises gas exchange can occur and is associated with increased mortality rates.[54]

Fluid removal is most commonly approached pharmacologically using diuretics. Loop diuretics (furosemide and bumetanide) require tubular secretion to be delivered to the site of action. Inadequate renal perfusion impairs delivery of diuretics to their target ion transporters, often necessitating higher dosing.[56] Optimal timing and dosing of diuretics in the pediatric CICU population remains undetermined. Of note, bumetanide may be safer in neonates with hyperbilirubinemia because displacement of bilirubin from albumin occurs less commonly than with furosemide. The side-effect profile of loop diuretics must be take into consideration, especially when reaching "ceiling doses." These include ototoxicity, nephrocalcinosis, electrolyte derangements (hyponatremia, hypocalcemia, hypokalemia, hypochloremia, hypomagnesemia), secondary metabolic alkalosis, and fever (rare).[57] Sequential nephron blockade through the addition of thiazide-type diuretics and aldosterone antagonists to a loop diuretic has been proposed as a means of increasing efficacy of diuretics by blocking distal tubule sodium reabsorption.[58,59] Aldosterone receptor antagonists, such as spironolactone, have weak diuretic effects but can augment potassium preservation when combined with other classes of diuretics. Additional aggressive forms of fluid removal and renal support may need to be employed in the postoperative period when fluid overload is refractory to medical management. Similarly, acute elevations in serum potassium level and/or inadequate clearance of nitrogenous wastes and medication metabolites affecting hemodynamic and neurologic status are additional indications for urgent RRT. Peritoneal dialysis (PD) is a form of RRT that is technically easier to accomplish in the neonate and infant population because there is no requirement for large intravascular catheters or anticoagulation, although control over fluid balance may be less precise when compared with continuous RRT (CRRT). The largest proportion of children requiring RRT (often in the form of PD) in the postoperative period are those infants less than 1 year of age and often less than 5 kg. Several single-center retrospective studies have demonstrated greater net negative fluid balance, decreased need for inotropic support, and lower levels of inflammatory mediators in neonates prescribed prophylactic PD in the postoperative period.[60,61] In contrast, a nonblinded randomized trial of neonates undergoing prophylactic PD after the Norwood procedure found no difference in vasoactive infusion score (maximum), time to sternal closure, time to extubation, or hospital length of stay.[62] Alternative forms of RRT that employ hematologic purification and fluid removal include continuous venovenous hemofiltration (± dialysis) and intermittent hemodialysis. Caution should be employed when dialyzing hemodynamically unstable patients, in particular those with significant preload requirements. Optimal vascular access is one of the most important technical factors determining success of CRRT and minimizing circuit failure. Internal jugular vein placement should be considered over femoral vein sites, and the largest-gauge catheter that can be safely placed is recommended to maximize blood flow.[63] Initiating CRRT must take into consideration overall fluid balance (extent of fluid overload), response to diuretics, hemodynamic status, and underlying anatomic candidacy for large-bore catheter insertion. Consideration for abnormal abdominal wall defects, residual hernias, and/or catheter dysfunction related to intraabdominal pathology should be weighed when placing PD catheters. Likewise, complications related to CRRT include bleeding (in particular when systemic heparin administration is indicated), thrombosis, and line infection. Patency of venous vessels may be required for long-term vascular access in patients who develop end-stage kidney failure, and thus avoidance of temporary subclavian vein catheters is recommended.[63]

Strategies to prevent AKI are limited, but current evidence supports maintenance of adequate intravascular volume and renal perfusion while minimizing venous congestion, administration of balanced salt as opposed to high-chloride intravenous fluids and avoiding or minimizing exposure to nephrotoxic medications. Particular vigilance must also be paid to electrolyte abnormalities during the period of active diuresis within the first 24 hours after CPB. Attention should be devoted to aggressive monitoring of serum potassium, calcium, and magnesium levels. Metabolic derangements secondary to renal failure such as metabolic acidosis, hyponatremia, hyperkalemia, and hypocalcemia should be avoided because they can exacerbate underlying myocardial dysfunction.

Gastrointestinal Complications and Postoperative Nutrition

Gastrointestinal complications occur commonly in the postoperative period, especially for neonates and infants. Necrotizing enterocolitis (NEC) remains one of the most severe gastrointestinal complications and is associated with significant morbidity and mortality. This condition exhibits a combination of intestinal inflammation, loss of mucosal integrity, epithelial necrosis, and bacterial translocation. Observed strictly in the neonate, NEC is most often seen in patients with CHD that includes diastolic runoff such as truncus arteriosus or aortopulmonary window and in ductal dependent single ventricle patients.[64] Cases of NEC may occur throughout the CICU admission with some reports suggesting a higher incidence in the preoperative period.[65] Though likely multifactorial, risk factors most likely associated with NEC in the CHD population include impaired splanchnic blood flow and mesenteric ischemia. Diastolic flow reversal related to aortopulmonary shunt runoff and Blalock-Taussig shunt size have been associated with increased incidence of NEC in the CHD population.[66,67] Although NEC may occur in as many as 18% of patients with HLHS,[68] the majority of cases require only supportive care and antimicrobial therapy, with a minority requiring surgical intervention.

The critically ill newborn and neonatal population often experiences difficulty with oral feeding postoperatively. Prolonged or complex hospitalizations, as well as recurrent laryngeal nerve injury, pose a risk for the development of oral feeding intolerance and possible aversion. Newborns denied oral feeds for weeks after birth require time to learn the oral-motor coordination required for successful oral feeding. These infants may need temporary supplemental or total NG tube feeding with high-calorie formulas. As the infant recovers at home with continued help from oral rehabilitation therapists, NG feeds are eventually weaned until feeding support is no longer needed.

Pain Management and Sedation

Pain, agitation, and anxiety are expected in the postoperative period and require an aggressive multidisciplinary approach with the goal of analgesic, sedative, and amnestic therapies to ensure hemodynamic stability, respiratory function in those spontaneously breathing, and overall well-being. Continuous or intermittent infusions of opioid and benzodiazepine agents, regional techniques (e.g., epidural anesthesia), patient-controlled analgesia, nonsteroidal antiinflammatory agents, child life therapy, and active family participation are key components of the multifaceted approach to postoperative pain management of the critically ill child.

Pain and agitation often coexist in the developmentally immature patient. Distinguishing between pain and agitation is an important challenge for the CICU care provider. This assessment should use previously validated pain and sedation scales to provide objective measurements and to guide therapies. Two scales have been formally validated to assess sedation in ventilated patients: State Behavioral Scale[69] and COMFORT Behavior scale.[70] These scales assess alertness, calmness/agitation, respiratory response, crying, physical movement, muscle tone, and facial tension. In an effort to optimize sedation and analgesia and avoid the development of opioid and benzodiazepine dependence, CICUs are increasingly adapting these pain/agitation scales into formalized sedation protocols to guide sedative/analgesic drug administration.[71]

The prescription of sedative/analgesic drugs in infants and children should be influenced by the developmental and physiologic changes that influence pharmacokinetics. Reduced gastric emptying, increased intestinal permeability, and increased intestinal transit time are observed in infants, whereas older children have greater adipose tissue and muscle bulk that may influence volumes of distribution. Critically ill children also have impaired renal and hepatic function, impairing medication clearance. Differences in pharmacokinetics between adults and children become negligible by 2 to 3 years of age because developmental changes are largely complete.

Please refer to Chapter 20 for further discussion of sedative and analgesic use in the CICU.

Infectious Complications

In children undergoing cardiac operations, hospital-acquired infections (HAIs) develop in 15% to 30% of admissions, often contributing to the length of stay and to higher morbidity and mortality.[72,73] Surgical site infections (SSIs) and bloodstream infections (BSIs) are the most common types of HAIs observed in the pediatric cardiac population, occurring in 3% to 8% and 2.3% to 10% of pediatric cardiac patients, respectively.[74] Risk factors associated with major postoperative HAIs include age (neonates), longer preoperative and postoperative hospitalizations, preoperative and postoperative mechanical ventilation, prolonged use of perioperative antibiotic prophylaxis, postoperative steroids, transfusion of blood products, surgical complexity, and open chest.[75,76]

Perioperative use of antibiotics, initiated intraoperatively within 1 hour before skin incision, have been demonstrated to reduce the incidence of postoperative wound infections by as much as fivefold.[77] Antibiotics given during the immediate recovery phase after surgery or until sternal closure have also demonstrated efficacy in reducing rates of SSIs, although prolonged use of prophylactic antibiotics may increase the risk of infection.[78] Low-grade fever (<38.5°C) during the early postoperative period is commonly observed after CPB and is rarely associated with an infectious cause. Early removal of indwelling catheters in the postoperative period may reduce the incidence of mediastinitis and sepsis. Mediastinitis occurs in 2% or less of patients undergoing cardiac surgery[79] and is characterized by persistent fever, purulent drainage from the sternotomy wound, sternal instability, and leukocytosis. *Staphylococcus* species are the most common offending pathogens, and risk factors include delayed sternal closure, early reexploration for bleeding, diabetes, obesity, and reoperation. As with sepsis after cardiac surgery in adults, delayed diagnosis of mediastinitis can lead to mortality rates as high as 25%. Treatment is primarily surgical with debridement, irrigation, use of negative pressure wound therapy (e.g., vacuum-assisted closure), and aggressive parenteral antibiotic therapy.

Appropriate antibiotic exposure has been the focus of national and international public health agencies concerned about the growing incidence of HAIs associated with drug-resistant organisms. Antimicrobial prophylaxis guidelines are available from both the Society of Thoracic Surgeons and the American Society of Health-System Pharmacists, which recommend the use of early-generation cephalosporins as first-line prophylaxis in the absence of confirmed allergies to β-lactam antibiotics.[77] Although significant variation in duration of prophylaxis exists across pediatric heart centers, current evidence suggests that the first dose should be administered before skin incision and continued for up to a maximum of 48 hours after cardiac surgery.[80]

The implementation of initiatives that focus on prevention of HAIs such as optimal antimicrobial prescription, infection control practice improvements, early removal of central lines and chest tubes, and bundling of processes of care may improve patient safety and frequency of HAIs. These initiatives involve grouped interventions that are focused on two to three evidence-based practice changes and have been shown to be successful in reducing rates of ventilator-associated pneumonia, central line–associated BSI, and SSI in adult and pediatric institutions. When performed routinely and appropriately, infection prevention bundles avoid variation in techniques (for example hand washing, central line maintenance), definitions, and surveillance practices, ultimately leading to reductions in HAIs.

Hemostatic Complications

Children with CHD present unique challenges to the management of hemostatic derangements. Abnormalities of coagulation, hemostasis, and fibrinolysis have all been reported in the CHD population. Cyanotic children, in particular those with polycythemia (hematocrit > 60%), are most severely affected. In addition, both quantitative and qualitative platelet defects have been described in the CHD population.[81] An immature coagulation system at birth, exposure to hypothermia, CPB-induced inflammatory response, increased fibrinolysis, and the hemodilutional effect of CPB all contribute to age-dependent differences in the concentration of coagulation factors, which predispose neonates to having higher rates of postoperative bleeding.[82] Furthermore, prostaglandin E infusions appear to also inhibit platelet activation. Children with noncyanotic CHD demonstrate platelet abnormalities as well, including the loss of von Willebrand factor. Additional hemostatic deficiencies present in the CHD population include increased fibrinolysis and decreased coagulation factor production. Perioperative inhibition of fibrinolysis produces a significant decrease in blood loss during palliative or corrective surgery for CHD.[83]

Postoperative bleeding is common in pediatric patients undergoing CPB and is associated with increased morbidity and mortality.[82]

CPB is a major thrombogenic stimulus that affects all aspects of the hemostatic system, although platelet dysfunction is the primary hemostatic abnormality. Prevention and treatment strategies have targeted the use of antifibrinolytic agents, modified ultrafiltration, adequate reversal of anticoagulation post CPB, transfusion of necessary blood components, and factor concentrates (recombinant factor VIIa, fibrinogen concentrates, and prothrombin complex concentrates). Inadequate heparin reversal, platelet dysfunction, and inadequate fibrinogen are most commonly associated with immediate postoperative bleeding. Chest tube volumes greater than 5 to 10 mL/kg/h should prompt multidisciplinary discussion with cardiothoracic surgery, anesthesia, and CICU teams regarding candidacy for reexploration versus continued medical management.

Blood products, including packed red blood cells, platelets, and fresh frozen plasma, should be administered when postoperative bleeding is prolonged or when abnormal coagulation laboratory values are observed. Recombinant factor VII should be administered in cases of significant postoperative hemorrhage resistant to routine blood product administration and repletion of fibrinogen with cryoprecipitate.[84] Off-label use of factor concentrates has been utilized in the pediatric cardiac population, although the evidence for their use is limited to retrospective and descriptive single-center reports. Recombinant factor VII and prothrombin complex concentrates should be reserved for refractory bleeding that is unresponsive to appropriate blood component replacement.

Sudden cessation of bloody output from a previously draining chest tube, in conjunction with tachycardia, rising intracardiac pressures, hypotension, and narrowing pulse pressure herald the clinical diagnosis of cardiac tamponade. Simple maneuvers to clear occluded chest tubes are required regularly to prevent fluid accumulation in the mediastinum and pericardial space. Ultimately, reexploration of the mediastinum is required to restore hemodynamic stability when there is suspicion of tamponade.

Quality Improvement Initiatives in Postoperative Care

In an effort to better understand the incidence and clinical impact of postoperative complications, including cardiovascular dysfunction/shock, several multi-center clinical registries have begun leveraging large amounts of surgical and postoperative clinical data with the intent to risk-stratify postoperative patients and better understand factors that contribute to morbidity and mortality in the CICU population.[85,86] The Pediatric Cardiac Critical Care Consortium is a volunteer quality improvement collaborative that collects clinical data from more than 30 CICUs across the United States (pc4quality.org). Consensus definitions for common complications have been used for data collection purposes. All of the postoperative complications tracked by the registry are documented by participating institutions with combined rates for all CICU encounters listed in Table 33.4 (abstracted as of April 17, 2017). Virtual Pediatric Systems LLC (VPS) is another registry of clinical outcomes providing benchmarking and novel risk adjustment tools designed specifically for the pediatric cardiac surgical population (www.myvps.org). The cardiac module within VPS has collected data on over 130,000 individual cases from 57 hospitals. Data from VPS Cardiac has led to the creation of a novel risk-adjustment scoring tool termed the *Pediatric Index of Cardiac Surgical Intensive Care Mortality*, an evolution of previous general pediatric ICU models (such as the

TABLE 33.4 Unadjusted Complication Rates Aggregated From All Participating PC⁴ Centers for All Postoperative Complications Occurring After Index Cardiac Surgical Procedures Between August 1, 2014, and December 31, 2017

CICU Postoperative Complications	All PC⁴ Centers (% [Unadjusted])	CICU Postoperative Complications	All PC⁴ Centers (% [Unadjusted])
Any Postoperative Complication	35.3	NEC	1.2
ARDS	0.4	Paralyzed diaphragm	1.3
Arrhythmia requiring therapy[a]	16.3	Pericardial effusion	1.1
Bleeding requiring reoperation	2.6	Pulmonary hypertension[c]	3.7
CA-BSI	1.0	Pleural effusion requiring drainage	3.9
Cardiac arrest	3.3	Pneumonia	1.0
Chylothorax requiring intervention[b]	3.7	Pneumothorax requiring intervention	2.2
CRRT for acute renal failure	1.0	Pulmonary embolism	0.1
Deep SSI	0.4	Pulmonary vein obstruction	0.2
ECMO	3.3	Seizure	1.7
Endocarditis	0.3	Sepsis	1.6
Hemothorax requiring intervention	1.0	Stroke	1.3
Hepatic failure	0.6	Superficial SSI	0.6
Intracranial hemorrhage	0.8	Systemic vein obstruction	1.3
IVH > Grade II	0.2	Unplanned reoperation or reintervention	6.9
Listed for heart transplant	0.4	UTI	0.9
LCOS	14.2	VAD	0.2
Mechanical circulatory support	3.4	Vocal cord dysfunction	2.1
Meningitis	0.01		

Abstraction date: April 24, 2018.

[a]Therapy must include pharmacologic (including electrolyte replacement) therapies, pacemaker, defibrillation, cardioversion, and/or cooling.

[b]Therapy defined as chest tube, medication, and/or change in diet.

[c]For any given CICU encounter, was therapy ever given for suspected or defined pulmonary artery hypertension or elevated pulmonary vascular resistance, excluding encounter in which nitric oxide was given for hypoxemia without any clear evidence of pulmonary hypertension.

ARDS, Acute respiratory distress syndrome; *CA-BSI,* catheter-associated bloodstream infection; *CICU,* cardiac intensive care unit; *CRRT,* continuous renal replacement therapy; *ECMO,* extracorporeal membrane oxygenation; *IVH,* intraventricular hemorrhage; *LCOS,* low cardiac output syndrome; *NEC,* necrotizing enterocolitis; *SSI,* surgical site infection; *UTI,* urinary tract infection; *VAD,* ventricular assist device.

Pediatric Index of Mortality-2 and Pediatric Risk of Mortality-3 scoring systems).[87]

Conclusion

The care of neonates, infants, children, and adults with acquired heart disease and CHD recovering from cardiac surgery presents one of the most complex and rapidly evolving challenges for the cardiac intensive care provider. Successful care of the pediatric cardiac surgical patient requires a comprehensive, well-coordinated team-based mode of care delivery that incorporates a broad knowledge base with efficient and sound clinical judgment.

References

A complete list of references is available at ExpertConsult.com.

34

Echocardiography in the Critically Ill Pediatric Patient

PRIYA SEKAR, MD; WILLIAM RAVEKES, MD

Since the end of the 20th century, noninvasive imaging techniques have assumed the primary role in the initial diagnosis of congenital and acquired heart disease in children. The majority of children with congenital heart disease safely proceed to surgical or transcatheter treatment on the basis of noninvasive testing alone (Tables 34.1 and 34.2).[1,2] Echocardiography remains the primary noninvasive tool because of its excellent resolution, ability to assess both anatomy and function, and lack of ionizing radiation. The examination can be performed at the patient's bedside with relative ease and expediency. When transthoracic acoustic windows are compromised by surgical dressings or chest tubes in the perioperative period, transesophageal echocardiography is very useful.[3-5] Other noninvasive techniques, including magnetic resonance imaging and computed tomography, are increasingly used and will be discussed elsewhere. This chapter reviews the basic principles of echocardiography and highlights applications and challenges of echocardiography in specific clinical settings.

Physical Principles

Pulse Transmission and Reflection

Before discussing details of image acquisition, it is useful to understand how echocardiographic images are generated.[6] Piezoelectric crystals are arranged at the tip of the imaging transducer. Piezoelectric crystals have an amazing property. When physically deformed, the crystals produce small amounts of electrical energy. Conversely, when electrical energy is applied to piezoelectric crystals, physical deformation occurs, and ultrasound waves are generated. Ultrasound is sound in frequencies ranging from 1 to 12 MHz (million cycles per second). Exciting the crystals with electrical energy, thereby producing ultrasound, is analogous to striking a gong with a mallet and producing audible sound.

Imaging systems do not send a single pulse of electrical energy to the crystals; rather, multiple, very short pulses are sent to the crystals. With each electrical pulse, a pulse of acoustic energy is produced. By pulsing the transducer repeatedly at very rapid rates, multiple acoustic pulses result.

If the transducer were simply placed on the patient's chest, most of the ultrasound energy would reflect back off the skin. Like light reflecting off a mirror, the ultrasound energy would never enter the patient. This is due to marked differences in impedance between the transducer and the skin. This impedance mismatch is markedly decreased by applying acoustic gel to the transducer head, thereby allowing acoustic energy to enter the patient.

Tissue properties determine how much of the acoustic energy penetrates into the tissues and how much reflects back to the transducer. Fat, for example, reflects little and transmits most energy. In contrast, bone and air reflect nearly all and transmit very little energy. This explains why it is so difficult to image the heart when there is air (e.g., pneumothorax or hyperinflated lungs) between the transducer and the heart. Air-containing structures prevent acoustic pulses from reaching the heart, like a curtain blocking an audience's view of actors on a stage. This also explains why the heart can be imaged from only a few select places on the body where the heart is near or in direct contact with the chest wall or diaphragm without intervening lung tissues. Often, repositioning the patient is required to achieve optimal echocardiographic images.

For an image of the heart to be displayed, the transmitted ultrasound pulse must reach the heart and reflect back to the transducer. As the received sound deforms the piezoelectric crystals in the transducer head, energy is converted back from acoustic to electrical energy. The imaging system can then display the returning signal as an illuminated pixel on a video monitor.

Signal Processing and Image Generation

Once the transducer converts the acoustic energy back into electrical energy, the imaging system performs complicated amplification and signal processing to optimize the signal-to-noise ratio. The returning signals are much weaker than the transmitted signal. Each reflector is assigned a velocity, a depth, and a density, which are detailed in the following paragraphs.

The system can accurately display a reflector's location on the monitor because the speed of sound is nearly constant through different tissue types. The distance of a reflector from the transducer is directly related to the time for sound to travel to, and from, the reflector. The imaging system calculates the distance of each reflector from the transducer using the time-distance formula:

$$D = c \times t/2$$

where D represents the distance to the target; c, the speed of ultrasound through tissue (1530 m/s); and t, the time for the pulse

TABLE 34.1   Lesions for Which Noninvasive Imaging Is Generally Sufficient Before Surgical or Transcatheter Intervention

Lesion	Features to Be Identified With Noninvasive Imaging	Associated Lesions to Identify/Exclude	Indications for Cardiac Catheterization
Shunts			
Atrial septal defect	Type of atrial defect, size, quantification of shunt (degree of right ventricular volume overload), pulmonary artery pressure, suitability for transcatheter closure.	Anomalous pulmonary venous return, pulmonary stenosis, pulmonary hypertension	Transcatheter closure commonly performed for secundum atrial septal defects. Catheterization usually unnecessary unless pulmonary hypertension or pulmonary vascular disease suspected and management depends on measure of pulmonary resistance.
Ventricular septal defect	Type, anatomic size, quantification of shunt (determined in part by left ventricular size), pulmonary artery pressure.	Multiple ventricular defects, coarctation	Catheterization usually unnecessary unless pulmonary vascular obstructive disease suggests inoperability. Some defects may allow transcatheter closure.
Patent ductus arteriosus	Anatomic size, pulmonary artery pressure, quantification of shunt (determined in part by left ventricular size), arch side and branching.	Coarctation of the aorta	Transcatheter closure.
Complete atrioventricular canal	Size of atrial and ventricular septal defects, atrioventricular valve morphology, balance, and function.	Outflow obstruction, patent ductus arteriosus	Only in rare patient for whom quantification of pulmonary resistance desired.
Cyanotic Lesions			
Transposition of the great arteries	Coronary artery origins and branching, intracardiac shunts, pulmonary artery pressure. Magnetic resonance imaging useful postoperatively to assess branch pulmonary arteries, ventricular function.	Outflow obstruction, arch obstruction, septal defects	Balloon atrial septostomy when needed, usually performed in intensive care unit.
Tetralogy of Fallot	Mechanism and severity of pulmonary stenosis, main pulmonary artery and branch pulmonary artery sizes, coronary artery origin and branching. Magnetic resonance imaging very useful postoperatively to image branch pulmonary arteries, quantify severity of pulmonary regurgitation, assess right ventricular function.	Multiple ventricular septal defects, aortic arch sidedness and branching	Uncommonly needed in older childhood left unrepaired and echocardiography unable to establish pertinent features. In rare cases, pulmonary balloon valvuloplasty performed to palliate and delay surgery.
Tricuspid atresia with normally related great vessels	Size of ventricular septal defect and severity of pulmonary stenosis, adequacy of foramen ovale, identification of other sources of pulmonary blood flow, branch pulmonary artery size and continuity, arch side and branching.	Pulmonary stenosis, left juxtaposition of the atrial appendages	Very rare need to perform balloon atrial septostomy to enlarge foramen ovale. Minority of surgeons prefer angiogram of branch pulmonary arteries before shunt. Catheterization commonly performed before potential Glenn or Fontan operation.
Ebstein anomaly	Morphology of tricuspid valve, severity of tricuspid regurgitation, right ventricular size and function.	Pulmonary valve or branch pulmonary artery stenosis, patent ductus arteriosus, pulmonary artery pressure	Usually not necessary.
Valvular pulmonary stenosis	Mechanism and severity of stenosis, tricuspid valve and right ventricular size and function, patent ductus arteriosus.	Can occur with more complex heart disease including heterotaxy syndrome	Balloon dilation is now treatment of choice.
Total anomalous pulmonary venous connection	Identification of individual pulmonary veins and their size and site of return, exclusion of pulmonary venous obstruction.	Can occur with other complex congenital heart disease, left heart hypoplasia	Generally not necessary and of significant risk when required to establish pulmonary venous return (potential for pulmonary hypertensive crisis).

TABLE 34.1 Lesions for Which Noninvasive Imaging Is Generally Sufficient Before Surgical or Transcatheter Intervention—cont'd

Lesion	Features to Be Identified With Noninvasive Imaging	Associated Lesions to Identify/Exclude	Indications for Cardiac Catheterization
Admixture Lesions			
Truncus arteriosus common	Morphology and function of truncal valve, branch pulmonary size and distortion.	Exclusion of multiple ventricular septal defects, ventricular hypoplasia (particularly right), aortic arch size	Generally unnecessary, rarely if pulmonary vascular obstructive disease is considered in an older infant or child.
Left Heart Obstructive Lesions			
Valvular aortic stenosis	Size of aortic annulus and morphology, severity of aortic obstruction, left ventricular size and function.	Mitral stenosis, coarctation, left heart hypoplasia	In most cases, used as initial choice for relief of obstruction, although there is controversy concerning superiority over surgical approach.
Aortic coarctation	Aortic arch anatomy and size, mechanism of aortic coarctation, aortic arch branching, left ventricular size and function. Magnetic resonance imaging or computed tomography excellent when echocardiographic visualization inadequate.	Mitral and/or aortic stenosis	Generally unnecessary before surgical repair. Some favor balloon dilation versus surgical treatment.
Hypoplastic left heart syndrome	Size of atrial septal defect, tricuspid valve function, right ventricular function, nature of mitral and aortic obstruction, left ventricular size, arch morphology. Postoperatively, magnetic resonance imaging useful in examining arch and branch pulmonary arteries.	Patent ductus arteriosus, partial anomalous pulmonary venous return	Not generally needed before Norwood procedure, but performed before Glenn and before Fontan for hemodynamics and visualization of branch pulmonary arteries.

TABLE 34.2 Lesions for Which Noninvasive Imaging Is Generally Insufficient Before Surgical or Transcatheter Intervention and for Which Cardiac Catheterization Is Generally Performed

Lesion	Features to Be Identified With Noninvasive Imaging	Associated Lesions to Identify/Exclude	Indications for Cardiac Catheterization/CT
Pulmonary atresia with intact ventricular septum	Tricuspid valve size and function, right ventricular size and function, right ventricular pressure, presence of coronary sinusoids or fistula.	Coronary artery stenoses, right ventricular dependent coronary artery anatomy	Coronary artery anatomy, stenoses, presence of right ventricular dependent coronary artery distribution
Tetralogy of Fallot with pulmonary atresia	Nature of pulmonary atresia (absent main pulmonary artery versus short segment valvular pulmonary atresia), branch pulmonary artery size, coronary artery anatomy. Magnetic resonance imaging may obviate need for catheterization especially when branch pulmonary arteries good size and collaterals absent.	Multiple ventricular septal defects, aortopulmonary artery collaterals, coronary artery abnormalities, branch pulmonary artery distortion, hypoplasia, or discontinuity	Establishment of pulmonary artery supply and branch pulmonary continuity, determination of overlap between antegrade pulmonary flow and collaterals, in some cases to allow balloon dilation of stenoses, in some cases to allow embolization of aortopulmonary collaterals
Glenn or Fontan shunt	Ventricular function, valvular function.	Very dependent on anatomy requiring Glenn shunt	Pulmonary artery anatomy and hemodynamics, exclusion of decompressing vertical vein from innominate vein

CT, Computed tomography.

of energy to travel to a reflector and back to the transducer. The longer it takes to travel to and from a reflector, the farther away the reflector is from the transducer. The process is analogous to airplanes localized with radar or submarines with sonar.

Once signal amplification occurs and the distance is calculated for each reflector, other postprocessing must take place before an image is displayed on the monitor. In brief, this postprocessing involves the conversion of an electrical voltage into a gray scale value. The brightness of an illuminated pixel on the monitor correlates directly with the strength of received energy. More powerful reflectors (e.g., fibrous tissue) are represented as a brighter gray scale value (i.e., closer to white), whereas weaker reflectors (e.g., pericardial fluid) are represented as darker values (i.e., closer to black).

This entire process occurs at rates between 50 and 150 times per second. The system has a processing capacity, and the system operator has considerable control over how that processing power is used. Though this control is very helpful and allows image optimization, there is always the possibility that incorrect system adjustment will diminish image quality and limit diagnostic information.

Determinants of Image Resolution

Image quality is quantified by spatial and temporal resolution. *Spatial resolution* refers to two-point spatial discrimination: how closely two adjacent structures can be located and correctly resolved as two separate structures rather than incorrectly as a single reflector. Imaging systems should be able to achieve spatial resolution along the plane of the imaging beam to 0.8 mm. This means that two structures as close as 1 mm or slightly less from one another can be resolved from one another. Spatial resolution is superior along the axial plane (i.e., the plane parallel to the imaging beam) compared to the lateral plane (i.e., the plane orthogonal to the imaging probe), where spatial resolution falls to between 1 and 2 mm.

Temporal resolution refers to the ability of the system to resolve accurately the position of a moving structure in time. Though temporal resolution is unimportant in imaging a static structure like the brain (because the structure being imaged does not change position from one moment to the next), it is obviously critically important when the goal is to accurately demonstrate cardiac motion. If, for example, a rapidly moving structure (e.g., a valve leaflet) moves from point A to point B and back to point A in 10 ms and the temporal resolution of the imaging system is 10 ms, the motion of the valve will not be displayed accurately. In this example the structure will not appear to move but will appear to remain at point A. Temporal resolution is particularly important when heart rates are faster, as in the fetus or neonate.

Transducer Selection: Tradeoff Between Resolution and Penetration

The sonographer chooses the optimal imaging probe, weighing the requirements for spatial and temporal resolution against the requirements for tissue penetration (Figs. 34.1 and 34.2).

Tissue penetration refers to the distance an acoustic pulse can reach. Penetration is indirectly related to probe frequency and directly related to beam transmission power. Higher-frequency transducers, covering frequencies between 8 and 12 MHz, provide superior spatial resolution but at the expense of lower penetration. Structures within 8 cm are typically imaged with high-frequency

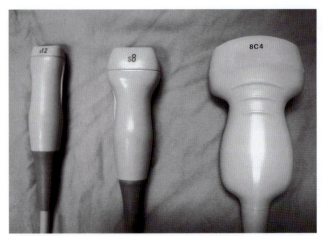

• **Figure 34.1** Transthoracic and abdominal imaging probes. The two probes on the left are phased array sector probes optimized for cardiac imaging. The smaller probe (S12), intended for neonatal imaging, is optimized to image at 12 MHz. Its smaller footprint allows the transducer to fit between narrower interspaces and shifts the acoustic focus closer to the transducer, resulting in an optimal imaging range of less than 6 to 8 cm. The 8-MHz probe (S8) in the middle has slightly inferior spatial resolution but has superior penetration. The latter is important in imaging the larger child. The probe on the right is a curvilinear probe (8C4) and is intended for fetal and abdominal imaging. The curved shape allows for a wider near field of view than the sector probes allow. When the fetus is in the near field, the wider near field of view is important.

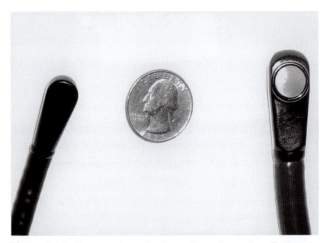

• **Figure 34.2** Transesophageal echocardiography probes. Both probes allow multiplane transesophageal imaging by electronically rotating the scan plane. The smaller probe on the left has a tip diameter of 8 by 10.7 mm and is optimized for neonates and children up to approximately 20 kg. The larger probe has a tip diameter of 14.9 mm and is intended for the larger child and the adult. The larger probe operates at a lower frequency, allowing for improved beam penetration but at some loss in image resolution.

probes. Lower-frequency transducers covering frequencies between 1 and 3 MHz penetrate farther into tissue (up to 15 to 20 cm) but sacrifice spatial resolution. The sonographer tends to use the highest-frequency transducer that provides adequate tissue penetration for the distance required, just as the golfer chooses the putter for short shots requiring more accuracy and the driver when shots require more power. The sonographer trades off the needs of spatial resolution against the requirements of tissue penetration.

Penetration is also directly related to transmission power. Just as a 100-watt lightbulb illuminates farther than a 15-watt bulb, increased beam power allows the ultrasound beam to penetrate farther. However, acoustic power is constrained by safety limitations. Tissue warming can occur if excessively high power is used. In addition, image resolution can decrease with higher power, another tradeoff for which the sonographer must accommodate.

Transducer "footprint," which is how the size of the transducer head is commonly described, is another practical consideration when imaging children. Higher-frequency transducers have a smaller footprint and therefore are ideal in imaging between rib spaces of neonates and small infants, compared with the lower-frequency transducers, which have larger footprints and may not physically fit in the intercostal spaces of a smaller pediatric patient. On occasion the sonographer will have to choose a higher-frequency transducer just to image in an intercostal space, compromising penetration for the footprint.

Transducers vary in other important ways, such as location of use. Transthoracic probes acquire images from the chest wall, whereas transesophageal probes are passed from the mouth and pharynx into the esophagus or stomach. Transesophageal probes must be smaller and more flexible. Transesophageal echocardiography should be considered when transthoracic images are poor or when transthoracic imaging is not possible due to logistics, such as a procedure being performed on the chest. Transesophageal imaging is contraindicated in the setting of esophageal varices, gastric bleeding, recent upper gastrointestinal surgery, or elevated intracranial pressure. Intravascular probes are mounted on catheters to allow intracardiac or intravascular imaging. Again, tradeoffs are present; miniaturization is achieved at the expense of some other imaging parameter, usually tissue penetration or resolution.

Doppler Analysis

Doppler analysis is a powerful complementary modality to two-dimensional imaging.[7] It is used primarily to quantify flow velocity and pressure gradients within the vascular system. Similar to the principles discussed concerning image generation, small packets of ultrasound energy are transmitted, but in this case to the blood pool. When ultrasound energy strikes a moving target such as the red cells, the returning signal frequency is shifted compared with the transmitted frequency. Blood flow toward the transducer shifts the returning frequency higher, whereas flow away shifts the frequency lower. This velocity causing the frequency change (referred to as the Doppler frequency shift) is characterized by the Doppler equation:

$$V = f_d \times 2c / f_o \times 1 / \cos\theta$$

where V represents the velocity of the reflector (i.e., red cell); f_d, the Doppler frequency shift; c, the speed of sound in tissue; f_o, the transmitted frequency; and θ, the angle between the direction of sound propagation and the direction of motion of the reflector.

Directionality of blood flow is determined by whether the frequency shift is higher (i.e., flow toward the probe) or lower (flow away from the probe). The speed of the red cells is related to the magnitude of the frequency shift. Fast-moving targets such as flow across a stenotic valve produce a larger frequency shift. Slower moving targets such as venous flow cause less of a frequency shift. The imaging systems routinely calculate the velocity from the measured frequency shift and then display that velocity for the sonographer.

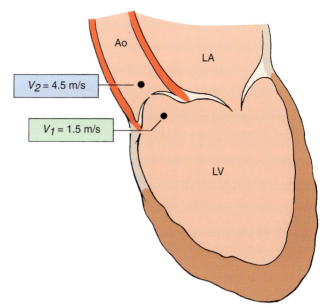

• **Figure 34.3** Calculation of the maximum instantaneous gradient across a stenotic aortic valve using the Bernoulli equation. In this example the aortic valve is doming due to the presence of severe aortic valve stenosis. Using Doppler interrogation, the velocity (V_1) is measured within the left ventricular outflow tract just proximal to the aortic valve, and V_2 is measured just distal to the doming aortic valve leaflets. Using the Bernoulli equation, $\Delta P = 4 (V_2^2 - V_1^2)$, where V_1 is 1.5 m/s and V_2 is 4.5 m/s, ΔP is 70 to 75 mm Hg. The valve gradient is a function of the orifice area and the flow across the area of interest. *Ao,* Aorta; *LA,* left atrium; *LV,* left ventricle.

The result of Doppler interrogation is a spectral display with velocity on the y-axis and time along the x-axis. The convention is to display flow away from the transducer as a positive value (i.e., above the zero baseline) and flow away from the transducer as a negative valve (i.e., below the zero baseline).

A very important relationship exists between the velocity and the pressure gradient producing this velocity. This is described by the Bernoulli equation:

$$\Delta P = 4(V_2^2 - V_1^2)$$

V_2 represents the velocity measured just distal to the site of interest, and V_1, the velocity just proximal to the site of interest. This can be used, for example, to measure the maximum instantaneous gradient across a stenotic valve (Fig. 34.3). If the velocity distal to the valve (V_2) is 4.5 m/s and velocity just proximal (V_1) is 1.5 m/s, then the pressure gradient resulting in this velocity increase would be:

$$\Delta P = 4(4.5^2 - 1.5^2)$$

or approximately 70 to 75 mm Hg.

Frequently V_1 is quite small, and when it is less than 1 m/s, it can be ignored. This results in the modified Bernoulli equation:

$$\Delta P = 4(V_2)^2$$

It is particularly important to include V_1 whenever the proximal velocity exceeds 1.5 m/s. This is typically the case, for example, when measuring the gradient across an aortic coarctation. Flow accelerates around the arch normally, and the velocity can reach or even exceed 1.5 m/s. Higher velocities occur when the arch is hypoplastic. Ignoring V_1 and using only the simplified Bernoulli equation would result in an overestimate of the maximum instantaneous gradient. There are important theoretical and clinical considerations in interpreting the calculated Doppler gradient, and these are discussed in the section concerning gradient assessment.

There are four different methods of Doppler interrogation: color, pulsed wave, continuous wave, and high pulse repetition Doppler. Each method has particular strengths and clinical applications.

Color Doppler. This is a very powerful technique allowing the velocity information to be overlaid across the two-dimensional image (see Video 3). Various color maps are used to encode this information, but a commonly used map displays blood flow toward the transducer in red and flow away in blue. Shades of blue are used to indicate the speed of flow away: Low-velocity flow away may be a darker blue and higher velocity a lighter shade of blue. Shades of red and yellow are used to indicate the speed of flow toward the transducer: Low-velocity flow toward the transducer may be a darker red and higher velocity a shade of yellow-red. Other encoding maps can display areas of turbulence, where the velocity at closely adjacent areas varies one to another in contrast to when flow is laminar.

Pulsed Wave Doppler. This is a commonly used Doppler technique and has the advantage of allowing velocity determination at a specific location in the heart (Figs. 34.4 and 34.5). Pulsed wave Doppler can be used, for example, to determine the gradient across a stenotic valve, vessel stenosis, or across a septal defect.

Whereas the strength of pulsed wave Doppler is its ability to measure velocity at a specific location, it has a very important limitation called *aliasing*. Aliasing occurs when pulsed Doppler cannot reliably calculate the speed and direction of the target. For pulsed Doppler to measure flow velocity accurately, the imaging system must sample (i.e., transmit acoustic packets) at a frequency

greater than twice the frequency shift produced by the flow being interrogated. When the interrogated flow velocity is quite fast, the sampling rate of the system may not be able to achieve the required sampling frequency, called the *Nyquist limit,* and if so, aliasing occurs.

Aliasing is analogous to the appearance of a spinning wheel illuminated in a dark room by a strobe light flashing at a frequency less than twice the spinning frequency. If the wheel is spinning more than twice as fast as the strobe rate, the wheel may appear to be spinning backward. If the strobe and spinning frequency are the same, the wheel may not appear to be moving at all! Aliasing becomes a clinically important limitation in cardiac imaging when blood flow is fast, such as across severely stenotic valves, vessels, or restrictive ventricular septal defects.

Continuous Wave Doppler and High Pulse Repetition Doppler. Fortunately, other Doppler techniques, including continuous wave and high pulse repetition frequency Doppler can accurately measure these higher-velocity events. They are able to do so by sampling at frequencies faster than traditional pulsed Doppler interrogation (in the case of continuous wave Doppler, sampling is "nearly continuous"). Though the higher sampling rate eliminates aliasing, another problem is introduced, called *range ambiguity.*

Range ambiguity is easily understood if the reader remembers back to the strength of pulsed Doppler interrogation: the ability to measure blood velocity at a specific location in the heart called a gate. When very high sampling frequencies are used with continuous wave Doppler or high pulse repetition frequency Doppler, returning signals are reaching the imaging system too fast to determine reliably the specific location from which the event is occurring (range ambiguity). An analogy is that of a police officer using a radar gun on passing motorists. If he "fires" the gun before waiting for the last "fire" to return, he will have difficulty determining from exactly which location (car in this case) the signal is returning.

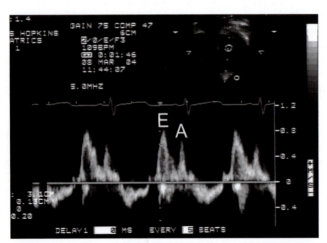

• **Figure 34.4** Pulsed Doppler interrogation of the mitral valve in a healthy 3-month-old infant. Mitral valve flow is displayed as a spectral display of instantaneous velocity against time. Flow is displayed above the baseline because flow is toward the transducer. Note the scale in meters per second (m/s) displayed at the right margin of the spectral display. For orientation, the gate of Doppler is displayed in the small image circled in the upper right corner. The gate is positioned just distal to the tips of the mitral valve leaflets within the left ventricle. Generally two filling waves are seen with mitral valve flow. The peak E velocity *(E)* occurs after mitral valve opening, and the peak A velocity *(A)* during atrial systole. In this young infant the E velocity is 0.8 m/s and A velocity, 0.6 m/s. The E/A ratio (peak E velocity/peak A velocity) is 1.3. Normal mitral and tricuspid valve velocities are displayed in Table 34.4.

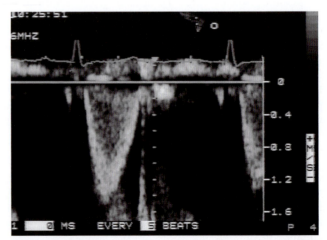

• **Figure 34.5** Pulsed Doppler interrogation of the aortic valve in a healthy 9-year-old child. Aortic velocity is displayed as a spectral display of instantaneous velocity against time. In this apical four-chamber view, flow is away from the transducer, so velocity is displayed below the baseline. Note the scale in meters per second (m/s) displayed at the right margin of the spectral display. For orientation, the gate of pulsed Doppler interrogation has been positioned just distal to the tips of the aortic valve leaflets within the ascending aorta. The maximum velocity ranges between 1.2 and 1.5 m/s. Normal aortic valve and pulmonary valve velocities are displayed in Table 34.3.

Fortunately, in clinical practice the problem of range ambiguity in interrogating high-velocity events is usually solved by applying clinical judgment and/or supplemental echocardiographic information. High-velocity events occur in specific clinical situations, so if locations that do make sense are suggested with continuous wave Doppler, the operator "knows" to interpret that information critically. In some situations the operator can use other information to assess for internal consistency. For example, if continuous wave Doppler suggests severe valvular pulmonary stenosis, the right ventricular pressure should be elevated. Usually, but not always, the operator can resolve range ambiguity.

Elements of the Transthoracic Echocardiogram

Clinicians in the intensive care unit caring for patients with cardiac disease should have familiarity with the elements of a two-dimensional transthoracic echocardiogram. The three basic elements of any examination include imaging sweeps for anatomic delineation, Doppler interrogation for blood flow velocity and direction, and measurement of systolic and diastolic function.

Imaging Planes and Sweeps for Anatomic Delineation

Two-dimensional images are typically obtained from four acoustic windows: subcostal (just inferior to the xiphoid process), apical (≈5th left intercostal space at the anterior axillary line), parasternal (2nd or 3rd left parasternal space, midclavicular line), and the suprasternal notch (Fig. 34.6).[8] Traditional echocardiography will display a thin tomographic two-dimensional image, but the heart is a complex three-dimensional moving organ. To best understand the anatomy, "sweeps" are required. Sweeps involve moving the ultrasound beam back and forth from multiple locations on the chest through the heart akin to surveying a room with a flashlight. At each location the sonographer images from two orthogonal planes and in each plane "sweeps" through the cardiac mass, generating multiple two-dimensional images. Common scan planes are

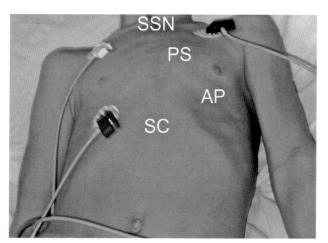

• **Figure 34.6** Orientation of scan planes in transthoracic echocardiogram. Normal scan positions. The patient is positioned with leads attached to allow electrocardiographic monitoring for timing. Four imaging positions or acoustic windows are commonly used: subcostal *(SC)*, apical *(AP)*, parasternal *(PS)*, and suprasternal sternal notch *(SSN)*.

illustrated in four figures: subcostal (Fig. 34.7), apical (Fig. 34.8), parasternal (Fig. 34.9), and suprasternal notch (Fig. 34.10).

Other imaging positions are less commonly used to image particular structures: right sternal border (atrial septum) and high left parasagittal (patent ductus arteriosus). Often in the postoperative patient, bandages or chest tubes may limit imaging from some of the standard locations, and nonstandard transthoracic or transesophageal windows are used.

Optimization of Imaging Conditions. The intensive care unit staff can be helpful in repositioning the patient. Subcostal images are generally obtained with the patient lying on his or her back and sometimes with knees bent. The apical and parasternal images are obtained with the patient in left lateral decubitus position so the left lung falls posterior to the imaging plane. Suprasternal notch images are best obtained with a pillow placed behind the patient's back so the neck is hyperextended. It is also helpful to the sonographer for the lights to be dimmed so the video monitor is more easily viewed.

Undergoing a transthoracic echocardiogram can be uncomfortable, particularly the subcostal and suprasternal notch imaging planes. For patients of certain ages or specific clinical conditions, sedation may be necessary to achieve adequate stillness and cooperation for image optimization. A transthoracic echocardiogram typically lasts 20 to 45 minutes (not as quick as a chest x-ray examination or computed tomography scan); this is important to recognize because this should guide the choice of sedative.

Doppler Interrogation

Color Doppler is performed of all valves (for regurgitation or stenosis), atrial and ventricular septum (for septal defects), main pulmonary artery (for patent ductus arteriosus), and branch pulmonary arteries and aortic arch (excluding peripheral pulmonary artery stenosis and coarctation). Small amounts of tricuspid and pulmonary regurgitation are common normal variants. Mild mitral regurgitation though less common is also a normal variant. A patent foramen ovale (PFO), allowing a small amount of left-to-right flow, is also a normal variant in the child younger than 1 year of age.

Pulsed wave Doppler is performed of each valve. The tricuspid valve and mitral valve have similar flow patterns (see Fig. 34.4). Filling generally occurs in two waves termed the *E wave* (during early diastolic filling of the ventricle) and the *A wave* (during atrial systole). Each wave has a peak velocity termed the *E velocity* and *A velocity*, respectively. In the fetus and neonate the peak A velocity typically exceeds the peak E velocity. The E velocity typically exceeds the A velocity after 1 year of age.

Normal reference values for pulmonary and aortic flow velocities in healthy children exist and are listed in Table 34.3. An example of pulsed wave Doppler signal across a semilunar valve is illustrated in Fig. 34.5. The normal aortic velocity exceeds that of the pulmonary velocity.[9] Accelerated flow usually indicates valve stenosis, although any condition that increases cardiac output will increase flow velocities to a mild degree. Anemia or any hyperkinetic state such as thyrotoxicosis, fever, or pain is an example.

Assessment of Left Ventricular Systolic and Diastolic Function

Theoretical Concepts. Myocardial contractility and systolic function should be distinguished from one another. Contractility is an intrinsic property of the myocardial fibers. Systolic function refers

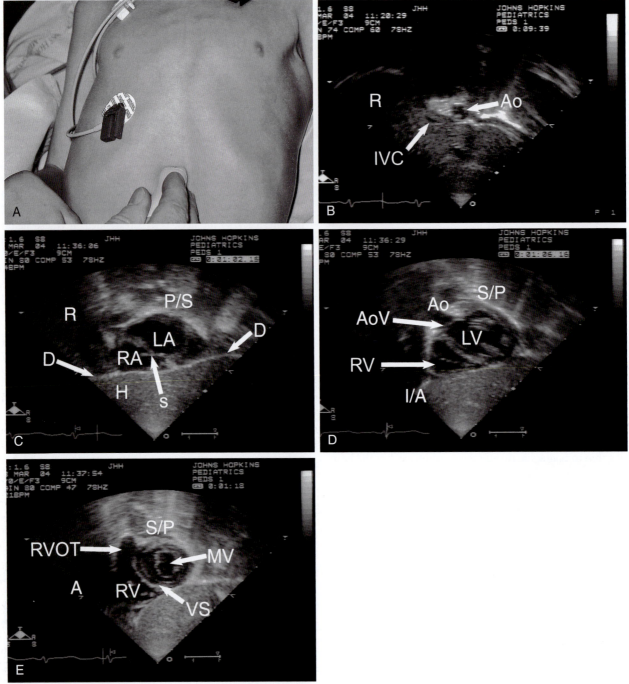

• **Figure 34.7** Subcostal imaging. Scans are illustrated at levels of interest. (A) Transducer position. The transducer is positioned just inferior to the xiphoid process. (B) Abdominal situs. The image is from anterior to posterior. The positions of the aorta and inferior vena cava are demonstrated. Often the location of the stomach is identified as well. (C) Atria and atrial septum. The *arrows* point to the atrial septum between right and left atrium. Both diaphragms are well seen. (D) Aortic valve, left ventricular outflow tract, and ascending aorta. The transducer is angled more anteriorly to demonstrate the left ventricular outflow tract and ascending aorta. (E) Short-axis cut at the level of the mitral valve. Note that the transducer is rotated 90 degrees clockwise from images in B to D. The mitral valve is open within the left ventricle in this diastolic frame. The ventricular septum is seen between the right and left ventricle and the proximal right ventricular outflow tract with the right ventricle. *A*, Anterior; *Ao*, aorta; *AoV*, aortic valve; *D*, diaphragm; *H*, liver; *I*, inferior; *IVC*, inferior vena cava; *LA*, left atrium; *LV*, left ventricle; *MV*, mitral valve; *P*, posterior; *P/S*, posterior-superior; *R*, right; *RA*, right atrium; *RV*, right ventricle; *RVOT*, right ventricular outflow tract; *s*, atrial septum; *S*, superior; *VS*, ventricular septum.

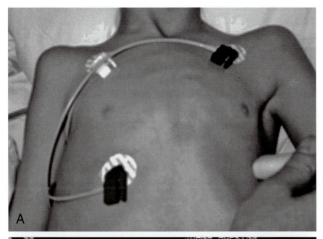

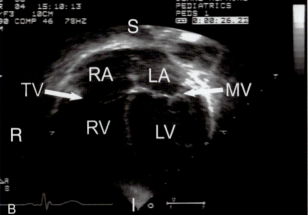

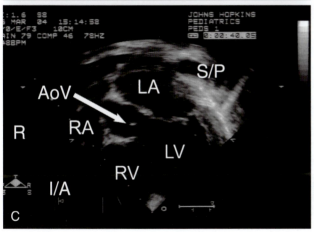

TABLE 34.3	Aortic and Pulmonary Valve Flow Velocities in Healthy Children	
	Peak Velocity	Mean Velocity
Aortic valve (adult)	1.35 ± 0.18 m/sec	
Aortic valve (child)	1.50 ± 0.15 m/sec	0.28 ± 0.05 m/sec
Pulmonary valve (child)	0.90 ± 0.10 m/sec	
Pulmonary valve (newborn)	0.80 ± 0.12 m/sec	

Values are displayed as mean ± one standard deviation from the mean.
m/sec, Meters per second.
From Snyder AR, Serwer GA, Ritter SB. The normal echocardiographic examination. In *Echocardiography in Pediatric Heart Disease.* St. Louis: Mosby; 1997:22-75.

• **Figure 34.8** Apical imaging. Scans are illustrated at levels of interest. (A) Transducer position. The transducer is positioned at the cardiac apex usually in the fourth or fifth intercostal space along the anterior axillary line. Often the patient is positioned in the left lateral decubitus position to minimize reflection of air from the left lung. (B) Four-chamber view. An excellent view for quickly assessing chamber size and atrioventricular valve function. The arrows point to the mitral valve and tricuspid valve. (C) Five-chamber view. The transducer is angled anteriorly from the four-chamber view to demonstrate the aortic valve *(arrow)* and ascending aorta (just distal to the aortic valve). The other cardiac chambers are also displayed. *A,* Anterior; *AoV,* aortic valve; *I,* inferior; *LA,* left atrium; *LV,* left ventricle; *MV,* mitral valve; *P,* posterior; *R,* right; *RA,* right atrium; *RV,* right ventricle; *S,* superior; *TV,* tricuspid valve.

to how well the fibers shorten when loaded. Though dependent on contractility, systolic function is affected by preload and afterload. Take, for example, a hypothetical patient in the intensive care unit who becomes hypovolemic. Function would decline due to reduced preload, not because of a change in myocardial contractility. If instead the patient became quite hypertensive, function would also decrease not because of any change in contractility but because of increased afterload. Finally, consider a patient in whom preload and afterload remain constant, but the ventricle becomes ischemic. In this last situation, both function and contractility decrease.

It is important for the intensivist to understand that though afterload is related to mean arterial pressure, afterload can also be increased without an increase in arterial pressure if the ventricle is dilated or wall thickness reduced. Adriamycin cardiomyopathy is a condition in which afterload is increased due to reduced wall thickness despite normal blood pressure and heart size.

Preload is defined as the stretch on the fibers at end-diastole. Preload is related to ventricular filling pressure but is not identical to that pressure because there is not a direct or constant relationship between filling pressure and fiber stretch (compliance). An example is the changes that occur with cardiopulmonary bypass. The changes may result in a "stiffer" (lower compliance) ventricle, so less fiber stretch occurs for the same filling pressure. Consequently, a higher filling pressure postoperatively does not necessarily mean that the ventricle is working at increased preload. It is important for the intensivist to remember this distinction when considering atrial pressure or mean capillary wedge pressure as a proxy for preload.

In children there is an age-dependent modulation of ventricular function with a decrease in function with age, in part related to increasing afterload.[10] The functional decrease, however, is also due to an age-dependent decrease in contractility (with higher levels of contractility seen in infants and children in the early years of life).

Diastolic function relates to the ability of the heart to relax and is an energy-consuming process. The importance of diastole is being increasingly recognized, in part because there is an improved theoretical understanding of diastole and because there are improved noninvasive tools for measuring diastolic function. Diastole has three phases: passive filling, diastasis, and atrial systole (sometimes called active filling). The timing and rate of ventricular filling are related to filling pressure, diastolic function, and pericardial constraint.

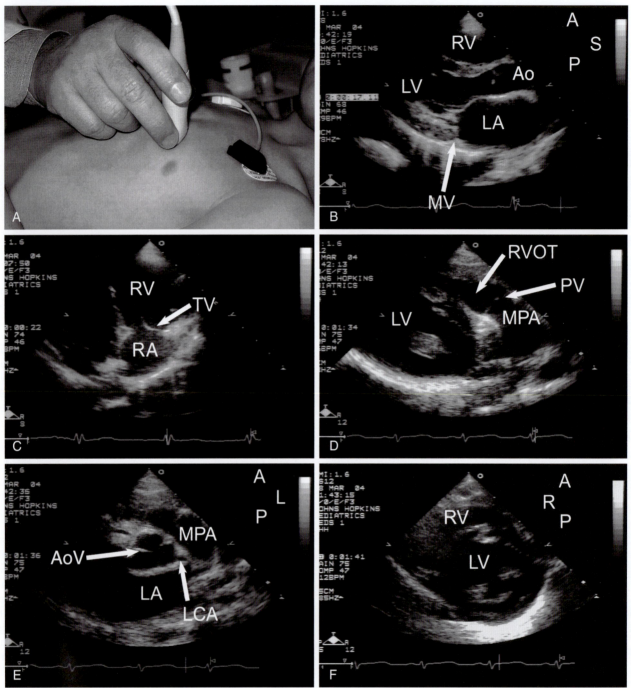

• **Figure 34.9** Parasternal imaging planes. Scans are illustrated at levels of interest. (A) Transducer position. The transducer is positioned in the second or third intercostal space in the midclavicular line. Left lung interference is often minimized by positioning the patient in the left lateral decubitus position. (B) Long-axis view at the level of the aorta. Demonstrates the left atrium and ventricle, aortic valve, mitral valve *(arrow)*, and ascending aorta. (C) Long-axis view angled to the tricuspid valve. Tricuspid valve *(arrow)* inflow, right atrium, and right ventricle are demonstrated. (D) Long-axis view angled to the left to the pulmonary valve. The right ventricular outflow tract *(arrow)*, pulmonary valve *(arrow)*, and main pulmonary artery are displayed. (E) Short-axis view at the aortic valve. The transducer is rotated to display the heart in its short axis. This view displays aortic valve *(arrow)* morphology, the proximal coronary arteries *(arrow)*, pulmonary valve, and main pulmonary artery well. (F) Short axis at ventricular level. Sweeping inferiorly from the aortic valve, a short-axis view of both ventricles is displayed. This is a standard view for assessing left ventricular function. The mitral valve is seen within the left ventricle. *A,* Anterior; *Ao,* aorta; *AoV,* aortic valve; *L,* left; *LA,* left atrium; *LCA,* left main coronary artery; *LV,* left ventricle; *MPA,* main pulmonary artery; *MV,* mitral valve; *P,* posterior; *PV,* pulmonary valve; *R,* right; *RA,* right atrium; *RV,* right ventricle; *RVOT,* right ventricular outflow tract; *S,* superior; *TV,* tricuspid valve.

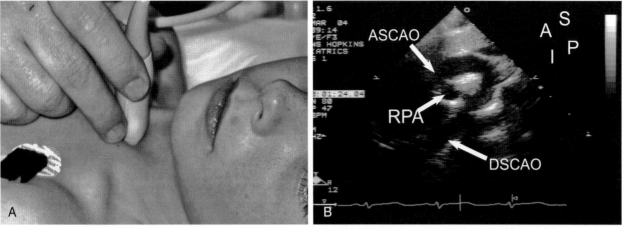

• **Figure 34.10** Suprasternal notch imaging plane. (A) Transducer position. The transducer is positioned in the suprasternal notch. (B) Aortic arch view. The aortic arch is seen in a long-axis view. The RPA is displayed posterior to the ASCAO and anterior to the DSCAO. The arch can be imaged in short axis by rotating the transducer 90 degrees. *A,* Anterior; *ASCAO,* ascending aorta; *DSCAO,* descending aorta; *I,* inferior; *P,* posterior; *RPA,* right pulmonary artery; *S,* superior.

Clinical Assessment of Systolic Function. Global systolic function is most commonly assessed in the intensive care unit using measures of ejection performance such as ejection fraction or shortening fraction. Ejection fraction is the percentage change in end-diastolic volume:

$$\frac{(\text{End-diastolic volume} - \text{end systolic volume})}{\text{end-diastolic volume}} \times 100$$

Volumes are most accurately measured using a biplane rather than single-plane method. Normative ranges for ventricular volumes are available for children[2] with normal left ventricular ejection fraction reported as 60.3% ± 6.7%.[11] Frequently apical views are used to assess ejection fraction, but it is possible to measure ejection fraction from other acoustic windows.

Often, shortening fraction is measured rather than ejection fraction. Shortening fraction, or percent change in ventricular diameter, is calculated using the following formula:

$$\frac{(\text{End-diastolic volume} - \text{end systolic volume})}{\text{end-diastolic volume}} \times 100$$

The shortening fraction is easy to measure and is a useful measure of systolic function when ventricular geometry is normal (Fig. 34.11). Normal values for shortening fraction range from approximately 29% to 41%,[10] with the higher range in neonates and younger children. When the normal left ventricular shape is altered (i.e., no longer round in the short-axis view), biplane methods such as ejection fraction provide a more accurate measure of systolic function. In addition, some studies have demonstrated considerable interobserver variability in the measurement.

As mentioned, both ejection fraction and shortening fraction are load dependent, and their interpretation must consider loading conditions. In addition, both are measures of global function. Any measure of systolic function must also consider whether there are regional wall motion abnormalities. Wall motion abnormalities in children are more commonly seen postoperatively after surgical incisions or placement of patches, with coronary artery abnormalities, or with cardiomyopathy.[12] The neonate may have systolic

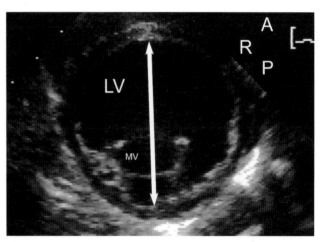

• **Figure 34.11** Motion mode (M-mode) examination of left ventricular function. Short-axis view of the left ventricle obtained in the parasternal short-axis view. The mitral valve *(MV)* is open within the left ventricle *(LV)* in this diastolic frame. The long arrow demonstrates the left ventricular endocardial dimension. By using the equivalent view in systole, the shortening fraction (or percentage change in short-axis diameter) can be calculated. This ventricle is dilated with increased dimension to wall thickness ratio. *A,* Anterior; *P,* posterior; *R,* right.

septal flattening due to normal newborn transition physiology and associated elevated pulmonary vascular resistance, making fractional shortening a less consistently reliable measure of systolic function.[13] Left ventricular strain analysis is being performed more routinely in certain populations, such as children who have received cardiotoxic chemotherapy or have genetic cardiomyopathies, as well as recovery from myocarditis. Strain is the mechanical deformation of any material. Myocardial strain imaging is a measure of left ventricular function that can be used segmentally or averaged to obtain global values for a region or the entire ventricle. For many diseases, strain imaging may be a more sensitive indicator of myocardial function than other conventional measurements such as ejection fraction. Other measures, including dP/dT and the myocardial performance index, have been described, and the interested reader is referred to other sources for more information.[14-16]

Left ventricular systolic dysfunction can be present in a wide spectrum of clinical conditions, including structurally normal hearts with genetic cardiomyopathy, myocarditis, and following cardiotoxic therapeutic agents such as chemotherapy; arrhythmias; and cardiac trauma, arrest, or sequelae of right ventricular dysfunction. Congenital heart defects can be associated with left ventricular systolic dysfunction preoperatively; common lesions with this association include, but are not limited to, the following: left ventricular obstructive lesions such as aortic valve stenosis, mitral valve disease, aortic coarctation, and anomalous coronary arteries. Postoperatively, transient left ventricular dysfunction often occurs due to effects of cardiopulmonary bypass regardless of the cardiac lesion.[17,17a]

Clinical Assessment of Diastolic Function. The assessment of diastolic function is best evaluated using atrioventricular valve inflow velocity and tissue Doppler analysis of the atrioventricular valve annular motion. The atrioventricular annulus moves away from the cardiac apex during diastole. Therefore when viewed from the apical four-chamber view, diastolic motion is away from the transducer. Similar to the E and A waves of mitral valve inflow, the atrioventricular annuli display an early diastolic (E′) and late diastolic (A′) motion. An example of normal mitral valve annular motion is displayed in Fig. 34.12, and normal tissue annular velocities are available for reference (Table 34.4). Annular motion varies significantly with age, with increasing E′ and E/E′ in the older child as compared with the infant.

There are three clinical stages of diastolic dysfunction.[18] The intensivist should be familiar with these stages. In mild diastolic dysfunction (stage 1, also called impaired relaxation), left ventricular relaxation is abnormal, but left ventricular filling pressure and compliance are still nearly normal. There is increased reliance on atrial systole to achieve left ventricular filling. Impaired relaxation is manifest by decreased early mitral inflow (E) and mitral annular velocities (E′), increased late mitral inflow (A) and mitral annular

velocities (A′), and so-called reversed E/A and E′/A′ ratios (in which these ratios are less than one).

With worsening diastolic dysfunction (stage 2, also called pseudonormalization or moderate diastolic dysfunction), left ventricular compliance is abnormal, and this results in elevated left ventricular end-diastolic pressure. Now the E/A ratio normalizes, whereas the E′/A′ ratio remains abnormal. The E/A ratio is preload dependent, whereas the E′/A′ is relatively less so.

With stage 3, or severe diastolic dysfunction (termed *restrictive pattern*), there is even worse ventricular compliance and even more elevated filling pressure. This stage is recognized by markedly elevated E and E′, and elevated E/A and E/E′ ratios. Stage 3 has been further differentiated into reversible and irreversible patterns based on the response to Valsalva maneuver. The irreversible pattern has a worse prognosis.

The E/E′ ratio is useful in estimating left ventricular end-diastolic pressure. Because E, mitral inflow velocity, is preload dependent, and E′, mitral annular velocity, is not preload dependent, the ratio increases with increased filling pressure. In an adult population[18]:

$$PCWP = 1.24 \, E/E' + 1.9 \text{ mm Hg}$$

where *PCWP* represents pulmonary capillary wedge pressure or left ventricular end-diastolic pressure. Tissue Doppler of mitral valve annular motion is increasingly being reported to detect diastolic dysfunction even in early or subclinical disease states.[19-23]

Assessment of Right Ventricular Systolic Function

The most common assessment of right ventricular systolic function is qualitative, typically using descriptors of mild, moderate, or severely depressed. Quantification of right ventricular systolic function is challenging due to the tripartite geometry of the normal right ventricle. Several methods exist to assess right ventricular function, but their use widely varies between centers. Tricuspid Annular Planar Systolic Excursion (TAPSE) is perhaps the most widely used, and normal values exist for children.[24,25] This method measures the longitudinal displacement of the tricuspid valve annulus in systole, recognizing that the right ventricular fiber orientation is more longitudinal than that of the left ventricle. Limitations of this method include load dependency; dependence on angle (and orientation of the heart within the chest); focus on only a small part of the right ventricular myocardium, specifically the basal lateral wall; and being affected by overall heart motion. Right ventricular shortening fraction is another method for assessment of right ventricular systolic function but is dependent on loading conditions, and there are currently no reference values for

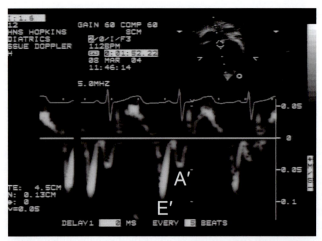

• **Figure 34.12** Pulsed tissue Doppler analysis of mitral annular motion in a healthy infant. Flow is below the baseline because the mitral valve annulus moves away from the transducer in this apical view. The early diastolic velocity (*E′*) is larger (9 cm/s) than the velocity during atrial systole (*A′* = 4 cm/s). Note that the motion of the mitral valve annulus is in the opposite direction to mitral valve inflow (flow is toward the apex during diastole).

TABLE 34.4	Mitral and Tricuspid Annular Tissue Doppler in Healthy Children		
	E′	A′	E/E′
Lateral mitral	16.0-17.1	6.2-6.6	5.9-6.4
Medial mitral	12.2-13.0	5.9-6.3	7.5-8.0
Tricuspid	15.6-16.7	9.9-10.5	3.6-4.0

From Eidem BW, McMahon CJ, Cohen RR, et al. Impact of cardiac growth on Doppler tissue imaging velocities: a study in healthy children. *J Am Soc Echocardiogr*. 2004;17:212-221.

right ventricular shortening fraction in children. Pulmonary artery acceleration time is a relatively new method proposed for right ventricular functional assessment, which inversely correlates with right heart catheterization based pulmonary hemodynamics, specifically mean pulmonary artery pressure and pulmonary vascular resistance. This method is also load dependent and heart rate dependent, and normative values for newborns are still being established.

Two other methods of right ventricular systolic function assessment include speckle tracking and right ventricular Tei index. Unfortunately, right ventricular Tei has not been found to be helpful in assessing right ventricular function during the newborn transition period.

General Applications of Echocardiography in the Intensive Care Unit

Gradient Assessment/Pressure Estimation

For congenital heart disease, as well as structurally normal hearts, echocardiography is routinely used to assess valve gradients and stenoses. As previously discussed, Doppler echocardiography is used to calculate the maximum instantaneous gradient and mean gradient across all cardiac valves (see Fig. 34.3). Doppler assessment does not measure pressures directly; peak velocity of blood is measured, which is converted to a pressure gradient using the modified Bernoulli equation. It is important to know that this Doppler-derived measurement is different from the peak-to-peak gradient typically measured in the catheterization laboratory. Peak velocity will be affected by cardiac function and other clinical factors such as loading conditions, anemia, and intrathoracic pressure. There is a good but imperfect correlation between the Doppler-derived maximum instantaneous gradient and the catheterization-derived peak-to-peak gradient.[26] Doppler mean gradient correlates well with catheter mean gradient across a broad range of gradients. One of the most important explanations for the differences between Doppler- and catheterization-derived maximum instantaneous gradients is related to pressure recovery. Immediately after a stenotic lesion, energy is converted back to pressure from kinetic energy. In the case of aortic stenosis the pressure in the ascending aorta is therefore higher compared with just distal to the stenotic leaflets. The catheter measurement of ascending aortic pressure is likely at the point where pressure recovery has occurred. Some have attempted to account for pressure recovery by correcting the Doppler-derived maximum instantaneous gradient to result in a better predictor of the catheter-based peak-to-peak gradient.[18,27,28]

Determination of Pulmonary Artery Pressure

In many situations in the intensive care unit, determination of pulmonary artery pressure is important. Echocardiography and Doppler provide several qualitative and quantitative measures of pulmonary artery pressure, which are detailed in Chapter 71. Briefly, the most common method for right ventricular pressure determination is tricuspid regurgitation velocity, using the modified Bernoulli equation. This estimates the pressure gradient between the right ventricle and the right atrium, and the right ventricular pressure can be determined by adding the right atrial pressure to this calculated gradient (Fig. 34.13). Many times patients in the intensive care unit have central venous catheters that afford the ability to

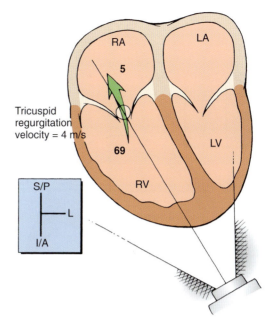

• **Figure 34.13** Estimation of right ventricular pressure from the velocity of tricuspid regurgitation. The velocity of tricuspid regurgitation is 4 m/s. Using the Bernoulli equation, one can calculate that the pressure gradient between right atrium and right ventricle is 64 mm Hg. Adding this gradient to the right atrial pressure, one can estimate right ventricular pressure. Estimated right ventricular pressure is 69 mm Hg. *I/A,* Inferior-anterior; *L,* left; *LA,* left atrium; *LV,* left ventricle; *RA,* right atrium; *RV,* right ventricle; *S/P,* superior-posterior.

get a "real-time" right atrial pressure estimate. In the absence of pulmonary stenosis the right ventricular systolic pressure estimate will equal the pulmonary artery systolic pressure. If there is a ventricular septal defect (Fig. 34.14) or a patent ductus arteriosus shunt (Fig. 34.15), the right ventricular pressure can be calculated using the systolic blood pressure and subtracting the gradient of the relevant shunt. Methods commonly used to quantify right heart pressure and right heart function by echocardiography are detailed in the chapter on pulmonary hypertension.[29]

Echocardiographic Indicators of Tamponade Physiology

Two-dimensional imaging is excellent for the visualization of pericardial effusion. The amount of fluid and its distribution should be imaged from multiple imaging windows and planes. One should determine if the effusion is loculated or not and whether it is circumferential or not. Noncircumferential effusions are generally small.

There are several echocardiographic signs of pericardial tamponade. When the pericardial pressure exceeds right atrial pressure, there will be a diastolic collapse of the right atrial free wall (Video 34.1A). One may see a similar finding for the right ventricular free wall. There are also changes in the Doppler inflow patterns of the atrial ventricular valves with pericardial tamponade. A sensitive finding is more than a 25% variation in peak inflow velocity during inspiration versus expiration. With increasing degrees of tamponade, there will be more variability in inflow velocity with the respiratory cycle. Pericardial effusions can occur in a variety of clinical scenarios in critically ill children.

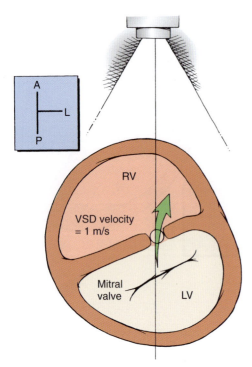

• **Figure 34.14** Estimation of right ventricular pressure in patient with large ventricular septal defect. Note in this systolic frame that the ventricular septum is flat (or neutral) in position without curvature into either ventricle. This occurs when right ventricular pressure is at least one-half left ventricular pressure. One can derive a quantitative measure of right ventricular pressure by measuring the velocity of the ventricular septal defect gradient using Doppler and then calculating the pressure difference between right and left ventricles. In this case estimated RV pressure is systemic in the absence of any significant gradient between the ventricles. *A,* Anterior; *L,* left; *LV,* left ventricle; *P,* posterior; *RV,* right ventricle; *VSD,* ventricular septal defect.

The size of the pericardial effusion is important but not always a reliable predictor of tamponade physiology. The rate of fluid accumulation can also influence when tamponade occurs. Two-dimensional motion mode (M-mode) and pulsed wave Doppler findings of tamponade have been described and are listed in Table 34.5. Of note, the echocardiographic findings associated with cardiac tamponade listed in Table 34.5 may not be applicable in the setting of single-ventricle physiology, large atrial septal defects, or severe respiratory distress, which can affect respiratory variation.

Echocardiographic Guidance of Procedures in the Intensive Care Unit

Pericardiocentesis

Once diagnosis of clinically important pericardial effusion has been made (reviewed earlier), pericardiocentesis can be performed under echocardiographic guidance at the bedside in the intensive care unit, obviating the transfer of the patient to the catheterization laboratory. Generally pericardiocentesis is performed from a subcostal or, less commonly, an apical approach. Before the procedure, images are obtained to measure the distance from the needle entry site to the proximal edge of pericardial fluid. One also measures the rim of pericardial fluid. In general, fluid

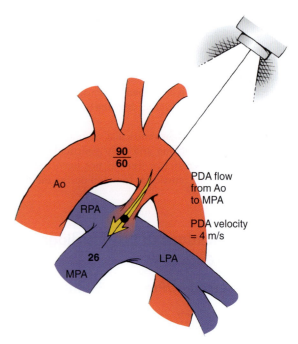

• **Figure 34.15** Estimation of pulmonary artery pressure from the velocity across the ductus arteriosus. The velocity across the ductus is 4 m/s. Therefore the pressure gradient is 64 mm Hg. The pulmonary artery pressure is therefore 64 mm Hg less than the systolic aortic pressure of 90 mm Hg. Estimated pulmonary artery pressure (26 mm Hg) is therefore normal. *Ao,* Aorta; *LPA,* left pulmonary artery; *MPA,* main pulmonary artery; *PDA,* patent ductus arteriosus; *RPA,* right pulmonary artery.

collections with rims less than 5 mm in dimension are difficult to tap, whereas those greater than 10 mm are generally relatively easy to drain. One can anticipate the appropriate angle of entry for the needle by considering the angle of the transducer at the appropriate plane (Fig. 34.16). This can be visualized online in Video 34.1B (subcostal imaging of pericardial imaging with injection of agitated saline contrast to ensure needle placement in the pericardial space) and Video 34.1C (subcostal image showing wire in good position inferior to the heart, entering the pericardial sac from the patient's left side). The transducer may need to be repositioned or temporarily removed depending on the interventionalist's approach, but imaging is typically resumed once fluid has been removed to confirm resolution of pericardial effusion and ventricular function.

Balloon Atrial Septostomy

In transposition of the great arteries, balloon atrial septostomy can increase the oxygen saturation by allowing for greater intracardiac mixing. This potentially lifesaving procedure, first described by William Rashkind, was initially performed under fluoroscopy.[29] Several studies have shown that the procedure can be performed safely and with equal efficacy in the intensive care unit under echocardiographic guidance, thereby avoiding patient transfer to the catheterization laboratory.

Imaging during the procedure is possible from either the apical or low parasternal acoustic windows. This allows the cardiologist performing the septostomy to work from either the umbilicus or the femoral vein without interference by the echocardiographer. Alternatively, balloon atrial septostomy can be performed under transesophageal echocardiographic guidance.

TABLE 34.5 Echocardiographic Findings Associated With Cardiac Tamponade

2D Findings	M-Mode Findings	Pulsed Wave Doppler Findings in Cardiac Tamponade
Pericardial effusion	Pericardial effusion	Marked respiratory variation of tricuspid and mitral peak velocities (increase with inspiration, decrease with expiration, >25%)
Presystolic collapse of the right atrium	Right ventricular compression (RVID <7 mm)	Marked respiratory variation of pulmonic and aortic peak velocities (increase with inspiration, decrease with expiration, >25%)
Right ventricular diastolic collapse in early diastole	Delayed mitral valve opening with inspiration	Marked respiratory variation of pulmonary vein peak velocities and velocity time integrals
Left atria diastolic collapse in late diastole and/or early systole	Decreased aortic valve opening with inspiration	Limitation of right heart filling by hepatic venous Doppler
Left ventricular diastolic collapse	Decreased LV ejection time with inspiration	
Dilated inferior vena cava with lack of collapse with inspiration		

2D, Two dimensional; *LV*, left ventricular; *M-mode*, motion mode; *RVID*, right ventricular internal dimension.
Modified from Anderson J, Kocis KC. Echocardiographic evaluation of pericardial effusions and cardiac tamponade in children. *Pediatric Ultrasound Today.* 11(8):137-152, 2006.

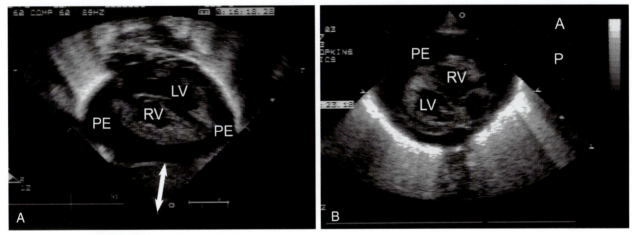

• **Figure 34.16** Pericardiocentesis performed under echocardiographic guidance. (A) Subcostal image before pericardiocentesis. In this premature infant with a large pericardial effusion the rim of fluid inferiorly measures 4 to 5 mm, and the distance from the skin to the anterior-inferior rim of fluid is 11 to 12 mm. Though this is a large pericardial effusion and the neonate was symptomatic, it was a complicated tap due to the tiny patient size. (B) Parasternal image before procedure. The effusion is nearly circumferential. *A,* Anterior; *LV,* left ventricle; *P,* posterior; *PE,* pericardial effusion; *RV,* right ventricle.

Images from a balloon atrial septostomy are illustrated in Fig. 34.17. As the catheter enters the right atrium, the echocardiographer may be able to help guide the positioning of the catheter in the left atrium. The catheter should be positioned well into the left atrium but not with the tip so far as to be in the left atrial appendage or touching the lateral wall. If the catheter is positioned too far within the left atrium, balloon inflation could tear the atrial wall. As the balloon is inflated, it should be noted to be free within the left atrium before the septostomy pull is performed. If the balloon is not free or is overinflated, atrial wall avulsion can occur with the pull. (Video 34.2 is a clip of appropriate echocardiographic guidance during a successful balloon atrial septostomy.) After the septostomy is performed, but before the catheter is removed, the echocardiographer should determine that the defect created is adequate (generally at least 4 mm) and that the defect margins

are clear. (Video 34.3 is a subcostal clip demonstrating an adequate postseptostomy atrial septal defect with red flow indicating left-to-right shunting across the newly created atrial septal defect.) Once the procedure is completed, the heart should be scanned to exclude any iatrogenic damage to the mitral valve, the tricuspid valve, or the inferior vena cava (IVC). Pericardial effusion should be excluded.

Assessment of Central Line Placement

When chest radiograph cannot adequately demonstrate the position of intravascular catheters, ultrasonography is quite good at doing so. One can also assess the presence of thrombus or vegetation on the line, but when a mass is identified, it may not be possible to distinguish one from the other echocardiographically. In some cases a line may dislodge and be in the pericardial or pleural

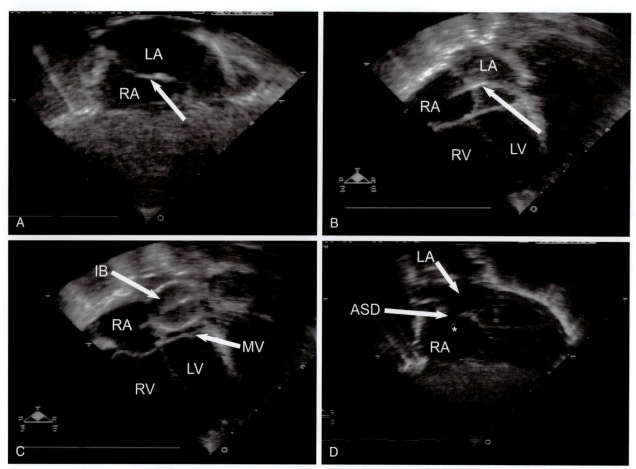

• **Figure 34.17** Echocardiographic visualization for balloon atrial septostomy. (A) Before septostomy. Subxiphoid view before patient is prepared and draped showing intact atrial septum. (B) Catheter across into the left atrium, balloon not yet inflated. Note that the catheter tip extends to the left atrial wall. Before balloon inflation the catheter should be pulled back so that the balloon is inflated within the left atrium and not within the left atrial appendage. (C) Balloon inflated within the left atrium. The balloon should not cross the mitral valve and be free within the left atrium before the septostomy is performed. If the balloon is overinflated and not free, it is possible to avulse the left atrial wall during septostomy. (D) Atrial septal defect after septostomy. Note the torn edges of the atrial septum. An adequate septostomy should create a defect with clear margins that is at least 4 mm in diameter. *ASD,* Atrial septal defect; *IB,* inflated balloon; *LA,* left atrium; *LV,* left ventricle; *MV,* mitral valve; *RA,* right atrium; *RV,* right ventricle.

space. When such a question arises, injection of a small amount of saline through the catheter, resulting in a contrast injection, is quite useful in demonstrating the position of the catheter. If contrast is seen in the pericardial space, then the catheter must have some communication with that cavity. Correspondingly, if contrast is seen in the pleural space, the catheter has extravasated into the chest.

Echocardiography and Extracorporeal Membrane Oxygenation

Extracorporeal membrane oxygenation (ECMO) is a form of mechanical cardiorespiratory support based on a modified cardiopulmonary bypass circuit. As discussed in Chapter 39, the use of ECMO has grown over the past two decades.

There are two major types of ECMO circuits, venoarterial (VA) and venovenous (VV). The indications for each type of ECMO circuit are also discussed in Chapter 39, but in brief, VA ECMO is used when there is cardiac dysfunction and/or cardiac and pulmonary dysfunction. VV ECMO is used when there is pulmonary dysfunction with preserved cardiac function. VA ECMO is more commonly used than VV ECMO. In VA ECMO there is a large-bore venous drainage cannula placed in the right atrium and an arterial reperfusion cannula placed in the aorta. In neonates and children the most common approach is to place the venous cannula via the right superior vena cava (SVC) into the right atrium and to place the arterial cannula in the right carotid artery into the aortic arch. Children going onto ECMO following open-heart surgery may also have direct cannulation of the right atrium and the ascending aorta from the front of the chest. Older children may also have cannulation via the femoral vessel, or a combination, such as with a right SVC venous cannula and femoral arterial cannula or any other combination of available arterial and venous vessels. VV ECMO is done by a single cannula that has both drainage and reperfusion portions placed in the right atrium. The VV cannula is designed for an SVC approach. Echocardiography for ECMO can be thought of in parts as follows: (1) the pre-ECMO

TABLE 34.6	Echocardiographic Evaluation on Extracorporeal Membrane Oxygenation
Pre-ECMO evaluation	Cannula placement evaluation • Continuous evaluation for VV ECMO, cannula placement and direction of outflow jet to tricuspid valve, ventricular function Immediately after cannula placement for VA ECMO, cannula position Valve abnormalities Intracardiac shunts: level, direction, and amount of shunt Left atrial and ventricular unloading Pericardial effusion/bleeding
Assessment while on VAD support	Biventricular size and function Left atrial and left ventricular size Valve abnormalities, aortic valve opening Cannula position Intracardiac thrombi Pericardial effusion/bleeding
Assessment during ECMO weaning	Ventricular size and function Right ventricle pressure New valve abnormalities Pericardial effusion/bleeding

ECMO, Extracorporeal membrane oxygenation; *VA,* venoarterial; *VAD,* ventricular assist device; *VV,* venovenous.

assessment, (2) echocardiography around the time of cannula placement, (3) surveillance on ECMO, and (4) weaning off the ECMO circuit. Table 34.6 summarizes the pertinent echocardiographic variables for each specific clinical time period.

Echocardiography Before Extracorporeal Membrane Oxygenation Placement

Whenever possible, detailed assessment of the cardiac anatomy and function by echocardiography is imperative before ECMO placement. A critical initial decision is whether to use VA or VV ECMO. If there is significant cardiac dysfunction (of either or both ventricles), then VA ECMO should be used. Detailed assessment should be done for both the right and left ventricular function. If this is the initial echocardiogram, careful evaluation of structural abnormalities that may account for the clinical picture (cyanosis or respiratory distress) should be excluded. Given the routes of cannulation, special care must also be taken to assess the systemic venous and aortic arch anatomy. Normal variants, such as a left superior vena cava (LSVC), to coronary sinus can adversely affect ECMO cannulation because the right superior vena cava is often smaller in patients with LSVC. Right aortic arch with mirror image branching or other aortic arch variants have similar concerns for the size of the right common carotid/innominate artery. Special care should be taken to look for all potential intracardiac shunts, including PFO, because these may be necessary to prevent left atrial hypertension and pulmonary edema. Unlike cardiopulmonary bypass or ventricular assist devices (VADs) (see later), VA ECMO circuits cannot typically provide complete bypass of the venous return; thus an atrial level shunt may be critical to allow the left atrium to decompress so that lungs do not become severely congested. For VA ECMO, detailed assessment of the aortic and mitral

valves is also very important. If there is greater than mild (or moderate plus) aortic valve regurgitation, the aortic reperfusion flow may go retrograde into the LV rather than providing adequate systemic perfusion. Mitral stenosis or regurgitation may lead to left atrial hypertension and poor pulmonary venous drainage. Pre-ECMO echocardiography may also show a reversible cause of cardiac distress such as unrecognized pericardial effusion with tamponade, for which the treatment would be pericardiocentesis rather than ECMO.

Echocardiography During Extracorporeal Membrane Oxygenation Cannulation

For patients going on VV ECMO, continuous echocardiography during the procedure is used as part of the cannula placement. Echocardiography is used to verify that the VV cannula outflow jet is directed toward the tricuspid valve and that the cannula is in good position within the right atrium (Video 34.4). The intraoperative echocardiogram should also assess for any changes in ventricular function that would require conversion to VA ECMO. The echocardiogram during cannula placement is usually done as a transthoracic study; it can be done as a transesophageal echocardiogram if the transthoracic images are inadequate.

The timing of echocardiography with VA ECMO cannulation varies in different centers. Some centers will use echocardiography to assess cannula placement before suturing cannulas in place, whereas other centers will use chest x-ray examination for initial cannula assessment and the echocardiography once the cannulas are sutured in place. Studies by Kuenzler and Thomas have shown that echocardiography is superior to chest x-ray examination for assessing cannula position.[30]

For neck cannulation the arterial cannula should be in the right innominate artery, with the tip of the cannula just extending into the aortic arch (Video 34.5). If the aortic cannula is in too far, it can extend down the ascending aorta and be on or very near the aortic valve, potentially limiting aortic valve excursion and even causing aortic insufficiency. The aortic cannula tip can also be inadvertently placed into the underside of the aortic arch, which would cause very high postcannulation pressures and damage the aortic arch. More rarely, the cannula will extend down the descending aorta, which may decrease the effective ECMO flow to the coronary arteries. An aortic cannula that is too high can be difficult to image. Using color flow Doppler to identify the outflow jet can be helpful. The venous cannula should be in the right atrium with the tip near the IVC/right atrial junction (Video 34.6A, two-dimensional image from right sternal border showing cannula in SVC with tip toward IVC/right atrium junction; Video 34.6B, color Doppler showing flow going into the SVC venous cannula). If the cannula is too high, it may not drain well because the side holes may abut against the wall of the SVC. If the cannula is in too far, it may damage the IVC or not drain well for the same reason as the cannula being too high (the side holes may be against the walls of the IVC).

Echocardiography on Extracorporeal Membrane Oxygenation

Patients on ECMO are inherently critically ill and need careful monitoring. Echocardiograms on ECMO should assess for changes in ventricular function and the right ventricular pressure.[31] Careful examination should be done for pericardial effusion/bleeding and also for any intracardiac thrombi. The cannula position can change, and the cannula should be reimaged whenever there is concern with the ECMO circuit flow and if there is a change in position on chest x-ray examination. Repeat assessment of the left atrial size, the mitral valve function, and the aortic valve function are also important components of echocardiography while on ECMO. If there is progressive left atrial dilation and no interatrial shunt, then the patient may need an atrial septostomy or a left atrial vent placed. The ventricular function may also decreased immediately after going onto ECMO (ventricular stunning). This transient worsening of ventricular function should improve within 24 to 48 hours. If the function does not improve, then the ventricular dysfunction is more likely secondary to the underlying pathology that initially required ECMO placement.

Echocardiography During Weaning of Support

ECMO is most commonly used as a bridge to recovery or definitive surgical procedure, such as in congenital diaphragmatic hernia. When the patient has recovered, echocardiography is used during weaning off ECMO. During an ECMO clamp trial, continuous echocardiographic assessment is done as the ECMO circuit flows are decreased and eventually the circuit is clamped. Echo assessment during the trials should include ventricular function, right ventricular pressure (if possible), and any new valve dysfunction. In patients who are on ECMO for cardiac support, echocardiography provides supportive data to determine the success or failure of the trial.

Echocardiography and Ventricular Assist Devices

In addition to ECMO, there has been a rapid increase in the use of VADs and other types of mechanical circulatory support in pediatric patients. As detailed in Chapter 40, VADs can be used for left ventricular support (left ventricular assist device [LVAD]), right ventricular support (right ventricular assist device [RVAD]), for both ventricles (biventricular assist device [BiVAD]), and also in univentricular hearts. Depending on the patient's size and the expected length of support, VADs can be extracorporeal (pump portion of the VAD outside of the body) or intracorporeal. Extracorporeal VADs for smaller pediatric patients include the Berlin heart, which is a pulsatile flow device, and the PediMag, a continuous flow device. The Berlin Heart is a durable, long-term device, and the PediMag is designed for short-term use. Intracorporeal VADs used in pediatric patients include the HeartWare and the HeartMate II. These are both continuous flow device, although the HeartWare is a rotational pump device and the HeartMate II uses an axial flow pump. Some patients may have both an intracorporeal LVAD and an extracorporeal RVAD if it is thought that the left ventricle will need long-term support and the right ventricle shorter-term help around the time of placement of the VADs. VADs in pediatric patients are used most commonly as a bridge to transplant and less commonly as a bridge to recovery. Other forms of mechanical circulatory support include the intraaortic balloon pump, Impella, and total artificial heart/SynCardia, but they are not commonly used in children.

All of the LVAD devices share a similar arrangement in that there is a large inflow cannula at the apex of the left ventricle that drains the blood out of the heart (Fig. 34.18, Video 7) and an outflow cannula in the ascending aorta. The extracorporeal pumps are placed on the patient's abdomen (Berlin Heart) or the bedside (PediMag). The HeartMate II has a longer inflow cannula, and

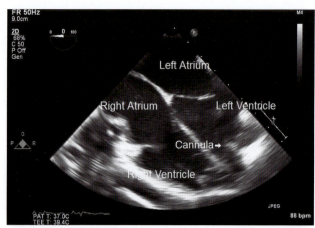

• **Figure 34.18** Apical four-chamber view of a heart being supported by a ventricular assist device (VAD). VAD cannula is in the left ventricular apex.

the pump is placed below the diaphragm, whereas the HeartWare has a very short outflow cannula, and the pump is placed on the ventricular apex above the diaphragm. For RVADs the inflow cannula is in the right atrium, and the outflow cannula is in the main pulmonary artery. (Of note, cannulas are named for the direction of blood flow relative to the VAD and not to the patient.) Because of this similar arrangement, echocardiographic assessment of patients before, during, and after VADs is almost identical for all of the different devices. The American Society of Echocardiography has published guidelines for assessment of adult patients' pre-VAD placement. There are no established protocols for VAD assessment in pediatric patients. Sachdeva et al. have published their single-center support approach to VAD imaging,[32] although all of their patients were using Berlin Hearts.

Echocardiography Before Ventricular Assist Device Placement

Detailed assessment of the cardiac anatomy by echocardiography is imperative before VAD placement (Table 34.7). In addition to looking for major structural anomalies, the clinician should take special care to look for all potential intracardiac shunts, including small PFOs because these should be closed at the time of LVAD placement. This is in contrast to a single-ventricle heart, in which the atrial septal defect needs to be widely patent with unobstructed flow. Detailed examination of the aortic and mitral valves is also very important in the most recent pre-VAD echocardiogram, especially for aortic regurgitation and mitral valve disease. If there is more than mild aortic regurgitation, the aortic valve may need to be "plastied" or closed completely at the time of VAD placement to prevent a circular shunt of VAD outflow into the ascending aorta retrograde flow across the aortic valve back into the VAD without adequate systemic flow. Mitral valve stenosis can affect VAD filling. For patients needing an RVAD or BIVAD, similar detailed examination of the pulmonary and tricuspid valves is needed. For smaller patients undergoing a HeartMate or HeartWare the distance from the LV apical endocardium to the mitral valve annulus should also be measured in the apical four-chamber view to see if the left ventricle is large enough to accommodate the inflow cannula.

Detailed assessment of right ventricular function is critical before LVAD implantation. The left ventricle is dependent on right ventricular function for pulmonary blood flow and left heart filling.

TABLE 34.7	Echocardiographic Evaluation for Ventricular Assist Devices
Pre-VAD evaluation	Cardiac anatomy Intracardiac shunts (PFO, ASD, VSD) • Level, direction, degree of shunt Valve abnormalities (leaflet appearance and coaptation, degree of regurgitation and/or stenosis, annular dilation) Chamber size and function • Measure distance from LV apex to mitral valve Intracardiac thrombus or spontaneous contrast Assessment of the ascending aorta
Intraoperative evaluation	RV size and function (if LVAD alone) Valve abnormalities Intracardiac shunts, level, direction, degree Left ventricular unloading Inflow and outflow cannula position and Doppler • LV inflow cannula in LV apex • Parallel to septum and aligned with mitral inflow • Unidirectional flow from LV into the cannula Outflow cannula in the ascending aorta Left ventricular decompression Repeat assessment of valve abnormalities
Assessment while on VAD support	Biventricular size and function Septal position New valve abnormalities Inflow cannula position and inflow Doppler Intracardiac thrombi Pericardial effusion and hematoma

ASD, Atrial septal defect; *LV*, left ventricular; *LVAD*, left ventricular assist device; *PFO*, patent foramen ovale; *RV*, right ventricular; *VAD*, ventricular assist device; *VSD*, ventricular septal defect.

If there is moderate to severe right ventricular dysfunction, the operative plan may need to be for a BiVAD or TandemHeart.

Transesophageal Echocardiography During Ventricular Assist Device Placement

Detailed analysis of the components listed earlier, including right ventricular function, intracardiac shunts, and aortic and mitral valve function, should be done on the prebypass portion of the transesophageal echocardiogram. Following placement and initiation of the pump, postimplantation transesophageal echocardiography should assess for the alignment of the VAD inflow cannula to the interventricular septum. The inflow cannula should parallel the septum. If the alignment is angled toward the septum, VAD inflow may be partially blocked. Similarly, if the alignment is too lateral, then the opening of the inflow cannula flow can be impinged by the lateral wall of the ventricle. This is often best seen in the midesophageal four-chamber view and the long-axis views.

Echocardiography After Placement of Ventricular Assist Device

Echocardiogram following VAD placement should include detailed analysis of the following: right ventricular function (for LVAD alone), biventricular size and function, position of the inflow cannula, and obstruction to flow into the inflow cannula.[33] There should be unidirectional, constant flow in the continuous flow devices and somewhat more pulsatile flow in the Berlin Heart. (Video 34.7 is an apical four-chamber clip showing an LVAD cannula entering the heart from the right of the screen with the tip in the left ventricular apex; Video 34.8 is an apical four-chamber view showing flow by color Doppler across the mitral valve into the LVAD apical cannula.) Any valve abnormalities, especially increasing aortic/semilunar valve regurgitation, should be critically assessed.

Thorough evaluation for intracardiac thrombus should be performed. Potential causes of decreased VAD filling include thrombus formation on the inflow cannula. Another potential cause is right ventricular dysfunction or pulmonary hypertension such that the septum shifts more leftward and over the VAD inflow. Repeat assessment of aortic valve opening and regurgitation should occur on follow-up studies. All studies should check for pericardial effusion and extracardiac hematoma. If the acoustic windows allow, examine the ascending aorta for thrombus or dissection. Special consideration should be given to the septal position and aortic valve opening. During adjustment of VAD flow rates the septum should be in neutral position. Shift of the interventricular septum leftward with increased VAD flow rates may be a sign of excessive VAD flow or inadequate filling of the left ventricle. Shifting of the septum rightward with decreased VAD flow rates can be a sign of inadequate VAD output and distention of the left ventricle.

Transesophageal and Intraoperative Echocardiography

Transesophageal probes are available for patients as small as 2 to 2.5 kg. Though single-plane probes exist, most imaging today is performed with multiplane probes and less commonly biplane probes. Single-plane imaging is inadequate for assessing outflow tract pathology. Multiplane imaging when possible is likely to improve imaging over biplane imaging but may not be possible in some smaller patients.

Besides the electronic control of the imaging plane, the operator can mechanically flex or extend the probe tip and shift the probe from right to left. The mechanical steering allows the operator to achieve nearly any plane desired. Occasionally contact with the esophagus or stomach is poor, or image quality is obscured by adjacent nasogastric tubes.

Indications

The most frequent indication for transesophageal echocardiography is in the operating room or in the perioperative period. The transesophageal approach does not compromise the operative field, and images are not obscured by chest tubes and dressings as with transthoracic imaging. Transesophageal echocardiography is also sometimes helpful in the outpatient setting in larger children or young adults in whom acoustic windows are limited. However, magnetic resonance imaging is frequently used as an alternative modality for this group of patients. Finally, transesophageal echocardiography is useful in the guidance of interventional catheterization procedures, such as the closure of atrial septal defect, or in the assistance of balloon atrial septostomy. There is also increasing experience with intracardiac probes as an alternative technique for guiding interventional procedures.

Summary

Echocardiography is an essential tool that is extensively used in the PCICU. Echocardiography can provide diagnostic information, guide clinical management, and assist in procedures. The PCICU clinicians should have a working knowledge of echocardiography because this tool should be a component of every patient's care.

Selected References

A complete list of references is available at ExpertConsult.com.

10. Brangenberg R, Burger A, Romer U, et al. Echocardiographic assessment of left ventricular size and function in normal children from infancy to adolescence: Acoustic quantification in comparison with traditional echocardiographic techniques. *Pediatr Cardiol.* 2002;23:394–402.

13. Colan SD, Borow KM, Neumann A. Use of the calibrated carotid pulse tracing for calculation of left ventricular pressure and wall stress throughout ejection. *Am Heart J.* 1985;109:1306–1310.

20. Eidem BW, McMahon CJ, Cohen RR, et al. Impact of cardiac growth on Doppler tissue imaging velocities: A study in healthy children. *J Am Soc Echocardiogr.* 2004;17:212–221.

29. Broderick-Forsgren K, Davenport CA, Sivak JA, et al. Improving on the diagnostic characteristics of echocardiography for pulmonary hypertension. *Int J Cardiovasc Imaging.* 2017;33(9):1341–1349.

31. Koth AM, Axelrod DM, Reddy S, et al. Institution of Veno-arterial Extracorporeal Membrane Oxygenation Does Not Lead to Increased Wall Stress in Patients with Impaired Myocardial Function. *Pediatr Cardiol.* 2017;38(3):539–546.

33. Iacobelli R, Di Molfetta A, Brancaccio G, et al. Acute and Long-Term Effects of Left Ventricular Assist Device Support on Right Ventricular Function in Children with Pediatric Pulsatile Ventricular Assist Devices. *ASAIO J.* 2017 May 12.

35

Bedside Ultrasonography in the Pediatric Intensive Care Unit

RENÉE WILLETT, MD; BECKY RIGGS, MD; ERIK SU, MD

With improving image quality and increasingly available portable machines, bedside ultrasonography has become central to the provision of high quality pediatric critical care. Bedside ultrasonography has been used for a number of years in the adult intensive care unit (ICU) and has become more common in pediatric ICUs (PICUs) for a variety of procedures. Ultrasonographically guided procedures, such as paracentesis and placement of arterial lines, have been shown to have lower complication rates and higher success rates.[1,2] Recently bedside ultrasonography has become increasingly widespread as a diagnostic tool that can be used emergently in the PICU. Bedside ultrasonography helps intensivists to make timely decisions without exposing children to radiation. Bedside ultrasonography also permits serial examinations, which are useful in the PICU, where a child's clinical status may be quickly evolving. With increasing exposure to bedside ultrasonography for a variety of different procedures and monitoring techniques, intensivists in the cardiac PICU can expand the use of this exceptionally valuable tool for patient management.

A spectrum of machines is available to the pediatric intensivist in the cardiac PICU. Full diagnostic platforms may have a variety of phased array transducers, transesophageal echocardiography capabilities, or advanced postprocessing features. In contrast, ultraportable handheld machines may be rapidly mobilized for emergencies even in confined spaces (Fig. 35.1). Each machine class possesses inherent benefits and limitations for PICU workflow, and decisions on which type to deploy in a PICU depend upon the anticipated clinical needs of the patient. For the applications described in this chapter the authors recommend an ultrasonography machine capable of good two-dimensional imaging with color Doppler and M-mode imaging capabilities. Recommended transducers include a pediatric phased array transducer primarily for diagnostic applications and a linear array transducer for procedural applications. Though the phased array transducer is best suited to cardiac imaging because of its sector-shaped imaging field, low frequency for deep structure imaging, and excellent temporal resolution of moving structures, alternatives may include curvilinear or microconvex transducers or a linear array probe with a trapezoid imaging feature to provide a wide field of view of deep structures (Fig. 35.2). The authors also recommend having multiple linear array transducers of different sizes to accommodate different procedural applications. A linear array that operates at frequencies toward 15 MHz and greater generates higher-resolution images of shallow structures for peripheral venous access in small children. A lower-frequency linear transducer capable of reaching 7 MHz

or lower may be used for imaging a deep femoral vessel in an adolescent with obesity or contractures.

Vascular Access

Obtaining central or peripheral access is a common procedure in any pediatric cardiac ICU. Although these procedures are performed daily, complications from failed attempts and delays in care remain a concern. Given the increasing availability of ultrasonography, many intensivists now obtain vascular access under ultrasonographic guidance, which decreases the rate of failure and complications in both pediatric and adult patients.[3,4] It is unclear how many intensivists use ultrasonography for vascular procedures in pediatrics, but in the adult population, estimates range from 28% to 73% depending on site.[5] Intensivists cite several barriers to more frequent use of ultrasonography, such as limited availability of the ultrasonography machine, perceived increased time required for the procedure, and concern that they will lose the skills required to place lines using only anatomic landmarks.[5]

Ultrasonography allows for direct visualization and facilitates the clinician's understanding of patient anatomy and physiology. With advances in image quality, arteries and veins are often distinct in appearance, even on portable ultrasonography. The walls of the artery appear thicker due to the muscular tunica media. The vessel resists compression and may pulsate. In contrast, the vein has a thinner wall and is easily compressible. In some clinical scenarios the vein may pulsate when the vessel runs in close proximity to an artery or in the setting of significant pulmonary hypertension. Compressibility is typically the most specific means of identifying the vein; however, if distinguishing the vessels remains difficult, the intensivist may use Doppler ultrasonography to determine the flow. Color Doppler information should be interpreted in context with other findings because inappropriate gain, scale, frequency, or other settings may affect the intensivist's ability to detect flow. It is important to remember that typically blue colors denote flow away from the probe and red colors denote flow toward the probe, not venous or arterial blood (Fig. 35.3). After determining the artery and vein, the intensivist should trace the vessels both distally and proximally to identify whether branching, tortuosity, stenosis, or thrombosis might interfere with cannulation.

Ultrasonography can be used for site selection, which is crucial in children with critical cardiac disease due to unique vessel anatomy either congenitally acquired or from prior procedures.

For example, ultrasonography may be used to locate vessels for instrumentation if the subclavian and jugular veins must be avoided to preserve the vascular architecture. In addition to traditional ultrasonographically guided cannulation in the internal jugular and femoral vein sites, use of ultrasonography has been described in identification of the axillary, subclavian, and peripheral upper extremity veins for cannulation with central venous catheters and peripherally inserted central catheters. An ultrasonographic survey of multiple sites before a vascular access procedure can help with site selection for a vessel that is patent and most easily accessible.

Ultrasonography may be used for either static evaluation of the vessel anatomy before cannulation or for real-time evaluation during needle insertion. There are two primary methods for real-time needle guidance. The first is to hold the probe transverse to the plane of the vessels to allow for continuous visualization of the vein and any neighboring arterial structures. However, this method requires the operator to repeatedly advance the needle and then find the needle tip. The inexperienced operator may be more likely to advance the needle too deeply using this method. A Pythagorean approach has been posited recommending that the operator first identify the depth of the target vessel, insert the needle at a 45-degree angle, then proceed from distal to proximal at an insertion site distal to the ultrasonography probe at a distance equivalent to the depth of the vessel from the probe face (Fig. 35.4). With this arrangement the operator could theoretically anticipate the needle intersecting the plane of the ultrasonography transducer in the vicinity of the vessel. The authors of this chapter recommend following the needle's tip to the vessel because this method facilitates active guidance of the needle for first-pass success. Another alternative is to hold the probe longitudinal to the plane of the vessel of interest, allowing for a continuous view of the needle entering the selected vessel. Although this method results in better visualization of the needle, there is a higher chance that the probe will come out of plane with the vessel. This may lead to frustration and cannulation of the inappropriate vessel and is recommended for a more advanced user.

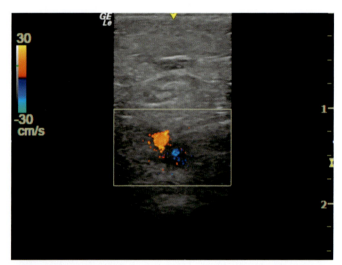

• **Figure 35.3** Color Doppler imaging of vessels. *Blue signal* denotes flow away from the transducer, and *red flow* is flow toward the transducer.

• **Figure 35.1** Ultraportable ultrasonography machine.

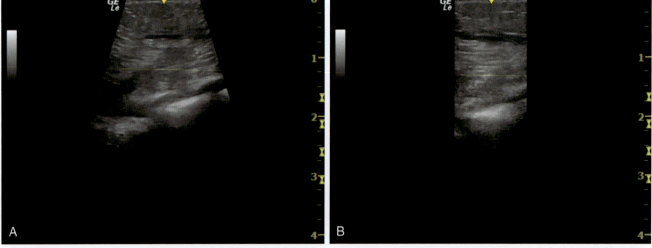

• **Figure 35.2** Trapezoid (A) versus standard (B) view using linear array transducer.

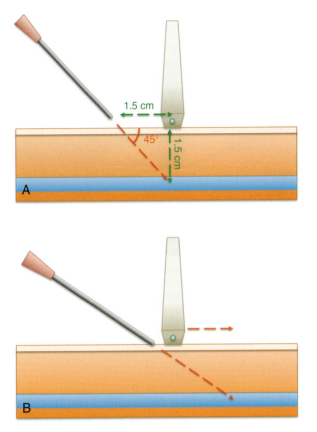

• **Figure 35.4** Pythagorean approach (A) to needle insertion versus following the needle (B).

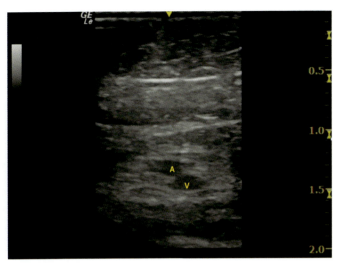

• **Figure 35.5** Transverse view of right femoral artery (A) and vein (V).

Site-Specific Considerations

Using ultrasonography during placement of a femoral central venous catheter allows direct visualization and may help the operator better position the leg to achieve separation of the two vessels (Fig. 35.5). Although there is limited data available in pediatrics, some studies have demonstrated decreased failure rates,[3,6] a reduction in arterial puncture,[6] and higher first-attempt success[7] when catheters are placed under ultrasonography. More data exist in the literature for adults. Although there is also slightly increased first-attempt success, a Cochrane Library review of available literature found no difference was appreciated in arterial puncture or other complications for adults or children.[8]

The data for internal jugular and subclavian venous catheters in pediatrics is similarly limited.[9] Ultrasonographic guidance has been shown to decrease the rate of failure and arterial puncture[6] but may increase the time to cannulation.[10] Unfortunately, there are no pediatric trials comparing ultrasonographically guided placement to using anatomic landmarks, but in adults ultrasonographic guidance has been shown to result in fewer failures,[6] fewer hematomas,[6,11] and a reduction in arterial punctures.[6,11]

In the pediatric cardiac ICU, umbilical arterial and venous catheters are common devices for vascular access in the newborn with congenital heart disease. During catheter placement a sector imaging transducer or linear array is placed over the subxiphoid region in the sagittal orientation to capture the inferior vena cava (IVC) longitudinally in the view of the transducer. The approach of the umbilical venous catheter is visualized through the umbilical

vein diagonally approaching the inferior cavoatrial junction from the surface. Insertion depth can be confirmed with the tip reaching the junction before the first verification radiograph (Fig. 35.6A). Similarly, insertion of an umbilical arterial catheter can be confirmed by aligning the probe with a longitudinal view of the descending aorta, allowing for simultaneous confirmation of tip placement at the level of the diaphragm (see Fig. 35.6B). Studies have demonstrated that ultrasonography is superior to x-ray examination when determining umbilical catheter position.[12-14] Use of real-time ultrasonographically guided placement decreases the average time required to place an umbilical catheter. Although cardiac patients were excluded from these studies, in the patient with normal abdominal vascular anatomy an operator could anticipate similar performance of ultrasonographic guidance for arterial or venous catheter placement.

Arterial Access

Arterial catheterization may also be performed with either static or real-time ultrasonographic guidance in a manner similar to venous catheterization. Studies have demonstrated decreased incidence of hematomas,[1,6,15,16] as well as decreased time to and increased success rate of cannulation compared with using palpation[15,16] or Doppler.[15] The usefulness of ultrasonographic guidance may be more pronounced in smaller children, who tend to be more difficult to cannulate.[15]

Although the literature remains complicated and somewhat conflicted on the benefits of ultrasonographic guidance during vascular access, ultrasonography remains a noninvasive means of potentially improving outcomes without significant associated risks.

Cardiac

Echocardiography is a mainstay of diagnosis and management in the pediatric cardiac patient, with an emphasis on detailed, highly optimized, and complete imaging of the heart. Bedside ultrasonography complements the physical examination and the formal echocardiogram, permitting the intensivist to have real-time, focused diagnostic imaging. Although bedside ultrasonography may never replace diagnostic echocardiography by a pediatric cardiology

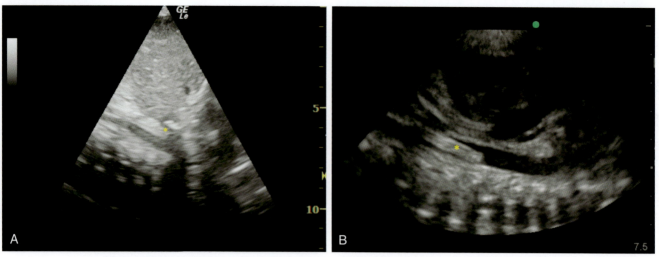

• **Figure 35.6** (A) Umbilical venous catheter tip *(*)* approaching the inferior cavoatrial junction visualized from the sagittal plane with the transducer in the subxiphoid position angled slightly to the patient's right. (B) Umbilical artery catheter tip *(*)* at the level of the diaphragm visualized from the sagittal plane with the transducer in the subxiphoid position angled slightly to the patient's left.

service, the focused cardiac ultrasonography examination[17] allows the intensivist to serially examine a patient and answer specific management questions, including evaluation of volume status, qualitative assessment of cardiac function, and evaluation of a pericardial effusion. In several limited series, bedside ultrasonography has modified the diagnosis and management of pediatric patients in the PICU.[18-20]

The tenets underlying cardiac evaluation using bedside ultrasonography are derived from diagnostic echocardiography. Selection of probe size may be important for visualization and may be limited by what is available in each cardiac PICU. When available, smaller, higher-frequency phased array probes are well suited for infants and small children because of their higher near-field image resolution and ability to maintain skin contact over a range of angles on a smaller thorax. Larger phased array probes are more likely to contain a single crystal advantageous for imaging, are capable of imaging deeper structures at lower frequency, and are appropriate for older children and young adults. Ultrasonography machines tend to use cardiac presets in which the screen indicator appears to the right of the screen, in contrast to the radiology conventions in which the indicator appears on the left of the screen. In this section on cardiac imaging, position will be described presuming screen indicator placement on the right side of the screen. The basic cardiac windows used by the cardiac intensivist are similar to those used by pediatric echocardiography services, including the parasternal, apical, and subcostal windows. Differences may occur between specialties in the orientation of the cardiac views. By convention, many pediatric echocardiography laboratories orient images obtained in the subcostal and apical position with the probe at the bottom of the screen, in contrast to parasternal and suprasternal views, in which the probe remains at the top of the screen. The pediatric intensivist, in keeping with many adult echocardiography services, may maintain the probe at the top of the screen in all transthoracic views for ease of operation among operators (Fig. 35.7). In the cardiac PICU, patient cardiac morphology naturally spans a wide spectrum of potential variants. Imaging of the heart is best performed when safe for the patient and the intensivist understands the patient's cardiac anatomy, has a clear clinical or academic question to

answer, and reviews the results collaboratively with diagnostic echocardiography services.

Qualitative Evaluation of Cardiac Function and Cardiac Views

The parasternal window offers the intensivist a qualitative means of assessing a variety of aspects of cardiac function. The parasternal view is generally obtained between the third and fourth intercostal space with the probe close to the sternum. In the short-axis view the indicator is pointed toward the patient's left shoulder. The parasternal short-axis view at the level of the papillary muscles (Fig. 35.8A) visualizes the ventricle at the point where radial myocardial movement is most apparent. This permits the intensivist to qualitatively evaluate ejection fraction and identify asymmetric movement of any areas of the circular left ventricle (LV). A noncircular, or D-shaped, LV during diastole or through the entire cardiac cycle suggests right ventricular (RV) dysfunction. Additionally, thickening of the RV wall may be appreciated. Visualization of other structures in the heart is possible by fanning the beam from the midpapillary region toward the mitral valve to the level of the aortic valve. At the aortic valve level, neighboring structures that can be visualized include the left atrium, the left coronary artery, the atrial septum at the 7 o'clock position, and the tricuspid valve at the 9 o'clock position (see Fig. 35.8B). Aortic valve opening in the setting of extracorporeal membrane oxygenation (ECMO) suggests that LV function is sufficient to overcome afterload and eject some quantity of stroke volume forward. Maintaining the same probe location and rotating the transducer counterclockwise 90 degrees such that the indicator is directed to the patient's right shoulder places the probe in the parasternal long-axis view. This view is aligned across the major axis of the LV, showing the left heart in continuity from the left atrium through the mitral valve, LV, aortic valve, and aortic root (Fig. 35.9). The parasternal long-axis view allows for qualitative evaluation of LV function. When the intensivist is concerned about poor cardiac output, the parasternal long-axis view allows the intensivist to rapidly evaluate the LV outflow tract, opening of the aortic valve, left atrium size, and excursion of the mitral valve leaflets. Additionally, pleural

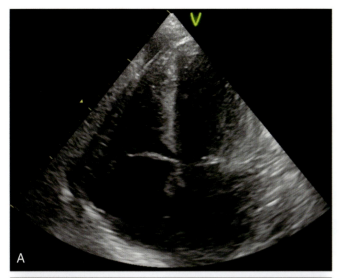

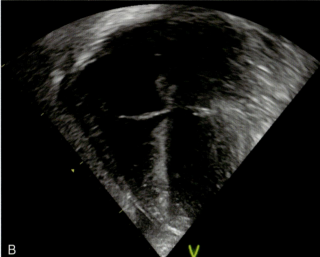

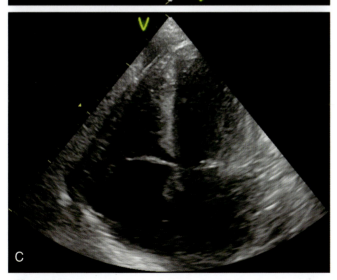

• **Figure 35.7** Comparison of some common cardiac view conventions for apical and subcostal views between specialties. (A) Adult cardiology and critical care medicine. (B) Pediatric cardiology. Apical and subcostal views are presented with the probe at the bottom of the screen. (C) Emergency medicine. In this convention the indicator appears on the left side of the screen and probe orientation on the patient is also correspondingly reversed in all views.

effusion versus pericardial effusion may be delineated based upon the presence of effusion below or above the descending aorta, respectively.

The apical four-chamber view is obtained with the probe placed in the area of the apex with the indicator directed toward the left flank, usually in the 2 to 3 o'clock position in patients with normal situs. Images of the heart are obtained with the transducer beam directed from the apex toward the atria. Optimally the view captures the four chambers of the heart with maximal visualization of the chambers and the semilunar valves (Fig. 35.10). Images may be difficult to obtain in a patient with large lung volumes, such as a person receiving positive pressure ventilation or who has lung hyperinflation. When available, this view permits qualitative assessment of relative chamber size, cardiac function, and aortic valve opening. In this view, regurgitation of the semilunar valves may be appreciated using Doppler modalities to assess flow on the atrial side of the mitral and tricuspid valve. Tilting the probe more shallowly so that the left ventricular outflow tract and aortic valve are visualized facilitates assessment of outflow tract blood velocity with pulsed wave or continuous wave Doppler. Aortic valve opening can be assessed in scenarios in which LV function is severely depressed, as in ECMO.

The subcostal view can also characterize the four chambers of the heart simultaneously and facilitates imaging of the atrial and ventricular septum. In a patient with normal situs the transducer is placed in the area below the xiphoid process and aimed at the left scapula. The indicator is oriented toward the patient's left flank or at the 3 o'clock position. The view is adjusted to optimize visualization of the four chambers of the heart (Fig. 35.11). Frequently an overhand grip and shallow angle of insonation facilitate positioning the probe nearly parallel to the skin. The view may be difficult to obtain in a child who has eaten or who has a gas-filled stomach from assisted ventilation or gastroparesis. However, the subcostal view may be the only view available in a child whose parasternal views are unobtainable due to an open chest or multiple bandages after cardiac surgery. Because the probe is oriented inferiorly to the heart, gravity dependent pericardial effusions are readily imaged here. Flow across septal defects is also more readily visualized from this plane because the ultrasonography beam is parallel to their flow.

Intravascular Volume Status

Intensivists have expended considerable effort to identify noninvasive ultrasonographic means of assessing fluid status and volume responsiveness. Within the pediatric cardiac population, assessing volume responsiveness before administration has broad applications because careful fluid management is critically important in these children. Adult studies have suggested that the collapsibility of the IVC is an effective surrogate for volume status. The IVC diameter is evaluated 2 to 3 cm distal to the cavoatrial junction in adults, and the variance between inspiration and expiration is compared (Fig. 35.12). Variance greater than 12% to 18% in an intubated, paralyzed patient has been correlated with volume responsiveness.[21] The effect of positive airway pressure on IVC dynamic changes reflecting volume status is also closely tied to intrathoracic pressures from positive pressure ventilation. A study performed by Lin and colleagues[22] revealed that anesthesia induction and intubation altered the performance of the IVC as a surrogate for fluid responsiveness. Induction itself increases venous capacitance and decreases apparent IVC diameter. However, increased intrathoracic pressures decrease respiratory variation in the IVC over the respiratory cycle and can

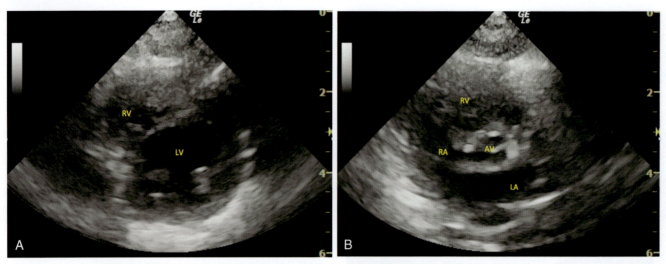

• **Figure 35.8** Parasternal short-axis view. (A) Midpapillary level. (B) Aortic valve level. *AV,* Aortic valve; *LA,* left atrium; *LV,* left ventricle; *RA,* right atrium; *RV,* right ventricle.

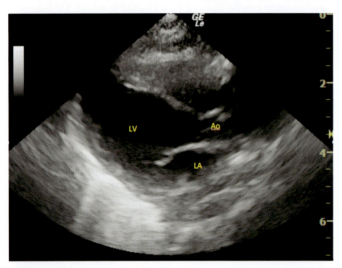

• **Figure 35.9** Parasternal long-axis view. *Ao,* Aorta; *LA,* left atrium; *LV,* left ventricle.

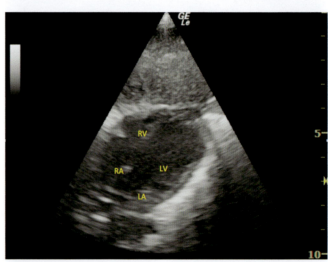

• **Figure 35.11** Subcostal four-chamber view. *LA,* Left atrium; *LV,* left ventricle; *RA,* right atrium; *RV,* right ventricle.

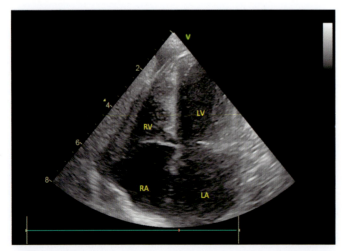

• **Figure 35.10** Apical four-chamber view. *LA,* Left atrium; *LV,* left ventricle; *RA,* right atrium; *RV,* right ventricle.

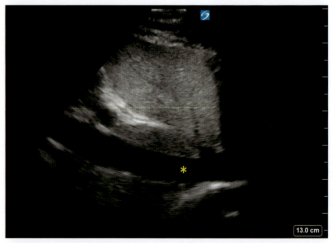

• **Figure 35.12** Longitudinal inferior vena cava view. Measurement site for inferior vena cava diameter is marked with an asterisk (*).

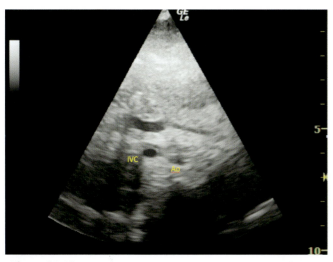

• **Figure 35.13** Transverse inferior vena cava view. *Ao,* Aorta; *IVC,* inferior vena cava.

increase the relative diameter of the IVC in relation to other intraabdominal structures. Additionally, pediatric IVC measurements have not been shown to consistently correlate with central venous pressure.[23] Therefore it is difficult to assess the functional utility of the measurement. The IVC to aorta ratio is another measure that can evaluate hypovolemia and hypervolemia (Fig. 35.13).[24-26] This ratio eliminates the issue of age-related size variability of the IVC. Intensivists rarely need another indicator of overall fluid status in addition to clinical and laboratory indicators, and the utility of the ratio to evaluate for volume responsiveness has not yet been studied. Although there is significant potential for both IVC collapsibility and the IVC to aorta ratio, there are factors affecting hemodynamics that may be more complex in the child with a congenital heart defect. A intensivist using ultrasonography for an examination of overall function should consider the absolute effects of cardiac dysmorphology in these assessments.

Pericardial Effusion and Pericardiocentesis

Effusion is recognized in the pericardial space as a dark anechoic area surrounding the heart that distends the pericardium and appears fluid and mobile relative to the beating heart (Fig. 35.14). Effusion is readily imaged from the subcostal region. The most specific sign of tamponade physiology is a distended IVC, but other signs include variability in aortic inflow, tricuspid inflow, or mitral valve inflow velocity of 25% or higher across the respiratory cycle or collapse of the RV free wall in diastole. Ultimately, the decision to drain a pericardial effusion is predicated on patient instability, and ultrasonography can help facilitate early intervention.[27]

The use of formal diagnostic echocardiography to identify the position of the insertion site and depth to a pericardial effusion has been well established in both the adult and pediatric literature,[28] but the intensivist may also use bedside ultrasonography to achieve the same views. Most commonly the phased array probe is held in the apical position, optimizing the view of the effusion at the base of the heart, and the needle is guided toward the visualized site. In a study by Tsang and colleagues,[28] the use of echocardiography during placement, generally from an apical view, was shown to infrequently identify the needle tip. Instead, the needle tended to be identified by guide wire or catheter

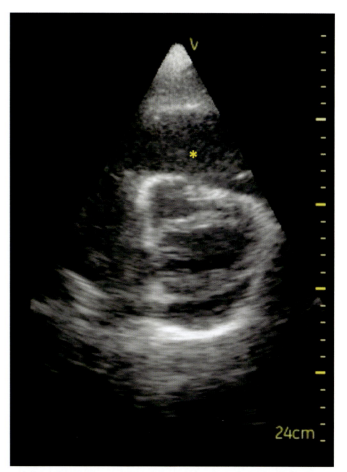

• **Figure 35.14** Pericardial effusion. Effusion space is marked with an asterisk (*).

insertion, drainage of fluid, or introduction of contrast. In a more recent study, interventional cardiologists use the linear probe in a long-axis position so that the effusion and the path of the needle are viewed concomitantly. This affords the intensivist the ability to watch the path of the needle continuously throughout the procedure.[29]

Cardiac Arrest

Within the cardiac PICU, an emerging use of bedside ultrasonography is during cardiac arrest, for which readily available bedside devices may identify potentially reversible arrest causes such as pericardial tamponade, pneumothorax, or hypovolemia. Echocardiography, in general, is mentioned within American Heart Association cardiac arrest algorithms as a potential adjunct for resuscitation guidance[30] and may be a useful adjunct to high-quality resuscitation. Effective bedside uses add diagnostic value without interfering with other ongoing activity. Generally, the subcostal window is the most readily available and avoids displacing compressors' hand placement. The view may be obtained during pauses for pulse checks and should never prolong the time during which compressions are being held. It is critical that the ultrasonography gel be fully removed between probe placement on the chest, especially if electrical defibrillation or cardioversion is performed because the gel conducts electricity.

Cardiac standstill, or the complete absence of cardiac contractility from severe biventricular dysfunction, has been correlated with near complete failure to achieve return of spontaneous circulation in the adult population.[31,32] A series of 14 pediatric emergency department patients who presented in cardiac arrest showed all 7 patients who presented in cardiac standstill did not experience return of spontaneous circulation (ROSC).[33] In settings where ECMO is available during CPR (ECPR) as a rescue modality, cardiac standstill may not portend ROSC failure. Three cases have been described in which patients manifested recovery of cardiac function after ECPR was deployed.[34] Though neurologic outcomes were varied, cardiac standstill is not independently predictive of ROSC and should not be used in isolation as a reason for terminating resuscitative efforts.

Extracorporeal Membrane Oxygenation

Bedside ultrasonography has significant utility for immediate decision making while a child is on ECMO. Although full formal echocardiography remains important for management, bedside ultrasonography allows for focused questions to be asked and answered rapidly. Standard cardiac views allow for evaluation of decompression of the LV and aortic valve opening, and serial examinations enable immediate, careful titration of the ECMO therapy parameters.[35,36] Placement of the ECMO cannulas should be formally evaluated by diagnostic echocardiography, but bedside ultrasonography may be used if emergent questions about cannula position arise. If the child was moved or received compressions or if the ability to achieve appropriate flows has changed, standard cardiac views can be used to immediately evaluate whether the cannula position has changed. Tracing superiorly from the IVC, the right atrium is easily visualized and permits the intensivist to quickly locate the tip of the cannula if the child is cannulated via the femoral vein (Fig. 35.15). If the child is cannulated via the internal jugular vein, the superior vena cava may be visualized via the parasternal long-axis view that is fanned toward the right atrium (Fig. 35.16). The arterial cannula may be evaluated via the aortic arch view by placing the probe on the right side of the sternum with the indicator pointed at the head and fanned toward the left scapula such that a view of the arch and its thoracic branches is captured.

Lung

Diagnosis of lung pathology in the clinical setting is largely dependent on imaging using ionizing radiation, such as chest x-ray examination and chest computed tomography. The impact of repeated radiographic examinations of critically ill pediatric cardiac patients in the PICU is unclear. Pulmonary ultrasonography presents a noninvasive, efficacious means of diagnosing lung pathology without radiation exposure and can easily be used for serial examinations. It has been described by multiple investigators in the inpatient setting and is readily performed at the PICU bedside. Pulmonary ultrasonography poses unique challenges when compared with ultrasound imaging of the rest of the body. Ultrasonography is not readily transmitted through air-filled spaces, and air in the lung obscures deeper structures. Interpretation of pulmonary ultrasonography hinges upon a growing literature on how pathology influences the appearance of lung ultrasonography artifacts.[37]

Infants are uniquely suited for ultrasonographic evaluation of the lungs. In the infant there is less ossification of the rib cage and higher body water content than in the older child. Together, these factors allow for better penetration of the ultrasound beam. However, the spaces between the ribs are smaller than in larger children, but this difficulty may be overcome by turning the probe parallel to the plane of the rib cage, placing the entirety of the beam directly between two ribs (Fig. 35.17). As the child ages, the intercostal space widens, rib ossification increases, and the water body content decreases. Although these changes may make obtaining adequate views more complicated, with small adjustments, most children may be appropriately evaluated.

When a linear probe is used, a standard thoracic view demonstrates soft tissue overlying the muscle layer and ribs and the intercostal space appearing farther from the probe. The ribs appear black and cast a shadow on deeper structures (Fig. 35.18A). Within the intercostal space the pleural line is appreciated as the visceral pleura slides over the parietal pleura. This pleural visceral interface appears as a shimmering bright line within the view similar to "ants on a log." Placing the M-mode cursor through this pleural visceral interface contrasts the more linear-appearing chest wall

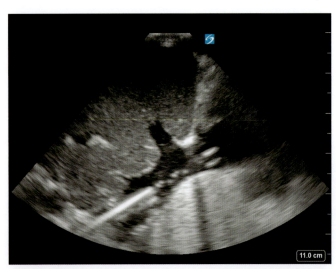

• **Figure. 35.15** Femoral extracorporeal membrane oxygenation cannula visualized from the sagittal inferior vena cava view in the subxiphoid position.

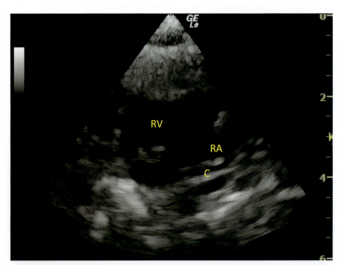

• **Figure 35.16** Right ventricular inflow view demonstrating cervical extracorporeal membrane oxygenation cannula entering the right atrium from the superior vena cava. *C,* Cannula; *RA,* right atrium; *RV,* right ventricle.

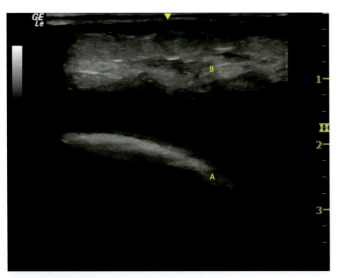

• **Figure 35.17** Intercostal view of normal lung using linear array transducer. Pleural line *(A)*. Intercostal muscles *(B)*.

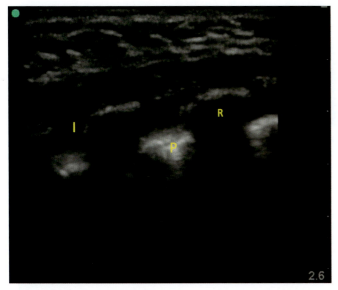

• **Figure 35.18** Sagittal view of normal lung using linear array transducer. *I,* Intercostal muscles; *P,* pleura; *R,* rib.

movement with the more granular movement of the lung surface. This relationship, which has a "seashore" appearance, denotes a nonpathologic interaction between the two pleura.

Although the ultrasound beam has difficulty penetrating air-filled lungs, certain artifacts are created that help elucidate normal and pathologic findings. A-lines are the parallel horizontal linear artifacts representing reverberation of the pleural line spaced at regular intervals down the screen (see Fig. 35.19B). A-lines are typically appreciated in the center of the ultrasound beam and are present irrespective of normal intraparenchymal physiology versus the presence of pathology. B-lines are parallel to the ultrasound beam, descend vertically from the pleural line, and obliterate A-lines as they traverse the lung parenchyma (see Fig. 35.19B). Although a few B-lines may indicate normal physiology, increased B-lines are suggestive of interstitial lung water or consolidation. Additionally, when consolidation is present, there may be hepatization of the

lung, when the appearance of the lung on ultrasonography approximates the appearance of liver. Finally, Z-lines appear similar to B-lines, but unlike B-lines they are shorter and do not reach the bottom of the screen. Within the neonatal population, lung ultrasonography is a useful adjunct for patient assessment in the newborn with respiratory failure, predicting need for intubation within 24 hours of birth depending independently on the extent of ultrasonographic findings.[38] Whether ultrasonography could have a similar impact on patients in the cardiac PICU is a topic of ongoing investigation.

Pneumothorax

In the setting of pneumothorax, ultrasonographic imaging of the lung takes on several characteristic findings. Because air does not permit transmission of ultrasound energy, intervening pneumothorax obscures anatomic structures distal to the parietal pleura. Therefore pleural sliding is abolished, and B-line and Z-line artifact, both of which originate on the visceral pleural line, disappear. Instead, the area where lung parenchyma typically appears is filled with mirror artifact of the intercostal musculature produced by internal reflection of the ultrasound beam between the skin and the pleural surface. Identification of pneumothorax hinges upon artifact recognition and may be challenging for novices because it is less intuitive. M-mode may help with recognition. Placement of the M-mode cursor over the pneumothorax space will not yield the "seashore" image described earlier but rather a "barcode" or "stratosphere" appearance of multiple parallel lines that does not reflect the movement of lung under the probe (Fig. 35.20A). As with any M-mode modality, it is crucial that the operator does not move. Identification of the point at which a pneumothorax ends and mobile lung appears is highly sensitive for pneumothorax and appears as a segment of sliding pleura that intermittently slides into the pneumothorax (see Fig. 35.20B).

Pleural Effusions

Pleural effusions appear as a dark anechoic area within the pleural cavity and appear and move similarly to other large collections of fluid under ultrasonography. Imaging of effusions can be important for planning thoracentesis, serial evaluation of effusions while the patient is receiving medical therapy (including chylothoraces), and monitoring for the formation of septations, particularly in sanguineous effusions. Pleural effusions are readily visualized in the areas where they come into contact with the parietal pleura, typically dependent areas of the chest or regions where the effusion may be trapped by septations or other intrathoracic barriers (Fig. 35.21A). Additionally, effusions can be visualized from areas below the costal margin through the diaphragm by aiming the probe up toward areas where the effusion comes into contact with the ultrasound beam (see Fig. 35.21B). Effusion imaging is performed with either sector probes (phased array and curvilinear) or linear array probes. Areas to visualize naturally include dependent areas on the affected hemithorax along the posterior axillary line or transhepatically from subcostal areas caudad to the anterior edge of the diaphragm, with the probe angled cephalad to image areas in the thorax. While visualizing effusions, it is helpful to set the machine to a depth of 4- to 10-cm penetration depending on the probe used. The trapezoid imaging feature is helpful for widening the field of view and aids in assessing the size of the effusion and planning for thoracentesis, if indicated.

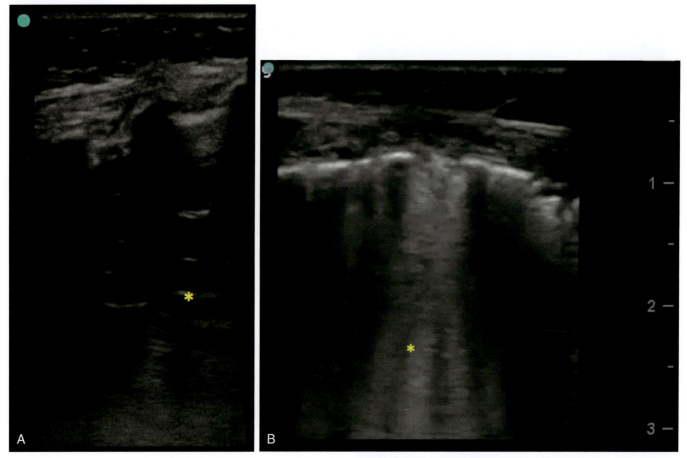

• **Figure 35.19** Artifacts seen in lung ultrasonography. (A) A-lines *(*)*. (B) B-lines *(*)*.

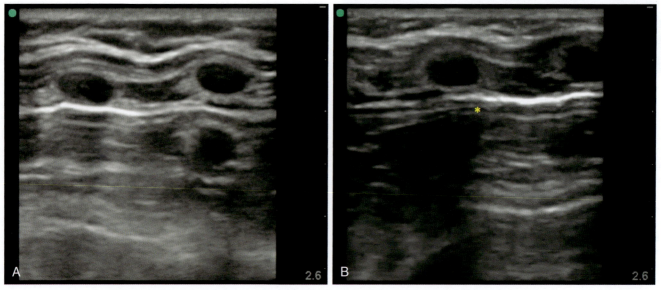

• **Figure 35.20** Pneumothorax detected by lung ultrasonography. (A) Two-dimensional image with lack of B-lines. (B) Lung point *(*)*.

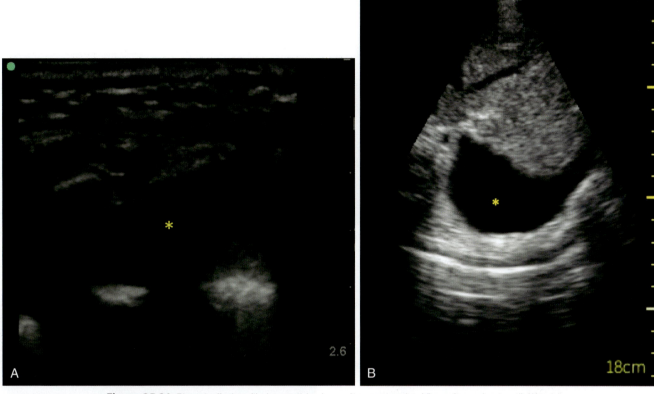

• **Figure 35.21** Pleural effusion *(*)* detected by lung ultrasonography. Views from chest wall (A) and subcostal position (B).

Pneumonia and Consolidation

Ultrasonography is particularly useful for identifying pathology that interferes with the normal distribution of air in the lung. In addition to the clinical examination, chest x-ray examination has been a mainstay for diagnosing pneumonia in children. However, ultrasonography allows for the diagnosis of pneumonia in many cases without radiation exposure. An increased number of B-lines may be present. Consolidated lung may be more visible than air-filled normal lung, leading to pneumonia being easily visualized with ultrasonography (Fig. 35.22). A study by Boursiani and colleagues[39] found that the specificity and sensitivity of chest x-ray and lung ultrasonography were similar, leading the authors to recommend the use of ultrasonography as a first-line examination. In another study by Zhan et al.,[40] pediatric residents with minimal ultrasonography experience were briefly instructed on how to perform a lung ultrasound examination to identify pneumonia. The sensitivity of the residents identifying pneumonia was 40%, but the sensitivity was 91% based upon prevalence by chest x-ray examination. Such findings reinforce the utility of ultrasonography in everyday practice and as a first-line test.

Diaphragm

Multiple authors have described imaging the diaphragm in children in the cardiac PICU as an assessment of diaphragmatic paresis following surgery or intrathoracic physiology.[41-46] Diaphragm imaging is accomplished from the subcostal region anywhere below

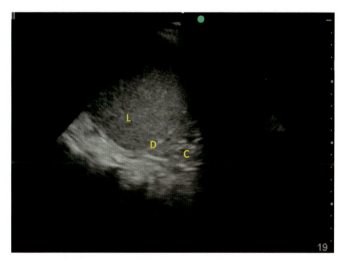

• **Figure 35.22** Lung consolidation detected by lung ultrasonography. *C,* Consolidated lung; *D,* diaphragm; *L,* liver.

the 12th rib using a sector imaging transducer. Typically, one hemidiaphragm is imaged at a time with the probe oriented in the sagittal (from the front of the chest) or coronal plane (from the flanks) such that the bright arc of the diaphragm is seen and its movement can be monitored (Fig. 35.23A). Some authors have described placing the probe in the subxiphoid area with a view transverse to the spine angled up toward the mediastinum, allowing

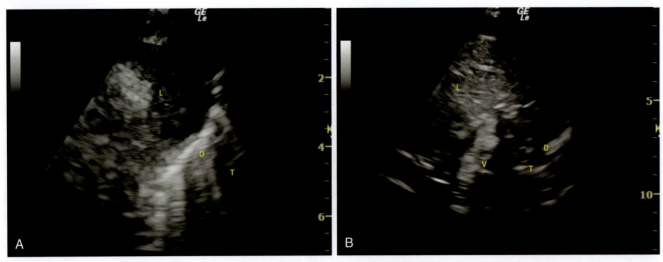

• **Figure 35.23** Views of the diaphragm obtained from the subcostal position (A) and subxiphoid transverse position (B). *D,* Diaphragm; *L,* liver; *T,* thorax; *V,* vertebral body.

the intensivist to image both leaflets simultaneously[41] (see Fig. 35.23B). From this vantage the movement of the diaphragm can be monitored, quantified with two-dimensional imaging or M-mode, and compared either between leaflets or across serial examinations. Additionally, the intensivist has full knowledge of the respiratory support the patient is receiving at the time of imaging. In the hands of intensivists, characterization of diaphragm movement from the subcostal position has similar accuracy to fluoroscopy and electromyography.[42,43] Another application for this assessment technique is the evaluation of intubation. Several authors have described imaging the diaphragm and confirmation of bilateral and symmetric hemidiaphragm leaflet movement as a means of rapid confirmation of intubation.[41,44-46] Differential movement of one leaflet might suggest mainstem intubation in the absence of prior bronchial obstruction or diaphragm pathology. Absence of diaphragm movement might suggest a misplaced endotracheal tube. In the realm of airway evaluation with ultrasonography, vocal cord dysfunction after extubation,[47] difficult airway assessment, and subglottic stenosis assessment in the area of the larynx and upper airway (Fig. 35.24) have been described but remain largely exploratory at this time.

Additional important factors influencing lung ultrasonography in critically ill pediatric cardiac patients include the fact that dressings and devices in the postoperative patient may influence lung visualization. An open chest in an infant with accompanying drains, pacing wires, and monitoring devices frequently leaves little thoracic space for visualization. In these situations, subdiaphragmatic transhepatic views of the lungs may be helpful, though pleural sliding is difficult to assess.

Abdomen

Abdominal evaluation using point-of-care ultrasonography has been well described in the emergency medicine literature as a means for rapid abdominal assessment of intraperitoneal bleeding after trauma.[48] In the PICU it is useful in identifying ascites as well. Evidence supporting use of abdominal ultrasonography in emergency medicine is not strong in children, with some series mustering a sensitivity for the examination at only 30% to 50%.[49] The low sensitivity may reflect variability in the technique among

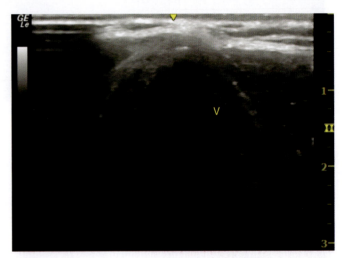

• **Figure 35.24** Ultrasonographic views of the vocal cords with the probe held transverse to the larynx over the cricothyroid membrane. *V,* True vocal fold.

operators and the vagaries of using ultrasonography in small children to identify small fluid collections. The performance characteristics of ultrasonography for evaluating ascites in the PICU are unclear. Because PICU patients are serially monitored and symptomatic fluid collections are likely to be larger than asymptomatic ones. Ultrasonographic imaging of ascites collections in the cardiac PICU may be easier.

Certain attributes of patients in the cardiac PICU present important considerations for abdominal imaging. Surgical patients may have subcostal dressings, drains, and pacing wires among other percutaneous devices that may influence available imaging windows. Intensivists examining patients with a history of abdominal heterotaxy should consider the patient's anatomy in image acquisition and interpretation. Though abdominal ultrasonography in the PICU is largely used for identification of free fluid, and discrimination of the liver and spleen is less important, providers should be prepared for variability in abdominal findings. Abdominal situs in the patient is important in ultrasonography primarily due to the location of the IVC and whether venous return from the lower extremities travels to the heart through an azygous continuation. Variations in vessel geometry at this level may make it more difficult to assess central venous catheter placement in the IVC, or IVC collapsibility in a patient with heterotaxy.

Abdominal Assessment of Free Fluid

Fluid in the abdomen, such as ascites, blood, or peritoneal dialysate, appears anechoic or dark. This evaluation is useful in the assessment of patients who have generated abdominal fluid collections from fluid overload, organ dysfunction, bleeding, or other causes. Fluid separates viscera in the peritoneal space and often appears irregular and compressible. Activating color Doppler over areas of ascites can often detect bulk movement of fluid with a corresponding Doppler signal.

Historically the Focused Assessment with Sonography for Trauma (FAST) was used to identify free abdominal fluid as an indication of hemorrhagic blunt thoracoabdominal injury. Visualization of this fluid was performed in two abdominal regions along the patient's flanks, the suprapubic region and the subcostal view of the heart. It is important to note that the FAST examination was performed on patients attached to backboards parallel to the floor or patients on an operating room table. In the PICU, patients often have their heads elevated for ventilator associated–event avoidance, and fluid often gravitates toward the lower quadrants of the abdomen. Therefore the authors recommend that intensivists also examine the bilateral lower quadrants in an evaluation of abdominal ascites.

The FAST examination can be performed using sector imaging probes, including cardiac phased array transducers, curvilinear/microconvex, or linear probes in trapezoid image mode if available. The right upper quadrant is visualized by placing the probe below the costal margin at the posterior axillary line aligned parallel to the bed (Fig. 35.25A) (coronal view) with the indicator pointing toward the patient's head and the corresponding ultrasonography screen indicator oriented to the left. The view should capture the right kidney, and in a patient with normal situs the liver and diaphragm cephalad to it. Free fluid in the abdomen separates the retroperitoneal kidney from the liver. Significant ascites may also separate the diaphragm from the liver, appearing both above and

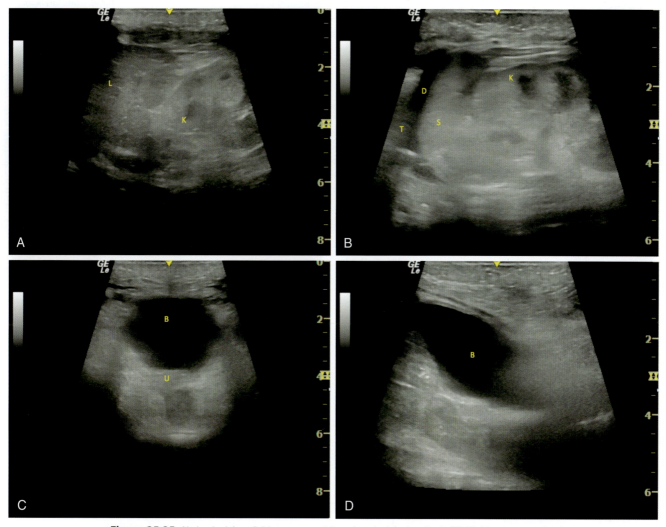

• **Figure 35.25** Abdominal free fluid assessment in a female infant patient. (A) Right upper quadrant view. (B) Left upper quadrant view. (C) Suprapubic transverse view. (D) Suprapubic longitudinal view. The last view typically incorporated into the abdominal Focused Assessment with Sonography for Trauma is a longitudinal subcostal view of the heart. *B*, Bladder; *D*, diaphragm; *K*, kidney; *L*, liver; *S*, spleen; *T*, thorax; *U*, uterus.

below the organ. The left upper quadrant is visualized similarly from the other side of the abdomen in the left subcostal region (see Fig. 35.25B), with the probe again oriented parallel to the bed with the indicator pointing toward the patient's head. The view should capture the left kidney, which will be located slightly more cephalad than on the right, and in the patient with normal situs splenic structures will appear cephalad and ventral to the left kidney. In both views the probe beam should be fanned ventrally and dorsally to successfully identify fluid.

The suprapubic region is the third abdominal view obtained in the traditional FAST examination. It is obtained by placing the probe in the suprapubic region above the pubic bone with the beam pointed toward the spine. The probe is oriented transversely across the bladder (see Fig. 35.25C) so that it appears as a round or trapezoidal dark fluid-filled structure. The bladder may be empty and difficult to visualize as a muscular spheroid containing limited fluid. The patient's uterus or prostate can sometimes be visualized dorsal to the bladder. The presence of an anechoic urinary catheter balloon can help identify the bladder. The probe can also be aligned sagittally with the indicator pointed toward the patient's head (see Fig. 35.25D). In this view, catheters and reproductive tract structures can be visualized longitudinally. Free fluid in this view appears outside the bladder, separating it from other structures.

Of note, this view may be used for evaluation of anuria in a patient with a urinary catheter. Identification of the catheter within the bladder confirms that it is not misplaced. Identification of a full bladder despite catheter placement suggests that the catheter is obstructed. An empty bladder indicates that the anuric patient is not producing urine.

The lower quadrants are visualized by placing the transducer along the anterior and lateral surfaces of the abdomen, sliding it medial-laterally with the probe indicator oriented toward the head and cephalad-caudad with the indicator oriented toward the patient's right. Below the abdominal musculature and peritoneal wall, fluid separates visceral structures.

Paracentesis

Drainage of abdominal fluid collections is readily accomplished with ultrasonographic guidance. Ultrasonography can identify fluid location and depth for needle insertion and plan needle trajectory. Needle insertion should occur 2 to 3 cm lateral to the inferior epigastric arteries that run along the lateral edge of the rectus abdominis muscles (Fig. 35.26). Needle placement is optimally performed with a linear probe aligned longitudinally over the needle to follow its path into the ascites fluid (Fig. 35.27). The trajectory of the needle should point caudad into an area of fluid. The orientation of the needle should be oblique enough to the skin surface so that the tissue track of the needle is long and reduces the risk of ascites leakage. Use of ultrasonography ensures that a short length of needle tip enters the peritoneal space. From this point, aspiration or drain placement using the Seldinger technique can occur. Use of a probe longer than 2.5 cm is recommended because the field of view is longer and better able to track needle insertion. If a longer probe is not available, the operator may slide the probe with the needle as it enters the abdomen. However, this may be technically difficult for a novice operator because it is challenging to stay over the needle while moving.

In instances in which a peritoneal dialysis catheter has been placed, evaluation of catheter malfunction can also be performed. In a series of 12 peritoneal dialysis catheter malfunctions, Esposito and colleagues[50] described cases of debris occlusion and catheter

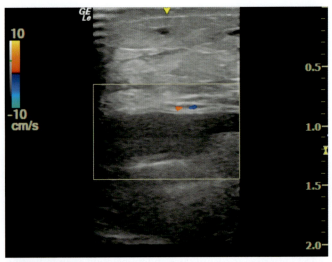

• **Figure 35.26** Inferior epigastric artery and corresponding vein identified with color Doppler in the abdominal wall.

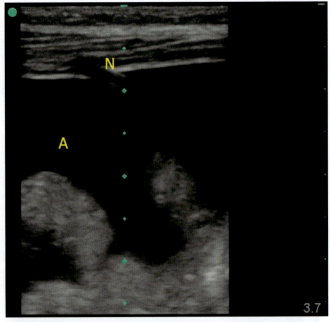

• **Figure 35.27** Paracentesis of ascites *(A)* performed with the probe oriented longitudinally over the needle *(N)*.

misplacement leading to catheter failure and proposed that bedside evaluation with ultrasonography facilitated resolution of the catheter issues.

Future Directions

In summary, ultrasound affords clinicians a broad array of diagnostic and procedural guidance modalities that augment clinical practice in the cardiac ICU. The fledgling field is rapidly evolving with increasing adoption of ultrasound in clinical practice and innovations in technology. Other authors in the anesthesiology setting have proposed the use of ultrasonography for identification of gastric content volume in anticipation of surgery.[51] Additionally, adult intensivists have proposed the use of ultrasonography for monitoring renal blood flow in hemodynamically unstable patients as a predictor of acute kidney injury.[52] The utility and accuracy of these techniques in the PICU setting remain investigational and may prove useful for intensivists in the future.

Selected References

A complete list of references is available at ExpertConsult.com.

8. Brass P, Hellmich M, Kolodziej L, et al. Ultrasound guidance versus anatomical landmarks for subclavian or femoral vein catheterization. *Cochrane Database Syst Rev.* 2015;(1):CD011447.

9. Brass P, Hellmich M, Kolodziej L, et al. Ultrasound guidance versus anatomical landmarks for internal jugular vein catheterization. *Cochrane Database Syst Rev.* 2015;(1):CD006962.

11. American Society of Anesthesiologists Task Force on Central Venous Access, Rupp SM, Apfelbaum JL, et al. Practice guidelines for central venous access: a report by the American Society of Anesthesiologists Task Force on Central Venous Access. *Anesthesiology.* 2012;116:539–573.

15. Aouad-Maroun M, Raphael CK, Sayyid SK, et al. Ultrasound-guided arterial cannulation for paediatrics. *Cochrane Database Syst Rev.* 2016;(9):Art. No.: CD011364.

20. Kutty S, Attebery JE, Yeager EM, et al. Transthoracic echocardiography in pediatric intensive care. *Pediatr Crit Care Med.* 2014;15:329–335.

22. Lin EE, Chen AE, Panebianco N, et al. Effect of inhalational anesthetics and positive-pressure ventilation on ultrasound assessment of the great vessels: a prospective study at a children's hospital. *Anesthesiology.* 2016;124:870–877.

38. Raimondi F, Migliaro F, Sodano A, et al. Use of neonatal chest ultrasound to predict noninvasive ventilation failure. *Pediatrics.* 2014;134:e1089–e1094.

42. Gil-Juanmiquel L, Gratacós M, Castilla-Fernández Y, et al. Bedside ultrasound for the diagnosis of abnormal diaphragmatic motion in children after heart surgery. *Pediatr Crit Care Med.* 2017;18:159–164.

44. Lin MJ, Gurley K, Hoffmann B. Bedside ultrasound for tracheal tube verification in pediatric emergency department and ICU patients. *Pediatr Crit Care Med.* 2016;17:e469–e476.

48. Fox JC, Boysen M, Gharahbaghian L, et al. Test characteristics of focused assessment of sonography for trauma for clinically significant abdominal free fluid in pediatric blunt abdominal trauma. *Acad Emerg Med.* 2011;18:477–482.

36

Imaging Modalities—Magnetic Resonance Imaging and Computed Tomography

LASYA GAUR, MD; CARA MORIN, MD, PHD; NICHOLAS MORIN, MD, PHD;
PHILIP SPEVAK, MD, MPH

Defining Imaging Modalities

Strengths and Weaknesses of the Various Imaging Modalities

Modality	Strengths	Weaknesses
Echocardiography	Spatial and temporal resolution Logistically simple Intracardiac visualization	Acoustic windows limited in some patients
Cardiac magnetic resonance	Biventricular function Tissue characterization	Logistically difficult Sedation requirements
Cardiac computed tomography	Spatial resolution Coronary imaging Extracardiac visualization	Radiation
Cardiac catheterization	Hemodynamic measurements Interventional options	Logistics and radiation

Spatial resolution is how close together in space two points can be differentiated from one another and is critical in imaging small and closely adjacent structures. The best spatial resolution is typically submillimeter.

Temporal resolution is how fast a moving structure can be imaged through time and is critical when structures are moving at high speeds (e.g., flail valve leaflet). Temporal resolution is typically less than 30 ms but can be as good as 10 ms. With improved temporal resolution one typically trades reduced spatial resolution.

Magnetic Resonance Imaging

The role of cardiac magnetic resonance (CMR) imaging in congenital heart disease (CHD) has expanded considerably in recent years. CMR is now routinely used for assessment of anatomy (especially in those with limited acoustic windows or to limit radiation exposure), quantification of ventricular function, valvular shunt fraction, and tissue characterization. Advantages of CMR include lack of ionizing radiation, wider field of view including extracardiac vascular structures, and noninvasive assessment of flow dynamics and cardiac output, obvious advantages for a pediatric population with complex cardiac anatomy and need for serial assessments over time. This section aims to provide a practical guide for the pediatric cardiac intensivist by including a basic description of commonly used CMR pulse sequences and their application to frequently encountered clinical case scenarios.

Basic Cardiac Magnetic Resonance Pulse Sequences

Conventional Spin Echo or "Black Blood" Imaging. In this sequence, flowing blood is suppressed and appears black while surrounding stationary structures appear gray or white to provide image contrast (Fig. 36.1). Images are acquired at a single phase in the cardiac cycle and are typically static. This sequence is especially useful for anatomic detail in the presence of magnetic field inhomogeneities, including metallic implants.[1-2] Breath-holds are required to limit blurring from cardiac motion.

Application: Anatomic definition, tissue characterization, cardiac tumors.

Gradient Echo. Gradient echo (GRE) sequences generate images in which blood appears white, surrounding structures gray (Fig. 36.2, Video 36.1), and any turbulence within the blood pool (indicating valve obstruction or regurgitation, shunt lesions) appears void of signal or dark. Images are acquired throughout the cardiac cycle and displayed in a "movie," or cine, format to illustrate dynamic cardiac motion.[2] Two types of GRE imaging are typically used: (1) steady-state free precession (SSFP) is widely used due to excellent contrast between the blood pool and surrounding structures, or (2) standard spoiled GRE sequences are used for phase contrast (PC), late gadolinium enhancement (LGE), and three-dimensional contrast-enhanced magnetic resonance angiography (CE-MRA) as defined below. GRE sequences are also used in the presence of magnetic field inhomogeneity

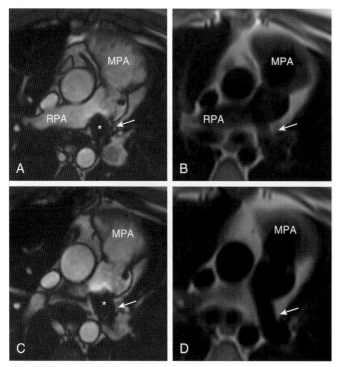

Figure 36.1 Bright blood images (A and C) with artifact in the stented proximal left pulmonary artery *(arrow)*. Location of the stent is indicated by an *asterisk*. Dark blood images show the left pulmonary artery in the same patient with improved definition (B and D). *MPA,* Main pulmonary artery; *RPA,* right pulmonary artery.

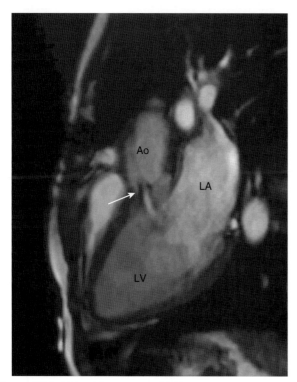

• **Figure 36.2.** Video 36.1 and cine SSFP image demonstrating aortic valve regurgitation *(arrow)* in the three-chamber view. Note dilation and myocardial thinning of the left ventricle. *Ao,* Aorta; *LA,* left atrium; *LV,* left ventricle; *SSFP,* steady-state free precession.

(endovascular metallic implants) because SSFP images are vulnerable to artifact.

Application: Quantification of ventricular volume and function, assessment of ventricular mass, visualization of cardiac motion (e.g., ventricular wall motion abnormalities), surgical conduits, or patches, as well as valve morphology.

Phase Contrast Imaging. This modified GRE sequence is used primarily for quantification of flow volume (in milliliters) and velocity (in meters per second) in vessels or across valves and to estimate cardiac shunts. When protons in motion in the blood pool are placed in a specific magnetic field gradient, they acquire a phase shift that is proportional to the velocity of flowing blood. A weighted average of the velocity through all the pixels within a designated slice in a vessel lumen is measured. The product of the velocity encoded and the cross-sectional area of the vessel or valve yields the flow at that instant in the cardiac cycle, which is integrated over time for flow rate over the entire cardiac cycle.[3-7] Similar to echocardiography, peak flow can be estimated by applying the Bernoulli equation: maximum instantaneous gradient = $4V^2$, where V^2 is the maximum instantaneous velocity.

Application: Quantification of valvular regurgitant fraction (e.g., aortic valve regurgitant fraction), intracardiac and extracardiac shunt flow (e.g., ratio of pulmonary blood flow [Q_p] to systemic blood flow [Q_s], or Q_p:Q_s, for ventricular septal defects, patent ductus arteriosus), flow across vessel stenosis, quantification of collateral flow, and cardiac output.

Late Gadolinium Enhancement. Late gadolinium enhancement (LGE) is used to delineate focal regions of myocardial fibrosis based on the principle that contrast washout is delayed in fibrosed or infarcted myocardium compared with normal myocardium. These are static images in which normal myocardium is black or nulled, whereas fibrosed or scarred regions appear bright or white.[8-10] Myocardial scar formation can be used for prognosis as well as anticipation of arrhythmia.

Application: Myocardial assessment for focal scar formation, cardiac tumor and thrombus assessment.

Three-Dimensional Contrast-Enhanced Magnetic Resonance Angiography. Three-dimensional contrast-enhanced magnetic resonance angiography (CE-MRA) is a fast spoiled GRE sequence performed using a single breath-hold to obtain a high-resolution three-dimensional data set of the heart. Data are displayed as two-dimensional images that can be visualized in any plane or volume rendered to a three-dimensional image (Fig. 36.3).[11] Gadolinium is typically used as the contrast agent (dose 0.1 to 0.2 mmol/kg). If multiple data sets are acquired over shorter acquisition time, dynamic contrast flow can be demonstrated in vascular structures, resembling contrast angiography via cardiac catheterization ("time-resolved" MRA).[12] This is useful when visualization of contrast passage in all phases of the cardiac cycle is important; however, spatial resolution is typically less than with CE-MRA, and artifact susceptibility is higher (Fig. 36.4, Video 36.2). Use of CE-MRA or time-resolved MRA can replace cardiac catheterization for some cases when delineation of the anatomy is the primary question.[13,14]

Application: Definition of extracardiac vascular structures (e.g., pulmonary arteries, anomalous pulmonary veins, aortic arch abnormalities, systemic veins, collateral vessels, surgical shunts, and conduits).

First-Pass Perfusion Imaging. First-pass perfusion imaging is used to visualize the passage of contrast through the myocardium. Poorly perfused areas are darker, whereas normally perfused regions

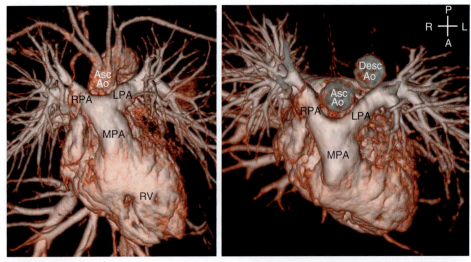

• **Figure 36.3** Magnetic resonance angiogram demonstrating postoperative anatomy after an arterial switch operation with the Lecompte procedure. *A*, Anterior; *Asc Ao*, ascending aorta; *Desc Ao*, descending aorta; *L*, left; *LPA*, left pulmonary artery; *MPA*, main pulmonary artery; *P*, posterior; *R*, right; *RPA*, right pulmonary artery; *RV*, right ventricle.

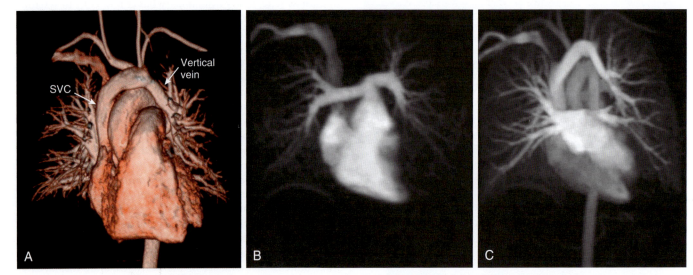

• **Figure 36.4** Triggered magnetic resonance angiogram (MRA) demonstrating supracardiac anomalous pulmonary venous return. (A) MRA showing the vertical vein to superior vena cava *(SVC)*. (B and C; Video 36.2) Contrast (via right arm injection) flows into the SVC and branch pulmonary arteries, with normal pulmonary venous return through the right and left lower pulmonary vein. The left upper pulmonary vein drains anomalously to the SVC via a vertical vein.

are brighter with contrast.[15] Images can be acquired at rest or during stress (via administration of adenosine or similar coronary vasodilator).

Application: Evaluate coronary perfusion if concern for coronary obstruction[16] following coronary reimplantation surgery (arterial switch operation or anomalous coronary repair), Kawasaki disease.

Parametric Mapping. T1 and T2 parametric mapping sequences are gaining importance in myocardial tissue characterization. T1 maps are useful for quantification of diffuse fibrosis (compared with regional scarring as depicted by LGE), whereas T2 maps can help distinguish areas of edema or hyperemia. Parametric mapping sequences provide a *quantitative* assessment of myocardial

involvement, compared with existing sequences such as T1- or T2-weighted imaging, which rely on visual estimates of signal intensity.[17] Application of these techniques are evolving for monitoring of disease progression, as well as therapy.

New Sequences

Four-Dimensional Flow Magnetic Resonance Imaging. Two-dimensional PC, as described previously, measures volume of blood flow in a single direction assigned perpendicular to direction of flow. An emerging technique in flow measurement encodes velocity in three spatial dimensions over time in the cardiac cycle.[18,19] Although it is not in broad clinical use currently, advantages include more comprehensive flow characterization, including those of complex flow patterns; characterization of beat-to-beat variability; and retrospective assessment of blood flow in any vessel within an acquired three-dimensional volume data set. Additional derived-flow parameters include wall shear stress, pulse wave velocity, and energy loss. Multicenter studies are necessary to validate and assess reproducibility of this technique for clinical use, as well as to continue to develop methodologic modifications for shorter scan times.

Frequently Asked Questions

1. When is contrast needed?

Contrast is required for specific pulse sequences as discussed earlier. In general, CE-MRA (for delineation of extracardiac vascular structures, including pulmonary arteries, veins, aortic arch, surgical shunts, and conduits), tissue characterization by LGE, and myocardial perfusion studies require contrast. Assessment of ventricular volumes, cardiac output, and quantification of valvar regurgitation do *not* require contrast administration. In some cases, use of three-dimensional SSFP with respiratory and cardiac gating can provide anatomic data without the use of a contrast agent.

2. My patient had a contrast reaction during computed tomography (CT). Can this patient receive contrast with magnetic resonance imaging (MRI)?

Yes. MRI requires use of gadolinium-based contrast agents (GBCAs), which are different than iodinated CT contrast agents, so allergy to one does not preclude use of the other. In general, most common reactions to GBCAs include nausea, cold sensation at the injection site, vomiting, or itching. Anaphylaxis is rare. The incidence of adverse events related to gadolinium is very low.[1] Patients with acute or chronic kidney disease are at risk for nephrogenic systemic fibrosis with highest risk in those with glomerular filtration rate at less than 30 mL/min/1.73 m².[2] Recent studies have shown preliminary effects of gadolinium deposition in the brain; however, long-term implications are unknown.[3,4]

3. When is anesthesia needed?

A successful CMR scan may require breath-holds to limit motion artifact, though new free-breathing sequences are available. Patients also have to lie still and to understand and comply with multiple breath-holding instructions over a 40- to 60-minute scan. In general, children 8 years and older without developmental delay do not require sedation if adequate preparation is performed before the scan. In some cases, infants may be fed and swaddled before the scan, and high-priority imaging can be accomplished quickly without sedation using free-breathing sequences with both cardiac and respiratory gating. When required, sedation is typically administered in the form of general anesthesia at the discretion of an experienced pediatric anesthesiologist to comply with breath-holding instructions. Complete cardiorespiratory monitoring is undertaken, with ongoing monitoring throughout the scan for adverse effects, including concerns for hypothermia or hyperthermia, rhythm abnormalities, or other anesthesia-related events. The electrocardiographic (ECG) tracing can be used to calculate the patient's heart rate and demonstrate changes in cardiac rhythm, but it cannot be used for diagnostic purposes because the MR signal alters the ECG signal. When need for sedation is unclear, goals of imaging should be discussed with the provider responsible for performance and interpretation of the MRI.

Case Examples

Case 1. *A previously healthy teenager presents with a 3-day history of dyspnea on exertion associated with chest pain at rest. This follows a recent viral illness. The echocardiogram shows poor ventricular function and pericardial effusion.*

Onset of cardiac symptoms and ventricular dysfunction following a recent acute viral illness are most consistent with a diagnosis of acute myocarditis. However, the differential diagnosis for ventricular dysfunction is broad and includes other cardiomyopathies. Dilated cardiomyopathy (DCM) and hypertrophic cardiomyopathy (HCM) are most common[20]; however, left ventricular noncompaction cardiomyopathy (LVNC), restrictive cardiomyopathy, arrhythmogenic right ventricular dysplasia (ARVD), and important coronary anomalies are also part of the differential and must be ruled out. CMR is an important noninvasive diagnostic tool in these cases.

CMR has a sensitivity of 82% in diagnosing pediatric myocarditis.[21] In acute myocarditis CMR can be used to detect inflammation and edema (T2-weighted imaging) in ventricular myocardium. Fibrosis (LGE) may be seen, especially in a patchy subepicardial noncoronary distribution (Fig. 36.5). SSFP imaging provides information about wall motion abnormalities. Right and left ventricular ejection fraction can be quantified in both acute and chronic myocarditis. Newer techniques such as parametric mapping may help quantify myocardial involvement without relying on visual estimation of signal intensity.[22]

DCM may be due to genetic or metabolic disease, cardiotoxic chemotherapy, associated with known neuromuscular disease, or idiopathic. Quantification of ventricular function and mass and serial assessments over time are useful. LGE, if present, is diagnostically useful because it has a characteristic midwall location and does not follow a coronary distribution. In some specific disease states such as Duchenne muscular dystrophy, diffuse fibrosis characterized by parametric mapping may allow for earlier detection and treatment of disease.[23] Acute myocarditis may be ruled out as described in association with clinical history.

For HCM, CMR identifies the pattern of myocardial hypertrophy (septal, concentric, apical, midventricular) with accurate quantification of left ventricular (LV) mass.[24] LGE is usually localized to regions of hypertrophy, and its presence may predict development of arrhythmia[25] (Fig. 36.6). Atrial enlargement (in the setting of ventricular diastolic dysfunction) can also be measured and serially assessed.

Diagnosis of other causes of myocardial dysfunction such as LVNC and ARVD are more challenging in children because criteria are less well defined. LVNC is a cardiomyopathy with presumed arrest of myocardial compaction. Myocardial trabeculae are well seen by CMR, especially when they exist in the apex; however, LGE may not be as useful. For ARVD, right ventricular (RV) wall motion abnormalities, including visualization of segmental thinning and quantification of RV function, are useful by CMR because this imaging can be limited on echocardiogram. RV fatty infiltration into normal myocardium can be assessed on directed T1-weighted spin echo imaging. Given that ARVD typically manifests in the second to fifth decade, criteria may not be sensitive in the pediatric population,[26] and progressive follow-up scans may be recommended to evaluate for onset of disease.

Case 2. *An adolescent who underwent transannular patch repair for tetralogy of Fallot (TOF) as an infant has had increasing exertional intolerance over the past year.*

CMR is ideally suited for postsurgical assessment in TOF in either the presence or absence of symptoms. Despite excellent

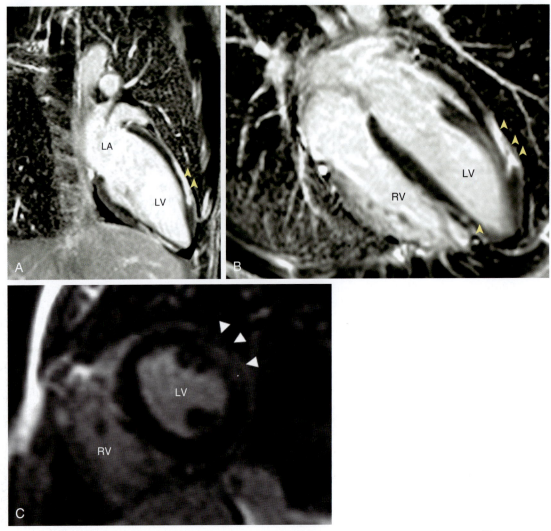

• **Figure 36.5** Delayed enhancement in the mid and inferolateral wall in a patient with myocarditis as seen in the two-chamber (A), four-chamber (B), and short-axis (C) views. Areas of hyperenhancement are indicated by *arrowheads*. *LV,* Left ventricle; *RV,* right ventricle.

long-term survival in repaired patients,[27] long-term morbidity due to hemodynamic and cardiac rhythm disruptions still exists. Chronic pulmonary insufficiency (due to disruption of pulmonary valve annulus at the time of surgery) can lead to RV volume overload with resultant dilation and dysfunction.[28] Follow-up of adult repaired TOF patients showed that severe RV or LV dysfunction (RV ejection fraction < 45%; LV ejection fraction < 55%) and RV dilation (z score > 7) as measured by CMR were independent predictors of major adverse clinical outcomes, including death and ventricular tachycardia.[29] Other long-term morbidities include LV dysfunction, arrhythmia, heart failure, presence of residual ventricular or atrial shunts, RV outflow tract (RVOT) aneurysms and diffuse myocardial fibrosis.[30-32]

Given these known morbidities, data from CMR are invaluable in assessing the cause of new-onset symptoms and determining criteria for further intervention.[33-36] PC sequences are used for quantification of pulmonary valvar regurgitant fraction, as well as differential pulmonary blood flow to each lung (Fig. 36.7, Videos 36.3 and 36.4). Pulmonary regurgitation is generally classified as mild (<20%), moderate (20% to 40%), or severe (>40%).

Proposed parameters for pulmonary valve replacement: RV diastolic volume index above 150 to 160 mL/m^2 or RV end-systolic volume index above 80 mL/m^2.

Morphology of branch pulmonary arteries, RVOT anatomic abnormalities, RV wall motion abnormalities, or abnormal RV ventricular geometry are well seen using customized imaging planes (Fig. 36.8, Videos 36.5 and 36.6). This is especially relevant to the older patient with limited echocardiographic windows. Location and hemodynamic impact of intracardiac shunts can be quantified (using Q_p:Q_s).

RV dimensions, function, and pulmonary regurgitant fraction are critical to decision making regarding surgical pulmonary valve replacement. Delayed gadolinium enhancement is useful in assessment of the adult with repaired TOF for prediction of arrhythmia burden, heart failure and exercise intolerance.[37,38]

Increasing interest in use of percutaneous pulmonary valves in a conduit or dynamic native RVOT underscores the importance of sizing the pulmonary valve annulus and high-resolution imaging of the dynamic RVOT, coronary arteries, and the branch pulmonary arteries.

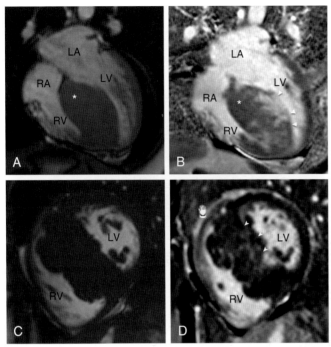

• **Figure 36.6** SSFP image in four-chamber (A) and short-axis (C) views showing severe septal hypertrophy *(asterisk)* in a patient with hypertrophic cardiomyopathy. Corresponding images show significant delayed enhancement in the area of the hypertrophied septum (B and D; *arrowheads*). *LA,* Left atrium; *LV,* left ventricle; *RA,* right atrium; *RV,* right ventricle.

Case 3. *An 8 year old was found to have hypertension on physical examination before sports participation.*

Initial cardiovascular assessment of hypertension in the older child warrants evaluation of aortic coarctation, a localized narrowing in aortic lumen generally at the aortic isthmus (Fig. 36.9). In general, echocardiography is the first choice for imaging and may be sufficient to determine the degree of coarctation and additional aortic arch anatomy. However, in the older child, imaging may be suboptimal or inadequate to delineate precise anatomy and presence and extent of collateralization.

Additional imaging choices include CMR or CT, which may be determined by the ability of this child to undergo a CMR study or clinical status. Both techniques should provide excellent data sets to resolve the anatomy. The specific advantage of CMR over CT is quantification of peak velocity at the level of the coarctation, as well as collateral burden, if suspected. Peak velocity at the level of stenosis can be used to estimate the hemodynamic gradient. Collateral flow is estimated by measuring the difference in flow at the level of the diaphragm and the aortic arch just distal to the obstruction.[39] Anatomic imaging of collaterals is well defined by MRA after gadolinium administration. Additional assessments relevant to aortic coarctation, including cardiac output, LV function and mass, and aortic valve stenosis and regurgitation, can be quantified by CMR.

Following intervention (surgery or balloon or stent angioplasty), CMR is performed to identify sequelae, including residual arch hypoplasia or coarctation and presence of aneurysms and dissections.

Case 4. *Over the past year, a 10-year-old status post non-fenestrated extracardiac Fontan operation at age 4 years has developed worsening cyanosis with an oxygen saturation of 82%.*

The total cavopulmonary connection (Fontan) operation is the final step in the three-step staged palliation for the functionally univentricular heart. The Fontan procedure involves redirection of systemic venous flow directly to the pulmonary arteries while ventricular output is pumped to the body, creating a circulation in series.[40] Variations in type of Fontan connection exist, and knowledge of these should inform assessment in the unknown adult patient with CHD (Fig. 36.10).

CMR is particularly suited to imaging complex postsurgical anatomy, especially in the case of single-ventricle anatomy with variable ventricular geometry.

The specific goals of CMR imaging:
1. *Assessment of anatomy and flow in the Fontan cavopulmonary connection:* Obstructions or baffle leaks can be seen on SSFP cine imaging. PC can be used to quantify blood flow into the superior and inferior vena cava, pulmonary veins, and branch pulmonary arteries, as well as to estimate $Q_p{:}Q_s$.
2. *Ventricular function and cardiac output:* SSFP cine stacks can accurately quantify right or left ventricular volumes and function with superior reproducibility compared with echocardiography.[41] Systemic cardiac output can be obtained by PC at the level of the systemic semilunar valves (or across both semilunar valves in a Damus-Kaye-Stansel type of arch reconstruction).
3. *Quantification of collateral burden:* Aortopulmonary (connection between systemic and pulmonary circulation) or venoatrial collaterals (connection between systemic venous and pulmonary venous circulation) can impose a volume load or cyanosis, respectively. Quantification of the collateral burden has been proposed by flow mapping in CMR by two separate methods with good agreement.[41-43]
    a. *Aortopulmonary collateral:* Flow in ascending aorta – flow in systemic cavae (inferior vena cava and superior vena cava)
    b. *Aortopulmonary collateral:* Total pulmonary venous flow – total flow in branch pulmonary arteries
4. *Presence of thrombi:* Thrombi may be present in up to 30% of the Fontan population with highest risk in the immediate postoperative period[44]; thrombi can be demonstrated by SSFP cine or other specialized black blood imaging.
5. Three-dimensional MRA with contrast or three-dimensional SSFP (noncontrast) sequences define the pulmonary arteries, including distortions or stenosis, aorta, and systemic venous connections.
6. LGE for myocardial fibrosis has been reported to be as high as 28% in the Fontan population and is associated with lower ejection fraction and higher frequency of arrhythmia.[45,46]

Case 5. *A 2 year old is found to have a large RV mass as an incidental finding on echocardiogram.*

Cardiac tumors are rare in children. Approximately 90% of pediatric cardiac tumors are benign. Rhabdomyoma is the most common type, followed by fibroma. The most common malignant cardiac tumor is a sarcoma.[47-49] If adequately imaged, fetal and transthoracic echocardiograms are typically sufficient to make a diagnosis of cardiac tumor; however, the tumor type is not easily characterized. Characterization of tumors by fat content, vascularity, fluid composition, and presence of fibrosis allows for noninvasive diagnosis.

Additional information includes tumor location (including obstruction to blood flow), size, and extent of tumor burden. LGE can also assist with diagnosis of intracardiac thrombi, a common differential in the workup of a cardiac mass. In a multicenter study, if a complete CMR was performed with good image quality,

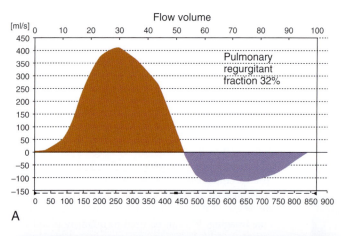

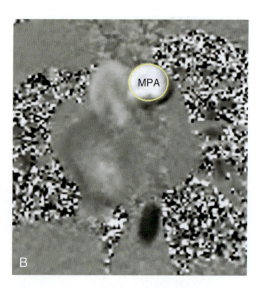

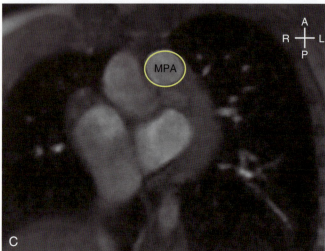

• **Figure 36.7** Main pulmonary artery flow-velocity curves with antegrade and reverse flow (A). (Video 36.3) Phase map representing different velocities (white or black depending on direction of flow) with stationary objects having a speckled appearance (B). (Video 36.4) Magnitude image demonstrating the anatomy of the region of interest (C). *MPA,* Main pulmonary artery.

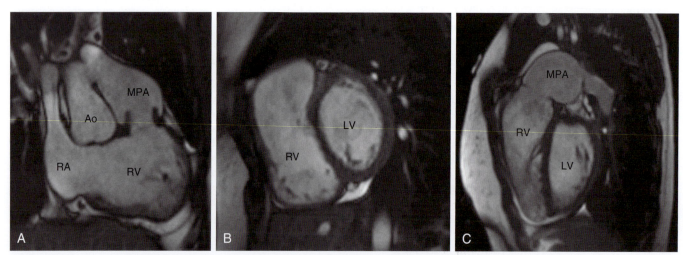

• **Figure 36.8** Dilated aneurysmal main pulmonary artery in a patient with tetralogy of Fallot as demonstrated in the RVOT SSFP image (A). (Video 36.5) Short-axis SSFP cine (B). (Video 36.6) Sagittal RV SSFP cine (C). *Ao,* Aorta; *LV,* left ventricle; *MPA,* main pulmonary artery; *RV,* right ventricle; *RVOT,* right ventricular outflow tract; *SSFP,* steady-state free precession.

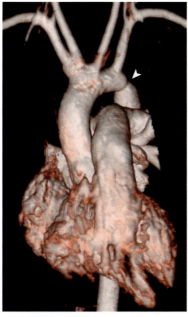

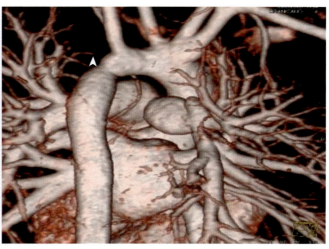

• **Figure 36.9** Aortic coarctation demonstrated on volume-rendered magnetic resonance angiogram just distal to the left pulmonary artery in descending aorta *(arrowhead)* in an adult. Right pulmonary artery stenosis also present (not shown).

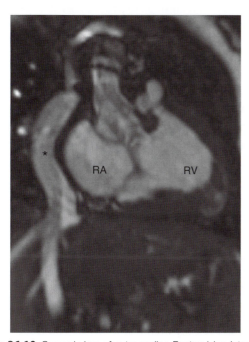

• **Figure 36.10** Coronal view of extracardiac Fontan lying lateral to the right atrium in a patient with hypoplastic left heart syndrome. *Asterisk,* Fontan; *RA,* right atrium; *RV,* right ventricle.

diagnosis of tumor type or a correct differential occurred in 97% of cases (confirmed by pathology).[50]

Typical assessment of tumor type by CMR involves use of specific sequences as outlined by Beroukhim et al.:

1. GRE cine imaging for size, location, and extent of cardiac mass, assessment of ventricular function and size
2. Spin echo (black blood sequences) with T1 and T2 weighting to bring out the properties of the tumor and use of fat suppression to increase diagnostic accuracy

3. Myocardial first-pass perfusion imaging to characterize vascular properties
4. Delayed enhancement imaging to improve recognition of thrombi

Of note, differentiation of malignant versus nonmalignant tumors remains limited using CMR. This is specifically true for vascular tumors in which vascularity can be classified; however, malignancy cannot be ruled out.

Noninvasive Calculation of Cardiac Output, Q_p/Q_s, and Valvar Regurgitated Fraction

Measurement of flow and velocity are integral to assessment and decision making in CHD. The principles outlined below can be applied to the breadth of congenital cardiac disease for simple or complex lesions.

Specific quantitative data provided by CMR include:

1. Stroke volume (milliliters per cardiac cycle) and cardiac output (liters per minute)
2. Shunt quantification (Q_p:Q_s): ratio of pulmonary blood flow (Q_p) to systemic blood flow (Q_s)
3. Valve regurgitant fraction (%)
4. Quantification of collateral flow

Cardiac Output and Stroke Volume. To assess flow by PC a cross-sectional region is defined and blood flowing perpendicular to the defined plane is quantified. In the case of cardiac output a plane perpendicular to blood flow is defined in the ascending aorta. Regions of interest are drawn around the vessel in systole and diastole to obtain a flow volume over time. This provides the stroke volume over one cardiac cycle and can be used to calculate cardiac output.

Estimation of Shunt Fraction (Q_p:Q_s). In the absence of shunts, pulmonary and systemic blood flow are equal (i.e., Q_p:Q_s = 1). In the presence of shunts, in right-to-left shunt, Q_p:Q_s is less than 1; in left-to-right shunt, Q_p:Q_s is greater than 1.

In general, flow measurements in the ascending aorta are quantified in this way (Q_s). A similar measurement is made in the main pulmonary artery (Q_p), including other sources of pulmonary blood flow if present (e.g., shunts). In the absence of significant semilunar or atrioventricular valve regurgitation or intracardiac shunts, RV and LV stroke volumes derived from short-axis cine images should be the same and may be used for confirmation and internal consistency. Quantification of shunt fraction by CMR has been shown to correlate well with angiographically derived measurements.[51,52]

Valve Regurgitant Fraction or Stenosis

Semilunar Valve Regurgitant Fraction. Blood flow is directly measured just distal to the pulmonary or aortic valve annulus and displayed using a flow curve representing antegrade and retrograde flow in the main pulmonary artery over time. The example shown for pulmonary regurgitant fraction (PRF) below is commonly used for surgical or interventional decision making in TOF (see Fig. 36.7).

$$PRF\ (\%) = Retrograde\ flow\ (mL)/Antegrade\ flow\ (mL)$$

Other techniques:

$$PRF\ (\%) = [RV\ volume\ (mL) - LV\ volume\ (mL)]/$$
$$RV\ volume\ (mL)$$

(assuming absence of intracardiac shunts or significant tricuspid insufficiency).

Atrioventricular Valve Regurgitant Fraction. Direct velocity mapping of the atrioventricular valve is limited by through-plane motion of the valve during the cardiac cycle. It is most reliably estimated by the difference in the ventricular stroke volume and forward flow. For example:

Mitral valve insufficiency (%)
$$= [LV\ stroke\ volume\ (mL) - Aortic\ stroke\ volume\ (mL)]/$$
$$LV\ stroke\ volume\ (mL)$$

Semilunar Valve Stenosis. Regions of interest drawn in a plane perpendicular to the stenotic jet provide information about peak velocity in the cardiac cycle, which can denote a pressure gradient. Of note, extra care must be undertaken in the assessment of stenotic lesions with eccentric flow to ensure that the PC plane is directly perpendicular to the direction of the jet. Also the site of stenosis must also be defined (subvalvar, valvar, or supravalvar) to correctly define the mechanism of stenosis. This can be accomplished by assigning the PC plane parallel to the flow (in-plane PC) and then assigning a through-plane PC acquisition to quantify the degree of stenosis.

Computed Tomography

When Computed Tomography Is Particularly Useful

Compared with CMR, CT can provide higher spatial resolution (<1 mm in all planes) but lower temporal resolution ($\approx$80 ms) and is particularly useful in assessing extracardiac anatomy (e.g., shunts, conduit and branch pulmonary arteries, aortic dissection, coronary artery abnormalities, vascular rings and slings) and pulmonary or airway pathology. Images are acquired rapidly over a few seconds, reducing the need for sedation or breath-holding in small children. Patients on support devices are more easily imaged

with CT than CMR. A limitation of CT is the radiation, which is particularly important in children and when multiple scans are needed.[53,54]

How the Computed Tomography Radiation Dose Can Be Reduced

The radiation dose can be reduced through modification of these components[54-57]:

Tube potential (kilovolt peak [kVp]): Systematic use of 70 to 80 kVp (as opposed to 120 kVp typically used in adults) reduces radiation and contrast dose.

Tube current (milliampere-second [mAs]): Adjustment is based on the child's size.

High pitch: Pitch is the table movement per rotation divided by the collimated beam width; increasing pitch results in decreased radiation dose.

Prospective gating (step-and-shoot): ECG-triggered acquisition timed for a specific portion of the cardiac cycle. Sometimes retrospective gating with radiation delivered throughout the cardiac cycle is needed for calculation of ventricular volumes and ejection fraction at the cost of a higher radiation dose.

"Ultra–low-dose" pediatric protocols allow effective doses of less than 1 mSv in comparison to portable chest radiographs, which have an effective dose of approximately 0.05 mSv, and cardiac catheterization, which ranges from 5 to 15 mSv (depending on many factors such as the age and size of the patient and the experience of the operator).

Other Changes in Computed Tomography Technology That Affect Image Quality and Radiation Dose

Dual-source CT: Two x-ray tubes and two detectors are arranged at a 90-degree angle, effectively doubling the temporal resolution of the scan at the same rotation speed.

Ultrawide detectors: Newer 4-cm detectors (compared to 2-cm) allow for decreased acquisition time and less sensitivity to respiratory motion.

Iterative reconstruction: Newly developed reconstruction algorithm, which improves image quality over traditional filtered back projection technique, compensating for noisier image data, which are often associated with using low kilovolt peak and milliampere-second. This method is a computationally intensive postprocessing technique and can be applied after image acquisition.

When Contrast Is Needed

Intravenous contrast is needed for imaging cardiovascular anatomy and vascular or graft patency and integrity. For nonvascular imaging, such as the airways, no contrast is necessary if the relationship with vascular structures is not important. Contrast is always necessary for cardiac imaging.

When Sedation Is Needed

For detailed coronary anatomy or ventricular function in children with high heart rates, imaging is obtained over several heartbeats and generally requires at least one breath-hold. For patients younger than 5 to 6 years of age, this may require general anesthesia. However, for noncoronary or only proximal coronary anatomy, imaging can be obtained without breath-holding. Thus most infants can be swaddled and imaged without sedation, patients 6 months to 3 years of age often require conscious sedation, and patients older than 4 years (depending on development) can often cooperate with holding still without any sedation.

Case Examples

Case 1. *How do I exclude a coronary artery abnormality in a previously healthy teenager who experiences a cardiac arrest while exercising and for whom echocardiography shows poor ventricular function?*

Congenital coronary artery anomalies of course or origin are typically identified using echocardiography in neonates and toddlers. In the emergent setting in this case of the teenager with exertional arrest, in which suspicion for coronary abnormality (such as abnormal aortic origin of the left coronary artery) is high, CT has excellent spatial resolution and is frequently superior to echocardiography outside the neonatal period. Coronary abnormalities diagnosed with CT include ostial atresia, anomalous origin from the pulmonary artery, and anomalous aortic origin with interarterial or intramural course. Coronary fistula would not typically result in exertional arrest. The evaluation of acute chest pain may include a broader differential diagnosis, including pulmonary embolism or aortic dissection, for which CT is also diagnostic. Sometimes multiple-phase acquisition is required (termed a *triple–rule-out scan*) (Fig. 36.11).

Case 2. *How do I exclude a vascular ring or sling in a 2 month old with worsening inspiratory stridor?*

Vascular ring or pulmonary sling is generally first diagnosed by echocardiography, but to image associated airway abnormalities, CT is useful and does not require anesthesia. MRI can also be used to evaluate for vascular ring or sling; however, MRI may provide a less detailed evaluation of the airways and has the disadvantages of longer scan time and the possible need for sedation in a patient with a compromised airway. New techniques in free-breathing MRI are also used in younger patients as a mean to avoid anesthesia (Fig. 36.12A).

Case 3. *How do I exclude aortic dissection in an adolescent with Marfan syndrome presenting with severe acute chest pain?*

Patients with aortopathies, including Marfan syndrome, are at increased risk of aortic dissection, aneurysm, and cardiac valve disease. Surveillance of asymptomatic patients is performed optimally with echocardiography in coordination with CMR (in patients old enough to not require sedation). In the emergent setting, CT is the modality of choice and requires ECG gating for evaluating coronary artery involvement. CT also allows for clear definition of extent of dissection and involvement of major aortic branch vessels, as well as the pleural and pericardial spaces. Additionally, ischemia of organs affected, such as renal infarction, can be assessed with CT (Fig. 36.13).

Case 4. *How do I exclude shunt thrombosis or distortion in the acutely cyanotic neonate status post placement of modified right Blalock-Taussig shunt or RV to pulmonary artery conduit?*

Acute obstruction of pulmonary blood flow can occur with systemic to pulmonary shunts or less commonly in ventricular to pulmonary artery conduits used in the staged palliation of single-ventricle lesions and requires immediate diagnosis. Although diagnosis and intervention by cardiac catheterization can be undertaken, rapid CT diagnosis of thrombus can allow urgent thrombolytic therapy and provide a "road map" before surgical or transcatheter therapy (Fig. 36.14).

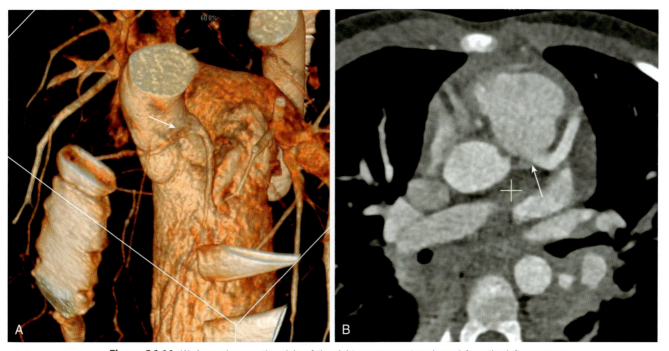

• **Figure 36.11** (A) Anomalous aortic origin of the right coronary artery *(arrow)* from the left coronary sinus immediately adjacent to the left coronary origin. (B) Anomalous origin of the left coronary artery *(arrow)* from the main pulmonary artery.

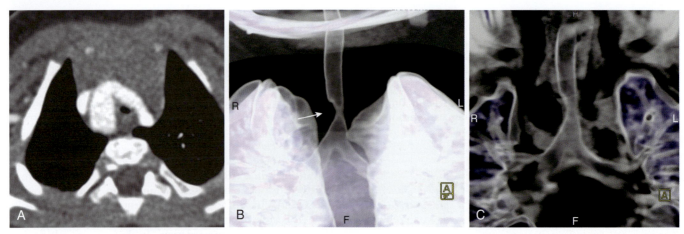

• **Figure 36.12** (A) Double aortic arch demonstrated in the axial plane showing a dominant right arch with smaller left arch encircling the trachea and esophagus. (B) Reformatting in the coronal plan shows that the tracheal narrowing is predominantly on the right aspect *(arrow)*. (C) Reformatting in coronal plane but with the windowing allowing visualization of the right *(R)* and left *(L)* arches.

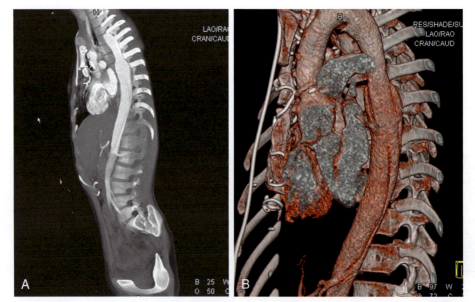

• **Figure 36.13** Stanford type B (DeBakey type III) dissection involving the thoracic and abdominal aorta. (A) Maximal intensity projection. (B) Rendered image, which provides an assisted visualization of the findings.

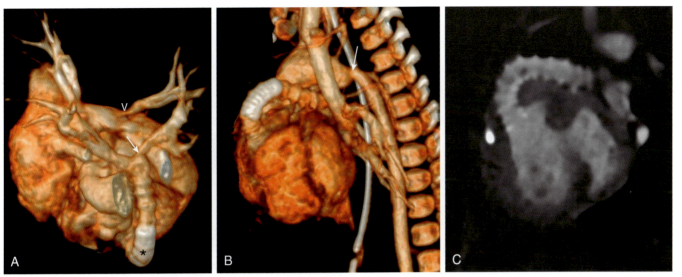

• **Figure 36.14** (A) Neonate with hypoplastic left heart syndrome with a Sano modification, including a right ventricular to pulmonary artery conduit *(asterisk)*. Note the moderate narrowing of the proximal left pulmonary artery *(arrow)* and possible mild narrowing at the left pulmonary vein *(V)*. (B) Same patient viewed in sagittal projection shows mild coarctation *(arrow)*. (C) Associated with gradually falling saturation, computed tomography demonstrated thrombus, which catheterization confirmed and where a stent was placed.

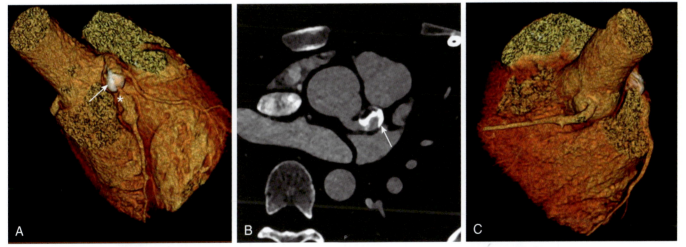

• **Figure 36.15** (A) Multiple saccular aneurysms of the left anterior descending coronary artery *(asterisk)*, and the proximal aneurysm is calcified *(arrow)*. (B) The calcification of the proximal aneurysm *(arrow)* is well seen in this reformatted axial image. Note the coronary narrowing immediately distal to the calcification. (C) Mild fusiform coronary aneurysm involving the proximal right coronary artery.

Case 5. *How should I best image coronary artery aneurysms seen on echocardiography in a toddler with Kawasaki disease?*

Kawasaki disease–related vasculopathy presents as coronary artery aneurysms, which can be complicated by progressive stenosis, leading to cardiac ischemia. Evaluation of the coronary arteries can be performed with conventional angiography, CT, or MRI. If intervention is suspected to be likely, angiography is the best choice in the emergent setting. CT is optimal for evaluating the degree of stenosis and calcification. Evaluation of the coronary arteries by MRI is less sensitive than CT, especially in the mid to distal coronary arteries and for identification of calcification (Fig. 36.15).

Case 6. *A newborn with totally anomalous pulmonary venous return where the anatomy of the individual pulmonary veins requires further delineation.*

Cyanosis was noted immediately after birth. Echocardiogram confirmed infradiaphragmatic totally anomalous pulmonary venous return, but all the pulmonary veins were not seen separately (Fig. 36.16).

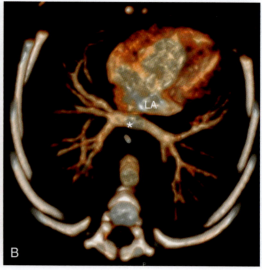

• **Figure 36.16** (A) Infradiaphragmatic totally anomalous pulmonary venous return. There is narrowing as the descending vein enters the liver *(arrow)*. (B) Axial image showing the pulmonary venous confluence *(asterisk)* including all 4 pulmonary veins as well as relationship to the left atrium *(LA)* for surgical planning

Selected References

A complete list of references is available at ExpertConsult.com.

1. Finn JP, Nael K, Deshpande V, et al. Cardiac MR imaging: state of the technology. *Radiology.* 2006;241:338–354.
4. Powell AJ, Geva T. Blood flow measurement by magnetic resonance imaging in congenital heart disease. *Pediatr Cardiol.* 2000;21:47–58.
10. Harris MA, Johnson TR, Weinberg PM, et al. Delayed- enhancement cardiovascular magnetic resonance identifies fibrous tissue in children after surgery for congenital heart disease. *J Thorac Cardiovasc Surg.* 2007;133:676–681.
11. Masui T, Katayama M, Kobayashi S, et al. Gadolinium-enhanced MR angiography in the evaluation of congenital cardiovascular disease pre- and postoperative states in infants and children. *J Magn Reson Imaging.* 2000;12:1034–1042.
15. Gebker R, Schwitter J, Fleck E, et al. How we perform myocardial perfusion with cardiovascular magnetic resonance. *J Cardiovasc Magn Reson.* 2007;9(3):539–547.
29. Knauth AL, Gauvreau K, Powell AJ, et al. Ventricular size and function assessed by cardiac MRI predict major adverse clinical outcomes late after tetralogy of Fallot repair. *Heart.* 2008;94:211–216.
41. Margossian R, Schwartz ML, Prakash A, et al. Pediatric Heart Network Investigators. Comparison of echocardiographic and cardiac magnetic resonance imaging measurements of functional single ventricular volumes, mass, and ejection fraction (from the Pediatric Heart Network Fontan Cross-Sectional Study). *Am J Cardiol.* 2009;104:419–428.
52. Hundley WG, Li HF, Lange RA, et al. Assessment of left-to-right intracardiac shunting by velocity-encoded, phase-difference magnetic resonance imaging. A comparison with oximetric and indicator dilution techniques. *Circulation.* 1995;91:2955–2960.

37

Cardiac Catheterization Laboratory

KEVIN D. HILL, MD, MSCI; JENNIFER ROARK, MSN, FNP-C;
GREGORY A. FLEMING, MD, MSCI

Diagnostic Cardiac Catheterization

The role of congenital cardiac catheterization has evolved since its introduction in the 1940s.[1] Advances in noninvasive imaging have decreased the role of catheterization as a primary diagnostic modality, yet the number of and indications for cardiac catheterization have increased substantially.[2] Partly this is attributable to a burgeoning number of transcatheter interventions that have markedly expanded the role of therapeutic cardiac catheterization.[2] However, diagnostic cardiac catheterization remains an important tool in the assessment of many different cardiac lesions and conditions. In contemporary reports from multicenter registries, approximately half of all congenital cardiac catheterizations are diagnostic procedures without any intervention.[3-5] This underscores the importance of thorough hemodynamic evaluation and accurate interpretation of data. However, it is also important to understand the limitations of cardiac catheterization, which provides only a snapshot assessment of physiology with hemodynamic data typically obtained under nonphysiologic conditions (e.g., general anesthesia, mechanical ventilation). Moreover, flow, shunt, and resistance calculations have several potential sources of error.[6,7] For these reasons, data obtained from a cardiac catheterization should always be interpreted cautiously and considered in the context of the patient's clinical course.

Assessment of Saturation Data

Saturation data are used to calculate flows and to estimate intracardiac shunting. Only four principal saturation data points are needed—a systemic and mixed venous saturation to calculate systemic flows, and a pulmonary arterial and pulmonary venous saturation to calculate pulmonary flows.[7] In a patient with no intracardiac shunting the pulmonary venous saturation and systemic arterial saturations are equivalent, and the mixed venous saturation is best represented by the most distal saturation, typically the right or left branch pulmonary artery (PA) saturation. Thus in the absence of an intracardiac shunt, only two saturations are needed. Despite this, congenitally trained interventional cardiologists will always obtain saturations (sometimes several) from multiple locations throughout the heart and lungs to overcome potential sampling errors, which are particularly prevalent when there has been inadequate mixing of blood from various sources.[6] Fig. 37.1 summarizes normal saturation ranges and demonstrates the expected range of sampling error at various locations throughout the heart. Sampling error is greatest in chambers receiving blood from multiple sources (e.g., the right atrium) and is lowest in the distal branch PAs due to more complete mixing of blood.

When there is a left-to-right shunt lesion (e.g., atrial septal defect [ASD] or ventricular septal defect [VSD]), there will be an increase (step-up) in saturations into the PAs reflecting the degree of shunting. In this scenario the pulmonary arterial saturation no longer accurately represents the mixed venous saturation. Instead the superior vena cava (SVC) saturation is typically used as the next best source for mixed venous saturation. In our opinion the SVC saturation is preferable to the inferior vena cava (IVC) saturation for estimating mixed venous saturation due to the wide variability in saturations in the IVC, which receives blood streaming from the low-saturation hepatic veins and from the higher-saturated renal circulation.[6,8] When systemic desaturation is present, it is important to obtain saturations directly from the pulmonary veins to determine whether desaturation is from right-to-left shunting, pulmonary venous desaturation, or a combination of the two.

Assessment of Pressure Data

Pressure measurements on the right side of the heart are typically obtained in bilateral branch PAs, the main PA, right ventricle, and right atrium. On the left side of the heart, a pulmonary capillary wedge pressure (PCWP) may be used to estimate left atrial pressures (unless there is an ASD or patent foramen ovale permitting direct assessment), and direct pressure measurements are obtained in the left ventricle, ascending aorta, and descending aorta. Any pressure gradient reflects a degree of obstruction across the vascular structure being evaluated. Fig. 37.2 summarizes the normal range of pressures in the various chambers of the heart and in the lungs. Fig. 37.2 demonstrates normal intravascular waveforms, and Fig. 37.3 provides select examples of abnormal pressure tracings in patients with obstructive lesions. Typically peak systolic or "peak-to-peak" gradients are used to estimate stenosis of the semilunar valves or arterial vascular structures (e.g., aortic stenosis, coarctation of the aorta), whereas mean gradients are used to estimate venous or atrioventricular (AV) valve stenosis. When AV valve stenosis is being evaluated, an estimate of the severity of stenosis can be obtained by comparing the atrial a-wave and the ventricular end-diastolic pressure. However, the most accurate measure of AV valve stenosis is obtained by measuring the area under the curve for simultaneously obtained atrial pressures (or PCWP in place of the left atrial pressure) and ventricular pressures (see Fig. 37.3C). When a patient is on the ventilator, pressure measurements are made at end expiration to minimize the effects of intrathoracic pressure on intracardiac pressures

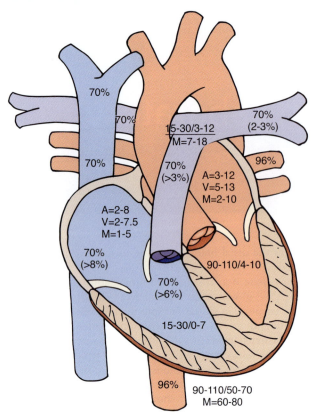

• **Figure 37.1** Range of normal pressure and saturations in children and adolescents. Saturations in parentheses represent the approximate sampling error in the various cardiac chambers. *A,* Atrial wave peak pressure; *M,* mean pressure; *V,* ventricular wave peak pressure.

TABLE 37.1	Equations Used for Catheterization Laboratory Calculations

$$Q_s = \frac{VO_2}{\text{Systemic arterial } O_2 \text{ content} - \text{mixed venous } O_2 \text{ content}}$$

$$Q_p = \frac{VO_2}{\text{Pulmonary venous } O_2 \text{ content} - \text{pulmonary arterial } O_2 \text{ content}}$$

$$Q_p{:}Q_s = \frac{\text{Systemic arterial saturation} - \text{mixed venous saturation}}{\text{Pulmonary venous saturation} - \text{pulmonary arterial saturation}}$$

$$Q_{ep} = \frac{VO_2}{\text{Pulmonary venous } O_2 \text{ content} - \text{mixed venous } O_2 \text{ content}}$$

$$Q_{es} = \frac{VO_2}{\text{Pulmonary venous } O_2 \text{ content} - \text{mixed venous } O_2 \text{ content}}$$

$$L \rightarrow R \text{ shunt} = Q_p - Q_{ep}$$

$$R \rightarrow L \text{ shunt} = Q_s - Q_{es}$$

$$PVRI = \frac{\text{Mean PA pressure} - \text{mean LA (PCW) pressure}}{Q_p}$$

$$SVRI = \frac{\text{Mean systemic pressure} - \text{mean RA pressure}}{Q_s}$$

O_2 content = [Hgb (g/dL) × 10 (dl/L) × 1.36 (mL O_2/g Hgb) × O_2 saturation] × [0.003 × PaO$_2$].

Hgb, Hemoglobin; *L,* left; *LA,* left atrium; *PA,* pulmonary artery; *PCW,* pulmonary capillary wedge; *PVRI,* pulmonary vascular resistance index; Q_{ep}, effective pulmonary blood flow; Q_{es}, effective systemic blood flow; Q_p, pulmonary blood flow; Q_s, systemic blood flow; *R,* right; *RA,* right atrium; *SVRI,* systemic vascular resistance index; *VO$_2$,* volume of oxygen utilization.

Calculations of Flows

Pulmonary (Q_p) and systemic (Q_s) blood flow is estimated in the catheterization laboratory using the Fick method, which requires measuring the rate of change of an indicator through the heart or across a vascular bed. The two most common indicators are cold saline and oxygen content. When cold saline indicator is used, the approach is known as thermodilution and requires a specific catheter (e.g., thermodilution or Swan-Ganz catheter) with a proximal side hole and a distal thermistor.[9] The side hole is positioned in the right atrium or a systemic vein while the thermistor is positioned in a branch PA. A known quantity of saline that is at least 10 degrees colder than the patient's body temperature (typically 5 to 10 mL) is injected rapidly through the side hole into the right atrium. If cardiac output is high, then the cold saline mixes with a relatively larger amount of blood, and the temperature change at the thermistor is therefore relatively small. If cardiac output is low, then the cold saline mixes with a smaller quantity of blood, and the temperature change at the thermistor is more dramatic. The thermodilution technique is not accurate whenever there is disruption of flow, for example, if there is significant tricuspid valve regurgitation, pulmonary valve regurgitation, or an intracardiac shunt. As an alternative to cold saline, oxygen content can be used as the indicator. If one knows the rate at which oxygen is being added or extracted from the vascular bed (estimated by the patient's volume of oxygen utilization [VO$_2$]), then flow can be estimated based upon the change in oxygen content.

Table 37.1 lists some of the important equations that are used in the cardiac catheterization laboratory to calculate flows using the Fick principle.

VO$_2$ represents the rate of oxygen consumption by the body, which is equivalent to the rate of oxygen delivery by the lungs. VO$_2$ can be directly measured but is more commonly estimated using heart rate and age-dependent tables published in 1970 by Lafarge and Miettinen.[10] Estimated VO$_2$ is a significant potential source of error in catheterization calculations. Rutledge and colleagues[11] demonstrated greater than 50% error when VO$_2$ estimates were applied to mechanically ventilated children less than 3 years of age, and Seckeler and colleagues[12] identified single-ventricle anatomy and critical illness as additional sources of substantial error. These limitations should be considered when evaluating cardiac catheterization data reliant upon VO$_2$ (e.g., Q_p, Q_s, and pulmonary vascular resistance [PVR]). Ratios such as $Q_p{:}Q_s$ and pulmonary to systemic vascular resistance (PVR:SVR) eliminate VO$_2$ from the equation and are helpful in evaluating catheterization data. It is also important to consider the entirety of the data without placing excess emphasis on any single measured, estimated, or calculated number.

Estimating Shunts

The ratio of pulmonary to systemic blood flow ($Q_p{:}Q_s$) is an important consideration in many congenital heart lesions. In a

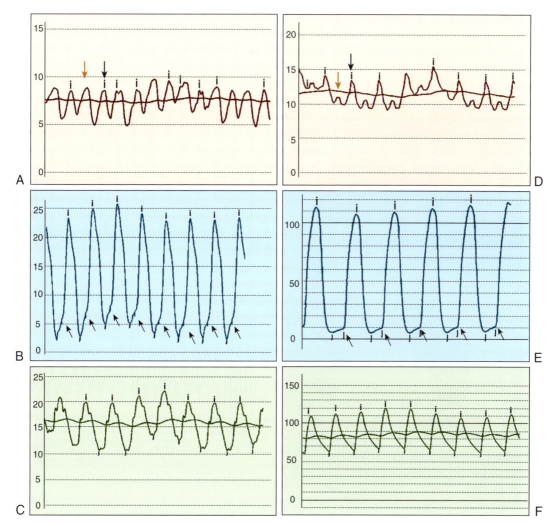

• **Figure 37.2** Intracardiac pressure waveforms: (A) Right atrium with an *a*-wave *(red arrow)* corresponding to atrial contraction, *v*-wave *(black arrow)* corresponding to ventricular contraction when the tricuspid valve bulges into the right atrium, and a mean atrial pressure of 7 to 8 mm Hg. (B) Right ventricle with a systolic pressure of 23 to 26 mm Hg and an end-diastolic pressure *(arrows)* of 5 to 8 mm Hg. (C) PA pressures with a systolic pressure of 20 to 22 mm Hg, diastolic pressure of 12 to 15 mm Hg, and a mean PA pressure of 16 to 17 mm Hg. (D) Pulmonary capillary wedge pressure demonstrating an *a*-wave corresponding to atrial contraction *(red arrow)*, a prominent *v*-wave *(black arrow)* secondary to moderate mitral regurgitation in this patient, and a mean pressure of 11 to 12 mm Hg. (E) Left ventricular pressure with a peak systolic pressure of 109 to 116 mm Hg and an end-diastolic pressure *(arrows)* of 8 to 11 mm Hg. (F) Descending aortic pressure demonstrating, systole, diastole, and a mean pressure.

patient breathing room air (21% fraction of inspired O_2 [FiO_2]) Q_p:Q_s can be easily estimated using the following equation:

$$Q_p{:}Q_s = \frac{\text{Systemic arterial saturation} - \text{mixed venous saturation}}{\text{Pulmonary venous saturation} - \text{pulmonary arterial saturation}}$$

This equation is not accurate when a patient is breathing a significantly higher FiO_2 because it does not consider dissolved O_2 (i.e., O_2 that is not bound to hemoglobin). In room air, dissolved O_2 contributes relatively little to the oxygen content of blood and can be ignored, but this is not the case when a patient is breathing a higher FiO_2. When a patient has bidirectional shunting, it is often helpful to estimate the magnitude of the right-to-left and

left-to-right shunts in addition to the Q_p:Q_s ratio. These can be obtained by calculating the patient's effective pulmonary blood flow, which represents the volume of desaturated blood flowing to the pulmonary vascular bed (i.e., excluding any left-to-right shunt), and the effective systemic blood flow, which represents the volume of fully saturated blood flowing to the systemic vascular bed (i.e., excluding any right-to left-shunt). Note from Table 37.1 that the equations for effective pulmonary and systemic blood flow estimation are identical. Fig. 37.4 documents catheterization data from a patient with transposition physiology, demonstrating a clinical scenario in which understanding effective pulmonary and systemic blood flow, as well as right-to-left and left-to-right shunting, may be useful. In this patient, and any patient with transposition physiology, the Q_p:Q_s is often high, but the effective pulmonary blood flow is low, leading to severe systemic desaturation.

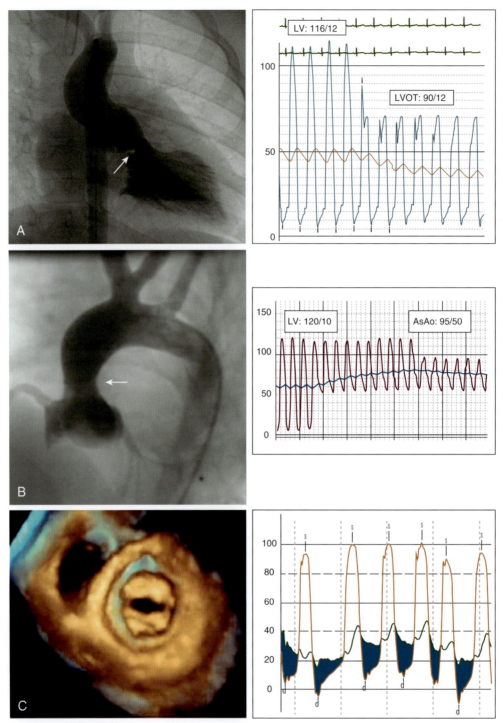

• **Figure 37.3** Examples of abnormal hemodynamic findings. (A) Subaortic stenosis. There is a systolic pressure gradient of 46 mm Hg as the catheter is pulled back across the left ventricular outflow tract. However, the pressure waveform continues to demonstrate a left ventricular trace consistent with subaortic stenosis. Angiography demonstrates the subaortic obstruction *(arrow)*. (B) Supravalvar aortic stenosis. There is no change in systolic pressure when the waveform initially changes from a ventricular trace to an aortic trace. As the catheter is retracted further into the distal ascending aorta, the systolic pressure drops, indicating mild supravalvar stenosis, which is demonstrated in the angiogram. (C) Mitral stenosis. The *shaded area* on the pressure trace demarcates a mean pressure difference of 12 mm Hg between the pulmonary capillary wedge pressure and the left ventricular pressure during diastole. The three-dimensional echocardiography image demonstrates a thickened, stenotic mitral valve. *AsAo,* Ascending aorta; *LV,* left ventricle; *LVOT,* left ventricular outflow tract.

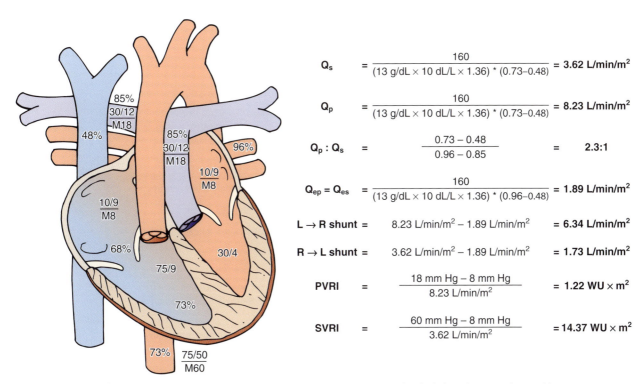

$$Q_s = \frac{160}{(13\ g/dL \times 10\ dL/L \times 1.36)\ *\ (0.73-0.48)} = 3.62\ L/min/m^2$$

$$Q_p = \frac{160}{(13\ g/dL \times 10\ dL/L \times 1.36)\ *\ (0.73-0.48)} = 8.23\ L/min/m^2$$

$$Q_p : Q_s = \frac{0.73 - 0.48}{0.96 - 0.85} = 2.3:1$$

$$Q_{ep} = Q_{es} = \frac{160}{(13\ g/dL \times 10\ dL/L \times 1.36)\ *\ (0.96-0.48)} = 1.89\ L/min/m^2$$

$$L \rightarrow R\ shunt = 8.23\ L/min/m^2 - 1.89\ L/min/m^2 = 6.34\ L/min/m^2$$

$$R \rightarrow L\ shunt = 3.62\ L/min/m^2 - 1.89\ L/min/m^2 = 1.73\ L/min/m^2$$

$$PVRI = \frac{18\ mm\ Hg - 8\ mm\ Hg}{8.23\ L/min/m^2} = 1.22\ WU \times m^2$$

$$SVRI = \frac{60\ mm\ Hg - 8\ mm\ Hg}{3.62\ L/min/m^2} = 14.37\ WU \times m^2$$

• **Figure 37.4** Case study demonstrating catheterization data and calculations in a newborn with d-transposition of the great arteries. Calculations are based upon the equations presented in the *right panel*. In this child there is severe systemic desaturation despite a $Q_p{:}Q_s$ of 2.1:1. This occurs because much of the pulmonary blood flow represents fully saturated blood from the pulmonary venous circulation. The effective pulmonary (Q_{ep}) and systemic (Q_{es}) blood flows, which respectively represent desaturated blood shunting right to left and saturated blood shunting left to right across the atrial septum, are low. In transposition this shunt is referred to as the "anatomic shunt," and the left-to-right versus right-to-left shunts are always equivalent. These values must be differentiated from "physiologic" left-to-right and right-to-left shunts, which respectively represent the amount of fully saturated blood that is recirculating back to the lungs (physiologic left-to-right shunt) and desaturated blood that is recirculating back to the body (physiologic right-to-left shunt).

Calculating Resistance

Resistance is calculated as the change in mean pressure divided by flow (see Table 37.1). The concept of resistance is particularly important in congenital heart disease because many shunt lesions can affect pulmonary or systemic pressures and blood flow. In patients with posttricuspid shunt lesions, PA pressures alone do not accurately reflect a patient's operative risk, and the PVR is more relevant. Importantly, however, standard PVR calculations are unreliable when there is branch PA stenosis because the relative right- versus left-sided flow and pressures will differ. In this scenario PVR can be reliably estimated only if the relative flow distribution and pressure in each lung segment is known. Because the lungs represent resistors in parallel, each individual lung actually has a higher resistance value than the combined resistance of the two lungs together. This is evident from the equation for calculating total resistance when there are multiple resistors in parallel:

$$\frac{1}{\text{Total lung resistance}} = \frac{1}{\text{Left lung resistance}} + \frac{1}{\text{Right lung resistance}}$$

Thus if a patient has a pulmonary vascular resistance index (PVRI) of 2 Wood units (WU)•m², one can appreciate that each individual lung will have a resistance of 4 WU•m² (assuming equal flow distribution). This concept is occasionally important in critically ill children with heart disease when it is necessary to understand if the patient might have underlying pulmonary vascular disease. For example, consider a patient with severe hypoplasia or complete agenesis of a lung (e.g., congenital diaphragmatic hernia). In such a patient a PVRI of 4 WU•m² would be normal for the single lung even though most would recognize a PVRI above 3.0 WU•m² as an abnormal value.

Indications for Diagnostic Catheterization

Guidelines from the American Heart Association on indications for cardiac catheterization and intervention in pediatric cardiac disease were published in 2011.[13] Specific diagnostic indications covered by these guidelines and directly relevant to the care of the critically ill child with congenital or acquired heart disease are summarized in Table 37.2. However, indications will vary depending on center expertise with catheterization and with other diagnostic imaging modalities such as cardiac magnetic resonance imaging (MRI) or computed tomography (CT).

Anytime diagnostic catheterization is considered, intervention may be required, and catheterization should be undertaken only by a team that is capable of performing any necessary interventions. Some common postoperative scenarios in which diagnostic

TABLE 37.2	Indications for Diagnostic Catheterization in Children With Critical Heart Disease	
Recommendation		**Level of Evidence**
Class I		
Conditions for which there is evidence and/or general agreement that a given procedure or treatment is beneficial, useful, and effective		
Cardiac catheterization recommended to assess pulmonary resistance and reversibility of pulmonary hypertension in patients with CHD or primary pulmonary hypertension when accurate assessment of pulmonary resistance is needed to make surgical and medical decisions		B
Cardiac catheterization is indicated in patients with complex pulmonary atresia for the detailed characterization of lung segmental pulmonary vascular supply, especially when noninvasive imaging methods incompletely define pulmonary artery anatomy		B
Cardiac catheterization is indicated in determination of coronary circulation in pulmonary atresia with intact septum		B
Cardiac catheterization indicated in patients being assessed for cardiac transplantation unless patient's risk for catheterization outweighs the potential benefit		C
Cardiac catheterization is recommended for surveillance of graft vasculopathy after cardiac transplantation		B
Cardiac catheterization with the potential for intervention is indicated early in the postoperative period in critically ill patients when there is high suspicion for the presence of a residual structural lesion(s) but noninvasive diagnostics fail to identify a cause for hemodynamic and/or clinical compromise		B
Cardiac catheterization with potential for intervention is indicated early in the postoperative period in any patient who requires mechanical cardiopulmonary support without a clear cause		B
Class IIa		
Conditions for which there is conflicting evidence and/or a divergence of opinion about the usefulness/efficacy of a procedure or treatment but the weight of evidence is in favor of usefulness/efficacy		
It is reasonable to perform a cardiac catheterization to determine pulmonary pressure/resistance and transpulmonary gradient in palliated single-ventricle patients before a staged Fontan procedure		B
Cardiac catheterization is reasonable in any CHD patient in whom complete diagnosis cannot be obtained by noninvasive testing or in whom such testing yields incomplete information		C
Cardiac catheterization is reasonable for the assessment of cardiomyopathy or myocarditis		B
Cardiac catheterization is reasonable for the assessment of coronary circulation in some cases of Kawasaki disease in which coronary involvement is suspected or requires further delineation or in the assessment of suspected congenital coronary artery anomalies		B
Cardiac catheterization is reasonable to perform for the assessment of anatomy and hemodynamics in postoperative cardiac patients when the early postoperative course is unexpectedly complicated and noninvasive imaging techniques (e.g., MRA, CT angiography) fail to yield a clear explanation		C
It is reasonable to perform cardiac catheterization with potential for catheter intervention early in the postoperative period in patients who are not pursuing a typical postoperative course (e.g., prolonged mechanical ventilation, systemic oxygen desaturation) and in whom noninvasive diagnostic testing does not determine a reason for this course		C

Level of Evidence A: Data derived from multiple randomized clinical trials or meta-analyses. Level of Evidence B: Data derived from a single randomized trial or nonrandomized studies. Level of Evidence C: Only consensus opinion of experts, cases studies, or standard of care.

CHD, Congenital heart disease; *CT,* computed tomography; *MRA,* magnetic resonance angiography.

Reprinted with permission. *Circulation.* 2011;123:2607-2652. Copyright 2011 American Heart Association, Inc.

catheterization is often needed but intervention might be expected include the following:

- Excessive desaturation following placement of a systemic to PA shunt when shunt or branch PA obstruction/occlusion should be anticipated
- Excessive systemic desaturation after superior or less commonly complete cavopulmonary anastomosis when desaturating (venovenous) collaterals may be anticipated
- In patients with suspected residual or recurrent arch obstruction following repaired coarctation of the aorta when balloon angioplasty or stent placement may be considered

- In patients with suspected or recurrent branch PA stenosis after patch pulmonary arterioplasty when balloon angioplasty or stent placement may be considered depending on the extent of obstruction and time since surgery

Diagnostic Cardiac Catheterization to Determine Surgical Candidacy: Special Considerations

To Assess Pulmonary Vascular Resistance. Although cardiac catheterization is no longer considered a necessary part of preoperative staging in the majority of patients with left-to-right shunt lesions, preoperative cardiac catheterization is still sometimes considered in patients felt to be at high risk for postoperative pulmonary hypertension. In general these are patients who have followed an atypical clinical course, for example, patients with late diagnosis of a shunt lesion. In such patients high PVR may contraindicate surgical intervention due to unacceptably high postoperative risk. In a patient referred for catheterization to assess surgical candidacy when there is baseline elevated PVRI, vasodilator testing is typically performed using 100% FIO_2 and/or inhaled nitric oxide. In patients with pretricuspid or posttricuspid shunt lesions, there is a general consensus that a decrease in PVRI below 4 WU•m^2 and/or a decrease in the PVR:SVR below 0.3 indicates that shunt closure may be undertaken safely.[14-18] Nonetheless, in patients for whom there is a baseline concern, care should be taken to avoid postoperative stimuli that may precipitate a pulmonary hypertensive crisis. When the PVRI is more significantly elevated (e.g., between 4 and 8 WU•m^2), greater consideration is warranted because the risk of postoperative pulmonary hypertensive crisis is increased. In these cases temporary balloon occlusion of the shunt, if possible, may provide additional useful information.[15,18] In some centers a decrease in PVRI to less than 6 to 8 WU•m^2 may be considered adequate to undertake complete or partial shunt closure (e.g., placement of a fenestrated patch), but this should be considered only in centers with the necessary expertise and resources to fully support the patient in the postoperative setting.[15,16] The decision to close a shunt should be made after considering the entirety of the patient's medical history and should not be dependent solely on the hemodynamics obtained at cardiac catheterization.

Pre-Glenn and Pre-Fontan Catheterization.
In many institutions cardiac catheterizations are a routine part of preoperative staging before superior cavopulmonary anastomosis (bidirectional Glenn) or complete cavopulmonary anastomosis (Fontan). These studies are performed first to evaluate for residual or recurrent lesions that may need to be addressed in the catheterization laboratory or in the operating room and second to evaluate for hemodynamic derangements that might place the patient at higher surgical risk. Common examples of anatomic or hemodynamic derangements that can be diagnosed with pre-Glenn or pre-Fontan catheterization include the following (Fig. 37.5):

- Previously unidentified pulmonary venous anomalies (especially pre-Glenn)
- A restrictive atrial septum
- A left SVC draining to the coronary sinus or similar venovenous collateral that might worsen post-Glenn desaturation
- Branch PA stenosis
- Residual or recurrent coarctation of the aorta
- Aortopulmonary collaterals (although opinions vary on whether to intervene on these)
- Elevated pulmonary arterial pressures or PVR
- Single-ventricle diastolic dysfunction (i.e., elevated ventricular end-diastolic pressure)

Despite the fact that these presurgical evaluations remain standard practice at most institutions, several have questioned whether an invasive test remains warranted following advances in noninvasive imaging such as cardiac MRI. In an analysis of the utility of pre-Glenn catheterization, Brown et al. randomized 82 standard-risk single-ventricle patients to pre-Glenn catheterization ($n = 41$) versus cardiac MRI ($n = 41$). They found that catheterization resulted in more minor adverse events (78% versus 5%; $P < .001$), longer

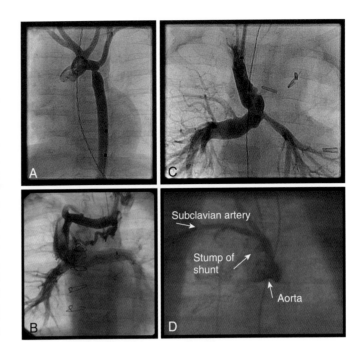

• **Figure 37.5** Select examples of residual or recurrent lesions sometimes identified in patients with single-ventricle physiology undergoing cardiac catheterization. (A) Recurrent coarctation after Norwood. (B) A desaturating (venous) collateral after bidirectional Glenn operation. (C) Left pulmonary artery stenosis after bidirectional Glenn operation. (D) An occluded modified Blalock-Taussig shunt.

preoperative hospital stays (median, 2 versus 1 day; $P < .001$), and higher hospital charges ($34,477 versus $14,921; $P < .001$). However, the frequency of successful bidirectional Glenn operation, frequency of postoperative complications, and long-term outcomes (median age at follow-up = 8.8 years) were all similar between the two groups.[19,20] Similarly, several retrospective analyses have failed to demonstrate a benefit of routine pre-Fontan catheterization in "standard"-risk patients without specific clinical indications for catheterization other than elective presurgical evaluation.[21-24] Clearly indications for these studies vary depending on center-level experiences and expertise.

To Evaluate Sources of Pulmonary Blood Flow in Patients With Pulmonary Atresia and Ventricular Septal Defect.
Patients with pulmonary atresia and VSD (PA/VSD) often have collateral sources of pulmonary blood flow that arise from the systemic circulation. On the most severe end of the spectrum they may not have any central PAs with various segments of the pulmonary vascular bed supplied by aortopulmonary collateral vessels. When echocardiography is able to identify central, confluent PAs supplied by a ductus arteriosus, our practice is to perform a systemic to PA shunt with the objective of encouraging growth of the PAs in anticipation of eventual definitive repair.[25] In this scenario cardiac catheterization can be deferred until the patient is bigger and potentially ready for definitive repair. When central PAs cannot be defined by echocardiography, then catheterization is necessary to determine if they are truly absent or potentially present but severely hypoplastic. This is critical because prognosis is directly related to the presence and size of these vessels. Angiography is also necessary to characterize additional systemic sources of pulmonary blood flow from aortopulmonary collaterals, which are most often supplied from the descending thoracic aorta but sometimes also from the subclavian arteries or the abdominal aorta (Fig. 37.6). These data are used

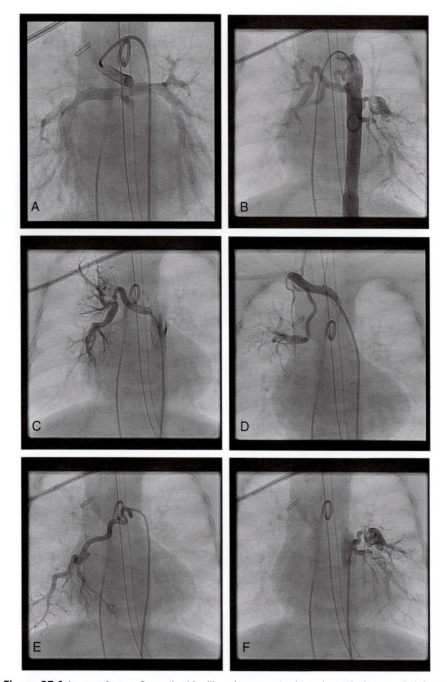

• **Figure 37.6** Images from a 3-month-old with pulmonary atresia and ventricular septal defect. (A) Angiography demonstrates central pulmonary arteries supplied by a central shunt. (B) Scout angiography in the aorta demonstrates multiple aortopulmonary collaterals. (C to F) Selective angiograms delineate each of the collaterals and the lung segments they supply. The collateral depicted in (D) arises from the subclavian artery, whereas the rest originate off the descending aorta. All of these collaterals supplied redundant flow to various segments of the lungs. They were all successfully occluded in the catheterization laboratory.

for surgical planning to determine whether the aortopulmonary vessels are a redundant source of pulmonary blood flow or the sole supply to a segment of lungs. In the former scenario the collaterals can be occluded with coils or plugs in the catheterization laboratory to reduce competitive flow to the lungs, and in the latter scenario unifocalization using the vessel(s) is typically performed. Angiographic data are also necessary to assess whether VSD closure can be safely performed. Two angiographic indices

taking into account the size of the PAs (i.e., the Nakata and McGoon indices) have been described to help with this decision.[26,27]

Therapeutic Cardiac Catheterization

Dr. William Rashkind ushered in the era of therapeutic cardiac catheterization in 1966 with the performance of the first balloon atrial septostomy for management of infants with transposition of the great arteries.[28] Since that time there have been significant advances in transcatheter interventions for patients with congenital heart disease. In addition, collaborations between surgeons and interventional cardiologists have sparked innovative hybrid approaches that provide potentially safer, faster, and less invasive alternatives to many procedures. This section is not intended as a comprehensive overview of all interventional cardiac catheterization procedures but provides an overview of some of the interventional approaches commonly needed in critically ill infants, children, and adolescents, including indications, procedural considerations, and safety concerns. We will also briefly discuss some of the novel transcatheter therapies that often require recovery and postprocedural management in the intensive care unit (ICU).

Atrial Septostomy

Indications for atrial septostomy have expanded since Rashkind first reported the potential utility of this intervention and now include management of patients requiring improved mixing or decompression of the left or right heart.[13] Septostomy can be performed at the bedside with echocardiographic guidance or in the catheterization laboratory under fluoroscopy. In our experience there are advantages to performing the procedure in the cardiac catheterization laboratory in patients with complex anatomy (e.g., hypoplastic left heart syndrome [HLHS]) or in higher-risk patients (e.g., requiring mechanical circulatory support). However, the bedside approach is preferred for the "straightforward" yet emergent septostomy (e.g., d-transposition of the great arteries) because it avoids transport and setup delays. Septostomy can be performed from the femoral venous approach or from the umbilical vein (if patent) through the ductus venosus. The latter approach avoids the potential for vascular injury and is often preferred when an umbilical venous line is in place (the line can be replaced after the procedure). Typically a septostomy balloon is advanced across the atrial septum and positioned in the left atrium. Care must be taken to position the balloon safely, avoiding inflation within or across important vascular structures such as the pulmonary veins, mitral valve, or the coronary sinus in patients with a left-sided SVC. The balloon is inflated with the appropriate volume of fluid (saline or a saline-contrast mixture) and then retracted so that the balloon is taut against the atrial septum. A forceful jerk/pull is applied to the catheter to bring the balloon to the junction of the right atrium and IVC. In patients with d-transposition of the great arteries, septostomy is indicated to improve atrial mixing and is usually considered in severely cyanotic neonates. The technique has low morbidity and mortality, and results are generally good with an immediate increase in preductal and postductal arterial oxygen saturation.

In severe mitral stenosis or atresia, alone or as part of HLHS, premature closure of the foramen ovale can result in left atrial hypertension with associated PA hypertension and lymphangiectasia. Decompression of the left atrium is necessary to lower PVR and improve oxygenation and cardiac output in these infants before surgical palliation. Balloon atrial septostomy may not be effective, and sometimes a blade septostomy or cutting balloon dilation is necessary to create an initial tear, followed by standard septostomy or static balloon dilation of the atrial septum. These procedures can be quite challenging, and the patients may be severely desaturated, requiring emergent left atrial decompression. To facilitate more rapid procedural completion, we have used a bedside hybrid approach with sternotomy, atrial septal puncture using an angiocatheter, and initial cutting balloon dilation followed by static balloon dilation of the atrial septum.[29]

Balloon atrial septostomy may also be required for decompression of the left atrium in patients requiring mechanical circulatory support who have severe left ventricular dysfunction resulting in left atrial hypertension, pulmonary edema, and pulmonary hypertension. These patients are often older and may have a thickened or intact atrial septum, in which case standard septostomy may be ineffective. Various techniques, including blade septostomy and/or cutting balloons, can be used.

Balloon atrial septostomy is rarely required in infants with tricuspid atresia. In some patients the foramen is restrictive, resulting in symptoms of right heart failure and poor cardiac output, and balloon septostomy may be helpful in enlarging the foramen. Often septostomy is ineffective in this setting, and surgical septectomy may be required.

Aortic Valve Stenosis

According to guidelines from the American Heart Association,[13] class I indications for aortic valvuloplasty include (1) newborns with isolated ductal dependent critical valvar aortic stenosis or isolated valvar aortic stenosis in the presence of depressed left ventricular systolic function, regardless of valve gradient; (2) resting peak systolic gradient across the valve of 50 mm Hg or higher by catheterization measurement; and (3) children with resting gradient of 40 mm Hg or higher in the presence of symptoms of angina or ST changes on exercise testing. In practice, findings from echocardiography are typically used to determine if intervention might be indicated. The echocardiogram mean Doppler gradient typically correlates best with the peak-to-peak gradient measured in the catheterization laboratory. Although many centers prefer a transcatheter approach to treat critical aortic stenosis due to the minimally invasive nature, some centers advocate primary surgical intervention.[30,31] Surgical options for treating critical aortic stenosis include surgical valvotomy, attempted primary repair of the aortic valve, or the neonatal Ross procedure. A recent meta-analysis comparing surgical intervention versus balloon valvuloplasty found no difference in mortality but higher rates of reintervention after balloon valvuloplasty.[32] The authors noted that reintervention is a suboptimal outcome measure that may be defined differently for surgical versus transcatheter approaches and argued for a prospective trial comparing the two approaches.

When transcatheter balloon valvuloplasty is performed in neonates with critical aortic stenosis, the procedure is best performed with the patient under general endotracheal anesthesia to reduce any metabolic demand. The approach can be retrograde from the femoral artery or umbilical artery, antegrade from the femoral or umbilical vein via a transseptal approach, or through a carotid artery approach by surgical cutdown or percutaneous puncture. Initial valvuloplasty is typically performed with a balloon that is 0.8 to 1.0 times the annulus size. Successful balloon aortic valvuloplasty reduces the peak systolic gradient to less than 30 mm Hg, ideally with minimal insufficiency. If a more significant gradient persists after the first dilation and the severity of aortic insufficiency is not prohibitive, valvuloplasty may be repeated with a slightly larger balloon.

Morbidity and mortality from aortic valvuloplasty are higher in neonates with critical aortic stenosis than when performed in older children, but outcomes have improved with better technology and equipment and proper selection of patients better suited for single-ventricle versus biventricular circulation. Although procedure-related mortality was up to 4.8% in early reports, advances in technique and equipment have improved this rate, and a multicenter study from the Congenital Cardiac Catheterization Project on Outcomes (C3PO) registry reported no procedure-related mortality.[33,34] Factors associated with decreased long-term survival include severe left ventricular dysfunction, a small left ventricle, and small aortic annulus.[33] The most common and feared complication with aortic valvuloplasty is creating more than moderate insufficiency, which has been reported in 14% to 22% of cases[33,35] and is sometimes unavoidable due to the morphology of the aortic valve. Increased aortic insufficiency is more likely in neonates with a unicommissural valve.[36] Some studies show a balloon to annulus ratio of greater than 0.9 to be associated with higher risk of insufficiency, but other studies have failed to show any definitive risk factors.[36,37]

Critical Pulmonary Valve Stenosis

Pulmonary balloon valvuloplasty was first performed in 1982[38] and remains the treatment of choice for valvar pulmonary stenosis. Neonates born with critical pulmonary stenosis typically present with a harsh murmur and may have some degree of cyanosis due to right-to-left shunt across the atrial septum. Rarely, there can be signs of right heart failure if the atrial septal communication is restrictive. There may be some degree of tricuspid valve hypoplasia and/or hypoplasia of the right ventricle. Neonates with critical pulmonary stenosis require prostaglandin E_1 (PGE$_1$) infusion to maintain ductal patency and allow for adequate pulmonary blood flow. Class I indications for pulmonary balloon valvuloplasty include ductal dependence (critical pulmonary valve stenosis) and/or a peak-to-peak catheter gradient or echocardiographic peak instantaneous gradient of greater than 40 mm Hg or clinically significant pulmonary valvar obstruction in the presence of right ventricular dysfunction.[13] When there is reduced transpulmonary valve flow, Doppler gradients are less reliable for evaluating the severity of obstruction. Reduced transpulmonary blood flow occurs when there is reduced right ventricular function or when the right ventricle is severely hypertrophied and has decreased compliance. Doppler gradients are also less reliable indicators of severity of obstruction if the PVR is elevated or there is a large patent ductus arteriosus. In these cases the Doppler gradient will be relatively lower because pressures in the main PA will be elevated. Occasionally in noncritical pulmonary stenosis the severity of obstruction may be difficult to estimate due to these factors, and it may be necessary to allow closure of the ductus arteriosus and/or for the PVR to fall to determine if there is an indication to proceed with balloon valvuloplasty in the neonatal period. When an intervention is indicated, it can be beneficial to maintain or reestablish patency of the ductus arteriosus because this will provide more stability during the balloon procedure and it provides a good route for stable wire position in the abdominal aorta.

Balloon pulmonary valvuloplasty is typically performed from a femoral venous approach. Initial valvuloplasty is typically performed with a balloon diameter that is 1 to 1.2 times the valve annulus and can be repeated with larger balloons up to 1.4 times the annulus diameter if the result is inadequate. Acute complications from balloon valvuloplasty are rare.[39] Some degree of pulmonary insufficiency is typically seen after valvuloplasty but is usually well tolerated acutely. Severe infundibular stenosis can occur immediately after valvuloplasty and is sometimes referred to as a "suicide right ventricle" when the infundibulum completely collapses upon itself. The significance of this is limited when the ductus arteriosus is patent, but when there is no ductus, this can severely impair cardiac output. Management includes fluid boluses to augment right ventricular filling with or without beta-blockers, which decrease contractility and reduce the severity of infundibular obstruction. When a patent ductus arteriosus is present, PGE$_1$ infusion may be needed after successful valvuloplasty until right ventricular compliance improves and allows sufficient antegrade pulmonary blood flow to maintain acceptable systemic oxygen saturation. Ductal patency can sometimes be needed for days after successful valvuloplasty. Infrequently, when there is very severe tricuspid valve or right ventricular hypoplasia, a modified Blalock-Taussig shunt or ductal stenting may be needed to augment pulmonary blood flow and allow for right ventricular growth and improved compliance.

Native and Recurrent Coarctation of the Aorta

Native coarctation of the aorta can present at any age and with a wide spectrum of severity. In the critical care setting coarctation is most commonly seen in neonates, who often present with cardiovascular collapse as the ductus closes. In this scenario there is no doubt that relief of the aortic obstruction is required, but most centers prefer surgical coarctation repair to transcatheter approaches.[40-43] Both surgical repair and balloon dilation of aortic coarctation are highly successful at acutely relieving the blood pressure gradient and heart failure produced by severe obstruction. However, balloon dilation of native coarctation is associated with a relatively high rate of early (within 6 to 12 months) recurrence, and there is an associated long-term risk of aneurysm formation along the segment of the aorta that is dilated.[44,45] Despite these concerns, the American Heart Association guidelines state that transcatheter balloon or stent angioplasty may be reasonable to consider in neonates who are deemed to be too critically ill or high risk for surgical intervention.[13]

In older patients (over 8 years of age) presenting with coarctation of the aorta and a peak systolic gradient greater than 20 mm Hg, stent placement is often the treatment of choice. Bare metal stents allow for relief of obstruction without the need to overdilate the aorta, thereby decreasing the risk of aortic wall injury, including the long-term risk of aneurysm formation.[46,47] Covered stents are increasingly being used to treat severe coarctations in which there is increased risk of aortic wall injury and to cover aneurysms or other aortic wall injuries created by previous catheter based or surgical management. Stents are less preferable in infants and neonates because they will require frequent dilation to accommodate for growth and because available stents that can be safely delivered in smaller children typically cannot be dilated to adult dimensions (>18 to 21 mm).[43]

In contrast to native coarctation, transcatheter approaches are the treatment of choice for recurrent coarctation. In these patients the risk of aneurysm formation is lower, presumably because the segment requiring dilation is protected by scar tissue. A peak systolic catheter gradient greater than 20 mm Hg is considered a class I indication for transcatheter balloon angioplasty in a patient with recoarctation, assuming favorable angiographic appearance.

Recurrent coarctation is a particular concern in patients with single-ventricle physiology after Norwood arch reconstruction because arch obstruction is poorly tolerated by the tenuous single-ventricle circulation. In the landmark Single Ventricle Reconstruction trial, recurrent coarctation occurred in 18% of survivors within the first year of life.[48] Median age at reintervention was 4.9 months with most interventions occurring at the time of stage II cardiac

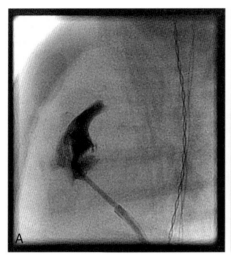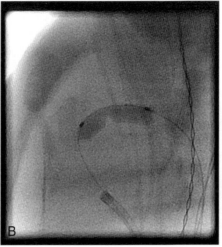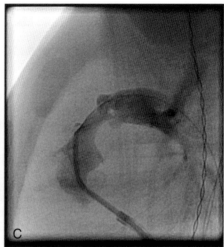

• **Figure 37.7** (A) Lateral angiogram demonstrates the infundibulum in a patient with pulmonary atresia with intact ventricular septum. (B) After radiofrequency perforation of the right ventricle a balloon is inflated across the right ventricular outflow tract. (C) Postintervention angiography demonstrates antegrade flow across the right ventricular outflow tract.

catheterization. In these patients Doppler echocardiography may underestimate severity of obstruction and for this reason cardiac catheterization should be considered in any patient with single-ventricle physiology with a history of arch repair and decreased systemic ventricular function and/or worsening tricuspid valve insufficiency to assess for recoarctation. Due to the significant adverse consequences of arch obstruction, many interventionalists advocate more aggressive thresholds for intervention in patients with single-ventricle physiology. A catheter gradient above 10 mm Hg is often considered as a reasonable threshold, and lower gradients may also warrant intervention when systolic function is decreased or when there is angiographic evidence of significant obstruction.

Pulmonary Atresia With Intact Ventricular Septum

Many infants born with pulmonary atresia with intact ventricular septum (PA/IVS) are candidates for perforation of the atretic pulmonary valve followed by balloon valvuloplasty in the catheterization laboratory. Determining candidacy for this approach requires a thoughtful and thorough analysis of the underlying anatomy with special attention to several key aspects of the anatomy. First, some of these patients may have severe right ventricular or tricuspid valve hypoplasia. In these patients there is also often muscular atresia of the pulmonary valve. In this scenario a single-ventricle strategy is usually preferred, and transcatheter intervention is neither feasible nor indicated.[49] Second, infants with PA/IVS often have extensive coronary sinusoids from the right ventricle, and sometimes the coronary circulation is considered "right ventricular dependent" due to severe proximal coronary artery stenosis or proximal coronary artery atresia. In these patients opening of the pulmonary valve is contraindicated because it will instantaneously reduce the right ventricular and therefore coronary perfusion pressure. For this reason coronary and right ventricular angiography is necessary in any patient with PA/IVS for whom a biventricular circulation is considered.

When valve perforation is deemed appropriate, a catheter is carefully positioned in the right ventricular infundibulum below the atretic pulmonary valve (Fig. 37.7). Perforation can be performed with a stiff wire or more commonly a radiofrequency wire. After valve perforation the radiofrequency wire is advanced into the main PA and then replaced with a floppy tipped wire so that balloon valvuloplasty can be performed. These patients often have poor right ventricular compliance, as well as right ventricular and tricuspid valve hypoplasia. After perforation and pulmonary valvuloplasty, there may initially be inadequate antegrade pulmonary blood flow, and many patients require continued ductal patency with PGE$_1$ infusion for days to weeks after the procedure. Sometimes ductal stenting or a systemic-to-PA shunt is required to augment pulmonary blood flow for a longer period of time. Depending on the degree of tricuspid valve hypoplasia and growth of the right ventricle after the procedure, some patients may ultimately require single-ventricle palliation or a "1.5-ventricle" repair, but many can achieve a biventricular circulation. Complications with pulmonary valve perforation are similar to those discussed with balloon pulmonary valvuloplasty; however, there is increased risk of perforation of the right ventricular outflow tract (RVOT) or main PA during attempts to perforate the pulmonary valve. This can lead to pericardial effusion or bleeding into the mediastinum.

Ductal Stenting

Many infants born with congenital heart disease have cyanosis due to ductal dependent pulmonary blood flow. Conventional management in these patients has been placement of a surgical aortopulmonary shunt as a bridge to further interventions. Stenting of the ductus arteriosus is an alternative that was first described in 1992 in two infants with PA/IVS after valve perforation and balloon valvuloplasty.[50] Since that time the procedure has been used as an alternative to a surgical shunt in infants with various congenital heart defects. Santoro et al.[51] reported that, compared to the modified Blalock-Taussig shunt, arterial duct stenting provided more balanced growth of the branch PAs. In situations in which there is antegrade pulmonary blood flow, the procedure can be performed from the femoral vein. More commonly, a retrograde femoral artery approach is used in patients with usual ductal anatomy, whereas in patients with a reverse-oriented ductus arteriosus an approach from the carotid or axillary artery, either by surgical cutdown or percutaneous access, is often required. The PGE₁ infusion is usually stopped several hours before the procedure to allow the ductus to contract so that the stent can be positioned. This makes the patient less stable and the procedure higher risk when there is ductal dependent pulmonary blood flow. Balloon-expandable coronary stents are typically used, and the entire ductus must be covered, sometimes requiring multiple telescoping stents, to avoid developing stenosis as the ductus contracts.

Branch Pulmonary Artery Stenosis

Transcatheter PA interventions to treat stenosis, including balloon angioplasty and stent placement, are some of the most common interventions in the cardiac catheterization laboratory.[8] The course of numerous cardiac lesions, including tetralogy of Fallot, PA/VSD, truncus arteriosus, transposition of the great arteries, and the broad spectrum of single-ventricle anomalies, can be complicated by PA disease. Balloon angioplasty is sometimes preferred to stent placement in younger children to avoid the need for serial stent dilations and due to the larger sheath sizes required for stent placement. Balloon angioplasty is also more effective for postoperative PA stenosis because these lesions are often caused by scar tissue that can be disrupted to allow improved growth of the vessel. However, balloon angioplasty is rarely able to relieve obstruction to the same extent that stents can[13]; therefore stents are often preferred in older patients. When balloon angioplasty is suboptimally effective and stent implantation must be considered in younger patients, sheath size limitations sometimes dictate the use of lower-profile "premounted" coronary, biliary, or peripheral vascular stents. A major drawback to many of these stents is that they cannot be dilated to adult dimensions and must either be "fractured" (depending on the stent this may or may not be feasible) or surgically removed when the patient has outgrown the stent.

With respect to the critical care setting, residual or recurrent PA stenosis is sometimes an issue in the immediate postoperative setting and may contribute to delayed convalescence. This is a particular concern in patients in whom right ventricular hypertension might be poorly tolerated (e.g., after tetralogy or truncus repair) or in whom unobstructed pulmonary blood flow is essential (e.g., single-ventricle palliation). Noninvasive diagnosis of PA stenosis in these settings is usually based on the presence of a Doppler-detected pressure gradient or evidence of narrowing by two-dimensional echocardiography. Unfortunately, Doppler gradients are flow dependent and may not accurately represent severity of stenosis. Other features, including evidence of right ventricular hypertension (more than one-half to two-thirds of systemic right ventricular pressures), significant flow discrepancy (discrepancy of 35%/65% or worse), or obstruction identified by CT angiography or cardiac MRI, may provide the impetus for proceeding to the cardiac catheterization laboratory. In children who are failing to convalesce as expected, and where there is concern for PA stenosis, transcatheter intervention should be considered to address the lesion. Traditionally it was felt to be unsafe to intervene on vessels that have undergone recent (within 6 weeks) surgical patching due to the risk of disrupting suture lines. However, reports have demonstrated that interventions, including PA angioplasty and stent placement, can be safely performed in the earlier postoperative period.[52,53] Intraoperative hybrid branch PA stenting can be performed under direct vision during open-heart surgery and may be preferred over percutaneous stent placement in the following situations: (1) the need for a concomitant surgical procedure such as

conduit replacement or VSD closure, (2) limited vascular access related to vascular occlusions, (3) low patient weight and/or age, and (4) as a "rescue" procedure for complications of percutaneous stent placement.

Complications after PA interventions are more commonly seen in younger patients and in the immediate postoperative setting and may include vessel dissection causing worse obstruction, vessel rupture causing bleeding into the chest, stent embolization or migration, stent obstruction of branches that must be "crossed," and reperfusion injury.[8]

Hybrid Stage I Palliation for Hypoplastic Left Heart Syndrome

The first report of a hybrid approach to stage I palliation for neonates with HLHS described a combination of surgical PA banding followed by percutaneous ductal stenting.[54] The goals of the hybrid procedure are to achieve restriction of blood flow to the lungs, unobstructed systemic blood flow, and unrestrictive flow from the left atrium to the right atrium without needing cardiopulmonary bypass. It is considered a class IIb indication as an alternative to conventional surgery in neonates with HLHS or complex single ventricle, in high-risk surgical candidates, and as a bridge to heart transplantation.[13] In 2005 Galantowicz and Cheatham described their approach (Fig. 37.8), which was performed through a median sternotomy and consisted of bilateral PA banding followed by insertion of a short sheath directly into the main PA to facilitate placement of the PDA stent. Treatment of the atrial septum was performed as a separate procedure in the catheterization laboratory from a femoral venous approach.[55] Many institutions use the hybrid approach to stage I palliation for high-risk surgical patients only; however, some institutions have adopted this as the primary approach for all neonates born with HLHS.[56] There is a significant learning curve, and complications remain an issue. Delayed or recurrent interatrial restriction can develop following the hybrid procedure requiring reintervention to the atrial septum.[57] Retrograde aortic arch obstruction, due to either

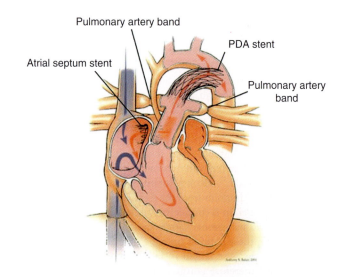

• **Figure 37.8** Schematic depicting a hybrid stage I procedure. *PDA,* Patent ductus arteriosus. (Reprinted with permission from Galantowicz M, Cheatham JP. Lessons learned from the development of a new hybrid strategy for the management of hypoplastic left heart syndrome. *Pediatr Cardiol.* 2005;26[3]:190-199.)

ascending aorta stenosis or ductal stent obstruction, is a significant concern with one study reporting a 24% incidence.[58] Any evidence of obstruction to the retrograde arch by echocardiogram has been considered a contraindication to proceeding with the hybrid approach.[13] The potential for decreased mesenteric blood flow exists, and studies have reported an increased risk of necrotizing enterocolitis compared to surgical Norwood.[59] Patients who have hybrid stage I palliation typically proceed to a comprehensive stage II surgical palliation at 4 to 6 months of age, which includes removal of PA bands and the ductal stent, Norwood type aortic arch reconstruction, atrial septectomy, and cavopulmonary anastomosis.

Transcatheter Pulmonary Valve Replacement

The first transcatheter pulmonary valve implantation was performed in 2000 by Bonhoeffer et al.[59a] Over the past decade, transcatheter pulmonary valve replacement (TPVR) has become widely used with the goal of reducing the number of surgeries required in a patient's lifetime. The current technology uses balloon expandable stent-valves (Fig. 37.9). The Melody valve (Medtronic Inc., Minneapolis, MN) is a bovine jugular venous valve sewn into a platinum iridium stent, and the SAPIEN XT valve (Edwards Lifesciences Corp., Irvine, CA) consists of bovine pericardial leaflets sewn into a stainless steel stent. Both valves have been approved by the US Food and Drug Administration for TPVR within preexisting right ventricular to PA conduits. The largest SAPIEN XT valve is 29 mm, which has allowed increased off-label use of TPVR for patients with "native right ventricular outflow tracts (RVOTs)," most commonly in patients with tetralogy of Fallot after transannular patch repair. TPVR requires placement of a large (16 to 22 Fr) venous sheath and a delivery system that can be difficult to maneuver into position from the percutaneous approach in younger patients and/or patients with complex anatomy. Hybrid periventricular approaches to TPVR have been reported. Many patients will require postprocedural recovery and monitoring in an ICU setting. The most severe procedural complications are tearing or rupturing of the conduit during ballooning and stenting and compression of the coronary arteries that can occur with placement of the stent in the RVOT. Heavily calcified and/or contracted conduits are at higher risk for having a tear while trying to expand the conduits with a balloon and/or stent. Most tears can be treated in the catheterization laboratory with placement of a covered stent, but surgical management is occasionally required. Coronary compression was found in 4.5% of patients in a multicenter study of patients presenting for TPVR.[60] It can be avoided by careful evaluation of the coronary anatomy with angiography during balloon inflation across the conduit before implantation of a stent. If balloon testing shows evidence of coronary compression, surgical management is typically pursued instead of TPVR. Long-term complications of TPVR include endocarditis and stent fractures leading to valve dysfunction, which sometimes requires surgical or catheter-based reintervention. Endocarditis has been a concern with the Melody valve, typically occurring greater than 6 months after valve implant, and has also been reported with the Sapien valve.[61,62]

Safety Considerations

Risk Scores

Appropriate use of cardiac catheterization in the critical care environment requires an understanding of the procedural risks associated with these procedures. Several attempts have been made to more accurately quantify procedural risks:

- Nykanen et al.[63] used data from 14,790 procedures (20 centers) in children and adolescents (<18 years of age) along with expert consensus, to develop the Catheterization RIsk Score for Pediatrics (CRISP) to predict risk of a procedurally related serious adverse event. The risk score is available as an online calculator (http://www.pmidcalc.org/?sid=26527119&newtest =Y) and assigns points based upon timing of the procedure (elective, emergent or postoperative), patient age/weight, need

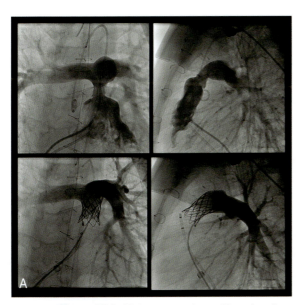
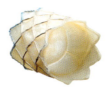
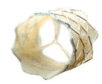
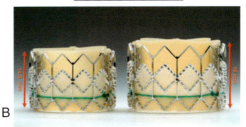

Melody valve

SAPIEN XT valve

• **Figure 37.9** (A) Anteroposterior and lateral angiograms *(top panels)* depict a right ventricle to pulmonary artery homograft with severe insufficiency. After transcatheter pulmonary valve replacement with a Melody valve, there is no insufficiency *(bottom panels)*. (B) The Melody and SAPIEN XT transcatheter pulmonic valves.

TABLE 37.3	Procedure Type Risk Categories			
	PROCEDURAL RISK CATEGORY			
	1	**2**	**3**	**4**
Diagnostic case	Age ≥1 year	Age 1 month to <1 year	Age <1 month	
Valvuloplasty		Pulmonary valve ≥1 month	Pulmonary valve <1 month, aortic valve ≥1 month, tricuspid valve	Mitral valve, aortic valve <1 month
Device or coil occlusion	Venous collateral/ left SVC	PDA, ASD, PFO, Fontan fenestration, systemic to PA collaterals	Systemic surgical shunt, baffle leak, coronary fistula	VSD, perivalvular leak
Balloon angioplasty	—	RVOT, aorta dilation <8 atm	PA <4 vessels PA ≥4 vessels all <8 atm Aorta >8 atm or cutting balloon, systemic artery (not aorta), systemic surgical shunt Systemic to pulmonary collaterals, systemic vein	Pulmonary artery ≥4 vessels, pulmonary vein
Stent placement	—	Systemic vein	RVOT, aorta, systemic artery (not aorta)	Ventricular septum, PA, pulmonary vein, systemic surgical shunt, systemic pulmonary collateral
Stent redilation	—	RVOT, atrial septum, aorta, systemic artery (not aorta), systemic vein	PA, pulmonary vein	Ventricular septum
Other	Myocardial biopsy	Snare foreign body, transseptal puncture	Atrial septostomy, recanalization of jailed vessel in stent, recanalization of occluded vessel	Atrial septal dilation and stent, any catheterization <4 days after surgery, atretic valve perforation

ASD, Atrial septal defect; *atm*, atmospheres; *PA*, pulmonary artery; *PDA*, patent ductus arteriosus; *PFO*, patent foramen ovale; *RVOT*, right ventricular outflow tract; *SVC*, superior vena cava; *VSD*, ventricular septal defect.
Modified from Bergersen L, Gauvreau K, Lock JE, et al. A risk adjusted method for comparing adverse outcomes among practitioners in pediatric and congenital cardiac catheterization. *Congenit Heart Dis.* 2008;3(4):230-240.

for inotropic support, presence of systemic illness, physiologic category, precatheterization diagnosis, and procedural risk category. In their analysis, serious adverse events occurred in 4.5% of all catheterization cases but in 14.4% of cases with a CRISP score of 10 to 14 and in 36.8% of cases with a CRISP score of 15 or higher.

- Bergersen et al.[64,65] used data from 9362 cardiac catheterizations (8 centers), along with expert consensus, to develop the Catheterization for Congenital Heart Disease Adjustment for Risk Method (Table 37.3). This risk model incorporates patient age, a hemodynamic vulnerability score, and type of intervention and can be useful to estimate risk to a patient before cardiac catheterization. In their analysis a high-severity adverse event, defined as any moderate (transient change in condition requiring monitoring), major, or catastrophic adverse event, occurred in 5% of all catheterization cases. The odds of death or a life-threatening adverse event were 4.8-fold higher for procedural risk category 4 versus 1, 1.8- and 2.0-fold higher for patients with one versus two hemodynamic vulnerability variables versus zero, and 1.5-fold higher for patients less than 1 year of age versus all others.

Although these analyses have used differing definitions of adverse events, differing methodology, and differing model covariates/risk predictors, several common factors have been consistently associated with increased risk, most notably, complexity of the intervention, younger age, presence of comorbid conditions (e.g., hemodynamic

vulnerability, respiratory failure, systemic illness), and timing of the procedure (e.g., elective versus emergent). These factors should be considered in evaluating the risk-benefit of catheterization for a patient in the critical care setting.

Cardiac Catheterization in Children Requiring Mechanical Circulatory Support

Children requiring mechanical circulatory support, including extracorporeal membrane oxygenation (ECMO), represent some of the highest-risk patients. Transport to and from the catheterization laboratory is itself an undertaking, and every precaution must be taken to prevent infection and/or hardware dislodgment. Moreover, catheterization introduces the potential for increased bleeding risks associated with systemic anticoagulation and thrombosis risk associated with holding anticoagulation for access. Other concerns include the potential for renal injury with the use of contrast agents and the obvious risks associated with performing interventions in such a vulnerable population. One must also consider that hemodynamic data may be of somewhat limited value in a patient receiving full cardiopulmonary support.

Despite all of these concerns and limitations, cardiac catheterization is often important in patients who require mechanical circulatory support. It is well documented that unrecognized anatomic lesions can contribute to failure to wean from mechanical circulatory support, and the diagnostic capabilities of other imaging modalities (e.g., echocardiography) may be limited by the indwelling hardware. For these reasons a class I recommendation from the American Heart Association is that "Cardiac catheterization with potential for intervention is indicated early in the postoperative period in any patient who requires mechanical cardiopulmonary support without a clear cause *(Level of Evidence: B)*."

Children With Williams-Beuren Syndrome

Williams-Beuren syndrome (WBS) is a multisystem disorder caused by deletion of the Williams-Beuren syndrome chromosome region of chromosome 7.[66] Although this is a rare condition, these children frequently require cardiac catheterization; WBS is associated with cardiac lesions, including supravalvar aortic stenosis, ostial stenosis of the coronary arteries, transverse arch hypoplasia and coarctation, branch PA stenosis, and renal artery stenosis. Cardiac arrest with induction of anesthesia, during transcatheter intervention, and during the postoperative period has been widely reported in children with WBS.[67] The exact cause is unknown, but coronary ostial stenosis has clearly contributed to some cases. We perform all catheterizations in children with WBS with an ECMO circuit in the laboratory and primed for immediate use if needed.

Radiation-Related Risks

Catheterization accounts for more cumulative radiation exposure to children with congenital and acquired heart disease than all other medical imaging procedures combined.[68,69] In some children multiple repeat cardiac catheterization procedures are expected, and the cumulative ionizing radiation burden can be substantial.[68,69] Children are particularly sensitive to the potential stochastic effects (e.g., those that lead to DNA mutations) of ionizing radiation, including cancer induction, because their rapidly dividing cells are more prone to DNA damage and because children have a longer anticipated life span during which these effects can develop.[70-72] For these reasons, as well as the safety concerns summarized previously, it is always important that the care team thoroughly consider whether a cardiac catheterization procedure is appropriately justified. This means that the procedure is both appropriately indicated and that the anticipated clinical benefits exceed all anticipated risks, including radiation.

Conclusion

Diagnostic and interventional cardiac catheterization procedures constitute an important part of the care of children with congenital and acquired heart disease. Providers caring for these children must understand the various indications for cardiac catheterization and how to appropriately interpret hemodynamic and angiographic data, and they must recognize both the anticipated benefits and safety concerns associated with these procedures.

Selected References

A complete list of references is available at ExpertConsult.com.

2. Beausejour Ladouceur V, Lawler PR, Gurvitz M, et al. Exposure to Low-Dose Ionizing Radiation From Cardiac Procedures in Patients With Congenital Heart Disease: 15-Year Data From a Population-Based Longitudinal Cohort. *Circulation.* 2016;133(1):12–20.

13. Feltes TF, Bacha E, Beekman RH 3rd, et al. Indications for cardiac catheterization and intervention in pediatric cardiac disease: a scientific statement from the American Heart Association. *Circulation.* 2011;123(22):2607–2652.

15. Del Cerro MJ, Moledina S, Haworth SG, et al. Cardiac catheterization in children with pulmonary hypertensive vascular disease: consensus statement from the Pulmonary Vascular Research Institute, Pediatric and Congenital Heart Disease Task Forces. *Pulm Circ.* 2016;6(1):118–125.

20. Brown DW, Gauvreau K, Powell AJ, et al. Cardiac magnetic resonance versus routine cardiac catheterization before bidirectional Glenn anastomosis: long-term follow-up of a prospective randomized trial. *J Thorac Cardiovasc Surg.* 2013;146(5):1172–1178.

29. Hill K, Fudge JC, Barker P, Jaggers J, Rhodes J. Novel transatrial septoplasty technique for neonates with hypoplastic left heart syndrome and an intact or highly restrictive atrial septum. *Pediatr Cardiol.* 2010;31(4):545–549.

32. Hill GD, Ginde S, Rios R, Frommelt PC, Hill KD. Surgical Valvotomy Versus Balloon Valvuloplasty for Congenital Aortic Valve Stenosis: A Systematic Review and Meta-Analysis. *J Am Heart Assoc.* 2016;5(8).

46. Meadows J, Minahan M, McElhinney DB, McEnaney K, Ringel R, Investigators C. Intermediate Outcomes in the Prospective, Multicenter Coarctation of the Aorta Stent Trial (COAST). *Circulation.* 2015;131(19):1656–1664.

69. Johnson JN, Hornik CP, Li JS, et al. Cumulative radiation exposure and cancer risk estimation in children with heart disease. *Circulation.* 2014;130(2):161–167.

38

Biomarkers in Care of Congenital Heart Disease Patients in the Intensive Care Unit

MELANIE NIES, MD; ALLEN EVERETT, MD

Pediatric congenital heart disease (CHD), as a heterogeneous group of rare individual diseases, with myriad anatomic variations and complicated medical and surgical management, is a prime target for biomarker discovery and applicability in perioperative patients in the intensive care unit (ICU). It is worthwhile for those involved in critical care management of patients to be familiar with common and promising biomarkers for CHD. This chapter will review the definition of a biomarker; describe challenges to discovery and validation of biomarkers in pediatric medicine; current biomarker use in CHD in the ICU; specific ICU situations, including nonsurgical and surgical care of patients with CHD and acquired pediatric heart disease in the ICU; and conclude with a literature review of biomarkers in critical care of patients with CHD.

The term *biomarkers* has a broad definition as "characteristics that are objectively measured and evaluated as indicators of normal biological processes, pathogenic processes or pharmacologic responses to therapeutic intervention."[1] For the purposes of this chapter we will use the term *biomarker* to refer to a protein and/or small molecule measured in a body fluid. As methods of discovery have become increasingly sophisticated, novel biomarkers are appearing with seemingly endless potential for clinical applicability. However, validation of biomarkers for everyday use in CHD is difficult. Barriers to development and validation of biomarkers include the difficulty in development of reliable, reproducible, clinically available assays; normative values in pediatrics, and developmental regulation. Biomarker discovery and validation, with the ultimate goal of creation of a high-quality assay that meets US regulatory approval, is a complex endeavor, with only the end product visible to the clinical practitioner ordering the test at the bedside.[2] From procuring pediatric patient samples and winnowing down long lists of biologically feasible proteins to finally developing and validating reliable bedside assays on large cohorts, the process can take years (Fig. 38.1)

Despite the complexities of validation, biomarkers enticingly offer enormous potential for screening, diagnosis, prognosis, and therapeutic monitoring. Currently the vast majority of research and practical experience on biomarkers in CHD is centered on two classes of biomarkers: (1) cardiac function/failure and (2) cardiac injury.

Cardiac Function/Failure Biomarkers

Cardiac function/failure biomarkers fall into two broad categories: (1) biomarkers of atrial/ventricular stretch (natriuretic peptides [NPs]) and (2) indicators of myocardial fibrosis and function, suppressor of tumorigenicity 2 (ST2), and galectin-3 (Gal3). Each of these biomarkers is discussed in detail in the following sections with emphasis placed on use in the ICU.

Natriuretic Peptides

The three natriuretic peptides (NPs) include atrial natriuretic peptide (ANP), brain natriuretic peptide (BNP), and natriuretic peptide C. BNP, although also contained in the brain, is predominantly secreted by cardiac ventricular myocytes as a means of physiologic adaptation to wall stress or volume overload. The NPs are almost exclusively cardiac expressed. They each contain a common 17–amino acid ring that is essential for binding to their cognate guanylyl cyclase receptors. NPs stimulate natriuresis and diuresis by attenuating the renin-angiotensin-aldosterone axis and relaxing pulmonary vasculature by elevation of cyclic guanine monophosphate (Fig. 38.2) BNP is the prototype for NPs, is the only NP studied in children, and will be the focus in the next section.

Cardiac Failure Biomarker Category 1: Natriuretic Peptides

Brain Natriuretic Peptide Structure. BNP is the biologically active cleavage product of prohormone proBNP, and NTproBNP is the biologically inactive N-terminal (Fig. 38.3). Plasma levels differ according to half-life; BNP has a half-life of approximately 22 minutes, whereas NTproBNP has a half-life of 1 to 2 hours, accounting for higher plasma levels of NTproBNP.[3] BNP has important characteristics as a biomarker of ventricular stress and dilatation, including clinical availability of point-of-care plasma assays, stability over freeze-thaw cycles,[4] and existing normative data for both healthy children[5-10] and those with structurally normal but failing hearts,[11] CHD,[11,12] and pulmonary hypertension (PH).[11,13] However, BNP is developmentally regulated, is affected by renal failure, shows wide variation between and within CHD

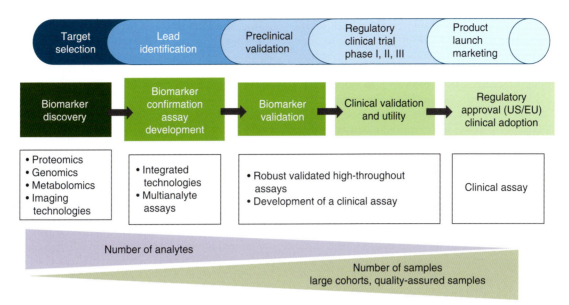

• **Figure 38.1** Biomarker Discovery and Validation Pipeline. The pipeline, leading from target selection and biomarker discovery from a vast possible number of analytes requiring a small discovery set to the product launch of a clinical assay that has been validated in large cohorts is a complex, expensive process, from which few clinically useful biomarkers have emerged. (Modified from Nies MK, Ivy DD, Everett AD. The untapped potential of proteomic analysis in pediatric pulmonary hypertension. *Proteomics Clin Appl.* 2014;8[11-12]:862-874. doi: 10.1002/prca.201400067.)

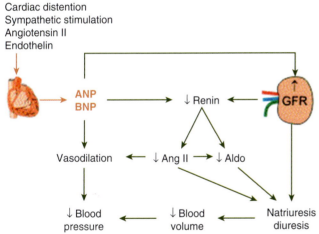

• **Figure 38.2** Natriuretic peptides are peptide hormones that are synthesized by the heart, brain, and other organs. The release of these peptides by the heart is stimulated by atrial and ventricular distention, as well as by neurohumoral stimuli, usually in response to heart failure. The main physiologic action of natriuretic peptides is to reduce arterial pressure by decreasing blood volume and systemic vascular resistance. Atrial natriuretic peptide (ANP) is a 28–amino acid peptide that is synthesized, stored, and released by atrial myocytes in response to atrial distention, angiotensin II *(Ang II)* stimulation, endothelin, and sympathetic stimulation (beta-adrenoceptor mediated). Therefore elevated levels of ANP are found during hypervolemic states (elevated blood volume), such as occurs in heart failure. A second natriuretic peptide (brain natriuretic peptide [BNP]) is a 32–amino acid peptide that is synthesized largely by the ventricles (as well as in the brain, where it was first identified). BNP is released by the same mechanisms that release ANP, and it has similar physiologic actions. *Aldo,* Aldosterone, *GFR,* glomerular filtration rate. (Modified from Fig. 2: Natriuretic Peptide Structure and Function, http://medicineforresidents.blogspot.com/2010/08/natriuretic-peptides-physiology.html.)

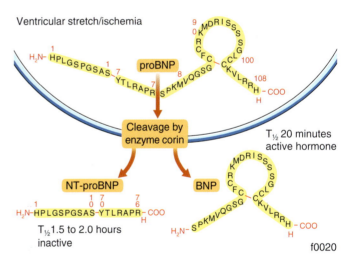

• **Figure 38.3** Protease corin cleaves proBNP108 into N-terminal-proBNP (NT-proBNP), a 76–amino acid biologically inert molecule, and brain natriuretic peptide (BNP), the biologically active counterpart.

subsets,[3,12,14] and is affected by age, gender, and pubertal stage.[10] The most notable developmental regulation is the log scale difference in NP levels in neonates during the physiologic transition within the first week of birth,[14] attributed to maturation of the kidney, decreasing pulmonary vascular resistance, and acute increase in ventricular afterload after birth. There is a generalized trend of decline after the first month; adult levels are reached around 6 years of age.[15,16]

Normative Pediatric Values. Assays for NTproBNP and BNP are US Food and Drug Administration (FDA) approved and available in most clinical laboratories. For NTproBNP, Albers et al.[17] established normative values based on review of combined data from four studies, encompassing 690 subjects from birth to 18 years of age, establishing 95th and 97.5th percentiles for healthy children. Normal values of BNP have also been established by meta-analysis[18] of 195 healthy infants, children, and adolescents admitted for minor procedures, from birth to 17.6 years of age. In all subjects older than 2 weeks, plasma BNP concentration was less than 32.7 pg/mL.[18] Of note, routine measurement of BNP versus NTproBNP varies by center, and even *within* centers because of vendor variability, further compounding the difficulty in comparison among small CHD subsets. BNP and NTproBNP are NOT interchangeable but do have excellent correlation between log BNP and log NTproBNP in adults and in children with CHD and PH.[19-21] For the purposes of this chapter, BNP and NTproBNP will be referred to collectively as BNP, except where different applications or plasma levels are important.

As a broad overview of BNP in the ICU and in CHD, there are both surgical and nonsurgical applications, both of which will be discussed in more detail in this chapter, with synopsis of the existing literature. In the realm of nonsurgical care, BNP can be used in the diagnostic workup of dyspnea from respiratory versus cardiac causes, cardiac failure in congenital and acquired heart disease, and PH crisis in nonsurgical patients with pulmonary arterial hypertension (PAH).[22] BNP is the only biomarker warranting mention in the most recent pediatric heart failure guidelines.[23] Regarding cardiothoracic surgical care, there are preoperative, perioperative, and postoperative applications of BNP, including as a prognostic marker for outcome and major postoperative events, including low cardiac output state and postoperative PH crisis, as discussed in the following sections.

Pattern of Natriuretic Peptide Release Before, During, and After Cardiac Surgery

Preoperative Levels. In their 2014 systematic review of the clinical utility of BNP in pediatric cardiac surgery, Afshani et al.[14] investigated the preoperative correlation of BNP with CHD severity and early postoperative outcome, including 20 peer-reviewed studies that evaluated immediate postoperative BNP levels. In the preoperative period they found that BNP levels were associated with cardiac failure. Preoperative BNP levels were higher in those being treated for cardiac failure than in those not being treated for cardiac failure. In univentricular hearts, BNP and NTproBNP predicted clinical cardiac failure by Ross score. After data amalgamation the authors determined the area under the curve (AUC) for receiver operating characteristic (ROC) analysis of 83% (95% confidence interval [CI], 71%-95%) for the prediction of clinical cardiac failure, with an NTproBNP screening cut point of 6.75 pg/mL (sensitivity 94%) and diagnostic cut point of 86.8 pg/mL (specificity 94%); Youden index was 25.1 pg/mL.[14] Although their systematic review showed that BNP levels predicted cardiac failure and were associated with adverse outcomes, including death, low cardiac output syndrome, length of stay, and duration of mechanical ventilation, postoperative levels were more predictive of early poor outcome (mortality <180 days after surgery).[14] Of note, the authors' attempted meta-analysis was unsuccessful due to difficulty in comparing results using different assays, small individual sample sizes, and heterogeneous outcome measures; ultimately, they did not seek to provide generalized cut points for diagnostic or prognostic classification in CHD.[14]

Perioperative and Postoperative Levels. BNP levels peak postoperatively between 6 and 24 hours.[12,14] In the first few hours after computed tomography (CT) surgery, NP levels are lower than baseline, attributed to breakdown without resynthesis,[14] removal

during ultrafiltration, and decreased filling of the heart. There is a second peak in BNP levels reported around postoperative day 5.[14]

In a prospective study of BNP levels in CHD in 221 patients undergoing CT surgery, Niedner et al.[12] evaluated BNP levels in patients with CHD undergoing both cardiac surgery and noncardiac surgery ("surgical stress" control arm). Patients were seen at a single center from 2003 to 2005, with 103 normative controls, 13 "surgical stress" controls, and 106 CHD repairs, ranging in age from 30 weeks' gestational age through 22 years. The purpose of the study was to identify circumstances in CHD of relative BNP deficit. They found progressively lower BNP expression in staged univentricular repair, speculated to be "perhaps from isolated cavopulmonary failure or impaired perioperative expression of natriuretic peptide" with the implication that BNP level may not be indicative of CHD severity in all types of single-ventricle physiology.[12] The authors speculated that, especially in patients with Fontan palliation, BNP insufficiency may exist with physiologic implications.[12] Alternatively, unloading of the systemic ventricle has also been proposed as a mechanism for BNP levels similar to those of controls.[15] In the "surgical stress" group there was no significant difference in preoperative and postoperative BNP level, confirming that the physiologic stress of surgery alone is not a confounder. They also noted a difference in baseline preoperative BNP levels between two groups of patients, based on age: (1) neonatal patients with CHD who were less than 44 weeks' gestational age (adjusted) and (2) nonneonatal patients with CHD who were more than 4 weeks of age plus older children. Median BNP levels in neonatal versus nonneonatal patients with CHD were 27 and 7 pg/mL, respectively. Median preoperative and postoperative BNP levels in neonatal CHD were 2370 versus 2140 pg/mL. Median preoperative and postoperative levels within the nonneonatal group were significantly different (22 versus 41 pg/mL with median change 19 pg/mL, $P < .001$). As mentioned earlier, postoperative BNP levels were more predictive of early poor outcome (<180 days) than preoperative or perioperative levels. However, due to small sample sizes, heterogenous outcome measures, and weak discriminatory power of AUC of ROC, ultimately cut points for diagnostic and prognostic classification are not provided in the literature.[12,14]

In essence, important trends in BNP levels in patients with CHD during and after CT surgery include the following:

- Clear demarcation in higher BNP levels in neonatal versus nonneonatal patients with CHD
- Preoperative BNP levels correlated to clinical severity of heart failure and length of therapy
- Postoperative levels correlated to early (<180 days) adverse outcome, but
- Progressively lower levels in staged univentricular repair subsequent to the Norwood procedure, regardless of clinical acuity, raise the concern that BNP level may not be indicative of CHD severity in all patients with single-ventricle physiology
- No significant increase in levels during noncardiac surgery ("surgical stress" control group)
- Wide variation between and *within* CHD subsets; due to small size, lesion-specific subsets lacked power for statistical analysis

In summary, although BNP levels appear to be valuable as a clinical adjunct marker preoperatively and postoperatively, at this time they are used only in conjunction and support of clinical measures of severity and echocardiographic parameters, without validated algorithms for changing clinical management. Further, for individual patients, levels should be followed for trends; random levels are meaningless at best and misleading at worst.

Brain Natriuretic Peptide in Pulmonary Hypertension. PH is an increasingly frequent cause for admission to the ICU, and PH crisis is a feared complication of postoperative management for patients with both CHD and structurally normal hearts with severe pulmonary disease. BNP is the best-studied PH biomarker in both pediatric and adult populations. However, for all the reasons described earlier, BNP has limitations, especially in the pediatric population, as have most biomarkers whose discovery has been from large-volume adult studies with results extrapolated to pediatric patients. Despite lack of a standardized catheterization laboratory protocol for pediatric PH,[24] cardiac catheterization remains the gold standard for diagnosis, prognosis, and therapeutic monitoring in PH. In adults with PH, BNP has been correlated with disease progression as a surrogate for invasive hemodynamics, including pulmonary vascular resistance and pulmonary artery pressure, with a negative correlation with cardiac index.[25,26] In pediatric PH, however, although elevated/rising BNP level is recognized as a means for high-risk versus low-risk stratification,[27] conclusive correlation with invasive hemodynamics has not been demonstrated. Three studies in pediatric patients that attempt to correlate BNP with invasive hemodynamics had mixed results. Bernus et al.[28] found no correlation with echocardiographic or hemodynamic data, whereas Lammers et al.[13] found optimal correlation between pulmonary vascular resistance index (PVRI) and BNP when PVRI is lowest and most stable. Finally, although Takatsuki et al.[21] demonstrated correlation of NTproBNP with invasive hemodynamics, the low magnitude of the correlations led the authors to recommend against using levels to replace clinical parameters. Finally, as noted earlier, BNP and NTproBNP are well correlated but not interchangeable, and different centers tend to collect either one or the other, rarely both, with more centers now collecting NTproBNP than in prior years. This is relevant given the assertion by Takatsuki et al. that although BNP was better correlated with real-time hemodynamics in the cardiac catheterization laboratory,[21] NTproBNP is preferable for longitudinal monitoring with longer half-life and stable levels.

Robust correlation with functional parameters and surrogates for clinical end points in pediatric PH would be highly valuable, but at best the data are conflicting. Lammers et al.[13] found in a retrospective cohort of 50 children with PH that BNP levels did not correlate with 6-minute walk distance (6MWD) testing, whereas Van Albada et al.,[29] in a cohort of 29 pediatric patients with idiopathic PAH (IPAH) and associated pulmonary arterial hypertension (APAH), found that NTproBNP levels correlated with functional class and 6MWD, and initiation of treatment resulted in decreased NTproBNP levels and increased 6MWD.

Further, in adult IPAH, BNP levels greater than or equal to 180 ng/mL predict worse survival outcomes,[26] but attempts in pediatric PH to identify a similar clinical cut point have proven more difficult, presumably due to smaller sample sizes, longer time until outcomes of interest, and poor sensitivity. Lammers et al.,[13] using AUC from ROC analysis of the UK Pulmonary Hypertension Service for Children, found that a BNP level of greater than 130 pg/mL predicted death or need for transplant with a sensitivity of 57.1% and specificity of 83.3%. Bernus et al.[28] when attempting to extrapolate the adult value of 180 ng/mL, had only 10 patients with BNP level of greater than 180 ng/mL. Finally, Van Albada et al. attempted to evaluate an adult PH cutoff value of NTproBNP level greater than 1400 pg/mL to identify patients with poor long-term prognosis (53% sensitivity and 88% specificity), but

only 6 pediatric patients had values of greater than 1400 pg/mL.[29] Using this cut point of greater than 1400 pg/mL, there was 83% mortality within 2 years; using a cut point of NTproBNP level greater than 1664 pg/mL gave 100% and 94% sensitivity and specificity, respectively, for mortality.[29]

In summary, in PH:
- Trends of BNP levels for individual patients appear more useful than a random absolute value at any given time.
- A threshold BNP value of BNP 130 pg/mL (NTproBNP >1664 pg/mL) is likely valuable for risk stratification.
- Despite mixed results and low-magnitude correlation with functional parameters and invasive hemodynamics, a rising/elevated value within the framework of developmental regulation implies higher risk of adverse outcome.

Currently there is no validated use of biomarkers specifically for PAH associated with CHD (APAH-CHD).[30] It will be especially difficult to generalize and/or create clinically useful cut points for APAH-CHD, given heterogeneity, small subsets of specific lesions, and the difference between elevation of pulmonary pressure in biventricular hearts and that in single-ventricle physiology. In a recent expert consensus statement on PH in children with CHD by the European Pediatric Pulmonary Vascular Disease Network, based on the 5th World Symposium on Pulmonary Hypertension in Nice in 2013 and the Pediatric Taskforce of the Pulmonary Vascular Research Institute (Panama, 2011), there is no mention of biomarker use to guide therapy. Thus extrapolation of the results discussed earlier to patients with CHD should be done carefully and with the understanding that no expert consensus or validated studies exist.

Cardiac Failure Biomarker Category 2: ST2 and Gal3

As described previously, the two general classes of cardiac failure biomarkers are those of ventricular stretch (NPs), and those of cardiac function and fibrosis, namely, ST2 and Gal3. Both ST2 and Gal3 are gaining widespread acceptance as adult biomarkers of myocardial function, fibrosis, and remodeling based on a growing body of literature and warrant discussion for anticipated future pediatric cardiology applications, particularly in heart failure and orthotopic heart transplant. Moreover, increased utility has been demonstrated as an adjunct to BNP in heart failure in adults[31] because both were included in the 2013 American College of Cardiology/American Heart Association guidelines as risk stratification biomarkers for acute and chronic heart failure in adults (class IIb recommendation).[32] However, increased concentrations of both biomarkers have been noted with concomitant noncardiac pathophysiologies such as chronic obstructive pulmonary disease and pneumonia, likely reflecting an inflammatory, and potentially confounding, milieu in patients with multiorgan system comorbidities.[31]

Soluble ST2 Structure and Function. ST2, a member of the interleukin-1 receptor family, is a receptor for interleukin-33 (IL-33). Two isoforms of ST2 are involved in cardiac signaling and pathogenesis: soluble ST2 (sST2) and a cell membrane–bound isoform (ST2L). Binding of the membrane-bound ST2 with its ligand IL-33 results in cardioprotective signaling. However, *soluble* ST2 functions as a scavenger receptor and competes for IL-33 binding with the membrane bound ST2. When sST2 levels are high, IL-33 binding to the cardiac membrane bound ST2 is reduced; in the absence of IL-33/ST2L cardioprotective signaling, there is resultant cardiac cellular death, tissue fibrosis, and reduced cardiac function.

sST2 has indeed been shown to be a marker of cardiac cellular death, tissue fibrosis, and reduced cardiac function in adult heart failure and transplant patients, as well as being predictive of hospitalization and mortality.[33]

Normative Pediatric Values. Normative median and 95 percentile ST2 values in children without heart failure were found to be similar to those of normal adults.[34] Although not statistically significant, higher levels were noted in males versus females when they were 15 years of age or older.[34]

Pediatric Use. ST2 shows promise as a potential biomarker of orthotopic heart transplant rejection in pediatric heart transplant recipients and hopefully in the overarching goal of eventual biopsy-free detection of rejection and therapeutic monitoring of antirejection medications. In a recent simultaneous biopsy and serum-based assessment of ST2 in both heart and small bowel transplant, Mathews et al.[35] showed that sST2 level was elevated in rejection and quiescent during rejection-free periods. The efficacy of this potential biomarker in two types of organ transplant supported claims that elevated sST2 level was a reflection of alloimmunity rather than just cardiac injury.[35] Immunostaining of endomyocardial biopsy specimens with marked increase in ST2 level during rejection, coupled with moderate discrimination by AUC of ROC analysis of serum at the time of rejection episodes, supports the circulating biomarker as a reflection of proximal graft rejection.[35] Further, serum levels of ST2 returned to rejection-free levels with effective treatment. Finally, given that sST2 does not require cardiomyocyte damage for secretion, such as other markers of cardiac injury, it is further proposed as a marker of early rejection.[35]

Galactin-3 Structure and Function. Gal3 is a carbohydrate-binding protein released by activated cardiac macrophages, resulting in the induction of cardiac fibroblasts, and is found to be upregulated in decompensated heart failure. This complex interplay, with progressive accumulation of myocardial collagen and alteration of the myocardial extracellular matrix, is hypothesized to link the inflammatory milieu of myocardial injury to fibrosis.[36] Gal3 is also implicated in apoptosis, which is speculated to be involved in the transition from compensated to decompensated heart failure.[36] Gal3 is an example of a biomarker that likely also plays an active role in the pathogenesis of heart failure and may have a future role as a therapeutic target or agent.

Normative Pediatric Values. In children without heart failure, Gal3 levels are similar to those in previous studies in normal healthy adults.[34] Levels varied according to which FDA-approved assay was used; as previously mentioned as a common weakness in biomarker validation, interassay variability impedes establishment of pediatric normative values and is a source of discrepancy among biomarkers.[34] Gal3 is not correlated with gender but does show a positive correlation with age.

Pediatric Use. As in adults, Gal3 has potential applicability in risk stratification for pediatric heart failure across causes, including CHD, but as of yet there is no current validation for its use in clinical management. Two studies (by Kotby et al.[36] and Mohammed et al.[37]) have evaluated serum Gal3 levels in children, including patients with preserved and reduced ejection fraction in dilated cardiomyopathy, CHD, and rheumatic heart disease. Both studies found a statistically significant difference in Gal3 levels between those with heart failure, whether with preserved or reduced ejection fraction, and control patients.[36,37] Analysis of AUC of ROC showed a cut-off value for differentiating patients with heart failure versus controls of greater than 3 ng/mL with sensitivity of 100%, specificity of 97.78%, positive predictive value of 97.8%, negative predictive value of 100%, and diagnostic accuracy of 100%.[36] Significant

differences were found in both studies between Gal3 levels and severity of heart failure by the Ross classification.[36,37] Kotby et al. also found a statistically significant increase in Gal3 levels of those not receiving spironolactone, whereas in adult patients receiving Aldactone, Gal3 levels were decreased. Thus an increase in Gal3 levels is speculated to be due to Gal3-mediated myocardial fibrosis.[35] Given the prevalence of Aldactone as an adjunct in heart failure in both pediatric and adult CHF patients, this is an unfortunate confounder, but it also indicates that elevated Gal3 levels may identify patients who would reap the most benefit from the antifibrotic effect of spironolactone.[35]

Biomarker of Cardiac Injury: Troponin

Due to unparalleled cardiac specificity, troponins serve as acute cardiac myocyte necrosis markers and are currently the best circulating measure of acute cardiac injury. As a broad overview, use of troponin in the ICU in CHD centers around identification of cardiac ischemia, postpericardiotomy syndrome, cardiac trauma, and myocarditis.

Troponin: Structure/Function. Cardiac troponin is the calcium-dependent regulator of the contractile apparatus of cardiac muscle, often thought of as the "switch" for cardiac muscle contraction and relaxation. Three subunits constitute troponin: troponin C (calcium-binding subunit [cTnC]), troponin T (thin filament that attaches to tropomyosin [cTnT]) and troponin I (inhibits actin-myosin interactions [cTnI]). The troponins are uniquely cardiac specific and are therefore specific cardiac necrosis biomarkers. Both cTnT and cTnI have been studied in pediatric and adult cardiac patients, and both are released with cardiac injury, with cTnI being unaffected by renal failure and thus the preferred of the two.[38]

Normative Pediatric Values. Assays for cTnI and cTnT are FDA approved and available in most clinical laboratories. Interassay variability exists, but generally the clinical upper limit of normal is considered the 99th percentile of the normal reference population. Based on the 2002 American College of Cardiology and European Society of Cardiology guidelines,[39] this is approximately 3 standard deviations from the mean of a normal adult population,[40] to maximize sensitivity while minimizing false-positives.[40] Typically the upper reference limit cutoff of 0.04 ng/mL is based on apparently healthy adults and used to risk stratify myocardial infarction in adults at The Johns Hopkins Hospital.[41] Normative values exist in pediatrics, with the highest concentrations immediately after birth, peaking on the third day of life, and decreasing toward adult values by the end of the first year of life.[42,43] Reported values in the literature tend to be more helpful to describing trends of developmental regulation, given the variety of assays used and increasing sensitivity of the assay over the decades since discovery. In an attempt to establish normal pediatric values, Hirsch et al.[42] evaluated two groups of children, the first of which included ambulatory pediatric patients with no apparent cardiac disease ($n = 120$) and patients in stable condition with known congenital or acquired cardiac abnormalities ($n = 96$), whereas the second group included 65 ICU patients with a variety of acute illnesses, with the results that cTnI levels were generally not elevated in group A. As will be further described later in the chapter, troponin levels are higher in infants than older children.[38,42,44]

Cardiac Ischemia in the Intensive Care Unit. In both surgical and nonsurgical patients, as well as those with and without structural heart disease, cTnI and cTnT are the preferred biomarkers of cardiac injury in both adults and children, with improved sensitivity and specificity for cardiac injury over creatine kinase (CK) and creatine kinase–myocardial band (CK-MB) assays.[38] cTnT is a sensitive and specific marker of myocardial injury, given that it is not expressed by skeletal muscle, either during development, as a result of skeletal muscle injury stimulus, or following noncardiac surgery.[45] In pediatric CHD, cTnI and cTnT are sensitive and specific for myocardial ischemia/infarction, although cTnI is often preferred because levels are not affected by renal failure.[38] In pediatric cardiology, cTnI is less likely to be elevated from myocardial ischemia due to coronary artery disease, given the much lower prevalence of coronary artery disease in pediatric patients.[46] As discussed previously, in patients in stable condition with known congenital or acquired cardiac abnormalities, troponin levels were within the same range as those in their apparently healthy, ambulatory pediatric peers.[42] In a recent study by Harris and Gossett[47] of 24 patients with elevated troponin levels, excluding recent cardiac surgery, "significant" CHD, neonates in the neonatal intensive care unit, or patients on extracorporeal membrane oxygenation (ECMO), only 3 had coronary-related diagnoses (anomalous origin of left coronary artery from pulmonary artery [ALCAPA] and Kawasaki disease), whereas the majority (17/24, or 71%) had myocarditis or cardiomyopathy. Although left heart catheterization was completed in nearly half the cases (10/24), in no case was the diagnosis made/changed, confirming the current standard of care among pediatric cardiologists that left heart catheterization and coronary angiography is reserved for a highly selective group, avoiding routine application of adult "door-to-balloon time" protocols.[47] Currently troponin is used as a clinical adjunct in the diagnosis of pediatric myocarditis; however, normal levels do not rule out the presence of myocarditis.[48] Further, in a retrospective review of patients presenting to the emergency department with chest pain over 7 years by Brown et al.,[49] only 48% of those with increased troponin levels were attributed to primary cardiac disease, although the yield increased to 87% when combined with abnormal ECG. The median troponin level of those with cardiac cause of chest pain differed from those with a noncardiac cause: 8.5 ng/mL (interquartile range 4.6-18.5) versus 0.34 ng/mL (interquartile range 0.12-1.3) (P = .02), respectively.[49] Two other important conclusions were drawn from this study: (1) less likelihood of noncardiac diagnoses in patients if troponin level is greater than or equal to 2 ng/mL and (2) no correlation between level of troponin elevation and morbidity and mortality.[49] Both of these conclusions were supported by a recent study evaluating the contribution of diagnostic modalities toward the final diagnosis after an elevated troponin level was demonstrated, as well as the contribution of the troponin level at various times during diagnosis and treatment to the final diagnosis and ventricular function.[50] This study found that troponin values within each subgroup did not distinguish between cardiac causes, with a wide range of values, among which levels in myocarditis patients were not the highest. Troponin absolute value and progression were also not helpful in differentiating between preserved versus depressed ventricular function.[50]

Although these studies were done in patients with no known history of CHD, given the findings of the study by Hirsch et al.[42] of comparable baseline troponin levels in normative versus stable cardiac disease, they can likely be extrapolated to CHD patients.

Thus, although the differential of cTnI elevation in both congenital and acquired heart disease is broad, including coronary artery aneurysm, injury, anomalous origin of the coronary arteries, anthracycline-induced cardiac toxicity, myocardial surgical injury, myocarditis, postpericardiotomy syndrome, and trauma, cTnI elevation in children is fundamentally different from that in adults, although adult cutoff values for normalcy are applied. As with

NTproBNP, knowledge of baseline values and/or trends over time are often more clinically relevant than a random value in time, especially given the demonstration, by increasingly sensitivity assays, that there is development/accrual of morbidity from structural and acquired heart disease, resulting in slowly rising troponin levels over time. This inherently decreases the utility of solitary cutoff values, even in adults.[40] Further, experts in the field have theorized that an early release of troponin may signify reversible injury, whereas sustained release may be associated with progressive cell death.[40] Values trended over time are therefore more informative, and an important future goal of risk stratification will be recognizing a pattern of troponin release that may distinguish acute disease/injury from chronic elevation.

Pattern of Troponin Release During Cardiac Surgery. Postoperative troponin levels can have value to explain poor cardiac function, especially in cases that require coronary reimplantation. Troponin release in CHD following cardiothoracic surgery and cardiopulmonary bypass (CPB) has been studied, with the following five themes: (1) cTnI and cTnT are of equal sensitivity and specificity for myocardial injury; levels behave similarly in the early postoperative phase (up to 28 hours).[51] cTnT has been described as peaking 30 minutes after termination of CPB with steady decline to baseline 4 to 5 days postoperatively[52]; (2) troponin I is preferable to cTnT as a biomarker of cardiac ischemia because it is unaffected by renal failure; (3) whereas infant myocardium is more resistant to hypoxia, congenitally abnormal myocardium is more sensitive to cardioplegic arrest,[52] with higher postoperative peak troponin levels in infants[38,42,44]; (4) higher postoperative values are associated with longer myocardial ischemia and extent of myocardial damage[44]; and (5) threshold levels for troponin as a marker of adverse outcome have been difficult to establish in children.[38]

Similar to BNP, troponin levels have been used in adults as a marker of poor outcome after CPB, with values above threshold levels being associated with severe cardiac event and/or death.[53] Similar thresholds have been proposed in pediatric cardiothoracic surgery for both cTnI and cTnT, with description of high troponin I release (especially ≥ 100 mcg/L) being associated with post-CPB mortality.[44,54] However, as discussed previously, as assays become increasingly sensitive, thresholds established using older assays become obsolete, and possible pitfalls of attempting to distinguish thresholds, especially across heterogeneous patterns of cardiac injury, has the potential to mislead. Further, in a contemporary study of troponin values in infants and children with CHD undergoing CPB, Gupta-Malhotra et al.[38] showed that, with the caveat of small sample size, for the 4 patients with cTnI values above this threshold (3 infants, 1 child), none had a severe cardiac event or death. Further, infants appear to have higher postoperative values of troponin, making thresholds difficult across age ranges.[38] Finally, differing results have been found in preoperative and postoperative troponin levels in cyanotic versus acyanotic patients, further complicating establishing a threshold value across the heterogeneous spectrum of CHD.[38] As described earlier, the adult cutoff value of cTnI less than 0.04 ng/mL is extrapolated to pediatric patients but does not account for developmental regulation, individual variance in cardiac injury, or presence of cyanosis.

Other Biomarkers

Evaluation of postoperative noncardiac organ system–related dysfunction in CHD is a burgeoning area of biomarker discovery; because this is addressed elsewhere in greater detail, only a brief overview is provided in this chapter. Two especially important areas of biomarker research and potential clinical utility are in postoperative acute kidney injury (AKI) and cerebral injury in CHD.

Biomarkers of Acute Kidney Injury Following CT Surgery

Postoperative AKI, defined by Kidney Disease Improving Global Outcomes (KDIGO) as serum creatinine level increase by 50% or more within 7 postoperative days, or 0.3 mg/dL within 48 postoperative hours from preoperative level,[55] has been estimated to complicate recovery in as many as 40% to 50% of children undergoing cardiac surgery,[56,57] underscoring the potential importance of an AKI biomarker for risk stratification in pediatric cardiac patients. In terms of markers of acute renal injury, pediatric studies and normative values continue to accrue; the most well studied markers are cystatin C (CysC) and neutrophil gelatinase-associated lipocalin (NGAL). CysC, similar to creatinine, is a marker of renal function, given its constant production by nucleated cells and filtration at the renal glomerulus.[58] CysC is unaffected by muscle mass or sex and has been proposed as a more accurate measure of glomerular filtration rate than creatinine, which rises late in the course of disease, potentially delaying diagnosis of AKI.[56] NGAL is a tubular protein that is upregulated with ischemia and best detected in the urine. CysC has been validated as a marker of cardiac surgery postoperative AKI and found to be more strongly associated with urine IL-18 or kidney injury molecule 1 (KIM1) biomarker.[56] This is an important finding given the significant limitation of serum creatinine in the timely diagnosis, treatment, and risk stratification of cardiac surgery postoperative AKI.[56] Other well-studied markers of renal injury associated with CT surgery postoperative AKI include three main classes: (1) markers of tubular injury, including NGAL, for which reference ranges are established, KIM1, IL-18, and liver-type fatty acid binding protein (L-FABP); (2) markers of inflammation, including IL-6; and (3) markers of cell cycle arrest, including tissue inhibitor of metalloproteinases-2 (TIMP-2) and insulin-like growth factor–binding protein 7 (IGFBP-7). As is the hope for future biomarker use in many clinical scenarios, biomarker combinations that harness the ability to evaluate functional markers (CysC) and tubular damage markers have been evaluated, with the ability to pinpoint timing of kidney injury.[59] As discussed by Bucholz et al.,[60] although AKI prevention studies are not currently even established, much less proven efficacious, possible interventions in pediatric patients undergoing cardiac surgery could include minimization of CPB time, avoidance of frequently used postoperative nephrotoxic medications, personalized optimization of hemodynamics/fluid management, and even possible postponement of elective procedures.

Much of the biomarker research regarding postoperative AKI has focused on markers of AKI, although the Translational Research Investigating Biomarker Endpoints in Acute Kidney Injury (TRIBE-AKI) consortium,[61] established to prospectively collect data on children undergoing cardiac surgery to validate novel kidney injury biomarkers, has also studied a panel of cardiac biomarkers. Bucholz et al.,[60] as part of the TRIBE-AKI consortium, evaluated five cardiac biomarkers (NTproBNP, troponin I, troponin T, h-FABP and CK-MB) on 106 children from the TRIBE-AKI cohort undergoing a Risk Adjustment for Congenital Heart Surgery (RACHS-1) cardiothoracic surgical procedure category of 2 to 4, finding that preoperative h-FABP and CK-MB levels are associated with the risk of postoperative AKI, providing good discrimination (AUC of

ROC curves analysis for h-FABP: AUC 0.70, 95% CI, 0.60-0.81, and for CK-MB: AUC 0.70, 95% CI, 0.60-0.81), with optimal cut points for detecting postoperative AKI for CK-MB of 2.9 mcg/L (sensitivity 64.2%, specificity 64.6%) and for h-FABP of 2.6 pg/mL (sensitivity 68%, specificity 68.8%) for preoperative h-FABP. This study notably excluded neonates and intentionally chose more complicated CT surgery by RACHS-1 score, acknowledging the subsequent limitations to generalizability. NTproBNP has not been found to consistently predict postoperative AKI after CT surgery in several pediatric evaluations,[60,62,63] nor did cardiac troponin I or T.[60]

Biomarkers of Brain Injury Following Computed Tomography Surgery

Estimates of abnormal neurodevelopmental outcomes are as high as one in three in congenital heart surgery.[64] Glial fibrillary acidic protein (GFAP), an astrocyte protein released after astrocyte injury or death, has been linked to neurologic outcomes in pediatric and adult patients after trauma and ECMO, as well as CHD.[65,66] GFAP is a promising potential biomarker of brain injury, levels of which have been shown to rise during CPB, especially during rewarming.[67]

In multivariate analysis controlling for CPB time, deep hypothermic circulatory arrest, and procedure risk category (RACHS), post-CPB GFAP has been shown to have a significant negative relationship with oxygen delivery nadir ($P < .03$), although no clinical neurologic outcomes could be documented in this retrospective study of 116 infants and children with CHD.[64] Given the multifactorial causes for white matter injury following congenital heart surgery, including likely preoperative intrinsically delayed brain development, potential compromise of cerebral oxygen delivery during CPB, as well as the proinflammatory cascade and capillary leak triggered by CPB, a brain injury biomarker such as GFAP could have potential utility in risk stratification, intraoperative modifications, and targeted developmental follow-up.[64]

Novel Biomarkers

The literature is replete with promising biomarkers, some of which may also prove to be therapeutic targets and active modifiers of the disease process. Biomarker discovery from urine and saliva, some of the least invasively obtained biofluids, is also becoming increasingly prevalent. As tempting as it is to incorporate some of these novel tests, care must be taken to avoid ordering tests without understanding pretest probability and the meaning of results and how the test results will change clinical management. Even validated adult biomarkers cannot yet be extrapolated to pediatric care without further testing and establishment of normative values.

Key Points and Conclusion

For the practitioner using biomarkers as a clinical adjunct, the following are key points and caveats that should be kept in mind:

1. There are no currently established pediatric guidelines for guiding any therapy solely based on biomarkers, although they can be used for risk stratification.
2. Establishing a baseline level is vital to utility.
3. The majority of research centers around two main classes of pediatric cardiac biomarkers: markers of cardiac function/failure and markers of cardiac injury.

4. For cardiac markers of function/failure:
   • BNP:
     • Postoperative BNP levels in CT surgery are correlated to clinical severity of heart failure, length of therapy, and adverse outcome but may not indicate severity across all types of single-ventricle physiology, especially in patients with Fontan palliation, with wide variation between and within CHD subsets.
     • In PH: no specific guidelines for APAH-CHD. NTproBNP is now preferred given longer half-life. Rising/elevated value within the framework of developmental regulation implies higher risk of adverse outcome.
   • ST2: promising potential biomarker of orthotopic heart transplant rejection.
   • Gal3: likely future utility in heart failure, use caution with concurrent spironolactone administration.
5. For cardiac markers of injury:
   • Troponin: both cTnT and cTnI are now preferred to CK and CK-MB given improved sensitivity and specificity; cTnI preferred because levels are not affected by renal failure. Levels peak after CPB and continue to fall over next 4 to 5 days.
6. Developmental regulation must be taken into account; the expectation should be for a changing baseline even in the same individual with age and accruing cardiac dysfunction/damage.
7. Interassay variability exists even in FDA-approved biomarkers.
8. As assay sensitivity improves, ranges are likely to change.
9. Multiorgan system failure can confound results; practitioners have a responsibility to understand potentially confounding factors before ordering tests with impunity.
10. Currently in cardiac intensive care, biomarker AUC of ROC analysis and clinical cut points for diagnosis are unlikely to be of as much practical use in the ICU as trends over time after a baseline is established, although these cut points may be useful for initial triage of diagnostic modalities.
11. In the future, using biomarkers as surrogate end points in clinical trials, markers of therapeutic response, and/or as a means of avoiding invasive procedures could revolutionize pediatric cardiac and ICU care.

Selected References

A complete list of references is available at ExpertConsult.com.

12. Niedner MF, Foley JL, Riffenburgh RH, Bichell DP, Peterson BM, Rodarte A. B-type natriuretic peptide: perioperative patterns in congenital heart disease. *Congenit Heart Dis.* 2010;5(3):243–255. doi:10.1111/j.1747-0803.2010.00396.x. [doi].
14. Afshani N, Schulein S, Biccard BM, Thomas JM. Clinical utility of B-type natriuretic peptide (NP) in pediatric cardiac surgery–a systematic review. *Paediatr Anaesth.* 2015;25(2):115–126. doi:10.1111/pan.12467. [doi].
22. Costello JM, Goodman DM, Green TP. A review of the natriuretic hormone system's diagnostic and therapeutic potential in critically ill children. *Pediatr Crit Care Med.* 2006;7(4):308–318. doi:10.1097/01.PCC.0000224998.97784.A3. [doi].
35. Mathews LR, Lott JM, Isse K, et al. Elevated ST2 Distinguishes Incidences of Pediatric Heart and Small Bowel Transplant Rejection. *Am J Transplant.* 2016;16(3):938–950. doi:10.1111/ajt.13542. [doi].
36. Kotby AA, Youssef OI, Elmaraghy MO, El Sharkawy OS. Galectin-3 in Children with Chronic Heart Failure with Normal and Reduced Ejection Fraction: Relationship to Disease Severity. *Pediatr Cardiol.* 2017;38(1):95–102. doi:10.1007/s00246-016-1488-2. [doi].
44. Immer FF, Stocker F, Seiler AM, et al. Troponin-I for prediction of early postoperative course after pediatric cardiac surgery. *J Am Coll Cardiol.* 1999;33(6):1719–1723. doi: S0735-1097(99)00061-3 [pii].
49. Brown JL, Hirsh DA, Mahle WT. Use of troponin as a screen for chest pain in the pediatric emergency department. *Pediatr Cardiol.* 2012;33(2):337–342. doi:10.1007/s00246-011-0149-8. [doi].
50. Thankavel PP, Mir A, Ramaciotti C. Elevated troponin levels in previously healthy children: value of diagnostic modalities and the importance of a drug screen. *Cardiol Young.* 2014;24(2):283–289. doi:10.1017/S1047951113000231. [doi].
60. Bucholz EM, Whitlock RP, Zappitelli M, et al. Cardiac biomarkers and acute kidney injury after cardiac surgery. *Pediatrics.* 2015;135(4):e945–e956. doi:10.1542/peds.2014-2949. [doi].

39

Extracorporeal Membrane Oxygenation

MELANIA M. BEMBEA, MD, MPH, PHD; ALLAN GOLDMAN, MRCP, MBBCH, MSC;
OSAMI HONJO, MD, PHD; RAVI R. THIAGARAJAN, MBBS, MPH

Extracorporeal membrane oxygenation (ECMO) is an established modality of extracorporeal life support (ECLS) for patients with severe, refractory cardiac and/or respiratory failure.[1] ECMO evolved as an extension of the cardiopulmonary bypass (CPB) technology developed in the 1950s.[2] The first use of ECMO in the intensive care unit was reported in 1972 in an adult with posttraumatic acute respiratory distress syndrome.[3] This was followed by the successful use of extracorporeal oxygenation in 1973 following surgical repair of tetralogy of Fallot[4] and in 1975 in a newborn with respiratory failure secondary to meconium aspiration syndrome.[5] Randomized controlled trials conducted in the 1980s showed superior outcomes in neonates with respiratory failure supported with ECMO compared with those supported with conventional mechanical ventilation.[6,7] Following these early successes, neonatal respiratory failure represented the main indication for ECMO in the pediatric age for the first 30 years that the technology was available.[1] However, the last 15 years have seen a dramatic increase in the use of ECMO for primary cardiac indications in neonates and older children alike.[8] The Extracorporeal Life Support Organization (ELSO) registry reported a total of 7243 neonatal cardiac ECLS cases and 9479 pediatric cardiac ECLS cases from inception in 1989 to December 31, 2015, of which 2849 neonatal cardiac cases and 3850 pediatric cardiac cases were reported between 2009 and 2015.[8] During the period from 2009 to 2015, yearly numbers of cardiac ECLS cases reported to the ELSO registry ranged from 310 to 470 for neonates, and from 439 to 673 for older infants and children.[8] Health care providers caring for children with cardiac disease should be knowledgeable about indications, management, and complications associated with ECMO because it is both a common and important treatment modality offered to these children.

General Indications and Contraindications

Cardiac indications for ECMO support include perioperative support and support for nonsurgical conditions. Increasingly in recent years ECMO has been used to support children with cardiac arrest failing to respond to conventional cardiopulmonary resuscitation (ECPR) (Box 39.1).

Perioperative Support

Indications for ECMO support surrounding cardiac surgery include preoperative stabilization, failure to wean a patient from CPB, postoperative low cardiac output syndrome (LCOS), and postoperative cardiopulmonary arrest (CPA).

Preoperative stabilization may be required in infants with profound cyanosis, cardiogenic shock, or severe pulmonary hypertension (e.g., infants with d-transposition of the great arteries).[9,10]

ECMO use for failure to wean from CPB typically entails direct cannulation of the right atrium and the aorta via the median sternotomy (central cannulation). Outcomes of patients who fail to wean from CPB have been shown to be worse than outcomes of those who are cannulated onto ECMO for LCOS or CPA occurring after a period of stability.[11] Reported rates of mortality reported after postcardiotomy ECMO in infants and children range between 29% and 61%.[11-16] Some of the risk factors for mortality in patients supported on ECMO postoperatively are peak serum lactate level within 24 hours of ECMO support initiation, renal failure requiring hemodialysis during the ECMO course, sepsis, increased blood transfusion requirements, and ECMO duration.[13,14,16]

Residual cardiac defects need to be considered as potential cause for postoperative low cardiac output. Transesophageal echocardiography, direct cardiac chamber pressure, and oxygen saturation measurements can assist in diagnosing residual cardiac defects. An intraoperative review of preoperative data and imaging can also be helpful.

Determining contraindications for perioperative ECMO support in infants and children who undergo cardiac surgery is a complex process and varies widely among centers providing cardiac surgical care. Some historically absolute contraindications have evolved into relative contraindications in recent years, including prematurity, pre-ECMO neurologic injury, multisystem organ failure, and severe coagulopathy. Heparinization of the circuit may worsen hemorrhage (e.g., intracranial hemorrhage, uncontrolled visceral bleeding), and thus ECMO may be deleterious in these cases. Weight less than 2 kg can pose technical challenges to ECMO cannulation and support. When health care teams are considering ECMO support, it is important to understand that ECMO is only a support modality and does not offer any therapeutic benefit. Thus children who benefit from perioperative ECMO support have a reversible reason for their acute refractory heart failure.

The mean duration of cardiac postoperative ECMO course was 6 days in neonates and 7 days in pediatric patients reported to the ELSO registry between 2009 and 2016.[8] Longer ECMO runs have been associated with higher mortality.[13,14,17] Patients unable to separate from ECMO after 5 to 9 days possibly have a nonreversible cause for cardiac failure and should be considered candidates for cardiac transplantation. Specialized care teams of surgeons, cardiologists, intensivists, nurses, and other providers need to thoughtfully evaluate options, consider patient and family values,

• BOX 39.1 | **Indications and Contraindications for Neonatal and Pediatric Extracorporeal Membrane Oxygenation for Cardiac Indications**

Indications
1. Refractory cardiogenic shock
   Acute myocarditis
   Cardiomyopathy
   Cardiac dysfunction in severe sepsis
2. Postoperative refractory cardiac failure
   Failure to wean from cardiopulmonary bypass
   Postoperative low cardiac output syndrome
   Refractory cardiac arrhythmias
   Pulmonary hypertension
3. Cardiac arrest refractory to conventional cardiopulmonary resuscitation
4. Procedural support
5. Bridge to lung or heart transplantation or ventricular assist device

Relative Contraindications
1. End-stage primary disease with poor prognosis
2. Severe neurologic injury or intracranial hemorrhage
3. Uncontrolled visceral bleeding
4. Prematurity (<34 weeks' gestation)
5. Small size (<2 kg)
6. Family or patient directive limiting ECMO use

ECMO, Extracorporeal membrane oxygenation.

and assess regularly the risks and benefits of continued extracorporeal support if there is no improvement in the patient's condition.[18]

Support for Nonsurgical Conditions

Nonsurgical cardiac conditions supported with ECMO include myocarditis and cardiomyopathy, refractory pulmonary hypertension, intractable arrhythmias with hemodynamic compromise (including from toxic ingestion), septic shock, cardiac trauma, and posttransplantation rejection.

Myocarditis and Cardiomyopathy. Neonates and children with acute myocarditis supported on ECMO have rates of survival to hospital discharge of 50% and 76%, respectively.[8,19] ECMO for acute myocarditis is used as bridge to recovery, ventricular assist device (VAD), or transplantation.[10] Although the use of VADs for acute myocarditis has increased in recent years, ECMO is still the support mode of choice for those patients presenting with fulminant acute myocarditis with severe cardiogenic shock or CPA that does not allow for sternotomy and VAD placement.[20-22]

Pulmonary Hypertension. Abnormal pulmonary vascular development in children with congenital heart disease and certain types of cardiac lesions (e.g., obstructed total anomalous pulmonary venous connection, truncus arteriosus, aortic origin of pulmonary artery) place postoperative patients at risk for acute pulmonary hypertension with pulmonary hypertensive crises and associated acute right ventricular failure.[23] The American Heart Association (AHA) and American Thoracic Society (ATS) 2015 guidelines recommend the use of mechanical cardiopulmonary support, including ECMO, for refractory pulmonary hypertensive crises in postoperative pediatric patients who undergo cardiac surgery (Class I; Level of Evidence B).[23] Residual lesions (e.g., residual pulmonary venous obstruction) should be ruled out as causes for pulmonary hypertension.[10]

Post–Cardiac Arrest Support

Use of ECMO for support of patients with CPA refractory to conventional CPR (ECPR) and of patients with profound cardiogenic shock following return of spontaneous circulation after CPA has been increasingly reported in the literature. The number of ECPR cases reported to the ELSO registry increased by 35% for neonates and 67% for children between 2009 and 2015, with a mean ECMO duration of 5 days.[8] The AHA 2015 guidelines state that CPR with ECMO (ECPR) may be considered for infants and children with cardiac diagnoses who suffer in-hospital cardiac arrest in settings that allow "expertise, resources, and systems to optimize the use of ECMO during and after resuscitation," with insufficient evidence to suggest for or against the routine use of ECPR for infants and children with noncardiac diagnoses who suffer in-hospital cardiac arrest (weak recommendation, very low-quality evidence).[24] In large national and international registries, survival rates to hospital discharge range from 40% to 43%.[8,25,26] In an analysis of the AHA Get With the Guidelines—Resuscitation (GWTG-R) registry, children with in-hospital CPR of 10 minutes or longer who underwent ECPR had improved survival to hospital discharge and survival with favorable neurologic outcomes (defined as Pediatric Cerebral Performance Category [PCPC] 1 to 3 or unchanged from admission), compared with children with in-hospital CPR of 10 minutes or longer who underwent continued conventional CPR.[25] Duration of CPR has been linked to mortality and neurologic injury after cardiac arrest in several studies, possibly due to decline in quality and effectiveness over time.[27-31] As such, many centers have implemented rapid-deployment ECMO or ECPR programs, to limit CPR duration and minimize no-flow or low-flow states. With creation of portable ECMO consoles and circuits and improved ultrasonography to facilitate cannula insertion, expansion of these programs in recent years has led to deployment strategies not only in intensive care units and operating rooms, but also in emergency departments and out-of-hospital settings.[32] Pediatric as well as adult ECPR studies suggest that the risk of mortality increases with longer CPR duration, as does the risk of poor neurologic outcomes.[27,33,34] On the contrary, even prolonged CPR events longer than 1 hour can be associated with favorable neurologic outcomes.[25-27] These issues illustrate that maintaining good quality of CPR while awaiting ECMO cannulation is essential to achieving good outcomes after ECPR.

Physiology of Blood Flow and Oxygenation During Extracorporeal Membrane Oxygenation

Biventricular Circulation

Pediatric cardiac ECMO patients have varying degrees of univentricular or biventricular failure, pulmonary hypertension, or pulmonary parenchymal disease. Thus as many as 97% of these patients are supported with venoarterial ECMO,[1] in which venous blood is drained from the right atrium and returned to the aorta, thus providing both cardiac and respiratory support. In contrast, in venovenous ECMO venous blood is drained from the venous circulation and returned to the right atrium. Thus in venovenous ECMO, normal cardiac function is essential. The total systemic blood flow (cardiac output) represents the sum of the extracorporeal flow and the native cardiac output. As opposed to CPB, in which all blood return to the heart is drained through cannulas in the superior and inferior vena cavae, in venoarterial ECMO, only ≈80% of venous return to the heart is drained through the circuit. As long as the heart can pump even small amounts of blood and the aortic valve continues to open, the pulse pressure (difference between the systolic and the diastolic blood pressures) is maintained at ≈10 mm Hg.[10] Severe heart failure without ventricular contractility can be complicated by accumulation of blood from bronchial and thebesian venous flow in the left chambers and subsequent increased pressure in the left ventricle, left atrium, and pulmonary circulation. When this problem is not addressed by an atrial septostomy or placement of a drainage cannula in the left atrium or pulmonary artery, there is increased risk for left ventricle distention, pulmonary edema, and pulmonary hemorrhage. Furthermore, stagnation of blood in the cardiac chambers and pulmonary circulation can lead to clot formation despite anticoagulation.

During venoarterial ECMO, pump flow and systemic vascular resistance are adjusted to maintain age-appropriate cardiac output and mean arterial pressure. Any increase in left ventricular afterload potentially impacting myocardial recovery can be mitigated by reducing systemic vascular resistance or by decreasing preload while maintaining coronary blood flow during venoarterial ECMO support.

In the postoperative cardiac patient requiring ECMO support the goal is to maintain lung inflation and function so that decannulation is not impeded by respiratory failure at the time of cardiac recovery. This may require higher levels of positive end-expiratory pressure and peak inspiratory pressure or alternate modes of ventilation such as high-frequency ventilation or airway pressure release ventilation (see Chapter 23). The oxygenator fraction of inspired oxygen (FiO_2) and sweep flow rates are adjusted to maintain normal oxygenation and normal PCO_2.

The Univentricular Circulation

ECMO has been used in single-ventricle circulations at all surgical stages. Generally the ECMO flow required for patients with single-ventricle physiology is higher than for patients with biventricular physiology, in an effort to maintain the systemic and the pulmonary parallel circulations. As such, patients with Blalock-Taussig (BT) shunt may require extracorporeal flows of 150 to 200 mL/kg/min.[10] The BT shunt is typically maintained open. Standard-sized shunts (3.5 to 4 mm) usually provide enough limitation to pulmonary blood flow that increasing ECMO flow rate most often provides adequate systemic blood flow. Occasionally the shunt needs to be surgically constricted, but this could lead to shunt thrombosis, and diminished flow through the shunt risks pulmonary parenchymal ischemia and potential irreversible lung injury. The position of the right common carotid cannula needs to be checked serially to avoid migration of the tip into the shunt and potential loss of extracorporeal cardiac output. Successful ECMO support in superior cavopulmonary (Glenn) and Fontan circulations has also been reported; these patients often require multisite venous cannulation to provide adequate venous decompression and pump flow.

Equipment

Typical venoarterial and single lumen venovenous circuits (Fig. 39.1) consist of a venous cannula, which drains blood from the right atrium, tubing connecting this cannula to a blood pump, an oxygenator, a heat exchanger, and then returned via the arterial cannula to the aorta in venoarterial ECMO and to the right atrium via the arterial limb of the cannula in venovenous ECMO. An optional venous reservoir can be inserted between the drainage cannula and the pump to serve as a compliance chamber and to allow for noninvasive pressure measurements. Contemporary pumps are mostly centrifugal (Fig. 39.2), although roller pumps continue to be used successfully, especially in small neonates and infants (Table 39.1). Centrifugal blood pumps are axisymmetric pumps that use an impeller assembly to produce a hydrodynamic pressure gradient through rotational kinetic energy. Roller blood pumps are peristaltic blood pumps that use compression of a circular segment of tubing with positive displacement of fluid. Most contemporary oxygenators use hollow fibers, with extracapillary blood flow and intracapillary gas flow. The sweep gas is the gas applied to the gas phase of the membrane lung. The sweep gas inlet oxygen fraction can range from 0.21 to 1.0 and is controlled by a gas blender. The heat exchanger transfers heat between the

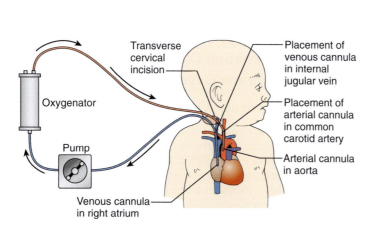

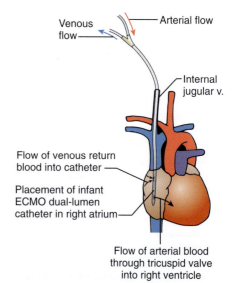

• **Figure 39.1** Venoarterial and venovenous extracorporeal membrane oxygenation circuit configurations. (From Ungerleider RM. Cannulation. In: Sabiston DC, ed. *Atlas of Cardiothoracic Surgery*. Coffman SM, Gordon RG, illustrators. Philadelphia: WB Saunders; 1995:537-8.)

Centrifugal Pump VAD

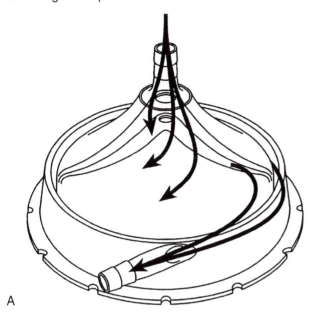

A

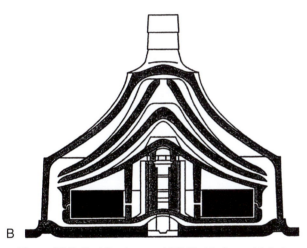

B

• **Figure 39.2** Centrifugal pump. *VAD,* Ventricular assist device.

TABLE 39.1	Differences Between Roller and Centrifugal Pumps	
	Roller Pump	**Centrifugal Pump**
Pump mechanism	Positive displacement	Centrifugal force
Pump inflow	Passive drainage	Active drainage
Pump occlusion	Occlusive pump	Nonocclusive pump
Retrograde flow	Not possible	Possible
Pump flow	Predictable	Varies
Factors affecting pump flow	Pump RPM Displacement volume	Pump RPM Preload and afterload
Risk of tubing rupture with outflow obstruction	Present	Not present
Hemolysis	Present	Present

RPM, Revolutions per minute

that helps detection and prevention of air embolization is a bubble sensor that is typically placed on the return or reinfusion side of the circuit. These devices shut down the ECMO pump when air bubbles are detected. Modern ECMO circuits can be equipped with noninvasive devices to continuously measure and display measurements such as blood flow rate, hemoglobin concentration, hematocrit, PO_2, PCO_2, and mixed venous saturation (SvO_2). Surface modification or coating (e.g., poly-2-methoxyethylacrylate, heparin, albumin), is applied to most ECMO circuits to improve biocompatibility and reduce thrombogenesis. Common technical problems encountered with ECMO circuits and potential solutions are presented in Table 39.2.

ECMO equipment, including circuits, surgical cart and instruments, cannulas, and connectors should all be stored in easily accessible locations. A mobile ECMO cannulation cart containing cannulas and equipment that can be rapidly mobilized to the bedside at the time of ECMO team activation can facilitate safe and rapid ECMO deployment.

Extracorporeal Membrane Oxygenation Cannulation and Initial Management

ECMO cannulation for failure to separate from CPB or in the immediate postoperative period is typically transthoracic. The arterial cannula in the ascending aorta may be already in place from CPB, and the venous cannula is inserted directly into the right atrium (usually through the right atrial appendage. *If possible, cannulas should be selected that are large enough to support 150 mL/kg/min flow with a pump inlet pressure of more than 20 mm Hg (for centrifugal pump ECMO) and an outlet pressure of less than 200 mm Hg.* Patients who cannot be successfully weaned from CPB often transition directly from CPB to ECMO and are usually completely heparinized (for their CPB circuit). This can result in a period of bleeding related to anticoagulation that can make the first few hours of ECMO challenging for the care team. In many cases, particularly with the coated and miniaturized circuits currently available, it is common to stop the heparin in these patients and perform the initial several

blood phase and a fully separated water phase and allows for blood flow returning to the patient to be warmed at a preset temperature. Modern oxygenators may have integrated heat exchangers. A bridge is an optional segment of tubing inserted between the drainage (venous) and the reinfusion (arterial) limbs of the circuit, close to the cannula connections, and can be opened when the venous and arterial ECMO cannulas inserted in the patient are clamped during a weaning trial. Although the clamping isolates the patient from the circuit, opening the bridge allows recirculation at the circuit level, thus allowing the circuit to be viable and the patient returned to ECMO support in case of weaning failure.

The ECMO circuit typically contains pump inlet, preoxygenator or premembrane, and postoxygenator or postmembrane pressure monitors (Fig. 39.3). The pressure gradient between the inlet and the outlet of the oxygenator is usually followed as an indicator for oxygenator clot formation. The ECMO circuit may also contain access ports for medication and blood product administration, for connection of ultrafiltration (including hemodialysis) devices, and for blood sampling for laboratory tests. An important safety feature

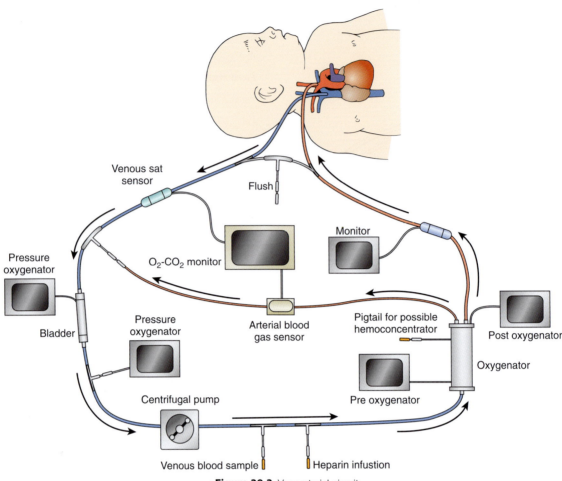

• **Figure 39.3** Venoarterial circuit.

hours of ECMO without anticoagulation to manage the bleeding. In the more common scenario, ECMO is initiated after a period off the CPB circuit, and during this time the surgical team is often able to achieve some control of bleeding by administering protamine to counteract the heparin in the CPB circuit. Achieving hemostasis in the operating room before implementing ECMO is extremely helpful. In these cases a bolus of 75 to 100 U/kg of unfractionated heparin (UFH) can be administered before ECMO initiation, although many surgical teams may still elect to perform the first several hours of postoperative ECMO support without heparin to reduce the likelihood of significant bleeding during the ECMO run. After hemostasis is achieved, all patients on ECMO require anticoagulation with heparin (or another agent if the patient has heparin sensitivity such as documented heparin-induced thrombosis and thrombocytopenia). Anticoagulation strategies are discussed in more detail later. If a prolonged ECMO course is anticipated, de novo neck cannulation or conversion from transthoracic to neck cannulation via the right common carotid artery and right internal jugular vein may be considered in an effort to minimize risk of infection with significantly delayed chest closure.

Following ECMO cannulation, correct position of the ECMO cannulas can be confirmed by x-ray examination, fluoroscopy, or echocardiography (Figs. 39.4 and 39.5). Radiographic confirmation of cannula position in patients cannulated through the neck is helpful and particularly important when cannulation is for veno-venous ECMO or when there are issues with venous drainage in

venoarterial ECMO. In general the tip of the venous cannula should be in the mid–right atrium or even down to the caval-atrial junction (just where the inferior vena cava [IVC] enters the right atrium), and the tip of the arterial cannula should be in the common carotid artery or in the aortic arch at the entrance of the innominate artery. It is important that the aortic cannula (when placed through the neck) is not inserted too far into the ascending aorta, because damage to the aortic valve from arterial cannulas positioned just above or at the valve level has been reported. If venous drainage is adequate, then it can be presumed that the venous cannula is in an adequate position. There are times that the tip of the venous cannula (when inserted from the neck) can lie against the eustachian valve at the floor of the right atrium, and this may cause intermittent obstruction to flow, requiring the cannula to be pulled back a centimeter or. If the cannula is across the tricuspid valve (often this is confirmed by echocardiography), flows may be adequate, but the cannula will need to be pulled back into the right atrium before the patient can be weaned from ECMO. For femoral venoarterial cannulations the tip of the venous cannula should extend to the mid–right atrium, and the tip of the arterial cannula should extend to the mid–descending aorta. ECMO providers should be familiar with their institution's cannula types (i.e., radiopaque to the tip or not) to correctly determine when examining radiographs where each cannula ends. In a single-center pediatric study published in 2009, echocardiography was found to be superior to chest radiographs for evaluating ECMO cannula position.[35]

TABLE 39.2 Common Technical Problems Encountered With Centrifugal Pump Extracorporeal Membrane Oxygenation in Children and Possible Solutions

Problem	Comments and Possible Solutions
1. Air in venous side of circuit (up to pump head): sources include IV cannulas, connectors, pressure monitoring line, and taps	a. Clamp arterial cannula and shunt, stop pump, ventilate patient, and attempt to maintain cardiac output. b. De-air with syringe via pump inlet pressure line.
2. Air in oxygenator: caused by membrane rupture, excess gas flow to blood flow ratio, air in venous line or pump head, entrainment from connectors or oxygenator shunt line infusions	a. Clamp ECMO lines between pump head and oxygenator, stop pump, ventilate patient, and attempt to maintain cardiac output. b. De-air with syringe via tap in shunt manifold. c. Reinstitute ECMO after securing point of air entry or adjusting gas flow; may require circuit change for oxygenator failure (see 6).
3. Air in arterial side of circuit (and patient): causes include membrane rupture (obstructed gas outlet port), entrainment from connectors or hemofilter, and major venous emboli	a. Clamp arterial cannula and shunt, stop pump, ventilate patient, and attempt to maintain cardiac output. b. Place patient head down. c. Replace blood volume. d. De-air arterial cannula with syringe, then clamp line. e. De-air circuit by aspirating via arterial cannula tap and/or oxygenator manifold. f. Secure air entry site or replace oxygenator if necessary. g. Reinstitute ECMO.

4. ↓ HbSO$_2$ (patient)
  a. Decreased flow
  b. Anemia
  c. Inadequate FiO$_2$ or ventilation
  d. Excessive shunt flow
  e. Pneumothorax
  f. Oxygenator failure (indicated by ↓ preoxygenator to postoxygenator pO$_2$ gradient)
	a. Adjust flow.
	b. Transfuse red cells.
	c. ↑ Ventilator FiO$_2$, optimize ventilation.
	d. Restrict shunt flow.
	e. X-ray, chest drain.
	f. ↑ Oxygenator FiO$_2$. If ineffective, replace oxygenator (see 6).

5. ↑ pCO$_2$ (patient)
  a. Inadequate ventilation of patient
  b. Pneumothorax
  c. Oxygenator failure (indicated by ↓ preoxygenator to postoxygenator pCO$_2$ gradient)
	a. Optimize ventilation.
	b. X-ray, chest drain.
	c. ↑ Gas sweep. If ineffective, replace oxygenator (see 6).

6. Oxygenator failure
  a. Inadequate anticoagulation
  b. Inadequate flow through oxygenator (high preoxygenator pressure indicates obstruction)
  c. Membrane rupture or perforation
  d. Plasma leak (hollow-fiber oxygenator)
	a. Clamp arterial cannula, stop pump.
	b Support patient with ventilation, inotropes, and fluids as required.
	c. New oxygenator and circuit can be connected across bridge in old circuit. De-air and recommence ECMO.
	d. Correct associated coagulation problems.
	e. Maintain adequate flow through oxygenator by high patient or shunt flow.

ECMO, Extracorporeal membrane oxygenation; *FiO$_2$,* fraction of inspired oxygen; *HbSO$_2$,* hemoglobin oxygen saturation; *IV,* intravenous.

When there is concern about cannula position, it is prudent to discuss those concerns with the surgical team. Most cardiac cases require venoarterial ECMO. In the rare instances of respiratory failure in a cardiac patient, venovenous ECMO may be appropriate. In these patients, correct catheter placement is essential and can be guided by fluoroscopy and/or echocardiogram (see Fig. 39.5).

Rapid-Deployment Extracorporeal Membrane Oxygenation

Institutions that use ECMO as the primary mechanical support device for emergent circulatory support have developed rapid-deployment strategies to decrease the time required to initiate ECMO support. One or two circuits primed with crystalloid are maintained sterile for a set period of time (usually no longer than 1 month), ready for use in the case of ECMO cannulation during CPR or ECPR.[36] Older children (usually above 20 kg) can be placed on ECMO emergently using the crystalloid-primed circuit, with subsequent typed and cross-matched blood transfusion to reestablish normal hemoglobin concentration if needed. Younger children may require a blood-primed circuit primed with type O, Rh-negative blood to reduce hemodilution. Availability of surgeons, in-house intensivists, and surgical team and equipment are requirements for successful and timely ECPR cannulation. High-quality CPR needs to be maintained for the entire duration of the cardiac arrest, with minimal interruptions for cannula placement, in an effort to avoid hypoxic injury. Team training through multidisciplinary simulations has been shown to decrease time from onset of cardiac arrest to time on ECMO in real patients in a pediatric cardiac intensive care unit.[37]

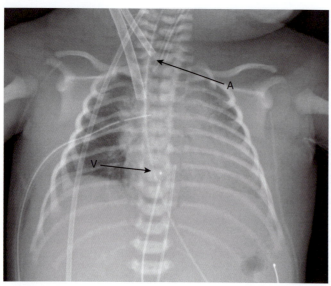

• **Figure 39.4** Correct cannula position in an infant cannulated through the right common carotid artery and the right internal jugular vein. Arrow *A* shows the position of the arterial cannula, and arrow *V* shows the correct position of the venous cannula with the dot representing the terminal cannula position. *ECMO*, Extracorporeal membrane oxygenation.

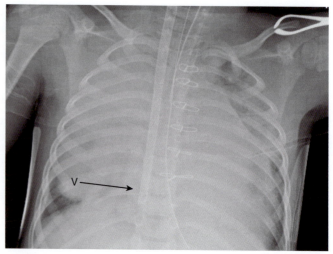

• **Figure 39.5** Correct cannula position of venovenous cannula in right internal jugular vein.

Critical Care Management During Extracorporeal Membrane Oxygenation Support

Extracorporeal Membrane Oxygenation Teams: a Multidisciplinary Approach

ECMO is a complex, high-risk, and resource-intensive process with unpredictable resource use. Cardiac ECMO centers maintain well-trained multidisciplinary teams, with a core set of cardiac surgeons, intensivists, ECMO specialists, nurses, and perfusionists, as well as consultants from areas such as cardiology, pharmacy, nutrition, transfusion medicine, hematology, pulmonology, and nephrology. Multidisciplinary ECMO training using medical simulation is gaining ground in many cardiac ECMO centers after growing evidence for improved technical skills and team performance.[37-41]

Neurologic Monitoring and Neuroprotection

Critically ill neonatal and pediatric cardiac ECMO patients are at high risk for neurologic injury surrounding their ECMO course. As many as 14% to 36% of ECMO patients suffer acute neurologic injury surrounding their ECMO course, including hypoxic-ischemic injury, thromboembolic stroke, and intracranial hemorrhage.[8,42-45] Neurologic injury during ECMO is associated with an 89% increase in risk of mortality.[46]

The mechanisms of neurologic injury in ECMO patients are not yet well understood. Profound cardiopulmonary failure and/or cardiac arrest lead to hypoxic-ischemic injury before ECMO, rendering the brain vulnerable. The profound inflammatory state associated with critical illness is then compounded by exposure to the foreign surfaces of the extracorporeal circuit, which triggers a profound global innate immune response by activating the contact and complement systems[47] and provokes perturbations in proinflammatory and prothrombotic pathways implicated in the pathogenesis

of neurologic injury during ECMO. The device-induced proinflammatory state and endothelial cell dysfunction increase thrombin generation and platelet activation.[48,49] Within the patient the device contributes to coagulation factor consumption, platelet exhaustion, and reduced platelet aggregation potential.[48,49] Added to that is the need for systemic anticoagulation to prevent circuit thrombus formation, creating the common paradox of thrombotic events in the device with simultaneous bleeding in the patient.[50] Thus patients are at risk for both thromboembolic and hemorrhagic intracerebral complications.

A recent systematic review of the literature found that neuromonitoring methods during ECMO are limited and supported primarily by grade 3B-4 evidence from small, single-center studies (median n = 28, interquartile range [IQR], 18-49).[51] Daily transfontanellar cranial ultrasonography for infants with open fontanels has entered routine clinical practice.[52-54] Near-infrared spectroscopy–based cerebral oximetry[55-60] and electroencephalography (EEG)[61-65] are used in many centers. The American Clinical Neurophysiology Society recommends the use of critical care continuous EEG in children on ECMO support.[66] A recent prospective quality improvement project conducted in a single quaternary care pediatric center showed that electrographic seizures occurred in 18% of consecutive neonates and children on ECMO support, were more common in patients with LCOS, and were associated with higher mortality and unfavorable neurologic outcome at hospital discharge.[67] Other neuromonitoring methods, including transcranial Doppler ultrasonography[68-70] and the serial monitoring or plasma brain injury biomarkers[71-75] are being investigated and showing early promising results for detection of impending neurologic injury during ECMO and for prediction of unfavorable neurologic outcomes.

The best neurologic monitoring strategy is to minimize the use of sedatives and neuromuscular blocking agents. Limiting sedation when possible (e.g., in the absence of severe pulmonary hypertensive crises) has many other advantages, including spontaneous breathing and ability to interact with family and staff.[10]

Respiratory Support

Respiratory management of neonatal and pediatric cardiac patients on ECMO is aimed at maintaining the lungs open and avoiding ventilator-induced lung injury, while taking into consideration cardiopulmonary and device-pulmonary interactions.[76] In general the goal for neonatal and pediatric cardiac patients on ECMO is to avoid atelectasis, mobilize secretions, and, if present, support resolution of pulmonary edema due to capillary leak after large-volume transfusions, post CPB, or post cardiac arrest. Pressure control ventilation is used with moderately high positive end-expiratory pressure of approximately 10 cm H_2O, rate of 10 breaths/min, and pressures adjusted to achieve 6 to 8 mL/kg tidal volume, limiting peak inspiratory pressures to 18 to 20 cm H_2O.[10,76] Limiting sedation and allowing for spontaneous respirations with pressure support or extubation on ECMO are becoming more common, especially in older children and adolescents, and may allow for improved cardiopulmonary interactions.[10,76]

Nutrition

There are few published articles on optimal nutrition during ECMO. Generally a combination of enteral and parenteral nutrition is provided based on the patient's nutritional requirements. The benefits of enteral nutrition have been well documented in critical illness at all ages, with recent data suggesting that early parenteral nutrition may be detrimental in critically ill children.[77] Enteral nutrition has been shown to be feasible during venoarterial ECMO in neonates and children, potentially rendering benefits and cost savings.[78,79] Some of the reported barriers for uninterrupted enteral nutrition during ECMO are ongoing vasopressor requirement, fasting for therapeutic or diagnostic procedures, and high gastric residual volumes.[80-83] None of the neonatal, pediatric, or adult studies of nutrition during ECMO have reported complications related to early initiation of enteral nutrition in these patients.[78,79,81-83] Antacids are commonly used for prophylaxis against acute gastritis.

Renal Supportive Therapy

Acute kidney injury is present at ECMO initiation in 60% to 74% of neonatal and pediatric patients and present by 48 hours of ECMO support in 86% to 93% of patients.[84] Renal support therapy, most commonly in the form of slow continuous ultrafiltration and continuous venovenous hemofiltration, is used in a majority of neonatal and pediatric ECMO centers.[85]

In neonates and children with critical cardiac disease, acute kidney injury may precede ECMO cannulation due to low cardiac output states, cardiac arrest, or exposure to nephrotoxic drugs. Acute kidney injury represents the most common indication for renal support therapy in cardiac ECMO centers[85] and can worsen during the ECMO course if diuresis or hemofiltration are employed aggressively in an effort to augment fluid clearance and advance the patient toward decannulation. Although fluid overload and acute kidney injury are associated with increased duration of ECMO support and with increased mortality before hospital discharge,[84,86] controversy remains as to the optimal rate of fluid removal and the optimal timing of initiation of renal support therapy during ECMO. If patients have adequate support on ECMO and can diurese adequately using their kidneys (with reasonable diuretic stimulation), then it may not be necessary to use forms of filtration. When there is impaired kidney function (usually heralded by decreased urine output despite adequate ECMO flow and often associated with rising levels of creatinine and blood urea nitrogen), then other forms of fluid management need to be considered. In some patients there is diffuse capillary leak resulting in third spacing, and in these patients, urine output may not be adequate despite reasonable ECMO

flows. Often these patients have normalizing lactates (suggesting appropriate systemic oxygen delivery from the ECMO circuit) and a low central venous pressure. As long as it is possible to maintain flows in these patients, the capillary leak should recover, and as they begin to mobilize their third-spaced fluid, their urine output should recover and respond to diuretics. In some institutions these patients are managed with peritoneal drainage catheters (simply to drain the ascites and take any potential "pressure" off the renal vessels). When ascites reaches the point that an abdominal "compartment syndrome" is present (which can be measured by an elevated bladder pressure), then insertion of a peritoneal drain is a good idea. Patients who have true renal failure with low urine output, rising creatinine level, and high central venous pressures will often require some other form of filtration and are good candidates for continuous ultrafiltration while on ECMO. The decision making around the best management of low urine output requires multidisciplinary collaboration because often these patients present with a variety of reasons for low urine output that may require differing management strategies—one "solution" does not necessarily fit all circumstances.

Infection Risk and Surveillance

The prevalence of hospital-acquired infections during ECMO support is estimated at 10% to 12%, higher than in non-ECMO critically ill patients.[87,88] Meticulous attention to hand hygiene and adherence to hospital-acquired infection prevention bundles is required to reduce risk of infection in ECMO patients.[89] Although there are no data to support the notion that antibiotic prophylaxis beyond the pericannulation period (24 to 48 hours post cannulation) reduces the risk of infections acquired during ECMO, prolonged courses of antibiotics are commonly used to provide infection prophylaxis in many ECMO programs.[90] Antibiotics commonly used for infection prophylaxis include cefazolin and vancomycin. Rarely antifungal agents are used as part of antibiotic prophylaxis.[90,91] Use of aminoglycoside antibiotics for infection prophylaxis has been shown to be associated with increased incidence of sensorineural deafness in ECMO survivors and should be avoided when possible.[92] Care of the skin to prevent pressure ulcers and preserving mobility of joints are important aspects of ECMO patient care.[93]

Anticoagulation and Blood Product Management

Upon initiation of ECMO support, exposure of blood to the foreign surfaces of the circuit triggers an inflammatory response with activation of the coagulation pathway and blood elements (leukocytes, platelets) and thrombin activation, leading to a hypercoagulable state in the device.[49] Anticoagulation to maintain patency of the circuit therefore needs to be balanced with the risk of bleeding within the patient.[49] Despite accumulating experience with anticoagulation management and ever-improving biocompatibility of ECMO circuits, hemorrhage and thrombosis remain important complications during ECMO support and can be life threatening.[1]

ECMO centers report large variability in anticoagulation monitoring and management. In an international survey conducted in 2012, 97% of respondents reported using activated clotting times (ACTs) to monitor UFH anticoagulation.[94] Typically heparin infusion rates range from 10 to 40 U/kg/h and are adjusted for ACT targets of 180 to 220 seconds. Studies have shown, however, that ACT is an indirect and often inaccurate reflection of heparin effect and can be outside the target range for many reasons. Therefore currently most centers also monitor activated partial thromboplastin time (aPTT) (94%), anti-factor Xa (aFXa) (65%), thromboelastography (TEG) (43%), and antithrombin activity (82%), at varying time intervals.[94] In addition, fibrinogen, D-dimers and platelet counts are measured serially to provide a more complete assessment of the patient's coagulation status.[94] aFXa is a reflection of actual heparin levels, and a target range is usually 0.3 to 0.7 to ensure adequate heparinization. Concomitant antithrombin III (AT III) levels can indicate the appropriate substrate for heparin to function, and when AT III levels are low, additional AT III (either as fresh frozen plasma or as a commercially available product [Thrombate III]) can be provided. Monitoring aFXa and AT III levels with adjustments as necessary has correlated with outstanding outcomes with respect to coagulation management in ECMO patients and is currently our preferred anticoagulation protocol.

ACT has several limitations; it is a global test of whole blood coagulation response, it has limited reproducibility, and results differ for different devices.[95-97] ACT can be influenced by factors such as the presence of heparin, platelet count, platelet dysfunction, hyperfibrinogenemia or hypofibrinogenemia, other coagulation factor deficiencies, hypothermia, or hemodilution.[49,96] In addition, ACT has poor correlation with aPTT and aFXa during neonatal and pediatric ECMO,[98-101] and some have proposed that aFXa may be preferable as a marker for degree of anticoagulation during ECMO.[102,103] In a single-center review comparing an anticoagulation protocol primarily driven by ACT versus aFXa and that included TEG and antithrombin measurements, Northrop et al.[103] demonstrated significant reductions in blood product transfusions, cannula and surgical site bleeding, as well as improved circuit life with the aFXa-driven protocol.

Antithrombin measurement and administration have become common practices in neonatal and pediatric ECMO, despite the lack of robust evidence on efficacy and safety of both pooled and recombinant formulations.[94,104-106] Antithrombin pharmacokinetics and pharmacodynamics during ECMO are poorly described.[107] Data from single-center studies suggest that, in selected populations, antithrombin replacement can decrease exposure to blood products[108,109] and improve efficiency of anticoagulation with unfractionated heparin (UFH) at least temporarily.[110,111] There is still significant debate and controversy, however, regarding the safety of antithrombin administration,[112] as well as contradictory reports of adverse events associated with antithrombin administration that will require further prospective study.[105,109-111,113,114]

Alternatives to UFH, including direct thrombin inhibitors such as bivalirudin and argatroban, are being increasingly used in ECMO patients of all ages; the use of these agents in pediatrics patients has been reported in those who develop heparin resistance or heparin-induced thrombocytopenia.[49,115,116] Some adult ECMO centers use bivalirudin as the first agent for anticoagulation, with significantly simplified anticoagulation management protocols.[117,118]

Postoperative neonatal and pediatric cardiac patients on ECMO are at high risk for bleeding. Minor local bleeding such as bleeding at the cannulation site can be controlled with local measures, correction of coagulopathy via plasma, cryoprecipitate, or platelet transfusions and reducing the level of anticoagulation used. Massive bleeding requires prompt blood product administration, including platelets for a goal of 75,000 to 100,000/mm^3, and administration of antifibrinolytics such as epsilon-aminocaproic acid.[119-121] UFH infusion rate can be decreased or interrupted in the contemporary era of surface-modified ECMO circuits in cases of severe bleeding, although the risks and benefits of doing so must be discussed at the bedside, taking into careful consideration the cause of bleeding, thrombus burden in the circuit, and each institution's circuit specification. The use of activated factor VII to control bleeding on ECMO has been reported from some centers.[122,123] Access to a fresh primed ECMO circuit should be readily available when ECMO bleeding management requires stopping anticoagulation and administration of prothrombotic agents.

Even in the absence of active bleeding, red blood cells and platelets may suffer shear injury during ECMO, with subsequent hemolytic anemia and thrombocytopenia. Thus transfusion of red blood cells may be needed to maintain hemoglobin concentrations that optimize oxygen delivery (typically 10 g/dL), and platelet transfusions may be needed to maintain platelet counts deemed safe for avoiding spontaneous hemorrhage in the face of ongoing anticoagulation (typically 75,000 to 100,000/mm^3). Plasma or cryoprecipitate is administered for goal fibrinogen concentrations of 100 mg/dL, or 150 mg/dL before surgical procedures.

Weaning From Extracorporeal Membrane Oxygenation

Indicators of cardiac function recovery (e.g., increasing pulse pressure, increasing end-tidal CO_2 and mixed venous saturations, echocardiographic evidence of improved contractility) guide readiness for weaning from ECMO. Mechanical ventilation is optimized, and inotropes or inodilators may be started before weaning. In venoarterial ECMO the extracorporeal flow is decreased gradually. The minimal flow rate is 200 mL/min for ¼- or ⅜-inch tubing and 500 mL/min for ½-inch tubing. Anticoagulation is increased to avoid thrombus formation at areas of stagnant flow. Patient ECMO flow is discontinued by clamping of the drainage and return cannulas above the bridge and opening of the bridge (shunt) in the circuit (see Fig. 39.3). Once the patient is isolated from the circuit and flow is only through the bridge, ECMO flow rates can be increased to reduce the risk of thrombosis in the circuit. Echocardiography, urine output, and serial blood gas and lactate levels are monitored carefully during the trial period off ECMO. The intravascular volume and vasoactive support are optimized based on these parameters. The ECMO cannulas are flushed every 5 to 10 minutes during the clamp trial to maintain patency. At the end of an appropriate time trial, which can vary from 30 minutes to several hours, depending on specific issues related to each individual patient (time from clamping to decannulation may vary by patient, diagnosis, and ECMO program), the patient is either decannulated from ECMO or placed back on ECMO should the clamp trial fail. A repeat weaning and clamp trial should be pursued only after potential reasons for failure have been evaluated and corrected.

When weaning from venovenous ECMO, the procedure is significantly different. Patients on venovenous ECMO have systemic venous return to the right atrium captured (in part) by the distal port of the dual-lumen cannula. This blood is returned to the oxygenator and then perfused back to the patient via the proximal cannula port (which is usually aimed toward the tricuspid valve). This oxygenated blood "mixes" with the systemic venous return to the right atrium that is not captured by the cannula and creates an oxygen saturation similar to what is seen following a Glenn procedure, in which the systemic venous return from the IVC mixes with the pulmonary venous return coming back to the heart from the pulmonary veins via the Glenn shunt. In this sense a patient on venovenous ECMO can be expected to have oxygen saturations similar to those of a patient following a Glenn procedure—saturations of approximately 80% (depending on the mixed venous saturations and the amount of venous blood being oxygenated by the circuit). As the lungs improve, they begin to oxygenate the blood that is flowing through them and the systemic saturations increase, indicating (along with the improving chest x-ray examination findings) that the patient may be ready to be separated from venovenous ECMO (which is actually a "liquid ventilator"). Separation from venovenous ECMO requires restoring adequate ventilation to the patient and then turning off the sweep gas to the circuit so that there is no oxygenation from the circuit. If the patient maintains adequate oxygenation and ventilation (removal of CO_2), then the patient is likely to be ready for cannula removal. Patients on venovenous ECMO usually do not have significant hemodynamic compromise requiring mechanical support, so evaluating their ability to be removed from ECMO is essentially related to how well their lungs function when the ECMO oxygenation and CO_2 regulation are removed.

Decannulation from ECMO can be done at the bedside or in the operating room. The timing of decannulation needs to be coordinated to ensure availability of the surgical team, surgical equipment, sedation and analgesia, blood products, and adequate patient monitoring. If cannulation is through the chest (as is typical following cardiac surgery), the surgical team occasionally elects to leave the sternum "open" for a few days after cannulation to ensure that the patient is stable, and when this is done, the sternum is typically closed at the bedside (or in the operating room) when the patient has made appropriate progress. If cannulation has been via neck vessels, they may or may not be reconstructed, depending on surgical preference, duration of ECMO, and quality of the vessels at the time of cannula removal. Adequate resources post-decannulation need to be available to address any complications that may arise and to be able to reinitiate ECMO should the need arise. A plan for potential recannulation should be made before decannulation, and equipment such as new appropriate-sized cannulas and a new circuit should be readily available if needed. In general, patients requiring recannulation after failed separation from ECMO have poor survival outcomes.

Cost

ECMO is a costly and resource-intensive technology. There are costs associated with the equipment itself and disposables such as cannulas and oxygenators. There are also personnel resources involved, including one ECMO specialist and one beside nurse per patient, as well as the specialized care team of intensivists, surgeons, and consultants. Training and certification need to be accounted for in the "work hours" of ECMO personnel. There are additional costs related to laboratory testing, imaging, blood products, and drugs. A systematic review of the literature conducted in 2015 evaluating the in-hospital cost of ECMO internationally found large variation in the cost of ECMO, ranging from $42,554 to $537,554 (in 2013 values).[124] In the United States the costs of ECMO were highest for congenital diaphragmatic hernia repair, followed by cardiac conditions, and lowest for respiratory conditions. The US charges were highest for cardiac conditions.[124] In a recent analysis of pediatric ECMO only, using the Healthcare Cost and Utilization Project Kids' Inpatient Database, the median inflation-adjusted inpatient costs for children requiring ECMO were $183,000, $240,000, and $241,000 in the years 2006, 2009, and

2012, respectively.[125] Analysis of the same database focused on children with single-ventricle disease found that the hospital length of stay in this patient population increased from 25.2 days in 2000 to 55.6 days in 2009 ($P < .001$) and that the total inflation-adjusted charges during the same time period increased from $358,021 (95% confidence interval [CI], $278,658-$439,765) to $732,349 (95% CI, $671,781-$792,917) ($P < .001$).[126] In a single-center study of children with congenital heart disease surgery, the calculated cost-utility for salvage ECMO was $24,386 per quality-adjusted life-year saved, which is within the range of accepted cost efficacy (<$50,000 per quality-adjusted life-year saved).[127]

Outcomes

Survival

Early survival outcomes after neonatal and pediatric cardiac ECMO are updated regularly in the ELSO registry. The ELSO registry is an international database started in 1989. As of July 2017, data from 87,366 ECLS cases in 329 centers have been reported to the registry.[128] Of these, 22,087 (25%) represented neonatal and pediatric cardiac and ECPR cases.[128] Overall survival to hospital discharge was 41% for neonatal cardiac cases, 51% for pediatric cardiac cases, and 41% for both neonatal and pediatric ECPR cases (Table 39.3).

In recent years in a pediatric ELSO registry report for 2009–2015, most neonates requiring ECMO for cardiac indications had congenital heart disease (81%), as did older infants and children (52%)[8] (Tables 39.4 and 39.5). Neonates and children with myocarditis and cardiomyopathy had higher survival rates to hospital discharge compared with congenital heart disease indications and with cardiac arrest.[8] For postoperative mechanical circulatory support for congenital heart disease, ELSO data are consistent with those reported by the Society of Thoracic Surgeons (STS). In a study published in 2014 that used data from 96,596 operations in 80 centers participating in the STS database, mechanical circulatory support was used in 2.4%.[129] Surgeries with the highest mechanical circulatory support rates were the Norwood procedure (17%), and complex biventricular repairs, including arterial switch, ventricular

TABLE 39.3	Extracorporeal Life Support Outcomes for Neonatal and Pediatric Cardiac and Extracorporeal Cardiopulmonary Resuscitation Cases				
	Total Runs	Survived ECLS		Survived to Hospital Discharge or Transfer	
Neonatal					
Cardiac	7266	4727	65%	2987	41%
ECPR	1613	1089	67%	666	41%
Pediatric					
Cardiac	9593	6620	69%	4941	51%
ECPR	3615	2078	57%	1508	41%

ECLS, Extracorporeal life support; *ECPR,* extracorporeal cardiopulmonary resuscitation.
From the Extracorporeal Life Support Organization, ECLS Registry Report, International Summary July 2017; with permission.

TABLE 39.4	Survival to Hospital Discharge and Mean ECLS Run Duration for Neonatal Cardiac ECLS, by Primary Diagnosis (2009–2015)		
	Proportion of Cases N (%)	Survival to Hospital Discharge (%)	Average Run Length, Days
Congenital heart disease	2301 (81)	44	6
HLHS	644 (23)	40	6
LVOTO	178 (6)	41	6
RVOTO	95 (3)	39	6
Septal defects	172 (6)	44	6
Cyanotic with decreased pulmonary flow	348 (12)	48	7
Cardiac arrest	41 (1)	41	7
Cardiogenic shock	57 (2)	39	5
Cardiomyopathy	44 (2)	59	9
Myocarditis	38 (1)	50	11
Other	368 (13)	50	7
Total	2849	45	6

ECLS, Extracorporeal life support; *HLHS,* hypoplastic left heart syndrome; *LVOTO,* left ventricular outflow tract obstruction; *RVOTO,* right ventricular outflow tract obstruction.
From Barbaro RP, Paden ML, Guner YS, et al. Pediatric Extracorporeal Life Support Organization Registry International Report 2016. *ASAIO J.* 2017;63(4):456-463; with permission

TABLE 39.5	Survival to Hospital Discharge and Mean ECLS Run Duration for Pediatric Cardiac ECLS, by Primary Diagnosis (2009–2015)		
	Proportion of Cases N (%)	Survival to Hospital Discharge (%)	Average Run Length, Days
Congenital heart disease	2010 (52)	54	6
HLHS	283 (7)	46	7
LVOTO	212 (5)	57	6
RVOTO	108 (3)	62	6
Septal defects	323 (8)	49	6
Cyanotic with decreased pulmonary flow	271 (7)	52	6
Cardiac arrest	128 (3)	45	6
Cardiogenic shock	175 (5)	61	6
Cardiomyopathy	317 (8)	65	8
Myocarditis	204 (5)	76	8
Other	1016 (26)	57	8
Total	3850	57	7

ECLS, Extracorporeal life support; *HLHS,* hypoplastic left heart syndrome; *LVOTO,* left ventricular outflow tract obstruction; *RVOTO,* right ventricular outflow tract obstruction.
From Barbaro RP, Paden ML, Guner YS, et al. Pediatric Extracorporeal Life Support Organization Registry International Report 2016. *ASAIO J.* 2017;63(4):456-463; with permission.

septal defect, and aortic arch repair (14%).[129] Survival to hospital discharge in the mechanical circulatory support group was much lower compared with children who did not require extracorporeal support (46.8% versus 97.1%, *P* < .0001).[129]

Survival after hospital discharge is also lower in children who underwent ECLS for cardiac indications, compared with those who did not. In a study published in 2014, Iguchi and colleagues[130] estimated that 5-year survival in children who required ECLS for congenital heart disease was 32.3% (95% CI, 25.1%-39.8%). Worse outcomes are seen in children with a single ventricle who require ECMO following a Norwood operation. In a single-center study also published in 2014, long-term survival to stage II palliation and stage III palliation in a cohort of 65 children was 35.9% and 25.4%, respectively.[131]

Neurofunctional and Quality-of-Life Outcomes

Interpretation of published neurofunctional and quality-of-life outcomes data for children who require ECMO for cardiac indications is somewhat limited by the heterogeneity of the populations of children with both congenital and acquired heart disease, heterogeneity in ages at the time of follow-up, and heterogeneity in the outcome measures used for evaluation.

Global tests such as the PCPC and Pediatric Overall Performance Category (POPC) have been used to determine outcomes at hospital discharge and up to 5 years later.[132-134] Several studies showed favorable outcomes in 81% to 91% of pediatric survivors who underwent ECMO for cardiac indications, where favorable outcome

was defined as PCPC/POPC of 2 or less or 3 or less at hospital discharge or no change from baseline PCPC/POPC.[132-134]

Neuropsychologic testing, including developmental and cognitive testing, at a median of 55 months, 53 months, and 43 months, respectively, following ECMO, in US and Canadian cohorts of children who underwent ECMO for cardiac indications, showed that 36% to 50% of survivors test within 1 standard deviation (SD) from the population mean, whereas 25% to 50% of survivors test in the severely disabled range of more than 2 SD below the population mean on a given test.[135-137]

Quality-of-life assessments in children who underwent ECMO for cardiac indications suggest that survivors experience diminished quality of life compared with age-matched, healthy peers.[138,139] In addition, in a cohort of 47 survivors who underwent ECMO for cardiac indications, physical, psychosocial, emotional, social domains, and school function assessed using the PedsQL health-related quality-of-life questionnaire, were all lower when compared with peers with chronic health conditions and with congenital heart disease who did not require ECMO support.[139]

Children who have undergone ECMO are also at risk for sensorineural hearing loss, which is seen in 5% to 28% of survivors during follow-up testing.[92,135,137,140-143] Any language delay should be considered for hearing testing.[144] Testing may need to be repeated as the child grows, because there is evidence that former ECMO patients may develop delayed or progressive hearing loss.[92,142,143]

In summary, neonates and children who require ECMO for cardiac indications are at risk for long-term neurofunctional disability. The 2012 AHA scientific statement on neurodevelopmental outcomes in children with congenital heart disease identified history of ECMO use as a high-risk factor for developmental disorders or disabilities.[144] It is therefore recommended that these children be frequently reevaluated at 12 to 24 months, 3 to 4 years, and 11 to 12 years and be counseled at high school and college age for educational or vocational options as they reach adulthood.[144]

Selected References

A complete list of references is available at ExpertConsult.com.

1. Thiagarajan RR, Barbaro RP, Rycus PT, et al. Extracorporeal Life Support Organization Registry international report 2016. *ASAIO J.* 2017;63(1):60–67.

10. Brogan TV, Lequier L, Lorusso R, MacLaren G, Peek G, eds. *Extracorporeal Life Support: The ELSO Red Book.* 5th ed. Ann Arbor, MI: Extracorporeal Life Support Organization; 2017.

84. Fleming GM, Sahay R, Zappitelli M, et al. The incidence of acute kidney injury and its effect on neonatal and pediatric extracorporeal membrane oxygenation outcomes: A multicenter report from the kidney intervention during extracorporeal membrane oxygenation study group. *Pediatr Crit Care Med.* 2016;17(12):1157–1169.

101. Kessel AD, Kline M, Zinger M, McLaughlin D, Silver P, Sweberg TM. The impact and statistical analysis of a multifaceted anticoagulation strategy in children supported on ECMO: Performance and pitfalls. *J Intensive Care Med.* 2017;32(1):59–67.

138. Costello JM, O'Brien M, Wypij D, et al. Quality of life of pediatric cardiac patients who previously required extracorporeal membrane oxygenation. *Pediatr Crit Care Med.* 2012;13(4):428–434.

40

Ventricular Assist Device Therapy

KRISTEN NELSON MCMILLAN, MD; ROBERT JAQUISS, MD

History and Current State of Ventricular Assist Device Support

Ventricular assist devices (VADs) are invaluable tools for the management of end-stage heart failure in children of all ages. Although development of such devices in adults has advanced substantially in the past few decades through several generations of VAD enhancements, the development of such devices for children has lagged behind. The slower development of pediatric devices has been due to a number of factors, such as the inherent differences in physiologic parameters in children, the variable anatomy in children whose heart failure is secondary to congenital heart disease (CHD), and the relatively small population in need of such devices, which creates much less economic incentive for industry-sponsored device development. However, the last 10 years have seen increased attention to VAD development and use in the pediatric population. Indeed, in the face of stable or only slightly increased numbers of pediatric donors, the number of pediatric heart transplants has increased significantly, in parallel with the increase in the number of children listed as heart transplant candidates. In part the ability to perform many more transplants with only slightly more donors is reflective of the use of VADs to bridge candidates to transplant who in the pre-VAD era would certainly have died.[1] Nonetheless, of all patients on the waiting list for solid-organ transplantation in the United Sates, children listed for heart transplantation face the highest waiting list mortality, an effect that is especially pronounced in the youngest and smallest children, in whom VAD solutions are least satisfactory.[2,3] It is anticipated that more children with CHD and cardiomyopathy-associated heart failure will require long-term VAD support in the coming decade as a bridge to transplantation or recovery.

For many years extracorporeal membrane oxygenation (ECMO) was the only readily accessible form of mechanical circulatory support (MCS) for both short-term (i.e., postcardiotomy) and medium-term support. However, use of ECMO beyond 10 to 14 days was limited by substantial rates of complications, particularly stroke, bleeding, and infection, greatly hampering its utility in patients requiring more durable support.[4] In North America there were limited options for other long-term assist devices in children smaller than adult size until 2000, when a Berlin Heart EXCOR pulsatile VAD was placed in a pediatric patient in the United States under compassionate use regulations.[5] Subsequently an investigational device exemption (IDE) study was conducted in the United States and Canada, leading to Food and Drug Administration (FDA) approval in late 2011.[6] In the past few years there has been wider use of the Berlin Heart device, increasing application of newer adult devices in ever smaller patients, "off-label" use of temporary devices for intermediate or longer-term support, and progress in initiatives to develop new devices for very small children.[7-11]

Pediatric Heart Failure

The number of children with heart failure has been increasing, resulting in growing demand for transplant and therefore for MCS in the pediatric population. Possible explanations include better recognition of pediatric cardiomyopathy with earlier intervention with medical therapy and advancements in surgery and perioperative care for children with CHD, leading to increased long-term survival of this patient population.[12] One of the inevitable consequences of improved survival of these patient groups will be an increased incidence of end-stage heart failure in children, adolescents, and young adults. A typical example of end-stage heart failure in the setting of operated CHD involves children whose morphologic right ventricle is sustaining the systemic circulation and who progress to failure of that systemic ventricle. Perhaps the largest group of patients who may become candidates for advanced heart failure management are those with single-ventricle physiology.

Although pediatric VAD therapy has been in recent rapid evolution, there has also been significant refinement of VAD therapy in adults over the last decade. The most significant change to have an impact on patient management strategy was the emergence of durable intracorporeal (implantable) continuous-flow devices such as the Thoratec HeartMate II (Abbott, Abbott Park, IL) and HeartWare HVAD (Medtronic, Dublin, Ireland). Owing to the impressive outcomes in patients supported with these devices, with relatively low-morbidity profiles, the indications for device placement have evolved, making the early institution of VAD therapy a reasonable option in preference to escalating medical management.[13] In adults VADs are used as a bridge to transplant, as a bridge to recovery, or as destination therapy (for patients who opt against transplantation or for whom transplantation is not an option). Although the use of destination therapy in pediatrics is evolving, the vast majority of pediatric VADs are currently still used as a bridge to transplant.

The applicability of the intracorporeal devices in the pediatric population is limited by body size, and therefore they are most commonly used for larger children and adolescents. However, there have been case reports of patients successfully implanted with HeartWare devices with a body surface area (BSA) of 0.6 m.[11,13] The advent of three-dimensional computed tomography mapping has also facilitated fit testing of such devices in children.[9,14]

Although miniaturized intracorporeal devices for smaller children are on the horizon, the Berlin EXCOR, a paracorporeal pulsatile device, is the only currently FDA-approved available option for infants.

Patient Selection

For patients with advanced heart failure, VAD implantation is indicated when the benefits of the device are deemed to outweigh the risks. Because patients, devices, and clinical settings represent infinitely variable (and changeable) combinations of risk and benefit, appropriateness and timing of device implantation are determined for each patient by the multidisciplinary team, the family, and where appropriate, the patient. Special consideration should be given to not only medical circumstances, but also social aspects. VAD selection should also be influenced by the institutional experience.

Beyond small size, other important confounding issues for children in whom VAD implantation is being considered may include the increased operative difficulty and potential complications inherent in patients who have had prior operations and have structurally abnormal hearts. Examples of the latter include anomalous anatomy intrinsic to their CHD (abnormalities of atrial situs, ventricular situs, great vessel arrangement, or systemic venous drainage). As well there may be "iatrogenic abnormalities" that must be accounted for during implantation (e.g., systemic to pulmonary shunts, cavopulmonary connections, and prior atrial septectomy). In addition to careful attention to the anatomy and circulatory physiology, a thorough understanding of the unique pathophysiologic features of pediatric heart failure is an absolute prerequisite to a successful outcome with VAD therapy.

At present, long-term VAD support in children generally requires candidacy for heart transplantation, or at least "candidacy for candidacy." When considering contraindications to VAD therapy in children, extreme prematurity, very low body weight (<2.0 kg), significant preexisting neurologic injury, a constellation of congenital anomalies with poor prognosis (unlikely survival beyond childhood), and major chromosomal aberrations are generally accepted contraindications for any form of MCS. Multisystem organ failure may be a relative contraindication but does not necessarily exclude patients from MCS if reversal of organ function is predicted with the achievement of hemodynamic improvement. Indeed, it has been well documented that liver, renal, and pulmonary dysfunction frequently improve after restoration of hemodynamic stability with MCS.

Device Selection

Because pediatric patients are so divergent in terms of size and cardiac physiology, appropriate device selection and good understanding of each device are keys to success.

Device selection for initial MCS in children with heart failure is ideally limited to cardiac support with VADs, which support the left ventricle (left ventricular assist device [LVAD]), right ventricle (right ventricular assist device [RVAD]), or both (biventricular assist device [BiVAD]), though pure RVAD support is extraordinarily rare. However, some children with acute decompensated heart failure also have significant pulmonary dysfunction, which is most often reversible and may require cardiopulmonary support. In such cases temporary support with ECMO may be indicated before LVAD implantation. In some cases of RVAD or BiVAD support an oxygenator can be added to the RVAD for temporary pulmonary support, and later removed with lung recovery. Moreover, if the patient is in cardiopulmonary arrest with ongoing cardiopulmonary resuscitation, then ECMO is the initial support of choice because this can be rapidly initiated (peripherally) and will provide support to both right and left heart as well as the lungs (Fig. 40.1).

Extracorporeal Membrane Oxygenation

ECMO is covered separately in Chapter 39, so we will limit the discussion here to the major differences between ECMO and VAD support.

ECMO is a temporary support strategy, and should be confined to short-term support for heart failure. Although it has previously been used as a bridge to transplant, ECMO is rarely used for this purpose in current practice given expectation of waiting times, which are likely to be measured in months. There is a significant survival benefit of long-term VAD support over ECMO support for patients waiting for heart transplantation.[6,15] In addition, posttransplant survival is higher in patients supported with VAD compared with those who had ECMO support, irrespective of diagnosis.[15,16]

Controversy exists, however, regarding the best mode of MCS if anticipated support duration is short (<2 weeks). Many pediatric heart centers use ECMO irrespective of the cause of heart failure. In addition to extracorporeal cardiopulmonary resuscitation, other potential applications of ECMO for circulatory support include the presence of significant pulmonary hypertension, hemodynamic instability due to septic shock, or severe pulmonary edema resulting from ventricular dysfunction. Thus ECMO is often preferred when the right heart is unable to provide "adequate" flow to fill the left heart (and therefore the systemic circulation). Suboptimal right heart output can be due either to inherent right ventricular dysfunction (e.g., severe cardiac allograft rejection), intractable ventricular arrhythmias, or pulmonary hypertension.

The advantages of short-term VADs compared with ECMO include the simplicity of the circuit and, more importantly, better decompression of the failing left ventricle, which may be crucial for optimizing recovery from pulmonary edema. The lack of an oxygenator and the simpler circuit configuration induce less inflammation and are likely less thrombogenic, which results in a lower level of anticoagulation requirement. Better ventricular decompression is critical in patients with acute heart failure in whom there is a reasonable chance of cardiac recovery (e.g., acute myocarditis). Short-term VAD support with a centrifugal pump provides excellent decompression of the left heart (or systemic ventricle), with immediate impact on left atrial pressure, pulmonary venous hypertension, pulmonary edema, and lung function. It is clear that short-term VADs that directly drain the left heart provide better decompression of a failing left ventricle than does a simple venoarterial ECMO strategy that has only indirect effect on the left heart. Left heart decompression during ECMO support can be enhanced if there is an adequate atrial septal defect (or if one can be created with possible stent implantation) either by transseptal flow[17] or the placement of a transseptal drainage cannula.[18] Conversely, with LVAD support, inflow comes from a cannula placed directly into the left side of the heart. Hence short-term VAD support may provide a better chance of pulmonary and cardiac recovery than ECMO support with or without direct left-sided decompression.[19]

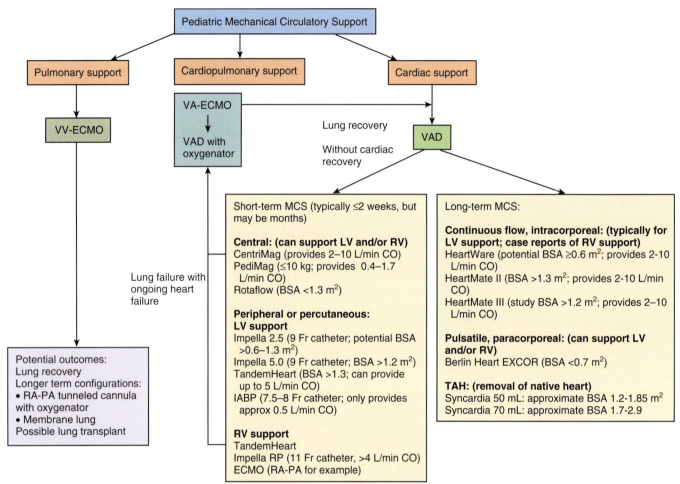

• **Figure 40.1** Pediatric mechanical circulatory support (MCS). Type of MCS support is determined by (1) type of organ support needed (heart and/or lungs), (2) anticipated duration of support, (3) patient's body size, and (4) the goal of MCS support (e.g., recovery, destination, or transplant). Listed BSAs for each device are approximate. *BSA*, Body surface area; *ECMO*, extracorporeal membrane oxygenation; *IABP*, intraaortic balloon pump; *LV*, left ventricle; *PA*, pulmonary artery; *RA*, right atrium; *RV*, right ventricle; *TAH*, total artificial heart; *VA*, venoarterial; *VAD*, ventricular assist device; *VV*, venovenous.

Other Temporary/Short-Term Ventricular Assist Devices

Left Ventricular Assist Device

Indication. Short-term VADs may be used in children with heart failure secondary to (1) acute, potentially reversible processes (e.g., acute myocarditis and acute rejection of a cardiac allograft), (2) acute exacerbation of chronic heart failure (e.g., acute worsening of dilated cardiomyopathy due to superimposed infection), or (3) postoperative ventricular dysfunction (e.g., following reimplantation of anomalous left coronary artery arising from the pulmonary artery and late arterial switch operation with deconditioning of the left ventricle). If the causes are acute processes, it is reasonable to anticipate that the cardiac function may recover with adequate left heart decompression, which would warrant a trial of temporary support.

Temporary Ventricular Assist Device Cannulation

The decision regarding when to discontinue or transition to other type of support warrants clinical judgment and varies considerably

between individuals. Outcomes for ECMO support in children with presumed acute myocarditis include survival rates of 63% in the Extracorporeal Life Support Organization registry[20] and 70% to 80% in single-center reports.[21-23] Most patients with acute myocarditis can be supported reasonably well with either mode of temporary MCS (ECMO or short-term VAD). The difference in left heart decompression, however, could make a difference in patients with the most severe form of the disease, those with such severe left ventricular (LV) dysfunction that the aortic valve does not open (fortunately a small proportion of the entire patient population).

In contrast to the goal of temporary VAD therapy in acute heart failure, which is recovery and explant, the goal of short-term VAD support in acute-on-chronic (AOC) heart failure is more modest. In the AOC setting the temporary VAD is used to optimize candidacy for placement of a durable (long-term) VAD and for ultimate transplantation. This approach is sometimes called a "bridge to decision," in that candidacy for durable VAD implant or transplantation may be indeterminate at the time of evaluation based on potentially reversible end-organ dysfunction. The use of a temporary VAD in this setting allows time for the clinical situation to stabilize and the determination of candidacy to be made conclusively. The rationale for this approach in children has been demonstrated in a recent multicenter analysis of children undergoing durable VAD implantation.[24,25] In this analysis, patients who were the most ill at the time of VAD implantation, Pedimacs category 1 (Box 40.1), had markedly worse survival than those in Pedimacs categories 2 and 3. Thus for the AOC patient in category 1 the implantation of the temporary VAD allows stabilization

---

• BOX 40.1 Pedimacs Patient Profile at Time of Implant

Pedimacs 1: "Critical cardiogenic shock" describes a patient who is "crashing and burning," in which a patient has life-threatening hypotension and rapidly escalating inotropic pressor support, with critical organ hypoperfusion often confirmed by worsening acidosis and lactate levels.

Pedimacs 2: "Progressive decline" describes a patient who has been demonstrated "dependent" on inotropic support but nonetheless shows signs of continuing deterioration in nutrition, renal function, hepatic function, respiratory function, fluid retention, tachyarrhythmia, or other major status indicator. Patient profile 2 can also describe a patient with refractory volume overload, perhaps with evidence of impaired perfusion, in whom inotropic infusions cannot be maintained due to tachyarrhythmia, clinical ischemia, or other intolerance.

Pedimacs 3: "Stable but inotrope dependent" describes a patient who is clinically stable on mild-moderate doses of intravenous inotropes (or has a temporary circulatory support device) after repeated documentation of failure to wean without symptomatic hypotension, worsening symptoms, or progressive organ dysfunction (usually renal). It is critical to monitor nutrition, renal function, fluid balance, and overall status carefully in order to distinguish between a patient who is truly stable at Patient Profile 3 and a patient who has unappreciated decline rendering them Patient Profile 2. This patient may be either at home or in the hospital. Patient Profile 3 can have modifier A, and if in the hospital with circulatory support can have modifier TCS.

Pedimacs 4: "Resting symptoms" describes a patient who is at home on oral therapy but frequently has symptoms of congestion at rest or with activities of daily living (ADLs). He or she may have orthopnea, shortness of breath during ADL such as dressing or bathing, gastrointestinal symptoms (abdominal discomfort, nausea, poor appetite), disabling ascites or severe peripheral edema (extremity or facial). This patient should be carefully considered for more intensive management and surveillance programs, which may in some cases reveal poor compliance that would compromise outcomes with any therapy.

Pedimacs 5: "Exertion Intolerant" describes a patient who is comfortable at rest but unable to engage in any activity, living predominantly within the house or housebound. This patient has no congestive symptoms, but may have chronically elevated volume status, frequently with renal dysfunction, and may be characterized as exercise intolerant.

Pedimacs 6: "Exertion Limited" also describes a patient who is comfortable at rest without evidence of fluid overload, but who is able to do some mild activity. ADLs are comfortable and minor activities outside the home such as visiting friends or going to a restaurant can be performed, but fatigue results within a few minutes of any meaningful physical exertion. This patient has occasional episodes of worsening symptoms and is likely to have had a hospitalization for heart failure within the past year.

Pedimacs 7: "Advanced NYHA Class 3" or "Ross Class III" describes a patient who is clinically stable with a reasonable level of comfortable activity, despite history of previous decompensation that is not recent. This patient is usually able to walk more than a block. Any decompensation requiring intravenous diuretics or hospitalization within the previous month should make this person a Patient Profile 6 or lower.

Pedimacs Patient Profile at Time of Implant. Reproduced with permission from The Society of Thoracic Surgeons. Copyright STS Pedimacs Users Guide. Retrieved from https://www.uab.edu/medicine/intermacs/pedimacs/pedimacs-documents.

---

and "downcategorization," potentially resulting in improved prognosis.

Temporary VAD support may be initiated via either peripheral access (either percutaneous or open surgical access) or centrally, via sternotomy. The advantage of the former approach is the rapidity with which support can be initiated in critically ill patients. The disadvantages include relatively large cannula size, which precludes this approach in small children, as well as the difficulty in providing biventricular support. The advantages of central cannulation include universal applicability, regardless of size. The disadvantages include the need to perform a sternotomy, or in some cases a redo sternotomy, which would obviously take longer than a peripheral approach. For both central and peripheral cannulation, flow is provided in a continuous fashion by either a centrifugal pump for a two-cannula system (see later) or an axial pump (see later) with one-cannula systems. For a two-cannula system an oxygenator can be inserted into the system to provide pulmonary support. This is not possible with a single-cannula system.

For peripheral cannulation, LVAD support may be accomplished with a single arterial cannulation site using the Impella system (Fig. 40.2) or with a left atrial (transvenous, transseptal) cannula in combination with arterial cannulation using the Tandem-Heart system (see Fig. 40.2). The Impella system is positioned retrograde across the aortic valve, under fluoroscopic (and often echocardiographic) guidance with the inflow to the system at the distal portion of the cannula and the outflow positioned above the aortic valve.[26,27] The inflow cannula for the TandemHeart is positioned across the atrial septum with either echocardiographic or fluoroscopic guidance with the arterial cannula being inserted into a femoral artery. Neither system has been used extensively in children, because of cannula size limitations (for TandemHeart 21 French [Fr] venous, 17 Fr arterial; for Impella 14 Fr arterial).[26,28] A recent comparison in an experimental animal model of acute heart failure suggested that the TandemHeart system may provide better left ventricular decompression than the Impella system at equivalent flow rates.[29] For RVAD support a right-sided version of the Impella has been developed, the so-called Impella RP. This has demonstrated significant efficacy in temporary right-sided support after durable LVAD implantation and right ventricular myocardial infarction,[30] but its use has not yet been reported in children.

For patients in whom central cannulation is elected, standard bypass cannulas are typically employed. For isolated LVAD support the inflow cannula may be placed via the left ventricular apex or via the left atrium. In the event that the latter approach is taken, care must be taken to avoid injury to the mitral valve in the event that recovery is hoped for. The outflow cannula for the LVAD may be placed directly into the aorta or attached to a graft sewn to the ascending aorta or one of its branches. If RVAD support is necessary, the inflow cannula is usually placed in the right atrium with the outflow cannula placed directly in the main pulmonary artery or into a graft anastomosed to the main pulmonary artery. Because the main pulmonary artery is quite short, great care must be taken to avoid rendering the pulmonary valve incompetent with cannula placement or positioning the cannula tip too distally so as to preferentially perfuse one lung (typically the left) at the expense of the other. In the event that pulmonary support is required in the setting of biventricular temporary VAD placement, an ECMO type of oxygenator can be inserted in the RVAD circuit, sometimes colloquially termed *RECMO*. With pulmonary recovery the oxygenator can easily be removed.[31-33] There are rare instances in

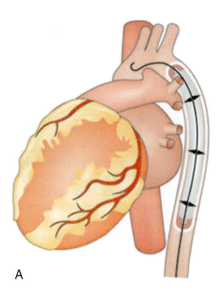
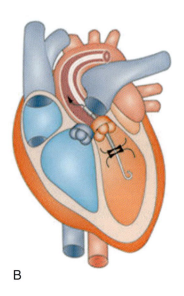
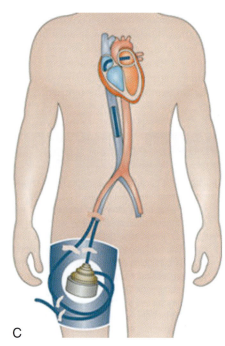

• **Figure 40.2** Percutaneous ventricular assist devices. (A) Intraaortic balloon pump; (B) Impella; and (C) TandemHeart. (From Westaby S, Anastasiadis K, Wieselthaler GM. Cardiogenic shock in ACS. Part 2: Role of mechanical circulatory support. *Nat Rev Cardiol.* 2012;9:195-208. doi:10.1038/nrcardio. 2011.205.)

which isolated RVAD support with an oxygenator may be necessary, such as in the case of severe pulmonary failure with right ventricular failure, as a means to unload the failing RV and allow recovery or bridge to lung or heart/lung transplantation.[34] Whether LVAD, RVAD, or BiVAD temporary support is elected, the sternum can typically be closed, and the patient may be able to be removed from mechanical ventilation in most cases within a relatively short time frame. For central cannulation one of several commercially available centrifugal pumps is employed depending on institutional preference and patient size, such as Thoratec PediMag or CentriMag (St. Jude Medical, St. Paul, MN), Rotaflow (Maquet, Wayne, NJ), or TandemHeart (Cardiac Assist, Inc./TandemLife, Pittsburgh, PA) (Table 40.1; see Fig. 40.2).

Intraaortic Balloon Counterpulsation

Although not technically a VAD, the intraaortic balloon pump (IABP) is discussed here for completeness. This device, which can be inserted peripherally or centrally, consists of a long balloon positioned in the descending aorta (see Fig. 40.2 and Fig. 40.3). The balloon is inflated and deflated with timing synchronized to provide inflation during ventricular diastole and deflation before ventricular systole. Thus the pump provides both enhanced coronary perfusion (diastole) and reduced ventricular afterload (systole). Though the IABP has greatly facilitated the management of adult patients with heart failure, its application in the pediatric population has been very limited for several reasons.[35] An important constraint is the size of the balloon (smallest currently is 7.5 Fr), making it too large for all but larger children and adolescents. Furthermore, heart failure in children is virtually never related to coronary insufficiency, rendering the enhancement of coronary perfusion by the IABP superfluous. Last, the compliance of the juvenile aorta is remarkably higher than in middle-aged and elderly adults, so the degree of diastolic unloading that the IABP can generate

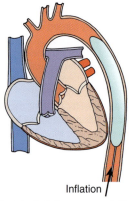
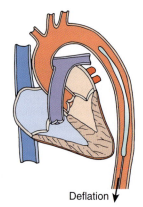

Inflation | Deflation

Diastole: inflation augmentation of diastolic pressure

↑ A. Coronary perfusion

Systole: deflation decreased afterload

↓ A. Cardiac work
↓ B. Myocardial oxygen consumption
↑ C. Cardiac output

• **Figure 40.3** Intraaortic balloon pump. An intermittently inflatable balloon placed into the descending aorta. On balloon inflation during diastole, there is augmentation of blood pressure and organ perfusion by pulsatile thrust; then on deflation it decreases the cardiac work with each systole (counterpulsation principle) by reducing cardiac afterload.

in children is minimal. Thus, although they may be reasonable for short-term support in larger children, IABPs have a very limited role in long-term mechanical support or bridging to transplantation.[36,37] In the event that a single arterial support apparatus is elected, the support provided by the Impella device is likely to be significantly superior in children to that provided by the IABP, though this proposition has been evaluated only in adults.[38]

							Labeled	Studied
Device	**Size Restrictions**	**Duration of Support**	**Type of Support**	**Pump Flow**	**Approved for Use by US FDA**	**Pathway of US FDA Approval**	**Excluding Use in Children**	**Protectively in Children**
Temporary								
ECMO	None	Days	Biventricular	Continuous	Yes	510K	No	No
CentriMag	None	Days-weeks	Univentricular or biventricular	Continuous	Yes	510K	No	No
Rotaflow	None	Days-weeks	Univentricular or biventricular	Continuous	Yes	510K	No	No
TandemHeart pVAD	N/A	Days	Univentricular	Continuous	Yes	510K	No	No
Impella 2.5/5.0	N/A	Days	Univentricular	Continuous	Yes	510K	No	No
Durable								
Berlin Heart EXCOR	Wt > 3 kg	Months-years	Univentricular or biventricular	Pulsatile	Yes	HDE	Labeled for children	Yes
HeartWare HVAD	Wt > ≈ 15 kg	Years	Univentricular or biventricular	Continuous	Yes	PMA	No	No
HeartMate II	Wt > ≈ 30 kg	Years	Univentricular	Continuous	Yes	PMA	No	No
SynCardia Total Artificial Heart	BSA > 1.7 m²	Years	Biventricular	Pulsatile	Yes	PMA	No	No

TABLE 40.1   Ventricular Assist Device Use in Pediatrics

BSA, Body surface area; *ECMO*, extracorporeal membrane oxygenation; *FDA*, Food and Drug Administration; *510K*, pathway of approval based on demonstrating equivalence to predicate device; *HDE*, humanitarian device exemption; *N/A*, not applicable; *PMA*, postmarket approval; *pVAD*, percutaneous ventricular device; *Wt*, weight.
From Vanderpluym CJ, Fynn-Thompson F, Blume ED. Ventricular assist devices in children: progress with an orphan device application. *Circulation.* 2014;129:1530-1537.

Durable Ventricular Assist Devices—Device Selection, Anatomic Considerations, Special Circumstances

Indication

When the cause of heart failure is chronic in nature and the patient is relatively stable with respect to secondary organ function and functional status (Pedimacs profile 2 or 3), then durable VADs are the devices of choice. In VAD selection the most important determinant is the size of a patient. For small children the only durable VAD that has achieved regulatory approval and widespread use worldwide is the Berlin Heart EXCOR (Berlin Heart, Inc., The Woodlands, TX) (Fig. 40.4). For larger children, adult-sized intracorporeal devices such as HeartMate II or the HeartWare HVAD may be employed (Figs. 40.5 and 40.6). The definition of "small" in the context of device selection is a moving target, but presently, the HeartWare, which is an intrapericardial device, has been used in children as small as a BSA of 0.6 m².[11,13] The Heartmate II, which is extrapericardial and larger than the HeartWare, is less often used in children, even in adolescents, because of its relatively large size.

Biventricular Failure and Evaluation of Ventricular Assist Device Support

Before making the decision regarding VAD implantation, it is essential to assess carefully the function of the right ventricle, because this will directly impact the device strategy (i.e., LVAD

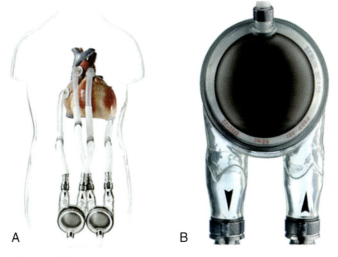

• **Figure 40.4** Berlin Heart. Pulsatile ventricular assist device for durable use. A, Device in situ. B, Individual pump. (Rossano JW, Jang GY. Pediatric heart failure: current state and future possibilities. *Korean Circ J.* 2015;45[1]:1-8. https://doi.org/10.4070/kcj.2015.45.1.1.)

versus BiVAD). It is frequently difficult to accurately assess the RV function in the setting of severe LV dysfunction, and some degree of RV dysfunction is almost inevitable in patients with chronic heart failure.[39] To this end, some centers have employed routine use of BiVAD for all patients, though this is becoming less common.[25] In general, outcomes have been worse for children

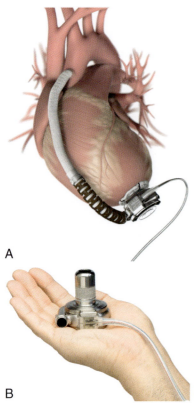

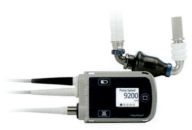

• **Figure 40.5** (A and B) HeartWare HVAD. Continuous-flow ventricular assist device for durable use. (Reproduced with permission of Medtronic, Inc.)

• **Figure 40.6** HeartMate II. Continuous flow ventricular assist device for durable use. (Courtesy Thoratec Image Library. http://www.thoratec.com/about-us/media-room/library.aspx.)

supported with a BiVAD strategy,[1] as is the case with adults.[40] Whether this reflects overtreatment of right ventricular failure with consequent poorer outcomes or an intrinsically sicker patient population (those requiring BiVADs) cannot be determined from available data. However, accumulating experience would suggest that an LVAD-only strategy can provide adequate circulatory support for most children with severe heart failure if right ventricular dysfunction is carefully managed post LVAD implant.[25] This approach requires the use of right ventricular afterload reduction (inhaled nitric oxide, phosphodiesterase inhibitors), inotropic support, and careful fluid management directed at avoiding overdistention of the impaired right ventricle. However, even in contemporary adult VAD practice, important RV failure complicates 25% to 40% of LVAD implantations,[41] and early, temporary RVAD support may be required.

Although avoidance of BiVAD implantation is desirable in most patients, this preference should not be used as justification for tolerance of severely compromised hemodynamics, because there are certainly circumstances in which durable BiVAD support is indicated. Examples of such circumstances include severe biventricular dysfunction early or late after cardiac transplantation, severe myocarditis involving both ventricles, or in patients with very elevated pulmonary vascular resistance.[39] Another specific population in which to consider BiVAD support rather than LVAD alone is in patients with restrictive cardiomyopathy, which is typically associated with biventricular dysfunction as well as elevated pulmonary vascular resistance.[42]

For small children requiring BiVAD implantation, whether a priori determined or elected during planned LVAD implantation, the durable device of choice is the Berlin Heart EXCOR. The EXCOR system includes cannulas specifically designed for right- and left-sided support, and the extracorporeal blood pump can serve both LVAD and RVAD configurations. For adults the HeartWare has been used in a BiVAD arrangement with either RV cannulation or RA cannulation, though this approach has rarely been used in children.[43-46] Furthermore, there have been reports of difficulty with RVAD configuration, resulting in higher rates of thrombosis.[47] For this reason some centers have opted for use of CentriMag for more long-term RVAD support. For larger (adult-sized) children with anatomy unsuitable for biventricular HeartWare implantation, long-term support has been accomplished with the total artificial heart (TAH) (SynCardia, Tucson, AZ) (Fig. 40.7).[48,49] The original device (70-mL capacity) is too large for many children, and a smaller device (50 mL) is currently in clinical trials in the United States, which may extend the use of the TAH in pediatrics.

Ventricular Assist Device for Right Heart Failure and Lung Failure

It is rare to require RVAD-only support, but there are case reports of pediatric patients requiring central cannulation (right atrium for drainage, right pulmonary artery for return as one example) for right ventricular failure due to severe lung failure. Such cases have typically utilized centrifugal pumps with an oxygenator in line to allow for both right heart and lung recovery, in essence creating a central ECMO circuit. Although in some cases this has been used as a bridge to transplant, there are now reports of extended right heart and lung recovery to decannulation without transplant.

Ventricular Assist Device for Single-Ventricle Hearts

One of the greatest advances in the care of children with CHD has been the development of a well-established surgical pathway for children born with univentricular hearts. For most such children the pathway involves three surgical steps: (1) an initial palliative operation resulting in parallel circulation (with the ventricle pumping to both the systemic circulation and pulmonary circulation), (2) conversion to an in-series arrangement by construction of a superior cavopulmonary anastomosis, and (3) completion of the in-series strategy by a completion of a total cavopulmonary connection (Fontan operation). Though this strategy is effective and durable for many patients, heart failure may develop at any point along the pathway, leading to the referral for transplantation and possibly for MCS.

The failure of univentricular palliation is relatively uncommon after either of the first two stages, and so there is much less experience with long-term MCS in those physiologic/anatomic states.

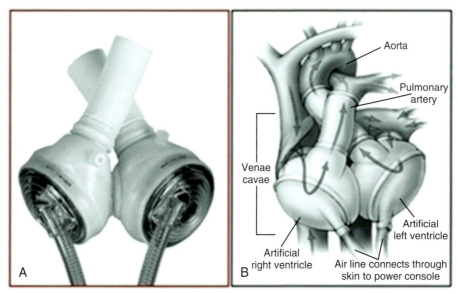

• **Figure 40.7** Total artificial heart. (A) Depiction of the SynCardia Total Artificial Heart. The TAH-t comprises two semi-rigid polyurethane ventricles of 70 ml volume with a flexible, multi-layered, polyurethane diaphragm separating the blood path from the pneumatic chamber. Quick-connect inflow sewing cuffs attach the artificial ventricles at the 27 mm mechanical valve to the remaining atria. Quick-connect outflow sewing grafts attach the artificial ventricles at the 25 mm mechanical valve to the pulmonary artery and aorta. Percutaneous conduits protrude from the pneumatic chamber, exiting through the upper right quadrant of the abdominal wall and attaching to 7-foot-long drivelines that connect the ventricles with the external driver and console. (B) Illustration of in situ implantation of the TAH-t complete with connection of the atrial cuffs and outflow graft to and from the ventricles and their respective anatomic structures, as well as the blood flow path. (From Park S, Sanders D, Smith B, et al. Total artificial heart in the pediatric patient with biventricular heart failure. *Perfusion*. 2014;29[1]:82-88. http://journals.sagepub.com/doi/full/10.1177/0267659113496580. doi: 10.1177/0267659113496580; Images courtesy syncardia.com.)

In general terms, VAD outcomes after the first stage have been quite poor and worse than after the second stage.[50] This is likely reflective of the inherent fragility of very young patients but also because of the technical complexity of managing a parallel circulation. Results of support in patients who have undergone superior cavopulmonary connection have generally been far better.[50-53]

The largest group of single-ventricle patients who are likely to be VAD candidates are those who have undergone Fontan completion. In general, failure of the Fontan circulation may occur from two causes: failure of the single ventricle itself ("left-sided" heart failure symptoms) or failure of the Fontan concept, wherein relative systemic venous hypertension is manifest as ascites, pleural effusions, obstructive hepatopathy, protein-losing enteropathy, plastic bronchitis, or some combination of these ("right-sided" heart failure symptoms).[54] By analogy to patients with biventricular circulation, these two forms of Fontan failure may be thought of as left-sided heart failure and right-sided heart failure, though it is important to understand that both forms may be present in a single patient at various times during the evolution of Fontan dysfunction.

The provision of MCS to failing Fontan patients has taken a variety of forms, with the specific type of support chosen guided by the perceived cause of the failure, based on anatomic considerations and the limited choice of available devices.[55] For example, patients with "pure" left-sided (heart/pump) failure have been successfully supported with a single LVAD placed in the systemic ventricle.[56,57] Interestingly, patients with apparently preserved pump function but with "right-sided" heart failure symptoms have also been successfully supported with a single LVAD.[24,55] In other patients with right-sided failure symptoms, imaginative surgical

reconstructions to permit BiVAD support have been undertaken.[55,58] In a similar way, successful use of the SynCardia TAH in a Fontan patient has been reported.[49] Dr. Mark Rodefeld has also been working for several years on a cavopulmonary assist device (Fontan blood pump) (Fig. 40.8), in which he ultimately hopes to be able to provide a modest pressure increase (2 to 6 mm Hg) to existing blood flow at the total cavopulmonary connection. This pressure change could potentially restore a more stable biventricular status, potentially impacting not only treatment of late Fontan failure, but also facilitating early surgical repair.[59]

At present, it is fair to say that no consistently successful single approach to the provision of MCS for failing Fontan circulation has emerged. A registry to accumulate experience with MCS in single-ventricle patients has been established,[60] but at present the experience remains too limited to provide firm guidance for the management of such patients. Given the relatively large and expanding size of the population with the Fontan circulation, it is likely that the urgency for finding MCS solutions for this group will increase markedly in the next few years and beyond.

Early Postoperative Management of Ventricular Assist Device Support

Left Ventricular Assist Device

At the time of arrival in the intensive care unit after either durable or temporary LVAD implantation, most patients will be on intravenous inotropic support and, typically, inhaled nitric oxide,

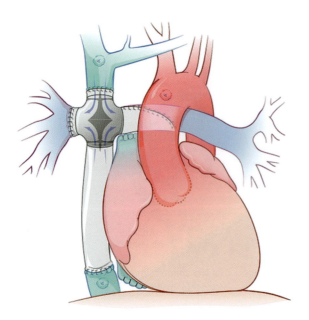

• **Figure 40.8** Cavopulmonary assist device. There is no right-sided ventricular power source in the Fontan circulation, such that venous return is profoundly altered and filling of the single ventricle is suboptimal. Dr. Rodefeld and his group have theorized that a means to modestly augment existing Fontan cavopulmonary flow (by 2 to 6 mm Hg) would address these problems by reproducing more stable two-ventricle physiology and permitting stabilization and/or compression of surgical stages. Gradual reduction in support would permit adaptation to the higher pressure needed (10 to 15 mm Hg) for a systemic venous source to independently perfuse the lungs. The functional parameters for a blood pump to provide low-pressure support in the complex four-way flow anatomy of a cavopulmonary connection are markedly dissimilar to any other circulatory assist application: No such pump currently exists. The goal of this pump would be to provide low-pressure, high-volume flow in four opposing directions without risk of venous pathway obstruction. (From https://www.fontanbloodpump.com/updates.)

both of which are intended to "support" the right ventricle. The duration of need for such support and therefore the optimum weaning strategy must be guided by a battery of physiologic and metabolic parameters. Beyond measures directed at supporting the right ventricle, initiation of vasodilator drugs is often necessary to achieve optimal mean arterial pressures because systemic vascular resistance is substantially elevated in most cases. Once full-flow perfusion is achieved on the VAD with the target mean arterial pressure, adequacy of systemic perfusion is confirmed by measures such as physical examination, urine output, clearance of lactate, reversal of acidosis, near-infrared spectroscopy saturations, mixed venous oxygen saturation, and end-organ function. Ventilation settings in patients on LVAD should be optimized to maintain a low pulmonary vascular resistance to maximize cardiac output from the native right ventricle and thus provide optimized preload for the LVAD. If a temporary VAD is used, unlike an ECMO circuit, the short-term VAD circuit does not contain a heat exchanger. Therefore desired temperature, usually normothermia, may not be always achievable, especially when the chest is left open in small children. In this setting, alternative strategies to maintain normothermia may be needed, such as an overhead radiant infant heater or an external convective warmer.

"Medical" Right Heart Support. If LVAD-only support is chosen, an important focus of postoperative care is directed at optimizing

the cardiac output of the right heart. The basic principles of preventing right heart failure on LVAD include optimizing cardiopulmonary interactions, minimizing pulmonary vascular resistance, and maintaining right heart cardiac output with the lowest possible central venous pressure. It is important to emphasize avoiding overdistention of the struggling right ventricle with injudicious administration of intravenous volume. If the ventricle is stretched beyond the peak of the Starling curve, right ventricular function may decrease and begin a downward spiral from which rescue without an RVAD may be impossible. The maxim that "a little bit of volume goes a long way" is worth remembering. Inotropes are usually required during the early postoperative period, and many centers would advocate the relatively routine use of inhaled nitric oxide and/or inhaled epoprostenol. Echocardiography is a very useful tool to assess right ventricle function in all VAD types. In the event that optimized management of right ventricular performance is inadequate, resort to a temporary (or durable) RVAD should be considered before the onset of end-organ dysfunction.

Bleeding. The surgical implantation of a durable VAD is fraught with the risk of postoperative bleeding in both adults and children.[61,62] Though postoperative bleeding is intrinsically undesirable, for several reasons it is particularly dangerous for patients who have undergone VAD implantation. The most acute consideration is the observation that postoperative bleeding is nearly always associated with a defect in normal coagulation, leading to the administration of so-called clotting factors—platelets, fresh frozen plasma, and cryoprecipitate—in addition to packed red blood cells to address acute posthemorrhagic anemia. In the aggregate, administration of blood products in large volumes may precipitate right ventricular dysfunction, as described previously. In addition, a longer-term consideration is the potential for transfused blood products to stimulate anti–human leukocyte antigen (HLA) antibodies, a process termed *sensitization,* which may make subsequent transplantation more difficult, though this has not been conclusively demonstrated.[63] In general terms the best approach to postoperative bleeding is to prevent it insofar as is achievable by meticulous intraoperative hemostasis. In the event that postoperative bleeding occurs, rational and targeted treatment of documented coagulopathy is indicated, with the addition of newer agents such as recombinant factor VIIa and prothrombin complex concentrates potentially playing a role[64] (see Chapter 24).

Device Management. Like the human ventricle, all VADs require adequate filling to function properly. Causes of inadequate LVAD preload include hypovolemia (including that caused by bleeding), right heart failure (or RVAD dysfunction in the event of BiVAD implantation), or cardiac tamponade. Assessment of adequacy of LVAD filling can be made directly with the extracorporeal Berlin Heart blood pump by inspection. For intracorporeal continuous-flow pumps (HeartWare and Heartmate II) the adequacy of filling can only be investigated with echocardiography. Because it is impractical to perform "continuous echocardiography" on a minute-to-minute basis, empirical volume adjustments must be guided by central venous pressure assessments. Pulsatile MCS devices (Berlin Heart and SynCardia) are not particularly afterload sensitive, or at least can be adjusted to eject against virtually any systemic vascular resistance, albeit at the risk of significant systolic hypertension. Continuous-flow devices such as the HeartWare, Heartmate II, and centrifugal pumps used for temporary VAD support are, by contrast, very afterload sensitive, so judicious use of vasodilators is particularly appropriate to optimize LVAD flow (Tables 40.2 to Table 40.4). There remains debate regarding

TABLE 40.2   HeartMate II Specific Patient Conditions/Events

| Differential Diagnosis | HEMODYNAMIC CHANGES | | | ECHO | Power | HM II | |
	CVP	MAP	SvO$_2$			Pulsatility Index	Flow
Hypovolemia	↓	↓	↓	Underfilled	↓	↓	↓
Tamponade	↑	↓	↓	RV compression	↓	↓	↓
Right HF	↑	↓	↓	Dilated RA/RV	↓	↓	↓
Hypertension	↔	↑	↔	Dilated LA/LV, Ao opening	↓	↑	↓
Thrombus on rotor	↑	↓	↓	Poss. dilated LA/LV, Ao opening	↑	↓	↑ Artificial reading
Thrombus on inflow/outflow	↑	↓	↓	Poss. dilated LA/LV, Ao opening	↓	↓	↓

Ao, Aorta; *CVP,* central venous pressure; *HF,* heart failure; *HM II,* HeartMate II; *LA,* left atrium; *LV,* left ventricle; *MAP,* mean arterial pressure; *Poss.,* possible; *RA,* right atrium; *RV,* right ventricle; *SvO$_2$,* mixed central venous oxygen saturation.

TABLE 40.3   HeartWare Specific Patient Conditions/Events: Decreased Pump Flow Index

| Differential Diagnosis | HEMODYNAMIC CHANGES | | | ECHO | HVAD | | |
	CVP	MAP	SvO$_2$		Power	Pulsatility	Trough
Hypovolemia	↓	↓	↓	Underfilled	↓	↓	↓
Tamponade	↑	↓	↓	RV compression	↓	↓	↓
RHF	↑	↓	↓	Dilated RA/RV	↓	↓	↓
Hypertension	↔	↑	↔	Dilated LA/LV, Ao opening	↓	↑	↑
Occlusion/Thrombus (on inflow/outflow)	↑	↓	↓	Dilated LA/LV, Ao opening	↓ Less than expected	↓	↑

Ao, Aorta; *CVP,* central venous pressure; *HM II,* HeartMate II; *LA,* left atrium; *LV,* left ventricle; *MAP,* mean arterial pressure; *RA,* right atrium; *RHF,* right heart failure; *RV,* right ventricle; *SvO$_2$,* mixed or central venous oxygen saturation.

TABLE 40.4   HeartWare Specific Patient Conditions/Events: Increased Pump Flow Index

| Differential Diagnosis | HEMODYNAMIC CHANGES | | | ECHO | HVAD | | |
	CVP	MAP	SvO$_2$		Power	Pulsatility	Trough
Hypervolemia	↑	↑	↑	Normal, possibly dilated	↑	↑	↑
Vasodilation	↔	↓	↑	Normal, underfilled	↑	↓	↑
Aortic Insufficiency	↑	↓	↓	AI, MR, Inc. LVEDD	↑	↔, ↓	↑
Thrombus (on rotor)[a]	↑	↓	↓	Dilated LA/LV, Ao opening, MR	↑	↓	↑

[a]With thrombus on the rotor, flow is erroneously elevated due to increased power needed to try and spin the rotor.
AI, Aortic insufficiency; *Ao,* aorta; *CVP,* central venous pressure; *Echo,* echocardiography; *HM II,* HeartMate II; *Inc.,* increased; *LA,* left atrium; *LV,* left ventricle; *LVEDD,* left ventricular end-diastolic dimension; *MAP,* mean arterial pressure; *MR,* mitral regurgitation; *SvO$_2$,* mixed or central venous oxygen saturation.

maintenance of some degree of pulsatility with native aortic valve opening. Potential benefits of pulsatility include prevention of aortic valve thrombosis, leaflet fusion, aortic valve insufficiency, better end-organ function, and possibly reduced gastrointestinal bleeding. However, using lower LVAD flows to achieve more

pulsatility may increase the risk of thrombosis. In the first few days after implantation, adjustments to pump settings may be necessary with some frequency, in response to changing patient conditions. However, after the acute postimplant phase the perceived need to adjust VAD settings, or changes in pump performance parameters, should provoke consideration of slowly developing problems such as pericardial effusions, pump thrombosis (which may be visible in the Berlin Heart), or the development of aortic valve insufficiency.

Anticoagulation

Anticoagulation With Durable Devices

All VADs are thrombogenic, and therefore all VAD patients require anticoagulation. The timing of initiation of anticoagulant therapy must be tailored to the clinical status of the patient. The mode and intensity of anticoagulation is variable, depending on which device is implanted. In general the Berlin Heart is thought to require higher levels of anticoagulation, with either warfarin or low-molecular-weight heparin or unfractionated heparin in combination with dual- or triple-antiplatelet therapy. For both continuous-flow devices (HeartWare and Heartmate II) anticoagulation is typically accomplished with warfarin in conjunction with aspirin,[65] although additional antiplatelet agents may be used. At present, thromboprophylaxis for both pulsatile and continuous-flow devices is based at best on expert guidelines[66,67] rather than based on evidence derived from randomized trials, and regimens are typically quite variable among centers.[65] For children in whom conventional anticoagulation is contraindicated, such as those with heparin-induced thrombocytopenia, or persistent coagulopathy, alternative strategies have been proposed, such as use of direct thrombin inhibitors.[68,69]

Anticoagulation With Temporary Ventricular Assist Devices

For temporary VADs there is very little published guidance about appropriate levels of anticoagulation. If the devices have been inserted peripherally, in patients for whom the perceived risk of bleeding is low, several heparin-based protocols have been suggested, employing activated partial thromboplastin time and/or anti-Xa monitoring.[70,71] For temporary systems implanted via sternotomy, with standard bypass cannulas connected to extracorporeal centrifugal pumps, there is essentially no guiding literature. In clinical practice, analogy is often made to the postcardiotomy ECMO circumstance, which is similar except that there is not an oxygenator in place (unless the patient requires RECMO). For such patients, early anticoagulation is often omitted until chest drainage has ceased. At that point, anticoagulation is initiated with unfractionated heparin, with anticoagulation targets similar to local practices with postcardiotomy ECMO. For the vast majority of patients on temporary VAD systems, whether peripherally or centrally inserted, there is not a need to transition to long-acting anticoagulant medications (warfarin or low-molecular-weight heparin) because the anticipated duration is short, terminated by either explantation in the event of cardiac recovery or conversion to a durable VAD system otherwise.

"Temporary" Durable Support

Because of the increased risk of thrombosis and stroke with the Berlin Heart device, the anticoagulation regimen required is perhaps the most intense for any population undergoing MCS. Furthermore, there is great reluctance to delay initiation of anticoagulation, so the risk of bleeding with the device is quite high as well. As a means of reducing the risk of thrombus, stroke, and bleeding, some centers have embraced a "hybrid approach" for small children.

In this strategy, durable Berlin Heart cannulas are attached to the patient surgically but initially connected to a continuous-flow device (rather than a Berlin Heart blood pump), based on the assumption that less early anticoagulation is required for such an arrangement. Later, when the risk of bleeding is thought to have subsided substantially, conversion to the Berlin Heart blood pump(s) is accomplished at the bedside, and full anticoagulation can be undertaken. In a similar vein, if there is a circumstance that would require prolonged reduction or cessation of anticoagulant medications for a patient supported with a Berlin Heart VAD, consideration can be given to temporarily converting back to a continuous-flow pump. It must be emphasized that these approaches are unapproved by any regulatory body, untested by any randomized trial, and potentially quite expensive. These considerations must be weighed against perceived risk of mandatory intense anticoagulation at a time of very high risk for hemorrhagic complications.

Complications of Ventricular Assist Device Support

Infection

Despite the use of strict aseptic techniques during both the insertion and maintenance of VADs, infections continue to be a major cause of morbidity and, more rarely, mortality.[62] LVAD implantation may result in an aberrant state of T-cell activation, heightened susceptibility of CD4 T cells to activation-induced cell death, and progressive defects in cellular immunity, all of which may contribute to an increased risk of opportunistic infection. Any suspicion of infection should be aggressively managed with immediate cultures and the administration of broad-spectrum antibiotics, followed by change to a more targeted regimen as soon as culture results and sensitivities are available. Little has been published regarding pediatric VAD infections; some have advocated antifungal prophylaxis in adults at least for the early perioperative period.[72,73] Adult studies have shown device-related infections to be very serious and often fatal.[73,74] Treatment must include timely antimicrobial therapy, surgical drainage or debridement, and sometimes device removal. As noted earlier, reevaluation of anticoagulation levels is necessary as well to ensure appropriate anticoagulation, given the potential for antimicrobial medications to alter the metabolism of anticoagulant medication, as well as the procoagulant effect of an inflammatory state. In addition, there is increasing recognition of a temporal association between infection and subsequent pump thrombosis, in which the inflammatory state is likely a contributing factor.[75,76] An excellent consensus guideline for the prevention, diagnosis, and management of VAD-related infection was recently published by the International Society for Heart and Lung Transplantation.[77]

Bleeding

For obvious reasons, bleeding is common in patients undergoing either temporary or durable VAD implantation, with the magnitude of risk related to the specific population under study. Bleeding after VAD implantation may be thought of as having two hazard phases. There is an early phase in the acute postoperative period in which the site of bleeding is related to the site of VAD implantation (local in the case of peripherally inserted temporary VADs; from the chest in the case of centrally inserted temporary VAD or any durable VAD). The later hazard phase is more constant and relates to intrinsic patient anatomic risk factors (e.g., prior stroke, mucosal ulceration) and VAD-related coagulopathy (over-anticoagulation and acquired von Willebrand syndrome). Although the acquired von Willebrand syndrome seems more common in adults supported with continuous-flow devices,[78] it has been reported in children as well, even those supported by the pulsatile Berlin Heart device and ECMO.[79] When bleeding does occur, it may be life threatening, as is the case with intracranial events or major gastrointestinal (GI) bleeding. GI bleeding in adults has been reported due to bleeding from arteriovenous malformations and is likely a complex process related to abnormal pulsatility, shear stress, and/or acquired von Willebrand factor deficiency; research in this area is ongoing. As pediatric patients are supported more frequently and for longer durations, this problem may become more prevalent in this population as well. Unless the bleeding is truly minimal, the only effective treatment is temporary cessation of anticoagulation for whatever period seems required, tempered with obvious attendant risk of device thrombosis or systemic thromboembolism—the proverbial rock and a hard place. Anemia in VAD patients may be multifactorial, and iron replacement may be helpful for those with iron deficiency related to blood loss. However, the use of erythrocyte stimulating agents is often avoided, given the thrombosis risk.

Thrombosis and Neurologic Complications

For children undergoing temporary VAD placement, there is no literature to assess the risk of thrombosis or thromboembolism. However, for children undergoing implantation of the Berlin Heart the risk is better studied. In the pivotal IDE trial the rate of cerebral thromboembolism (presumed to be from the pump) approached 30% and was not less in the postapproval study[7,75] These finding were disappointing in that the patients were relatively intensely anticoagulated.[68] Recent single-center reports have been more encouraging, with reduction in stroke related in part to the use of antiinflammatory medications[80] and perhaps also to the longer durations of support, given that the risk seems highest in the first few weeks of support.[68] Some centers have reported success with the use of steroids in decreasing the initial postoperative inflammatory response without increasing infection risk.[80] Pentoxifylline has also been used to decrease the fibrinogen levels and improve the rheology of the red cell. In children undergoing implantation of a continuous-flow device the stroke rate was remarkably less at 7%,[10] though clearly the population getting the Berlin Heart pump is younger, smaller, more likely to have CHD, and more likely to have a BiVAD implant. The risk associated with current continuous-flow LVADs is likely related to nonphysiologic hemodynamics with abnormal pulsatility as previously discussed, as well as turbulence at anastomotic sites and vascular shear stress much greater than physiologic values. Shear stress in particular is a known potent activator of thrombogenesis. In general, pump thrombosis and systemic thromboembolism, which is predominantly to the central nervous system, are more common in pulsatile devices than in continuous-flow devices.[62,68] For both continuous and pulsatile devices, pump thrombosis and systemic thromboembolism continue to be problem areas in need of better solutions.

The Future

Destination Therapy in Pediatrics

In adults it is relatively common to employ long-term VAD support for patients who have been deemed not to be transplant candidates

and whose cardiac function is unlikely to recover. This strategy, termed *destination therapy*, is now increasingly being considered for certain pediatric populations. For example, destination therapy has been employed in patients with certain forms of muscular dystrophy and in selected patients whose skeletal myopathy is far exceeded by their cardiomyopathy.[82,83] In patients with malignancy for whom cure is either unlikely or unproven, destination therapy or VAD therapy as a bridge to decision is increasingly performed. In some patients with graft failure late after transplant, destination therapy is also not unreasonable, particularly in a patient who may wish to reduce or minimize immunosuppressive therapy or in whom compliance has been an issue.

Novel Devices

At the time this chapter is being written, a new centrifugal "adult" device is currently undergoing clinical trials for both bridge-to-transplant and destination therapy indications (HeartMate 3, Abbott, Abbott City, IL) (Fig. 40.9). Preliminary results with the device, which is smaller than existing devices and provides full magnetic levitation to improve blood flow paths, are encouraging,[84] and FDA approval for use in bridge applications (to transplant or to recovery) was granted in August 2017. A novel axial flow device (Jarvik 2015) is also about to begin evaluation as part of the PumpKIN program, in a prospective trial in children between 8 and 20 kg.[9] Additional devices are in various stages of development, as are novel anticoagulation strategies, novel battery designs, and novel energy transfer systems (which with improved batteries may permit completely implantable VAD systems). The population with heart failure is large, and there is a great unmet need for smaller and more biocompatible devices.

Ventricular Assist Device Weaning

Although the vast majority of pediatric patients remain on VAD support until transplantation, there may be potential for weaning to explantation (i.e., recovery) for some patients. Because traditional oral heart failure therapy is typically continued during VAD therapy in addition to the mechanical unloading provided by the VAD itself, it is not surprising that improvement in cardiac function occurs. How to define adequate functional recovery to permit explantation, particularly regarding LVAD therapy, which is likely to be even more complicated in small children, has yet to be unanimously agreed upon. Explantation has much more commonly been demonstrated for temporary RVAD support, which is usually needed for only 1 to 2 weeks following LVAD implantation. The explantation of an LVAD has been achieved much less commonly. One such published set of criteria used for explantation for adult

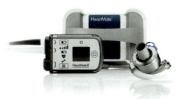

• **Figure 40.9** HeartMate 3. Fully magnetically levitated left ventricular assist device, allowing for wide and consistent blood flow paths and an artificial pulse designed for enhanced hemocompatibility. (From Thoratec Image Library. http://www.thoratec.com/about-us/media-room/library.aspx.)

LVAD patients includes an left ventricular ejection fraction of more than 40% to 45%, LV end-diastolic dimension (LVEDD) less than 55 mm, and approximately normal cardiothoracic ratio. Patients with LVEDD of 40 to 50 mm had the most long-term success with the least need for reimplantation or transplantation.[86,87] Many protocols obtain baseline stress testing and right heart catheterization before any weaning and perform short VAD stops during catheterization to assess hemodynamics without support for brief periods to assist with determination of candidacy for explantation.[87,88]

The cause of heart failure is obviously an important factor in determining the likelihood of recovery. Dilated cardiomyopathy secondary to acute myocarditis or tachyarrhythmias may have potential for complete recovery of cardiac function, making these patients the ideal candidates for VAD explantation. Much more research is needed in this area, but with the increase in VAD support across all ages and stable heart transplantation donor availability over the past decade, it is likely that evaluation for potential explantation may become more common.

Conclusion

The parallel growth of pediatric cardiac surgery and VAD technology has led to the development of mechanical support specifically tailored to the management of pediatric heart failure. Pediatric VADs are used for heart failure refractory to conventional medical therapy and act as a bridge most often to transplantation but may also act as a bridge to recovery, or even, in rare cases, as destination therapy. Each currently available device has specific advantages and disadvantages, and so device selection must be tailored to anatomic and clinical circumstances. Anticoagulation and infection prophylaxis remain major targets for improvement in the management of pediatric patients undergoing VAD placement. Furthermore, protocolized management across institutions will allow us to further study the complex interactions between inflammation, immunity, and use of VADs in the pediatric population. The field of MCS in children has come a great distance but has a great distance yet to travel.

Selected References

A complete list of references is available at ExpertConsult.com.

Adachi I, Burki S, Zafar F, Morales DL. Pediatric ventricular assist devices. *J Thorac Dis.* 2015;7(12):2194–2202. doi:10.3978/j.issn.2072-1439.2015.12.61. PubMed PMID: 26793341. Review, PubMed Central PMCID: PMC4703653.

Almond CS, Morales DL, Blackstone EH, Turrentine MW, Imamura M, Massicotte MP, et al. Berlin Heart EXCOR pediatric ventricular assist device for bridge to heart transplantation in US children. *Circulation.* 2013;127(16):1702–1711. doi:10.1161/CIRCULATIONAHA.112.000685. [Epub 2013 Mar 28]; PubMed PMID: 23538380.

Almond CSD, Thiagarajan RR, Piercey GE, Gauvreau K, Blume ED, Bastardi HJ, et al. Waiting list mortality among children listed for heart transplantation in the United States. *Circulation.* 2009;119(5):717–727. doi:10.1161/CIRCULATIONAHA.108.815712. [Epub 2009 Jan 26]; PubMed PMID: 19171850. PubMed Central PMCID: PMC4278666.

Baldwin JT, Adachi I, Teal J, Almond CA, Jaquiss RD, Massicotte MP, et al. Closing in on the PumpKIN Trial of the Jarvik 2015 Ventricular Assist Device. *Semin Thorac Cardiovasc Surg Pediatr Card Surg Annu.* 2017;20:9–15. doi:10.1053/j.pcsu.2016.09.003. PubMed PMID: 28007073. Review, PubMed Central PMCID: PMC5189910.

Blume ED, Rosenthal DN, Rossano JW, Baldwin JT, Eghtesady P, Morales DL, et al; PediMACS Investigators. Outcomes of children implanted with ventricular assist devices in the United States: First analysis of the Pediatric Interagency Registry for Mechanical Circulatory Support (PediMACS). *J Heart Lung Transplant.* 2016;35(5):578–584. doi:10.1016/j.healun.2016.01.1227. [Epub 2016 Feb 10]; PubMed PMID: 27009673.

Bulic A, Maeda K, Zhang Y, Chen S, McElhinney DB, Dykes JC, et al. Functional status of United States children supported with a left ventricular assist device at heart transplantation. *J Heart Lung Transplant.* 2017;36(8):890–896. doi:10.1016/j.healun.2017.02.024. [Epub 2017 Mar 2]; PubMed PMID: 28363739.

Eghtesady P, Almond CS, Tjossem C, Epstein D, Imamura M, Turrentine M, et al; Berlin Heart Investigators. Post-transplant outcomes of children bridged to transplant with the Berlin Heart EXCOR Pediatric ventricular assist device. *Circulation.* 2013;128(11 suppl 1):S24–S31. doi:10.1161/CIRCULATIONAHA.112.000446. PubMed PMID: 24030413.

Fraser CD Jr, Jaquiss RD. The Berlin Heart EXCOR Pediatric ventricular assist device: history, North American experience, and future directions. *Ann N Y Acad Sci.* 2013;1291:96–105. doi:10.1111/nyas.12144. [Epub 2013 Jun 10]; PubMed PMID: 23750961. Review.

Massicotte MP, Bauman ME, Murray J, Almond CS. Antithrombotic therapy for ventricular assist devices in children: do we really know what to do? *J Thromb Haemost.* 2015;13(suppl 1):S343–S350. doi:10.1111/jth.12928. PubMed PMID: 26149046. Review.

Morales DLS, Zafar F, Almond CS, Canter C, Fynn-Thompson F, Conway J, et al. Berlin Heart EXCOR use in patients with congenital heart disease. *J Heart Lung Transplant.* 2017;36(11):1209–1216. doi:10.1016/j.healun.2017.02.003. [Epub 2017 Feb 8]; PubMed PMID: 28259596.

Rosenthal DN, Almond CS, Jaquiss RD, Peyton CE, Auerbach SR, Morales DR, et al. Adverse events in children implanted with ventricular assist devices in the United States: Data from the Pediatric Interagency Registry for Mechanical Circulatory Support (PediMACS). *J Heart Lung Transplant.* 2016;35(5):569–577. doi:10.1016/j.healun.2016.03.005. [Epub 2016 Mar 17]; PubMed PMID: 27197775. PubMed Central PMCID: PMC5113942.

Rosenthal DN, Lancaster CA, McElhinney DB, Chen S, Stein M, Lin A, et al. Impact of a modified anti-thrombotic guideline on stroke in children supported with a pediatric ventricular assist device. *J Heart Lung Transplant.* 2017;36(11):1250–1257. doi:10.1016/j.healun.2017.05.020. [Epub 2017 May 20]; PubMed PMID: 28606584.

Rossano JW, Lorts A, VanderPluym CJ, Jeewa A, Guleserian KJ, Bleiweis MS, et al. Outcomes of pediatric patients supported with continuous-flow ventricular assist devices: A report from the Pediatric Interagency Registry for Mechanical Circulatory Support (PediMACS). *J Heart Lung Transplant.* 2016;35(5):585–590. doi:10.1016/j.healun.2016.01.1228. [Epub 2016 Feb 10]; PubMed PMID: 27056612.

Vanderpluym CJ, Fynn-Thompson F, Blume ED. Ventricular assist devices in children: progress with an orphan device application. *Circulation.* 2014;129(14):1530–1537. doi:10.1161/CIRCULATIONAHA.113.005574. PubMed PMID: 24709867.

Zafar F, Castleberry C, Khan MS, Mehta V, Bryant R 3rd, Lorts A, et al. Pediatric heart transplant waiting list mortality in the era of ventricular assist devices. *J Heart Lung Transplant.* 2015;34(1):82–88. doi:10.1016/j.healun.2014.09.018. [Epub 2014 Oct 14]; PubMed PMID: 25447574.

41

Cardiopulmonary Bypass

STEVE BIBEVSKI, MD, PHD; LLOYD FELMLY, MD; MINOO N. KAVARANA, MD, FACS

Until the advent of hypothermia and the heart lung machine, cardiac surgery was limited to palliative operations performed "outside" the heart. Tetralogy of Fallot was palliated with a subclavian artery to pulmonary artery shunt that was pioneered by Alfred Blalock, Vivien Thomas, and Helen Taussig in 1943.[1] In 1952 F. John Lewis performed an atrial septal defect (ASD) repair by direct suture using hypothermia (28°C) and inflow occlusion.[2] Shortly thereafter in May 1953, John Gibbon performed the first successful open-heart operation using a pump-oxygenator, repairing an ASD in a young girl.[3] Unfortunately, all his subsequent attempts were met uniformly with failure. The following year, C. Walton Lillehei at the University of Minnesota performed the first of 45 successful intracardiac repairs using controlled cross-circulation by using adult volunteers as live cardiopulmonary bypass (CPB) circuits during the repair of congenital intracardiac defects.[4] Although this technique provided the ability to perform intracardiac repairs with significant success, the pump times were 6 to 40 minutes and cardiotomy times 4 to 14 minutes, which highlights the speed with which these repairs were performed. This speed was driven in part by surgeons not truly knowing the "safe period" for bypass and in part by the relative simplicity of their understanding of congenital heart defect anatomy. Further, the risk to both donor and patient seemed unreasonably high, and for these reasons the technique of cross-circulation with volunteer "heart-lung bypass donors" did not gain popularity. In 1954 John Kirklin at the Mayo Clinic modified the existing heart-lung machines and went on to perform the world's first successful, reproducible *series* of open-heart operations using a heart-lung machine.[5] The modifications he and his colleagues made to the original pumping and oxygenator system revolutionized cardiovascular surgery, and CPB circuits in use today have evolved into more elegant, technologically superior, and significantly smaller versions of his original model.

Cardiopulmonary Bypass in Neonates and Infants

CPB in neonates and infants has significant differences in comparison to CPB in adolescents and adults. Depending on a wide range of variables, some patient specific (e.g., age, weight, underlying condition being repaired) and some specific to the system (such as oxygenator type, circuit size and prime volume, timing and need for additional blood products, target temperature during CPB, flow rates, use of and type of cardioplegia, use of reduced flow or circulatory arrest), the response to CPB in neonates and infants can contribute in important ways to their postoperative intensive care unit (ICU) course (Box 41.1). Compared with the typical use of CPB in adults, neonatal (and infant) cardiac repairs often require more profound levels of hypothermia (including temperatures <28°C), hemodilution (and the need for blood prime), and low perfusion flow rates (including extended periods of low flow or even interrupted [circulatory arrest] flow). Anatomic abnormalities like aortopulmonary collaterals or interrupted aortic arch require alteration of bypass strategies and/or cannulation techniques. Furthermore, the reality is that unlike coronary bypass grafting, which is a procedure performed on the surface of the heart, most congenital heart repairs are truly intracardiac, and this influences cannulation such that bicaval cannulation—often of extremely small caval vessels—is the norm rather than the exception. Significant hemodilution in neonates and small infants is unavoidable due to large circuits and prime volume relative to their intravascular volume. Hemodilution results in lower hematocrits and dilution of clotting factors and plasma proteins, increasing the risk for dilutional coagulopathy. Immature organ systems have an impact as well (i.e., the production of vitamin K–dependent clotting factors by the liver is diminished, increasing the patients' propensity for coagulopathy and postoperative bleeding).

Neonates and infants require much higher flow rates per body surface area to meet metabolic demands. Neonates are often perfused at flow rates up to 200 mL/kg/min. As temperature is reduced, flow rates can be decreased. This has the benefit of producing less blood in a small and complicated surgical field. Furthermore, in some instances patients are cooled to profoundly hypothermic temperatures (e.g., 15°C to 18°C), and the pump is then turned off (deep hypothermic circulatory arrest [DHCA]). This provides the surgeon with the opportunity to remove the cannulas from the patient and to perform a precise repair in an operative field unencumbered by blood, cannulas, or other apparatus related to CPB. Small children, however, have impaired thermoregulation that requires significant attention to temperature monitoring. When CPB is resumed, patients are rewarmed to their normal temperature, but the effects of profound hypothermia on enzyme systems and on the immediate convalescence of the patient cannot be underappreciated.

In general the immature brain tolerates oxygen deprivation better than the mature brain. This supports the clinical observations that infants tolerate longer periods of DHCA better than older children or adult patients. The lungs are also immature at birth, and lung development proceeds up to approximately 8 years of age.[6] At birth the number of alveoli present is approximately one-tenth of what it is in the adult. The lungs of the neonate are quite fragile and have increased potential for pulmonary edema and hypertension.[7] The kidneys of neonates and infants have high vascular resistance with preferential blood flow away from the outer cortex. Sodium reabsorption and excretion, concentrating and diluting mechanisms, and acid-base balance capacity are limited. These characteristics all influence the response of neonates and infants to CPB. Finally, the immune system of the neonate is immature. Complement generation is impaired, and neonatal mononuclear cells are dysfunctional.[8] These differences and many more make CPB in the infant and neonate a specialized endeavor that requires great attention to detail and the ability to adapt to unexpected situations. As more experience and understanding has been gained with regard to the conduct of CPB, the impact that it has on postoperative patients and their outcomes has become increasingly evident.[9]

In contrast to the previous editions of this textbook, this chapter will characterize specific postoperative challenges faced in the ICU following exposure to CPB, the CPB-specific factors that contribute to the development of these challenges, and the treatment options (preoperative, intraoperative, and postoperative) available to mitigate and minimize some of these potentially deleterious effects of CPB.

Basic Cardiopulmonary Bypass Terms, Conditions, and Strategies

To better understand the relationship between CPB and postoperative convalescence, it is helpful to have a basic understanding of how CPB is provided and of some of the common CPB strategies used by the surgical team. For patients to be placed on CPB, they require anticoagulation. This is usually accomplished with heparin and is managed by following indicators during surgery of adequate heparinization. In the past many centers monitored anticoagulation during CPB using the activated clotting time (ACT), but there have been numerous published reports demonstrating the lack of correlation between heparin levels and the ACT. The ACT can be affected by clotting factor abnormalities and is only a reflection of the ability of the blood to clot, not directly of heparin levels. In recent years many centers have shifted to measuring heparin levels (most often by monitoring Anti Xa levels) and antithrombin III (AT III) levels. Neonates in particular may have low AT III levels, and AT III is essential for heparin to work. Consequently, augmentation of the AT III levels (with exogenously administered AT III—either as thrombate or by fresh frozen plasma [FFP]) is now commonly employed before heparin dosing. During CPB the heparin level is monitored at regular intervals, and if AT III

levels are adequate, then management of heparin levels can ensure adequate anticoagulation during exposure to the extracorporeal circuitry.

Placing a patient on CPB is similar to the application of veno-arterial (VA) extracorporeal membrane oxygenation (ECMO) in the ICU—there needs to be an arterial "inflow" cannula (most frequently placed directly into the aorta, but in some circumstances it is placed in a femoral artery or even into a side graft sewn to a vessel like the innominate artery) and a venous "return" cannula. (CPB cannot be supported with venovenous cannulation!) In many circumstances for repair of congenital heart defects, it is necessary to enter the cardiac chambers, so venous return needs to recover venous blood from both the superior vena cava and the inferior vena cava directly (two separate cannulas) as opposed to simply one cannula placed into the right atrium. Once the patient has been anticoagulated and cannulated, CPB commences, and flow rates are adjusted to provide adequate tissue perfusion. For neonates and infants these flow rates can be as high as 200 mL/kg/min, so cannulas need to be of sufficient size to support adequate perfusion.

Depending on the size of the patient, as well as on the patient's starting hemoglobin level, and the amount of solution needed to "prime" the pump, blood products may need to be added to the pump or during CPB. Today it is commonplace for surgical teams to use a "cell saver" that returns any excessive blood loss either to the pump for reinfusion during CPB or into a system where the blood can be processed for reinfusion, thus minimizing the need for additional blood products and blood exposure.

The surgical team can then choose from numerous strategies that can present challenges in the postoperative setting. Unlike ICU-based ECMO, various degrees of cooling might be employed. Many surgical teams will cool patients to a temperature between 25°C and 32°C. This will allow the team to turn down flow rates, if necessary, to improve exposure of the surgical field while decreasing metabolism so that it can tolerate the periods of decreased perfusion. In some situations the team may use more "profound" cooling (employing temperatures as low as 15°C). The team may elect to do this if they are anticipating a more prolonged period of diminished perfusion (such as during aortic arch repair or repair of pulmonary arteries, in which bronchial flow can create interference with the surgeon's ability to visualize fragile structures and perform delicate suture reconstruction). At these profoundly low temperatures, surgeons may even turn off the CPB flow for periods of time (using DHCA). This can enable them to perform a cardiac repair in a surgical field that is not flooded with blood. They can even remove the cannulas, if their presence hampers surgical repair, because during DHCA there is no CPB, and the cannulas are not needed. Of course, the consequence of DHCA is NO perfusion to vital organs (e.g., kidney, brain), and despite the decreased oxygen need provided by profound hypothermia, there is a risk for subtle to severe levels of organ ischemia and injury depending on the duration of DHCA. Many teams now use DHCA only sparingly and for relatively short duration (exposure times less than 30 minutes between periods of reperfusion).

In many cases the heart chambers need to be opened, and it is helpful for the team to "arrest" the heart so that it is not beating. An open, beating heart is a risk for ejecting air into the circulation. To provide this arrest a cross-clamp is placed on the aorta, and a solution designed to arrest (and protect the heart) is infused proximal to the clamp so that it can enter the coronary arteries. This solution, called cardioplegia, contains a high potassium level, to create diastolic arrest, among other compounds to help decrease the heart's metabolic need for substrate. Current solutions can help support cardiac arrest for up to 3 to 4 hours (or more)—usually more than enough time for the surgical team to complete the cardiac repair. However, the consequence of cardioplegic arrest is still a period of ischemia (albeit somewhat "protected") to the heart, from which it will need to recover.

To protect the heart during the period of aortic cross-clamping, ice or iced saline is sometimes placed over the heart. Likewise, ice packs are often placed around the head of infants who are undergoing periods of altered cerebral perfusion (e.g., DHCA). More recently, carbon dioxide (CO_2) is often added to the pump during cooling because cooling tends to make blood alkalotic, and this can decrease flow to the brain. Adding CO_2 (called pH-stat strategy) can improve cerebral blood flow (and protection) when periods of DHCA are anticipated.

For patients undergoing repair of the aortic arch, DHCA used to be a common strategy because it was difficult to continue perfusion through an aortic cannula with the aorta wide open. In recent years it has been popular to sew a side graft for arterial perfusion onto the innominate artery. At cold temperatures the flow rate can be decreased to 25 to 50 mL/kg/min, and with a snare on the proximal innominate, flow will not enter the aorta but instead perfuse the cerebral circulation and return through numerous collaterals to the other head vessels and the descending aorta. With clamps or snares selectively placed on the other head vessels and on the descending aorta, it is possible for the surgical team to provide perfusion to the brain and to the organs in the abdomen (e.g., kidney, mesentery) while working on a widely opened aorta. This technique is often called "selective" or "regional" cerebral perfusion and has contributed to less frequent use of complete DHCA.

The effects of all of these strategies, and others, on the neonate or infant are discussed later. Suffice it to say that infants exposed to CPB are generally exposed to varying degrees of hypothermia, some periods of cardiac (and occasionally whole body) ischemia, and dilution of their blood and clotting factors from the pump prime (sometimes requiring transfusion of blood, platelets, and other clotting factors). In the ICU handoff it is commonplace for the surgical team to communicate the total CPB time (although they do not commonly communicate the temperature that the neonate or infant was cooled to). They will generally communicate the aortic cross-clamp time or the DHCA time (but they may communicate the total clamp or DHCA time and not specify how often cardioplegia was reinfused or how often reperfusion was employed during the period of DHCA).

In general the quality of the cardiac repair is probably more relevant than the total CPB time or whether or not the neonate or infant needed additional CPB to revise the repair. However, there is a correlation between length of CPB and convalescent complications or difficulty. (If CPB duration itself were detrimental, then we would likely expect more CPB-related issues from prolonged ECMO; however, even in those circumstances, the outcome is usually related to underlying adequacy of repair or severity of residual disease rather than to duration of exposure to extracorporeal circulation). Rather than focus on actual CPB time, duration of aortic cross-clamping, or whether or not periods of DHCA were used, it may be more helpful to the ICU team to know the following: (1) What is the quality of the repair? Any residual lesions or anatomic problems that might influence convalescence? (2) Were there any problems noted during CPB that might be important to know about in the convalescent period (e.g., arrhythmias, acidosis, poor urine output, difficulty ventilating)? (3) What seems to be most helpful (and most harmful) to this particular patient (such as "the

patient respond well to calcium, but not to volume"; or "the patient is being atrially paced for junctional rhythm")? Although there is certainly an exposure "cost" to patients for CPB, when it is performed well, with adequate perfusion flow rates, attentiveness to cerebral, cardiac, and whole body protection, appropriate circuitry and use of various strategies; and no overt issues related to injury of vessels or other structures from the CPB instrumentation, the influence of CPB on convalescence should be minimal.

Postoperative Low Cardiac Output Syndrome

Low cardiac output syndrome (LCOS) is a well-recognized, common postoperative complication seen following CPB in neonates and infants with a predictable constellation of hemodynamic and physiologic aberrations. Approximately 25% of children experience a decrease in cardiac index of less than 2 L/min/m^2 within 6 to 18 hours after cardiac surgery.[10] Inappropriately managed LCOS is a risk factor for increased morbidity and death and may occasionally be progressive and refractory, requiring a period of "myocardial rest" with extracorporeal life support (ECLS).[11] The approach to managing LCOS should therefore be proactive and preemptive and involve early detection and early institution of therapy to mitigate and reverse its negative effects. Factors associated with the development of myocardial dysfunction include the inflammatory response associated with CPB (from exposure of blood to foreign surface), myocardial ischemia from aortic cross-clamping with inadequate myocardial protection (despite the use of cardioplegia, each heart may be "biologically" different and respond in unpredictable ways to routine application of well-accepted cardioplegia regimens), reperfusion injury (particularly to areas that were hypoperfused preoperatively, such as areas of lung), hypothermia, and ventriculotomies (which can impose actual injury to heart muscle) when performed. Further compromise in cardiac output may occur due to residual or undiagnosed structural lesions or in instances of late presentation with preexisting right ventricular, left ventricular, or biventricular dysfunction.[12] The risk is greatest for neonates and young infants undergoing complex surgical repairs presenting in circulatory collapse, and those infants and children with preexisting ventricular dysfunction.[12]

Certain preoperative, intraoperative, and postoperative strategies have been successfully instituted to prevent or minimize LCOS and involve addressing the metabolic and endocrine response to CPB, preload optimization, inotropic support, judicious afterload reduction and lusitropy, exclusion of structural defects with precise transesophageal echocardiography, mechanical ventilation strategies, and pulmonary vasodilator therapy for pulmonary hypertension.

LCOS is usually reflected by low blood pressure and (when there is normal sinus rhythm) tachycardia—typical hallmarks of "shock." However, blood pressure can be normal if low cardiac output is associated with increased systemic vascular resistance, and heart rhythm can be deceptive, particularly if there is heart block. Sometimes LCOS can be perpetuated by cardiac rhythm abnormalities. For example, patients in junctional rhythm may lose their "atrial kick," and this can result in a diminished cardiac output. The ICU team can monitor evidence for tissue perfusion, and in the current era a downward trend on the near-infrared spectroscopy (NIRS) or an upward trend in lactic acidosis (or increasing base deficit) are important signs that cardiac output may not be normal. Typical management strategies are related to improving preload (if appropriate), decreasing afterload (when possible), or improving contractility (with a variety of pharmacologic agents). Making certain that the cardiac rhythm is not abnormal (or in need of pacing) and that the hemoglobin level is adequate to optimize oxygen delivery are also important. In the face of requiring escalating inotropic support, consideration for early placement on ECLS is warranted. It is also imperative to know of (and to investigate for) the presence of any important residual anatomic defects needing revision.

Preoperative and Intraoperative Strategies

Endocrine Response

CPB is associated with tremendous increases in native catecholamines, particularly epinephrine and norepinephrine. This is due partly to surgical stress but also to peripheral vasoconstriction with relative ischemia, lack of pulsatile blood flow, and acidosis.[13,14] This elevation of catecholamines extends into the postoperative period.[15] It seems that the initial increases in catecholamine levels fall considerably upon reperfusion of the lungs, likely related to the uptake and metabolism of the catecholamines in the lungs. When the lungs are excluded from the circulation (total CPB), there is significant accumulation of norepinephrine. Hypothermia also has the effect of raising the serum catecholamine levels not only by increasing production, but also by decreasing the metabolism and the downregulation of catecholamine receptors. Circulatory arrest also results in increases of catecholamine levels, but it is likely the rewarming, reperfusion phase of circulatory arrest that is most associated with catecholamine surge.[16,17] Catecholamine levels tend to fall rapidly once normothermia is achieved and bypass is discontinued. It is clear that the level of anesthesia has a great influence on the surge of catecholamines associated with CPB and surgery. The anesthetic management of neonates has been shaped largely based on the findings of Anand and Hickey.[18] High-dose narcotic induction and maintenance can result in reduction of catecholamine levels and reduced postoperative complications. However, there is a rise in serum cortisol levels after induction of anesthesia and surgery. Initiation of CPB causes the cortisol levels to fall secondary to hemodilution. After separation from CPB, levels again begin to rise, and this continues for 24 hours, after which they gradually fall to normal. The effect of ultrafiltration on the levels of glucocorticoids is not known. Preoperative and postoperative steroids have been shown to mitigate the effects of the LCOS after CPB.[19,20]

It appears that hypothermia and CPB result in a decrease in the level of insulin, as well as decreased peripheral response to the insulin. The net result is an increase in the serum glucose level. The level of insulin increases after reperfusion and rewarming.[21] Glucagon and human growth hormone are released as part of the general stress response. Growth hormone is an anabolic hormone that tends to rise in both adults and children during and after CPB. A few studies show an increase in glucagon level during the CPB period, and there is clearly a gradual rise in glucagon levels after surgery that peaks at approximately 6 hours.[8]

Thyroid hormone levels decrease during the CPB period and into the first several days after surgery.[22,23] The reasons for this include hemodilution, decrease in thyroxine-binding globulin, and increased glucocorticoid levels. The lowest levels of thyroid hormones seem to be associated with poor outcome. For this reason, triiodothyronine administered intravenously after CPB can be a useful inotropic agent.

Myocardial Protection

Neonatal repair is the preferred approach to many congenital heart defects. As the complexity of and time required for repair increases, so does the need for effective and optimal myocardial protection. There is some laboratory evidence that the immature myocardium has different structural and functional characteristics than the adult myocardium.[24] The immature heart is less compliant, resulting in a very limited range of the Starling curve. The normal neonatal heart is operating at maximal saturation of adrenergic stimulation, and there is an exaggerated negative inotropic response to anesthetic agents and therefore a requirement for greater doses of inotropic agents when they are needed.[25] The immature myocardium relies heavily on glucose as its major substrate and also has a greater reliance on extracellular calcium for calcium-mediated excitation-contraction coupling.[26,27] It is widely accepted that the immature heart has a greater tolerance to ischemia than the adult or mature heart. However, most of this laboratory data has been obtained with normal hearts. It is unclear what the ischemic tolerance is when there are preexisting conditions such as cyanosis, hypertrophy, or acidosis. Many of these conditions may be present in neonates and infants who require surgical correction of their heart defect and may compromise myocardial protection. Infants and children with chronic cyanosis as a result of inadequate pulmonary blood flow often have increased bronchial collateral flow. This increased blood return to the left heart can result in insufficient myocardial protection by warming the heart and washing out cardioplegia.[28] Hypertrophied ventricles may also have inadequate myocardial protection and suffer from subendocardial ischemia during prolonged cardioplegic arrest periods.

Hypothermia remains the most important factor for successful myocardial protection in infants.[29] Electromechanical arrest, ventricular decompression, and hypothermia all work together to decrease the myocardial oxygen consumption. Topically applied iced saline may be helpful; however, it often interferes with the operative procedure and may result in phrenic nerve palsy. Therefore many groups use topical cooling intermittently. Typically, cardioplegia is delivered through a catheter or needle in the aortic root after the cross-clamp has been applied. Retrograde cardioplegia delivery (via the coronary sinus), however, has received significant attention and is gaining in popularity in neonates. It is particularly useful in neonates requiring prolonged aortic cross-clamp time and in whom delivery of cardioplegia into the aortic root may not be possible (e.g., aortic valve replacement, arterial switch operation). Blood cardioplegia may be superior to crystalloid cardioplegia, especially for longer (>1 hour) myocardial ischemic times.[29]

Typically, cardioplegia solutions should have a calcium concentration that is below the serum concentration.[30] Despite the potential for excessive calcium influx secondary to hyperkalemia-induced membrane depolarization, potassium remains the most widely used cardiac arresting agent in all of cardiac surgery. Magnesium helps to maintain that negative resting membrane potential and also inhibits sarcolemmal calcium influx.[31] The addition of magnesium to blood cardioplegia results in significantly improved functional recovery. Magnesium enrichment of hypocalcemic cardioplegic solutions can result in near complete functional recovery, but even high-dose magnesium supplementation cannot reverse dysfunction in severely stressed hearts that receive normocalcemic cardioplegia.[32] Typically an induction dose of 30 mL/kg cardioplegia solution at 4°C is delivered. Although there is no conclusive evidence either to support or refute the practice, many surgeons will use multiple doses of cardioplegia at approximately

20- to 30-minute intervals during the ischemic period. This practice may be helpful when there are significant bronchial collaterals, or in operations performed using mild or moderate hypothermia, both of which may result in premature warming of the heart. Single-dose or reduced frequency del Nido cardioplegia, which has a higher concentration of magnesium and lidocaine, has been gaining acceptance in many pediatric cardiac surgery programs. The reduced need to halt the flow of the surgical repair helps reduce the cross-clamp time while maintaining excellent myocardial protection.[33]

In selected operations on the right side of the heart in which the septa are intact, that is, tricuspid valve repair or pulmonary valve repair or replacement (or when aortic cross clamping with administration of cardioplegia may not be feasible, such as when there is significant scarring around or thinning of the aorta), a technique referred to as "empty beating" may be employed, in which case little myocardial ischemia occurs and a cross-clamp is not employed. This is a reasonable technique as long as there is no communication between the right and left sides of the heart through which air can pass and result in air embolus to the systemic circulation. Mild hypothermia with fibrillatory arrest can be used in operations on the right side of the heart, especially when a significant intracardiac communication exists, such as an ASD. This technique is not recommended when there is significant aortic valve regurgitation because severe left ventricular distention will occur.

Intramyocardial air has also been suggested as a contributing factor for myocardial dysfunction after pediatric cardiac surgery.[34,35] In 4% of 350 consecutive pediatric patients undergoing repair of congenital cardiac defects, intramyocardial air was detected in the immediate postbypass period using intraoperative echocardiography, despite aggressive "deairing" maneuvers before removing the aortic cross-clamp.[35] Hemodynamic instability was apparent in some of these patients, but in many cases the intramyocardial air produced no clinical signs. None of the patients had clinical evidence of air embolism to other organs (e.g., brain). Echocardiographic imaging demonstrated increased echogenic areas localized to the right ventricular free wall and along the inferior portion of the intraventricular septum, suggesting the distribution of air was localized to the area supplied by the right coronary artery. The right coronary artery is a likely source for embolization of retained left ventricular air because of the location of the ostium of the right coronary artery on the anterior aspect of the aorta. Therefore residual left ventricular air is more likely to enter the right coronary artery and result in right ventricular ischemia and dysfunction, except in patients undergoing an arterial switch procedure for d-transposition in which the left coronary artery and left ventricle may be involved. (Following an arterial switch operation, *both* coronary arteries are anterior, and thus the risk of air embolism to either the right or left coronary distribution is increased.) Deairing is performed with the aortic cross-clamp left in place, and the cardioplegia needle is used to vent air from the left ventricle. Therapy for myocardial air embolism is directed at increasing perfusion pressure to propel air through the arterioles and capillary bed. Dramatic hemodynamic and echocardiographic improvements have been demonstrated in patients with intramyocardial air after the administration of phenylephrine or reperfusing the heart with high pump flow rates and high perfusion pressures on CPB.[35] Some groups "blow" carbon dioxide (CO_2) over the operative field to limit the risk of significant air embolus and reduce the risk of neurologic events.[36] (Carbon dioxide is heavier than air, so it displaces air from the pericardial sac during surgery. Carbon dioxide also dissipates from the

circulation more readily than air, so it is less likely to cause an air embolus.)

Other adverse effects of CPB include increased capillary permeability and increased total body water (TBW), which often results in tissue edema and multiple organ dysfunction. Intraoperative techniques that have been developed for reversing tissue edema and hemodilution after CPB include conventional ultrafiltration (CUF) during CPB and modified ultrafiltration (MUF), which is performed in the immediate post-CPB period and removes excess water from the patient, as well as providing a method for salvaging blood from the circuit. MUF has been shown to modulate the inflammatory response to CPB by removing inflammatory mediators, including interleukin (IL-6, IL-8), and tumor necrosis factor. A prospective randomized trial of MUF showed improved hemodynamics with a reduction in TBW and decreased need for blood transfusion when compared with nonfiltered controls. MUF has been shown to improve left ventricular systolic function after CPB, resulting in increased systolic blood pressure and cardiac index.[37]

Postoperative Strategies

Postoperative strategies that may be used to manage patients at risk for or in a state of low cardiac output include the use of hemodynamic monitoring, enabling a timely and accurate assessment of cardiovascular function and tissue oxygenation; optimization of ventricular loading conditions; the judicious use of inotropic agents; afterload reduction and lusitropy; an appreciation of and the use of positive pressure ventilation for circulatory support; and in some circumstances mechanical circulatory support. All interventions and strategies should culminate in improving the relationship between oxygen supply and demand, ensuring adequate tissue oxygenation.[10]

NIRS has now become a standard monitoring tool in postoperative ICU assessment and provides a reasonable measure of tissue oxygen delivery and its response to resuscitation.[38] Arterial lactate levels and myocardial oxygen consumption trends are also useful for monitoring hemodynamic optimization.

Maximizing oxygen delivery preload optimization is achieved by correcting the hemoglobin level with packed red blood cells transfusions; positive inotropic support is improved with epinephrine, dobutamine, or dopamine and lusitropy; and afterload reduction is achieved with phosphodiesterase inhibitors such as milrinone. In patients with the vasodilatory form of LCOS, vasopressin and norepinephrine can be judiciously used to normalize afterload. Pulmonary hypertension, right ventricular dysfunction, and cyanosis can be treated with inhaled nitric oxide (iNO) and hyperventilation to reduce arterial CO_2. Postoperative steroids have been shown to reduce the inflammatory vasodilatory shock seen in LCOS.[20] Calcium infusions have recently received some attention in the management of LCOS in children undergoing CPB.[39] Neonates undergoing cardiac surgery for various univentricular heart staging strategies receive the maximum hemodynamic benefit from calcium, likely due to the fact that the immature myocardium with structurally underdeveloped sarcoplasmic reticulum is most dependent on extracellular calcium levels.[39] Occasionally, however, despite all of these measures persistent lactic acidosis and poor tissue perfusion necessitate ECMO or mechanical support. Early institution of mechanical support before end-organ failure has set in has been shown to improve outcomes in some neonates undergoing the Norwood procedure.[40]

Postoperative Acute Kidney Injury and Fluid Management

Children undergoing CPB tend to develop severe tissue edema from a capillary leak syndrome secondary to the inflammatory response seen during CPB. This increased capillary permeability leads to tissue and subsequent organ dysfunction, particularly myocardial and pulmonary edema. Acute kidney injury, which is common postoperatively and carries substantial morbidity and mortality, complicates postoperative fluid management. Strategies to reduce TBW focus on reducing hemodilution intraoperatively and removing excess volume with diuresis or renal replacement therapy postoperatively.

Intraoperatively, hemodilution may be addressed prebypass, during CPB, and in the postbypass period. Prebypass strategies include circuit miniaturization and the use of colloid or blood prime as opposed to crystalloid. The use of blood versus asanguineous prime is often debated; however, recent evidence suggests that asanguineous prime followed by transfusion as needed may decrease the inflammatory response associated with CPB when compared with blood prime.[176] There is some suggestion in recent studies that circuit miniaturization may obviate the need for MUF and lead to decreased transfusions while on CPB.[41] This, however, is in the setting of substantial evidence that MUF leads to decreased perioperative blood transfusions.[42-44] Continuous removal of fluid in the venoarterial direction while on CPB is referred to as CUF, as opposed to MUF, which involves a short period of ultrafiltration in the arteriovenous direction immediately after separating from bypass. CUF can be an effective technique; Thompson et al.[45] noted that when amounts of fluid removal are standardized, CUF and MUF resulted in equivalent outcomes measures such as hematocrit, ventricular function, and postoperative transfusions. However, CUF is complicated by the inability to remove large amounts of fluid without having to administer replacement fluid to maintain reservoir levels, whereas MUF has the advantage of filtering the entire circuit and delivering blood filtered to a desired hematocrit back to the patient, resulting in greater hemoconcentration.[46] MUF, with or without preceding CUF while on CPB, has been shown in several studies to be superior to CUF alone with regard to increasing hematocrit, decreased inotrope usage, decreased chest tube output and blood transfusion, and decreased duration of mechanical ventilation.[42,47,48] There is some discrepancy in the literature as to the superiority of MUF over CUF; however, outcomes may be affected by technique, circuit arrangements, and the heterogeneity of the studied populations. Flow rates require careful monitoring during MUF, however, because aggressive ultrafiltration can lead to increased runoff from the aorta, compromising cerebral blood flow.[49]

The postoperative mainstay of fluid balance in the ICU remains diuresis; however, standard loop diuretic therapy is usually limited in the first 48 hours due to a blunted response due to a diuretic-refractory oliguric phase. Neonates undergoing complex congenital cardiac surgery commonly develop some mild to moderate acute kidney injury and demonstrate a positive fluid balance in the first 24 to 48 hours with an elevated pressor and inotrope requirement. There is increasing evidence that early peritoneal dialysis (PD), traditionally reserved for patients in renal failure, is a safe and effective way to manage fluid balance. Renal failure is common after pediatric cardiac surgery, and renal failure requiring PD is associated with a high mortality.[50-52] However, early application of PD by identifying patients at high risk for renal failure per the

RIFLE (Risk, Injury, Failure, Loss, End Stage) criteria leads to more net negative fluid balance and decreased mortality,[53-55] and usage has therefore been expanded in some centers to include those at high risk of renal failure or prophylactically in those with signs of fluid overload. PD was recently compared to diuresis in a randomized trial and found to be superior in reducing fluid overload, ventilator duration, and inotrope requirements.[56] Serious complications of PD catheter placement include hydrothorax, peritonitis, and bowel perforation[57]; however, these are uncommon, and catheter placement may be accomplished intraoperatively in a transdiaphragmatic fashion, which may be safer than transabdominal placement at a later time.[58] Instillation of dialysate into the abdomen has been shown to be well tolerated, with minimal to no effect on cardiac or pulmonary dynamics.[59,60]

PD has been shown to reduce the inotrope and pressor need and maintain an even or slightly negative fluid balance during this critical first 24 to 48 hours postoperative period.[56] However, as with any intervention during this critical phase of instability, PD has been shown to be associated with increased morbidity in neonates with hypoplastic left heart syndrome undergoing the Norwood procedure. Acute fluid shifts in some situations may result in worsening hemodynamic instability and outcomes if not carefully monitored.[61]

Hemostasis and Cardiopulmonary Bypass

Bleeding is the Achilles' heel of complex neonatal congenital cardiac surgery repairs. CPB exerts intended and unintended effects on the enzymatic and formed elements of the coagulation and inflammatory systems. Compared with adults, children are at special risk for known, and unknown, differences in their hemostatic systems. CPB leads to a whole body inflammatory response involving the formed blood elements, coagulation, complement, and kallikrein/kinin systems.[62] Hemodilution is directly related to the volume of crystalloid and colloid required to prime the circuit and the patient's own blood volume and can dilute blood components by as much as 40%.[4] Although children have relatively larger circulating blood volumes when compared with adults (e.g., preterm infants have an estimated blood volume of 90 to 100 mL/kg compared to 70 to 80 mL/kg in an adult),[5,6] their low absolute blood volume accentuates their dilutional coagulopathy. Further, their small blood volume creates practical limitations on the use of certain blood conservation strategies such as autologous donation and cell saver. A profound thrombotic reaction involving both the extrinsic and intrinsic coagulation pathways is initiated by continuous exposure of heparinized blood to the perfusion circuit and to the wound during cardiac surgery. Despite large doses of heparin during CPB, heparin does not block thrombin generation but partially inhibits thrombin after it is produced. Thrombin is continuously generated, and a consumptive coagulopathy is initiated.[7-9] If thrombin formation could be completely inhibited during CPB, the consumption of coagulation proteins and platelets could largely be prevented.

The coagulopathy induced by CPB affects children more profoundly than adults. Neonates are particularly affected, as a result of their unique cardiac lesions, immature hematopoietic and coagulation systems, and small blood volumes.[63] After birth, erythropoiesis profoundly decreases, accompanied by the cessation of fetal hemoglobin production. This physiologic anemia results in hemoglobin nadirs of 9 to 11 g/dL at 8 to 12 weeks of age. Neonates have inherent deficiencies in vitamin K–dependent factors II, VII, IX, and X, which may be corrected by administering vitamin K at birth.[64] Deficiencies in contact factors XI, XII, prekallikrein, and high-molecular-weight kininogen are also present at birth.[65,66] Hepatic immaturity leading to decreased factor synthesis and accelerated clearance of factors through higher metabolic rates also play a role. Levels of coagulation inhibitors are also low. Protein C, protein S, heparin cofactor II, and AT III levels are 40% to 60% of adult values, slowly achieving adult levels by 180 days.[66] Platelet aggregation may be impaired,[67] and fibrinogen exists in a dysfunctional fetal isoform.[66] Notably fibrinogen level, platelet counts, and levels of factors V, VIII, von Willebrand factor, and XIII are normal at birth.[66] In spite of the preceding, prothrombin time and thrombin clotting time are normal within a few days of birth.[66] Thromboelastography has shown that neonates and infants actually develop faster and stronger clots than adults.[68]

Following surgery, bleeding that persists after the patient is brought to the ICU can be a major contributor to morbidity. The surgical team can likely comment on the possibility that bleeding is mechanical and might require reexploration. Bleeding that exceeds a rate of 10 mg/kg/h is significant. Factor replacement therapy (platelets, fresh frozen plasma, cryoprecipitate, and occasionally recombinant factors IX or VII) has utility, and a thromboelastogram can be helpful in directing therapy. Most important to the management of these patients is close communication between the surgical and ICU teams. It is critical to replace blood loss in the immediate postoperative period, usually milliliter for milliliter to maintain hemodynamics and hemoglobin levels.

Pulmonary Dysfunction

Pulmonary injury can manifest in several ways because the lungs have both a parenchymal and a vascular component. Parenchymal effects of CPB are reflected by alterations in pulmonary compliance most commonly related to an increase in lung water. The impact of this on the patient is a diminished ability of the lungs to perform their function in gas exchange, which may result in a requirement for increased ventilatory support. Endothelial cell dysfunction is exacerbated by CPB, cardioplegic arrest, and hypothermia. The vascular effects are manifested by changes in pulmonary vascular resistance, which in turn affects function of the right ventricle. The lungs are in a unique position in the circulation and may be vulnerable to different mechanisms of injury.

There are multiple specialized cells within the lung, including many cells of inflammation. The lung is an important source and target of the inflammatory response to CPB. Part of the pulmonary derangement that occurs is related to the inflammatory response from CPB. This is manifest as decreased functional residual capacity, compliance, and gas exchange, as well as increased pulmonary vascular resistance and pulmonary artery pressure.[69] Post-CPB acute respiratory distress syndrome can occasionally impair oxygenation and ventilation to a severe degree, eventually requiring temporary ECMO support.[91]

Inflammation is not the only factor that produces impairment of pulmonary function from CPB. When patients are placed on bypass, the lungs have a sudden and significant decrease in antegrade flow via the pulmonary artery. During "total" bypass the lungs receive only "nutrient" flow from their bronchial supply. This relative ischemia of the lungs, in addition to the inflammatory effect of CPB, may result in significant clinical pulmonary dysfunction.[70] It seems that low-flow CPB produces worse pulmonary injury than circulatory arrest,[71,72] suggesting that the interaction between the inflammatory and ischemic components is complex. Both the inflammatory and ischemic factors produce damage to the

pulmonary endothelium,[70,73-75] and this leads to increases in post-CPB pulmonary vascular resistance and pulmonary artery pressure, both of which can have significant implications in neonates and small infants, especially after certain types of procedures, such as the Norwood procedure for hypoplastic left heart syndrome.

A number of suggestions have been made for limiting this pulmonary dysfunction. Some intriguing work with Perflubron (liquid ventilation) infused into the lungs before bypass demonstrate that the antiinflammatory and oxygen-carrying capabilities of this compound can have a dramatic effect on postbypass pulmonary parenchymal and vascular function.[76,77] The use of steroids may lessen the inflammatory response to CPB. Steroids given before exposure to CPB reduce lung water accumulation, improve post-CPB pulmonary compliance, and limit post-CPB pulmonary hypertension.[78] MUF after CPB seems to immediately improve pulmonary function compared with function in patients who do not undergo ultrafiltration.[69,79-86] All of this suggests that some significant advances can be made with respect to the pulmonary response to CPB.

Following CPB, patients are at particular risk for life-threatening pulmonary hypertensive crisis (PHC). iNO has been shown to reduce pulmonary hypertension and improve postoperative outcomes in children with pulmonary hypertension undergoing congenital heart surgery with CPB.[87] At low doses iNO has been shown to improve ventilation/perfusion matching, decrease the intrapulmonary shunt fraction, and often increase the systemic arterial saturation.[88] Further, a randomized controlled trial using iNO in the postoperative period after surgery for congenital heart disease demonstrated decreased time to meet criteria for extubation and decreased incidence of PHC.[87,89] Empiric NO infused into the CPB circuit has also been shown to improve postoperative outcomes.[90]

In patients with significant lung dysfunction following exposure to CPB, increased ventilator requirements can create a form of "pulmonary tamponade" with decreased filling of the heart due to the increased peak ventilator pressures. These patients may benefit from having the surgical team reopen the sternum (if it is closed) to provide less impairment of hemodynamics from temporarily increased ventilation requirements.

Neurologic Injury

In the patient with congenital heart disease, neurologic injury continues to play a significant role in quality of life over the patient's entire life span. Although historically there were clear causes for severe neurologic injury, they have since been better understood and significantly reduced from the routine treatment of our patient population.[92]

Profound hypothermia with DHCA was historically associated with choreoathetosis, seizures, and other forms of immediately recognizable neurologic dysfunction.[93] With advances in management strategies for hypothermic CPB and more sophisticated use of DHCA (including acid/base blood gas management strategies—particularly for high-risk groups such as those with prominent aortopulmonary collaterals, reduced exposure duration to altered flow and reperfusion techniques, and use of higher hemoglobin during CPB) prominent clinically evident neurologic injury following CPB has become uncommon. Part of the problem in developing strategies to improve the impact of neurologic injury is that it is difficult to separate patient- and disease-related risk factors (over which we have little control) from risk factors related to controllable CPB management strategies.

The actual incidence of neurologic injury after infant cardiac repair, 10% to 25% of patients in some series,[94-97] highlights the importance of attention to detail in factors affecting the infant brain. This risk of injury can be viewed in three components: (1) preexisting risk associated with various congenital heart lesions and with each individual child's own unique brain substrate, (2) injury induced by CPB and the various CPB strategies that can be employed by the surgical team, and (3) injury sustained during the "vulnerable" period after exposure to CPB when the patient is in the ICU. When neurologic injury is manifest in a patient after CPB, it is often impossible to determine which of these elements played the most prominent role.

The risk for abnormal neurologic development, even without exposure to CPB or repair of the lesion, is significant and ranges from 2% to 10% for a variety of congenital heart lesions.[98] This may relate to abnormal cerebral perfusion patterns or to actual associated structural anomalies within the brain. Certain cardiac defects associated with syndromes (i.e., atrioventricular septal defects and trisomy 21) have an even higher incidence of abnormal brain development irrespective of whether the patient is exposed to CPB. The natural history of neurologic development without cardiac surgery is not known and is unlikely ever to be known for several serious and life-threatening congenital cardiac lesions because it is rare to leave these lesions unrepaired or for these children to survive without surgery long enough to provide an adequate "control" group. Nevertheless, there is literature to show that cerebral flow patterns are extremely abnormal in infants with congenital heart disease before they are placed on CPB.[98-100]

Finally, the condition of infants at the time of presentation greatly affects their neurologic outcome.[101] Perhaps the greatest impact on the reduction of neurologic injury in the preoperative period comes from prenatal diagnosis and subsequent delivery of the child in a center equipped to handle the fragile infant with severe heart disease.[100] Nonetheless, careful attention to detail with regard to adequate systemic perfusion, cerebral perfusion pressures, avoidance of hypoxia and perhaps just as importantly hyperoxia, as well as glucose levels and temperature control, are all critically important. Some groups now recommend routine magnetic resonance imaging spectroscopy in neonates scheduled to undergo repair under CPB, especially in infants born preterm, to look for preexisting neurologic injury or substrate for injury such as small intraparenchymal bleeds, immature myelination, or other structural abnormalities. Although the utility of this strategy is yet to be determined, infants with significant presurgical abnormalities can be delayed from cardiac repair, or the increased risk can be communicated to the parents and appreciated by the care team.

The physiology of CPB produces many "alterations" that might relate to neurologic injury. During CPB, microembolic events commonly occur and can contribute to end-organ injury.[102] Alteration in cerebral blood flow can be demonstrated by middle cerebral artery transcranial Doppler, retinal angiography, echocardiography, and infrared spectroscopy, although monitoring with any of these methods has not been clearly shown to be clinically beneficial. Direct evidence of air embolism to the brain can possibly be suggested by visualization of air in the coronary vessels, electrocardiographic changes of ST-segment elevation, and blanching of the skin of the head.[35,103,104] Neurologic events have been correlated with the presence of focal dilations of the microvasculature or very small aneurysms in terminal arterioles and capillaries within the cerebral circulation. The use of membrane oxygenators, arterial filters, and adequate heparinization (ACT >400 seconds) for CPB decreases the number of microemboli and may reduce the incidence

of embolic events during CPB.[105-107] Yet despite these methods, air embolism remains an important factor in postoperative neurologic dysfunction.

During pediatric CPB the frequency in which the left side of the circulation is exposed to air increases the likelihood of systemic air embolization. In a report of perioperative neurologic effects in neonates undergoing the arterial switch operation for transposition of the great arteries, the presence of a VSD was associated with an increased incidence of postoperative seizure activity.[108] Although this could be related to longer periods of DHCA (in a historical series when DHCA was used more frequently), the data could also suggest a higher incidence of air embolism as a cause for neurologic dysfunction. When recognized, cerebral air embolism can be treated by attempts to reduce gas bubble size by reestablishing hypothermic CPB or through the use of hyperbaric oxygen therapy in the early postoperative period.[109] Major cerebral air embolism has also been treated with retrograde cerebral perfusion in adult patients, although experience with this modality in children is limited. Both hypothermia and hyperbaric therapy reduce the size of gaseous microbubbles and allow them to pass through the arterial and capillary beds, resulting in reduced ischemia.

Hypothermic Injury to the Brain

Early experience with deep hypothermia suggested that using extremely low temperatures (esophageal temperatures of less than 10°C) resulted in a dramatic increase in neurologic and pulmonary injury. Neurologic sequelae, especially choreoathetosis, were commonly reported.[25,93,110] Neuropathologic examination of the brain of animals undergoing profound levels of hypothermia revealed microvascular lesions compatible with the no-reflow phenomenon.[111,112] Similar histologic brain lesions were observed in children who died after cardiac surgery using circulatory arrest.[113] These early reports diminished the enthusiasm for profound levels of hypothermia, and most institutions "increased" target hypothermic temperatures for DHCA to between 18°C and 20°C.

More recent, and probably more accurate, information suggests that some of these early fears are unfounded. Profound hypothermia does not seem to create cerebral injury[114,115] and in fact may correlate with improved cerebral protection during periods of DHCA. However, risk for injury may be affected by the type of blood gas management strategy used during DHCA (pH-stat versus alpha-stat), the duration of the time spent cooling, the duration of the period of DHCA, or the presence of significant aortopulmonary collaterals.[111,115-122]

The lower limit at which hypothermia causes significant end-organ damage is not known. Current clinical practices suggest, however, that temperatures of 15°C and below are probably no worse than temperatures of 18°C to 20°C. It seems clear that at hypothermic temperatures (<22°C) autoregulation of cerebral blood flow is lost and decreases in a linear fashion with decreases in mean arterial pressure.[123]

It is now well recognized that cerebral blood flow decreases in a linear relationship to decreasing temperature, whereas cerebral metabolism is reduced exponentially as temperature is decreased (Fig. 41.1). This provides most of the cerebral protection afforded to the brain by cooling because cerebral metabolic needs for oxygen are significantly lowered and cerebral blood flow becomes "luxurious." Nevertheless, cerebral metabolism persists, even at very low temperatures, and the brain is therefore susceptible to ischemic injury despite hypothermia if cerebral blood flow is eliminated (e.g., DHCA) for prolonged periods of time. It is

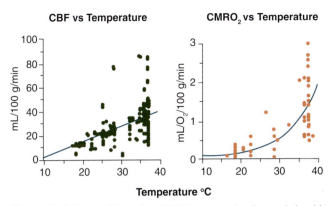

• **Figure 41.1** Cerebral blood flow *(CBF)* decreases in a linear relationship to decreasing temperature, whereas cerebral metabolism is reduced exponentially as temperature is decreased. *CMRO₂*, Cerebral metabolic rate of oxygen consumption. (From Nichols DG, Cameron DE, Ungerleider RM, et al. *Critical Heart Disease in Infants and Children.* 2nd ed. Philadelphia: Mosby; 2006.)

TABLE 41.1	Recommended Pump Flow Rates for Normothermic Cardiopulmonary Bypass
Patient Weight (kg)	**Pump Flow Rate (mL/kg/min)**
<3	150-200
3-10	125-175
10-15	120-150
15-30	100-120
30-50	75-100
>50	50-75

From Nichols DG, Cameron DE, Ungerleider RM, et al. *Critical Heart Disease in Infants and Children.* 2nd ed. Philadelphia: Mosby; 2006.

possible to predict the amount of cerebral blood flow required to support cerebral metabolic needs at decreasing temperatures, and this is the rationale behind continuous low-perfusion CPB (Table 41.1).[123-125]

Cerebral blood flow is regulated by several adjustable parameters. Although cerebral blood flow seems to be "autoregulated" at normothermic and moderately hypothermic temperatures,[126] autoregulation is lost at temperatures below 22°C,[123,127-129] and cerebral flow is more dependent on mean arterial pressure. Fortunately, at these cold temperatures the brain needs very little blood flow.[124] The acid-base strategy employed during cooling also affects cerebral blood flow and metabolism. Alpha-stat is a more commonly used method, but there has recently been enthusiasm in some centers for more routine use of pH-stat strategies.[130,131] pH-stat requires addition of CO_2 to the circuit during cooling, so the blood gases are "corrected" for the alkalosis that occurs with hypothermia. CO_2 is a potent cerebral vasodilator, and addition of CO_2 to the circuit significantly increases blood flow to the brain.[115,132] Although this might promote more homogeneous cerebral cooling, the addition of CO_2, especially at temperatures below 15°C, creates significant acidosis (pH <6.9) in the circulating blood and at the cellular level. This acidosis at the time of circulatory arrest may be the reason for substantial impairment in cerebral metabolic recovery in animals subjected to these conditions

experimentally.[115] However, if pH-stat is used for cooling and then the CO_2 is removed from the circuit (the patient is returned to alpha-stat blood gas management for a few minutes before establishing DHCA), the acidotic effects of pH-stat with respect to cerebral metabolic recovery may be alleviated.[122] Recent work suggests that hyperoxygenation on CPB in combination with pH-stat cooling can produce enhanced cerebral protection and extend the "safe period" of DHCA.

One group of patients that seems to be at increased risk for neurologic injury, and especially for choreoathetosis, is the group with significant aortopulmonary collaterals (such as older, cyanotic patients).[133,134] This has been demonstrated in an elegant experimental model by Kirshbom et al.,[119] who also demonstrated how use of pH-stat cooling protected the brains of these particular animals.[118] It is important to note, however, that neither alpha-stat nor pH-stat strategies protect the brain from significant structural or metabolic derangement after prolonged periods (60 minutes) of DHCA, with either strategy associated with indistinguishable damage.[120]

There may be some relatively simple interventions that can limit injury from DHCA. Intravenous methylprednisolone (30 mg/kg) given at least 8 hours before CPB exposure significantly improves cerebral metabolic recovery and renal function recovery after DHCA.[135] There is also evidence that aprotinin[136] (unfortunately, no longer clinically available), thromboxane A_2 receptor blockade,[137] platelet activating factor inhibitors,[138] or free radical scavengers[139] might improve cerebral recovery after DHCA, but none of the these, except for steroids, is currently clinically used in the United States. Recognition of high-risk groups (severe cyanosis, substantial aortopulmonary collaterals) might prompt use of pH-stat cooling, and in light of recent clinical work it might be warranted to use hyperoxygenation if a period of circulatory arrest is planned. It may also be helpful to switch to alpha-stat before inducing DHCA. It is important to cool for an adequate duration before using DHCA. Some authorities suggest that cooling duration be around 20 minutes. However, cooling duration needs to be considered as only one element in preparing the patient for DHCA and exists against a complex backdrop that includes target temperature, pH strategy used for cooling, hematocrit, patient's individual and unique biologic risk for DHCA, and, probably most importantly, the duration of uninterrupted circulatory arrest before cerebral reperfusion. In general, long periods of uninterrupted circulatory arrest at "warmer" temperatures would benefit from a longer duration of prearrest cooling. Patients cooled for less time have a higher likelihood of brain injury,[116,117,123,140,141] and if jugular venous oxygen saturations can be measured, it is probably unwise to use prolonged periods of DHCA if jugular venous oxygen saturations remain below 95%.[117,123] If continuous low-flow CPB can be used, this might be better for cerebral protection, although the effects of continuous low-flow perfusion on the lung and on the microvasculature might be deleterious compared with DHCA.[71,72]

DHCA should be used for only the period of time necessary to benefit from its advantages because brain injury does seem to relate to the duration of the arrest period.[121,140,142-144] The effect of 60 minutes of DHCA on the brain's microvasculature involves a loss of normal architecture, extraluminal edema and protein deposition, leukocyte accumulation, and vacuolization of surrounding neuron cytoplasm. Although no significant differences have been demonstrated between a prolonged single period of DHCA or intermittent reperfusion, interesting data were provided by Langley et al.[120] and by Mault,[145] who separately demonstrated that periods of DHCA up to 60 minutes can be associated with

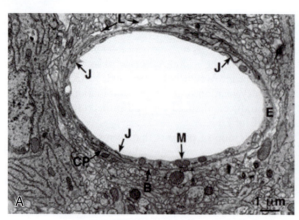
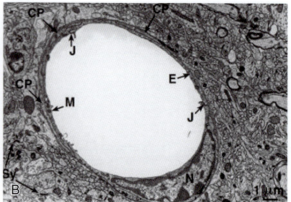

• **Figure 41.2** Electron micrographs of cerebral architecture (A) before and (B) after 60 minutes of deep hypothermic circulatory arrest with intermittent reperfusion periods every 15 minutes at 25 mL/kg/min. There is no alteration in architecture when intermittent perfusion is employed. *CP,* Small cellular projection; *E,* endothelial layer; *J,* junctional complex; *M,* mitochondria. (From Nichols DG, Cameron DE, Ungerleider RM, et al. *Critical Heart Disease in Infants and Children.* 2nd ed. Philadelphia: Mosby; 2006.)

absolutely normal recovery of cerebral metabolism and preservation of neural microarchitecture if the brain is perfused from the pump for 1 to 2 minutes (25 to 50 mL/kg/min) every 15 to 20 minutes (Fig. 41.2). This means that sequential periods of DHCA can be used as long as they are not prolonged beyond 15 to 20 minutes. If the brain is perfused between periods of DHCA, the duration of the DHCA periods may not be additive.[146] Similar findings have been alluded to by Miura et al.[147] and Robbins et al.[148] Currently the use of reperfusion between "short" (less than 15-minute duration) periods of circulatory arrest with the time of reperfusion determined by return of the cerebral NIRS to baseline values has been recommended as a prudent strategy to guide circulatory arrest periods. It is important for the surgical team to prevent infusion of air into the arterial cannula when reperfusion is provided.

Even when planning aortic arch reconstruction, such as with a Norwood procedure, it is possible to provide intermittent or continuous low-flow cerebral perfusion by first placing the proximal shunt on the innominate artery and then by moving the arterial cannula to the shunt.[149] During the period of DHCA the head should be packed in ice.[121] Although little can be done during reperfusion to improve cerebral recovery,[140] use of MUF after weaning from CPB may improve recovery of cerebral metabolism.[85,150] After DHCA, cardiac output and cerebral oxygen delivery should be maintained because this is the period when the brain is most vulnerable to injury.[151,152] There is also information that the brain might be better protected after DHCA if the patient is removed from CPB at rectal temperatures of 34°C as opposed to 36°C or warmer.[153]

As mentioned earlier, most recent data regarding DHCA versus continuous low-flow hypothermic CPB suggest that at 8-year follow-up there are no significant differences between groups.[154-156] Both groups are impaired compared with normal, but it is difficult to impugn DHCA as a cause of long-term neurologic outcome as it compares with continuous low flow. The patients exposed to DHCA seem to have more issues with motor skills, whereas those exposed as infants to primarily hypothermic low-flow strategies have more problems with attention deficit and other learning disabilities. Even more intriguing are the data reported by the group from Children's Hospital of Philadelphia suggesting that neonates may be at risk for brain injury during CPB, *regardless* of

which strategy is used.[157] It is certainly clear that the neurodevelopmental outcome for infants who undergo repair of congenital heart disease is multifactorial and relates only in part to the CPB strategies that are used. There are numerous other issues that involve preoperative risk factors, genetic predisposition, postoperative factors, and many more that are also important and need to be considered when evaluating the impact of CPB strategies on long-term neurologic outcome.[155,158]

Hematocrit During Cardiopulmonary Bypass

Hemodilution during CPB is a widely applied strategy based upon the notion that increased viscosity is detrimental during periods of hypothermia. Data from human studies have confirmed earlier findings in animal studies suggesting that higher hematocrit levels lead to better cerebral protection.[159,160] The results of these two clinical trials indicated that hematocrit levels during bypass below 24% were associated with lower scores on psychomotor development index on the Bayley scales. These studies also suggested that there was no improvement in neurologic outcome with higher levels of hematocrit. Therefore there appears to be a minimum recommended hematocrit during bypass, especially for longer bypass runs with deeper hypothermia.

Monitoring During Cardiopulmonary Bypass

Cerebral Oximetry

Cerebral oximetry with NIRS is a noninvasive, continuous assessment of brain oxygen delivery and use. NIRS-based cerebral oximeters quantitate a venous-weighted ratio of oxygenated and deoxygenated hemoglobin in the region of cerebral cortex underlying the sensors, usually placed on the forehead and sometimes overlying the kidney. By comparison with pulse oximetry, cerebral oximeters trend venous-weighted measurements because the entire returned signal is measured rather than just the pulsatile measurements that make pulse oximetry specific to arterial blood oxygen saturation.[161] Because cerebral oximetry interrogates all hemoglobin in the reflectance arc (including arterial, venous, and capillary hemoglobin), the resulting number is biased toward the larger venous hemoglobin mass, which is consistently higher than, but correlated with jugular venous oximetry.[161,162] Whereas the pulse oximeter is a useful trend of pulmonary function and the a-A gradient, cerebral oximetry trends the ratio of regional oxygen delivery and use to detect cerebral ischemia.

A comprehensive review of the evidence for the use of cerebral oximetry was performed by Hirsch et al.,[163] concluding, "Although near-infrared spectroscopy has promise for measuring regional tissue oxygen saturation, the lack of data demonstrating improved outcomes limits the support for widespread implementation." Although there is no standard of care for the use of NIRS-based cerebral oximetry, the technology has a strong presence in pediatric cardiac anesthesia. Unfortunately, what should be done with the data generated remains somewhat unclear, and this has resulted in some centers adopting the technology and others deferring its use.

In a cross-sectional survey of NIRS use, Hoskote et al.[164] aimed to explore the use of NIRS in pediatric cardiac ICUs in the United Kingdom, Ireland, Italy, and Germany. NIRS use varied considerably with 35% of centers reporting that NIRS was not used at all, and only some of the centers using the technology believed that NIRS added value to standard monitoring. Although most responding units used NIRS for high-risk patients, the majority (88%) did not have any protocols or guidelines for intervention. As mentioned earlier, a large part of the variable use of the technology likely lies in the lack of target thresholds and defined intervention algorithms to support the use of NIRS in the pediatric cardiac operating room and ICU.

For the intensive care doctor the NIRS data can be useful in a number of ways. Postoperatively the information obtained (particularly the trend in both cerebral and renal saturations) can signal significant changes in hemodynamic status before the patient shows outward changes. In a study by Gil-Anton et al.[165] in which the authors looked at spectroscopy after congenital heart surgery, it was demonstrated that combined cerebral and renal monitoring was correlated with central venous oxygen saturation and cardiac output; low cardiac output detection was associated with a different spectroscopy pattern. Spectroscopy probes were placed on the forehead and renal area, and serial cardiac output measurements were obtained by femoral transpulmonary thermodilution over the first 24 hours after surgery. In the 15 patients studied, central venous oxygen saturation ($ScvO_2$) was correlated with cerebral and combined measurements. Likewise, the systolic index was correlated with the NIRS signals. Statistically significant differences were found in the NIRS measures registered in the 29 low cardiac output events detected by thermodilution.

Goal-Directed Therapy and Near-Infrared Spectroscopy

Cerebral oximetry provides a target for support of oxygen delivery to the brain that is similar to strategies for shock treatment, collectively termed *goal-directed therapy*.[166,167] Therapies promoted by NIRS monitoring of the brain are best understood by examining the determinants of oxygen delivery to the brain. For most organs, oxygen delivery is a function of cardiac output and arterial oxygen saturation. The uneven application of systemic vasoconstriction makes the brain relatively immune to decrements in cardiac output, so cerebral blood flow is a function of cerebral perfusion pressure, not cardiac output.[168] Oxygenation delivery to the brain can thus be expressed as a function of the cerebral perfusion pressure, the arterial resistance, arterial hemoglobin concentration, the saturation

	TABLE 41.2	Goal-Directed Therapy by Near-Infrared Spectroscopy
Variable	**Clinical Scenario Causing Cerebral Desaturation**	**Intervention**
O_2 delivery	Depressed ventricular function, reduced ABP	Increased inotropic support
CPP	Hypotension, elevated ICP, elevated central venous pressure	Maintain ABP above the lower limit of autoregulation; check venous drainage cannula
r4	Hypocarbia, vasospasm, malpositioned arterial cannulas	Decrease minute ventilation, pH-stat management; check aortic cannula position
[Hb]	Anemia	Transfusion
% Sat	Cyanosis	Lung recruitment maneuvers, increase FiO_2, manage Q_P/Q_S ratio
η	Polycythemia, sickle cell disease	Partial exchange transfusion, permissive anemia
O_2 consumption	Fever, seizure, arousal	Cooling, sedation

ABP, Arterial blood pressure; *CPP*, cerebral perfusion pressure; *η*, blood viscosity; *FiO₂*, fraction of inspired oxygen; *[Hb]*, blood concentration of hemoglobin; *ICP*, intracranial pressure; *% Sat*, arterial oxygen saturation; *Qₚ*, pulmonary blood flow; *Qₛ*, systemic perfusion; *r*, resistance vessel radius.

of hemoglobin, and the blood viscosity. Table 41.2 shows examples of how the understanding of oxygen delivery and consumption can prompt interventions when cerebral oximetry is low.

Goal-directed therapy guided by cerebral oximetry monitoring is expected to result in higher pump flow rates during bypass, higher CO_2 levels, a tendency for pH-stat management, and more blood transfusions.[169] Further, centers that favor the use of cerebral oximetry are more likely to adopt regional cerebral perfusion techniques as an alternative to DHCA.[170,171] These shifts in practice have been shaped in part by the inclusion of cerebral oximetry monitoring in the congenital cardiac operating suite over the last decade as part of a more global effort at goal-directed therapy specific to pediatric CPB. The impact of these changes on neurologic outcome is the subject of ongoing trials that require long-term neurologic follow-up.

The ICU clinician can also use information obtained during the CPB period. Zulueta et al.[172] looked at the role of intraoperative regional oxygen saturation using NIRS in the prediction of LCOS after pediatric heart surgery. They assessed the applicability of intraoperative regional oxygen saturation (rSO_2) desaturation score by NIRS in the early detection of postoperative LCOS in infants with congenital heart disease who underwent cardiac surgery. The intraoperative cerebral and somatic rSO_2 were measured and a rSO_2 desaturation score calculated (by multiplying the rSO_2 below 50% of the threshold by seconds). The aim of the study was to evaluate the applicability of intraoperative rSO_2 desaturation score in the early detection of postoperative LCOS. Thirteen of 22 patients (~60%) had an intraoperative cerebral rSO_2 desaturation score greater than 3000% per second. Patients with a rSO_2 desaturation score greater than 3000% per second had a significantly lower intraoperative central venous saturation (SvO_2; $P = .002$), cardiac index (confidence interval [CI], $P = .004$), oxygen availability index (DO_2I; $P = .0004$), and a significantly higher extraction of oxygen (ERO_2; $P = .0005$) when compared with patients with a rSO_2 desaturation score less than 3000% per second. Nine patients had postoperative LCOS; all of them had an intraoperative rSO_2 desaturation score greater than 3000% per second (9 of 13 patients, 69%; $P = .001$), requiring prompt treatment with major inotropic support, surface hypothermia, or ECMO support ($n = 4$). Their conclusion was that the intraoperative use of NIRS provided an early warning sign of hemodynamic or metabolic compromise, enabling early and rapid intervention to prevent or reduce the severity of potentially life-threatening complications.

Perhaps one of the most compelling reasons to use NIRs in the operating room and in the ICU lies in the rapid identification of important changes in perfusion that can affect end-organ viability. In an interesting report, Scholl et al.[173] describe the rapid diagnosis of cannula migration by cerebral oximetry in neonatal arch repair. This report's contention is that continuous monitoring of the rSO_2 permits early detection of cerebral ischemia, allowing for prompt intervention; in their case, continuous cerebral oximetry assisted with the positioning of the arterial cannula, avoiding a prolonged episode of cerebral ischemia. Likewise, changes in the trend of cerebral NIRS in the ICU (or in the renal NIRS) can provide an early warning sign that the patient may be having problems, and often this information precedes the elevation of lactic acid level or other signs of LCOS.

Postoperative Electroencephalography

There are emerging data that suggest monitoring electroencephalography (EEG) post CPB is worthwhile and may identify patients at risk for worse neurodevelopmental outcomes.[174] In a study by Latal et al., which aimed to evaluate the predictive value of preoperative and postoperative amplitude-integrated electroencephalography (aEEG) on neurodevelopmental outcomes, the authors evaluated a prospectively enrolled cohort of 60 infants with congenital heart disease who underwent cardiac surgery with CPB in the first 3 months of life. Infants with a genetic comorbidity were excluded. aEEG was assessed for 12 hours preoperatively and 48 hours postoperatively. Background pattern was classified by the use of standard categories, and the presence of seizures and sleep-wake cycles (SWCs) was noted. Outcomes at 1 and 4 years of age were assessed with standardized developmental tests. Postoperatively, abnormal background pattern (flat trace, burst suppression, or continuous low voltage) was detected in 7 (12%), discontinuous normal voltage in 37 (61%), and continuous normal voltage in 16 (27%) infants. Nineteen infants (32%) did not return to normal SWCs within the recording period. Seizures were detected in 4 infants preoperatively and in another 4 postoperatively. Abnormal postoperative background pattern and lack of return to SWCs independently predicted poorer intelligence quotient at 4 years ($P = .03$ and $P = .04$, respectively) but was not related to motor outcome. They concluded that abnormal postoperative background pattern and lack of return to SWCs are markers for subsequent impaired cognitive development.

Although the American Clinical Neurophysiology Society recommends continuous EEG monitoring after neonatal cardiac surgery, this is not common practice in many programs. It is probably fair to claim that with EEG monitoring the actual incidence of postoperative seizure activity is higher than clinically apparent because seizures are often subclinical. Postoperative seizures, even when subclinical, are associated with worse neurocognitive outcomes. In a study by Naim et al.,[175] subclinical seizures identified by postoperative EEG monitoring are common after neonatal cardiac surgery. Naim et al. implemented routine continuous EEG monitoring and reviewed the results for an 18-month period. Clinical data were collected by chart review, and continuous EEG tracings were interpreted using standardized American Clinical Neurophysiology Society terminology. A total of 161 patients underwent continuous EEG monitoring. Electrographic seizures occurred in 13 neonates (8%) beginning at a median of 20 hours after return to the ICU after surgery. Neonates with all types of congenital heart disease had seizures. Seizures were clinically detected in only 2 of those 13 neonates (15%), and status epilepticus occurred in 8 neonates (62%). In separate multivariate models, delayed sternal closure or longer DHCA duration was associated with an increased risk for seizures. Mortality was higher among neonates with than without seizures (38% versus 3%; $P < .001$).

It is difficult to recommend continuous EEG monitoring in all children who undergo repair using CPB because this prospective study identified seizures in only 8% of neonates after cardiac surgery with CPB. The majority of seizures had no clinical correlate and would not have been otherwise identified. Seizure occurrence is, however, a marker of greater illness severity and increased mortality, and EEG monitoring can be indicated for selected patients.

Conclusion

CPB in neonates, infants, and children undergoing cardiac surgery creates extensive alterations to physiology that can significantly impact the ICU course. A variety of strategies, including variations in (1) circuit size (which alters foreign surface exposure, dilution effects from prime, and need for blood in the prime); (2) target temperatures (from profound cooling [less than 22°C] to moderate cooling [32°C to 34°C]); (3) flow rates—from full flow (up to 200 mL/kg/min), to decreased or low flow (25 to 50 mL/kg/min), to no flow (DHCA); and (4) myocardial protection techniques, can influence postoperative convalescence. Patients can present with increased TBW, temporary decreased renal function, impairments to ventilation, neurologic abnormality, or diminished cardiac function—and all of these issues can relate in part to exposure to CPB. It is critical that surgeons and intensivists caring for these children are familiar with all available invasive and noninvasive diagnostic tools in both the operating room and the ICU. These will help them to recognize early the impact that CPB has on specific organ systems and incorporate the various prophylactic and therapeutic strategies into their management plan.

References

A complete list of references is available at Expertconsult.Com.

42

Initial Management and Stabilization: Emergency Department Transport

CORINA NOJE, MD; KELLY A. SWAIN, MSN, CPNP-AC; AUTUMN K. PETERSON, BSN, MSN, CPNP-AC; EDD SHOPE, ADN; JENNIFER L. TURI, MD

Infants and children with congenital and acquired heart disease can present with a myriad of nonspecific findings, including poor feeding, cyanosis, tachypnea, respiratory distress, shock, and altered mental status. A thorough knowledge of cardiac physiology is required to accurately evaluate and effectively stabilize these patients, including an understanding of the typical age and pattern of presentation.

The diagnosis of ductal dependent congenital heart disease (CHD) has continued to evolve over the last decade. Although nearly universal screening ultrasound examinations have increased prenatal diagnosis of critical CHD (those requiring intervention within the first year of life),[1] the majority of these patients continue to be diagnosed postnatally.[1,2] For this reason, most US states now mandate that pulse oximetry screening for critical CHD be completed before a newborn is discharged from the hospital.[3,4] Such screening consists of a single measurement in the lower extremity after 24 hours of age.[5] In the United States it is estimated that pulse oximetry screening will detect almost 1200 neonates with critical CHD and prevent 20 neonatal deaths each year.[3]

On the other side of the spectrum, more patients are surviving into adulthood with CHD.[6,7] Although many of these patients have minimal or no residual defects, patients with more complex lesions may have progressive evolution of their altered physiology or residual disease, thus requiring an understanding of the long-term complications of residual defects and surgical repairs.

Goals of Management

The primary goal in caring for all infants and children with cardiac disease is to ensure adequate oxygen delivery (DO_2). The heart must provide sufficient blood flow (cardiac output) to preserve organ function. The amount of blood flow required is dependent on tissue oxygen demand and blood oxygen supply. Conditions that increase demand, such as elevated metabolism from fever or infection, or that decrease supply, such as hypoxemia or anemia, can affect the amount of cardiac output required to sustain normal organ function. Patients with heart defects may have difficulty providing adequate cardiac output if they have inefficient pump function (e.g., intracardiac or extracardiac shunts, valvular insufficiency, arrhythmias) or depressed pump function (e.g., diminished ventricular contractility). Further, conditions of the vasculature, such as hypovolemia or decreased peripheral vascular resistance, may affect the ability of the heart to generate adequate cardiac output. To effectively manage patients with inadequate DO_2, it is critical to understand the basic factors that constitute it.

DO_2 is a function of systemic cardiac output and arterial O_2 content. Because DO_2 normally far exceeds the amount of O_2 actually consumed during periods of homeostasis, evidence of inadequate DO_2 can be assessed by the amount of O_2 that is extracted during circulation. Fractional O_2 extraction represents the difference between the O_2 content of the arterial versus venous blood. Practically, it can be measured as arterial oxygen saturation (SaO_2)–central venous oxygen saturation (SvO_2)/SaO_2, with less than 0.3 representing normal extraction and greater than 0.5 demonstrating inadequate delivery. As DO_2 falls below the critical threshold, aerobic metabolism can no longer be maintained. Anaerobic metabolism will generate lactic acid as a by-product. Therefore measurement of acidosis or lactate can provide a very useful measure of the severity and duration of inadequate DO_2.

Understanding the components of DO_2 provides the opportunity to augment supply. Cardiac output is directly related to heart rate and stroke volume. Stroke volume is dependent on preload, afterload, and myocardial contractility. Both pulmonary blood flow (Q_p) and systemic blood flow (Q_s) are determined by these fundamental forces. In the patient with two ventricles, ventricular interdependence, or the effect of one ventricle on the other, may play a role in pulmonary or systemic blood flow. In some situations the pericardium and restriction by the pericardial space may also play a role in cardiac output by altering preload.

Oxygen content is primarily a function of hemoglobin concentration and arterial oxygen saturation. Thus patients who are chronically hypoxemic can improve DO_2 at any given cardiac output by maintaining a higher hemoglobin concentration. Arterial oxygen saturation may be affected by pulmonary parenchymal abnormalities with increased ventilation/perfusion (V/Q) mismatch or by the mixing of systemic and pulmonary venous return. Low mixed venous oxygen content contributes to desaturation and suggests increased oxygen extraction due to inadequate DO_2. This in turn is due either to systemic cardiac output that is insufficient to meet metabolic needs or to inadequate hemoglobin concentration.

Presentation

Many infants and children with congenital heart defects and heart disease will present to health care providers in a nontertiary care center or one that does not have specialized pediatric cardiac care or intensive care units. These patients may have a known congenital cardiac lesion or may have an unknown or an evolving cardiac process. Recognition and diagnosis of cardiac disease in these patients can be challenging due to their complex physiology, age-dependent presentation, and nonspecific clinical findings[8] and may frequently be misdiagnosed as sepsis or respiratory failure. It is essential that an infant or child who presents with shock, acidosis, or respiratory insufficiency due to a cardiac cause is quickly recognized and stabilized. A thorough understanding of the anatomy and pathophysiology of the congenital cardiac lesions and their impact on DO_2 is necessary to help direct initial stabilization, transport, and subsequent management of such patients.

CHD generally can be categorized as cyanotic or acyanotic. Cyanotic heart disease is caused by insufficient blood flow to the lungs or ineffective mixing of oxygenated and deoxygenated blood in parallel circulations. Acyanotic heart disease is due to (1) inadequate systemic blood flow due to obstruction either into or out of the left ventricle (LV), (2) myocardial dysfunction, or (3) maldistribution of pulmonary blood flow.

Cyanotic Heart Disease

Cyanosis occurs in patients with inadequate Q_p or those in whom the pulmonary and systemic circulations occur in parallel with inadequate mixing of oxygenated and deoxygenated blood. Neonates whose Q_p is dependent on a patent ductus arteriosus (PDA) may present hours to days after birth, with severe hypoxemia and acidosis as the ductus closes. Decreased Q_p may be due to obstructed flow from the inlet of the pulmonary ventricle (e.g., tricuspid atresia) or from its outlet (e.g., severe pulmonary stenosis, pulmonary atresia [PA] with intact ventricular septum, or tetralogy of Fallot). The PDA allows blood to bypass the level of obstruction. An atrial or ventricular septal defect is also required to "decompress" the systemic venous return to the systemic side of the circulation and allow mixing of oxygenated and deoxygenated blood. The blood in the systemic ventricle therefore consists of desaturated systemic venous blood (via the septal defect) and a smaller volume of saturated pulmonary blood depending on the degree of pulmonary obstruction (Q_p:Q_s <1). Although Q_s may initially be normal, with ductal closure systemic DO_2 falls rapidly due to both decreasing Q_p:Q_s and greater O_2 extraction. This results in anaerobic metabolism, acidosis, and myocardial dysfunction.

Neonates may also present with significant cyanosis in the presence of inadequate mixing of parallel pulmonary and systemic blood flow as is seen with d-transposition of the great arteries (d-TGA) or with obstructed pulmonary vein outflow as seen with total anomalous pulmonary venous return (TAPVR). Patients with d-TGA with intact ventricular septum will present at birth with severe cyanosis but with preserved Q_s. Acidosis and myocardial dysfunction will develop over time as O_2 saturations fall, though the rapidity will depend on the presence and size of an atrial shunt to provide mixing. Patients with obstructive TAPVR also present with cyanosis but may demonstrate significant respiratory insufficiency due to pulmonary hypertension with increased transmural pressure across the pulmonary vasculature and pulmonary edema formation.

The differential diagnosis of a neonate who presents with severe cyanosis must include the possibility of a ductal dependent pulmonary circulation with a closing ductus arteriosus. For neonates with suspected CHD the initial evaluation should include the following:

- Four-extremity blood pressure measurements (e.g., upper and lower limb systolic blood pressure difference >10 mm Hg usually indicates aortic arch abnormalities).
- Preductal and postductal oxygen saturation measurements (oxygen saturation as measured by pulse oximetry [SpO_2]) to identify differential cyanosis (i.e., preductal SpO_2 > postductal SpO_2) and reverse differential cyanosis (i.e., postductal SpO_2 > preductal SpO_2). A preductal-postductal SpO_2 difference of more than 10% usually indicates ductal dependent CHD.[9] Reverse differential cyanosis is usually observed in TGA but was also described in supracardiac total anomalous pulmonary venous connection.[10]
- Hyperoxia test to differentiate between CHD and non-CHD (e.g., SpO_2 <85% on both room air and 100% oxygen usually indicates CHD).

Other causes of central cyanosis in a neonate should be evaluated concurrently with initiating prostaglandin E_1 (PGE_1) while establishing a definitive diagnosis. These causes include pulmonary causes such as persistent pulmonary hypertension, congenital diaphragmatic hernia, pneumothorax, or pleural effusion, as well as central nervous system depression due to perinatal asphyxia, neurologic disorder, or maternal sedation. In addition to four-extremity blood pressure measurements, preductal and postductal saturation levels, and hyperoxia testing, the diagnosis can be further elucidated by physical examination; chest x-ray examination to evaluate cardiac size, position, and shape and vascular markings; electrocardiogram to assess ventricular hypertrophy, conduction defects, or arrhythmia; and arterial blood gas measurement to assess gas exchange and acidosis. Ultimately, an echocardiogram will be required but will not always be available on presentation.

Acyanotic Heart Disease

Children with acyanotic heart disease will present emergently when Q_s is inadequate. This may represent (1) ductal dependent systemic circulation with obstructed flow into or out of the LV (e.g., mitral stenosis, aortic valve disease, aortic coarctation), (2) myocardial dysfunction (e.g., cardiomyopathy, anomalous coronaries), or (3) maldistribution of pulmonary blood flow with left-to-right shunts (e.g., ventricular septal defect [VSD]). These lesions result in inadequate systemic DO_2 either by actual obstruction to flow through the left heart or by excessive Q_p with a functional decrease in blood flow to the systemic circulation. As the pathophysiology for each of these defects worsens, the ability of the lungs to oxygenate blood is impaired due to increased intravascular and extravascular lung water and elevated pulmonary vascular resistance (PVR).

Ductal Dependent Systemic Circulation. Limitation to Q_s can occur at a number of levels along the left ventricular outflow tract (i.e., hypoplastic left heart syndrome, interrupted aortic arch, critical coarctation of the aorta). Systemic blood flow in these patients, as in those with ductal dependent pulmonary blood flow, depends on flow through a PDA to bypass the level of obstruction, as well as a septal defect to allow adequate egress from the pulmonary circulation. The neonate, if not diagnosed prenatally or before discharge home, is likely to present following ductal closure with progressive increase in LV afterload, a decrease in myocardial function, and acidosis due to inadequate DO_2. Clinically this is manifested by poor perfusion with decreased pulse rates in the lower extremities and pulmonary edema due to increased afterload to the pulmonary vascular bed and transudation of fluid. Ultimately, complete closure of the ductus will cause profound cardiovascular collapse.

As in the case of severe cyanosis, the differential diagnosis of a neonate who presents with circulatory collapse must include the presence of a ductal dependent lesion with a closing ductus arteriosus. This evaluation should also include four-extremity blood pressure measurements, preductal and postductal saturation levels, and a hyperoxia test in addition to physical examination, chest x-ray examination, electrocardiogram, and cultures. This presentation is frequently mistaken for severe sepsis. Although this diagnosis must also be considered and empirically treated, the use of PGE_1 should not be delayed while confirming the diagnosis.

Myocardial Dysfunction. Inadequate O_2 delivery due to significant myocardial dysfunction may be due to cardiomyopathy, coronary anomalies, arrhythmias, or progressive cardiac dysfunction due to other lesions. Cardiomyopathy may represent primary defects due to mitochondrial or metabolic disorders or to inflammatory heart diseases such as myocarditis. Patients with structural congenital heart defects may also develop myopathic changes in the heart due to volume or pressure overload.[11] Significant myocardial dysfunction may present as severe hypoxemia, acidosis, and/or ventricular failure. Specific clinical signs depend on age and cause. Neonates and infants are more likely to present with failure to thrive and feeding intolerance, diaphoresis, tachycardia, mottling, and respiratory distress. In addition to these findings, infants with cardiomyopathy due to anomalous origin of the left coronary artery from the pulmonary artery (ALCAPA) may present with extreme irritability, particularly during feeds due to intermittent cardiac ischemia caused by coronary steal with the drop in PVR over the first weeks of life. The coronary anatomy of any infant who presents with cardiogenic shock of unknown cause must be assessed to rule out the presence of ALCAPA or other anomalies of the left coronary artery. Older children tend to present with more overt signs of LV failure, including tachycardia, decreased peripheral perfusion, pulmonary edema, dyspnea, and abdominal pain. These ultimately may progress to cardiogenic shock.

Maldistribution of Pulmonary Blood Flow. Infants with large left-to-right shunts are likely to develop maldistribution of pulmonary blood flow or pulmonary overcirculation (Q_p:Q_s >1). As PVR decreases after birth, the pressure gradient across the shunt increases and augments the degree of shunting. These patients are likely to present at greater than 1 month of age with tachypnea, increased work of breathing, hepatomegaly, diaphoresis, and poor feeding. The increased metabolic requirement associated with excessive respiratory and cardiac work also leads to poor weight gain and typically a history of failure to thrive. If Q_p is markedly increased, particularly with left-to-right shunts distal to the tricuspid valve, such as a large VSD or aortopulmonary window, Q_s will decrease. This occurs both by overcirculation of the pulmonary vasculature with reduced ejection of blood from the systemic ventricle and by an overall decrease in myocardial function due to LV volume overload. Each of these mechanisms results in pulmonary congestion with increased V/Q mismatch. Over time, increased Q_p leads to a series of pulmonary microvascular changes that first produce reversible pulmonary vasoconstriction and later fixed pulmonary vascular disease.

Initial Stabilization and Management

The initial stabilization and management of infants and children with cardiac disease must focus on establishing adequate DO_2. To do this effectively there must be adequate and balanced output to both pulmonary and systemic circulations. Manipulating cardiac output and O_2 carrying capacity may also be necessary depending on the nature and severity of the lesion and the degree to which the lesion has affected myocardial function. In addition to cardiac considerations, initial stabilization should take into account abnormalities of other organ systems that occur as comorbid conditions or may be due to the effects of inadequate DO_2 on end-organ function.

Ensure Adequate Pulmonary and Systemic Output

Intravenously administered PGE_1 dilates the ductus arteriosus to provide Q_p or Q_s to neonates with ductal dependent lesions. An infusion of PGE_1 should be initiated for any clinically unstable neonate with severe cyanosis or cardiovascular failure to reestablish flow. This should be done before confirming the presence of a ductal dependent lesion. Patients who may benefit from early PGE_1 initiation include (1) those with right-sided cardiac lesions who need to maintain Q_p (tricuspid atresia, PA, tetralogy of Fallot with PA, Ebstein anomaly), (2) those with left-sided cardiac lesions that need to maintain Q_s (hypoplastic left heart syndrome, critical aortic coarctation, interrupted aortic arch), and (3) those with parallel circulations (d-TGA) to augment effective mixing of circulations, though this is likely to be insufficient without an atrial septal defect (ASD) of adequate size. However, PGE_1 administration may be not helpful in d-TGA with intact ventricular septum with a small ASD because there is limited mixing and critical aortic stenosis because the ductus is distal to the area of obstruction and the LV is still subjected to outflow; PGE_1 administration may be relatively contraindicated for patients with obstruction of the blood flow into or out of the left atrium (e.g., TAPVR with obstruction). In those conditions the benefits of PGE_1 outweigh the risks, and PGE_1 should be started pending definitive diagnosis. Consideration must also include the serious side effects of PGE_1 infusion, which may be dose related. Up to 38% of patients may develop one or more adverse reactions, the most common being apnea (18%), hypotension (13%), and fever (11%).[12] The starting dose for the PGE_1 infusion is 0.01 to 0.03 mcg/kg/min, though this should be initiated at a higher dose (0.05 to 0.1 mcg/kg/min) if the ductus has closed and the patient is in extremis. To decrease the risk of side effects, once patency is established, the dose should be minimized if possible. In addition to the presence of a PDA, lesions with obstructed Q_p or Q_s also require a site of mixing of Q_p and Q_s, typically an ASD. As described earlier in the case of a minimal ASD, reestablishing patency of the ductus is unlikely to provide adequate mixing of the circulations, and an atrial septostomy may be required. This should be considered before transport so that the accepting team can have the necessary personnel and equipment present on the infant's arrival.

Once ductal patency has been restored, cardiac output must be optimized and balanced between pulmonary and systemic circulations. In the absence of a fixed obstruction the distribution of total cardiac output to the pulmonary and systemic circulation is determined by the relative resistance of each vascular bed (Table 42.1). PVR is affected by pH, pCO_2, pO_2, lung volume, noxious stimuli, hematocrit, and a number of medications. Patients with excessive Q_p and consequent low DO_2 to the systemic circulation can be managed by increasing PVR to decrease Q_p and increase Q_s. Conversely, decreasing PVR will increase Q_p and decrease the relative flow to the systemic circulation. Therefore significant care should be taken with overventilation or oxygenation of patients

TABLE 42.1	Factors That Influence Pulmonary Vascular and Systemic Ventricular Afterload	

↑PVR	↑ Systemic Ventricular Afterload
• ↑ $PaCO_2$ • ↓ Ventilatory rate • ↓ Vt • ↓pH • ↑ PEEP (overdistention) • Atelectasis (hypoxia) • Pain/agitation • Catecholamines	• ↑ SVR • High-dose catecholamines • Pain/agitation • Negative intrathoracic pressure

↓ PVR	↓ Systemic Ventricular Afterload
• ↓ $PaCO_2$ • ↑ Ventilatory rate • ↑ Vt • ↑ pH • O_2 • iNO • Milrinone • PGE_1 • Analgesia/sedation • Muscle relaxation	• ↓ SVR • Milrinone • Captopril/enalapril • ↓ Pain/agitation • Positive pressure ventilation

iNO, Inhaled nitric oxide; *PEEP,* positive end-expiratory pressure; *PGE_1,* prostaglandin E_1; *PVR,* pulmonary vascular resistance; *SVR,* systemic vascular resistance; *V_t,* tidal volume.

with ductal dependent systemic circulation. In discussing this with the transport team, it is essential that the communication be concise and goal directed.

Similarly, alterations in PVR can help improve hemodynamics in other cardiac lesions. Minimizing PVR can decrease RV afterload to encourage more forward flow out of the RV to increase LV preload and possibly cardiac output *as long as the LV is compliant.* Manipulation of PVR also provides some control over intracardiac shunting and effective cardiac output. Shunting through large intracardiac shunts is affected by the relative resistances of the downstream circuits. In the case of an ASD the compliance of the ventricle will determine its filling pressure and therefore the pressure gradient across the ASD. Shunt flow across an ASD is typically left to right because the right ventricle (RV) is typically more compliant than the LV. However, in newborn infants with an ASD the RV may be relatively stiff or noncompliant, and the direction of shunt flow may be right to left, resulting in some arterial oxygen desaturation. For VSDs and extracardiac shunts the downstream resistance is provided by the systemic and pulmonary vasculature. Decreased PVR will increase Q_p:Q_s and reduce effective systemic perfusion. In most cases the PVR is substantially less than the systemic vascular resistance (SVR), and shunt flow will be toward the pulmonary circuit.

Stabilize Hemodynamics

Myocardial function is determined by both the contractile function and the loading conditions of the heart. The general approach to improving cardiac output is to augment contractility with inotropic support, to optimize preload with careful titration of fluid resuscitation or diuretic therapy, and/or to minimize afterload of the RV and/or LV with vasodilators or by altering PVR as described earlier.

Additional support of LV function can be achieved with positive pressure ventilation by decreasing wall stress with resultant decrease in the afterload on the LV. The adequacy of DO_2 can also be improved by minimizing O_2 consumption with temperature control, sedation, and mechanical ventilation.

Myocardial contractility is controlled by the presence of intracellular calcium and therefore can be improved by increasing ionized calcium or infusing inotropic medications, such as catecholamines or phosphodiesterase inhibitors. Calcium supplementation plays an essential role in augmenting LV function in children.[13-15] The underdeveloped sarcoplasmic reticular system in the neonatal myocyte causes the myocardium to be more dependent on extracellular calcium concentration than the adult myocardium. Because intracellular calcium plays a central role in myocardial contractility in neonates, blood levels of ionized calcium should be normalized to augment stroke volume. Infants with chromosome 22q11 deletions (velocardiofacial syndrome, DiGeorge syndrome) are particularly susceptible to low calcium levels.[16]

Catecholamines, or beta-adrenergic agents, represent a class of agents that provide varying effects on contractility, heart rate, and vascular resistance depending on the specific receptors stimulated. The more frequently used agents include epinephrine, dopamine, dobutamine, and isoproterenol. Epinephrine is typically used at a dose of 0.03 to 0.3 mcg/kg/min, with predominant beta-1 effects and increased contractility at lower doses. At higher doses, alpha-1 effects predominate with vasoconstriction. Dopamine is used at doses of 3 to 10 mcg/kg/min, though its use may be limited because it is associated with a greater incidence of arrhythmias, as well as increased PVR at higher dosing.[17] Dobutamine is an effective positive inotropic agent but frequently produces unacceptable degrees of tachycardia.[18] Isoproterenol is used predominantly for its chronotropic effect. Inotropic drugs increase contractility by increasing cytosolic Ca^{2+} concentration, which may also impair relaxation of the heart, decrease ventricular compliance, and limit preload.[19] In addition, augmenting inotropy will increase myocardial energy utilization. Milrinone is an inotropic agent that works through an alternative mode of action. As a phosphodiesterase-3 inhibitor, it potentiates the action of cyclic adenosine monophosphate (cAMP) to provide inotropic effects, as well as vasodilation. Data suggest that milrinone minimizes low cardiac output syndrome in some postoperative patients.[20] Milrinone may serve an important role in patients with decompensated heart failure and preserved blood pressure by reducing afterload, particularly given that beta-adrenergic receptors are desensitized in these patients, resulting in a blunted response to catecholamines.[21-24] It should be remembered, however, that the half-life of milrinone is relatively long at 2 to 3 hours, and its use can cause persistent hypotension and should be used in caution with patients with renal insufficiency. Vasopressor agents such as norepinephrine and vasopressin that increase afterload should be used with great caution in patients with poor myocardial function.[25] These agents do, however, serve an important role in increasing diastolic blood pressure to maintain myocardial perfusion, as well as in the treatment of severe vasoplegia with hypotension due to sepsis or systemic inflammation.

Preload, or the amount of blood that distends the ventricle before contraction, determines the effectiveness of contraction as described by the Frank-Starling law. The impact of preload on output will depend on the compliance of the ventricle. In a compliant ventricle, enhancing preload will increase stroke volume and cardiac output. However, in a poorly compliant ventricle, augmenting preload will negatively impact the strength of contraction, elevate venous pressure, and generate pulmonary edema. The neonatal myocardium is stiffer than that of older children; therefore it both requires a greater than normal preload to maintain output and is less tolerant of excess preload.[26] An infant presenting with congestive heart failure, pulmonary edema, and a stable systemic blood pressure may respond to diuretics to reduce ventricular wall stress and relieve pulmonary edema without compromising ventricular output. However, an infant with a myopathic ventricle presenting with hypoperfusion, hypotension, and acidosis is more likely to require carefully titrated fluid administration to optimize preload and augment cardiac output. Chest x-ray examination and liver size can aid in determining fluid and diuresis requirements. When titrating fluid, careful monitoring of central venous pressure (CVP) is crucial because small changes in volume can cause overdistention in a noncompliant ventricle. In the absence of a CVP, which is typical on transport, we recommend administering smaller-volume boluses (5 mL/kg to 10 mL/kg) with frequent reassessment of the effectiveness of the fluid bolus(s). If there appears to be a positive response with a reduction in heart rate and/or improved blood pressure and perfusion, volume augmentation of preload should continue. However, if there is a worsening of vital signs and/or signs of fluid overload, one should consider stopping volume augmentation and administer diuretics instead.

Reducing afterload may improve myocardial function by decreasing ventricular wall tension and myocardial oxygen consumption and improving stroke volume. Afterload can be optimized by using agents that vasodilate (nicardipine, nitroprusside, milrinone, dobutamine), as well as by avoiding medications (high-dose dopamine, epinephrine, norepinephrine) or situations (pain, agitation) that raise SVR. Patients with left-to-right shunts and LV volume overload have shown improved function with cautious reduction of systemic afterload. Children with LV outflow tract obstruction and pressure overload, such as severe aortic stenosis, may have massively increased, fixed afterload. Administering vasodilators in these patients will not increase Q_s but rather may cause shock, myocardial ischemia, or life-threatening arrhythmias. In this situation, afterload reduction is accomplished by relief of the fixed obstruction using surgical or cardiac catheterization techniques.

Mechanical ventilation may be needed to support respiratory failure and decrease O_2 utilization in the case of poor DO_2. In addition, positive pressure ventilation impacts preload, contractility, and afterload of the right and left ventricles to directly alter cardiac output. During spontaneous ventilation, inspiration generates negative intrathoracic pressure, which enhances venous return to the heart. The increase in preload to the RV augments stroke volume. Positive pressure, on the other hand, increases intrathoracic pressure and reduces preload to the RV.[27] This will be further accentuated by other factors that impact preload, such as hypovolemia or sepsis. Mechanical ventilation augments LV output primarily by altering its transmural pressure. The change in pleural pressure from negative to positive decreases the transmural pressure and lowers the afterload against which the LV must pump. Although this may have minimal impact on a normally functioning myocardium, it can provide significant support to a dysfunctional LV.

Changes in lung volumes also can impact RV afterload by altering PVR. Pulmonary vasculature resistance is determined by the resistance of the alveolar and extraalveolar vessels. When the lung is hyperinflated beyond functional residual capacity (FRC), the small alveolar vessels become compressed, and PVR is increased. Conversely, hypoventilation (with resultant atelectasis) distorts and collapses the larger extraalveolar vessels and increases PVR. Further, atelectasis may also decrease alveolar pO_2 and cause hypoxic pulmonary vasoconstriction. Therefore maintaining lung volume at FRC without overdistention or atelectasis results in optimal PVR. Because minor changes in lung volume and ventilation can have significant effects on hemodynamic function, transitioning from negative pressure to positive pressure ventilation during resuscitation can significantly destabilize a patient, particularly in the presence of hypovolemia or vasodilation from sedative agents or sepsis. Preload should be optimized in such patients to compensate for increased intrathoracic pressure with initiation of positive pressure ventilation. These effects can be exacerbated in patients with significantly decreased cardiac function. In such cases it is prudent to be prepared for cardiovascular collapse, including the ability to rapidly mobilize extracorporeal membrane oxygenation (ECMO) support if readily available.

Transport

The approach to transporting neonates and children with suspected or known heart disease requires not only thorough knowledge of pediatric cardiac pathophysiology and strong clinical skills, but also clear understanding of the transport environment's unique features and thoughtful appreciation of the significant heterogeneity that characterizes the field of critical care transport.

Transport Hazards

By virtue of its mobile and underresourced nature, transport is a hostile environment with a multitude of potential hazards that can affect both the patient and the crew: noise, vibration, and poor lighting; exposure to gravitational forces; extreme heat/cold with alterations in thermoregulation; changes in barometric pressure (leading to hypoxia and gas expansion with altitude); limited resources (e.g., personnel, equipment, supplies, therapies); difficulties monitoring patient status; and communication and interpersonal challenges. The safe completion of every transport is contingent upon thorough assessment of these possible risks.

Overview of Critical Care Transport

Critical care transport (CCT) is a unique discipline whose goal is to take critical care services to the patient and rapidly begin advanced care. CCT borrows the use of ambulances, stretchers, and monitors from the prehospital environment and adds critical care–trained personnel and specialized equipment (e.g., isolette, ventilator, intraaortic balloon pump, ECMO pump).

Each CCT has its own variables related to the patient (e.g., age, weight, comorbidities); disease process (e.g., severity of illness, complications, treatments); referring and receiving institutions (e.g., resources, interfacility distance); time of day, geographic and environment conditions (e.g., inaccessible area, traffic, weather); and the transport team's resources (e.g., personnel, vehicles, equipment, medications, supplies) and communication skills (e.g., interactions with referring staff, patient, family).

Transport Modes

Mode of transport (ground versus air) is determined based on resource availability, transport specifics, and the characteristics of each transport vehicle: ground, rotor-wing, and fixed-wing ambulance (Table 42.2).

TABLE 42.2	Characteristics of Transport Vehicles Used for Pediatric Interfacility Transport		
Transport Vehicle	**Advantages**	**Disadvantages**	**Comments**

Ground ambulance	• Larger work space for crew
	• No equipment restrictions
	• No altitude-related hazards/physiologic risks
	• Able to board large medical teams
	• Able to transport very large patients
	• Able to carry heavy equipment
	• Able to stop/pull over
	• Able to divert to another facility
	• Readily available
	• Low cost
		• Subject to traffic and road conditions that may:
		  • Delay arrival time
		  • Increase out-of-hospital time
		  • Increase risk for tubes/lines dislodgment
		• Limited gas availability over longer distances
			• Should be considered for:
			  • Stable patients
			  • Short interfacility distance (e.g., urban transports)
			  • Patients likely to require assessments/interventions difficult to perform in flight (e.g., intubation, CPR)
			  • Transports with anticipated need for large medical teams (>3-4 crew members), and/or heavy equipment
			  • Situations when air transport is unavailable (e.g., weather restrictions, lack of resources, cost-prohibitive)
			  • Situations when air transport may be hazardous (e.g., PPHN, tension pneumothorax)

Rotor-wing ambulance	• Reduces transport time to the referring facility
	• Reduces total out-of-hospital time
	• Reduces time to diagnostic/therapeutic procedure
	• Able to land at:
	  • Referring facility's helipad
	  • Remote landing sites (e.g., road, field, parking lot)
	• Able to land immediately if the aircraft malfunctions
	• Able to quickly divert to another facility
		• Very small work space
		• Staff/patient weight and habitus restrictions
		• Environmental exposure (e.g., extreme heat/cold)
		• Unpressurized cabin leads to altitude-related hazards/physiologic risks (e.g., hypobaric hypoxia, expanding gases)
		• Equipment requires FAA approval
		• Not all programs have IFR capability (most fly under VFR conditions)
		• Weather restrictions
		• Not readily available
		• High cost
			• Should be considered for:
			  • Unstable patients
			  • Patients requiring emergent transport for time-sensitive diagnostic/therapeutic procedures
			  • Long interfacility distance (e.g., rural transports)

Fixed-wing ambulance	• High speed over long distances
	• IFR capability
	• Pressurized cabin
	• Able to land at alternate airport
	• Compared with rotor-wing:
	  • Less-restrictive weight requirements
	  • Usually smoother flight
	  • Lower cost
		• Requires:
		  • Flight plan
		  • Airport-to-airport destinations
		  • Ambulance rides to and from the airport
		  • Insurance preauthorization
		• Involves multiple transfers:
		  • Bedside to stretcher
		  • Stretcher to ambulance
		  • Ambulance onto tarmac
		  • May need transition to/from aircraft-specific stretcher
		  • Tarmac into airplane
		  • Airplane to tarmac
		  • Tarmac into ambulance
		  • Stretcher off-loaded from ambulance
		  • Stretcher to bedside
		• Equipment requires FAA approval
		• Similar weather restrictions as rotor-wing
		• May not be able to pressurize cabin at sea level, hence risking altitude-related hazards
		• Diversion takes longer:
		  • May not be able to land at closest airport (depending on the type of aircraft and required runway)
			• Should be considered for:
			  • Very long interfacility distance (including international transports)
			  • Stable patients
			  • Patients susceptible to altitude-related risks who are unlikely to tolerate flight in unpressurized cabin (i.e., rotor-wing)

CPR, Cardiopulmonary resuscitation; *FAA,* Federal Aviation Administration; *IFR,* instrument flight rules; *PPHN,* persistent pulmonary hypertension; *VFR,* visual flight rules.

TABLE 42.3	Presentation of Patients With Unknown Cardiac Diagnosis			
Age	Signs and Symptoms	Cardiac Diagnosis	Initial Considerations and Interventions	Transport Concerns
Neonates	• Cyanosis	• Ductal dependent pulmonary circulation • TAPVR with obstruction • d-TGA	• Ensure ductal patency: PGE₁ • Ensure adequate mixing: atrial septostomy	• PGE₁ side effects (e.g., apnea, hypotension)
	• Acidosis • Poor perfusion • Irritability • Shock • Cardiac arrest	• Ductal dependent systemic circulation • Anomalous left coronary artery	• Ensure ductal patency: PGE₁ • Ensure adequate mixing: atrial septostomy • Assess coronary arteries	• PGE₁ side effects (e.g., apnea, hypotension)
• Infants	• Respiratory distress • Failure to thrive • Hepatomegaly	• Pulmonary overcirculation	• Optimize preload • Balance Q_p:Q_s	• Oxygen (i.e., worsens pulmonary overcirculation)
• Neonates/Infants	• Tachycardia • Tachypnea • Failure to thrive • Feeding intolerance • Cardiogenic shock	• Cardiomyopathy	• Optimize preload • Consider inotropic support • Consider PPV: noninvasive or invasive (with appropriate support) • Assess coronary arteries	• Respiratory support (i.e., risks and benefits of PPV) • Arrhythmias • Cardiac arrest
Children	• Fatigue • Edema • Abdominal pain • Poor appetite • Poor weight gain • Tachycardia • Cardiogenic shock	• Cardiomyopathy	• Optimize preload • Consider inotropic support • Consider PPV: noninvasive or invasive (with appropriate support)	• Respiratory support (i.e., risks and benefits of PPV) • Arrhythmias • Cardiac arrest

d-TGA, d-Transposition of great arteries; *PGE₁,* prostaglandin E₁; *PPV,* positive pressure ventilation; *Q$_p$,* pulmonary blood flow; *Q$_s$,* systemic blood flow; *TAPVR,* total anomalous pulmonary venous return.

Transport Team Compositions

Neonatal and pediatric critical care transport teams are as unique as the institutions they represent. The teams usually consist of two or more members at their core, but depending on the specifics of each transport, they may flex to add specialists in airway management, intravenous access, or, in extreme conditions, a mobile ECMO team. A national survey of 229 unit-based and 106 dedicated neonatal transport programs in the United States identified 26 different team compositions routinely used in neonatal transport.[28]

When neonatal or pediatric critical care transport teams arrive at referring institutions, they bring not only equipment, medications, and technology that may be unavailable at the community hospital, but also skills and training to manage a difficult situation. Once at the bedside, all team members must work and communicate well with each other and with the referring institution's staff to resuscitate, stabilize, and safely retrieve the patient in a timely manner.

Transport Process

Interfacility transports for neonates and children generally follow a standardized path. This begins with the transport intake, which initiates the triage process by collecting demographic and clinical information. It continues with the pretransport planning phase to determine the urgency of dispatch, anticipated level of care, transport mode, and team composition. Finally, it concludes with the retrieval process itself.

Transport Intake. Transport intakes for neonates and children with heart disease are particularly challenging because the patients' initial presentation varies vastly depending on age and disease process. As stated earlier, it is not uncommon for these patients to be misdiagnosed at the referring institution. Patients with previously undiagnosed cardiac disease often present with a myriad of nonspecific findings; therefore triaging such patients requires a heightened suspicion for a possible cardiac cause (Table 42.3). Patients with known cardiac disease usually present with complications arising from either their underlying disorder or the medications, surgeries, and interventions received (Table 42.4). Therefore a thorough transport intake process is paramount to the appropriate triage of any patient with heart disease, whether known or previously undiagnosed. During the intake process it is important to obtain detailed information regarding the initial presentation, physical examination and diagnostic testing, interventions performed at the referring institution, and the patient's responses to those interventions.

Whether using a general transport intake form or a cardiac-specific one, a full set of vital signs, a focused cardiac examination (e.g., murmurs/gallops, pulses, perfusion), and the results of laboratory work (e.g., blood gas, lactate, and glucose levels, complete cell blood count, metabolic panel, coagulation studies) and diagnostic workup (e.g., 12-lead electrocardiogram, chest radiograph) should be elicited. An emphasis on 12-lead electrocardiogram

TABLE 42.4	Presentation of Patients With Known Cardiac Diagnosis
Cardiac Diagnosis	**Presentation/Complications**
Single-ventricle palliation	• Occluded shunt • Pleural effusion • Arrhythmias • Thromboembolic events (e.g., ischemic or hemorrhagic stroke) • Hepatic dysfunction
Residual intracardiac shunt or valvular disease	• Congestive heart failure
Recent cardiac surgery or catheterization	• Postpericardiotomy syndrome • Cardiac tamponade • Infections/mediastinitis • Thromboembolic events (e.g., ischemic or hemorrhagic stroke)
Heart transplant	• Rejection • Infections • Renal dysfunction • Graft coronary artery disease • Gastrointestinal disorders
Ventricular assist device recipient	• Equipment failure • Thromboembolic events (e.g., ischemic or hemorrhagic stroke)

should be amplified because this can be performed easily in most referring sites, can be sent to the transport team quickly, and can provide significant information. Additionally, a thorough physical examination should specifically evaluate for presence of hepatomegaly, pulmonary edema, peripheral edema, or jugular venous distention (in older children/adolescents). For neonates with suspected CHD the initial evaluation should also include four-extremity blood pressure measurements, preductal and postductal saturation levels to identify differential cyanosis and reverse differential cyanosis, and a hyperoxia test for cyanotic neonates to differentiate between CHD and non-CHD.

Generally, if CHD (cyanotic or acyanotic) is suspected based on the initial presentation, physical examination can offer important diagnostic clues. However, a definitive diagnosis cannot be made unless an echocardiogram is available at the referring institution; hence the importance of timely recognition and rapid stabilization, followed by expedited transfer to a tertiary care center with pediatric cardiac expertise.

Pretransport Planning. Planning for interfacility transport of a critically ill neonate or child with congenital or acquired heart disease is a complex and usually time-sensitive process. Ideally, the transport team should collaborate with the receiving medical/surgical team (e.g., intensivist, pediatric cardiologist, cardiothoracic surgeon) and the referring team to accomplish four major goals before dispatch:

1. Assess the patient's severity of illness and clinical stability before transport.
2. Determine what interventions and/or therapies are required to stabilize the patient, and weigh the risks and benefits of their initiation before transport (e.g., oxygen; PGE₁; inhaled nitric oxide; noninvasive respiratory support; intubation and mechanical ventilation; inotropic support; fluid administration; blood product transfusion; diuretics; management of arrhythmias with medications, cardiac pacing, cardioversion, or defibrillation; or ECMO).
3. Determine if the patient requires emergent life-saving procedures or surgical interventions upon arrival at the receiving facility (e.g., cardiac catheterization, pericardiocentesis, cardiac surgery, ECMO/extracorporeal cardiopulmonary resuscitation).
4. Identify the most appropriate transport mode and team composition needed to retrieve the patient safely and expeditiously.

Stabilization and Management in Transport. Transport management of critically ill neonates and children with cardiac disease should be tailored to their individual needs based on the disease process, severity of illness, and the specifics of each transport (e.g., transport mode, duration, anticipated hazards, skills of transport personnel, and available resources).

Resuscitation should ideally occur before transport because it generally includes stabilizing the airway, obtaining reliable venous access, and correcting various electrolyte abnormalities (hypoglycemia and hypocalcemia) and metabolic acidosis. Furthermore, volume resuscitation, blood product transfusion, initiation of inotropic support, and/or disease-specific therapies (e.g., PGE₁) may be indicated in select cases to optimize the Q_p:Q_s balance and improve DO_2 and end-organ perfusion. Management should be continued throughout transport to the tertiary care center. Given the complexity of these high-acuity transports, CCTs may follow cardiac-specific transport protocols under close guidance from medical control. Several sample pediatric cardiac transport protocols are included in Boxes 42.1, 42.2, and 42.3 (heart failure, blocked cardiac shunt, and cardiac tamponade, respectively).

Special consideration should be given to the transport management of neonates with suspected CHD, particularly with regard to the risks and benefits of PGE₁ administration, elective intubation, and O_2 therapy during transport.

Prostaglandin E₁ Initiation Before Transport: Indications, Dosing, Risks, and Adverse Effects. The early initiation of PGE₁ therapy may be life-saving to patients with ductal dependent CHD, whereas lack of PGE₁ availability at outside hospitals is associated with increased morbidity.[29] Ideally, the PGE₁ infusion is titrated to the lowest dose that maintains ductal patency to minimize the risk of side effects. Some transport programs recommend at least 30-minute monitoring for apnea after initiation of PGE₁ infusion before transporting a nonintubated neonate.[30] In practice the benefits of starting PGE₁ (i.e., establishing ductal patency for cyanotic neonates who failed the hyperoxia test and young neonates who present in shock) are generally weighed against the risks of complications, in particular, apneic spells requiring intubation. This is especially true if securing the airway may be technically challenging or if preexisting hemodynamic instability may increase the risk of cardiopulmonary arrest.

Elective Intubation Before Transfer: Risks and Benefits. Endotracheal intubation for neonates with CHD carries a number of risks related either to the patient's limited ability to tolerate the procedure or to technical difficulties, such as tube occlusion, displacement, and equipment failure during transport. The common practice of elective intubation for otherwise stable neonates receiving PGE₁ before transport has been shown to significantly increase the odds of major transport complications.[12] However, pretransfer intubation should be performed for neonates with apnea following PGE₁ initiation, particularly with rotor-wing transports, long ground transports, or bad weather forecast. Other patients likely to benefit from pretransport intubation may be those with hypotension and significant metabolic acidosis, given the decrease in LV afterload with transition from spontaneous to mechanical ventilation, as

---

• BOX 42.1   Heart Failure Transport Protocol

Johns Hopkins Hospital Bloomberg Children's Center Pediatric Transport Team
Heart Failure

I.   Indications for Use

A. Patients with known heart failure of any etiology.

B. Patients with known or suspected myocarditis.

C. Patients with known or suspected cardiomyopathy.

D. Patients with unrepaired congenital heart disease.

E. Patients with shunt-dependent cardiac anatomy/physiology at any of the stages of palliation (Norwood/Damus-Kaye-Stansel procedure, Glenn, Fontan, right ventricle-to-pulmonary artery conduits).

F. Patients with ventricular assist devices.

G. Patients post heart transplant.

II.   Responsibilities

A. When heart failure is suspected during the intake call, team configuration should include: paramedic, transport nurse, respiratory therapist, and transport fellow.

- Note that Stat Medevac may dispatch a nurse, instead of a paramedic, to accompany the transport nurse and fellow. A respiratory therapist should join the team if inhaled nitric oxide needs to be administered.

B. Nurses and paramedics with the Pediatric Transport Team will perform urgent interventions for patients with heart failure.

C. Transport fellow to perform the following:

1. Will review the patient's most recent echocardiogram, if one is available.

2. Will review the patient's current EKG or rhythm strip from the referring hospital.

3. Will bring anatomical drawing when possible, for the team to review en route.

4. Will inform the team of goal saturations based on patient's anatomy.

5. Will inform cardiology of reason for transport.

III.   Assessment

A. All patients with suspected heart failure will have continuous cardiac, NIBP, pulse oximetry, and quantitative ET CO_2 monitoring.

B. Physical examinations should include capillary refill and liver size, both before and after medical interventions.

IV.   Interventions

A. If patient has suspected or known heart failure:

1. Maintain patent airway.

2. Assist breathing if necessary.

3. Establish IV/IO access.

4. Review chest x-ray to evaluate cardiac silhouette and lung fields.

B. If patient with suspected or known heart failure is **hypoxic**:

1. Place patient on supplemental oxygen with FiO_2 concentration to achieve goal saturations for the patient.

2. Consider administration of **Furosemide 0.5-1 mg/kg IV** if chest x-ray suggests pulmonary interstitial edema and fluid overload.

3. Consider **PRBC transfusion** to achieve goal hemoglobin for the patient.

4. **Consult Medical Control** regarding initiation and titration of **Nitric Oxide (iNO)**.

5. For shunt-dependent patients with more profound hypoxemia (SaO_2 <70%), follow appropriate algorithm to improve pulmonary blood flow through the shunt according to the **Blocked Cardiac Shunt protocol**.

C. If patient with suspected or known heart failure has **poor cardiac output** (poor perfusion, hepatomegaly, poor urine output, altered mental status):

1. Administer **5 mL/kg NS (0.9%) or 5% albumin** if hypotensive or liver edge <2–3 cm below right costal margin.

2. Consider initiation of **noninvasive positive pressure ventilation** to lower the afterload on the systemic ventricle, using a Mapleson circuit or traditional bag mask.

3. Defer intubation during transport, given high risk of cardiac arrest on induction.

4. Consider initiation and titration of **Milrinone** infusion **in consultation with Medical Control**.

5. For shunt-dependent patients with pulmonary over circulation (SaO_2 >90%), aim to improve systemic blood flow by:

   a. Placing patient on **21% FiO_2** (room air).

   b. Allowing hypercarbia with $PaCO_2$ 45–50 mmHg.

D. If hypoxemia or poor perfusion persists, be prepared for **hemodynamic compromise**:

1. Consider initiation and titration of vasopressor therapy (**Dopamine or Epinephrine**) in consultation with Medical Control.

2. Treat supraventricular and ventricular dysrhythmias (SVT, VT, torsades de pointes, VF) following the appropriate therapeutic algorithm (according to individual protocols).

3. **Consult Medical Control** for airway plan; ideally, intubation should be performed with ECMO back-up available.

E. **Consult Medical Control** for further medical directions and to discuss ECMO eligibility.

V.   Reportable Conditions

A. Unable to manage airway or obtain IV access.

B. Worsening clinical status with interventions.

C. No response to treatment protocol.

VI.   Documentation

A. Physical assessments and vital signs.

B. All interventions and patient responses.

C. Medical consults and directions.

ECMO, *Extracorporeal membrane oxygenation;* EKG, *electrocardiogram;* ET CO_2, *end-tidal carbon dioxide;* FiO_2, *fraction of inspired oxygen;* iNO, *inhaled nitric oxide;* IO, *intraosseous;* IV, *intravenous;* NIBP, *noninvasive blood pressure;* NS, *normal saline;* PRBC, *packed red blood cells;* SaO_2, *arterial oxygen saturation;* SVT, *supraventricular tachyarrhythmia;* VF, *ventricular fibrillation;* VT, *ventricular tachycardia.*

---

well as those with ductal dependent lesions and severe hypoxemia or clinically significant pulmonary overcirculation who may require tight control of oxygenation and ventilation to balance Q_p:Q_s. If patients are at high risk for cardiac arrest on induction, noninvasive respiratory support may be attempted during transport, with planned intubation to be performed upon arrival at the tertiary care center, ideally with ECMO backup available.

Oxygen Therapy During Transport: Goal Oxygen Saturation and Safety of Oxygen Administration During Transport. Oxygen is a potent pulmonary vasodilator. Its administration to neonates with suspected ductal dependent CHD may be both beneficial (in case of hypoxemia) and harmful (because pulmonary overcirculation may lead to circulatory collapse). Neonates with suspected CHD receiving greater than 70% O_2 are at greatest risk of metabolic acidosis and critical hypoxemia; therefore supplemental O_2 should be cautiously weaned to maintain SpO_2 above 75%.[31] In practice, if CHD is suspected, goal O_2 saturations are generally maintained between 75% and 85% to optimize patient stability during transport.

Transport Complications

Given the high-risk nature of transporting critically ill neonates and children with heart disease, complications are not uncommon.

• **BOX 42.2** **Blocked Shunt Transport Protocol**

Johns Hopkins Hospital Bloomberg Children's Center Pediatric Transport Team
Blocked Cardiac Shunt

I. Indications for Use

A. Patients with shunt-dependent cardiac anatomy/physiology (including, but not limited to: hypoplastic left heart syndrome, post Norwood procedure; tricuspid atresia, post Blalock-Taussig shunt; or pulmonary atresia, post Blalock-Taussig shunt) who:
   1. Sustain a significant prolonged oxygen desaturation (SaO_2 <70%), or
   2. Sustain a sudden oxygen desaturation and a shunt murmur is no longer audible on auscultation.

II. Responsibilities

A. When blocked cardiac shunt is suspected during the intake call, team configuration should include: paramedic, transport nurse, respiratory therapist, and transport fellow.
   • Note that Stat Medevac may dispatch a nurse, instead of a paramedic, to accompany the transport nurse and fellow. A respiratory therapist should join the team if inhaled nitric oxide needs to be administered.

B. Nurses and paramedics with the Pediatric Transport Team will perform urgent interventions for patients with blocked cardiac shunt.

C. Transport fellow to perform the following:
   1. Will review the patient's most recent echocardiogram, if one is available.
   2. Will bring anatomical drawing when possible, for the team to review en route.
   3. Will order **Heparin 100 units/kg (MAXIMUM PEDIATRIC DOSE: 2000 units)** to bring on transport.
   4. Will designate a physician to contact pediatric cardiac surgery and pediatric cardiology.

III. Assessment

A. All patients with suspected blocked cardiac shunt will have continuous cardiac, NIBP, pulse oximetry and quantitative ET CO_2 monitoring.

IV. Interventions

A. If suspected blocked cardiac shunt:
   1. Maintain patent airway.
   2. Assist breathing if necessary.
   3. Establish IV/IO access.
   4. Avoid hypoglycemia (goal glucose 90–150 mg/dL).
   5. Maintain normothermia (goal temperature 36–37.5°C).

B. To improve pulmonary blood flow through the shunt:
   1. Reduce pulmonary vascular resistance (PVR):
      a. Place on **100% FiO_2** concentration and titrate to achieve goal SaO_2 = 75%–85%.
         • Accurate pulse oximetry reading may be difficult to obtain due to poor peripheral perfusion.
         • Wean FiO_2 if patient develops pulmonary over-circulation (can occur when SaO_2 >90%).

   b. Begin bag mask ventilation (BMV) with continuous ET CO_2 in place aiming to achieve goal $PaCO_2$ 35–40 mmHg.
      • ET CO_2 will likely be low, reflective of diminished blood flow through the shunt.
      • Obtain blood gas when possible to determine gradient between $PaCO_2$ and ET CO_2.
      • Use of sodium bicarbonate may worsen acidosis as CO_2 generated from bicarbonate metabolism cannot be exhaled through the lungs.
   c. If hypoxemia continues, consider inhaled nitric oxide (iNO) use and prepare for intubation according to the **Intubation Protocol**.
   d. Once intubated, consider ongoing sedation and paralysis.

   2. Improve shunt patency (if presumed clotted):
      a. Administer **Heparin 100 units/kg IV bolus. (MAXIMUM PEDIATRIC DOSE: 2000 units)**
         • Heparin dose and medication calculation must be double-checked by two qualified providers prior to administration.

   3. Increase systemic vascular resistance (SVR):
      a. Administer **NS (0.9%) or 5% Albumin 5 mL/kg**; may repeat with medical direction, while monitoring liver size after each bolus.
      b. **Consult Medical Control** for choice of vasopressor therapy:
         • **Phenylephrine 1–5 micrograms/kg IV** bolus followed by initiation of infusion starting at **1 microgram/kg/minute**; may titrate according to medical directions. (Note that Phenylephrine will increase cardiac afterload without inotropic support and should be used with either low dose Dopamine or Epinephrine infusion.)
         • **Dopamine infusion,** starting at **5 micrograms/kg/minute**; may titrate according to medical directions.
         • **Epinephrine 1–5 microgram/kg IV** bolus followed by initiation of infusion starting at **0.05 micrograms/kg/minute;** may titrate according to medical directions.

C. If hypoxemia persists, be prepared for hemodynamic compromise (bradycardia or tachycardia with poor end-organ perfusion, PEA, asystole, VT, VF) and follow the appropriate therapeutic algorithm (according to individual protocols).

D. **Consult Medical Control** as soon as feasible.

V. Reportable Conditions

A. Unable to manage airway or obtain IV access.
B. No response to treatment protocol.
C. Cardiac arrest (for determination of ECMO activation).

VI. Documentation

A. Physical assessments and vital signs.
B. All interventions and patient responses.
C. Medical consults and directions.

ECMO, Extracorporeal membrane oxygenation; ET CO_2, end-tidal carbon dioxide; FiO_2, fraction of inspired oxygen; IO, intraosseous; IV, intravenous; NIBP, noninvasive blood pressure; NS, normal saline; PEA, pulseless electrical activity; SaO_2, arterial oxygen saturation; VF, ventricular fibrillation; VT, ventricular tachycardia.

They may include malpositioned endotracheal tubes, dislodgment of tubes and lines, equipment malfunction, hypothermia, hypoglycemia, respiratory decompensation (apnea, hypoventilation, desaturation), cardiovascular complications (hypotension, arrhythmias), and cardiopulmonary arrest. A mechanism must be in place at each institution to report, review, and analyze all transport-related complications to identify all preventable events and mitigate further patient safety risks.

Summary

Patients with cardiac disease frequently present with nonspecific complaints, and therefore it is essential to have a high index of suspicion for a cardiac cause. The goal of therapy for all patients with known or suspected cardiac disease is to ensure adequate DO_2. This entails establishing unobstructed and balanced flow to the pulmonary and systemic circulations, with adequate mixing if needed, as well as supporting cardiac output and O_2 carrying capacity. The

• BOX 42.3 Cardiac Tamponade Transport Protocol

Johns Hopkins Hospital Bloomberg Children's Center Pediatric Transport Team

Cardiac Tamponade

I. Indications for Use

A. Patients with penetrating or blunt chest trauma, patients who underwent recent cardiac surgery, or patients without preexistent cardiac pathology who have:
 1. Tachycardia for age, decreased systolic blood pressure (SBP) for age, distant heart tones, distended neck veins (not always present due to hypovolemia).
 2. Pulsus paradoxus (fall in SBP >10 mmHg during the inspiratory phase):
  a. High sensitivity for detection of cardiac tamponade in a spontaneously breathing patient.
  b. Can be detected on pulse oximetry tracing or BP reading.
  c. Extent of pressure variation may help predict the degree of cardiovascular compromise.
  d. Pattern of pulsus paradoxus is reversed in a mechanically ventilated patient (SBP is higher during inspiration and lower during expiration) due to positive intra-pleural pressure.

II. Responsibilities

A. When cardiac tamponade is suspected during the intake call, team configuration should include: paramedic, transport nurse, and transport fellow. Stat Medevac may dispatch a nurse, instead of a paramedic, to accompany our nurse and fellow.

B. Nurses and paramedics with the Pediatric Transport Team will perform urgent interventions for patients with cardiac tamponade.

C. Transport fellow will inform CT surgery and cardiology of patient's name, diagnosis, reason for suspicion, and clinical condition, with estimated transport time.

III. Assessment

A. All patients with suspected cardiac tamponade will have continuous cardiac, NIBP, pulse oximetry, and quantitative ET CO_2 monitoring.

IV. Interventions

A. If patient has suspected cardiac tamponade:
 1. Ensure airway patency and administer **100% oxygen** unless otherwise contraindicated based on patient's underlying medical condition.
 2. Assist breathing with bag mask ventilation (BMV) if necessary, however be mindful that positive pressure ventilation will further decrease venous return and therefore may compromise an already tenuous patient and increase the risk of cardiac arrest.
 3. Establish IV/IO access.
 4. Administer **20 mL/kg NS IV bolus**.
 5. If patient remains hypotensive despite initial volume resuscitation and exam not concerning for tension pneumothorax, continue fluid resuscitation according to the **Shock Protocol**.

B. Notify receiving facility of patient's condition and possible need for immediate intervention upon arrival.

C. **Consult Medical Control** as soon as feasible.

D. If patient with suspected cardiac tamponade develops **cardiac arrest**:
 1. Initiate/continue CPR.
 2. Intubate (if not already done), according to the **Intubation Protocol**.
 3. Establish IV/IO access (if not already done) and fluid resuscitate.
 4. Treat cardiac dysrhythmias per appropriate protocol.
 5. Fellow will perform emergent **needle pericardiocentesis**:
  a. Place patient at a 30° angle (reverse Trendelenburg).
  b. Insert a 16G, 18G, or 20G 5–8 cm long needle attached to a 10 mL syringe just to the left of the xiphoid process, 1 cm inferior to the bottom of the rib at about a 45° angle to the skin.
  c. While gently aspirating, advance needle toward the patient's left shoulder until pericardial fluid is obtained.
  d. Upon entering the pericardial sac, clamp the needle at the skin edge with hemostat to prevent further penetration, attach a 30 mL syringe with a stopcock and gently and slowly remove the pericardial fluid.

V. Reportable Conditions

A. Unable to manage airway or obtain IV access.
B. Need to perform emergent pericardiocentesis.
C. Worsening clinical status with interventions.
D. No response to treatment protocol.
E. Cardiac arrest.

VI. Documentation

A. Physical assessments and vital signs.
B. Print-outs of rhythm and pulse oximetry tracing strips.
C. All interventions and patient responses.
D. Medical consults and directions.

BP, Blood pressure; CPR, cardiopulmonary resuscitation; CT, cardiothoracic; ET CO_2, end-tidal carbon dioxide; IO, intraosseous; IV, intravenous; NIBP, noninvasive blood pressure; NS, normal saline.

---

safe transport of these patients requires a strong understanding of cardiac physiology, as well as appreciation for the unique challenges posed by transport as a function of limited resources and numerous variables encountered. For that reason, effective triage is paramount to determining what interventions and/or therapies will be needed on arrival to the referring facility, during transport itself, and immediately upon return to the receiving institution.

Selected References

A complete list of references is available at ExpertConsult.com.

4. Kemper AR, Mahle WT, Martin GR, et al. Strategies for implementing screening for critical congenital heart disease. *Pediatrics.* 2011;128(5):e1259–e1267.

9. Gupta N, Kamlin CO, Cheung M, Stewart M, Patel N. Improving diagnostic accuracy in the transport of infants with suspected duct-dependent congenital heart disease. *J Paediatr Child Health.* 2014;50(1):64–70.

12. Meckler GD, Lowe C. To intubate or not to intubate? Transporting infants on prostaglandin E₁. *Pediatrics.* 2009;123(1):e25–e30.

14. Mahony L. Calcium homeostasis and control of contractility in the developing heart. *Semin Perinatol.* 1996;20(6):510–519.

19. Slinker BK, Wu Y, Green HW 3rd, Kirkpatrick RD, Campbell KB. Overall cardiac functional effect of positive inotropic drugs with differing effects on relaxation. *J Cardiovasc Pharmacol.* 2000;36(1):1–13.

22. Nakano SJ, Miyamoto SD, Movsesian M, Nelson P, Stauffer BL, Sucharov CC. Age-related differences in phosphodiesterase activity and effects of chronic phosphodiesterase inhibition in idiopathic dilated cardiomyopathy. *Circ Heart Fail.* 2015;8(1):57–63.

27. Marini JJ, Culver BH, Butler J. Mechanical effect of lung distention with positive pressure on cardiac function. *Am Rev Respir Dis.* 1981;124(4):382–386.

31. Shivananda S, Kirsh J, Whyte HE, Muthalally K, McNamara PJ. Impact of oxygen saturation targets and oxygen therapy during the transport of neonates with clinically suspected congenital heart disease. *Neonatology.* 2010;97(2):154–162.

43

Patent Ductus Arteriosus

GRAHAM D. UNGERLEIDER, MD; DEREK A. WILLIAMS, DO;
ROSS M. UNGERLEIDER, MD, MBA

The ductus arteriosus is a vascular connection between the systemic and pulmonary circulations, which although vital during fetal development, can lead to severe morbidity and mortality when persistent postnatally. Paradoxically, the ductus arteriosus can also be essential for survival in some congenital heart defects. Typically the ductus arteriosus is a communication between the main pulmonary trunk and the descending aortic arch, distal to the left subclavian takeoff. A patent ductus arteriosus is essential for survival during fetal development to divert pulmonary flow into the systemic circulation (because there is no need during fetal development for pulmonary perfusion). After birth, pulmonary artery flow is typically directed toward the lungs, and the ductus normally closes during the first day after birth. Failure of the ductus to close in this timely fashion (within 15 to 24 hours) is given the nomenclature of a *patent ductus arteriosus* (PDA). Although a PDA is an associated finding in numerous congenital lesions (and occasionally necessary for life after birth), this chapter will concentrate on the isolated form of PDA in infants, children, and young adults.

Fetal Circulation

During gestation the ductus arteriosus and foramen ovale provide necessary right-to-left shunts of blood returning from the placenta into the fetal systemic circulation. This systemic perfusion from the ductus exists in the fetus because the lungs (during fetal development) are not ventilated and thus pulmonary vascular resistance (PVR) is high. Additionally, anatomic positioning of the foramen ovale preferentially causes a shunt of blood with the highest oxygen saturation returning from the inferior vena cava to the head vessels on ascending aortic arch. The ductus arteriosus, however, shunts a significantly higher volume of relatively desaturated blood returning from the superior vena cava to the descending aortic arch. As a result, those tissues with the highest metabolic demand, the brain and myocardium, preferentially receive more oxygenated blood than the rest of the developing organ systems. After birth, spontaneous ventilation begins, PVR drops, and with the right-to-left shunt across the ductus into the aorta no longer vital, spontaneous closure of the ductus arteriosus begins.[1]

Mechanism of Spontaneous Closure

The spontaneous closure of the ductus arteriosus starts proximally and moves distally toward the aorta, occurring in two stages:

functional and anatomic. Although the ductus arteriosus may appear similar to the aortic and pulmonary arteries, it differs in that it has a media composed primarily of circumferentially layered smooth muscle cells and minimal elastin fibers. Additionally, mucoid lakes, which consist of subintimal pools of a poorly characterized mucoid substance, help to distinguish the ductal tissue as unique from surrounding pulmonary artery and aortic tissue.[2] Functional ductal closure typically occurs within the first 10 to 15 hours after birth. This first stage occurs due to medial smooth muscle contraction, which is stimulated by exposure to four principal postnatal changes: (1) increased arterial oxygen tension, (2) decreased mean ductal pressure, (3) decreased circulating prostaglandin E_2 (PGE_2), and (4) decreased density of PGE_2 receptors in the ductal intima and media. As the smooth muscle cells of the ductus arteriosus contract, ductal wall thickness increases, and the intimal cushions shorten and protrude, resulting in the functional closure of the ductus arteriosus.

The second, anatomic phase of closure occurs as a result of ischemia to the medial tissue, induced by the functional closure, and is generally completed in a few days to weeks after birth. The resultant hypoxia in the ductal wall from contraction of the media induces medial cell necrosis and transcription of various growth factors. These growth factors promote proliferative subendothelial deposition of extracellular matrix and concomitant neointimal thickening. Additionally, extensive wall hypoxia inhibits endogenous production of prostaglandins and nitric oxide, permanently preventing any dilatation of ductal wall. The end result is a constricted, fibrous structure known as the ligamentum arteriosum. Failure of spontaneous closure results in the persistent patency of the ductus arteriosus.

It is also important to note that ductal closure is also highly affected by gestational age. As previously mentioned, increased oxygen tension promotes ductal constriction, whereas prostaglandins promote ductal dilatation. In the full-term infant the ductus arteriosus is much more sensitive to the partial pressure of oxygen; however, in the preterm infant the ductus arterious is more sensitive to prostaglandin E_1 (PEG_1). This helps to explain why decreased gestational age at birth (i.e., *prematurity*) is an inherent risk factor for PDA.

Anatomy and Embryology

The ductus arteriosus develops from the distal portion of the sixth aortic arch (Fig. 43.1), and in the majority of persons connects

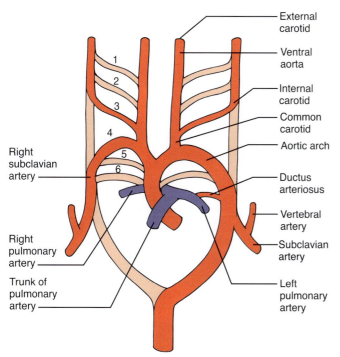

External
carotid

Ventral
aorta

Internal
carotid

Common
carotid

Aortic arch

Ductus
arteriosus

Vertebral
artery

Subclavian
artery

Left
pulmonary
artery

Right
subclavian
artery

Right
pulmonary
artery

Trunk of
pulmonary
artery

• **Figure 43.1** This diagram shows the fate of the embryologic aortic arches. Typically, the sixth aortic arch becomes the ductus arteriosus. (From Burke RP. Patent ductus arteriosus and vascular rings. In: Sellke FW, del Nido PJ, Swanson SJ, eds. *Sabiston & Spencer Surgery of the Chest.* 7th ed. Philadelphia: Elsevier; 2005.)

the main pulmonary trunk or proximal left pulmonary trunk to the isthmus of the descending aortic arch, approximately 5 to 10 mm distal to the takeoff of the left subclavian artery. The shape, length, diameter, and course of the ductus arteriosus can be highly variable, which is important to consider when selecting the best interventional therapy. Typically, though, the ductus is somewhat conical in shape, being broader at the base of the aorta than at the pulmonary trunk. The ductus may also exist as left, right, or bilateral in projection, where the connection may occur from the proximal left or right pulmonary trunk to any position on the aortic arch or, rarely, brachiocephalic vessels. In a right aortic arch the ductus travels in a retroesophageal fashion and can create a vascular ring[3] (see Chapter 44).

Perhaps the most important anatomic relationship for the surgeon to be aware of is the nearness of the ductus to the left recurrent laryngeal nerve, which controls the left vocal cord. During its course into the thoracic cavity, the left recurrent laryngeal nerve separates from the vagus nerve anterior to the aorta and then wraps around the ductus, anterior to posterior, before ultimately slinging superiorly into the tracheoesophageal groove. In the event that the ductus connects to the aorta more proximally along the arch, the recurrent nerve may separate and double back under the aorta in a retrograde fashion. Damage to the nerve can result in temporary or permanent ipsilateral vocal cord paralysis, which can be associated with feeding difficulties postoperatively such as aspiration.

Risk Factors

The incidence of isolated PDA in the United States is approximately 1 in 2000 to 2500 live births and is believed to constitute approximately 7% to 10% of all congenital heart defects. There is a 2:1 incidence among females compared with males. By far the greatest

risk factor for PDA, however, is prematurity. The incidence of PDA increases with lower gestational age (77% at 28 weeks) and also with low birth weight (30% of infants weighing less than 2500 g). A proposed explanation for this is that in the preterm infant circulating PEG_2 is more prevalent due a lack of first-pass metabolism as a result of lung immaturity. Additionally, it has been demonstrated that first-trimester exposure to rubella of nonimmunized mothers produced cardiovascular anomalies in 60% of infants, the most common of which was PDA. Other associations include fetal hydantoin syndrome, warfarin exposure in utero, Down syndrome, and trisomy 13.[4] A PDA may also be more common in babies born at high altitude.

Pathophysiology

As previously mentioned, the ductus arteriosus typically closes within the first day after birth. In the event patency persists, the pathophysiology relates directly to the degree of flow reversal (from the aorta through the ductus into the pulmonary arteries) as a consequence of the decline in PVR that occurs naturally with a newborn's first breath. Because systemic vascular resistance (SVR) is much higher than PVR, a left-to-right shunt will commonly occur across the patent ductus. Thus the degree of left-to-right shunting across a PDA is primarily affected by PVR, as well as by the size of the PDA, because SVR is usually high. Blood travels along the path of least resistance, and, as a result, oxygenated blood from the aorta can flow retrograde across the patent ductus into the pulmonary circulation, where it is recirculated back to the left side of the heart. This results in an increased volume and subsequent workload for both the left atrium and ventricle. Over time this recirculation of cardiac output causes left atrial enlargement and left ventricular dilatation and hypertrophy. Ultimately, depending on the degree of shunting, irreversible pulmonary hypertension can ensue, leading to right-sided heart failure.

Although the degree of left-to-right shunting via the patent ductus is largely dependent on the relationship between SVR and PVR, not all PDAs are created equal, and the impact of a PDA on the physiology and clinical condition of the patient during the first weeks to months of life can be quite variable.

Large PDAs with a substantial left-to-right shunt (usually characterized by a $Q_p:Q_s$ >2:1) can result in left heart failure, manifested by pulmonary overcirculation and edema (with tachypnea), left atrial and left ventricular dilatation, and increased cardiac work. Large PDAs are inherently less restrictive to flow from the systemic to pulmonary circulations, and, as a result, the degree of left-to-right shunting can be severe. In addition to left atrial dilatation and left ventricular strain, this additional blood volume can permanently alter the pulmonary vascular bed. Histologic studies have demonstrated that with the persistent increased blood flow there is increased medial smooth muscle in the pulmonary arterial vessels. Irreversible pulmonary vascular disease ensues when subendothelial cellular proliferation and deposition leads to intimal damage, resulting in both thrombosis and fibrosis of the smaller pulmonary arterioles. This may result in severe pulmonary hypertension and, ultimately, right-sided heart failure. Although this sequelae of consequences is unusual in the modern era, it can occur if a large PDA is left untreated. In patients with severe and irreversible pulmonary hypertension, closure of the PDA is contraindicated.

In medium-sized PDAs, a moderate left-to-right shunt ($Q_p:Q_s$ of 1.5-2.0) may be well compensated for by the left ventricle and produce minimal symptoms. In these patients, pulmonary artery pressures may be only mildly to moderately elevated, and it is primarily the size (length and diameter) of the ductus that regulates the degree of shunting rather than the ratio of SVR to PVR. These patients may be completely asymptomatic, or they may experience poor feeding, dyspnea, and growth retardation as sequelae of failing to meet the body's metabolic demand.

The natural course of small PDAs (Q_p:Q_s <1.5) is typically uneventful. The additional workload of the net left-to-right shunt is slight and is well compensated by the left ventricle. Left ventricular failure and pulmonary hypertension do not occur. Patients may be asymptomatic their entire lives, and the discovery of a PDA may simply be an incidental finding if a murmur is investigated later in life and results in obtaining an echocardiogram.[5]

Infants and children with large PDAs, if symptomatic, tend to present with signs and symptoms of congestive heart failure. This can range from a murmur heard on physical examination to tachypnea and signs of pulmonary overcirculation on chest x-ray examination. Premature neonates with a significant PDA may present on days 3 to 4 of life with unexplained respiratory distress and metabolic acidosis that is recalcitrant to ventilator support. There are large PDAs that are vital for survival in certain complex congenital heart defects (either as a source of pulmonary blood flow in patients with restricted pulmonary flow or for systemic blood flow in cases of restricted aortic flow). These large PDAs, because they are critical for survival, are not the focus of this chapter. The most common presentation for a PDA (outside the neonatal period) is a murmur being heard in an otherwise asymptomatic child.

Other known complications of a persistent ductus, although rare, are worth mentioning. Endocarditis, although now rare in patients with PDA, was a leading cause of mortality before the widespread adoption of prophylactic antibiotics and surgical repair. When endocarditis does occur, vegetations can typically be visualized on the pulmonic end of the ductus, and, consequently, septic emboli ejected to the lungs may form pulmonary abscesses. Such cases are initially managed conservatively with antibiotics and then referred for surgery. Another exceedingly rare but emergent complication of a persistent ductus is aneurysm. Ductus arteriosus aneurysm can occur either spontaneously or secondarily as a complication of prior intervention. Aneurysm of the ductus is an immediate indication for surgical repair due to the high risk of rupture[6] and infection; unrepaired, the mortality has been reported as high as 91%.[7] There have been only limited case studies of ductal aneurysm in patients with inherited collagen vascular disease.[8] Additional complications, such as laryngeal nerve palsy, have been also reported.[9]

Diagnosis

Diagnosis of PDA in the newborn and infant starts with a good history and physical examination. In preterm newborns there must be a high index of suspicion for any patient with respiratory deterioration despite adequate ventilator support. Failure to gain weight adequately is common. Although systolic pressure is typically maintained, patients with a hemodynamically significant shunt may present with a widened pulse pressure due to diastolic runoff. A murmur may be present also: classically, a III/VI+ crescendo-decrescendo, "machine-like" murmur, which is best auscultated at the left upper sternal border. Electrocardiogram may be normal or demonstrate left ventricular hypertrophy. Chest x-ray examination can show increased pulmonary vascular markings and interstitial fullness but is also frequently unremarkable.

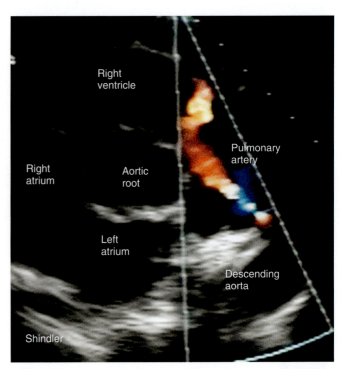

• **Figure 43.2** Diagnosis of a patent ductus arteriosus (PDA) is easily achieved with echocardiography. This image demonstrates flow through a PDA with relevant adjacent structures labeled. (http://rwjms1.umdnj.edu/shindler/pdacf1.gif.)

The hallmark for diagnosis is ultrasonography. Two-dimensional echocardiography with color flow and Doppler can be used to diagnose a majority of PDAs in the newborn (Fig. 43.2). Cardiac catheterization is rarely indicated for diagnosis (unless pulmonary hypertension is suspected), although it is becoming the preferred method for treatment of PDAs in appropriately selected patients. Likewise, other imaging modalities such as computed tomography scan or magnetic resonance imaging, although they can demonstrate a PDA, are usually not necessary. Once the diagnosis is made, and this is usually easily done by echocardiography, the team can decide from numerous options on the best plan of management.

Management of the Patient With Patent Ductus Arteriosus

Medical Management

A PDA is a common diagnosis in premature neonates. It is advisable to involve a cardiology team in the diagnosis to ensure that there are no other important associated heart defects or aortic arch anomalies that make management decisions more complex. In the case of the isolated PDA in a premature neonate, anticongestive therapy (such as Lasix) can help to manage the consequences of pulmonary overcirculation, but in most cases it is beneficial to get the ductus to close. Prostaglandin inhibition (most often with nonsteroidal antiinflammatory drugs [NSAIDs] such as indomethacin) is the typical treatment of choice. In most cases this will promote closure of the ductal tissue in the functional and anatomic sequence described earlier in this chapter. The ductus may occasionally reopen, but for responsive patients this has proven to be the most favorable method for encouraging ductal closure. In some

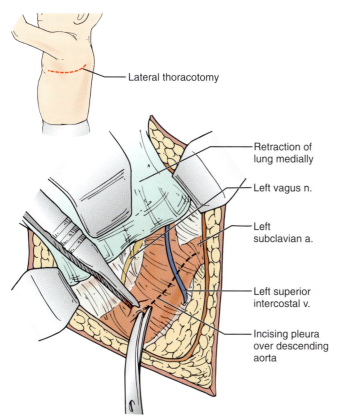

• **Figure 43.3** The ductus arteriosus is generally exposed through a small, left lateral thoracotomy. Once the lung has been retracted anteriorly, the posterior parietal pleural overlying the descending aorta is incised to guide subsequent dissection. As depicted in this illustration, the left superior intercostal vein is often a reliable marker for the location of the ductus arteriosus, which is usually just inferior to this vein. *a.,* Artery; *n.,* nerve; *v.,* vein. (From Ungerleider RM. Patent ductus arteriosus. In: Sabiston DC, ed. *Atlas of Cardiothoracic Surgery.* Philadelphia: WB Saunders; 1995.)

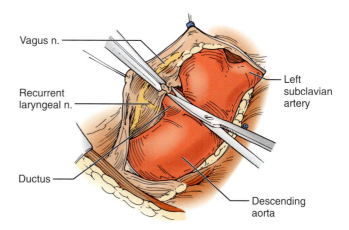

• **Figure 43.4** Once the parietal pleura overlying the aorta has been incised, dissection is carried out medially, pushing the adventitial tissue carefully off the ductus, which can be positively identified by the recurrent laryngeal nerve encircling it. *n.,* Nerve. (From Ungerleider RM. Patent ductus arteriosus. In: Sabiston DC, ed. *Atlas of Cardiothoracic Surgery.* Philadelphia: WB Saunders; 1995.)

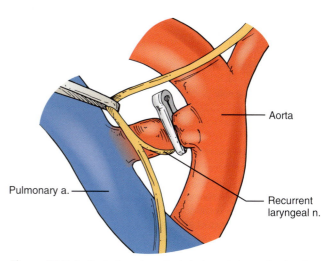

• **Figure 43.5** An illustration of a patent ductus arteriosus that has been successfully obliterated with a hemoclip. *a.,* Artery; *n.,* nerve. (http://accesssurgery.mhmedical.com/data/books/963/hop002_fig_63-03.png.)

patients, indomethacin is contraindicated, often due to renal insufficiency or to gastrointestinal bleeding, and, in those patients, surgical ligation of the PDA is warranted.

Open Surgical Approach

Surgical ligation remains the most common method used for closure of a persistent PDA in newborns, whereas percutaneous device closure is more typically used in older patients. The standard surgical approach has been well described and involves a left lateral thoracotomy for exposure. A short incision is made in the third or fourth intercostal space just below the scapula. (Fig. 43.3) In older infants and children, outside the neonatal age, some surgeons recommend sparing the latissimus and serratus muscles. In premature infants, however, the tissue is often edematous and the babies can be critically ill, and muscle sparing incisions are not as common. Once the pleural cavity is open (it is not necessary to use an extrapleural approach, although some surgeons do use this technique), the lung is retracted inferomedially, and the posterior pleura overlying the descending aorta is incised (see Fig. 43.3). The surgeon should identify the anatomic landmarks that help to positively identify the ductus, including the left subclavian artery, the area between the left subclavian artery and the ductus when it exists, the aortic arch, and the descending aorta. Careful sharp

and electrocautery dissection along the superior and inferior edges of the ductus can help to isolate it, and the surgeon should be able to identify the vagus nerve and the recurrent laryngeal nerve branch, which wraps around the left-sided ductus (Fig. 43.4). The left recurrent laryngeal nerve is carefully pushed away from the main part of the ductus so that it is less likely to be injured during the ligation. Most typically in premature neonates, many of which weigh between 500 and 900 kg, the ductus is occluded with a single hemoclip (Fig. 43.5). This clip ligation technique has become the preferred surgical management strategy for PDA ligation in this patient population and has been associated with a lower incidence of complications, including recurrent laryngeal nerve injury and chylothorax (compared with surgical ligation with ligatures). The PDA in a premature neonate can be large, and many times can be the size of the aorta! It is important for the surgical team to choose an appropriate-sized clip to completely occlude the PDA, because use of a clip that is too small can lead

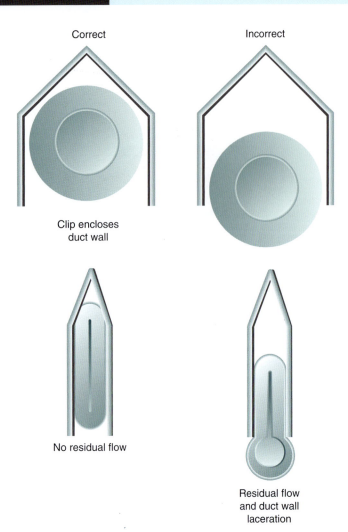

Correct   Incorrect

Clip encloses
duct wall

No residual flow

Residual flow
and duct wall
laceration

• **Figure 43.6** An appropriate-sized hemoclip is required to ensure complete occlusion of the patent ductus arteriosus (PDA). If the hemoclip is not applied across the entire ductus, a persistent PDA can be present. If the hemoclip is not securely applied, it can be extruded in part off the ductus, also resulting in persistent flow. Too large a hemoclip can encroach on underlying structures such as the esophagus or left bronchus. (From Burke RP. Patent ductus arteriosus and vascular rings. In: Sellke FW, del Nido PJ, Swanson SJ, eds. *Sabiston & Spencer Surgery of the Chest*. 7th ed. Philadelphia: Elsevier; 2005.)

to persistent PDA shunt (or even extrusion of the clip off the ductus with recurrence of ductal shunt), and a clip that is too large can push on underlying structures, such as the esophagus or left bronchus (Fig. 43.6). In premature neonates, clip ligation is quick, effective, and has very little long-term disadvantage (other than the presence of a hemoclip on the patient's future chest x-ray examination). It is critical for the surgeon to feel confident about the anatomy because there are reports of inadvertent ligation of the aortic isthmus or of the left pulmonary artery—both of which can have disastrous consequences. It is now common practice to then carefully close the thoracotomy in layers, and use of a chest tube is no longer considered necessary unless there has been injury to the lung or there is some residual bleeding. Bleeding is uncommon, but blood should always be available for patients undergoing PDA occlusion, even tiny premature neonates. These patients can be extremely edematous, and there can be a substantial amount of fluid in the very fragile tissue, so the surgical team may need to

be patient and careful during the dissection. Likewise, in babies with severe lung disease, even the slightest retraction of the lung can cause hemodynamic compromise, and the surgical team may need to periodically allow the anesthesia team to reinflate the lungs. Use of a pulse oximeter is standard to help guide this part of the intraoperative management. It is also now common practice to ligate the PDA of a premature neonate at the bedside in the neonatal intensive care unit (NICU) because transportation of these often critically ill neonates to the operating room (OR) risks dislodgment of the endotracheal tube or temperature variation and just increases the complexity of the logistics for this otherwise straightforward surgical procedure. The movement of the surgical team to the patient's bedside is an example of how medical care has progressed, to the patient's advantage, over the last decade, and there are essentially no complications related to bringing the OR to the intensive care unit (ICU) for these procedures. It is likely that this experience with PDA ligation in the NICU (which began in the late 1980s) has led to the application of other operative procedures being done at the bedside of critically ill or unstable patients (such as cannulation for extracorporeal membrane oxygenation [ECMO], chest closure, and exploration for bleeding).

Larger patients (over 2 kg) should generally have their PDAs ligated in the OR, although this size recommendation is arbitrary and is dependent on the patient's condition and the environment available for performing these procedures at the bedside in each institution. At some point, however, the better lighting and access to supplies in the OR makes the OR a more suitable environment for PDA ligation. Although some surgeons in the past have recommended division of the PDA, division is rarely practiced today because it carries with it more risk, including risk of exsanguinating hemorrhage. Ligation has become the preferred surgical procedure for the PDA in the older infant and young child (when interventional catheterization laboratory closure is not available or possible). In older children the PDA can be quite large, and with the increased blood pressure in these older children, simple clip ligation may be more hazardous and risks tearing the ductus, which can be fatal. (As in any comment, it is important to understand that there are variations in opinion. For example, some surgeons recommend video-assisted techniques for PDA ligation, and hemoclips are commonly applied in these circumstances, so it is not contraindicated to use a clip, although as described later, proponents of this technique would be less likely to use it on a patient with a large PDA greater than 10 mm in diameter). The preferred technique for most surgical groups is "suture obliteration" (Fig. 43.7), in which three to four suture ligatures are placed around the PDA and sequentially tied. The sutures are often placed gently through some of the adventitial tissue at the aortic and pulmonary ends of the PDA to prevent them from sliding toward each other, and a third ligature is often securely tied between these two, creating complete obliteration of ductal flow. Suture obliteration and even video-assisted ductal closure are becoming less common because most children who have PDAs are now referred for catheterization laboratory closure.

Finally, there is the occasional patient with a very large PDA that is too large for catheterization laboratory closure and that may be associated with significant flow and pulmonary hypertension. These ductus can be daunting for a surgeon, and ligation of these large PDAs through a sternotomy incision with the patient on cardiopulmonary bypass (CPB) is an option. In these cases the patient can be placed on CPB, and with the flows decreased the large PDA can be more safely encircled and securely tied while it

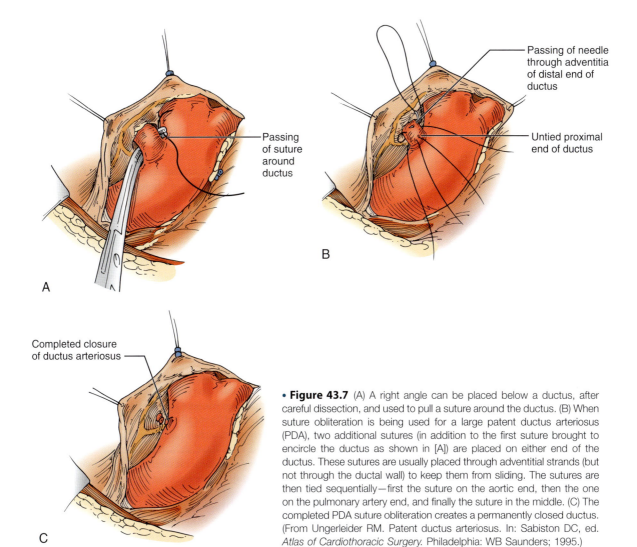

Passing of suture around ductus

Passing of needle through adventitia of distal end of ductus

Untied proximal end of ductus

A

B

Completed closure of ductus arteriosus

C

• **Figure 43.7** (A) A right angle can be placed below a ductus, after careful dissection, and used to pull a suture around the ductus. (B) When suture obliteration is being used for a large patent ductus arteriosus (PDA), two additional sutures (in addition to the first suture brought to encircle the ductus as shown in [A]) are placed on either end of the ductus. These sutures are usually placed through adventitial strands (but not through the ductal wall) to keep them from sliding. The sutures are then tied sequentially—first the suture on the aortic end, then the one on the pulmonary artery end, and finally the suture in the middle. (C) The completed PDA suture obliteration creates a permanently closed ductus. (From Ungerleider RM. Patent ductus arteriosus. In: Sabiston DC, ed. *Atlas of Cardiothoracic Surgery.* Philadelphia: WB Saunders; 1995.)

is not under as high a pressure (Fig. 43.8). This technique with open closure through the pulmonary artery is also indicated when there is calcium in the PDA (making it a risk for ligation), as can be the case in older patients.

Video-Assisted Thoracoscopic Surgery

Endoscopic intervention via video-assisted thoracoscopic surgery (VATS) is a relatively new technique for ligation of PDAs (as well as division of some vascular rings [see Chapter 44]). Proponents of VATS ductal division cite the potential for decreased post-thoracotomy pain and decreased long-term risk of scoliosis (from thoracotomy incisions), as well as improved cosmesis, as benefits of an endoscopic approach.[10]

The standard surgical technique for VATS closure of a patent ductus has been well described by Burke et al.[11] In the VATS approach a series of three to four keyhole incisions is made for both camera visualization and instrumentation with the patient in the right lateral decubitus position. This technique does not make use of standard rib retraction. Another difference is the use of a dual-lumen or single-lumen endotracheal tube with a bronchial blocker (in selected patients who are large enough to accommodate this technique) to allow for selective isolation of the left lung while gaining exposure to the relevant anatomy. This is another reason why this approach may be better reserved for older patients (and many of those are now being treated with catheter-based therapy).

Contraindications to VATS closure include a ductal diameter greater than 1.0 cm, ductal calcification, dense adhesions due to prior surgery or infection, as well as concomitant oscillating ventilation.[11]

Surgical Complications

Acute complications of both conventional and VATS ligation of PDA include pneumothorax, chylothorax, bleeding, aortic and pulmonary artery obstruction, recanalization, vocal cord dysfunction, and infection. The most common of these complications is left recurrent laryngeal nerve damage, which can result in ipsilateral vocal cord paresis. Patients weighing less than 1000 g at the time of closure have the greatest relative risk for nerve damage. In a series published by Clement et al.,[11a] neonates and infants with vocal cord paralysis following repair had a longer duration of tube feeding, supplemental oxygen, and ventilator support. In a separate series by Truong et al., 65% of patients with recurrent nerve damage at a median follow-up of 16 months had persistent paralysis.[11b]

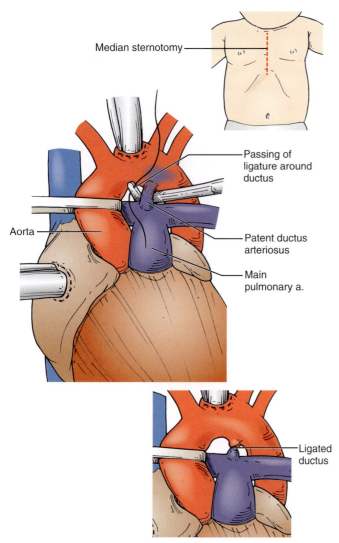

Median sternotomy

Passing of ligature around ductus

Aorta

Patent ductus arteriosus

Main pulmonary a.

Ligated ductus

• **Figure 43.8** For a large ductus, or when the ductus exists as a part of another cardiac lesion requiring simultaneous surgical repair, the patent ductus arteriosus (PDA) can be approached through a median sternotomy. The PDA is the vessel between the right and left pulmonary arteries, which should be definitively identified. With the patient of cardiopulmonary bypass the pump flows can be decreased, allowing even large ductus to be securely tied under low pressure. *a.,* Artery. (From Ungerleider RM. Patent ductus arteriosus. In: Sabiston DC, ed. *Atlas of Cardiothoracic Surgery.* Philadelphia: WB Saunders; 1995.)

Transcatheter Patent Ductus Arteriosus Closure

In 1967 Porstmann et al.[12] introduced transcatheter closure of the PDA, but it was not until 20 years later that the PDA occlusion trial by Rashkind et al.[13] increased attention to this option's merit and described a reproducible technique. Over the ensuing 30 years, many devices, and newer generations of devices, have been designed, showing great occlusion success with minimal complications. These devices have further expanded the treatment range of patent ages and sizes such that for the isolated PDA, transcatheter occlusion has become an accepted standard of care.

The primary indication for transcatheter PDA closure is the same as that for surgical closure, which is essentially a patent ductus with left heart volume load (dilation). Up until 2007, when the American Heart Association released its guideline revisions for the prevention of infective endocarditis, small, audible, non–volume loading PDAs were being routinely occluded in the catheterization laboratory. The revised guidelines no longer limited transcatheter closure to prophylaxis for patients with a small PDA[14] and expanded the use of this technique to all patients with PDA. Since 2007, patients with PDAs are being commonly referred for transcatheter occlusion, and this is becoming the primary method for PDA occlusion. Although use of this technique is related to provider, patient, and family preference, it is also the case that these patients are generally seen by cardiologists who offer transcatheter PDA occlusion as the method of choice, and surgical closure is rarely selected.

Diagnosing volume load from a PDA is usually achieved through echocardiography. The narrowest portion of the PDA, the pulmonary and aortic dimensions, and the length of the PDA are important data for a successful occlusion. Some institutions have had success with measurement of the minimal diameter and aortic end diameter from two-dimensional echocardiographic images.[15] Others have found a poor correlation between the measurement performed from an angiogram compared with that from echocardiography.[16] Angiography continues to be the gold standard for measurement of the ductal components necessary to guide safe transcatheter closure.

The most common approach to PDA occlusion is antegrade from the femoral artery, but the retrograde approach from the venous system has become equally successful with the newer devices on the market. Classically, coil occlusion was the cheapest and most widely used technique. Coils come in many diameters and lengths and even have detachable options. Nondetachable coils seem to carry a higher risk of embolization when compared with other detachable device options. Presently in the United States the most widely used device for occlusion is the AMPLATZER Duct Occluder (ADO) by St. Jude Medical. This device is composed of nitinol and interwoven polyester and is a self-expanding device. It has an occlusion success rate of 98.4% at 6 months. The newer generation, the ADO II, has eliminated the polyester and comes in smaller sizes, allowing PDA occlusion in smaller patients. The ADO II reports a 98% successful occlusion rate.[17] Gudausky et al.[18] reported a significant procedure success rate if the proper occlusion strategy is used. They suggested a coil occlusion for a minimal PDA of 1 mm or less or an ADO if the PDA exceeded 1 mm. Other AMPLATZER devices (e.g., vascular plugs, ventricular septal defect occluder) have been used with success as well. Newer devices such as the Medtronic Micro Vascular Plug and the Occlutech PDA Occluder are now showing up in the literature. Interventionalist preference still guides much of device selection. Despite the many device choices, transcatheter occlusion continues to offer excellent rates of occlusion with low complication rates.[19]

Now that newer and small devices are available, transcatheter occlusion is being offered to neonates, for whom occlusion has historically been solely a surgical approach. A recent study reported mean procedure weight of 1249 g and a success rate of 88% without any procedural deaths plus a survival to discharge of 96%.[20] Time and new device design will tell if low-birth-weight patients will achieve equal procedure success.

Conclusion

A patent ductus is a common congenital heart defect. It can exist in isolation or as an associated defect with numerous other congenital heart lesions. Occasionally a congenital heart defect *requires* the persistence of patency of the ductus arteriosus for survival, and these "ductal dependent" lesions can require the ductus for either pulmonary or systemic blood flow. When the ductus arteriosus exists as a sole defect, it may present (commonly) as a part of the respiratory insufficiency or hemodynamic insufficiency of a premature neonate, or it may be relatively asymptomatic and be diagnosed later in infancy or childhood by a murmur or subtle signs of left heart failure.

PDA is generally an easy diagnosis by echocardiography. Once diagnosed, indication for treatment is usually left heart volume overload (with left atrial or left ventricular dilation). Pulmonary overcirculation on chest x-ray examination is helpful in prompting a decision for treatment.

Initial treatment may be medical (in premature neonates) using nonsteroidal antiinflammatory agents such as indomethacin. Occlusion of a PDA is now being performed in the catheterization laboratory as a common catheterization laboratory intervention and is typically successful. Although the ability to close a PDA in the catheterization laboratory is moving toward smaller patients, premature neonates (often weighing less than 1000 g) are typically referred for surgical closure if medical management fails. In this patient group, closure is commonly performed in the NICU using hemoclip ligation. Surgical ligation of a PDA in older patients is generally performed in an OR using suture ligation as an option.

Postoperative management is usually related to pain control (if surgical thoracotomy was employed). Hemodynamics are typically excellent with elevation of the diastolic blood pressure. When catheterization laboratory closure is employed, a small residual defect may be present and should close over time as the device creates complete thrombosis in the PDA. Embolization of the device into the pulmonary artery is rare but has been reported. Following surgical closure, left vocal cord paralysis (which can lead to aspiration with feeding), chylothorax, bleeding (rare), paralyzed left hemidiaphragm, and pneumothorax are potential complications.

Finally, and of importance to the growth of future ICUs, the ability to successfully and safely close a PDA at the bedside in a NICU has led to more enthusiasm for extending bedside treatment in an ICU to other indications in critically ill neonates and infants (including ECMO cannulation, chest closure, and exploration for bleeding).

References

1. Gournay V. The ductus arteriosus: physiology, regulation, and functional and congenital anomalies. *Arch Cardiovasc Dis.* 2011;104:578–585.
2. Gittenberger-de Groot AC, Strengers JLM. Histopathology of the arterial duct (ductus arteriosus) with and without treatment with prostaglandin E$_1$. *Int J Cardiol.* 1988;19:153–166.
3. Quinn D, Cooper B, Clyman RI. Factors associated with permanent closure of the ductus arteriosus: a role for prolonged indomethacin therapy. *Pediatrics.* 2002;110(10):2002.
4. Hajj H, Dagle JM. Genetics of patent ductus arteriosus susceptibility and treatment. *Semin Perinatol.* 2012;36:98–104.
5. Driscoll DJ. Left-to-Right Shunt Lesions. *Pediatr Clin North Am.* 1999;46:355–368.
6. Day JR, Walesby RK. A spontaneous ductal aneurysm presenting with left recurrent laryngeal nerve palsy. *Ann Thorac Surg.* 2001;72:608–609.
7. Lund JT, Jensen MB. Aneurysm of the ductus arteriosus a review of the literature and the surgical implications. *Eur J Cardiothorac Surg.* 1991;5:566–570.
8. Siu BL, Kovalchin JP, Kearney DL, Fraser CD, Fenrich AL. 2001. Aneurysmal Dilatation of the Ductus Arteriosus in a Neonate. *Pediatr Cardiol.* 2001;22:403–405.
9. Benjamin JR, Smith PB, Cotten CM, Jaggers J, et al. Long-term morbidities associated with vocal cord paralysis after surgical closure of a patent ductus arteriosus in extremely low birth weight infants. *J Perinatol.* 2010;30:408–413.
10. Nezafati MH, Soltani G, Vedadian A. Video-assisted ductal closure with new modifications: minimally invasive, maximally effective, 1,300 cases. *Ann Thorac Surg.* 2007;4:1343–1348.
11. Jacobs JP, Giroud JM, Quintessenza JA, Morell VO, Botero LM, Van Gelder HM, et al. The modern approach to patent ductus arteriosus treatment: complementary roles of video-assisted thoracoscopic surgery and interventional cardiology coil occlusion. *Ann Thorac Surg.* 2003;76:1421–1428.
11a. Clement WA, El-Hakim H, Phillipos EZ, Cote JJ. Unilateral vocal cord paralysis following patent ductus arteriosus ligation in extremely low birth weight infants. *Arch Otolaryngol Head Neck Surg.* 2008;134(1):28–33.
11b. Truong MT, et al. Pediatric vocal fold paralysis after cardiac surgery: rate of recovery and sequelae. *Otolaryngol Head Neck Surg.* 2007;137(5):780–784.
12. Portsmann W, Wierny L, Warnke H. Der Verschluss D.a.p. ohne Thorakotomie (1 Mitteilung). *Thoraxchirurgie.* 1967;15:199.
13. Rashkind WJ, Mullins CE, Hellenbrand WE, Tait MA. Nonsurgical closure of patent ductus arteriosus: clinical application of the Rashkind PDA Occluder System. *Circulation.* 2002;75:583–592.
14. Wilson W, et al. Prevention of infective endocarditis: guidelines from the American Heart Association: a guideline from the American Heart Association Rheumatic Fever, Endocarditis and Kawasaki Disease Committee, Council on Cardiovascular Disease in the Young, and the Council on Clinical Cardiology, Council on Cardiovascular Surgery and Anesthesia, and the Quality of Care and Outcomes Research Interdisciplinary Working Group. *J Am Dent Assoc.* 2007;138:739–745.
15. Ramaciotti C, Lemler MS, Moake L, Zellers TM. Comprehensive assessment of patent ductus arteriosus by echocardiography before transcatheter closure. *J Am Soc Echocardiogr.* 2012;15:1154–1159.
16. Carmo Mendes I, Heard H, Peacock K, Kransemann T, Morgan GJ. Echocardiographic versus angiographic assessment of patent arterial duct in percutaneous closure: toward X-ray free duct occlusion? *Pediatr Cardiol.* 2017;38:302–307.
17. Gruenstein DH, Ebeid M, Radtke W, Holzer R, Justio H. Transcatheter closure of patent duct arteriosus using the AMPLATZER duct occlude II (ADO II). *Cather Cardiovasc Interv.* March 4, 2017.
18. Gudausky TM, Hisrch R, Khoury PR, Beekman RH. Comparison of two transcatheter device strategies for occlusion of the patent ductus arteriosus. *Catheter Cardiovasc Interv.* 2008;72:675–680.
19. Jin M, Liang YM, Wang XF, Guo BJ, Zheng K, Gu Y, et al. A Retrospective Study of 1,526 Cases of Transcatheter Occlusion of Patent Ductus Arteriosus. *Chin Med J.* 2015;128:2284–2289.
20. Zahn EM, Peck D, Phillips A, Nevin P, Basaker K, Simmons C, et al. Transcatheter closure of patent ductus arteriosus in extremely premature newborns: early results and midterm follow-up. *JACC Cardiovasc Interv.* 2006;9:2429–2437.

44

Vascular Rings and Pulmonary Artery Sling

WILLIAM S. RAGALIE, MD; MICHAEL E. MITCHELL, MD

Clinical Background

The term *vascular ring* refers to a spectrum of congenital aortic arch anomalies that can cause compressive symptoms of the aerodigestive tract. "True" or "complete" vascular rings completely encircle the trachea and esophagus, whereas "incomplete" vascular rings do not. The term itself was first coined in 1945 by Gross after successful repair of a double aortic arch in a 4-year-old patient,[1] although the anatomy of a double aortic arch had been described as early as 1737 by Hommell. Numerous variations have been described, and several authors have grouped vascular rings under various schema. An early report from the Mayo Clinic divided vascular rings into seven types (types A through G) and is of historical interest.[2] Backer and Mavroudis[3] proposed a simplified grouping system with the following subcategories:

- Double aortic arch
  - Dominant right arch
  - Dominant left arch
  - Balanced or codominant arches
- Right arch with left ligamentum
  - With retroesophageal or "aberrant" left subclavian artery
  - With mirror-image branching
- Innominate artery compression
- Pulmonary artery sling (PAS)

Left aortic arch with aberrant right subclavian artery, although not always a true vascular ring (dependent on a right-sided ligamentum), is often included in the discussion of vascular rings because the management of symptomatic patients follows many of the same principles. Left aortic arch with aberrant right subclavian artery is the second most common aortic arch anomaly and is present in 0.5% to 2% of humans. The most common aortic arch anomaly is bovine arch, in which all four vessels arise from a common trunk. Symptoms—either respiratory distress or dysphagia—are caused by extrinsic compression of the trachea and/or esophagus by the vascular ring, although respiratory symptoms in patients with vascular rings may also be compounded by intrinsic airway disease such as tracheomalacia or congenital tracheal stenosis (CTS) with complete tracheal rings. CTS has a particularly strong association with PAS. Because of the potential complicating features of tracheal pathology, a good understanding of the pathophysiology and management of pediatric tracheal disease is extremely useful in approaching the patient with a vascular ring who has respiratory symptoms. All symptomatic patients with vascular ring should be considered for surgical correction. In fact, it is estimated that over 70% of patients with a vascular ring eventually become symptomatic.[4,5] The principles of surgical correction are ligation and division of the vascular ring to relieve extrinsic compression, preservation of distal blood flow, and tracheal repair or reconstruction as necessary. Incidentally diagnosed individuals should be considered on a case-by-case basis, but generally patients with complete vascular rings should be offered repair, whereas asymptomatic patients with incomplete rings may be initially observed. Knowledge of the natural history of unrepaired vascular rings is limited to a few small series of patients with mild or no symptoms.[6,7]

Prevalence and Associations

The estimated prevalence of true vascular rings is 0.05% to 0.1% of the general population. In a study by Yu and colleagues,[8] the authors performed two-dimensional echocardiography on 186,213 newly registered school-aged children as part of a pre–sports participation screening program. They diagnosed 1088 patients with vascular ring, the majority (992) having a right aortic arch with an aberrant left subclavian artery. Similarly, in a review of 18,347 pregnant women whose fetuses were screened for congenital heart disease over a 10-year period in Israel, 18 cases (0.1%) of vascular rings were diagnosed and confirmed postnatally.[9] In a large series of 4850 consecutive autopsies in England, there were 10 reported vascular rings that had not been diagnosed premortem.[10] The most common genetic anomaly associated with vascular rings is 22q11 microdeletion, although others include 3q29 duplication, and 16p13.3 deletion.[11] Specifically, haploinsufficiency of the genes *CRKL, TBX1,* and *ERK2,* which are located on chromosome 22, has been implicated experimentally in abnormal neural crest cell migration, leading to abnormal development of the aortic arch and great vessels.[12] Intracardiac defects associated with vascular rings include tetralogy of Fallot, ventricular septal defect, and truncus arteriosus.[13] Associated extracardiac anomalies include DiGeorge syndrome, given the association with 22q11 microdeletion, and also tracheomalacia, aortic coarctation, interrupted aortic arch, Pierre Robin sequence, brain ventriculomegaly, and cleft lip and palate.[14,15]

Embryology

Initially, cranial neural crest cells migrate within the human embryo to form six paired pharyngeal arches, as well as paired left and

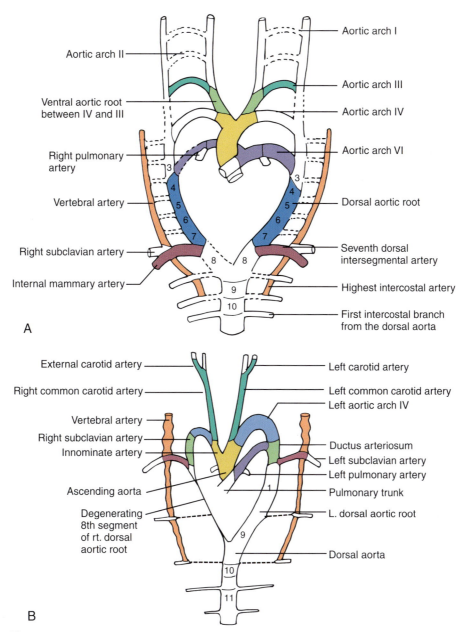

Aortic arch I

Aortic arch II

Ventral aortic root
between IV and III

Right pulmonary
artery

Vertebral artery

Right subclavian artery

Internal mammary artery

Aortic arch III

Aortic arch IV

Aortic arch VI

Dorsal aortic root

Seventh dorsal
intersegmental artery

Highest intercostal artery

First intercostal branch
from the dorsal aorta

A

External carotid artery

Right common carotid artery

Vertebral artery

Right subclavian artery
Innominate artery

Ascending aorta

Degenerating
8th segment
of rt. dorsal
aortic root

Left carotid artery

Left common carotid artery
Left aortic arch IV

Ductus arteriosum
Left subclavian artery
Left pulmonary artery
Pulmonary trunk

L. dorsal aortic root

Dorsal aorta

B

• **Figure 44.1** Primitive aortic arches in (A) early stage of embryonic development and (B) after involution of the right aortic arch. (From Ziegler MM, et al. Vascular compression syndromes. In: *Operative Pediatric Surgery.* 2nd ed. New York, McGraw Hill, 2014. Reprinted with permission from McGraw Hill, Inc.)

right dorsal aortae and ventral aortae, and their systematic regression and remodeling contribute to the mature human aorta[15] (Fig. 44.1). The paired right and left dorsal aortae are present at approximately 3 weeks of intrauterine growth. Typically the left dorsal aorta persists to form a left-sided descending aorta, and the right dorsal aorta largely regresses but does contribute to the mature right subclavian artery. Abnormal regression patterns of the pharyngeal arches result in vascular ring anatomy. The first and second arches regress to form part of minor facial arteries and do not contribute to the mature aorta. The third aortic arch forms the common and proximal internal carotid artery. The fourth arches become the innominate artery on the right and the ascending aorta and transverse arch on the left. The fifth arch regresses, and the sixth arch becomes the pulmonary artery and the ductus

arteriosus on the left. Complete rings result from a failure of regression of a paired aortic arch, resulting in two mature aortic structures on either side of the aerodigestive tract. The "sidedness" of the aortic arch is determined by its relationship to the trachea, whereas the "sidedness" of the descending aorta is determined by its relationship to the vertebral bodies.

Presentation and Diagnosis

Patients with vascular rings range in presentation from the incidentally diagnosed asymptomatic patient to those with life-threatening respiratory failure and/or intractable feeding intolerance. Anterior anatomic variations (e.g., innominate artery compression) tend to cause respiratory symptoms, whereas posterior pathology (e.g., aberrant subclavian artery) tends to cause dysphagia. Complete vascular rings (e.g., balanced double aortic arch) tend to cause symptoms of both tracheal and esophageal compression. Respiratory symptoms include apparent life-threatening event (ALTEs), in which a previously asymptomatic child may suffer a respiratory arrest without any significant prodrome. Other respiratory symptoms range in severity from cough ("seal bark" has been used to describe the cough associated with vascular ring), stridor, recurrent pneumonias, hyperinflation, migrating atelectasis, and ventilator dependence. The more severe cases will tend to present within the first few months of life. Apneic events are more common in patients with innominate artery compression and tracheomalacia. Symptoms of esophageal compression tend to present later, classically when the infant progresses from liquid to more solid foods. The term *dysphagia lusoria* ("from an unknown source") has been used to describe the dysphagia due to compression from an aberrant subclavian artery. The range of dysphagia is broad, from a neonate who is intolerant of enteral nutrition to a nearly asymptomatic child who has learned to slowly and thoroughly chew his or her food.

A variety of imaging modalities are used in the workup of patients with vascular rings. On fetal ultrasonography, vascular rings can be diagnosed by the presence of a U-shaped configuration of the aorta and ductus arteriosus, with the trachea located in between.[6] Initial respiratory symptoms will usually prompt a chest radiograph, on which right-sided or double aortic arch may be noted. Dysphagia may prompt a contrast esophagram, which will classically demonstrate posterior indentation of the esophagus when due to a vascular ring, and anterior esophageal indentation when due to a PAS. Once the diagnosis of a vascular ring has been made in a symptomatic patient, high-quality cross-sectional imaging should be strongly considered to aid in operative planning. Computed tomography (CT) also has the advantage of providing more detailed rendering of the trachea and mainstem bronchi, which can be especially helpful in cases with associated CTS and tracheomalacia. However, intravascular contrast agents will not opacify atretic portions of a nondominant side of a ring.[13] Magnetic resonance (MR) imaging, on the other hand, will better display soft tissue, such as atretic portions of a nondominant arch or the ligamentum. Cardiac gating is usually not required and can be performed with respiratory pauses or quiet breathing.[16] Whereas CT and MR imaging can delineate important subtleties that will influence operative planning, their use should also take into account the clinical status of the patient, specifically that in a critically ill neonate the risk of a contrast load for CT or difficulties with time and sedation required in the MR scanner may outweigh the benefit of the additional anatomic detail this affords. Catheter angiography is of historic interest and is currently rarely used in the workup of patients with vascular rings. Echocardiography is extremely useful to evaluate for the presence of intracardiac defects.

Bronchoscopy, both preoperatively and postoperatively, plays an important role in the management of the child with a vascular ring. This can confirm the diagnosis of tracheal stenosis and tracheomalacia and can accurately document the length of involved trachea. Bronchoscopy can also rule out other causes of respiratory distress, such as subglottic stenosis, and it can also determine whether the bronchi have an abnormal branching pattern. However, severely hypoplastic tracheas may not be able to be traversed at all, and moderately stenotic tracheas may not be safely traversed without compromising ventilation. Inflammation and edema following bronchoscopy can also compromise an already stenotic

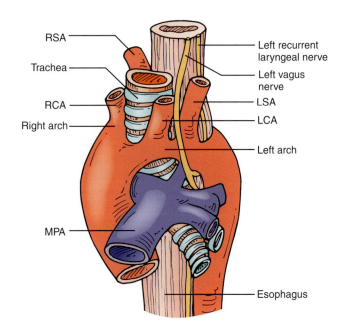

• **Figure 44.2** Balanced double aortic arch. *LCA,* Left common carotid artery; *LSA,* left subclavian artery; *MPA,* main pulmonary artery; *RCA,* right common carotid artery; *RSA,* right subclavian artery. (From Backer CL, Mavroudis C, Stewart RD, et al. Congenital anomalies: vascular rings. In: Patterson GA, Cooper JD, Deslauriers J, et al., eds. *Pearson's Thoracic and Esophageal Surgery.* Churchill Livingstone, Philadelphia, 2008. Reprinted with permission from Elsevier.)

trachea. External compression patterns seen with bronchoscopy may also give a clue as to the type of vascular ring. Innominate artery compression is usually discrete, and compression is noted anterior and to the right. Double aortic arch tends to cause a more complex pattern of distal tracheal compression and may be seen affecting the carina as well.

Specific Anatomic Variations of Vascular Rings

Double Aortic Arch

In double aortic arch the right aortic arch gives rise to the right common carotid and right subclavian arteries, and the left arch gives off the left common carotid and left subclavian arteries (Fig. 44.2). The arches then converge posteriorly to form one descending thoracic aorta. The ring created encircles both the trachea and esophagus. Either arch may be the largest or "dominant" vessel. Right-dominant arch is more common, accounting for approximately 75% of cases. Left-dominant aortic arch accounts for approximately 20% of cases, with the remaining 5% of cases having right and left aortic arches of equal caliber. Surgical correction requires the division of the nondominant vessel. Division of the dominant vessel may result in the development of a pressure gradient between the ascending and descending aorta. It is often useful to measure simultaneous pressure gradients intraoperatively to ensure division of the correct vessel and avoidance of coarctation. An additional pitfall is injury to the recurrent laryngeal nerve. The right recurrent laryngeal nerve passes underneath the right aortic arch itself rather than the right subclavian artery.

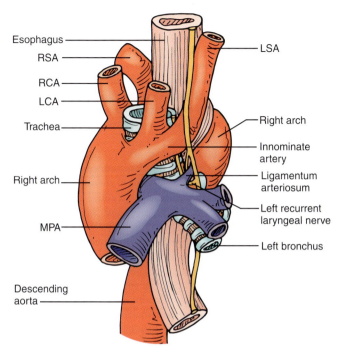

• **Figure 44.3** Right aortic arch. In this example there is mirror-image branching of the common carotid and subclavian arteries, and a left-sided ligamentum "completes" the vascular ring. *LCA,* Left common carotid artery; *LSA,* left subclavian artery; *MPA,* main pulmonary artery; *RCA,* right common carotid artery; *RSA,* right subclavian artery. (From Backer CL, Mavroudis C, Stewart RD, et al. Congenital anomalies: vascular rings. In: Patterson GA, Cooper JD, Deslauriers J, et al., eds. *Pearson's Thoracic and Esophageal Surgery.* Churchill Livingstone, Philadelphia, 2008. Reprinted with permission from Elsevier.)

Right Aortic Arch With Left Ligamentum

In right aortic arch variants of vascular ring the aortic arch is positioned to the right of the trachea and the left-sided ligamentum arteriosum either attached to the descending aorta or the left subclavian artery, thereby "completing" the vascular ring (Fig. 44.3). There are two main variants of right aortic arch: (1) Right aortic arch with retroesophageal left subclavian and (2) right aortic arch with mirror-image branching. In right aortic arch with retroesophageal left subclavian artery—which accounts for approximately 65% of cases—the left subclavian is the most posterior artery on the arch and crosses midline by passing posterior to the esophagus.[17] When a bulbous, aneurysmal deformity of the origin of an aberrant subclavian artery is present, it is termed a *Kommerell diverticulum,* after the German radiologist who first described the anatomy.[18] It is a remnant of the fourth aortic arch and, as such, can be present in a right or left aortic arch and can cause compression of the aerodigestive tract similar to those caused by other vascular rings. In addition to the dysphagia that it causes, there is also risk of further aneurysmal degeneration and rupture.[19] If resection of a Kommerell diverticulum is performed, the subclavian artery can be reimplanted to the ipsilateral common carotid in an end-to-side fashion to avoid upper extremity ischemia.[20] The aberrant subclavian artery can often be sacrificed in the neonatal period without reimplantation, but in older children reimplantation is required to avoid limb ischemia. Mirror-image branching is almost universally associated with congenital heart defects, including tetralogy of

Fallot, transposition of the great arteries, truncus arteriosus, and tricuspid atresia.[15]

Principles of Surgical Repair of Vascular Rings

Approach is typically via thoracotomy on the side opposite the dominant arch. Single lung isolation with a double-lumen endotracheal tube or mainstem bronchus intubation with a single-lumen endotracheal tube on the nonoperative side is performed if possible. The lung is retracted anteriorly, exposing the aortic arch and ductus or ligamentum. A longitudinal incision is made along the parietal pleura overlying the descending aorta and ipsilateral subclavian artery, and this flap is reflected anteriorly. The ductus or ligamentum is sharply dissected, ligated, and divided. Division of the ductus or ligamentum allows the aortic arch to retract cephalad away from the pulmonary artery, relieving some compression of the trachea and esophagus. The surgeon should be aware of the recurrent laryngeal nerve; its course will lie closer to the ductus or ligamentum because the anteriorly reflected pleural flap will place tension on the vagus nerve. The smaller of the two aortic arches is then dissected in preparation for ligation and division. As stated previously, high-quality cross-sectional imaging should allow the surgeon to plan the thoracotomy ipsilateral to the smaller arch. Test occlusion of the smaller arch is performed, and blood pressures are measured from cuffs placed on both arms and one leg as a precautionary measure to rule out any pressure gradient. Each end of the arch is then doubly ligated with purse-string permanent monofilament sutures and then oversewn with a running stitch. After the clamp is released, the two ends should naturally separate as evidence of relief of compression on the trachea and esophagus. The hemostasis of the two divided ends of the ring must be excellent because the distal aspect will retract posteriorly behind the esophagus, and any persistent hemorrhage will be difficult to expose and control.

Several authors have reported success with a video-assisted thoracoscopic surgery (VATS) approach to vascular rings. In 2005 Koontz and colleagues[21] reported an initial experience of VATS division of vascular rings in 13 patients with no complications and only one conversion to an open approach. Kogon and colleagues[22] reported on 47 patients with vascular ring treated with either open or VATS approach in which 14 of 16 cases attempted with VATS approach were successful in dividing the vascular ring, and there was no difference in procedure time, intensive care unit length of stay, or survival between the two approaches.

Pulmonary Artery Sling

PAS is characterized by an aberrant origin of one main pulmonary artery from the contralateral main pulmonary artery. The aberrant pulmonary artery courses between the trachea and esophagus, often causing tracheobronchial compression at the level of the carina (Fig. 44.4). A left pulmonary artery arising from the superior and posterior aspect of the right main pulmonary artery is the more common phenotype. The first successful repair was performed by Potts and colleagues[23] in 1953. The incidence of PAS is much less common than aortic arch anomalies and is estimated at 59 per million live births.[8] Patients with PAS tend to present earlier and with more severe symptoms than patients with vascular rings. Respiratory symptoms in PAS may be due to posterior compression of the trachea by the aberrant pulmonary artery; however, the most severe distress is caused by primary tracheal stenosis with

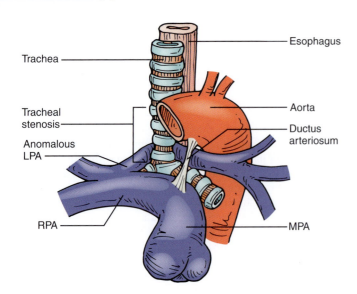

• **Figure 44.4** Pulmonary artery sling. The aberrant left main pulmonary artery courses posterior to the trachea. *LPA,* Left pulmonary artery; *MPA,* main pulmonary artery; *RPA,* right pulmonary artery. (From Fiore AC, Brown JW, Weber TR, et al. Surgical treatment of pulmonary artery sling and tracheal stenosis. *Ann Thorac Surg.* 2005;79[1]:38-46, Fig. 1. Reprinted with permission from Elsevier.)

complete tracheal ring, which can be seen in conjunction with PAS. Therefore a thorough understanding of the management of CTS and tracheal reconstruction is mandatory in the approach to a patient with PAS. PAS is associated with tracheal stenosis and complete tracheal rings in up to 80% of cases and with intracardiac defects in approximately 30% of cases.[24] Interestingly, the extent of tracheal stenosis and complete rings is variable and not limited to the area where the PA sling passes around the trachea. The etiology of PAS and the relation to CTS is not fully understood at this time. CT imaging plays a key role in decision making because this modality can accurately document both the length of tracheal stenosis and the relation to the PAS. If the stenosis is severe and presents in the neonatal period, it can be the case that the lumen is so small that it cannot be safely traversed with a bronchoscope. Presentation may require urgent intervention because ventilation with the endotracheal tube positioned above the stenosis may be extremely tenuous in the most severe cases. In general, symptoms include respiratory distress, recurrent respiratory tract infections, intermittent air trapping, migrating atelectasis, and ALTEs. Ultimately, almost all patients with PAS and CTS become symptomatic; however, some patients with isolated PAS may present late if at all. Repair is recommended in all patients with PAS and tracheal stenosis at the time of diagnosis. Age at presentation is typically determined by the degree of tracheal stenosis.

The principles of surgical repair of PAS with tracheal stenosis are translocation of the aberrant pulmonary artery to an anatomically normal course and reconstruction of abnormal trachea. If tracheal stenosis is present, approach is via median sternotomy. However, isolated PA sling can be repaired without cardiopulmonary bypass via thoracotomy. In children with PA sling and CTS, the patient is placed on cardiopulmonary bypass with moderate hypothermia by cannulating the ascending aorta and right atrial appendage. The aberrant artery is harvested at its origin and then reimplanted in the normal position on the main pulmonary trunk. Great care is taken to avoid kinking. There is some evidence that

cardiopulmonary bypass reduces the rate of late occlusion of the translocated pulmonary artery because initial attempts at repair were performed without cardiopulmonary bypass with high rates of late occlusion.[25] Cardiopulmonary bypass also facilitates tracheal reconstruction in neonates and infants. Options for tracheal reconstruction include resection of the stenotic segment with end-to-end anastomosis for short-segment disease and slide tracheoplasty for long-segment disease. Generally, a few tracheal rings can be resected and still allow for a tension-free end-to-end anastomosis.[26]

Cases of longer-segment stenosis are approached with slide tracheoplasty. When slide tracheoplasty is performed, the trachea is transected horizontally at the midpoint of the stenotic segment. Then a vertical incision is made along the anterior side of one end and the posterior side of the other end, and the two segments are anastomosed together with a long elliptical suture line (Fig. 44.5). This may be performed with a running absorbable suture. Detailed initial work by Grillo and colleagues, who popularized the technique in adults, demonstrated that slide tracheoplasty doubles the circumference and quadruples the cross-sectional area of the stenotic trachea.[26-28] Outcomes following slide tracheoplasty have improved over time and are now considered excellent at major centers even with neonatal cases. However, a multidisciplinary approach including otolaryngology and CT surgery is often required, and inflammation and granulation tissue at the suture line of the tracheal reconstruction can prove challenging and require multiple bronchoscopic interventions. Mortality is increased in the presence of other comorbid conditions, particularly congenital heart disease. In a series of 101 pediatric patients undergoing slide tracheoplasty for long-segment CTS in a 17-year single-center experience, Butler and colleagues reported an overall survival of 88.2%.[29] Other earlier described techniques of tracheal reconstruction, such as augmentation with autologous pericardium or cartilage,[30] were challenged by significant postoperative complications such as dehiscence and in the current era are now reserved primarily for the salvage setting.

PAS may also present with tracheal stenosis that has abnormal bronchial bridging patterns, such as bridging bronchus, which complicates standard tracheal reconstruction techniques. Alterations of slide tracheoplasty have been described to conform to these abnormal branching patterns.[24,29] The technique of side-to-side tracheobronchoplasty has also been described for patients with tracheal stenosis and a bridging bronchus and can be safely performed in neonatal patients as a one-stage procedure, along with repair of PAS.[31] In this procedure the edges of the trachea and right upper lobe bronchus are opened longitudinally, then anastomosed in a side-to-side fashion, which preserves the length of the native trachea without placing tension on the anastomosis (Fig. 44.6).

Innominate Artery Compression

External compression of the trachea from a posteriorly displaced, crossing innominate artery can cause respiratory symptoms and deformation of the trachea similar to that seen in true vascular rings.[32] Historically, many patients with innominate artery indentation of the trachea did not require surgery. In a 1969 review of 285 patients with the diagnosis of innominate artery compression of the trachea, Mustard and colleagues[33] reported that only 13.7% ultimately required surgical repair. Today, patients who are clinically symptomatic are recommended for anterior innominate artery pexy or aortopexy, as initially described by Gross. The principle

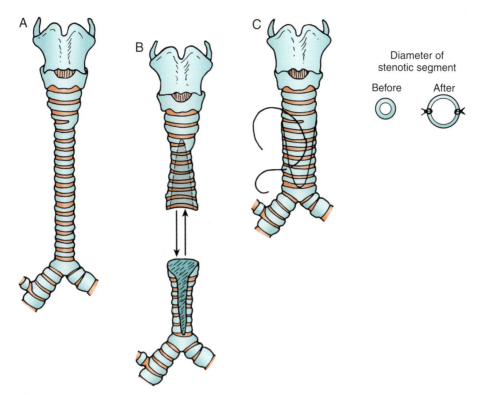

• **Figure 44.5** Technique of slide tracheoplasty, as popularized by Grillo. The stenotic trachea (A) is transected at its midpoint. The two cut ends are incised longitudinally on opposite ends (B). Then the two ends are brought together using an elliptical anastomosis (C). (From Fiore AC, Brown JW, Weber TR, et al. Surgical treatment of pulmonary artery sling and tracheal stenosis. *Ann Thorac Surg.* 2005;79[1]:38-46, Fig. 4. Reprinted with permission from Elsevier.)

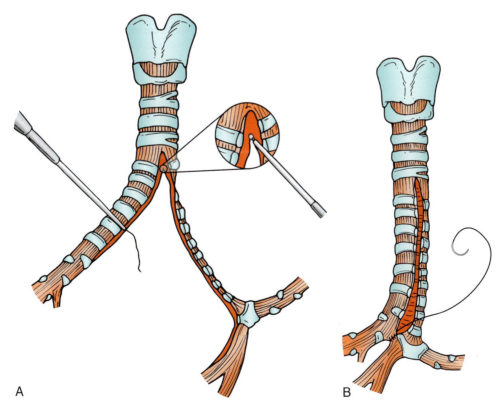

• **Figure 44.6** Side-to-side tracheobronchoplasty. When tracheal stenosis occurs in abnormal bronchial patterns, such as bridging bronchus, the bronchi are opened longitudinally (A) and anastomosed in a side-to-side fashion (B). (From Ragalie WS, Chun RH, Martin T, et al. Side-to-side tracheobronchoplasty to reconstruct complex tracheobronchial stenosis. *Ann Thorac Surg.* 2017;104[6]:666-673, Fig. 1. Reprinted with permission from Elsevier.)

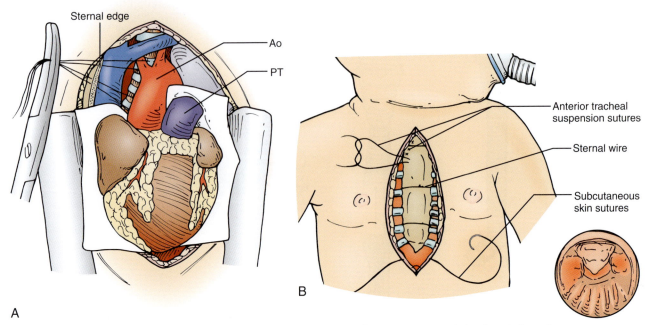

• **Figure 44.7** Anterior tracheal suspension. Pledgeted monofilament sutures are tied to the anterior wall of the trachea and passed through the right sternal plate (A). With the sternum closed, the sutures are tied (B) while simultaneously looking with the bronchoscope *(inset)*. *Ao,* Aorta; *PT,* pulmonary trunk. (From Mitchell ME, Rumman N, Chun RH, et al. Anterior tracheal suspension for tracheobronchomalacia in infants and children. *Ann Thorac Surg.* 2014;98[4]:1246-1253, Fig. 2. Reprinted with permission from Elsevier.)

of aortopexy is to bring the vascular structures away from the trachea. Aortopexy has been described by both right and left thoracotomy, mini–anterior thoracotomy, or thoracoscopy, and full or partial median sternotomy. Pledgeted permanent monofilament sutures are passed through the edges of the sternal plate, and the sternum is closed. The sutures are then tied down to suspend the aorta anteriorly from the trachea.

Tracheomalacia

The technique of anterior tracheal suspension has been described as a surgical treatment for directly addressing tracheomalacia.[34] In this technique the trachea is exposed often via median sternotomy, and pledgeted permanent monofilament sutures are placed on the anterior surface of the malacic trachea. The sutures are passed through the right sternal plate and the sternum is closed (Fig. 44.7). Then, with the use of simultaneous fiberoptic bronchoscopy, the sutures are tied down with just the right amount of tension to ensure optimal luminal enlargement without distortion. This technique can be added to other procedures involving tracheal and great vessel reconstruction without significantly increasing the operative time. We have found that it is a particularly useful adjunct to tracheal reconstruction for CTS because these patients often have distal malacia as well. Other experimental surgical treatments that have shown promise for treating tracheomalacia include bioresorbable airway splinting.[35] Stem cell–based, tissue engineered tracheal replacement for severe unrepairable long-segment tracheal stenosis has been described.[36] Further reports will define the role that these exciting new therapies will play in the management of tracheomalacia and tracheal stenosis.

Conclusion

Vascular rings and PAS represent a challenging and potentially rewarding spectrum of congenital heart disease. Knowledge of the management of the tracheal diseases associated with vascular rings is crucial to caring for these patients, as is close collaboration with ancillary pediatric specialties.

Selected References

A complete list of references is available at ExpertConsult.com.

3. Backer CL, Mavroudis C. Congenital Heart Surgery Nomenclature and Database Project: vascular rings, tracheal stenosis, pectus excavatum. *Ann Thorac Surg.* 2000;69:S308–S318.
8. Yu JM, et al. The prevalence and clinical impact of pulmonary artery sling on school-aged children: a large-scale screening study. *Pediatr Pulmonol.* 2008;43:656–661.
17. Backer CL, et al. Vascular rings. *Semin Pediatr Surg.* 2016;25:165–175.
22. Kogon BE, Forbess JM, Wulkan ML, Kirshbom PM, Kanter KR. Video-assisted thoracoscopic surgery: is it a superior technique for the division of vascular rings in children? *Congenit Heart Dis.* 2007;2:130–133.
24. Backer CL, et al. Pulmonary artery sling: current results with cardiopulmonary bypass. *J Thorac Cardiovasc Surg.* 2012;143:144–151.
26. Backer CL, Mavroudis C, Gerber ME, Holinger LD. Tracheal surgery in children: an 18-year review of four techniques. *Eur J Cardiothorac Surg.* 2001;19:777–784.
34. Mitchell ME, et al. Anterior tracheal suspension for tracheobronchomalacia in infants and children. *Ann Thorac Surg.* 2014;98:1246–1253.
36. Elliott MJ, et al. Stem-cell-based, tissue engineered tracheal replacement in a child: a 2-year follow-up study. *Lancet.* 2012;380:994–1000.

45

Coarctation of the Aorta

JENNIFER S. NELSON, MD, MS; MATTHEW L. STONE, MD, PHD; JAMES J. GANGEMI, MD

Coarctation of the aorta (CoA) is a heterogenous lesion that generally refers to a congenital narrowing of the thoracic aorta, directly opposite, proximal, or distal to the ductus arteriosus, resulting in a pressure gradient. True coarctation is a distinct, shelf-like thickening or infolding of the aortic media into the lumen of the aorta, although coarctation has also been used to describe a long-segment narrowing, or hypoplasia of a segment of the aorta.[1-7]

CoA is relatively common. The estimated prevalence is approximately 3 cases per 10,000 live births worldwide. Aortic coarctation is recognized in 5% to 8% of patients with congenital heart disease excluding mitral valve prolapse or related bicuspid aortic valve. The male to female ratio is between 1.27:1 and 1.74:1.[8]

CoA was first described in 1760 by Morgagni, but it was not until the 1920s that it became recognized as a cause of shortened life span, hypertension, endocarditis, and congestive heart failure (CHF).[9] Of the patients with CoA who survived infancy, mean life expectancy in the presurgical era was only three decades.[10] A pivotal time in the evolution of the treatment of infants with CoA and other aortic arch anomalies was the late 1970s, when prostaglandin E_1 (PGE_1) became available to maintain patency of the ductus arteriosus.[11] This drug allowed preoperative stabilization of critically ill neonates presenting with shock.

Surgical repair was pioneered by Craford and Gross in the 1940s. In the decades that followed, various surgical and interventional techniques have been developed, leading to dramatically improved patient outcomes.[12-14]

Anatomy, Embryology, and Classification Systems

An aortic coarctation usually lies in close proximity to the ductus arteriosus or ligamentum arteriosum, commonly just distal to the left subclavian artery (Fig. 45.1). An isolated coarctation is more commonly found in older children. In infants, CoA is commonly associated with hypoplasia of the aortic isthmus and other cardiac anomalies.[3,15,16] Aortic hypoplasia is defined as a narrowed external diameter of an aortic segment with a normal aortic media. Proximal and distal transverse arch hypoplasia are defined as 60% and 50%, respectively, of the diameter of the ascending aorta; isthmic hypoplasia is defined as less than 40% of the diameter of the ascending aorta.[17] Some degree of arch hypoplasia is present in most normal neonates.[18,19]

There are two main embryologic theories to explain the development of coarctation. Some investigators have suggested that ductus smooth muscle tissue migrates into the periductal aorta and subsequently causes constriction after birth as the ductus closes.[19,20] A second theory to explain the development of CoA cites decreased aortic flow secondary to associated cardiac defects. The flow theory is supported by the fact that constellations of intracardiac anomalies with decreased aortic flow patterns have an increased incidence of CoA and other arch anomalies and that constellations with increased aortic flow (because of decreased pulmonary flow) rarely are associated with CoA.[17,19,21,22] Lymphatic obstruction and related aortic compression is another theory described in Turner syndrome.[23]

Historically coarctations were classified as either adult (postductal) or infantile (preductal). The adult form referred to a discrete narrowing, which was more properly described as juxtaductal in location.[1] The infantile or preductal form was characterized by more diffuse narrowing of an aortic segment in addition to the juxtaductal narrowing. A more modern classification from the Congenital Heart Surgery Nomenclature and Database Project, which guides the surgical approach, recognizes three categories: (1) isolated coarctation, (2) coarctation with ventricular septal defect (VSD), and (3) coarctation with complex intracardiac anomaly.[7]

Associated Defects

Coarctation is often associated with other defects. Bicuspid aortic valve and VSD represent the two most common associated defects, present in 40% to 50% and 25% to 40%, respectively.[15,24,25] CoA is also frequently associated with complex heart disease and other left-sided obstructive lesions. For example, Shone's syndrome describes multilevel left-sided obstruction consisting of CoA, supravalvular mitral stenosis, parachute mitral valve, and subaortic stenosis.[26] Right-sided obstructive lesions such as tetralogy of Fallot, tricuspid atresia, pulmonary stenosis, and atresia are rarely associated with CoA. Intracranial aneurysms represent a potentially life-threatening associated extracardiac abnormality.[27]

CoA has a known association with several chromosomal abnormality syndromes, in particular trisomy 13 and 18, Turner, Noonan, Jacobsen, Williams-Beuren, Ellis-van Creveld, and PHACES syndrome.[28-30]

Newborns and Infants

Pathophysiology

Among patients with CoA, young age at presentation closely correlates with severity of obstruction and associated defects. This

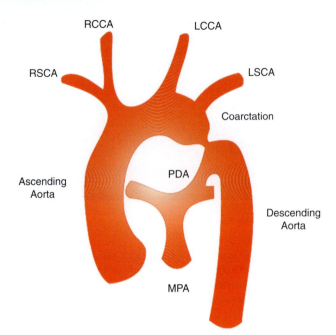

• **Figure 45.1** Isolated coarctation of the aorta with preductal coarctation. *LCCA,* Left common carotid artery; *LSCA,* left subclavian artery; *MPA,* main pulmonary artery; *PDA,* patent ductus arteriosus; *RCCA,* right common carotid artery; *RSCA,* right subclavian artery.

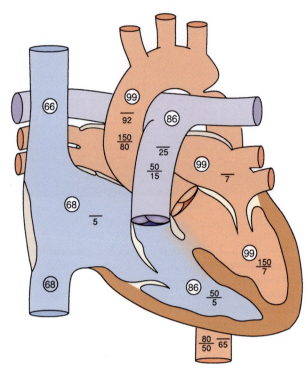

• **Figure 45.2** Pathophysiology of coarctation of the aorta and ventricular septal defect in infancy. There is a step-up in oxygen saturation between the right atrium (68%) and the right ventricle (86%), indicating a left-to-right shunt at the ventricular level, which increases pulmonary blood flow and pressure (50/15). Left ventricular pressure (150/7) and ascending aortic pressure (150/80) are elevated compared with descending aortic pressure (80/50) because of the coarctation.

correlation may be explained by the predictable timing and process of ductal closure.[31] When ductal closure causes aortic obstruction, a severe increase in left ventricular (LV) afterload results. LV ejection fraction decreases acutely in response to the higher afterload, because there is no time for compensatory development of muscle hypertrophy. Such increased afterload results in elevated ventricular wall tension, decreased myocardial perfusion pressure, and, in extreme cases, ischemic myocardium.

The increased LV end-diastolic pressure and increased left atrial pressure cause a left-to-right shunt at the foramen ovale and hence increased pulmonary blood flow (Q_p) that leads to clinical heart failure. Pulmonary hypertension occurs secondary to (1) increased Q_p and (2) increased pulmonary venous pressures secondary to left atrial hypertension.[32] The volume- and pressure-loaded right ventricle often demonstrates depressed function.

This pattern of CHF is exaggerated in the presence of severe CoA with a large VSD (Fig. 45.2). LV blood is ejected into the right ventricle and pulmonary circulation at systemic pressures, leading to a substantially increased pulmonary-to-systemic blood flow ratio (Q_p:Q_s). As the ductus closes, Q_s decreases further, and Q_p:Q_s may become much greater than 1:1. Systemic hypoperfusion leads to the oliguria and metabolic acidosis observed in many infants on presentation.[32]

Other associated cardiac lesions may influence the hemodynamic burden. For example, in cases in which the ductus remains patent, the right ventricle is able to support systemic perfusion. In cases of severe coarctation in neonates, "critical coarctation," adequate systemic cardiac output can be maintained by the right ventricle only across a patent ductus arteriosus. These infants present in profound shock with systemic hypotension, acidosis, and tachypnea (from pulmonary hypertension) when the ductus closes. They emergently require intravenous PGE₁ to open the ductus and restore systemic perfusion. Hypertrophy and volume overload help the

right ventricle to maintain adequate cardiac output, especially in the presence of a VSD. Infants with atrioventricular septal defects and coarctation can experience more severe heart failure for equivalent degrees of aortic obstruction than infants without atrioventricular septal defects because of the addition of atrioventricular valve regurgitation to the left-to-right shunting described previously.

Presentation

Infants under 3 months of age with CoA have characteristic presenting signs (Box 45.1). CHF is often present. Poor peripheral perfusion, acidosis, tachypnea, and failure to thrive are common.[33,34] The physical examination reveals an ejection murmur along the left sternal border and in the left subscapular area. The precordial impulse is prominent and often accompanied by a systolic thrill if the infant has intracardiac defects. Hepatomegaly and a gallop rhythm point to CHF. Femoral pulses are diminished in most, but not all, cases. CoA is difficult to diagnose prenatally due to flow across the ductus arteriosus in utero.[35] Less than 25% of neonates in the United States requiring neonatal surgery for coarctation are diagnosed prenatally.[36,37] It is a diagnosis that is also frequently missed in the newborn period. Patients are often not referred until they are in shock or renal failure. Less than 30% of infants with physical findings of CoA are referred with the correct diagnosis.[38,39] Most infants are thought to have other diagnoses despite decreased femoral pulses in 88% of cases because decreased femoral pulse can also be a sign of shock from other

Tachypnea
Cyanosis
Poor perfusion
Difficulty feeding
Failure to thrive
Hepatomegaly
Cardiomegaly
Decreased femoral pulses
Murmur
Metabolic acidosis
Respiratory failure

Data from Goldman S, Hernandez J, Pappas G. Results of surgical treatment of coarctation of the aorta in the critically ill neonate. Including the influence of pulmonary artery banding. J Thorac Cardiovasc Surg. 1986;91:732-737; Yee ES, Soifer SJ, Turley K, et al. Infant coarctation: a spectrum in clinical presentation and treatment. Ann Thorac Surg. 1986;42:488-493.

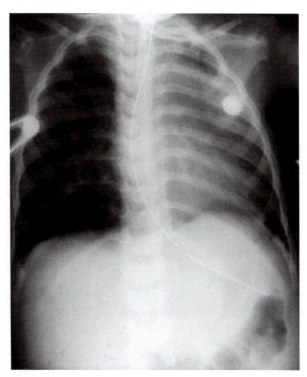

• **Figure 45.3** Chest radiograph of an infant with coarctation of the aorta, showing hallmark signs of cardiomegaly and pulmonary congestion.

causes (such as neonatal sepsis).[39] Conversely, patients may be erroneously suspected of having a coarctation when they are in shock. Even in patients over 1 year of age, the diagnosis is usually delayed despite classic findings of murmur and upper extremity hypertension.[40] In contrast to older children, infants presenting before 5 days of age rarely have upper extremity hypertension due to depressed cardiac output. After 5 days, hypertension becomes more common, and after 15 days the incidence is 86%.[39] Aortic obstruction is the most likely diagnosis when these physical findings are accompanied by a gradient between upper and lower extremity pulses and systolic pressure. However, the absence of such a gradient does not rule out the diagnosis of aortic obstruction, and, in fact, when distal (systemic) perfusion is maintained by a patent ductus arteriosus, the pressures in the lower extremities may be equal to or even higher than those in the upper extremities.

The absence of a systolic pressure gradient in patients with CoA usually has one of three anatomic or physiologic explanations: (1) The ductus may be patent such that the right ventricle provides flow to the lower body. These patients may have differential cyanosis with lower oxygen saturations recorded from the toe than the preductal hand. (2) LV function may be so poor that systemic hypotension makes it impossible to detect a gradient between upper and lower extremities. (3) Finally, in rare instances the right subclavian artery has an aberrant origin distal to the coarctation, thus eliminating any gradient. The physician should never exclude the diagnosis of CoA solely because of failure to detect a gradient in pulse volume or systolic pressures between upper and lower extremities.

Evaluation

Electrocardiographic (ECG) findings are influenced by the presence of associated intracardiac anomalies and the age at presentation. Infants most commonly show right ventricular hypertrophy and later develop biventricular hypertrophy. A minority of patients have LV hypertrophy alone. ST-segment depression and T-wave inversion in V_5 and V_6 can also be found.[41]

The chest radiograph of infants with CoA is different from that of older patients with isolated CoA. In infancy, cardiomegaly and pulmonary congestion are hallmarks (Fig. 45.3).[41] Two-dimensional echocardiography with Doppler (echo Doppler) is a sensitive and

specific diagnostic method for infants with CoA (Fig. 45.4) and associated intracardiac anomalies.[25,42,43] In experienced hands, diagnosis of CoA by echo Doppler achieved 95% sensitivity and 99% specificity.[44] Prenatal diagnosis of CoA based on normal fetal aortic arch growth curves has evolved significantly.[45-47]

The role of cardiac catheterization in CoA continues to develop in light of the greater use of noninvasive diagnostic techniques. Cardiac catheterization and angiography are desirable if echocardiography fails to delineate the anatomy completely or where balloon angioplasty or stent placement offers definitive treatment (Fig. 45.5).

Medical Management

The primary objective in the medical management of neonates with critical CoA is to maintain ductal patency with PGE_1. It is our practice to administer PGE_1 to every newborn in shock until critical coarctation, interrupted aortic arch, or other ductus-dependent lesions have been excluded.

Although shock and CHF usually improve after PGE_1 administration, some infants will require inotropic support and mechanical ventilation in addition to PGE_1. Hyperoxia and hypocarbia should be avoided to minimize pulmonary overcirculation.

PGE_1 is given initially in doses of 0.05 mcg/kg/min to 0.1 mcg/kg/min but can be increased gradually to 0.2 mcg/kg/min if it is not effective at the lower dose. Maximal response occurs 15 minutes to 4 hours after the start of the infusion.[48] Side effects and complications of PGE_1 include cutaneous vasodilation, hypotension, rhythm or conduction disturbances, respiratory depression and apnea, fever, jitteriness or seizure activity, increased infection, diarrhea, necrotizing enterocolitis, metabolic derangements, and (rarely) coagulopathy.[49,50] Many side effects are related to high doses, longer infusion periods, and poorer general medical condition at the start of therapy.[49]

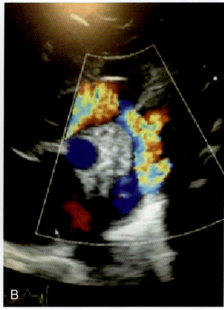
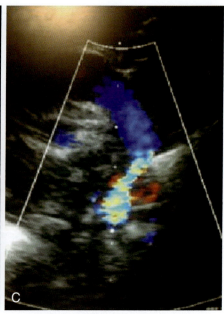

• **Figure 45.4** Echocardiography in infants with coarctation of the aorta demonstrating characteristic flow acceleration and discrete narrowing in the setting of nonductal and ductal dependent circulations. A, Discrete aortic coarctation without patent ductus arteriosus (PDA). B, Discrete aortic coarctation with PDA in an infant who was prostaglandin dependent preoperatively. C, Recurrent coarctation.

McElhinney and coworkers[51] found an elevated risk of necrotizing enterocolitis in neonates whose highest dose of prostaglandin was greater than 0.05 mcg/kg/min. It is common practice to decrease the dose to 0.01 to 0.02 mcg/kg/min as soon as the desired effect has been achieved.[52]

Endotracheal intubation and mechanical ventilation are frequently required in the newborn with critical coarctation because of CHF, shock, and the risk of apnea from PGE_1 therapy. If PGE_1 is begun in the absence of shock and apnea, ventilatory support is not mandatory, provided that resources for intubation are immediately available. In newborns with isolated CoA the expected decrease in the pulmonary vascular resistance from ventilation and PGE_1 does not affect the hemodynamics. Conversely, in those with CoA and VSD, more blood will be shunted left to right as the pulmonary vascular resistance falls. Ventilation must be carefully controlled to help balance Q_p:Q_s in patients with arch obstruction and left-to-right intracardiac shunt. This requires a ventilation strategy designed to increase pulmonary vascular resistance by lowering the fraction of inspired oxygen (FiO_2) to maintain O_2 saturations of approximately 85% and adjusting minute ventilation to achieve a pCO_2 of 40 to 50 mm Hg. Maintaining Q_p:Q_s as close to 1:1 as possible is a necessary strategy for maintaining adequate systemic blood flow. Normal acid-base balance with lactate levels below 2 mmol/L can provide an indication of adequate oxygen delivery. Mixed venous oxygen saturation is not useful as a measure of systemic oxygen delivery if the measurement is obtained from the right atrium in the presence of a significant atrial shunt, which raises right atrial saturation.

Fluid and electrolyte balance should also be optimized before surgery. Severe metabolic acidosis (pH < 7.2) from systemic hypoperfusion is corrected with bicarbonate administration (0.5 to 1 mEq/kg), given slowly. Bicarbonate doses can be repeated until the metabolic acidosis has resolved; however, inability to correct the acidosis with multiple doses of bicarbonate suggests persistent acid production. This could be associated with poor myocardial function or ischemic tissue, such as ischemic bowel. Severe anemia can also contribute to persistent acidosis.

Although it is appropriate to correct dehydration, fluid volume expansion, even in the hypotensive infant with critical coarctation, may be hazardous. Hypotension is usually not caused by hypovolemia in this setting but rather by aortic obstruction, ductus closure, and ventricular failure. During the initial resuscitation in the emergency department, a small fluid bolus (normal saline, 5 mL/kg) may be useful as a therapeutic trial. An additional bolus is justified only if there is a favorable response to the first bolus. Infants with prolonged shock and acidosis who develop fluid loss from capillary leak syndrome may require repeated fluid boluses. Some infants develop systemic vasodilation after PGE_1 and require titrated isotonic fluid administration (5 mL/kg per dose).

Conversely, the newborn with an established diagnosis of CoA and CHF who is responding to PGE_1 therapy should receive fluid restriction (70% to 80% of maintenance requirements) to limit the salt and water load in the face of heart failure. Another scenario involves the newborn who remains hypotensive despite restoration of ductal patency with PGE_1. Poor ventricular function is the likely cause of persistent hypotension in this setting, and the infant may benefit from inotropic support rather than volume expansion. Low-dose dopamine (5 to 7 mcg/kg/min) may be useful in this situation. With a patent ductus, balanced circulation, and necessary inotropic support the infant should be readily stabilized during the preoperative period. Table 45.1 summarizes preoperative management strategies for infants with critical CoA.

Most infants can be adequately stabilized with the measures described herein, and surgery should be delayed for 12 to 24 hours until metabolic derangements have been corrected. Symptomatic infants who are unresponsive to PGE_1 have a high mortality. The options for these patients include emergency repair of CoA with or without cardiopulmonary bypass. Additional diagnoses should be sought if the patient is difficult to stabilize.

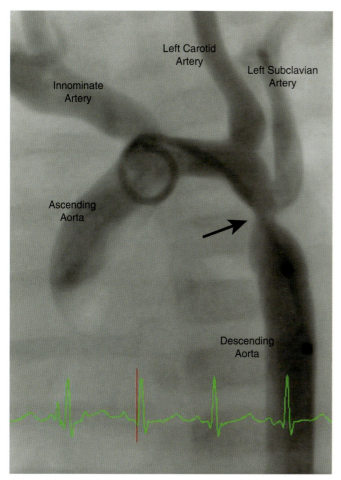

Left Carotid Artery

Left Subclavian Artery

Innominate Artery

Ascending Aorta

Descending Aorta

• **Figure 45.5** Angiogram of aortic coarctation in an infant. The solid line black arrow denotes discrete coarctation just distal to the takeoff of the left subclavian artery in what is commonly the juxtaductal position. (From Vergales JE, Gangemi JJ, Rhueban KS, et al. Coarctation of the aorta—the current state of surgical and transcatheter therapies. *Curr Cardiol Rev.* 2013;9:211-219, with permission.)

TABLE 45.1	Preoperative Management Strategies for Infants With Critical Coarctation
Drugs	PGE_1 0.05-0.2 mcg/kg/min Calcium supplementation Correction of acidosis by $NaHCO_3$ administration Inotropic support as needed for poor ventricular function (e.g., dopamine 5 mcg/kg/min)
Ventilation	Controlled ventilation with avoidance of hyperoxia or hypocarbia to maintain balanced circulation (Q_p:Q_s 1 : 1)
Fluid management	Fluid bolus administration as indicated by urine output in 5 mL/kg aliquots of isotonic solution Decreased maintenance requirement in normotensive patient
Laboratory studies	Serial electrolytes Calcium Creatinine Type and cross-match CBC Arterial blood gas Liver function tests
Imaging	CXR Echocardiogram (evaluate cardiac function, aortic and ductal anatomy, and concomitant intracardiac defects)

CBC, Complete blood count; *CXR*, chest x-ray; *PGE_1*, prostaglandin E_1.

Timing of Intervention

The objective of surgical treatment of CoA is relief of aortic obstruction with minimal risk of repeat stenosis. The debate surrounding the ideal age for repair has focused on the issues of operative mortality in infancy, the risk of restenosis, and the likelihood of persistent hypertension after repair. Neonates presenting with CHF should undergo repair as soon as they are metabolically stable. Nonetheless, the optimal surgical technique and whether single- or two-stage repair of associated defects is appropriate are still debated.[53]

Anesthetic Management

A preoperative understanding of concomitant congenital anomalies is critical to the anesthetic management of the infant with CoA. Transthoracic echocardiography is used to detect the potential presence of concomitant intracardiac anomalies and to assess biventricular function. Initial evaluation of the airway should focus on the presence of structural facial abnormalities that may influence management of the airway. For CoA repair approached via median sternotomy using cardiopulmonary bypass, a transesophageal echocardiogram probe should be placed in addition to standard monitors.

Routine monitoring for off-pump repair of CoA includes ECG leads, a urinary catheter, temperature probe, and arterial and central venous access. Central venous access is important for drug administration and pressure monitoring, particularly with more complex intracardiac lesions. Large-bore peripheral intravenous catheters are placed for volume infusion as needed. Packed red blood cells are available in the operating room during the repair of CoA in the event of hemorrhage. Irradiated blood products should be used to prevent graft-versus-host disease in all infant CoA repairs unless DiGeorge syndrome has been specifically excluded. Antibiotic prophylaxis (cefazolin 30 mg/kg, or 2 g for patients >60 kg, or cefuroxime 50 mg/kg, or 1.5 g for patients >50 kg) is administered preoperatively, within 60 minutes of skin incision. To ensure consistent antibiotic administration, it is our standard practice to give antibiotics at the time of skin preparation.

For systemic pressure monitoring, and to monitor acid-base status, hemoglobin, and calcium levels, a radial arterial line is placed. Use of the right radial artery allows for monitoring of coronary and cerebral perfusion because the right subclavian artery is typically proximal to the aortic cross-clamp during surgical repair. Infants with an aberrant right subclavian artery arising distal to the site of CoA may necessitate placement of a proximal aortic catheter for pressure monitoring. If sacrifice of the left subclavian artery is necessary during the repair, intraoperative and postoperative assessment of left upper extremity perfusion is imperative. A femoral arterial line is not routinely placed; however, a blood pressure cuff is placed on the lower extremity to evaluate adequacy of perfusion during and after cross-clamp.

Induction of anesthesia for neonates and infants is usually via the intravenous route with additional inhalational supplementation as needed. For maintenance of anesthesia, volatile agents (typically isoflurane or sevoflurane) are used throughout the operation and may be titrated to assist with blood pressure control. Intravenous narcotics are used for analgesia. A caudal block or epidural is an option in select patients. Neonates and infants are usually kept intubated at the end of the surgical procedure.

Nicardipine is used first line for blood pressure management because it provides direct pharmacologic action on the vascular smooth muscle with minimal myocardial depression.[54] Acidosis and hypotension may immediately follow cross-clamp removal, necessitating aggressive correction of acid-base balance and management of mean arterial pressures with alpha-adrenergic agents to ensure adequacy of end-organ perfusion. This phenomenon is rare and minimized by thoughtful communication between surgeon and anesthesiologist to coordinate a slow cross-clamp removal with empiric supportive measures. Although spinal cord perfusion is a significant concern through the cross-clamp period, prevention of hypotension and acidosis, use of passive cooling, and minimization of cross-clamp times has resulted in a very rare incidence of ischemic spinal cord complications.[55]

Surgical Repair of Coarctation

In general, we approach repair of CoA in neonates and infants with surgery. Four operative procedures are commonly used: (1) resection of the stenotic segment and end-to-end aortic anastomosis (EEA), (2) CoA resection with extended EEA, (3) patch augmentation, and (4) subclavian flap aortoplasty (Fig. 45.6). The optimal procedure depends on the age of the patient, the need for growth of the repair, the length and complexity of the stenosis, and the surgeon's preference. Table 45.2 shows the frequency of coarctation repair techniques used in 2474 patients (75% neonates or infants) with isolated CoA or hypoplastic aortic arch between 2006 and 2010.[55]

Resection with EEA is a surgical technique that was historically used in neonates via a left thoracotomy. Advantages include removing all ductal tissue from the repair site and preserving the left subclavian artery. Unfortunately, many neonates have some degree of hypoplasia of the aortic arch as well as extensive ductal tissue in the periductal aorta, making simple resection and EEA insufficient to provide adequate relief from the coarctation. A modification of that technique, called extended EEA, uses a beveled end-to-side anastomosis of the descending aorta to a separate incision extended onto the underside of the aortic arch, proximal to the hypoplastic segment (see Fig. 45.6B). This approach provides superior relief from the various levels of obstruction found in neonatal coarctation.[56,57] The incidence of recurrent coarctation may be decreased with this approach because all ductal tissue and tissue with tubular hypoplasia is excised. Extended EEA repair has become the procedure of choice for neonatal coarctation in most centers.[55] Extended EEA repair is usually performed through a left thoracotomy but can be performed via a median sternotomy on cardiopulmonary bypass when associated defects are repaired at the same setting (e.g., VSD closure).[58]

The subclavian flap repair uses the ipsilateral subclavian artery as a fold-down flap to enlarge the coarctation site (see Fig. 45.6B).[59] It is performed via a left thoracotomy approach. The use of viable native tissue allows growth of the repaired segment, and tension is avoided at the anastomosis. Criticisms of the technique include the obligatory sacrifice of the subclavian artery, inability to correct

arch hypoplasia in some cases, the low but constant risk of extremity ischemia, subtle impairment of arm temperature, strength or length over time, as well as late cerebral ischemic syndromes by a steal mechanism.[58-60] The subclavian flap technique has fallen out of favor due to the higher late recurrence rate of coarctation following use of the subclavian flap compared with extended EEA.[61] If a subclavian flap repair is contemplated, arterial monitoring lines, blood pressure cuffs, and even blood gas sampling should be avoided on the repair side to avoid ischemic complications.

Prosthetic patch augmentation is a third surgical option that has been used successfully in neonates.[62] A longitudinal incision opens the coarcted segment, which is then covered with a Dacron (polyester) or polytetrafluoroethylene patch (see Fig. 45.6B). This approach avoids an extensive dissection and the attendant risk of sacrificing intercostal collaterals. Unfortunately, long-term follow-up shows that children with a prosthetic patch aortoplasty are at risk for aneurysm development on the aortic wall opposite the patch (particularly if the posterior shelf is resected, thus theoretically weakening the aortic wall opposite the patch). This approach has generally been reserved for coarctation repair in selected circumstances.[63,64]

When concomitant cardiac procedures or transverse arch repairs are performed, CoA should be repaired by the median sternotomy approach. In neonates in particular the proximal descending aorta can be mobilized and brought cephalad and anterior to join the undersurface of the arch. Alternately, the lesser curve of the aorta may be opened and the underside of the arch augmented with patch material such as pulmonary homograft in a Norwood-style arch reconstruction.[65] Patch augmentation may be accomplished with or without coarctectomy and reanastomosis of the back wall. The incision in the descending aorta should extend 10 to 15 mm beyond the ductal insertion site, and the toe of the patch should be broad to create a wide anastomosis that will prevent recoarctation. Hypothermic circulatory arrest is generally used for these procedures, although novel selective perfusion techniques have been described.[66]

Surgical Complications and Postoperative Critical Care Management

Surgical morbidity after repair of CoA includes anastomotic bleeding, cardiac arrest, chylothorax, gastrointestinal bleeding, phrenic nerve injury, postcoarctectomy hypertension, recurrent laryngeal nerve injury, seizures, and spinal cord injury (Fig. 45.7). In the landmark review by Brewer and associates,[67] 12,532 coarctectomies were described, and spinal cord ischemic injury occurred in 51 cases (0.41%), but rarely in infants and neonates. There was no association with cross-clamp time. Lack of collaterals and the intrinsic anatomy of the anterior spinal artery may contribute. A 2012 study of the STS Congenital Heart Surgery Database found no occurrences of spinal cord injury out of 973 coarctation repairs.[55]

Respiratory Complications. Newborns and infants with CoA and VSD may have a reactive pulmonary circulation and pulmonary hypertension. Patients at risk should receive intravenous sedation and controlled ventilation during the first 12 to 24 hours after surgery. Documented pulmonary hypertension should be initially treated with inhaled nitric oxide. Thereafter these patients can usually be weaned from mechanical ventilation and extubated.

Stridor may become evident at the time of extubation secondary to recurrent laryngeal nerve manipulation or injury, leading to

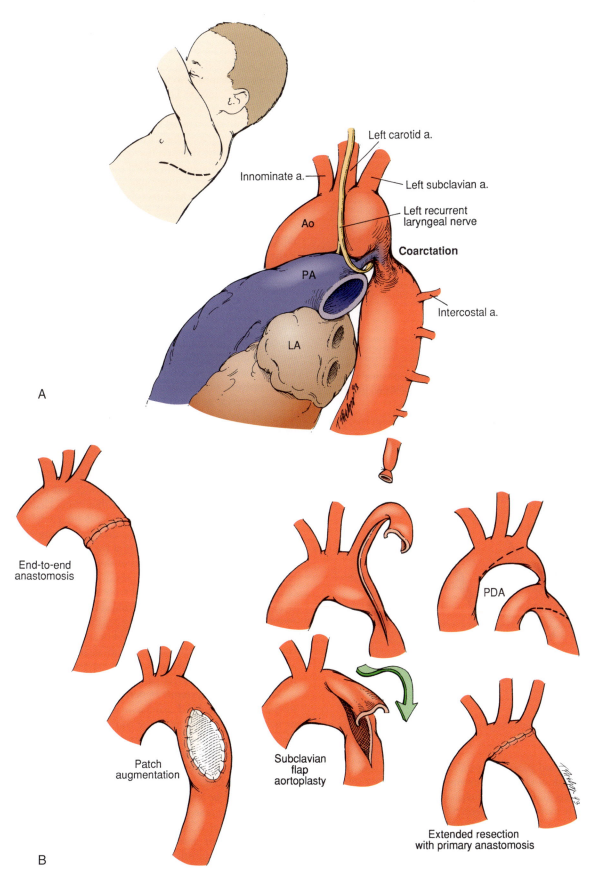

Left carotid a.

Innominate a.

Left subclavian a.

Left recurrent laryngeal nerve

Coarctation

Ao

PA

Intercostal a.

LA

A

End-to-end anastomosis

PDA

Patch augmentation

Subclavian flap aortoplasty

Extended resection with primary anastomosis

B

• **Figure 45.6** Surgical approach to coarctation of the aorta. (A) Placement of a typical surgical incision and surgical anatomy. (B) Four operative procedures commonly used in repair of coarctation of the aorta: resection of the stenotic segment and end-to-end aortic anastomosis, patch augmentation, subclavian flap aortoplasty, and extended resection with primary anastomosis. *a,* Artery; *Ao,* aorta; *LA,* left atrium; *PA,* pulmonary artery; *PDA,* patent ductus arteriosus.

TABLE 45.2	Frequency of Coarctation Repair Techniques for 2474 Patients With Isolated Aortic Coarctation or Hypoplastic Aortic Arch Undergoing Coarctation Repair 2006–2010	
Repair Technique		**Frequency (%)**
Extended end-to-end anastomosis		56
End-to-end anastomosis		33
Patch aortoplasty		4
Subclavian flap repair		3
Interposition graft		3
Other		0.4

Modified from Ungerleider RM, Pasquali SK, Welke KF, et al. Contemporary patterns of surgery and outcomes for aortic coarctation: an analysis of the Society of Thoracic Surgeons Congenital Heart Surgery Database. *J Thorac Cardiovasc Surg.* 2013;145:150-158, with permission.

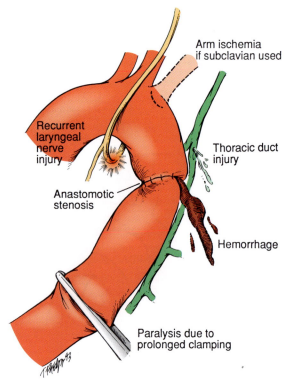

• **Figure 45.7** Complications following repair of coarctation of the aorta.

unilateral vocal cord paresis or paralysis. Newborns and infants are at greatest risk of clinical compromise because the compliant chest wall retracts during partially obstructed inspiration and poor lung expansion may result. Patients with significant respiratory distress should be reintubated. If there is evidence of obstruction in a newborn, nasal continuous positive pressure can be tried. If the nerve was traumatized but not severed, function may return after several days. Nutrition should be optimized in preparation for another extubation attempt. Repeated failed extubation secondary to recurrent laryngeal nerve dysfunction warrants airway evaluation by an otolaryngologist.

Phrenic nerve injury leading to hemidiaphragmatic paralysis may be diagnosed initially by chest radiograph. Typically the hemidiaphragm is elevated, although this can be masked by positive pressure ventilation. Diagnosis is made by fluoroscopy or ultrasound study of the diaphragm, with the patient momentarily removed from positive pressure ventilation and breathing spontaneously. Older children are usually asymptomatic with hemidiaphragmatic paralysis, and intervention is not necessary. However, a paralyzed hemidiaphragm may prohibit separation of the infant from mechanical ventilation. In that setting, definitive management involves plication of the diaphragm, which some surgeons perform immediately on diagnosis. Others may optimize nutrition and offer a second attempt in several days. If the second extubation fails, a diaphragmatic plication may be indicated.

Lymphatic injury leading to chylothorax usually presents as a milky pleural effusion after the initiation of postoperative feeds. If the diagnosis is unclear, triglyceride levels (generally >1.1 mmol/L with fat intake) or lipoprotein electrophoresis looking for chylomicrons is diagnostic.[68] Chylothorax may require prolonged chest tube drainage, which can improve lung function and enable monitoring of the amount drained. In addition to compromised lung function, persistent chylothorax may lead to hypoproteinemia, hypogammaglobulinemia, and lymphopenia with resultant nutritional debilitation. There is debate over whether chylothorax after CoA repair is best treated by immediate thoracic duct ligation or conservatively with dietary maneuvers alone, but institution of clinical practice guidelines has been shown to decrease hospital length of stay and use of mechanical ventilation.[69,70] Conservative treatment with dietary manipulation alone excludes long-chain fatty acids in favor of medium-chain fatty acids, which can be absorbed directly by the portal system and bypass the thoracic duct. If necessary, flow through the thoracic duct can be further reduced by resting the gastrointestinal tract and providing total intravenous nutrition. Enteral feeds without long-chain fatty acids may resume after 1 to 2 weeks of rest. If the chyle recurs with restarting enteral feeds, the thoracic duct can be surgically ligated, or sometimes simple reexploration of the thoracotomy will reveal the area (most often in the region of the superior intercostal vein; just above the area of coarctation repair) that is oozing chyle, and this area can be easily controlled with a few ligatures. Nutrition is an important consideration during this process. If the patient's nutritional status deteriorates during persistent chylothorax, surgical ligation of leaking lymphatics should be undertaken earlier in the course. Novel interventional techniques such as lymphangiography and obliteration of leaking chylous channels with embolization may be an option in select patients.[71]

Postoperative Systemic Hypertension. The cardiac problems for patients with isolated coarctation generally involve hypertension or ischemia. Early postoperative control of hypertension protects the aortic anastomosis, minimizes the risk of aneurysm formation in the dilated poststenotic segment, and alleviates postcoarctectomy syndrome. Hence mean arterial pressure should be rigidly maintained in the normal range for age. During the immediate postoperative period this may be achieved by titration of nitroprusside and esmolol infusions, nicardipine, or labetalol alone and adequate pain relief.[54,72] Once the patient is ready for discharge from the intensive care unit, intermittent doses of propranolol, atenolol, labetalol, or captopril may be substituted. CoA repair before 1 year of age has been associated with a low incidence of late hypertension; relief after 1 year of age results in a sixfold increase in occurrence.[73]

Management strategies for infants following surgical coarctation repair are shown in Table 45.3.

Results of Surgery

Survival. Early (perioperative), intermediate, and long-term morbidity and mortality define the outcomes of CoA. The operative mortality for coarctation depends primarily on the complexity of coexisting lesions. In a 2013 study of the Society of Thoracic Surgeons Congenital Heart Surgery Database (STS CHSD), Ungerleider and colleagues[55] reported outcomes for 5025 patients undergoing primary repair of CoA at one of 95 participating centers between 2006 and 2010. They found that mortality was 1%, 2.5%, and 4.8% for patients with isolated CoA, CoA plus VSD, and CoA plus other cardiac diagnoses, respectively (Table 45.4). When the group of infants with CoA and other major cardiac defects was further stratified into CoA plus Shone's syndrome and CoA plus non-Shone's other complex cardiac defects, the mortality rates were much higher for the non-Shone's group (1.5% vs. 6.8%, respectively).

The management of the VSD does not appear to have a significant impact on the early and intermediate results, and this has led to considerable controversy. Some have argued for coarctation repair only with the expectation for spontaneous VSD closure. Opponents of this approach contend that it will leave some infants with persistent CHF and possible ventilator dependency. Others advocate for repair of CoA and banding of the pulmonary artery during a first stage. This prevents CHF from pulmonary overcirculation but commits the infant to a second-stage operation for debanding alone (if the VSD has closed spontaneously) or debanding plus VSD closure. The third option entails a single-stage repair via median sternotomy in which the VSD is closed and the CoA repaired. This approach also permits reconstruction of a hypoplastic proximal aortic arch or repair of subaortic stenosis, if necessary. Opponents of this approach have worried about neurologic complications if the single-stage repair is carried out under deep hypothermic circulatory arrest. Because current data suggest that both single- and two-stage approaches have low early and intermediate mortality rates (<5%), the approach depends on institutional preference, the size of the VSD (i.e., the likelihood of spontaneous VSD closure), the presence of proximal arch hypoplasia, and the presence of subaortic stenosis.[55]

Prematurity and low birth weight have been reported as risk factors for coarctation repair. With advancing techniques, survival in small infants has improved. Bacha and associates[74] reported a series of 18 patients with median weight of 1.33 kg, with one early and two late deaths. In an STS CHSD study of 594 infants by Curzon[75] in 2008, the discharge mortality for low-weight infants

---

TABLE 45.3   Postoperative Management of Infants Following Repair of Aortic Coarctation

Drugs	Infants with compromised ventricular function: dopamine, milrinone Postoperative hypertension: nicardipine, esmolol
Ventilation	Typically controlled ventilation out of operating room Inhaled nitric oxide for infants at risk for pulmonary hypertension
Fluid management	⅔ maintenance rate NPO for 48 hours secondary to risk of postoperative mesenteric arteritis/postcoarctectomy syndrome
Laboratory studies	Serial electrolytes Serial hematocrit Creatinine Serial ABG
Imaging	CXR (pneumothorax, chest tube placement) Echocardiogram (evaluate cardiac function, aortic and ductal anatomy, and concomitant intracardiac defects)

ABG, Arterial blood gas; *CXR,* chest x-ray; *NPO,* nil per os.

TABLE 45.4   Outcomes of Surgical Coarctation Repair for 5025 Patients 2006–2010

Variable	Overall	CoA/HAA-Isolated	CoA/HAA–VSD	CoA/HAA–Other Major Cardiac Defects	P value
n	5025	2705	840	1480	< .0001
In-hospital mortality, %	2	1	3	5	< .0001
LOS; days; mean ± SD (median)	14 ± 22 (7)	10 ± 16 (5)	20 ± 24 (11)	19 ± 28 (9)	< .0001
Any complication, %	36	25	55	46	< .0001
Cardiac arrest, %	1	0.4	2	2	< .0001
Chylothorax, %	3	2	4	5	< .0001
RLN injury, %	4	2	9	4	< .0001
Phrenic nerve/paralyzed diaphragm, %	1	0.4	1	2	< .0001
Unplanned cardiac reoperation, n/N (%)[a]	33/973 (3)	7/479 (1)	9/177 (5)	17/297 (6)	.002
Spinal cord injury, n/N (%)[a]	0/973 (0)	0/499 (0)	0/177 (0)	0/297 (0)	N/A

All based on total group population and rounded to nearest whole percent, unless otherwise specified.
[a]Some complications in this database were only coded since 2010, and denominator is specified.
CoA/HAA, Coarctation or hypoplastic aortic arch; *LOS,* length of stay; *N/A,* not applicable; *RLN,* recurrent laryngeal nerve; *SD,* standard deviation; *VSD,* ventricular septal defect.
Modified from Ungerleider RM, Pasquali SK, Welke KF, et al. Contemporary patterns of surgery and outcomes for aortic coarctation: an analysis of the Society of Thoracic Surgeons Congenital Heart Surgery Database. *J Thorac Cardiovasc Surg.* 2013;145:150-158, with permission.

was 7.1% compared with 2.7% for infants weighing 2.5 to 4 kg at the time of coarctation surgery.

Recoarctation. Recoarctation is one of the most common complications of CoA surgery. It can be due to several mechanisms: (1) incomplete initial repair, (2) residual abnormal aortic tissue that may proliferate, (3) failure of the anastomotic site to grow, (4) thrombus formation at the suture line, or (5) intimal and medial hyperplasia at the anastomotic site.[76] Recoarctation rates have been highest in patients repaired during infancy. Use of the EEA has also been implicated. It is generally felt that with the best techniques available, restenosis occurs in approximately 20% of neonatal repairs, 10% to 15% of infant repairs, and 5% of childhood repairs.[77] When significant restenosis occurs (resting gradient >20 mm Hg), balloon dilation has become the intervention of choice.[6] When necessary, surgical repair of recurrent CoA usually involves prosthetic patch enlargement of the stenotic site or bypass of the segment with a tubular graft.

Older Children and Adolescents

Pathophysiology

In older children and adolescents, discrete CoA is most common, and the fixed aortic obstruction leads to excessive pressure work of the LV. Two major compensatory mechanisms arise in this setting: (1) LV hypertrophy to increase systolic pressure without increasing wall stress and (2) aortic collateralization to decrease LV afterload. Consequently, patients develop varying degrees of LV hypertrophy, depending on the coarctation gradient and the presence of collateral circulation.

Presentation

Coarctation in the older child is usually an isolated and asymptomatic lesion frequently discovered following an evaluation for a murmur or upper extremity hypertension. Occasionally, headaches and epistaxis may be presenting complaints. Murmurs are present in most patients with CoA who are over 1 year of age. The murmurs tend to be systolic and at least grade 3/6 in intensity. Most are heard best in the left upper sternal border, are crescendo-decrescendo in quality, and can be accompanied by an apical diastolic rumble.

Among children over 1 year of age with CoA who are otherwise asymptomatic, 89% to 92% have upper extremity hypertension.[38,78] Hypertension in children should be assessed by obtaining four-extremity blood pressures. However, in most cases it is the gradient between right arm and lower extremity pressure that is most revealing, because the left subclavian artery (and hence the left arm) may be involved in the coarcted segment. Collateral circulation may decrease the gradient across the stenotic area, leading to misinterpretation regarding the degree of stenosis. Other patients do not have a gradient at rest but develop one upon exercise. Therefore stress testing is recommended preoperatively and postoperatively to reveal occult gradients.[79] A delay in the femoral pulse compared to the radial pulse is a hallmark for coarctation and is an important part of the physical examination.

A minority of symptomatic older children with CoA show signs of ischemia or hypertensive organ damage. Patients with long-standing CoA have arteriolar tortuosity of the retinal vessels, a finding not seen in patients with early coarctation repair.[80] Some children complain of dyspnea on exertion or claudication. An

aneurysmal anterior spinal artery compressing the spinal cord or a branch compressing a nerve root is a rare cause of lower extremity pain, paresthesia, and muscle weakness.[81] Subarachnoid hemorrhage and coma from a ruptured intracranial aneurysm represent a devastating presentation of CoA in the older child.

Evaluation

Results of a chest x-ray examination may be nonspecific in children. Later in life, classic findings of isolated CoA include LV enlargement, irregularity or notching of the aortic arch (prestenotic and post-stenotic dilation on either side of the coarctation, causing the classic "3 sign," and rib notching on ribs 4 to 8).[82] Rib notching, which is created by tortuous collaterals, correlates directly with age and inversely with the diameter of the coarctation.[40] ECG findings may appear normal in older children with isolated coarctation, but the most common ECG abnormality in older children is LV hypertrophy. ST-segment depression and T-wave inversion can also be seen.

Echocardiography is the diagnostic gold standard for CoA. In older children and adolescents with suboptimal windows, computed tomography angiography and magnetic resonance imaging are valuable modalities for evaluating anatomic detail (Fig. 45.8).

Although used more frequently for therapeutic intervention than diagnosis in contemporary practice, cardiac catheterization remains a useful modality in patients with CoA. Hemodynamic data, including pressure gradients across the coarctation, are easily obtained, and aortic measurements may be taken for surgical or interventional planning. The introduction of newer stents, including covered stents, that can be ultimately enlarged to adult sizes has increased enthusiasm for catheterization laboratory treatment of CoA in older children and adolescents in some programs. This strategy has increased the use of catheterization in the diagnosis of CoA because intervention can be provided at the same time.

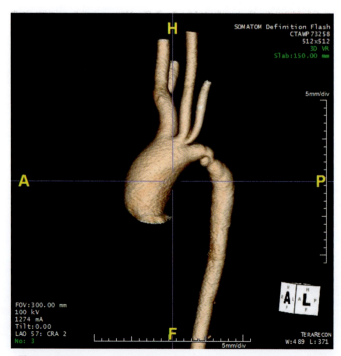

• **Figure 45.8** Three-dimensional reconstruction of a computed tomography angiogram in a 14-year-old girl with a native coarctation of the aorta.

Medical Management

When an older child with coarctation presents for surgical repair, preoperative management is important. Preexisting hypertension occurs in many patients with CoA and may be exacerbated by aortic cross-clamping, which carries the risk of myocardial failure, dysrhythmia, reflex cardiac arrest, or cerebral hemorrhage. All such patients should receive beta-adrenergic–blocking drugs to control hypertension before surgery. Successful control of perioperative hypertension has been reported with the use of propranolol 1.5 mg/kg/d for 2 weeks preoperatively and 1 week postoperatively.[83] Failure to provide preoperative beta-blockade may lead to marked hypertensive responses to intubation. Vasodilators are contraindicated before surgery in the hypertensive child with CoA. LV function may not increase cardiac output sufficiently to compensate for vasodilation because of the relatively fixed obstruction from CoA. Furthermore, tachycardia associated with vasodilation may lead to myocardial ischemia.

Timing of Intervention

The ideal age for repair of isolated CoA is debatable. The discussion has focused on risk of restenosis, and the likelihood of persistent hypertension after repair. Long-term outcome studies suggest that residual hypertension and cardiovascular morbidity and mortality are increased when repairs are made later in life.[73] A series by Seirafi and coworkers[73] reported a 4% incidence of late hypertension in the group repaired during infancy, compared with 17% in the group that underwent later repair.

In general, indications for surgery for isolated coarctation in children and adolescents include a peak-to-peak gradient of 20 mm Hg or higher, although treatment may still be indicated with a lower gradient in the presence of significant collateral flow, left ventricular hypertrophy, hypertension, and elevated LV end-diastolic pressure.[84-86]

Anesthetic Management

Standard monitors are used in addition to one or more arterial lines, a central venous line, temperature probe, and a urinary catheter. Large-bore IVs are placed for purposes of volume administration as needed. An intravenous or mask induction may be used for older children and adults who present for elective CoA repair. In larger patients, lung isolation with a double-lumen endotracheal tube or bronchial blocker can facilitate exposure when the procedure is done through a thoracotomy. No single anesthetic technique has been universally advocated because both inhaled and intravenous agents have been used with success. Recently isoflurane has been used for both anesthetic and blood pressure titration, and fentanyl has been used for pain control.

Vasoactive agents should be available to treat sudden alterations in the blood pressure associated with clamping and unclamping of the aorta. On release of the cross-clamp, metabolic acidosis and acute hypotension may ensue. In anticipation of this "declamping syndrome," blood loss should have been replaced and normovolemia ensured. Any metabolic acidosis should be corrected. An alpha-adrenergic infusion and bolus doses (e.g., phenylephrine) should be immediately available in the event of hypotension. Calcium administration can treat the hypotension associated with declamping. Finally, and most importantly, the surgeon must release the aortic cross-clamp slowly.

In older patients, well-developed collaterals increase the risk of blood loss, which can be minimized by a controlled hypotensive technique. This technique also makes an otherwise tense aorta easier to mobilize. Consideration should also be given to the use of drugs that can be titrated, such as sodium nitroprusside, nitroglycerin, and esmolol. Given the increased ventricular wall tension that occurs during aortic cross-clamping, control of heart rate with esmolol may be desirable to limit myocardial oxygen consumption because increased wall tension limits myocardial perfusion pressure. The risk of spinal cord ischemia due to hypoperfusion during aortic cross-clamping must be weighed against the level of controlled hypotension.

For patients at greater risk of spinal cord ischemia, several strategies have been suggested for preservation of spinal cord blood flow, including use of temporary vascular heparin-bonded shunts, left-heart bypass, femoral-femoral venoarterial cardiopulmonary bypass, and mild systemic hypothermia. The anterior spinal artery is the sole blood supply to the motor portion of the spinal cord and receives several collateral branches from intercostal arteries. The largest branch is the artery of Adamkiewicz, which arises in the lower thoracic region. During clamping of the aorta, this artery becomes the sole source of collateral circulation to the cord. In general, retrograde flow is much less efficient than caudally directed flow. Some teams place a femoral arterial catheter to ensure an adequate distal mean arterial pressure of at least 50 mm Hg. A lumbar drain can also be used to augment the perfusion pressure. In cases in which a lumbar drain is placed, we typically drain cerebrospinal fluid (CSF) to maintain CSF pressures of 10 mm Hg. In the absence of neurologic deficits, drains are capped at 24 hours and removed 48 hours postoperatively. For late-onset deficits, drains may be kept longer.

Older or asymptomatic children are frequently extubated in the operating room or relatively quickly after CoA repair. Postoperative care must include adequate pain management. Cardiac catheterization patients typically have mild pain, which can be treated with acetaminophen or ibuprofen when hemostasis is adequate. In the surgical repair of CoA, thoracotomy incisions are more painful than sternotomy incisions. Regional techniques include epidural or intrathecal narcotics, epidural local anesthetics, or intercostal blocks. Thoracic epidurals remain controversial due to potential risks associated with heparinization and spinal cord injury. With a small risk of paraplegia associated with CoA repair, some providers opt to place epidurals or other regional blocks after the procedure is completed when the patient has moved his or her lower extremities. If lower extremity movement is questionable, any local anesthetic infusion should be stopped to permit assessment. Narcotics can cause respiratory depression by any route, and patients receiving narcotics should be closely monitored. Another option for older children is patient- or nurse-controlled analgesia in a monitored setting.

Surgical Repair

Children 1 to 10 years of age are usually treated by resection and EEA. As in neonates, the approach is via a left thoracotomy. Children presenting at this age typically have focal stenoses without tubular hypoplasia of the distal transverse arch or isthmus. Large collaterals are frequently seen. Hemorrhage can be difficult to control if one of these enlarged vessels is damaged during the dissection.

Repair in the adolescent age-group is usually accomplished by prosthetic patch aortoplasty, tubular graft replacement of the stenotic segment, or prosthetic graft bypass of the coarctation. With these patients, growth of the repair is not necessary, and mobilization and clamping of the aorta for EEA can be dangerous because of the presence of extensive arterial collaterals and the greater risk of paraplegia in the mature central nervous system. Cross-clamping of the aorta in some patients in whom collaterals are not well developed will produce unacceptable hypotension in the distal aorta (<50 mm Hg), raising the risk of paraplegia.

Complications of Surgery and Postoperative Management

Bleeding and the Collateral Circulation. Postoperative bleeding can be a problem following CoA repair. The aortic repair itself, by definition, is a high-pressure suture line that is relatively extensive. Loss of integrity of the suture line results in catastrophic bleeding. In older children with long-standing CoA, collaterals may have formed. The collateral system has an anterior and posterior collateral circulation. The anterior connects the internal mammary arteries and the external iliac arteries via the epigastric system. The posterior connects the thyrocervical arteries and the descending aorta via retrograde flow through dilated intercostal arteries. The intercostals can cause significant bleeding after a CoA repair because it takes time for the collaterals to regress. Heparin is frequently given for CoA repair in older children and is not always antagonized with protamine. The intensive care management of bleeding involves careful blood pressure control and correction of a heparin-induced coagulopathy with protamine or fresh frozen plasma. The surgeon should be notified when a patient is bleeding after coarctation repair.

Postoperative Hypertension. Postoperative hypertension is seen in patients with persistent stenosis or recoarctation but can also be found in the absence of a significant residual postoperative gradient, and the hypertension can last for variable lengths of time. The study of postcoarctectomy hypertension suggests a biphasic and multifactorial etiology. Postrepair hypertension may be explained by surgical stimulation of sympathetic nerve fibers located between the media and adventitia of the aortic isthmus; this stimulation causes release of norepinephrine with consequential blood pressure elevation. This sympathetic stimulation also causes the juxtaglomerular cells to release renin.[87] Benedict and colleagues[88] demonstrated a 750% increase in norepinephrine concentrations in the first 12 postoperative hours, a finding unique to coarctectomy patients.

A second blood pressure change has been observed 2 to 3 days postoperatively, consisting primarily of increased diastolic blood pressure. This second blood pressure response has been associated with mesenteric arteritis. Rocchini and colleagues[89] showed an elevation in plasma renin activity in the first postoperative week, compared with a non-CoA control surgical group. Elevated renin activity is important in early postoperative hypertension but not in chronic postrepair hypertension because renin levels return to normal by the seventh postoperative day. Therefore it is postulated that manipulation of the aorta during surgical repair causes sympathetic discharge, resulting in immediate postoperative hypertension. This in turn leads to renin release, which causes secondary hypertension.[90] The hypertensive response to surgical repair is not seen after balloon angioplasty, nor is there a rise in plasma catecholamine levels or plasma renin activity.[91]

Altered baroreceptor function was reported in a group of children with mild arm systolic hypertension despite good surgical repair. Their baroreflex was reset to operate at a higher arterial pressure with reduced sensitivity to changes in arterial pressure compared with control children.[92] Clarkson and associates demonstrated that most patients were normotensive 5 to 10 years after their repair, but blood pressure increased in later years. This observation was independent of age of repair (study population had repair at >1 year of age).[93]

Postcoarctectomy Syndrome. Postcoarctectomy syndrome is a well-described complication of CoA repair occurring 2 to 3 days after surgery. The primary symptom is severe abdominal pain, accompanied by hypertension, fever, abdominal tenderness, vomiting, ileus, melena, and leukocytosis. There is a higher incidence of postcoarctectomy syndrome in patients with severe aortic constriction and hypertension, and it is rare in neonates.[94] It has been suggested that the sudden increase in blood pressure to vessels below the CoA causes postcoarctectomy syndrome, resulting in necrotizing arteritis of the small arteries of the mesentery and small intestine. Alternatively, the increased postoperative renin levels in some patients might cause abdominal pain by shunting blood from mesenteric vessels.[90] These changes have been demonstrated by angiography, laparotomy, and autopsy. The changes are reversible, and the syndrome is treated and/or prevented by control of postoperative hypertension and bowel rest.[95-97] It is our practice to keep all patients nil per os after surgical coarctation repair for 48 to 72 hours. Interestingly, postcoarctectomy syndrome is generally not seen after endovascular treatment of CoA.[76]

Long-Term Outcomes of Surgery

Follow-up now spanning several decades has illuminated the long-term health outlook for patients after coarctation repair. Toro-Salazar and coworkers analyzed 50-year outcomes for 252 patients who survived to hospital discharge after repair of isolated CoA from 1948 to 1976.[98] Cumulative long-term survival for isolated coarctation decreased over time from 95% at 10 years to 89% at 20 years, 82% at 30 years, and 79% at 40 years. The major explained causes of late death in this population included coronary artery disease, intraoperative death during a second cardiac operation, and aortic dissection. Ninety-two of the 207 long-term survivors were examined, and 31% were found to have an undiagnosed cardiovascular abnormality, of which systemic hypertension was most common. The cause of chronic hypertension in the absence of recoarctation may relate to increased stiffness of the repaired aorta; the proximal aortic wall is more rigid than the postcoarctation wall and typically has more collagen and less smooth muscle.[99]

Interventional Therapy

Alternatives to surgical repair for some patients with CoA include balloon angioplasty and stenting. Both procedures are approached percutaneously. Devices such as dilating balloons are positioned over a wire via a sheath in the femoral artery. Immediate results can be evaluated by angiography and pressure measurements. Potential complications include aortic rupture, cerebrovascular accidents, femoral vessel trauma, and aortic aneurysm formation in the long term.

For infants and young children, surgery is generally used to treat native coarctation; however, balloon angioplasty is a reasonable palliative strategy for neonates in extremis who are considered too unstable for urgent surgery.[85] For recurrent coarctation in infants and young children, angioplasty is first-line therapy because aneurysm development over time is far less common than following angioplasty for native coarctation.[85] Where elastic recoil may limit

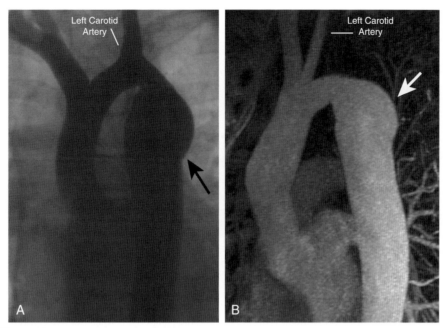

• Figure 45.9 (A) Angiogram demonstrating aneurysm development *(black arrow)* in a 13-year-old patient who previously underwent subclavian flap aortoplasty for coarctation of the aorta. (B) Magnetic resonance imaging of a 30-year-old patient also demonstrates aneurysm formation *(white arrow)* after subclavian flap aortoplasty. Note the absence of the left subclavian artery in both images. (From Vergales JE, Gangemi JJ, Rhueban KS, et al. Coarctation of the aorta—the current state of surgical and transcatheter therapies. *Curr Cardiol Rev.* 2013;9:211-219, with permission).

the effectiveness of angioplasty for longer segment coarctations, balloon-expandable stents have been successfully used in children and adults for both native and recurrent coarctation. In children, selecting a stent that can be dilated to adult size is ideal.

Angioplasty for Native Coarctation. The use of balloon angioplasty in *native* CoA has been evolving since it was first described, but it remains controversial due to high rates of recoarctation and risk of aneurysm formation.[100] Reported rates of recoarctation range from 8% to 32%.[101-104] In a study by Kaine and colleagues,[105] patients who had early angioplasty failures and those who developed recoarctation during follow-up were younger at angioplasty. However, infants with a hypoplastic aortic isthmus appear to be the most high-risk group.

Aneurysm formation after balloon angioplasty is likely related to progression of disease from small tears in the aortic intima and media (Fig. 45.9).[106] In a 2014 Congenital Cardiovascular Interventional Study Consortium (CCISC) study, 8 of 34 (24%) patients developed aneurysms at intermediate follow-up.[104]

Angioplasty for Recoarctation. Balloon angioplasty has evolved as the procedure of choice for recoarctation.[85] Recurrent CoA after surgical EEA, patch angioplasty, and subclavian flaps have all been successfully treated with angioplasty, and success rates range from 80% to 93%.[107] It has been hypothesized that the scar and fibrosis surrounding the anastomotic site are protective for patients with recoarctation because rates of injury to the aortic wall in this cohort are less than 2%.

Need for reintervention is a more common problem. Yetman and coworkers[108] reported on long-term follow-up of 90 patients for 3 to 144 months (median, 39 months); repeat angioplasty or surgical repair was required for recurrent aortic arch narrowing in 33% of their patients over the 12-year period. They found no relationship between time to reintervention and type of initial surgery, age or weight at balloon angioplasty, and percent increase

in coarctation diameter. Predictors of time to reintervention included transverse arch diameter less than 2 standard deviations below the mean and higher preangioplasty and postangioplasty pressure gradient.[108] In a study of 22 infants, Maheshwari and colleagues[109] reported that the risk of restenosis with growth in childhood is low and can be successfully treated with repeat angioplasty. Long-term follow-up (median, 56 months) revealed a restenosis rate after initial optimal results of 16%. With reintervention the success rate was 95%. Lower infant weight correlated with a suboptimal long-term outcome.

Stents. Advances in endovascular stent technology have enabled the use of stents in congenital heart disease, including CoA (Fig. 45.10). In 1991 O'Laughlin and coworkers reported the first use of a bare metal stent to treat CoA.[110] Subsequent reports have focused on the indications and benefits of the stent. In a 2010 study of early and mid-term outcomes of coarctation patients undergoing stent placement using the CCISC[111] registry, stent placement successfully relieved the blood pressure (BP) gradient in 249 of 260 (96%) of cases. Recoarctation was seen in 20% by 60 months; need for reintervention was seen in 4%; and aortic wall complications, including dissection or aneurysm, were seen in 1%.[112] The Coarctation of the Aorta Stent Trial[113] was a prospective, multicenter, single-arm clinical study designed in 2007 to evaluate the safety and efficacy of the Cheatham-Platinum (CP) stent (NuMED, Hopkinton, NY) in the treatment of CoA. In the trial, 105 patients (ages 8 to 52 years) underwent attempted stent placement. In 104 patients, implantation was successfully completed with no significant adverse events and no significant postprocedure gradient. At 1 month, 99% had a gradient less than 20 mm Hg, and at 2 years (with 86% follow-up), 90% had a BP gradient less than 20 mm Hg. In the same series, 22% had stent fracture, 6% were diagnosed with aortic aneurysm, and by 2015 a total of 19 patients had undergone repeat percutaneous intervention (for

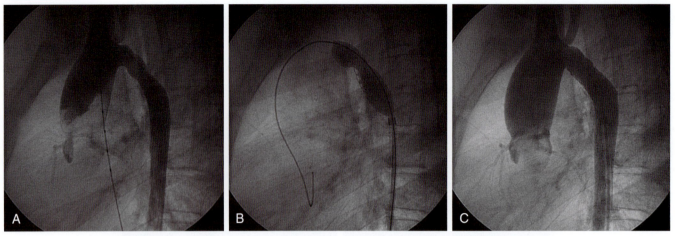

• Figure 45.10 (A) Angiogram demonstrating discrete coarctation in a 14-year-old girl with hypertension. (B) Stent deployment over a 15-mm Z-med balloon (B. Braun Interventional Systems Inc., Bethlehem, PA). C, Angiogram following placement of a Palmaz 3910B stent. Pressure gradient was relieved.

treatment of aortic injury or for dilation of the original stent).[113] No patient required surgical reintervention.

Although intermediate results from the use of stents have been promising, patient selection remains important. For example, patients with Turner syndrome may have a higher risk of adverse outcome from endovascular stenting of CoA.[114] The use of stents is infants and small children is also challenging and controversial due to the desire to accommodate somatic growth, the paucity of approved devices, and the need for relatively large sheaths for stent placement. Endovascular techniques and devices such as "growth stents" that enable repeat dilation continue to develop, but further research and longer follow-up is needed.[115]

Another developing area of interest is in the use of covered stents. Because covered stents use a fabric covering over the stent framework, they can create a new lining to the aorta at the site of deployment and have been useful as a rescue therapy for procedure-related aortic disruption. Initial safety and efficacy studies are promising, but covered stents are not yet widely available for the treatment of coarctation in children.[116]

Critical Care Management After Angioplasty or Stent Placement

After angioplasty or stent placement, patients are generally observed in the intensive care unit. Care is similar to that of postoperative surgical patients, although monitoring is less invasive. Commonly patients after interventional procedures are breathing spontaneously and extubated. Fluid balance must be assessed. Difficult access in the catheterization laboratory or multiple laboratory evaluations can result in significant blood loss during the procedure. Pneumothorax is possible if access was obtained from the internal jugular or subclavian vein. Bleeding can occur at the site of the stent or balloon dilation, the puncture site of the access, or any place along the course of the catheter. Retroperitoneal bleeding associated with catheter access is difficult to detect initially because a large volume of blood may fill the space before any obvious signs except for falling hematocrit. Therefore we recommend routine measurement of the hematocrit 6 hours post procedure.

Special attention should be paid to evaluation of the groin puncture site and circulation in the corresponding limb. If pulses are diminished on the affected side (assuming that they are present elsewhere), attempts should be made to ensure perfusion to the affected limb. If the leg is cold and poorly perfused, surgical intervention, including clot removal and vessel repair, should be considered. If the leg is cool, less-invasive measures, including tissue plasminogen activator, heparin, or low-molecular-weight heparin can be considered. The uncomplicated poststent or postballoon patient is monitored overnight in the intensive care setting and discharged to home the next day.

Conclusion

CoA is a heterogeneous lesion whereby the treatment strategy is heavily influenced by the age, size, and clinical status of the patient at the time of presentation. There is no comprehensive evidence-based algorithm for the management of coarctation. Surgical and percutaneous interventions are both low-risk options in the modern era. Lifelong follow-up is required to evaluate for late complications and recoarctation.

References

A complete list of references is available at ExpertConsult.com.

46

Repair of Interrupted Aortic Arch With Ventricular Septal Defect

ANDREW C. FIORE, MD; RENUKA E. PETERSON, MD; CHARLES B. HUDDLESTON, MD

Interrupted Aortic Arch

Classification and Anatomy

Interrupted aortic arch (IAA) is a rare but highly lethal form of congenital heart disease, carrying a mortality rate higher than 90% in the neonatal period if not treated. The incidence of IAA is 1% of all congenital heart defects. Celoria and Patton[1] described the currently used anatomic definitions, in which type A is interrupted distal to the left subclavian artery (LSCA); type B is interrupted between the left subclavian and left carotid arteries; in type B1 the origin of the right subclavian artery (RSCA) is on the descending thoracic aorta; and type C is interrupted proximal to the left carotid artery. Type B IAA is the most common (78%), followed by type A (20%) and type C (2%) (Fig. 46.1). All patients have a patent ductus arteriosus, and most have a ventricular septal defect (VSD). Also seen are aortic valve anomalies, truncus arteriosus, and double-outlet right ventricle (RV). The VSD is typically conoventricular in origin and is associated with posterior malalignment of the conal septum and varying degrees of left ventricular outflow tract obstruction (LVOTO) at the subvalvar and/or valvar level. In rare cases, when IAA is not associated with VSD, aortopulmonary window should be suspected. In nearly all patients the aortic arch sidedness is left, but rarely the IAA can be right sided with the descending aorta in the right hemithorax. This has been observed in patients with single-ventricle anatomy.

Many patients with IAA have extracardiac anomalies. Unlike those with coarctation, the predominant extracardiac abnormality in these patients is DiGeorge syndrome. The association of DiGeorge syndrome with type B IAA suggests that both are part of a causally heterogeneous developmental field defect. Using fluorescence in situ hybridization (FISH) analysis, Lewin and colleagues[2] demonstrated that 50% to 80% of patients with IAA type B have 22q11.2 chromosomal deletions. IAA is usually a rare anomaly, but in DiGeorge syndrome it is a common defect.

Conley and associates reported that 36% of their patients with DiGeorge syndrome had type A IAA, and all of their autopsied patients had congenital heart disease.[3] Reports of IAA type A with DiGeorge syndrome are rare. The presence of IAA type B with or without DiGeorge phenotype is an indication for genetic screening for the 22q11 deletion in the patient.

The aortic valve is usually bicuspid (80% to 90%) with varying degrees of commissural fusion and annular hypoplasia. In addition to posterior malalignment of the conal septum relative to the ventricular septum, Jonas[4] has pointed out a prominent muscle bundle on the left ventricular (LV) free wall that can project into the left ventricular outflow tract (LVOT) (muscle of Moulaert), significantly contributing to outflow obstruction (Fig. 46.2).

Embryology

The normal embryology of the aortic arch is a complex interaction of tissues arising from the primitive aortic arches, truncus arteriosus, and left dorsal aorta. Schematic drawing of the postnatal aortic arch illustrates the origins of the various portions of the arch complex (Fig. 46.3). The fourth aortic arch is of particular interest in the pathogenesis of IAA type B. As shown in Fig. 46.3, aortic arch tissue between the left carotid and left subclavian arteries is derived from the fourth primitive aortic arch. The RSCA, also derived in part from the fourth arch, is often malposed in patients with IAA. This anomaly is especially prevalent in patients with IAA type B, but it can also be associated with coarctation or can be an independent anomaly. When anomalous, the origin of the RSCA is distal to the LSCA, and the artery courses posteriorly to the esophagus, potentially causing esophageal or tracheal compression. When an aberrant RSCA arises distal to the interruption or coarctation, the patient may have decreased blood pressure in the right arm or right vertebral-subclavian steal. It is also noteworthy that an aberrant RSCA is associated with greater degrees of LVOTO because in utero more blood must pass through the ductus and less through the ascending aorta. The LSCA is usually not malposed and takes origin from the descending thoracic aorta, but on rare occasions either SCA can take origin from the ipsilateral pulmonary artery (PA) and require ligation and reimplantation at the time of surgical repair.

Decreased aortic flow potentially leads to atresia or interruption. However, not all children with obstructive arch lesions have intracardiac lesions that decrease aortic flow. Freedom and associates[5] studied this issue in patients with IAA and VSD and found no definitive mechanism for decreased aortic flow, although 50% had LV outflow tract narrowing that was characterized as conoventricular malalignment.

Left-sided outflow tract and arch anomalies may be due to neural crest migratory problems. Cranial neural crest gives rise to ectomesenchyme, which populates pharyngeal arches III, IV, and VI. These primitive vessels contribute to the formation of the carotid arteries, a portion of the aortic arch, the RSCA, and the ductus arteriosus. The tunica media of the aortic arch consists

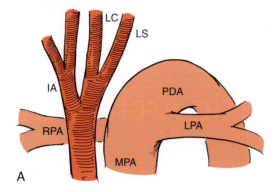

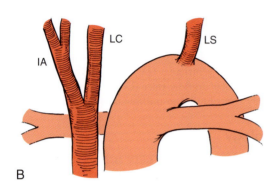

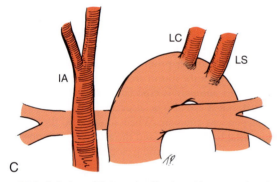

• **Figure 46.1** Celoria and Patton classification of interrupted aortic arch. Type A is interrupted distal to the left subclavian artery, type B between the left subclavian and left carotid arteries, and type C proximal to the left carotid artery. *IA,* Innominate artery; *LC,* left carotid artery; *LPA,* left pulmonary artery; *LS,* left subclavian artery; *MPA,* main pulmonary artery; *PDA,* posterior descending artery; *RPA,* right pulmonary artery.

entirely of cranial neural crest cell derivatives. Thus abnormal migration of neural crest cells may have structural consequences and change blood flow patterns. Chromosomal abnormalities may induce abnormalities of the neural crest cells. There is also experimental evidence that fibronectin plays a role in neural crest cell migration and that fibronectin deficiency might result in obliteration of the fourth arch artery in the chick embryo.

Associated Anomalies

Associated cardiovascular anomalies are always present with IAA. The most common is VSD (70% to 80%) and atrial septal defect (ASD) or stretched patent foramen ovale (PFO), which can be quite large and hemodynamically important. Other commonly

TABLE 46.1   Anomalies Seen in Association With Interrupted Aortic Arch

Associated Cardiac Anomalies	n	TYPE OF INTERRUPTED AORTIC ARCH N (%)		
		Type A	Type B	Type C
VSD (isolated)	44	7 (35)	35 (71)	2 (100)
"Single ventricle"	8	5 (25)	3 (6)	NA
Truncus arteriosus	7	2 (10)	5 (10)	NA
DORV	5	2 (10)	3 (6)	NA
TGA + VSD	2	2 (10)	NA	NA
Complete AV canal	2	1 (5)	1 (2)	NA
DOLV	1	NA	1 (2)	NA
Isolated v. inversion + VSD	1	1 (5)	NA	NA
None (PDA present)	1	NA	1 (2)	NA
Total	71	20 (100)	49 (100)	2 (100)

AV, Atrioventricular; *DOLV,* double-outlet left ventricle; *DORV,* double-outlet right ventricle; *NA,* not applicable; *PDA,* posterior descending artery; *TGA,* transposition of the great arteries; *VSD,* ventricular septal defect.
Reprinted with permission from Jonas RA. *Comprehensive Surgical Management of Congenital Heart Disease.* 2nd ed. Boca Raton, FL: CRC Press; 2014:622.

associated lesions include truncus arteriosus, transposition of the great arteries (TGA) with VSD, aortopulmonary window, and various forms of single ventricle. The frequency of these associated anomalies is shown in Table 46.1.

Pathophysiology

The pathophysiology of IAA is similar to neonatal coarctation of the aorta (CoA) with VSD. Systemic blood flow is dependent on ductus patency. As the ductus closes, the infant develops shock, acidosis, and renal failure. The increasing systemic resistance redirects blood flow to the pulmonary circulation, which ultimately results in volume and pressure overload of the heart with resulting pulmonary edema and biventricular failure.

Diagnostic Assessment

IAA presents in a fashion similar to critical coarctation in the newborn. In cases in which prenatal diagnosis was not established, the infant develops tachypnea and poor peripheral perfusion as the ductus closes, generally within the first 7 to 10 days of life. Physical examination reveals tachypnea, tachycardia, a single second heart sound, and hepatomegaly and decreased femoral pulses. There may not be a significant murmur due to the large VSD, though with increasing pulmonary blood flow, a systolic murmur may be noted. Differential cyanosis between the upper and lower body is usually difficult to appreciate because of left-to-right shunting at the VSD level leaving some *oxygenated* blood traveling to the descending aorta *via* the ductus arteriosus. However, pulse oximetry may show higher oxygen saturation levels in the preductal arm (usually the right arm) compared with the lower body if the great vessels are normally related. If the great vessels are transposed, the oxygen saturation may be higher in the lower body (reversed differential cyanosis).

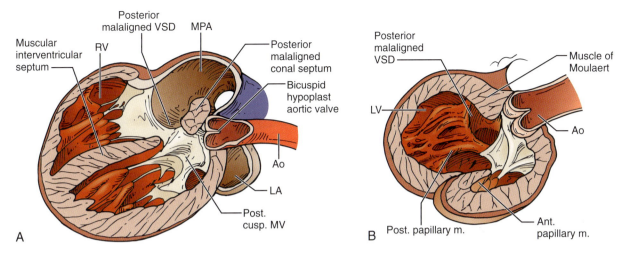

• **Figure 46.2** Morphologic factors contributing to left ventricular outflow tract obstruction. (A) The conal septum is usually posteriorly malaligned relative to the muscular interventricular septum, thereby creating a posterior malaligned ventricular septal defect (VSD), as well as contributing to left ventricular outflow tract obstruction. (B) The muscle of Moulaert is a prominent muscle bundle that extends from the left ventricular free wall into the outflow tract, also contributing to the left ventricular outflow tract obstruction. *Ao,* Aorta; *LA,* left atrium; *LV,* left ventricle; *MPA,* main pulmonary artery; *MV,* mitral valve; *RV,* right ventricle.

Given the common association between IAA type B and DiGeorge syndrome, every infant with suspected IAA should be examined for the DiGeorge stigmata. These include a broad nasal bridge, malar hypoplasia, narrow palpebral fissures, hypertelorism, low-set posteriorly rotated ears, retrognathia, small mouth, and submucosal cleft palate. Given that the stigmata may be difficult to appreciate in the newborn, FISH testing, which probes for submicroscopic deletions in chromosome 22q11.2, should be used. Because patients with DiGeorge syndrome have thymic and parathyroid deficiency of variable degree, the physician must anticipate the possibility of T-cell deficiency and hypocalcemia. The major risk of T-cell deficiency in this patient population is developing graft-versus-host disease after transfusion with nonirradiated blood.

The electrocardiogram (ECG) and chest x-ray findings do not establish a specific diagnosis, but the ECG shows RV hypertrophy, and the chest x-ray demonstrates cardiomegaly with increased pulmonary circulation, suggesting congenital heart disease.

Echocardiography establishes the specific diagnosis. The suprasternal aortic arch view shows the absence of continuity between the ascending aorta and descending aorta, and the ductus is seen connecting to the descending aorta. The LSCA may often be seen arising from the descending aorta. The presence of coexisting defects should be carefully explored. Imaging with computerized tomographic angiography and subsequent three-dimensional model building is extremely useful, especially in cases of suspected abnormal arch anatomy. Cardiac catheterization is rarely helpful unless further ambiguity exists.

Of particular importance is the diagnosis of LVOTO, which may be underrecognized preoperatively. Several echocardiographic indices may identify LVOTO, including the indexed cross-sectional area of the LV outflow tract, the subaortic diameter index, and the aortic valve diameter z score. Salem and associates showed that patients with aortic valve diameter less than 4.5 mm (z score < −5) subsequently developed LVOTO, whereas those with aortic valve diameter greater than 4.5 mm (z score > −5) did not.[6] Failure

to diagnose and correct significant LVOTO surgically is likely to result in persistent heart failure in the postoperative period.

Preoperative Critical Care Management of Interrupted Aortic Arch

The preoperative critical care management of IAA is similar to that of neonatal CoA. The primary objective is to maintain ductal patency with PGE_1. Shock and congestive heart failure usually improve after PGE_1 administration, but some infants will require inotropic support and mechanical ventilation. Hyperoxia and hypocarbia should be avoided to lessen the chances of pulmonary overcirculation. It is extremely important that any end organ injury to the brain, kidney, lungs, and heart in the early neonatal period be given adequate time to fully recover with medical treatment before surgery is undertaken. Before operation, all patients should have normal blood gas levels and end-organ indices.

Hypocalcemia is a common finding in patients with IAA, even those who do not have DiGeorge syndrome. These infants require calcium replacement because they are at increased risk for symptomatic hypocalcemia during hyperventilation and transfusion of citrated blood products. Irradiated blood products should be used to prevent graft-versus-host disease in all infant IAA repairs unless DiGeorge syndrome has been specifically excluded. Currently at most institutions all pediatric blood products are irradiated as an extra safety precaution.

Indications and Timing of Surgery

The presence of IAA is an indication for operation in most patients once end-organ evaluation is complete and is typically performed in the first 5 to 10 days of life. In the term infant (above 35 weeks) with a birth weight above 1.5 kg and in the absence of significant irreversible end-organ injury or coexisting noncardiac abnormalities, we prefer primary single-stage repair. This includes amalgamation

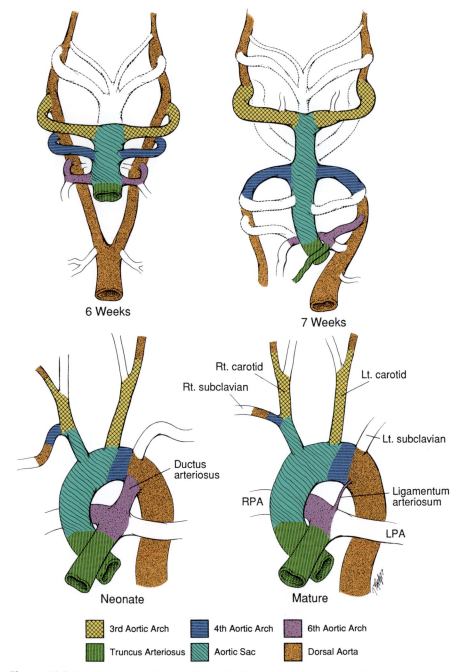

6 Weeks

7 Weeks

Rt. carotid

Rt. subclavian

Lt. carotid

Ductus arteriosus

Lt. subclavian

RPA

Ligamentum arteriosum

LPA

Neonate

Mature

| | 3rd Aortic Arch | | 4th Aortic Arch | | 6th Aortic Arch |
| | Truncus Arteriosus | | Aortic Sac | | Dorsal Aorta |

• **Figure 46.3** The postnatal aortic arch, illustrating the embryologic origins at the sixth and seventh gestational weeks of the various portions of the arch complex. *LPA*, Left pulmonary artery; *Lt.*, left; *RPA*, right pulmonary artery; *Rt.*, right.

of the ascending and descending aorta with patch augmentation and closure of atrial and ventricular septal defects.

The preterm infant (less than 35 weeks; less than 1.5 kg) or term newborn with severe coexisting noncardiac abnormalities such as diaphragmatic hernia, genetic syndromes, necrotizing enterocolitis requiring operation, severe but reversible neurologic injury, or end-organ damage requiring months to recover may instead be a candidate for hybrid strategy. In rare case, we have successfully used bilateral PA banding with or without ductal stenting to achieve a stable balanced circulation during the extended recovery period.

Another alternative palliative strategy in these circumstances is IAA reconstruction employing the left common carotid artery with PA banding.

Primary Repair of Interrupted Aortic Arch With Ventricular Septal Defect

Following placement of a nasopharyngeal temperature probe and a Foley urinary catheter, arterial monitoring is achieved with right radial and femoral lines. Venous access is via umbilical or femoral vein, but access in the neck is avoided if the patient is less than

5 kg because of potential superior vena cava thrombosis. A blood pressure cuff is placed appropriately, and cerebral and lower extremity near-infrared spectroscopy monitoring is employed.

Following midline sternotomy and thymus removal (if present) the innominate vein and artery and left common carotid artery (LCCA) are circumferentially and extensively dissected cephalad. The pericardium is opened, and a segment is harvested and treated in glutaraldehyde for VSD closure (alternatively 0.4-mm Gore-Tex is used). The ductus is encircled, and the right PA can be temporarily occluded for hemodynamic stability. We prefer bicaval cannulation, LV venting through the right superior pulmonary vein, and regional cerebral perfusion (30 to 50 mL/kg/min). Heparin is administered, and the innominate artery is cannulated directly or a 3.5-mm Gore-Tex tube is sewn to the innominate artery (right common carotid artery if aberrant RSCA is present) and an 8-mm arterial cannula inserted. A Y adapter is placed on the arterial line, and the ductus is cannulated with an 8-French cannula and snared following bicaval cannulation and vent insertion. Alternatively (not our usual preference), the second cannula can be placed in the descending thoracic aorta at the diaphragm level for retrograde perfusion.

Cardiopulmonary bypass is initiated, ice is placed around the head, and cooling to 18°C is accomplished with systemic vasodilation employing milrinone to achieve homogeneous body temperature. Importantly, a minimum cooling duration of 20 to 30 minutes is used regardless of when the desired temperature is reached.

During this period the arch vessels and descending thoracic aorta are extensively mobilized. The aberrant RSCA is ligated and divided, and intercostal arteries are ligated with clips and divided to allow for a tension-free anastomosis. Care is taken to complete the dissection on the aorta without cautery to avoid left recurrent nerve injury. Head vessel snares are placed appropriately.

With cooling complete the ductal cannula is removed, the purse-string tied, and the ductus ligated. With brain and heart fully perfused, the descending thoracic aorta is clamped first, the ductus divided, and a second suture ligature of 6-0 polypropylene placed beyond the ductal tie. The ascending aorta is now cross-clamped very proximally, cardioplegia infused in the proximal ascending aorta (del Nido, 20 mL/kg), and regional cerebral perfusion commenced. Alternatively, cardioplegia can be delivered through a side port on the aortic cannula during a short period of circulatory arrest.

All residual ductal tissue is completely excised from the descending aorta, mindful that the origin of the LSCA is usually at the level of normal aortic tissue. An incision is made leftward in the ascending aorta and extended onto the LCCA and proximally onto the ascending aorta. A counterincision is made for 5 to 8 mm in the LSCA. The posterior aortic anastomosis is completed starting superiorly at the apex of the LSCA and the LCCA incisions and both corners turned with continuous 6-0 polypropylene (Fig. 46.4). A cutback incision of 5 to 8 mm is now made anteriorly in the descending thoracic aorta. The corners are trimmed and the anastomoses augmented with a hemicone-shaped patch of pulmonary homograft or autologous treated pericardium (Fig. 46.5). Upon completion of the arch anastomosis the descending clamp is removed first, followed by the LSCA, and lastly the LCCA for arch air evacuation. Cold reperfusion of the brain and body is now maintained for 3 to 5 minutes, and then full rewarming is begun.

During rewarming the ASD is closed and the VSD assessed through the right atrium. If significant subaortic obstruction is present, the conal septum is resected following the technique of Bove.[7]

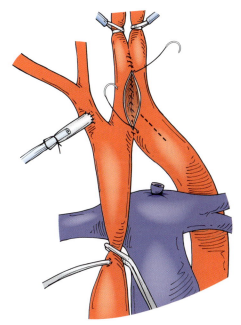

• **Figure 46.4** The arch reconstruction is performed with regional cerebral perfusion. The posterior anastomosis is completed amalgamating the carotid and subclavian arteries, followed by a cutback incision in the descending aorta.

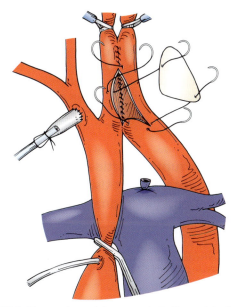

• **Figure 46.5** The anastomosis is augmented with a patch of autologous pericardium or homograft material.

The VSD is closed with autologous treated pericardium and continuous 6-0 polypropylene or 0.4-mm Gore-Tex. Alternatively, if the VSD is anterior with leftward extension or in the absence of the conal septum, closure is performed through a transverse main PA incision.

The cross-clamp is removed, epicardial pacing wires are inserted, and transesophageal or surface echocardiography is employed during bypass weaning. After separation from the extracorporeal circuit, a double-lumen right atrial line is inserted, and either sternal closure over mediastinal drain is performed or alternatively the skin is closed and sternal closure delayed 2 to 4 days if there is any evidence of hemodynamic instability or edema.

Alternatively, the arch reconstruction can be accomplished without regional cerebral perfusion, employing a brief period of circulatory arrest at 18°C, provided the anastomosis can be completed in less than 20 to 30 minutes to avoid the potential of early or late neurologic injury. At present there are no unequivocal data to suggest a superior benefit with either technique.

Repair of Interrupted Aortic Arch With Ventricular Septal Defect Following Hybrid Procedure

The procedure is identical to the procedure for primary repair with the following exceptions.

1. During the final phase of cooling with the brain and heart perfused, the descending thoracic aorta is clamped and the ductus cannula removed. The main pulmonary artery (MPA) proximal to the stent is temporarily snared, and the stent is completely divided and cut anteriorly on the descending aorta until normal aorta is reached. With the use of a Freer elevator the stent is shelled out and all intimal flaps on the descending aorta repaired. Regional cerebral perfusion, aortic cross-clamping, and cardioplegia are now instituted, and the arch is reconstructed followed by reperfusion of the brain and body as previously described. Subsequently the VSD and ASD and right atrium are closed as noted earlier.

2. During rewarming with the heart beating the residual stent in the main PA and bands are removed. If the branch pulmonary arteries easily admit a Hegar dilator and have a Z score of −1, then no band site reconstruction is performed; band site reconstruction is usually not necessary if the banding was performed within 2 to 3 months. Otherwise the band sites and the main PA are patched with autologous *nontreated* pericardium or pulmonary homograft. Alternatively, intraoperative balloon dilation of the band sites can be performed.

Repair of Interrupted Aortic Arch With Ventricular Septal Defect Using Left Common Carotid Artery and Pulmonary Artery Banding

Preincisional monitoring is described under primary repair. Following a third or fourth interspace thoracotomy (usually left) the LCCA is extensively and circumferentially mobilized cephalad, and the aberrant RSCA (if present) is ligated and divided. The LSCA and ductus are circumferentially mobilized as is the descending thoracic aorta for three to five pairs of intercostals. Following heparinization (not used in all centers) the ductus is divided and all residual ductal tissue removed from the descending aorta. The LCCA is marked on its left lateral side, doubly ligated distally, and divided cephalad after temporarily occlusion with a small vascular clamp proximally. The artery is now rotated down, spatulated, and sewn to the descending thoracic aorta with monofilament suture. Following clamp removal the pericardium is opened anterior to the left phrenic nerve and PA banding performed using established techniques.

Postoperative Surgical Complications

Early Complication. Any significant residual lesion, including anastomotic stenosis (arm to leg gradient of greater than 20 to 30 mm Hg), LVOTO (LV-aorta peak gradient > 30 mm Hg), or residual atrial or ventricular level shunt (pulmonary-to-systemic blood flow ratio [Q_p:Q_s] > 1.3 : 1.0) should be corrected before intensive care unit transfer. We keep all patients pharmacologically paralyzed 12 to 24 hours to reduce bleeding and to accommodate for the usual low cardiac output syndrome 6 to 12 hours postoperatively. Persistent bleeding may suggest inadvertent residual ductal tissue or tension at the aortic anastomosis and should prompt immediate reoperation.

Low cardiac output resulting in generalized edema secondary to capillary leak, low urine output requiring continuous furosemide (Lasix) infusion, and the need for volume with multiple inotropic drugs usually resolves at 36 to 48 hours postoperatively. Inability to extubate within 2 to 4 days of sternal closure should stimulate an aggressive search for residual hemodynamic, neurologic, or airway lesions.

Late Complications. Recurrent nerve paralysis may require a gastrostomy tube before discharge to avoid the dangers of home nasogastric feedings causing aspiration in the neonate. Phrenic nerve paralysis with diaphragm elevation and the inability to extubate should prompt early plication. Chylothorax is treated with a nonfat diet (e.g., Monogen), total parenteral nutrition, and occasionally pleurodesis with thoracic duct ligation. Residual arch obstruction is addressed with balloon dilation, stent placement, or reoperation with patch enlargement.

LVOTO is rarely sufficient to require intervention in the neonatal period, but 20% to 40% of patients will require LVOT surgery within 10 years postoperatively.

Strategies for Treatment of Left Ventricular Outflow Tract Obstruction at the Time of Interrupted Aortic Arch Repair

1. In our practice for a 2- to 3-kg baby, if the echocardiographic aortic annulus diameter is greater than or equal to 4 mm, we do not intervene on the LVOT.
2. Guidelines based on the patient's weight and echocardiographic aortic annulus diameter:
   Aortic annulus diameter is less than the weight in kilograms plus 1.0: Norwood/Rastelli or Yasui
   Aortic annulus diameter is weight plus 1 to 1.5: no intervention or subaortic resection
   Aortic annulus diameter is greater than the weight plus 1.5: no intervention
3. Guidelines based on the aortic annulus z score and indexed cross-sectional area of the aortic valve[8]:
   Aortic annulus z score is greater than −3: no intervention
   Aortic annulus z score is less than −4: Norwood/Rastelli or Yasui
   Aortic Valved Index Area is greater than 0.9 cm²/m²: no intervention
   Aortic Valved Index Area is less than 0.6 cm²/m²: Norwood/Rastelli or Yasui

If the aortic valve annulus is below these guidelines, then we prefer IAA repair and a modified Norwood procedure with an RV-PA Gore-Tex conduit (usually 5 mm) in the neonatal period. The IAA operation is modified according to Mosca and associates.[9] The proximal MPA is divided, and the aortic incision is carried proximally to a point adjacent to the divided MPA. The Damus-Kaye-Stansel (DKS) connection is made, and the homograft patch is cut longer and wider to extend from the IAA repair to cover the opening in the ascending aorta and MPA (DKS connection).

At 4 to 6 months of age, following cardiac catheterization, a Rastelli operation with VSD enlargement is our preferred strategy because it allows for a larger RV to PA conduit insertion. In very rare instances a patient with IAA and VSD would at this stage (4 to 6 months of age) follow a univentricular palliation pathway of bidirectional Glenn shunt and later completion of extracardiac Fontan.

In some centers, patients with IAA and VSD and LVOTO that fall below the guidelines discussed earlier will receive a Yasui operation as the primary single-stage neonatal palliation (not our preference). The Yasui combines the features of the Norwood operation (aortic arch reconstruction with DKS connection) and the Rastelli operation (VSD closure to the DKS connection and RV to PA conduit insertion).[10] The VSD patch is the roof of the tunnel that permits the LV blood to pass through the VSD under the patch to the pulmonary valve and then into the reconstructed ascending aorta, bypassing the LVOTO. Recently a report demonstrated that early mortality following the Yasui procedure was significantly less than following the Norwood operation, but this has not been universally observed.[11]

It is important to keep in mind that these are only guidelines for intervention on the LVOT and that each individual patient must be carefully evaluated by the cardiologist and cardiovascular surgeon. We emphasize a word of caution in interpreting subaortic echocardiographic measurements in the newborn when there is reduced flow across the LVOT in the presence of a large VSD because the patient's volume status and the dynamic phase of systole and diastole profoundly impact the measurements and can lead to inconsistent data. Therefore we rely on the diameter of the aortic valve annulus and the guidelines outlined earlier. We favor a conservative policy with respect to the LVOT in newborns, recognizing that at a later time reoperation will frequently be required, but now in an older patient.

Postoperative Critical Care Management

Cardiovascular Function. Cardiovascular events after IAA repair are anticipated with invasive monitoring. Central venous, right atrial, and arterial lines in the right radial and femoral artery are useful monitors. In the presence of LVOTO or hypoplasia of the left heart structures a left atrial line is inserted. The operation involves significant aortic suture lines that are at risk for bleeding. Blood pressure control with sedation or low-dose milrinone is employed and guided by arterial pressure monitoring. However, systemic vasodilators should be avoided in the face of residual LVOTO or anastomotic stenosis because vasodilation in this setting leads to refractory hypotension. Right radial and femoral arterial pressure monitoring identifies an aortic pressure gradient, which would suggest a stenosis at the site of repair if beyond 20 to 30 mm Hg. Elevations in left atrial pressure beyond 15 to 20 mm Hg may point to residual LVOTO or LV dysfunction. Milrinone, dopamine, epinephrine, and calcium are useful as the initial therapy for ventricular dysfunction and for systemic vasodilation postoperatively. An arterial pressure gradient or left atrial pressure elevation should be further investigated with echocardiography. Pulmonary hypertension diagnosed echocardiographically is treated with inhaled nitric oxide.

Respiratory Function. Respiratory management is similar to that in patients undergoing other complex congenital heart operations. Left mainstem bronchus compression and malacia from tension at the arch repair site is a rare complication. The patient presents with left lung hyperinflation or complete atelectasis, which may become evident immediately or several months to years postoperatively. The diagnosis is made with bronchoscopy or computed tomographic scan of the chest.

Management is individualized. Various operative approaches have been attempted, including descending thoracic aortopexy or bronchial wall suspension.[12] If pexy procedures fail, then our preference is interposition graft placement to elongate the descending thoracic aorta, which is highly effective but may require future reoperations in growing children. In children and young adults, graft insertion is performed using a lateral thoracotomy on the appropriate side, employing left heart bypass (left atrial to descending thoracic aortic cannulation) with mild hypothermia to prevent potential spinal cord and lower body ischemia. We believe that patch augmentation to enlarge the arch anastomosis at the initial repair also reduces tension on the descending aorta to avoid this complication.

DiGeorge Syndrome. Patients with IAA and DiGeorge syndrome usually require calcium supplementation in the postoperative period. However, there is a wide spectrum, ranging from normal calcium and parathyroid hormone levels to frank hypoparathyroidism and hypocalcemia. Late-onset hypoparathyroidism is also possible. Therefore calcium levels should be monitored very closely in the postoperative period and periodically after discharge from the hospital.

Immunodeficiency represents the other concern in the DiGeorge syndrome population. In addition to the need for blood product irradiation to prevent graft-versus-host disease, there may be an increased risk for pneumonia and sepsis in this population. Schreiber and associates[13] have shown that nearly 50% of the late deaths after IAA repair result from pneumonia and sepsis.

Outcomes

IAA is a lifelong disease that is associated with late morbidity and the need for reoperation primarily centered on the progression on LVOTO. In the current era the hospital or 30-day operative mortality for single-stage repair is 2% to 4%, whereas the 8- to 10-year actuarial survival is 75% to 85%.[14] Despite this superior early survival, reoperation for LVOTO continues to be required in 20% to 40% of patients by 10 years.[15] The hazard risk is increased in the presence of bicuspid aortic valve, type B interruption with aberrant left LSCA, and the need for multiple reoperations on the LVOT. The actuarial freedom from any reoperation at 10 years is only 60%.

The recurrence of LVOTO can be anatomically variable. If the subaortic obstruction is discrete and the aortic valve annulus is adequate, then resection with myomectomy through the aortic valve is advised. If obstruction recurs, another option is septoplasty (modified Konno; see Chapter 51), provided the aortic valve and annulus are normal without significant stenosis or insufficiency. Complex LVOTO that is recurrent and multilevel is best treated with the Ross-Konno operation (see Chapter 51).

The early and midterm results of the hybrid procedure for high-risk neonates with IAA and VSD are continuing to emerge. Recent reports have demonstrated that substantial growth of the aortic valve and the LVOT occurs at 2 to 4 months following PA banding (with or without ductal stent placement), permitting either conventional aortic arch reconstruction with VSD closure or Norwood/Rastelli (or Yasui) pathway to achieve biventricular repair.[16]

References

A complete list of references is available at ExpertConsult.com.

47

Atrial Septal Defects

GRAHAM D. UNGERLEIDER, MD; THARAKANATHA R. YARRABOLU, MD;
ROBERT D. STEWART, MD

Atrial septal defects (ASDs) are a group of anatomic abnormalities that result in shunting of blood between the atria (Fig. 47.1). ASD is the second most common congenital heart lesion after ventricular septal defect and occurs in 5 to 6 infants out of 1000 live births.[1,2] The most common ASD, representing approximately 80% of ASDs, is the secundum ASD, which is essentially a hole in (or deficiency of) the septal tissue in the region of the fossa ovalis. The ostium primum ASD (10% of ASDs), a hole in the septum near the atrioventricular (AV) valves, is typically associated with a cleft in the left AV valve. It is more appropriately referred to as a partial atrioventricular septal defect (AVSD), and a partial AVSD is the least extreme defect among the spectrum of AVSDs because it only creates shunting at the atrial level. The sinus venosus ASD is a communication above the level of the atrial septum due to override of the embryologic sinus venosus. Sinus venosus ASD almost always occurs in the superior portion of the heart and typically involves partial anomalous pulmonary venous (PAPVR) drainage of the right upper and middle lobes. Very rarely a sinus venosus defect may be situated in the inferoposterior portion of the atrial septum, this time overriding the inferior vena caval orifice. Finally, unroofed coronary sinus (CS), the least common of these four types of ASD, is an opening in the inner wall or "roof" of the CS within the left atrium (LA), thus shunting the blood in or out of the CS and then draining into the right atrium (RA) through the ostium of the CS.

This chapter will describe each of these ASDs, including their embryology, evaluation, natural history, intervention, and outcomes.

Embryology and Anatomy

Secundum Atrial Septal Defect and Patent Foramen Ovale

During the fourth week of embryonic development the septum primum forms at the superior portion of the common atria and grows inferiorly toward the endocardial cushion. The inferior opening is called ostium primum, which closes with the fusion of endocardial cushions. The ostium secundum forms in the superior portion of the atrium during the fifth and sixth embryonic weeks. Anterior superior infolding of common atria to the right of septum primum results in closure of ostium secundum and formation of fossa ovalis.[3] This muscular portion of the septum is termed the *septum secundum* (Fig. 47.2). The rim of the thickened muscular portion is called the *limbus*. Most of this structure is not a true "wall" between the left and right atria but rather opposition of two separate atrial walls. If

a surgeon were to cut into the limbus superiorly or medially to enter the LA, that incision would likely create a hole outside the heart. The area of the oval fossa and the muscular septum immediate anterior and inferior is the only "true" septal wall. The oval fossa is covered by a thin-walled tissue called the *septum primum.* The septum primum is anchored at the inferior edge and not at the superior margin of the limbus, thus forming a flap valve. This flap valve in gestational life allows the oxygen-rich blood from the placenta via the ductus venosus and inferior vena cava (IVC) to flow into the left atria (Fig. 47.3A). This left atrial blood then travels through the left ventricle (LV) and ascending aorta, allowing the maximal oxygenated blood to be delivered to the brain. Immediately after a neonate begins spontaneous breathing, flow of blood increases to the lungs and drains into the LA. This increases the left atrial pressure and pushes the septum primum against the septum secundum, closing the oval fossa (see Fig. 47.3B).[4] In the majority of people the septum primum fuses closed; however, in up to 25% of people the septum primum is fully covering the oval fossa but can be opened in the conditions when right atrial pressure increases, the so-called patent foramen ovale (PFO) (see Fig. 47.2). The significance of the PFO is described later. Any deficiency in the normal septum primum, whether it is too small to fully cover the oval fossa, contains one or more holes ("fenestrations"), or is absent, leads to persistent communication between the atria at the level of the oval fossa. This is the secundum ASD and understandably is also referred to as an oval fossa ASD (Fig. 47.4A-D).

Ostium Primum Atrial Septal Defect

The septum primum originally develops as a ridge of muscular tissue that grows toward the endocardial cushion tissue of the developing AV valves. It eventually fuses with the cushion and closes the primordial hole, the ostium primum, between the AV valves and the septum primum. Arrest of complete formation of the endocardial cushion and the septum primum leaves a spectrum of AVSDs. The AV septum is that portion of the septum that in the normal heart actually separates the LV from the RA. This is due to the higher attachment of the normal mitral valve to the septum compared to the attachment of the tricuspid valve (Fig. 47.5)—a feature that is helpful in distinguishing the morphologic *right* from the morphologic *left* ventricle. In AVSDs the absence of this AV septum can be identified by the attachment of the mitral and tricuspid valves at the same level (see Fig. 47.5). When the ventricular portion of the endocardial cushion is intact, the resulting septal defect is only at the atrial level (see Fig. 47.5). The vast majority are associated with a persistent cleft or "zone of

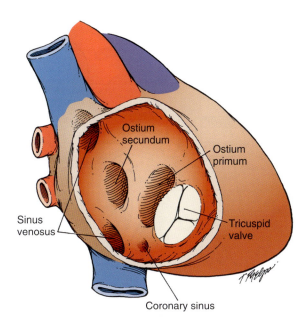

• **Figure 47.1** Various types of atrial septal defects (ASDs) viewed through the right atrium (ostium secundum, ostium primum, sinus venosus). An unroofed coronary sinus may also act as an ASD.

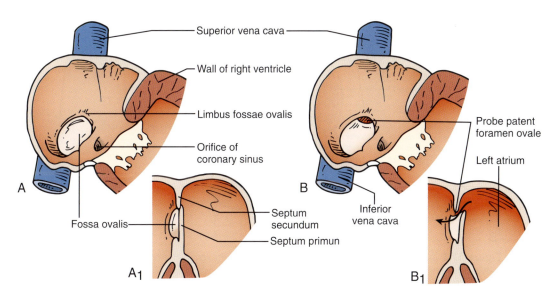

• **Figure 47.2** Embryology of the atrial septum. (A) The fossa ovalis is created by upward growth of the septum primum that attaches to the left superior aspect of the septum secundum. (B) When the septum primum does not attach completely to the underside of the septum secundum, a patent foramen ovale may result. (Redrawn from Moore KL. *The Developing Human.* 2nd ed. Philadelphia: WB Saunders; 1977.)

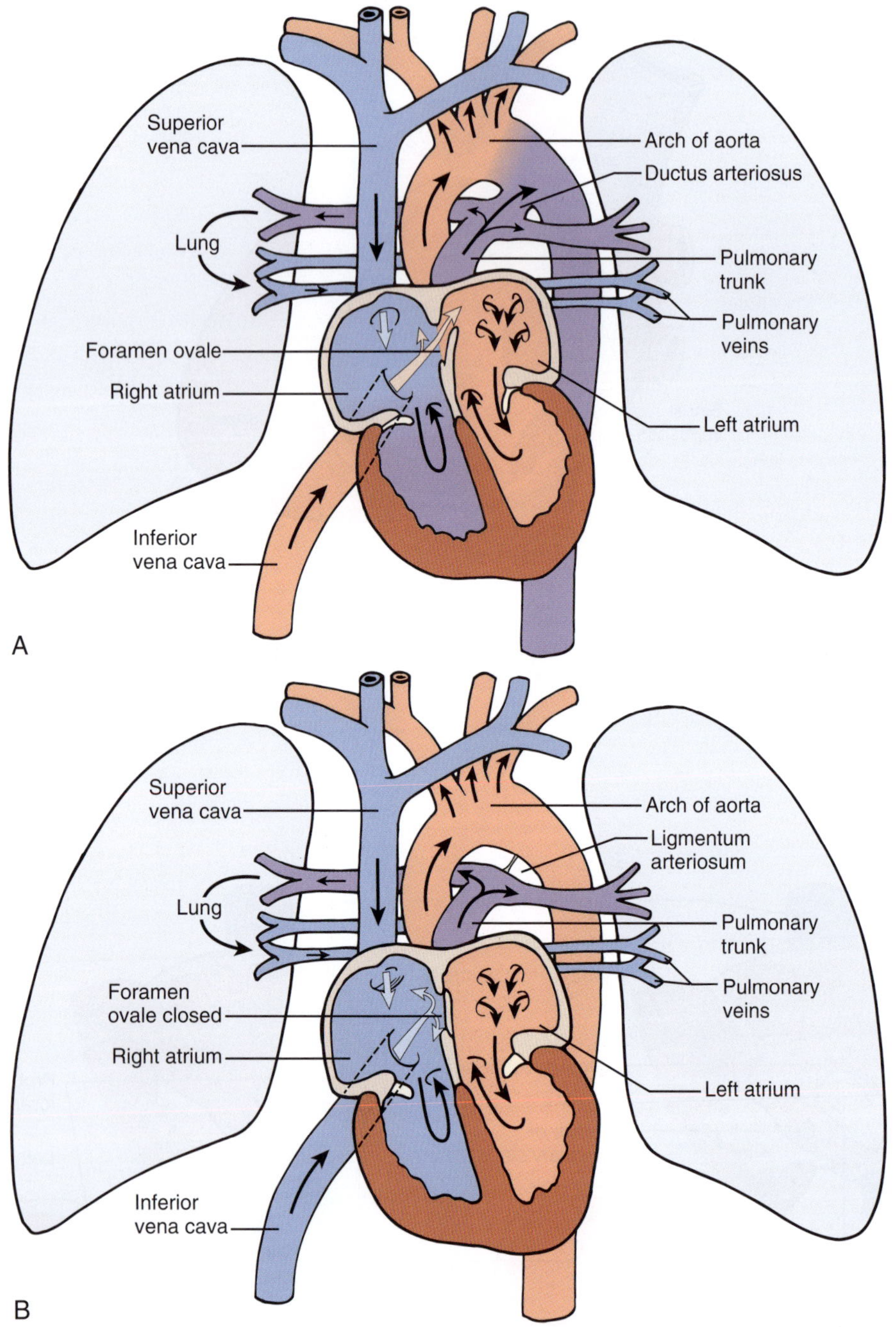

Superior vena cava

Arch of aorta

Ductus arteriosus

Lung

Pulmonary trunk

Pulmonary veins

Foramen ovale

Right atrium

Left atrium

Inferior vena cava

A

Superior vena cava

Arch of aorta

Ligmentum arteriosum

Lung

Pulmonary trunk

Pulmonary veins

Foramen ovale closed

Right atrium

Left atrium

Inferior vena cava

B

• **Figure 47.3** (A) Fetal circulation favors systemic venous return *across* the open foramen ovale from the inferior vena cava (IVC) (oxygenated blood from placenta, shown as red). This oxygenated blood is made available for left heart output to the head vessels and developing brain. Less oxygen-rich blood (depicted as blue, and mixing with some of the IVC return to create moderately saturated blood, depicted as maroon) fills the right ventricle and is ejected by the right heart across the patent ductus arteriosus for distal systemic perfusion. (B) After birth, right heart ejection to the lungs of desaturated *(blue)* blood occurs, resulting in oxygenation of the blood by the baby's lungs so that it can return to the left heart for ejection to the body. At this point the foramen ovale generally closes (from left atrial pressure) to prevent mixing of the two circulations. Thus the foramen ovale and atrial septal defect (ASD) is a normal fetal structure that should obliterate in the postnatal period. (Redrawn from Moore KL. *The Developing Human.* 2nd ed. Philadelphia: WB Saunders; 1977.)

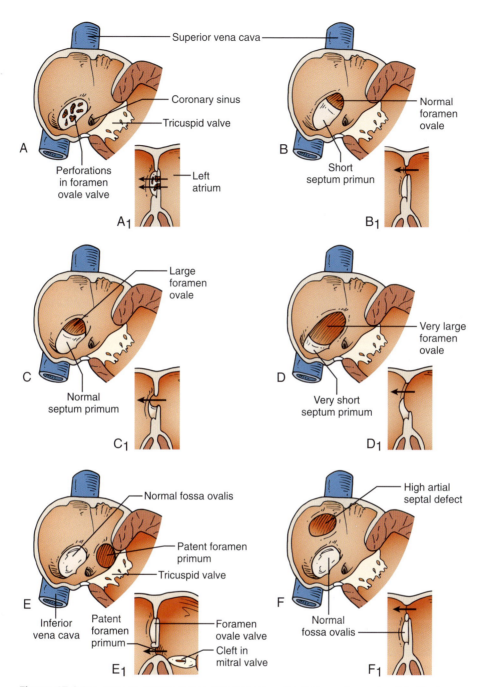

• **Figure 47.4** The primum septum that is meant to cover the fossa ovalis can be defective in many ways, including having multiple fenestrations (A), not being adequately large to attach to the septum secundum (B-D). Any of these defects will result in a "secundum" atrial septal defect (ASD). When there is absence of the atrioventricular septum (E), the result is an ostium primum ASD, and these are generally associated with a "cleft" in the mitral valve. In these circumstances the septum primum may be completely closing the fossa ovalis, and there may be little or no defect of the secundum variety. It is potentially confusing that a "secundum" ASD results from deficiency of the septum primum, and an "ostium primum" ASD is actually deficiency of the atrioventricular septum. (F) A sinus venosus defect occurs above the fossa ovalis in the tissue that actually constitutes the common wall between the roof of the left atrium and the back of the superior vena cava (SVC) (see Fig. 47.6). (Redrawn from Moore KL. *The Developing Human.* 2nd ed. Philadelphia: WB Saunders; 1977.)

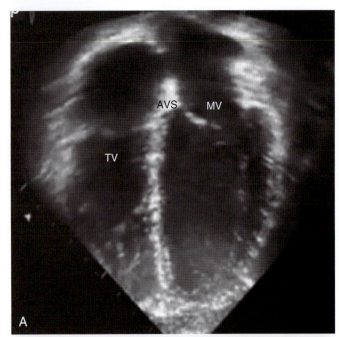

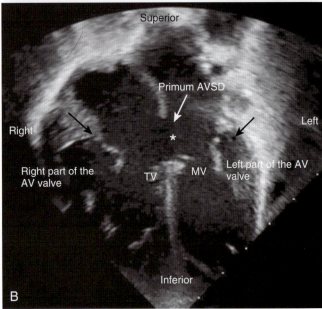

• **Figure 47.5** (A) A four-chamber echocardiogram of a normal heart demonstrates that the mitral valve (MV) attaches at a higher point on the septum than the tricuspid valve (TV). This results in a septum that separates the left ventricle from the right atrium, and this septum is called the *atrioventricular septum* (AVS). (B) In atrioventricular septal defects (AVSDs), the AVS is absent, and this can be diagnosed by noting that the mitral and tricuspid valves will attach at the same level. In this image, there is a large atrial communication (*)—a "partial" or "primum" AVSD or ostium primum atrial septal defect.

apposition" in the anterior leaflet of the left AV valve (see Fig. 47.4E). Current nomenclature regards this lesion more commonly as a partial AVSD.

Sinus Venosus Atrial Septal Defect

The right horn of the sinus venosus is embryologically connected to the primitive atria and eventually forms the inflow of the superior

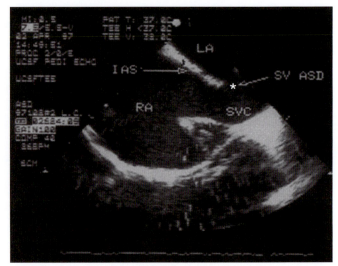

• **Figure 47.6** An echocardiogram that demonstrates a high sinus venosus (SV) atrial septal defect (ASD) (*). The septum primum is intact (IAS) closing the fossa ovalis, so there is no true secundum ASD. This echocardiogram demonstrates that the abnormality in an SV defect is *absence* of the structure that is the common wall separating the posterior superior vena cava (SVC) from the roof of the left atrium (LA). *RA,* Right atrium.

vena cava (SVC) where it enters into the RA. When this confluence is malpositioned toward the LA, it forms an override of the left and right atria, thus creating a connection, the sinus venosus ASD, that lies superior to the true atrial septum (see Fig. 47.4F; Fig. 47.6). Because of this leftward orientation of the sinus venosus, the right upper and right middle lobe pulmonary veins get incorporated with the SVC in the majority of sinus venosus ASDs, creating PAPVR return (Fig. 47.7). This creates two levels of left-to-right shunt, from LA to RA and from pulmonary vein to RA. A less common defect involves the ostia of IVC and right inferior pulmonary vein and is called *inferior sinus venosus ASD.*

Unroofed Coronary Sinus

The embryologic origin of the CS is the left horn of the sinus venosus that merges with the RA around the time of atrial septation. The regression of the roof of this structure happens after that point of development, explaining why the ostium of the CS remains in the typical location despite the opening into the LA. Many of the unroofed CSs are associated with a persistent left superior vena cava (LSVC). For this reason, shunting can be right to left from the LSVC to the LA, as well as left to right from the LA into the CS and into the RA through the normal ostium.

Natural History

Secundum type of ASDs can close spontaneously, but other types do not. A report by Campbell[5] noted that mean age of death was 37.5 ± 4.5 years with 75% dying by the age of 50 years and 90% dying by the age of 60 years.[5] The primary pathophysiologic result of any isolated ASD is left-to-right shunting. The degree of shunting is related to both the size of the actual defect and the relative difference in the compliance of the right ventricle (RV) compared to the LV. Compliance is defined as the "distensibility" of a ventricular chamber, with stiffer chambers being less compliant. Physiologically, compliance is measured as $\Delta P/\Delta V$, where P is pressure and V is

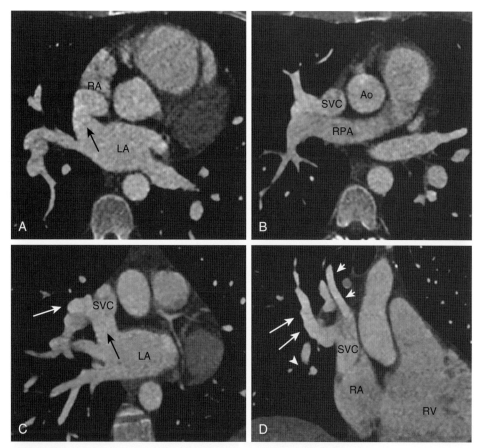

• **Figure 47.7** A magnetic resonance image of a sinus venosus atrial septal defect (ASD) demonstrates the communication between the superior vena cava (SVC) and the left atrium (LA) (*black arrow,* A). Pulmonary venous return to the side of the SVC at the level of the pulmonary artery (B) is nicely appreciated. This pulmonary venous return to the side of the SVC continues at a level superior to the right pulmonary artery (*white arrows,* C and D). The *black arrow* in (C) is the sinus venosus ASD. *Ao,* Aorta; *RA,* right atrium; *RPA,* right pulmonary artery; *RV,* right ventricle. (Courtesy Dr. Shi-Joon You, The Hospital for Sick Children [SickKids], Toronto.)

volume. In compliant chambers, large increases in volume result in chamber distention (much like a well-inflated balloon can easily increase in size when air is blown into it) with minimal increases in pressure. In noncompliant chambers (much like a small noninflated balloon), wall stiffness resists distention with volume infusion, and instead the intracavitary pressure increases as volume is added. Noncompliance, or wall stiffness, is a hallmark of "diastolic dysfunction" (as is often seen in some forms of congenital heart disease—like tetralogy of Fallot), and in these patients the noncompliance of the RV compared with the LV can result in right-to-left shunting across an ASD. Shortly after a baby is born, the RV is stiff and less compliant than the LV, and it is common for newborns to be mildly cyanotic from right-to-left shunting across the foramen ovale. As the lungs fill with air and the RV begins to pump against lower pulmonary resistance, the RV compliance improves, the atrial level shunt reverts to left to right, and this typically will close the foramen ovale by pushing the top of the septum primum against the top of the septum secundum (see Fig. 47.3). Although the direction of the shunt across an ASD is determined primarily by the differential compliance of the downstream chambers (RV and LV; with the RV generally being more compliant than the LV), other factors can also influence this downstream "compliance," such as severe stenosis or hypoplasia of the inlet (tricuspid or mitral) valve. The direction of the atrial shunt can also be influenced by "streaming" of blood

from the IVC that might be directed along the atrial septum and across a PFO or secundum ASD. Additionally, because shunting between atria occurs at low pressure, the development of pulmonary vascular disease is a late process if it occurs at all. Even in the sixth and seventh decade of life, many ASDs will continue to present without fixed pulmonary hypertension.[6] The enlargement of the right atrium and ventricle, however, do cause late atrial arrhythmias, tricuspid regurgitation, and RV dysfunction. These changes are slow to occur, and the precise window for surgical intervention remains poorly defined.

Presentation and Evaluation

The typical presentation of a child with an ASD is that of a completely asymptomatic child with a murmur noted on routine examination. Some children present with shortness of breath, easy fatigue, or other vague symptoms. In a child with profound symptoms or congestive heart failure, other causes, including concomitant cardiac defects, must be excluded.[7] Older children and adults may present with symptoms of mild fatigue and exercise intolerance, which gradually worsen with the age. Palpitations (due to atrial arrhythmias) are a common complaint. Patients who develop Eisenmenger syndrome (reversal of the left-to-right shunt secondary to pulmonary hypertension) present with cyanosis and syncope, although this is an uncommon occurrence from isolated ASD. Due to the low velocity/low pressure, shunting at the ASD per se does not produce a murmur. However, the volume overload in the RV produces a pulmonary systolic ejection murmur heard at the left sternal border due to relative pulmonary stenosis. The long ejection time of the RV due to this volume overload also creates the fixed split second heart sound associated with significant ASDs from delayed closure of the pulmonary valve. A large ASD may also have a diastolic murmur of relative tricuspid stenosis as a result of increased flow across the AV valve. A chest x-ray examination may demonstrate right heart enlargement, most notably a right atrial bulge. An electrocardiogram (ECG) can show P-wave changes and large R waves consistent with RA and RV enlargement. Other ECG findings common in ASDs include incomplete right bundle branch block and RSR′ in the V_1 lead. This latter finding is associated with an increased likelihood of needing closure of the ASD.[8,9]

The fundamental diagnostic tool is the echocardiogram. Transthoracic echocardiography can quickly, painlessly, noninvasively, and with relative cost efficiency diagnose an ASD and quantify the degree of right atrial and ventricular enlargement (Fig. 47.8). Perhaps more critically, the size and margins of the defect can be assessed, which helps determine the preferred mode of intervention, surgical versus transcatheter device. In older patients with questionable pulmonary hypertension the relative left-to-right versus right-to-left shunting, the estimation of RV pressure calculated by tricuspid regurgitation velocity, and any degree of RV dysfunction can also be determined with echocardiography. In the typical pediatric patient with an uncomplicated ASD, no other diagnostic studies are warranted outside of preprocedural laboratory studies, including an electrocardiogram. However, in older patients a history of palpitations requires an electrophysiologic evaluation with a minimum of 24-hour Holter monitoring. Any further concerns for arrhythmias may warrant an electrophysiologic study to determine the need for catheter-based or surgical antiarrhythmia ablations.[10] The role of cardiac catheterization for diagnosis of this condition is extremely limited in the pediatric population.[11] In the older patient with a large ASD and any question of elevated pulmonary pressures a cardiac catheterization can ascertain if closure of the ASD will prompt risk of RV dysfunction following closure. Cardiac magnetic resonance (CMR) imaging is often used to define the levels of PAPVR into the SVC in sinus venosus ASDs when not clearly defined on echocardiogram.[12] CMR is also valuable in older patients with long-standing ASDs to assess RV size and function.[13] Gated computed tomographic imaging is an emerging and potentially useful alternative to CMR, particularly for patients with complex ASDs.

Indication for Closure

Classically the primary indication for closure of an ASD is a calculated shunt fraction, described as the relative flow through the pulmonary system (Q_p) to the flow through the systemic system (Q_s), that is, a Q_p:Q_s of greater than 1.5:1. However, because few pediatric patients with an ASD undergo a cardiac

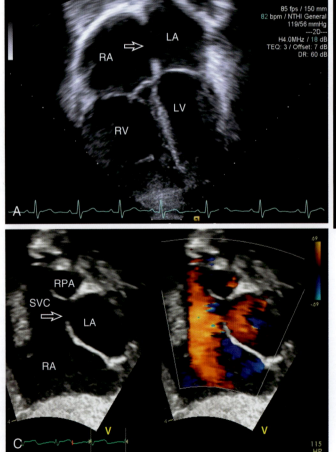

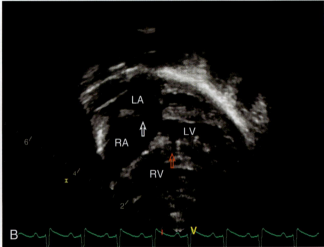

• **Figure 47.8** (A) Transthoracic echocardiogram in apical four-chamber view shows secundum type of atrial septal defect (ASD; *arrow*) with mildly dilated right atrium (RA) and right ventricle (RV). (B) Transthoracic echocardiogram in subcostal view shows primum type of ASD *(white arrow)* and inlet type of ventricle or septal defect *(red arrow)* in a patient with common atrioventricular canal defect. (C) Transthoracic echocardiogram in two-dimensional and color subcostal views shows sinus venosus type of ASD *(arrow)*. An intact septum primum covering the fossa ovalis can be appreciated, and the sinus venosus defect is superior to this region. In this patient the fossa ovalis is intact, and there is no secundum component. *LA*, Left atrium; *LV*, left ventricle; *RPA*, right pulmonary artery; *SVC*, superior vena cava.

catheterization,[13] the primary indication for closure of a secundum ASD is echocardiographic evidence of a significant left-to-right shunt and some degree of right heart enlargement. This is a relatively qualitative judgment but is the most typical path for pediatric patients. Alternatively, in some children and many adult patients there are a variety of indications, including symptoms (progressive dyspnea), arrhythmias, significant tricuspid regurgitation, RV dysfunction, and embolic stroke. These sequelae of ASDs are uncommon before the third to fourth decade of life and progressively become more common with advancing age.[14] Although the same criteria for secundum ASDs can apply to sinus venosus ASDs and ostium primum ASDs (partial AVSD), it is arguable that the presence of sinus venosus and ostium primum ASDs constitutes an indication for closure. Sinus venosus ASDs include PAPVR and have two levels of shunting, so many authorities would recommend closure regardless of right heart size.[15] Similarly, because partial AVSD includes a cleft in the left AV valve, only a very small ostium primum defect with no left AV valve regurgitation would be managed without intervention. If a patient presents with any degree of cyanosis or pulmonary hypertension, the patient must be evaluated by right heart catheterization, including the patient's response to pulmonary vasodilators, typically oxygen and nitric oxide. Only in the case of irreversible elevated pulmonary vascular resistance is closure of the ASD an absolute contraindication. Many patients with a response to the vasodilators will be helped with removal of the shunts if predominantly left to right.[6] The timing of surgery for the typical pediatric patient is based on medical and psychosocial issues. The operation can be performed without blood products when the patient is larger, certainly if the weight is above 15 kg. So waiting until that point is a reasonable consideration. Despite the fact that the right heart remodels even at older ages, completing the repair before school age may decrease the psychosocial input on the child. For those reasons, 3 to 5 years of age is an ideal time frame. However, early closure during infancy should be considered in those patients with compromised lung function, chronic lung disease, or diaphragmatic hernia or in those who are ventilator dependent for any other reasons.[16]

Catheter-Based Device Closure of Atrial Septal Defects

The majority of secundum ASDs (including PFOs) can be safely closed with a transcatheter technique in the cardiac catheterization laboratory. The first transcatheter device closure was introduced in 1976 by Mills and King.[17] Since then, there have been several devices introduced to close ASDs. Currently the most commonly used devices in the United States are the Amplatzer septal occluder device and the Gore Cardioform septal occluder device (Fig. 47.9). Current technology has developed catheter-based ASD devices that are able to close only secundum ASDs and PFOs. There is no role for catheter-based closure of CS ASDs, sinus venosus ASDs due to the PAPVR, or ostium primum ASDs because the device would interfere with the AV valves and place the conduction system at risk.

The indication for closure of a secundum ASD should be the same for surgical closure or catheter-based device closure. Careful echocardiographic assessment can usually determine the two anatomic qualifications for device closure: the size of the defect relative to the total length of the atrium and the size of the atrial rims.[18] The atrial rims are needed to hold the device around the entire defect. Deficient rims of atrial septal tissue near the aorta

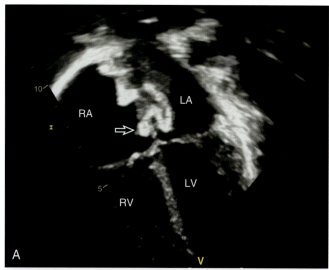

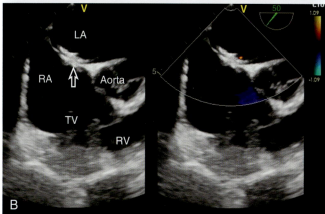

• **Figure 47.9** (A) Transthoracic echocardiogram in apical four-chamber view shows Amplatzer device across the secundum type of atrial septal defect (ASD; *arrow*). (B) Transesophageal echocardiogram in short axis view shows Gore Cardioform device across ASD *(arrow)*. *LA,* Left atrium; *LV,* left ventricle; *RA,* right atrium; *RV,* right ventricle; *TV,* tricuspid valve.

or near the IVC are the common reasons for referring patients for surgical closure (Fig. 47.10).[19] Transthoracic echocardiography is typically sufficient, but in questionable cases, transesophageal echocardiography[20] and three-dimensional echocardiography[21] can help with assessment of appropriate anatomy for device closure in the catheterization laboratory. Balloon sizing and intracardiac echocardiography both can assist in making such a determination in the catheterization laboratory.[22] Device closure of secundum ASDs has become the standard, and the overall success is well established.[23]

Even though this technique is safe and feasible in many patients, it is not free from complications. Complications of device closure include embolization of the device, device malalignment, thrombosis, conduction abnormalities, residual shunts, impingement of device on adjacent structures such as AV valves, SVC, CS, pulmonary veins, or aorta.[24] The long-term complication of erosion of the device into the aorta or atrial wall has also been described, so patients who undergo device closure, particularly with large devices, should receive periodic follow-up to ensure that the device is stable in the atrial septum. Oversized devices have eroded through the atrial wall, and so the absolute size of the device is limited, especially in smaller children requiring larger devices.[25,26] The technology

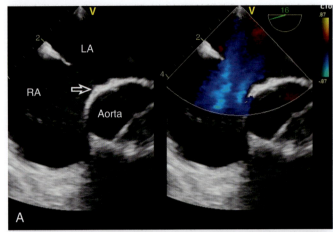

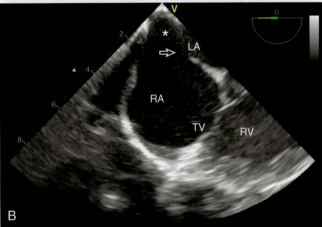

• **Figure 47.10** (A) Transesophageal echocardiogram in short axis view shows deficient retroaortic rim with atrial septal defect *(arrow)*. (B) Transesophageal echocardiogram shows absent superior rim *(*)* in secundum type of ASD *(arrow)*. *LA,* Left atrium; *RA,* right atrium; *RV,* right ventricle; *TV,* tricuspid valve.

continues to evolve, and there are more opportunities for device closure with later-generation devices. In cases in which a family is interested in device closure of a "borderline" defect, operating room (OR) backup can be used if the defect is determined to be not amenable to closure in the catheterization laboratory, and the patient can go to the OR under the same anesthetic for surgical closure. Any signs of clinical change, especially tachyarrhythmia, must be investigated. A change in the murmur must be evaluated with echocardiography and prompt intervention pursued. Although some devices can be retrieved percutaneously if embolized in the catheterization laboratory, consideration must be made for prompt surgical intervention for device retrieval and ASD closure.[27]

Another consideration in the choice of device closure is the potential need for other interventions. The presence of arrhythmias or important tricuspid regurgitations for which a maze procedure and/or a tricuspid annuloplasty would benefit the patient, a surgical approach likely outweighs the "ease" of the percutaneous procedure. This is more typical in older patients.

Patent Foreman Ovale

PFOs are extremely common but have little or no hemodynamic consequence, and so routine closure is never warranted. PFOs

have been implicated in cryptogenic strokes, and closure after one of these events is a controversial issue. Results from several studies suggest that in high-risk patients with recurrent cryptogenic stroke, known venous thrombosis, or an aneurysmal septum, device closure is likely beneficial. However, for the cryptogenic stroke population with standard PFO, clear evidence for closure by transcatheter device is lacking.[28,29]

Surgery for Atrial Septal Defects

Secundum Atrial Septal Defect

Surgery for the secundum ASD represents our congenital heart surgery history more than any other lesion. Secundum ASD was the first intracardiac lesion repaired on cardiopulmonary bypass as well as by multiple ingenious methods before that sentinel procedure performed by John Gibbon in 1953.[30] Multiple improvements in pump and oxygenation technology and vast surgical experience now make it one of the simplest and safest operations we perform. For this reason, multiple limited-access cosmetic approaches have been developed to conduct the operation. The gold standard remains the full median sternotomy (Fig. 47.11A), and it is the safest approach, particularly when there are complicating factors involving questionable venous anatomy or any secondary lesions. Limited skin incisions with partial sternotomy, submammary incisions with right anterolateral thoracotomy, and axillary incisions with small lateral thoracotomy approaches have all been proven to be safe and effective.[31,32] Femoral cannulation, placing the IVC cannula through a preplaced chest tube site, and avoiding the aortic cross-clamp by using controlled fibrillation have all aided in making smaller and smaller scars. Along the same lines, robotic-assisted surgery for closure of secundum ASDs has been accomplished at many centers.[33] The fundamentals of the operation include aortic and bicaval cannulation with cardioplegic arrest. No vent is required because the left heart is amply drained through the defect. The RA is opened and suctioned clear with cardiotomy suction to expose both cavae, and the lack of any pulmonary venous connections to the RA is confirmed. Avoiding suctioning the blood from the LA prevents air getting to the left heart. The margins of the defect are inspected, especially at the inferior aspect near the IVC. If there is septal tissue that can be approximated without tension at the inferior portion of the ASD, it can almost always be closed primarily with a 5-0 or 4-0 polypropylene suture run from the inferior and superior points toward the middle (Fig. 47.12B). The left heart is extensively deaired with the Valsalva breath and the suture tied (see Fig. 47.12D). Some surgeons recommend blowing carbon dioxide over the operative field during these open procedures. Carbon dioxide displaces air in the incision, and any CO_2 retained in the heart after cardiotomy is usually readily absorbed, thus reducing the risk of air embolism. A subsequent Valsalva breath can test for any residual leaks, including unseen fenestrations in the septum primum. If there is minimal septal tissue near the IVC, then a patch of autologous pericardium, with or without glutaraldehyde, or Gore-Tex should be used to close the defect (see Fig. 47.11AB). A similar continuous suture technique is employed with careful deairing performed. With either closure technique, one must avoid the error of mistaking the eustachian valve for the margin of the defect, thus closing the IVC into the LA. Although this should be primarily avoided by noting the IVC above the level of ASD closure, it must be immediately considered, and promptly corrected, if there is systemic desaturation upon separating from bypass.

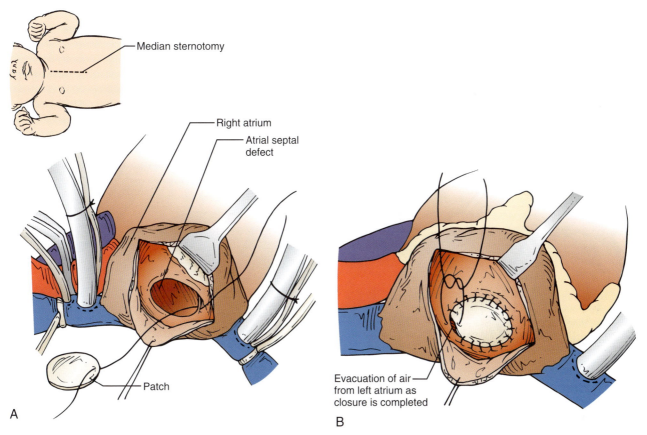

Median sternotomy

Right atrium

Atrial septal defect

Patch

A

Evacuation of air from left atrium as closure is completed

B

• **Figure 47.11** (A) The surgical approach to atrial septal defect (ASD) closure is typically through a median sternotomy. Both the superior vena cava (SVC) and the inferior vena cava (IVC) are cannulated for venous return so that the right atrium can be entered to expose the defect. In most circumstances the defect is closed with a patch. (B) Before the suture line is completed, the left heart is completely deaired to limit potential ejection of air into the systemic circulation. In most cases these procedures are performed under cardioplegic arrest so that the heart cannot eject during the time the defect is being repaired. (Redrawn from Ungerleider RM. In: Sabiston DC Jr. *Atlas of Cardiothoracic Surgery.* Philadelphia: WB Saunders; 1995.)

Because the conduct of this operation, even with very limited incisions, is so straightforward, the need for any inotropic agents or pressor support is extremely rare. For this reason many surgical and anesthesia teams will perform this operation with an arterial line and two good intravenous lines and forego a central line. The expectation should be extubation in the OR or shortly after the patient has been returned to the intensive care unit (ICU). The use of local anesthetics in the wound, typically 0.25% Marcaine, may help limit the need for narcotics post-operatively.

Sinus Venosus Atrial Septal Defect

Sinus venosus ASDs, ostium primum ASDs, and unroofed CS ASDs can be approached through similar incisions to the secundum ASD, but the incisions are more likely performed through a standard midline sternotomy due to a greater variability in their anatomy. Aortic and bicaval cannulation is the same as in secundum ASD closure. Cardioplegic arrest without a vent is standard. A key element for repair of the sinus venosus defect is high cannulation of the SVC near the innominate vein with a right-angled cannula to allow maximal exposure of all anomalous pulmonary veins.

Differentiation between the pulmonary veins and the azygos vein is important.

There are multiple surgical techniques for repair of the sinus venosus ASD. When the anomalous pulmonary veins enter the SVC close to or at the SVC-RA junction, then a single patch of pericardium, with or without glutaraldehyde, or of Gore-Tex is used to close the ASD, including the pulmonary veins, thus baffling the flow of the veins into the LA through the defect (Fig. 47.13). This technique is effective in a majority of cases.[34] However, when the anomalous veins enter higher into the SVC, a single-patch technique will likely compromise the pulmonary vein drainage, the SVC drainage, or both because the baffle has limitations of the size of the SVC for both systemic and pulmonary venous drainage.

A two-patch technique involves the opening of the SVC with a lateral incision and subsequent augmentation of the SVC after an appropriate baffle patch is sewn from the high pulmonary vein through the ASD. A variation of the two-patch technique is a lateral caval flap where the wall of the SVC and RA is cut out as an in situ baffle that includes the orifices of the ASD, creating an autologous baffle.[35] The resulting defect in the side of the SVC and RA is then patched with autologous pericardium (Fig. 47.14).

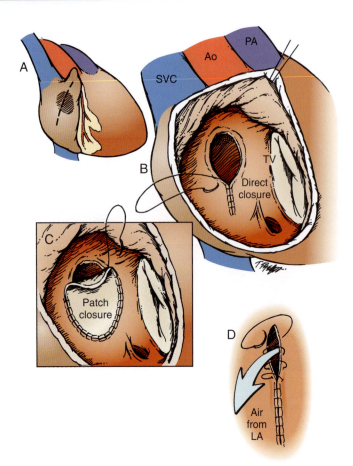

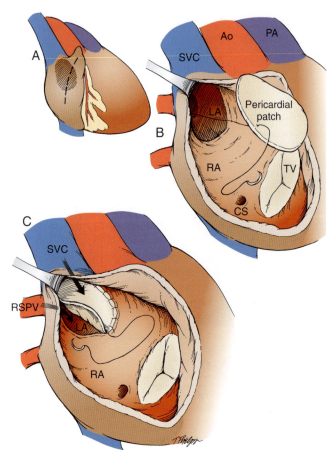

• **Figure 47.12** Surgical procedure for atrial septal defect (ASD) closure. (A) Orientation of right atriotomy, avoiding area of sinoatrial node. (B) Direct suture closure of secundum ASD. (C) Patch closure of secundum ASD. (D) Deairing of the left atrium. *Ao,* Aorta; *CS,* coronary sinus; *LA,* left atrium; *PA,* pulmonary artery; *SVC,* superior vena cava; *TV,* tricuspid valve.

• **Figure 47.13** Surgical correction of sinus venosus defect using a pericardial patch to direct the pulmonary venous blood across the atrial septal defect and into the left atrium. (A) Right atriotomy *(dashed line)* for repair of sinus venosus defect. In many cases it is our preference to make the same kind of oblique atriotomy that would be made for closure of a secundum defect to avoid the sinoatrial node, which is generally near the junction between the superior vena cava (SVC) and the right atrium. (B) Right atrium (RA) opened to expose subcaval sinus venosus defect through which the left atrium (LA) is viewed. (C) Anomalous right superior pulmonary vein (RSPV) enters at the SVC–right atrium (RA) junction. The defect is closed with a pericardial patch so that blood from the RSPV is baffled into the LA and blood from the SVC enters the RA. When this type of oblique atrial incision is used, it is not necessary to augment the atriotomy with additional patch material. *Ao,* Aorta; *CS,* coronary sinus; *PA,* pulmonary artery; *TV,* tricuspid valve.

Another popular alternative for high-lying anomalous pulmonary veins is the Warden procedure[36] (Fig. 47.15). In these cases the anomalous pulmonary veins enter "high" along the lateral border of the SVC and would require a long lateral tunnel to baffle them into the LA. The Warden procedure provides an option that can reduce the risk of baffle obstruction from long tunnels. The SVC is divided immediately proximal ("above") the entry of the highest pulmonary vein. The distal SVC is patched closed on the transected end and therefore drains only pulmonary blood. The entire orifice of the SVC is then closed with a patch from inside the RA, including the ASD with the patch. Therefore all of the anomalous pulmonary venous blood is directed to the LA (Fig. 47.16). The proximal end of the SVC is then anastomosed to the right atrial appendage. Three key elements to the success of this operation are full mobilization of the SVC, including division of the azygous vein if necessary to create a nontense anastomosis between the SVC and RA, meticulous excision of the pectinate muscles of the atrial appendage, and augmentation of the anastomosis with a pericardial patch if there is any question of tension.

In any approach to the sinus venosus ASD, attention must be paid to the sinoatrial node. The node can be seen as a yellow slightly thickened area of the RA just above the SVC junction. Even if not directly injured, division of the SA nodal artery, which may happen with the two-patch technique, can cause SA node

dysfunction, which will manifest as a low atrial or junctional rhythm.[37,38] Late stenosis of the pulmonary venous pathway is very uncommon, but narrowing of the SVC can occur rarely due to scarring or the bulging of the pulmonary venous baffle into the lumen of the SVC.

Ostium Primum Atrial Septal Defect

Surgical closure of the ostium primum ASD requires exposure of the left AV valve through the defect and is most typically achieved with sternotomy and similar cannulation strategy as for the secundum ASD. A left atrial vent placed through the right superior pulmonary vein will allow a clear field for closure of the cleft. A 5-0 or 6-0 polypropylene suture placed at the base

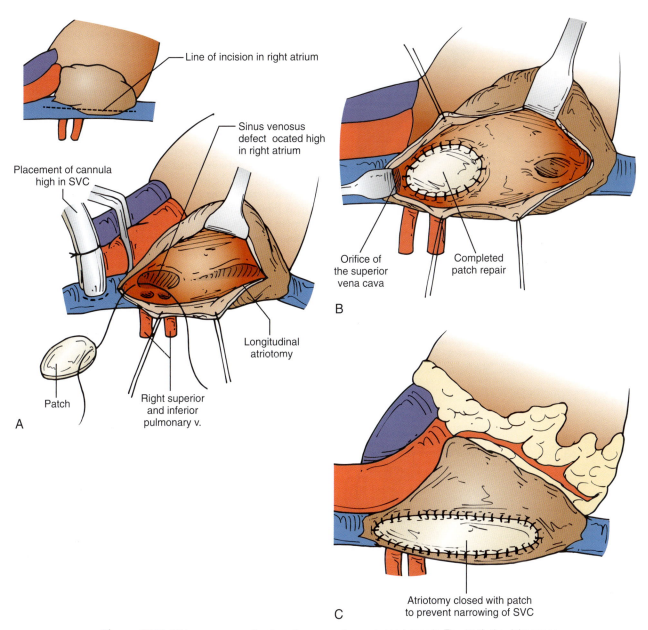

Line of incision in right atrium

Sinus venosus defect ocated high in right atrium

Placement of cannula high in SVC

Patch

Longitudinal atriotomy

Right superior and inferior pulmonary v.

A

Orifice of the superior vena cava

Completed patch repair

B

Atriotomy closed with patch to prevent narrowing of SVC

C

• **Figure 47.14** (A) In some cases (such as the magnetic resonance image in Fig. 47.7), the right upper lobe pulmonary veins enter the side of the superior vena cava (SVC) higher than can be reached through an oblique atrial incision. In these cases a longitudinal incision extending from the right atrium up the lateral aspect of the SVC has been used (historically). This incision can be very close to the location of the sinoatrial node. It does provide excellent exposure of the anomalous pulmonary veins so that they can be directed below a patch into the left atrium (B), but simply closing the atrial incision primarily risks narrowing the SVC, so typically a pericardial patch is used to augment the size of the SVC (C), especially considering that the underlying patch to close the atrial septal defect (ASD) may also be bulging a bit into the lumen of the SVC. (Redrawn from Ungerleider RM. In: Sabiston DC Jr. *Atlas of Cardiothoracic Surgery.* Philadelphia: WB Saunders; 1995.)

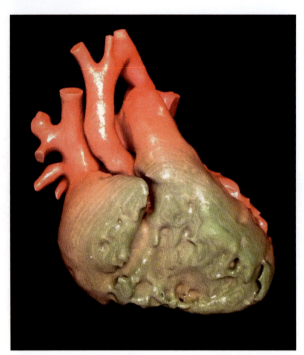

• **Figure 47.15** A magnetic resonance image reconstruction of sinus venosus atrial septal defect with partial anomalous pulmonary venous return. Note the right upper lobe pulmonary veins draining into the high superior vena cava (SVC), above the level of the right pulmonary artery (which crosses below the SVC). This anatomy may be best repaired with a Warden procedure (see Fig. 47.16). (Courtesy Dr. Shi-Joon You, The Hospital for Sick Children [SickKids], Toronto.)

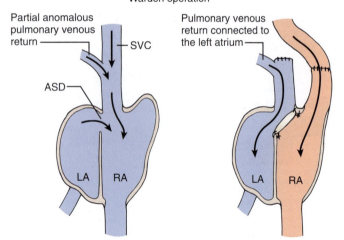

• **Figure 47.16** When the drainage of the right upper lobe pulmonary veins is high above the superior vena cava (SVC)–right atrial junction, we prefer a Warden procedure. In this procedure the SVC is divided (and closed) cephalad to the most superior pulmonary vein. This converts the SVC into an extension of the pulmonary venous return. The entry of the SVC into the atrium is then baffled across the sinus venosus atrial septal defect (ASD), directing all pulmonary venous return from the right veins to the left atrium. The divided end of the SVC is then attached to the right atrial appendage to restore systemic venous return to the right side of the circulation.

of the cleft and retracted to the left followed by a suture at the leading edge of the cleft, as noted by chordal attachments, and retracted to the right perfectly displays the entire cleft, which is closed with a series of interrupted sutures (Fig. 47.17A). The valve is tested, and then the vent can be placed through the valve into the LV to assist with deairing (see Fig. 47.17B). The ostium primum defect is closed with an autologous pericardial patch. A continuous suture along the raphe between the left and right AV valves begins the closure. Rounding the inferior edge close to the CS, the AV node, and His bundle are dangerously close. Great care to take suture bites at the very margin of the defect will protect from potential conduction block (see Fig. 47.16C). An alternative strategy is to run the patch high around the CS. This protects the AV node and His bundle at the expense of CS blood draining to the LA with very mild desaturation. This latter technique is contraindicated when there is a persistent left SVC because shunting the left SVC blood along with CS blood into the LA would create a significant right-to-left shunt. The upper suture line is brought around the atrial tissue near the root of the aorta. Obvious care not to take large enough bites to affect the aortic valve is employed. The left heart is deaired and the suture line closed. The presence of a PFO or secundum ASD is noted and closed as well (see Fig. 47.17D).

The closure of the unroofed CS involves patch closure of the extent of the defect or in cases in which the opening is immediately proximal to the ostium of the sinus, the edge of the unroofed wall can be sutured to the free edge of the CS ostium. If a left SVC is present, it must be cannulated or snared to allow exposure free of excessive drainage from the LSVC.

For all repairs of ASDs, regardless of type, postoperative transesophageal echocardiography is essential because it allows for the assessment of residual leak, venous pathway obstruction, AV valve regurgitation, and ventricular function.[39]

Result of Surgery and Long-Term Prognosis

ICU care should be streamlined with monitoring continuous vital signs, urine output, and chest tube bleeding. Necessary tests include arterial blood gas levels, including electrolytes, a chest x-ray examination, and an ECG. All other testing should be guided by clinical indication. Generally these patients are very stable. Hypotension and tachycardia almost always represent some degree of hypovolemia. Because the RV has been volume loaded since birth, it is not unusual to need to give intravenous fluid boluses for mild hypotension. Because these patients generally have fairly normal hearts, we try to avoid the use of blood transfusion. Hypertension and tachycardia almost always represents inadequate pain and/or anxiety control. ICU stay should typically be overnight at most, and total hospital stay ranges from 2 to 4 days. Pain control, early mobilization, and diuresis with furosemide are the essential components of care. An echocardiogram before discharge or in early follow-up to assess for any degree of pericardial effusion is standard. Postpericardiotomy syndrome can occur with any congenital heart operation but may be more prevalent after ASD closure. It manifests as pleural effusion with some combination of fever, chest pain, pericardial rub, and irritability. Standard therapy consists of nonsteroidal antiinflammatory drug and diuretic for any effusion. Occasional patients may require percutaneous pericardial drainage for persistent effusions.

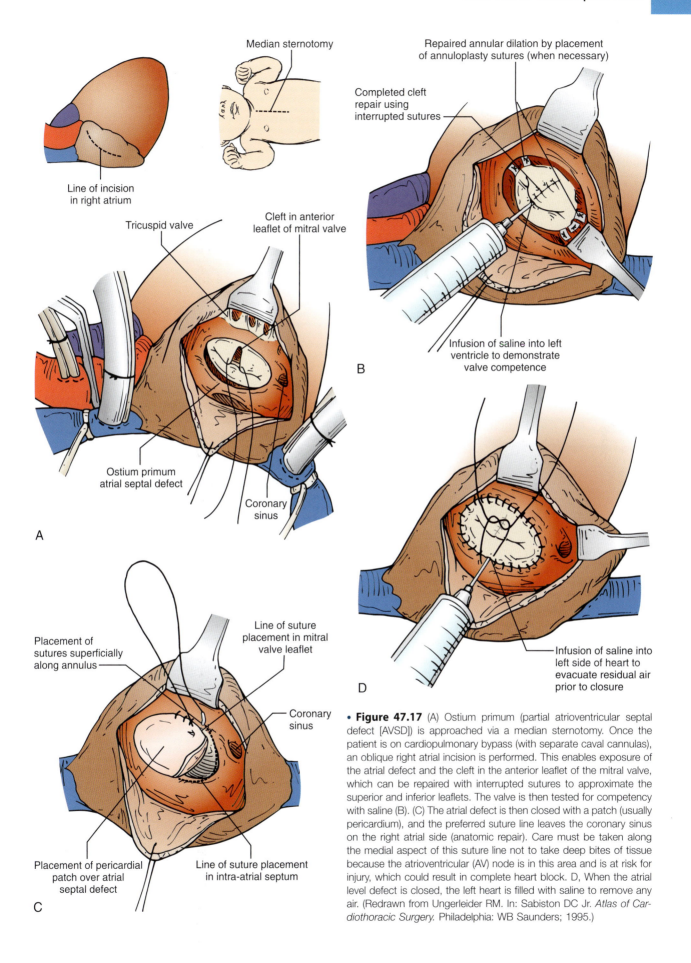

• **Figure 47.17** (A) Ostium primum (partial atrioventricular septal defect [AVSD]) is approached via a median sternotomy. Once the patient is on cardiopulmonary bypass (with separate caval cannulas), an oblique right atrial incision is performed. This enables exposure of the atrial defect and the cleft in the anterior leaflet of the mitral valve, which can be repaired with interrupted sutures to approximate the superior and inferior leaflets. The valve is then tested for competency with saline (B). (C) The atrial defect is then closed with a patch (usually pericardium), and the preferred suture line leaves the coronary sinus on the right atrial side (anatomic repair). Care must be taken along the medial aspect of this suture line not to take deep bites of tissue because the atrioventricular (AV) node is in this area and is at risk for injury, which could result in complete heart block. D, When the atrial level defect is closed, the left heart is filled with saline to remove any air. (Redrawn from Ungerleider RM. In: Sabiston DC Jr. *Atlas of Cardiothoracic Surgery.* Philadelphia: WB Saunders; 1995.)

Outcomes

Short-term results for ASD closure in children are excellent. The mortality should be essentially zero in isolated defects. Long-term outcomes at 35 years in patients who had ASDs closed as children show survival, exercise capacity, and quality of life were equivalent to the normal population. There is a higher incidence of atrial arrhythmias, as well as RV dysfunction and enlargements. Of course, the patients in these longitudinal series were operated on in a different era (1965–1980), and so numerous advances in our current era, including much improved myocardial protection, would suggest that these excellent results should only be better with current surgery and interventional ASD closure.

References

A complete list of references is available at ExpertConsult.com.

48

Total Anomalous Pulmonary Venous Return

JAMES ST. LOUIS, MD; ERICA MOLITOR-KIRSCH, MD; SANKET SHAH, MD, MHS;
JAMES O'BRIEN, MD

Total anomalous pulmonary venous return (TAPVR) is a rare lesion, making up approximately 2% of all patients who present with a congenital cardiac anomaly. The anatomy most often consists of the all the pulmonary veins connecting to a common confluence that drains to the systemic venous circulation and eventually empties into the desaturated atrial chamber. Patients will most often present with a large left-to-right shunt resulting in pulmonary overcirculation and heart failure. Less frequently, the pulmonary venous connection is obstructed, leading to cardiopulmonary collapse shortly following birth. Medical management is essentially ineffective for these patients, making TAPVR one of the few defects requiring emergent surgical intervention in a congenital cardiac practice. Mortality following operative correction has improved over the last several decades, although certain subsets have persistently worse survival.[1-4]

Embryology

Near the end of the first month of fetal life the primordial pulmonary buds have developed from the foregut. At this stage these structures are surrounded by the splanchnic plexus of the foregut and share drainage to the cardinal and umbilicovitelline veins. It is also at this time that this plexus begins the process of differentiation into the final pulmonic phenotype (Fig. 48.1). Initially there is no direct connection of the pulmonary vascular plexus to the heart, but a common pulmonary vein eventually emerges from a combination of the evagination of left atrial tissue, the pulmonary venous plexus itself, and the surrounding mesoderm.[5-7] The plexus of parenchymal pulmonary veins will eventually connect with this common pulmonary vein, which in turn connects with the sinoatrial portion of the heart. This connection will be incorporated into the left atrial wall, with the individual pulmonary veins draining independently into the chamber. The original connection to the systemic venous system will eventually involute, leaving the richly oxygenated blood draining directly to the systemic atrium. An anatomic defect occurs when the pulmonary venous plexus fails to connect to the systemic atrium and there is persistence of one or more of the early connections to the systemic venous circulation.

Classification

The most commonly used classification scheme was proposed by Craig, Darling, and Rothney.[8] They classified this anomaly based on the drainage pattern of the pulmonary venous return to the systemic venous circulation. The supracardiac type occurs most frequently, occurring in 50% of cases in most published series.[1,3,7] In supracardiac TAPVR all pulmonary veins enter a common confluence that subsequently connects to either the innominate vein or directly to the superior vena cava (Fig. 48.2). The second most frequent type, termed infracardiac, occurs when the common confluence drains inferiorly to below the diaphragm to enter either the portal vein or the inferior vena cava directly (Fig. 48.3). This type occurs approximately 25% to 30% of the time. The cardiac type occurs when the drainage of the confluence is to the coronary sinus or directly into the right atrium. Finally, the mixed type of TAPVR consists of a variable number of connections that drain directly to the heart or to an additional extracardiac structure.[9] This classification scheme is most practical because it helps in surgical planning, postoperative management, and long-term care. An alternative classification scheme is that of Burroughs and Edwards,[10] in which the anatomy is classified according to the embryologic basis of abnormal connection.

Associated Defects and Genetics

TAPVR may present as either an isolated anomaly or in association with another congenital cardiac defect. Sadiq and colleagues described a series of patients with right atrial isomerism and found that 70% had some form of TAPVR. All these patients had an additional congenital anomaly, with the most common being an atrioventricular septal defect, double-outlet right ventricle (RV), double-inlet left ventricle (LV), transposition of the great arteries, or pulmonary artery (PA) atresia.[11] In the series by St. Louis et al., 27% of patients with TAPVR had an associated cardiac lesion. The majority consisted of functionally single-ventricle anatomy, with more than half being diagnosed with heterotaxy syndrome.[1] The population-based study reported by Seale showed that in patients with TAPVR, excluding those with heterotaxy and complex single-ventricle anatomy, 14% had associated cardiac lesions. These lesions consisted of ventricular septal defects, coarctation of the aorta, interruption of the aortic arch, tetralogy of Fallot, and double-outlet RV.[3]

Whereas most cases of TAPVR are sporadic, with a recurrence risk of approximately 2.5%, reports have described familial occurrences.[12] Paz and Castilla[13] reported a family in which three of the children had TAPVR. Based on chromosomal evaluation, the authors

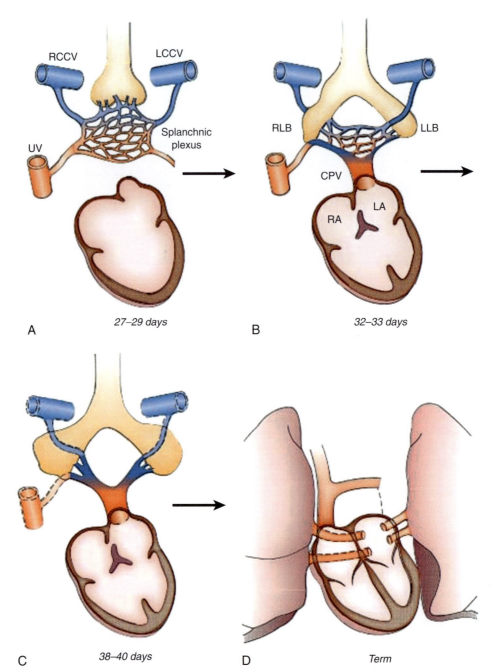

RCCV   LCCV

Splanchnic
plexus

UV

A   *27–29 days*

RLB   LLB

CPV

RA   LA

B   *32–33 days*

C   *38–40 days*

D   *Term*

• **Figure 48.1** Normal development of pulmonary veins. (A) At approximately 4 weeks of gestation, the primordial lung buds are enmeshed by the vascular plexus of the foregut (the splanchnic plexus). At this stage there is no direct connection to the heart, with all the drainage to the splanchnic plexus. (B) By the end of the first month of gestation the common pulmonary vein (CPV) establishes a connection between the pulmonary venous plexus and the sinoatrial portion of the heart. (C) Next, the connections between the pulmonary venous plexus and the splanchnic venous plexus involute. (D) The CPV incorporates into the left atrium (LA) so that the individual pulmonary veins connect separately and directly to the LA. *LCCV,* Left common cardinal vein; *LLB,* left lung bud; *RA,* right atrium; *RCCV,* right common cardinal vein; *RLB,* right lung bud; *UV,* umbilical vein. (From Allen HD, Shaddy RE, Penny DJ, et al. Anomalies of the pulmonary veins. In: *Moss and Adams' Heart Disease in Infants, Children, and Adolescents: Including the Fetus and Young Adult.* 9th ed. Lippincott Williams & Wilkins, 2016:882.)

concluded that the most likely mechanism for this occurrence could be attributed to either a small chromosome translocation or a single autosomal dominant gene mutation. Bleyl and colleagues[14] reported a large Utah-Idaho family in which TAPVR segregated as an autosomal dominant trait. The gene in this family was localized to the centromeric region of the fourth chromosome using linkage mapping. They suggested that a vascular endothelial growth factor receptor (VEGFR), thought to have a role in vasculogenesis, maps near the pericentric region of chromosome four and is a candidate gene for both familial and sporadic cases of

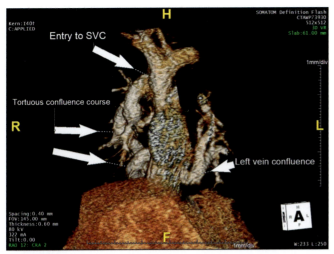

• **Figure 48.2** A volume-rendered image from a contrast-enhanced computed tomography angiogram of the chest as viewed from the anterior and slightly rightward projection. Most of the cardiac mass, except the right atrium, has been cropped out to easily visualize venous anatomy. Left superior and inferior pulmonary veins come to a confluence posterior to the left atrium. The confluence courses rightward posterior to the right atrium to enter the right chest. Here, after a tortuous course and picking up drainage from the right lower, middle, and upper veins, the venous confluence drains into the superior vena cava (SVC) from a posterior and lateral aspect.

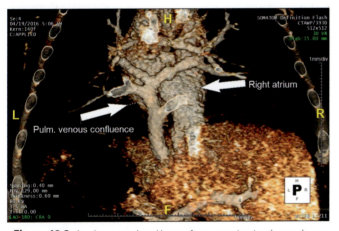

• **Figure 48.3** A volume-rendered image from a contrast-enhanced computed tomography angiogram of the chest as viewed from the posterior projection. Right and left superior pulmonary veins come to a confluence posterior to the left atrium. As the confluence courses inferiorly, right and left inferior pulmonary veins drain into the confluence, which ultimately drains into portal circulation in the liver.

TAPVR. Le Cras and colleagues,[15] using a transgenic animal model, showed that with a VEGFR inhibitor, pulmonary vascular growth and postnatal alveolarization were arrested.

Clinical Presentation

In a comprehensive, population-based study from several European countries the most common signs and symptoms at the time of presentation in children with TAPVR were cyanosis (43%), respiratory distress (31%), failure to thrive (11%), circulatory collapse (4.5%), a murmur (0.5%), or supraventricular tachycardia (0.5%).[3] Patients not diagnosed prenatally will often present early with findings similar to those observed with a large atrial septal defect (ASD), although mild cyanosis is present. The infants initially appear well. Over time they will develop signs of congestive heart failure such as tachypnea, tachycardia, and hepatomegaly. They may present with recurrent pneumonias and failure to thrive. Physical examination will reveal a hyperactive RV impulse, split and fixed S_2, systolic ejection murmur at the upper left sternal border, and a middiastolic rumble at the left lower sternal border. Electrocardiograms will demonstrate right axis deviation, RV hypertrophy, and right atrial enlargement. Chest radiography will show cardiomegaly with increased pulmonary venous markings. In children greater than 4 months of age a prominent vertical vein may create the appearance of the "snowman" sign on chest radiographs.[16]

For children with pulmonary venous obstruction (PVO), rapid progression to metabolic acidosis, cardiac failure, and death may occur shortly following birth. If the child survives the initial 24 hours, tachycardia, poor peripheral perfusion, and hypotension can occur. They may develop lactic acidosis, arrhythmias, and end-organ dysfunction related to cardiogenic shock. Cardiac auscultation findings are minimal and may include a loud S_2 and gallop rhythm. Chest radiography reveals pulmonary edema with a small heart. Electrocardiograms will show right axis deviation and RV hypertension.

Diagnostic Assessment

The diagnosis of TAPVR can be difficult on prenatal ultrasonography. In the series by Seale and colleagues,[3] only 1.9% of cases were diagnosed prenatally. This observation suggests that an increased awareness of this diagnosis should occur at the early stages of evaluation of any child with suspected congenital heart disease. A recent paper from Tongsong and colleagues[17] presented a comprehensive set of guidelines for increasing the number of accurate prenatal diagnoses at the time of initial imaging. In this work the authors recommend further imaging studies when the initial ultrasonogram does not depict the entry of the pulmonary veins into the left atrium when one of these additional conditions is met: (1) the presence of a vascular confluence in the space behind the heart, (2) abnormal spectral waveforms in the pulmonary veins, (3) a smooth posterior wall of the left atrium, (4) increased retroatrial space, (5) a dilated coronary sinus, or (6) a dilated superior vena cava. In a review of 26 fetuses with a prenatal diagnosis of TAPVR, Ganesan and colleagues[18] described several consistent ultrasonographic findings, including the lack of visible pulmonary venous connections to the left atrium and the presence of a visible venous confluence on axial four-chamber views. The presence of an additional vertical venous channel on three-vessel or axial abdominal views was also sometimes noted. A high index of suspicion is required to avoid a false-negative or false-positive echocardiographic study. When there is doubt, it may help to have an experienced cardiologist review echocardiographic images.

The differential diagnoses of these children can be grouped according to the child's age at presentation.[19] Patients with severe obstruction are first seen as neonates and will often be mistaken for having other more common severe illnesses of the newborn associated with acidosis and hypoxia, including persistent pulmonary hypertension of the newborn, sepsis with pneumonia, and hyaline membrane disease. For this reason it is recommended that all such critically ill newborns undergo careful echocardiography to rule out structural heart disease. Neonates beyond the first few days of life will have clinical findings similar to those seen with a large ventricular septal defect, atrioventricular septal defect, truncus arteriosus, or patent ductus arteriosus. Children beyond the neonatal period must be distinguished from patients with a large ASD, a common atrium, and partial anomalous pulmonary venous return.

Echocardiography is an important initial diagnostic tool for patients with suspected TAPVR. The distinguishing echocardiographic features include RV diastolic volume overload, an absence of the pulmonary venous connections to the left atrium, and identification of an alternative drainage site of the pulmonary veins. The objectives of preoperative echocardiography are to do the following[20]:

- Identify the drainage of individual pulmonary veins
- Identify the position of the confluence in relation to the left atrium
- Identify the presence and degree of obstruction to pulmonary venous flow
- Assess if there is obstruction at the level of the atrial septum
- Estimate RV pressure
- Identify any associated cardiac lesions

Multiple echocardiographic views and methods should be used to comprehensively evaluate suspected TAPVR. Two-dimensional echocardiography provides good anatomic information and can be validated by color Doppler side-by-side comparison (Fig. 48.4). The pulsed Doppler technique provides important physiologic information before surgical intervention.[20] A transthoracic echocardiogram is the starting point and should suffice in most situations. Use of transesophageal views for diagnosis has been described, but at most institutions this is limited to intraoperative evaluation.[21]

With the advent of multidetector computed tomography (CT) scanning, detailed images of the pulmonary venous drainage, including inflow and runoff vessels from the confluence, can be

achieved. Image interpretation is aided by the use of advanced postprocessing techniques. Volume-rendered three-dimensional reconstruction of the vascular bed provides a global overview for rapid identification of pathology. The combination of axial and three-dimensional images in helical CT angiography (CTA) is helpful in the assessment of TAPVR containing the individual pulmonary vein.[22] Maximum-intensity projection and multiplanar reformat images provide views similar to or better than traditional angiography. Measurements on CTA may be used for objectively assessing the degree of stenosis. In an adult coronary artery disease model, high interreader, intrareader, and interstudy reproducibility for a given scanner has been established.[23] Distortion-free detailed interrogation is performed with thin-section multiplanar reformats, which can be oriented to any desired plane. Axial two-dimensional source data are used when other techniques are inconclusive. In the setting of TAPVR, CTA is ideal when surgically pertinent anatomic and physiologic information cannot be obtained by echocardiography. CTA helps in surgical planning by delineating stenosis or obstruction, the site(s) of abnormal connections, and the course of the anomalous vein in relation to the left atrium. CTA provides accurate diagnosis with very short scan times, obviating the need for sedation, and has become the modality of choice in critically ill neonates.[24] Recurrent pulmonary vein obstruction is a common postoperative morbidity associated with early repair of TAPVR. CTA can demonstrate the type of stenosis and the entire course of the individual veins to better effect than echocardiography.

Currently available magnetic resonance imaging (MRI) scanners and cardiovascular imaging software from all manufacturers provide high-resolution angiographic images without patient exposure to radiation. In TAPVR with PVO, when emergent intervention is required, CTA is preferred for these reasons. Patients undergoing MRI for pulmonary venous assessment and evaluation of associated cardiovascular anomalies must remain still in the scanner for up to 20 to 60 minutes to minimize motion artifact; therefore children under 6 years of age typically require sedation or anesthesia.[25] Infants younger than approximately 6 months may fall into a natural sleep after being fed and swaddled comfortably. For children greater than 6 months of age, some institutions prefer to employ general anesthesia with mechanical ventilation via endotracheal intubation or laryngeal mask airway.[26] Respiratory motion artifact can be eliminated by holding breaths for brief periods (8 to 15 seconds) after a few seconds of hyperventilation. It is important to have communication of expected anatomy, duration of study, and cardiorespiratory risk factors between the anesthesiologist and the radiologist before the start of and throughout the MRI.

Measurement of quantitative flow to each lung, the fractional flow to each lung in patients with pulmonary vein stenosis, can be obtained with phase-contrast imaging. It is worth noting that the US Food and Drug Administration has not yet approved the use of gadolinium (Gd)-based contrast agents for pediatric cardiac MRI. However, judicious off-label use of different Gd-based MRI contrasts is used at most centers, with a reasonably good safety profile. Dynamic-contrast MR angiography with a Gd-based contrast agent under sedation is very useful for evaluation of the thoracic vessels of infants and small children in the preoperative and postoperative states.[27]

Diagnostic cardiac catheterization is reserved for patients in whom echocardiography or CT imaging is not satisfactory or when associated lesions need to be further defined. Cardiac angiography is performed after direct cannulation of the anomalous pulmonary vein or selective PA angiography. A delay in contrast transit through

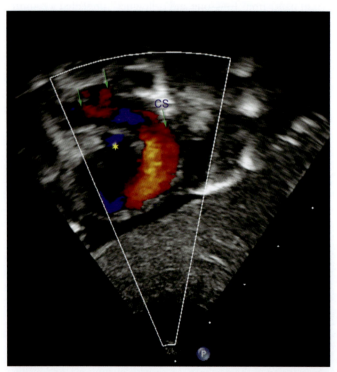

• **Figure 48.4** Two pulmonary veins, one from either side (*green arrows*), drain into the coronary sinus (CS), as visualized from subcostal coronal echocardiographic view. This appearance has sometimes been likened to the tail of a whale ("whale tail sign"). The yellow star shows right-to-left flow across the foramen ovale.

the pulmonary bed and small caliber of the pulmonary veins at insertion suggest obstruction to pulmonary venous return. Catheterization can be particularly helpful in case of atresia of the common pulmonary vein when echocardiography and CT are not able to visualize pulmonary veins. Pulmonary arteriograms in this situation show persistence of contrast medium in the pulmonary arteries, and the left atrium, the great veins, and the right heart chambers are not opacified.[28] Another diagnostic hallmark of TAPVR is that oxygen saturations from the right and left atria are nearly the same as those in the PA and aorta, because the right atrium is a common mixing chamber. Because of streaming of blood flow along fetal patterns, there could be minor differences in the left and right oxygen saturations depending on the type of TAPVR. Again depending on the drainage site, high oxygen saturations can be noted in the portal vein, coronary sinus, superior vena cava, and innominate vein.[29]

Preoperative Pathophysiology

Children with TAPVR have an obligatory left-to-right shunt from the pulmonary veins to the right heart and an intracardiac right-to-left shunt across an atrial communication. The specific physiology will depend on the degree of PVO, which can be severe in up to 25% of the cases, and on the amount of pulmonary blood flow. When the obstruction is severe, significant pulmonary edema and pulmonary hypertension will occur immediately. This will result in an increase in the right-to-left intracardiac shunt and subsequently worsening systemic cyanosis. The condition will rapidly progress with worsening acidosis and low cardiac output.

In children with no obstruction to the pulmonary venous connection the physiology is similar to that of other patients with significant left-to-right shunts and will likely go undetected in the neonate if not diagnosed on routine prenatal ultrasound examinations or postnatal screening. With time, as pulmonary vascular resistance (PVR) decreases, pulmonary blood flow will increase, resulting in right heart enlargement and clinical signs of heart failure including tachypnea, tachycardia, and failure to thrive. Mild cyanosis will occur but is often not noticeable, especially in children with darker skin complexions.

Children frequently present with a combination of excessive pulmonary blood flow and mild PVO. These findings are often seen in the supracardiac type with drainage of the confluence to the left side of the innominate vein via a vertical venous connection. In a number of these cases there could be an increase in pulmonary blood flow to three to five times systemic levels, leading to obvious symptoms and signs of congestive heart failure. Pulmonary artery pressure may range from mildly to severely elevated depending on the degree of PVO and PA blood flow. PVO most often occurs at the level of the vertical vein as it courses between the left PA and left bronchus. These children can become critically ill from viral respiratory infections and often demonstrate failure to thrive.

When PVO is severe, neonates are critically ill with pulmonary venous hypertension resulting in pulmonary edema, reflex pulmonary arterial vasoconstriction, and pulmonary arterial hypertension with associated decreased pulmonary blood flow. Right-to-left shunting occurs at the ductal and atrial levels. This physiology causes marked hypoxemia. Additionally, decreased pulmonary venous return to the left atrium and impingement of the septal wall on the LV cavity by the RV result in impaired LV filling and function with decreased cardiac output. Severely affected neonates present with cyanosis, respiratory distress, and hemodynamic compromise with hypotension and poor perfusion.

Preoperative Critical Care

The level of preoperative support required will reflect the pathophysiologic state of the patient and depends on the degree of PVO and pulmonary blood flow. Critical care management of infants with TAPVR and severe PVO is supportive and focuses on stabilization, optimization of oxygen delivery, and prevention of pulmonary hypertensive crisis. Of neonates and infants presenting with TAPVR, approximately one-third have severe PVO requiring mechanical ventilation and inotropic support, and 2% to 4% are moribund upon presentation.[4,30-32] Due to tenuous and potentially inadequate oxygen delivery, intubation and mechanical ventilation should be instituted promptly. Deep sedation and neuromuscular blockade may be beneficial to decrease metabolic demands and agitation-related elevations in PVR, as well as to promote stable minute ventilation and avoid hypercarbia-related elevations in PVR. Inotropic support with dopamine or epinephrine may be useful to improve cardiac output while awaiting surgery. Initially, sodium bicarbonate may be of benefit to mitigate severe metabolic acidosis while the interventions discussed previously are instituted to improve perfusion. This should be used as a temporizing measure while the operating room (OR) is being prepared and the patient is being transported for operative correction.

Standard lines and monitoring include umbilical artery catheter, umbilical venous catheter (UVC), and regional oxygen saturation monitoring via near-infrared spectroscopy (NIRS). In infants with infracardiac TAPVR, one may prefer to avoid UVC placement in favor of alternative central venous access. Therapeutic goals include normoventilation without excessive ventilator pressures or volumes and adequate oxygen delivery and cardiac output as indicated by central venous oxygen saturation and regional oxygen saturations, lactate levels, and end-organ function. Though an increasing percentage of neonates with TAPVR are diagnosed prenatally, others present in a shock-like state and may initially be treated for sepsis, respiratory distress syndrome, or other conditions before TAPVR diagnosis. It is important to be aware that previously implemented therapies may not be indicated for TAPVR. Pulmonary vasodilators such as inhaled nitric oxide (iNO) have not been of demonstrated benefit preoperatively and may result in increased pulmonary edema.[33] Similarly, attempts to increase pulmonary blood flow with hyperoxygenation, aggressive hyperventilation, or sodium bicarbonate–induced alkalosis are not indicated. Prostaglandin E_1 (PGE_1) is not routinely recommended due to similar risks, though some authors have described the cautious use of PGE_1 in select patients with low cardiac output syndrome (LCOS) in an attempt to provide right-to-left shunting to the systemic circulation or to relax the ductus venosus in infracardiac TAPVR.[34] Diuretic use should be employed with caution because the noncompliant RV may benefit from higher filling pressures

Surgical Intervention

For neonates with severe PVO, surgery is performed as soon as possible after stabilization, typically within the first 24 hours of life. In those with lesser degrees of PVO, surgery is performed electively depending on the infant's physiologic state. However, even infants without PVO are at increased risk for prolonged postoperative mechanical ventilatory support when elective repair is delayed, suggesting that decreasing the duration of the abnormal preoperative pathophysiologic state may result in improved postoperative physiology.[35]

The goal of surgical intervention for the repair of TAPVR is simply to reestablish the communication that nature had intended between the pulmonary veins and the left atrium. This requires an anastomosis between the confluence of the pulmonary veins or the posterior pericardium in the posterior wall of the left atrium. Due to the positioning of this anastomosis and the relatively inconvenient location of the posterior pericardium, there have been multiple approaches described. Common to all the more frequently employed approaches is a median sternotomy incision. A subtotal thymectomy is then performed, and the pericardium is opened anteriorly just to the right of midline. This preserves the anterior portion of the pericardium should it be needed to reconstruct the atrial septum. The aorta is then cannulated. A single-stage venous cannula can be used in the right atrium or, especially in somewhat larger babies, a bicaval cannulation technique can be used, which then allows one to limit the period of deep hypothermic circulatory arrest. The patient is then placed on cardiopulmonary bypass and cooled, typically to a temperature of 18°C.

There are three general approaches to the posterior pericardium: (1) via the right atrium and across the atrial septum, (2) via the left side by rotating the right apex of the heart toward the right shoulder, and (3) a superior access obtained by retracting the superior vena cava and the aorta laterally. Our preferred approach is via the right atrium. A transverse atriotomy is made, which is carried down across the atrial septum onto the posterior wall of the left atrium and extended toward the base of the left atrium, carefully avoiding encroaching on the area adjacent to the mitral valve annulus. This allows for an excellent exposure to the posterior pericardium. If the pulmonary venous confluence is oriented in the horizontal position, then an incision parallel to that on the left atrium is made in the posterior pericardium. Typically for infracardiac TAPVR, the confluence of the pulmonary veins is oriented in a vertical (superior to inferior) direction. Thus the incision in the posterior pericardium would be overlying this confluence and almost perpendicular to the left atrial incision. Regardless of which direction the incision in the posterior pericardium is made, it allows for a generous anastomosis with the posterior wall of the left atrium. A direct anastomosis from the pulmonary venous confluence to the left atrium is performed with fine 7-0 or 8-0 polypropylene suture.

Recently, in an effort to decrease the incidence of recurrent pulmonary venous stenosis, we have begun to use a so-called sutureless technique for reestablishing communication from the pulmonary venous confluence to the left atrium. This technique involves creating a pericardial well encasing the pulmonary venous confluence. The pericardial walls of this well are then anastomosed to the back wall of the left atrium (Fig. 48.5). With this technique the incision in the posterior pericardium is made parallel to the orientation of the pulmonary venous confluence, and the anastomosis is likewise performed with fine (7-0) polypropylene suture. The anastomosis is taken from the left lateral side toward the surgeon on the right. A secondary advantage of this technique is that the pulmonary venous confluence does not have to be incised initially, and thus one can maintain cardiopulmonary bypass during this portion of the anastomosis, limiting the use of deep hypothermic circulatory arrest. Before completing the rightward side of the circumferential anastomosis of the pericardium, the pulmonary venous confluence is opened. At this time one can decrease the bypass flow to minimal flow to allow good visualization and complete the anastomosis of the posterior pericardium to the back wall of the left atrium.

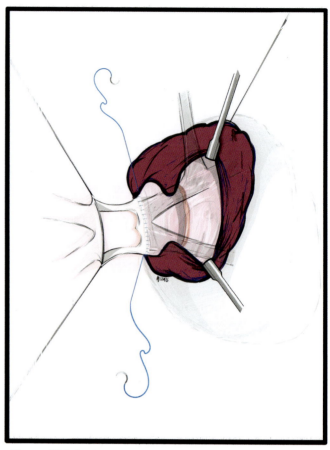

• **Figure 48.5** Surgical view illustrating a transatrial approach to supracardiac total anomalous pulmonary venous connection. The right and left atria are open, and a "no-touch" anastomosis encircling the open pulmonary venous confluence has been started. (Courtesy Richard McComas.)

Upon completion of this anastomosis reestablishing communication from the pulmonary veins to the left atrium, the ASD is then closed (Fig. 48.6). Occasionally the left atrium is found to be diminutive in association with TAPVR and could benefit from augmentation. This is accomplished by patching the atrial septum using a piece of autologous pericardium, which then enlarges the capacity of the left atrium and decreases the potential for significant left atrial hypertension. If the left atrium is of sufficient size, then the atrial septum can be closed primarily. The decision to leave a small patent foramen ovale as a "pop-off" may be made in cases in which there is concern about significant pulmonary vascular reactivity postoperatively. While the patient is rewarmed, the right atrium is then closed with a 6-0 polypropylene suture in a running fashion (Fig. 48.7).

There has been some controversy concerning the issue of leaving the vertical communicating vein open after the repair. The theoretical benefit of leaving the vertical vein open is that it may increase the capacitance of the left atrium by including the vertical vein in the volume of the confluence. If the communicating vein is not ligated, there is certainly the potential for the development of a left-to-right shunt that may need to be closed in the future. With the advancement in interventional techniques this can almost always be performed in the cardiac catheterization laboratory without the need for additional surgery.

Standard surgical practice for both elective and emergent repair, combined with improved perioperative definition of the anatomy

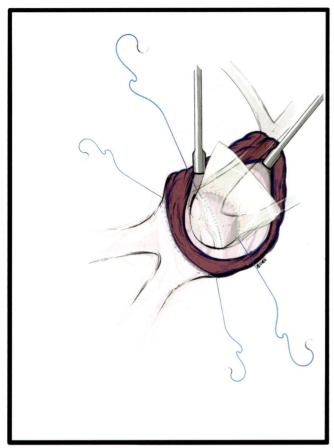

• **Figure 48.6** With the anastomosis between the left atrium and the posterior pericardial reflection surrounding the open pulmonary venous confluence, the atrial septal defect is being closed with a patch of bovine pericardium. (Courtesy Richard McComas.)

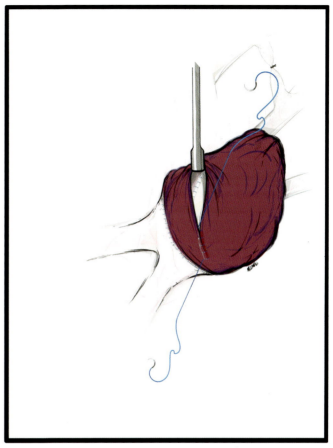

• **Figure 48.7** Final closure of the right atrium with ligation of the vertical communicating vein inserting into the left aspect of the innominate vein. (Courtesy Richard McComas.)

and advanced postoperative management, has resulted in significant improvement in overall operative mortality. The persistence of several common morbidities has shifted the current emphasis in surgical practices in attempts to avoid these issues. A particularly vexing postoperative morbidity involves the occurrence of recurrent pulmonary venous stenosis at either the anastomotic site or involving the individual pulmonary veins. Recent studies have documented an incidence of postoperative pulmonary venous stenosis of up to 25% in TAPVR patients.[34] Several modifications of the surgical techniques during the initial operative correction of TAPVR have been implemented to decrease the incidence of this problematic complication.

Surgical techniques that ensure the adequate relief of pulmonary venous stenosis while effectively reducing the incidence of continued recurrences have evolved over the last decade. Most early surgical procedures relieved the stenosis but often failed to maintain patency over even short periods. Techniques have varied from bypassing the obstructed vessels with vascularized left atrial tissue to incising and directly suture patching the affected segments.[34] Numerous materials have been used with these procedures, including autologous pericardium, in situ rotational atrial flaps, Gore-Tex, bovine pericardium, and synthetic extracellular matrix scaffolds. Regardless of the material used, recurrence rates continue to remain significant when direct suturing to the incised vessels is attempted. Caldarone and colleagues presented a limited number of patients with recurrent pulmonary venous stenosis (PVS) following correction of TAPVR.

The majority of these patients underwent reconstruction with direct augmentation with a significant recurrence rate and mortality.[36] It is interesting to note that two patients with recurrent PVO underwent a no-touch reconstruction of the affected area with no recurrence and improved overall outcomes when compared with the other patients in the series.

The so-called sutureless repair of recurrent pulmonary venous stenosis was first reported by Lacour-Gayet and colleagues[37] in 1996. The technique was initially used in a 3-year-old boy who had developed recurrent pulmonary venous stenosis following an initial attempt to relieve recurrent PVS after the neonatal repair of TAPVR. These same authors subsequently reported on a small series of patients who underwent repair using these techniques.[38] The original technique involved a combination of a simple incision through the affected vessels and complete excision of all disease tissue. A vascularized flap of native pericardium was then anastomosed to the atrial wall, creating a pouch of in situ pericardium that passively drained the pulmonary veins into the open left atrium.

Various techniques and materials based on these original descriptions of the so-called sutureless repair have been used to treat patients with recurrent disease. Several key factors common to all the various techniques are important to note and are described nicely by Caldarone and colleagues.[36] Adequate decompression of the affected pulmonary vein is of utmost importance. Whether the access to the diseased segment is achieved from within the left atrium or through an incision from the outside of the heart, the incision needs to be carried completely through the scarred segment until distensible, nonsclerotic pulmonary veins are reached. This task may require incision deep into the hilum of the lung. It should be stressed that it is important to maintain the incision anteriorly so as not to violate the pleuroparietal reflection because violation will ultimately result in hemorrhage into the pleural space.

Postoperative Critical Care

The postoperative course is highly predicated by the degree of preoperative pathophysiology and the intraoperative course. Preoperative PVO is associated with increased morbidity and mortality.[a] Knowledge of the infant's preoperative state and a detailed handoff from both the surgeon and the anesthesiologist, particularly with regard to episodes of preoperative or intraoperative pulmonary hypertension, arrhythmia, and respiratory or hemodynamic concerns, optimize a smooth transition of care. Optimal monitoring includes arterial, central venous, left atrial, and PA lines. Pulmonary artery line monitoring has been associated with decreased postoperative mortality.[41] Temporary arterial and ventricular pacing wires are standard. NIRS monitoring of cerebral and flank regional saturations is commonly employed. Infants are routinely transported receiving both ventilation via an endotracheal tube and inotropic infusions such as dopamine, epinephrine, or milrinone. Additionally, iNO is commonly instituted in the OR before transfer. Maintaining deep sedation and neuromuscular blockade (NMB) is prudent during the transition from the OR to the intensive care unit (ICU). Infants who required extracorporeal membrane oxygenation (ECMO) preoperatively or who were unable to safely separate from cardiopulmonary bypass will arrive to the ICU on ECMO support. The major postoperative concerns include severe respiratory insufficiency, pulmonary hypertension, and low cardiac output. Postoperative arrhythmias and recurrent pulmonary venous stenosis can also occur in the postoperative period (Box 48.1).

Severe respiratory insufficiency occurs due to preoperative pulmonary edema and pulmonary hypertension, which are exacerbated by cardiopulmonary bypass. Management strategies mirror those of preoperative care. Because infants remain at risk for pulmonary vasoreactivity, continuous analgesia, sedation, and NMB

are routinely employed in the first 24 to 48 hours to prevent stimuli-induced increases in PVR that can occur due to pain, agitation, routine care, suctioning, or other procedures. Though center variation exists, analgesia with fentanyl (5 to 10 mcg/kg/min), sedation with versed (0.05 to 0.2 mg/kg/h) or dexmedetomidine (0.3 to 1 mcg/kg/h), and NMB with vecuronium (0.1 to 0.2 mg/kg/h) are commonly used. If the infant is hemodynamically stable without labile PVR, NMB is typically discontinued on postoperative day 1 to 2 with subsequent weaning of analgesic and sedative infusions as dictated by the clinical course. Mechanical ventilation is provided to promote adequate oxygenation and normoventilation and decrease oxygen consumption. Ventilatory support is weaned as tolerated once the infant is off NMB. Postoperative mechanical ventilation times vary relative to the degree of preoperative PVO, ranging between 5 and 13 days with a median of 7 days.[35]

Postoperative pulmonary hypertension is common and is associated with death in the postoperative period.[31,42-44] iNO has been demonstrated to be of benefit in the OR, and initiation of this therapy before transfer to the ICU is not uncommon. A concentration of 20 ppm is sufficient in the majority of cases without concern for toxicity. In moderate- to high-risk patients, iNO at similar concentrations is routinely used postoperatively to prevent pulmonary hypertensive (PHTN) crisis.[39] In addition to monitoring sedation, analgesia, and NMB, critical care management includes close attention to acid-base status with avoidance and correction of respiratory acidosis, bicarbonate administration to acutely correct metabolic acidosis, and optimization of hemodynamics to prevent and correct lactic acidosis, all of which are important in preventing pulmonary hypertensive crisis. Continuous monitoring of right atrial, PA, and left atrial pressures are helpful in recognizing PHTN and determining the cause of PHTN and LCOS.

Pulmonary hypertensive crisis is an acute elevation of PVR to systemic or suprasystemic levels with resultant RV failure, which in turn compromises LV function and leads to hypoxemia, hypotension, and LCOS. This life-threatening event can occur despite the preventative measures described earlier. Infants typically initially exhibit tachycardia with an elevated PA pressure and central venous pressure (CVP) followed by hypotension and desaturation, which may progress to bradycardia followed by cardiac arrest. Because tachycardia, hypotension, and desaturation may be caused by hypovolemia, assessment of PA and CVP tracings (elevated in PHTN and low in hypovolemia) provides an important clue for diagnosis. Tamponade can mimic pulmonary hypertensive crisis. If pulmonary hypertensive crisis is suspected, immediate intervention to reverse the process is paramount in preventing cardiac arrest. Administration of 100% oxygen and intravascular volume should be provided quickly. Additional doses of sedation, analgesia, and NMB should be considered. Transient modest hyperventilation via increased ventilator rate or hand ventilation may be employed with caution while avoiding excessive hyperventilation that could adversely impact cerebral perfusion. Bolus dose epinephrine should be readily available for administration in case the situation is not quickly reversed. Because metabolic acidosis is a potential cause or consequence of a pulmonary hypertensive crisis, it is reasonable to administer sodium bicarbonate presumptively. Confirmed acidosis should be corrected. If not already in use, iNO should be implemented.[33] Transient escalation of ongoing iNO to concentrations of 40 to 80 ppm may be of benefit. Emergent cannulation for ECMO has been used to rescue infants from cardiac arrest related to pulmonary hypertensive crisis. Additionally, elective ECMO

---

[a]References 1, 3, 4, 31, 39, 40.

initiation may be warranted in infants with labile PVR or tenuous hemodynamics before development of, during, or after successful reversal of an acute pulmonary hypertensive crisis.

Postoperative LCOS results from decreased left atrial and LV compliance due to abnormal preoperative filling, which may be exacerbated by cardiopulmonary bypass.[40,45-49] Underfilling of the left heart can be exacerbated by PHTN and RV dilation. Occasionally the increased blood return to the left atrium after the removal of PVO further elevates left atrial pressure (LAP), causing a vicious cycle of worsening pulmonary edema, PHTN, and subsequent RV and LV dysfunction. Critical care management includes monitoring and maintaining optimal filling pressures, which are often as high as 12 to 15 mm Hg in the initial postoperative period. Caution must be taken to avoid overaggressive volume administration because this may lead to LAP elevation and PHTN. Inotropic support is typically required for the first 24 to 48 hours. Typical inotropic support includes dopamine (3 to 10 mcg/kg/min) and/or epinephrine (0.02 to 0.15 mcg/min) in addition to milrinone (0.5 to 1 mcg/kg/min) for afterload reduction. In addition, maintaining an optimal heart rate via temporary pacing or the use of medications, such as isoproterenol (to increase) or esmolol, dexmedetomidine, or amiodarone (to slow) heart rates to target levels may be helpful in improving cardiac output. In case reports of infants with vasodilatory shock with associated pulmonary HTN after repair of TAPVR, vasopressin infusion at doses of 0.0003 to 0.0012 U/kg/min has been demonstrated to increased systemic blood pressure, decrease PA pressures, and allow weaning of epinephrine.[50]

Dysrhythmias, primarily supraventricular tachycardias, occur in 2% to 20% of patients.[51,52] Routine measures such cardioversion for atrial fibrillation, overdrive pacing for atrial flutter, adenosine, esmolol, or amiodarone for reentrant SVT, or amiodarone with associated pacing as needed to control junctional ectopic tachycardia are used to optimize cardiac output.

Persistent LCOS, marked respiratory insufficiency, or desaturation may be due to multiple causes, including severe PHTN, ventricular dysfunction, abnormal lung parenchyma or atelectasis, and PVO. In patients with hemodynamic instability, investigation with chest x-ray examination to assess lung status and echocardiogram to assess for cardiac function, evidence of pulmonary HTN, pericardial effusion, and PVO is indicated. Transesophageal echocardiography may allow better imaging of the pulmonary venous anastomoses. If these studies are unrevealing, timely cardiac catheterization to assess for recurrent PVO is crucial. When PVO occurs in the early postoperative period, it is typically due to a technical problem with the anastomosis and requires immediate repair.

Recent series report ECMO use in 5% to 12% of infants after TAPVR repair, with higher utilization (up to 21%) in those with preoperative PVO. Of infants who require ECMO, up to 85% have preoperative PVO. The most common indications for ECMO are PHTN or LCOS. Survival of infants requiring ECMO ranges from 42% to 50%, with lower survival in those with PHTN compared with those for whom LCOS is the indication for ECMO.[3,35] The length of ECMO support varies in relation to the indication and the degree of lung disease present. Once ECMO is initiated, it is our practice to discontinue iNO and discontinue or wean inotropes to minimum levels. Milrinone is typically continued to aid in diastolic relaxation and minimize excessive systemic vascular resistance. iNO and low-dose inotropic support are reinstituted at the time of weaning. If the indications for ECMO are unclear or the infant is unable to wean from ECMO despite

reasonable pulmonary and cardiac function and an apparent lack of pulmonary vasoreactivity, cardiac catheterization is routinely performed on ECMO.

Weaning of support, whether conventional or extracorporeal, should proceed with caution. Stimuli for pulmonary hypertensive crises increase with weaning of sedation and iNO. Weaning of sedation and mechanical ventilation place increased demands on the heart, which may not be well tolerated. Thus close monitoring and a high level of vigilance must be maintained throughout the weaning period. In some cases, reinitiation of earlier supportive measures is required, and weaning must be delayed until the patient exhibits improved stability.

Outcomes

Surgical outcomes have continued to improve over the last several decades for most complex congenital heart defects. Using data from a large registry of congenital heart disease collected over a 30-year period, St. Louis et al.[1] showed a significant improvement in operative mortality for neonates who underwent correction of TAPVR before 1 month of age. In this study the overall surgical mortality for patients without associated congenital heart defects (except patent ductus arteriosus and ASD) was 13%. These results improved over the period from 1980 to 2013, with a mortality in the later decades of 4%. This observation corroborated several small, single-center experiences, all showing a period-dependent improvement in survival.[2,53-55] Several preoperative and intraoperative morbidities continue to have a negative impact on overall survival. Preoperative PVO has a significant impact on operative mortality, as shown in the study by St. Louis as well as others.[54] Several other studies have refuted these results, concluding that the presence of preoperative PVO has been neutralized with the advancements in preoperative diagnostic imaging and improvements in postoperative management.[4]

Regardless of the controversy surrounding certain risk factors in this population, patients with heterotaxy and functional single-ventricular anatomy warrant special attention because their operative mortality is significantly greater. Gaynor and colleagues reported on a group of 72 patients with functional single-ventricle anatomy and TAPVR. The outcomes were poor for the group as a whole; they were particularly poor if repair of TAPVR was required at initial palliation, usually for PVO along with aortopulmonary shunt.[56] Overall mortality was 63% at 1 year and 81% at 5 years. Sixteen percent died preoperatively, and 38% died in the OR. Hashmi and colleagues reported their experience over a 26-year period with a series of 91 patients with right atrial isomerism. Overall mortality was 69%.[57]

Even with the improvement in immediate operative survival, long-term morbidities must still be considered and monitored in this patient population. The occurrence of postoperative pulmonary venous stenosis has proven to be a formidable challenge. The incidence of this disease has been reported as 18% to 25% of patients in recent literature.[3] Management must be aggressive because mortality in patients left untreated exceeds 50%. Another less common but important complication is the lifelong risk of rhythm disturbances. A review from Tanel at al.[58] showed that survivors of TAPVR repair appeared to have a significantly higher incidence of sinus node dysfunction and recommended ongoing follow-up for arrhythmia surveillance.

Long-term functional status in patients with simple TAPVR appears to be excellent. Most series report these patients as growing normally and being asymptomatic. Paridon et al.

reported the only study of exercise tolerance in this group. He studied nine patients at an average of 10 postoperative years; he documented small diminutions in aerobic exercise capacity and a heightened chronotropic response, although all patients were asymptomatic.[59]

Summary

The last several decades have seen an extraordinary evolution in the diagnosis and management of children with the most complex congenital heart disease. Outcomes have continued to improve, with the expectation that even the sickest infants will survive. With these outstanding operative results, emphasis has shifted to addressing the long-term morbidities that are inevitable following the successful repair of the smallest children. The increased effort to address neurologic and developmental deficits in these patients has also proved to be successful, increasing the quality of life for adults who have undergone these types of repairs. Constant and accurate follow-up is critical and presents an ongoing hurdle to achieving outcomes similar those of the general population.

For patients with TAPVR, correction in the newborn period is associated with low mortality and excellent mid-term outcomes. Diagnostic advances have allowed the visualization of these defects as never before, providing accurate and detailed preoperative definition of the anomalous anatomy and physiology. Surgical technique has continued to evolve, although the approach that will best mitigate long-term complication remains controversial. The development of postoperative pulmonary vein stenosis is the most serious long-term complication. For patients with heterotaxy syndrome and functional single-ventricular anatomy, outcomes have improved but are still far short of those seen with other patients with TAPVR.

Selected References

A complete list of references is available at ExpertConsult.com.

1. St. Louis JD, Harvey BA, Menk JS, et al. Repair of "simple" total anomalous pulmonary venous connection: a review from the Pediatric Cardiac Care Consortium. *Ann Thorac Surg*. 2012;94(1):133–137.
3. Seale AN, Uemura H, Webber SA, et al. Total anomalous pulmonary venous connection: morphology and outcome from an international population-based study. *Circ*. 2010;122(25):2718–2726.
4. Bando K, Turrentine MW, Ensing GJ, et al. Surgical management of total anomalous pulmonary venous connection: thirty year trends. *Circ*. 1996;94(supplII):II 12–II 16.
9. St. Louis JD, Turk EM, Jacobs JP, O'Brien JE Jr. Type IV total anomalous pulmonary venous connection outcomes following surgical correction. *World J Pediatr Congenit Heart Surg*. 2017;*in press*.
25. Geva T, Powell AJ. Allen HDS, Robert E, Penny Daniel J, Feltes Timothy F, Cetta Frank, eds. *Moss and Adams' Heart Disease in Infants, Children, and Adolescents: Including the Fetus and Young Adult*. 9th ed. Philadelphia, PA: Lippincott Williams & Wilkins; 2016:373–412.
36. Caldarone CA, Najm HK, Kadletz M, et al. Surgical management of total anomalous pulmonary venous drainage: impact of coexisting cardiac anomalies. *Ann Thorac Surg*. 1998;66:1521–1526.
53. Karamlou T, Gurofsky R, Al Sukhni E, et al. Factors associated with mortality and reoperation in 377 children with total anomalous pulmonary venous connection. *Circ*. 2007;115(12):1591–1598.
56. Gaynor WJ, Collins MH, Rychik J, et al. Long-term outcome of infants with single ventricle and total anomalous pulmonary venous connection. *J Thorac Cardiovasc Surg*. 1999;117:506–514.

49

Ventricular Septal Defects

ASHOK MURALIDARAN, MD; IRVING SHEN, MD

Definition

A ventricular septal defect (VSD) is an opening in the interventricular septum resulting in direct communication between the left and right ventricles. VSDs can be single or multiple. It is the most commonly diagnosed congenital heart anomaly, present in 20% of patients with congenital heart disease.

Embryology

Traditionally the ventricular septum is thought to be derived mostly from three sources. The primary fold arising from the apex of the primitive ventricle, eventually becoming the trabecular septum, fuses with the inlet septum, which originates posteroinferiorly, and with the infundibular or conal septum, which extends downward from the conal ridge. Some evidence, however, points to the inlet and the apical trabecular septa originating from the same source.[1] The conal ridge fuses with the endocardial cushions to form the membranous portion of the interventricular septum. Fig. 49.1 shows the various components contributing to the formation of the interventricular septum.

Anatomy

There are several schemes for classifying VSDs. The traditional classification describes four types based on the location of the VSD: type 1 or supracristal/subarterial/conal, type 2 or perimembranous/paramembranous, type 3 or inlet/atrioventricular canal, and type 4 or muscular[2] (Fig. 49.2). A separate classification of "malaligned" defects is often employed to describe VSDs that are part of lesions like tetralogy of Fallot or interrupted aortic arch, in which the conal septum and the other components of the septum are fully formed but are displaced anterior or posterior with respect to each other. Perimembranous defects constitute 80% of the defects with the other types being 5% to 10% each.

Subarterial defects are also known as outlet, conal septal, supracristal, or subpulmonary VSDs. They are located beneath the pulmonary valve, and their superior edge is a fibrous ridge between the two semilunar valves. They can be associated with prolapse of the right coronary leaflet of the aortic valve with associated regurgitation. This type of defect is more common in the Asian population.

Perimembranous (paramembranous) defects are also known as membranous or infracristal defects. They are located between the anterior and posterior divisions of the septal band and between the conal and trabecular interventricular septum. The lateral border is formed by the tricuspid annulus; the superior border is usually the aortic annulus. There may be a variable amount of muscular rim at the superior and lateral borders. The defect can extend into the inlet, trabecular, or outlet portions of the interventricular septum. Extension of the defect to the base of the noncoronary leaflet of the aortic valve may cause aortic regurgitation (AR). The conal septum may be anteriorly malaligned as in tetralogy of Fallot, causing right ventricular outflow tract obstruction, or, less commonly, it may be malaligned posteriorly, causing left ventricular outflow tract obstruction.

Inlet defects are also called atrioventricular canal-type defects. The posterior margin of the defect runs along the septal leaflet of the tricuspid valve. The anterior leaflet of the mitral valve often has a cleft. The defect extends superiorly to the membranous septum.

Muscular defects are located anywhere in the muscular septum. The margins are characteristically muscular. They are frequently multiple. They may be anterior, midmuscular, apical, or in the inlet septum. The latter differs from the inlet or atrioventricular canal-type VSD in that it is separated from the tricuspid valve and membranous septum by muscle tissue. Infundibular or outlet muscular VSDs differ from subarterial VSDs because of the presence of a rim of muscle separating the defect from the annuli of the aortic and pulmonary valves.

Associated Anomalies

VSDs can be isolated lesions or part of a variety of major congenital malformations such as tetralogy of Fallot, double-outlet right ventricle, transposition of the great vessels, and truncus arteriosus. Fifty percent of patients with VSDs requiring repair have associated cardiovascular anomalies, most commonly patent ductus arteriosus, atrial septal defect (ASD), aortic coarctation, aortic stenosis, and pulmonary stenosis.[3]

Pathophysiology and Natural History

The dimension of the defect and pulmonary vascular resistance (PVR) determine the blood flow across a VSD (shunt).[4] Smaller VSDs are said to be restrictive because there is a pressure gradient across the defect with a greater left ventricular pressure than right ventricular pressure. The left-to-right shunt depends primarily on the pressure differences. Larger defects approximate the size of the aortic annulus and are nonrestrictive with equal right and left ventricular pressures. In these cases the relative resistances in the systemic and pulmonary vasculature determine the left-to-right shunting.

PVR is high in the immediate postnatal period and begins to decrease within the first 2 weeks of life.[5] For babies with large

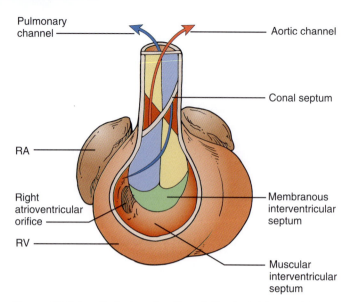

Pulmonary channel

Aortic channel

Conal septum

RA

Right atrioventricular orifice

RV

Membranous interventricular septum

Muscular interventricular septum

Figure 49.1 Longitudinal section through the fetal right ventricle and outflow tract displaying the components contributing to the formation of the interventricular septum. *RA,* Right atrium; *RV,* right ventricle.

nonrestrictive VSDs the drop in PVR accentuates the left-to-right shunt, leading to a large volume load in the pulmonary circulation, increasing left atrial pressure, and causing left ventricular volume overload. Congestive heart failure (CHF) develops with decreased peripheral perfusion and increased work of breathing, associated with a drop in stroke volume and tissue oxygen delivery. This results in activation of the renin-angiotensin system, which further increases systemic vasoconstriction and the left-to-right shunting, exacerbating the CHF.[6-8]

If infants with nonrestrictive VSDs remain untreated, the pulmonary overcirculation can eventually lead to a fixed elevation of PVR and pulmonary vascular disease. These changes are not reversible after VSD closure. Eisenmenger complex develops when PVR becomes greater than systemic resistance, reversing the shunt and causing cyanosis.

Infants and children with smaller restrictive VSDs remain asymptomatic. Those with larger nonrestrictive VSDs develop increasingly severe CHF within the first several months of life. This manifests as respiratory symptoms and failure to thrive. These infants have an appreciable mortality within the first year if left untreated.[9] Children with moderate shunting develop a gradual increase in PVR over time, and as the PVR approaches systemic levels, the degree of shunting decreases with improvement in symptoms. If untreated, such patients go on to develop Eisenmenger complex and die in the third or fourth decade of life. The development of Eisenmenger physiology increases the risk of death 10- to 12-fold and carries a 25-year survival of only 42%.[10]

Spontaneous closure of VSDs is well documented and is more likely to occur within the first several months of life in patients with smaller defects. Muscular defects are the most likely to close by further septal muscular development. This is based mostly on autopsy studies in which most of the postmortem reports of spontaneously closed defects are of the muscular type.[11] Perimembranous VSDs have the next highest rate of spontaneous closure. The mechanism of spontaneous closure of these defects frequently involves the adherence of excess (aneurysmal) tricuspid valve tissue. Before the description of this mechanism in 1970, septal aneurysms were often presumed to be congenital in origin.[12] A recent natural history study from the Belgian registry on adult congenital heart disease documented a 13% incidence of spontaneous closure of perimembranous VSDs.[13] The authors also noted a 3% incidence of infective endocarditis, 3% incidence of progression to moderate to severe aortic valve insufficiency, and a low rate of atrial arrhythmia and heart block in the unrepaired perimembranous VSD group. Of note, the unrepaired patients had a significantly smaller VSD and left-to-right shunt compared with the repaired group.

Diagnosis

Symptoms

Infants with small defects are usually asymptomatic, and the detection of a murmur results in their diagnosis. Moderate defects result in a predisposition to pulmonary infection and varying degrees of growth retardation during the first few years of life but without severe signs of CHF. Larger defects, particularly nonrestrictive VSDs, produce signs and symptoms of CHF early in the first year of life, including tachypnea, poor feeding, sweating, irritability, failure to thrive, and poor weight gain. This symptom complex results from the increased work of breathing and energy expenditure associated with pulmonary overcirculation and poor peripheral perfusion.

Physical Signs

Children with smaller defects may present with a harsh holosystolic murmur with no overt signs of CHF. Those patients with larger defects and shunts (pulmonary-to-systemic blood flow ratio [Q_p:Q_s]; see subsequent discussion) in excess of 2:1 may have signs of CHF, including poor growth, tachypnea, poor perfusion with reduced peripheral pulses, a palpable thrill along the left sternal border, and a harsh holosystolic murmur loudest over the fourth intercostal space. There may be a diastolic murmur related to increased blood return to the left atrium. There is accentuation of the second heart sound. Hepatomegaly and pulmonary congestion may be present. Resting oxygen saturation less than 90% before surgical repair is a sign of significantly elevated PVR and portends an increased risk of pulmonary hypertension and death after surgical closure.

Electrocardiography

Typical findings on the electrocardiogram include left ventricular hypertrophy and left atrial enlargement reflected in bifid P waves and prominent R and T waves in the inferior leads and V_6, particularly with larger defects. Findings of right ventricular hypertrophy with an RSR′ pattern in lead V_1 occur later in the disease process.

Chest X-Ray Examination

Radiographic findings include cardiomegaly and an enlarged main pulmonary artery shadow. Left atrial enlargement and prominence of the pulmonary vasculature are also seen. These radiographic findings are more notable with larger defects and may be absent or more subtle with small VSDs.

Echocardiography

The type, size, number, and location of medium and large VSDs can be accurately defined by two-dimensional transthoracic

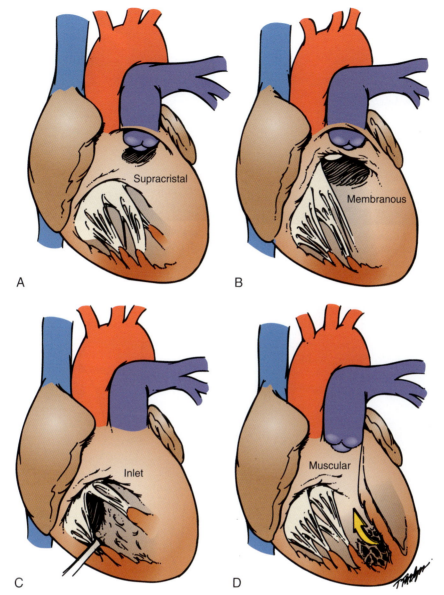

Figure 49.2 Various types of ventricular septal defects viewed from within the right ventricle. (A) Supracristal or subarterial. (B) Membranous, perimembranous, or paramembranous. (C) Inlet or atrioventricular (AV) canal type. (D) Muscular or trabecular.

echocardiography. Figs. 49.3 to 49.6 demonstrate the four common VSD types based on their location. Left atrial and ventricular dimensions can be measured and may be important in determining the management of a particular defect. Estimates of pulmonary artery pressure can be made using Doppler imaging of the velocity of a tricuspid regurgitant jet, if present. Other associated cardiac anomalies and the relationship of the VSD to the surrounding structures and valves can also be delineated with this modality. In the majority of cases echocardiography provides sufficient information to proceed with closure of the defect or to follow it expectantly. Transesophageal or epicardial echocardiography is particularly important for providing an intraoperative assessment of VSD closure. Small defects can be missed, especially if they are in the apex of the heart or in the vicinity of larger ones, and often reveal themselves after closure of the bigger VSD.

Cardiac Catheterization

Cardiac catheterization may be indicated when echocardiographic data are unsatisfactory, in patients with large defects and significant pulmonary hypertension, or if there is doubt about the anatomy of associated lesions. Recent American Heart Association and American Thoracic Society (AHA/ATS) guidelines for pediatric pulmonary hypertension recommend cardiac catheterization to measure PVR index (PVRI) if early repair has not been performed in the first 1 to 2 years of life for a significant VSD.[14]

Cardiac catheterization can demonstrate the location, size, and number of defects, along with associated cardiac anomalies. It facilitates direct measurement of left and right heart pressures and oxygen saturations (Fig. 49.7), from which quantification of the intracardiac shunt and PVR may be derived.

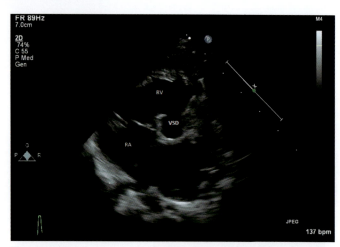

Figure 49.3 Transthoracic two-dimensional echocardiogram showing the short-axis view of a supracristal ventricular septal defect (VSD). Note the defect in the 1- to 2-o'clock position at the right ventricular outflow tract. *RA,* Right atrium; *RV,* right ventricle.

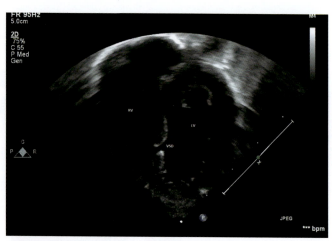

Figure 49.6 Four-chamber view of a midmuscular ventricular septal defect (VSD). *LV,* Left ventricle; *RV,* right ventricle.

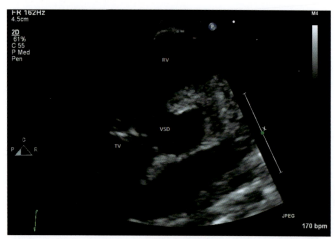

Figure 49.4 Short-axis view in a transthoracic echocardiogram of a perimembranous VSD. The defect is seen at the 10-o'clock position close to the tricuspid valve, in contrast to the position of the supracristal defect shown in Fig. 49.3. *RV,* Right ventricle; *TV,* tricuspid valve; *VSD,* ventricular septal defect.

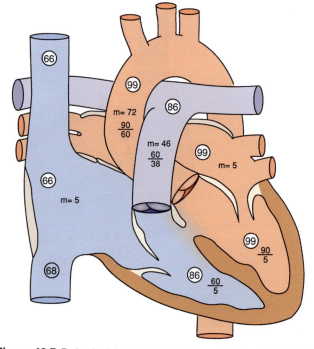

Figure 49.7 Pathophysiology of ventricular septal defect (VSD). Note step-up in O_2 saturation from the right atrium (66%) to the right ventricle (86%), indicating left-to-right shunt at the ventricular level. Right ventricular pressure (60/5 mm Hg) is elevated compared with the normal right ventricular pressure but is less than the left ventricular pressure (90/5 mm Hg), indicating that the VSD is *restrictive.* The pulmonary artery pressure is elevated as well. *m,* Mean pressure.

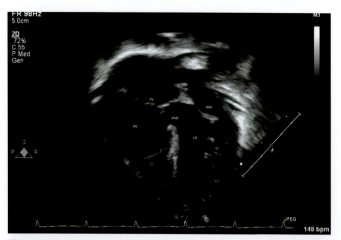

Figure 49.5 Four-chamber view of an inlet ventricular septal defect (VSD), displaying its posterior location at the level of the tricuspid and mitral valves. *LV,* Left ventricle; *MV,* mitral valve; *RV,* right ventricle; *TV,* tricuspid valve.

The shunt fraction is the ratio of pulmonary blood flow (Q_p) to systemic blood flow (Q_s). It is calculated according to the following formula:

$$Q_p:Q_s = [(AO_2 - MVO_2)/(PVO_2 - PaO_2)]$$

where AO_2 is the aortic oxygen saturation, MVO_2 is the mixed venous oxygen saturation, PaO_2 is the pulmonary arterial saturation, and PVO_2 is the pulmonary venous saturation.[14]

One can calculate the PVR using the formula:

$$PVR = \frac{(Mean\ PAP - PCWP\ or\ LAP) \times 80}{Cardiac\ Output}$$

where PAP is the pulmonary artery pressure, PCWP is the pulmonary capillary wedge pressure, and LAP is the left atrial pressure.

Surgical repair of the VSD is considered safe for PVRI less than 6 Wood units (WU) $\times$ m^2 (WU $\cdot$ m^2) or if the ratio of pulmonary to systemic vascular resistance (PVR/SVR) is less than 0.3.[14] The AHA/ATS guidelines recommend testing for vascular reactivity during catheterization using inhaled nitric oxide and oxygen to assess for reversibility of pulmonary hypertension for PVRI that is greater than 6 WU $\cdot$ m^2 and for PVR/SVR that is 0.3 or higher. Repair can be beneficial if the vascular bed is reactive but is contraindicated if it is not. In one study, for example, patients with a PVRI of less than 8 WU $\cdot$ m^2 had a greater than 90% survival after surgery, whereas patients with a PVRI of greater than 8 WU $\cdot$ m^2 had a survival of less than 45%.[15] Heart-lung transplantation or lung transplantation with VSD closure is the only surgical option for this group of patients.[16]

With the availability of newer agents for managing pulmonary hypertension, it is not unreasonable to treat patients with single or multiple pulmonary vasodilators for a period of time and reassess the hemodynamics with cardiac catheterization to revisit candidacy for surgical repair.

Indications for Surgical Repair

Infants with a large defect and significant CHF in whom spontaneous closure is unlikely are candidates for early closure, regardless of the patient's size. A trial of diuretic therapy with or without the addition of digoxin may control the symptoms of CHF and allow the infant to grow. The addition of an angiotensin-converting enzyme (ACE) inhibitor to reduce SVR may be helpful in selected cases. In these cases, surgical repair is typically performed between 3 and 6 months of age. If medical therapy fails, surgical repair should be undertaken promptly and can be done safely even in neonates.

Children with moderate-sized defects and shunts greater than 1.5:1 generally have mild to moderate elevations of pulmonary artery pressure and resistance. They can be followed until they are up to 5 years of age to maximize the chance of spontaneous closure. Failing the latter, surgical repair may be performed.

Patients with subarterial or supracristal VSDs can develop progressive AR due to prolapse of the adjacent aortic valve leaflet caused by Venturi forces associated with left-to-right flow across the defect.[17] The risk of aortic valve prolapse increases with increasing defect size. Surgical closure of these defects is usually recommended because the rate of spontaneous closure is low and the risk of developing aortic valve insufficiency is common. These defects should be repaired as soon as there is echocardiographic evidence or physical findings of AR and definitely before significant AR

develops. Simultaneous aortic valvuloplasty should be considered if the AR has progressed beyond a moderate degree. One study has shown that lesser degrees of AR remained stable after simple defect closure, and more severe regurgitation was associated with a significant need for reintervention despite aortic valvuloplasty at the time of VSD repair.[18] A recent study on adults, however, showed that patients older than 40 with unrepaired supracristal VSDs have a lower risk of AR progression than younger patients, questioning the need for routine prophylactic repair in this specific population.[19]

Some patients with pressure-restrictive VSD by Doppler criteria can still develop progressive left heart dilation due to the "volume unrestrictive" nature of the defect. Although such patients are referred for surgical closure, this practice has been questioned by some based on observations that the left heart dilation often regresses spontaneously over time.[20]

Children with small VSDs and left-to-right shunts less than 1.5:1 generally have no symptoms. Although they are at risk of bacterial endocarditis, close follow-up and prophylactic antibiotic therapy may be considered as an alternative to surgical repair.[21] A report from the Swedish registry for congenital heart disease noted a 20- to 30-fold higher incidence of infective endocarditis among adults with small unrepaired VSDs compared with the general population.[22] Some would hence recommend surgical closure of small VSDs after an episode of VSD-associated infective endocarditis. Preemptive surgical closure for such small VSDs is controversial.

A special situation in the neonatal period occurs when an infant is diagnosed with an aortic coarctation and a concomitant VSD. The optimal management strategy for neonates with this combination of lesions is controversial. A two-stage approach, involving coarctation repair with or without pulmonary artery banding via a left thoracotomy, followed by VSD closure and removal of the band 6 to 12 months later, has been demonstrated to be safe and effective.[23,24] A single-stage approach of simultaneous VSD and coarctation repair via a median sternotomy can be performed with comparably low morbidity and mortality.[25] A single-stage, two-incision approach is another alternative whereby the coarctation repair is performed via a thoracotomy followed immediately by the VSD repair via sternotomy.[26] It is also a reasonable strategy to repair the coarctation through a left thoracotomy and leave the pulmonary artery unbanded. If the infant remains in severe CHF, even after "unloading" of the systemic output with coarctation repair, the VSD can be closed through a sternotomy with a short period of cardiopulmonary bypass (CPB).

Pulmonary artery banding is rarely indicated for the treatment of VSD except in some infants with multiple or complex defects and/or contraindications for being placed on CPB (sepsis, intracranial hemorrhage). Banding in this situation controls the heart failure and allows the resolution of comorbid conditions before surgical VSD closure and pulmonary artery debanding.

Operative Management

With the patient in supine position a median sternotomy is performed and the thymus subtotally resected to facilitate exposure. The pericardium is opened and suspended. Ascending aortic and bicaval venous cannulation are performed after heparinization. Purse-string sutures should all be elongated and narrow. CPB is established, and, depending on the anticipated complexity of the procedure, cooling anywhere from 34°C to 30°C is begun. The left heart can be decompressed by placing a vent through the left

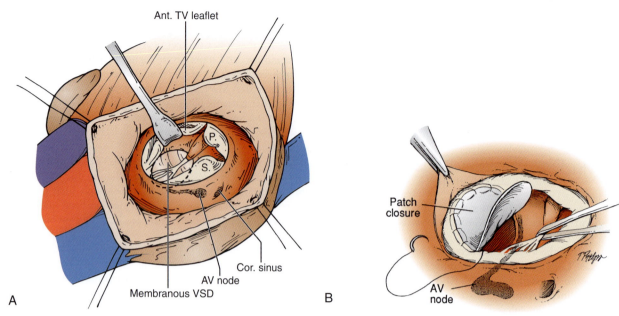

Figure 49.8 Ventricular septal defect (VSD) closure via the transatrial approach. (A) A right atriotomy has been performed, and the VSD is seen across the tricuspid valve (TV). Note the position of the atrioventricular node (AV node) and the conduction system that runs along the posterior and inferior border of the VSD. (B) A Dacron or PTFE patch is used to close the defect. A portion of the TV suspensory apparatus is being retracted. *P.,* Posterior leaflet; *PTFE,* polytetrafluoroethylene; *S.,* septal leaflet of the tricuspid valve.

atrial appendage or, more commonly, the right superior pulmonary vein. Cardioplegia is administered in antegrade fashion after cross-clamping the aorta and redosed at regular intervals if necessary. For neonates, another option is to use single venous cannulation through the right atrial appendage and perform the repair under hypothermic circulatory arrest at a rectal temperature of 18°C.

An oblique right atrial incision is made after the caval snares are secured. Retractors are positioned after placement of stay sutures. The anatomy is inspected through the tricuspid valve. VSDs are ordinarily closed with a patch (usually polytetrafluoroethylene [PTFE], Dacron, bovine, or glutaraldehyde-treated autologous pericardium) unless they are quite small. Patch material can be sewn into place with either interrupted sutures or a continuous technique. Particular care is required with the superior sutures to avoid injury to the aortic valve; inferiorly, sutures are placed away from the margins of the VSD to avoid the conduction tissue. Occasionally exposure of the defect may be compromised by the tricuspid valve or supporting apparatus. In these cases it may be helpful to partially detach the septal leaflet of the tricuspid valve to facilitate exposure of the lateral and inferior borders. The septal leaflet is then repaired with a running polypropylene suture.

After repair of the VSD is complete, the tricuspid valve is tested for competence and repaired as necessary. An ASD or patent foramen ovale, if present, is closed. The right atrium is closed, and after deairing the heart the cross-clamp is removed. When deairing and rewarming are complete, the patient is separated from CPB. Ultrafiltration can be undertaken either during CPB or after cessation of CPB but before decannulation and protamine administration. Ideally, intraoperative transesophageal or epicardial echocardiography is used to rule out a residual VSD. Information about tricuspid and aortic valve competence and ventricular function is also obtained using this modality. If there is a question about the significance of a residual VSD, direct measurement of pulmonary artery pressure and simultaneous measurement of oxygen saturations

in the superior vena cava and pulmonary artery can be made, and the $Q_p{:}Q_s$ can be estimated. A decision can then be made to go back on bypass to repair the residual defect if the $Q_p{:}Q_s$ remains significant ($\geq 1.5 : 1$). Rarely, if it is felt that further attempts at repair may be unsuccessful, a pulmonary artery band can be placed to restrict the pulmonary blood flow with plans to repair the residual defects in the future, allowing time for spontaneous regression of the defects and somatic growth.

For infants with moderate to severe pulmonary hypertension, placement of a pulmonary artery catheter, left atrial line, and even a peritoneal dialysis catheter should be considered to aid in postoperative management. Inhaled nitric oxide can also be helpful in the postoperative management of this subgroup of patients.

The vast majority of membranous and inlet VSDs are closed via the transatrial approach (Fig. 49.8) but can be closed through a ventriculotomy in selected cases. Supracristal defects must be closed through either a ventriculotomy or an incision in the pulmonary artery, with sutures anchored to the pulmonary valve annulus.

Muscular VSDs, especially multiple/complex defects remain a surgical challenge. Whereas inlet and midmuscular defects can be repaired through the tricuspid valve, anterior defects are sometimes approached via a right ventriculotomy and apical VSDs through an apical left ventriculotomy. To enhance exposure of these defects, transection of crossing muscle bundles or even the moderator band has been suggested.[27] Other described techniques include placing an "oversized patch" on the left ventricular side of the defect and the "sandwich" technique, in which sutures are passed along the inferior rim of an anterior muscular VSD and brought out of the epicardial surface of the right ventricle and tied down, hence obliterating the defect.[28] A cardioscope, introduced through the aortic root, can aid in visualization of the muscular defects, permitting direct inspection of the left side of the ventricular septum and illuminating the defects from the right ventricular aspect.

Alternatively, a right-angle clamp introduced through an aortotomy to probe the septum from the left side can be helpful in identifying the defects. Multiple apical defects can be effectively repaired with the septal obliteration technique, in which the defects are excluded from the right ventricular cavity with a pericardial patch.[29] A simpler technique involves primary closure of the muscular defects after identifying each VSD with a silk suture passed through the defect from the right ventricle and fished out of the left heart via an incision in the interatrial septum.[30]

The intraoperative placement of devices designed for transcatheter closure of ASDs or VSDs is another option for muscular defects.[31] Periventricular device deployment without the use of CPB has been described by multiple groups—initially in muscular VSDs but more recently also in perimembranous and supracristal defects.[32-35] The periventricular approach is usually through a median sternotomy. After placement of a purse-string suture on the right ventricle, a guide wire is introduced through the purse-string suture across the VSD under transesophageal echocardiography guidance. A sheath that is introduced into the right ventricle over the guide wire is used to deploy the closure device across the defect. Extreme care must be taken to avoid a transmural injury to the left ventricular free wall by the guide wire or the introducer.

Postoperative Care

Extubation in the operating room for older uncomplicated patients is appropriate. Neonates and infants may require ventilatory support and aggressive diuresis for 24 to 72 hours before safe extubation. If postoperative inotropic support is required, diuresis may not be effective in the initial 24 hours after surgery.

On the patient's admission to the intensive care unit a baseline measurement of hemodynamic parameters is performed. The heart rate and rhythm, arterial blood pressure, central venous pressure, and core and peripheral temperatures are monitored. Left atrial or pulmonary artery pressures may also be monitored in complicated cases or in patients who are at risk for or have exhibited signs of pulmonary hypertension. Admission hematocrit, serum chemistries, serum lactate level, arterial blood gas values, and coagulation parameters are checked. In addition to an electrocardiogram, chest radiography to check support equipment position and the pleural spaces is performed.

Estimates of cardiac output are made on the basis of peripheral perfusion and temperature, strength of pedal pulses, urinary output, serum lactate, and acid-base status. Some programs also use near-infrared spectroscopy routinely or selectively to monitor the adequacy of tissue oxygenation. Volume replacement may be required for low filling pressures. For elevated filling pressures (>10 mm Hg) and low cardiac output, inotropic support is required. A vasodilating agent is used to treat inadequate cardiac output associated with an elevated mean arterial blood pressure. Milrinone works well in this situation. The majority of patients undergoing straightforward VSD closure require minimal if any inotropic support postoperatively and can be extubated fairly promptly. Most benefit from diuresis instituted within 12 hours of surgery and continued until after the institution of enteral feedings. In patients with a large VSD and significant left-to-right shunt, it is not uncommon to find depressed left ventricular function by echocardiography in the immediate postoperative period, especially if their repair was delayed.[36] It is felt that an acute change in loading conditions—decreased preload from closure of the defect and an increased afterload from excluding the relatively low-resistance pulmonary circulation—contributes to this finding. Plasma levels of brain natriuretic peptide are elevated in the postoperative period compared with their preoperative values and seem to continue to rise for at least 3 days following repair.[37]

Patients who have long-standing pulmonary overcirculation or preoperative evidence of elevated PVR are prone to pulmonary hypertensive crises early in their postoperative recovery. A pulmonary artery line may be helpful in these patients. A typical pulmonary hypertension protocol to maintain pulmonary vasodilation involves full sedation and paralysis, hyperventilation, strict acid-base control, and fastidious pulmonary toilet. Use of inhaled nitric oxide and inhaled prostacyclin analogues is highly recommended in addition to conventional measures mentioned earlier with transition to oral pulmonary vasodilatory agents if the pulmonary artery pressures remain elevated.[14]

Early postoperative dysrhythmias occur in up to one-third of patients.[38] Supraventricular and junctional ectopic tachycardias are usually accompanied by marked deterioration in cardiac output and must be aggressively treated. Cooling the patient to 33°C or 34°C is effective with simple topical cooling. A peritoneal dialysis catheter, if present, may also be used for this purpose. These interventions require sedation and frequently neuromuscular blockade. Amiodarone, procainamide, dexmedetomidine, or a combination of these agents can be used to treat these tachycardias should the response to cooling be insufficient.

Complete heart block is another complication of VSD closure. It is often transient in nature, due to surgical trauma or edema associated with suture placement adjacent to the conduction tissue. Heart block usually resolves in 24 to 48 hours. Disruption of the conduction pathway results in permanent heart block. A contemporary series quoted a 5% incidence of combined temporary and permanent heart block and a 2% incidence of complete heart block requiring a pacemaker implantation.[39] All patients undergoing VSD repair should have temporary atrial and ventricular epicardial pacing wires placed at the time of surgery. These temporary wires are useful in both the diagnosis and treatment of dysrhythmias during the early postoperative period. If there is postoperative complete heart block, a transvenous or epicardial permanent pacemaker system is required if sinus rhythm is not restored within 7 to 10 days.

Outcome

Mortality rates for isolated VSD closure are less than 1%. For closure of multiple VSDs the rate may be as high as 7%.[40] The incidence of residual shunting due to patch dehiscence is very small. On the contrary, it is common to have some degree of residual shunting from small residual defects around the patch, with an incidence reported to be approximately 33%.[41] The same study noticed that two-thirds of these residual defects closed by the time of hospital discharge. Fig. 49.9 shows a residual patch leak on echocardiography with color Doppler imaging. Morbidity rates in infants seem to be higher with decreasing operative weight. In patients with postoperative right bundle branch block, there is a tendency toward left ventricular dilation in the long term, which confirms the need for long-term follow-up of these patients.[42] Long-term survival is excellent after successful VSD repair.

Interventional Therapy

Percutaneous transcatheter closure of VSDs with devices is less well established than device closure of ASDs. This technology has most commonly been used in the treatment of muscular

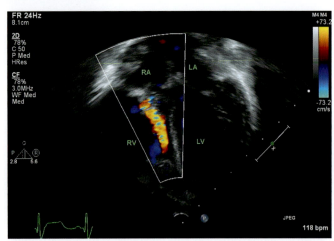

Figure 49.9 Two-dimensional echocardiogram with color Doppler revealing a residual defect at the border of a patch following closure of a perimembranous defect. *LA,* Left atrium; *LV,* left ventricle; *RA,* right atrium; *RV,* right ventricle.

VSDs with acceptable results.[43] The proximity of vital structures such as the aortic valve and the septal leaflet of the tricuspid valve to the paramembranous VSD makes device closure of this defect more challenging, although newer modifications have been developed.

The only US Food and Drug Administration–approved phase I clinical trial for device closure of hemodynamically significant perimembranous VSDs was reported in 2006.[44] This multicenter study used the Amplatzer Membranous VSD Occluder (AGA Medical Corp., Golden Valley, MN) in 32 of 35 patients in whom it was attempted. The median age was 7.7 years, and patients under 8 kg were excluded from the study. Although the rate of complete closure by echocardiography was 96% by 6 months, 2 patients required permanent pacemaker implantation at 3 and 16 months post procedure. New AR developed in 53% of patients within 24 hours of the procedure, deceasing to 39% by 6 months. Of the 35 patients, 4 were referred to surgery for either device placement–related significant AR, inadequate device positioning, or difficulty with device retrieval causing entanglement in the tricuspid valve chordae. A total of 6 out of 35 (17%) patients eventually needed a surgical intervention either for pacemaker placement or for VSD closure.

A later multi-institutional study narrowed the device closure to a subpopulation of membranous defects that had an associated aneurysm.[45] The investigators used the Amplatzer Duct Occluder I device, positioning it within the aneurysm and hence away from the aortic valve and from the crest of the ventricular septum, which correlated with a reduced incidence of new AR and heart block. The authors selected patients with a "wind-sock" appearance of the aneurysm, with very specific inclusion criteria based on the geometry of the aneurysm, the details of which are beyond the scope of this chapter. The device was successfully placed in 19 of 21 selected patients, whose weights were all above 8 kg with a median age of 5 years.

A recent meta-analysis of published studies comparing device closure with surgical closure of perimembranous VSDs showed comparable rates of successful closure and short-term complication rates.[46] The mean age in the device group was 12.2 years, whereas that of the surgical cohort was 5.5 years. An important current limitation to the application of percutaneously placed devices is

patient size because most patients with hemodynamically significant VSDs present with failure to thrive during infancy. Currently in the United States, percutaneous closure of perimembranous VSDs in the cardiac catheterization laboratory is not a recommended or commonly performed procedure.

A staged approach to treating infants with multiple VSDs involving initial pulmonary artery banding followed by delayed catheter-based closure of the muscular VSDs that have failed to close spontaneously in the intervening period may prove effective in the management of these challenging patients. As discussed earlier, a combined approach in the operating room could also be effective. As the technology improves, the indications for these procedures will expand. Patient follow-up will be important because the long-term outcomes of these procedures are still being accrued.

Selected References

A complete list of references is available at ExpertConsult.com.

1. Lamers WH, Wessels A, Verbeek FJ, et al. New findings concerning ventricular septation in the human heart. Implications for maldevelopment. *Circulation*. 1992;86(4):1194–1205.
2. Jacobs JP, Burke RP, Quintessenza JA, Mavroudis C. Congenital heart surgery nomenclature and database project: ventricular septal defect. *Ann Thorac Surg*. 2000;69(suppl 4):S25–S35.
12. Misra KP, Hildner FJ, Cohen LS, Narula OS, Samet P. Aneurysm of the membranous ventricular septum. A mechanism for spontaneous closure of ventricular septal defect. *N Engl J Med*. 1970;283(2):58–61.
13. Gabriels C, De Backer J, Pasquet A, et al. Long-term outcome of patients with perimembranous ventricular septal defect: results from the Belgian registry on adult congenital heart disease. *Cardiology*. 2017;136(3):147–155.
14. Abman SH, Hansmann G, Archer SL, et al. Pediatric pulmonary hypertension: guidelines from the American Heart Association and American Thoracic Society. *Circulation*. 2015;132(21):2037–2099.
19. Egbe AC, Poterucha JT, Dearani JA, Warnes CA. Supracristal ventricular septal defect in adults: Is it time for a paradigm shift? *Int J Cardiol*. 2015;198:9–14.
20. Kleinman CS, Tabibian M, Starc TJ, Hsu DT, Gersony WM. Spontaneous regression of left ventricular dilation in children with restrictive ventricular septal defects. *J Pediatr*. 2007;150(6):583–586.
22. Berglund E, Johansson B, Dellborg M, et al. High incidence of infective endocarditis in adults with congenital ventricular septal defect. *Heart*. 2016.
26. Kanter KR, Mahle WT, Kogon BE, Kirshbom PM. What is the optimal management of infants with coarctation and ventricular septal defect? *Ann Thorac Surg*. 2007;84(2):612–618, discussion 618.
27. Seddio F, Reddy VM, McElhinney DB, Tworetzky W, Silverman NH, Hanley FL. Multiple ventricular septal defects: how and when should they be repaired? *J Thorac Cardiovasc Surg*. 1999;117(1):134–139, discussion 139–140.
28. Kitagawa T, Durham LA 3rd, Mosca RS, Bove EL. Techniques and results in the management of multiple ventricular septal defects. *J Thorac Cardiovasc Surg*. 1998;115(4):848–856.
30. Talwar S, Bhoje A, Airan B. A simple technique for closing multiple muscular and apical ventricular septal defects. *J Card Surg*. 2015;30(9):731–734.
32. Bacha EA, Cao QL, Starr JP, Waight D, Ebeid MR, Hijazi ZM. Perventricular device closure of muscular ventricular septal defects on the beating heart: technique and results. *J Thorac Cardiovasc Surg*. 2003;126(6):1718–1723.
33. Omelchenko A, Gorbatykh Y, Voitov A, Zaitsev G, Bogachev-Prokophiev A, Karaskov A. Perventricular device closure of ventricular septal defects: results in patients less than 1 year of age. *Interact Cardiovasc Thorac Surg*. 2016;22(1):53–56.

34. Hongxin L, Wenbin G, Liang F, Zhang HZ, Zhu M, Zhang WL. Perventricular device closure of a doubly committed juxtaarterial ventricular septal defect through a left parasternal approach: midterm follow-up results. *J Cardiothorac Surg.* 2015;10:175.

35. Zhang S, Zhu D, An Q, Tang H, Li D, Lin K. Minimally invasive periventricular device closure of doubly committed sub-arterial ventricular septal defects: single center long-term follow-up results. *J Cardiothorac Surg.* 2015;10:119.

36. Pacileo G, Pisacane C, Russo MG, et al. Left ventricular mechanics after closure of ventricular septal defect: influence of size of the defect and age at surgical repair. *Cardiol Young.* 1998;8(3):320–328.

37. Mainwaring RD, Parise C, Wright SB, Juris AL, Achtel RA, Fallah H. Brain natriuretic peptide levels before and after ventricular septal defect repair. *Ann Thorac Surg.* 2007;84(6):2066–2069.

39. Anderson BR, Stevens KN, Nicolson SC, et al. Contemporary outcomes of surgical ventricular septal defect closure. *J Thorac Cardiovasc Surg.* 2013;145(3):641–647.

41. Preminger TJ, Sanders SP, van der Velde ME, Castaneda AR, Lock JE. "Intramural" residual interventricular defects after repair of conotruncal malformations. *Circulation.* 1994;89(1):236–242.

42. Veeram Reddy SR, Du W, Zilberman MV. Left ventricular mechanical synchrony and global systolic function in pediatric patients late after ventricular septal defect patch closure: a three-dimensional echocardiographic study. *Congenit Heart Dis.* 2009;4(6):454–458.

43. Holzer R, Balzer D, Cao QL, Lock K, Hijazi ZM. Amplatzer muscular ventricular septal defect I. Device closure of muscular ventricular septal defects using the Amplatzer muscular ventricular septal defect occluder: immediate and mid-term results of a U.S. registry. *J Am Coll Cardiol.* 2004;43(7):1257–1263.

44. Fu YC, Bass J, Amin Z, et al. Transcatheter closure of perimembranous ventricular septal defects using the new Amplatzer membranous VSD occluder: results of the U.S. phase I trial. *J Am Coll Cardiol.* 2006;47(2):319–325.

45. El Said HG, Bratincsak A, Gordon BM, Moore JW. Closure of perimembranous ventricular septal defects with aneurysmal tissue using the Amplazter Duct Occluder I: lessons learned and medium term follow up. *Catheter Cardiovasc Interv.* 2012;80(6):895–903.

46. Saurav A, Kaushik M, Mahesh Alla V, et al. Comparison of percutaneous device closure versus surgical closure of peri-membranous ventricular septal defects: A systematic review and meta-analysis. *Catheter Cardiovasc Interv.* 2015;86(6):1048–1056.

50

Atrioventricular Septal Defects

PETER SASSALOS, MD; MING-SING SI, MD; RICHARD G. OHYE, MD;
EDWARD L. BOVE, MD; JENNIFER C. ROMANO, MD, MS

Definition

Atrioventricular septal defects (AVSDs), also referred to as atrioventricular (AV) canal defects, endocardial cushion defects, and AV communis, represent a spectrum of congenital heart disease. They account for approximately 4% of congenital heart defects and are strongly associated with Down syndrome.[1] They are characterized by a variable deficiency of the AV septum and abnormal AV valves (AVVs). The specific type is determined by the septal defects, AVVs, and the relationship to the ventricles.

Classification and Anatomy

The embryologic cause of AVSDs is the failure of endocardial cushions to properly develop. They derive from mesenchymal origin and migrate to septate the heart, ultimately contributing to the lower portion of the atrial septum, division of the AVV, and the inlet portion of the ventricular septum. When this does not completely occur, the result is an AVSD.

The pertinent anatomy of AVSDs includes the size and type of the atrial (ASD) and ventricular septal defects (VSD), the characteristics of the AVV(s), the left ventricular outflow tract (LVOT), and the location of the conduction system. The ASD is an ostium primum defect located in the lower portion of the atrial septum directly superior to the AVVs. The VSD is an inlet-type defect located directly inferior to the AVVs. The AVV(s) in AVSDs can have either a single or two separate orifices. In either case they are in the same plane, in contrast to a normal heart, where the mitral valve attaches to the septum more superiorly than the tricuspid valve (Fig. 50.1). The leaflets constituting these valves are termed the *anterior or superior bridging leaflets* (SBLs), *posterior or inferior bridging leaflets* (IBLs), and *mural or lateral leaflets* (LLs) (Fig. 50.2). The SBL is toward the surgeon's left hand in a typical surgeon's view from the right atrium. There are typically five to six total leaflets, consisting of the SBL, which may be divided into left and right components, the left and right IBL, and the left and right LL. The left (LAVV) and right AV valve (RAVV) components are often incorrectly described as the mitral and tricuspid valve, respectively.[2] The LVOT is elongated with AVSDs. The aortic valve becomes displaced anterior and superiorly. This increases the outlet portion of the LVOT in comparison to the inlet portion, producing the classically described "gooseneck" deformity on angiography. It is postulated that this contributes to the predisposition of AVSD patients to develop LVOT obstruction (LVOTO) in the future (Fig. 50.3). Last, because of the absence of the AV septum, the conduction system is not at the usual apex of the triangle of Koch.[3,4]

It is displaced posterior and inferior toward the coronary sinus (CS) in the nodal triangle defined by the CS, rim of the ASD, and posterior attachment of the IBL. The bundle of His then courses under the IBL to travel anterior and superior on the leftward aspect of the crest of the ventricular septum.

Classification of AVSDs includes incomplete, transitional, and complete.[5] They should be distinguished on the basis of the AVV. If there is a common AVV orifice, the defect is complete, and if there are two separate AVV orifices, then the defect is incomplete. Incomplete AVSDs are also known as partial AVSDs or ostium primum ASDs.[5] They consist of an ostium primum ASD, no VSD, and two separate AVV orifices with typically a cleft in the LAVV between the SBL and IBL (see Fig. 50.1). Of note, some prefer zone of apposition to cleft because it is thought to instead be a commissure and is not considered a true mitral valve.[2,6] Throughout the chapter the term *cleft* will be used preferentially. A complete AVSD consists of an ostium primum ASD, a typically large and nonrestrictive VSD, and a common AVV orifice (see Fig. 50.1). Transitional or intermediate AVSDs have been described as an additional subtype, which is not used primarily by our center.[5] They consist of an ostium primum ASD, a common AVV (single orifice), and no ventricular level shunting (either due to the absence of a VSD or closure of the VSD by aneurysmal tissue). Others have defined transitional AVSD (also known as intermediate AVSD) as an AVSD with two distinct left AVV and right AVV orifices and also both an ASD just above and a VSD just below the AV valves.[5] Although these AV valves in the intermediate form do form two separate orifices, they remain abnormal valves.[5] The VSD in this lesion is often restrictive.[5]

Complete AVSDs are also subcategorized based on the SBL using the Rastelli classification.[7] Type A has a SBL that is divided and attached to the crest of the ventricular septum. Type B has straddling chordae from the left SBL to right ventricular (RV) papillary muscles. Type C is a free-floating SBL that is not divided or attached to the crest (Fig. 50.4). Type A is the most common, type B is rare and more likely associated with single-ventricle anatomy, and type C is more commonly associated with conotruncal anomalies.

Complete AVSDs are then further distinguished as balanced or unbalanced. This is determined not by the size of each ventricle but the proportion of the common AVV orifice distributed over each ventricle.[8] This becomes an important determinant of surgical repair. Balanced and some unbalanced AVSDs (uAVSDs) are amenable to biventricular repair, whereas severely uAVSDs are treated with single-ventricle palliation. This is particularly important in patients with Down syndrome, who are not considered for

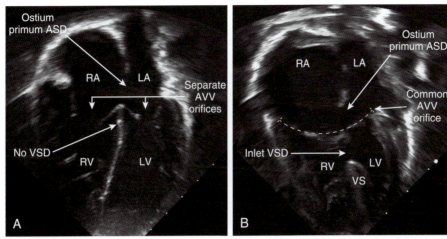

• **Figure 50.1** Transthoracic echocardiogram apical four-chamber views. (A) Incomplete AVSD consisting of an ostium primum ASD, no inlet VSD, and two separate AVV orifices. (B) Complete AVSD consisting of an ostium primum ASD, a large inlet VSD, and a common AVV orifice. *ASD,* Atrial septal defect; *AVSD,* atrioventricular septal defect; *AVV,* atrioventricular valve; *LA,* left atrium; *LV,* left ventricle; *RA,* right atrium; *RV,* right ventricle; *VS,* ventricular septum; *VSD,* ventricular septal defect. (Courtesy Dr. Gregory Ensing, Department of Pediatrics, University of Michigan C.S. Mott Children's Hospital.)

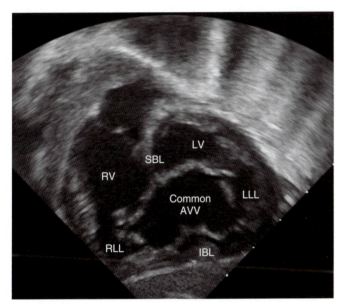

• **Figure 50.2** Transthoracic echocardiogram subcostal view demonstrating common AVV anatomy in diastole. *AVV,* Atrioventricular valve; *IBL,* inferior bridging leaflet; *LLL,* left lateral leaflet; *LV,* left ventricle; *RLL,* right lateral leaflet; *RV,* right ventricle; *SBL,* superior bridging leaflet. (Courtesy Dr. Gregory Ensing, Department of Pediatrics, University of Michigan C.S. Mott Children's Hospital.)

single-ventricle palliation by many institutions given their poor outcomes with a Fontan procedure.[9,10]

Associations

There is a strong association with Down syndrome. Approximately 30% to 40% of cardiac abnormalities in patients with Down syndrome are AVSDs.[1] Other cardiac defects are also associated with AVSDs. A left superior vena cava (LSVC) can be present. Additional ASDs can be seen. Abnormalities of the AVV, such as a single papillary muscle with parachute left AV valve (PLAVV)

(2% to 6%) or double-orifice left AV valve (DOLAVV) (8% to 14%) can be seen.[11] There is an association with conotruncal anomalies, either tetralogy of Fallot (TOF) (10%) or double-outlet right ventricle (DORV) (2%).[12] A patent ductus arteriosus (PDA) is commonly present but not always recognized on preoperative studies in the setting of a nonrestrictive VSD. Other defects can also be seen rarely.

Pathophysiology and Natural History

The pathophysiology of AVSDs is similar regardless of the type. The mechanism is left-to-right shunting across the septal defects, which can be exacerbated by AVV regurgitation (AVVR). The degree of left-to-right shunting at the ASD and VSD levels is dependent on the ventricular compliance and the pulmonary (PVR) and systemic vascular resistance (SVR), respectively. Initially after birth the PVR is high, and the degree of shunting (relative pulmonary and systemic blood flow; Q_p:Q_s) is less. As the PVR falls, there is increased pulmonary blood flow, leading to a higher Q_p:Q_s. If left unrepaired, this increased pulmonary blood flow will induce vascular changes that lead to pulmonary vascular occlusive disease. The result is an increase in the PVR, leading to pulmonary hypertension. The Q_p:Q_s will decrease or can even reverse, leading to cyanosis, as in Eisenmenger syndrome.

The presence of AVVR further worsens the pathophysiology. It creates ventricular volume overload and can lead to congestive heart failure (CHF). The regurgitant jet can also create an obligate left ventricle (LV)-to-right atrial (RA) shunt via the left atrium (LA).

The presentation therefore varies depending on these factors. Incomplete AVSDs can present similarly to other ASDs and may be well tolerated for several decades. Complete AVSDs present earlier during infancy. Those with Down syndrome may have a delayed presentation due to higher PVR and decreased Q_p:Q_s. In contrast, those with a large VSD, AVVR, or left-sided obstruction such as subaortic stenosis (sub-AS) or coarctation of the aorta (CoA), have an accelerated presentation. However, the natural history in all cases leads to progressive CHF and associated sequelae.

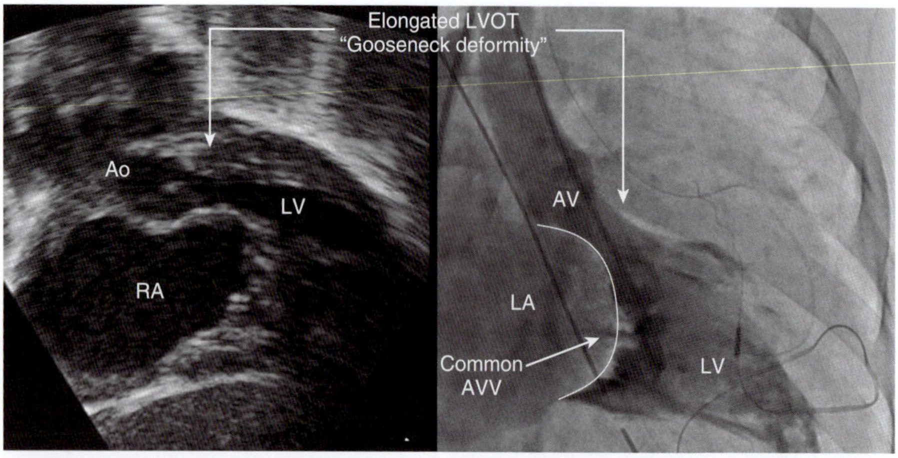

• **Figure 50.3** Transthoracic echocardiogram subcostal view and a left ventriculogram, both demonstrating the elongated LVOT, or "gooseneck deformity," seen in AVSDs. *Ao,* Aorta; *AV,* aortic valve; *AVSD,* atrioventricular septal defect; *AVV,* atrioventricular valve; *LA,* left atrium; *LV,* left ventricle; *LVOT,* left ventricular outflow tract; *RA,* right atrium. (Courtesy Drs. Gregory Ensing and Jeffrey Zampi, Department of Pediatrics, University of Michigan C.S. Mott Children's Hospital.)

Advanced stages can also lead to irreversible pulmonary vascular obstructive disease. In this setting, CHF symptoms will improve, which is an ominous sign. It has been reported that up to 90% of patients with complete AVSDs will have pulmonary vascular disease at 1 year of age.[13] If left untreated, AVSDs are ultimately fatal.

Diagnostic Assessment

Patients with AVSDs warrant a thorough diagnostic evaluation, including a birth history and physical examination, laboratory studies, electrocardiogram (ECG), chest radiograph (CXR), and transthoracic echocardiogram (TTE). In select cases, additional evaluation such as transesophageal (TEE) or three-dimensional echocardiography, cardiac catheterization, and cardiac magnetic resonance imaging may be indicated to answer specific clinical questions.

Physical examination may reveal stigmata of Down syndrome. Patients may have overt CHF signs. There is typically an active precordium and possibly a prominent thrill. There can be a pulmonary outflow murmur and a fixed, widely split second heart sound. A regurgitant systolic murmur may be heard in cases of AVVR. An ECG will have left axis deviation and may also demonstrate atrial enlargement and a prolonged PR interval. A CXR may demonstrate cardiomegaly and increased pulmonary vascular markings.

A TTE is the mainstay of diagnosis (see Figs. 50.1 and 50.2). Pertinent details to guide preoperative planning include the type of systemic venous connections, the size and location of ASD(s) and VSD, AVV anatomy and function, the degree of balance, size and function of the ventricles, the presence of systemic outflow tract obstruction, presence of a PDA, and any other associated cardiac defects.

The degree of unbalance in complete AVSDs can be challenging to evaluate. The anatomy of an AVSD makes standard measurements difficult and often unreliable.[14] For example, z scores are not applicable, and ventricular size is not a consistent marker for unbalance because often the RV is larger than usual given the presence of a large atrial level shunt. Therefore a left-dominant uAVSD may have a nondominant RV that appears normal in size.

In cases of right-dominant uAVSDs with LV hypoplasia, attempts have been made to apply similar diagnostic algorithms used in other cardiac anomalies with hypoplastic left-sided structures to guide management.[14] For example, the Rhodes score[15] and the Congenital Heart Surgeons Society (CHSS) score[16] used to assess LV adequacy in critical aortic stenosis have been used without success. Likewise, with left-dominant uAVSDs with RV hypoplasia, measures used for lesions such as pulmonary atresia with intact ventricular septum have not correlated well either.[14]

It is therefore important to look at additional variables. In an effort to better guide these decisions specifically in patients with uAVSDs, extensive work has been done at Children's Hospital of Philadephia.[8,14,17-20] They have studied morphometric analysis of AVSDs in a retrospective fashion in an effort to use echocardiographic variables to estimate the degree of unbalance, guide surgical management, and predict outcomes. They first described the atrioventricular valve index (AVVI).[8] Using a subxiphoid or subcostal left anterior oblique view, they bisect the common AVV by a line connecting the conal septum to the crest of the muscular septum. The smaller orifice area is then divided by the larger orifice area to give a ratio. A value equal to 1 is a balanced defect. An AVVI value of 0.67 was found retrospectively to distinguish those defects determined clinically to be balanced or unbalanced. Furthermore, in their series all patients with an AVVI less than 0.27 were found to undergo single-ventricle palliation. More recently, to eliminate ambiguity associated with this index, the modified AVVI was introduced.[17] This is calculated as the LAVV area divided by the total AVV area. A value equal to 0.5 is a balanced defect. A modified AVVI less than or equal to 0.4 is right dominant and greater than or equal to 0.6 is left dominant. In retrospective analysis it was found that all patients with modified AVVI less than 0.19 underwent single-ventricle palliation, and all those with values between 0.4 and 0.6 underwent biventricular repair.[17]

Other echocardiographic variables studied have included RV/LV inflow angle, LV inflow index (LVII), the amount of LA overriding the RAVV, VSD size, and the presence of retrograde flow in the transverse aortic arch.[8,14,19-21] The RV/LV inflow angle is described as the angle between the base of the RV and LV free walls using the crest of the ventricular septum as the apex of the angle.[20] The LVII is the assessment of the LV color Doppler inflow

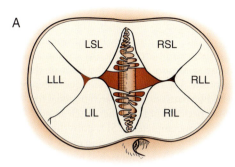

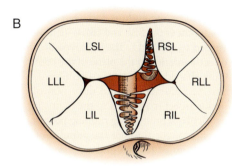

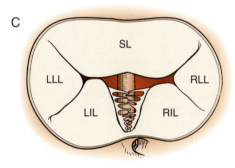

• **Figure 50.4** Rastelli classification of complete AVSDs. (A) Type A has a SBL that is divided and attached to the crest of the ventricular septum. (B) Type B has straddling chordae from the left SBL to RV papillary muscles. (C) Type C is a free-floating SBL that is not divided or attached to the crest. *AVSD,* Atrioventricular septal defect; *LIL,* left inferior leaflet; *LLL,* left lateral leaflet; *LSL,* left superior leaflet; *RIL,* right inferior leaflet; *RLL,* right lateral leaflet; *RSL,* right superior leaflet; *RV,* right ventricle; *SL* or *SBL,* superior bridging leaflet. (From Jacobs JP, Burke RP, Quintessenza JA, et al. Congenital Heart Surgery Nomenclature and Database Project: atrioventricular canal defect. *Ann Thorac Surg.* 69(4 suppl):S36-S43, 2000 with permission.)

jet.[19] Used together, these variables help stratify patients into appropriate surgical management.

In patients who present late or with cyanosis a diagnostic cardiac catheterization is indicated to determine the PVR. If the PVR is elevated, pulmonary vasoreactivity testing should be performed. Surgical closure of septal defects is contraindicated with a fixed PVR of greater than 10 U/m^2.

Preoperative Critical Care Management

The management of all AVSDs follows the same principles. Treatment is directed at management of the underlying pathophysiology of left-to-right shunting and AVVR. Digoxin will increase cardiac inotropy. Afterload-reducing agents will decrease the SVR to decrease left-to-right shunting and improve AVVR. Diuretics will optimize

the patient's fluid status and preload. The goal is to control associated symptoms, avoid the complications of disease, and optimize the patient for anticipated surgery.

Down syndrome poses multiple management challenges with important implications. These patients are more difficult to sedate, they may have cervical spine instability that requires special precautions, and they are at increased risk of advanced pulmonary vascular disease. This is due in part to a combination of small airways, macroglossia with obstructive symptoms, chronic hypoventilation, and hypercarbia. This predisposition therefore affects clinical presentation, timing of surgical repair, and their candidacy for single-ventricle palliation in the setting of uAVSDs.

For patients who can be medically optimized, timing of surgical management of incomplete AVSDs is similar to that for secundum ASDs at approximately 2 to 4 years of age. Recommended timing for complete AVSDs is 4 months of age, earlier than for isolated VSD closure due to increased risk of advanced pulmonary vascular disease due to combined atrial and ventricular level shunting. However, in cases in which patients are unable to be managed medically and present symptomatic growth failure, earlier surgical management is recommended. The decision of complete repair or palliation is dependent on each patient. In general, complete repair is favored except in cases when contraindicated by comorbidities impacting surgical risk. Examples include patients not suitable for cardiopulmonary bypass due to poor clinical state or comorbidities such as prematurity, end-organ dysfunction, extracardiac anomalies, or neurologic factors. Additional reasons are those patients with complex congenital heart disease requiring more complex operations and uAVSDs that require single-ventricle palliation.

Surgical Correction

The first successful repair of an AVSD was by C. Walton Lillehei using cross-circulation in 1955.[22] This was followed with repair using cardiopulmonary bypass by Kirklin, McGoon, and Cooley.[23-25] The single-patch technique was then reported by Maloney et al.[26] in 1962, the two-patch technique by Trusler et al.[27] in 1976, and the modified single-patch technique by Wilcox et al.[28] in 1997, followed by Nicholson et al.[29] in 1999.

The goal of surgical repair of AVSDs is to create normal anatomy and physiology by septation of the heart with no residual intracardiac shunts and normal function of the AVVs. Depending on the type of AVSD, various techniques are employed. In addition, some types of anatomy and associated defects warrant special consideration and will be discussed separately.

Incomplete Atrioventricular Septal Defects

A standard median sternotomy is performed. We use autologous pericardium, which is harvested and placed in dilute glutaraldehyde solution, although other patch materials can be used. Polyethylene terephthalate (Dacron) is generally avoided because the roughness of the material can lead to hemolysis in the setting of an AVVR jet impacting the surface of the patch. Bicaval cannulation with aortic inflow is established with mild hypothermia and an LV vent. Antegrade cardioplegia is administered. A right atriotomy is performed close to and parallel to the AV groove to provide maximal exposure. The anatomy is inspected. The ostium primum ASD is closed by placing a series of horizontal mattress sutures on the rightward aspect of the crest of the ventricular septum, through the midpoint of the two AVV orifices, and then through the autologous pericardial patch. The sutures are then tied down. Before the patch closure is completed, attention is directed to the LAVV. The cleft between the SBL and IBL of the LAVV is tested by injecting saline into the LV to assess for coaptation and the degree of regurgitation. Identifying the last chords on the SLB and the IBL also assists with alignment of the cleft. The cleft is then closed with interrupted polypropylene sutures. The valve is again tested. The RAVV is then tested for competence. The pericardial patch is trimmed to appropriate size and sutured to the rim of the ASD using a running polypropylene suture. Care is taken to place superficial sutures in the area of the conduction system. It is our practice to leave the CS on the RA side, although others choose to place it on the left. The left heart is deaired before completion. The aortic cross-clamp is removed, the right atriotomy is closed, and the patient weaned from cardiopulmonary bypass.

Complete Atrioventricular Septal Defects

The exposure, harvesting of autologous pericardium, and cannulation strategy are the same as discussed earlier. The anatomy is inspected. The size and type of ASD and VSD are confirmed. The Rastelli type is determined. The LAVV papillary muscle configuration and adequacy of the left lateral leaflet are noted (Fig. 50.5A). The common AVV is then tested with cold saline to identify the central point of apposition of the SBL and IBL. This is the critical step of the operation. This location is marked with fine polypropylene suture to define the plane for septation of the common AVV into the left and right components.

There are three different techniques then used to close the VSD. These are the single patch, modified single patch or so-called Australian technique, and the two-patch technique. The theoretical advantages and disadvantages of each summarized in Table 50.1. The single-patch technique involves dividing the SBL and IBL into left and right components. A single patch is then used to

close both the ASD and VSD. The divided edges of the SBL and IBL are then reattached to the patch. The modified single-patch technique closes the VSD primarily by sandwiching the common AVV between the crest of the ventricular septum and ASD patch. This brings the common AVV to the level of the crest of the ventricular septum. The two-patch technique uses a polytetrafluoroethylene (PTFE) patch or other patch material to close the VSD and autologous pericardium or other patch material to close the ASD. As with an incomplete AVSD, polyethylene terephthalate should be avoided because in the setting of AVVR, hemolysis can occur. The common AVV is sandwiched between the two patches, thereby partitioning the valve into left and right components. This technique is favored by the authors and described in more detail.

Once the midpoint of the SBL and IBL is identified and marked, attention is turned to the VSD. The inlet type of VSD is crescent shaped and directly inferior to the plane of the common AV valve. A corresponding shaped PTFE patch is fashioned. The height of the patch must be accurate to avoid distortion of the common AVV. The inferior aspect is attached to the rightward aspect of the crest of the ventricular septum using running polypropylene suture. Each end is then brought through the annulus of each bridging leaflet at the midpoint of the left and right components. Care is taken under the IBL to avoid injury to the bundle of His as it penetrates to travel along the leftward aspect of the ventricular septum (see Fig. 50.5B).

Horizontal mattress sutures are then passed through the free superior edge of the VSD patch, then through the SBL and IBL along the line demarcating the right and left components, and last through the fixed autologous pericardial patch. The sutures are tied down, sandwiching and partitioning the common AVV into left and right components (see Fig. 50.5C).

The LAVV is then inspected. The cleft is closed with interrupted polypropylene sutures, although running sutures have also been described (see Fig. 50.5D). The valve is tested with saline. If there is additional regurgitation following closure, advanced valve repair techniques can be used, such as partial suture annuloplasty. Next, the RAVV is tested in a similar fashion. If there is regurgitation, the SBL and IBL are often attached to the autologous pericardial patch at the midpoint or partially closed to each other to improve competency. In general the extra leaflet tissue is favored over the LAVV because right AVVR (RAVVR) is better tolerated.

Following the repair of each valve, the autologous pericardial patch is cut to size and used to close the ostium primum ASD with running polypropylene suture. As previously mentioned, the AV node is displaced in AVSDs and located in the nodal triangle adjacent to the CS ostium. As a result, to minimize the risk of complete heart block (CHB), many surgeons prefer to suture around the CS ostium, placing it on the left side of the heart and creating an obligate right-to-left shunt. Our preference is to suture to the rim of the ostium, maintaining it on the correct right side of the heart. Any additional secundum ASDs can be closed primarily (see Fig. 50.5E). The remainder of the operation is completed in a similar fashion as described previously. In addition, a transthoracic LA line is typically placed for postoperative management.

Special Considerations

Palliative Procedures

In some cases, as described earlier, palliative procedures are necessary. The main procedure is pulmonary artery (PA) banding, which is used to decrease left-to-right shunting, avoid heart failure, protect

TABLE 50.1	**Theoretical Advantages and Disadvantages of Each Type of Complete Atrioventricular Septal Defect Repair[a]**		
Variable	Single Patch	Modified Single Patch	Two Patch
Applicability	All patients	Less feasible with large VSD	All patients
CPB/XC	Longer	Shorter	Longer
VSD closure	Easier	Easier	More difficult
AVV leaflets	Divided	Not divided	Not divided
AVV geometry	Maintained	Displaced inferiorly to ventricular septum	Maintained
AVV damage or distortion risk	Higher	Higher	Lower
LVOTO risk	Lower	Higher	Lower

[a]Of note, these are believed by those who advocate each approach without well-supported data in the literature. There is no clear consensus on the best type, and therefore technique varies by institutions.

AVV, Atrioventricular valve; *CPB,* cardiopulmonary bypass; *LVOTO,* left ventricular outflow tract obstruction; *VSD,* ventricular septal defect; *XC,* aortic cross-clamp.

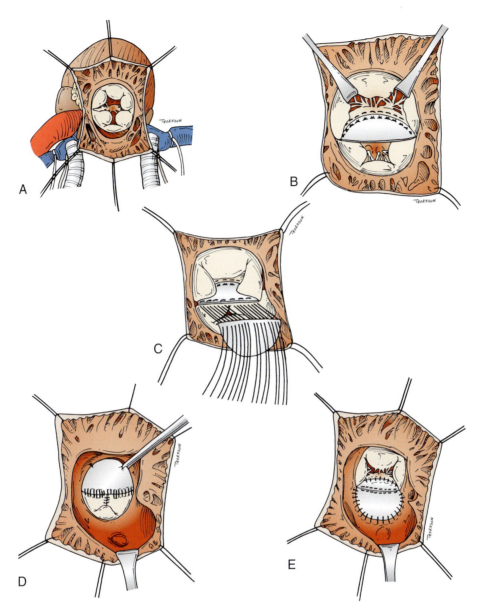

• **Figure 50.5** Complete AVSD repair using the two-patch technique. (A) Typical surgeon's view through a right atriotomy. The SBL is toward the surgeon's left hand, corresponding to the leaflet at the 9-o'clock position in this illustration. Rastelli type A anatomy is shown. (B) VSD closure using a crescent-shaped PTFE patch. The inferior aspect is attached to the rightward aspect of the crest of the ventricular septum. (C) Horizontal mattress sutures are then passed through the free superior edge of the VSD patch, then through the SBL and IBL at the defined midpoint of each leaflet, and last through the fixed autologous pericardial patch. The sutures are tied down, sandwiching and partitioning the common AVV into left and right components. (D) The ASD patch is retracted anteriorly. The LAVV is then inspected. The cleft is closed with interrupted polypropylene sutures. (E) Following the repair of each valve, the autologous pericardial patch is cut to size and used to close the ostium primum ASD with running polypropylene suture. The completed repair is shown with the coronary sinus maintained on the correct right side of the heart. An additional small secundum ASD was also closed primarily. *ASD,* Atrial septal defect; *AVSD,* atrioventricular septal defect; *AVV,* atrioventricular valve; *IBL,* inferior bridging leaflet; *LAVV,* left atrioventricular valve; *PTFE,* polytetrafluoroethylene; *SBL,* superior bridging leaflet; *VSD,* ventricular septal defect. (Courtesy Dr. Thor Thorsson, Department of Pediatrics, University of Michigan C.S. Mott Children's Hospital.)

the pulmonary vasculature, allow somatic growth, and to delay complete biventricular repair or staged single-ventricle palliation. When the patient presents with CoA, it can be combined with this repair and performed through a thoracotomy. Otherwise, a median sternotomy is the preferred approach. Caution should be taken when PA banding is performed in the setting of a restrictive VSD or AVVR to avoid suprasystemic RV pressure or worsened regurgitation due to increased afterload, respectively.

Left Superior Vena Cava

The presence of an LSVC impacts both cannulation strategy and closure of the ostium primum ASD. Various cannulation strategies can be used. If there is a single LSVC, it must be cannulated. If there are bilateral SVCs with a bridging vein, the larger SVC can be cannulated and the other controlled with a tourniquet between the bridging vein and heart. If there is no bridging vein, options include cannulation of both SVCs, cannulation of the larger SVC and control of the smaller SVC with CVP monitoring, or placement of a flexible cardiotomy suction into the CS to drain the LSVC. In the case of an AVSD repair the latter may compromise exposure and visualization, and the other techniques are preferred.

In the absence of an LSVC the CS can drain to either atrium with minimal shunt as described earlier. However, in the presence of an LSVC, the CS must be placed on the RA side during closure of the ostium primum ASD to avoid a large obligate right-to-left shunt. Last, if the LSVC is unroofed, more complex baffling must be performed to allow drainage to the RA. This can be done using standard techniques described elsewhere in this book.

Left Atrioventricular Valve Abnormalities

The AVV tissues and geometry in AVSDs have known abnormalities. However, two distinct abnormalities can make repair even more challenging. These include parachute LAVV (PLAVV) and double-orifice LAVV (DOLAVV). The incidence is estimated to be approximately 10%.[30]

PLAVV is defined as unifocal attachment of chordae tendineae to the LAVV. A true PLAVV has a single papillary muscle to which both leaflets are attached via chordae.[31] Another variant can be an asymmetric valve with two papillary muscles, one of which is dominant and reaches to the valve leaflets.[32] The effect is restricted valve opening and potential for LAVV stenosis. The mural or LL are usually deficient or absent in this scenario. Parachute-type valves can be isolated, associated with AVSD, or part of Shone's complex as part of the constellation of supravalvar mitral ring, sub-AS, and CoA.[33]

With AVSDs a PLAVV can lead to potential LAVV stenosis with cleft closure. The degree of cleft closure must be carefully evaluated based on preoperative imaging and intraoperative findings. If possible, complete closure is preferred even at the expense of mild stenosis. In a single-center retrospective study the most common reason for reoperation was progressive left AVVR (LAVVR) through an incompletely closed cleft. Those patients with stenosis tended to improve with time. For those patients who do require intervention for stenosis, other techniques include division of the papillary muscle between the chordae to each leaflet, chordal fenestration, or leaflet augmentation.[32]

DOLAVV is the presence of two separate orifices of the LAVV. It is a defect in the leaflet tissue rather than bridging tissue across a single orifice. As with PLAVV, it requires special attention during AVSD repair. Based on the largest single-center experience, the

recommendation for complete cleft closure was made when feasible based on the valve characteristics. If the AVV orifices appear inadequate, partial closure can be performed. The intervening tissue should never be divided to create a single orifice because it will lead to significant regurgitation. In cases in which there is regurgitation through the accessory orifice, it can be closed with a patch, and the cleft should then be partially closed to maintain an adequate-size dominant orifice.[34]

Unbalanced Atrioventricular Septal Defects

uAVSDs represent a complex subset of patients accounting for approximately 10% of AVSDs.[14] There is a spectrum of unbalance and, depending on the severity and the dominant ventricle, various surgical strategies may be used. These include primary or staged biventricular repair, one-and-a-half ventricle repair, or single-ventricle palliation.

For those with moderate imbalance, a biventricular repair can be attempted. However, if the hemodynamics are not favorable in the operating room or early postoperative period, it is critical to convert these patients early to single-ventricle palliation.[14] For example, with a right-dominant uAVSD, if left-sided structures appear inadequate, the patient may present with LA hypertension, pulmonary venous congestion, and pulmonary vascular changes. If not addressed, these changes can be irreversible and make the patient an unsuitable candidate for single-ventricle palliation. Another option described in a small case series for marginal candidates is a staged repair.[35] The first stage is ostium primum ASD closure, partial VSD closure, and septation of the common AVV in such a way as to create balance over both ventricles. A PA band is placed along with snare-controlled secundum ASD closure. The rationale is to increase blood flow to the left side of the heart to promote growth and enable staged completion in the future.

For left-dominant uAVSD, if the RV is felt inadequate to support the entire systemic circulation, a one-and-a-half ventricle repair can be performed.[14,36] In this case a complete AVSD repair is performed in conjunction with a bidirectional Glenn procedure. However, long-term advantages over a single-ventricle approach are not well defined. Another option is to leave an ASD.[37] If the right heart is inadequate, cardiac output can be maintained through right-to-left shunting at the expense of hypoxemia. This does not work as well with right-dominant uAVSD because the left-to-right shunting does not increase cardiac output and further volume loads the marginal left heart.[14]

Last, if the techniques described are not feasible, the patient undergoes staged single-ventricle palliation. Depending on the associated anatomy, stage I procedures are variable. However, patients will ultimately culminate with a Fontan circulation. This is discussed elsewhere in the book.

Complete Atrioventricular Septal Defect With Tetralogy of Fallot

Conotruncal abnormalities, such as TOF, are commonly associated with AVSDs. These patients were historically managed with a systemic-to-pulmonary artery shunt followed by complete repair. However, multiple centers have shown promising results with primary complete repair.[38,39]

The conduct of the operation is similar to a complete AVSD repair except in VSD closure and management of right ventricular outflow tract obstruction (RVOTO). The VSD is an inlet type with outlet extension. The typical crescent-shaped patch used in the two-patch technique must therefore be modified into a comma shape that allows closure of the outlet portion. In some cases a second VSD patch can be used and then the patches sutured to each other. VSD closure can typically be done through a transatrial approach for AVSD with TOF; however, a right ventriculotomy is usually necessary for AVSD with true DORV. Standard techniques for TOF repair are used to address RVOTO, including division of infundibular muscle bundles, pulmonary valvotomy, and transannular patch if necessary. Of note, it is very important to avoid both significant pulmonary insufficiency and RAVVR. This is very poorly tolerated. Extra attention must be paid to the RAVV in these cases to ensure competence. If this is not achievable and a transannular patch is required, creation of a monocusp valve or instead placement of an RV-to-pulmonary artery conduit should be considered to provide a competent pulmonary valve.[36]

Reoperation for Left Atrioventricular Valve Repair or Replacement

Despite advances in the surgical techniques and management of AVSDs, LAVVR continues to be problematic. Indications for operation include symptoms, moderate to severe regurgitation with LV dilation, decreased ventricular function, or need for concomitant cardiac surgery.

Valve repair is favored over replacement at reoperation, however, with variable success depending on the underlying cause. Repair techniques may include primary or repeat cleft closure, various forms of annuloplasty, Alfieri-type repair, valvotomy, or leaflet augmentation. Saline testing and intraoperative TEE are used to assess the adequacy of repair.

When valve repair is not successful, LAVV replacement is warranted. Unfortunately, mitral valve replacement (MVR) carries the highest morbidity and mortality of any valve replacement in pediatric patients.[40] A large, multicenter review analyzed 139 patients less than 5 years of age who underwent 176 MVRs for any cause with a mean follow-up of 6.2 years. The incidence of CHB, endocarditis, thrombosis, and stroke were 16%, 6%, 6%, and 2%, respectively. The 10-year survival was 74%.[41] The 40-year experience of two centers also showed similar findings. The hospital mortality was 6%. The 35-year actuarial survival and freedom from reoperation were 71% and 63%, respectively.[42] In both studies there was an increased risk of mortality associated with AVSDs.

Replacement of the LAVV poses many challenges. First, options are limited, and all have disadvantages. Bioprosthetic valves and xenografts have limited durability in the systemic circulation, and the smallest bioprosthetic valve currently available is 19 mm in diameter. Mechanical valves have better durability; however, there are risks of anticoagulation. These risks are magnified as children become more active with involvement in higher-risk activities, teenagers gain autonomy and become less compliant, and females enter child-bearing years. On-X (CryoLife Inc., Kennesaw, GA) valves are pure pyrolytic carbon mechanical valves that are thought to be less thrombogenic. Studies have shown comparable results with a lower international normalized ratio goal of 1.5 to 2.0 in the aortic position.[43] Studies have not been completed in the mitral position. The smallest mechanical valve currently available is 15 mm in diameter; however, the smallest On-X valve is 23 mm in diameter in Europe and 25 mm in diameter in the United States.

Second, implantation can be technically challenging. The goal is to place an adequate size, or potentially larger size, valve if possible to allow growth of the patient and minimize reoperations. However, this must be balanced with the risk of CHB, compression of the left circumflex coronary artery, and development of LVOTO. If an appropriate-size valve is unable to be placed, supraannular positioning is an option.[44] Care must be taken to avoid pulmonary venous obstruction in this case. Alternatively, if aortic valve replacement will also be required, a Manougian root enlargement can increase the size of the mitral valve annulus. Last, contrary to adults who undergo MVR with preservation of the subvalvar apparatus, resection is usually required to avoid mechanical leaflet obstruction in children.

As a result of these limitations in neonates and smaller infants, off-label use of different valves has been investigated with limited long-term outcomes available. Melody (Medtronic, Minneapolis, MN) valves have been implanted in the mitral position. They are bovine jugular veins in a stent that can be expanded to as little as 9 mm in diameter. They then have the potential for serial balloon dilation and future growth.[45] Extracellular matrix of porcine small intestinal submucosa (CorMatrix, Roswell, GA) has been fashioned by hand or factory produced into a cylinder valve as small as 12 mm in diameter for use in the AVV position. The ends of the cylinder are then sutured to the papillary muscles and annulus.[46,47] Last, the Ross II MVR has been favored by some institutions, using a pulmonary autograft inserted into a pericardial-wrapped synthetic graft for the benefit of avoiding anticoagulation.[48-50]

Reoperation for Left Ventricular Outflow Tract Obstruction

Patients with AVSDs are at risk for LVOTO, which accounts for the second most common indication for reoperation. Multiple surgical techniques have been described to address LVOTO. Initial techniques include a sub-AS resection of any membrane and fibromuscular tissue, a septal myectomy, and resection of anomalous secondary or tertiary AVV chords. Advanced techniques include resuspension of the LAVV, conversion of a Rastelli type A SBL into type C by dividing chordal attachments to the crest of the ventricular septum,[51,52] SBL augmentation to enlarge the LVOT,[53,54] and LAVV replacement. Other options may include a Konno-type procedure, Ross-Konno procedure if there is associated valvar aortic stenosis, and an apical-to-aortic conduit, which is rarely performed today.[53,55]

Postoperative Critical Care Management

The general management following any AVSD repair is similar to that of most cardiac surgical patients. However, tailored care is required based on the particular risks of these operations. Baseline knowledge of intraoperative ventricular function, residual lesions, and the degree of AVVR is important. Patients typically have some degree of early LV dysfunction, which is also seen in isolated VSD closure. This is presumably from the removal of left-to-right shunts leading to increased LV afterload. This can also manifest as low cardiac output. Hemodynamic monitoring, including LA pressures, lactic acid measurements, and mixed venous oxygen saturations, can help guide management.

The median ventilator days, intensive care unit length of stay, and postoperative hospital length of stay are 2, 4, and 7 days, respectively.[56] If a patient is not progressing appropriately and demonstrates signs of cardiorespiratory failure, a suspicion for worsening AVVR should prompt further evaluation. Efforts to decrease SVR may be beneficial and will also decrease the stress on the LAVV repair. Other considerations include CHB and arrhythmias, which must be addressed appropriately. Last, for patients at high risk for pulmonary vascular disease, placement of a transthoracic PA line and leaving a small ASD can be helpful. Appropriate measures should be taken to minimize PVR and the risk of a pulmonary hypertensive crisis. Optimal pain and sedation control, which may be more difficult in patients with Down syndrome, must be maintained. Ventilatory maneuvers to maintain adequate oxygenation and normal pCO_2 are important. Pulmonary vasodilator therapy, including either inhaled nitric oxide or oral sildenafil, may be required.

Outcomes

The mortality following complete AVSD repair is generally slighter higher than for incomplete or transitional AVSD repairs. However, surgical mortality has dramatically improved over time with advances in the understanding and management of these patients. Early series reported short-term mortality for complete AVSDs as high as 10% to 20%.[57,58] More contemporary series report this mortality as less than or equal to 3%.[56-63] The Society of Thoracic Surgeons Congenital Heart Surgery Database reported an aggregate mortality rate of 3.2% for 3116 AVSD operations performed across centers from 2011 to 2014.[64] Excellent results and similar survival have been achieved with each of the various types of surgical repairs.[a]

A number of risk factors for death are suggested in the literature. They are not consistent and do not all achieve statistical significance; however, they have been demonstrated to contribute by many authors. These include operations performed in an earlier era, previous palliative procedures, age less than 3 months or late presentation with evidence of pulmonary vascular obstructive disease, weight less than 3.5 kg, chromosomally normal patients, heterotaxy syndrome, uAVSDs, complex AVSDs, significant preoperative LAVVR, need for LAVV replacement, and need for future reoperation.[58,60,62] Down syndrome was historically associated with worse outcomes. This may have been related to delayed repair and the presence of pulmonary hypertension. It has been shown that irreversible pulmonary hypertension can develop in these patients by 6 months of age.[67] However, recent studies have shown a trend toward increased survival in patients with Down syndrome, except in cases of uAVSDs that undergo single-ventricle palliation.[9]

Despite these improvements the morbidity has not significantly changed. The incidence of CHB has decreased with better understanding of the surgical anatomy,[3] reported as 0% to 4% in most recent series.[57-63] However, the incidence of both LAVVR and LVOTO has remained unchanged, providing the greatest source of morbidity and most common indications for reoperation.

Risk of reoperation for LAVVR is approximately 10%.[30] The median time to reoperation is usually within the first few years.[58,62,68] Risk factors for reoperation include younger age, given fragility of tissues, or older age secondary to chronic leaflet and annular changes; chromosomally normal patients; complex AVSDs; LAVV abnormalities such as PLAVV, DOLAVV, or dysplastic leaflets; deficient lateral leaflet; significant preoperative LAVVR; incomplete or partial AVSDs; and partially closed or left open cleft at original operation.[57,58,62,68-72] Based on author experience, patients with Down syndrome tend to have more favorable AVVs versus chromosomally normal patients related to more consistent anatomy

and better size and leaflet tissue quality. They have also been found to have larger LAVV and aortic valve areas by echocardiogram.[73]

Risk of reoperation for LVOTO is approximately 5% to 10%.[30,62] The median time to presentation and reoperation is delayed at approximately 5 years.[36,58,62] Of those, approximately 35% to 45% will require another reoperation.[53] This predisposition is due to a multitude of factors. These include an elongated outflow tract, septal hypertrophy, the anterolateral muscle bundle of the LV, papillary muscle displacement, abnormal chordal attachments between the common AVV and the muscular or conal septum, redundant AVV tissue, displacement of the AVV leaflet tips into the LV, and intrinsic LVOT hypoplasia.[14,55,74-76] The literature has also suggested an increased risk associated with Down syndrome, incomplete or transitional AVSD,[77] and Rastelli type A complete AVSD.[53] Last, there has been concern that the modified single-patch technique creates anatomy similar to incomplete AVSDs that provides the substrate for LVOTO. Single-center experiences have not demonstrated an increased risk[29,59,63]; however, the delayed presentation may become more evident as longer-term follow-up becomes available for this technique.

In summary, the surgical treatment and perioperative management of patients with AVSDs has led to excellent survival for this complex congenital heart defect. However, continued efforts to improve the associated morbidity are necessary in the future.

Selected References

A complete list of references is available at ExpertConsult.com.

5. Jacobs JP, Burke RP, Quintessenza JA, et al. Congenital Heart Surgery Nomenclature and Database Project: atrioventricular canal defect. *Ann Thorac Surg.* 2000;69(4 suppl):S36–S43.
7. Rastelli G, Kirklin JW, Titus JL. Anatomic observations on complete form of persistent common atrioventricular canal with special reference to atrioventricular valves. *Mayo Clin Proc.* 1966;41(5):296–308.
14. Cohen MS, Spray TL. Surgical management of unbalanced atrioventricular canal defect. *Semin Thorac Cardiovasc Surg Pediatr Card Surg Annu.* 2005;135–144.
26. Maloney JV Jr, Marable SA, Mulder DG. The surgical treatment of common atrioventricular canal. *J Thorac Cardiovasc Surg.* 1962;43:84–96.
27. Trusler GA. Discussion of Mills NL, Ochsner IL, King TD. Correction of type C complete atrioventricular canal. Surgical considerations. *J Thorac Cardiovasc Surg.* 1976;71(1):20–28.
29. Nicholson IA, Nunn GR, Sholler GF, et al. Simplified single patch technique for the repair of atrioventricular septal defect. *J Thorac Cardiovasc Surg.* 1999;118(4):642–646.
38. Najm HK, Van Arsdell GS, Watzka S, et al. Primary repair is superior to initial palliation in children with atrioventricular septal defect and tetralogy of Fallot. *J Thorac Cardiovasc Surg.* 1998;116(6):905–913.
53. Van Arsdell GS, Williams WG, Boutin C, et al. Subaortic stenosis in the spectrum of atrioventricular septal defects. Solutions may be complex and palliative. *J Thorac Cardiovasc Surg.* 1995;110(5):1534–1541, discussion 1541–1532.
62. Suzuki T, Bove EL, Devaney EJ, et al. Results of definitive repair of complete atrioventricular septal defect in neonates and infants. *Ann Thorac Surg.* 2008;86(2):596–602.
63. Nunn GR. Atrioventricular canal: modified single patch technique. *Semin Thorac Cardiovasc Surg Pediatr Card Surg Annu.* 2007;28–31.

---

[a]References 29, 57, 59, 62, 65, 66.

51

Left Ventricular Outflow Tract Obstruction

BAHAALDIN ALSOUFI, MD; ALAA ALJIFFRY, MBBS; ROSS M. UNGERLEIDER, MD, MBA

Left ventricular outflow tract obstruction (LVOTO) is a complex congenital cardiac defect that interferes with the ejection of blood from the left ventricle into the ascending aorta.[1-4] LVOTO is a heterogeneous defect in which the timing and mode of clinical presentation vary based on multiple factors, including the degree and levels of obstruction, associated hypoplasia of the left ventricle and mitral valve, and the presence of concomitant cardiac and extracardiac anomalies such as aortic arch obstruction, patent ductus arteriosus, and atrial or ventricular septal defect.[1-4] Subsequently, the timing and type of intervention differ based on those factors, with the initial procedure ranging from an extreme of neonatal single-ventricle palliation to isolated adolescent aortic valve intervention.

The classification of LVOTO is typically based on the level of obstruction and includes valvar, subvalvar, and supravalvar stenosis. Valvar stenosis is the most common type and constitutes approximately 65% to 75% of cases, whereas subvalvar and supravalvar stenosis constitute approximately 15% to 20% and 5% to 10% of cases, respectively.[1-4]

Valvar Aortic Stenosis

Valvar aortic stenosis is the most common form of LVOTO, occurring in 65% to 75% of patients. Bicuspid aortic valve occurs in 1% to 2% of the population and represents 3% to 5% of all congenital heart anomalies, with the incidence in males being three to five times higher than that in females.[5,6] Valvar aortic stenosis is an anatomic and clinical spectrum that ranges from one extreme of critical neonatal aortic stenosis that is associated with ductal-dependent systemic circulation (almost 10% of those patients) to another extreme of mild aortic stenosis in asymptomatic children with the only finding being an incidental murmur on physical examination.[1,3,4]

Critical Neonatal Aortic Stenosis

The aortic valve pathology is most commonly bicuspid associated with thickened dysmorphic cusps and fused commissures. Less commonly, the valve is tricuspid with thickened cusps and fused commissures. When the valve is unicuspid, there might be a single commissure or no commissure, and the small orifice might be central or eccentric.[7]

During fetal development, severe LVOTO exposes the left ventricle to increased afterload that results in ventricular hypertrophy with subsequent systolic and diastolic myocardial dysfunction. Ventricular hypertrophy and higher intracavitary pressure lead to decreased coronary perfusion pressure and chronic in utero subendocardial ischemia with consequent development of endocardial fibroelastosis that further impairs ventricular function. Additionally, reduced in utero antegrade blood flow through the aortic valve leads to underdevelopment of the left heart structures and hypoplasia of the mitral valve, left ventricle, subvalvar area, ascending aorta, and aortic arch.[1,8,9] Clinical presentation varies based on the severity of LVOTO and the degree of associated ventricular hypoplasia and dysfunction. Neonates with critical aortic stenosis often have a rapidly developing and dramatic presentation after birth. As the ductus arteriosus closes, they experience decreased systemic and coronary perfusion, acute hemodynamic deterioration with cardiovascular collapse, metabolic acidosis, end-organ injury, and shock.[1,8,9] Neonates and infants with lesser degrees of obstruction may gradually develop symptoms secondary to persistent high left ventricular afterload, left atrial hypertension, myocardial dysfunction, and poor systemic cardiac output. Symptoms such as failure to thrive, irritability, and tachypnea and increased work of breathing might necessitate early intervention during the first few months of life.[9]

Diagnostic studies include electrocardiography (ECG), which might demonstrate evidence of left ventricular or biventricular hypertrophy, with common evidence of strain. The chest x-ray examination might show cardiomegaly and evidence of pulmonary congestion in neonates with critical aortic stenosis, but findings might be normal in those with less severe stenosis. Echocardiography is the primary form of diagnosis, and it delineates the level of obstruction, gradient across the LVOT, presence of endocardial fibroelastosis, hypoplasia of left heart structures, mitral valve anomalies, ascending aorta or aortic arch, and associated cardiac anomalies such as atrial and ventricular septal defects and patent ductus arteriosus. The direction of flow across the transverse arch and ductus might help to determine whether or not the left heart is capable of supporting the systemic circulation after biventricular repair. Of note, the LVOT gradient may be underestimated in those neonates due to severe left ventricular dysfunction, frequent presence of mitral regurgitation, and existence of patent ductus arteriosus or distal arch obstruction. Cardiac catheterization for diagnosis is usually not required but can be helpful to measure LVOT gradient directly (in older patients with less severe LVOTO) and to evaluate associated anomalies that may not be apparent on echocardiography. The role of cardiac catheterization in neonatal aortic stenosis is mainly for intervention rather than diagnosis. It

615

is important to mention the role of fetal echocardiography in the prenatal diagnosis of neonates with critical aortic stenosis. Prenatal identification of LVOTO and associated intracardiac and extracardiac anomalies can result in better planning of the care following delivery (both for the medical team and for the family) and avoidance of circulatory collapse in patients with unrecognized pathology as a result of ductal closure and can offer the possibility of fetal intervention with aortic valvuloplasty, which, in selected cases, can be associated with better growth of left heart structures and higher likelihood of achieving biventricular repair.[10]

In neonates with ductal-dependent systemic circulation, urgent neonatal intervention is indicated. In those with less severe stenosis, surgery is indicated when the infants develop symptoms such as failure to thrive, respiratory distress, and irritability, in conjunction with peak Doppler-derived LVOT gradient that is greater than 40 mm Hg or a peak-to-peak catheter-derived LVOT gradient that is greater than 30 mm Hg.[9]

The medical management of neonates with postnatal diagnosis of ductal-dependent critical aortic stenosis involves rapid restoration of ductal patency with the use of prostaglandin E_1 infusion. This will restore systemic perfusion by shunting blood right to left across the ductus and can help reduce pulmonary hypertension seen with severe left ventricular dysfunction (Fig. 51.1). Intubation and mechanical ventilation may also be required to aid in correction of severe acidosis and control of pulmonary hypertension. The use of inotropic drugs improves the poor ventricular contractility. Judicious administration of intravenous fluids and correction of metabolic and electrolyte anomalies are important in the resuscitation of these critically ill patients.[1,9] In neonates with very severe LVOTO or in those with severely depressed left ventricular function or inadequate left ventricle or mitral valve sizes, balloon atrial septostomy might be needed to allow unobstructed pulmonary venous egress to the right side of the heart, which is supporting

the systemic circulation. In the absence of atrial communication, severe pulmonary hypertension and respiratory compromise might be very rapid, necessitating extracorporeal membrane oxygenation (ECMO) support for stabilization before any intervention. On the other hand, when the degree of aortic valve stenosis seems to be less severe, and the left heart structures seem to be well developed, especially in those who seem to have adequate cardiac output generated from the left ventricle with mainly left-to-right shunt across the ductus arteriosus, a trial of discontinuation of prostaglandin can be undertaken, and intervention can be deferred if the child is growing and having no symptoms of poor cardiac output or respiratory compromise.

The most important aspect in the management of infants with critical aortic stenosis is to determine whether the left heart structures are capable of supporting the systemic circulation.[1,11-15] Although the decision is obvious in patients with well-developed left heart structures (who should be amenable to a two-ventricle repair pathway) or in patients with severe hypoplasia of the left ventricle or mitral valve (who will require staging toward single-ventricle palliation), the middle of the spectrum is more complex in terms of clinical decision making. The most difficult decisions revolve around patients who have borderline development of the left ventricle and the mitral valve.[1,11-15] In those patients, single-ventricle palliative options, although possible, would forfeit the opportunity for appropriate candidates to undergo biventricular repair. Conversely, aggressive attempts to attain biventricular status could come at the relative cost of greater risk of death and higher subsequent morbidity and reoperation.[1,11-15] The importance of proper treatment selection is reflected by the higher mortality reported in older series due to failure to address the heterogeneity of this disease and to tailor the treatment to specific patient anatomy. The significance of appropriate initial triage cannot be overestimated because multiple reports have shown universally poor results in patients requiring a crossover between strategies.

Several studies have attempted to identify preoperative predictors of suitability for single-ventricle versus biventricular repair in neonates with critical aortic stenosis.[1,11-15] Rhodes identified several clinical risk factors for successful biventricular repair, including mitral valve area less than 4.75 cm^2/m^2, long-axis dimension of the left ventricle relative to the long-axis dimension of the heart less than 0.8, diameter of the aortic root less than 3.5 cm/m^2, and left ventricular mass less than 35 g/m^2. The presence of more than one of those risk factors predicted high mortality following biventricular repair.[11] Subsequently he proposed a score that is derived from a multivariable regression equation with a discriminating score less than −0.35 predictive of death after a biventricular repair. However, the Rhodes score was based on retrospective data from a small group of 65 patients with critical aortic stenosis who were preselected for biventricular repair, and subsequent investigation from multiple different studies has shown poor discrimination with the Rhodes score when applied to neonates with multiple levels of left-sided obstruction or whose primary pathology is other than critical aortic stenosis.[1,11]

The Congenital Heart Surgeons' Society (CHSS) reported a multi-institutional study of 320 neonates with critical aortic stenosis enrolled between 1994 and 2000.[12] Biventricular repair was performed in 116 patients, whereas an initial Norwood procedure was performed in 179 patients. Five-year survival was 70% for neonates who underwent biventricular repair and 60% for those who underwent a Norwood procedure. Complex statistical techniques were then used to model the magnitude and direction of the survival benefit for the Norwood procedure over biventricular

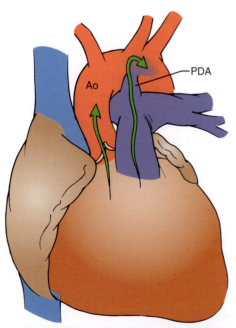

• **Figure 51.1** In neonates with severe left ventricular outflow tract obstruction, cardiac output across the aortic valve may be limited. In these patients, prostaglandin infusion can augment distal systemic perfusion across a patent ductus arteriosus. This dependency of the patent ductus arteriosus for systemic perfusion is usually observed as a right-to-left shunt across the ductus arteriosus.

repair pathway. Independent factors associated with greater survival benefit with the Norwood pathway included younger age at entry, higher grade of endocardial fibroelastosis, lower z score of the aortic valve at the level of the sinuses of Valsalva, larger ascending aortic diameter, absence of moderate or severe tricuspid regurgitation, and lower z score of the left ventricular length.[12] Subsequently a regression equation was formulated to predict patient's survival benefit, with a positive number representing improved survival with a Norwood procedure, a negative number representing improved survival with a biventricular repair strategy, and the magnitude of the number representing the degree of predicted survival benefit. Importantly, the CHSS demonstrated that commonly used selection criteria resulted in inappropriate patient triage in a significant number of neonates. Predicted survival benefit favored the Norwood procedure in 50% of patients who had biventricular repair, and it favored biventricular repair in 20% of patients who had the Norwood procedure. Choosing the correct management strategy could have resulted in a substantial survival advantage for patients in the cohort in whom the incorrect management option was chosen.[12] Further analysis of the CHSS data showed that inappropriate pursuit of biventricular repair in borderline candidates was more frequent and more consequential in survival terms than inappropriate pursuit of a single-ventricle palliation strategy.[13] The final updated form of the CHSS equation is available through the CHSS website (http://www.chssdc.org/content/chss-score-neonatal-critical-aortic-stenosis).

The single-ventricle palliation strategy using the Norwood operation or the hybrid approach is discussed in Chapter 66.[14] Heart transplantation can be an alternative strategy, although that is reserved usually for patients who fail initial single-ventricle or biventricular repair strategies.[15,16]

The focus for the remainder of this chapter will be on biventricular repair options.

Percutaneous balloon valvuloplasty is considered the initial procedure of choice at most centers.[17-20] However, it is relatively contraindicated in the rare patients with preexistent moderate and severe aortic valve regurgitation. Vascular access is usually obtained with an antegrade (venous) transseptal approach using the umbilical or femoral veins; however, a retrograde approach using the carotid, femoral, or umbilical artery is also common (Fig. 51.2). Advantages of percutaneous valvuloplasty include avoidance of surgical morbidity associated with cardiopulmonary bypass. Disadvantages include vascular access complications, inability to precisely determine where the leaflets will tear with resultant potential for aortic valve insufficiency, and rarely, mitral valve injury.[17-20] It is important not to overdilate the aortic valve because the goal of intervention in these critically ill patients is improvement, and not complete elimination, of LVOT gradient until the patient is older and bigger, at which point a more precise intervention can be planned. The initial balloon size is usually chosen at 80% to 90% of the diameter of the aortic valve annulus because there is evidence that the incidence of new-onset or worsening aortic regurgitation increases as the balloon to annulus ratio increases. During the procedure the balloon is positioned across the valve with half or more of its length below the annulus. During balloon inflation, observation of the "tight waist" is important. In older patients, ventricular pacing during balloon inflation might be required to avoid balloon malposition. After the first balloon inflation the LVOT gradient is remeasured and angiogram is repeated to assess the degree of aortic regurgitation. It is acceptable to reinflate the balloon or use the next balloon size up for inadequate relief of an LVOT gradient as long as significant iatrogenic aortic regurgitation is nonexistent. Nonetheless, it is

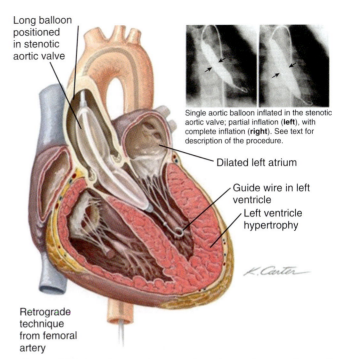

Single aortic balloon inflated in the stenotic aortic valve; partial inflation (**left**), with complete inflation (**right**). See text for description of the procedure.

Long balloon positioned in stenotic aortic valve

Dilated left atrium

Guide wire in left ventricle

Left ventricle hypertrophy

Retrograde technique from femoral artery

K. Carter

• **Figure 51.2** A balloon catheter can be advanced across the aortic valve via the femoral artery (or in infants from a femoral venous approach, across the patent foramen ovale, through the left atrium, and antegrade out the aortic valve). Under both echocardiographic and angiographic guidance, the properly sized balloon can be inflated to dilate a stenotic aortic valve. It is important not to oversize the balloon to limit the risk of aortic insufficiency from tearing the leaflets off their annular attachments. (Copyright Elsevier, Inc. - NETTERIMAGES.COM.)

still important not to exceed the annular diameter with the larger balloon. At the end of the intervention an exit angiogram and another set of hemodynamic measurements, including cardiac output, should be obtained. Following the percutaneous intervention and removal of the arterial and venous sheaths, hemostasis is obtained while carefully monitoring limb perfusion and distal pulses. Acute occlusive arterial injury is a well-known complication following cardiac catheterization in neonates and small infants, and the reported incidence is 0.6% to 9.6%. The risk of vascular injury increases in smaller children, with the need to perform an intervention via the artery, exchanging arterial catheters and the use of larger catheters, a longer procedural time, and a final activated clotting time of less than 250 seconds. Following percutaneous intervention, patients are transferred back to the intensive care unit. Their convalescence following the intervention varies based on several factors, including preprocedure cardiac function, preexistence of other organ dysfunction, and the degree of residual LVOTO or iatrogenic aortic regurgitation. Although the optimal intervention goal is to achieve adequate relief of LVOTO with minimal iatrogenic aortic regurgitation, this objective is not always attained. In patients with significant residual lesions (LVOTO or aortic regurgitation), cardiac output and systemic perfusion are severely affected, requiring significant inotropic support, mechanical ventilation, and careful fluid management as described later for postoperative care following surgical intervention.[18]

Before the evolution of percutaneous balloon valvuloplasty as the standard first intervention of choice, surgical valvotomy was the mainstay of treatment of critical aortic stenosis in neonates and infants.[1,3,21-33] Different approaches such as transventricular closed aortic valvotomy and open valvotomy with inflow occlusion or with cardiopulmonary bypass were developed. The current surgical technique, when surgery is considered the best option, uses cardiopulmonary bypass and cardioplegic arrest of the heart. In neonates and infants the goal is to perform a valvotomy that will decrease LVOTO and prevent significant aortic insufficiency. An aortotomy that is directed toward the noncoronary aortic sinus is performed to allow adequate exposure of the valve. Aortic valvotomy is then completed by dividing the fused commissures to within 1 to 2 mm of the aortic wall only. In neonates, given that small increases in valve opening are associated with significant reduction in LVOT gradient, conservative valvotomy is recommended to avoid the risk of aortic regurgitation (Fig. 51.3).

The goal of intervention for neonates and infants with critical aortic stenosis is to improve LVOTO by opening the aortic valve

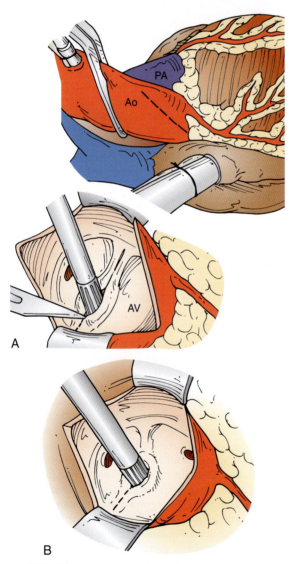

• **Figure 51.3** Transaortic surgical valvotomy provides direct visualization of the aortic valve pathology and can allow more precise opening of a congenitally stenotic aortic valve. Most valves are bicuspid (A) and can be opened across the entire fused portion, although when the valve is unicuspid (B), a more limited commissurotomy must be performed. (From Stark J, de Leval M. *Surgery for Congenital Heart Defects.* 2nd ed. Philadelphia: WB Saunders; 1994.)

as much as possible, without tearing it or creating significant aortic insufficiency. In most patients, aortic valvotomy, whether it is performed percutaneously or surgically under direct vision, will restore enough outflow from the left ventricle to support systemic circulation. However, it is important to emphasize that the condition of these infants can be extremely critical, and it may take some time (several days) for the left ventricle to begin functioning more normally. Many of these patients present for intervention with significant left ventricular dysfunction caused by a combination of intrauterine flow abnormalities as well as from critical LVOTO. Simply opening the aortic valve does not always result in immediate return of normal cardiac output. The left ventricle may still be "stiff" (noncompliant), and, in neonates with significant left ventricular dysfunction and associated pulmonary hypertension, it may sometimes be helpful to maintain ductal patency with prostaglandin infusion for a few days following percutaneous or surgical valvotomy to help support the systemic circulation and decompress pulmonary artery hypertension until the left ventricular compliance and systolic function improve (see Fig. 51.1). If the patient is an appropriate candidate for biventricular pathway, left ventricular recovery should occur within a few days following intervention.

Intensive care unit management centers around ensuring that the infant has adequate systemic perfusion. An echocardiogram following valvotomy can indicate the quality of left ventricular function and ensure that there appears to be adequate flow across the LVOT. When left ventricular dysfunction is severe, the infant may be tachycardic (with heart rates approaching 180 beats/min). Because cardiac output = stroke volume × heart rate, when stroke volume is limited by poor left ventricular function, heart rate will generally increase to maintain output. Therefore, in the absence of a primary arrhythmia such as junctional ectopic tachycardia, tachycardia following aortic valvotomy is a sign of compromised left ventricular function. These babies should remain ventilated because adding the work (and increased oxygen demand) of breathing to an already compromised cardiac output might be enough to result in hemodynamic collapse. Perfusion should be monitored by physical signs (such as pulses and skin temperature, near-infrared spectroscopy), as well as by chemical signs (such as lactate level, signs of acidosis on blood gas and mixed venous saturation if available). Babies with decreased perfusion may need to have escalated management with afterload reduction and/or inotropes. As the parameters of perfusion stabilize, the infant can be carefully followed with the expectation that the patient will recover. In extremely compromised patients, ECMO support might be needed to provide adequate systemic perfusion to the kidneys and other vital organs while waiting for the left ventricle function to recover.

When neonates fail to improve, it is important to reevaluate the adequacy of the aortic valve and aortic annulus. If the left ventricle is adequate and there is no significant inflow obstruction (congenital mitral valve abnormality), the neonate may be a candidate for neonatal aortic valve replacement. Although a primary Ross procedure with annular enlargement (Ross-Konno) may be a lifesaving initial operation in selected patients with severe multilevel LVOTO, more commonly it is used later in patients who continue to have persistent poor systemic perfusion and pulmonary hypertension associated with persistent LVOTO or significant aortic regurgitation following percutaneous or surgical intervention.[34-39] The details of this operation will be described later in this chapter. Persistent postoperative poor systemic perfusion and pulmonary hypertension due to inadequate left ventricle or mitral valve size to support the systemic circulation suggests that a single-ventricle palliation strategy was likely the correct choice for that patient, and usually a crossover to that strategy is associated with high mortality.[1,11-13] The alternative option of listing for heart transplantation is restricted by the long time needed until a donor heart is available and the high risk of waiting list mortality.[15,16]

The choice between percutaneous valvuloplasty and surgical valvotomy is largely institution dependent. Few studies have compared outcomes between the two approaches, although it is worthwhile to note that outcomes with both surgical and percutaneous approaches have improved recently due to technical advances, improved perioperative care, and most importantly improved patient selection and more proper patient triage to undergo single-ventricle palliation versus biventricular repair strategy.[28,32,40] There are no prospectively randomized studies comparing outcomes between the two approaches. Numerous reports cited the early and late outcomes of either one approach or the other, but few compared surgical versus percutaneous approaches, and those that did are limited by the lack of adjustments between the two groups. In a retrospective multi-institutional study by the CHSS, 110 patients underwent either surgical aortic valvotomy ($n = 28$) or percutaneous balloon valvuloplasty ($n = 82$).[40] The study demonstrated that, while controlling for preprocedure morphology, percutaneous balloon valvuloplasty was more effective in relieving stenosis than surgical aortic valvotomy as evidenced by greater mean percentage reduction in systolic gradient (65% versus 41%) and lower residual median gradients (20 mm Hg versus 36 mm Hg). However, percutaneous balloon valvuloplasty was also associated with greater likelihood of important aortic regurgitation (18% versus 3%). Freedom from reintervention was similar for the two groups (91% at 1 month and 48% at 5 years). Significant factors for reintervention included preprocedural use of inotropic agents, the presence of postprocedural moderate to severe aortic regurgitation, and a lower weight at initial intervention. Risk-adjusted freedom from death was also similar between the two groups and was 82% at 1 month and 74% at 1 year. Risk factors for death included preprocedural mechanical ventilation and anatomic factors such as smaller aortic valve diameter at the level of the annulus, sinotubular junction, or subaortic region, indicating that many of those patients might have been inappropriately triaged into the biventricular tract and that they might have been better served by a single-ventricle palliation approach.[40] Both surgical and percutaneous outcomes have improved with better selection, and some centers have reported operative mortality of 5% to 10% and freedom from reintervention of 85% at 5 years from surgical aortic valvotomy in neonates and infants. At the end, careful evaluation of patients' characteristics along with understanding institutional expertise should help determine the first-line procedure.

Valvar Aortic Stenosis in Older Children

Children with LVOTO that is not critical enough to require care during infancy represent the other end of the spectrum of valvar aortic stenosis. In older patients there is typically adequate development of left heart structures, and their pathology is mainly confined to the aortic valve itself. Aortic valve anatomy in this group of patients is most commonly bicuspid (>70% of patients). In the remaining patients the valve is tricuspid, although a unicuspid valve can be occasionally seen in these older patients.

The pathophysiology of valvar aortic stenosis is related to increased afterload on the left ventricular myocardium with subsequent left ventricle hypertrophy. Ultimately, symptoms may occur related to the associated decreased left ventricular compliance and increased left ventricular end-diastolic pressure. Left ventricular hypertrophy can lead to consequent subendocardial ischemia and predisposition to sudden death from ventricular arrhythmias.[9]

Most children are asymptomatic in the early years of life and have normal growth. The stenosis is often identified during routine physical examination due to the presence of a murmur. Symptoms of congestive heart failure (such as shortness of breath and decreased exercise tolerance), angina, and syncope or even sudden death are indications that the LVOTO is becoming severe. Occasionally, spontaneous endocarditis is the presenting manifestation of valvar aortic stenosis.[9]

The diagnosis is mainly with echocardiography. The correlation between the Doppler-derived and cardiac catheterization gradients is usually reliable in older patients; cardiac catheterization is more often used for those patients in whom balloon valvuloplasty is being considered. Occasionally, diagnostic cardiac catheterization is performed to validate a significant LVOT gradient when echocardiogram data are confusing, to evaluate coronary anatomy and to measure end-diastolic pressures. The role of magnetic resonance imaging for the diagnosis of those patients is increasing as a noninvasive modality that provides valuable information about the size of the aortic annulus, ascending aorta, and aortic arch. It can also delineate coronary origins and allow measurement of systolic function, left ventricular mass, and LVOT gradients. Finally, myocardial perfusion can be assessed during rest and stress induced by adenosine and dobutamine for better understanding of hemodynamic effects of LVOTO. In younger patients, magnetic resonance imaging might require sedation and at times general anesthesia, but in older children that is not required.

Indications for intervention in these older patients include (1) the presence of symptoms such as angina, syncope, or congestive heart failure, ischemic or repolarization changes on rest or exercise ECG, associated with resting peak systolic LVOT gradient of greater than 40 mm Hg; (2) the presence of depressed left ventricular function (even with LVOT gradient <40 mm Hg); or (3) resting peak systolic LVOT gradient of greater than 50 mm Hg. Asymptomatic patients with LVOT gradient of less than 40 mm Hg are generally followed at regular intervals (every 6 to 12 months) by outpatient cardiology.[9]

Both percutaneous balloon valvuloplasty and surgical aortic valvotomy are viable options in this age-group and can be done successfully as initial management strategies. In older patients with significant valvar LVOTO, most centers continue to prefer percutaneous balloon valvuloplasty. However, surgical valvotomy can often be performed with more precision in older patients, with incision in the areas of commissural fusion carefully extended to, but not into, the aortic valve annulus. The risk of aortic insufficiency is less with surgical valvotomy than with balloon valvuloplasty, and surgical options for aortic valve repair are possible. In addition, thinning of the aortic cusps and excision of thickened nodules may increase the mobility of the valve and decrease residual LVOT gradient. Although it is usually recommended not to incise the false raphe, a few groups have reported an improved experience with creation of a tricuspid valve from a bicuspid valve or a bicuspid valve from a unicuspid valve by incising the raphe and resuspending the incised cusps with neocommissures created from triangular patches of glutaraldehyde-treated autologous pericardium.[29,31] The experience of aortic valve repair is small, and the lowest age limit to allow these techniques is not very clear. Nevertheless, aortic valve repair may become a more common option in the years ahead.

All forms of LVOTO create pressure loading to the left ventricle that can result in varying degrees of left ventricular hypertrophy. In more severe instances this can lead to an increase in left ventricular end-diastolic pressures and a less compliant ventricle. In the preoperative period these patients may be extremely volume sensitive and in fact preload dependent, although they remain at risk of developing pulmonary edema as well. Therefore they require very judicious and careful management of their preload status to preserve their cardiac output. Excessive inotropic therapy may increase cardiac oxygen demand and tachycardia, which may lead to decreased ventricular volume, increased LVOTO, and ventricular ischemia.

Although these patients often have preserved systolic function after relief of their LVOT obstruction, they may have some degree of diastolic dysfunction that can manifest as pulmonary edema or tachycardia (related to low stroke volumes and rate-dependent cardiac output). Because of the challenged cardiac output, particularly in neonates and infants, maintenance of adequate hemoglobin (to increase oxygen delivery capability) is reasonable. Postoperative maintenance of cardiac output can be monitored by measurement of oxygen delivery (mixed venous oxygen saturation, arteriovenous oxygen difference, lactate levels) and intubation to decrease systemic oxygen demand. It is prudent to mechanically support ventilation until oxygen delivery is normal (normal indices of perfusion), with normal heart rate trend without tachycardia and recovering left ventricular function on echocardiogram.

Naturally the postoperative convalescence in older patients is typically less complicated and the risk of death is very low, approaching 1%. Following percutaneous balloon valvuloplasty or surgical aortic valvotomy, almost 35% of patients will require reintervention on the aortic valve within 10 years.

When aortic valvuloplasty or repair fails or is not successful, aortic valve replacement may become necessary. The goal of aortic valvuloplasty or repair is to delay the need for aortic valve replacement, and it is likely that many patients with aortic valve interventions will ultimately require a valve replacement. There are numerous options for aortic valve prostheses, and none of them are "perfect." An optimal choice for an aortic valve prosthesis would include (1) ready availability in different sizes, (2) durability, (3) excellent (normal) hemodynamic profiles, (4) minimal thromboembolic risk (without the need for lifelong anticoagulation), (5) growth potential, (6) low incidence of structural valve degeneration, and (7) minimal risk for needing reoperation. No such choice is currently available, and all alternatives are associated with important drawbacks.

Mechanical prostheses come in different styles, although the bileaflet design has become the most widely used. Size is limited by the properties of the material, and, although these valves can be made in small sizes (15 to 17 mm) that can be placed in young patients, they are often not suitable for infants and very small children. The hemodynamic profiles vary with size, and smaller prostheses have inferior flow properties.

Annular enlargement techniques could be used to allow placement of larger prostheses in small patients. To enlarge the aortic annulus, it is critical to appreciate the important anatomic constraints imposed by the conduction system, mitral valve, and coronary arteries (Fig. 51.4). Before the more widespread application of the pulmonary autograft procedure in infants and children, annular enlarging procedures that allowed placement of larger prosthetic valves were more common (Fig. 51.5). Those techniques include the Nicks, Manougian, and Konno procedures. In the Nicks procedure the aortic incision is extended to the area between

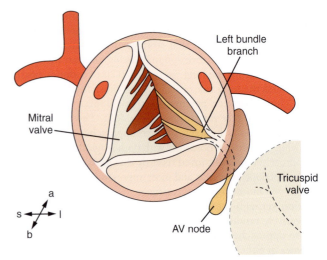

• **Figure 51.4** The anatomic features of the aortic root demonstrate the location of the conduction system below the commissure between the right and noncoronary sinus, the attachment of the mitral valve to the area under the left and noncoronary sinus, as well as the typical location of the right and left coronary artery ostia. These anatomic structures determine some of the limitations for surgical incisions. (From Pigula FA. Surgery for congenital anomalies of the aortic valve and root. In: Sellke FW, del Nido PJ, Swanson SJ. *Sabiston and Spencer Surgery of the Chest.* Philadelphia: Saunders; 2005.)

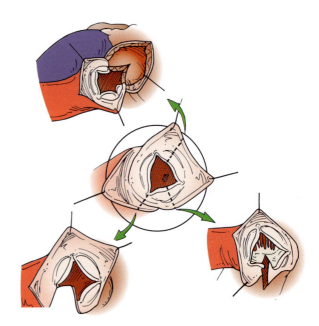

• **Figure 51.5** The locations around the aortic annulus where it is safe to make an incision for annular enlargement. An incision in the commissure between the left and noncoronary cusps *(lower left)* will extend onto the anterior leaflet of the mitral valve. This Manougian annular enlargement can be repaired with a patch and enlarges the annulus by 2 to 3 mm. Likewise, the Nicks enlargement *(lower right)* extends into the roof of the left atrium and, once repaired with a patch, enlarges the annulus by 2 to 3 mm. The Konno-Rastan aortoventriculoplasty *(upper left)* is created with an incision across the interventricular septum, between the right and left coronary arteries, and can create annular enlargement of 1 cm when necessary.

the left noncoronary commissure and the base of the noncoronary cusp into the area of intervalvular fibrosa without cutting into the anterior mitral valve leaflet.[41] In the Manougian procedure the incision is the same as in the Nicks procedure, but the cut is extended across the intervalvular fibrosa into the center of the anterior mitral leaflet.[42] In the Konno procedure the aortic annulus is incised between the right and left coronary cusps extending into the ventricular septum with patch reconstruction of the septum and ascending aorta.[43]

Operative mortality of aortic valve replacement with a mechanical prosthesis in children is 2% to 13%, and survival ranges between 75% and 88% at 15 years.[44-51] Importantly, lifelong anticoagulation is required, which is challenging due to poor compliance and activity restrictions, in addition to complicated pregnancy in females.[44] Reported freedom from bleeding is 96% to 100% at 10 years, and reported freedom from thromboembolism is 90% to 100%, better than in adults.[44-51] The different hemodynamic properties in children with faster heart rate and less incidence of arrhythmias, atrial dilation, or myocardial dysfunction might all contribute to the relatively lower thromboembolism risk. Despite the lack of structural valve degeneration, reoperations are not uncommon, and freedom from reoperation is 55% to 90% at 15 years, usually related to pannus formation (fibrous ingrowth across the valve mechanism) or development of patient-prosthesis mismatch as the child grows in the presence of fixed prosthesis sizes, in addition to occasional reoperations for valve thrombosis, perivalvular leak, or endocarditis.[44-51]

Tissue prostheses most typically are manufactured using bovine or porcine valves mounted on rigid struts. They are unavailable in sizes below 19 mm, and therefore they are not suitable for small children, even using annular enlargement techniques. The hemodynamic profiles vary with size, and smaller prostheses have inferior flow properties, particularly due to the large size of the sewing ring compared to the actual orifice size of the valve opening. Stentless bioprosthetic valves are glutaraldehyde-prepared porcine aortic roots. Although they have the hemodynamic advantage of not needing rigid stents for mounting the valve tissue, and thus have hemodynamic superiority at any comparable size, they are still subject to structural degeneration, calcification, and need for early reoperation, particularly in younger patients. All bioprosthetic valves have low thromboembolic risk and thus do not require anticoagulation. Nonetheless, their use in children is associated with decreased valve longevity due to lack of growth potential and, most importantly, from structural valve degeneration that is faster than that seen in adults and is inversely related to patient age and prosthesis size. For the most part, bioprosthetic valves are not a good choice for aortic valve replacement in young patients. In children and young adults, reported survival is almost 85% at 10 years, whereas reported freedom from reoperation is only 15% to 30% at 10 years.[52]

Homografts (or allografts) are cadaver human valves. Both aortic and pulmonary homografts are available for human implantation. Homografts are harvested from human donors and cryopreserved for implantation. Hospitals using homografts will usually have specially made liquid nitrogen storage containers in the operating room for maintaining a homograft stock, and selected homografts can be thawed in the operating room at the time of implantation. Aortic homografts are most commonly used for aortic valve replacement. Early techniques used a "freestyle" form of placing the homograft valve into the aortic annulus, but more commonly the homograft is now used as a complete aortic root replacement with reimplantation of the coronary arteries (Fig. 51.6). Aortic homografts provide

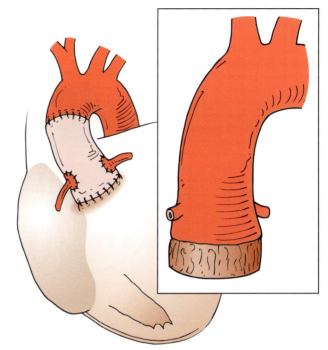

• **Figure 51.6** Aortic homografts are harvested as aortic roots containing an aortic valve. They are cryopreserved and maintained in the operating room in a specially designed freezer until chosen for implantation. Currently most surgeons prefer sewing in the valve as a root replacement with reattachment of the coronary arteries, as demonstrated in this illustration. (Reprinted from Stelzer P, Adams DH. Surgical approach to aortic valve disease. In: Otto CM, Bonow RO, eds. *Valvular Heart Disease: A Companion to Braunwald's Heart Disease.* 3rd ed. Philadelphia: Elsevier Science; 2009:187–208.)

excellent hemodynamic profiles that are similar for larger and smaller sizes; hence they are suitable for small children. However, homograft availability, especially in the smallest ranges, varies due to a limited donor pool. They have a negligible thromboembolic risk and thus do not require anticoagulation. Nonetheless, as is the case for all nonviable tissue prostheses, their use in children is associated with decreased longevity and frequent reoperation due to rapid degeneration, ultimately leading to deterioration of their hemodynamic properties. Homograft longevity varies with type (aortic versus pulmonary) and patient age, and reported freedom from reoperation is 15% to 88% at 10 years. Their use in children is very limited except in very small children unable to undergo the Ross procedure or those with invasive endocarditis.[52,53]

The Ross procedure (named after Donald Ross, who first performed this procedure in the 1967) uses the pulmonary autograft (the patient's own pulmonary valve, which is "harvested" during the surgical procedure) that is transplanted into the aortic position and therefore can be applied to all patient ages (Fig. 51.7). Because the pulmonary autograft is the patient's own living pulmonary valve, the Ross procedure is associated with an excellent hemodynamic profile in all sizes,[45,54] and growth potential of this living valve replacement allows maintenance of this superior hemodynamic profile throughout life.[55] Furthermore, the Ross procedure is a versatile operation that can be used in patients with various LVOT pathologies. The addition of Konno-type aortoventriculoplasty (Ross-Konno) allows successful management of patients with significant annular hypoplasia or complex multilevel LVOTO.[34-37,39,56-59] The original Ross-Konno description involved a large incision into the septum, creating a ventricular septal defect

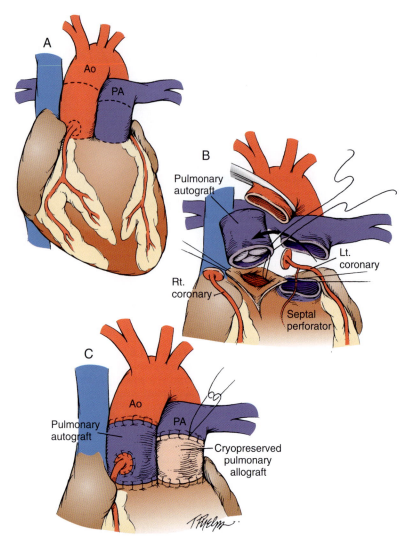

• **Figure 51.7** Ross procedure. A, Great arteries are transected above the sinotubular ridge. Aortic sinuses are excised, and coronary arteries are mobilized. B, Pulmonary autograft is excised from the right ventricular outflow tract to avoid injury to the septal perforator branches of the left coronary artery. The proximal end of the autograft is anastomosed to the annulus with interrupted or continuous sutures. C, The coronary arteries are anastomosed to the pulmonary autograft. Autograft-to-aorta (Ao) anastomosis is completed, and the right ventricular outflow tract is reconstructed usually with a cryopreserved pulmonary allograft.

that is closed with patch. The modified Ross-Konno involves an incision across the aortic annulus into the septum, extensive septal myectomy and LVOT enlargement without a patch, using a portion of the infundibular muscle from the right ventricular outflow tract that can be harvested with the pulmonary autograft[59] (Fig. 51.8). In children the autograft is implanted most commonly as a full root; alternatively, subcoronary or inclusion techniques could be used in older patients but not in young children with small aortic roots.[60] Anticoagulation is not required after Ross due to negligible thromboembolic risk.

Despite technical complexity, the Ross procedure can be performed safely in experienced hands with operative mortality of less than 2.5%.[3,39,45,54,58,60-63] Infants (patients <1 year old) have a higher mortality risk, approaching 15% to 20%, likely due to the more common association of other important cardiac lesions. Mortality risk can be highest in neonates, particularly those with complex LVOTO needing simultaneous arch or mitral procedures. Mortality risk is also increased in emergency surgery, when longer bypass time is required, or in those patients with preoperative ventricular dysfunction.[34-39] These findings suggest that prior palliation with surgical or percutaneous aortic valvuloplasty might decrease mortality risk and that neonates with concomitant significant mitral pathology or arch obstruction might benefit from other surgical alternatives, which may include single-ventricle palliation. Time-related survival of children following Ross is stable with meager attrition risk beyond the perioperative period.[3,39,45,54,58,60-63] Long-term survival after Ross is superior to other valve substitutes, likely due to an excellent autograft hemodynamic profile and trivial thromboembolic or bleeding risks.[3,45]

Despite its numerous advantages, recommendation for Ross has waned due to concerns about late neoaortic root dilation and subsequent autograft regurgitation.[64-71] In addition, some argue that the Ross procedure creates "two-valve disease" because it requires

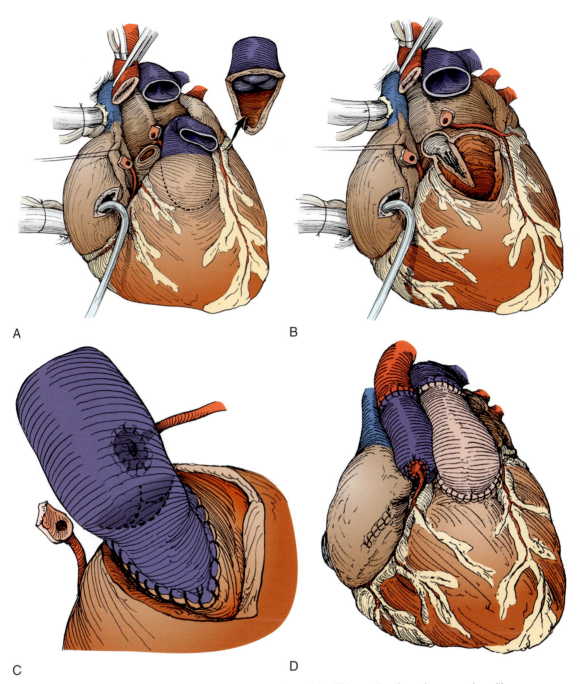

A

B

C

D

• **Figure 51.8** The Ross-Konno procedure is performed by (A) harvesting the pulmonary valve with an extra "tongue" of infundibular muscle after the aorta has been divided and the coronary arteries removed as buttons. B, An incision is then made across the infundibular septum by cutting into the septum between the right and left coronary arteries. This is especially easy to visualize after the pulmonary autograft has been removed. C, The pulmonary autograft is then anastomosed to the aortic root using the infundibular muscle to repair the interventricular septal defect. The coronary arteries are placed into this neoaorta. D, The procedure is completed with a pulmonary homograft to repair the right ventricular outflow tract.

a replacement for the pulmonary valve in addition to the aortic valve. It is debatable if neoaortic annulus and root dilation following Ross is growth proportional to somatic enlargement or disproportionate pathologic remodeling.[55,64,65] In general, neoaortic root dimensions immediately after Ross are larger than in healthy children, the annulus grows in proportion to the child's somatic growth, whereas the root at sinuses and sinotubular junction levels

dilate disproportionately with time. Autograft regurgitation can develop in association with neoaortic dilation, more so with dilation of the sinotubular junction than the sinus.[64-71]

Several factors increase the risk for late autograft reoperation due to autograft dilation, such as older age, bicuspid aortic valve pathology with predominant regurgitation, dilated sinotubular junction, dilated aortic annulus, and geometric mismatch between semilunar valves (aortic larger than pulmonary).[62,65-71] Freedom from autograft reoperation in children with congenital aortic stenosis is 75% to 95% at 10 years, and this freedom from needing reoperation is highest for those with aortic stenosis or mixed (stenosis and insufficiency) disease and worse for patients with primary aortic insufficiency or those with annular-aortic ectasia (often seen as part of bicuspid aortic valve disease).

Children undergoing Ross-Konno are an interesting group because most patients have stenosis and a small aortic annulus and thus are potentially at lower risk of root dilatation.[59] Conversely, annular incision in Ross-Konno and patch placement could result in loss of native annular support to the autograft, with subsequent higher root dilation risk.[65] A recent report showed that, after Ross-Konno, both the neoaortic annulus and the root increased in size proportionately to somatic growth with little risk of late autograft regurgitation or reoperation.

Several technical modifications have been described aiming to reduce autograft dilation risk.[72,73] These techniques include thinning of the muscle rim below the valve, suturing the autograft within the native aortic annulus, autograft shortening, proximal and distal suture line enforcement, or ascending aorta replacement with Dacron graft. Moreover, some surgeons suggested encasing the entire autograft in Dacron tube to prevent dilation, a technique that is suitable only for patients who will not need autograft growth, and further follow-up is necessary to confirm the hypothetical advantages of this modification.[72,73]

Management of failing autograft depends on failure mode, cusp status, and neoaortic root size.[74-77] Patients with reasonably preserved cusps and regurgitation due to dilation with poor coaptation are candidates for aortic valve–sparing root replacement.[75,76] Right ventricle to pulmonary artery conduit longevity following Ross is higher than for those conduits placed following repair of other congenital anomalies due to several factors, such as anatomic conduit position and infrequent incidence of branch pulmonary stenosis. Reported freedom from conduit reoperation is 90% to 95% at 10 years and 75% to 85% at 15 years.[3,39,45,54,58,60-63] Factors associated with increased conduit reoperation include smaller conduit size, longer follow-up, and fresh or aortic homograft use. Of note, recent experience in percutaneous pulmonary valve replacement has allowed cardiologists to address this problem without surgical intervention with good immediate and mid-term results.[78] Recent use of handmade polytetrafluoroethylene (PTFE) valved conduits in the right ventricle–pulmonary artery position has garnered some enthusiasm by selected providers (see Chapter 60).

Subvalvar Aortic Stenosis

Subvalvar aortic stenosis is defined as LVOTO below the level of the aortic valve. It represents the second most common form of LVOTO, occurring in 15% to 20% of patients.[2,4] More than 50% of the cases will have associated cardiac defects like ventricular septal defect, coarctation, atrioventricular septal defect, valvular aortic stenosis, and mitral valve anomalies. Subvalvar aortic stenosis can be either fixed or dynamic obstruction due to apposition of the anterior mitral valve leaflet against the hypertrophied interventricular septum in patients with hypertrophic obstructive cardiomyopathy (HOCM). Other less frequent causes include organic obstruction due to other cardiac structures such as a posteriorly deviated conal septum, abnormal attachments of the mitral valve chordae or papillary muscles to the interventricular septum, accessory mitral valve tissue, and abnormal muscle bundles within the LVOT.[79-81]

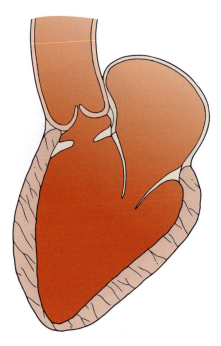

• **Figure 51.9** Discrete subaortic stenosis appears as a ridge of tissue below the aortic valve. Attachments are typically to both the septum and the anterior leaflet of the mitral valve. (From Karamlou T, Cohen GA. Left ventricular outflow tract obstruction and valvar aortic stenosis. In: Kaiser LR, Kron IL, Spray TL. *Mastery of Cardiothoracic Surgery*. 3rd ed. Philadelphia: Wolters Kluwer; 2014.)

Fixed obstruction is most common and is seen in almost 85% of cases. It is usually classified as discrete obstruction in 70% of patients and diffuse tunnel-like obstruction in the remaining 10% to 15%. However, the reality is that there is likely a continuous spectrum of fixed fibromuscular LVOTO.[79-84]

In the discrete form a ridge of fibromuscular tissue exists just below the aortic valve (Fig. 51.9). This membrane is circular or crescentic in shape, extends around the LVOT, and attaches to the interventricular septum on one side and the anterior leaflet of the mitral valve on another side. Unlike valvar stenosis, discrete subvalvar stenosis is rarely present in infancy. A debate exists whether this lesion is truly congenital or an acquired form of LVOTO. In these patients there is echocardiographic evidence that the angle between the long axis of the left ventricle and the aorta is more acute than usual. The turbulent flow as a result of this abnormal angulation forms the substrate for this lesion by sustaining a shear process leading to injury, fibrosis, and membrane formation.[85] The aortic valve is commonly affected by this lesion because of the turbulent flow that leads to cusp thickening and fibrosis, in addition to the extension of the fibrous membrane onto the undersurface of the aortic valve cusps, all interfering with cusp coaptation and contributing to subsequent aortic regurgitation. Those changes to the aortic valve cusps and subsequent aortic regurgitation are commonly evident before the development of significant LVOT gradients.

The less common diffuse form of subvalvar aortic stenosis consists of a long fibromuscular tunnel that extends toward the apex of the left ventricle. Although diffuse subvalvar aortic stenosis can be present as part of complex congenital anomalies that affect the left heart structures, such as Shone's anomaly and hypoplastic left heart complex, it can also be seen as a secondary lesion following earlier resection of a discrete membrane. It is believed that scarring from the initial resection, in combination with an abnormal angulation between the left ventricle and aorta, can lead to progressive fibromuscular proliferation and subsequent tunnel-like obstruction.

HOCM creates dynamic LVOTO. It usually presents during the second or third decade of life and is rarely seen in children. It can present at a younger age, less than 1 year of age, in patients with inborn errors of metabolism or malformation syndromes in combination with other cardiomyopathy phenotypes. It is characterized by asymmetric ventricular septal hypertrophy that affects the upper septum more than the middle or apical septum. Although it can be sporadic, it is often familial and follows an autosomal dominant transmission.[83]

Histologically it is characterized by myocardial fiber disarray with the existence of disorganized and bizarrely shaped hypertrophied myocytes. The mechanism of LVOTO has a fixed component due to the hypertrophied septum and a dynamic component due to the systolic anterior motion of the anterior leaflet of the mitral valve as a result of coexisting anterior displacement of the mitral papillary muscles. The systolic anterior motion of the anterior leaflet of the mitral valve can also lead to failure of mitral valve coaptation and consequent regurgitation.

The pathophysiology of subvalvar aortic stenosis is similar to that of valvar aortic stenosis. In the presence of increased afterload on the left ventricular myocardium, left ventricular hypertrophy develops, although it is notable that the degree of ventricular dysfunction is often more pronounced than that of valvar stenosis. This hypertrophy can lead to consequent subendocardial ischemia and predisposition to sudden death from ventricular arrhythmias.[9] The frequently associated involvement of the aortic valve cusps (as described earlier) often leads to early development of aortic regurgitation, and this aortic regurgitation often presents earlier than significant ventricular dysfunction as a result of LVOTO. In the rare patients with HOCM who are symptomatic during childhood, the most common presentation is congestive heart failure followed by arrhythmia-related sudden death.

In patients with subvalvar stenosis, the ECG will demonstrate evidence of left ventricular hypertrophy. Echocardiography is the principal modality for diagnosis, and it delineates the level of obstruction, gradient across the LVOT, presence of aortic insufficiency, and the existence of concomitant structural anomalies of the mitral valve and septum. Although cardiac catheterization can provide direct measurement of LVOT gradient, it is usually not necessary.

Whereas percutaneous intervention is often an appropriate option for the management of valvar aortic stenosis, surgery is the primary management strategy for subvalvar aortic stenosis. Medical treatment is often ineffective and is limited to the treatment of the rare children with mild dynamic obstruction due to HOCM. In those patients, medical management often includes beta-blockers, calcium channel blockers, and dual-chamber ventricular pacing.

Surgery for subvalvar aortic stenosis is indicated for (1) patients with symptoms of LVOTO such as shortness of breath, angina, syncope, or diminished exercise tolerance; (2) patients with the onset of newly appearing aortic regurgitation (on echocardiogram), even in the presence of lower LVOT gradients; and (3) patients with LVOT gradient more than 40 mm Hg for discrete stenosis or more than 50 mm Hg for diffuse stenosis. In asymptomatic children with LVOT gradient of less than 30 to 40 mm Hg and no evidence of left ventricular hypertrophy or aortic regurgitation, surgery can be deferred. In children with HOCM, surgery is indicated in symptomatic children, especially in high-risk patients with a strong family history of sudden death, a history of ventricular

tachycardia and syncope, or in those with septal hypertrophy measuring 30 mm or greater.[9]

Surgical management of discrete subvalvar aortic stenosis involves resection of the membrane via an aortotomy. The discrete fibrous membrane is typically apparent approximately 5 mm below the right coronary artery cusp and usually extends "counterclockwise" below the right/left coronary commissure and around to the surface of the anterior leaflet of the mitral valve. The membrane is removed using a combination of sharp and blunt dissection, including the attachments to the mitral valve and extensions into the aortic cusps. Care should be taken to avoid injury to the adjacent structures, such as the mitral and aortic valves, and the conduction system that is located below the right/noncoronary commissure. Following removal of the membrane, septal myectomy is generally performed by resecting a 2- to 3-mm wedge of muscular septum beneath the intercoronary commissure (the commissure between the right and left coronary artery cusps) (Fig. 51.10). This supplemental myectomy is believed to decrease the incidence of LVOTO recurrence by reducing LVOT turbulence, although some argue that scarring itself can increase the risk of LVOTO recurrence.[86-89]

Diffuse tunnel-like obstruction can be relieved by transaortic resection of the obstructing muscle, although that is associated with a higher risk of injury to adjacent structures, iatrogenic ventricular septal defect, or permanent heart block. The modified Konno operation is an alternative effective procedure. An incision is made to the right ventricular outflow tract below the pulmonary valve. A right-angle clamp is passed through the aortic valve to guide the incision on the interventricular septum. The ventricular septal defect that is created is then closed with a prosthetic patch. The right ventriculotomy can be closed primarily or with a patch[86,90,91] (Fig. 51.11). In patients with concomitant aortic valve disease, a Ross-Konno operation or aortic valve replacement with Konno annular enlargement may be necessary.[59]

Children with HOCM are managed with a substantial septal myectomy designed to remove a significant portion of the hypertrophied septum from below the aortic valve. When adequate muscle is removed, the LVOTO is diminished because of increased outflow for the left ventricle, even in the presence of systolic anterior motion of the mitral valve (Fig. 51.12). Alternatively, a modified Konno operation similar to that described previously for diffuse tunnel-like obstruction could be used (see Fig. 51.11).[92-94] Because the LVOTO in HOCM is often created by billowing of the anterior leaflet of the mitral valve into the left ventricular outflow tract during systole, some surgical groups have historically advocated for treating this disease with mitral valve replacement.

The postoperative convalescence is usually uncomplicated in patients with discrete subvalvar aortic stenosis.[86,88,89,95-99] Operative mortality is low and ranges between 0% and 3% in the current era. Reported late mortality has also been low, averaging approximately 0.2% (range 0.1% to 0.6%) per year following surgery. Surgical repair of discrete stenosis is effective, and the usual average postoperative gradients range between 5 and 10 mm Hg. The reported need for reoperation is on average 2% (range 1% to 4%) per year following surgery.[86,88,89,95-99] Factors associated with recurrent LVOTO requiring reoperation include younger age (<10 years) at surgery, higher preoperative gradient, postoperative gradient of greater than 10 mm Hg, not performing septal myectomy, and increased complexity of LVOTO. Reoperation for progressive aortic regurgitation might be necessary, especially in patients with a more severe degree of preoperative regurgitation or residual regurgitation. The results of the modified Konno operation are also good, although naturally surgery for the more complex diffuse tunnel-like stenosis

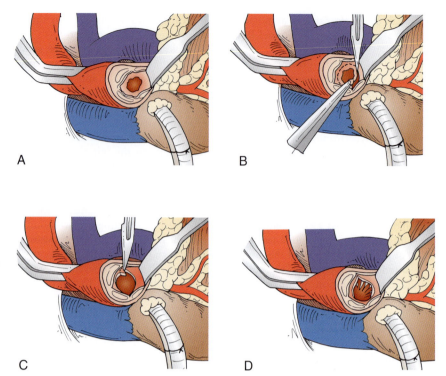

• **Figure 51.10** Resection of discrete subaortic stenosis is performed through an aortotomy on cardio-pulmonary bypass. (A) The aortic valve leaflets are gently retracted. (B) The underlying membrane is then carefully resected, beginning near the conduction area below the right and noncoronary commissure and extending around toward the anterior leaflet of the mitral valve. (C) A myomyectomy is then performed in the interventricular septum below the commissure between the right and left coronary cusps. (D) The final result is removal of the membrane, preservation of the aortic valve leaflets, and a disruption of the fibrous ring with the septal incision. (Redrawn from Ungerleider RM, Shen I. Left ventricular outflow tract obstruction. In: Gardner TJ, Spray TL. *Operative Cardiac Surgery.* 5th ed. New York: Arnold; 2004.)

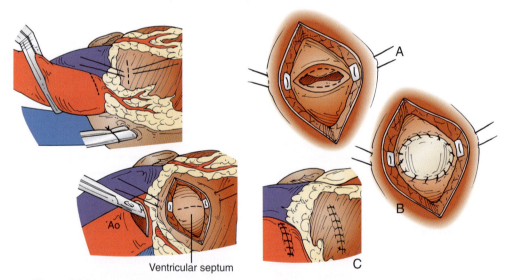

Ventricular septum

• **Figure 51.11** A modified Konno operation can be performed when the subaortic stenosis is below the aortic valve and the aortic valve is normal enough to warrant being preserved and not replaced. An incision is made in both the aorta and in the infundibulum of the right ventricle. A right-angle clamp is then passed safely below the aortic valve and can be used to push up against the interventricular septum in the area that is chosen for resection. A ventricular septal defect (VSD) is created in this portion of the septum (A), and muscle from below the aortic valve is resected. This VSD is then patched (B), and the aortic and right ventricular incisions are closed (C). This procedure removes muscle from the interventricular septum below the aortic valve and can relieve subaortic stenosis while preserving the aortic valve. (From Stark J, de Leval M. *Surgery for Congenital Heart Defects.* 2nd ed. Philadelphia: WB Saunders; 1994.)

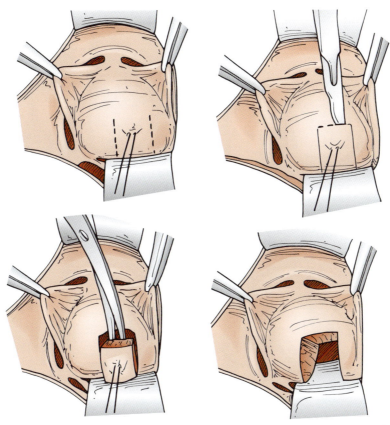

• **Figure 51.12** A large amount of muscle can be resected from the interventricular septum by working through the aortic valve. Muscle is generally removed from the septum in the area below the commissure separating the right and left coronary sinuses. For patients with hypertrophic obstructive cardiomyopathy, a significant amount of muscle can be removed and create an enlarged left ventricular outflow tract. (From Stark J, de Leval M. *Surgery for Congenital Heart Defects.* 2nd ed. Philadelphia: WB Saunders; 1994.)

is associated with higher postoperative gradients and reoperation and mortality risks.[86,90,91] The experience with surgical management of HOCM in children is limited; however, it is usually successful with average postoperative LVOT gradient of 15 to 20 mm Hg and survival above 90% at 10 years.[83,92-94]

Supravalvar Aortic Stenosis

Supravalvar aortic stenosis represents the least common form of LVOTO, occurring in 5% to 10% of patients.[2,4] This can present as a sporadic form, as part of Williams syndrome due to deletion of 1.6 Mb of chromosome 7q11.23 containing the elastin gene, or in a familial form.[100-102]

As a result of the deletion in the elastin gene, the great vessels are less elastic and thus are exposed to more shear stress than usual, with subsequent development of progressive medial thickening and fibrosis and gradual narrowing of those vessels.

In approximately 75% of cases, supravalvar aortic stenosis is discrete and localized to the area of the sinotubular junction and proximal ascending aorta. In the remaining 25% of cases it is diffuse with involvement of the entire ascending aorta, aortic arch, and arch vessels. In several case, there may be narrowing of the main pulmonary artery that can extend into the peripheral branch pulmonary arteries[102,103] (Fig. 51.13).

In the discrete form a thick membranous ridge exists, forming an obstructing ring just above the commissures of the aortic valve. Histologically this sinotubular ridge displays intimal hyperplasia,

medial thickening, and dysplasia with multiple areas of calcifications and necrosis. This ridge often creates the characteristic hourglass appearance of the ascending aorta. As a result, the aortic commissures are increasingly drawn more closely together. This causes a gradual decrease in the opening of the aortic valve cusps, and in the most severe form the free edges of the cusps adhere almost totally to the sinotubular junction.

The coronary arteries in supravalvar aortic stenosis are affected in several ways. The free edges of the aortic valve cusps that are adherent to the sinotubular ridge can lead to impediment of the blood flow into the sinuses of Valsalva and accordingly to the coronary arteries. Additionally, the proliferative thickening process at the sinotubular ridge can extend into the coronary ostia, creating coronary artery obstruction, more so in the left coronary artery. Moreover, given that the coronary ostia originate below the ridge level, this exposes the coronaries to continued high pressures due to the systolic hypertension of the aortic root proximal to the ridge. This is associated with accelerated degenerative changes in the coronary arteries, including intimal hyperplasia, fibrosis, medial hypertrophy, and adventitial fibroelastosis. There is often a marked dilation and tortuosity of the coronary arteries due to the fact that they are filling during systole, and in some cases accelerated atherosclerosis and focal dissections are noted.[102-105]

In general the aortic valve is morphologically normal, and the annulus is of normal size. Nonetheless, there can be significant systolic hypertension of the aortic root proximal to the ridge (which also creates significant left ventricular hypertension despite normal

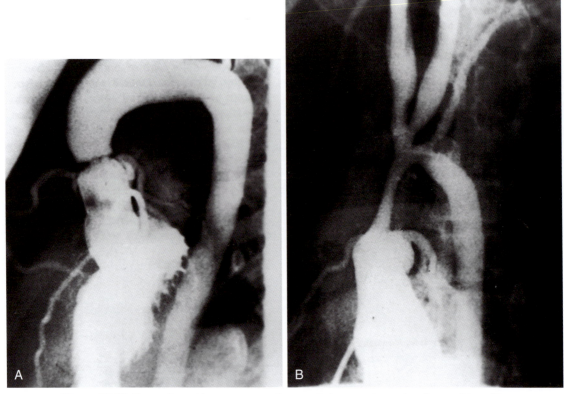

• **Figure 51.13** The angiographic appearance of supravalvular stenosis can be discrete (A) or diffuse (B). In B the stenosis continues to the innominate, carotid, and subclavian arteries. (From Kirklin JW, Barratt-Boyes BG: *Cardiac Surgery*. 2nd ed. New York: Wiley; 1986:1226-1227, with permission.)

peripheral blood pressure). Thickening of the aortic cusps and even aortic insufficiency, usually mild to moderate in severity, can be present in almost 30% to 40% of patients.

As a result of increased afterload on the left ventricular myocardium, left ventricular hypertrophy develops, similar to other forms of LVOTO. In addition, the prevalence of coronary artery flow obstruction in supravalvar aortic stenosis can lead to ischemic myocardial damage that can be distinctive to this type of LVOTO.

The cardiac symptoms emerge with progression of LVOTO, usually in the early first or sometimes second decade of life. However, earlier presentation in infants and young children is not uncommon, especially in cases associated with familial history of the disease. Those symptoms include reduced exercise tolerance, syncope, and angina-like chest pain. In some advanced cases, patients present with sudden death from ventricular fibrillation associated with severe myocardial dysfunction. In patients with associated involvement of the pulmonary arteries or aortic arch branches, the medical picture might be further complicated by clinical manifestation of those other obstructive lesions. External manifestations in patients with Williams syndrome that include elfin facies, mental retardation, and unreserved hypersociable persona should warrant the evaluation of cardiac involvement, even in asymptomatic patients.[9,105]

In patients with supravalvar stenosis, the ECG will demonstrate evidence of left ventricular hypertrophy, and, if coronary flow is restricted, there may be signs of left ventricular strain. As in other forms of LVOTO, diagnosis is usually provided by echocardiography, which can delineate the level of obstruction, gradient across the LVOT, coronary artery flow, and degree of left ventricular hypertrophy. However, echocardiography may not be able to clarify the

presence of obstruction of the distal aortic arch or the origins of the arch vessels. Cardiac catheterization is useful to better delineate the status of the coronary arteries, although care must be exercised during the imaging of those coronary arteries, especially when there is echocardiographic evidence of coronary artery flow restriction. Cardiac catheterization will also allow precise measurement of LVOT gradient, end-diastolic pressures in the ventricles, and description of obstructive lesions in the aortic arch, arch vessels, and branch pulmonary arteries. Magnetic resonance imaging is gaining an increased role in the assessment of those patients and is useful demonstrating coronary artery involvement and obstructive lesions in the aortic arch, arch vessels, and branch pulmonary arteries. Magnetic resonance imaging has replaced cardiac catheterization at many cardiac centers as a less invasive diagnostic modality although it can still be associated with important anesthesia risk.

There is essentially no role for catheter-based treatment of discrete supravalvar aortic stenosis, and surgery is the primary management strategy. Medical treatment is often ineffective, and afterload-reducing agents should be avoided because they can result in reduced coronary perfusion. Similarly, balloon dilation of the supravalvar aortic stenosis is unsuccessful, and the role of percutaneous interventions is usually limited to addressing peripheral branch pulmonary artery stenosis (and, occasionally, distal aortic branch stenosis) as part of a collaborative approach in patients with severe cases.[9,106]

Surgery is indicated in patients with symptoms of LVOTO or decreased coronary perfusion. Surgery is also indicated in patients with LVOT gradient of 40 to 50 mm Hg in association with echocardiographic evidence of a significant narrowing of the sinotubular junction. In asymptomatic children with LVOT

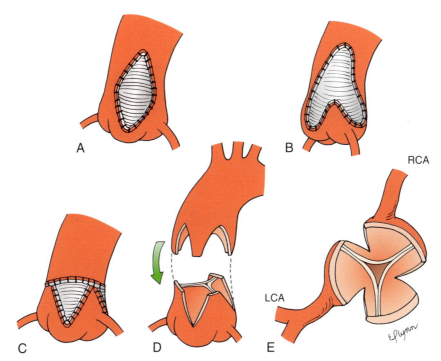

• **Figure 51.14** A variety of techniques have been described for the treatment of supravalvar aortic stenosis including (A) the single-patch technique, (B) the double (or pantaloon) patch, (C and E) incisions into all three sinuses (E) with a three-patch repair (C) or (D) reverse flap repair using the ascending aorta. (Redrawn from Pigula FA. Surgery for congenital anomalies of the aortic valve and root. In: Sellke FW, del Nido PJ, Swanson SJ. *Sabiston and Spencer Surgery of the Chest.* Philadelphia: Elsevier Saunders; 2005.)

gradients less than 30 to 40 mm Hg and no evidence of left ventricular hypertrophy, surgery can be deferred, and the patient can be followed semiannually with serial echocardiograms and office visits.

The goals of surgical treatment of supravalvar aortic stenosis should be the relief of LVOTO and coronary artery obstruction and preservation of the aortic root geometry and aortic valve function. In patients with more diffuse disease the extent of surgery should be tailored to the level of distal involvement of the ascending aorta and aortic arch.[9,105-107]

In 1961 McGoon, Starr, and their associates individually described the single-patch repair technique. A longitudinal aortotomy in the ascending aorta is extended across the sinotubular ridge and into the noncoronary sinus. Additionally, the thickened membranous ridge is excised. The longitudinal aortotomy is then closed using a teardrop-shaped patch[108] (Fig. 51.14A).

In 1976 Doty and associates described an extended aortoplasty that comprises the creation of an inverted Y-shaped incision across the sinotubular ridge and into the middle of the noncoronary sinus as well as into the right coronary sinus to the left of the right coronary ostia. The aortic root is then reconstructed with the use of a generous pantaloon-shaped patch that is sutured into the two sinuses of Valsalva[109] (see Fig. 51.14B).

In 1988 Brom described a more extensive aortoplasty that involves complete transection of the ascending aorta above the sinotubular junction (see Fig. 51.14C; Fig. 51.15). Following that, three longitudinal incisions are extended into the three sinuses of Valsalva to fully open the area of supravalvar narrowing while preserving symmetric geometry of the aortic root. Following excision of the membranous ridge, the reconstruction of the root is accomplished with three separate triangular patches. Finally, an end-to-end

anastomosis is created between the ascending aorta and the reconstructed aortic root. The theoretical advantage of this technique is the effective relief of LVOTO while simultaneously restoring aortic root geometry.[110]

Using a similar concept, Myers described the sliding aortoplasty technique in 1993. In this procedure, three longitudinal incisions are extended into the three sinuses of Valsalva. The sliding aortoplasty is carried out by cutting out corresponding triangular patches in the ascending aorta and then advancing the ascending aorta to augment each sinus of Valsalva (see Fig. 51.14D). The theoretical advantage of this technique is the exclusive use of autologous tissue, thus maintaining the potential for growth.[111] However, in neonates and infants this technique has the potential disadvantage of shortening the aorta, and when there is concomitant pulmonary artery stenosis (as is commonly the case), this technique may create pressure on the posterior right pulmonary artery (which courses posterior to the aorta) and lead to right pulmonary artery stenosis. In a recent demonstration, Ungerleider and colleagues described a technique that combines the Brom and Myers techniques to create longer patches to repair the incisions into the coronary sinuses and use the height of these patches to fit into contralateral incisions on the ascending aorta (Fig. 51.16). At this time the three-sinus repair is the preferred technique for supravalvar stenosis in neonates and infants at many centers.

Different patch materials have been used, ranging from autologous pericardium homograft to PTFE. Obviously, in patients with evidence of coronary artery involvement the thick membrane should be peeled off the coronary artery ostia. In some cases, coronary osteoplasty is needed with the use of patch enlargement of the proximal coronary artery. Very rarely, coronary artery bypass grafting is necessary. Of note, the surgeon should be very careful during

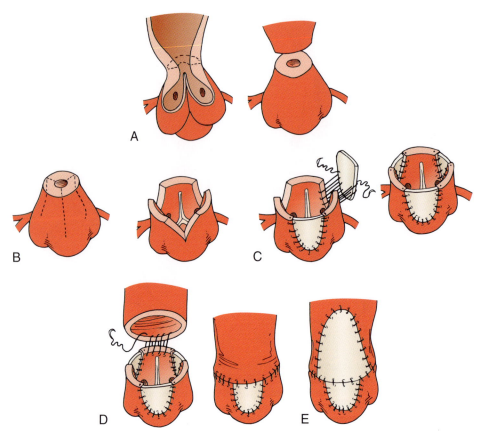

• **Figure 51.15** The three-patch repair (Brom technique) requires transection of the aorta (A), which is usually thickened, and incisions into each of the three sinuses (B). The sinus areas are then enlarged with individual patches (C), and the reconstructed aortic root is then reattached to the ascending aorta (D). It is often necessary to augment the ascending aorta with a patch (E). (Redrawn from Hazekamp MG, Kappetein AP, Schoof PH, et al. Brom's three-patch technique for repair of supravalvular aortic stenosis. *J Thorac Cardiovasc Surg.* 1999;118:252.)

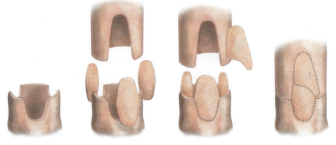

• **Figure 51.16** A technique for reconstruction of the aortic root in supravalvar stenosis employing a three-patch augmentation. The patches are left long so that they extend above the sinuses and are fit into contralateral incisions in the ascending aorta. An additional patch can be used anteriorly to augment the size of the connection. This technique combines the Brom and Myers technique and is preferred when there is concomitant repair of the pulmonary artery so that the reconstructed aorta will not put pressure posteriorly on the right pulmonary artery. (Courtesy Dr. Ross M. Ungerleider.)

patch enlargement of the right and left coronary sinuses because distortion of the coronary arteries might occur with resultant coronary artery ischemia. Naturally, patients with more distal ascending aorta or arch involvement might require a more extensive patch augmentation with the use of selective cerebral perfusion or deep hypothermic circulatory arrest. In general a single patch that extends from the noncoronary sinus into the proximal arch or a Brom three-patch aortoplasty in conjunction with ascending aortoplasty with an extended patch and subsequent end-to end anastomosis is performed.

The postoperative convalescence is typically uncomplicated in older patients with discrete supravalvar aortic stenosis, although it can be more complicated in neonates and infants who present with severe preoperative myocardial dysfunction, those with concomitant severe pulmonary artery stenosis and elevated right heart pressures, and those with diffuse disease requiring extended distal aortoplasty. Operative mortality following surgical repair of discrete supravalvar aortic stenosis is low and ranges between 0% and 5% in the current era.[102,107,112-117] On the other hand, mortality following surgical repair of diffuse supravalvar aortic stenosis is higher, with some reports showing operative mortality as high as 40%. Late mortality has varied in the reported literature and ranged between 5% and 25% at an average 20 years of follow-up. Factors that have been identified in the literature to be associated with late mortality include diffuse form, age less than 2 years, male gender, concomitant valvar stenosis, and residual postoperative gradient of greater than 40 mm Hg. All techniques are associated with immediate relief of LVOTO, and the average reported residual postoperative gradients have ranged between 15 and 30 mm Hg.[102,107,112-117] Some of the reported series have shown a benefit for the multiple-patch techniques over the single-patch technique, whereas others have shown comparable results.[102,107,112-117] The presence of concomitant valvar stenosis was also associated with significant residual gradients, defined as mean gradient more than 40 mm Hg. The incidence of aortic valve regurgitation has been very low in all the techniques. The need for reoperation ranges between 0% and 32%. Aortic valve surgery is the most commonly performed reoperation. Additional reasons for reoperation include distal aortic obstruction, recurrent supravalvar stenosis, and less commonly pulmonary artery stenosis. Factors associated with increased reoperation need include concomitant valvar stenosis, age less than 2 years, and diffuse supravalvar stenosis. Although the single-patch technique was associated with increased reoperation risk in some series, that has not been uniform, and many studies have reported comparable early and late outcomes between the various patch repair techniques.[102,107,112-117]

References

A complete list of references is available at ExpertConsult.com.

52

Mitral Valve Disease

JOSEPH R. NELLIS, MD, MBA; NICHOLAS D. ANDERSEN, MD; JOSEPH W. TUREK, MD, PHD

Isolated congenital mitral valve disease is rare.[1-6] More commonly, it is associated with complex and challenging congenital cardiac conditions like Shone's complex and connective tissue disorders. In these situations the abnormal mitral valve continues to serve as the systemic atrioventricular valve. In patients with conotruncal abnormalities a tricuspid valve or an Ebstein anomaly (positioned low in the ventricle with displaced and dysplastic valve leaflets) may be found in the systemic atrioventricular valve position. In the most severe cases, congenital mitral valve disease can occur with single-ventricle pathologies.

Hypoplastic left heart syndrome affects the mitral apparatus, left ventricle, aortic valve, and ascending aorta. The mitral valve is not the primary focus of this presentation, and the goals of care are focused on single-ventricle palliation. However, atrioventricular valve insufficiency may influence long-term morbidity and mortality.[7] Similarly, complete atrioventricular septal defects involve the mitral valve, and complex repairs are often required to septate the ventricles and restore atrioventricular valve function.

Complex congenital cardiac presentations like these are discussed in greater detail elsewhere. This chapter will focus on isolated mitral valve diseases of the infant and child, in which the mitral valve is the primary concern.

History

Mitral valve stenosis was the first mitral valve lesion to be addressed surgically. Elliot Cutler performed the surgery on an 11-year-old girl in 1923 at the Brigham Hospital in Boston.[8] Although this patient survived for 4 years, she was the only survivor of Cutler's transapical valvotomy technique. In 1947 Dwight Harken, a protégé of Cutler's at the Brigham, proposed a mitral valve repair with "selective insufficiency." He believed performing serial resections of the commissures and preserving the anterior leaflet would prove successful. Unfortunately, 6 of his first 10 patients died.[9]

At the same time Charles Bailey was working on a simple commissurotomy approach in Philadelphia.[10] He successfully conducted trials of his technique in the laboratory before applying it clinically. His desire to advance the treatment for this dreaded condition was not without resistance, resulting in the nickname "The Butcher of Hahnemann Hospital," following the deaths of his first two patients. Learning from his earlier mistakes, he developed an overlapping glove technique to safely slip a hooked knife into the heart. On June 10, 1948, Bailey booked three mitral valve procedures in three different hospitals across Philadelphia—knowing his surgical privileges would be revoked if another patient died. Following the death of the first patient that day, Bailey rushed to the second case and successfully performed the first hook-knife commissurotomy. His patient, a 24-year-old woman with a 2-year history of mitral stenosis, lived another 38 years.

In 1964 Young and Robinson[11] performed the first mitral valve replacement in a 10-month-old child. Shortly thereafter, in 1976 Carpentier and colleagues[12] proposed a systematic way of categorizing and describing congenital mitral disease, thereby uniting the field and laying the foundation for many of today's surgical repairs.

Embryology

Mitral valve formation begins during the fourth week of gestation and continues through the sixth month.[13-16] Endocardial cushions begin to advance from the anterior and posterior endomyocardium during the fourth week and merge during the fifth and sixth weeks—dividing the heart into a common atrium and ventricle, as well as two rudimentary atrioventricular canals. The cushions continue to expand laterally, forming early leaflets by the seventh week. Over the next 5 weeks the early leaflets undergo epithelial-to-mesenchymal transition—replacing early endomyocardial tissue with muscle. As the early leaflets transition into muscle, they merge inferiorly with a myocardial ridge that runs from the anterior wall of the left ventricle, through the apex, to the posterior atrioventricular canal. This ridge begins to delaminate from the ventricular wall at approximately 7 weeks' gestation and can be recognizable as the anterolateral and posteromedial papillary muscles by 10 weeks. By 12 weeks the papillary muscles are only connected to the left ventricle inferiorly and the early leaflets superiorly. As the leaflets thin during the 14th week, chordae begin to appear, and the mitral apparatus is recognizable by the 15th week. Over the next 2 months, the muscular tissue of the leaflets and primitive chordae is slowly replaced by thin collagen, and the mitral apparatus is complete by 6 months.[17,18]

Isolated malformations of the mitral valve may occur due to irregularities in development at any one of these steps.

- Endocardial cushions fail to migrate—mitral atresia
- Incomplete endocardial cushion differentiation—mitral valve stenosis
- Incomplete endocardial cushion thinning—supramitral or intramitral rings
- Union of the early papillary muscles—parachute mitral valve
- Incomplete myocardial ridge delamination—parachute-like asymmetric mitral valve
- Incomplete chordae development—hammock or arcade mitral valve

Although this list is not exhaustive, it depicts the common isolated mitral valve diseases seen in clinical practice. This chapter will describe each of these conditions, as well as others, in much greater detail. However, before discussing these pathologic findings, it is important to recognize normal mitral valve anatomy and physiology.

Anatomy

Diagnosis and management of mitral valve disease demands a thorough understanding of mitral valve anatomy and physiology (Figs. 52.1 and 52.2A).[19] The mitral valve, or mitral apparatus, is made of four distinct parts—a fibromuscular annulus, two leaflets,

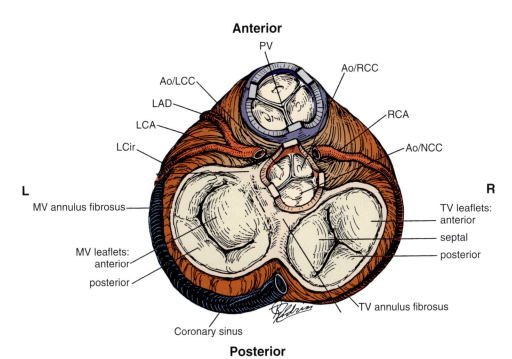

• **Figure 52.1** Cross-sectional anatomy showing the mitral valve (MV) and surrounding structures. *Ao/LCC,* Left coronary cusp aortic valve; *Ao/NCC,* noncoronary cusp aortic valve; *Ao/RCC,* right coronary cusp aortic valve; *LAD,* left anterior descending coronary artery; *LCA,* left coronary artery; *LCir,* left circumflex coronary artery; *MV,* mitral valve; *PV,* pulmonary valve; *RCA,* right coronary artery; *TV,* tricuspid valve. (From Lamberti JJ, Mitruka SN: Congenital anomalies of the mitral valve. In Mavroudis C, Becker CL, eds. *Pediatric Cardiac Surgery.* Philadelphia: Mosby; 2003; with permission.)

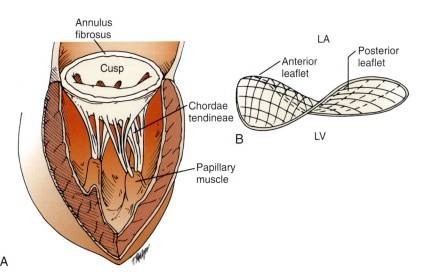

• **Figure 52.2** Mitral apparatus and annular geometry. (A) The mitral apparatus includes the annulus, leaflets, chordae, and papillary muscles. (B) The mitral annulus is not a planar structure. It is saddle shaped with the anterior and posterior commissures representing the low points of the saddle. *LA,* Left atrium; *LV,* left ventricle. (From Levine RA, Handschumacher MD, Sanfilippo AJ, et al. Three-dimensional echocardiographic reconstruction of the mitral valve, with implications for the diagnosis of mitral valve prolapse. *Circulation.* 80:589-598, 1989; with permission.)

multiple chordae, and two papillary muscles. The mitral valve separates the left atrium and ventricle. During diastole it acts as a funnel for blood entering the left ventricle, and during systole it acts as a barrier preventing retrograde flow from the left ventricle into the left atrium.

The anterior aspect of the mitral valve is located behind the left main coronary artery slightly below the level of the aortic valve. The anterior border is continuous with the left fibrous trigone, subaortic curtain at the junction of the left coronary and non-coronary sinuses, and the right fibrous trigone more medially. The atrioventricular node is located within the right fibrous trigone, adjacent to the posteromedial commissure of the mitral valve. The posteromedial commissure separates the anterior and posterior leaflets along their posterior margins, whereas the anterolateral commissure defines these leaflets along their anterior margins. The posterior leaflet and remaining annulus share a continuous border with the atrioventricular groove along the posterior and lateral aspects of the valve. The circumflex coronary artery and coronary sinus run within this groove and are intimately involved with the mitral annulus along these borders. Failure to acknowledge the proximity of these important structures may dramatically impact an otherwise successful mitral valve surgery, particularly during valve replacement.

The valvar portion of the mitral apparatus is composed of the annulus and leaflets. The annulus is a D-shaped fibromuscular structure to which the leaflets and surrounding myocardium attach. In three dimensions the annulus more closely resembles a saddle (see Fig. 52.2B).[20] The anterior third of the annulus is continuous with the left and right fibrous trigones and is attached to the fibrous skeleton of the heart. It supports the anterior leaflet and is the fixed portion of the annulus. The remaining annulus is a dynamic structure that contracts 20% to 40% during systole. It supports the posterior leaflet and is the portion of the annulus that dilates with valvar and ventricular dysfunction.

The anterior leaflet is triangular to trapezoid in appearance and is easily distinguishable from the crescent-shaped posterior leaflet. By definition the posterior leaflet contains three standard clefts, or scallops, but additional deviant clefts are observed in over a third of patients.[21] The anterior leaflet does not contain standard clefts and carries deviant clefts in less than 10% of patients. Standard posterior scallops and their associated anterior leaflet regions are labeled numerically front to back (e.g., P1 : A1 being the anterior-most leaflets and P3 : A3 the posterior-most). The anterior leaflet occupies 150 degrees of the mitral annulus anteriorly, and the posterior leaflet occupies the remaining 210 degrees. The lateral borders of the leaflets are defined by the anterolateral and postero-medial commissures. Commissures are differentiated from clefts by the presence of fanning chordae that span both leaflets inferiorly. False commissures, or clefts, are supported by chordae that do not cross adjacent leaflet margins. Despite their differences, the anterior and posterior leaflets occupy the same surface area and together, in their entirety, measure more than twice that of the primary mitral orifice. Mitral coaptation occurs below the level of the annulus and is dependent on a balanced subvalvar apparatus to prevent incompetence.

The subvalvar apparatus is made of chordae and two papillary muscles. The anterolateral papillary muscle anchors chordae to both leaflets and the anterolateral commissure, and it receives its blood supply from the first diagonal branch of the left anterior descending coronary artery and the obtuse marginal branches of the circumflex coronary artery.[22,23] The posteromedial papillary muscle anchors chordae to both leaflets and the posteromedial

commissure, and it receives 85% of its blood supply from the right coronary artery and 15% from the posterolateral branch of the circumflex coronary artery.[22,23] Chordae are fibrous thread-like bands that connect the papillary muscles to the leaflets. Approximately 9 chordae originate from the apical portion of each papillary muscle and branch to make over 30 distinct attachments on the leaflets.[24] The area in which the chordae course from the papillary muscles to the leaflets represents the secondary mitral orifice. Chordae are classified into four broad categories based on their origin and insertion.

True chordae originate from the papillary muscle and insert onto the mitral valve leaflet.[24] True chordae can be divided into first-order and second-order chordae. True first-order chordae insert onto the margin or free edge of the leaflet—they are responsible for preventing mitral valve prolapse during systole. A special subset of true first-order chordae are commissural chordae. Commissural chordae are straight chordae that fan distally and insert on the anterior- and posterior-most aspects of both mitral leaflets. True second-order chordae insert further back on the leaflet, closer to the annulus in the rough zone. They tend to be thicker and play a variable role in left ventricular function. False chordae are structural and do not follow the traditional papillary muscle–leaflet pattern.[24] False chordae can lie between adjacent papillary muscles, papillary muscles and the ventricle, or the rough zone of the leaflet and the ventricle.

Classification of Mitral Valve Disease

Valvar disease is often divided into obstructive and regurgitant processes. Unfortunately, congenital mitral valve diseases affecting the infant and child are not always as clear-cut. These pathologies commonly present as pure obstructive or regurgitant processes, but a substantial subset can display a mixed presentation or even be completely asymptomatic.

Following convention, this chapter will divide mitral valve disease into obstructive and regurgitant processes. Diseases with variable presentations will be listed under their most common presentation.

Obstructive Mitral Valve Disease

Congenital Mitral Stenosis

Congenital mitral stenosis is largely a catch-all diagnosis for obstructive lesions involving the mitral valve. These lesions often involve multiple aspects of the mitral apparatus and include diagnoses such as mitral rings, parachute mitral valves, and mitral arcade.

Examples of less characteristic pathologies include tethered commissures and hypoplastic leaflets. These lesions are often associated with larger syndromes or infectious causes, although isolated cases have been reported. Transthoracic echocardiogram with Doppler demonstrates a triangular-to-trapezoid, or funnel-like, acceleration across the mitral valve. Three-dimensional echocardiogram has helped differentiate these obstructive pathologies preoperatively, but meticulous intraoperative investigation remains the gold standard.

Mitral Rings

Mitral rings are composed of redundant annular tissue, classified as either supramitral or intramitral, based on proximity to the mitral leaflets and involvement with the subvalvar apparatus. Mitral rings interrupt transvalvar flow to varying degrees based on their size. They commonly present with obstructive symptoms, but they can also present asymptomatically as an incidental murmur.[6] The etiology of mitral rings is uncertain, although it is believed to involve inadequate separation or thinning of the endocardial cushions during development.

Intramitral rings are thin, fibroelastic rings in direct contact with the mitral leaflets. They restrict the ability of the leaflets to open and always affect the subvalvar apparatus. Supramitral rings are characterized by excess fibrous tissue between the leaflets and the left atrial appendage, sparing the leaflets and the subvalvar apparatus (Fig. 52.3A and B).[25,26] These rings represent progressive lesions that can be completely or partially circumferential. The median age of diagnosis is 3 years, although the presentation is variable and often related to the size of the ring or the presence of additional cardiac conditions (e.g., Shone's syndrome or ventricular septal defects).[6,27,28] Diagnosis with transthoracic echocardiography remains difficult and is made in only 50% to 70% of cases preoperatively.[29] Doppler echocardiography may show a convex acceleration above the mitral valve that arcs superiorly toward the atrium, as compared with the inferiorly orientated acceleration

seen with classic congenital mitral stenosis.[30] Supramitral rings should not be confused with cor triatriatum sinistrum.

Cor triatriatum sinister contains a fibromuscular ring located above the level of the left atrial appendage, thereby dividing the left atrium into two compartments (see Fig. 52.3C and D).[31] Cor triatriatum sinister forms when a left pulmonary vein fails to properly incorporate into the left atrium. Like supramitral rings, these rings can present as obstructive processes or asymptomatically, based on the extent of the disease and activity level of the individual. Often cor triatriatum sinister is associated with atrial septal defects.

Parachute Mitral Valve

The leaflets in parachute mitral valves are anchored to a single papillary muscle by short, thick, hypoplastic chordae—giving the mitral apparatus a parachute-like appearance (Fig. 52.4).[1,6,32] The single papillary muscle is often centrally located, as opposed to the anterolateral and posteromedial arrangement seen with normal mitral anatomy. As a consequence, the leaflets are restricted during diastole, taking on a funnel-like appearance and obstructing transvalvar flow. In the apical four-chamber view this funnel-like appearance has been described as pear shaped—a pathognomonic

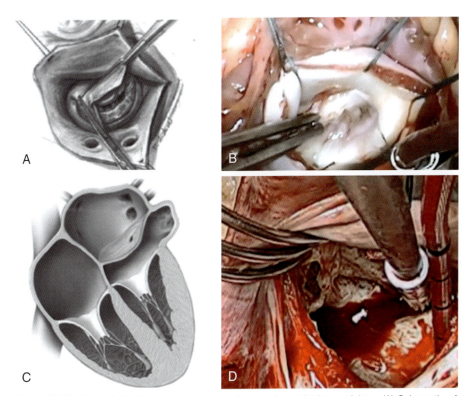

• **Figure 52.3** Differentiating between supramitral rings and cor triatriatum sinister. (A) Schematic of a supramitral ring with the leaflets visible. (B) Intraoperative view into the left atrium showing a supramitral ring that is being grasped and a visible mitral valve. (C) A schematic of cor triatriatum sinister. (D) Intraoperative view into the left atrium showing the opening of the membrane immediately inferior to the valve retractor. The mitral valve is located below this membrane. For blood to go from the left atrium to the left ventricle it has to go through the small opening in the membrane. ([A] From Baird CW, Myers PO, del Nido PJ. Mitral valve operations at a high-volume pediatric heart center: evolving techniques and improved survival with mitral valve repair versus replacement. *Ann Pediatr Card.* 5:13-20, 2012; with permission. [C] From Saxena P, Burkhart HM, Schaff HV, et al. Surgical repair of cor triatriatum sinister: the Mayo Clinic 50-year experience. *Ann Thorac Surg.* 5:1659-1663, 2014; with permission.)

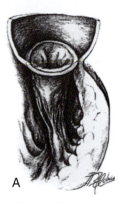
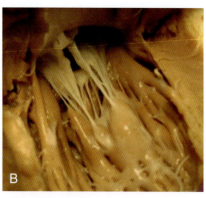

• **Figure 52.4** Parachute mitral valve with the chordae anchoring to a single papillary muscle on the posterolateral ventricular wall. (A) Schematic. (B) Autopsy specimen. ([A] From Lamberti JJ, Mitruka SN. Congenital anomalies of the mitral valve. In: Mavroudis C, Becker CL, eds. *Pediatric Cardiac Surgery.* Philadelphia: Mosby; 2003 with permission. [B] From Baird CW, Marx GR, Borisuk M, et al. Review of congenital mitral valve stenosis: analysis, repair techniques, and outcomes. *Cardiovasc Eng Technol.* 2:167-173, 2015; with permission.)

finding in this disease entity. Parachute mitral valves are believed to be the result of papillary muscle fusion between the 5th and 10th week of gestation. Diagnosis is made with three-dimensional echocardiography.

Parachute-like asymmetric mitral valve disease is a similar condition to parachute mitral valve disease but contains two asymmetric papillary muscles. Whereas the posteromedial papillary muscle appears normal, the anterolateral papillary muscle is often positioned higher in the ventricle, with fewer chordae, and in contact with the mitral annulus. Parachute-like asymmetric mitral valve disease arises between the 5th and 15th week of gestation when the early papillary muscle fails to delaminate from the ventricular wall and form appropriate chordae with the valvar apparatus.

Parachute mitral valve can often be managed medically throughout the first decade of life, delaying surgery until the child is substantially larger.

Mitral Valve Atresia

Mitral valve atresia involves the constellation of a small annulus, short chordae, and closely associated papillary muscles. In essence the mitral apparatus never finished growing. Eighty percent of cases are seen in association with larger ventricular anomalies, including hypoplastic left heart syndrome, left ventricular outflow tract obstruction, and double-outlet right ventricle. Infants with mitral valve atresia present with severe obstructive symptoms early in life, often requiring an immediate operation.

Mitral valve function is often inferred in the context of coexisting cardiac malformations. Large ventricular septal defects or single-ventricle pathologies may compensate for decreased forward flow across an atretic mitral valve. In these settings the mitral valve should be interrogated closely and appropriately addressed to minimize the need for subsequent operations.

Pathophysiology of Mitral Valve Obstruction

Mitral valve obstruction, from any cause, results in the restriction of blood flow from the left atrium to the left ventricle. As the left atrial filling pressure increases, the force of contraction increases, and a pressure gradient develops across the obstruction. When the impedance of the obstruction is greater than the contractile strength of the left atrium, left ventricle filling is compromised, and volume backs up into the pulmonary veins. Often in patients with pure mitral valve stenosis, this decrease in left ventricular filling is compounded by a decreased ejection fraction and abnormal contractility.[33] Together, these findings result in diminished cardiac output.

The increase in left atrial, pulmonary venous, and pulmonary capillary wedge pressures results in an increase in interstitial and alveolar fluid. The increase in interstitial fluid along with the pulmonary venous congestion compresses the small airways, restricts ventilation, and contributes to the increased work of breathing that is associated with left atrioventricular obstruction. Simultaneously hypoxemia and hypercapnia develop secondary to alveolar shunting and impaired gas exchange. Late signs and symptoms of mitral valve obstruction include pulmonary artery hypertension, right ventricular hypertrophy, and ultimately right ventricular dysfunction with or without tricuspid insufficiency. At this point, left ventricular filling is affected by both the mitral valve obstruction and the increased pulmonary vascular resistance. In the setting of right-sided failure, cardiac output is further reduced, and peripheral signs of heart failure, including end-organ damage become evident.

Left ventricular filling across the obstructed mitral valve occurs during diastole. With an increasing heart rate the diastolic time decreases, and left atrial contractility normally increases to maintain cardiac output. Due to the increased demands on the left atrium at baseline in severe mitral obstruction, it fails to compensate for the decreased diastolic times during tachycardia, resulting in acute pulmonary congestion. Prolonged mitral valve obstruction increases the risk of atrial dilation and dysrhythmias. Atrial fibrillation is particularly bad for these patients due to the loss of atrial contractility and the decreased diastolic filling times that are seen with rapid ventricular response.[34]

Diagnosis of Mitral Valve Obstruction

The presentation of mitral valve obstruction varies depending on the severity of the obstruction, the presence of additional comorbidities, and the metabolic demands of the child.[5] Evidence of mitral obstruction is not apparent in the fetus, as evident in patients with hypoplastic left heart and complete mitral atresia who develop normally until birth. Signs and symptoms thereafter depend on the degree of obstruction and range from asymptomatic to fulminant heart failure. With increasing obstruction, fatigability, irritability, feeding difficulties, tachypnea, and chronic cough become more apparent. Pulmonary hypertension is often associated with peripheral edema, recurrent lower respiratory infections, and ultimately failure to thrive. As the child grows older, activity will be limited by the obstruction. This is not always noticeable to the patient or parents, particularly if the child has adapted his or her activities to avoid feeling fatigued or has grown up in a sedentary household.

The physical examination in mitral valve obstruction once again depends on the severity of the obstruction. Often the symptoms are subtle and may only be associated with decreased peripheral pulses. The first heart sound is quiet, whereas the second is more pronounced and split to a varying degree based on the magnitude of the underlying pulmonary hypertension. When the left atrium can no longer compensate for the obstruction, children develop left and later right-sided heart failure. As in adults, this presents with wet crackles on auscultation, increased jugular venous distention, pulsus paradoxus, and dependent edema.

Noninvasive testing is central to diagnosing and differentiating the alternative forms of mitral valve obstruction. The electrocardiogram will show left atrial dilation, right axis deviation, and if advanced, right ventricular hypertrophy. Left atrial enlargement is seen on chest x-ray examination along with prominent pulmonary vasculature that has been redistributed to the upper middle and upper lobes.

Echocardiography provides all of the necessary information for the management of mitral valve stenosis.[35,36] Two-dimensional and Doppler echocardiography can be useful in measuring mitral valve anatomy and function, including flow velocities, gradients, and annular areas.[37,38] With improvements in acquisition quality, three-dimensional echocardiography has been more widely used in diagnosing and managing congenital heart disease, particularly mitral valve pathologies.

Cardiac catheterization provides a direct measure of the left- and right-sided pressures but is often unnecessary in this patient population given the advances in echocardiography.

Medical Management

Successful medical management of mitral valve stenosis relies on diuretics and nutritional supplementation. Ventricular dysfunction is common with pure mitral valve stenosis, and digoxin is often employed to improve cardiac output. Beta-adrenergic antagonists can be used for patients who develop symptoms with exertion, although they should be used cautiously in the setting of congestive heart failure.[39-41]

Atrial fibrillation is common in patients with progressively worsening mitral valve stenosis. Atrial fibrillation is approached similarly in children and adults, with the primary goal being rate control. Due to the obstructive pathology of these patients, the loss of organized atrial contractility may cause them to rapidly decompensate. The threshold for electrical cardioversion with anticoagulation before, during, and after should be low. Pretreatment and continued maintenance therapy with amiodarone has been shown to improve the effectiveness of cardioversion when required, making amiodarone a favored first-line rate-limiting agent in the hemodynamically stable child with atrial fibrillation.[42-44]

Episodes of acute respiratory failure often precede heart failure and represent the earliest hospitalizations for children with isolated mitral valve obstruction. Increased interstitial edema presents as wheezing. These episodes may worsen with increases in cardiac output due to decreased diastolic times, resulting in a presentation much like that of an asthmatic. However, beta-adrenergic bronchodilators will worsen the clinical picture for these children. Furthermore, beta-adrenergics increase the likelihood of reflexive tachycardia and atrial fibrillation, both of which are poorly tolerated by children with mitral valve obstruction. The best treatment for respiratory symptoms in these children is diuretics and/or antibiotics, if a concomitant respiratory infection is suspected.

Endotracheal intubation and mechanical ventilation may be needed to alleviate increased work of breathing and cardiac workload. Lung-protective ventilatory strategies, including increased positive end-expiratory pressure, decreased tidal volume, and permissive hypercapnia, should be used cautiously in this population. The concern with these strategies includes increasing pulmonary vascular resistance with increasing positive end-expiratory pressure and reducing myocardial contractility with increasing acidosis. Patients should be gradually introduced to a protective lung strategy to avoid acute rises in carbon dioxide levels. Further, respiratory rates should be used to counter acidosis, and positive end-expiratory

pressures should be minimized to support right ventricular function. Children requiring ventilatory support should be considered for endovascular and surgical intervention.

Endovascular interventions are continually improving and present a less invasive alternative to surgery for infants and children for whom medical management fails. The most common approach is single- or double-balloon transseptal valvuloplasty, depending on the degree of stenosis and threat of procedure-induced mitral regurgitation. Complications following endovascular intervention include atrial perforation, cardiac tamponade, and cerebrovascular events. Children with concomitant mitral regurgitation are not good candidates for balloon valvuloplasty. Currently, endovascular approaches for mitral stenosis are palliative procedures, allowing children to grow before undergoing definitive mitral valve surgery.

Surgical Management

Mitral valve obstruction is rarely an isolated diagnosis; surgical repair is challenging and reserved for those who have failed medical management and early endovascular options. Valve repair is preferred over valve replacement due to the dynamic advantages a repair confers to a growing child. In cases of severe obstruction that are refractory to endovascular palliation, mitral valve replacement may be unavoidable. Outcomes for mitral valve replacement improve with age, although recent surgical advancements are promising.

The threshold to offering open-heart surgery depends on the pathology that is present and patients' response to nonsurgical options. Classically, mitral valve operations in the infant and child are reserved for those presenting with refractory congestive heart failure and pulmonary hypertension secondary to mitral obstruction. Other indications include the development of structural or electrical changes. Less complex operations, such as procedures to address isolated supramitral ring, are offered earlier, whereas complex operations with less predictable outcomes are approached more conservatively.

Open surgical repair of the mitral valve involves cardiopulmonary bypass and often proceeds through a left atrial or transseptal approach. Once the mitral apparatus can be visualized, the surgical repair is specific to the underlying pathology. Supramitral rings are amenable to sharp or blunt dissection and have a quite favorable prognosis. Parachute valves are less straightforward and involve papillary muscle division with or without papillary muscle reimplantation. Mitral atresia and severe mitral stenosis can be complex and may require chordal fenestration, leaflet extension, or any of the earlier techniques (Fig. 52.5).

The completed repair is immediately assessed under direct visualization and later off bypass using transesophageal echocardiography. The degree of residual obstruction and/or iatrogenic regurgitation is measured, and if it is unacceptable, the valve is either revised or replaced. Traditional prosthetics may suffice in the immediate postoperative period but carry a higher morbidity and mortality rate. Recently, externally stented bovine jugular vein valves placed into the mitral position as hybrid valves have shown promising results.[45] As the patient grows and experiences patient-prosthesis mismatch, the valve is expanded using catheter-based balloon dilation.

Postoperative Critical Care

Postoperative care is dictated by patient anatomy and physiology following repair. The management of children with residual postoperative mitral valve obstruction and little to no regurgitant

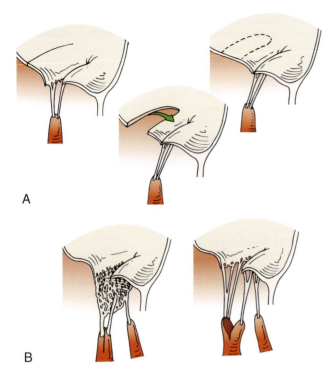

• **Figure 52.5** Surgical management of obstructive mitral pathologies. (A) Leaflet extension. (B) Chordal fenestration and papillary muscle splitting. (From Oppido G, Davies B, McMullan DM, et al. Surgical treatment of congenital mitral valve disease: midterm results of a repair-orientated policy. *J Thorac Cardiovasc Surg.* 6:1313-1320, 2008; with permission.)

flow follows the guidelines discussed earlier in "Medical Management." The primary goals of care are focused on pain management, optimizing volume status, and preventing both tachycardia and atrial arrhythmias. Benzodiazepines and fentanyl analgesics are standard during the first 24 hours postoperatively. Neuromuscular blockade may be necessary for stabilization in cases of reactive pulmonary circulation. Based on the degree of residual obstruction, left atrial pressures may remain elevated to facilitate left ventricular filling and cardiac output. Afterload reduction should not be used to increase cardiac output in this population. Forward flow is limited at the level of the atrioventricular orifice, not the aortic orifice. Afterload reduction is more likely to cause reflex tachycardia, which leads to decreased diastolic filling times, acute pulmonary congestion, and a further reduction in cardiac output. Maintaining sinus rhythm is essential for patients with mitral valve obstruction and may require the use of temporary epicardial pacing.

Complications specific to the surgical correction of mitral valve obstruction include arrhythmias and decreased cardiac output syndrome. As discussed earlier, these children are susceptible to arrhythmias due to left atrial dilation, increased left atrial pressures, and normal postoperative stress. Temporary epicardial pacing leads should be placed intraoperatively for all children. Low cardiac output syndrome is a constellation of symptoms that may include decreased cardiac index, oliguria, hypotension, lactic acidosis, and pulmonary congestion. This entity exists on the continuum with cardiogenic shock and is often caused by decreased left ventricular filling across a residual obstruction or right ventricular dysfunction secondary to pulmonary hypertension. A pulmonary artery catheter or Doppler echocardiography may help differentiate these two causes. Inotropes and/or pacing may be used for obstructions,

whereas interventions aimed at improving right ventricular function consist of correcting the underlying acidosis (hyperventilation), decreasing positive end-expiratory pressure if the patient is on mechanical ventilation, or adding nitric oxide.

If severe right heart dysfunction is observed in the operating room after repair, the sternum may be left open. The open chest decreases intrathoracic pressures and prevents direct myocardial compression in the setting of surgical edema. An open sternum also decreases the pulmonary vasculature resistance and facilitates gentler ventilatory settings while the heart recovers.

Regurgitant Lesions of the Mitral Valve

Mitral Valve Prolapse

Mitral valve prolapse occurs when the mitral leaflets coapt above the level of the annulus during systole. It is a rare condition in the newborn or child and is often associated with connective tissue disorders—classically Marfan syndrome—when present. Although simple mitral valve prolapse represents a benign finding, the condition may deteriorate to a regurgitant process with disease advancement or decreased left end-diastolic volume. The P2 leaflet is the most likely area to prolapse and is amenable to resection of the prolapse leaflet and primary repair with or without ring annuloplasty.

Mitral valve prolapse is often misdiagnosed in the child. Historically the mitral valve annulus was believed to be a planar two-dimensional structure. Because it is actually a three-dimensional nonplanar structure, the apparent level of the annulus changes with each echocardiogram window.[20] To prevent these errors, mitral valve prolapse is now defined as leaflet coaptation 2 mm above the annular plane in the parasternal long-axis view.[46] Mitral valve prolapse may also be misdiagnosed in cases of large atrial septal defects or other causes of decreased left end-diastolic volume. In these cases the left ventricular walls become unusually close, which positions the papillary muscles closer to the valvar apparatus, and adds slack in the chordae, resulting in the leaflets rising above the annulus. Correcting end-diastolic volumes usually corrects the perceived prolapse.

Cleft of the Mitral Valve

Clefts are abnormal divisions of the leaflets that rarely occur in isolation. The anterior leaflet is more commonly affected than the posterior leaflet and often presents with severe regurgitant flow. Transthoracic echocardiography with three-dimensional reconstruction helps differentiate clefts from prolapsed leaflets (Fig. 52.6). Surgical intervention is indicated for mitral clefts and relies on direct closure of the cleft with or without posterior annuloplasty (Fig. 52.7A).

Double-Orifice Mitral Valve

Double-orifice mitral valve occurs when a bridge of tissue divides the normal mitral annulus into two distinct left-sided atrioventricular canals.[47] Complete subtypes are characterized by a thick fibrous band that divides the orifice and makes contact with the annulus, whereas incomplete subtypes involve a thin membrane isolated to the free margins of the leaflets. Double-orifice mitral valve should not be mistaken for duplicate mitral valve, which involves duplication of the mitral apparatus (annuli, leaflets, chordae, and papillary muscles). Double-orifice mitral valve is usually discovered secondary to more immediate congenital cardiac defects. When it is found in isolation, 43% of cases present with progressively worsening regurgitation due to hypoplastic chordae and leaflets, 37% are asymptomatic, 13% have obstructive symptoms, and 7% have both obstructive and regurgitant symptoms.

Double-orifice mitral valve is best diagnosed through the visualization of two antegrade jets during diastole. Transthoracic echocardiography looking from the apex of the left ventricle to the base of the heart in the short axis serves as the most reliable window for making the diagnosis. Advancing the handle toward the base in the short axis or using three-dimensional reconstitution aids in categorization of the two subtypes. Operative intervention is indicated for symptomatic patients or those experiencing left atrial remodeling. Simple resection of the bridge worsens the regurgitant process and is not advised.[48] Each orifice should

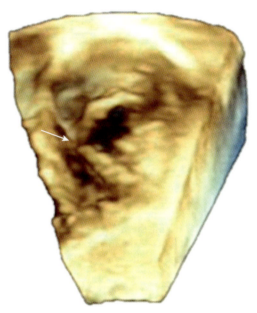

• **Figure 52.6** Three-dimensional echocardiogram image from a patient with partial atrioventricular canal and a large cleft in the anterior leaflet of the mitral valve *(arrow)*.

be repaired as if it were an independent valve. If in doubt, a residual regurgitant lesion is favored over iatrogenic stenosis. The majority of isolated double-orifice mitral valves can be managed medically.

Mitral Arcade or Hammock

Mitral arcade or hammock—given its intraoperative appearance—occurs when the chordae are thickened, fused, or completely absent. Mitral arcade stems from irregularities in chordae development at the early papillary muscle–leaflet interface. Unlike parachute or parachute-like asymmetric mitral valves, this pathology maintains a normal papillary muscle structure. Due to the underdeveloped chordae, the leaflets are restricted and primarily present as a regurgitant process. Patients may also have additional obstructive patterns on Doppler due to impeded flow through the chordae in the secondary mitral orifice. Surgical repair, when necessary, aims to relax the leaflets through chordae fenestration, papillary muscle division, and leaflet augmentation (see Fig. 52.5).

Pathophysiology of Mitral Insufficiency

In mitral regurgitation a fraction of the left ventricular end-diastolic volume is lost across the mitral valve during systole. To compensate for the decrease in cardiac output, heart rate, stroke volume, and ejection fraction increase. Because of the increase in stroke volume, there is a proportionate increase in regurgitation. This creates a positive feedback loop, accelerating heart failure in mitral insufficiency at an exponential rate. Chronic mitral regurgitation leads to left ventricular hypertrophy and dilation, left atrial dilation, pulmonary hypertension, and ultimately right ventricular dysfunction. Acute-onset mitral insufficiency due to chordae or papillary muscle rupture is not well tolerated and presents with flash pulmonary edema and reduced cardiac output.

Diagnosis of Mitral Insufficiency

The clinical diagnosis of mitral insufficiency and obstruction are somewhat similar, although distinguishable based on the presence of key physical examination findings. Both obstructive and regurgitant lesions present with the same chief complaints—fatigability,

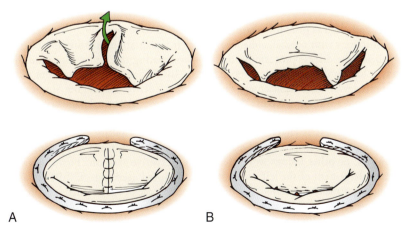

A   B

• **Figure 52.7** Surgical management of mitral insufficiency. The top figure represents the pathology and the bottom figure the corrected repair. (A) Cleft closure with or without a posterior annuloplasty ring. (B) Dilated annulus with reduction annuloplasty.

difficulty feeding, recurrent respiratory infections, and ultimately failure to thrive (see "Diagnosis of Mitral Valve Obstruction"). Mitral regurgitation can be identified by the characteristic high-pitched apical pansystolic murmur that radiates to the left axilla. There may also be a lower-frequency diastolic murmur and third heart sound in chronic cases when the left ventricle is dilated. In severe cases of acute-onset mitral regurgitation, cardiac output may dramatically fall and become refractory to medical management (afterload reduction, inotropes), requiring urgent surgical intervention.

The electrocardiogram often demonstrates signs of left ventricular hypertrophy and left atrial dilation. Chest radiography may reveal cardiomegaly, a third mogul or double-density sign, bronchial cuffing, and superior distribution of the pulmonary vasculature. In acute exacerbations, pulmonary edema with blunting of the phrenic angles may be present.

Echocardiography is the gold standard for diagnosing and monitoring mitral regurgitation. Measurement of the vena contracta provides insight regarding regurgitant volume. Furthermore, two-dimensional echocardiography plays an important role in measuring intracardiac pressures, determining the leaflet motion abnormalities, and identifying associated cardiac abnormalities. Three-dimensional echocardiography provides a complete view of the entire mitral apparatus, including planes that would otherwise be difficult to reach in two dimensions. Doppler facilitates characterization of the regurgitant waveform. Cardiovascular magnetic resonance imaging provides the finest anatomic and functional data but is less often used because it typically requires sedation or general anesthesia.

Medical Management

Medical management of mitral regurgitation is based on promoting cardiac output and preventing pulmonary edema. These goals are achieved through afterload reduction, inotropes, and diuresis. If the patient requires hospitalization for an acute exacerbation, intravenous inotropes and afterload-reducing antihypertensive medications should be used. Children who become refractory to outpatient management or who develop signs of end-organ damage, a left ventricular end-systolic z score greater than 5, or a shortening fraction of less than 33% should be considered surgical candidates.[49]

Surgical Management

Mitral regurgitation in the infant and child is primarily classified into three broad categories—insufficiency with normal, enhanced, or restricted leaflets. Conceptualizing the disease processes in this way helps explain the pathophysiology and guide surgical repair. Valve repair continues to be preferred over valve replacement due to reduced mortality and the dynamic advantages repairs confer to a growing child.

Mitral regurgitation with normal leaflets is characterized by annular dilation with an otherwise normal mitral apparatus. Dilated cardiomyopathies, ischemic injuries, or other lesions associated with systolic heart failure lead to enlargement of the left ventricle and annulus. The posterior annulus is normally a dynamic structure that contracts 20% to 40% during systole, helping the leaflets coapt. In the setting of dilated mitral regurgitation the annulus can no longer provide the centrally directed force it once did, and a central regurgitant jet develops. Surgical repair is focused on downsizing the annulus, bringing the leaflets closer together, and

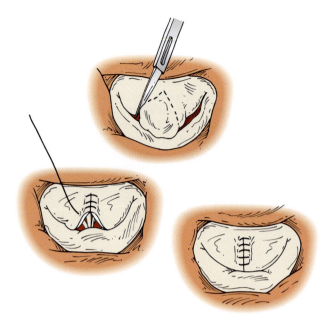

• **Figure 52.8** Primary surgical management of anterior or posterior mitral prolapse in an infant and child using triangular resection and direct reapproximation. (From Baird CW, Myers PO, del Nido PJ. Mitral valve operations at a high-volume pediatric heart center: evolving techniques and improved survival with mitral valve repair versus replacement. *Ann Pediatr Cardiol.* 5:13-20, 2012; with permission.)

increasing the area of coaptation. This is often accomplished with a posterior annuloplasty ring or annular plication, depending on the size of the patient and the degree of insufficiency (see Fig. 52.7B). If the ventricle has expanded sufficiently, the papillary muscles will follow, and the leaflets may display signs of a restricted pathology as well.

Enhanced mitral leaflet motion or prolapse results in coaptation above the mitral annulus. At that level the leaflets experience decreased surface area contact as well as perpendicular or normal forces during coaptation, resulting in mitral insufficiency. In the pediatric patient, anterior and posterior leaflet prolapse is reliably repaired through triangular leaflet resection (Fig. 52.8). A partial posterior annuloplasty ring may or may not be used to support the repair. In older children, anterior leaflet prolapse may not be amendable to simple resection, and polytetrafluoroethylene can be used to reapproximate the leaflet (Fig. 52.9).[50] Isolated mitral cleft, or an abnormal division of the leaflets, is repaired by reapproximating the leaflet edges and directly suturing them.

Insufficiency stemming from restricted leaflet motion presents a particularly challenging surgical scenario. When insufficiency stems from abnormal papillary muscles, as in the case of parachute mitral valve, the muscles are first split. If additional length is needed, the papillary muscles can be relocated. Cases of insufficiency that stem from fused or shortened chordae are again treated in a conservative fashion. First, chordal fenestration and freeing is attempted (see Fig. 52.5B). If additional length is desirable, neochordae or leaflet extensions may be performed (see Figs. 52.5A and 52.9).

Many of the principles discussed in the surgical management of obstructive mitral lesions can also apply to regurgitant lesions. The goal of early surgical repair, particularly in complex cases, is often palliative. When repairs become unsalvageable, hybrid valves

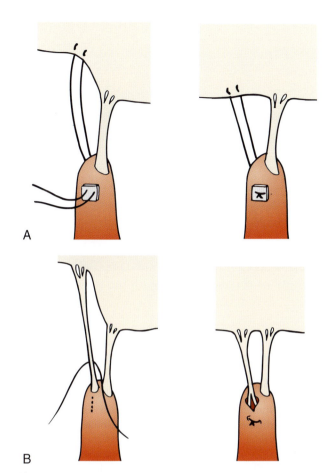

• **Figure 52.9** Advanced surgical management of mitral insufficiency using loop polytetrafluoroethylene (A) and chordal shortening (B). These techniques are reserved for older patients due to the risk of papillary muscle ischemia and restricted chordal growth. (From Oppido G, Davies B, McMullan DM, et al. Surgical treatment of congenital mitral valve disease: midterm results of a repair-orientated policy. *J Thorac Cardiovasc Surg.* 6:1313-1320, 2008; with permission.)

sewn into the mitral position may be used.[45] Definitive treatment in these cases is often mechanical valve replacement at a later time.

Postoperative Critical Care

Principles of postoperative care following operative treatment of regurgitant mitral valve pathology are similar to those for obstructive mitral disease as outlined earlier in the chapter.

Results

Mitral valve repair, when possible, remains preferable to replacement, due to improved survival and the dynamic nature that repairs confer. Five-year mortality and rate of reoperation following mitral repair are 4% to 7% and 10% to 37%, respectively, with only 8% to 10% of reoperations being replacements.[51,52] Five-year mortality

and rate of reoperation following initial mitral valve replacement are 11% to 27% and 10% to 42%, respectively.[53-56] Younger age at operation, mixed stenotic and regurgitant pathologies, and concomitant left ventricular outflow tract obstructions were all associated with the need for reoperation.[53,57]

Mitral Valve Replacement

Admittedly, mitral valve repair is not always possible. If a mechanical valve is placed in a child, prophylactic upsizing of the annulus to delay patient-prosthesis mismatch is generally not recommended. Evidence suggests that the mitral annulus continues to grow at the same rate with or without the introduction of a prosthetic valve.[58] Annular upsizing is associated with coronary artery stretching and an increased risk of complete heart block, which may require permanent pacemaker placement.[59] Collectively, these risks should warrant serious consideration when upsizing is being considered.

The threat of a thromboembolic events and stroke associated with valve replacement is not negligible. Reported incidences following mitral valve replacement in the infant are as high as 8% to 16%.[56,60-62]

Conclusion

Congenital mitral valve disease is rarely seen in isolation. It is more commonly associated with complex congenital defects, including Shone's complex, hypoplastic left heart syndrome, transposition of the great arteries, and connective tissue diseases. Symptoms vary based on the degree of obstruction or regurgitation. Obstructive pathologies are treated with diuretics and rhythm management, whereas insufficient pathologies depend on afterload reduction, inotropes, and diuretics. Operative intervention is indicated when medical management fails. Valve repair, not replacement, is the primary goal for congenital mitral valve disease based on the dynamic advantages it confers.

Selected References

A complete list of references is available at ExpertConsult.com.

30. Hertwig C, Haas NA, Habash S, et al. The "Polar Light Sign" is a useful tool to detect discrete membranous supravalvular mitral stenosis. *Cardiol Young.* 2015;25:328–332.
45. Emani SM, Piekarski BL, Zurakowski D, et al. Concept of an expandable cardiac valve for surgical implantation in infants and children. *J Thorac Cardiovasc Surg.* 2016;152:1514–1523.
49. Johnson JT, Eckhauser AW, Pinto NM, et al. Indications for intervention in asymptomatic children with chronic mitral regurgitation. *Pediatr Cardiol.* 2015;36:417–422.
51. Baird CW, Marx GR, Borisuk M, et al. Review of congenital mitral valve stenosis: analysis, repair techniques and outcomes. *Cardiovasc Eng Technol.* 2015;6:167–173.
56. Brown JW, Fiore AC, Ruzmetov M, et al. Evolution of mitral valve replacement in children: a 40-year experience. *Ann Thorac Surg.* 2012;93:626–633.

53

Heart Disease and Connective Tissue Disorders

CHARLES D. FRASER III; DUKE E. CAMERON; KRISTEN NELSON MCMILLAN;
LUCA A. VRICELLA

The genetic basis for heart and vascular conditions is heterogeneous and includes both heritable and de novo mutations. More than 100 genes associated with congenital or progressive cardiovascular abnormalities have thus far been identified. In recent years there has been a growing awareness of and focus on connective tissue diseases (CTDs) and associated cardiovascular pathology, particularly in children. These diseases are hereditary disorders of the connective tissues of the body.[1] Connective tissues are biologic tissues with an extracellular matrix (ECM) that serve to support and bind structures and organs across numerous systems. The ECM is a highly organized multimolecular structure that is essential for normal arterial tortuosity and aneurysm formation, with a risk of subsequent vascular (i.e., aorta and carotid artery) dissection and rupture. Furthermore, many CTDs also impose risk of structural heart defects, including patent ductus arteriosus (PDA), bicuspid aortic valve, coarctation of the aorta, and atrioventricular valve disease.

Children with CTDs are prone to aortic dissection, aneurysm, and aortic rupture.[2-5] In fact, aortic dissection is the primary cause of morbidity and mortality in the most common CTDs. Although incidences of cardiovascular manifestations vary by disease type, mortality following aortic catastrophe in these patients is exceptionally high, with up to 40% of pediatric patients dying immediately and 1% to 3% expiring every hour in the first 24 hours following the initial event. Should the child reach the operating room alive, operative mortality as high as 25% has been reported.[2] In response to these devastating statistics, various medical and surgical strategies have been developed to mitigate the risk of cardiovascular catastrophe by means of prophylactic intervention.

Advances in genetic analysis have had a significant impact on the identification and management of children with CTDs, providing a better understanding of the cause and phenotypes of disease, improving management strategies, and offering insights into long-term prognosis.[1] In this chapter we provide a description of the most common CTDs that affect the pediatric population and their associated cardiovascular pathology. We will focus on the most common forms of cardiovascular phenotype (namely proximal aortic pathology and mitral valve disease) to define surgical indications and operative management.

Diagnostic Syndromes and Associated Heart Disease

The most common CTDs affecting the cardiovascular system include Marfan syndrome (MFS), Loeys-Dietz syndrome (LDS), Ehlers-Danlos syndrome (EDS), osteogenesis imperfecta (OI), and other nonsyndromic conditions such as familial thoracic aortic aneurysmal disease. All CTDs carry varying degrees of risk for aortic dissection and other cardiovascular pathology and, as such, require close surveillance and management to avert the risk of cardiovascular catastrophe. Patients with CTDs and proximal aortic aneurysms will often require aortic root replacement (ARR) to prevent aortic dissection or rupture, often warranting surgical intervention at an early age. Although children and young adults with bicuspid aortic valves, conotruncal abnormalities, Turner syndrome, and other anomalies may need surgical replacement of the proximal aorta, they do not fall into the CTD syndromes described herein.

Marfan Syndrome

First described in 1896,[6] MFS is an inherited disorder resulting from mutations in the *FBN1* gene and most commonly affects the ocular, skeletal, and cardiovascular systems.[7,8] Although the syndrome is most commonly inherited in an autosomal dominant pattern, approximately 25% of cases result from de novo mutations.[8] MFS has a prevalence of 1 in 5,000 to 10,000. The syndrome is characterized by a high degree of clinical variability, although ocular, cardiovascular, and skeletal manifestation are the true hallmark of this disorder.

Up to 90% of patients with a clinical diagnosis of MFS have mutations in *FBN1,* a gene that codes for fibrillin 1.[1] Fibrillin 1 is a structural component of ECM microfibrils that provide mechanical stability and critical elastic properties to connective tissues.[9] Furthermore, more recent studies suggest that the fibrillin-deficient state of MFS leads to upregulation of the effects of the cytokine transforming growth factor beta (TGFβ), which then results in dysregulation of this signaling cascade. This derangement in signaling is thought to be responsible for the diverse and variable phenotypic expression of the disease.[10] Several hundred *FBN1*

Criteria for Marfan Syndrome Diagnosis From Revised Ghent Criteria

In the Absence of Family History

1. Ao z score ≥2 AND ectopia lentis = MFS
2. Ao z score ≥2 AND fibrillin 1 mutation = MFS
3. Ao z score ≥2 AND systemic score ≥7 = MFS
4. Ectopia lentis AND fibrillin 1 mutation = MFS

In the Presence of Family History

1. Ectopia lentis and a family history of MFS = MFS
2. Systemic score ≥7 and family history of MFS = MFS
3. Ao z score ≥2 (above 20 years of age), ≥3 (below 20 years of age) and family history of MFS = MFS

Ao, Aortic diameter at the sinuses of Valsalva above the indicated z score or aortic dissection; MFS, Marfan syndrome.

mutations responsible for altered fibrillin 1 structure have been reported, although no major correlation between the specific mutation and subsequent phenotypic manifestations have been identified. Furthermore, clinical variability exists even in patients with identical genotypic mutations, suggesting a potential role of modifier genes in the phenotypic expression of MFS.[10]

The clinical diagnosis of MFS is based on the revised Ghent criteria (Box 53.1).[11] These diagnostic criteria place a greater emphasis on cardiovascular manifestations than was done previously. The cardinal features of MFS based on the Ghent nosology are aortic root aneurysms and ectopia lentis. In the absence of family history the presence of these two clinical manifestations is alone sufficient for the diagnosis of MFS. In the absence of either aortic root aneurysm or ectopia lentis the presence of an *FBN1* mutation or a combination of systemic score of 7 or higher and family history of FMS is sufficient for diagnosis.[9,11] With a positive family history an isolated finding of ectopia lentis, aortic root enlargement, or a systemic score of 7 or higher suffices for diagnosis.[11]

Cardiovascular pathology is the leading cause of morbidity and early mortality in MFS.[1,12] The most prominent cardiovascular manifestations of MFS are mitral valve prolapse and aortic dilation. Mitral valve prolapse in MFS is thought to develop as a result of fibromyxomatous changes in the leaflets and chordae tendineae, calcification of the annulus, abnormal annular compliance and distensibility, and, in some cases, mitral valve enlargement.[13] These abnormalities result in prolapse of leaflets followed by mitral regurgitation (MR) and in severe cases, rupture of chordae tendineae.[14] Mitral valve pathology is the most common structural heart pathology encountered in MFS, but tricuspid valve prolapse, dilation of the proximal pulmonary artery, (supra)ventricular arrhythmias, and impaired systolic and diastolic left ventricular (LV) function are not uncommon.[1,10] *FBN1* mutations also lead to arterial aneurysm formation, particularly of the ascending aorta. Although the walls of the entire arterial tree are weakened, dilation most commonly occurs at the sinuses of Valsalva.[1,10,13] As the weakened proximal aorta dilates, aortic valve leaflet coaptation diminishes, and central regurgitation ensues. Eccentric regurgitation is seen when asymmetric enlargement of the root or cusp prolapse develops. These changes in the proximal aorta make aortic pathology the leading cause of mortality in MFS.[13]

Although most patients with MFS present in late childhood or adolescence, a more severe form of MFS (infantile MFS) has been described.[15] Infantile MFS typically presents with early onset of cardiovascular disease as well as severe skeletal manifestations, chest wall deformities, arachnodactyly, hyperextensible joints, micrognathia, and various ocular pathologies.[15] The most salient and life-threatening feature of infantile MFS is its aggressive vascular phenotype. As many as 61% of infants with this syndrome will have substantial cardiac abnormalities, with the most common being mitral valve prolapse and annular enlargement; these can in turn result in severe congestive heart failure, with failure to thrive and ventilator dependance.[15] In early series investigating infantile MFS, mitral valve prolapse was identified on echocardiography in the majority of these children, with almost all of these progressing to various degrees of MR. Thirty percent of these children will also manifest substantial proximal aortic root dilation.[15]

Nonsurgical cardiovascular management of MFS typically focuses on close follow-up of the vascular tree, aimed at monitoring of aortic diameters and prevention of dissection or rupture. In addition, medical management with losartan and beta-blockers is part of the routine long-term nonsurgical management strategy. Longitudinal imaging, afterload reduction, and congestive heart failure management are the cornerstone of medical therapy of mitral valve regurgitation, which remains the most common structural abnormality in these patients.[5,13] Guidelines for cardiovascular surveillance, indications for surgical intervention, and clinical follow-up strategies will be discussed later.

Over the past five decades, the life span of patients with MFS has markedly improved largely due to advances in both medical and surgical management of the cardiovascular manifestations of the disease.[12] With appropriate medical and, when necessary, surgical intervention the life expectancy of patients with MFS approaches that of the general population. However, this improvement in outcome is maximized when the patient receives comprehensive cardiovascular care by a multidisciplinary team with extensive knowledge and experience in the care of patients with CTDs.[1]

Loeys-Dietz Syndrome

LDS is an autosomal dominant CTD characterized by aortic aneurysms and generalized arterial tortuosity, hypertelorism, and bifid/broad uvula or cleft palate. It was first described in 2005.[16-18] Although the clinical features of this disorder share some similarities with MFS, LDS is caused by mutations in the genes encoding the transforming growth factor beta receptor 1 (*TGFBR1*) or 2 (*TGFBR2*).[19,20] Additional syndromic features may include craniosynostosis, Chiari malformation, clubfeet, PDA, and the potential for aneurysmal enlargement or dissection throughout the arterial tree.[10] In contrast to MFS, LDS less commonly presents with long bone overgrowth or lens dislocation. Additionally, aortic aneurysms in LDS tend to have accelerated growth when compared to those observed in MFS. As a consequence of this highly malignant vascular phenotype, children with LDS tend to present for surgical intervention at a younger age.

LDS results from mutations in the mothers against decapentaplegic homolog 3 (*SMAD3*) gene and the transforming growth factor beta 2 ligand gene (*TGFB2*), which lead in turn to anomalies of *TGFBR1* and/or *TGFBR2*. Chromosome deletions are responsible for these malformations, and the size of the microdeletion is thought to correlate with the broad spectrum of clinical presentation in LDS.[16] Although LDS can be divided into four types based on the specific mutation, significant clinical variability exists within and between individuals of each type, and therefore guidelines for management and treatment are similar across all types.

TABLE 53.1 Loeys-Dietz Syndrome (LDS) Subgroup Classification System

LDS Subtype	Gene	Other Disorders Reported
1	TGFBR1	Thoracic aortic aneurysm and dissection
2	TGFBR2	Thoracic aortic aneurysm and dissection, Marfan syndrome type 2
3	SMAD3	Aneurysms-osteoarthritis syndrome
4	TGFB2	Aortic and cerebral aneurysm, arterial tortuosity, and skeletal manifestations

• **BOX 53.2** Guidelines for Routine Clinical Care in Children With Loeys-Dietz Syndrome

Yearly echocardiography; shorter intervals depending on the extent of aortic disease

Angiotensin-receptor blockade, beta-blocker, or angiotensin-converting enzyme inhibitor for strict blood pressure control

Avoidance of contact/competitive sports, isometric exercises, strenuous exercise, blows to head/chest

Avoidance of stimulants and vasoconstrictors

Subacute bacterial endocarditis prophylaxis in those with artificial valves

Cardiac surgery consultation when surgical thresholds for intervention are approaching

Modified from Patel ND, Alejo D, Crawford T, et al. Aortic root replacement for children with Loeys-Dietz syndrome. Ann Thorac Surg. 2017;103(5):1513-1518. doi:10.1016/j.athoracsur.2017.01.053.

The main organ systems affected in LDS include skeletal, craniofacial, cutaneous, and cardiovascular. Indications for surgical intervention will be detailed in subsequent sections, but as compared to MFS, arterial dissection can occur at diameters smaller than those observed in MFS, implying a need for earlier surgical intervention in LDS.[1,10] Arterial tortuosity is observed throughout the entire arterial tree, and resulting complications may occur at any location. As a result, frequent and comprehensive surveillance as well as early surgical intervention is warranted.

Originally LDS patients were categorized into two types, depending on the prevalence and severity of craniofacial (type 1) or cutaneous (type 2) features. However, more recently, four types of LDS have been described based on genotype (Table 53.1). LDS types 1 and 2 have significant craniofacial anomalies and also the most severe cardiovascular manifestations of disease. Type 4 is the least severe form of LDS in terms of risk of cardiovascular catastrophe. The various subtypes of LDS, associated genetic mutations, and phenotype characteristics are summarized in Table 53.1.

Rapidly progressive aortic aneurysmal disease is a distinctive feature of LDS and can involve the ascending or descending aorta.[16] Aortic dissection has been reported in children as young as 3 months.[17] In fact, the initial reports of LDS types 1 and 2 described a mean age of death of 26.1 years, with aortic dissection and cerebral hemorrhage as the primary causes of death.[20] Although improvements in diagnosis, surveillance, and early interventions have improved the life span of affected individuals, the severity of the cardiovascular manifestations of LDS cannot be overstated. Congenital heart defects such as bicuspid aortic valve, atrial septal defects, and PDA are more commonly seen in children with LDS types 1 and 2 when compared with the general population. In addition to mitral valve prolapse and dysfunction, pulmonary root dilation and tricuspid valve regurgitation have been observed. Of note, children with LDS may require aortic or mitral valve interventions even without presence of aortic root dilation, given the severity of structural valve disease.[16] Atrial fibrillation, ventricular hypertrophy, ventricular arrhythmias, and heart failure have also been described.

In view of the vast cardiovascular expressions of disease, individuals diagnosed with LDS require echocardiography at frequent intervals (every 6 to 12 months) to monitor the status of heart valves, aortic root, and ascending aorta.[16] Additionally, frequent imaging with magnetic resonance angiography (MRA) or computed tomography angiography (CTA) with three-dimensional reconstruction is recommended to monitor the entire arterial tree for aneurysmal enlargement and dissection. Although MRA and CTA may expose the patient to ionizing radiation and anesthesia, serial imaging is critical to prevention of cardiovascular catastrophe. Many advocate for surveillance CTA or MRA every 1 to 2 years depending on severity of disease. Cameron et al. reported that 33% of their originally reported surgical cohort of LDS 1 and 2 required multiple vascular surgical interventions, highlighting the need for judicious, lifelong surveillance.[17]

Management of children with LDS mirrors that of children with MFS and is summarized in Box 53.2. However, given the aggressive nature of disease, thresholds for intervention tend to be lower than with MFS. Well-defined guidelines for surgical intervention are limited and vary slightly based on the type of LDS and the severity of disease. Aortic dissections have been reported in individuals with maximal aortic diameters of less than 4.0 cm in LDS types 1, 2, or 3 and at less than 5.9 cm in LDS type 4. Therefore, given the aggressive nature of the disease and relatively low rate of complications with proximal aortic surgery in experienced centers, ARR is indicated when the root diameter reaches a threshold of 4.0 cm for LDS types 1 and 2. In children with LDS type 3, which is caused by mutations in *SMAD3* and is moderately aggressive, ARR is recommended for aneurysms between 4.0 and 4.5 cm in size. LDS type 4 is the mildest phenotype, and therefore the threshold for intervention is slightly higher at 4.5 cm. Additionally, aneurysmal growth of greater than 0.5 cm/y warrants surgical intervention. However, regardless of type in these children, those with a concerning family history of aortic catastrophe and severe craniofacial features may warrant earlier intervention.[21]

Ehlers-Danlos Syndrome

EDS is inherited in an autosomal dominant pattern, affecting collagen synthesis with an estimated prevalence of 1 in 5000.[22] To date, six major subtypes of EDS have been described (Villefranche nosology).[10] Vascular EDS, also known as type IV EDS, results from mutations in the *COL3A1* gene, which affects type III collagen synthesis. Characteristic features of vascular EDS include thin, translucent skin; characteristic facial appearance (large eyes, small chin, sunken cheeks, thin nose and lips, lobeless ears); vascular fragility demonstrated by extensive bruising; easy bleeding; and spontaneous arterial, intestinal, or uterine rupture.[1,2,22-24] Cardiovascular manifestations of EDS include arterial aneurysms at any location throughout the arterial tree, mitral valve dysfunction, and venous malformations. The diagnosis of type IV EDS is based on clinical findings and confirmed by genetic analysis for the causative mutation or by identification of abnormal type III collagen synthesis.

The most common cause of death in EDS is secondary to aortic aneurysms and subsequent dissection or rupture, typically occurring in adulthood, with nearly 50% of all deaths in patients with type IV EDS attributable to aortic aneurysms.[25] Similar to MFS and LDS, management strategies are dictated by the presence of aortic aneurysms and/or structural heart disease. Indications for surgical intervention are discussed later and are similar to those for patients with MFS. Given the severity of this subtype of EDS, long-term follow-up is required, with frequent imaging surveillance of the heart, aorta, and arterial tree.

Osteogenesis Imperfecta

OI is a group of CTDs caused by a defective synthesis of collagen type I. Cardinal clinical features include blue sclerae, pathologic long bone fractures, conductive and sensorineural hearing loss, and dental abnormalities. Although cardiovascular involvement is a less common feature of OI, up to 12% of patients may have pathology of the left-sided heart valves and enlargement of the proximal aorta.[1] Mitral valve prolapse, for example, is present in up to 7% of patients with OI, and aortic regurgitation has been documented in up to 10% of these patients.[26] Although data are limited, cardiac surgery in OI patients portends worse outcomes compared with patients without CTDs, with mortality rates as high as 15% to 25% in some series.[26] Furthermore, as with other CTDs, tissue fragility leads to excessive bleeding and increased transfusion requirements in these patients as well as increased difficulty with valve repair. Screening with echocardiography in patients with OI should be considered to identify patients with valvular pathology or enlarged proximal aortas. Medical and surgical intervention guidelines are not well defined, but, given the nature of the disease, management guidelines similar to those previously described for CTDs are recommended.

Surgical Indications

Clinical indications for surgical interventions in children with CTDs vary based not only on type of disease but, in some cases, also on institutional guidelines. Although evidence exists for the management of more common CTDs, many have ill-defined surgical indications, and as such, surgeon- and center-specific preferences have emerged. In this section, indications for surgical intervention in proximal aortic aneurysms as well as mitral valve pathology in children with CTDs will be described.

Aortic Root Aneurysms

Indications for ARR in asymptomatic children are summarized in Table 53.2. Clearly these indications change in those children who present with symptoms, aortic dissection, rupture, or substantial pathology of the aortic valve.

The indications listed for MFS are in accordance with the 2010 multisociety guidelines.[11] Rupture and dissection are rare in prepubescent patients with MFS, so delaying intervention until later in childhood is reasonable. This is beneficial for many reasons, including that it allows annular growth to achieve a size of at least 2.0 cm; this diameter would accommodate a prosthetic valve compatible with adult life should a valve-sparing technique not be feasible.[27] Conversely, as described previously, patients with LDS (type 1 in particular) are at risk of aortic catastrophe earlier

TABLE 53.2	Summary of Indications for Valve-Sparing Aortic Root Replacement in Children
Diagnosis	**Criteria for VSRR in Children**
Marfan syndrome	Max diameter >5.0 cm or increase of >0.5 cm/y Diameter of 4.5-5.0 cm if: • Family history of or rupture • Aortic valve regurgitation • Need for mitral valve repair and aortic root 4.0-5.0 cm
Loeys-Dietz syndrome	
• LDS type I and II	Maximal diameter of >3.5-4.0 cm Increase in diameter of >0.5 cm/y Severe craniofacial features
• LDS type III	Maximal diameter of >4.0-4.5 cm Increase in diameter of >0.5 cm/y
• LDS type IV	Maximal diameter of >4.5 cm Increase in diameter of >0.5 cm/y
Bicuspid aortic valve	Maximal diameter >5.5 cm
Nonsyndromic thoracic aortic aneurysms	Maximal diameter >5.5 cm

LDS, Loeys-Dietz syndrome; *VSRR,* valve-sparing aortic root replacement.

in life and at smaller aortic diameters (<4.0 cm) and therefore require earlier surgical intervention. Indications for intervention in children with congenital heart disease are much more nebulous, given the extremely rare incidence of dissection and rupture in patients with conotruncal abnormalities. These patients will often present for surgical intervention because of aortic or neoaortic valve disease, rather than for progressive isolated enlargement of the aortic root.[27]

Mitral Valve Disease

Indications for intervention of mitral valve pathology in children with CTD are nebulous and with limited data support, particularly in asymptomatic children with mitral valve prolapse and/or MR. Signs and symptoms of heart failure in children with mitral valve disease and CTD indicate surgical intervention. Children with infantile MFS will often develop early evidence of heart failure as a result of the early onset of mitral valve dysfunction, and in many of these young children, mitral valve pathology will precede aortic dilation.[15] However, in many children with CTD, mitral valve disease will be discovered during longitudinal surveillance imaging and may not be symptomatic. In these patients, indications for surgery are less well understood, and many adapt strategies used in adults for the management of MR. Johnson et al. studied asymptomatic mitral valve regurgitation in children to identify risk factors for morbidity and mortality in this population. In their study the risk of late LV dysfunction and subsequent heart failure increases with preoperative LV end-systolic z score (LVESZ) and decreased LV function. To reduce the risk of progression to ventricular dysfunction and heart failure, they concluded that surgery should be pursued before LVESZ is 5 or higher and LV ejection fraction is 33% or lower. Serial echocardiography is therefore critical in these patients to identify disease progression.[28]

Aortic Root Procedures in Connective Tissue Diseases

Surgical intervention for aortic root aneurysms has evolved over recent decades. Historically, ARR with concomitant aortic valve replacement (the Bentall procedure) has been the universally accepted technique of choice for management of aortic root pathology. However, valve preservation by means of valve-sparing aortic root replacement (VSRR) is an attractive alternative to mechanical prostheses, particularly in children. Avoidance of anticoagulation, low risk of thromboembolism, endocarditis, and promising results at long-term follow-up make VSRR the ideal prophylactic procedure to limit the risk of aortic catastrophe, while avoiding the risks associated with prosthetic valves.[2,27,29-31]

As mentioned earlier, the gold standard treatment of patients with aortic root pathology has traditionally been aortic root and valve replacement. This technique, originally described by Bentall and De Bono in 1968,[32] eliminates the portion of aorta at greatest risk of aortic catastrophe with low operative complications and excellent long-term outcomes.[33] However, the limitations of this procedure are related to the adverse events associated with either the mechanical or bioprosthetic valves associated with these conduits. Operative techniques for valve preservation can be broadly categorized into either remodeling or reimplantation procedures, which denote whether the ARR Dacron graft sits atop the valve annulus (remodeling) or contains the entire valve complex starting just below the ventricular-aortic junction (reimplantation) (Fig. 53.1).[34,35] The remodeling technique (also known as Yacoub technique or David II) creates neoaortic sinuses that are theoretically advantageous

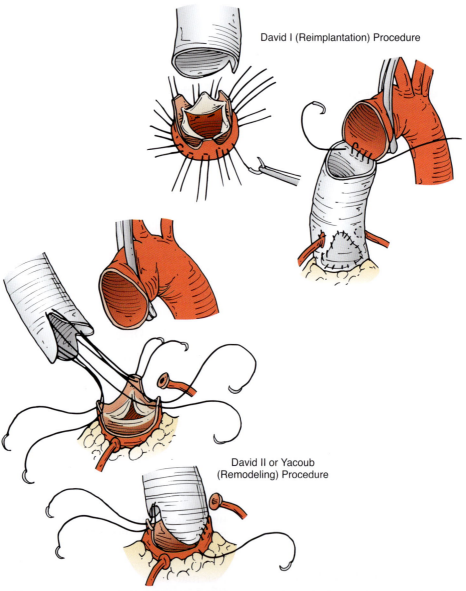

David I (Reimplantation) Procedure

David II or Yacoub (Remodeling) Procedure

• **Figure 53.1** Remodeling versus reimplantation techniques for valve-sparing aortic root reconstruction. In the aortic root remodeling procedure a scalloped Dacron graft is anastomosed to the sinus remnants, leaving the annulus unsupported. Conversely, in the reimplantation procedure the annulus and the aortic valve are contained and supported by the graft. (From Cameron D, Vricella L. Valve-sparing aortic root replacement with the Valsalva graft. *Oper Tech Thorac Cardiovasc Surg.* 2005;10[4]:259-271. doi:10.1053/j.optechstcvs.2005.11.001.)

to leaflet integrity but do not stabilize the annulus. This propensity for late enlargement of the aortic sinus remnants and annulus leads to aneurysmal dilation and aortic regurgitation. Subsequent modifications to remodeling techniques aimed at preventing the occurrence of this late complication, buttressing the annulus by suture or prosthetic strips to aid in annular stabilization.[36] Despite these modifications in technique, the outcomes following aortic root remodeling were mixed, and attention turned toward reimplantation strategies as a better technique, particularly for patients with CTDs.

Reimplantation VSRR techniques have evolved over many iterations and modifications of the original techniques pioneered by Tirone David. In the early iterations the reimplantation procedure used a straight Dacron tube graft (David I). This provides the annular stabilization lacking in remodeling techniques. The straight grafts lacks, however, sinuses that could relieve stress on the aortic valve following prosthetic ARR. The technique originally described by Dr. David has now been modified into its fifth iteration, the so-called David V procedure. To allow for annular stabilization and to reduce stress on the aortic valve, custom-designed prostheses have been used with sinuses incorporated into the proximal graft. The Valsalva graft (Gelweave Valsalva graft; Vascutek, Renfrewshire, Scotland, UK) is a commercially available aortic root prosthesis with three components: a collar with horizontally oriented crimps or pleats, a skirt with vertically oriented pleats that make the sinus segment more compliant, and a long tubular segment with horizontal pleats. Graft sizes range from 20 to 34 mm, which meets size requirements for most patients.

The technical aspects of the reimplantation VSRR strategy we employ have been described previously.[34] We approach repair via standard median sternotomy and initiate cardiopulmonary bypass via bicaval venous and distal ascending aortic cannulation. We routinely explore the right atrium in pediatric patients to evaluate for a patent foramen ovale. The patient is cooled to 28°C, and, as most patients in our experience have competent aortic valves, cold blood cardioplegia is administered in antegrade fashion after cross-clamping. The aorta is transected just above the sinotubular junction (STJ), and the ascending aorta is excised up to within 1 to 1.5 cm of the aortic cross-clamp. Stay sutures are placed 4 to 5 mm cephalad to the top of each of the aortic valve commissures, and the root is mobilized from the right ventricular outflow tract with care to also avoid injury to the left main coronary artery and right branch pulmonary artery.

After aortic root mobilization, valve sizers are used to assess optimal STJ diameter for prosthesis sizing. Most pediatric patients in our experience have CTD and will present with dilated sinuses and competent aortic valves. Our approach is to preserve or slightly reduce the STJ diameter to maintain leaflet apposition and valve competence. The sinuses are excised leaving 4 to 5 mm remnant along the annulus. It is important for the surgeon to leave enough rim of aortic wall above the valve to facilitate subsequent reimplantation of the valve onto the graft. Three subanular pledgetted horizontal mattress sutures are placed from within the LV outflow tract directly below the nadir of each leaflet and out through the subannular level of the LV outflow tract. It is crucial that the dissection around the base of the aorta enable the graft to effectively contain the ventriculoaortic junction. These three sutures are then brought through the base of the Valsalva graft (Fig. 53.2). The commissural posts are reimplanted at equal distance along the distal circumference of the pseudosinuses, recreating the ideal geometry of the root-valve aortic complex. In the authors' experience, only three subannular sutures are needed for aortic root fixation within

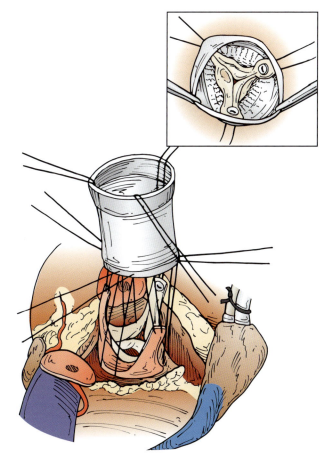

• **Figure 53.2** In the reimplantation technique (Johns Hopkins modification), three subannular sutures are placed through the base of the graft. (From Cameron D, Vricella L. Valve-sparing aortic root replacement with the Valsalva graft. *Oper Tech Thorac Cardiovasc Surg.* 2005;10[4]:259-271. doi:10.1053/j.optechstcvs.2005.11.001.)

the graft (although some other experts use six such sutures, with the additional three placed below the nadir of each commissure), avoiding the complexity of a circumferential subanular interrupted suture line.

Next (Fig. 53.3) the sinus remnants are reimplanted within the base of the graft with a running suture, constituting the hemostatic, internal suture line. (Some have suggested "marking" the location for the sinus implantation on the inside of the graft with a marking pen to provide a guide for preserving symmetric height of each valve within the conduit). Valve competence should then be assessed because malposition of the commissure or distortion of the annulus can lead to poor leaflet coaptation and regurgitation. The right and left coronary artery buttons are then anastomosed to corresponding sites within the left and right pseudosinuses (Fig. 53.4). We use circumferential Teflon strips to reinforce these suture lines and the distal graft-aortic anastomosis (Fig. 53.5) to minimize bleeding and late pseudoaneurysm formation.

Postoperatively patients are treated with low-dose aspirin for 2 months, whereas patients with CTD are usually maintained on beta-blockers and angiotensin receptor blockers (ARBs) indefinitely (see additional considerations later). A predischarge echocardiogram is obtained, followed by annual examinations thereafter. Additionally, antibiotic prophylaxis for endocarditis is often indicated because many children will have trivial or mild aortic insufficiency.[34]

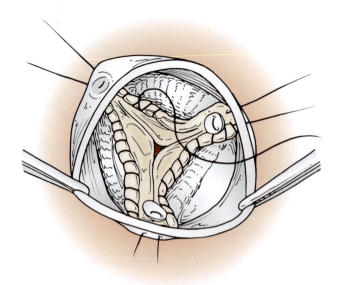

• **Figure 53.3** A running monofilament suture is used to resuspend the sinus remnants within the Dacron prosthesis with pseudosinuses as the hemostatic suture line. (From Cameron D, Vricella L. Valve-sparing aortic root replacement with the Valsalva graft. *Oper Tech Thorac Cardiovasc Surg.* 2005;10[4]:259-271. doi:10.1053/j.optechstcvs.2005.11.001.)

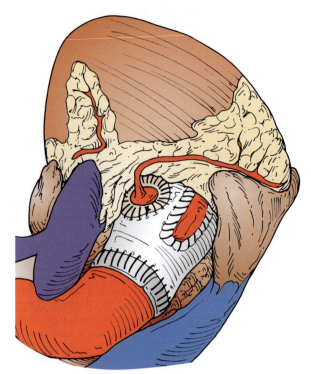

• **Figure 53.5** Completed reimplantation valve-sparing root replacement. (From Cameron D, Vricella L. Valve-sparing aortic root replacement with the Valsalva graft. *Oper Tech Thorac Cardiovasc Surg.* 2005;10[4]:259-271. doi:10.1053/j.optechstcvs.2005.11.001.)

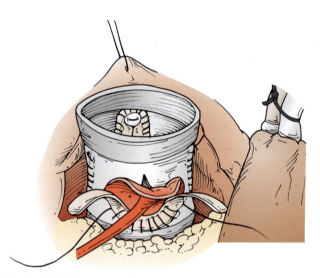

• **Figure 53.4** The coronary artery buttons are reimplanted on corresponding sites on the graft. The suture line is reinforced with circumferential Teflon felt strips to aid in hemostasis and possibly in the prevention of late pseudoaneurysms. The size of the buttons is kept to a minimum, to prevent late true aneurysmal dilation. (From Cameron D, Vricella L. Valve-sparing aortic root replacement with the Valsalva graft. *Oper Tech Thorac Cardiovasc Surg.* 2005;10[4]:259-271. doi:10.1053/j. optechstcvs.2005.11.001.)

Bicuspid Aortic Valves and Valve Repair

In pediatric patients requiring VSRR a small portion will present with bicuspid aortic valves. Our approach in children has been that of pursuing VSRR in the absence of significant calcifications and stenosis or if a complex repair is not necessary to address regurgitation.[27] When reimplanting bicuspid aortic valves, maintenance of valve geometry is critical when the posts are suspended within the graft (Fig. 53.6). In regard to valve repair, we do not

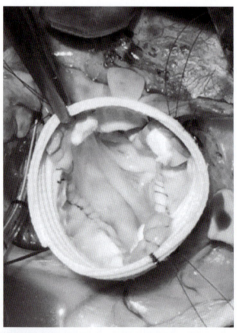

• **Figure 53.6** Completed reimplantation valve-sparing root replacement in a child with a competent bicuspid aortic valve. (From Vricella LA, Cameron DE. Valve-sparing aortic root replacement in pediatric patients: lessons learned over two decades. *Semin Thorac Cardiovasc Surg Pediatr Card Surg Annu.* 2017;20:56-62. doi:10.1053/j.pcsu.2016.10.001.)

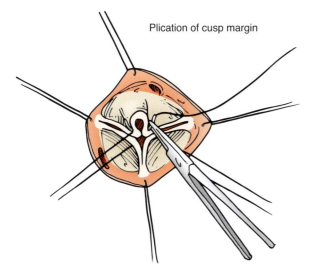

Plication of cusp margin

• **Figure 53.7** Bicuspid aortic valve plication in valve-sparing aortic root replacement. (From Vricella LA, Cameron DE. Valve-sparing aortic root replacement in pediatric patients: lessons learned over two decades. *Semin Thorac Cardiovasc Surg Pediatr Card Surg Annu.* 2017;20:56-62. doi:10.1053/j.pcsu.2016.10.001.)

advocate VSRR when a complex bicuspid valvuloplasty is indicated. However, when necessary, we have used plication of the free margin at the midpoint (Fig. 53.7) with a Gore-Tex suture to achieve rise in the height of the cusp and of the coaptation in the case of prolapse. This is performed following completion of the internal suture lines so that valve geometry can be fully assessed.[27]

Aortic Arch Repair

Most children will not require aortic arch repair at the time of VSRR. However, some children with more severe CTD phenotypes and large arches may require both aortic root and arch replacements. Arch replacement is typically performed with the patient under deep hypothermia (<24°C) with selective antegrade cerebral perfusion, and if needed, limited periods of circulatory arrest. We have not performed and do not advocate prophylactic aortic arch replacement for children with CTD undergoing ARR who do not meet aortic arch replacement criteria because only a minority of children in our experience go on to develop significant late arch enlargement following VSRR.[27]

Simultaneous Repair of Pectus Excavatum

When physiologically and cosmetically important, pectus excavatum deformities can be addressed at the time of aortic root intervention. We have performed concomitant modified Nuss procedure in a small number of children undergoing VSRR. A Gore-Tex membrane is interposed between the anterior cardiac structures and the Nuss bar before chest closure.[27] In these children, postoperative pain management is crucial, and a thoracic epidural may be beneficial to avoid pulmonary complications and aid in early mobilization.

Outcomes Following Valve-Sparing Aortic Root Replacement

Published data on long-term outcomes following VSRR in children with CTD are limited. Recently our institution completed its 100th pediatric VSRR. Within this cohort of patients, nearly 80%

of children had confirmed CTD. Perioperative mortality was 3%. Of 100 children, only 8 required subsequent aortic surgery due to progressive aortic arch dilation at an average of 7.2 years after VSRR. Additionally, only 5.9% of patients who underwent a reimplantation VSRR developed late aortic insufficiency requiring late aortic valve replacement. Six children developed pseudoaneurysms of their aortic grafts requiring reoperation, with 4 of these children having CTD. One child developed pseudoaneurysms at the coronary button anastomoses requiring revision of the anastomoses without complication. The reimplantation VSRR is a safe and effective surgical strategy in children with CTD and avoids the potential adverse effects associated with prosthetic aortic valves. Late aortic insufficiency and pseudoaneurysm formation remain a late concern, and as such, diligent postoperative follow-up with multidisciplinary care teams is warranted.

Mitral Valve Procedures in Connective Tissue Diseases

Pediatric patients with CTDs will often present in early childhood with aortic root enlargement, MR, or both.[45] MR is often the mode of early clinical presentation in patients with severe infantile MFS,[15,38] whereas patients with LDS and other CTDs will more frequently present with aortic root enlargement.[17,20] Whereas aortic disease is the known culprit of premature sudden death in the majority of CTDs, mitral valve dysfunction is the most common cause of morbidity and mortality in infantile MFS.[14,39] In these children, mitral valve pathology usually manifests with severe bileaflet mitral valve prolapse and annular and LV enlargement.

Data investigating outcomes following mitral valve surgery in children with CTDs are limited. Mitral valve replacement in children with CTD has been associated with high rates of reoperation, complications resulting from chronic anticoagulation, and mortality at both short- and long-term follow-up.[40] Rates of reoperation for subsequent mitral valve replacement and long-term mortality are as high as 20% and 40%, respectively, in previous reports.[40,41] Mitral valve repair, rather than replacement, is intuitively the preferred surgical approach in these growing children for many of the reasons discussed earlier regarding the disadvantages of prosthetic valves.[37,42]

Several techniques have been used to correct MR in the setting of bileaflet prolapse in children, this being the main structural abnormality in children with CTD and MR.[43] In children with CTDs, repairs involving the valve leaflets or subvalvular cordal apparatus are often difficult and require a substantial learning curve, particularly for surgeons who primarily focus on congenital heart disease.[44] Consequently, employing these more complex techniques may result in a higher rate of repair failure or a lower threshold for valve replacement.[39] Our group has therefore used a simplified approach to mitral valve repair in this particular group of young patients. This experience has been recently published, with 18 children with CTD undergoing mitral valve repair, with 1 death and 94.4% of patients experiencing resolution of MR at median follow-up time of 2.4 years (range, 0 to 13.9 years).[37]

All operations are performed with conventional cardiopulmonary bypass, mild to moderate hypothermia, aortic cross-clamping, and cardioplegic arrest. Because some patients with CTD will require additional intervention on the aortic root/valve or arch, mitral valve repairs are performed before intervening on other structures. If the mitral valve is in fact unrepairable, the option of then sparing the aortic valve becomes less imperative. The preferred technique

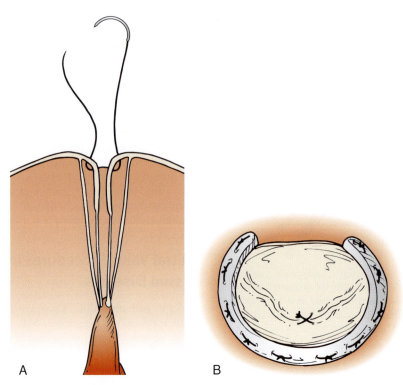

A   B

• **Figure 53.8** Edge-to-edge mitral valve repair and ring annuloplasty. (A) Sagittal view: the anterior and posterior leaflets are brought together by a figure-of-eight full-thickness suture across the zone of apposition between the two leaflets and away from their free margin. (B) En face view of the mitral valve following a completed ring annuloplasty edge-to-edge valve repair. (From Vricella LA, Ravekes WA, Arbustini E, et al. Simplified mitral valve repair in pediatric patients with connective tissue disorders. *J Thorac Cardiovasc Surg.* 2017;153[2]:399-403. doi:10.1016/j.jtcvs.2016.09.039.)

for mitral valve repair at our institution consists of a ring mitral annuloplasty and an edge-to-edge valvuloplasty, first described by Alfieri and colleagues.[45,46] The combination of edge-to-edge repair and anuloplasty stabilizes and moderately downsizes the annulus, corrects the prolapse, and typically prevents systolic anterior motion (SAM), while avoiding mitral stenosis (Fig. 53.8).[37,46,47] It is important (see Fig. 53.8A) to place the full-thickness suture away from the free margin of the leaflets to allow for downward displacement of the zone of apposition between anterior and posterior leaflets, preventing prolapse while avoiding SAM.[37]

Following correction of MR, children with CTDs may demonstrate some initial hemodynamic limited tolerance to the correction of regurgitation and resulting acute increase in LV afterload, often requiring substantial inotropic support and afterload reduction in the immediate postoperative period. The intermediate-term results of this simplified approach are promising; we have observed a significant reduction in LV end-diastolic dimension, from a mean z score of 4.9 to 1.3 at approximately 2 years post repair. Furthermore, over 90% of patients with severe preoperative MR had documented mild or less MR on follow-up echocardiography.[37] Comparatively, results of mitral valve replacement in children have inferior outcomes with a high incidence of reoperation and higher mortality rates.[39,40]

Although there are limited long-term data on mitral valve repair in children with CTDs, the technique described herein offers a simplified strategy for effective correction of MR from complex mitral valve prolapse. It avoids SAM of the anterior mitral leaflet with resultant LV outflow obstruction and postoperative mitral stenosis and allows the surgeon to effectively and quickly address MR in this unique group of pediatric patients, who will often require concomitant cardiovascular interventions in the setting of often-limited cardiopulmonary reserve.[37]

Preoperative and Postoperative Considerations

To prevent progression of aneurysm formation, patients with LDS and MFS in particular are placed on ARB agents, such as losartan or irbesartan. These agents block TGFβ activity, which has been implicated in vascular aneurysm formation. For mildly affected older children and adults, losartan by itself is often used. For very severely affected young children, it is often routine now to use ultra–high-dose irbesartan.

Beta-blocker therapy may also be part of the regimen as a means to decrease aortic wall stress. Atenolol is a beta-blocker that is commonly used; however, it has a number of potential side effects. Therefore it is usually added to the medication regimen only when ARB therapy has been maximized and ongoing aneurysm or root dilation progression is documented or if it is needed to address a rhythm issue. Preoperatively, discontinuation of ARB therapy for 3 to 5 days before surgery may decrease postoperative hypotension. If ARB and/or beta-blocker therapy is continued up until the time of surgery, postoperative hypotension may be due to residual medication effect.

For patients who require repair of descending aortic aneurysms, an additional anesthetic consideration is placement of a lumbar drain for thoracic or thoracoabdominal aneurysm repair, which may be performed (often by an anesthesiologist) the night before surgery or just before the repair. Aortic cross-clamping can increase cerebrospinal fluid (CSF) pressure, potentially decreasing spinal cord perfusion pressure. Draining CSF from the lumbar region may lessen the CSF pressure, improve blood flow to the spinal cord, and reduce the risk of ischemic spinal cord injury during repair of descending aortic aneurysms.

Postoperative Management in the Intensive Care Unit

Surgery for CTDs treats the manifestations of the disease and does not treat the disease. Patients with aortic, aortic valvar, or mitral pathology due to CTDs will bring their repaired heart to the intensive care unit (ICU) and still have the underlying challenges of CTD. They may be even more susceptible than non-CTD patients to variations in blood pressure, afterload, and force of LV contraction. Blood pressure management is often advised to control the risk of bleeding, particularly in the immediate postoperative period. Consideration of choice of vasoactive infusions for these patients to control hypertension should take into account the impact on wall stress. For example, in MFS mice treated with calcium channel blockers (CCBs), accelerated aneurysm expansion, rupture, and premature death occur. Furthermore, patients with MFS and other forms of inherited thoracic aortic aneurysm taking CCBs display increased risk of aortic dissection and need for aortic surgery compared with patients taking other antihypertensive agents. Therefore the most common antihypertensive infusions used in the cardiac ICU for these patients are esmolol or nitroprusside. The use of beta-blockers in particular can be useful to control the force of LV contraction and may be more prudent than afterload reduction (if cardiac output is otherwise normal). For patients with hypotension, use of vasopressin or low-dose catecholamine infusion may improve blood pressure without significant increase in vessel wall stress through avoidance of tachycardia. Following mitral valve repair for severe mitral insufficiency, afterload reduction for the LV is typically helpful (most often in the form of milrinone in the ICU), and many of these patients with CTDs should be managed in the intermediate and long term with losartan or beta-blockers as noted earlier.

It is imperative to assess postoperative extremity movement in patients who have had descending aortic aneurysm repair. For those patients with a lumbar drain, complications from lumbar drainage, such as hematoma formation, may also mimic signs of iatrogenic spinal cord ischemia. Computed tomography (CT) or magnetic resonance imaging (MRI) may be necessary to differentiate between ischemia and hematoma-induced neurologic injury.

Because of the relative fragility of the tissue, "late" bleeding can result in pseudoaneurysm, and this can require careful surgical reintervention. Follow-up surveillance with chest x-ray examination that demonstrates an enlarging mediastinal shadow can be an indication for a CT or MRI scan to evaluate for a contained but expanding false aneurysm.

Heart block and other rhythm disturbances are unusual in the immediate postoperative period, although any time there is major aortic root reconstruction, the risk of heart block needs to be considered, and the use of prophylactic pacing wires is typical. Bleeding, when it persists after the patient is returned to the ICU, needs to be conveyed in a timely manner to the surgical team because they will be most familiar with potential "troublesome" areas in the suture lines that might warrant reexploration. In general, these patients can be extubated early and will have normal hemodynamics (or return of normal hemodynamics in a short time frame), and with appropriate pain management they can be moved quickly through their hospital course.

Summary

Children with CTDs will often present with cardiovascular disease necessitating intervention, most commonly in the form of aortic aneurysms. Management of proximal aortic disease in these patients has evolved over the past three decades, and in current practice, valve preservation can be achieved with excellent results. Additionally, children with CTDs may also develop structural heart disease, including mitral valve pathology. When indicated, surgical management of valvular disease in children with progressive valve incompetence is critical to reducing morbidity and mortality. Valve preservation should be performed when possible to avoid the associated complications of prostheses in either the aortic or mitral positions. Finally, children with CTDs require long-term, longitudinal follow-up with both serial imaging and a multidisciplinary treatment team because these are systemic diseases with numerous affected organ systems.

References

A complete list of references is available at ExpertConsult.com.

54

Aortopulmonary Window; Hemitruncus

INDER D. MEHTA, MD; PRASHOB PORAYETTE, MD, MSC; RAMON JULIO RIVERA, MD;
AMULYA BUDDHAVARAPU, MD; CHRISTOPHER MEHTA, MD

Epidemiology

Aortopulmonary (AP) window, also known as AP septal defect, is a persistent communication between the walls of the intrapericardial aorta and pulmonary trunk due to failure of closure of the embryonic AP foramen. AP window was first described by J. Elliotson in 1830.[5] This abnormality occurs during septation of the truncus arteriosus into the pulmonary artery and aorta[1,2] and is associated with two separate semilunar valves. It is a rare congenital anomaly representing only 0.1% to 0.2% of all congenital heart disease.[3] Some studies have shown a male preponderance (2 : 1).[3] It is associated with additional congenital heart anomalies in approximately 50% of cases, the most common being an interrupted aortic arch (IAA).[4] The first successful surgical closure of AP window was reported by Robert Gross[6] in 1952.

Classification

According to the classification by Mori et al.,[7] there are three subtypes of AP window. Type I consists of a proximal defect close to the sinotubular junction, with very little inferior rim above the semilunar valves. Type II defines a distal defect toward the margins of the pericardial reflection, with absence of a superior rim at the pulmonary artery bifurcation. Type III refers to a large defect that extends from the semilunar valves to the pulmonary artery bifurcation. In 1979 Richardson et al.[4] proposed a classification similar to Mori's classification. Types I and II remained the same. The Richardson type III describes the anomalous origin of pulmonary artery (AOPA) directly from the ascending aorta. This type is erroneously referred to as "hemitruncus" but is no longer recognized as a morphologic variant of truncus arteriosus because there are two semilunar valves. The Society of Thoracic Surgeons Congenital Heart Surgery Database Committee accepted the original Mori classification with the addition of a fourth subtype, an "intermediate" defect, consisting of a smaller, central defect with a circumferential rim of tissue, and proposed that aortic origin of either pulmonary artery be classified as a separate defect[8] (Figs. 54.1 to 54.4).

Embryology

The septum dividing the truncus is formed proximally by the fusion of the distal right and left truncal wall cushions forming two channels (aortic and pulmonary) and distally by the contributions from the fourth and sixth aortic arches. The aortic channel aligns distally with the fourth arch to form the aorta, and the sixth aortic arch aligns with the other channel to form the pulmonary artery. This results in complete septation of the truncus arteriosus with separate aorta and pulmonary artery and with two separate semilunar valves. AP window and anomalous origin of pulmonary artery from the aorta occur due to deficiency in the septation of the truncus arteriosus during embryologic development.[9]

Some authors have suggested that it is incorrect to describe the lesions as "aortopulmonary septal defects" due to the separate nature of formation of the walls of the intrapericardial arterial trunks. There is no known stage in embryogenesis, with a complete septum formed between the cavities of the arterial trunks.[10] Hence, the AP window is described as a persistence of the embryonic AP foramen from a failure of fusion of distal cushions with each other, or the arterial spine formed from the fourth and sixth aortic arches.

Proximal AP window (type I) can occur due to failure of fusion of the truncal wall cushions, whereas distal defect (type II) and AOPA can result from abnormal migration of the sixth aortic arch.[3,9,11-14]

Morphology

AP window is most commonly a single communication between the intrapericardial portions of the aorta and the pulmonary artery and usually is located a few millimeters above the two separate semilunar valves.[3,13] It may be round, oval, or spiral and may vary in size from a few millimeters to over a centimeter. It is characterized by the presence of proximal separate walls of aorta and pulmonary artery with two distinct roots.[2]

In AOPA a single pulmonary artery (most commonly the right pulmonary artery) arises anomalously from the ascending aorta, most often from the posterior or posteromedial aspect of the ascending aorta, a short distance above the sinotubular junction. This anomaly is associated with two separate semilunar valves, and therefore the term *hemitruncus* is misleading because this is not a lesion with a common arterial "trunk" but rather simply an anomalous origin of a branch pulmonary artery from the aorta.[12]

Associated Lesions

Additional congenital heart lesions are present in up to 50% of patients with AP window[15] and commonly are related to obstruction to systemic or pulmonary outflow. The most common associated defect is interrupted aortic arch (most commonly type A). The

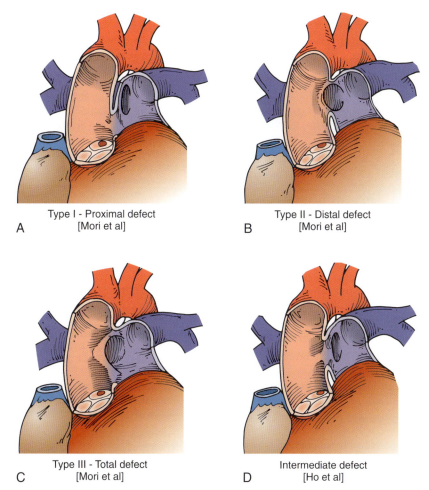

Type I - Proximal defect
[Mori et al]
A

Type II - Distal defect
[Mori et al]
B

Type III - Total defect
[Mori et al]
C

Intermediate defect
[Ho et al]
D

• **Figure 54.1** Types of aortopulmonary window, according to the Society of Thoracic Surgeons Congenital Heart Surgery Nomenclature and Database Project. (A) Type I consists of a proximal defect with very little inferior aortopulmonary septum above the semilunar valves. (B) Type II is a distal defect with absence of the superior septum. (C) Type III is a large defect that spans from the semilunar valves to the pulmonary artery bifurcation. (D) An intermediate aortopulmonary window is a central defect with proximal and distal septal rims. (From Jacobs JP, Quintessenza JA, Gaynor JW, et al. Congenital heart surgery nomenclature and database project: aortopulmonary window. *Ann Thorac Surg.* 2000;69:S44-S49.)

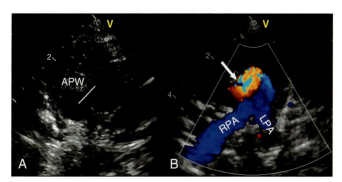

• **Figure 54.2** Echocardiographic assessment of aortopulmonary window. (A) Suprasternal view showing the aortopulmonary window (*APW*) type I visualized as a "dropout" (*white line*) between the ascending aorta and main pulmonary artery. (B) Color shows the turbulent antegrade systolic flow into the main pulmonary artery (*white arrow, red flow*) and branch pulmonary arteries (*blue flow*). *LPA,* Left pulmonary artery; *RPA,* right pulmonary artery.

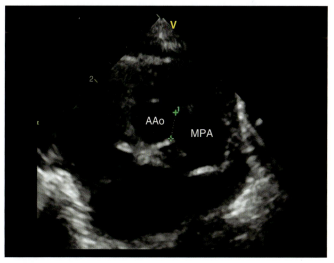

• **Figure 54.3** Echocardiographic assessment of aortopulmonary window. Suprasternal view showing the aortopulmonary window type I visualized as a "dropout" (*green dashed line*) between the ascending aorta (*AAo*) and main pulmonary artery (*MPA*).

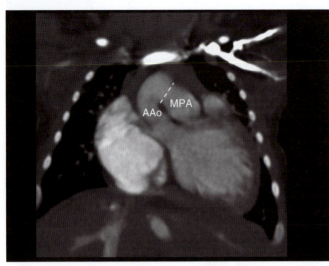

• **Figure 54.4** Aortopulmonary window. Cardiac computed tomography angiogram shows aortopulmonary window type II between the ascending aorta *(AAo)* and bifurcation of main pulmonary artery *(MPA)*.

TABLE 54.1	Associated Spectrum of Congenital Cardiovascular Anomalies With Aortopulmonary Window		
Anomaly		*n*	**% of All Patients**
Anomalies of aortic arch		21	51
Interrupted aortic arch at isthmus		5	12
Interrupted aortic arch between left common carotid and left subclavian artery		1	2
Aortic coarctation		4	10
Aortic isthmal hypoplasia		3	7
Aortic atresia		1	2
Right aortic arch		4	10
Double aortic arch		1	2
Anomalous origin of right subclavian artery		1	2
Left subclavian artery from pulmonary trunk		1	2
Ventricular septal defect		7	17
Atrial septal defect		15	36
Patent arterial duct		16	38
Anomaly of pulmonary outflow		8	19
Stenosis of pulmonary arteries		3	7
Tetralogy of Fallot (1 with nonconfluent pulmonary arteries)		2	5
Pulmonary valvar stenosis		1	2
Aortic origin of right pulmonary artery		1	2
Isolated left pulmonary artery from duct		1	2
Left ventricular outflow obstruction		4	10
Subaortic stenosis		3	7
Aortic valvar stenosis		1	2
Persistent left superior caval vein to coronary sinus		3	7
Superior-inferior ventricular relationship		2	5
Coronary arterial anomaly		2	5
Right coronary artery from pulmonary trunk		1	2
Absent left coronary orifice		1	2
Mitral valvar and pulmonary venous stenosis		**1**	**2**

Modified from Bagtharia R, Trivedi KR, Burkhart HM, et al. Outcomes for patients with an aortopulmonary window, and the impact of associated cardiovascular lesions. *Cardiol Young.* 2004;14(5):473-480

combination of distal AP window, AOPA, intact ventricular septum, and IAA is described as Berry syndrome.[18,19]

1. Some other commonly associated lesions that have been reported include patent ductus arteriosus, septal defects, Tetralogy of Fallot, coronary abnormalities, and transposition of great arteries.[13,15,18,20-23]

2. AP window has also been reported with extra cardiac anomalies as part of the VATER association (vertebral defects, imperforate anus, tracheoesophageal fistula with esophageal atresia, radial and renal dysplasia).[28,29]

3. The spectrum and frequency of association of cardiovascular lesions with AP window was well studied by Bagtharia et al[23] as shown in Table 54.1.

4. Of note, Tetralogy of Fallot[20] can be difficult to diagnose because AP window allows a significant amount of blood to shunt into the pulmonary circulation, providing adequate palliation for tetralogy of Fallot until significant pulmonary vascular disease develops. Right aortic arch is commonly present in patients with AP window with tetralogy of Fallot, and the presence of a right aortic arch with AP window should alert providers to rule out tetralogy.

Extracardiac anomalies associated with AP window have rarely been reported with VATER association (vertebral defects, imperforate anus, tracheoesophageal fistula with esophageal atresia, radial and renal dysplasia).[28,29]

The AOPA may be associated with AP window, as mentioned above, or may individually be associated with other cardiac anomalies such as PDA, IAA, septal defects, and Tetralogy of Fallot.

Physiology

The left-to-right shunt across the AP window depends on the size of the defect and the relative resistances in the pulmonary and systemic circuits. This physiology is similar to that found in PDA but differs from PDA because AP window generally causes flow reversal in the entire thoracic aorta and not just the descending aorta (Figs. 54.5 and 54.6). This diastolic runoff can have deleterious consequences on both systemic and coronary perfusion.

Anomalous origin of a pulmonary artery from the ascending aorta also results in a large left-to-right shunt and exposes the affected lung to high flow and systemic pressure, making it vulnerable to the early development of pulmonary vascular obstructive disease. The contralateral lung receives the entire right heart output, which may lead to pulmonary hypertension, although this is not likely due to the flow but rather from poorly understood humoral mechanisms related to the presence of pulmonary hypertension in the contralateral lung.

Clinical Features

History

The presentation of these patients will depend on the size of the defect, the relative pulmonary and systemic vascular resistances,

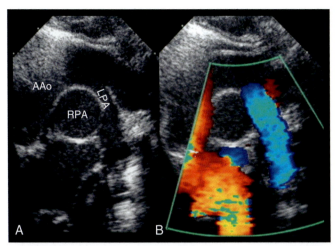

• **Figure 54.5** Echocardiographic assessment of anomalous origin of left pulmonary artery *(LPA)* from the ascending aorta *(AAo)*. (A) Suprasternal sagittal view showing the origin of the left pulmonary artery from the distal ascending aorta. (B) Echocardiogram with color shows the diastolic antegrade systolic flow into the left pulmonary artery *(blue flow)* with diastolic flow reversal in the transverse arch *(red flow)*. *RPA,* Right pulmonary artery.

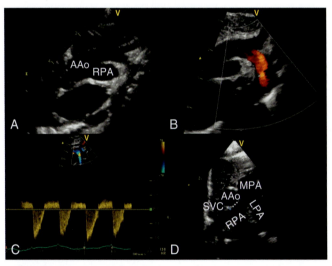

• **Figure 54.6** Echocardiographic assessment of anomalous origin of right pulmonary artery from the ascending aorta. (A) Suprasternal aortic arch view showing the origin of the right pulmonary artery from the ascending aorta *(AAo)*. Echocardiogram with (B) color *(red flow)* and (C) Doppler show the diastolic flow reversal in the transverse arch. D, Suprasternal three-vessel view showing the origin of the right pulmonary artery *(RPA)* from the AAo *(dashed white line)*. *LPA,* Left pulmonary artery; *MPA,* main pulmonary artery; *SVC,* superior vena cava.

associated lesions, and the age at diagnosis. When the defect is small, there is a small left-to-right shunt with minimal or no symptoms. More commonly, this defect is large, and there is a significant left-to-right shunt. Patients typically present with severe congestive heart failure manifested by tachypnea, poor feeding, delayed growth, and often repeated respiratory infections but with normal oxygen saturations. These patients usually have pulmonary hypertension and are at risk for developing early-onset pulmonary vascular obstructive disease, which can lead to cyanosis from right-to-left shunting across the defect. Although the symptoms may be similar to those of an untreated patient with a large VSD,

Patients with AP window may present earlier due to additional diastolic runoff at the expense of systemic perfusion and may even develop coronary perfusion steal.

Patients with a large AP window typically do not survive infancy. Occasionally, those who survive and are encountered as children and young adults frequently have significant pulmonary vascular obstructive disease with its right heart sequelae.

Physical Examination

Physical examination reveals bounding peripheral pulses with a widened pulse pressure. Cardiomegaly is common. There are congestive heart failure symptoms with increased left ventricular impulse. Right heart failure presents with hepatomegaly and peripheral edema. Findings of increased left-to-right shunt include diastolic rumble and systolic murmur in the left third and fourth intercostal space.

Diagnosis

Chest x-ray shows signs of increased pulmonary blood flow such as an enlarged cardiac silhouette and increased pulmonary blood flow markings.

Electrocardiogram reveals left atrial enlargement due to increased pulmonary blood flow, seen as widened P waves. There may be signs of left ventricular enlargement. Prominent R waves in the anterior precordial leads may represent right ventricular hypertrophy. Occasionally, ST segment changes from ischemia may be seen in the presence of significant diastolic runoff.

Echocardiography is usually sufficient for diagnosis in most cases of children with AP window and can show the location and size of the defect (see Figs. 54.2, 54.3, 54.5, and 54.6). It is also useful for evaluation of associated anomalies, flow reversal in the entire thoracic aorta with diastolic flow in branch pulmonary arteries (see Figs. 54.5, 54.6). Left heart chamber enlargement can be seen due to left-to-right shunt. High parasternal short-axis view shows a "dropout" defect between the aorta and the main pulmonary artery (see Figs. 54.2 and 54.3). The right pulmonary artery may have anomalous origin from the ascending aorta. The origin of the left coronary artery has to be defined due to associated coronary anomalies.

Magnetic resonance imaging (MRI)/computed tomography (CT): These imaging techniques (see Fig. 54.4) can help if echocardiography is not clearly able to demonstrate the AP window. Additionally, MRI may also be helpful in determining pulmonary versus systemic blood flow distribution (Qp:Qs ratio).

Cardiac catheterization: It is usually not necessary to make the diagnosis and is typically reserved to evaluate associated cardiac anomalies. In older children or adults with AP window, cardiac catheterization is helpful for assessment of pulmonary vascular resistance (Fig. 54.7). When a cardiac catheterization is performed, it is important to determine if the elevated pulmonary resistance is fixed or reversible by measuring the responsiveness of the pulmonary vascular bed to oxygen and/or other vasodilators. If the resistance is reactive, timely repair of the defect should be considered.

Differential Diagnosis

Lesions that should be differentiated from AP window are PDA, VSD, truncus arteriosus, and ruptured aneurysm of the sinus of Valsalva. Rarely, AP window may be associated with aortic or

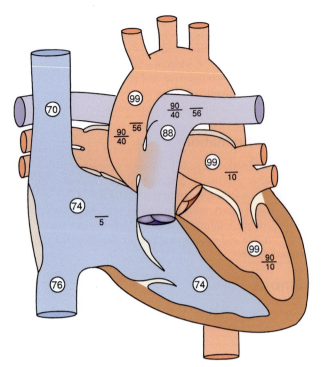

• **Figure 54.7** Pathophysiology of aortopulmonary septal defect. Hemodynamic measurements during cardiac catheterization reveal the communication between the main pulmonary artery and the aorta. Both right and left atrial and ventricular saturations are normal; however, there is an increase in saturation in the main pulmonary artery, indicating a left-to-right shunt. This is accompanied by systemic or near-systemic pressure in the main pulmonary artery. In this example pressures are equal, indicating a large defect.

pulmonary atresia. This lesion can be very difficult to differentiate from truncus arteriosus, but the differentiation is that there are two arterial trunks arising from the heart (one from the right ventricle and one from the left ventricle) in AP window and from anomalous origin of the pulmonary artery from the aorta, whereas in truncus arteriosus there is only one semilunar valve and one arterial trunk with a large underlying VSD. Additionally, it can also be challenging to differentiate it from a solitary aortic trunk with complete absence of intrapericardial pulmonary arteries.[2]

Management

The treatment of AP window is closure of the defect and should be performed soon after the diagnosis is established. Preoperative management of heart failure should be instituted while the patient is awaiting closure of AP window. Diuretics and afterload reduction are the mainstay of medical treatment. Sometimes inotropic support may be needed if there is significant left ventricular dysfunction. Mechanical ventilation with maneuvers to decrease the degree of pulmonary overcirculation may be required in the preoperative period. When AP window is associated with an aortic obstructive lesion such as an IAA, preoperative stabilization is challenging, given the increase in systemic resistance from the obstructive lesion and the decrease in pulmonary vascular resistance from the obligatory alprostadil (prostaglandin E_1) to maintain ductal blood flow to the descending aorta.

Transcatheter Closure of Aortopulmonary Window

Transcatheter closure of AP window may be considered in some older children and adults in whom certain criteria are met: (1) small defects located very distal to the semilunar valves, (2) coronary arteries can be adequately visualized, (3) left-to-right shunt without evidence of shunt reversal, and (4) no evidence of advanced pulmonary vascular obstructive disease. Some reports of successful closure in older children and adults are documented in the literature[30-37]; however, in general these defects are most appropriately managed with surgical closure.

Surgical Treatment

Repair is indicated in all patients with AP window or AOPA, and should be done at the time of diagnosis due to the risk of developing pulmonary vascular obstructive disease.

Isolated Aortopulmonary Window. Patch closure is the preferred surgical treatment for AP window.[13,38,39] It is performed through median sternotomy on cardiopulmonary bypass (CPB). In small infants the repair may necessitate the use of deep hypothermic circulatory arrest. Inflow cannulation is high on the ascending aorta, well above the defect so that an aortic cross-clamp can be placed below the arterial cannulation site but far enough above the AP window that it will not limit exposure for repair. A single-stage venous cannula is usually satisfactory for repair of AP window, although bicaval venous cannulation may be needed for concomitant repair of associated cardiac defects.

Anterior Approach (Fig. 54.8). After the aortic cross-clamp is applied, the anterior wall of the AP window is opened vertically, and the coronary ostia are inspected. Repair is usually performed using an anterior sandwich patch technique with either native pericardium or a prosthetic material (polytetrafluoroethylene [PTFE], bovine pericardium, or homograft). The patch is sewn to the inferior, posterior, and superior rim of the defect. Anteriorly the incision is closed incorporating the patch in the suture line (Video 54.1). A variation of this technique is to separate the aorta and pulmonary artery and to close each resultant arterial defect with patch material. Although this decreases the risk of recanalization or residual defect, it is more time consuming and carries a greater risk of distortion of the repaired arteries. Nevertheless, this technique is preferred by some, particularly for defects that are between the ascending aorta and the main pulmonary artery (proximal to the right pulmonary artery)

Transaortic Approach (Fig. 54.9). Transaortic patch closure of AP window is an acceptable alternative technique for repair of this defect. This technique is more useful for variations that include involvement of a more extensive portion of aorta than can be approached by the anterior technique, such as involvement of the right pulmonary artery along the posterior portion of the aorta.

Transpulmonary Approach. Due to difficulty in the visualization of the coronary ostia and even the AP window defect itself, this approach of opening the pulmonary artery and either placing a patch through it or repairing the defect with a pulmonary artery flap is not recommended for typical forms of this defect. In addition, it is associated with a higher prevalence of reintervention due to subsequent pulmonary artery stenosis.[13,23]

Following repair, an intraoperative transesophageal echocardiogram is recommended to confirm the absence of any residual defects and to rule out the creation of important pulmonary arterial stenosis resulting from the repair.

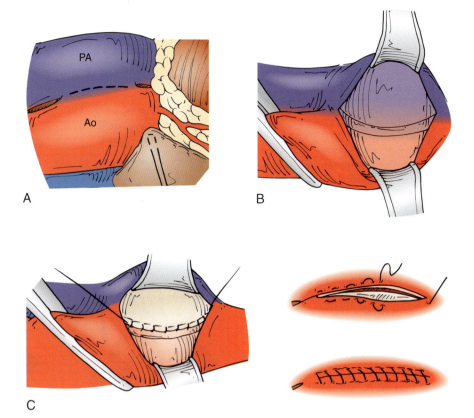

• **Figure 54.8** Surgical correction of aortopulmonary (AP) window. (A) Incision on the septum over the AP window. (B) AP window defect is seen. Coronary arteries are visualized to protect them during patch placement. (C) Placement of patch. Suturing is started posteriorly, and, as the repair is continued anteriorly, the patch is sandwiched between the aorta and the pulmonary artery.

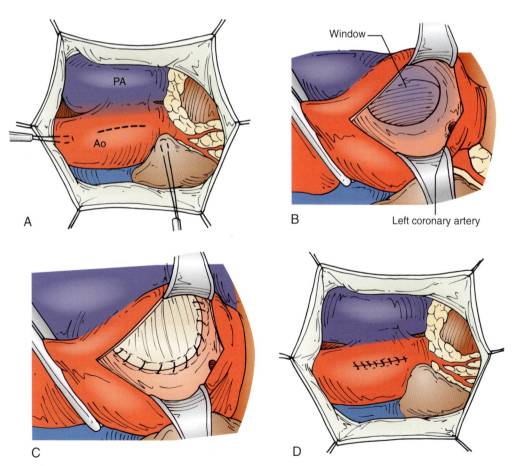

• **Figure 54.9** Transaortic approach for repair of aortopulmonary (AP) window. (A) Longitudinal incision on the anterior aspect of the aorta. (B) AP window defect is visualized, and the coronary arteries are visualized to protect them during patch placement. (C) Patch closure of AP window defect. (D) Closure of the aortic incision.

Other Techniques. Techniques other than patch closure are of historical interest and should be avoided. These include (1) simple ligation of the AP window, which can cause fatal intraoperative bleeding, incomplete closure, and recanalization; and (2) division or suture without CPB. Although division and direct suture closure of "small" defects might be contemplated (without using CPB), this technique is generally not preferred, and historical application of this technique (using partial occlusion clamps off CPB) ran the risk of resulting in fatal hemorrhage and/or distortion and narrowing of the pulmonary artery or the aorta.

Repair of Aortopulmonary Window With Interrupted Aortic Arch

AP window with IAA needs to be distinguished from truncus arteriosus with IAA. When there is simply an AP window with IAA, distinguished by the presence of two separate outflow tracts and semilunar valves, the repair requires closing the AP window and repairing the aortic arch[40] (Fig. 54.10). We prefer cannulating the aorta using a PTFE graft placed on the innominate artery because the distal ascending aorta is usually small, and there is very little space above the AP window for cannulation. Once CPB is commenced, there will be flow through the window and across the ductus arteriosus into the descending aorta, but the branch pulmonary arteries must be occluded to promote systemic perfusion. The patient is typically cooled to a more significant degree of hypothermia (18°C to 25°C) depending on the preferred strategy of the surgical team. Once the patient has been cooled to the target temperature, selective cerebral perfusion with distal collateral perfusion can be accomplished by snaring the innominate artery proximal to the arterial infusion PTFE graft, as well as the other head vessels. The heart can be arrested with cardioplegia. The PDA is then divided, and the ductal tissue can be trimmed from the descending aorta. A vascular clamp on the distal descending aorta prevents collateral circulation from obscuring the operative field. With the distal aorta trimmed the back wall of the descending aorta can be attached to the underside of the ascending aorta—usually this can be done at the site of the AP window, although frequently the AP window defect can be extended cephalad to create a more appropriate neoaorta. The defect in the pulmonary artery is patched—we typically use a piece of pulmonary homograft. Finally, the neoaorta is repaired by extending an incision down the descending aorta and patching over the anterior aspect of the new aorta with homograft. This is an extensive repair, but the technique of connecting the back of the descending aorta to the underside of the ascending aorta and patching the anterior surface with homograft (similar to neoaortic reconstruction in a Norwood arch reconstruction) usually results in a very nicely repaired aorta with minimal distortion or obstruction.[40]

Anomalous Origin of a Pulmonary Artery From the Ascending Aorta

The cannulation strategy is similar to that of the AP window with an aortic cannula placed high in the ascending aorta. The anomalous pulmonary artery is controlled with a snare when CPB is initiated. Typically the right pulmonary artery is the one that arises anomalously from the side of the aorta. We have found that it can be best excised by making a transverse incision in the aorta and taking the orifice of the pulmonary artery out as an "island" with a substantial cuff of aorta to make it easier to sew to the pulmonary artery. With the aorta divided by this maneuver, it is fairly simple to find a site on the main pulmonary artery to anastomose the right pulmonary artery using fine monofilament suture. With the pulmonary artery repaired, it is then necessary to repair the ascending aorta. Because removing the pulmonary artery with a substantial "cuff" of aortic wall creates a significant defect in a tiny aorta (when this procedure is performed in infants),

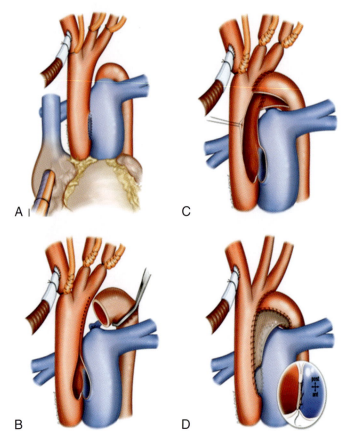

• **Figure 54.10** Schematic illustration of surgical repair of aortopulmonary window with interrupted aortic arch. (A) The aortopulmonary window *(dashed line)* is associated with a type A interrupted aortic arch. The pulmonary artery trunk is dilated compared with the ascending aorta. A single aortic cannula is placed through a 3.5-mm polytetrafluoroethylene graft anastomosed to the right innominate artery. (B) The arch vessels are occluded with snares after selective cerebral perfusion is performed. (C) A partial anastomosis is carried out between the descending aorta and the aortic arch, then an incision (1.5 cm long) is made on the descending aorta. (D) An autologous pericardial patch is used to enlarge the descending aorta, the arch concavity, and the ascending aorta. When the suture reaches the anterior-superior edge of the aortopulmonary window, a continuous mattress suture incorporates the wall of the pulmonary artery, the patch, and the aortic wall (the "sandwich" patch technique, used to close the aortopulmonary window, can be seen in the magnified insert). *Ant,* Anterior; *Post,* posterior. (Modified with permission from Roubertie F, Kalfa D, Vergnat M, et al. Aortopulmonary window and the interrupted aortic arch: midterm results with use of the single-patch technique. *Ann Thorac Surg.* 2015;99[1]:186-191.)

a direct connection can create shortening of the aorta and compression of the posterior pulmonary artery. For this reason, we augment the posterior aorta with a generous patch of homograft. This creates a neoaorta that lies nicely over the newly repaired right pulmonary artery without any tension and with potential for future growth (because the anterior portion of the repair is all native tissue) (Fig. 54.11; Video 54.2).

Following repair of AP window or of anomalous origin of a pulmonary artery from the aorta, intraoperative echocardiography should be employed to ensure that the defect is repaired (e.g., no residual shunting across a repaired AP window or compression of the right pulmonary artery by the aorta in isolated anomalous origin of the pulmonary artery). Intraoperative echocardiography

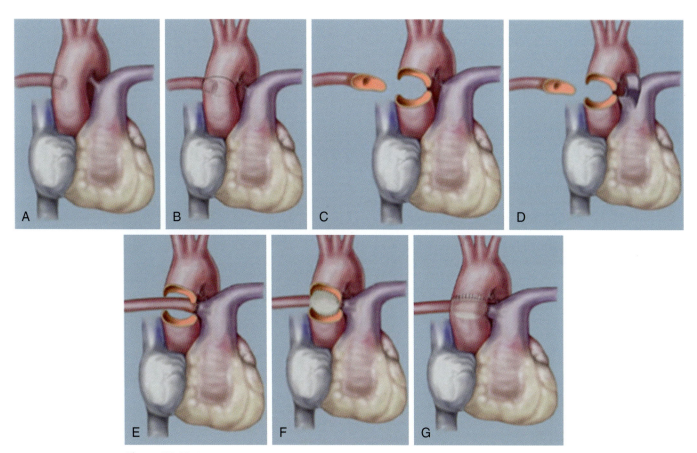

• **Figure 54.11** Schematic illustration of repair of anomalous origin of the right pulmonary artery (RPA) from the ascending aorta. (A) Morphology, showing only the left pulmonary artery being connected to the main pulmonary artery (MPA) and the right ventricle. Separate origin of the RPA from the ascending aorta. (B) Transverse incision on the anterior aspect of the ascending aorta. Margins of the RPA origin are clearly visualized. (C) Excising a generous button of RPA along with part of the posterior wall of the aorta. (D) Cruciate incision is made on the main pulmonary artery in preparation for anastomosis with the RPA. (E) Large anastomosis is created between the RPA button and the MPA. (F) Repair of posterior wall defect in the ascending aorta using a homograft patch. This patch is made patulous to avoid compression of the RPA running posterior to the repaired ascending aorta. (G) Repair is completed by closing the anterior aortic incision.

can also be used to evaluate ventricular function and help guide the use of inotropic therapy.

Postoperative Management

Infants after repair of AP window are at risk for the development of severe pulmonary hypertensive crises, especially in the presence of pain, hypoxia, or acidosis. These episodes can occur suddenly and are related to an acute severe increases in pulmonary vascular resistance. These events manifest with an acute increase in pulmonary artery pressure, a sudden drop in cardiac output with hypotension, a sudden decrease in end-tidal CO_2 detection and arterial oxygen saturation, and acute worsening in perfusion. If this condition is not rapidly reversed, it can lead to a cardiac arrest. Immediate sedation and paralytics should be given, and the patient should be hyperventilated with 100% O_2. In refractory cases inhaled nitric oxide or even temporary support with extracorporeal membrane oxygenation may be required.[9] Attention to warning signs postoperatively can prevent this complication from occurring. We recommend leaving a pulmonary artery pressure monitoring

line in place to assist in the postoperative management, and we transport these patients to the ICU deeply sedated, neuromuscularly blocked, ventilated with high inspired fraction of oxygen, and occasionally on inhaled nitric oxide because the rigors of transfer from operating room to ICU may be enough to cause a crisis. Lung mechanics are abnormal in infants and children with large left-to-right shunts due to increased extravascular lung water resulting in decreased lung compliance and increased resistance to expiratory flow.[41,42] Therefore we advocate using volume-controlled mode of ventilation to maintain a tight control of minute ventilation and acid-base status. The pharmacologic support usually consists of inotropic support with milrinone and pressor support with low-dose dopamine or epinephrine. Much of the postoperative support will be determined by the preoperative condition of the patient. Diuretics are resumed postoperatively to facilitate removal of excess extravascular water. Depending on the patient's age and degree of preoperative pulmonary resistance, deescalation from nitric oxide, oxygen, and ultimately ventilatory support can take several days. Occasionally the use of phosphodiesterase type 5 inhibitors in patients with rebound pulmonary hypertension can successfully wean them off inhaled nitric oxide.[43] If patients undergo repair in the first few months of life, the convalescence can be fairly uncomplicated, unlike older patients who may require more thoughtful and prudent management due to their increased baseline pulmonary vascular resistance and increased pulmonary artery reactivity.

Outcomes

Operative mortality of isolated AP window and AOPA is low in the current era and low birth-weight children (<2.5 kg) and those with associated congenital anomalies are at higher risk of operative mortality. Long-term survival as well as late results of surgical correction of AP window without associated anomalies are excellent.

McElhinney et al.[13] reported on outcome of repair of AP window in patients younger than 6 months of age. Of the total 24 patients, 12 had isolated AP window, and 12 had associated lesions (9 of 12 had associated IAA, and 3 of 12 had other significant cardiac anomalies). There were no early or late deaths of patients with isolated AP window but 5 out of 12 with associated lesions died early. Follow-up of survivors revealed recurrent aortic arch obstruction in all patients who had AP window and IAA, but only 2 out of the 9 needed reintervention at the time of follow-up.

Backer and Mavroudis[22] reported outcomes of surgical repair of AP window at a single center over a 40-year period (1961–2001). Of the 22 patients in their series the median age was 0.3 years, ranging from 11 days to 13 years. The associated lesions were IAA in 4, right PA origin from the aorta in 4, VSD in 3, ASD in 1, TOF in 1, and TGA in 1. Of these patients, 2 had attempted ligation without CPB, and 1 patient had division and oversewing of AP window between clamps on CPB. AP window was divided on CPB with primary aortic closure in 10 patients. Circulatory arrest was used with associated IAA repair, and anastomosis of the right PA to the main PA in 3 patients. Toward the latter part of their experience, 6 patients had open transaortic patch closure, 1 of whom had simultaneous arterial switch and another simultaneous IAA repair. Patients were followed up from 1 month to 26 years, with a median of 8 years. They reported 5 early deaths and 1 late death from pulmonary hypertension in the first 16 patients, for whom the primary strategy was AP window division, with a mortality rate of 37%. There were no deaths in the 6 patients who underwent transaortic patch closure, with normal PA and aortic growth observed over a maximum follow-up period of 8 years.

Bagtharia et al.[23] have reported the outcomes of management of AP window among 42 patients with a median age at presentation being 62 days, ranging from birth to 6 years, between 1969 and 1999. Associated cardiac defects were present in 34 of these patients, 6 of whom had IAA. The correct diagnosis was initially missed in 13 patients, 6 of whom died without surgical repair, and 1 was lost to follow-up. Repair was performed in 35 patients: subsequent to repair of other defects in 4; along with repair of other defects in 17, of whom there were 3 mortalities; and as an isolated procedure

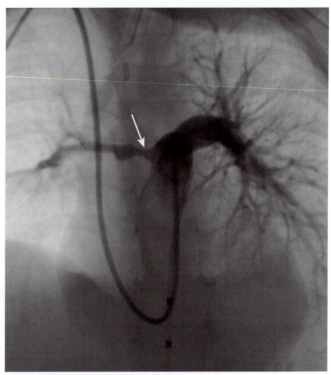

• **Figure 54.12** Postoperative complication. Right pulmonary artery proximal stenosis *(arrow)* and diffuse hypoplasia after surgical repair of anomalous origin of the right pulmonary artery from the ascending aorta.

in 14 patients, with 1 of them having a transcatheter closure. There were 9 deaths in total, all in patients with complex defects, except 1 with a missed AP window after repair of coarctation of aorta. Survival rates by Kaplan-Meier estimates were 81% at 3 months until 11.5 years, and 69% up to 21 years. Increased time-related mortality was associated independently only with the presence of an IAA, hazard ratio being 5.87 ($P = .009$). The outcomes for isolated lesion were excellent, concurring with similar results from other study populations.

For repair of AOPA, Limited data are available on long-term outcome and reintervention rate on development of pulmonary artery stenosis. Prognosis is also determined by the presence of associated anomalies and on the pulmonary vascular resistance at the time of repair, especially for older patients. The most commonly expected complication is stenosis of the repaired pulmonary artery (Fig. 54.12), which is identified by echocardiogram and is typically amenable to stent repair in the cardiac catheterization laboratory.

References

A complete list of references is available at ExpertConsult.com.

55

Truncus Arteriosus

JAMES JAGGERS, MD; CHARLES R. COLE, MD

Persistent truncus arteriosus is a relatively rare cardiac anomaly, occurring in 0.4% to 4% of individuals with congenital heart disease.[1-3] The condition is characterized by a single arterial trunk arising from the heart, overriding the ventricular septum and receiving blood from both ventricles. This persistent truncal artery supplies blood to the systemic, coronary, and pulmonary circulations. This chapter will discuss the natural history, embryology, anatomy, and physiology of truncus arteriosus as well as the clinically relevant aspects of classification, presentation, diagnosis, surgical correction, and postoperative management.

Natural History

The prognosis of unrepaired persistent truncus arteriosus is poor, with mortality rates in the first year of life exceeding 70%.[4] The majority of deaths that occur during infancy result from severe congestive heart failure (CHF).[5] As pulmonary vascular resistance (PVR) decreases shortly after birth, excessive pulmonary blood flow results, leading to pulmonary edema, left ventricular (LV) volume overload, and ultimately death from CHF in most patients. Rarely, sudden cardiac death has been reported in preoperative patients with truncus arteriosus. Some of these cases are linked with significant truncal valve stenosis,[5,6] whereas ventricular arrhythmia induced by myocardial ischemia has been implicated in others.[4,7] Unrepaired patients who survive infancy generally develop severe pulmonary vascular occlusive disease early in childhood.[4] Case reports have documented patients with unrepaired truncus arteriosus surviving into adulthood. Survival in these patients has been attributed to pulmonary artery stenosis or increased PVR, which limits the pulmonary blood flow and slows the development of CHF.[8]

Embryology

Truncal ridges form in the truncus arteriosus during week 5 of gestation and become continuous with the conal septum superiorly. These ridges eventually fuse to separate the truncus arteriosus into two channels, the aorta and pulmonary trunk. The spiral formation of these ridges results in the normal orientation of the aorta and pulmonary artery (PA), with the aorta positioned posteriorly and to the right of the PA. The conus cordis gives rise to the LV and right ventricular (RV) outflow tracts when the conal septum is complete. The truncal and conal septa then fuse, creating RV-to-PA and LV-to-aortic continuity. Persistent truncus arteriosus results from failure of the truncal ridges and aortopulmonary septum to develop and divide into the aorta and pulmonary trunk.[9]

The mechanism for failure of the truncal septation remains unclear. Deficiencies in neural crest development and migration have been implicated as a possible mechanism for conotruncal anomalies.[10,11] Truncus arteriosus and other arch anomalies have been associated with deletion of chromosome 22q11. DiGeorge syndrome (velocardiofacial syndrome), a monoallelic microdeletion of chromosome 22q11, is characterized by conotruncal heart defects, hypoplasia of the thymus and parathyroid gland, craniofacial dysmorphisms, and developmental delay.[12] A microdeletion of chromosome 22q11 has been identified in 20% to 40% of cases of truncus arteriosus.[13]

Anatomy

The anatomy of truncus arteriosus is best described by failure of the PA to separate from the aorta during development, leading to a large common arterial trunk that serves as outflow for both ventricles. The systemic, coronary, and pulmonary blood flow all arise from this common arterial trunk (Fig. 55.1). The segmental anatomy of truncus arteriosus can be described as situs solitus with a D-looping ventricle (Fig. 55.2). The common artery arises from a common semilunar valve that overrides a large ventricular septal defect (VSD), frequently with malalignment to the right. The common semilunar valve, or truncal valve, may have a variable number of cusps, with three cusps occurring most frequently.[14]

Collett and Edwards[15] established a classification system based on the origins of the PAs from the truncal artery in 1949. Van Praagh and Van Praagh[9] classified truncus arteriosus based on the morphology of the conotruncal septum and the presence of associated anomalies. Russell et al.[16] recently proposed a "simplified" categorization for the common arterial trunk that places emphasis on the nature of the systemic pathways. In this system, groups are assigned with either aortic or pulmonary dominance of the common arterial trunk.

Classification

The system established by Collett and Edwards[15] describes type I as an arterial trunk originating from the common semilunar valve with its immediate bifurcation into a PA and ascending aorta (Fig. 55.3). Collett and Edwards type I therefore has common origin of the right and left PAs. Type II defects refer to the separate origin of the left and right PAs from the posterior wall of the truncal artery. Type III describes anatomy similar to that of type II but with the right and left PAs originating farther apart. In type IV, often referred to as pseudotruncus, the main PA is absent, with the lungs receiving their blood supply through aortopulmonary

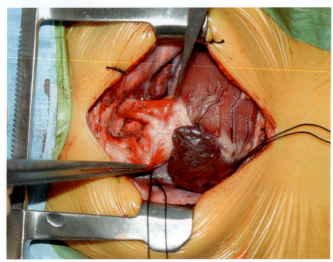

• **Figure 55.1** Truncus arteriosus in an infant undergoing surgical correction in the neonatal period. The picture is displayed from the surgeon's view, with the patient's head on the left side of the image. (Courtesy Max Mitchell, MD.)

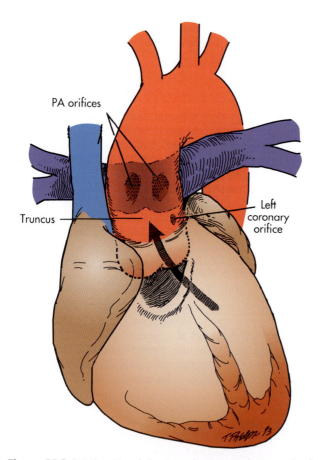

• **Figure 55.2** Relationship of the truncal artery to the truncal valve *(boldface dotted line)*, left coronary ostium, and ventricular septal defect *(arrow)*. *PA,* Pulmonary artery.

collaterals. Most would agree that this entity should not be described as a truncus defect but rather is a form of pulmonary atresia with VSD and major aortopulmonary collateral arteries.

Richard Van Praagh and Stella Van Praagh classified truncus arteriosus based on the presence or absence of the conotruncal

septum. When the conal septum fails to form, a conal-type VSD results. The system uses the designation A to represent the presence of a VSD and B for the absence of a VSD. The variable development of the truncal septum defines their specific category. In Van Praagh type 1 the truncal septum is partially developed so that a PA and aorta coexist. Type A1 is identical to type I of Collett and Edwards. In Van Praagh type 2, complete absence of the truncal septum is seen, with the main PAs originating from the truncal artery separately. This includes Collett and Edwards type II and most cases of type III. Van Praagh type 3 is characterized by the absence of one PA originating from the truncal artery. Most commonly, type 3 will include the right PA originating from the common trunk, with pulmonary blood supply to the left lung provided by a PA arising from the aortic arch (a subtype of Collett and Edwards type III) or by systemic to pulmonary collaterals. The term *hemitruncus* is sometimes used when one PA takes origin from the ascending aorta (Fig. 55.4). Van Praagh type 4 describes any type of truncus associated with an interrupted arch defect. The arch anomaly is usually a type B interruption with the descending aorta receiving its blood supply from a large patent ductus arteriosus (PDA) and the PAs originating from the truncal artery. The Van Praagh system allows a clearer anatomic description of the defect, allowing better preoperative planning for repair. It also eliminates those defects without at least one PA originating from the truncus.

The classification system proposed by Russell et al. assigns groups with either aortic or pulmonary dominance (Fig. 55.5). In this system, truncus arteriosus with aortic dominance describes hearts with a common arterial trunk with both PAs coming from truncus and an unobstructed aortic arch. Therefore truncus arteriosus with aortic dominance includes Collett and Edwards types 1, 2, and 3 and also includes Van Praagh types 1, 2, and 3. Meanwhile, truncus arteriosus with pulmonary dominance describes hearts with an obstructed aortic arch, including hearts with coarctation, hypoplastic aortic arch, and interrupted aortic arch (Van Praagh type 4). Russell et al. therefore describe that pulmonary dominance is found only when the aortic component of the trunk is hypoplastic and an arterial duct supplies the majority of flow to the descending aorta.[16] In this setting (with pulmonary dominance) the aortic component is discrete from the pulmonary component within the pericardial cavity, and the PAs arise from the sides of the major pathway. In cases with aortic dominance the common trunk itself supplies the arch vessels and descending aorta; the PAs arise close together from the dorsal surface of the arterial trunk.[16]

Associated Anomalies

Various cardiovascular anomalies have been described in association with truncus arteriosus, many of which have important implications in management and outcome. Variations in coronary artery anatomy can add significant complexity and risk to repair and are relatively common, occurring in 15% to 49% of cases.[17,18] Coronary ostia can originate in various positions from within the truncal artery or as a single coronary with a variable epicardial course. There is a strong tendency for the left coronary artery to arise from a more posterior level than it does normally from the aorta.[18] Anomalous origin of the left coronary artery from the right coronary will cross the RV outflow tract (RVOT). This is of particular importance when planning the construction of the RV-to-PA conduit. When the left main coronary ostium originates more superiorly in the commissure, care must be taken to avoid injury during separation of the PAs.

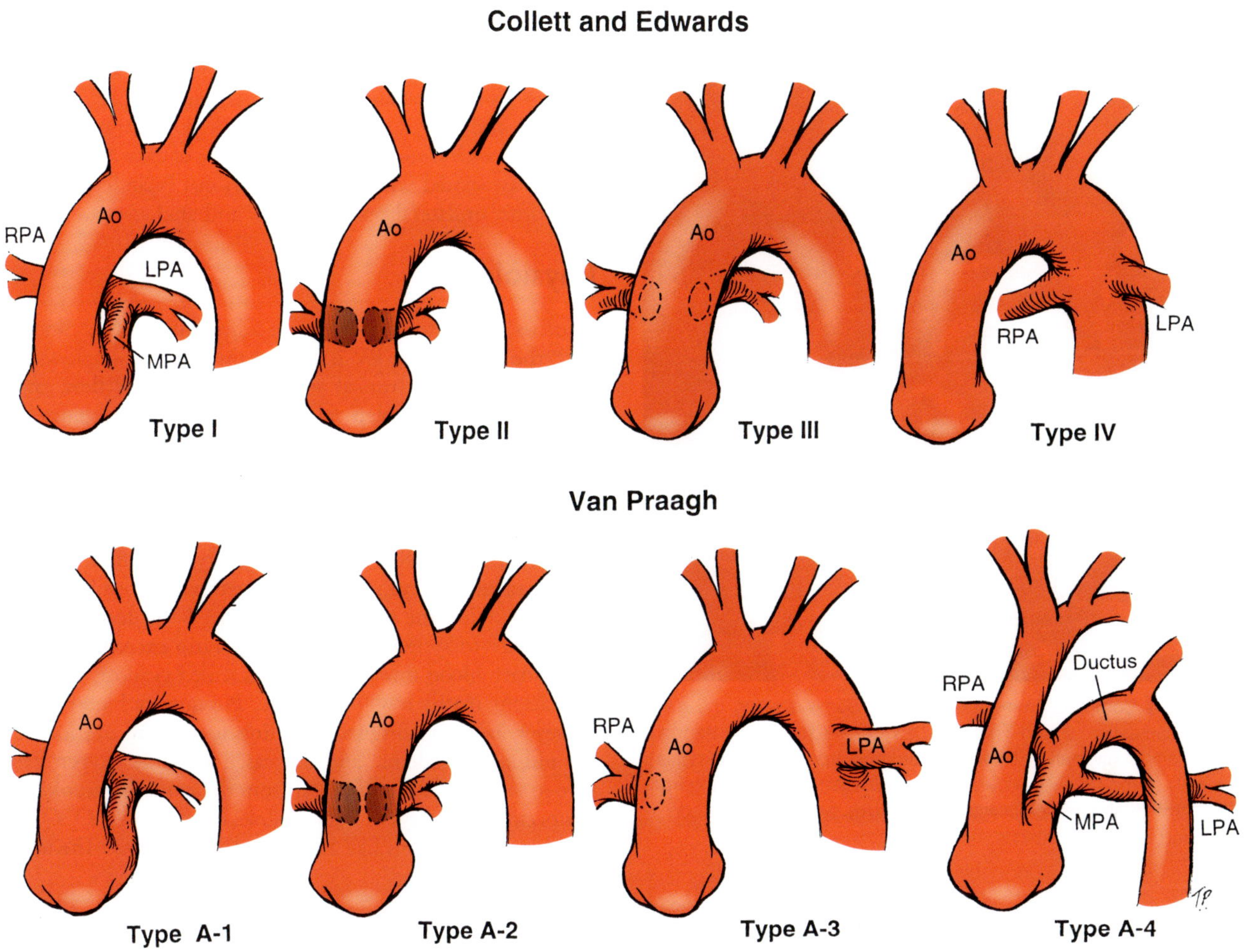

Collett and Edwards

Van Praagh

• **Figure 55.3** Collett and Edwards and Van Praagh classifications (see text for details). Collett and Edwards types I, II, and III and Van Praagh types A1 and A2 are similar. Collett and Edwards type IV is now considered a variant of tetralogy of Fallot with pulmonary atresia. Van Praagh type A3 has the right pulmonary artery originating from the truncus and the left pulmonary artery from a ductus off the descending aorta. In the Van Praagh type A4 the truncus arteriosus occurs with interrupted aortic arch. A patent ductus arteriosus supplies the descending aorta. Pulmonary arteries originate from the posterior aspect of the truncal root. *Ao,* Aorta; *LPA,* left pulmonary artery; *MPA,* main pulmonary artery; *RPA,* right pulmonary artery.

Structural abnormalities of the truncal valve may have significant clinical implications and must be considered during management. The truncal valve may have a variable number of cusps, with three cusps reported in 64% of cases, four cusps in 27%, and two cusps in 8%.[14] Truncal valve incompetence has long been linked to poor outcomes, and a recent analysis of Congenital Heart Surgeons' Society data confirms this in a series of 572 patients in which mortality for repair of truncus arteriosus with truncal valve repair was 30% versus 10% for isolated truncus repair.[19] Truncal valve insufficiency leads to ventricular dilation and low diastolic coronary perfusion. Truncal valve stenosis is often mild or even exaggerated because of the excessive left-to-right shunt and volume overload. It is unusual to have severe truncal valve stenosis that requires intervention at the time of initial repair. These scenarios in combination with increased diastolic pulmonary runoff can lead to significant myocardial ischemia.

The VSD in truncus arteriosus is similar to the malalignment defect of tetralogy of Fallot and results from the failure of the conal septum to develop and rotate. The defect is often large,

nonrestrictive, with the superior border being formed by the truncal valve. The inferior and anterior borders are formed by the two limbs of the septomarginalis trabeculation (SMT). In two-thirds of cases the posterior arm of the SMT and the ventriculoinfundibular fold join to separate the VSD from the septal leaflet of the tricuspid valve. This separation places the conduction system away from the inferior border of the VSD and less likely to be injured during repair. In one-third of cases, a deficiency of the ventriculoinfundibular fold and posterior division of the SMT exists, with the defect extending to the annulus of the tricuspid valve. This leaves the conduction system close to the inferior edge of the VSD and vulnerable to injury during closure.[20]

Another abnormality associated with truncus arteriosus is interruption of the aortic arch; most commonly type B. Approximately 10% of patients with truncus arteriosus will have an interruption of their aortic arch. The highest-mortality group for truncus arteriosus repair was among patients who underwent concomitant repair of interrupted aortic arch and truncal valve repair (60% mortality).[19] Other defects of surgical significance

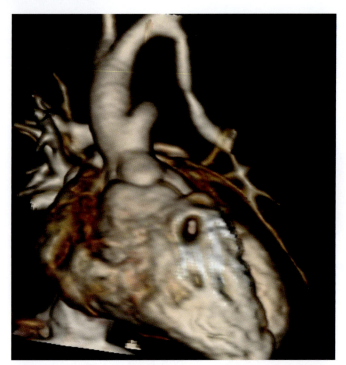

• **Figure 55.4** Computed tomography image demonstrating the most common presentation of Van Praagh type 3, characterized by the right pulmonary artery originating from the common trunk, with pulmonary blood supply to the left lung provided by a pulmonary artery arising from the aortic arch (a subtype of Collett and Edwards type III). This is sometimes referred to as hemitruncus.

occurring with truncus arteriosus include right aortic arch (18% to 36%), left superior vena cava, aberrant subclavian artery, and atrial septal defect.[2,21] Pulmonary artery branch stenosis can also occur.[22] Noncardiac anomalies are present in approximately 20% of cases and may contribute to death. DiGeorge syndrome is associated with truncus arteriosus in 30% of cases.[23] Less common defects associated with truncus arteriosus include tethered-cord syndrome, unilateral renal agenesis, and anal atresia.

Physiology

Truncus arteriosus is a complete admixture lesion. Blood from both the LV and the RV is ejected through the single semilunar valve and into the truncal artery. Relative blood flow, and thus oxygen saturation, is dependent on the relative resistance of each circulation. Pulmonary blood flow may be limited by stenosis of the PAs, but this is uncommon. In most instances, pulmonary blood flow (and thus arterial oxygen saturation) is determined by the resistance to flow in the pulmonary vascular bed. In the perinatal period, elevated PVR will limit pulmonary blood flow, and patients will frequently be cyanotic with oxygen saturations between 75% and 80%. After the second week of life, PVR decreases, and the pulmonary-to-systemic (Q_p:Q_s) flow ratio exceeds 1. Increased pulmonary blood flow results in decreased cyanosis with oxygen saturations in the low 90% range. Pulmonary blood flow may, however, become torrential, leading to volume overload of the LV, pulmonary edema, and decreased systemic oxygen delivery. Left-to-right shunting of blood from the common trunk into the PAs occurs both in systole and diastole, increasing the Q_p:Q_s relative to other shunt lesions like an isolated large VSD.[24] The increased

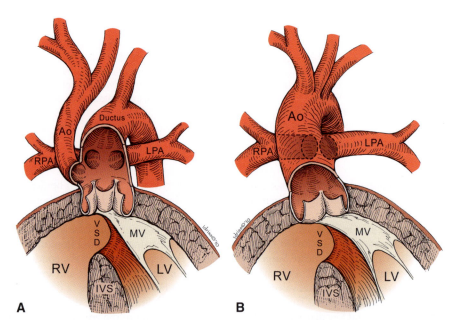

• **Figure 55.5** The illustration shows the essential features of pulmonary versus aortic dominance as observed in our autopsied specimens with common arterial trunk. Panel A shows interruption of the aortic arch. Only in this setting, and in hearts with severe aortic coarctation, did we find origin of the pulmonary arteries from either side of the intrapericardial pulmonary trunk. Panel B shows the salient features of aortic dominance, with the pulmonary arteries arising separately but next to each other from the leftward and dorsal aspect of the common trunk. We also found pulmonary arteries arising more anteriorly and then crossing as they extended toward the pulmonary hilums.[16] *Ao,* Aorta; *IVS,* interventricular septum; *LPA,* left pulmonary artery; *LV,* left ventricle; *MV,* mitral valve; *RPA,* right pulmonary artery; *RV,* right ventricle; *VSD,* ventricular septal defect. (Used by permission, Russell HM, Jacobs ML, Anderson RH, et al. A simplified categorization for common arterial trunk. *J Thorac Cardiovasc Surg.* 2011;141[3]:645-653.)

pulmonary diastolic runoff may also contribute to decreased coronary artery perfusion as well as the development of intestinal ischemia and necrotizing enterocolitis. The development of CHF is accelerated in the presence of an insufficient truncal valve. In most cases of truncus arteriosus signs of CHF are present by the second to third weeks of life. Over time the continued exposure of the pulmonary vascular bed to excessive blood flow leads to the development of pulmonary vascular obstructive disease. The PVR increases, and the pulmonary-to-systemic ratio approaches 1 or less. A point is reached at which these changes become irreversible.

Clinical Presentation

Truncus arteriosus is generally diagnosed in the neonatal period, with a presenting sign of mild cyanosis. As the child develops CHF, symptoms of dyspnea, diaphoresis, and failure to thrive will become apparent. Physical examination usually reveals a systolic thrill and murmur over the left third and fourth intercostal spaces parasternally. The patient has a jerky, collapsing arterial pulse due to the rapid runoff from the truncal artery into the pulmonary circulation. The apical impulse is prominent, and signs of cardiomegaly are noted. The second heart sound is single and accentuated. When truncal valve incompetence is present, a diastolic murmur follows the second heart sound. Hepatomegaly is often present.

Diagnosis

The first diagnostic test usually obtained is a chest radiograph, which reveals cardiomegaly with biventricular enlargement and increased pulmonary vasculature. The aortic arch is to the right in 20% of patients, and the left PA may be elevated from the normal position. The superior mediastinum may be narrow due to the absent main PA. The electrocardiogram findings are nonspecific and usually indicate biventricular hypertrophy.

Echocardiogram is currently the gold standard for diagnosis of truncus arteriosus. In most cases, echocardiogram will detail all relevant anatomy for surgical planning.[25] The parasternal long-axis views will demonstrate a single great vessel overriding the ventricular septum (Videos 55.1 and 55.2). The parasternal short-axis views allow evaluation of truncus valve morphology, whereas apical and subcostal views will give the best assessment of truncal valve stenosis and insufficiency. Characterization of truncal valve function using color and spectral Doppler to evaluate for insufficiency or stenosis is critical. In addition to evaluating the outflow VSD, a diligent search for any additional VSDs must be performed. The origin of the left and right PAs must be established and investigation for pulmonary stenosis performed. Coronary artery anomalies are frequent in truncus arteriosus, and thus coronary anatomy must be fully delineated. The origin of the coronary ostia is of particular importance because the left main ostia may originate more superiorly in the common trunk and must be avoided when separating the PAs. Additionally, anomalous origin of the left coronary artery from the right coronary will cross the RVOT and is susceptible to injury during construction of the RV-to-PA conduit. Finally, the aortic arch through the proximal descending aorta must be evaluated for interruption

Cardiac catheterization (Fig. 55.6) is reserved for cases in which anatomy could not be clearly defined on echocardiogram, additional information is needed concerning the truncal valve, or the PVR warrants further assessment. Pulmonary vascular resistance is usually only mildly elevated (2 to 4 Wood units/m^2) in infants younger than 3 months. In the setting of elevated or fixed PVR, operative correction may not be tolerated.

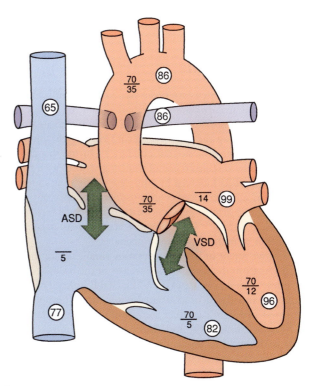

• **Figure 55.6** Pathophysiology of truncus arteriosus. Excessive pulmonary blood flow leads to volume overload of the ventricles. Mixing at the ventricular and arterial level produces similar pulmonary and systemic arterial saturations (*circled values*). Pressure in the right ventricle is at systemic levels to maintain truncal flow. *ASD,* Atrial septal defect; *VSD,* ventricular septal defect.

Preoperative Management

In the modern era, complete repair of persistent truncus arteriosus is recommended during the neonatal period. This approach minimizes the risk of developing CHF and increased PVR. Many patients require little preoperative management. As previously discussed, mild cyanosis is present at birth with saturations in the 70s to 80s. Supplemental oxygen is not necessary in this setting and may actually worsen volume overload due to its action as a pulmonary vasodilator. Severe cyanosis in the early neonatal period may indicate branch pulmonary stenosis or parenchymal lung disease.

In patients with an interrupted aortic arch, maintaining a PDA for distal perfusion using prostaglandin E$_1$ therapy is necessary. If a PDA is identified in the absence of an interrupted aorta, evaluation for discontinuous PA should be undertaken.[26] If there is not an interrupted aortic arch or discontinuous PA, then prostaglandin E$_1$ infusion is unnecessary and may worsen pulmonary overcirculation.

One must be careful with the institution of enteral nutrition in patients with truncus arteriosus. The presence of a substantial pulmonary overcirculation and lower diastolic blood pressure may contribute to necrotizing enterocolitis. If operation is delayed past the first week or two of life, then slow initiation of feeding is justified.

If truncus arteriosus is diagnosed in the prenatal period or immediately after birth, obtaining central access and arterial access using the umbilical vessels is preferred if surgical correction is planned in the following few days. This will spare the femoral vessel for interventional procedures that may be needed later in life. Additionally, genetic evaluation of 22q11 deletion is an important part of the diagnostic and preoperative evaluation.

Surgical Technique

Surgical repair of truncus arteriosus has evolved significantly since the first complete correction was reported in 1968.[27] As detailed by McGoon and associates, the successful repair of truncus arteriosus consisted of closing the VSD and reconstructing the pulmonary outflow graft using a homograft conduit.[27] During this era many surgeons employed staged repair of truncus arteriosus with palliative banding of the PAs followed by complete repair at an older age.[28] Currently, most experienced centers maintain a policy of complete repair of truncus arteriosus as a neonate, regardless of birth weight, with excellent results.[29,30] It is, however, acceptable to delay surgical intervention in markedly preterm neonates.

Definitive repair of truncus arteriosus entails separation of the branch PAs from the truncal artery, repair of the residual defect in the common trunk, closure of the VSD, establishment of RV-to-PA continuity, and repair of associated anomalies. The operation is performed through a median sternotomy with standard aortic and bicaval cannulation and routine cardiopulmonary bypass (CPB) under mild to moderate hypothermia. In the presence of an interrupted aortic arch, deep hypothermic circulatory arrest or hypothermic selective antegrade cerebral perfusion may be employed. If deep hypothermic circulatory arrest is used, intermittent cerebral perfusion may also be used as a neurologic protective strategy. Following sternotomy, subtotal thymectomy is performed if present. The thymus is often small, and its absence is suggestive of DiGeorge syndrome. The pericardium is opened, and a pericardial patch is harvested for later construction of the RVOT with a homograft. The patient is then heparinized, and at the initiation of CPB the pulmonary arteries are snared to prevent pulmonary overcirculation.

Once the child is appropriately cooled, the aortic cross-clamp is applied, and antegrade cardioplegia is administered. Great care must be taken to ensure adequate initial delivery of cardioplegia during the conduct of the operation. Because the cross-clamp is placed distal to the PAs, standard delivery of cardioplegia into the truncal root will allow cardioplegia to run off into the pulmonary circulation and result in inadequate myocardial protection. To ensure cardioplegia delivery to the coronary arteries the PA branches must be occluded. In the setting of significant truncus valve insufficiency, retrograde or direct ostial delivery of cardioplegia may be required. The choice of cardioplegia solution is at the discretion of the surgeon. An LV vent is then inserted through the right upper pulmonary vein or through the right atrium if a patent foramen ovale is present.

Once the heart is completely arrested and cardioplegia delivered, the PAs are detached from the truncal artery with an elliptical incision (Fig. 55.7). A generous cuff of tissue surrounding the orifice of the PAs should be harvested if possible. Visualization of the PA origins may be facilitated by an anterior aortotomy, and in some cases it may be advantageous to completely transect the aorta to facilitate visualization of the PA and coronary origins. The position of the left main coronary artery ostium, usually just inferior to the PAs, must be identified to prevent injury during separation of the main trunks. Transection of the aorta also facilitates repair of the truncal valve if indicated. The aorta may often simply be repaired primarily, but prosthetic material may be necessary to avoid distortion of the semilunar valve pillars.

Next, an anterior right ventriculotomy is made in the RVOT. Care must be taken to avoid injury to the truncus valve because

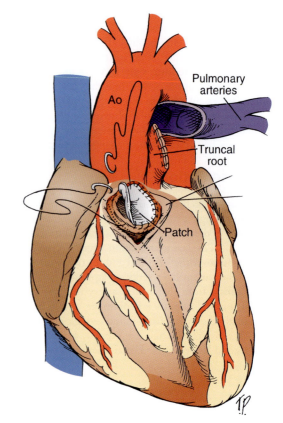

• **Figure 55.7** Repair of truncus arteriosus. The pulmonary arteries are detached from the truncal root. Through the longitudinal infundibulotomy, the malaligned ventricular septal defect is baffled with a prosthetic patch with the base of the truncal root directing left ventricular blood to the aorta (Ao).

it is often located more inferiorly than the external view of the truncus root would suggest. The subarterial VSD is closed through the ventriculotomy. If the septal defect is restrictive, the anterior extension of the SMT can be resected. This will prevent substantial outflow tract obstruction with closure of the VSD. When the inferior border of the VSD is separated from the septal leaflet of the tricuspid valve by the posterior-division SMT, the conduction system is safely behind the margin of the repair. If this muscular rim is absent, the conduction tissue resides close to the inferior border. Complete heart block is avoided by the meticulous placement of sutures in this area. Closure of the VSD is usually accomplished with a Dacron or expanded polytetrafluoroethylene (ePTFE [GORE-TEX]) patch (Fig. 55.8). If there is an atrial-level defect, it is closed at this time using a right atriotomy incision. Once the atrial and ventricular defects are closed, the heart is deaired and the cross-clamp removed.

Next, reconstruction of the RVOT is performed. This is usually accomplished with a valved conduit such as a pulmonary or arterial homograft or a bovine jugular valved conduit (Fig. 55.9). Most surgeons prefer a valved conduit to prevent RV dysfunction from significant pulmonary insufficiency in the early postoperative period because PVR may be elevated and possibly reactive in the early postoperative period. Often homograft is chosen because of the small size of the distal PA bifurcation and the relatively short distance between the RVOT and the PA, which makes the jugular venous valved conduit difficult to fit. However, it has been shown that small homograft size is associated with earlier necessity of

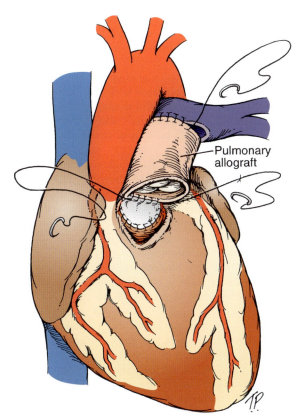

• **Figure 55.8** Repair of truncus arteriosus *(continued)*. Right ventricle to pulmonary artery continuity is established by interposition of valved conduit (usually cryopreserved pulmonary allograft).

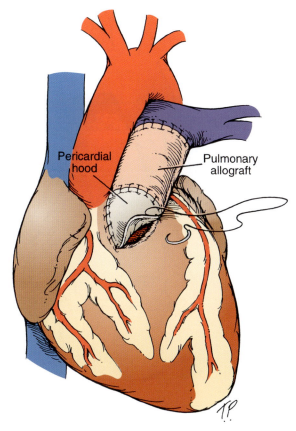

• **Figure 55.9** Repair of truncus arteriosus *(continued)*. Use of pericardial patch as proximal hood extension for pulmonary allograft.

reoperation for conduit replacement.[31] In patients who have demonstrated low PVR and favorable anatomy, direct anastomosis of the PA bifurcation to the RVOT with reconstruction of the RVOT with a monocusp or simple pericardial patch may be an acceptable alternative to the use of a valved conduit.[32]

Truncus Valve Dysfunction

One of the most difficult challenges surgeons face in treating patients with truncus arteriosus is correction of a stenotic or regurgitate truncus valve. In general a conservative approach to truncus valve repair is warranted. Because of the excessive cardiac output going through the truncal valve, gradients across a truncus valve of up to 3 m/s may be insignificant following complete repair. If necessary, conservative commissurotomy can be performed.[24] Additionally, truncus valve insufficiency should be addressed only if severe. Severe truncal valve regurgitation is a poor prognostic indicator for long-term survival,[19] but mild to moderate truncus valve regurgitation is often well tolerated and will improve postoperatively. However, failure to address significant truncal insufficiency, necessitating early reoperation with truncus valve surgery, has uniformly bad outcomes on a recent review of the Society of Thoracic Surgeons Congenital Heart Surgery Database (100% mortality, n = 4).[19] Specific anatomic features associated with the need for truncus valve surgery include an abnormal number of truncus valve cusps, the presence of valve dysplasia, and the presence of an anomalous coronary artery pattern.[33] Repair of the truncus valve is preferred over replacement due to the long-term risk and frequency of repeated truncus valve replacement. Recent reports have indicated that in

the appropriate cohort, truncus valve repair can be safely performed with reasonable and durable results.[34-36] In the setting of severe truncus valve regurgitation or stenosis, when repair is not an option, replacement can be performed using a cryopreserved aortic or pulmonary homograft and standard root replacement techniques (Fig. 55.10).

Truncus Arteriosus With Interrupted Aortic Arch

When truncus is associated with interrupted arch, repair proceeds differently from the previous description. These neonates have ductal-dependent systemic circulation and require prostaglandin therapy until surgical repair, usually in the first week of life and with generally good results.[37,38] In this subset of patients the interrupted arch is addressed with resection of the PDA and direct anastomosis of the distal descending aorta to the ascending aorta. This anastomosis may be augmented with a prosthetic patch, usually homograft patch material. Closure of the VSD and reconstruction of the RVOT are accomplished in a fashion similar to that of simple truncus.

Postoperative Management

The postoperative issues of infants after complete repair of a persistent truncus arteriosus are generally similar to those of neonates following repair of other lesions, with a few notable exceptions. Myocardial dysfunction and systemic inflammation post

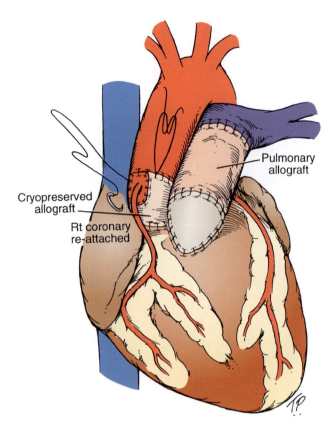

• **Figure 55.10** Repair of truncus arteriosus in the setting of severe truncal insufficiency. The truncal root is replaced with a second cryopreserved allograft, and coronary arteries are reimplanted to the allograft root.

Cryopreserved allograft

Rt coronary re-attached

Pulmonary allograft

cardiopulmonary bypass should be expected. Most infants will require some degree of inotropic support for the first 24 to 48 hours. Milrinone is commonly used in the immediate perioperative period to prevent low cardiac output syndrome and also because it can provide pulmonary afterload reduction. Central venous pressure (CVP) should be maintained at relatively high levels because of the decreased compliance of the RV. A protective ventilation strategy with lower mean airway pressure should be used. Because the RV is usually relatively noncompliant, only moderate increases in stroke volume can be achieved at any given preload. To optimize cardiac output, pacing at heart rates of 140 to 160 beats/min can be accomplished with epicardial pacing leads placed at the time of repair. Calcium chloride infusion may also be beneficial in cases of refractory hypotension due to the differences in calcium metabolism, particularly in patients with DiGeorge syndrome.[39] Relative adrenal insufficiency may contribute to postoperative hypotension and low cardiac output states, and high-dose corticosteroid administration may be needed in the setting of refractory hypotension.[40] Extracorporeal membrane oxygenation (ECMO) may be indicated if adequate perfusion cannot be achieved in spite of maximal medical efforts.

Pulmonary hypertension, both sustained and paroxysmal, can be anticipated in infants with preoperative elevation of PA pressures and those who undergo delayed repair. Pulmonary hypertensive crisis and low cardiac output are particularly prevalent in infants who are repaired after the neonatal period. Avoidance of these potentially fatal events has been paramount in the decrease in mortality and morbidity associated with repair.[41] RV function is typically compromised following cardiopulmonary bypass, and

even modest elevations of PVR are poorly tolerated. Events that trigger pulmonary hypertensive crisis, such as hypoxia, hypercapnia, acidosis, pain, airway stimulation, and LV failure, must be avoided. A mild respiratory alkalosis may be beneficial if pulmonary hypertensive crisis is suspected. The diagnosis should be suspected in the setting of acutely increased CVP and decreased cardiac output. A PA catheter can be useful in cases in which pulmonary hypertension is expected. Transthoracic echocardiography can also facilitate diagnosis through analysis of tricuspid and pulmonic regurgitant jet velocities.

The most common complication following truncus repair is pulmonary stenosis at the distal anastomosis. This is especially common in type 2 and type 3 truncus. It is not uncommon for patients to require catheter-based interventions on the PAs to delay the necessity of conduit replacement. RV-PA conduit insufficiency is common after a truncus repair but is usually well tolerated.

Severe truncus valve insufficiency can have a profound effect on postoperative recovery. Moderate to severe truncus valve insufficiency will decrease cardiac output and is poorly tolerated in patients with postbypass ventricular dysfunction. Additionally, ECMO may not be tolerated in the setting of severe truncus valve insufficiency because it will lead to LV dilation and further worsen ventricular function. If truncus valve insufficiency is significant, afterload reduction may aid in increasing cardiac output.

Coronary injuries and mechanical obstructions to coronary flow may lead to ventricular compromise following repair. Injury to the left coronary artery is possible during separation of the PAs from the arterial trunk. Additionally, in the setting of anomalous origin of the left coronary artery from the right coronary artery, coronary injury is possible when constructing the RV-PA conduit. Furthermore, coronary artery compression by the RV-PA conduit may lead to impaired cardiac perfusion. ST changes on electrocardiogram or inability to demonstrate flow in both coronary arteries on postoperative transesophageal echocardiography, particularly in the presence of impaired ventricular function, should alert the surgeon to myocardial ischemia.

Multiple arrhythmias may be encountered in the postoperative period following truncus arteriosus repair. Truncus arteriosus is a high-risk operation for the development of junctional ectopic tachycardia (JET),[42] likely related to the VSD repair.[43] Management of JET includes cooling, reduction of beta-adrenergic stimulation, antiarrhythmic medication, or overdrive pacing. Ventricular arrhythmias are less common following truncus repair and may be an indication of coronary injury or coronary compression. Right bundle branch block is nearly always present postoperatively. Complete heart block occurs in 3% to 5% of patients. Temporary epicardial pacing wires can be used to support the patient until the atrioventricular conduction system recovers or a permanent pacemaker is placed.[24]

There is also an impact of 22q11 deletion on the postoperative course of children following cardiac surgery. In a recent publication it was found that children with 22q11 deletion had an increased amount of unplanned noncardiac operations, increased incidence of fungal infection and wound infection, and an increased need for dialysis in the postoperative period compared with children with no chromosomal abnormalities.[44] Mortality did not differ between age-matched controls, and there was no difference in the length of mechanical ventilation, intensive care unit length of stay, or hospital length of stay. Upper and lower airway abnormalities common in DiGeorge syndrome, including subglottic stenosis, glottis webs, and laryngotracheomalacia, may complicate attempts at extubation.[45,46] Immune deficiencies may be present in patients with 22q11 deletion, and blood transfusion poses an increased risk of cytomegalovirus (CMV) infection and graft-versus-host disease in this population. For this reason, CMV-seronegative blood and irradiated blood should be considered until genetic testing is complete.[47]

Results

The mortality rate for truncus arteriosus repair has improved significantly since the early series, with current mortality, as reported by the Society of Thoracic Surgeons Congenital Heart Surgery Database, ranging from 0% to 27.3%.[48] Much of this improvement is attributed to the emphasis on repair during the neonatal period, before the development of irreversible pulmonary vascular disease. Historical reports have documented mortality of children repaired between the ages of 2 and 5 years ranging from 25% to 85%.[49] Modern single-institution reports have documented in-hospital survival of greater than 95% with greater than 90% survival at 1 year and beyond.[30,38] Operative factors significantly associated with poorer survival over time are operative weight of 2.5 kg or less, truncus valve replacement,[30] truncus valve dysfunction,[38] interrupted aortic arch, and coronary artery anomalies. The highest mortality for truncus arteriosus repair is among those who underwent concomitant repair of interrupted aortic arch and truncus valve repair (60% mortality).[19] Much emphasis now focuses on long-term outcomes related to truncus valve insufficiency and conduit restenosis.[19,29,37,50,51]

The major late complication after truncus arteriosus repair is obstruction or stenosis of the conduit. A variety of techniques to achieve RV-PA continuity have been devised, and the method used is often determined by patient-specific anatomy or surgeon preference.[52] Given the variable and increased PVR in the newborn period, many surgeons prefer using homograft conduits, rather than transannular patch or valved bovine jugular vein, in truncus arteriosus repair.[53] Rajasinghe et al.[51] performed a retrospective review to assess long-term outcomes among 165 patients who underwent truncus arteriosus repair in infancy. In this review, patients were followed for up to 20.4 years (median 10.5 years), with 25 patients lost at cross-sectional follow-up. There were 23 late deaths, 8 of which occurred within 6 months of repair and 13 of which occurred in 1 year. Ten of the late deaths were related to reoperations. Actuarial survival among all hospital survivors was 90% at 5 years, 85% at 10 years, and 83% at 15 years. A significant independent risk factor for poorer long-term survival was truncus with moderate to severe truncus valve insufficiency before repair. During the follow-up period, 107 patients underwent 133 conduit reoperations. Median time to conduit reoperation was 5.5 years, and the only factor significantly associated with shorter time to conduit replacement was smaller conduit size at initial repair.[54] Actuarial freedom from truncus valve replacement among patients with no prerepair truncus valve insufficiency was 95% at 10 years. Actuarial freedom from truncus valve replacement was significantly lower among patients with truncus insufficiency before initial repair (63% at 10 years). At follow-up all patients, except 3, were in New York Heart Association functional class 1.[51] Although 10- and 20-year survival has dramatically improved with improved conduit material, the need for future conduit replacement adds lifetime risk to these patients, and replacement or revision is almost inevitably necessary in this group of patients.[51]

Surgical repair of truncus arteriosus associated with interrupted aortic arch is a rare combination of complex anomalies and has been evaluated independently for long-term outcomes. Bohuta et al. evaluated 16 patients with truncus arteriosus and interrupted aortic arch (TA-IAA) who underwent one-stage repair. Mean follow-up duration was 18.2 years (13 of 14 patients). There were 2 (12.5%) early deaths and no late deaths. Functional status in all patients was good. Thirteen patients underwent 25 surgical reoperations and 5 interventional procedures (3 aortic arch balloon angioplasties and 2 PA balloon angioplasties). Overall freedom from any reoperation was 69.2% at 1 month, 54.5% at 3 years, 30% at 5 years, 11.1% at 10 years, and 0% at 15 years after the initial operation. Freedom from aortic reoperation was 76.9% at 1 month, 72.7% at 3 years, 70% at 5 years, 66.7% at 10 years, and 57.1% at 15 years. Freedom from RV-to-PA conduit replacement was 84.6% at 1 month, 63.6% at 3 years, 40% at 5 years, 11.1% at 10 years, and 0% at 15 years. Finally, freedom from truncus valve reoperation was 100% at 5 years, 88.9% at 10 years, and 85.7% at 15 years. The study documents that one-stage repair of TA-IAA can be undertaken with good long-term results. Despite a significant reoperation rate, functional status remains good at long-term follow-up.[55] RV-PA conduit replacement was the most common reason for reoperation in the study, with isolated RVOT reoperations, consisting of 56% of all surgical reoperations, demonstrating that improved conduits are still needed.

Surgical repair of truncus arteriosus in the neonatal period has led to good short-term and long-term outcomes. Truncus arteriosus with truncal valve dysplasia or with interrupted aortic arch remains a challenging lesion. Additionally, reoperation for conduit restenosis or outgrowth remains high.

Selected References

A complete list of references is available at ExpertConsult.com.

9. Van Praagh R, Van Praagh S. The anatomy of common aorticopulmonary trunk (truncus arteriosus communis) and its embryologic implications. A study of 57 necropsy cases. *Am J Cardiol.* 1965;16(3):406–425.
14. Anderson RH, Thiene G. Categorization and description of hearts with a common arterial trunk. *Eur J Cardiothorac Surg.* 1989;3(6):481–487.
15. Collett RW, Edwards JE. Persistent truncus arteriosus; a classification according to anatomic types. *Surg Clin North Am.* 1949;29(4):1245–1270.
16. Russell HM, Jacobs ML, Anderson RH, et al. A simplified categorization for common arterial trunk. *J Thorac Cardiovasc Surg.* 2011;141(3):645–653.
19. Russell HM, Pasquali SK, Jacobs JP, et al. Outcomes of repair of common arterial trunk with truncal valve surgery: a review of the society of thoracic surgeons congenital heart surgery database. *Ann Thorac Surg.* 2012;93(1):164–169, discussion 169.
29. Bove EL, Lupinetti FM, Pridjian AK, et al. Results of a policy of primary repair of truncus arteriosus in the neonate. *J Thorac Cardiovasc Surg.* 1993;105(6):1057–1065, discussion 1065–1056.
48. Jacobs JP, Mayer JE Jr, Mavroudis C, et al. The Society of Thoracic Surgeons Congenital Heart Surgery Database: 2016 update on outcomes and quality. *Ann Thorac Surg.* 2016;101(3):850–862.
51. Rajasinghe HA, McElhinney DB, Reddy VM, Mora BN, Hanley FL. Long-term follow-up of truncus arteriosus repaired in infancy: a twenty-year experience. *J Thorac Cardiovasc Surg.* 1997;113(5):869–878, discussion 878–869.

56

Coronary Artery Anomalies

JULIE A. BROTHERS, MD; MARSHALL L. JACOBS, MD

This chapter focuses on the medical and surgical management of coronary artery anomalies in the pediatric patient without other congenital heart defects. The vast majority of aberrant coronary arteries are without functional consequence and are not clinically significant. However, there are a few anomalies of which the practitioner should be aware because they may lead to ventricular arrhythmia, myocardial ischemia, left ventricular (LV) dysfunction, and, in some, sudden cardiac death (SCD). This chapter will focus on the following coronary anomalies: anomalous origin of a coronary artery from the pulmonary artery, anomalous origin of a coronary artery from the wrong sinus of Valsalva, and coronary artery fistulae.

Normal Coronary Anatomy

In the structurally normal heart the two coronary arteries arise from the center of the right and left aortic sinuses of Valsalva. The right aortic sinus of Valsalva gives rise to the right coronary artery (RCA), which directly enters the right atrioventricular groove and frequently terminates as the posterior descending artery. The left aortic sinus of Valsalva gives rise to the left main coronary artery (LMCA), which usually bifurcates into the left anterior descending (LAD) and circumflex coronary arteries a short distance from the origin. The LAD subsequently courses in the anterior interventricular groove, whereas the left circumflex coronary artery runs in the left atrioventricular groove (Fig. 56.1). When coronary arteries arise normally, the coronary ostia are round, and the proximal portion of the coronary artery exits the aortic wall perpendicularly.[1] More rarely, the ostium may be located in the correct sinus but somewhat eccentrically, closer to one of the valve commissures. As well, on occasion one or both coronary ostia may originate above the aortic sinuses (i.e., above the sinotubular junction). Although this particular abnormality of coronary origin is usually a benign condition, a high takeoff of a coronary artery may be relevant in the context of planned surgery to address other cardiac abnormalities.

Anomalous Origin of a Coronary Artery From the Pulmonary Artery

Anomalous origin of a coronary artery from the pulmonary artery is a rare congenital anomaly that is associated with a high risk of death in the first year of life if not diagnosed and treated appropriately.[2,3] This anomaly was first described by Krause[4] in 1865 followed by Brooks[5] in 1885. However, it became known as the Bland-White-Garland syndrome in 1933 after Bland and colleagues[6]

reported clinical and autopsy findings of an infant who died from anomalous origin of the LMCA from the pulmonary artery.

The most prevalent form of anomalous origin of a coronary artery from the pulmonary artery is anomalous left coronary artery from the pulmonary artery (ALCAPA). Most commonly the LMCA arises from the pulmonary artery (Fig. 56.2). The RCA may also arise from the pulmonary artery (ARCAPA), but this is approximately 10 times less common than ALCAPA. Very rarely, other coronaries may arise from the pulmonary artery, such as the LAD, circumflex, or both RCA and LMCA; the latter being quite rare and almost always fatal. ALCAPA is the most common cause of myocardial infarction in the pediatric population, and this diagnosis should be high on the differential if a child of any age, but notably an infant, presents with evidence of myocardial infarction or otherwise unexplained severe LV dysfunction. The incidence of ALCAPA ranges from 1 in 30,000 to 1 in 300,000 people, making up 0.25% to 0.5% of congenital heart disease diagnoses. ALCAPA is not considered an inheritable disease, and there is no racial or ethnic predilection; however, there is a 3:1 male to female ratio of occurrence.[7] By 1 year of age, approximately 85% of patients will have presented with clinical symptoms of congestive heart failure, although there are rare cases of patients presenting later in childhood and even into adulthood. There is a 90% mortality rate in infancy if not quickly diagnosed and appropriately managed. Although ALCAPA usually occurs in isolation, other known associated cardiac defects include patent ductus arteriosus (PDA), ventricular septal defect (VSD), coarctation of the aorta, and tetralogy of Fallot.

Anatomy and Embryology

There are different theories regarding the embryologic development of ALCAPA. In one very early theory, Abrikosoff[8] proposed that ALCAPA occurs when there is abnormal aorticopulmonary septation of the conotruncus. Alternately, according to Hackensellner,[9] a persistence of the pulmonary buds, along with involution of the aortic buds that form the coronary arteries, together could lead to ALCAPA formation in utero. Most recently, Sharma et al. studied normal cardiac embryogenesis in the mouse embryo and observed that *VEGF-C* stimulates vascular growth near the outflow tract while a vessel-free zone directly surrounds the aorta and pulmonary artery. Coronary vessels develop around the outflow tracts but do not invade the vessel-free zone. Wild-type islet 1 gene expression levels in the embryo allow cardiomyocytes to differentiate specifically in the aortic wall, where they support vessel growth and facilitate connections between coronary vessels and luminal endothelium. The result is correctly positioned coronary

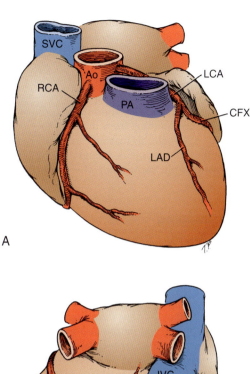

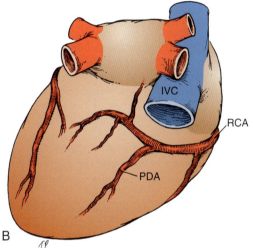

• **Figure 56.1** Normal coronary anatomy. (A) Anterior aspect. (B) Posterior aspect. The posterior descending artery originates from the right coronary indicating a dominant right coronary system. *Ao,* Aorta; *CFX,* circumflex coronary artery; *IVC,* interior vena cava; *LAD,* left anterior descending coronary artery; *LCA,* left coronary artery; *PA,* pulmonary artery; *RCA,* right coronary artery; *SVC,* superior vena cava.

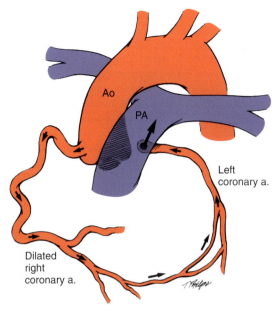

• **Figure 56.2** Schematic representation of a dilated, tortuous right coronary artery *(a)* associated with anomalous left coronary artery. *Arrows* indicate coronary "steal," with direction of blood flow from right coronary to left coronary, ultimately draining into the pulmonary artery *(PA). Ao,* Aorta.

artery stems on the aorta. They also demonstrated in murine models that *VEGF-C*–deficient hearts exhibited severely hypoplastic peritruncal vessels, resulting in delayed and abnormally positioned coronary stems. Mice heterozygous for islet 1 *(Isl1)* exhibited decreased aortic cardiomyocytes and abnormally low coronary artery stems. In hearts with outflow tract rotation defects, misplaced stems were associated with shifted aortic cardiomyocytes and myocardium-induced ectopic connections, including abnormal connections of a coronary artery with the pulmonary artery. These data support a model in which coronary artery stem development first requires *VEGF-C* to stimulate vessel growth around the outflow tract. Then, aortic cardiomyocytes facilitate interactions between peritruncal vessels and the aorta. Derangement of either step can lead to mispatterned coronary artery stems.[10,11]

In ALCAPA the LMCA arises from the main pulmonary artery (MPA) but on occasion may arise from one of the branch pulmonary arteries. Although the ALCAPA usually originates from the rightward aspect of the posterior (facing) sinus of the MPA, it may also arise from the leftward portion of the posterior (facing) sinus. In ARCAPA the anomalous RCA most often arises from the anterior portion of the pulmonary artery. In ALCAPA the anomalous LMCA takes its usual course but is often much smaller in caliber, resembling a vein more than an artery. The RCA arises normally, but, notably in those who have survived infancy and are diagnosed later in childhood or adulthood, the RCA is quite dilated, and there are significant collateral branches from the RCA to the LMCA.

Pathophysiology

During fetal life there are similar systemic and pulmonary circulation pressures secondary to an unrestrictive PDA; as well, there are similar oxygen concentrations in the MPA and aorta, resulting in adequate myocardial perfusion despite the anomaly of coronary origin. At this stage there is no need for RCA collateralization to occur. After birth, in the neonatal period, the pulmonary artery resistance and pressure remains elevated, thereby maintaining perfusion of the LV myocardium through the anomalous coronary artery. Soon after birth, with the transition to postnatal circulation (systemic and pulmonary circulations in series, rather than parallel), there is a decrease in MPA pressure, pulmonary vascular resistance (PVR), and oxygen content in the pulmonary artery. With the LV being perfused with desaturated blood at a low pressure and in the face of inadequate collateral circulation from right coronary artery to left, myocardial ischemia and ventricular dysfunction result from insufficient myocardial perfusion.[12]

At first, myocardial ischemia occurs only during periods of increased myocardial demands, for instance, when the infant is feeding or crying. Further increases in myocardial oxygen consumption with inadequate collateral circulation lead to infarction of the anterolateral LV free wall, which results in mitral valve papillary muscle dysfunction, significant mitral valve regurgitation, and LV volume overload. Flow reversal occurs from the LMCA into the pulmonary trunk during diastole due to the low PVR. If some intercoronary collaterals are present, this may set up left-to-right shunting and coronary steal. Because of this, the LV myocardium continues to be underperfused. Congestive heart failure, with elevated LV end-diastolic and left atrial pressure, is the outcome from a combination of LV systolic dysfunction, left-to-right shunt, and significant mitral valve insufficiency.

Interestingly, in the presence of another cardiac defect, such as a PDA or VSD, the pulmonary artery pressure will remain elevated, and there may be adequate LV perfusion pressure to prevent ischemia. A thorough investigation of the coronary arteries should be done before attempting surgical or catheter closure of these cardiac defects because the diagnosis will become apparent shortly after closure due to the abrupt drop in pulmonary arterial pressure, usually with a fatal outcome. Alternatively, a small number of patients develop significant collateralization. If this occurs, then perfusion of the left coronary system is maintained. However, as the PVR starts to drop, a left-to-right (coronary-pulmonary) shunt develops from the RCA to the MPA, with the LMCA acting as a conduit from the RCA to the MPA, leading to a pulmonary-coronary steal. This leads to progressive dilation of the RCA and left coronary artery systems. Patients who have LMCA ostial stenosis are somewhat protected because it reduces the coronary steal phenomenon. Although the left-right shunt is relatively small compared with overall cardiac output, it is significant because it pertains to coronary blood flow. Although children with extensive collaterals may survive past infancy, there is commonly progressive LV dysfunction.[13] In a small number of patients the collateralization is enough to ensure adequate myocardial perfusion at rest and potentially even with exercise, and these patients may not be diagnosed until adulthood.[14] When this occurs, the most common presentations are angina, dyspnea, palpitations, or fatigue.[15]

Clinical Presentation

Children with ALCAPA are born healthy and often do not come to medical attention until approximately 6 to 8 weeks of age, when the physiologic consequences of the decrease in PVR become apparent.[16] However, many infants may not be diagnosed until closer to 3 months of age, when symptoms have invariably increased in frequency and severity. Approximately 85% of infants will present with signs and symptoms of myocardial ischemia and congestive heart failure, including sweating and pain (crying or restlessness) with feeding, nursing, or stooling; tachypnea; poor weight gain; and pallor. In fact, the chest pain from myocardial ischemia may initially be mistaken for infantile colic, which may delay parents seeking medical attention.

The remainder of the patients may present in either childhood or adulthood. In childhood they come to attention due to the loud murmur of mitral regurgitation or exercise-induced symptoms. A small percentage may remain asymptomatic until adulthood, when they may present with exertional chest pain, presyncope, or syncope. These patients remain at risk of SCD.[13] Their late presentation is believed to be due to early formation of adequate collateralization to the LV myocardium. The symptoms associated with ARCAPA are less severe, and patients generally present later in childhood or into adulthood; however, myocardial ischemia and SCD can still occur.

Physical examination of the infant with ALCAPA will likely show signs of congestive heart failure, including tachypnea, tachycardia, and hepatomegaly. The left heart is usually enlarged, often with associated mitral regurgitation. The LV precordial impulse may appear prominent and displaced inferiorly and laterally. The first heart sound is either normal or diminished (from the mitral

regurgitation), and the second heart sound is normal or closely split with a loud P_2, if pulmonary hypertension is present. An S_3 gallop rhythm is commonly present. In infants with significant mitral regurgitation a pansystolic murmur at the apex may be audible. In older children, adolescents, and adults a continuous murmur may be audible at the left upper sternal border due to continuous retrograde blood flow from the left coronary artery to the pulmonary artery, resulting from the intercoronary collateral communication. Although this may be hard to differentiate from a PDA, this murmur does not peak around the second heart sound and has a louder diastolic component when compared to a PDA murmur.

Diagnostic Imaging

Infants with ALCAPA generally have cardiomegaly on chest radiograph, especially from the enlarged left atrium and LV, with or without pulmonary venous congestion. However, this is not sensitive or specific for ALCAPA. However, the electrocardiogram (ECG) can be useful when an infant presents with congestive heart failure. There may be classic findings of an anterolateral infarct pattern with deep and narrow (>3 mm) Q waves in leads I, aVL, V_5, and V_6, poor R wave progression across the precordial leads, and ST-segment depression or inversion in the inferior and lateral leads (Fig. 56.3). Although this pattern can be found in other causes of myocardial infarction or cardiomyopathy, if these ECG abnormalities are seen in an infant or child in congestive heart failure, the diagnosis of ALCAPA needs to be strongly considered. Certainly, any infant with dilated cardiomyopathy should be evaluated for ALCAPA, and the diagnosis should also be in the differential in older patients presenting with dilated cardiomyopathy.

Echocardiography usually demonstrates a dilated LV with global or regional hypokinesis, decreased LV function, and severe mitral regurgitation with left atrial dilation. These findings may also be seen in young patients with dilated cardiomyopathy as well as those with myocarditis. Careful attention should be paid to the origins of both coronary arteries, including the possibility of abnormal origin of the LMCA from the pulmonary artery. The short-axis view should demonstrate the coronary origins. In ALCAPA

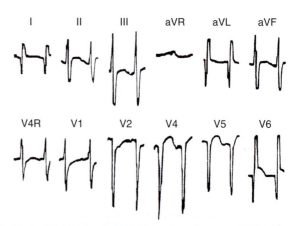

• **Figure 56.3** Electrocardiogram with anterolateral myocardial infarction pattern in a 2-month-old infant with anomalous origin of the left coronary artery. Note deep Q waves in I, aVL, and V6, as well as the QS pattern in V2 through V5. (From Park MK. *Pediatric Cardiology for Practitioners*. Chicago: Mosby–Year Book; 1988:280; with permission.)

the LMCA will not be seen arising from the aorta but rather from the pulmonary artery. Color flow Doppler should reveal retrograde flow from the coronary artery to the pulmonary artery and is pathognomonic for ALCAPA.[17] As well, in the absence of retrograde flow from the coronary artery into the pulmonary artery, ALCAPA can be distinguished from ostial atresia of the left coronary artery, because retrograde flow in both branches of the LMCA (i.e., LAD and circumflex coronaries) will be seen with ALCAPA, whereas retrograde flow in the LAD coronary along with antegrade flow in the circumflex coronary suggests LMCA atresia.[18] Additionally, an enlarged RCA is almost always present and should raise suspicion of this diagnosis. Another echocardiographic finding is increased echogenicity (or echo brightness) of the LV papillary muscles due to infarction. Although echocardiographic imaging of coronary artery origins has improved significantly over the past several years, identifying coronary origin and course can be challenging in some cases. Therefore, if any question remains about visualization of both coronary ostia, then further evaluation is mandatory to rule out ALCAPA.

Magnetic resonance imaging (MRI) is a useful noninvasive diagnostic tool for delineating congenital coronary anomalies.[19,20] Although there are case reports of using MRI in diagnosing ALCAPA, there are no case series with this anomaly. Computed tomography angiography (CTA) has been used extensively for coronary artery delineation in adults. Advantages of this technique include rapid acquisition time and high resolution, but the disadvantages include radiation exposure and the need for a slower heart rate with ECG gating, largely precluding its use in infants.

For diagnosis of ALCAPA the gold standard remains cardiac catheterization with angiography and should be performed before surgery. Cardiac catheterization in these patients will demonstrate elevated filling and pulmonary artery pressures along with a low cardiac output. In those patients diagnosed at an older age, it may show only mildly elevated pulmonary artery pressures but with normal filling pressures and cardiac output. An aortogram should be performed to delineate the coronary artery origins. The aortogram will demonstrate a dilated RCA arising normally from the aorta but no LMCA arising from the aorta. If collaterals are present, it should show blood flow from the RCA through the collaterals providing late, retrograde filling of the left coronary artery and a blush of contrast into the MPA. A step-up in oxygen saturation may be noted in the MPA in the presence of a significant left-to-right shunt from the collaterals. If any doubt remains, a main pulmonary arteriogram with distal balloon occlusion should clearly demonstrate the anomalous left coronary artery.[21]

Treatment and Management

Medical Management. Initial medical management of ALCAPA is stabilization, mechanical ventilation, and treatment of congestive heart failure before surgical repair. This includes diuretics, afterload reduction medications, and inotropic agents. Mechanical ventilator support may be required. Delivery of oxygen at high fraction of inspired oxygen (FiO_2) should be done judiciously because this may further decrease the PVR, increasing the coronary steal from the RCA to the MPA. As well, caution should be taken with aggressive afterload reduction because that may decrease RCA perfusion, which subsequently leads to decreased left coronary artery blood flow and increased ischemia. Inotropic medication should also be used judiciously because it may increase myocardial oxygen consumption, thereby worsening the ongoing ischemia due to decreased myocardial blood flow. Occasionally, mechanical

circulatory support (extracorporeal membrane oxygenation [ECMO]) may be required, but this is usually in the setting of delayed diagnosis with the misconception of idiopathic dilated cardiomyopathy.

Surgical Management. All patients diagnosed with ALCAPA should undergo surgical repair. In infants presenting with congestive heart failure, surgery should occur as soon as possible after stabilization due to ongoing risk of myocardial ischemia and death.[22] In patients who are older and are asymptomatic, surgery can be performed electively. Because infants requiring surgery are usually critically ill, centers that perform ALCAPA surgery should have the ability to use LV assist devices and ECMO; if not, the child should be transferred to a hospital with these abilities.[23]

The goal of surgical repair is the creation of a two-coronary system. Simple ligation of the anomalous coronary is now of historical interest only; it should not be performed.[24] Indeed, even patients who present with severe LV dysfunction and mitral insufficiency should undergo repair that establishes two-coronary antegrade circulation because significant recovery of function may be expected and improvement in mitral regurgitation often occurs. Because the degree of mitral valve regurgitation nearly always improves after surgery, LV aneurysmectomy and mitral valve repair or replacement are rarely indicated at the time of initial procedure.

Surgical Techniques

Historically the first successful operation for ALCAPA was simple ligation of the anomalous LMCA at the pulmonary artery (Fig. 56.4). The ligation prevents the left-to-right shunt, which allows perfusion of the LV through collateral vessels from the RCA. However, this procedure is no longer recommended because myocardial perfusion remains solely from the RCA and its collateralization, leading to increased risk of early mortality and late SCD events. Instead, a variety of techniques were developed to create a dual coronary artery system.

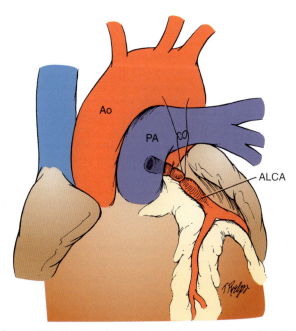

• **Figure 56.4** Ligation of anomalous left coronary artery (ALCA). *Ao,* Aorta; *PA,* pulmonary artery.

era, bypass grafting is usually used to create a dual coronary artery system after previous ligation or if previous repair has resulted in coronary artery stenosis or occlusion. If this technique is used, the internal mammary artery is the conduit of choice, even in neonates and infants.[29-31] The saphenous vein or the left subclavian artery should not be used because of the risk of anatomic stenosis or occlusion and poor long-term results.[32,33]

Direct Reimplantation. In most patients with ALCAPA, direct reimplantation of the anomalous coronary artery onto the aorta can be performed (Fig. 56.6).[34,35] When the anomalous coronary ostium is in the posterior-facing sinus, the procedure is fairly straightforward. Direct implantation is possible even if the ostium is located in the nonfacing sinus by excising a large button or flap of pulmonary artery wall in continuity with the coronary artery. Such a flap of autologous tissue may be converted to a cylinder to extend the coronary artery, thus minimizing tension on the anastomosis to the aorta.[36]

After induction of anesthesia and placement of monitoring lines, a median sternotomy is performed. Because of the risk of ventricular fibrillation from myocardial ischemia and LV dysfunction, the heart should be manipulated or disturbed as little as possible before the patient is placed on cardiopulmonary bypass. This operation may be performed using either continuous low-flow bypass with moderate hypothermia (25°C to 28°C) or deep hypothermic circulatory arrest (18°C) in very small infants. The pulmonary artery and course of the left coronary artery are visualized on the epicardial surface. If the anomalous left coronary artery originates far leftward in the posterior-facing sinus or on the anterior nonfacing sinus, direct reimplantation may be more challenging, requiring special techniques to establish connection to the aorta. An alternative technique that may be necessary if the coronary arises anteriorly from the pulmonary artery or from a branch pulmonary artery is extending the coronary artery with a tube constructed from pulmonary artery wall to allow reimplantation. The pulmonary artery can be repaired primarily with a continuous suture of 7-0 polypropylene (Prolene), or, more commonly, the pulmonary artery is repaired with a patch of autologous pericardium.

Modified Takeuchi Operation. The Takeuchi operation, or intrapulmonary artery tunnel, is an alternative surgical strategy for repair of ALCAPA. Takeuchi and colleagues originally described creating an aortopulmonary window with a portion of the anterior pulmonary artery wall that would baffle blood from the aorta to the anomalous coronary artery ostium.[26] Alternatively, the baffle is constructed using an expanded PTFE (Gore-Tex) patch in the modified Takeuchi operation.

Postoperative Management

The management issues expected after surgical repair are usually related to the child's preoperative medical status, including low cardiac output, LV dysfunction, and hypotension. Care should be taken to optimize the patient's hemoglobin level and normalize the electrolyte levels, acid-base and fluid status and provide adequate inotropic support. In those with severe cardiac dysfunction preoperatively, placement on ECMO support or use of an LV assist device may be temporarily needed. Bleeding is commonly encountered, more often in small infants and those who require mechanical support. Whenever necessary, platelets and fresh frozen plasma should be used to replace ongoing loss. Delayed sternal closure may be necessary in those patients with continued low cardiac output or bleeding issues. Cardiac dysrhythmia due to preoperative

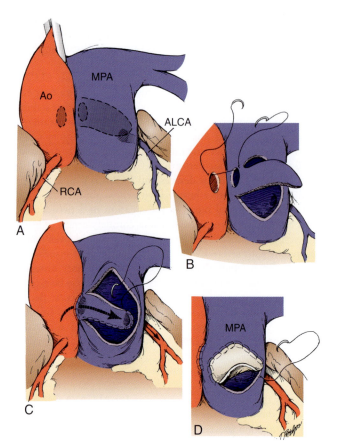

• **Figure 56.5** Technique of intrapulmonary aortocoronary tunnel (Takeuchi repair). (A) Initial incisions *(dotted lines)* in aorta *(Ao)* and main pulmonary artery *(MPA)* in preparation for tunnel to anomalous left coronary artery *(ALCA)*. (B) Anastomosis of Ao to MPA, creation of flap within MPA. (C) MPA flap becomes anterior wall of tunnel between the aorta and the ALCA. (D) Closure of MPA defect with pericardium. *RCA,* Right coronary artery.

In 1968 Meyer and colleagues[25] reported the first successful left subclavian artery–to–left coronary artery bypass. This technique is rarely used today in patients with ALCAPA (Fig. 56.5). The Takeuchi operation, or intrapulmonary artery tunnel, is an alternative surgical strategy for two-vessel coronary repair of ALCAPA. Originally Takeuchi and colleagues described the creation of an aortopulmonary window and used a portion of anterior pulmonary artery wall to form the roof of a tunnel directing blood from the aorta to the abnormally placed ostium of the anomalous coronary artery within the pulmonary artery. The MPA must then be augmented with a patch of pericardium or prosthetic material.[26] This technique, which does not involve excision and reimplantation of the origin of the left coronary artery, has been modified by constructing a baffle using a polytetrafluoroethylene (PTFE) patch rather than the flap of MPA anterior wall. The main complications of the modified Takeuchi operation include baffle leak, baffle occlusion, and supravalvar pulmonary artery stenosis. Finally, the procedure of choice for most surgeons is direct reimplantation of the anomalous coronary onto the aorta, especially as experience with coronary mobilization and transfer has increased over the years based on the arterial switch operation for transposition of the great vessels.[27,28]

Coronary Artery Bypass Grafting. Coronary artery bypass grafting is rarely used in patients with ALCAPA. In the current

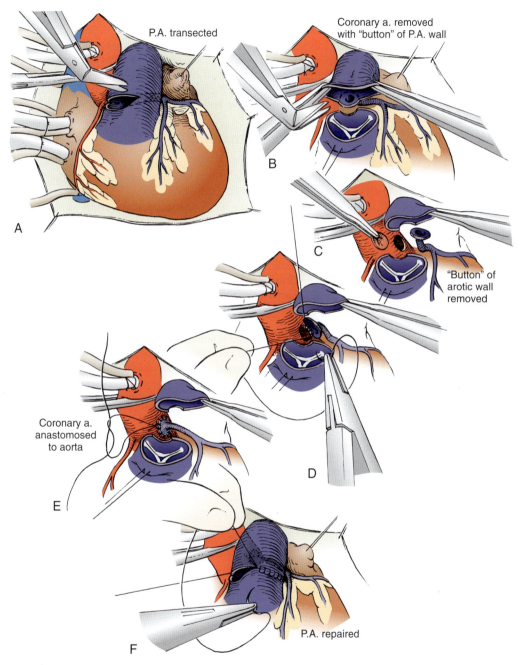

• Figure 56.6 Technique of direct coronary transfer for anomalous left coronary artery *(a.)*. (A) Transection of pulmonary artery (PA). (B) Removal of coronary artery ostial button. (C) Preparation of aorta. (D) Coronary anastomosis. (E) Completion of coronary anastomosis. (F) Repair of the main PA. (From Hallman GL, Cooley DA, Gutsesell HP. *Surgical Treatment of Congenital Heart Disease.* 3rd ed. Philadelphia: Lea & Febiger; 1987; with permission.)

LV myocardial ischemia or infarction remains a concern, and patient should be monitored expectantly.

Outcomes. As discussed previously, simple ligation for ALCAPA has unacceptable early and late mortality rates. In general, survival after establishment of a dual coronary system is excellent.[37-40] Vouhe and colleagues[40] from France reported on 31 consecutive patients who underwent reimplantation of the anomalous coronary. In the short term, there were 3 hospital deaths and 2 additional deaths within the first 3 months. There were no late deaths. Of the 23 who were studied at more than 1 year after repair, all had normal LV function; in the 5 who had severe mitral regurgitation preoperatively, the severity had decreased to mild or no regurgitation. The reimplanted anomalous coronary artery was patent in all patients. In another study of 23 infants who underwent ALCAPA repair, 16 underwent aortic reimplantation, and 7 underwent trapdoor flap or tubular extension technique repair. Four patients died early in the postoperative period, but LV function was improved in all of the remaining patients. However, only 1 of 5 infants with preoperative severe mitral valve regurgitation had significant improvement, and 2 patients ultimately underwent mitral valve replacement.[39] This differs from a report by Lange and colleagues,[41] who evaluated the long-term results of 56 patients with ALCAPA who underwent either subclavian artery anastomosis or coronary artery transfer. There was no early mortality in those who underwent repair in the current decade. Late mortality was similar in each group, with 1 patient each. At final follow-up, 95% of patients had normal LV function, and 84% had less than grade 2 severity mitral regurgitation.

Anomalous Aortic Origin of a Coronary Artery With Course Between the Aorta and the Pulmonary Artery

Anomalous aortic origin of a coronary artery (AAOCA) consists of either an anomalous aortic origin of the LMCA (AAOLCA) or the RCA (AAORCA). The anomaly of origin most often consists of an origin that is *not* within the expected or "appropriate" sinus of Valsalva. The proximal course of the anomalous coronary artery is important and should be determined because this largely serves to determine the clinical significance and potential risk of SCD to the patient. When the anomalous coronary courses anterior to the pulmonary artery (prepulmonic) or posterior to the aorta (posterior/retroaortic), these have generally been considered benign, although there are a couple of case reports of SCD with retroaortic AAOLCA. Additionally, the anomalous LMCA or LAD can course through the conal septum, termed *intraseptal* or *intraconal* or *intramyocardial*, and this is also generally believed to not be clinically significant; however, the importance of the anomalous intraseptal coronary is differentiating it from the interarterial AAOLCA. Interarterial AAORCA or AAOLCA occurs when both coronary arteries arise from, or above, the same aortic sinus with either a single ostium or two separate ostia and the anomalous coronary courses between the aorta and pulmonary artery. Several population and autopsy series have identified both interarterial AAORCA and AAOLCA as the subtypes that lead to increased risk of SCD, notably in young otherwise healthy athletic individuals, with the risk much greater with AAOLCA than AAORCA.

The prevalence of congenital coronary anomalies in the general population is difficult to ascertain. A number of studies have attempted to quantify this value, with estimates ranging between 0.1% and 1% in both the adult and pediatric populations.[42-47]

The differing rates are likely a combination of differing definitions of coronary anomalies, imaging modality, and patient population studied.[48-51]

When looking specifically at the prevalence of interarterial AAOCA, which is the subtype of greatest clinical concern, a recent MRI study evaluating several thousand middle school children found this anomaly in 0.7% of this population, of which 0.5% were AAORCA and 0.2% AAOLCA. This prevalence of interarterial AAOCA is larger than the previously cited of 0.1% to 0.3%.[47] In most studies, interarterial intramural AAORCA occurs three to six times more often than AAOLCA. AAOCA appears to be more prevalent in males than females at approximately a 3:1 ratio.[52] Although no specific genetic abnormality has been found, there have been several reports of familial occurrences.[53]

Anatomy

When there are two separate coronary ostia, either the RCA or the LMCA may arise from, or above, the "wrong" sinus of Valsalva with a subsequent course of the aberrant coronary artery between the aorta and pulmonary artery (Fig. 56.7). The interarterial anomalous coronary artery also frequently has an intramural (i.e., shared wall with the aorta) proximal segment of varying lengths before exiting from the aorta onto the epicardium. When the two ostia arise from the same sinus, the ostium of the anomalous coronary artery is commonly elliptical and slit-like with an acute-angle takeoff.[54] Much more rare is when there is a single coronary artery origin within or above the right aortic sinus and the single coronary artery gives rise to an LMCA or LAD that runs between the aorta and pulmonary artery, or the single coronary artery origin within or above the left aortic sinus gives rise to an RCA that courses between the great vessels.[55,56] In the cases with the single coronary artery, the anomalous coronary almost always has a round orifice and does not have an intramural component when it arises from the proximal portion of the single coronary.

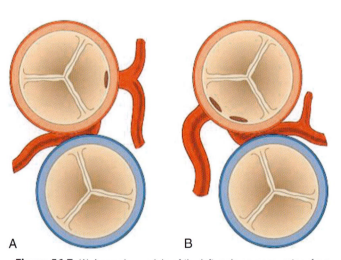

• **Figure 56.7** (A) Anomalous origin of the left main coronary artery from the rightward aspect of the posterior-facing sinus of the pulmonary artery. (B) Anomalous origin of the left main coronary artery from the leftward aspect of the posterior-facing sinus. Anomalous origin of the left main coronary artery from the nonfacing sinus of the pulmonary artery. (Reprinted with permission from Gaynor JW. Coronary artery anomalies in children. In: Kaiser LR, Kron IL, Spray TL, eds. *Mastery of Cardiothoracic Surgery*. Philadelphia: Lippincott-Raven; 1998:882.)

Pathophysiology

When the anomalous coronary courses interarterially and commonly intramurally, this is associated with an increased incidence of SCD.[57-61] The greatest danger of sudden death appears to be during or just after maximal exertion in young athletes, mainly between the ages of 12 and 22 years. Both interarterial AAOLCA and AAORCA are associated with sudden death, but the former, although much less prevalent than AAORCA, carries a significantly higher risk of an adverse event. Based on autopsy studies of patients with AAOCA, SCD is hypothesized to occur from a mismatch between myocardial demand (which is increased during exertion) and myocardial oxygen delivery, which is dependent upon the anomalous coronary blood flow, which may fail to increase in relation to demand or may even decrease during exertion. This results in myocardial ischemia or ventricular tachyarrhythmias (or both). This limited or diminished coronary blood flow is probably the result of one or many anatomic and physiologic factors, including an initial intramural course of the anomalous coronary that leads to a variable degree of stenosis and hypoplasia that can be stretched out and flattened as the aorta dilates during exercise, an acute-angle takeoff from the aorta with a slit-like orifice, vasospasm of the anomalous vessel, intussusception of the proximal intramural segment, and myocardial scar that can lead to arrhythmogenic foci. The risk of ischemia is greatest with vigorous exercise, when there is a significantly greater cardiac output and oxygen demand placed on the heart.[62-64]

Clinical Presentation

Patients commonly are asymptomatic, and the coronary anomaly is found serendipitously when an echocardiogram is performed for an unrelated reason, such as for a cardiac murmur, abnormal ECG, or a family member with a coronary anomaly or other congenital cardiac disease.[52,65] For a small number of patients the initial diagnosis is made after they experienced sudden cardiac arrest or SCD. Others may be diagnosed due to a variety of symptoms, commonly related to exercise, including chest pain, palpitations, dizziness, presyncope, or syncope. Although these symptoms are commonly seen in children without coronary anomalies, this will prompt a visit to a pediatric cardiologist, where an echocardiogram is often performed and the coronary anomaly is found. Given the prevalence of up to 0.7% of interarterial AAOCA in the screened population, echocardiograms performed on children and adolescents with symptoms that are not likely to be ischemia in this low-risk population are going to yield the diagnosis of AAOCA, even though the symptoms are unrelated.[47]

There are no specific physical findings in patients with AAOCA. The results of physical examination and resting ECG are almost always normal. Because of this, young athletes with AAOCA will not be diagnosed through a screening program that uses history, ECG, and physical examination alone. This can generally be diagnosed only with an imaging study, most commonly echocardiography. Indeed, the diagnosis should be entertained in any young person with exercise-induced complaints suggestive of myocardial ischemia or arrhythmia, notably syncope with exercise, or in those presenting with sudden cardiac arrest or SCD.

Diagnostic Testing

In the evaluation of a young person with concern for a coronary anomaly, a resting ECG should be obtained to evaluate for arrhythmias and evidence of prior or evolving myocardial infarction, the latter of which would be concerning in someone presenting with sudden cardiac arrest.

Transthoracic Echocardiography. Transthoracic echocardiography with color flow Doppler should be performed to ensure normal intracardiac anatomy and to evaluate heart function, especially focusing on areas of abnormal wall motion signifying possible history of ischemia.[66-68] This technique has evolved as the preferred initial diagnostic modality due to its availability, ease of performing in children, cost-effectiveness, and lack of radiation.[66-69] Close attention should be paid to the coronary artery origins and proximal course. In the majority of young people, both the coronary artery origins and proximal course are able to be visualized, especially when combined with color flow Doppler mapping. Color Doppler should always be used when imaging coronary anatomy. In patients with an intramural anomalous coronary, two-dimensional imaging alone may not adequately distinguish the intramural component, and the vessel may appear to arise normally where it exits the aorta. The addition of color Doppler imaging can also help demonstrate the abnormal direction of blood flow within the aortic wall.[66,68] However, echocardiographic imaging does have limitations, such as the need for different frequency transducers, patient size, inadequate echocardiographic windows, and patient cooperation.[69] Because of these issues, the majority of children are referred for a confirmatory CTA or cardiac MRI.

Computed Tomography Angiography and Magnetic Resonance Imaging. Coronary CTA is one option for diagnostic confirmation of suspected coronary anomalies. Current-generation scanners can be used with high spatial and temporal resolution within the duration of a single breath hold.[69-72] CTA is useful in delineating the shape of the anomalous ostium, the angle of takeoff, and the proximal and distal course.[71] Three-dimensional intraluminal reconstruction can reveal the relationship between the leaflets of the aortic valve and the anomalous coronary vessel, which may be important for preoperative evaluation.[72] Limitations of the CTA include heart rate and rhythm control, proper timing of the scan relative to introduction of intravenous contrast, minimization of patient motion, and radiation exposure.[73] Improvements in MRI techniques have enabled accurate detection of anomalous coronary artery origin while eliminating exposure to radiation.[73-75] Postprocessing of the three-dimensional images can be performed in a manner similar to that for coronary CTA. Limitations of MRI include the length of time needed for imaging and sedation needed for younger children. The decision for use of CTA versus MRI in assessment of coronary anomalies in children is largely provider and institution dependent, based on access to each imaging modality.

Coronary Angiography. Occasionally, cardiac catheterization with angiography is used to visualize the coronary anatomy; however, this is not the first choice in children because it is invasive and exposes children to ionizing radiation. Noninvasive imaging as described earlier has largely replaced this modality. However, it may be used in older adult patients to evaluate for atherosclerotic coronary artery disease before undergoing surgical intervention.

Cardiopulmonary Exercise Testing. After the diagnosis of a coronary anomaly has been established, cardiopulmonary exercise testing (CPET) is almost always used to evaluate for ischemia and inducible arrhythmias. Postoperatively, it is also used before allowing the patient to return to competitive sports.[76] The authors recommend combining CPET with an additional imaging modality, such as a nuclear perfusion scan or stress echocardiogram to optimize the sensitivity of identifying ischemia.[77] Yet, basing management decisions on a single CPET is difficult because ischemia is intermittent and the positive predictive value of ischemia in this population is quite low.[78] At the author's institution, if a traditional CPET does not elicit the patient's symptoms, an individualized approach with a nontraditional exercise testing protocol may be used in an attempt to reproduce symptoms.

Surgical Management

Indications for Surgery. Surgical intervention is indicated in any patient with AAOLCA or AAORCA with an interarterial, intramural course who has signs and/or symptoms of myocardial ischemia or potentially lethal ventricular arrhythmias. Furthermore, most would agree that surgery is indicated in asymptomatic patients with interarterial, intramural AAOLCA because of the imprecisely estimated but significant risk of sudden death. Surgery for asymptomatic young patients with AAORCA who have no evidence of inducible ischemia or arrhythmia remains controversial.[76]

Surgical Techniques

Unroofing Procedure. The unroofing procedure is the most commonly performed operation for patients with AAOCA with an interarterial and intramural course.[79-82] After the median sternotomy is performed, the pericardium is opened, and the anatomy is inspected. Conventional cardiopulmonary bypass is established. External features of the heart and aorta are examined. After cardioplegic arrest of the heart, the ascending aorta is opened by means of an oblique aortotomy. Alternatively, the ascending aorta may be transected well above the origin of the coronaries. The orifice(s) from which the coronary arteries arise are identified, and the course of the coronary arteries is ascertained. To enlarge the often slit-like ostium of the coronary artery with anomalous origin and course, it is opened longitudinally starting at the anomalous coronary os and continuing toward the correct sinus (Fig. 56.8). The entire intramural segment of the artery is unroofed, to the point where the coronary artery exits the aortic wall from within the appropriate sinus of Valsalva. If the anomalous coronary ostium arises close to a commissure of the aortic valve, it may be necessary to take down the apex of the commissure in to achieve unroofing into the appropriate sinus. If that is necessary, the aortic valve commissure is resuspended with a pledgeted suture. Some surgeons prefer to approximate the intima of the unroofed segment using fine monofilament sutures. The aortic incision is then closed, and the heart is reperfused. As the patient is rewarmed, close attention should be paid to the ECG to evaluate for signs of myocardial ischemia, and transesophageal echocardiography should be performed to assess aortic valve function.

Creation of a Neo-ostium. An alternative technique that may be used when the anomalous coronary ostium is proximal to the level of the adjacent aortic valve commissure and the intramural segment passes behind the aortic valve commissure is the creation of a neo-ostium in the correct sinus. This technique avoids the takedown and resuspension of the commissure, which can lead to postoperative aortic valve insufficiency. After a probe is passed through the intramural segment of the anomalous coronary, the anomalous vessel is opened from within the "appropriate" sinus at the location where it exits the aorta, and a neo-ostium is created. The intima is sewn to the aortic wall with interrupted sutures.

Other Techniques. When there are two separate coronary ostia within a single sinus, and the anomalous coronary artery has an interarterial course but not an intramural course, coronary artery translocation with reimplantation may be used.[83,84] Some advocate pulmonary artery translocation, which may be considered when the anomalous coronary course is not intramural but the ostia are close together.[84] Pulmonary artery translocation does not alter the origin or course of the anomalous coronary artery but opens the space between the aorta and pulmonary trunk, thus diminishing the possibility of compression of the interarterial segment of coronary artery. Although surgery is most often performed on patients with an intramural segment, and although unroofing is the most prevalent surgical procedure performed for AAOCA in the United States, alternative approaches have found favor elsewhere. Vouhe, in Paris, has advocated what he refers to as an "anatomical" repair that creates an enlarged neo-ostium into the appropriate sinus, eliminates completely the intramural segment, and restores a normal angle of takeoff. This does not involve unroofing. Rather, it involves incision into the "appropriate" sinus and extension of that incision into the proximal coronary artery on the epicardial surface. Patch enlargement of the neo-ostium completes the repair. Vouhe suggests that reimplantation of the anomalous coronary artery may be indicated in variants without an intramural course.[85] Coronary artery bypass grafting using saphenous vein or internal mammary artery grafts may be an option in the older adult, but this is not a desirable procedure for children and young adults due to concerns with long-term graft patency.[86]

Surgical Results

No data exist regarding long-term neo-ostia patency rates after the unroofing procedure. Short-term to midterm results have overall been reassuring, although there have been rare anecdotal and published reports of SCD or sudden cardiac arrest after surgical repair.[87] These patients appear to be those whose initial presentation was sudden cardiac arrest or syncope with exertion. There have been reports of aortic valve insufficiency, ranging from mild to necessitating aortic valve replacement in one patient.[81,88] There have also been reports of subclinical evidence of postoperative myocardial ischemia despite patent neo-coronary ostia by echocardiography.[78] Because the long-term surgical results are unknown, these patients should continue to be followed with clinical evaluations throughout their lifetime.

Coronary Artery Fistula

A coronary artery fistula is a communication between a coronary artery and either a cardiac chamber (known as coronary-cameral fistula) or a vessel in the pulmonary or systemic vasculature (known as a coronary arteriovenous fistula).[89-92] Runoff via the fistulous connection results in blood from the involved coronary artery bypassing the myocardial capillary bed and entering the cardiac chamber into which the fistula connects. Alternatively, a coronary artery fistula can connect a high-pressure cardiac chamber to a coronary artery; these types of fistulae are also known as right ventricular myocardial sinusoids or LV myocardial sinusoids and have the potential to result in ventricular dependent coronary circulation. This type of fistula is seen in some hearts with pulmonary atresia and intact ventricular septum and in some hearts with aortic atresia and mitral stenosis.

The majority of coronary artery fistulae are congenital. Although they are quite rare, representing only 0.2% to 0.4% of all congenital

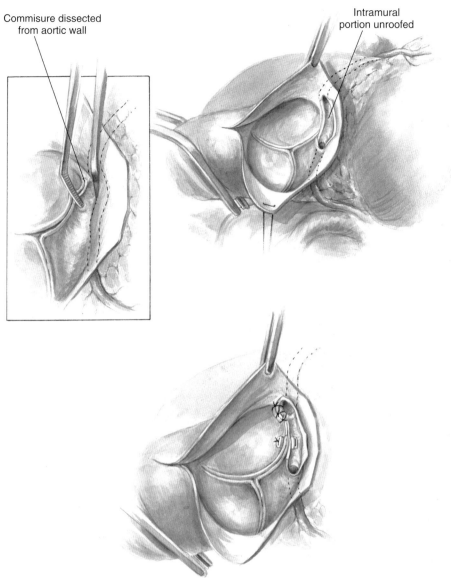

Commisure dissected from aortic wall

Intramural portion unroofed

• **Figure 56.8** In the modified unroofing procedure, the intramural segment of the anomalous coronary is incised from within the lumen of the aorta up to the point at which the coronary artery leaves the aortic wall in the appropriate sinus. If the origin of the anomalous coronary artery is at a level distal to the commissure, there is very little risk to simply unroofing that segment. In patients in whom the intramural course is at or proximal to the commissure, the commissure may require detachment and reflection into the lumen of the aorta so that unroofing can be accomplished. The commissure should then be secured to the aortic wall at the appropriate level to prevent prolapse of the aortic leaflets and aortic insufficiency. Fine monofilament suture is used to secure any ragged edges of the intima. (From Jaggers J, Lodge AJ. Surgical therapy for anomalous aortic origin of the coronary arteries. *Semin Thorac Cardiovasc Surg Pediatr Card Surg Annu.* 2005;122-7.)

heart defects, coronary artery fistulae constitute nearly half of all congenital coronary anomaly diagnoses. There are no known gender or racial/ethnic differences. Coronary artery fistulae may present at any age but are commonly identified due to a cardiac murmur in an asymptomatic child; alternately, they may be diagnosed due to symptoms of congestive heart failure or coronary insufficiency. Congenital coronary artery fistulae may be found in isolation or along with other congenital heart disease, most commonly atrial septal defect, VSD, PDA, and tetralogy of Fallot.[90,92] Acquired fistulae may occur after a penetrating trauma, cardiac catheterization, or surgery or due to complications from Kawasaki disease.[91]

Anatomy

Coronary artery fistulae may originate from either the right or the left coronary artery; it is rare to have both coronary arteries involved.[92,93] The majority of fistulae arise from a coronary artery with an otherwise normal anatomic course. A fistula can arise in the midsection of the coronary artery with a normal coronary continuing after the fistulous communication or at the termination of the vessel as an end artery. Proximal to the fistula the coronary is often dilated and elongated in proportion to the shunt size across the fistulous communication. Distal to the fistula the vessel usually returns to a normal size.

The RCA and LAD are the most common coronary sites of origin. Most fistulous connections end in a venous chamber or vessel on the right side of the heart, followed by the LV, left atrium, and coronary sinus. Lowe and colleagues reviewed 286 patients and found the most common site of origin was the RCA followed by the left coronary artery system.[94,95] The right side of the heart was the most common site of drainage, in the following descending order: right ventricle (39%), right atrium (33%, including the coronary sinus and superior vena cava), and pulmonary artery (20%). The left atrium or LV was the termination site in the remaining 8%.

Pathophysiology

Coronary fistulae result in a left-to-right or left-to-left shunt. Small fistulae are not of hemodynamic significance. However, larger fistulae can lead to hemodynamic compromise through a coronary steal phenomenon, which occurs from decreased myocardial blood flow distal to the site of the fistulous connection. This occurs due to the diastolic pressure gradient between the coronary artery and the low-pressure receiving vessel. With a large fistula the diastolic perfusion pressure inside the coronary vessel progressively decreases. The ostium and section proximal to the fistula progressively enlarges over time, which may lead to aneurysm, calcification, thrombosis, and rupture. The hemodynamic consequences of the shunt are related to the amount of blood flow from the fistula to the chamber and the resistance of the chamber into which the fistula drains.

When a fistula drains to the right side of the circulation, there is usually a small- to moderate-size shunt. For instance, those that drain to the right atrium will have physiology similar to an atrial septal defect, and those that drain to the pulmonary arteries will have physiology similar to a PDA. When the fistula drains into a left-sided chamber, the physiology would either be a volume load similar to mitral regurgitation if there is drainage into the left atrium or an aortic runoff with physiology similar to that of aortic regurgitation with drainage into the LV.

Clinical Presentation

Patients with a coronary artery fistula are usually asymptomatic and rarely present in infancy. However, those with large fistulous connections may present in infancy in congestive heart failure. Many patients are diagnosed when a murmur is heard during a physical examination. When symptomatic from a moderate to large fistula, the most common complaints are palpitations, fatigue, syncope, angina, and shortness of breath with exertion. When there is a coronary to right atrium fistula, atrial fibrillation may be present from right atrial enlargement.

On physical examination, often there are no pertinent findings. However, a continuous murmur may be auscultated, which can be confused for a PDA. The murmur of a coronary artery fistula is heard lower on the left sternal border, which is not the typical location for a PDA murmur. Left-to-left shunts that are large may cause a widened pulse pressure, as is commonly seen with significant aortic valve regurgitation.

Natural History

The natural history of congenital coronary artery fistulae is gradual progression in size over many years. Despite the progressive enlargement, spontaneous rupture is rare. Rupture generally occurs due to aneurysmal dilation and coronary wall weakening from a congenital defect or atherosclerotic plaque buildup. Bacterial endocarditis may occur secondary to turbulent flow, but infective endocarditis prophylaxis is no longer recommended. Small fistulae may spontaneously close.

Diagnostic Imaging

Commonly the ECG findings are normal, or there may be evidence of LV volume overload and, rarely, myocardial ischemia. In an older patient with a coronary to right atrium fistula, atrial fibrillation may be present. Results of chest radiographs are usually normal, but there may be cardiomegaly or evidence of congestive heart failure.

Two-dimensional echocardiography can usually delineate the coronary anatomy, including where the fistula originates, into which chamber it drains, and any chamber enlargement or hypertrophy. Color Doppler will help demonstrate flow through the fistulous connection. Cardiac MRI and CTA are promising additional noninvasive imaging techniques to provide detailed coronary anatomy. However, cardiac catheterization with selective coronary angiography remains the primary modality used to define the coronary anatomy, fistula size, origin and drainage site, and presence of any stenosis; it can also be used to perform a hemodynamic evaluation. In some cases an experienced interventional cardiologist will embolize the coronary artery fistula using a coil or other device without needing open heart surgery.[95] Use of transcatheter device closure is reserved for those fistulae with favorable characteristics, such as a nontortuous coronary artery, a fistula with distal narrowing limiting the chance of device embolization, and no additional heart defects that would necessitate surgical intervention.[96,97] However, because the transcatheter approach can be fairly complicated and the anatomy has to be amenable, many patients continue to undergo surgical closure as the preferred therapy.

Surgical Management

Indications for Surgery. Any patient who presents with a symptomatic fistula should undergo closure. As well, anyone who is asymptomatic with a moderate or large fistula should undergo surgical closure on an elective basis. Patients with small fistulae may not need surgical closure; however, because the natural history is to enlarge over time, patients with small fistulae should be followed closely with echocardiography, MRI, or CTA, and potentially repeat coronary angiography.

Surgical Techniques. Before surgical closure the coronary artery fistula anatomy must be clearly defined. After the coronary anatomy is carefully inspected, the fistula may be ligated without cardiopulmonary bypass if it is located at the terminal portion of the coronary artery and if there is no viable myocardium distal to the fistula (Fig. 56.9). Intraoperative transesophageal echocardiography may be useful to verify that the fistula is closed. Cardiopulmonary bypass should be used for fistulae with tortuous pathways, multiple communications or terminations, if the fistula arises from the middle of a coronary artery, if aneurysm formation is present, or if another cardiac lesion needs to be repaired simultaneously.

A variety of techniques can be used to close the fistula. Multiple pledgeted sutures can be placed to close a fistula that ends in the midportion of the coronary artery, using caution to avoid compromising distal perfusion (Fig. 56.10). Another technique is to longitudinally open the coronary along the epicardial surface and oversew the origin of the fistula from within the coronary artery (Fig. 56.11). The coronary artery can then be closed primarily. If

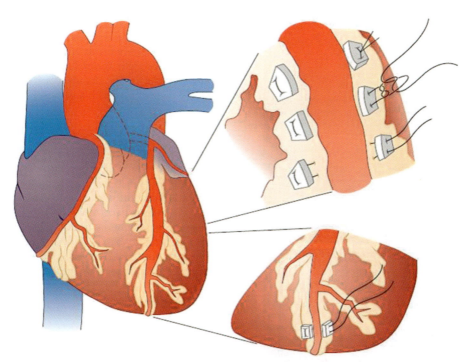

• **Figure 56.9** If the termination site of the fistula is at the distal aspect of the coronary and no significant myocardium is in jeopardy, the coronary may be ligated proximal to the termination site. If the fistula terminates in the midportion of the left anterior descending coronary artery, the fistulous communication may be closed with multiple pledgeted sutures placed underneath the coronary artery so as not to impair distal perfusion. (Reprinted with permission from Gaynor JW. Coronary artery anomalies in children. In: Kaiser LR, Kron IL, Spray TL, eds. *Mastery of Cardiothoracic Surgery.* Philadelphia: Lippincott-Raven; 1998:888.)

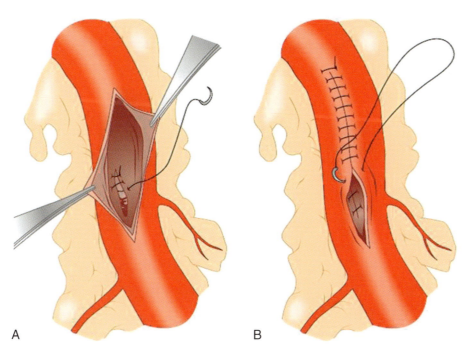

A   B

• **Figure 56.10** (A) When the fistulous communication arises from the midportion of the dilated coronary, the coronary may be opened longitudinally and the origin of the fistula oversewn from within the coronary. (B) The coronary artery is closed primarily. (Reprinted with permission from Gaynor JW. Coronary artery anomalies in children. In: Kaiser LR, Kron IL, Spray TL, eds. *Mastery of Cardiothoracic Surgery.* Philadelphia: Lippincott-Raven; 1998:889.)

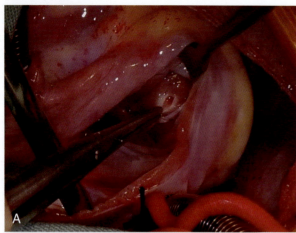
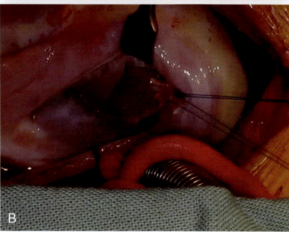

• **Figure 56.11** Intraoperative images showing the transcameral closure technique. (A) Identification of the fistula orifice inside the right ventricle through the right atrium and tricuspid valve. (B) The fistula is closed by suture ligation with pads. (From Zhang W, Hu R, Zhang L, et al. Outcomes of surgical repair of pediatric coronary artery fistulas. *J Thorac Cardiovasc Surg.* 2016;152[4]:1123-1130.e1. Copyright 2016 The American Association for Thoracic Surgery.)

distal perfusion of the coronary bed is affected after fistula closure, the use of coronary artery bypass grafting may be needed. Finally, if the coronary artery fistula ends in a right-sided chamber (e.g., right atrium or right ventricle), then the fistula may be closed from within the cardiac chamber itself. The termination site may be closed primarily or with a pericardial patch.

Surgical Results

The operative mortality for coronary artery fistula repair remains low with rare reports of perioperative myocardial infarctions.[98,99] Late results are overall encouraging, with only a handful of patients with residual small fistulae or who experience a recurrence of the fistula. Pediatric patients also have excellent long-term outcomes as reported by Mavroudis and colleagues. Eight patients, with an average age of 5.5 years, underwent fistula closure with complete closure, and none had recurrences of their fistulae, and there were no reported perioperative or late deaths.[98]

References

A complete list of references is available at ExpertConsult.com.

57

Transposition of the Great Arteries and the Arterial Switch Operation

ALEXIS L. BENSCOTER, DO; AMY RYAN, MSN, RN, CPNP-AC;
JAMES S. TWEDDELL, MD

Transposition of the great arteries (TGA) makes up 5% to 7% of all congenital heart disease. It occurs in 3 per 10,000 live births.[1] Without surgery, TGA is fatal, with a mortality rate of 30% in the first week and 90% within the first year of life.[35] Severity of illness varies depending on anatomy, degree of mixing at the atrial and ventricular levels, and presence of systemic ventricular outflow tract obstruction, with some infants requiring emergent balloon atrial septostomy (BAS) and/or extracorporeal membrane oxygenation (ECMO) immediately after birth.

Embryology and Genetics

There are two prominent theories regarding the development of TGA. The original theory, proposed by Goor and Edwards and supported by Anderson and colleagues, is known as the "conal development hypothesis." Per Goor and colleagues, normal absorption of the bulboventricular ledge allows the aorta to rotate to the left during normal development of the heart and become oriented over the left (or primitive) ventricle.[2,3] If this absorption does not occur, there is persistence of a subaortic conus, underdevelopment of the subpulmonary conus, and dextroposition of the aorta occurs.[4]

A second theory by del la Cruz and colleagues proposes that TGA is the result of linear, as opposed to normal, spiraling of the aortopulmonary septum. This results in the fourth aortic arch remaining in contact with the anterior conus, in alignment with the right ventricle (RV).[4]

Animal studies have linked nodal signaling pathway genes to TGA, with *ZIC3* being associated with X-linked heterotaxy and familial d-TGA. Additionally, genes *CFC1, FOXH1,* and *PROSIT240* have been associated with isolated and syndromic d-TGA.[5]

Anatomic Features

Mathew Baillie first described TGA in 1797, although the term *transposition* was not coined until 1814 by Farre.[1] TGA describes any heart in which there is ventriculoarterial (VA) discordance. In simple terms the morphologic RV is primarily connected to the aorta, whereas the morphologic left ventricle (LV) is connected to the pulmonary artery (PA). TGA can be further subdivided based on if the morphologic right and left atria are connected to the morphologic right and left ventricles. When the atria are connected to the appropriate ventricles, they are said to have atrioventricular

(AV) concordance. The atrium and ventricles usually have normal configuration, and the conduction system is also usually normal.

In simple transposition the atria are connected to the correct ventricles (AV concordance), but the RV is connected to the aorta, and the LV is connected to the main PA (VA discordance). Isolated VA discordance occurs in 50% of cases.[1] Congenitally corrected transposition refers to both AV and VA discordance. The remainder of this chapter will focus primarily on d-TGA.

Associated Anomalies

Ventricular Septal Defects. Ventricular septal defects (VSDs) are found in 50% patients with d-TGA.[6,7] When a VSD is present, there can be malalignment of the outlet septum. Anterior displacement of the septum results in hypoplasia of the right ventricular outflow tract (RVOT) and in the case of d-TGA is associated with aortic valve hypoplasia, coarctation, hypoplastic aortic arch, and interrupted aortic arch. Posterior malalignment of the outlet septum results in LV outflow tract obstruction (LVOTO) with pulmonary valve and subpulmonary stenosis and is present in 12% to 33% of cases.[1]

Coronary Artery Variations. Coronary artery variations are associated with TGA, and it is imperative to know the correct anatomy before the surgery.[8] In almost all cases the coronary arteries arise from the aortic sinuses facing, or adjacent to, the PA.[7] Leiden convention remains the most commonly used classification system for describing coronary anatomy in TGA[7,8] (Fig. 57.1). Early in the experience with the arterial switch operation (ASO), atypical coronary patterns, such as a retropulmonary left coronary artery, were associated with increased risk in some series. In the current era it appears that most coronary artery patterns can undergo an ASO with acceptable risk, but the presence of a single coronary ostium or an intramural coronary artery have both been shown to contribute significantly to risk of mortality.[8]

Pathophysiology and Clinical Presentation

In d-TGA, pulmonary and systemic circulations are acting as two closed circuits in parallel to each other. As a result, there is a higher oxygen saturation in the main PA than in the aorta. This is the basis for "transposition physiology." Deoxygenated blood returns to the right heart and is pumped into the aorta and out to the body, while oxygen-rich blood returns from the lungs to the left heart and is pumped, once again, into the pulmonary arteries. For

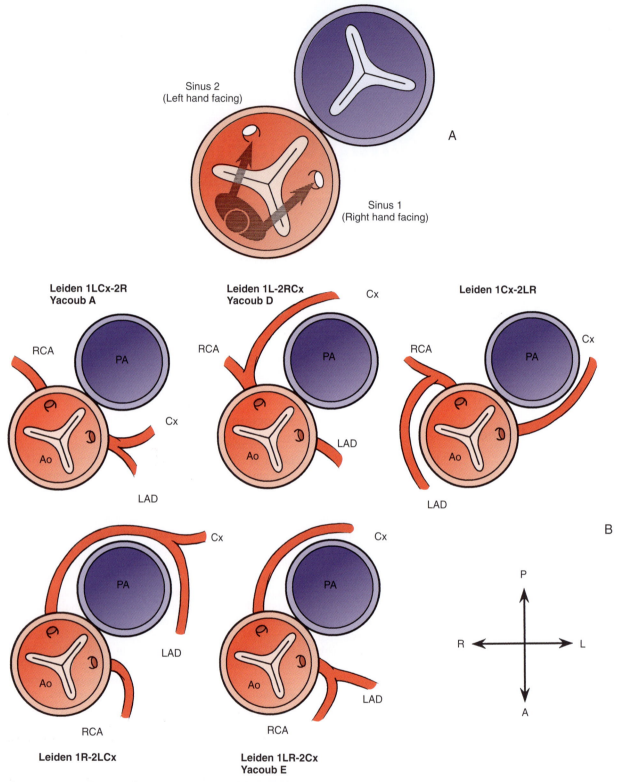

• **Figure 57.1** Coronary artery patterns seen in transposition of the great arteries. Upper panels show coronary artery distribution as visualized by two-dimensional echocardiography and caudally angulated aortography. Lower panels show the same coronary artery distribution as viewed from the front. *Ant,* Anterior; *Cx,* circumflex coronary artery; *Inf,* inferior; *L,* left; *LAD,* left anterior descending artery; *Post,* posterior; *R,* right; *Sup,* superior. (From Pasquali AK, Hasselblad V, Li JS, et al. Coronary artery pattern and outcome of arterial switch operation for transposition of the great arteries: a meta-analysis. *Circulation.* 2002;106:2575-2580.)

the patient to survive there must be adequate systemic oxygen delivery. A patent ductus arteriosus (PDA) will result in increased pulmonary blood flow, increased left atrial pressure, and increased shunting across whatever atrial septal defect (ASD) is present. A VSD will also result in some mixing, but a PDA or VSD alone may be inadequate. In a newborn the most reliable strategy to increase systemic oxygen delivery is left-to-right shunting at the atrial level, and therefore a BAS is indicated in the newborn with d-TGA and excessive cyanosis.

The rate of prenatal diagnosis of d-TGA historically has been low, but with the recommendation of obtaining an outflow tract view on fetal ultrasonography this rate has improved.[9] Because of the low rate of prenatal diagnosis, an understanding of the clinical findings of the neonate with d-TGA is essential. Presentation varies greatly based on the degree of mixing at the ductal, atrial, and ventricular levels and if there are other anatomic lesions present, such as any degree of LVOTO. All neonates will be cyanotic to some degree, but the degree of cyanosis and hypoxemia can range from very subtle, going unnoticed until the infant fails the pulse oximetry screen in the nursery, to rapidly progressive cyanosis and hypoxemia that may become life-threatening within an hour of birth. The remainder of the physical examination may be relatively unrevealing as to the diagnosis of d-TGA. A systolic murmur, respiratory distress, and signs of heart failure may be present. The cardiac silhouette has been classically described as an "egg-on-a-string" on chest radiography, in which the heart is globular in appearance and the superior mediastinum is narrow with hyperinflated lungs and small thymus.[10] However, chest radiography results may be normal. Electrocardiogram (ECG) findings may also be normal or show right ventricular hypertrophy depending on age of the patient. Echocardiogram should be obtained as soon as possible to make the diagnosis.

Reverse differential cyanosis higher saturations in the postductal circulation compared with the preductal circulation (right arm saturation that is lower than the lower extremities) can be seen with TGA with VSD and arch hypoplasia or interrupted arch. Reverse differential cyanosis can also occur with simple TGA when there is elevated pulmonary vascular resistance with a PDA.[6]

Preoperative Management

Prostaglandin E$_1$

Most hypoxic neonates will benefit from prostaglandin E$_1$ (PGE$_1$). PGE$_1$ maintains ductal patency, increases pulmonary blood flow resulting in increased left-to-right shunting at the atrial level, and results in improved systemic oxygen saturation. PGE$_1$ should be initiated when d-TGA is suspected or has been diagnosed.[11,12] In the setting of a closed PDA, PGE$_1$ may need to be started at higher doses to reopen the ductus.[13]

PGE$_1$ causes systemic vasodilation, which can result in flushing of the skin and hypotension. It does have effect on the gastrointestinal system and has been associated with necrotizing enterocolitis, and long-term use has been associated with pyloric stenosis.[14] It also penetrates the central nervous system and can cause jitteriness and seizure-like activities. One of the most common side effects in the neonatal population, especially at higher doses, is apnea. Apnea may require intubation and mechanical ventilation but has been overcome with noninvasive positive pressure with use of continuous positive airway pressure or high-flow nasal cannula. Aminophylline is effective in preventing apnea related to PGE$_1$, but side effects include tachycardia, decreased cerebral blood flow, and an increased risk of necrotizing enterocolitis, and it has a narrow therapeutic window.[15]

Balloon Atrial Septostomy

BAS, or the Rashkind procedure, is used for patients with persistent cyanosis after initiation of PGE$_1$.[16] BAS is generally viewed as a safe procedure and can be performed at the bedside under echocardiographic guidance or in the cardiac catheterization laboratory. BAS typically results in immediate improvement of mixing and arterial oxygen levels (PaO$_2$ and arterial oxygen saturation [SaO$_2$]). Additionally, in some cases PGE$_1$ can be stopped after BAS. Whether or not the procedure has been successful is determined by the clinical status of the patient and hemodynamics.[17]

Risks of BAS include vascular injury, arrhythmia, atrial perforation, and tamponade. Recently the potential for stroke as a consequence of BAS was raised in a study by McQuillen et al.,[17] who showed increased risk of focal brain injury in neonates with TGA who underwent BAS versus those who did not. However, in a similarly powered study, Petit et al.[18] showed no incidence of stroke in neonates who underwent BAS. Finally, in a large database review by Mukherjee et al.,[19] comparing neonates who had undergone BAS to those who had not, the infants who had undergone BAS were two times more likely to have had a stroke perioperatively. This being a retrospective chart review, one of the largest limitations to the study was timing of head imaging and inability to determine when the stroke occurred in relation to repair.

Because neonates with d-TGA and a highly restrictive ASD are at increased risk, prenatal diagnosis would identify patients at immediate need for intervention. The fetal diagnosis of an intact or restrictive atrial septum should be suspected if the atrial septum is not freely mobile and when the septum appears thick with limited or no visible shunting on color Doppler imaging with two-dimensional echocardiography.[20] Additionally, recent studies by Divanovic et al. have demonstrated that an RAS can also be diagnosed using two-dimensional echocardiography when there is a small or absent interatrial communication and the pulmonary venous Doppler forward/reverse velocity time integral ratio is 3 or less. Punn and Silverman[21] have also shown that a hypermobile septum with reverse diastolic PDA flow also predicts the presence of an RAS and need for urgent BAS postnatally.

It is recommended that infants with d-TGA and an intact atrial septum or RAS be delivered with a neonatologist and a cardiac specialist in the delivery with a plan for intervention and urgent transport as needed. Most centers are now recommending delivery by cesarean section in the cardiac catheterization laboratory with planned intervention at birth for infants who are expected to be hemodynamically unstable. Interventions include cardiac catheterization with BAS, possible immediate surgical intervention, and ECMO available in the catheterization laboratory if necessary.[22] These deliveries require attendance of a neonatology team, an interventional cardiology team, a cardiologist specializing in echosonography, a cardiac intensive care specialist, and a cardiovascular surgeon with full operating team, including cardiac anesthesia and perfusion specialists.

Surgical Treatment of the Infant With Transposition of the Great Arteries

The Arterial Switch Operation

Timing of Surgery. The ASO will restore the LV as the systemic ventricle, and it is essential that the LV be prepared for systemic work. In the fetus, both ventricles do systemic work and therefore are equally prepared for systemic work at birth. In the preoperative neonate with d-TGA and an intact ventricular septum the LV will become deconditioned as the pulmonary vascular resistance drops and LV-generated pressure decreases. Therefore to ensure that the LV is adequately prepared, the arterial switch should be performed before the LV becomes deconditioned, within the first 3 weeks of life. Furthermore, repair by 6 days of age for the uncomplicated patient with d-TGA and intact ventricular septum has been shown to be associated with decreased hospital charges and was not associated with increased mortality or worse outcome.[23,24] For individuals with a nonrestrictive VSD and without obstruction to pulmonary or systemic blood flow, surgery can be safely delayed up to 90 days of age.[25] For patients with ductal dependent systemic or PA blood flow, neonatal intervention is required.

The ASO is performed through a median sternotomy incision. The most commonly encountered anatomy of TGA is that with the great vessels oriented anterior-posterior, and the most common coronary pattern has the left anterior descending coronary and the circumflex arising from the left-facing sinus and the right coronary artery arising from the right-facing sinus (Fig. 57.2). Before cannulation for cardiopulmonary bypass the aorta is separated from the main PA, and the branch pulmonary arteries are mobilized to their first branches. Marking sutures are placed in the pulmonary root at the anticipated implantation sites for the coronary arteries.

The arterial cannula is placed in the distal ascending aorta near the origin of the innominate artery. Placing the aortic cannula as far cephalad as possible provides the greatest exposure of the base of the heart. Typically, both cava are separately cannulated. With commencement of cardiopulmonary bypass the ductus arteriosus is ligated proximally and distally and then divided. A vent is placed into the LV, and an antegrade cardioplegia cannula is placed in the ascending aorta. The aorta is cross-clamped, and cardioplegia is delivered via the aortic root for initial arrest, after which the ASD and/or VSD are repaired through a right atriotomy.

Coronary Transfer Techniques

The aorta is transected 2 to 3 mm cephalad to the sinotubular junction (Fig. 57.3). The coronary ostia are examined and excised with a button of adjacent sinus aorta. For an adequate button to be obtained, the aortic wall is incised close to the leaflet attachment of the aortic valve. The proximal coronary arteries are mobilized to allow transfer of the coronary buttons to the pulmonary root.

Medially based trapdoor incisions are created at the sites identified by the marking sutures (Fig. 57.4A and B). The marking sutures help ensure proper alignment of the reimplanted coronary arteries. The trapdoor incisions minimize the rotation of the proximal coronary arteries. The coronary buttons are sewn in place using 7-0 or 8-0 polypropylene sutures. It should be noted that

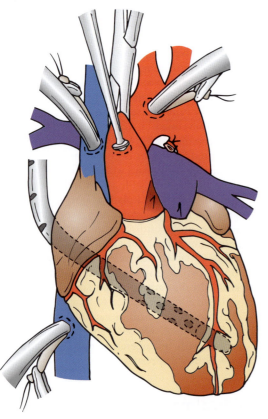

• **Figure 57.2** Typical anatomy and cannulation for the arterial switch operation for simple transposition of the great arteries. The aorta is cannulated near the base of the innominate artery, and both the superior and inferior vena cava have been separately cannulated. The ductus arteriosus has been divided. A cross-clamp has been applied, and a left ventricular vent has been placed. The sites of implantation of the coronary arteries have been marked with sutures.

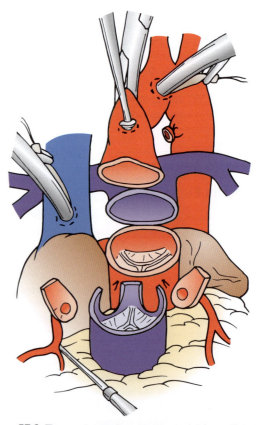

• **Figure 57.3** The great vessels are transected a few millimeters above the sinotubular junction. Coronary ostia are examined and excised with a button of adjacent sinus aorta. To obtain an adequate button the aortic wall is incised close to the leaflet attachment of the aortic valve. The proximal coronary arteries are mobilized to allow transfer of the coronary buttons to the pulmonary root.

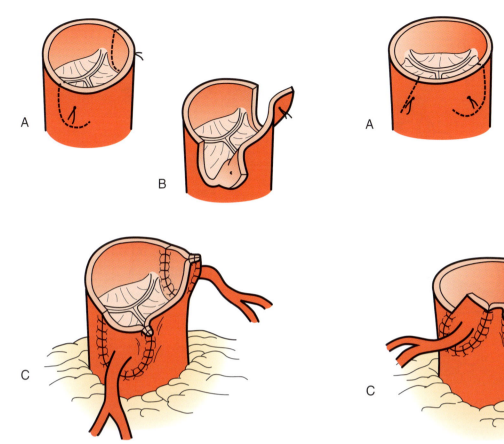

• **Figure 57.4** The sites for implantation of the coronary buttons were marked before initiation of bypass (A). Medially based trapdoor incisions are created (B). The marking sutures help ensure proper alignment of the reimplanted coronary arteries. The trapdoor incisions minimize the rotation of the proximal coronary arteries. The coronary buttons are sewn in place using 7-0 or 8-0 polypropylene sutures (C).

• **Figure 57.5** In cases in which the implantation site of the coronary is close to the facing commissure of the pulmonary valve and a medially based trapdoor cannot be created, an oblique incision can be used.

the reimplanted coronary ostia will occupy a more cephalad position, with respect to the neoaortic valve, than they occupied in the native aorta. Furthermore, in cases in which the proximal coronary artery has a redundant course, the coronary button may be placed even more cephalad than shown to prevent kinking of the proximal coronary artery. In situations in which the implantation site is close to the facing commissure of the pulmonary root, an oblique incision can be used rather than a medially based trapdoor incision (Fig. 57.5).

When both coronary arteries arise from a single sinus of Valsalva, an intramural course of the proximal coronary artery is nearly always present (Fig. 57.6A). The intramural coronary will exit the aorta as though it were arising from the correct sinus of Valsalva. When the button is excised, the external course of the intramural coronary must be identified, and likely the button will include a large portion of the sinus aorta from which the coronary would normally arise. To obtain an adequate cuff of sinus aorta, separating the commissure of the aortic valve from the aortic wall may be necessary. An intramural coronary will typically have a slit-like ostium. Cutting back the origin and unroofing the common wall between the aorta and the coronary artery enlarges the ostium of the intramural coronary (see Fig. 57.6B). It is usually possible to separate the two ostia and implant them individually (see Fig. 57.6C). Enlargement of the slit-like ostium and unroofing can be challenging in a small neonate, and rotating the button through

the vertical axis may result in a kink or buckle of the coronary. To prevent proximal coronary obstruction, it may be preferable to transfer the coronary button by rotating it in the horizontal plane (see Fig. 57.6D). A hood of autologous pericardium or pulmonary homograft patch is used (see Fig. 57.6E).

The closed technique is useful when a single coronary is encountered or the great vessels lie side by side and the right posterior sinus gives rise to the right and circumflex coronary arteries (Fig. 57.7A). The coronary button is excised as in the open technique. The PA is divided, and the superior extent of the commissures of the PA are marked externally with a suture. The Lecompte maneuver is performed, then the distal ascending aorta is anastomosed to the proximal pulmonary root (see Fig. 57.7B). The marking suture helps prevent injury to the pulmonary valve during subsequent coronary artery reimplantation. The root is then distended with cardioplegia or by unclamping the aorta. The appropriate site for implantation of the coronary artery is then determined by positioning the coronary button over the distended root (see Fig. 57.7C). The optimal site should allow reimplantation without kinking of either branch of the coronary artery. Often some rotation of the button is required (see Fig. 57.7D). The coronary artery button is implanted with fine polypropylene suture.

A patch extension of the coronary artery button can be helpful when the great arteries lie side by side and the right-facing sinus gives rise to a large coronary artery that includes the circumflex and right coronary artery with early branching, also in cases of a single coronary artery. The PA is transected, and the incisions for

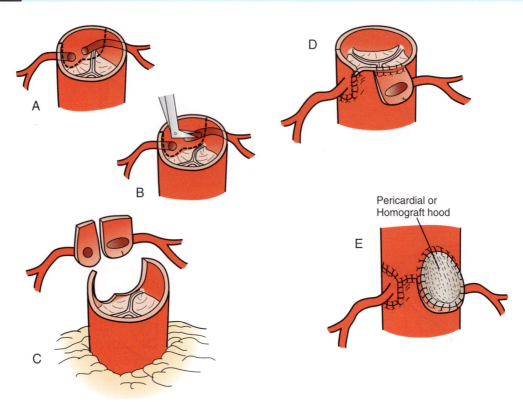

• **Figure 57.6** If both coronary ostia are seen to originate from a single sinus of Valsalva, an intramural coronary artery should be suspected (A). The exit point of the intramural coronary artery should be identified, and the coronary frequently exits the aorta from the correct sinus of Valsalva. The commissure may need to be taken down and care taken to avoid damaging the coronary when excising the button (B). The intramural portion of the coronary should be unroofed. Two separate buttons are created (C). Typical rotation through the vertical axis may result in kinking of the coronary, and instead the coronary can be rotated through the horizontal plane (D). To prevent twisting or kinking of the coronary a hood of pericardium or homograft can be created to complete the reimplantation (E).

reimplantation of the coronary buttons are made as usual (Fig. 57.8A). Medially based trapdoor incisions are created (see Fig. 57.8B). The patch extension, using either homograft or autologous pericardium, of the coronary ostial button reduces the rotation of the coronary artery (see Fig. 57.8C) and prevents kinking of either branch.

The Lecompte maneuver is performed, and the neoaortic root and ascending aortic anastomosis is completed (Fig. 57.9). The defects in the proximal aortic root that result from excision of the coronary artery buttons are repaired with a generous "pantaloons"-shaped patch of homograft or autologous pericardium (Fig. 57.10). Finally, the neopulmonary root is anastomosed to the distal main PA (Fig. 57.11). With side-by-side great vessels the anastomosis may need to be positioned under the right PA to prevent branch PA obstruction.

d-Transposition With Arch Hypoplasia and a Ventricular Septal Defect

Significant arch hypoplasia occurs in 5% to 9% of patients presenting with d-TGA. Primary complete repair or a staged repair strategy can be used.[26,27] With a complete repair, a sternal incision is made and the arch is repaired using either deep hypothermic circulatory arrest or continuous antegrade cerebral perfusion. The ASO and VSD closure are performed using standard techniques. The VSD may be remote from the tricuspid valve and more easily approached through a ventriculotomy. Repair through the

pulmonary root should be avoided because this is associated with an increased risk of neoaortic valve regurgitation.[28] The great vessels are more commonly side by side, and both coronary transfer and neopulmonary artery reconstruction will be more complicated. Mortality is increased compared with simple d-TGA.

d-Transposition With Left Ventricular Outflow Tract Obstruction

Significant hypoplasia of the LV outflow tract that precludes the use of the pulmonary valve as a neoaortic valve occurs in up to a third of patients with d-TGA.[29] Repair options include baffling the LV outflow through the VSD to the aorta, either the Rastelli procedure or the REV procedure *(réparation à l'étage ventriculaire)*, combined with connection of the RV to the PA either via a direct connection or with a valved conduit. An alternative approach is aortic root translocation (Nikaidoh or Bex procedure), in which the aortic root is excised and repositioned posteriorly over the LV by opening up the outflow septum and the hypoplastic pulmonary valve annulus. Timing of repair depends on the degree of cyanosis. Those neonates with severely limited pulmonary blood flow will require a neonatal repair of a systemic to PA shunt, whereas those with milder degrees of LVOTO will be able to be managed without neonatal intervention. The choice of definitive procedure is frequently based on institutional experience and surgeon preference.[30] Aortic root translocation is suitable for those with moderate degrees of pulmonary annular hypoplasia and may decrease the late risk

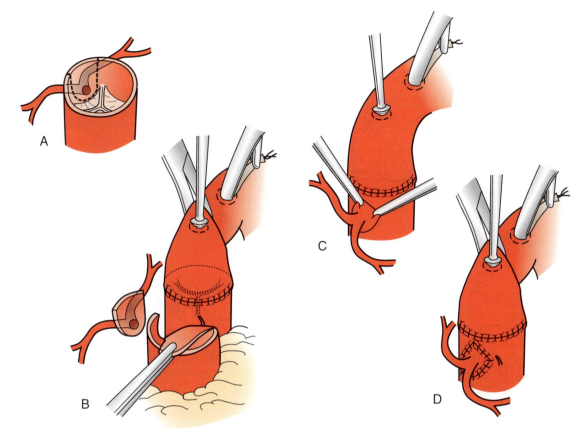

• **Figure 57.7** The closed technique may be useful for challenging coronary transfers in cases of single coronary artery or in cases of a large coronary from the right-facing sinus that gives rise to the right coronary artery and circumflex. The coronary ostial button is excised in the usual way (A). The ascending aorta is anastomosed to the neoaortic root, and the top of the commissure of the pulmonary valve is marked externally (B). The neoaortic root is distended, and the best implantation site for the coronary button is determined (C). Finally, the coronary is implanted, taking care to avoid injury to the neoaortic valve (D).

of recurrent LVOTO.[31] Aortic root translocation adds the risk of coronary insufficiency because the proximal coronaries require mobilization and potentially reimplantation. Postoperative concerns include residual VSD, conduction abnormalities, LVOTO, and RVOTO. The risk of LVOTO may be lower after the REV compared with the Rastelli procedure. All three procedures will require late reintervention on the RVOT for either regurgitation or conduit stenosis.

Atrial Switch Operations

Redirection of blood flow at the atrial level, either a Senning or Mustard operation, was the first successful surgical approach for patients with d-TGA. These operations are rarely used for isolated d-TGA in developed countries today, although they are used for late presentation in some parts of the world and as part of anatomic correction of corrected transposition. Acute complications include baffle obstruction, most commonly compromising flow from the superior vena cava, resulting in superior vena cava syndrome, or pulmonary veins, resulting in pulmonary edema that will require reintervention.[32,33] Late complications of the atrial-level switch include systemic right ventricular dysfunction and tricuspid regurgitation, baffle obstruction, and arrhythmias. There does not seem to be a clear advantage of the Senning or Mustard procedure, and similar long-term results have been reported with both operations.

Postoperative Critical Care Management

Most infants recover quickly following an uncomplicated ASO. Postoperative transesophageal echocardiogram before return to the intensive care unit (ICU) is routine and permits early detection and repair of residual lesions before returning to the ICU. Standard monitoring includes continuous ECG, invasive arterial and central venous pressure, pulse oximetry and capnography. While left atrial pressure lines were common in the past these are no longer routine unless LV dysfunction is anticipated. Continuous venous saturation monitoring or even the use of PA catheters has been reported and could be useful in selected cases.[34] An ECG and chest radiography should be obtained on arrival to the ICU.[5]

Low Cardiac Output Syndrome and Left Ventricular Dysfunction

Low cardiac output syndrome can occur after any operation requiring cardiopulmonary bypass and cardioplegic arrest from either inadequate myocardial protection, long ischemic time, or postbypass inflammation.[14,35] Infants with d-TGA are at particular risk. Even the neonate undergoing an ASO in the first few days of life may have an LV that is less than ideally prepared to do work against systemic afterload, and this may lead to LV dysfunction and mitral valve regurgitation.[14,35] Inotropic agents should be used to increase contractility and improve LV ejection fraction. The use

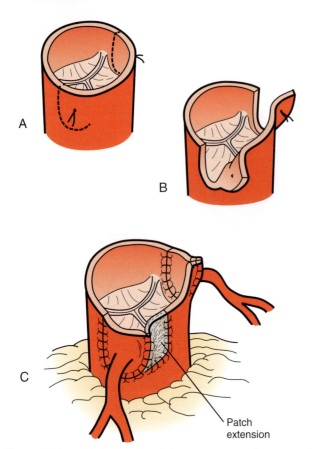

• **Figure 57.8** A patch extension of the coronary artery button can be helpful when the great arteries lie side-by-side and the right-facing sinus gives rise to a large coronary artery that includes the circumflex and right coronary artery with early branching. It can also be useful in cases of a single coronary artery. The pulmonary artery is transected, and the incisions for reimplantation of the coronary buttons are made as usual (A). Medially based trapdoor incisions are created (B). The patch extension, using either homograft or autologous pericardium, of the coronary ostial button reduces the rotation of the coronary artery (C) and prevents kinking of either branch.

of afterload-reducing agents, sodium nitroprusside, alpha-blockade with phentolamine, or in the past phenoxybenzamine or the use of the phosphodiesterase 3 inhibitor milrinone is common strategy to maximize systemic output. The LV of newborns with d-TGA may have systolic pressure limitations and may be able to generate pressures of only 50 to 60 mm Hg. Afterload reduction, by lowering systemic vascular resistance, will, as explained by Ohm's law (Pressure = Flow × Resistance), maximize cardiac output despite the inability of the LV to generate high pressure. Although afterload reduction can result in lower blood pressure, a degree of moderate hypotension is well tolerated in the postoperative ASO patient. Identification of the development of low cardiac output through close monitoring of perfusion, urine output, and filling pressures, as well as objective laboratory measures, including arterial and venous blood gas evaluation, near-infrared spectroscopy, and lactate level trend, is essential because it may be a sign of LV dysfunction.[36,37] Although some degree of diastolic dysfunction is anticipated if the echocardiogram shows decreased systolic function, especially with regional wall motion abnormalities, coronary insufficiency is the most likely cause, and prompt evaluation of the coronary arteries, including cardiac catheterization, is indicated.

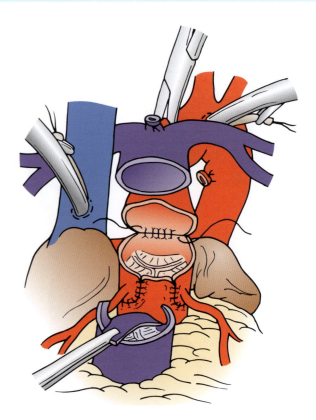

• **Figure 57.9** The Lecompte maneuver is performed, placing the pulmonary arteries anterior to the aorta, and the neoaortic root is anastomosed to the ascending aorta.

Timing of Extubation

In the early experience with the ASO, deep sedation and neuromuscular blockade were routine in the early postoperative management.[34] With increasing experience and improved preoperative and intraoperative management there has been a trend toward earlier extubation. The benefits or earlier extubation include shorter hospital length of stay, a lower risk of pneumonia, and decreased cost.[38] A recent meta-analysis confirms these benefits, demonstrating that this is associated with more rapid recovery and fewer complication.[39]

Coronary Artery Insufficiency or Obstruction

Specific to the ASO is reimplantation of the coronary arteries. Coronary artery obstruction due to distortion or kinking of the proximal coronary arteries is the leading cause of early postoperative mortality after the ASO. Certain coronary artery patterns are more technically challenging to transfer, but coronary insufficiency can occur with the most typical arrangement. A baseline ECG should be obtained when the patient arrives to the ICU after surgery. Coronary artery insufficiency may present as low cardiac output syndrome with ventricular dysfunction; therefore if the patient appears to be in low output or to have acute or developing ventricular dysfunction, a bedside ECG should be performed and echocardiogram to evaluate both functions, looking specifically for regional wall motion abnormalities and the proximal coronary arteries. The threshold for coronary angiography should be low. If possible, continuous ST segment

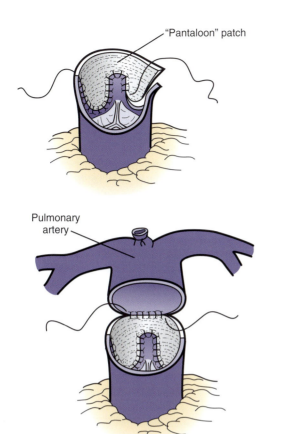

• **Figure 57.10** The defects in the aortic root created as a consequence of excising the coronary buttons are repaired using a generous "pantaloons"-shaped patch.

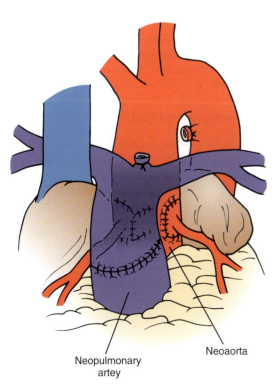

• **Figure 57.11** The completed arterial switch operation.

monitoring should be started on arrival to the ICU. In addition to ventricular dysfunction, coronary obstruction may cause arrhythmia or cardiac arrest.[6,35]

Late Presentation of d-TGA

Late presentation of d-TGA, beyond 3 weeks of age, occurs occasionally in North America and is common in the developing world. Options include a primary ASO, ASO after LV preparation with a PA band plus or minus a systemic to PA shunt, or an atrial-level correction. Several single-center series have shown reasonable results with primary ASO in patients up to 8 weeks of age with only a modest increase in mortality, but mechanical circulatory support should be available in the case of LV failure. For the patient beyond 8 weeks of age another option is to prepare the LV by placing a PA band.[40-44] This is commonly combined with a systemic to PA shunt to both relieve cyanosis and add volume load to the LV as a further stimulus to hypertrophy. Echocardiography can be used to assess the LV preparation, and a suitable hypertrophic response can occur in 1 to 2 weeks.[45] Single-center series have shown good results.[46] Long-term results appear to be good for survivors of late ASO. A recent study from China reports that children with d-TGA above 6 months of age at the time of ASO had quality-of-life scores indistinguishable from their normal peers.[47] Management of the patient with d-TGA presenting beyond 3 weeks of age will depend on the specific patient's anatomy and institutional ability and experience, particularly the availability of mechanical circulatory support. Although late arterial switch may be accomplished primarily or after LV preparation, an atrial-level switch operation should be considered for patients who do not respond to or tolerate PA banding or presenting beyond 6 months of age.

Early Reoperation After the Arterial Switch Operation

Early intervention for complications are necessary in approximately 3.3% of patients, with pacemaker insertion being the most common early reoperation.[48] Residual, sometimes multilevel, obstruction of the RVOT is also a common postoperative finding that may require return to the operating room within the first year after ASO.[49] Lastly, revision of the coronary anastomosis site may be indicated if stenosis and/or obstruction occurs. Freedom from reoperation decreases from 95% to nearly 80% from 1 to 20 years after surgery.[48]

Outcomes

Mortality After the Arterial Switch Operation

Currently, overall mortality rates after ASO are less than 5%, with early mortality (less than 30 days after surgery) reported between 2.2% and 3.4%.[48,50,51] Patients with VSDs or aortic arch obstruction have higher early mortality rates when compared with those with intact ventricular septum, and mortality after late ASO repair (>1 month old) in the patient with simple d-TGA increases to 5.4%.[5,24] Other risk factors for mortality include resection of LVOTO, need for ECMO, and weight less than 3 kg. Myocardial ischemia is the most common cause of early death; 2.9% of patients with specific coronary artery variations, namely a single coronary ostium or an intramural coronary artery, are at increased risk for early mortality.[48]

Long-Term Outcomes After the Arterial Switch Operation

Late survival following the arterial switch is excellent with 15-year survival in excess of 95%.[48,50,51] Reintervention is sometimes required, for RVOT obstruction (RVOTO), neoaortic valve regurgitation, and coronary insufficiency. The freedom from later reoperation has been reported to be between 75% and 85% at 15 years of follow-up.[48,50,51]

Right Ventricular Outflow Tract Obstruction. The incidence of RVOTO is 7% to 40%, making it the most common cause of late reoperation after ASO. Although there can be multilevel obstruction of the RVOT, the main pulmonary trunk and the right branch PA are the most frequent sites of obstruction. Other areas of obstruction include stenosis at the pulmonary bifurcation, left pulmonary branch artery, and RV infundibulum. Valvar stenosis is less common and is reported in only 7.7% of patients. Risk factors include the technique for reconstruction of the neopulmonary root in which coronary buttons were excised and possibly the Lecompte maneuver. There are mixed findings regarding history of PA banding. Interventions to relieve obstruction include balloon valvuloplasty with or without stent placement, patch enlargement, or valved conduit replacement of the PA. Freedom from intervention was 68% at 1 year and 42% at 5, 10, and 15 years.[49]

Neoaortic Root Dilation and Neoaortic Valve Regurgitation. Neoaortic root dilation occurs to some degree in more than two-thirds of patients after ASO and is a risk factor for development of neoaortic valve regurgitation. Risk factors for dilation include Taussig-Bing anatomy, history of PA banding or arch obstruction, and length of follow-up. The probability of being free from neoaortic root dilation (z score >2.5) was reported at 84%, 67%, 47%, and 32% at 1, 5, 10, and 15 years postoperatively, respectively. It is estimated that the root diameter increases at a rate of 0.16 cm per year, and the z score increases 0.08 per year.[52]

The development of significant neoaortic valve regurgitation requiring late reoperation is not rare with need for reoperation in 5% to 22% of patients at a median follow-up of 14.5 years (maximum of 27 years).[53] A retrospective study found the incidence of at least moderate neoaortic regurgitation to be 0.5%, 5.6%, and 41.6% at 5-, 15-, and 25-year follow-up, respectively.[51] Freedom from moderate to severe neoaortic valve regurgitation decreases from 96%, 92%, and 89% at 1, 5, and 10 years after surgery to 75% at 15 years.[52] Ideally, timing of valve repair should be before the development of severe aortic regurgitation, so a valve-sparing root replacement can be entertained. Once severe, valve replacement is recommended.[53]

Long-term follow-up should aim to monitor progression of the LV outflow tract. An echocardiogram every 1 to 2 years to evaluate the neoaortic valve and root is recommended. Indications for surgery are the development of symptomatic neoaortic regurgitation and/or progressive dilation of the LV.[54]

Coronary Artery Obstruction. Coronary obstruction is present in 5% to 7% of late survivors. The incidence of coronary-related myocardial ischemia, infarction, or mortality diminishes significantly after the first 3 months after surgery. Freedom from coronary events is 88% at 20-year follow-up.[5] Exercise stress testing is more beneficial than clinical examination for recognition of ischemia and risk for coronary events. Cardiac catheterization is the gold standard for detection, because ECGs and echocardiograms are not sensitive.[55]

Arrhythmias. The occurrence of arrhythmias following ASO is low. Arrhythmia-free survival is found in over 94% of patients at up to 25 years of follow-up.[5,55] Late postoperative arrhythmias beyond 30 days occur in 2.4 to 9.6% of patients. These are most frequently associated with residual hemodynamic lesions or coronary artery occlusion. Atrial arrhythmias, particularly atrial flutter, are most common and are often associated with RVOTO. Tachycardias arising from the LV are most commonly due to ischemia or may be related to scarring.[5]

Unlike patients who are status post ASO, those who have undergone the atrial switch (Mustard/Senning) procedure are at significantly higher risk for arrhythmia. Atrial arrhythmias are seen most frequently secondary to intraatrial baffle placement and atrial scarring. Surgical placement of the baffle can affect both the AV node and the coronary sinus ostium. Additionally, the long-term use of the RV for systemic output can place these patients at greater risk. The incidence of atrial tachyarrhythmias continues to rise with increasing patient age. Atrial flutter and atrial fibrillation are predictors of sudden cardiac death in those who are status post Senning/Mustard. Intraatrial reentry tachycardia, AV nodal reentry tachycardia, and focal atrial tachycardia are also common. Medical therapy and cardioversion are the first-line treatments for maintenance of normal sinus rhythm. It has been reported that the intervals between successful cardioversion for atrial tachycardias become shorter as the number of events increases.[56] Fifteen percent of atrial switch patients have pacemakers, although these are more frequently implanted for systemic RV dysfunction leading to low cardiac output rather than for arrhythmia control. Pacemaker insertion in this population is associated with increased risk of mortality.[57]

Postoperative Outcomes Specific to the Rastelli Procedure

After the Rastelli procedure, patients are at risk for reoperation due to RV to PA conduit stenosis and LVOTO due to stenosis of the LV to aortic baffle.[58] Less common causes for reintervention include tricuspid regurgitation and residual aortic arch obstruction. Risk for late reintervention is increased in patients with history of VSD, aortic arch obstruction, prolonged length of cardiopulmonary bypass, and post-ASO neopulmonary stenosis and neoaortic regurgitation at discharge.[48,50,51] Freedom from reintervention was significantly worse in d-TGA with Taussig-Bing anatomy.[50]

Neurodevelopmental Outcomes

Multiple studies have shown that patients who are have undergone ASO have, on average, IQs within the normal range.[59-61] Despite a normal IQ, ASO survivors have concerning and consistent neurodevelopmental impairment. In a landmark study, Bellinger et al. followed d-TGA patients who underwent ASO up to 16 years of age. The study found that these children performed below average in academic achievement (both in reading and math skills), fine motor function, sustained attention, high-order language skills, and social cognition. Additionally, they found that these adolescents had impaired visual-spatial skills and working memory ability. By the age of 16, one-third received tutoring; one-quarter had received special education, occupational therapy, or psychotherapy services; and one in six had been retained in a grade at least once.[60] More recent studies have continued to demonstrate changes in language, visual-spatial skills, executive function, and social cognition.[59] Additionally, children are significantly less proficient in identifying facial expressions and mental emotions, dealing with desires, and understanding concealed emotions of others.[61]

The acquired and intrinsic causes of neurodevelopmental impairment and therefore those factors that may be under the control of care providers remain unknown. In addition to hypoxia in the immediate neonatal phase, patients with d-TGA physiology have low PaO_2 levels in utero. It is hypothesized that these factors in addition to cardiopulmonary bypass and low cardiac output can have long-lasting effects on neurodevelopment.[62,63] There is wide variation in preoperative, intraoperative, and postoperative care without a clear difference in neurodevelopmental outcome among late survivors, suggesting that some of the neurodevelopmental burden may be intrinsic. Importantly, the fetal blood flow pattern is distinctly abnormal, and whereas in the normal fetus the most fully saturated blood is directed to the brain, in the fetus with transposition the opposite is true, and abnormal brain development, including delayed maturation and decreased head size, have been identified.[64,65] There is evidence that the postnatal, preoperative condition of the patient impacts neurodevelopment outcome. Prenatally diagnosed infants with d-TGA who have early resuscitation and short time to initiation of prostaglandin infusions performed significantly higher in executive functions and social cognition tests than those who were diagnosed postnatally. Those who were undiagnosed at birth were more likely to be at high risk for ductal closure, acidosis, hypoxemia, and hypoxic-ischemic injury.[59] Andropoulos and colleagues[63] found that 18% of postnatally diagnosed TGA patients had a pH of less than 7.2 compared with only 3% of those who were prenatally diagnosed. The American Heart Association and the American Academy of Pediatrics recommend that all patients with d-TGA undergo a neurodevelopmental screen in early childhood.[66]

Closing Remarks

The management of TGA is one of the great success stories in the history of congenital heart disease. Over a 70-year period we have progressed from the bleak natural history, through palliative procedures, to the atrial-level correction and ultimately, the ASO with excellent long-term survival. This diagnosis has arguably created the modern congenital heart surgery unit capable of complex neonatal correction as well as originating the field of interventional cardiology. In the current era, postoperative management of d-TGA has become almost routine. Nevertheless, long-term follow-up is needed to identify problems requiring late reintervention directed at coronary insufficiency, neoaortic regurgitation, and right ventricular outflow obstruction. Nevertheless, we have entered the era of lifelong follow-up for a diagnosis that was once lethal in the neonatal period.

References

A complete list of references is available at ExpertConsult.com

58

Double-Outlet Right Ventricle

DAVID BICHELL, MD

Double-outlet right ventricle (DORV) includes an array of ventriculoarterial arrangements in which both great arteries associate primarily with the right ventricle (RV). Corrective strategies are varied, aimed at repatriating the aorta to the left ventricle (LV) and providing unobstructed biventricular outflow tracts. Though DORV is only a description of the ventriculoarterial associations, it can occur also with various combinations of atrioventricular arrangement, including atrial isomerism and complex heterotaxy, which can additionally challenge the correction or palliation. In most clinical series, DORV strategies and outcomes have been subgrouped into the typical, more common, biventricular versus the more complex because the latter has different expectations and treatment strategies.

Definition

By simplest definition, DORV refers to both aorta and pulmonary artery (PA) arising from the RV, almost always in combination with a ventricular septal defect (VSD). Association with the RV is commonly defined as an aorta that overrides the septal crest by more than 50% and therefore lies principally over the RV. The great arteries can be positioned in any configuration around one another, and the VSD can be variably positioned beneath the great vessels to result in the phenomenon of both great arteries mostly aligned with the RV. Depending on the configuration of the great arteries and their relationship with the VSD, DORV anatomy and physiology may resemble that of a simple VSD, that of tetralogy of Fallot (TOF), or that of transposition of the great arteries (TGA). An anterior or rightward aorta may put the PA in closer association with the LV, producing transposition-type physiology, whereas a more posterior aorta is associated with the LV and tetralogy-type or VSD-type physiology results, depending on the degree of pulmonary stenosis (PS). Tetralogy of Fallot (anteriorly malaligned VSD and aortic override of the septum) overlaps with DORV and is called DORV if the aortic override of the septum is 51% favoring the RV. At the other end of the rotational spectrum, transposition of the great vessels is instead called DORV if the PA is principally affiliated with the LV.

Historical Perspective

An autopsy specimen with both great vessels arising from the RV was described in the 18th century.[1,2] Until the 20th century, considered among variations of TGA, DORV-like pathology was referred to as "partial transposition," in which the aorta is transposed and the PA is not.[3] The Taussig-Bing variant of transposed aorta with leftward malposed PA was described 1949.[4]

The anomaly was first called double-outlet ventricle by Braun in 1952, and Witham is credited with first referring to the lesion as double-outlet right ventricle in 1957.[1,5,6] The earliest operative repair was performed by John Kirklin in 1957.[7] Landmark descriptions with clinical correlations, with or without PS followed, as survivable pathways of correction were devised and described.[8]

Embryology

As aquatic organisms climbed out of the sea, a separation into pulmonary and systemic circulations required the septation of a formerly single ventricular outflow tract. In embryogenesis, crest cells migrate from neural folds to the forming conotruncus to direct the septation of the ventricles and of the great arteries. In addition to a separation into two distinct vessels, the great arteries reposition around each other as their associated subvalvar conus grows or recedes, leading the arteries to associate with their respective destination ventricles.[9] D-looping of the primitive heart tube places the aorta rightward of the PA. In normal cardiac development a subsequent resorption of the subaortic conus tows the aorta posteriorly and leftward, to achieve fibrous continuity with the mitral valve and proximity with the LV. Persistence of the subaortic conus leaves the aorta rightward or ventral to the PA, muscle maintains separation between the aortic and mitral valves, and the aorta associates with the RV.[10] In DORV, aortic and pulmonary coni rotate incompletely around one another to join the advancing septal crest, and resultant ventriculoarterial alignment can range from concordant ("VSD-type," "TOF-type") to discordant (Taussig-Bing, "TGA-type").[11] The Taussig-Bing arrangement is very similar to arrested progression with bilateral conus and rightward aorta (Fig. 58.1).[4,12] Attractive as the concept of bilateral persistent conus is in describing DORV development, in fact there is heterogeneity of actual anatomy that defies a single morphogenic explanation.[13,14] But the bilateral conus serves as a useful heuristic to visualize the relationships.

Genetics

Conotruncal dysmorphogenesis is a consequence of an interplay between multiple partially understood gene pathways.[15] Gene alterations in animal models elucidate some mechanisms and identify points where mutation can produce the DORV phenotype. Among genes with demonstrated involvement in the formation of DORV are *BMP2* and *BMP4,* implicated in directing neural crest cell migration,[16] *TGFB2,* when knocked out, produces DORV in mice,[17]

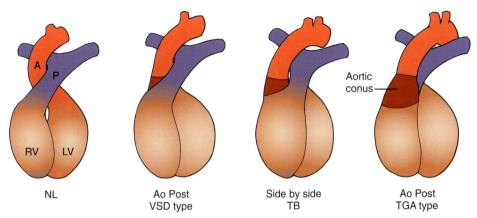

• **Figure 58.1** Variants of double-outlet right ventricle according to the relative orientations of the great arteries. Depicted are various degrees of persistence of the subaortic conus and the implications for aortic position relative to the pulmonary artery. *Left,* The normal heart has no residual subaortic conus, with aorta-mitral continuity and aorta (A) connected directly to the left ventricle (LV). *Middle left,* With near complete resorption of the subaortic conus the aorta is delivered posterior to the pulmonary artery (P); with less conal resorption the aorta is close to the LV. *Middle right,* Side-by-side aorta and pulmonary artery. *Right,* The subaortic conus is intact, there is no mitral-aortic continuity, and the aorta is anterior to the pulmonary artery and more closely associated with the right ventricle (RV).

and *GATA4*, interacting with *FOG2* (cardiac cofactor), if inhibited, also yields DORV in an animal model.[18]

Retinoic acid, a vitamin A metabolite, plays a role in cardiac morphogenesis, and gene mutations affecting its ligand-receptor complex can cause DORV, among other defects.[19,20]

Though TOF is commonly associated with syndromes, DORV is much less so, though some associations of DORV with trisomy 21, trisomy13, trisomy18, and 22q11 deletion have been described.[21]

Surgical Anatomy and Classification

Irrespective of controversies about the mechanisms behind the development of DORV, a classification based on clinical pathology is important to direct patients onto the most successful corrective pathways and expectations. A majority of DORVs are situs solitus with concordant atrioventricular connection. The position of the VSD with respect to the great arteries and the presence or absence of PS, are the relationships most relevant to designing the corrective approach.[22,23]

Ventricular Septal Defect Position

The VSD can be *subaortic, subpulmonic, doubly committed,* or *uncommitted* (Fig. 58.2). Commonest is the subaortic VSD, with a rightward malposed aorta. The relative incidence of subaortic VSD is 42% to 59%, subpulmonary is 21% to 37%, uncommitted is 11% to 26%, and doubly committed is 3% to 9%.[1,24-29] The original Taussig-Bing variant includes the combination of subpulmonary VSD, side-by-side great arteries, and bilateral subarterial conus, with or without subaortic stenosis. The term *Taussig-Bing* is loosely used as synonymous with any DORV with subpulmonary VSD and transposition-like physiology.[4,30]

Great Artery Position

In normal cardiac development the aorta is positioned posterior to the PA, in continuity with the more posterior LV. In the case

of DORV the aortic position can be posterior or rightward and still remain in reach of the LV, but when it is found to lie farther rightward or anterior, the aorta is farther from the LV, the PA closer to the LV, and TGA physiology ensues. Incomplete growth of the pulmonary infundibulum yields stenosis or atresia of the pulmonary valve.[31] Underdevelopment of the subaortic conus may produce aortic stenosis, and downstream effects include coarctation or arch hypoplasia.

Outflow Tract Obstruction

Rightward or leftward deviation of the conal septum determines VSD commitment and affects either outflow tract.[11] Commonest is an anterior and leftward conal septum deviation, defining subaortic VSD, crowding, and PS. In cases of doubly committed VSD, PS is common. With uncommitted VSD, PS is uncommon (see Fig. 58.2).

Atrioventricular Abnormalities

Atrioventricular canal defect (AVC) occurs with DORV, is usually unbalanced, and is usually associated with a subpulmonary VSD and with malformed elements of the left heart, including mitral stenosis, mitral atresia, or straddling mitral valve.[11,32-36]

AVC with DORV should raise suspicion of heterotaxy. Heterotaxy polysplenia is most commonly associated with AVC and is accompanied by LV hypoplasia and systemic venous anomalies such as interrupted inferior vena cava with azygos continuation.[23,37] Heterotaxy asplenia is more commonly associated with subpulmonary stenosis, common atrioventricular valve, common atrium, and anomalous pulmonary venous connection.[11]

Associated Obstructive Lesions

Sixty-six percent of patients with a subaortic VSD have PS, with favored flow through the aorta, and subaortic stenosis or arch

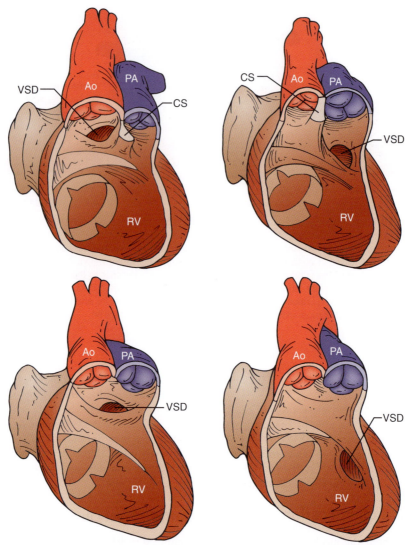

• **Figure 58.2** Characterization of double-outlet right ventricle according to ventricular septal defect (VSD) types. Upper left, Subaortic VSD with anterior and leftward conal septum deviation, crowding, and stenosis of the pulmonary valve. Upper right, Subpulmonary VSD, with posterior and rightward deviation of the conal septum and crowding of the rightward malposed aorta. Lower left, Doubly committed VSD with absent conal septum. Lower right, Noncommitted VSD: VSD remote from the great arteries.

obstruction is rare. Conversely, among those with a subpulmonary VSD, 30% have arch obstruction, 14% have PS, and 6% have subaortic stenosis. With doubly committed VSD, 59% have PS, 14% have subaortic stenosis, and 9% have arch obstruction, and with uncommitted VSD, 32% have PS, 6% have subaortic stenosis, and 10% have arch anomalies.[1,27,29,38]

Other Anatomic Considerations

Coronary anomalies occur in 50% of DORV cases.[11,30] Most clinically relevant are cases with the left coronary artery crossing a pulmonary or neopulmonary outflow tract, posing challenges to its enlargement.

With discordant atrioventricular connection, the aorta is anterior and leftward of the PA, and the VSD position is subpulmonary more commonly than subaortic.[39] Juxtaposed atrial appendages, Ebstein malformation of the tricuspid valve, tricuspid atresia,

double-inlet RV, and double-chamber RV have all been described in association with DORV.[37,40,41]

Classification

A current and widely accepted system of classification for DORV, based on clinical presentation and treatment strategy, was developed by the Society of Thoracic Surgeons–European Association for Cardio-Thoracic Surgery (STS-EACTS) Congenital Heart Surgery Nomenclature and Database Project and consists of four types of DORV. In the absence of PS, DORV with a subaortic VSD is termed *VSD-type*. In the presence of PS, it is *TOF-type*. In variants where the PA associates more closely with the LV, it is considered *TGA-type*, and when the VSD is remote from both semilunar valves, it is *noncommitted VSD-type*. Relative prevalence by type is VSD-type, 25%; TOF-type, 35%; TGA-type, 20%; and noncommitted VSD-type, 20%.[42]

Pathophysiology

Perfusion Balance

A spectrum of physiologies matches the spectrum of anatomic variants of DORV. An unrestrictive VSD means equivalent pressures in the LV and RV and pulmonary blood flow that is gated by the degree of PS. In the absence of PS the balance between pulmonary and systemic circulations is dictated by the pulmonary vascular resistance (PVR). In the neonate, postnatal changes in PVR exacerbate or ameliorate pulmonary blood flow extremes, producing a moving target for management. All influences taken together, DORV physiology can range from congestive heart failure in cases of unrestricted pulmonary blood flow, to cyanosis from pulmonary hypoperfusion. In TGA-type DORV the presence of subaortic stenosis may further exacerbate congestive failure and systemic hypoperfusion.

Mixing/Oxygenation Balance

The commitment of the VSD determines streaming. Whereas in TOF-type DORV, hypoxia may result from PS, the TGA-type DORV, with subpulmonary VSD, will also exhibit hypoxia but due instead to inadequate mixing and RV-aorta streaming. In the single-ventricle variants, mixing is more complete, and oxygenation is more reflective of relative pulmonary and systemic flows.

Patent Ductus Arteriosus

A patent ductus arteriosus (PDA) may circumvent PS to produce pulmonary overcirculation and congestive failure despite the presence of PS. Conversely, severe PS or pulmonary atresia may require maintenance of ductal patency to achieve adequate pulmonary blood flow. Aortic stenosis or arch obstruction may render the systemic circulation dependent on ductal patency. In transposition physiology, ductal patency represents one of three levels where mixing can improve hypoxia.

Presentation and Preoperative Management

The infant with VSD-type DORV (subaortic VSD and no PS) will have excessive pulmonary blood flow and symptomatic congestive failure in the first weeks of life, worsening along with the fall of PVR. Examination may reveal tachypnea, tachycardia, a holosystolic murmur, and a mid-diastolic rumble (mitral flow murmur). Cardiomegaly and prominent pulmonary vascularity is seen on chest x-ray examination. The mainstay of nonoperative, anticongestive management includes diuretics and afterload reduction, escalating as necessary to mechanical ventilation and pulmonary vasoconstrictive strategies such as permissive hypercapnia and low inspired O_2 concentration. When conservative measures fail, operative management can include a palliative PA band or definitive operative repair (Table 58.1).

The infant with TOF-type DORV (subaortic VSD with PS) will have restricted pulmonary blood flow and a balance of circulation governed by the degree of PS. Presentation may range from asymptomatic to cyanotic, and hypercyanotic spells may occur with dynamic, muscular sub-PS. The physical examination reveals the harsh systolic murmur of PS and a single second heart sound. The chest x-ray examination may show a small cardiac silhouette and dark lung fields. Medical management includes hydration, sedation, and mechanical ventilation. When present, a PDA can circumvent the effects of PS to result in balanced or excessive pulmonary blood flow. Cyanotic infants or those with ductal dependent pulmonary blood flow are maintained on prostaglandin (PGE$_1$) and may additionally undergo palliative ductal stenting, operative aortopulmonary shunt construction, or definitive operative repair (Table 58.2).

A patient with TGA-type DORV (subpulmonary VSD) will exhibit hypoxia from inadequate mixing. The physical examination will reveal cyanosis, tachypnea, a systolic murmur if stenosis is present, and a diastolic rumble if the patient is primarily congested. The chest x-ray examination may reveal cardiomegaly and prominent pulmonary vascular markings. Preoperative management is directed at optimizing intracardiac mixing, which can occur at the VSD, atrial septal defect (ASD), and PDA levels. Therapies may include PGE$_1$ infusion, mechanical ventilation, and balloon atrial septostomy.

DORV with absent VSD is rare, and adequate systemic circulation will depend on mitral insufficiency and an ASD that can produce enough left-to-right shunting to support the RV and its dual output.[43,44] A restrictive VSD can cause the physiologic equivalent of aortic stenosis.[45] Preoperative management may include PGE$_1$ infusion and balloon atrial septostomy.

Diagnostic Imaging

An echocardiogram is often obtained prenatally or perinatally, and the diagnosis is confirmed often even before a physical examination. The subxiphoid short-axis view shows two great arteries with predominant commitment to the RV. A parasternal long-axis view may confirm discontinuity between the mitral valve and aorta. The size and commitment of the VSD is characterized from subxiphoid views, along with the LV to aorta pathway. Great arteries that are parallel, seen in the same plane, with bilateral conus characterize the Taussig-Bing or TGA-type DORV. Arch and ductal anatomy is viewed in suprasternal notch view. Coronary anatomy is commonly well characterized by echocardiography. Additional important information includes an evaluation of the relative size of the ventricles, atrioventricular valve abnormalities, presence of additional VSDs, degree of pulmonary or aortic stenosis, and tricuspid to pulmonary distance (to accommodate an intracardiac baffle). The pathway for planning an intracardiac tunnel can be challenging, and three-dimensional echocardiography has an expanding role.[46,47]

Determining the feasibility of an intraventricular tunnel repair for DORV can be difficult from echocardiography alone, and three-dimensional modeling from computed tomography or magnetic resonance angiography has found an expanding role in surgical planning. The construction of physical three-dimensional printed models from individual patient data may inform operative surgical strategies to prevent improvisational approaches and intraoperative error (Fig. 58.3).[1,48-50]

Angiography has largely been supplanted by echocardiography in the diagnosis of DORV. Coronary artery and arch anatomy is more definitively imaged by angiography, but surgical correction seldom requires the information obtainable by angiography, the criteria for which were established in 1965.[51]

Surgical Procedures

As many as one-third of patients presenting with DORV will have unbalanced ventricular size, straddling atrioventricular valve chordae, or an unworkable biventricular pathway to connect the LV to the systemic circulation and will need to undergo a palliative single-ventricle approach.[52]

TABLE 58.1   Double-Outlet Right Ventricle: Characteristics and Treatment Strategies

| ANATOMY | | | | | PALLIATION | | |
VSD Position	PS/No PS	AS/No AS	STS-EACTS Classification	Physiology	Medical	Interventional/ Surgical	Surgical Corrections
Subaortic or doubly committed VSD	No pulmonary stenosis	No aortic stenosis	VSD-type	Congestion ($Q_p > Q_s$)	Diuretics, afterload reduction, mechanical ventilation, hypercapnia	Pulmonary artery band	VSD baffle to aorta, Kawashima
	Pulmonary stenosis	No aortic stenosis	TOF-type	Cyanosis ($Q_p < Q_s$)	Beta-blockade, hydration, sedation, PGE_1	Aortopulmonary shunt, ductal stent	VSD baffle to aorta, RVOT procedure (Rastelli or REV)
Subpulmonary VSD	No pulmonary stenosis	No aortic stenosis	TGA-type	Cyanosis (streaming)	PGE_1, mechanical ventilation	Balloon atrial septostomy	VSD baffle to pulmonary valve, arterial switch VSD baffle to pulmonary valve, arterial switch + RVOT procedure (Rastelli or REV)
		Aortic stenosis					
	Pulmonary stenosis	No aortic stenosis		Cyanosis ($Q_p < Q_s$)	PGE_1, mechanical ventilation	Aortopulmonary shunt, ductal stent	Yasui, Nikaidoh, Yamagishi truncal switch
Noncommitted VSD	No pulmonary stenosis	No aortic stenosis Aortic stenosis	Non-committed VSD-type	Congestion ($Q_p > Q_s$)	Diuretics, afterload reduction, mechanical ventilation, hypercapnia	Pulmonary artery band	Any of above, depending on pathway between VSD and suitable great artery, ± RVOT procedure
	Pulmonary stenosis	No aortic stenosis		Cyanosis ($Q_p < Q_s$)	PGE_1, mechanical ventilation	Aortopulmonary shunt, ductal stent	

AS, Aortic stenosis; *PGE₁,* prostaglandin E₁; *PS,* pulmonary stenosis; *Qₚ,* pulmonary blood flow; *Qₛ,* systemic perfusion; *REV, réparation à l'étage ventriculaire; RVOT,* right ventricular outflow tract; *STS-EACTS,* Society of Thoracic Surgeons–European Association for Cardio-Thoracic Surgery; *TGA,* transposition of the great arteries; *TOF,* tetralogy of Fallot; *VSD,* ventricular septal defect.

TABLE 58.2   Surgical Corrections for Double-Outlet Right Ventricle

Procedure Name	Description	Conditions
IVR	Intraventricular LV-aorta tunnel	Aorta posterior, sufficient TV-PA separation to accommodate baffle
Rastelli	Intraventricular LV-aorta tunnel after VSD enlargement, with RV-PA reconstruction	Aorta posterior, rightward or anterior, pulmonary stenosis
Kawashima	Intraventricular LV-aorta tunnel, circumnavigating the pulmonary valve	Aorta anterior or rightward (TGA), no pulmonary stenosis
Jatene arterial switch (IVR-ASO)	Intraventricular LV-PA tunnel with coronary transfer to pulmonary artery	
Double root translocation	Aortic root translocation to LV with pulmonary root translocated to RV	
REV	Intraventricular LV-aorta tunnel after resection of conal septum, with direct RV-PA connection	Aorta anterior or rightward (TGA), pulmonary stenosis, Taussig-Bing
Nikaidoh (aortic root translocation)	Aortic root translocation to LV with RV- PA conduit	
Yamagishi (half-turn truncal switch)	En bloc rotation of aorta and PA, coronary reimplantation	
Yasui	Intraventricular LV-PA tunnel, Damus-Kaye-Stansel anastomosis, RV-PA conduit	

ASO, Arterial switch operation; *IVR,* intraventricular baffle repair; *LV,* left ventricle; *PA,* pulmonary artery; *REV, réparation à l'étage ventriculaire; RV,* right ventricle; *TGA,* transposition of the great arteries; *TV,* tricuspid valve.

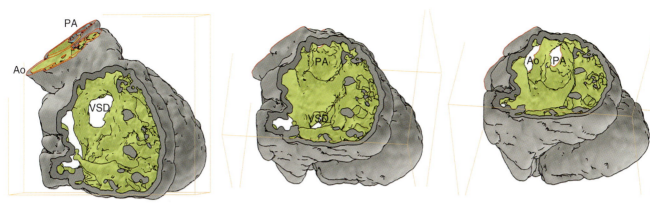

• **Figure 58.3** Three-dimensional images of double-outlet right ventricle with noncommitted (remote) ventricular septal defect (VSD), reconstructed from computed tomography angiogram. Various views are depicted showing the relationship of the VSD to the aorta (Ao) and pulmonary artery (PA). (Courtesy Jason Christensen, MD, Vanderbilt University.)

The timing for repair for biventricular variants is affected by the clinico-anatomic classification and its attendant physiology. In general, VSD-type and TOF-type DORV are repaired at approximately 3 months of age, unless excessive pulmonary blood flow (congestive heart failure) or compromised pulmonary blood flow (PS) drives an earlier intervention. Patients with subpulmonary VSD, the TGA-type, generally require repair or palliation earlier. A palliative approach might be taken for patients whose risk is improved with time, such as those born prematurely, those with multiple VSDs, or those with concomitant extracardiac problems that need resolution. The goals of complete repair are to septate the heart while creating unobstructed pathways from the LV to the aorta, and from the RV to the PA. There are numerous surgical approaches to achieving these goals, illustrating the complex spectrum of geometries that DORV represents.

VSD-type (Subaortic VSD, No PS)

The VSD-type DORV presents anatomy closest to normal, usually with a posterior aorta, in closest association with the LV. A definitive repair is achieved with an intraventricular baffle repair (IVR) to direct LV flow through the VSD to the rightward displaced aorta (Fig. 58.4). The pathway is feasible if sufficient distance separates the tricuspid and pulmonary valves, where the tunnel is constructed (Fig. 58.5). The baffled VSD closure can often be achieved through a right atriotomy, though exposure sometimes requires an RV infundibulotomy. Creating an unobstructed pathway may require enlarging the VSD, which can be safely achieved by resecting septal muscle anteriorly and leftward, remote from the His bundle, left and right bundle branches. VSD enlargement is required if the VSD diameter is less than that of the aortic valve (see Fig. 58.5).

Concomitant anomalies to consider at repair include ASDs, PDA, and coarctation of the aorta.[53-55]

In addition to heart block and residual VSD, perioperative complications importantly include LV-aorta baffle obstruction or RV outflow obstruction.

TOF-Type (Subaortic VSD With PS)

With a more rightward or anteriorly malposed aorta and right infundibular narrowing, establishing continuity of the LV and aorta is through an intracardiac baffle as with the VSD-type, but additional attention is applied to creating an unobstructed RV outflow tract. The Rastelli procedure includes an intraventricular LV-aorta baffle, possible VSD enlargement, and a conduit reconstruction of the pulmonary outflow tract (Fig. 58.6).[56] The REV procedure *(réparation à l'étage ventriculaire)* is a modification that repositions the main PA in direct connection with the RV, avoiding a conduit.[57-59]

TGA-Type (Subpulmonary VSD, No PS)

With the aorta positioned more anteriorly, the PA more posteriorly, and in the absence of PS, a neonatal single-stage repair can usually be achieved with a baffled closure of the VSD to the PA and a Jatene arterial switch (arterial switch operation [ASO]) procedure (Fig. 58.7).[60-62] The ASO is commonly performed with a Lecompte maneuver to move the pulmonary arteries anterior to the aorta. When the aorta is rightward malposed, there are special challenges to repositioning the pulmonary arteries that may require additional arterioplasty, and that should heighten vigilance for obstruction postoperatively. Alternatively, the Kawashima intraventricular tunnel, an intracardiac LV-aorta baffle, is applied, sometimes requiring two patches to accommodate an indirect pathway to the aorta.[63-65]

TGA-Type (Subpulmonary VSD, With PS)

With transposition physiology and a pulmonary valve that is of insufficient size to be reassigned as a neoaortic valve, the ASO approach is not feasible. The Nikaidoh aortic root translocation includes opening the stenotic pulmonary annulus to accommodate the leftward shift of the aortic root to a new position over the LV.[66-69] A double root translocation is similar to the Nikaidoh but preserves the integrity of the pulmonary root in addition to the aortic root, shifting it toward the RV and obviating the need for a conduit to reconstruct the RV outflow tract.[67] The half-turned truncal switch reassigns the transposed great vessels to achieve ventriculoarterial concordance by en bloc rotation of both great arteries on a single pedicle.[70,71] When the aorta is too small or too remote for an intracardiac baffle and an ASO is not feasible, the Yasui operation combines the great vessels as one in a Damus-Kaye-Stansel anastomosis, the VSD is baffled to

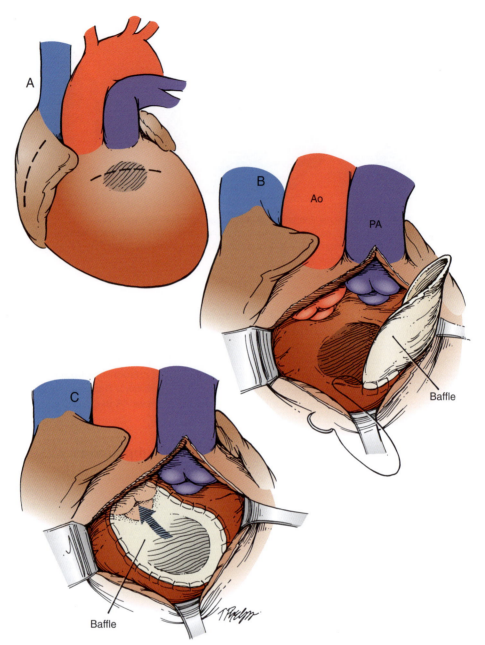

• **Figure 58.4** Intraventricular baffle repair of VSD-type double-outlet right ventricle. (A) The approach can be transatrial or by ventriculotomy *(dashed lines)*. (B) A baffle is constructed to direct the ventricular septal defect (VSD) to the aorta (Ao). (C) Completed, the baffle directs left ventricular outflow to the aorta, without obstructing the right ventricular egress to the pulmonary artery (PA).

the PA, and a separate RV outflow tract conduit is constructed (Fig. 58.8).[72]

In general, though many operations have been devised, the choice of operation follows simple principles and a simple decision tree. If sufficient ventricular volume and atrioventricular connections exist for a biventricular repair, and at least one semilunar valve is adequate, the repair strategies are prescribed by the answers to two questions: (1) Can the best unobstructed pathway be constructed from the LV to the aorta? If so, the repair will include an LV-aorta baffle. If not, then the best repair may include an LV-PA baffle in combination with ASO or aortic root translocation. (2) Is the resultant pulmonary outflow tract adequate? If not, then

the addition of an RV outflow tract enlargement procedure is necessary.

Postoperative Critical Care Management

Residual Anatomic Defects

Residual intracardiac shunts or obstructions are important contributors to morbidity. Even as routine intraoperative echocardiography has reduced the number of patients arriving in the intensive care unit with unexpected anatomy, it is incumbent on the intensivist to maintain vigilance to rule out residual lesions that could

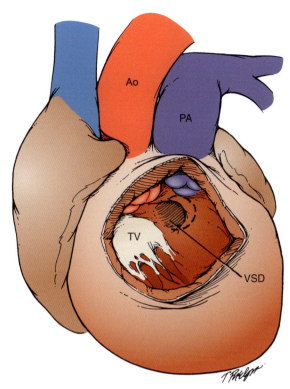

• **Figure 58.5** Relationship of the ventricular septal defect (VSD) to the tricuspid valve (TV), the aorta (Ao), and the pulmonary artery (PA). The distance between the TV and PA must be sufficient to provide a pathway for the intraventricular baffle. When necessary, an enlargement of the VSD can be carried out on its rightward aspect, remote from the His bundle.

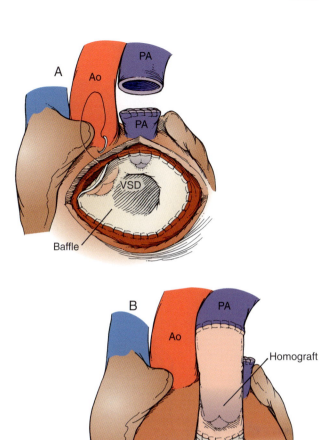

• **Figure 58.6** Rastelli procedure. The baffled ventricular septal defect (VSD) closure directs the left ventricle (LV) to the aorta (Ao), and the stenotic pulmonary artery (PA) is excluded. Continuity between the right ventricle (RV) and the PA is achieved with placement of a conduit.

need to be addressed early.[28,73] Echocardiography can detect most residual anatomic problems and assess function, atrioventricular valve competence, effusion, tamponade, and other important evolving issues in the early postoperative period. Early diagnostic catheterization and even interventional procedures are shown to be safe and can reduce early postoperative morbidity.[74] The commonest reason for early reoperation is residual VSD, and a patient with a pulmonary-to-systemic blood flow ratio (Q_p:Q_s) above 2 will likely need to return to the operating room. Intracardiac baffle obstruction can result from an insufficiently enlarged VSD or a fold or distortion of the baffle construct itself. Especially prone to baffle obstruction is the noncommitted VSD-type DORV, with a long pathway between the LV and the aorta. An RV-occupying intraventricular baffle decreases RV ejection fraction, even in absence of obstruction.[75]

Aortic insufficiency can result from conal septal resection near the valve or from VSD sutures placed near the valve. Aortic insufficiency after a Yasui operation can constitute a left-to-right shunt if the aorta remains in continuity with the RV. Tricuspid insufficiency is common at the VSD patch margin and should also be ruled out with a high index of suspicion. Right ventricular outflow tract obstruction and branch PS are all common postoperative residual burdens that contribute to low cardiac output, high filling pressures, and high inotropic requirement. Coronary compromise, especially when the corrective procedure included coronary transfer or reimplantation, can present late, potentiated by cardiac edema, RV distention, PA pressure elevation, and atrial distention, all of which can exert progressive distortion, stretch, or extrinsic compression to formerly patent coronaries.

Hemodynamic Monitoring and Support

Patients returning from the operating room after complex repairs typically have a transthoracic right atrial line, an arterial line, and sometimes a left atrial line. Near-infrared spectroscopy (NIRS) is used intraoperatively and postoperatively with indirect measure of cerebral mixed venous oxygen saturation (SvO_2) and relative somatic versus cerebral oxygen delivery when somatic NIRS is additionally applied. Post–cardiopulmonary bypass (CPB) inflammatory effects and the myocardial preservation effects produce a low cardiac output state to some extent in every patient, commensurate usually with the degree of tissue injury incurred, both incisive and by duration of CPB and myocardial ischemic time. The nadir in cardiac output and cardiac reserve is 8 to 12 hours post CPB. Principles of hemodynamic support during this critical period include appropriate preload titrated to optimize ventricular filling in the setting of diastolic dysfunction, combined with afterload reduction and judicious inotropy, titrated to optimize systolic function without imposing excessive myocardial oxygen demand. To varying degrees, all will suffer biventricular dysfunction in the early postoperative period, and the nature and duration of surgery will produce particular RV or LV dysfunction. Low SvO_2,

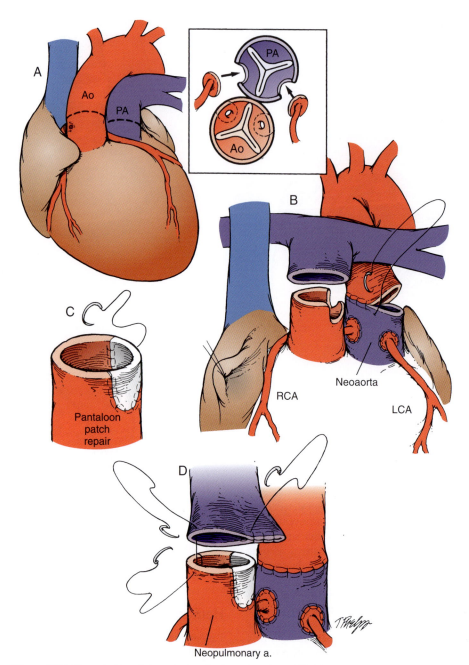

• **Figure 58.7** The arterial switch procedure for the correction of TGA-type double-outlet right ventricle. (A) The aorta (Ao) and pulmonary artery (PA) are transected and coronary arteries transferred, transforming the PA into a neoaorta. (B) The pulmonary artery is repositioned anterior to the neoaorta (Lecompte maneuver). (C) The aorta is reconstructed and reassigned as the neopulmonary artery. (D) The neopulmonary artery to pulmonary artery anastomosis is completed. *LCA,* Left coronary artery; *RCA,* right coronary artery.

evidenced by low NIRS values, in the presence of other acceptable-appearing measures is early warning of biochemical shock, and SvO_2 goal-directed management improves outcomes over conventional monitoring alone.[76]

Left Ventricular Dysfunction

Low cardiac output, the imbalance of tissue O_2 supply and demand, is common after complex cardiac corrections. Oliguria, peripheral

vasoconstriction, and metabolic acidosis are signs of anaerobic metabolism, oxidative stress, and inadequate tissue O_2 delivery.

The strained LV, with escalating end-diastolic pressure and escalating preload requirement for adequate filling, can enter a narrow window where the difference between therapeutic maneuvers and detrimental maneuvers narrows. A rapid infusion of volume to the strained LV can increase preload and result in increased endocardial wall tension, compromising coronary blood flow, and diastolic flow reversal that exacerbates pulmonary edema upstream

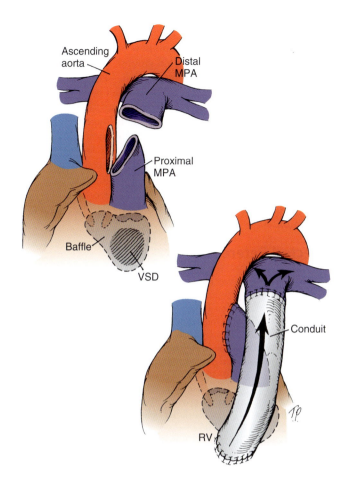

• **Figure 58.8** Damus-Kaye-Stansel construction. The aorta (Ao) and the pulmonary artery (PA) are anastomosed together to form a single route of egress from the left ventricle (LV), which is achieved by baffled ventricular septal defect (VSD) closure. Continuity between the right ventricle (RV) and the PA is established with the placement of a conduit.

from the stiff LV.[77] Pulmonary edema strains the RV, converting LV failure into biventricular failure.

The typical postoperative decline in cardiac output is supported by the judicious balance of preload, afterload reduction, and inotropy. When atrial pressure rises, SvO_2 declines, and metabolic acidosis progresses, more aggressive maneuvers to support recovery may be necessary, such as opening the sternum and instituting mechanical support.

Right Ventricular Dysfunction

Right heart failure can be a consequence of LV failure or can be from isolated right heart problems. Right heart failure is heralded by systemic venous congestion, hepatomegaly, ascites, pleural effusions, pericardial effusions, and edema. Sources of impaired right heart function can be a fixed anatomic obstruction, which must be suspected and corrected early, or intrinsic myocardial dysfunction. Corrections for DORV variants that have pulmonary or neopulmonary augmentations can suffer residual obstruction as described earlier in "Residual Anatomic Defects." Further, sternal compression of an RV-PA conduit can produce RV obstruction that eludes echocardiographic detection in the operating room. The resultant pressure load on the RV adds to the effects of

myocardial compromise from ventriculotomy, retraction, and myocardial preservation injury. Anticipated perioperative RV dysfunction is treated with a combination of balanced preload management and inotropy, pacing, pulmonary vasodilation, and a low threshold for reopening the sternum. Rapid volume infusion to a failing RV can elevate atrial pressure, in turn elevating coronary sinus pressure, and, in a low output state, acutely compromising coronary perfusion. Even in the absence of coronary compromise, acute right heart distention changes interventricular septal geometry and overall pericardial space constraint, thereby negatively affecting LV function.[78,79]

Pulmonary hypertension, often a result of vasoreactivity from the effects of cardiopulmonary bypass, exerts an afterload pressure on the RV. Patients with lesions characterized by excessive pulmonary blood flow preoperatively are especially vulnerable to postoperative reactive pulmonary hypertension. Pulmonary hypertensive episodes can be precipitated in the early postoperative period by suctioning, hypercarbia, and hypoxia. Acute treatment strategies may include paralysis, inhaled nitric oxide, and hyperventilation. Anticipated pulmonary hypertension prompts the surgeon to leave a patent foramen ovale so that LV filling and cardiac output is supported even as the transit of pulmonary blood flow is reduced.

Arrhythmia

Heart Block. The surgical repair of DORV requires VSD closure and additionally may require VSD enlargement, and heart block is a risk of any such surgical manipulation of the myocardium in the area of the atrioventricular node and bundle of His. The incidence of postoperative complete heart block (CHB) is more common after the Rastelli procedure than after simpler VSD closures. Postoperative heart block with placement of a permanent pacemaker is an independent risk factor for late mortality.[80]

Transient postoperative CHB is not uncommon, and temporary pacing in the immediate perioperative period allows controlled time to assess recovery. The probability of recovery from transient postoperative heart block plateaus after 10 days, and it is customary to place a permanent pacemaker after 7 to 10 days of unrecovered postoperative CHB.[81] It is concerning that more than one-third of patients with CHB have no onset until after the 30th postoperative day. Also concerning is the evidence that resolved transient postoperative heart block is a risk for late-onset heart block.[82]

Atrial Tachyarrhythmia

Procedures that require muscle resection to enlarge the outflow tract are common among DORV repairs and may incite enhanced automaticity of the His bundle or junctional ectopic tachycardia (JET) in the early postoperative period. JET reduces the atrial contribution to diastolic filling of the ventricle and can have a profound effect on cardiac output, especially in the early postoperative period when diastolic dysfunction demands optimal preloading conditions to support a low cardiac output. The implications of JET include a prolongation of mechanical ventilation time and increased length of stay, but it is not demonstrated to increase mortality.[83] Procedures employing myectomy are more arrhythmogenic than those with myotomy, presumably producing more tissue injury or infiltrative hemorrhage that affects the His bundle.[84] Other factors contributing to postoperative tachyarrhythmia include longer ischemic time, shown to be an independent predictor of JET in a prospective study.[85] Patients on a milrinone infusion may be more predisposed to tachyarrhythmia postoperatively.[86]

Outcomes

Mortality

Overall early mortality for all biventricular DORV repairs is 4% to 8%.[25,27,28,87] Intraventricular baffle repairs with ASO have the highest early mortality, independently of anatomic subtype.[28] Noncommitted VSD is the only anatomic subgroup with higher early and late moratlity.[28,88,89] Fontan outcomes are better than biventricular repairs for patients with complex DORV, with subpulmonary VSD, suggesting the importance of choosing the correct pathway early.[90] A bad biventricular repair may be worse than a good single-ventricle palliation.

Overall survival for complex DORV, including heterotaxy, atrioventricular canal defects, unbalanced ventricles, and total anomalous pulmonary venous return is 84% at 1 year and 81% at 5 years.[90] Atrioventricular valve insufficiency, pulmonary venous obstruction, and neonatal presentation are independent risk factors for mortality in patients with complex DORV with heterotaxy and atrioventricular canal defects.[90]

Late mortality is low for all repair types. Overall reported 10-year and 15-year survival is above 85% for biventricular repairs.[24,25,28,91] Ninety-five percent 15-year survival is reported for the most favorable patients (atrioventricular concordance, subaortic VSD, and no major PA anomalies).[25] Late survival is lower if inclusive of prerepair attrition and complex variants.[24] Restrictive VSD, mitral anomalies, and small left-sided features predict poor outcome.[24,28,91,92] Late age at repair is an independent predictor of late sudden death, presumably because of myocardial damage and hypertrophy incurred by late or palliative strategies.[93]

Reintervention

The overall freedom from reoperation for all DORV repairs is 86.5% at 1 year, 74.1% at 5 years, and 61.4% at 10 years.[28] For patients with atrioventricular concordance, subaortic VSD, and no major PA anomalies, 100% 15-year freedom from reintervention is expected. With subpulmonary VSD, freedom from reintervention is 85%.[25]

Baffle obstruction causing LV outflow obstruction is the commonest cause of reoperation for IVR groups.[28,91] A restrictive VSD and IVR repair are risks for late reoperation.[28] Long or convoluted intraventricular pathways are at highest risk for reobstruction, and freedom from such reoperation is worst for patients with noncommitted VSD, in which the baffle pathway is longest. Aortic valve reoperation and arch reconstruction is a common reintervention in the IVR-ASO group.[28]

Acquired RV outflow tract obstruction is the commonest reason for reintervention in the subpulmonary VSD group in general.[28,94] In long-term follow-up after the REV repair, reoperation is commonly required for RV outflow tract obstruction but not for LV obstruction.[59]

Selected References

A complete list of references is available at ExpertConsult.com.

24. Bradley TJ, Karamlou T, Kulik A, et al. Determinants of repair type, reintervention, and mortality in 393 children with double-outlet right ventricle. *J Thorac Cardiovasc Surg.* 2007;134:967–973.e6.
25. Brown JW, Ruzmetov M, Okada Y, et al. Surgical results in patients with double outlet right ventricle: a 20-year experience. *Ann Thorac Surg.* 2001;72:1630–1635.
28. Villemain O, Belli E, Ladouceur M, et al. Impact of anatomic characteristics and initial biventricular surgical strategy on outcomes in various forms of double-outlet right ventricle. *J Thorac Cardiovasc Surg.* 2016;152:698–706.e3.
42. Walters HL, Mavroudis C, Tchervenkov CI, et al. Congenital Heart Surgery Nomenclature and Database Project: double outlet right ventricle. *Ann Thorac Surg.* 2000;69:S249–S263.
87. Li S, Ma K, Hu S, et al. Surgical outcomes of 380 patients with double outlet right ventricle who underwent biventricular repair. *J Thorac Cardiovasc Surg.* 2014;148:817–824.
90. Takeuchi K, McGowan FX Jr, Bacha EA, et al. Analysis of Surgical Outcome in Complex Double-Outlet Right Ventricle With Heterotaxy Syndrome or Complete Atrioventricular Canal Defect. *Ann Thorac Surg.* 2006;82:146–152.

59

Tetralogy of Fallot With and Without Pulmonary Atresia

STEPHANIE S. HANDLER, MD; SALIL GINDE, MD; CHARLES P. BERGSTROM, MD;
RONALD K. WOODS, MD, PHD

The treatment of tetralogy of Fallot (TOF) exemplifies both the remarkable success and the questions and challenges associated with "successful repair" and long-term survival. Although TOF was once uniformly lethal, current operative mortality is less 2%, and it is estimated that more than 90% of infants with TOF repaired in the current era will survive to the fifth and sixth decades of life.[48] Improvements in perioperative care and longer-term management enabled this success, as well as an appreciation of the fact that the postrepair right ventricle (RV) remains a potential source of morbidity throughout life.

TOF occurs without gender predilection in approximately 0.3 of every 1000 live births and accounts for 3% to 4 % of all infants with congenital heart disease.[6,86,125] The cause of TOF is unknown. Neils Stenson[112] first described this defect nearly 350 years ago (1671); however, it was two decades later (1888) that Etienne-Louis Fallot[33] formalized the defining features of TOF: (1) ventricular septal defect (VSD), (2) RV hypertrophy, (3) overriding aorta, and (4) right ventricular outflow tract obstruction (RVOTO). These features were later termed *tetralogy of Fallot* by Maude Abbott (1924).[1]

Surgical intervention began with the systemic to pulmonary artery shunt (SPAS) by Blalock, Taussig, and Thomas in 1944.[56] Lillehei et al.[74] reported the first repair in 1954. By the early 1980s, surgeons were introducing primary repair in infancy.[a] In the past decade most major centers have converged to a practice of repair in the first 3 to 6 months of life with greatly diminished use of palliative shunting.

Anatomy

The segmental anatomy in patients with TOF is typically normal, with normal abdominal and atrial situs and concordant atrioventricular and ventriculoarterial connections. The right ventricular outflow tract (RVOT), pulmonary valve, and main/branch pulmonary arteries (PAs) constitute the most variable anatomic feature of TOF. Stenosis can occur at one or more levels and can range from mild to complete atresia of the pulmonary valve, dependent on the degree of anterior and cephalad deviation of the infundibular septum.[72,121]

---

[a]References 30, 43, 59, 67, 97, 117, 126.

Tetralogy of Fallot With Pulmonary Stenosis

The more common variety of TOF with pulmonary stenosis (TOF/PS) consists of moderate stenosis of the RVOT, pulmonary valve, and main PA with branch PAs of adequate caliber (Fig. 59.1). The pulmonary valve is bicuspid in approximately 75% of patients, unicuspid in less than 10%, and tricuspid in the remainder.[124] Valve dysplasia occurs in 50% of bicuspid valves. The VSD is characterized by a large, nonrestrictive interventricular communication in the membranous septum created by the anterior and cephalad deviation of the infundibular (conal or outlet) septum relative to the crest of the ventricular septum. Additional muscular VSDs can occur but are infrequent. The malalignment of the infundibular and ventricular septa creates the aortic override, whereby a portion of the aortic valve exists on the right side of the projected septal plane and the aortic valve forms the "roof" of the interventricular communication. The aortic valve and root demonstrate variable degrees of clockwise rotation such that the right coronary sinus is more leftward. A right aortic arch is common (20% to 25%) as are an aberrant subclavian artery (10%) and persistence of a left superior vena cava (SVC) (7% to 10%).[90]

Coronary artery abnormalities include an origin of the left anterior descending coronary artery (LAD) from the proximal right coronary or a duplicated LAD (approximately 5% to 7% cases) with the aberrant or additional vessel crossing the RVOT at variable distances from the pulmonary valve annulus.[28,34] Less common is a single coronary artery from the left sinus giving rise to all major branches with the right coronary artery crossing the RVOT. A patent foramen ovale (PFO) or atrial septal defect is routinely present. Other concomitant anomalies include atrioventricular septal defect[122] (5% of cases) or absent pulmonary valve (approximately 3% of cases).[53]

Tetralogy of Fallot With Pulmonary Atresia

In addition to the usual anatomic features of TOF/PS, TOF with pulmonary atresia (TOF/PA) is defined by atresia of the pulmonary valve with variable hypoplasia of the main PA, ranging from a cord-like structure to a patent vessel (Fig. 59.2). There is a higher likelihood of (1) additional muscular VSDs, (2) right aortic arch (25% to 50%), and (3) aberrant subclavian artery (15% to 20%).[3,46,113] To avoid confusion with nomenclature and the terms

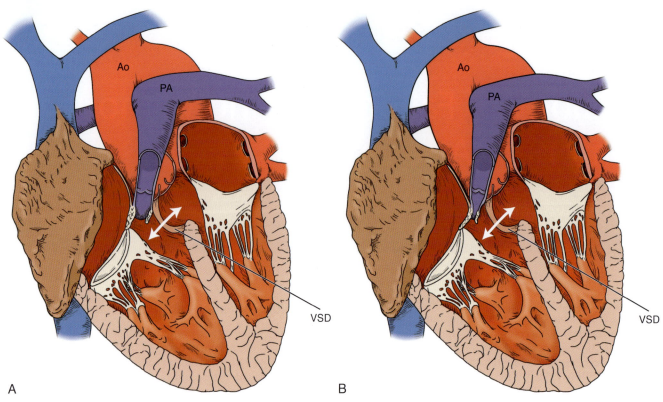

A

B

• **Figure 59.1** Anatomy of tetralogy of Fallot with pulmonary stenosis with unrestrictive perimembranous ventricular septal defect (VSD), aortic override, and right ventricular outflow tract (RVOT) stenosis. (A) More typical anatomy with mild to moderate RVOT obstruction stenosis. (B) More severe RVOT stenosis. *Arrows* indicate direction of shunting across VSD. *Ao,* Aorta; *PA,* pulmonary artery.

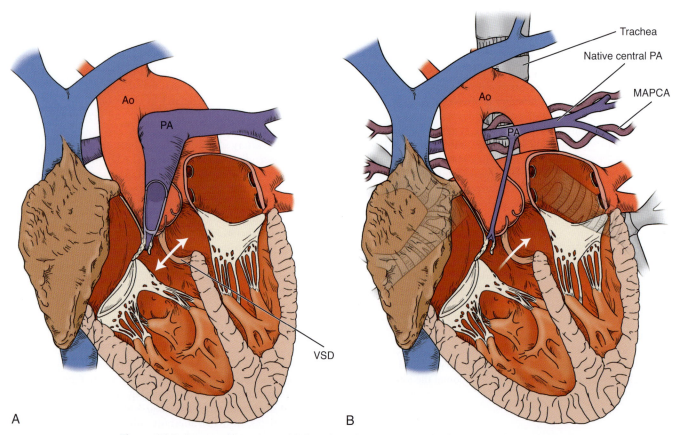

A

B

• **Figure 59.2** Anatomy of tetralogy of Fallot with pulmonary atresia. (A) Confluent central pulmonary arteries (PAs) supplied by patent arterial duct. (B) Small native central PAs and major aortopulmonary collateral arteries (MAPCAs). *Arrows* indicate direction of shunting across VSD. *Ao,* Aorta; *PA,* pulmonary artery; *VSD,* ventricular septal defect.

PA/VSD versus TOF/PA, we use the classification of TOF/PA in reference to all forms of PA/VSD with concordant segmental anatomy in which the RV is developed and the goal is a two-ventricle circulation.[113]

The hallmark and complicating feature of this diagnosis is the variable anatomy of the native central PAs and the presence of major aortopulmonary collateral arteries (MAPCAs) providing variable segmental pulmonary blood flow (see Fig. 59.2).[3,46,99,101,108] In more than half of cases, native central PAs are well developed, supplied by a large ductus arteriosus, and provide flow to all bronchopulmonary segments. However, one-third of patients with TOF/PA do not have a ductus arteriosus.[3] Patients with confluent native PAs may have MAPCAs providing either single or dual supply to respective segments. If central PAs are nonconfluent, MAPCAs will invariably be present, with the number of MAPCAs having an inverse relationship to the distribution of blood flow from the native central PAs.[108] MAPCAs typically arise from the descending thoracic aorta in the region of the left bronchus or carina but can arise from the subclavian arteries, ascending aorta or the aorta below the diaphragm, or even the coronary arteries.

Genetics

Approximately 25% of patients with TOF have chromosomal abnormalities.[6,125] Trisomy 21 and microdeletions of chromosome 22q11.2 constitute the majority, with trisomy 13 and 18 being much less common. Chromosome 22q11.2 microdeletions occur in approximately 20% of patients with TOF/PS and 40% of patients with TOF/PA. DiGeorge syndrome, a result of a more significant deletion, is associated with craniofacial abnormalities, immune deficiencies, hypocalcemia, and neurocognitive delay. Velocardiofacial syndrome is a less extensive deletion without the immune deficiencies or hypocalcemia. Chromosome 22q11 deletions have been reported to be associated with more severe abnormalities of the pulmonary vasculature in TOF/PA, longer duration of intensive care unit (ICU) stay, airway malacia, and an alarmingly high association with long-term neuropsychiatric disorders.[6,23,50,76,84] In TOF/PS there has not been a uniform relationship with mortality.[83,84]

Other associative or causative mutations include those of the jagged 1 gene (Alagille syndrome), NK2 homeobox 5 gene, *GATA4, GATA6,* forkhead box transcription factor 1, nodal, teratocarcinoma-derived growth factor 1, and growth differentiation factor 1.[125] TOF-associated copy number variants have been linked to chromosomes 22q11.2, 3p25.1, 1q21.1, and 7p21.3 and the plexin A2 gene.[109]

Overall, the risk for TOF recurrence in a family is approximately 3%. Screening may include fluorescence in situ hybridization or microarray with more specific or extensive analysis pending preliminary results. Programs with dedicated cardiac geneticists are currently developing testing panels to optimize utility and minimize cost. Results have implications for not only prognosis but also screening related family members.

Physiology

Tetralogy of Fallot With Pulmonary Stenosis

Because the VSD is nonrestrictive, the relative resistances to systemic and pulmonary blood flow dictate the amount and direction of flow across the VSD. With severe RVOTO, flow will be right to left, resulting in cyanosis. With mild RVOTO, flow will be left to right, resulting in pulmonary overcirculation. The more typical situation is somewhere between these two extremes. As the intrinsic pulmonary vascular resistance decreases in the first 1 to 2 weeks of life, and with dynamic narrowing of the RVOT, the physiology may change over time.

Hypercyanotic episodes or "Tet" spells occur because of a marked decrease in the ratio of pulmonary to systemic blood flow (Q_p:Q_s) and concomitant increase in right-to-left shunting across the VSD. Episodes can be provoked by a decrease in systemic vascular resistance or an increase in resistance to pulmonary blood flow. The desaturation and resulting metabolic acidosis can increase the pulmonary vascular resistance, thereby worsening the right-to-left shunting. Thresholds for defining hypercyanosis vary (arterial oxygen saturation [SaO_2] <70% to <80%), and a severe episode can be associated with irritability, hyperpnea, marked cyanosis, pallor, and lethargy or loss of consciousness. Fortunately, the classic Tet spell is uncommon in developed health care settings where patients with severe RVOTO at risk for hypercyanotic episodes undergo surgical correction at a young age.

Tetralogy of Fallot With Pulmonary Atresia

In contrast to TOF/PS, in which a portion of the systemic venous blood passes antegrade through the RV and into the pulmonary bed, in TOF/PA all pulmonary blood flow is from the aorta—either from a patent ductus arteriosus (PDA) supplying central PAs, MAPCAs, or a combination of the two. Systemic venous blood passes through the VSD from the RV to the left ventricle (LV) to mix with pulmonary venous blood before ejection into the aorta. As such, pulmonary arterial and systemic arterial oxygen saturations will be equal. Oxygen saturation levels greater than 85% indicate a Q_p:Q_s of 2:1 or greater, whereas saturations in the 70% range indicate a Q_p:Q_s of 1 or less. As in TOF/PS, patients with TOF/PA may have evidence of inadequate, adequate, or excessive net pulmonary blood flow depending on the size of the PDA and/or size and number of MAPCAs.

In the presence of MAPCAs, systemic oxygen saturations may not reveal the variable local physiology occurring in various bronchopulmonary segments. Certain segments may receive high-flow, high-pressure blood from nonstenotic MAPCAs, whereas other segments may receive substantially lower flow due to various degrees of MAPCA origin stenosis or intrinsic limitations of the native PAs. The net oxygen saturation may be "acceptable," despite the deleterious physiology occurring in local segments.

Diagnosis

Clinical Manifestations

If TOF/PS is left unrepaired, mortality rates for patients with TOF/PS reach 30% by 6 months and 50% by 2 years with fewer than 10% expected to reach age 21 years. The rare adult patient who survives with unrepaired TOF is at high risk for morbidity and mortality due to complications related to severe cyanosis, exercise intolerance, arrhythmias, cerebral abscess, and congestive heart failure due to long-standing RV hypertension.[12] Patients with unrepaired TOF/PA have a worse prognosis, with a mortality rate of 50% by 1 year and 85% by 5 years. Fortunately, it is now rare for children to go unrepaired beyond infancy, and due to advances in fetal echocardiography, a greater percentage of patients with TOF/PS or TOF/PA are diagnosed prenatally.

In patients with TOF/PS and mild RVOTO the presentation is similar to that of a VSD with symptoms dependent on the degree of pulmonary overcirculation. Patients with an intermediate degree of RVOTO may not be symptomatic with a relatively balanced Q_p:Q_s and no significant right-to-left shunting at baseline to cause cyanosis. If RVOTO is more significant, right-to-left shunting across the VSD will result in cyanosis. In the most severe form of RVOTO, antegrade blood flow across the pulmonary valve is not sufficient, and pulmonary blood flow is dependent on a PDA supplying the central PAs.

For TOF/PA most neonates with MAPCAs are asymptomatic, with adequate pulmonary blood flow resulting in acceptable oxygen saturations without congestive heart failure. Over time the MAPCAs tend to develop stenoses, which may limit pulmonary blood flow and result in cyanosis. In addition, if untreated for years, pulmonary vascular disease may develop in segments supplied by unobstructed MAPCAs, leading to a net decrease in pulmonary blood flow. More rarely, MAPCAs result in excessive pulmonary blood flow over the first few weeks of life as the pulmonary vascular resistance drops, resulting in congestive heart failure symptoms of tachypnea and failure to thrive.

Physical Examination

Infants with TOF/PS and TOF/PA are generally full sized and normal in appearance in the absence of an associated genetic anomaly. Growth failure or progressive cyanosis may develop over time if there is congestive heart failure or inadequate pulmonary blood flow. Hypertrophic osteoarthropathy may be present in the unrepaired older child with long-standing cyanosis. Auscultation of the chest typically reveals a harsh systolic ejection murmur along the left upper sternal border, reflecting flow across the stenotic outflow tract. Absence of a systolic ejection murmur should raise suspicion of pulmonary atresia, and the murmur may decrease in intensity or become absent if there is little to no flow across the RVOT (such as during a hypercyanotic spell). The second heart sound is usually single and of normal intensity and may be accompanied by an ejection click. A continuous murmur may be present in TOF/PA over the site of a large MAPCA or PDA, which may increase in intensity as the pulmonary vascular resistance decreases.

Diagnostic Tests

Chest radiographic findings depend on the degree of pulmonary blood flow because pulmonary vascular markings may be decreased, normal, or increased, depending on the degree of RVOTO in TOF/PS and collateral circulation in TOF/PA. The great vessel shadow is diminished in the superior mediastinum because of the diminished caliber of the main PA. The hallmark of TOF is a boot-shaped heart with a prominent upturned cardiac apex related to the RV hypertrophy and concavity in the region of the main PA. The electrocardiogram should reflect the degree of RV hypertrophy and demonstrate right axis deviation, upright and peaked T waves in the right precordial leads, and reversal of the R/S ratio.

Echocardiography is the mainstay of diagnosis for intracardiac anatomy. Improvements in two-dimensional echocardiography and color flow Doppler have significantly reduced the need for cardiac catheterization. The intracardiac anatomy, aortic arch sidedness, presence of a PDA, and coronary anatomy can accurately be determined with echocardiography. The parasternal and subcostal windows best demonstrate the characteristic features of TOF, including anterior, cephalad deviation of the infundibular septum

and the VSD (Fig. 59.3). Interrogation of the blood flow across the RVOT in these views with color and spectral Doppler provides both qualitative and quantitative assessment of the degree of RVOTO. Measurements of the pulmonary valve annulus and main PA help determine the need for patch augmentation of the pulmonary annulus during surgical repair.

For patients with TOF/PA, echocardiography with color flow imaging can be used to demonstrate the lack of continuity between the RV and the main PA. There is an inverse relationship between the size of native branch pulmonary arteries and the presence of MAPCAs, such that MAPCAs are more likely to be present when native branch pulmonary arteries are severely hypoplastic (echocardiographically derived PA diameter z score < −2.5).[75] Branch pulmonary arteries may also be discontinuous with bilateral PDAs supplying the right and left pulmonary arteries.[3] The limitation of echocardiogram in TOF/PA is the inability to accurately delineate all sources of pulmonary blood supply when MAPCAs are present.

Cardiac catheterization and angiography are necessary in the majority of cases of TOF/PA. Angiography provides a thorough anatomic description of the native PAs and MAPCAs and the source of flow to each lung segment (Fig. 59.4). Surgical planning relies upon this information to determine which MAPCAs should be unifocalized to preserve flow to a given segment. Catheterization may not be necessary if there are confluent central PAs supplied by a PDA without MAPCAs seen on ancillary imaging studies.

Angiographic assessment of the central PA size has been used as a predictor for postoperative RV pressures and mortality. The McGoon ratio is the summed diameters of the right and left PA divided by the diameter of the lower thoracic aorta. A McGoon ratio of greater than 1.2 predicts that postoperative RV systolic pressure will be acceptable, and a ratio of less than 0.8 suggests inadequate PA size for complete intracardiac repair.[96] The Nakata index is determined by the summed cross-sectional areas of the right and left PA relative to body surface area, with an index of greater than 150 mm^2/m^2 acceptable for a complete intracardiac repair.[91] However, both the McGoon ratio and Nakata index may not apply to patients with multiple sources of pulmonary blood flow from unrepaired MAPCAs, and their usefulness in infants is unclear.

Computed tomography and magnetic resonance imaging (MRI) are increasingly used to clarify anatomy before surgical repair. These modalities are specifically useful to demonstrate coronary artery anatomy and the three-dimensional relationship of MAPCAs to other structures in the mediastinum. Also, for TOF/PA MRI-determined flows may help determine suitability for VSD closure.[42]

Laboratory analysis of the patient with TOF is similar to that of other patients with congenital heart disease (see Part IV), with particular emphasis on genetic and calcium abnormalities.

Initial Medical Management

Initial medical management of a patient with TOF depends on the severity of the anatomic defects. In patients with TOF/PS and mild to moderate RVOTO with adequate systemic oxygen saturation, no specific medical therapy is necessary. If there is more severe RVOTO, preoperative stabilization and maintenance of adequate pulmonary blood flow may be necessary. Neonates presenting with ductal dependent pulmonary blood flow require prostaglandin infusion (prostaglandin E_1 [PGE_1]) to maintain

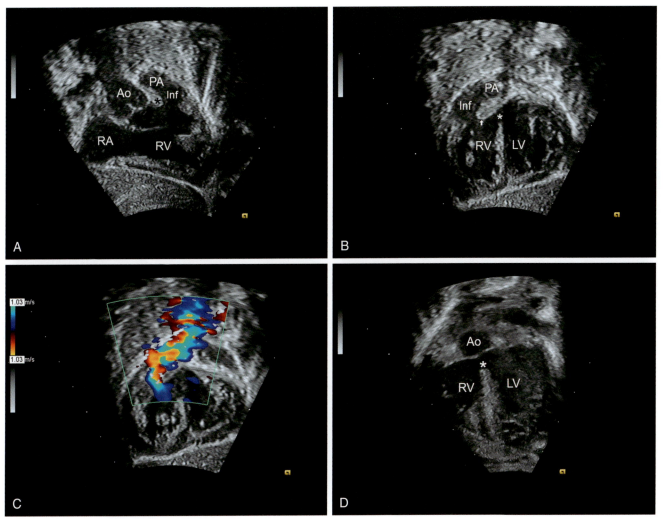

• **Figure 59.3** Echocardiographic images of tetralogy of Fallot. (A) Subcostal coronal view of tetralogy of Fallot showing the anteriorly deviated infundibular septum *(*)*, narrowed subpulmonary infundibulum *(Inf)*, and main pulmonary artery (PA). Subcostal sagittal view without (B) and with (C) color Doppler showing anterior-superior malalignment of the infundibular septum *(arrow)* from the interventricular septum resulting in the ventricular septal defect *(*)* and subpulmonary infundibular stenosis *(Inf)*. (D) Apical view demonstrating the ventricular septal defect *(*)* and the overriding ascending aorta (Ao). *LV,* Left ventricle; *RA,* right atrium; *RV,* right ventricle.

ductal patency. Management of infants with TOF/PA depends on the degree and stability of pulmonary blood flow. Patients without a ductal dependent circulation will likely not require any specific medical intervention before surgical palliation or repair unless there is excessive pulmonary blood flow causing congestive heart failure, in which case management with diuretics as well as provision of adequate calories to maintain somatic growth preoperatively would be appropriate. Patients with ductal dependent circulation would be treated with prostaglandin infusion to maintain ductal patency while awaiting surgical palliation or repair.

Whereas classic palliation of ductal dependent TOF usually includes a surgically placed aortopulmonary shunt (SPAS), palliation of RVOTO with pulmonary valve balloon valvuloplasty or RVOT stent placement in selected cases may relieve significant cyanosis and allow for somatic growth and growth of PAs before definitive surgical correction.[69,110] In addition, coiling of aortopulmonary collaterals providing dual-source pulmonary blood flow may also be performed to promote native PA growth.

Surgical Management

Intraoperative Monitoring

As for most cardiac procedures in the current era, access and monitoring include the following: (1) one to two peripheral intravenous lines, (2) central venous line, (3) arterial line, (4) pulse oximetry, (5) multilead electrocardiogram (ECG) monitoring, (6) Foley catheter, (7) esophageal and rectal or Foley catheter temperature probes, and in many centers (8) two-site near-infrared spectroscopy (NIRS) monitoring—cerebral and flank somatic.[118] Preoperative and postoperative transesophageal echocardiography (TEE) is routinely performed for complete repair but may not be necessary for palliative SPAS.

Tetralogy of Fallot With Pulmonary Stenosis

Eventually, all patients will require surgical intervention. The major issues are (1) the timing of intervention and (2) whether to first

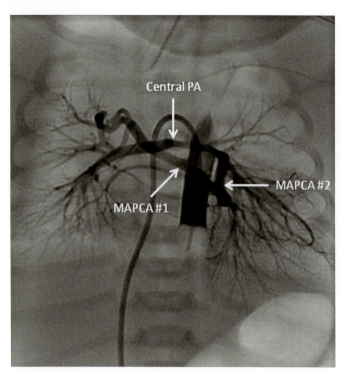

• **Figure 59.4** Angiographic depiction of major aortopulmonary collateral arteries (MAPCAs) and moderate-size native central branch pulmonary arteries (PAs).

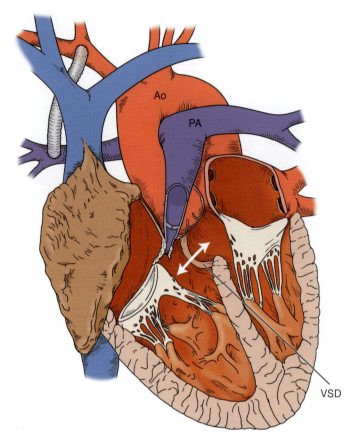

• **Figure 59.5** Modified Blalock-Taussig shunt. *Arrow* indicates direction of shunting across VSD. *Ao,* Aorta; *PA,* pulmonary artery; *VSD,* ventricular septal defect.

palliate or to perform a complete repair. Patient condition determines the timing of intervention. The neonate dependent on PGE$_1$ to maintain adequate oxygen saturations should undergo intervention with either complete repair, SPAS, or stenting of the duct or RVOT. On the other hand, if oxygen saturations off PGE$_1$ are reasonable (>85%), repair may be deferred until the child is approximately 3 to 6 months of age or sooner if progressive cyanosis ensues. Timing of repair for the patient with minimal RVOT or PA stenosis (pink tetralogy) is identical to that for a patient with an unrestrictive VSD, preferably by 6 months of age.

Opinion or preference for initial palliation with SPAS versus complete repair varies among surgeons and institutions.[b] In general, most would currently agree that an older nonneonatal patient who requires intervention should undergo primary repair, rather than palliation, with exception perhaps for unusual circumstances.[36]

Opinion is more variable for the neonatal age group.[36] Proponents of primary repair cite a noninferior operative mortality, avoidance of acute shunt complications, benefits of earlier restoration of normal oxygen saturations, and the need for only one operation. Proponents of initial palliation cite a noninferior overall mortality with two procedures and less morbidity and shorter length of neonatal stay. The belief that a SPAS decreases the use of transannular patching at the time of subsequent complete repair has not been established as fact. Although opinion varies, various patient factors might favor an initial palliative approach—prematurity, low patient weight, an LAD arising from the right coronary artery in a context in which a transannular or ventricular incision is anticipated, and/or significant comorbid medical conditions that would render cardiopulmonary bypass (CPB) excessively high risk.

Based on a large cohort from the Society of Thoracic Surgeons (STS) database spanning the interval of 2002 to 2007, approximately 10% of patients received a shunt—53% of neonates and 15% of patients in the age-group of 30 days to 3 months.[4] By 6 months of age 61% had undergone repair. According to a more recent STS data report, the median age (interquartile range) at repair was 0.4 years (0.3 to 0.6).[115] Although neonatal repair was associated with a somewhat higher discharge mortality compared with SPAS (7.9% versus 6.2%), this multicenter data does not address the overall mortality or morbidity of a particular strategy. Because convincing data and guidelines do not exist, it is reasonable to proceed with either strategy, taking into account the local expertise and infrastructure and what works best for a given care team.[36]

Systemic to Pulmonary Artery Shunt. In contrast to historical management, currently patients undergo a SPAS with the intent of complete repair within the next 4 to 8 months. Types of SPAS include a modified Blalock-Taussig shunt (MBTS), which connects the subclavian artery to the ipsilateral branch PA, and a central shunt, which connects the ascending aorta with the main PA (Fig. 59.5).[129] (For TOF/PS the latter would typically be a Gore-Tex shunt.) In the more recent era there is trend to do the SPAS procedure through a median sternotomy (required for central shunt) because it does not require partial or complete lung collapse, CPB can easily be implemented if required, and it leaves the child ultimately with one chest incision. Opinion on optimal shunt size varies, but in general for a 3.5-kg baby most would place either a 3.5- or 4-mm MBTS or a 3-mm central shunt. A heparin bolus is given before creating the shunt—dosing varies from 50 U/kg

[b]References 4, 7, 8, 10, 30, 43, 57, 67, 82, 97, 111, 117.

to in excess of 100 U/kg. Anticoagulation and antiplatelet management after surgery vary considerably among institutions. It is our bias to start a heparin drip in the operating room, if feasible, at approximately 20 U/kg/h. We also prefer to initiate aspirin in the first 12 hours after admission to the ICU and adjust dosing based on objective measures of platelet inhibition.

Management options for the PDA include ligation after completing the shunt or no ligation and simply discontinuing the PGE₁. There are no data proving superiority of a particular approach. Ligation eliminates competitive flow, which may enhance flow through the shunt and reduce the risk of thrombosis, whereas spontaneous closure preserves the option of restarting PGE₁ to reopen the duct if there is concern for shunt thrombosis later in the ICU.

Repair. The goals of repair are to (1) close all septal defects, (2) provide a durable and reasonably patent and competent outflow tract, (3) avoid or correct branch PA stenosis, and (4) result in normal sinus rhythm with good ventricular function, cardiac output, and oxygen delivery. We would consider leaving a small (2 mm) PFO only in a higher-risk neonate. Repair is done using bicaval venous drainage for CPB at temperatures ranging from 28°C to 34°C. Cardioplegic arrest is used for the intracardiac portion of the repair. Surgical options include (1) transatrial and trans-PA repair with the combined exposure allowing resection of RVOT muscle, VSD closure, pulmonary valvotomy, if needed, and patch enlargement of the main PA; (2) in addition to a pulmonary arteriotomy, use of a ventriculotomy for both exposure and patch closure of the VSD and to relieve RVOTO; and (3) transannular patching in which the incision on the main PA is extended across the annulus onto the RV for a variable distance (Fig. 59.6). Limited transannular incision (<5 to 10 mm of ventricular incision) has been advocated to reduce the potential long-term negative impact on RV function; however, longer-term data supporting this approach are not yet available.[71] In the context of a transannular patch, creation of a monocusp valve may improve early hemodynamics; however, this speculation and the long-term competence of the valve have not been confirmed. Branch PA stenosis may be addressed either by a separate patch or extension of the patch on the main PA. In general, small branch PA expand adequately after repair and do not require patch reconstruction. Postoperative TEE is used routinely in the operating room to evaluate ventricular systolic function and assess for residual intracardiac defects.

There are no data demonstrating clear superiority of a particular inotrope strategy in the operating room. We typically wean from CPB using epinephrine (dose range 0.02 to 0.1 mcg/kg/min) and consider a low-dose milrinone infusion without a loading dose if blood pressure is generous. For the sake of this discussion we presume the TEE demonstrates no residual VSD and at most mild tricuspid regurgitation. Although the TEE provides important information about the RVOT and pulmonary valve, in the absence of clearly unacceptable findings, we would obtain direct pressure measurements in the RV and PA before making a decision to return to CPB for further relief of RVOTO. In general we would accept a gradient of 25 to 30 mm Hg with an RV to systemic systolic pressure ratio of up to 0.6:1, acknowledging the variation in thresholds that may be suitable for a particular patient and circumstance.

A residual VSD further complicates decision making and should be avoided using vigilance at the time of repair. The interplay between a VSD and residual RVOTO may mask the significance of the VSD and/or imply a worse degree of RVOT stenosis. Although a high shunt fraction (calculated from blood samples

from the SVC and PA) is informative, a low shunt fraction is not necessarily reassuring. Unless the residual VSD is very small (estimated by TEE at approximately 1 mm) and the RVOT gradient low, our bias is to attempt to close the defect.

The debated issue with repair is the significance of a transannular or ventricular incision.[36] First, a transannular patch ultimately will leave the child with pulmonary insufficiency. Second, an incision on the RV may impair function, and the resultant scar may be a source for future dysrhythmia. These concerns are played against (1) a desire to provide adequate relief of RVOTO; (2) in some circumstances, perhaps better exposure to the cephalad aspect of the VSD afforded by a ventriculotomy and no need to manipulate the tricuspid valve (in our opinion, transatrial neonatal VSD repair can be a very challenging procedure, due solely to the meticulous care of the tricuspid valve required for a perfectly competent postrepair valve); and (3) need for less muscle resection afforded by a ventriculotomy and/or a transannular patch. Moreover, the threshold for defining adequate relief of RVOTO varies. Most would agree that an RV to systemic systolic pressure ratio of 0.7 with a gradient across the RVOT by direct intraoperative measurement of 45 is unacceptable. However, it is less clear what to do with a pressure ratio of 0.6 or 0.7 and a gradient of 35 mm Hg, particularly if the valve is perfectly competent and expected to remain so. The risks of progressive RVOTO and need for reoperation are weighed against the potential longer-term risk of pulmonary insufficiency and RV dysfunction. Most would agree, however, that the younger patient, particularly the neonate, may not tolerate residual RVOT stenosis, VSD, or tricuspid insufficiency. The main point is that the surgical decision should be individualized and take into account the overall condition of the heart and the patient. There is no single correct RVOT gradient threshold or RV to systemic pressure ratio. The driving principle is achieving a good repair, not avoiding a ventricular or transannular incision.

According to recent multicenter data from the United States only one in five patients were repaired without a ventriculotomy or a transannular patch (46% were repaired with a transannular patch).[115] In contrast to programs in the United States, there may be greater willingness to tolerate residual outflow tract gradients in other parts of the world, with the belief that a certain threshold of residual gradient is well tolerated and may reduce the long-term consequences of pulmonary insufficiency and the need for pulmonary valve replacement (PVR).[131] However, it is also possible that patient characteristics and age at presentation are relevant factors. In the United States, for example, the percentage of patients undergoing transannular patching ranges from approximately 80% in neonates to 50% in the 3- to 6-month age-group.[4,115] Very few surgeons desire to make an incision in the RV of a neonate unless absolutely necessary. Therefore, if done in 80% of patients, it more realistically reflects the fact that a neonate requiring surgery likely has a degree of RVOTO that requires transannular patching to achieve an adequate repair.

Tetralogy of Fallot With Pulmonary Atresia

Practical constraints preclude a full description of the rationale and technical considerations for the various approaches to surgical management of patients with TOF/PA. Therefore we will describe the primary concerns and decision making and refer the reader to several references for additional detail.[c] Management of a baby

[c]References 11, 17-19, 26, 29, 32, 55, 66, 73, 81, 96, 98, 101, 104, 114.

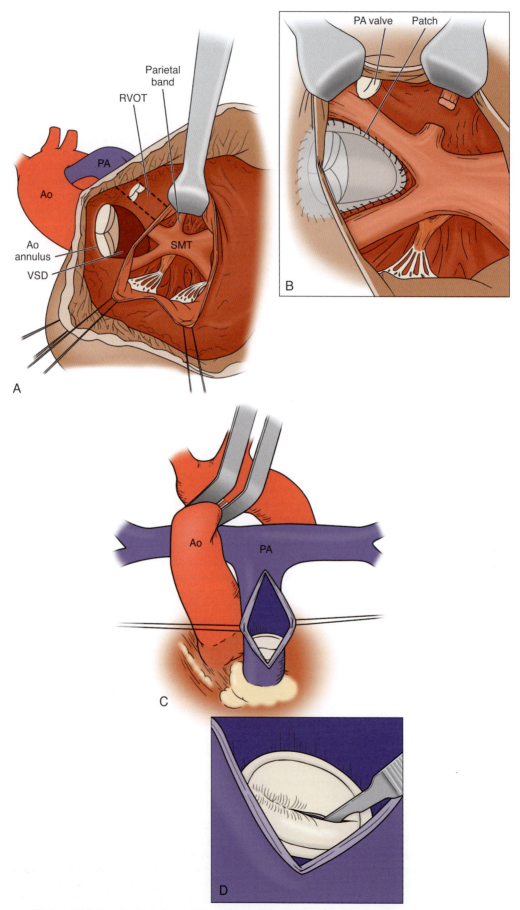

• **Figure 59.6** Repair of tetralogy of Fallot with pulmonary stenosis. (A) Transatrial view of ventricular septal defect (VSD) and right ventricular outflow tract (RVOT). (B) Patch closure of VSD and view of RVOT and pulmonary valve after division of parietal band and resection of RVOT muscle. Incision of main pulmonary artery (PA) (C) for commissurotomy of bicuspid valve (D).

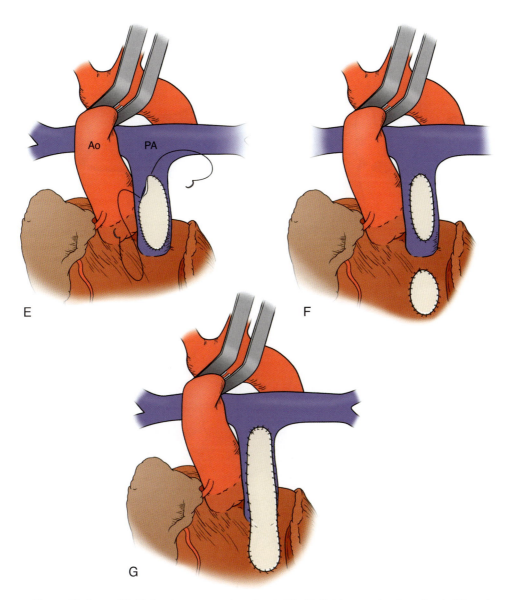

• **Figure 59.6, cont'd** (E) Patch reconstruction of main PA. (F) Patch reconstruction of main PA and infundibulum after limited ventriculotomy to better enlarge RVOT. (G) A transannular patch. *Ao,* Aorta; *SMT,* septomarginalis trabeculation.

with confluent, good-size or mildly hypoplastic central PAs is identical to that of the TOF/PS patient, with the added step of establishing continuity between the RV and PAs, either with patch augmentation of the native RVOT if feasible or more often with placement of an RV to PA valved conduit. The one exception may be the need to eliminate the infrequent MAPCA to normalize the volume load on the heart.

For the patient with MAPCAs and either severely hypoplastic or nonconfluent central PAs, the strategy is to develop a suitable pulmonary vascular bed leading ultimately to an arrangement with VSD closure and an RV to PA conduit. The specific strategy for developing the pulmonary vasculature depends on what view one takes of the embryologic origin of MAPCAs and their suitability as long-term sources of pulmonary blood flow. One view is that MAPCAs are not suitable or effective in the long term, and surgical strategy should focus on the native PAs.[26,73] In contrast, another view is that MAPCAs are very suitable, in many cases essential to

establishment of an adequate pulmonary vascular bed, and should be unifocalized early in the first few months of life for their benefit to be fully realized.[18,29,32,81] Unifocalization refers to a surgical procedure that reduces multiple origins of pulmonary blood flow to ultimately one origin—the RV (Fig. 59.7). Regardless of the viewpoint, it is paramount to define the native PA and MAPCA anatomy early in life, the number of segments supplied solely by native PAs, the number supplied solely by MAPCAs, and those with dual supply. The ultimate goal is to establish a pulmonary vascular bed with sufficient surface area to permit VSD closure with an acceptably low RV pressure and good gas exchange.

In the anti-MAPCA view the only option is to do various forms of SPAS or an RV to PA conduit to develop the native PAs—the latter may afford better access for interval catheter-based rehabilitation of the PAs, if needed, with replacement and upsizing of the conduit at the time of VSD closure. With the pro-MAPCA view, unifocalization is done to incorporate the MAPCAs into the

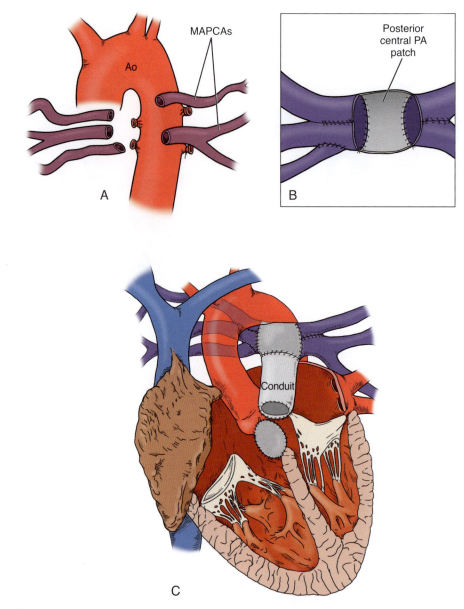

• **Figure 59.7** Repair of tetralogy of Fallot with pulmonary atresia. (A) Major aortopulmonary collateral arteries (MAPCAs). (B) Unifocalization using patch material to reconstruct central pulmonary artery (PA) confluence. (C) Completed repair with ventricular septal defect patch and right ventricle to PA valved conduit. *Ao,* Aorta.

pulmonary circulation. This is done by anastomosing MAPCAs to the native PAs either centrally, at the hilum, or more distally as needed. For absent central PAs, patch material may be needed to reconstruct the central PA (see Fig. 59.7). Depending on circumstances and institutional preference, this may be done in a single stage, typically via a median sternotomy (CPB as needed for the unifocalization), or in two stages via sequential thoracotomies. With the latter approach the two procedures can be separated by a few days during the same hospital admission or the child discharged and readmitted a few weeks later for the second procedure. For either approach, once the PAs are unifocalized, the source of pulmonary blood flow can be a SPAS or an RV to PA conduit. The latter may provide greater ease of access for catheter-based intervention for stenosis and rehabilitation of the vascular bed. For the sequential approach, SPASs (one for each side) are placed, with the bilateral circulations unifocalized centrally during a later procedure, typically requiring patch material to complete the unifocalization. If not placed at this time, an RV to PA conduit would be placed at the time of VSD closure and the SPASs taken down.

In general, patient condition drives timing of the first intervention. If there is profound cyanosis, ductal dependent central or branch PA blood flow, or dual-supply central PA/MAPCA flow amenable to shunt for growth of the central PAs, neonatal intervention may be required. Otherwise, the goal is to perform unifocalization in the first 3 to 6 months of life to preserve blood flow to all lung segments and prevent the development of pulmonary vascular disease from unrestrictive pulmonary blood flow.

Timing of VSD closure is variable—it may be possible at the initial single-stage unifocalization or may require weeks to months of PA growth and rehabilitation. Criteria to determine suitability have been described and continue to be used but remain imperfect.[42,133] In several series, septation has been achieved in 60% to 80% of patients; however, reports of 15- to 30-year follow-up are lacking. If septation results in an RV to systemic pressure ratio of greater than 0.5, options are VSD patch takedown or fenestration. Unless the PA bed is further improved, this leads to the difficult circumstance of a cycle of repeated upsizing of SPAS or conduit replacements and the chronic effects of cyanosis, potentially ultimately palliated only with heart-lung transplantation.

This condition highlights the relevance of skilled, multidisciplinary teams with good judgment based on the primary principle of achieving a good pulmonary vascular bed. There is no need to rush to VSD closure in the context of a borderline vascular bed. Even with a seemingly good single-stage repair early in life, patients remain at risk for requiring further surgical or catheter-based interventions.

Postoperative Care

We will limit our focus to postoperative care after complete repair of TOF/PS and assume that an excellent repair has been done—acceptably low RV pressure and outflow gradient, no or trivial tricuspid regurgitation, sinus rhythm, and no residual VSD or PFO. In TOF, closure of the VSD volume loads the RV. Also, the RV is intrinsically less compliant than it is with many other diagnoses, and coronary flow may be more dependent on systolic pressure. These factors underlie many of the challenges that may be encountered in postoperative management.

Monitoring established in the operating room is continued in the cardiac ICU. There is a growing trend to use cerebral and somatic NIRS on all ICU patients.[118] We strongly endorse this approach. It provides a noninvasive measure of regional balance of oxygen delivery and consumption and allows early detection of impaired oxygen delivery. It is an important basis of goal-directed therapy that has been shown to improve survival in pediatric heart patients. Central venous pressure (CVP) monitoring with at least a right atrial line or central venous line is mandatory. Many centers also place a left atrial line to assist in fluid management because the restrictive right heart may limit the ability to use CVP for that purpose.

Management is based on principles applicable to any postoperative cardiac patient—adequate oxygen delivery based on good cardiac output and oxygenation, adequate perfusion pressure, appropriate pain management, and provision of appropriate energy substrate. One feature somewhat specific to the TOF patient is a focus on optimizing right heart function due to the factors listed earlier. This includes early extubation, consideration of pharmacologic heart rate control, provision of adequate intravascular volume, and judicious use of inotropes.

Despite extensive evidence that extubation improves cardiac output,[14,15,60,105,106] institutional rates for early extubation are variable but low. A recent Pediatric Heart Network study demonstrated efficacy in promoting early extubation using a collaborative learning model.[77] Airway pressure release ventilation and negative pressure ventilation have been successfully used with noted augmentation in cardiac output.[106,107,127] In the presence of bleeding, hemodynamic instability, or junctional ectopic tachycardia (JET), extubation may need to be delayed.

Biventricular systolic function is usually preserved. Right heart diastolic dysfunction is present in varying degrees, with more severe dysfunction being associated with longer ICU stay.[21,25,102] Although inodilator (milrinone) therapy is a mainstay in the cardiac ICU, it is our opinion that it should be used less aggressively in TOF patients. The original trial of this drug was not designed to evaluate efficacy in TOF (approximately 25% of study cohort), which was the only diagnostic group with a propensity for postoperative RV diastolic dysfunction. Our bias is based on the potentially uniquely harmful effects of hypotension on coronary perfusion in patients with TOF and the longer half-life of the drug. Our typical regimen includes epinephrine (0.02 to 0.08 mcg/kg/min) and if blood pressure is appropriate, a low-dose infusion of milrinone (0.25 mcg/kg/min). We will further increase epinephrine as needed but have a low threshold for adding vasopressin (0.2 to 0.8 mU/kg/min) as needed to maintain appropriate blood pressure. Some centers avoid beta agonists and even titrate beta-adrenergic antagonist therapy (beta-blockers) to achieve a lower heart rate and improve preload. In contrast, others view the sinus tachycardia typical of TOF patients as compensatory to maintain cardiac output in the context of reduced RV stroke volume and rely on improvement in tachycardia as an indicator of improved RV compliance and readiness to progress with weaning of various support measures. As with any postoperative cardiac patient, the TOF patient may experience a period of lower cardiac output beginning in the first 12 to 18 hours. However, for the majority of patients, the decline in cardiac output is mild and resolves within 12 hours.

There are a variety of pain management regimens that may be used. Our typical regimen is a balance of dexmedetomidine and fentanyl infusions while the patient is intubated, transitioning to lower-dose infusion or fentanyl as needed once extubated. Scheduled dosing of acetaminophen and/or ketorolac may limit the opiate requirement. Enteral feeding with a bowel regimen is begun once vasoactive medications have been weaned to low doses. Transthoracic lines are typically removed by the first or second postoperative day, before removal of chest drains. Pacing wires may also be removed at this time if rhythm has been normal; however, we often conservatively maintain pacing wires for an additional day or two given the potential for late-onset JET. Removal of the arterial line occurs once the patient is extubated and inotropes are no longer needed—typically by postoperative day 2 or 3. The central venous line may be removed 12 to 24 hours after cessation of inotropes. Discharge from the ICU typically occurs on postoperative day 3 to 5. Before the patient is discharged from the hospital, a transthoracic echocardiogram is done. It is recognized that timing for these various events varies across institutions.

When it comes to various details of postoperative management, there is not a single correct approach. However, two practices are important for all teams to follow. The first is the team handoff. Congenital heart care is inherently complex. Seamless continuation of care in the ICU requires knowledge of the operative course and an updated assessment of the patient. It is imperative that the surgical team and critical care team engage in a systematic, checklist style of communication to ensure transfer of all relevant information. However, this process should not supersede a focus on the patient. Both teams should work together to transfer monitoring and establish an acceptably stable condition of the patient before engaging in the formal handoff. Second, programs should practice routine quality assessment and modify management as indicated and likewise share knowledge and learning with other programs.

A subset of patients will demonstrate more challenging postoperative courses. We will address only the more significant or common issues in the following subsections.

Arrhythmias and Low Cardiac Output

JET may occur in 5% to 14.6% of neonates and infants after repair of TOF.[31,52,85,132] It occurs more frequently in younger patients, typically in the first 24 hours but as late as 72 hours after surgery. Because JET rarely occurs before repair, it is thought to be related to a surgical action (e.g., retraction, direct injury) and/or medication initiated in the operating room or ICU. One definition of JET is a narrow QRS complex, nodal or infranodal tachycardia with atrioventricular dissociation and a ventricular rate greater than the atrial rate, typically greater than 170 to 180 beats/min, and associated with hemodynamic compromise. As with all automatic rhythms, it does not initiate or terminate abruptly but rather has a progressive warm-up phase. Diagnosis is suspected with absent or retrograde P waves along with obvious cannon A waves and/or continuous variability in the CVP tracing and is easily confirmed with a bipolar ECG using the temporary epicardial atrial leads.

Because the cause is not known, effective prevention remains elusive. Options include minimizing intraoperative tissue tension/trauma, avoiding high doses of inotropes, and avoiding hyperthermia. Some have shown effective prevention using magnesium, amiodarone,[5,54] or dexmedetomidine.[58] Liberal sedation, mild hypothermia (35.5°C to 36°C), and lowering inotropic dosage are first-line treatments to slow the rate. The primary goal is to slow the rate sufficiently to permit either atrial pacing or dual-chamber pacing and atrioventricular synchrony, which is important to maximize filling of the restrictive RV. Although other agents may be used, amiodarone is typically the antiarrhythmic agent of choice to provide more aggressive rate reduction. For a 3-month-old a reasonable goal would be a JET rate sufficiently low to permit sequential pacing at a rate of approximately 140 to 150 beats/min. Typically, normal sinus rhythm ensues after 1 to 5 days of treatment. Opinion on duration of antiarrhythmic medication varies. We typically continue it for a few days after rhythm control is achieved.

A subset of these patients can become very sick—hypotension, oliguria, capillary leak, and need for additional intravenous fluid to maintain filling of a progressively stiffer RV. Even with rhythm control, it may take several additional days for renal recovery and elimination of body water sufficient to permit improvement of chest wall and pulmonary compliance appropriate for extubation. Although low cardiac output syndrome can occur in any patient, in our experience severe declines in output in the TOF patient are uncommon in the absence of JET.

Hypoxia

The systemic blood should be fully saturated after repair. Desaturation therefore requires prompt attention. Although it may be due to ventilation/perfusion (mismatch from atelectasis or edema, a residual atrial-level shunt should be ruled out with echocardiography. A very small residual atrial-level shunt can lead to a surprising degree of hypoxia in a TOF patient, depending on the degree of RV diastolic dysfunction. Regardless of whether the surgeon intentionally left a small atrial-level shunt, it is important to evaluate the overall impact on oxygen delivery. Although a PFO may help preserve cardiac output in the context of a noncompliant RV, excessive desaturation may impair overall oxygen delivery. If measures of oxygen delivery and the overall condition of the patient are adequate, expectant management is appropriate. As the RV compliance improves, the right-to-left shunt decreases or reverses, and saturations return to normal. If oxygen delivery is inadequate with no other explanation, the shunt should be reduced or eliminated.

Another source of hypoxia in the repaired TOF/PA patient is reperfusion injury. Reperfusion injury is defined as local pulmonary edema seen by chest radiograph resulting from increased perfusion after relief of obstructed pulmonary blood flow, particularly in patients with MAPCAs who undergo PA rehabilitation. This injury may occur in 50% or more of patients undergoing unifocalization and is associated with bilateral unifocalization and relief of more severe MAPCA origin stenoses.[80] However, it seems to be self-limited and has not been associated with increased morbidity or long-term vascular changes.[9]

Residual Defects and Tamponade

Although uncommon, residual lesions can be missed on the postrepair TEE, or a residual VSD can occur after the TEE secondary to patch dehiscence. Therefore if low cardiac output persists beyond the usual period a residual VSD should be ruled out. Patients typically do not tolerate residual VSDs and unless diminutive (less than 2 mm) and asymptomatic, consideration should be given for surgical closure. Moderate or worse tricuspid regurgitation is uncommon following repair but can be another source of poor hemodynamics. Neonates in particular do not tolerate this well. Because reoperation on an unstable neonate to repair a delicate valve can be challenging, it is best avoided with meticulous attention to detail at the time of repair.

Global cardiac tamponade typically occurs early in the context of a patient known to be bleeding, and presentation may be insidious, marked by rising atrial pressures, increasing fluid requirement, hypotension, and/or a sudden decrease in chest drainage. In this clinical setting there should be a low threshold for echocardiographic assessment to rule out tamponade because progressive RV diastolic dysfunction may have similar clinical features. Focal tamponade can have equally significant impact on output and be more difficult to diagnose with transthoracic echocardiography. Consideration may be given to TEE or chest computed tomography with contrast. As with global tamponade, surgical drainage is indicated for focal tamponade causing low cardiac output.

Considerations for the Challenging Neonate

Because there is no uniformly accepted definition of "complex," we will consider a specific clinical scenario that exemplifies factors that may challenge decision making and management. Consider the following patient: ductal dependent TOF/PS, 5 days old born prematurely at 28 weeks' gestation, intrauterine growth restriction with a weight of 1.1 kg, 22q11.2 deletion, and a lower genitourinary anomaly—all negative prognostic factors. The parents are capable, fully informed, engaged in care, and desire maximal therapy. Complete repair is a valid option as are various palliative approaches, including RVOT patch enlargement with VSD left open, systemic to PA shunt, ductal stent, RVOT stent, or prolonged prostaglandin infusion followed either by repair or one of the listed palliative procedures. Complete repair done correctly, although associated with higher upfront risk, has the advantage of restoring normal circulation and oxygenation and removing the cardiac aspect of subsequent decision making.[100] Although some form of palliative procedure may seem more appealing or safe, none are without risks and limitations. For example, in our experience the risk of an acute SPAS complication is approximately 17% in patients under 3 kg and 37% if these patients receive a 3-mm shunt.[89] Various stenting procedures may be considered, though patient size may require direct surgical cardiac access.[24,68,70] Our experience with RVOT stenting has been mixed, with variable durability, and in one case, challenging stent removal at the time of repair. At present we would be slightly more inclined to proceed with an outflow tract/PA patch but recognize that stenting, chronic prostaglandin infusion, and even repair are reasonable options. We acknowledge there is no single correct approach, and we continue to manage these patients in a very individualized manner.

Outcome

Tetralogy of Fallot With Pulmonary Stenosis

According to a formal analysis of STS multi-institutional data (2010), discharge mortality for infant primary repair of TOF/PS was 1.3% and for neonatal repair was 7.8%.[4] For neonatal palliation with SPAS, discharge mortality was 6.2%. For patients with prior palliation, mortality with repair was 0.9%. In a second report of multi-institutional data from the Pediatric Health Information System, Steiner et al.[111] reported both mortality and various measures of morbidity versus age at repair. Discharge mortality was 6.4% for neonatal repair, 1.9% for repair at age 30 to 90 days, and 0.7% for repair at age 90 to 180 days; hospital length of stay was 18, 8, and 7 days; duration of mechanical ventilation was 3, 1, and 0 days; duration of inotropes/pressors was 4, 3, and 2 days; need for extracorporeal membrane oxygenation was 4%, 1%, and 1%; and total charges were approximately $240,000, $140,000, and $112,000, respectively. Single centers with mature infrastructure and high-performing teams have reported series with very low to zero mortality, even with neonatal repair. In the current era, mortality would be considered very rare except in circumstances with significant comorbidity and/or an extracardiac malformation. Freedom from reintervention at 5 years varies depending on age at repair, ranging from as high as 95% for infant repair to as low as 35% to 50% for neonatal repair.[d]

There has been growing concern about the long-term impact of pulmonary insufficiency and/or a ventricular incision. This in turn led to a focus on various valve-sparing approaches and ventricular incision–sparing approaches.[36,71,123,124] Various authors have reported excellent early results, and it remains possible that these approaches will improve the long-term outcome; however, convincing data are not yet available. Longer-term data were provided by Hickey et al.[48] in a very interesting follow-up of a cohort of 1181 patients, evaluating major outcomes versus type of initial repair—no ventricular patch, ventricular patch, transannular patch, and conduit. Twenty- and 30-year survival and freedom from reintervention were not related to type of initial repair. Eighty-five percent of patients were alive at 18 years and 80% alive at 30 years, with half of surviving patients having undergone reintervention (predominantly pulmonary valve or conduit surgery). Not surprisingly, pulmonary atresia was predictive of worse outcomes. Another 10- to 15-year study of a cohort of patients 2 to 3 years of age compared a standard transannular patch approach with one using a more limited (<1 cm) ventricular incision. Although 10 years may not be sufficient follow-up, there was no difference in various measures of RV size or performance.[71]

It is perhaps not surprising that the pulmonary valve annulus diameter (z score) is an important predictor of need for reintervention, typically a z score of less than −2 being the transition point.

In an analysis of technical performance score (TPS), Nathan et al.[92] demonstrated a strong relationship between a class III (worst score) TPS and need for reintervention, with preoperative pulmonary annulus z score of less than −2 being a strong correlate with poor TPS score. Hoashi et al.[49] reported 20-year follow-up of a cohort of 222 patients with a valve- and annulus-preserving approach and no ventricular incision. Freedom from moderate or greater pulmonary regurgitation was 36%, with a bicuspid valve and annulus z score of less than −2 being most predictive of developing regurgitation.

Although a specific z score transition might be related to the use of transannular patching, it could potentially be an inherent characteristic of smaller pulmonary valves, for two reasons. First, the valve could be such that any procedure to achieve a valve opening equal to that of the annulus results (eventually) in insufficiency. Second, depending on the actual diameters under consideration, residual stenosis would result even with a perfect pulmonary valve repair based on consideration of cross-sectional area alone (e.g., typically more than a 50% reduction in cross-sectional area can lead to important stenosis). Consider this in practical terms. For a 4.5-kg infant with a pulmonary valve annulus of 5 mm, normal would be approximately 9 mm; typical standard deviation is approximately 1.5 mm. In this case the lower cutoff would be approximately 6 mm, which is close to the value of 5 mm. Yet a perfect valve procedure (aperture of 5 mm) yields a cross-sectional area of 19.6 mm^2 versus 63.6 mm^2 for the normal value.

To summarize the results:

1. It is important to keep in mind there is inherent selection bias in all retrospective studies. Higher-grade RVOT or pulmonary valve stenosis will necessitate more aggressive surgical techniques. It would be inappropriate to draw firm conclusions based on a comparison of patients who remain asymptomatic out to 3 to 6 months of age with those requiring surgery in the first week of life.

2. Data suggest that valve-sparing approaches are appropriate for patients with pulmonary annulus diameter z scores above −2. This does not ensure long-term pulmonary competence because most valves require some degree of surgical manipulation, which can impair long-term function. Moreover, a majority of patients have bicuspid valves, and half of these are thickened and dysplastic to varying degrees. It would be optimistic to expect these valves to function well for 30 to 50 years. However, if an adequate diameter annulus and valve aperture can be achieved, there appears to be little downside to this approach because the chronic impact on the RV would be expected to be similar or better compared with a transannular approach.

3. There are clearly perceived pros and cons of a ventricular incision. At one end of the spectrum the view is that any ventricular incision should be avoided, yet it is acceptable to do an aggressive transatrial intracardiac resection of RVOT muscle. At the other extreme is the view that a ventricular incision affords complete relief of RVOT stenosis and lessens the long-term stimulus for fibrosis as well as the incidence of tricuspid valve dysfunction and early to intermediate need for RVOT reintervention. It is unlikely this variability in viewpoint will be resolved in the near future. However, an adequate valve-sparing approach at the level of the annulus does not guarantee that the subvalve RVOT will be adequate after muscle resection. In other words,

---

[d]References 2, 7, 30, 36, 57, 59, 67, 82, 88, 93, 117, 119.

a limited ventricular incision may still be needed despite a valve-sparing procedure.

4. Outcomes have improved dramatically over the past decades. Focus has now shifted to improving both long-term results and quality of life of the patients.

5. Regardless of initial method of repair, patients remain at risk long term for both mortality and need for reintervention. Guidelines on when to intervene and the type of intervention exist and continue to be refined. Patients merit regular interval evaluation throughout their lives.

Tetralogy of Fallot With Pulmonary Atresia

For TOF/PA, short to intermediate term outcomes are more variable and inferior to those of standard TOF/PS. Overall, complete repair with VSD closure has been attained in 60% to 80% of patients. Most studies report early survivals of 80% to 90%.[e] Using a standardized approach to early single-stage repair, the group at Stanford reported complete unifocalization and intracardiac repair in 88% of 458 patients and a survival of 88%.[11] An RV to systemic pressure ratio of more than 0.35, initial surgery type (palliation or revision worse than complete repair), and chromosomal abnormalities (most commonly 22q11 deletion or Alagille syndrome) were associated with worse survival over time. In the report by Zhu et al,[133] the intraoperative flow study was highly predictive of 5-year survival. There were no cardiac-related deaths in patients with mean pulmonary artery pressure (PAP) of less than 25 mm Hg and flow at 3 L/min/m^2, whereas 5-year survival was as low as 60% in patients with higher mean PAP. Many of these deaths were attributed to RV dysfunction as a result of VSD closure. Although VSD closure has been labeled a favorable prognostic factor,[29] this more likely reflects the importance of the adequacy of the pulmonary vascular bed for long-term survival.

There is nontrivial attrition over longer-term follow-up. Zhu et al.[133] reported a 5-year survival of 78%. Carotti et al.[19] reported a 14-year survival of 75%, and d'Udekem et al.[27] reported survival of 58% at 30 years of age. There is debate about the longer-term fate of unifocalized MAPCAs. D'Udekem et al.[26] evaluated 60 MAPCAs and noted thrombosis of 26 vessels and greater than 50% stenosis in 12. However, the mean age of patients in this series at the time of initial surgery was 1.4 years. In contrast, Mainwaring et al.[78,79] reported durable function of MAPCAs and stable hemodynamics in a cohort of 80 patients who achieved low PA pressures with initial repair. Multiple interventions are the norm for these patients, either in staging to complete repair or maintaining the pulmonary vasculature after repair, primarily with balloon angioplasty to relieve peripheral stenoses. Davies et al.[29] reported a reintervention rate of approximately 40% at 5 years after repair. Duncan et al.[32] reported a 50% reintervention rate, again primarily to either maintain or further rehabilitate the pulmonary vascular bed.

Longer-term data are lacking for the subset of patients who after exhaustive efforts fail to achieve an acceptable vascular bed. Patients may do reasonably well with pulmonary flow driven by systemic pressures via the VSD or alternatively with an appropriately sized shunt. However, it is reasonable to expect long-term prognosis to be poor. Repeated shunt upsizing, frequent catheter interventions, and/or RV failure will leave heart-lung transplantation as the only final palliative intervention for this small subset of patients.

In our opinion the following are important summary points for outcomes in TOF/PA:

1. Achieving an adequate vascular bed is paramount and requires good flow to at least 10, and preferably more, bronchopulmonary segments.

2. Earlier unifocalization will likely lead to more favorable performance of MAPCAs and preservation of an adequate vascular bed.

3. Ultimately, complete repair can be expected in more than two-thirds of patients with excellent short-term outcomes.

4. Ongoing attrition leads to worse intermediate to long-term outcomes with survivals of approximately 70% at 10 or more years of age.

5. Multiple reinterventions are the norm—achieving good outcomes requires a multidisciplinary team approach to comprehensively manage these patients.

Longer-Term Follow-Up and the Adult With Tetralogy of Fallot

Despite good long-term survival after TOF repair, patients are at risk for late cardiac complications, including exercise intolerance, heart failure, arrhythmias, and sudden death. After adjusting for early mortality, Murphy et al.[88] reported a 32-year survival of 86%, which was significantly lower compared with 96% survival in a matched control population. Similarly, Nollert et al.[93] reported an adjusted 36-year survival of 85% in 490 patients that survived initial TOF repair, with a significantly increased risk for sudden death and congestive heart failure 20 years after repair.

Since these initial reports, there has been tremendous focus on understanding the impact of residual hemodynamic and electro-physiologic abnormalities on the risk for morbidity and mortality long-term after TOF repair. Chronic, severe pulmonary valve insufficiency is the most common residual hemodynamic lesion and is a result of transannular patch and/or pulmonary valve disruption during TOF repair.[128] Although well tolerated in the first two to three decades of life, chronic severe pulmonary valve insufficiency when left untreated eventually results in progressive RV dilation, RV dysfunction, exercise intolerance, congestive heart failure, tachyarrhythmias, and death.[f] RV dilation and dysfunction also negatively impact LV systolic and diastolic function.[13,40,61]

Surgical PVR results in a reduction in RV volumes, as well as improvements in symptoms and functional status in patients with severe pulmonary insufficiency after TOF repair.[35] PVR is typically performed with either a homograft or heterograft and can be performed with low discharge mortality of 2% or less at experienced centers.[35,94] In general, PVR is indicated in patients after TOF repair with chronic severe pulmonary insufficiency associated with exercise intolerance and/or RV systolic dysfunction.[128]

Timing of PVR in asymptomatic patients with RV dilation and normal RV systolic function is less well defined. A number of studies using cardiac MRI have demonstrated that there may be a threshold at which normalization of RV volumes after PVR may not always occur (i.e., indexed RV end-diastolic volume >150 to 170 mL/m^2 and RV end-systolic volume >82 to 90 mL/m^2).[16,95,116] Other factors that may contribute to decision for PVR in asymptomatic patients include sustained tachyarrhythmias, significant functional tricuspid insufficiency resulting from RV

---

[e]References 18, 26, 29, 32, 51, 55, 66, 98, 104.

[f]References 40, 47, 61, 62, 103, 128.

dilation, large RV outflow tract aneurysm, QRS duration of more than 140 ms, or in women before pregnancy.[39,130] Percutaneous PVR is an alternative option for select patients with existing bioprosthetic pulmonary valve dysfunction after TOF repair.[22]

In addition to pulmonary insufficiency, patients after TOF repair are at risk for other hemodynamic lesions that may require percutaneous or surgical reintervention.[48] Residual RVOTO can occur at any level, including subvalvar, valvar, or branch pulmonary arteries. Reintervention for residual RVOTO is indicated in the setting of severe RV hypertension associated with exercise intolerance and/or RV dysfunction. Residual atrial or ventricular septal defects can occur. Aortic root dilation with or without aortic valve insufficiency is also a growing concern in adults with repaired TOF.[87] Other cardiac and noncardiac comorbidities, including obesity, lung disease, chronic kidney disease, and coronary artery disease, are increasingly prevalent in the adult with repaired TOF and can increase the risks associated with cardiac reinterventions.

Scar from atrial and ventricular incisions and residual hemodynamic lesions after TOF repair predispose to development of late arrhythmias.[37,63] Risk factors for ventricular arrhythmia and sudden death include older age at repair, QRS duration on electrocardiogram of more than 180 ms, LV dysfunction, RV dysfunction, RV hypertrophy, and atrial arrhythmias.[37,41,120] Although severe pulmonary insufficiency may be an important driver for the risk for ventricular arrhythmias, it is unclear if PVR reduces the risk of sudden death and mortality in this setting.[38,44] Patients with several risk factors for ventricular tachycardia and sudden death may benefit from electrophysiologic study, arrhythmia surgery at the time of PVR, and/or implantation of a cardioverter-defibrillator.[64,65] Atrial arrhythmias occur in up to 20% of adult patients after TOF repair.[63] Intraatrial reentrant tachycardia, also known as atrial flutter, is the most common atrial arrhythmia, although atrial fibrillation is becoming more common in patients over 45 years of age. Antiarrhythmias and electrophysiologic ablation can be effective to treat atrial arrhythmias, but recurrence rate is higher than in patients with structurally normal hearts.[65]

Summary

Improvements in all aspects of perioperative management of congenital heart disease have led to dramatic improvements in outcomes for patients with TOF. There is a clear trend to attempt to preserve the pulmonary valve/annulus in TOF/PS with the goal of preserving long-term function of the RV. The validity of this approach remains to be verified by long-term follow-up. Despite this focus, more than half of contemporary repairs entail either a ventriculotomy or transannular incision. The latter is particularly true for neonatal repair, an approach advocated by select groups.

Although neonatal repair is a valid option for the symptomatic neonate, there are no randomized studies comparing neonatal repair versus a staged approach. For TOF/PA, repair strategies vary based upon the ability to achieve unifocalization of MAPCAs with the primary focus of attaining an adequate pulmonary vascular bed suitable to permit low RV pressures after VSD closure. Each institution should carefully evaluate the maturity of their infrastructure and their data and pursue an approach that provides the best outcomes in their hands.

Long-term follow-up is critical to detecting and managing issues that may arise, such as pulmonary insufficiency, RV dilation and dysfunction, arrhythmias, and peripheral pulmonary stenoses, among others. Transition of care to adult congenital cardiology providers enhances care as patients progress through adulthood.

Selected References

A complete list of references is available at ExpertConsult.com.

4. Al Habib HF, Jacobs JP, Mavroudis CM, et al. Contemporary patterns of management of tetralogy of Fallot: data from The Society of Thoracic Surgeons Database. *Ann Thorac Surg.* 2010;90:813–820.
6. Apitz C, Webb G, Redington AN. Tetralogy of Fallot. *Lancet.* 2009;374:1462–1471.
18. Carillo SA, Mainwaring RD, Patrick WL, et al. Surgical repair of pulmonary atresia with ventricular septal defect and major aortopulmonary collaterals with absent intrapericardial pulmonary arteries. *Ann Thorac Surg.* 2015;100:606–614.
36. Fraser CD, Bacha EA, Comas J, et al. Tetralogy of Fallot. *Semin Thorac Cardiovasc Surg.* 2015;27:189–204.
48. Hickey EJ, Veldtman G, Bradley TJ, et al. Late risk outcomes for adults with repaired tetralogy of Fallot from an inception cohort spanning four decades. *Eur J Cardiothorac Surg.* 2009;35:156–166.
54. Imamura M, Dossey AM, Garcia X, et al. Prophylactic amiodarone reduces junctional ectopic tachycardia after tetralogy of Fallot repair. *J Thorac Cardiovasc Surg.* 2012;143:152–156.
84. Michielon G, Marino B, Formigari R, et al. Genetic syndromes and outcome after surgery for correction of tetralogy of Fallot. *Ann Thorac Surg.* 2006;81:968–975.
105. Shekerdemian LS, Penny DJ, Novick W. Early extubation after surgical repair of tetralogy of Fallot. *Cardiol Young.* 2000;10(6):636–637.
111. Steiner MB, Tang X, Gossett JM, et al. Timing of complete repair of non-ductal-dependent tetralogy of Fallot and short-term postoperative outcomes, a multicenter analysis. *J Thorac Cardiovasc Surg.* 2014;147:1299–1305.
121. Van Praagh R. The first Stella Van Praagh memorial lecture: the history and anatomy of tetralogy of Fallot. *Semin Thorac Cardiovasc Surg Pediatr Card Surg Annu.* 2009;12:19–38.
125. Villafane J, Feinstein JA, Jenkins KJ, et al. Hot topics in tetralogy of Fallot. *J Am Coll Cardiol.* 2013;62:2155–2166.

60

Pulmonary Valve Replacement: Indications and Options

YOSHIO OOTAKI, MD, PHD; DEREK A. WILLIAMS, DO

Survival after surgical repair of congenital heart defects has continuously improved over the last several decades with advances in surgical techniques, cardiopulmonary bypass, and perioperative care. This has created the need to address the emerging long-term issues of older children and young adults with "repaired" congenital heart disease. Half of the patients who survive tetralogy of Fallot repair require pulmonary valve replacement (PVR) within 30 years. As a result, PVR or right ventricular outflow tract (RVOT) reconstruction is becoming the most frequent congenital heart surgical procedure performed on adolescents and young adults. More recently there is growing enthusiasm for percutaneously inserted bioprosthetic valves in the pulmonary position. In this chapter we will review the current indications and approach for PVR.

Indications

PVR is required in various situations such as isolated pulmonary valvular disease or pulmonary insufficiency after repair of tetralogy of Fallot (Box 60.1). Current indications for PVR include symptomatic and asymptomatic patients with increased risk for right ventricular (RV) dilation, RV failure, exercise intolerance, arrhythmia, and sudden cardiac death (Box 60.2). Numerous studies have demonstrated the benefits of PVR, and guidelines for PVR in adults with CHD have been published by the American,[1] Canadian,[2] and European[3] cardiac societies. These guidelines are clear in symptomatic patients with severe pulmonary regurgitation recommending PVR. However, they are less clear in asymptomatic patients with severe pulmonary regurgitation. PVR offers improvement in symptoms and RV function, but the sickest patients receive the least benefit and carry higher surgical risks.

Given the limitations of echocardiography to accurately assess the RV, magnetic resonance imaging (MRI) has become the more preferable approach to assess pulmonary regurgitation fraction, RV volume, and RV ejection fraction. Several MRI studies have reported that RV volumes return to the normal range if the preoperative RV end-diastolic volume (RVEDV) index is less than 150 to 170 mL/m^2 or the RV end-systolic volume is less than 80 to 90 mL/m^2.[4-6] Additional findings such as an RV pressure more than two-thirds systemic, a pulmonary-to-systemic flow ratio of more than 1.5 : 1, residual shunt, severe tricuspid regurgitation, an RVOT aneurysm, and reduced left ventricular function are also factors promoting a need for PVR. Maximal benefit from PVR seems to occur with earlier intervention before the RV suffers irreversible change. Although aggressive application of PVR to younger children may result in a higher likelihood of reintervention within 10 years,[7] waiting to perform PVR for preoperative RV end-systolic volume (RVESV) greater than 95 mL/m^2 has an increased risk for suboptimal hemodynamic outcomes and adverse clinical events.[5]

Common candidates for PVR include patients with transannular patches for repair of tetralogy of Fallot, congenital pulmonary valve stenosis, repaired truncus arteriosus, and other anomalies requiring placement of an RV–pulmonary artery (PA) conduit. RV function is more successfully preserved in patients after repair of pulmonary stenosis compared with patients with pulmonary insufficiency following repair of tetralogy of Fallot.[8] Patients with residual pulmonary insufficiency after congenital pulmonary stenosis repair had superior RV remodeling after PVR when compared with tetralogy of Fallot patients with residual pulmonary insufficiency after PVR.[9] In patients requiring PVR, significant tricuspid regurgitation is more common in patients with pulmonary atresia and intact ventricular septum compared with patients with tetralogy of Fallot.[10] Therefore complete knowledge of the original congenital heart defect is extremely important before PVR. In addition to the recommended indications for PVR, the optimal timing for PVR requires a thorough workup and discussion based on the individual patient.

There is agreement that PVR is recommended in symptomatic patients with severe pulmonary insufficiency (particularly with RV dilation), heart failure, and new-onset arrhythmia. However, PVR is still controversial in asymptomatic patients. There is no randomized trial to prove PVR reduces long-term adverse clinical outcomes compared with medical treatment. Multicenter clinical registries will be necessary to assess long-term clinical benefit after PVR.

Pulmonary Valve Replacement Options (Box 60.3)

Surgical PVR is becoming one of the most common operations in adult congenital heart disease. The mortality is reassuringly low, reported as 0.9% from the Society of Thoracic Surgeons Congenital Heart Surgery Database (STS CHSD) and 4.1% from the Adult Cardiac Surgery Database (STS ACSD).[11] The risk of a major complication (temporary or permanent renal failure at discharge requiring dialysis, neurologic deficit persisting at discharge, atrioventricular block or arrhythmia requiring a permanent pacemaker, postoperative mechanical circulatory support, phrenic

BOX 60.1 Primary Disease

- Pulmonary valve stenosis
- Tetralogy of Fallot with or without pulmonary atresia
- Pulmonary atresia with intact ventricular septum
- Truncus arteriosus and other congenital heart defects repaired with an RV-PA conduit
- Post Ross procedure

PA, Pulmonary artery; RV, right ventricle.

BOX 60.2 Indications for Pulmonary Valve Replacement

Moderate or severe pulmonary regurgitation (regurgitation fraction ≥25%)
I. Asymptomatic patient with two or more of the following criteria
  a. RV end-diastolic volume index >150 mL/m² or z score >4. In patients whose body surface area falls outside published normal data: RV/LV end-diastolic volume ratio >2
  b. RV end-systolic volume index >80 mL/m²
  c. RV ejection fraction <47%
  d. LV ejection fraction <55%
  e. Large RVOT aneurysm
  f. QRS duration >140 ms
  g. Sustained tachyarrhythmia related to right heart volume load
  h. Other hemodynamically significant abnormalities:
    - RVOT obstruction with RV systolic pressure ≥2/3 systemic
    - Severe branch pulmonary artery stenosis (<30% flow to affected lung) not amenable to transcatheter therapy
    - ≥ Moderate tricuspid regurgitation
    - Left-to-right shunt from residual atrial or ventricular septal defects with pulmonary-to-systemic flow ratio ≥1.5
    - Severe aortic regurgitation
    - Severe aortic dilation (diameter ≥5 cm)
II. Symptomatic patients with one or more of the above criteria
III. Special considerations
  a. In patients who underwent TOF repair at ≥3 years of age, PVR may be considered if fulfill ≥1 of the quantitative criteria in section I.
  b. In women with severe pulmonary regurgitation and RV dilation and/or dysfunction, PVR may be considered if fulfill ≥1 of the quantitative criteria in section I due to pregnancy-related complications.

LV, Left ventricle; PVR, pulmonary valve replacement; RV, right ventricle; RVOT, right ventricular outflow tract; TOF, tetralogy of Fallot.
From Geva T. Repaired tetralogy of Fallot: the roles of cardiovascular magnetic resonance in evaluating pathophysiology and for pulmonary valve replacement decision support. J Cardiovasc Magn Reson. 2011;13:9.

BOX 60.3 Pulmonary Valve Replacement Options

- Allograft
- Bioprosthetic stented valve
- Bioprosthetic stentless valve (Contegra, Freestyle)
- Mechanical valve
- ePTFE valve (monocusp, bicuspid, tricuspid)
- Transcatheter pulmonary valve (Melody, Sapien)

ePTFE, Expanded polytetrafluoroethylene.

nerve injury, or any unplanned reintervention before discharge) is reported as 2.2% from the STS CHSD and 20.9% from STS ACSD. PVR carries higher morbidity and mortality in the adult population compared with the pediatric population, possibly secondary to a higher prevalence of other preoperative risk factors such as endocarditis. There is also an increasing volume of literature suggesting that the risk for PVR is significantly higher when performed by non–congenital heart surgeons and when patients are cared for in intensive care units that are not accustomed to caring for congenital heart patients.[12,13] The difference between the mortality for PVR in the STS CHSD and the STS ACSD is likely not due to patient comorbidity alone.

Surgical Approach

In the majority of PVR surgeries a repeat sternotomy is necessary. The risk of a reentry injury during repeat sternotomy is low (0.3% to 1.3%)[14,15]; however, major injury requires emergent cannulation to initiate cardiopulmonary bypass (CPB). There are clear risk factors that increase the risk of PVR in certain patients such as the existence of a transannular patch, a prior RV-PA conduit, or an enlarged and aneurysmal aorta; however, reentry injury is not associated with an increased risk of operative mortality in the current era.

Typically CPB at normothermia or mild hypothermia is common for PVR. In the case of a residual atrial or ventricular level shunt, aortic cross-clamping with cardioplegic arrest of the heart is preferred over techniques such as "empty, beating" right heart surgery to reduce the risk of systemic air embolism. In general the favored recommendation is to avoid "empty, beating" heart surgery for congenital heart surgery due to the possibility of unrecognized residual shunts, and we recommend aortic cross-clamping and cardioplegic arrest unless the anatomy makes this more dangerous (e.g., a calcified, enlarged, or heavily scarred aorta). Ventricular fibrillation using an electric fibrillator is an alternative technique to avoid "empty, beating" heart surgery, which carries a risk for embolic brain injury in some patients. The pulmonary annulus is visualized through a longitudinal incision to the RVOT. An appropriate-size valve or valved conduit can be chosen, and the selected valve can be placed using a wide variety of surgical techniques.

Allograft. Allografts (Fig. 60.1A) have been widely used for more than 50 years. Early outcomes with allografts have been excellent, especially in neonates and infants; however, valve deterioration over time has been an issue, especially in smaller allografts.[16] Decellularized pulmonary homografts have better early to midterm results when compared with conventional homografts or to bovine jugular vein (BJV) conduits.[17] Freedom from conduit dysfunction was significantly better at 10 years in decellularized pulmonary homografts (83%) compared with conventional pulmonary homografts (58%).[18] However, long-term outcomes beyond 10 years have been discouraging, especially in small children. In some countries such as Japan, allografts are not widely available.

Bioprosthetic Stented Valve. The durability of bioprosthetic stented valves (see Fig. 60.1B) in the aortic position over time have greatly improved. When a stented, bioprosthetic valve is used, a patch pulmonary arterioplasty to augment the size of the RVOT can be used to allow placement of an adequate-size prosthesis (Fig. 60.2).

Comparison of results with the use of stented bioprosthetic valves in the pulmonary position demonstrate that the durability in the pulmonary position in young patients is suboptimal, mainly

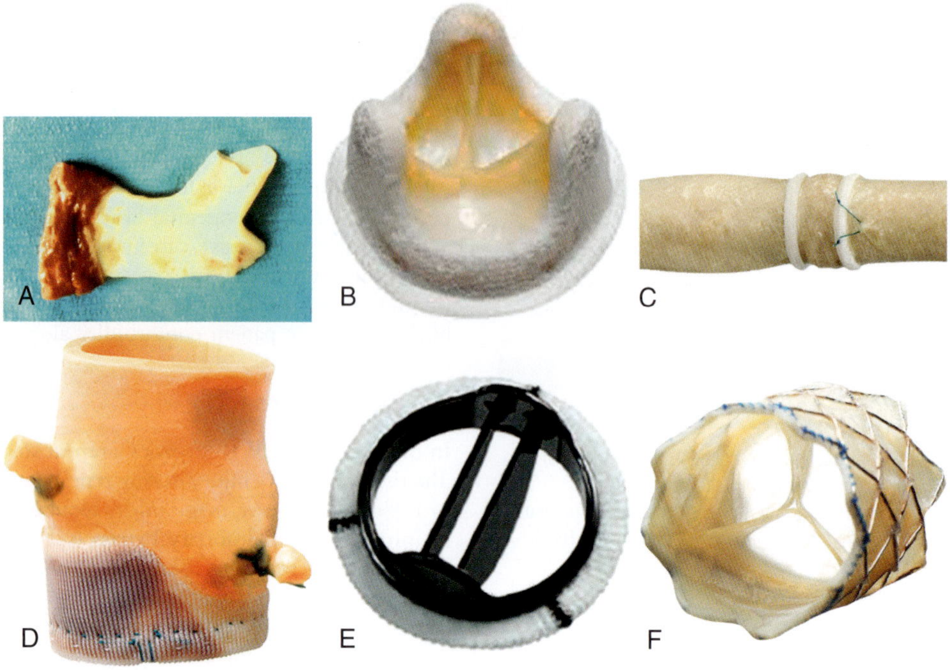

• **Figure 60.1** Various types of commercially available valves that can be inserted into the pulmonary position. (A) Cadaver allograft pulmonary valve. (B) Stented bioprosthetic valve (bovine and porcine). (C) Contegra (bovine jugular vein) bioprosthesis. (D) Medtronic stentless porcine root. (E) Mechanical (St. Jude). (F) Melody stented bioprosthesis (transcatheter insertion).

due to dystrophic calcification and relative stenosis of the valve opening with changes in body size via somatic growth over time. Kwak and associates[19] reported that patients more than 20 years of age showed no valvular dysfunction during nearly 14 years of follow-up. However, patients less than 20 years of age showed a 98.5% freedom from valvular dysfunction at 5 years, but this decreased to 68.2% at 10 years, and only 24.7% at 14 years, thus indicating significantly worse outcomes compared with patients more than 20 years of age.

Lee and associates compared the performance of three types of bioprostheses (stented porcine, stented bovine pericardial, and stentless porcine valves). They reported freedom from repeat PVR at 10 years at 84.6% for stented bovine pericardial valves, 48.5% for stented porcine valves, and 31.2% for stentless porcine valves.[20] Buchholz and associates could not identify any differences between the durability of stented biologic valves with bovine pericardial or porcine leaflets. However, considering that the pressure gradient across the valve increased sooner in the pericardial group, these results suggest that bovine valves might be preferred over porcine valves.[21] Chen and associates[22] reported that freedom from reintervention was similar for the porcine and bovine pericardial valves and the reintervention-free survival rate at 5 and 10 years was 94% and 36%, respectively. Of note, these studies were not randomized trials comparing one valve over others. A prospective randomized trial would be necessary to investigate the best stented pulmonary valve to be used in the pediatric population. However, the available data have led most practitioners to choose stented bovine pericardial valves as the current stented bioprosthesis of choice and in fact to use these preferentially over stentless porcine bioprostheses as well.

Bioprosthetic Stentless Valve. The BJV (Contegra, Medtronic Inc., Minneapolis, MN) was introduced into clinical practice as an alternative to the use of homografts in 1999[23] (see Fig. 60.1C).

The recognized advantages of the BJV include (1) the structural continuity between the wall of the jugular vein of the conduit and valve leaflets, which provides optimal hemodynamics because of the ideal effective orifice area; (2) the unlimited availability in sizes from 12 to 22 mm in diameter, representing a good alternative to the homograft shortage, particularly for the smaller sizes; and (3) the availability of a long inflow and outflow length, which obviates the need for either proximal or distal augmentation, thus facilitating conduit tailoring and positioning, helping to avoid potential distortion and sternal compression.

BJVs are associated with a significantly greater risk of late endocarditis. The reintervention-free survival rate is concerning and has been reported at 5, 10, and 15 years as 73%, 45%, and 26%, respectively.[24] BJVs might have advantages for small children (less than 2 years of age) because of availability in small sizes and the expected need for replacement making long-term durability less of a factor.[7]

The Medtronic Freestyle valve is a stentless bioprosthesis derived from the porcine aortic root (see Fig. 60.1D) and decellularized using glutaraldehyde and then treated with alpha-amino oleic acid to minimize xenograft calcification. Potential advantages of the Freestyle valve include the availability of a range of larger sizes (19 to 29 mm) and the flexible nature of the bioprosthesis, allowing for easy implantation in curved RVOTs. The reintervention-free survival rate was reported as 85% at 5 years and 71% at 10 years.[25] Long-term durability is an issue, though it performs equally well compared with the homograft.

Mechanical Valve. The vast majority of patients, especially children who require PVR, obtain a tissue valve because of the relatively good durability and the lack of a need for anticoagulation. Although the thromboembolic risk after PVR with mechanical valves is presumed to be high, recent studies suggest promising midterm results.[26] Freedom from PVR reoperation after 5 and 10

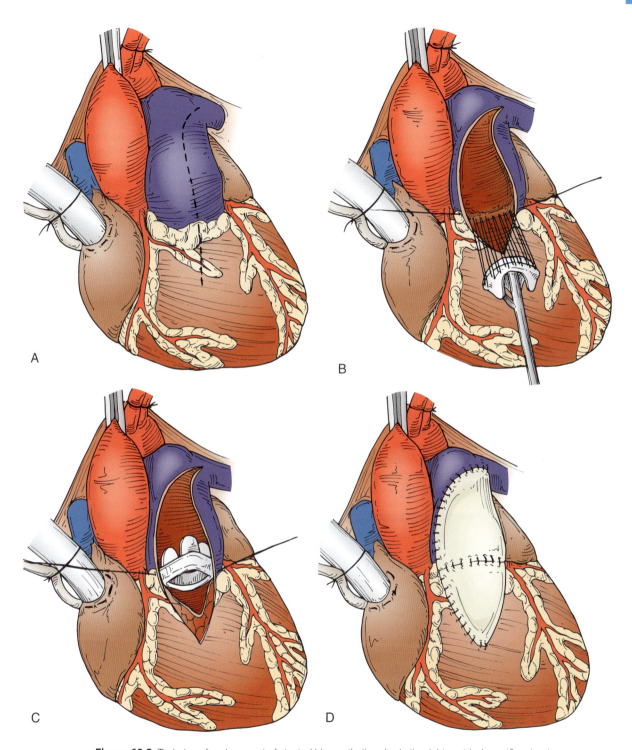

• Figure 60.2 Technique for placement of stented bioprosthetic valve in the right ventricular outflow tract (RVOT). (A) A longitudinal incision is made in the RVOT extending out to the pulmonary bifurcation. (B) After sizing for the appropriate valve, it is retained on its "handle," and a continuous suture line is placed along the posterior portion of the RVOT and the top part of the valve sewing ring. Notice that the valve is oriented "backward," but when the sutures are tightened, the valve will "flip" into its desired orientation. (C) The valve is seated into position, and the posterior suture line is continued to the edge of the incision in the RVOT. (D) A prosthetic patch is then used as a "roof" over the valve and RVOT incision. This allows placement of a large valve into the RVOT. Notice that the anterior portion of the valve sewing ring is secured to the outflow patch.

years was reported as 96% and 89%, respectively. Performance of mechanical prostheses (Fig. 60.1E) in the pulmonary position may improve when valvular thrombosis is prevented by prudent patient selection, avoiding mechanical valves in patients at increased risk of valvular thrombosis, and by strict compliance to anticoagulation therapy. An important disadvantage of the mechanical valve in the pulmonary position is its interference with permitting catheter intervention to the distal pulmonary arteries—the mechanical disks and architecture of the valve impose a formidable impediment to floating catheters into the distal pulmonary arteries. The mechanical valve in the pulmonary position, although not a commonly preferred option, can be a reasonable choice for complex patients who may be receiving one final procedure aimed at providing a durable PVR, who have normal distal pulmonary arteries, and for whom long-term anticoagulation is acceptable.

Expanded Polytetrafluoroethylene Valve. Expanded polytetrafluoroethylene (ePTFE) has been reported for PVR. Monocusp valves were reported in 2002,[27] and bicuspid valves have been created in situ and more recently in conduits.[28,29] Tricuspid valves have been created primarily in Japan, where allografts have not been widely available.[30] The follow-up now exceeds 10 years, and freedom from reoperation has been 100% at 5 years and 95.4% at 10 years. Ootaki and associates[31] described a simplified technique to create a tricuspid ePTFE valved conduit, which consists of commercially available ePTFE graft and 0.1-mm thick ePTFE membrane (WL Gore & Associates, Flagstaff, AZ) (Fig. 60.3), and have shown similar, excellent results with freedom from valve replacement at 100% at 4 years. The trileaflet ePTFE valve is shorter than the bicuspid valve (because valve height is related to leaflet length, trileaflet valves have shorter leaflets and thus a shorter valve height, resulting in shorter conduit length). The

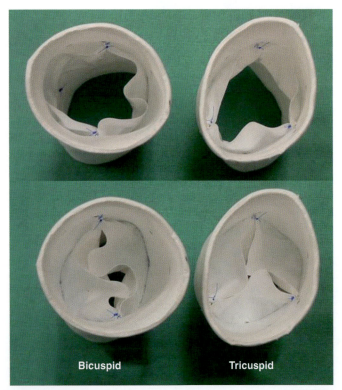

• **Figure 60.3** A bicuspid and tricuspid polytetrafluoroethylene valve. The potential advantages of the tricuspid valve versus the bicuspid valve are discussed in the text.

Bicuspid   **Tricuspid**

trileaflet valve potentially has superior hemodynamics to a bileaflet valve, although this has not yet been demonstrated in human recipients.

Homografts or BJVs, even available for small children who require RVOT replacement, have potential problems with durability as described earlier. When they are used in small sizes (for smaller patients), conduit replacement is an expected eventuality. However, compared with homografts and BJV options, ePTFE valved conduits have a more optimistic outlook. Yamashita and associates[32] reported that freedom from conduit replacement and reintervention at 5 years was 90.1% and 77.2%, respectively, after implantation of an ePTFE valved conduit less than or equal to 16 mm in diameter.

Transcatheter Pulmonary Valve Replacement

Transcatheter PVR was first reported in humans in 2000.[33] Since then transcatheter PVR has emerged as a variable alternative to surgical PVR in patients with RVOT dysfunction. The Medtronic Melody transcatheter pulmonary valve (TPV) (Medtronic, Minneapolis, MN) is composed of a BJV valve sutured within a platinum iridium stent (see Fig. 60.1F). The multicenter US trial was completed in 2009 and showed favorable results.[34,35] Although there was an issue of stent fracture, altering the implant approach with bare metal prestenting of the preexisting conduit reduced this risk significantly.[36] The Food and Drug Administration (FDA) approved its full commercial issue in 2015. The Melody TPV is marketed for failing conduits 16 mm or larger at the time of surgical placement. The valve comes in two sizes (16 mm and 18 mm) with the 16-mm valve achieving a maximal diameter of 20 mm and the 18-mm valve achieving a maximal diameter of 22 mm. Cheatham and associates[37] reported successful maximal dilation of the 18-mm valve up to 24 mm with only mild residual regurgitation. The Edwards Sapien system is widely used in the aortic position, and it was first reported in the pulmonary position in 2006.[38] The Edwards Sapien XT valve is a bovine pericardial tissue valve mounted within a cobalt chromium stent and comes in diameters of 20, 23, 26, and 29 mm. The Sapien XT valve received FDA approval for implantation in the pulmonary position in 2016. The Sapien 3 is the newest generation and awaits FDA approval for the pulmonary position.

Presently the primary usage of the transcatheter approach is for patients with a failing RVOT conduit and an RVOT diameter (or previous conduit size) of less than 28 mm. With the availability of the Sapien valve, which can reach 30 mm in diameter, case reports are emerging showing successful implantation in the native RVOT primary in patients with a transannular patch repair for tetralogy of Fallot. Additionally, a trial in under way studying new valve designs for the native RVOT.

Coronary artery compression is one of the main concerns at the time of transcatheter PVR. The incidence of coronary artery compression has been found to be 5% during test balloon inflation[39] and should be checked for before finalizing inflation of a stented valved conduit in the RVOT.

Conduit tear has been another concern during implant. A retrospective review of the multicenter US trial revealed a rate of 6%. The commercially available NuMED Covered Cheatham-Platinum Stent was 98% effective in preventing or repairing these tears.[40]

Endocarditis is one of the main concerns after transcatheter PVR. Freedom from endocarditis at 5 years was 89%[36] and has been reported as a frequent midterm outcome in numerous series.

Outcomes after transcatheter PVR are comparable with the surgical approach in the short-term and midterm follow-up. Long-term data are needed to make a final judgment on the most appropriate patient selection for transcatheter PVR.

Hybrid Approach

Several hybrid approaches have been reported using the RV approach for smaller-size patients[41] or performing main PA plication.[42] These approaches can prevent the exposure to CPB and reduce transfusions, which have resulted in reducing surgical morbidity and mortality. However, there are no long-term data to support any benefits to this approach. Surgical mortality and morbidity after surgical PVR have been minimal in the current era. Presently the hybrid PVR approach is best suited for patients with higher risks for surgery employing CPB and should be based on the individual factors involved. This is a team dynamic between the surgeon and the interventionist that allows for creative approaches to complex patients.

Summary

Currently there are multiple options for PVR, and the future will undoubtedly provide more. Longevity of the various valves is dependent upon the type of conduit and age/size of the patient at implantation. The ePTFE valved conduit shows particular promise as a preeminent valve in children and adolescents. For adolescents and young adults there exist several options with proven durability of each valve. To date there is no "perfect" valve for providing a permanent solution in pulmonary position, though presently surgical PVR followed by transcatheter PVR is the preferred option to limit future surgical intervention.

References

A complete list of references is available at ExpertConsult.com

61

Pulmonary Atresia With Intact Ventricular Septum

MICHELLE A. GRENIER, MD; FRANK SCHOLL, MD

In 1783, Hunter described membranous or muscular atresia of the right ventricular outflow tract. This deformity was revisited by Peacock in 1869 and then again by Robert Freedom in 1989.[1] They described remarkable heterogeneity of the right ventricular inlet and functional size, as well as the subepicardial connections between the diminutive RV chamber and the coronary artery circulation. The span of almost 100 years between these published investigations speaks to the difficulty in understanding this particular form of heart disease. Pulmonary atresia with intact ventricular septum (PA/IVS) is anatomically and functionally a left-sided heart with normal atrial relations (situs solitus), concordant atrioventricular and ventriculoarterial connections presenting with obstruction to RV outflow that can range from a relatively normal RV chamber and tricuspid valve size with an imperforate membrane in the location of the pulmonary valve at one end of the spectrum, to "hypoplastic right heart syndrome" with a diminutive tricuspid valve, a tiny RV cavity and often RV to coronary artery connections associated with a long area of muscular infundibular atresia at the other end of the spectrum. The ventricular septum is intact. Because of the absence of antegrade flow across the RV outflow tract, PA/IVS is a "ductal dependent" lesion. The patent ductus arteriosus (PDA) supplies pulmonary blood flow, and multiple aortopulmonary collaterals and nonconfluent pulmonary arteries are uncommon. Approximately 20% of patients have subendocardial fistulous connections, frequently called "sinusoids." Infants born with this disease usually present with cyanosis shortly after birth when their PDA begins to close.

Poor development of the tricuspid valve is a result of the abnormal, highly pressured right ventricle (that has no outlet), and the degree of tricuspid regurgitation appears to correlate with the severity of the defect. Fetal loss may account for an underestimated incidence and prevalence of the defect, which is estimated at 0.6/10,000 live births. Consequently, the real incidence of this defect is speculated as being up to ten times higher. The prenatal echo is a postnatal prognosticator, with an emphasis on the tricuspid valve Z score as well as on the anatomy of the RV chamber—with attention to the presence of a well-developed inlet, apical trabecular, and outlet (tripartite) portions of the right ventricle. There have been attempts to characterize muscular hypertrophy with the proposal that intervention may cause regression of the hypertrophy with a real versus perceived growth of ventricle. This has been the rationale for fetal intervention for this disease. Figure 61.1 provides a schematic representation of the spectrum of defects in PA/IVS.

Because of this wide spectrum and variability in disease severity, mainly related to tricuspid valve size, RV chamber anatomy, and coronary artery anomalies, complex algorithms for treatment are required to ensure optimum outcomes for these often fragile patients. These algorithms have resulted in improved survival in patients diagnosed with PA/IVS, particularly in the more severe forms of the spectrum.

This chapter reviews the embryology, anatomy, physiology, treatment strategies, and outcomes for this diverse group of patients.

Embryology

The embryologic cause of PA/IVS to this day remains unknown. Identifiable genetic syndromes and other cardiac and noncardiac malformations are less common in PA/IVS than in other forms of congenital heart disease. There are currently no known genetic causes, although there are reports of familial cases of PA/IVS with an autosomal dominant inheritance pattern with incomplete penetrance.[2] A single-gene theory has also been proposed in a sibling pair, suggesting that an autosomal recessive pattern may have a role.[3] However, based on these somewhat conflicting sources, evidence is insufficient to establish a consistent genetic association for PA/IVS

The failure of the separation of the pulmonary valve leaflets leads to decreased flow through the tricuspid valve and RV, which leads to RV muscular hypertrophy and hypoplasia of the RV cavity in utero. It has been proposed that this perturbation in fetal blood flow may occur after cardiac septation, which may explain the normal size of the proximal main pulmonary artery in most cases of PA/IVS when compared with pulmonary atresia with ventricular septal defect (PA/VSD).[4]

The later fusing of the pulmonary valve leaflets may be related to viral infection or inflammatory disease in midterm gestation, as opposed to the atresia occurring in PA/VSD, which is felt to be an early developmental event. However, there has been no relationship established between PA/IVS and maternal rubella, despite the suggested association between pulmonary stenosis and maternal rubella.[4-6] Additionally, there are most often no other associated findings of cardiac inflammation that would indicate this is a systemic or at the very least cardiac inflammatory process.

The development of coronary fistulae (sinusoids) does not appear to be an inflammatory process but rather seems to be due to myointimal hyperplasia in the presence of a rich background of glycosaminoglycans. There are mild degrees of medial-intimal

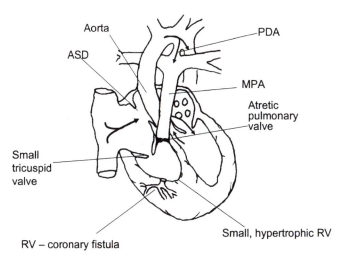

• **Figure 61.1** Native anatomy of pulmonary atresia with intact ventricular septum. The atretic pulmonary valve prevents exit of blood from the small, hypertrophic right ventricle (*RV*). As a result, the elevated right heart pressures drive systemic venous blood through the atrial septal defect (*ASD*) to mix with pulmonary venous blood in the left heart. This desaturated blood is ejected into the aorta to supply both the systemic circulation and the pulmonary circulation via the patent ductus arteriosus (*PDA*). Coronary blood supply to the RV is maintained in part by an RV–coronary fistula. Note also the small tricuspid valve and the normal caliber of the main pulmonary artery (*MPA*).

thickening due to a loss of normal wall with replacement of the wall by fibrocellular material. Of note, this process does not occur in thin-walled low pressure systems.

Anatomic Considerations

Pulmonary Artery Anatomy

Complete fusion or absence of the pulmonary valve cusps is the hallmark of PA/IVS. Often the main pulmonary artery is only mildly hypoplastic, and frequently it is normal in size. The pulmonary valve sinuses are often normally developed, and the leaflets may, in milder forms, be fairly thin. However, usually the cusps are quite misshapen and even cartilaginous in their appearance.

Ventricular Anatomy

The RV ranges in size and form from a well-developed tripartite RV (with an inlet, trabecular, and outlet portion) to a severely hypoplastic diminutive inflow chamber. Bull et al.[7] in 1982 showed that RV hypertrophy led to decreased apical trabecular chamber and inflow size. Both by angiography and autopsy they showed that hearts with obliterated infundibular and trabecular cavities had thicker walls and smaller tricuspid valves than those in which the normal three portions of the ventricular cavity were represented.[7] This original tripartite classification is helpful in determining treatment strategy for these patients. Typically the left ventricular anatomy is normal in size and geometry.

Tricuspid Valve Anatomy

The tricuspid valve itself exhibits a high degree of variability in form and function, ranging from severe stenosis to massive

regurgitation. The anatomic size of the tricuspid valve also determines or is correlated with RV morphology. The patients with the smallest tricuspid valves tend to have absence or attenuation of the trabecular and outlet portions of the ventricle. These patients are the ones least likely to have a tripartite RV.[7,8]

Ebstein anomaly of the tricuspid valve is an unusual component of PA/IVS seen in approximately 10% of cases. It can pose a significant challenge in the management of patients who present with this tricuspid valve anatomy.[9]

Coronary Artery Anomalies

Coronary artery anomalies represent the most likely reason for patients succumbing to this disease entity. Ischemic events related to abnormal coronary anatomy and abnormalities in the arterial wall are common in the more severe forms of the disease. Coronary artery anomalies in patients with PA/IVS include (1) RV-to-coronary artery fistulae, (2) coronary artery stenoses, and (3) coronary occlusions. In some, a substantial part of the coronary blood supply may depend on the RV. This RV-dependent coronary circulation may determine survival after RV decompression (RVD): RVD may cause RV "steal" in the presence of fistulae alone and ischemia, coronary isolation, or myocardial infarction in the presence of coronary stenoses (Fig 61.2).[10]

Microstructural abnormalities of the coronary arterial wall are also common and can lead to ischemic areas of myocardium with subsequent fibrosis even if aorta coronary continuity exists.

Fetal Diagnosis

PA/IVS can be diagnosed in utero and this can help with educating the family and preparing the medical and surgical team for eventual treatment options, including having the baby delivered at a center where prostaglandins can be started and transfer to a cardiac center initiated.

The true value of fetal echocardiography in the diagnosis of PA/IVS lies in predictive factors, and the ability to develop postnatal plans. Some of the morphologic and physiologic predictors for the postnatal surgical pathway include a combination of z-scores of fetal cardiac measurements and tricuspid/mitral valve (TV/MV) ratios, the presence of coronary fistulae, the right atrial pressure (RAP) based on the patent foramen ovale, the tricuspid valve dimension and competency and the ductus venosus Doppler. The combination of these variables can predict a biventricular circulation (at 26 weeks gestation) with a 92% specificity. The tricuspid valve z-score is a good predictor at all gestation. The best predictive scores for specific gestations include the pulmonary z-score (23 weeks) and the median tricuspid z-score (26 weeks) with a combination of median PV z-score and TV/MV ratio (26 to 31 weeks), and a combination of median TV z-score and median TV/MV ratio (31 weeks). The RAP score and the presence of coronary fistulae are good independent predictors with a RAP score >3 predicting a biventricular repair (83%) and the presence of coronary artery fistulae usually predicting a single ventricle route.[11]

Physiology

Due to the atretic pulmonary valve and absence of flow from the RV to the pulmonary arteries, the physiology is dependent on left-to-right ductal flow for pulmonary circulation. Prostaglandin infusion is the mainstay of medical treatment in these newborns and allows time for further workup and planning. Systemic venous

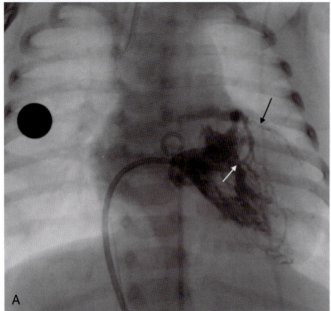

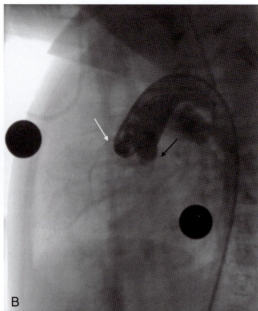

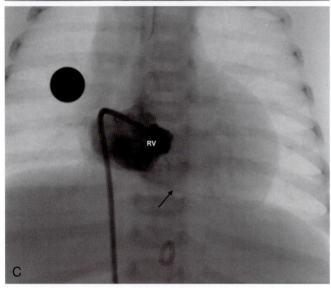

• **Figure 61.2** (A) RV angiogram in AP projection demonstrating an abnormal right ventricle with RV sinusoidal connections to the coronary arteries *(white arrow)*. Notice the opacification of the LAD *(black arrow)* and the suggestion of proximal stenosis of the left coronary artery system, which would define this coronary artery flow as dependent on the right ventricle. (B) Lateral aortogram of the above patient demonstrating absence of antegrade filling of the left coronary artery system from the aorta. *Black arrow* denotes the area where a left main coronary artery should be seen. The right coronary artery *(white arrow)* is demonstrated arising from its typical location off the right coronary sinus. (C) This angiogram of an infant with PA/IVS demonstrates a diminutive RV chamber. There is opacification of the distal right coronary artery *(black arrow)* filling from the RV, but additional injections showed no indication of RV dependent coronary circulation (RVDCC).

return to the right atrium requires a nonrestrictive ASD to allow right to left shunting to support cardiac output.

Treatment Strategies

Preprocedural Care and Evaluation

Patients are maintained on prostaglandin infusion after birth, and standard workup for newborns with complex congenital heart disease is undertaken. Imaging with echocardiogram and cardiac catheterization, including aortic root injection to determine aortocoronary continuity, is standard. This allows adequate and accurate categorization of risk, as well as surgical planning.

PA/IVS is a rare form of complex congenital heart disease with significant morphologic heterogeneity. Because of the significant morphologic heterogeneity seen in PA/IVS, repair or palliation strategies have a wide variation, from single-ventricle palliation to complete biventricular repair. The likelihood of significant

coronary artery abnormality is related to tricuspid valve Z score (Figure 61.3). the smaller the tricuspid valve, the greater the likelihood of need for staging to the single ventricle or transplant pathways.

Infants with PA/IVS are diagnosed initially with an echocardiogram to determine size of the tricuspid valve, size of the RV chamber, and presence of important RV sinusoids or suggestion of RV–coronary artery communication. In addition, the echocardiogram can define the adequacy of the atrial septal communication. Because of the lack of antegrade flow across the RV outflow tract, infants with PA/IVS have an obligate right to left shunt across the atrial septum in order to support systemic cardiac output. In some instances, the ASD may appear restrictive (Fig. 61.4) and inadequate to support increasing cardiac output demands, and it may benefit from the addition of an atrial septostomy at the time of cardiac catheterization.[12,13,14]

Infants with small tricuspid valves, small RV chamber size, a need for an atrial septostomy, or any concern regarding the anatomy

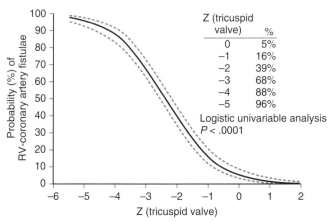

• **Figure 61.3** The relationship between tricuspid diameter (Z value) and the likelihood of having ventriculo-coronary artery fistulae. (Reproduced from Hanley FL, Sade RM, Blackstone EH, et al. Outcomes in neonatal pulmonary atresia with intact ventricular septum. A multi-institutional study. *J Thorac Cardiovasc Surg*. 1993;105:406-427, with permission.)

of the coronary circulation, especially if there is a concern that the anatomy has RV dependent coronary circulation (RVDCC), should be brought to the cardiac cath lab for angiography. Angiography can define the nature and severity of any coronary artery abnormalities and at this time, an atrial septostomy can be performed if indicated (in as many as 25% of patients in one series).[12]

Patients who do not have RV-dependent coronary circulation are assessed by echocardiography as to the adequacy of the RV to support a biventricular treatment strategy.[15] Echocardiographic assessment of the ventricular morphology has replaced angiography at our institution for anatomic delineation of RV morphology. Angiography is, however, still used as the definitive test to evaluate the coronary artery anatomy.

If the patient has RVDCC, we recommend that they be sent for heart transplant evaluation and, if accepted as a candidate for transplant, proceed down this pathway. These patients do experience some attrition due to coronary ischemic events during the waiting-list period; however, outcomes have generally been good. Survival for pediatric patients undergoing primary transplantation approaches

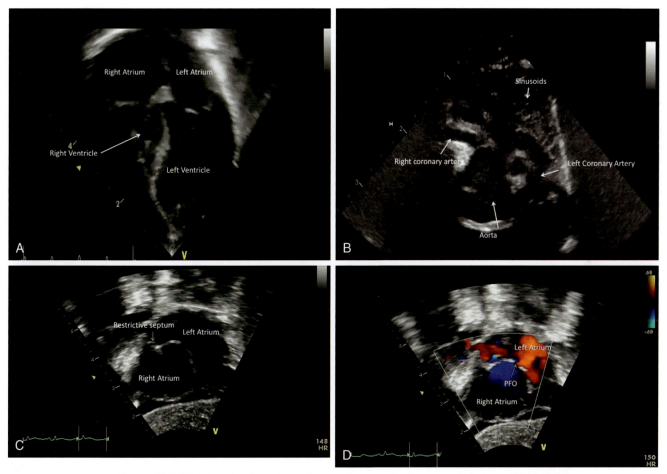

• **Figure 61.4** (A) A four-chamber echocardiogram demonstrates the anatomic features of PA/IVS with a small right ventricle, a small tricuspid valve (compare the tricuspid valve size to the size of the mitral valve), and relatively normal left-sided heart structures. (B) Echocardiogram of infant with PA/IVS demonstrating extremely abnormal coronary arteries. Both coronary arteries are dilated and there are prominent sinusoids in the right ventricle. These abnormalities would be an indication for cardiac cath with angiography to delineate the anatomy and severity of the coronary artery abnormalities and to distinguish if there is RV-dependent coronary artery circulation. (C and D) Two-dimensional echocardiogram (C) of infant with restrictive atrial septum in PA/IVS. Color flow (D) confirms the small right-to-left shunt across the ASD. This atrial septum appears restrictive and a potential limitation for access of systemic venous return to the left ventricle, and it should be treated with atrial septostomy at the time of preoperative cardiac cath.

85% at 5 years[16] in what would otherwise be a uniformly fatal condition in patients with PA/IVS and RVDCC.

Anesthesia Considerations

In general, these infants should be considered severely ill and potentially unstable. Physiologic monitoring in the operating room should include an arterial line in the left upper extremity (avoiding, if possible, the ipsilateral side of the planned aortopulmonary shunt), a central venous line, and near infra-red spectroscopy. Umbilical arterial and venous lines may be used if available. Transesophageal echocardiography (TEE) allows for assessment of myocardial function and the results of surgical intervention.[14]

Surgical Considerations

Single-Ventricle Palliation

Patients with clearly defined RV hypoplasia that is unlikely to support a two-ventricle approach and who do not have RV-dependent coronary circulation will follow the single-ventricle pathway. Due to the obligate duct dependent physiology to maintain pulmonary blood flow, the initial step for these patients is to establish a stable source of blood flow to the lungs. This has been traditionally performed with a modified Blalock-Taussig shunt or a central shunt. Over the past several years we (FS) have worked with our interventional cardiology colleagues on a ductal stenting protocol for these patients and have been pleased with this technique as well. If the patients have a circuitous ductal course, this is often best approached via a right common carotid artery cutdown in the hybrid suite. Using this technique, we have been able to successfully establish stable pulmonary blood flow. In those rare patients for whom we are unable to provide adequate pulmonary blood flow via stenting of the arterial duct, a central shunt from ascending aorta to main pulmonary artery is used.

There has been some controversy regarding whether or not to ligate the PDA when performing a shunt for PA/IVS. Currently, the majority of surgical procedures for shunts reported to the Society of Thoracic Surgeons Congenital Heart Surgery Database (STS CHSD) report leaving the PDA open (not ligated) indicating that leaving the PDA open following a shunt is generally the preferred option for most surgeons.[17] The advantages of leaving the PDA open include the ability to resuscitate the infant in the ICU (with PGE) in the event of shunt thrombosis in the postoperative period, the decreased intraoperative risk of shunt construction without needing to dissect a fragile ductus arteriosus, and a reported decrease in morbidity and mortality associated with leaving a PDA open following Blalock-Taussig shunt,[18] especially in infants with PA/IVS.[19]

Two-Ventricle Palliation

In those patients with anatomy favorable for a biventricular repair strategy based on non-RVDCC, adequacy of the tricuspid valve and RV anatomy, the initial steps in palliation focus on creation of a patent RV outflow tract (RVOT) to allow decompression of the RV and development of anterograde pulmonary blood flow.

Patients who have a tripartite RV and simple plate-like atresia of the valve, with a near normal infundibulum, undergo percutaneous radiofrequency perforation of the outflow tract in the cardiac catheterization laboratory. This is frequently the only procedure required, and they can then be followed over time for the development and severity of pulmonary insufficiency and the need for pulmonary valve placement later in life.

Traditionally we elected to perform this procedure with an open surgical approach. However, we (FS) have shifted our approach since 2007 to a hybrid approach in the newborn period. Although other centers have adapted an "either/or" approach using a percutaneous or surgical approach with sternotomy and cardiopulmonary bypass, we have a true hybrid model. This is similar to the approach described by others,[20,21] with some important differences.

Procedures are done in the hybrid operating suite. A median sternotomy incision is made, and the anterior portion of the RV is exposed. A purse-string is placed toward the inferior margin of the heart, and through this a needle is passed under direct vision, with echocardiographic and fluoroscopic guidance, from the RV cavity to the main pulmonary artery crossing the valve plate. A guide wire is then advanced across the ductus arteriosus and the tip left in the descending aorta. The RV to pulmonary artery connection is then made using a balloon sized to approximate the diameter of the main pulmonary artery. Most often a stent is left in the newly created RVOT to prevent its closure due to infundibular hypertrophy. Postprocedure echocardiography is used to assess ventricular function and tricuspid valve function. Fluoroscopy and completion angiography are used to assess final stent placement and infundibular and pulmonary anatomy.

This technique requires that the surgeon and interventional cardiologist work side by side to achieve the best outcome. It allows the creation of an unobstructed pathway for blood exiting the RV to the lungs and in most cases avoids the need for an alternate source of pulmonary blood flow. If necessary, as measured by oxygen saturations at the time of the procedure, this is easily accomplished at the same setting either with ductal stenting or central aorto-to-pulmonary shunt. Temporary snaring of the ductus at the time of the procedure has been described to allow for assessment of oxygen saturations in patients with tenuous RVOTs.[21] However, we have not found this necessary or useful with the addition of outflow tract stenting.

Patients are followed serially and may require dilation of the RVOT stent. Eventually, usually late in the first year of life, they undergo removal of the stent with patch augmentation of the RVOT and creation of a monocusp, or more recently bicuspid, pulmonary valve along with tricuspid valve repair if necessary.

As described earlier, this technique avoids the need for neonatal cardiopulmonary bypass to establish a surgical RVOT augmentation, along with its accompanying morbidity. Additionally, it avoids the complications of percutaneous intervention with radiofrequency perforation of the outflow tract, particularly in patients with poorly defined infundibulum, including inadvertent extracardiac infundibular perforation. Our experience with this hybrid technique suggests a reduced need for alternate sources of pulmonary blood flow.

One-and-One-Half-Ventricle Palliation

In those patients with questionable RV anatomy and function for a two-ventricle repair, the initial course is identical to that described earlier. Should the RV fail to declare itself as adequate to support the entire cardiac output, a one-and-one-half-ventricle approach is considered. These patients undergo a bidirectional superior cavopulmonary connection to off-load the RV volume load and provide adequate pulmonary blood flow. The inferior caval flow is still directed through the RV in this situation. The ASD can be closed at the time of creation of the one-and-one-half-ventricle circulation or it can be left open and closed at a later time in the cath lab.

Ebstein Malformation and Pulmonary Atresia and Intact Ventricular Septum

We (FS) have used a similar technique in neonates with Ebstein malformation of the tricuspid valve and pulmonary atresia and intact septum. An RV-to-pulmonary artery connection is established without the use of a stent, a central aortopulmonary shunt is created, and the tricuspid valve competence is improved with a DeVega type of annuloplasty, rather than a complex tricuspid repair. The goal of this initial palliation is a more stable circulation that will allow for somatic growth. The patients are then brought back at 5 to 7 months of age, when the RV cavity has grown, and converted to a biventricular physiology with creation of a transannular patch with pulmonary valve creation, takedown of the central shunt, and cone type of tricuspid valve repair.

Summary of Surgical Options

In general, infants with PA/IVS are staged according to their tricuspid valve and RV size, potential for growth of right-sided structures, and presence of coronary artery abnormalities that might preclude RVOT decompression procedures. An algorithm for this is presented in Fig. 61.5 generated from data from the Congenital Heart Surgeons Society (CHSS). Fig. 61.6 shows our treatment algorithm from Joe DiMaggio Children's Hospital.

Postoperative Considerations in the ICU

The postoperative management for patients with PA/IVS is determined by both the procedure as well as by the anatomic burden of the defect. The underlying issues that can complicate postoperative management in the ICU include the severity of the coronary artery disease and the adequacy of the interatrial communication. Infants with severe forms of PA/IVS who have small

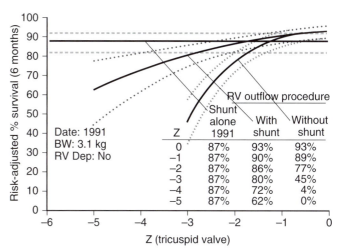

• **Figure 61.5** The effect of tricuspid valve diameter (Z value) and 6-month survival for neonates treated by systemic-to-pulmonary shunt alone versus right ventricular (RV) outflow procedure (pulmonary valvotomy or transannular patch), with or without the addition of a systemic-to-pulmonary shunt. (Reproduced from Hanley FL, Sade RM, Blackstone EH, et al. Outcomes in neonatal pulmonary atresia with intact ventricular septum. A multi-institutional study. *J Thorac Cardiovasc Surg.* 1993;105:406-427, with permission.)

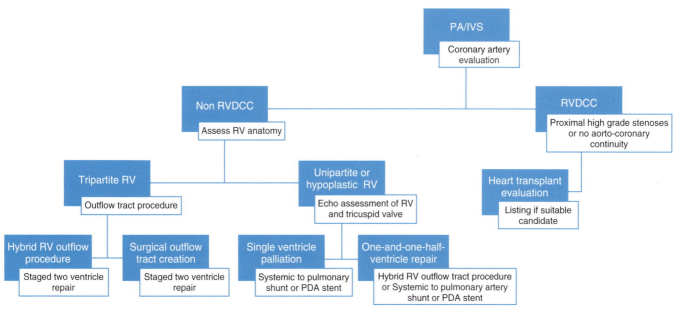

• **Figure 61.6** Treatment algorithm for patients with pulmonary atresia with intact ventricular septum (PA/IVS). *PDA,* Patent ductus arteriosus; *RV,* right ventricle; *RVDCC,* right ventricular–dependent coronary circulation.

(unipartite) RV cavities and who receive an aortopulmonary artery shunt depend on all of the systemic venous return having unobstructed access to the left atrium. When the ASD is no greater than a patent foramen, it can limit cardiac output since restriction at the ASD creates obstruction to increasing systemic venous return. In the presence of a shunt, this can contribute to increased shunt flow into the pulmonary artery with diminished forward cardiac output, presenting with increasing acidosis and pulmonary over-circulation. There is no medical treatment for this condition and an emergent atrial septostomy may be required. A central venous catheter in the right atrium may demonstrate elevated right atrial pressures, but in the presence of severely impaired cardiac output, with diminished return to the right atrium, the CVP may not be as important as a clinical suspicion of this possibility.

If the infant has significant RV to coronary artery connections, an RVOT patch may decompress the right ventricular pressures (which are typically suprasystemic prior to surgery) and create coronary steal with potential for ischemia. This may be heralded by ST segment changes, arrhythmias, or even cardiac arrest. Placing a baby on ECMO following palliation for PA/IVS is a tricky venture, since emptying the right heart has the potential to create even greater decrease in RV pressures with consequent coronary artery steal. This can be true even for babies who have been treated with a shunt alone, and the risk of ECMO is the potential for creating coronary artery ischemia and infarction of affected myocardial beds. However, ECMO (as a bridge to transplant) can be considered as a salvage in otherwise hopeless situations, and it may be important to leave the right heart "full" and not empty it completely.

A decrease in systemic oxygen saturation in the postoperative period requires evaluation. Although shunt thrombosis is possible, systemic oxygen desaturation can also be caused by low cardiac output (with low mixed venous O2 bringing down the mixed systemic saturations—see Chapter 62 on palliative procedures), atelectasis or hemothorax (ruled out by CXR), or low hemoglobin. When shunt thrombosis is suspected, it may be possible to restart prostaglandins (if the ductus was left untied) and to increase shunt (and total body) perfusion with epinephrine until the baby stabilizes. Evaluation of the shunt can be by echocardiogram, but CT or angiography is more definitive. Because of the potential for shunt thrombosis, many centers maintain the infants on low dose heparin for a few days postoperatively, and then switch them to aspirin prior to hospital discharge.

Outcomes

Overall, regardless of anatomic subtype, modern era survival for patients with PA/IVS is in the 70% to 90% range at 10 years[22]; this has improved since the 1980s, when survival rates were reported to be as less than 50% at 5 years.[23-25] Technical improvements in neonatal congenital heart surgery and cardiac catheterization, as well as improvements in the care of patients with single-ventricle physiology, are likely responsible for this improved survival.

Quality of life for patients with PA/IVS has been studied. In a single-institution study, children and adolescents with favorable anatomy for biventricular repair appear to have a normal exercise capacity and cardiac reserve when compared with those with single-ventricle palliation.[26] However, as shown in a multi-institutional study, in patients with smaller initial tricuspid valve z scores, survival with a biventricular repair may be at a cost of late deficits in exercise capacity. These authors emphasized that outcomes may be better in using a one-and-one-half or even a single ventricle strategy in these patients.[27]

Conclusion

PA/IVS is a highly variable continuum of severe congenital heart disease. The severity of disease ranges from patients with simple plate-like pulmonary atresia with relatively normal RV anatomy and geometry who can undergo a biventricular treatment pathway, to those patients with "hypoplastic right heart syndrome" who must undergo single-ventricle palliation. Patients with RV sinusoids and coronary artery fistulae with RV-dependent coronary circulation have an associated high rate of early mortality. Our program has adopted a primary transplant strategy for these fragile patients. For those patients whose anatomy allows for potential one-and-one-half- or two-ventricle pathways we have adapted a hybrid treatment strategy for early palliation with excellent early and midterm results. Quality of life for these patients is subjectively good; however, when measured objectively, many of them continue to have limited exercise capacity.

References

A complete list of references is available at ExpertConsult.com.

62

Palliative Procedures: Deciding on Clinical Pathway; One Versus Two Ventricles

IMMANUEL I. TURNER, MD; RICHARD G. OHYE, MD, CS

Overview

Biventricular repair requires two ventricles, each fully capable of supporting the systemic and pulmonary circulation.[1] Septation has been interpreted as the pursuit of biventricular circulation rather than single-ventricle track.[2] Although successful biventricular repair is preferable, the improvement in neonatal staged palliation has improved single-ventricle prognosis. Recent studies have shown the two-ventricle options that subject both the child and family to multiple surgical procedures and lengthy hospitalizations, as well as low cardiac output, should be avoided.[2] Others argue that an aggressive approach to biventricular or one-and-one-half-ventricle surgical management should be the goal with two ventricles and more complex intraventricular anatomy.[3]

Atrioventricular valve size, ventricular size and volume, chordal configuration, systemic and pulmonary venous return, location of ventricular septal defect(s), and anatomy of intraventricular connections are all components that go into the decision. There are several tools and calculators to help with determining which pathway a patient should ultimately follow based on anatomy and physiology (see Chapter 51 on left ventricular [LV] outflow tract obstruction).

Even after the decision has been made and the patient placed into a single-ventricle pathway, some of these patients may be converted to a one-and-one-half-ventricle or biventricular repair. Although it is preferable to accurately triage appropriate patients to biventricular repair, later conversion is an option. This chapter reviews the decision making for clinical pathway single-ventricle versus biventricular repair, as well as the initial palliative procedures that are requisite for single-ventricle repair. Importantly, the decision-making process described within this chapter addresses the choice of single ventricle versus biventricular based only on the adequacy of the anatomy. The discussion is not relevant to those cases in which the patient can clearly be a biventricular candidate but is felt to be too complex surgically to be accomplished. A patient with two adequate ventricles and two adequate atrioventricular (AV) valves, in the absence of absolute contraindications, such as significant AV valve straddle, should be a candidate for biventricular repair.

Decision Making

Perhaps the most important and likely the very first decision that needs to be made for patients who present with congenital heart disease is "whether the patient will be a complete (two ventricle) repair or need to be staged to palliation (single ventricle—Fontan—or possibly one-and-one-half-ventricle reconstruction). Morphologic information that influences this decision includes concerns about ventricular imbalance (mainly related to the size of the ventricles), septal malalignment, valvar morphology, and the presence of the components of the ventricles.[1] This ventricular imbalance at the ends of the spectrum represent a relatively simple surgical decision. The challenges concerning decision making arise for those subtypes that fall within the borderline position on the spectrum, often resulting in a choice between a "straightforward" single-ventricle palliation or a more complex two-ventricle repair. Decision making can be further complicated by the fact that some patients present with extremely complex anatomy and numerous diagnostic studies may be required to inform the best decisions. Fortunately, it is usually possible to stabilize patients with complex congenital heart disease using a variety of tools, including prostaglandins (to preserve pulmonary or systemic blood flow in ductal dependent lesions), ventilation, and inotropic support in dedicated intensive care units (ICUs) with consolidated and collaborative expertise in managing critical heart disease. This often provides additional time for critical decision making, and the need to make hasty determinations is less usual in the current era. Palliation in unstable or critical patients is often tricky and carries high risk, and the advent of a sophisticated multidisciplinary team approach to these patients has created great benefit. Amid these challenges it is important to remember that, although the outflow obstruction can be related to ventricular imbalance, it is the inflow in the ventricular cavity that may represent the biggest challenge to determining the feasibility of two-ventricle repair.[4]

We will review diagnosis-specific issues for decision making. Many of the following studies give a specific surgical approach to a specific anatomy and physiology, along with decision-making guidelines for selecting between a biventricular or single-ventricle repair. The risk factors that have an impact on early mortality or survival, which are outlined later, are provided with the hope that they might be helpful for application to practice at an individual center. However, there are no data to support a particular pathway that is applicable to all centers. Multi-institutional studies that identify guidelines or calculators may be more broadly applicable. The final decision for univentricular versus biventricular is patient specific and also depends on the experience of the surgeon and the institutional resources.

Left Ventricular Hypoplasia and Outflow Obstruction

The crux for neonates born with systematic outflow obstruction is whether or not the LV is adequate to support systemic circulation. The relationship between LV hypoplasia and outflow obstruction has been related to flow, as well as shear stress at an intraventricular level.[5] At one end of the spectrum there is such severe hypoplasia of the LV, as in hypoplastic left heart syndrome (HLHS), that transplant or a single-ventricle pathway with Fontan completion is required for survival. At the other end of the spectrum the hypoplasia can be mild enough and the LV capable of supporting the systemic circulation. However, it is the gray zone with moderate LV hypoplasia that includes the "borderline" patients where the decision making can be a challenge. The decision making with this anatomy is further complicated by the need to proceed with therapy when the systemic perfusion may be ductal dependent and the pulmonary blood flow unrestricted. It is difficult to determine, based on hemodynamics, if the LV is adequate while the ductus is patent. Consideration is given not only to the size of the LV, but also to the size of the mitral valve, the presence of any secondary obstruction across the mitral valve (as might occur in some forms of parachute mitral valve or other congenital mitral anomalies), the presence of significant endocardial fibroelastosis, the size of the LV outflow tract, the anatomy and size of the aortic valve, and the presence of an aortic coarctation. In addition, the presence of intracardiac shunts at the atrial and/or ventricular level can influence hemodynamics, and this impact needs to be considered when making critical determinations regarding potential for two-ventricle versus one-ventricle pathways. Once the ductus is closed, the values of the cardiac index, LV end-diastolic pressure, and LV outflow gradient can be considered in the determination.[2]

Currently there is no set of defined criteria to identify which patients are more likely to benefit from biventricular repair. Systemic cardiac output obstruction can occur at different levels, including at the level of the mitral valve, LV, LV outflow tract obstruction (LVOTO), aortic valve, or aorta. Several scores and calculators have been developed to try to identify preoperative risk factors for choosing the biventricular pathway (see Chapter 51). The Rhodes score analyzes the LV size, aortic valve area, and mitral valve size.[6] Its application is only for those patients with obstruction at the level of the aortic valve. The Rhodes score evaluation was subsequently updated by Colan et al., with the important caveat that, as with the Rhodes score, it is specifically for critical aortic stenosis and not for the borderline LV. The Colan modification also assumes a mitral valve annulus z score of less than 2, assuming that any mitral valve of that size likely requires univentricular palliation.[7]

The Congenital Heart Surgeons' Society (CHSS) conducted a large prospective multi-institutional trial looking at preoperative characteristics to determine biventricular versus single-ventricle repair.[8] The question they set out to answer was which demographic, morphologic, and functional factors help predict survival benefit for a biventricular repair pathway versus univentricular palliation in neonates with LVOTO. The initial intended biventricular repair

with either balloon dilation or surgical valvotomy was indicated in 116 patients. An initial Norwood procedure was performed in 179 patients. The survival at 5 years for the biventricular repair and Norwood were 70% and 60%, respectively. The study used multivariable hazard models for survival with each of the two pathways. Incremental risk factors for death in patients undergoing biventricular repair included lower z score of aortic valve at sinuses, younger age at entry, and higher-grade endocardial fibroelastosis. Risk factors for death in patients with Norwood as their initial procedure were lower ascending aorta diameter and moderate to severe tricuspid valve regurgitation. Based on these risk factors, a prediction of survival could be calculated for all patients. The predictions for survival for the biventricular repair versus the Norwood pathway were compared with the differences representing predicted survival benefit. The investigators found that although discordant treatment selection (i.e., a patient predicted to benefit from a univentricular repair who underwent a biventricular repair and vice versa) resulted in a worse survival for both univentricular and biventricular repair, the cost of a discordant biventricular repair in a patient who would have been predicted to benefit from a univentricular approach was much more significant.

Conclusions drawn from the CHSS study included the following: mortality is high for neonates with critical LV outflow obstruction, survival is improved with more appropriate selection of the repair pathways, and the pathway predicting survival benefit relates to the adequacy of the left-sided structures. The final result of this study was a multiple linear regression equation that predicted both magnitude and direction of the survival benefit for the optimal pathway based on characteristics of individual patients. The calculator can be found at www.chssdc.org. Follow-up studies have shown reintervention in patients selected inappropriately, as determined by the CHSS score, for biventricular repair tended to have poorer outcomes.[9] This suggests that in borderline cases, univentricular palliation may be the safer strategy based on early to midterm follow-up.

Left ventricular outflow obstruction can occur at multiple levels, allowing for numerous and different options to provide systemic outflow, as well as to address the aortic valve. The Yasui operation, for example, is designed for the unusual patient with arch hypoplasia, severe aortic stenosis, and two well-formed ventricles, two well-formed inlet (AV) valves, and a large ventricular septal defect (VSD). When this combination of lesions is present, the Yasui procedure has shown (whether performed in one or two stages) a lower mortality rate than the Norwood operation.[10] This procedure includes a Damus-Kaye-Stansel connection (detailed later in the chapter), a baffle of the VSD to the systemic outflow, and a conduit for right ventricle (RV) to pulmonary artery (PA) (Fig. 62.1) continuity. Another option for a patient with the combination of defects described earlier is the Ross-Konno procedure, which has been used for enlarging the LV outflow tract and repairing the aortic valve annulus in neonates.[11] Many of the studies aimed at addressing LV outflow obstruction in the neonate have developed parameters to help with the decision making. Some of these criteria include LV outflow tract dimension (subaortic area and valve) greater than or equal to the weight of the patient in kilograms to proceed with standard repair of aortic arch hypoplasia and VSD. Additional criteria include aortic annular dimension greater than 4.5 mm or z score greater than −5.

In combination with any of these procedures the resection of endocardial fibroelastosis can be helpful with long-term ventricular compliance.[12] Both the Yasui and the Ross-Konno are procedures to provide a two-ventricle outcome for complex congenital heart

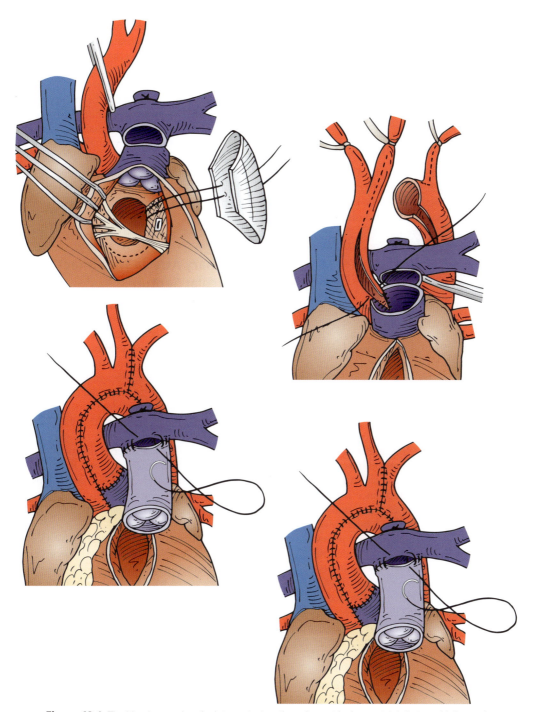

• **Figure 62.1** The Yasui procedure for interrupted aortic arch, ventricular septal defect, and left ventricular outflow tract obstruction. The figure delineates the baffle of the ventricular septal defect to the systemic outflow, the Damus-Kaye-Stansel (DKS) anastomosis, the arch reconstruction, and the right ventricle to pulmonary artery conduit placement. (Modified from Kanter KR. The Yasui operation. *Oper Tech Thorac Cardiovasc Surg.* 2010:206-222.)

disease. However, in some institutions, patients with the defects described earlier may be staged to a single-ventricle pathway, and unique features of the anatomy (disease-specific factors) and of the patient (patient-specific factors) may have critical influence on which pathway is chosen—this field is, unfortunately, that complicated!

Another study looked at echocardiographic parameters to determine independent risk factors for failure of biventricular repair for patients with multiple left heart lesions.[13] By multivariate analysis the predictors of failure identified included moderate/large VSD,

unicommissural aortic valve, and lower mitral valve lateral dimension z score. In the subset of patients with mitral valve involvement (including those with stenosis, hypoplasia, or parachute morphology) the univariate analysis showed failure of biventricular repair was associated with lower LV mass z score and lower mean LV/RV long-axis ratio. Hypoplastic mitral valve annulus was an independent risk factor for failure of the biventricular approach. One caution in determining the degree of mitral stenosis must be taken as it pertains to the transmitral Doppler velocity. The gradient may be underestimated in the presence of an atrial septal defect with left-to-right shunting. It may in fact be the mitral valve that constitutes the bigger difficulty when deciding if biventricular repair is feasible in a patient with multiple left heart obstructive lesions. In addition, following such biventricular repairs such as a Ross-Konno procedure, it is often the mitral valve that contributes significantly to long-term morbidity.[14]

Unbalanced Atrioventricular Septal Defect

Decision making for an unbalanced complete AV septal defect (UCAVSD) is dependent on which ventricle has the majority of the inflow, the percentage of unbalance, and the adequacy of the AV valves. Several studies have identified echocardiographic data aimed at determining parameters that are successful at biventricular repair. Cohen et al. expressed the AV valve index (AVVI) as the ratio of the smaller AV valve component of the divided common AV valve over the larger component. Thus the numerator and denominator could be left or right AV valve area depending on the dominance. More recently to simplify the usage and understanding, the modified AVVI is a ratio of the relative area of the left AV valve in relation to the entire common AV valve.[15] Therefore an AAVI between 0.4 and 0.6 identifies the balanced range of the spectrum. Patients with an AVVI between 0.2 and 0.4 with unbalance to the left (meaning that the RV is larger than the LV) who were treated with a multitude of operative management strategies, including single-ventricle palliation, were found to have poor outcomes. Additional studies have suggested the use of a standard criteria of at least 40% of the common AV valve should overlie the LV to favor a biventricular approach. These data suggest that at the extreme end of the spectrum, patients with severe imbalance and straddling chords are better managed by following the Fontan track.[16] This also holds true when the unbalance is to the right (with a smaller RV compared with the LV) because when one ventricle (and often the size of the potential inlet valve) is too small, it may be better to choose the single-ventricle pathway over a two-ventricle repair. In some circumstances in which the RV is marginal, a one-and-one-half-ventricle pathway could be selected in which the RV is used for the inferior vena cava (IVC) return and the superior vena cava (SVC) return is diverted into the pulmonary arteries directly with a bidirectional Glenn procedure. It is also reasonable to consider a two-ventricle repair, leaving a fenestrated atrial septal defect that can be evaluated and closed at a later time in the catheterization laboratory.

Other reports argue that there is high risk associated with single-ventricle palliation in this particular anatomic condition.[17] It is suggested that a more aggressive surgical approach to parachute mitral valve or closely spaced papillary muscles in right-dominant UCAVSD patients via the splitting of a single papillary muscle head and the elongation of a papillary muscle with release off the LV free wall can be used for biventricular repair. For a left-dominant UCAVSD the tethering attachments to the anterior papillary muscle can be mobilized and the sinus/trabecular portion of the right ventricle enlarged to allow for biventricular repair. More recent studies have examined the inflow angle between the right and left atrioventricular valves and the septum (right ventricle/left ventricle inflow angle) angle in determining right ventricular dominance, which showed promise in guiding early operative decision-making.[18] MRI is extremely helpful for better analysis of ventricular volumes to help guide decision on treatment and should be considered as critical for many of these patients.[19] A major discriminator for proceeding with a biventricular circulation was a measured ventricular volume of the hypoplastic (left) ventricle of greater than 20 mL/m2 by

any imaging (two or three dimensional echocardiography, cardiac MRI, and cardiac catheterization) modalities.[17] That discriminator contrasts with prior reports that argued a volume less than 40 mL/m2 was considered hypoplastic for the LV. The authors caution that the volumes must be measured in the face of equal ventricular pressures and with the septum in the midline position. They expected and observed that the septum shifts rightward in two-ventricular septation in right-dominant lesions. With left-dominant lesions an increase in RV volume was thought to be secondary to papillary muscle mobilization and increased RV inflow. It has been noted that patients with trisomy 21 with severe ventricular hypoplasia as a subgroup have been reported to have poor outcomes with single-ventricle palliation, regardless of whether they have a dominant right or LV, and therefore may benefit from a more aggressive approach at achieving a biventricular repair.

Pulmonary Atresia With Intact Ventricular Septum

The tricuspid valve is the key determinant for successful biventricular repair of pulmonary atresia with an intact ventricular septum, which would generally include an initial procedure of a transannular patch and a systemic to PA shunt. The size of the tricuspid valve is linked to development of a tripartite RV. Outcomes following biventricular repair are significantly worse when the tricuspid valve z score is less than −4.[20] Continued evaluation of the adequacy of the right heart is necessary to determine if the biventricular approach can be successful long term. If the right heart is determined to be inadequate for borderline cases, the one-and-one-half-ventricle pathway, which places a superior cavopulmonary connection while leaving antegrade pulmonary blood flow through the pulmonary valve from the IVC, has been successful. However, the benefit of a one-and-one-half-ventricle repair is theoretical because follow-up studies suggest that exercise capacity and cardiac reserves are similar to univentricular patients.[21]

Biventricular repair with tricuspid valve z score greater than −2.5 and a tripartite RV have improved outcomes with or without a shunt in the early neonatal period. The decision-making process for pulmonary atresia with an intact ventricular septum can be further complicated by the presence of coronary fistulae, particularly in the setting of RV dependence of the coronary circulation (Fig. 62.2). When there are two of three main coronary arteries dependent on the high-pressure RV for coronary supply, it is not prudent to decompress the RV and pursue a biventricular approach. In these patients single-ventricle palliation also carries a higher risk, not only initially, but also during subsequent staged palliation. Primary transplantation has been suggested as a preferred option for this population.[22]

Congenitally Corrected Transposition of the Great Arteries

The anatomic correction of congenitally corrected transposition of the great arteries with the "double switch" operation has been well studied. The aim of this approach is to allow the LV to function as the systemic ventricle. More recently there have been some risk factors identified, such as the need for LV retraining, whereby single-ventricle palliation may lead to better outcomes than a two-ventricle approach. If the VSD is restrictive, then LV pressure can be less than the RV (systemic) pressure at the time of presentation, depending on the presence of important subpulmonary stenosis (which is often present in this lesion. The LV outflow tract connects to the PA, and the combination of LV outflow

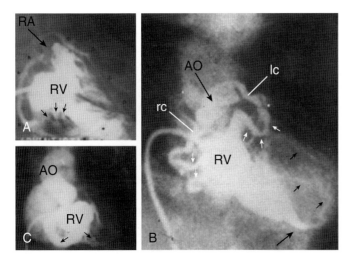

• **Figure 62.2** Right ventriculography in the anteroposterior projection of pulmonary atresia with intact ventricular septum. (A) Pulmonary atresia with imperforate valve. Note great development of coronary-cavitary connections *(arrows)* originating from the inlet and trabecular portions with right and left coronary arteries opaque. (B) Infundibular pulmonary atresia and reduced tricuspid valve dimensions. *White arrows* point to coronary-cavitary connections which communicate with the right *(rc)* and left coronary *(lc)* arteries. (C) Right ventricle is reduced in the inlet portion. Tricuspid valve dimensions are reduced. The aorta is densely opaque due to huge myocardial sinusoid/right coronary communication. *Ao,* Aorta; *RA,* right atrium; *RV,* right ventricle. (Modified from Santos MA, Azevedo VM. *Arq Bras Cardiol.* 2004;82[5]:420-425.)

obstruction—pulmonary stenosis—and VSD is common). When there is no LV outflow obstruction, the LV will need training to help prepare it to accommodate the systemic circulation. If the patient is older, as in a teenager or young adult, the results of training followed by the double switch procedure have been disappointing. Other studies have shown that age greater than 12 years is associated with a greater probability of LV failure and higher operative mortality at anatomic correction.[23] Survival in subsequent studies was 84.9% at 7 years. Twelve percent had new LV dilation or impaired systolic ventricular function, and 14% developed aortic regurgitation after the double switch.[24] Patients in that series who required LV training had moderate to severe LV dysfunction (39% compared with 6% who required no LV training).

Anatomic factors complicating a double switch include dextrocardia (especially when a Senning/Rastelli procedure is required to complete the conversion to anatomic repair, and this risk is most likely secondary to conduit compression under the sternum), anomalous coronaries, and predominant inlet rather than conoventricular VSD. Although the majority can be overcome to allow an anatomic repair, a physiologic repair can be considered. However, the outcomes of a traditional physiologic repair of congenitally corrected transposition of the great arteries with VSD closure, leaving the RV as the systemic ventricle, have been disappointing. This traditional approach of VSD closure versus Fontan procedure was evaluated. The best long-term outcomes were found with the Fontan procedure.[25] Risk factors for death at any time were RV end-diastolic pressure greater than 17 mm Hg, complete heart block after surgery, subvalvar pulmonary stenosis, and Ebstein malformation of the tricuspid valve.

Heterotaxy Syndrome

The complex ventricular relationships and positioning associated with heterotaxy syndrome may complicate biventricular repairs in

this patient population. These can be complex operations, and venous abnormalities (for both the systemic and pulmonary venous return) have been identified as risk factors for repair (either univentricular or biventricular) with the need for complex intraatrial baffles (in two-ventricle repairs) or the presence of progressive pulmonary venous stenosis (in one-ventricle pathways) carrying a late risk of obstruction. In general it is our opinion that essentially any patient with two adequate ventricles and two adequate AV valves should be considered a candidate for a biventricular repair. Despite that goal, many patients in this category are still treated with single-ventricle palliation, and the following information is included for completeness. The single-ventricle pathway results in this population have been less than ideal, although they have improved more recently.[26] Hemodynamics are critical to consider in decision making for these patients if a single-ventricle palliation is undertaken. Many of these patients may have abnormal and obstructed pulmonary venous drainage, and in these cases the single-ventricle pathway is not likely to lead to a satisfactory outcome. A single-ventricle pathway may be applied to patients with good ventricular compliance and function, well-developed pulmonary arteries, and low pulmonary resistance (implying unobstructed pulmonary venous drainage).

Palliative Procedures

Once the decision is made to proceed with a single-ventricle pathway, the most critical factors include both when the patient should receive the initial palliation and what that palliation should be. The four keys to optimal palliation include (1) a precise diagnosis before palliation, (2) an initial operation that prevents potential late problems (such as progressive ventricular outflow obstruction), (3) adequate, controlled pulmonary blood flow, and (4) timely ventricular unloading with either bidirectional superior cavopulmonary anastomosis (bidirectional Glenn) or hemi-Fontan procedure.[27]

Accurate preoperative evaluation is essential to planning the optimal initial palliation. Initial procedures may have to be adapted in the presence of complicating factors, such as systemic outflow obstruction (intracardiac, aortic arch, coarctation) and pulmonary venous obstruction (anomalous pulmonary venous connection and restrictive atrial septal defect). The first palliation is performed with the eventual goal of normalization of the volume and pressure work of the functional ventricle, while supplying blood adequately saturated with oxygen to the systemic circulation, regardless of the underlying cardiac anatomy.[27] Pulmonary vascular resistance (PVR) in the early neonatal period precludes obtaining this goal in one step; therefore the palliation needs to be provided in stages that are all compatible with an ultimate plan for each individual patient.

The initial postnatal palliation requires that the pulmonary and systemic circulation remain in parallel, while pulmonary blood flow is controlled, allowing for proper development and maturation of the pulmonary vascular bed. The following stages of the palliation are to create a gradual conversion to Fontan physiology, first with superior venocavopulmonary connection and subsequently to complete cavopulmonary connection (Fontan), which then alters the circulation from being in parallel to one connected in series.

The early postnatal medical management is directed at determination of the anatomy and management of the volume and pressure load on the ventricle while maintaining adequate oxygen delivery. Underlying the stabilization is the delicate balance between the systemic and pulmonary vascular resistance with the understanding that over the first 4 to 6 weeks the PVR will fall and adjustments may have to be made accordingly.[28] This initial time period is one of continued evaluation and adjustment to maintaining the patient's clinical stability. The evaluation is directed at answering the following questions: (1) Is there a reliable source of systemic blood flow? (2) Is there a reliable source of pulmonary blood flow? (3) Is there any impediment to pulmonary venous return? and (4) Is there an appropriate balance between the systemic and pulmonary circulations?[28] For complex patients, and many of these patients present complex anatomic challenges, there may be obstruction (or potential for late development of obstruction) to systemic or pulmonary blood flow. For these patients the ductus arteriosus can often be maintained with prostaglandin to support both systemic and pulmonary blood flow while decisions are made regarding the most appropriate surgical staging.

Prostaglandin E_1 (PGE_1) was initially described by Olley and colleagues[29] in 1976. Patients benefiting from PGE_1 can be divided into ductal dependent pulmonary (i.e., pulmonary atresia with intact ventricular septum, or tricuspid atresia) and systemic (HLHS) circulation. Both of these groups require PGE_1 soon after birth to maintain adequate systemic oxygen delivery. When ductal patency is part of the management, the balance between systemic and pulmonary blood flow can initially be challenging. When the circulations are in parallel (meaning ventricular output can distribute through the ductus to either the systemic or pulmonary bed), the relative blood flow to each circulation depends predominantly on relative balance between pulmonary and systemic vascular resistance. Because pulmonary resistance is generally much lower than systemic resistance, flow across the ductus, presuming "normal" vascular beds to the pulmonary and systemic circulation, is typically increased to the pulmonary vascular bed, including diastolic "runoff" from the systemic circulation into the pulmonary circulation. Manipulation of the inspired gases can help manage the balance of systemic and pulmonary circulation by changing the vascular resistance in the pulmonary bed.[30] Oxygen is a potent pulmonary vasodilator. Hypercarbia is a significant vasoconstrictor and cerebral vasodilator. Even with optimal medical management, there may still be an imbalance between the pulmonary and systemic blood flow. This relative imbalance can ultimately adversely affect the patient from a hemodynamic and systemic oxygen delivery standpoint. Thus earlier surgical palliation may be necessary when medical manipulations are inadequate to overcome the resulting imbalance in circulation.

The goals of initial palliation are to provide unobstructed systemic blood flow, controlled pulmonary blood flow with well-balanced pulmonary and systemic circulations, and unobstructed pulmonary and systemic venous return.[4] The primary surgical options for initial palliation include (1) PA band, (2) systemic to PA shunt, (3) Damus-Kaye-Stansel (DKS) procedure, (4) Norwood/hybrid Norwood, and (5) early bidirectional Glenn or hemi-Fontan procedure. The optimal procedure to accomplish these goals will depend on the anatomy (disease-specific factors) and on the age, size, and condition of the patient at the time of presentation (patient-specific factors). Timing of initial palliation depends on the severity of the flow imbalance at baseline with regard to the pulmonary circulation. In patients with reduced pulmonary blood flow the degree of cyanosis (<70%) is the best indicator to proceed with surgical palliation with systemic to PA shunting or other appropriate form of palliation. Excessive pulmonary blood flow and the onset of signs and symptoms consistent with volume overload and heart failure (growth failure, tachycardia, tachypnea, and the need for mechanical ventilation) suggest the need for intervention. These signs will worsen as the PVR decreases. Common

methods to control pulmonary blood flow include PA banding or PA ligation and a systemic to PA shunt. Control of excessive pulmonary blood flow will also be important to control the pressure and volume overload to the pulmonary circulation and to protect the lungs from the development of pulmonary vascular obstructive disease. When the patient has obstruction (or potential for obstruction) to systemic outflow, conversion of systemic outflow to the pulmonary outflow tract with a DKS type of procedure (including a Norwood reconstruction) should be considered. In these circumstances in which the pulmonary outflow tract is converted to become the systemic outflow, a source of pulmonary blood flow (either an aortopulmonary shunt or an RV-PA conduit) may need to be incorporated into the plan.

Historically, congenital heart surgery was linked to palliation because complete repair of heart defects in infancy was technically challenging. Therefore the early history of palliation included staged repair of heart defects. The lessons learned from and the techniques that evolved from these procedures that were intended to keep patients alive until more definitive surgery could be performed have greatly influenced the current methods for palliation.

Pulmonary Artery Banding

Neonatal presentation with excessive pulmonary blood flow and signs of heart failure require control of the pulmonary blood flow to allow adequate somatic growth, to eliminate the volume load on the ventricle, and to protect the pulmonary vascular bed from the development of pulmonary vascular obstructive disease as the normal post- decrease in PVR occurs.[28] The strategy of PA banding is an attempt to optimize the pulmonary-to-systemic blood flow ratio (Q_p:Q_s) to avoid the potential for resultant multiorgan system dysfunction.[31] PA banding, first described by Muller and Danimann in 1952, is the creation of "controlled" pulmonary stenosis to prevent pulmonary hypertension and excessive pulmonary blood flow.[27,32] The approach previously included left thoracotomy or median sternotomy. We more commonly perform PA banding through a median sternotomy to allow for better positioning of the band and to minimize distortion of the branch pulmonary arteries. Furthermore, median sternotomy provides excellent and flexible access to virtually any anatomic arrangement, and it also becomes the only incision many of these patients need, even for future repairs, thus limiting the number of incisions. A variety of materials (polytetrafluoroethylene [PTFE], umbilical tape, silk ligature) can be used to make the band at the discretion of the surgeon.

The Trusler formula for PA banding is a calculation used to estimate the starting band circumference: 24 mm +1 mm/kg in weight for a total admixture defect (single ventricle).[33] The formula has been modified by Baslaim[34] to place a band that is 2.25 mm more narrow in the single-ventricle patient population. This affords effective protection of the PA bed so that the PVR at the time of the stage II and Fontan procedures is as low as possible.

After circumferential dissection the PA is encircled by a subtraction technique or direct around the PA. The band is then tightened with clips or sutures sequentially placed through the band. Historically PA bands were commonly used to control excessive PA blood flow in infants with symptomatic VSDs until they grew larger and were more amenable to surgical VSD closure. When banding for patients with VSDs (who would ultimately become candidates for a two-ventricle repair), the goal of the band was to drop the PA pressure to approximately one-half the systemic pressure. A tighter band often created less pulmonary blood flow and significant hypoxemia. The goal for single-ventricle patients is somewhat different because it is essential to protect the pulmonary vascular bed from high pressure to enable conversion to cavopulmonary physiology in a timely fashion. For this reason we generally band the PA as tightly as we can—often dropping the PA pressure distal to the band to a "normal" PA pressure (20 mm Hg). We pay attention to the arterial oxygen saturation that results and aim to have the PA pressure as low as possible with oxygen saturations in the 75% to 85% range. When placing a band, the systemic pressures may increase. However, concomitant with this is an increase in afterload because the ventricle no longer has the low-resistance pulmonary circuit as an unobstructed "pop off," so some of these patients may require brief (1 to 2 day) therapy with low-dose inotropes. Postoperatively it is important to make sure that the patient has adequate systemic oxygen delivery (meaning the patient has adequate systemic oxygen saturations), as noted previously, along with adequate systemic cardiac output, which can usually be monitored by following the lactic acid levels. In some cases the heart cannot manage this change in afterload, and the band may need to be adjusted in the few days following initial banding.

The PA pressure can be measured distally by direct pressure catheter to assess band tightness. Transesophageal echocardiography is helpful to determine placement and ensure no encroachment on the valve and minimal distortion of the branch pulmonary arteries. Echocardiography can also provide a Doppler flow measurement across the band site, which can be useful in measuring PA pressure. A more normal PA pressure facilitates interpretation of the PA pressure distal to the band, as well as the gradient measured by echocardiography. Pulmonary artery banding is more commonly used in single-ventricle patients with tricuspid atresia, double-inlet LV, and unbalanced AV septal defect with unrestricted pulmonary blood flow.

Caution should be used in placing PA bands in single-ventricle patients with discordant ventricular-arterial connections and reliance on a VSD or bulboventricular foramen for systemic output because this anatomic substrate can lead to systemic outflow obstruction.[4] The postoperative course after banding a patient with this anatomy can involve significant myocardial hypertrophy and obstruction in as many as 70% of patients.[35] These patients would be better served with a DKS or a modified Norwood procedure with pulmonary blood flow provided by a systemic to PA shunt to provide reliable systemic outflow.[36]

Hybrid palliation consisting of bilateral PA banding and ductal stenting and a modified hybrid approach with bilateral PA banding and continuation of PGE_1 are strategies that have been used for HLHS and other complex congenital cardiac defects until second-stage palliation can be performed.[37] This has been shown to be an effective method of resuscitation for high-risk single-ventricle neonates. The second surgery can include conventional Norwood (rapid stage) or primary transplantation.[31] Caution should be used with ductal stenting in the presence of a diminutive ascending aorta secondary to the increased risk of compromised coronary perfusion.[38]

Systemic to Pulmonary Artery Shunt

Shunts connecting the systemic to pulmonary circulation trace back to the early history of congenital heart surgery. Originally these shunts provided lifesaving pulmonary blood flow to patients with cyanotic heart defects at a time when there simply was no technology to allow for complete repair of the underlying defect.

There are many who believe that the field of cardiac surgery was launched with the creation of the first shunt by Alfred Blalock that connected the divided subclavian artery to the side of the right PA in an infant with severe tetralogy of Fallot. The success of this procedure (a Blalock-Taussig [BT] shunt), an outcome from research in Dr. Blalock's animal laboratory with help from surgical technician Vivien Thomas and innovative encouragement from his cardiology colleague, Helen Taussig, opened the possibility for surgeons to treat a spectrum of congenital heart defects characterized by inadequate pulmonary blood flow. Soon other types of shunts were created, including the Waterston shunt and the Potts shunt. Although the Waterston and Potts shunts are of only historical interest, the classic BT shunt, which is a direct end-to-side anastomosis of the transected subclavian artery to the PA, is still used in some centers.[39] The Waterston shunt involves an aortopulmonary connection with anastomosis between the posterior aorta and the anterior right PA.[40] The Potts shunt involves a connection between the descending thoracic aorta and the left PA (Fig. 62.3).[41]

For the most part, due to a variety of issues associated with the shunt described previously, a modified BT shunt has become the one most commonly used in initial palliation in the current era. The original description of the modified BT shunt was by de Leval et al in 1981. The modification involved the interposition of a polytetrafluoroethylene (PTFE) graft between the subclavian artery and the PA.[42] The modified BT shunt can be approached through a right or left thoracotomy and median sternotomy. The approach can depend on subclavian and PA anatomy, the presence and location of the ductus arteriosus, the great vessel relationship, and surgeon preference. There has been an increasing trend toward use of the median sternotomy for this procedure. The sternotomy approach is technically more flexible (enabling shunt placement from and to a variety of locations to connect the systemic circulation to the pulmonary circulation regardless of the variation in anatomy) and is associated with fewer shunt failures than thoracotomy.[43]

Advantages of the sternotomy include the availability of using cardiopulmonary bypass if necessary, no compromise to the lung function affecting the oxygen saturation, decreased intrathoracic collateral formation from adhesions if the pleural space is not opened, more central placement on the pulmonary arteries, flexibility despite unusual anatomic challenges, and access for ligation of the ductus arteriosus should the surgical team feel this is helpful. The anastomosis is performed with occlusion clamps on the subclavian artery and the PA and can be done with or without cardiopulmonary bypass depending on the patient's degree of desaturation. The diameter of the PTFE interposition graft acts as a resistor to control pulmonary blood flow. The amount of flow through the shunt is determined by Poiseuille's law.[44] All factors being constant, the flow of blood through the shunt will be determined by the diameter of the shunt to the fourth power (r^4). As a result, shunt selection is a critical point in the decision-making process. Shunt size selection can be guided by the patient's weight (in kilograms) and an approximate guide is (1.5 to 2.0 kg) 3.0-mm shunt, (2.0 to 4.0 kg) 3.5-mm shunt, (4.0 to 5.0 kg) 4.0-mm shunt. Other changes that can play a role include alteration in the length of the graft and changes in position on the systemic arterial tree.

The postprocedural oxygen saturation goal should be 75% to 85%, indicating an appropriate-size shunt and Q_p:Q_s close to 1. The shunt can be heparin bonded to minimize risk of thrombosis.[45] Both anastomoses are usually created with 7-0 polypropylene suture. A thrill can be palpated in the shunt and distal PA. Transesophageal echocardiography can be used to assess the shunt if desired. Adequate systemic perfusion must be maintained and may initially

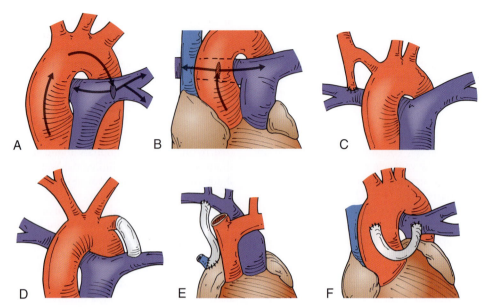

• **Figure 62.3** Shunt types. (A) Potts shunt. (B) Waterston shunt. (C) Blalock-Taussig shunt (classic). (D) Left Blalock-Taussig shunt (usually this is performed when there is a right aortic arch—not as depicted here for a left aortic arch). (E) Modified Blalock-Taussig shunt (using Gore-Tex). (F) Central shunt (using Gore-Tex). (From Ungerleider RM, Sabiston DC Jr. The tetralogy of Fallot. In: Sabiston DC Jr, ed. *Textbook of Surgery: The Biological Basis of Modern Surgical Practice.* Philadelphia: WB Saunders; 1991.)

require additional inotropic support. As in the preoperative setting, balancing systemic and pulmonary vascular resistances can be used, although it may have less effect due to the fixed resistance of the graft.

Anticoagulation with heparin is frequently used over the first postoperative night in the ICU to help reduce the risk for shunt thrombosis. Many surgeons leave the ductus open at the time of shunt placement (historically, through a thoracotomy the ductus was never ligated because it was often inaccessible from the surgical site) and allow it to close spontaneously after prostaglandins are stopped. That way, in the unusual advent of shunt thrombosis, the ICU staff may be able to regain stability of the patient by restarting prostaglandins. Aspirin 1–5 mg/kg/dose orally daily is often started postoperative day 1. Aspirin for shunt thrombosis prophylaxis is commonly used, although evidence for efficacy is mainly based on observational data. A retrospective study evaluated the impact of aspirin on preventing shunt thrombosis and improving survival.[46] Researchers concluded that there was a beneficial effect on both shunt thrombosis and survival rates. A recent randomized controlled trial showed that clopidogrel coupled with aspirin is no better than aspirin alone. A subgroup analysis showed a 40% relative risk reduction in the incidence of primary outcomes with aspirin alone (death, transplantation, or shunt thrombosis).[47]

Takedown of the shunt, at the time of the next stage, involves dividing the shunt and preserving the subclavian and pulmonary arteries. Failure to divide the shunt can result in tenting of the PA and possible PA stenosis.

Another challenge with the creation of a systemic-to-PA shunt is the management of preexisting antegrade pulmonary blood flow. Preservation of antegrade blood flow can contribute to pulmonary overcirculation and volume overload, which is further worsened in a patient with AV valve regurgitation. The preservation is sometimes related to the desire to provide protection in the event of shunt thrombosis. However, the presence of competitive flow has been associated with trends toward increased shunt thrombosis

and mortality.[48] The decision to maintain a patent native pulmonary outflow tract remains at the discretion of the surgeon.

The modified BT shunt is frequently considered to be a simple procedure and low-risk solution to complex defects. However, there is still associated important morbidity and mortality. The Society of Thoracic Surgeons Congenital Heart Surgery Database recently reported a 7.2% hospital mortality after modified BT shunt. In subgroup analysis they identified the diagnosis of pulmonary atresia with intact ventricular septum and a functionally univentricular heart as being predictive for early mortality and for composite morbidity defined as the need for reoperation or mechanical circulatory support.[49] Other risk factors for survival after a modified BT shunt included weight less than 3 kg and a larger shunt size-to-weight ratio. This decreased early survival underscores the risk of oversizing the shunt or maintaining a patent pulmonary outflow tract, in addition to the effect of overcirculation on late survival.[50]

Central shunts have also been performed with PTFE interposition grafts between the aorta and the main PA.[51] The central shunt can be approached through a median sternotomy. The main PA and branches are mobilized. The procedure can be performed with or without cardiopulmonary bypass. If performed without cardiopulmonary bypass, heparin 1.5 mg/kg or 100 U/kg can be administered. A side-biting clamp is placed on the main or branch PA, a longitudinal incision is made, and an end-to-side anastomosis is performed with 7-0 polypropylene running suture. The aorta can be clamped with a side-biting clamp, and either incision or hole punch can be used for aortotomy. The graft is cut to an appropriate length and anastomosed to the aorta, end to side, with 7-0 polypropylene running suture.[51] Shunt sizing ranges from 3.0 to 6.0 mm based on weight: (<3.0 kg) 3.0 mm, (<6.0 kg) 3.5 mm, and (>6.0 kg) 4.0 mm. The exact configuration of the shunt is at the discretion of the surgeon and will depend on the specific anatomy of the patient. Stretch PTFE can be particularly useful when a curve is necessary (see Fig. 62.3).

Damus-Kaye-Stansel Procedure

Functional single-ventricle anomalies that may have systemic ventricular outflow tract obstruction due to restriction at a VSD or bulboventricular foramen include those with tricuspid atresia and double-inlet LV and ventriculoarterial discordance and d- or l-transposition of the great arteries with hypoplasia of the RV. The obstruction may be evident at the time of birth, and these univentricular patients require an initial palliation that includes a DKS procedure. Even when no obstruction is present at the time of presentation, these patients remain at risk for developing obstruction over time at the level of the VSD or bulboventricular foramen, so strong consideration of a DKS should be given to any patient with these diagnoses.

The DKS procedure has contributed to improved clinical outcomes following the Fontan completion by addressing the systemic outflow obstruction, if present at birth, or preventing its potential development later as restriction develops at the VSD or bulboventricular foramen. Damus, Kaye, and Stansel originally described an end-to-side anastomosis between the main PA and the ascending aorta to achieve a biventricular repair in patients with d-transposition of the great arteries.[52] The original DKS procedure was an end-to-side anastomosis between the main PA and ascending aorta with or without a prosthetic patch to roof the anastomosis (Fig. 62.4). Since the original there have been many modifications. Laks et al.[52a] reported on the aortic flap technique as a modification that involves an incision for the posteriorly based triangular flap along with a prosthetic patch (see Fig. 62.4).

The operation can be performed with conventional continuous-flow cardiopulmonary bypass with mild to moderate hypothermia (24°C to 34°C). The end-to-side anastomosis is then performed with a 7-0 polypropylene suture and, if necessary, a prosthetic patch to enlarge the ascending aorta. Waldman and colleagues[53] reported technical modifications of the DKS in which the aorta was sutured to create a new bivalve single aorta known as the "double-barrel method." The double-barrel or side-to side anastomosis is performed after both the aorta and pulmonary trunk are divided above the level of the sinus and sutured together, involving approximately half of the circumference of the pulmonary trunk.[54] The common orifice of both great arteries is then anastomosed to the divided ascending aorta using polypropylene sutures.

In both operations the semilunar valve is evaluated at the time of anastomosis. Semilunar valve distortion resulting in aortic or pulmonary regurgitation has been evaluated in several studies. The double-barrel technique has been shown to less frequently be associated with deterioration in pulmonary regurgitation when compared to the end-to-side technique.[55] For patients undergoing pulmonary artery band placement before DKS, the duration of the band placement was the only risk factor identified on subgroup analysis as contributing to postoperative semilunar valve regurgitation.[56] Ultimately, the decision for surgical technique will be based on the anatomy and surgeon preference. If the relationship of the great arteries is anterior-posterior, the double-barrel technique can be performed. Likewise, if the relationship of the great arteries is side by side, the double-barrel or ascending aortic flap technique can be performed. The discrepancy between the aorta-to-pulmonary anastomosis and the ascending aorta may require patch augmentation to prevent stenosis.

In cases in which systemic outflow obstruction is associated with aortic arch hypoplasia or coarctation of the aorta, a Norwood procedure is recommended. The Norwood reconstruction is essentially an "extensive Damus-Kaye-Stansel." It creates a single outflow from the heart using the pulmonary outflow tract. In cases in which there is a stenotic and hypoplastic aortic valve, the aortic valve is a secondary outlet, and the net result is that all cardiac output is directed into a single, newly constructed aorta. When necessary, this reconstructed aorta extends around the aortic arch and past any area of juxtaductal aortic coarctation. The reader is referred to Chapter 66 to learn more about this procedure.

In both the DKS and the Norwood procedure the PA becomes a systemic outflow tract, and a subsequent source of pulmonary flow needs to be created. Typically this is either an aortopulmonary shunt or an RV-PA conduit. In cases with a hypoplastic RV or a RV that is supplied with blood across a VSD (bulboventricular foramen), an RV-PA conduit may be contraindicated. An in-depth discussion regarding the most appropriate source of pulmonary blood flow, techniques of intraoperative management, and cerebral protection are beyond the scope of this chapter. In brief, the Norwood operation was initially described in 1981 and involved a modified BT shunt as the source of pulmonary blood flow. A modification to the Norwood procedure included the RV to PA conduit as the source of pulmonary blood flow. Some centers use a central shunt as the source of pulmonary blood flow. The technique for pulmonary blood flow is related to stability of the patient postoperatively given the potential for coronary steal from diastolic runoff with both the central and modified BT shunt. A multicenter randomized trial comparing the modified BT shunt and RV-PA (in patients with HLHS) conduit was performed.[57] There was a 10% reduction in mortality at 1 year in patients with the RV-PA conduit. However, there was no significant difference in transplant-free survival at 2 years following the Norwood procedure between the two groups.[58]

The Hybrid Procedure

An alternative to the surgical Norwood procedure, particularly for very high-risk patients, is the hybrid procedure, which involves stenting of the ductus arteriosus and banding of the branch pulmonary arteries in the catheterization laboratory. Gibbs et al.[59] initially described the hybrid approach for HLHS patients in 1993. The motivation for performing the hybrid procedure was to move the high-risk Norwood procedure out of the neonatal period with the hopes of improving both neurodevelopmental outcomes and survival. Follow-up studies looking at subsequent surgical palliation have shown that delaying the surgical palliation with a comprehensive stage II (a combination of an arch reconstruction and a cavopulmonary connection) did not mitigate the impact of early risk factors.[60] Fontan candidacy and transplant-free survival were similar between the two groups undergoing a Norwood stage I or comprehensive stage II. Overall, survival rates of standard palliation at experienced centers remain higher than those published for the hybrid procedure.[61] The selection of a hybrid or a Norwood procedure should depend on individual center outcomes and resources. The other caveat with the hybrid procedure is the potential for distortion of the central pulmonary arteries and decreased pulmonary arterial growth, resulting in an increased rate of pulmonary arterial interventions.[62] A more recent study has shown that the risk factor for PA intervention is duration of bilateral PA bands, with patients having bands longer than 90 days at the highest risk.[63] Due to this finding, as well as to avoid the dilation of the proximal main PA that complicated the aortic reconstruction portion of the comprehensive stage II operation, an evolving strategy is the rapid stage I Norwood. With this strategy the hybrid procedure is initially performed for higher-risk patients, and after improvement

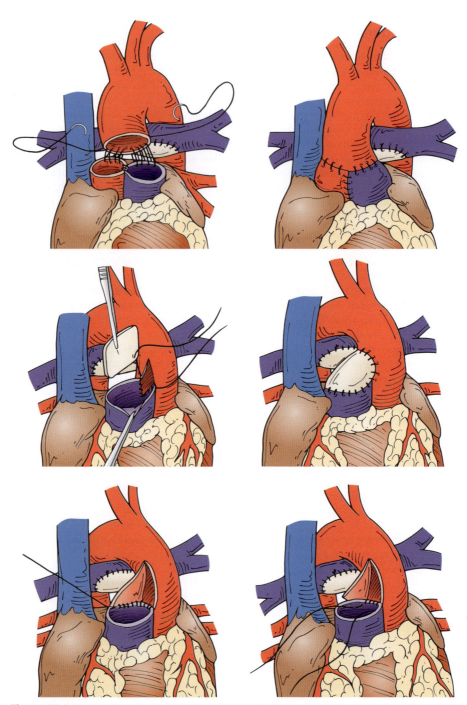

• **Figure 62.4** Damus-Kaye-Stansel (DKS) procedure. The figure depicts (top to bottom) the double-barrel technique, the standard DKS technique, and the modified flap technique. (Modified from Laks H, Gates RN, Elami A, et al. Damus-Stansel-Kaye procedure: technical modifications. *Ann Thorac Surg.* 1992;54:169-172.)

in clinical status a traditional Norwood is performed, which avoids both the challenges of long-term PA banding and subsequent comprehensive stage II (Fig. 62.5).

Superior Cavopulmonary Anastomosis

First described by Jacobs and Norwood in 1996 in a series of over 400 patients undergoing the hemi-Fontan procedure, the addition of a stage II operation is considered to be one of the most significant advances in the care of the functionally univentricular heart.[27,64]

This interim stage allows for the elimination of the shunt-dependent physiology of the Norwood procedure. This in turn removes the volume overload on the single ventricle, allowing it to remodel and decrease the ventricular end-diastolic pressure before the Fontan procedure.[65] Another advantage is that other anatomic or physiologic abnormalities (e.g., PA stenosis/distortion or AV valvar regurgitation) can be addressed at the time of this stage, thus promoting the patient to become a better candidate for ultimate completion Fontan. The operation is well tolerated in patients as early as 3 months of age, and typical timing between 4 and 6 months of age

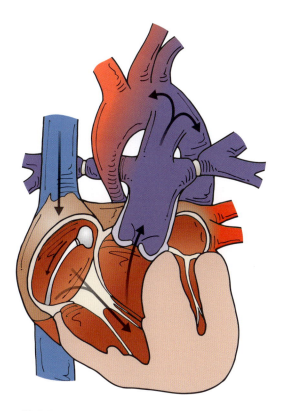

• **Figure 62.5** The hybrid procedure. This procedure involves enlargement of atrial-level communication (if necessary), bilateral pulmonary artery band placement, and ductal stent insertion. (Modified from Galantowicz M, Cheatham JP, Phillips A, et al. Hybrid approach for hypoplastic left heart syndrome: intermediate results after the learning curve. *Ann Thorac Surg.* 2008:85:2063-2070.)

has been shown to increase survival and progression to Fontan completion in some subsets of patients.[65,66] In patients with bilateral SVCs, delay of movement to bilateral, bidirectional Glenn procedures has been recommended, and this makes sense because resistance to flow through a tube (as described earlier) is related to the fourth power of the radius of the tube. In bilateral SVC, each SVC is "smaller" than the normal single SVC and therefore will produce more resistance to flow, which might be a factor in adaptation to cavopulmonary circulation. The type of superior cavopulmonary connection has been shown to have little influence on long-term outcomes. The hemi-Fontan is technically more complex; however, those who prefer it argue that it provides superior flow characteristics and less energy loss in computer flow modeling, improves flow to the central pulmonary arteries, and facilitates a lateral tunnel Fontan (Fig. 62.6). Operative details have been extensively published previously.[67]

The bidirectional Glenn procedure is less complex from a technical standpoint and is more appropriate for a subsequent extracardiac Fontan (Fig. 62.7). Although performance of a bidirectional Glenn anastomosis without cardiopulmonary bypass has also been described, most centers describe using continuous cardiopulmonary bypass with a small right-angle cannula in the high SVC or SVC/innominate vein junction. In either case it is important to ligate the azygous vein (unless the azygous is a continuation of an interrupted IVC) to prevent pop off of cavopulmonary flow to the IVC, which would result in decreasing pulmonary flow.

It is imperative that the ICU team appreciate the unique requirements of postoperative management in the patient following a Glenn or hemi-Fontan (superior cavopulmonary anastomosis) procedure. First of all, these patients will remain mildly hypoxemic and usually have systemic oxygen saturations in the 80% range. Despite these saturations the Glenn procedure provides a important hemodynamic advantage. Before this stage, many patients are surviving from an aortopulmonary shunt. In a shunted patient there is a need for additional cardiac output (a cardiac output for the body and additional output to supply the shunt). The heart needs to eject one output that goes to the body and additional output that perfuses the shunt for pulmonary blood flow. In a patient with 1:1 shunt flow versus systemic flow, this would predict a double cardiac output! Once the patient is converted to a Glenn procedure, the cardiac output drops to normal. One output is ejected from the heart into the aorta. This output is distributed to the body. The portion returning from the upper body traverses through the SVC and through the Glenn connection into the lungs before returning to the heart with oxygenated blood. This oxygenated blood mixes with the portion of the cardiac output that is distributed to the lower body and that returns to the heart via the IVC. This means that conversion from a shunted physiology to cavopulmonary physiology can cut cardiac output demands substantially.

The oxygen saturations, however, are the product of "mixing" of the blood return from the upper body (which returns via the pulmonary vascular bed) with blood return from the lower body. In most infants the SVC is approximately one-third of systemic venous return, and the IVC has approximately two-thirds of systemic venous return. If the SVC return is fully oxygenated by the lungs, this one-third of blood returns to the heart with 100% oxygen saturation. A "normal" IVC saturation is approximately 70%. The math predicts a saturation of 80%—one part returning at 100%, two parts at 70% = 240/3 = 80%!

When the patient following conversion to a Glenn procedure has a low oxygen saturation, there are numerous factors that can influence this equation. For example, if the IVC return is 60% saturated (from low cardiac output; more extraction if hemoglobin is low), then even if the lungs are fully oxygenating the SVC return, the systemic saturations, after mixing in the heart, will be one part 100% and two parts 60% = 220/3 = 71%. A chest x-ray examination in this patient might look completely normal, and increased ventilation will not improve these saturations. Instead, the patient needs to be managed with increasing cardiac output to raise the IVC saturations back up toward 70%. When there is obstruction to the Glenn connection, pulmonary flow may be compromised, and perhaps this will be evident from an increased central venous pressure (CVP). If the Glenn connection provides only 20% of venous return to the heart (with the rest popping off through collaterals to the IVC), then the saturations may be one part 100% plus four parts 70% (because the Glenn connection is now only 20% of return, 80% is through the IVC) = 380/5 = 76%. If the cardiac output is also slightly low, or IVC saturations are diminished a bit by the pop off from the SVC, then the saturations may be lower: one part 100%, four parts 60% is 100 + 240 = 340/5 = 68%. Apparent from these calculations is the enormous effect that low IVC saturations have on systemic saturations following a Glenn procedure. Decreases in pulmonary flow may not have as much effect on systemic oxygen saturation as decreases in systemic blood flow, and it is critical for the ICU team to appreciate this. However, diminished Glenn flow (with high CVPs) may need to be evaluated (and repaired). If the high Glenn pressure is related to PVR, it can be treated with oxygen or pulmonary vasodilators. Maintaining a higher PCO_2 can augment Glenn flow by increasing flow to the

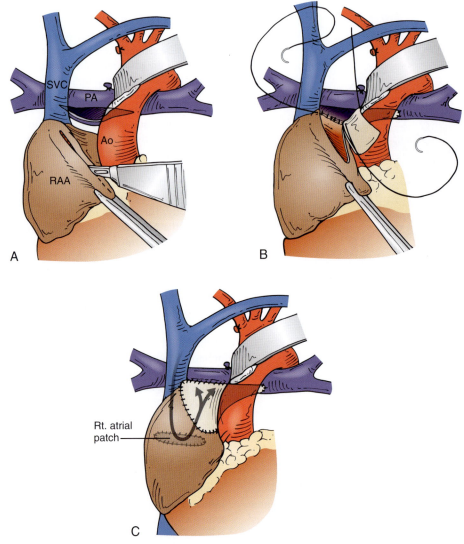

• Figure 62.6 Hemi-Fontan procedure. (A) Central pulmonary arteries (PAs) are opened anteriorly from posterior to the superior vena cava (SVC) to distal to insertion of the ligamentum arteriosum. An incision is made in the base of the right atrial appendage extending up to the SVC/right atrium (RA) junction. (B) The inferior aspect of the pulmonary arteriotomy is sutured to the outside of the SVC. (C) A patch of polytetrafluoroethylene (PTFE) is sutured within the RA at the level of the limbus. (Figure reproduced with permission from Hirsch-Romano J, et al. Modified Hemi-Fontan procedure. *Oper Tech Thorac Cardiovasc Surg.* 2013:117-123.)

brain that will return via the Glenn connection. Likewise, placing the patient in a 30-degree head-up position can theoretically improve flow from the Glenn connection into the pulmonary arteries. All of these factors should be considered when caring for a patient following a Glenn procedure. For the most part in well-selected patients with normal pulmonary resistance, low ventricular end-diastolic pressures, and good cardiac function, and in the setting of an unobstructed anastomosis with ligation of the azygous vein and no distortion of the pulmonary arteries, patients following a Glenn procedure should have oxygen saturations of approximately 80% and CVPs in the range of 12 to 18 cm H20. Over the long run, patients with Glenn procedures will need to be converted to Fontan.

The lack of "hepatic factor" (blood from the hepatic circulation getting to the pulmonary circulation) can lead to the development of pulmonary arteriovenous connections that can result in hypoxemia (right-to-left shunt at the pulmonary parenchymal level), and when this occurs, as heralded by decreasing oxygen saturations months to years following a Glenn procedure, consideration for conversion to Fontan (to restore hepatic factor to the pulmonary circulation) needs to be a part of the plan. Venovenous collaterals that direct blood from the (high pressure) SVC to the (low pressure) IVC can also lead to systemic desaturation following a Glenn procedure and are often amenable to occlusion in the catheterization laboratory.

Summary

Patients with a variety of complex congenital heart defects may undergo palliation as a primary therapy. In some cases palliation is performed for patients with correctable heart defects who present a challenge for repair and for whom staging to later repair provides

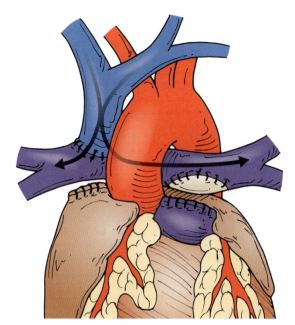

• **Figure 62.7** Bidirectional Glenn procedure. The superior vena cava (SVC) is anastomosed in an end-to-side fashion to the pulmonary artery. It is important to ligate the azygous vein (to limit decompression of SVC blood via the azygous to the intact inferior vena cava [IVC] circulation). The atrial junction from the SVC site is oversewn. When performed on cardiopulmonary bypass (CPB), it is often possible to complete an atrial septectomy through the atrial junction before oversewing it. Cannulation of the SVC must be performed meticulously to prevent stenosis to the Glenn circuit after the cannula is removed at the completion of the case. (Modified from Backer CL, Russell HM, Deal BJ. Optimal initial palliation of patients with functionally univentricular hearts. *World J Pediatr Congenit Heart Surg.* 2012;3[2]:165-170.)

a perceived benefit. For the most part palliation in the current era is part of the strategy for patients whose underlying cardiac anatomy is not compatible with two-ventricle repair and for whom staging to Fontan is preferred.

Palliation is aimed at providing pulmonary blood flow to patients with restricted pulmonary flow, controlling (reducing) pulmonary blood flow for patients with excessive pulmonary flow, and eliminating the potential for systemic ventricular outflow obstruction. In the case of those patients being staged to the Fontan pathway an intermediary step of superior cavopulmonary anastomosis is commonly included.

Palliation for single ventricle is part of a staging toward Fontan, whereas palliation for patients with repairable (two-ventricle) anatomy may be a temporizing procedure to enhance the safety of the surgical repair. In all cases the eventual goal for the patient should be well communicated.

Conversion of Patients Initially Treated With Single-Ventricle Palliation

As we have reviewed previously, the decision making to determine the single-ventricle versus biventricular pathway is critical. Currently, excellent early and midterm results can be achieved with single-ventricle palliation culminating with a Fontan.[68] However, late complications after Fontan completion still remain a concern. In patients with complex intraventricular anatomy

and two adequate ventricles and AV valves, the single-ventricular pathway is sometimes chosen. Although we feel that these patients are best served with a biventricular repair, factors that present a challenge to many surgeons and centers with regard to septation in these patients include technical difficulty, risk of heart block, postoperative LVOTO, iatrogenic AV valve regurgitation, and the need for RV-PA conduit.[3] A portion of these patients may present with serious complications related to their Fontan physiology (i.e., plastic bronchitis, protein-losing enteropathy) and require conversion to a biventricular repair. Others may present for elective takedown. We have used a strategy of one-and-one-half-ventricle and biventricular repair for these patients with acceptable outcomes.[3]

Similarly, the group at Boston Children's Hospital showed that conversion from failing single-ventricle palliation to biventricular conversion could also be performed with acceptable morbidity and mortality in selected patients with unbalanced atrioventricular septal defect.[17]

Recruitment of the Borderline Left Ventricle

There has been recent interest in the recruitment of the borderline LV, whether borderline with respect to size or function. The overall results have been mixed but encouraging. The rehabilitation generally consists of initial single-ventricle palliation with concurrent and staged resection of endocardial fibroelastosis, aortic and/or mitral valvuloplasty, and maintenance of a restrictive atrial septal defect. There exists an anecdotal case report by Hammel et al.[69] of a patient with true HLHS who underwent staged rehabilitation to a biventricular repair. However, this is balanced by a small case series of attempted rehabilitations by the same group with a 50% mortality (2 of 4).[70]

The group at Boston Children's Hospital has undertaken a policy of attempted LV conversion in patients with a borderline LV. Their initial publication in 2009 outlined the results of nine patients with endocardial fibroelastosis and a borderline LV. All nine underwent successful biventricular repair. Follow-up at a median of 5.6 months (range, 1 to 38 months) revealed one death from noncardiac causes (motor vehicle accident) and two reoperations. One important caveat is that the mean LV end-diastolic dimension z score was only -0.2 ± 1.7, indicating relatively mild ventricular hypoplasia, and three of the nine would have been expected to do well with a biventricular repair based upon the CHSS calculator mentioned earlier.[71]

A second publication from 2013 reviewed the outcomes of 34 subjects undergoing staged LV recruitment. These subjects had smaller LV end-diastolic volume z scores (-2.5 ± 1.2). There were 4 deaths (12%) and 11 successful biventricular repairs (32%).[72]

Their most recent publication outlines the outcomes of 51 subjects and attempted to define preoperative factors that were related to poor outcome. It is important to note that these patients were enrolled conditionally on surviving their initial palliation and demonstrating LV growth. The composite primary end point was death, transplantation, or biventricular repair takedown, which occurred in 11 of 51 subjects (22%). Of the 11 failures, 10 had HLHS. One-third of the patients with HLHS met the primary end point, whereas only 1 of 18 UCAVSD subjects did. On analysis for risk factors an LV end-diastolic pressure of greater than 13 mm Hg was associated with a poor outcome. The transplant-free biventricular survival was therefore 78%. This can be compared to the survival from the single-ventricle reconstruction trial. To form a similar group, one can look at the 3-year transplant-free survival conditional on surviving to 1 year, which is 90% to 95%.[58] Thus, although biventricular physiology is certainly desirable, ongoing efforts at improving outcomes for both univentricular and biventricular repair and defining which patients will ultimately benefit from one pathway or the other remain important.

Selected References

A complete list of references is available at ExpertConsult.com.

1. Anderson RH, Ho SY. Which hearts are unsuitable for biventricular correction? *Ann Thorac Surg.* 1998;66(2):621–626.
2. Jonas RA. Fontan or septation: when I abandon septation in complex lesions with two ventricles. *Semin Thorac Cardiovasc Surg Pediatr Card Surg Annu.* 2009;94–98.
3. Hoashi T, Bove EL, Devaney EJ, Hirsch JC, Ohye RG. Outcomes of 1(1/2)- or 2-ventricle conversion for patients initially treated with single-ventricle palliation. *J Thorac Cardiovasc Surg.* 2011;141(2):419–424.
4. Davies RR, Pizarro C. Decision-making for surgery in the management of patients with univentricular heart. *Front Pediatr.* 2015;3:61.
6. Rhodes LA, Colan SD, Perry SB, Jonas RA, Sanders SP. Predictors of survival in neonates with critical aortic stenosis. *Circulation.* 1991;84(6):2325–2335.
29. Olley PM, Coceani F, Bodach E. E-type prostaglandins: a new emergency therapy for certain cyanotic congenital heart malformations. *Circulation.* 1976;53(4):728–731.
32. Muller WH Jr, Danimann JF Jr. The treatment of certain congenital malformations of the heart by the creation of pulmonic stenosis to reduce pulmonary hypertension and excessive pulmonary blood flow; a preliminary report. *Surg Gynecol Obstet.* 1952;95(2):213–219.
37. Galantowicz M, Cheatham JP. Lessons learned from the development of a new hybrid strategy for the management of hypoplastic left heart syndrome. *Pediatr Cardiol.* 2005;26(3):190–199.
42. de Leval MR, McKay R, Jones M, Stark J, Macartney FJ. Modified Blalock-Taussig shunt. Use of subclavian artery orifice as flow regulator in prosthetic systemic-pulmonary artery shunts. *J Thorac Cardiovasc Surg.* 1981;81(1):112–119.
54. Yamauchi S, Kawata H, Iwai S, et al. Risk factors for semilunar valve insufficiency after the Damus-Kaye-Stansel procedure. *Ann Thorac Surg.* 2015;100(5):1767–1772.
57. Ohye RG, Sleeper LA, Mahony L, et al. Comparison of shunt types in the Norwood procedure for single-ventricle lesions. *N Engl J Med.* 2010;362(21):1980–1992.
58. Newburger JW, Sleeper LA, Frommelt PC, et al. Transplantation-free survival and interventions at 3 years in the single ventricle reconstruction trial. *Circulation.* 2014;129(20):2013–2020.
64. Jacobs ML, Rychik J, Rome JJ, et al. Early reduction of the volume work of the single ventricle: the hemi-Fontan operation. *Ann Thorac Surg.* 1996;62(2):456–461, discussion 461–452.
70. Hammel JM, Duncan KF, Danford DA, Kutty S. Two-stage biventricular rehabilitation for critical aortic stenosis with severe left ventricular dysfunction. *Eur J Cardiothorac Surg.* 2013;43(1):143–148.
72. Emani SM, McElhinney DB, Tworetzky W, et al. Staged left ventricular recruitment after single-ventricle palliation in patients with borderline left heart hypoplasia. *J Am Coll Cardiol.* 2012;60(19):1966–1974.

63

Fontan Procedure

THOMAS S. MAXEY, MD; JAMES R. HERLONG, MD; LAURA N. JANSEN, PA-C;
PAUL M. KIRSHBOM, MD

Single-ventricle (SV) heart disease describes a spectrum of congenital heart malformations in which the ventricular mass is not capable of being septated into a systemic and pulmonary circulation. Atresia of an atrioventricular or semilunar valve typically results in SV anatomies that have complete mixing of the systemic and pulmonary venous circulations. Structural defects that are generally managed with a staged palliation include variations of single left ventricle (e.g., tricuspid atresia with normally related great arteries or transposition of the great arteries, double-inlet left ventricle with normally related great arteries or transposition of the great arteries, malaligned atrioventricular canal with hypoplastic right ventricle, and pulmonary atresia with intact ventricular septum) and variations of single right ventricle (e.g., hypoplastic left heart syndrome [HLHS], double-outlet right ventricle with mitral atresia, malaligned atrioventricular canal with hypoplastic left ventricle, and heterotaxy syndromes). Children with SV anatomy generally undergo a series of palliative surgeries resulting in unobstructed systemic blood flow and a separate, low-pressure, nonpulsatile pulmonary blood flow. To best tolerate this type of circulation, patients must be (or have):

- Free of arch obstruction
- Minimal semilunar valve pathology
- Normal ventricular function (with left ventricular end-diastolic pressure <12 mm Hg)
- Minimal atrioventricular valve regurgitation
- Unobstructed pulmonary venous return
- Undistorted pulmonary arteries (PAs) with normal PA pressures (<15 mm Hg mean) and resistance (<2 indexed WU × m²)

Although the surgical palliation for SV heart disease does not create an anatomic or physiologic long-term solution, it does foster the anatomic substrate needed for what is known as *Fontan physiology.*

There are approximately a thousand Fontan operations performed yearly. Unfortunately, transplant-free survival is only 50% at 30 years. Long-term survival in the Fontan population is primarily dictated by the inherent heart defect and ventricular performance. There are, however, performance characteristics of the Fontan circuit that clearly play a role in long-term outcome. A thorough understanding of the Fontan circuit, along with improved surveillance to detect and treat subtle disturbances, offers the only possibility of improving both transplant-free survival and quality of life.[1,2] This chapter covers the surgical indications, techniques of various Fontan modifications, postoperative physiology, and expected issues for the modified Fontan procedures. Gaining an appreciation for the surgical history of this procedure is helpful in understanding the more contemporary perspective of managing SV heart disease.

Preoperative Assessment

Fontan's initial description of the procedure for tricuspid atresia listed specific criteria for selecting patients known as the "10 commandments" (see Chapter 65, Box 65.2). The significant advances in surgical technique and critical care have broadened the Fontan patient population to numerous other SV anomalies. Although Fontan's original selection criteria form the foundation of the physiologic characteristics needed for good long-term outcome, the original commandments are not as rigid as once thought. With few exceptions, contemporary criteria for Fontan completion now include normal ventricular function, absence of significant atrioventricular valve regurgitation, normal systemic and pulmonary venous drainage, absence of PA distortion, and low pulmonary vascular resistance (PVR). Various modifications to the Fontan procedure have decreased the occurrence and potential impact of these risk factors. PA stenosis and/or hemodynamically significant atrioventricular valve regurgitation can be addressed at the time of the superior cavopulmonary anastomosis or Fontan completion. Discrete pulmonary vein stenosis can be addressed, typically with a sutureless type of technique, simultaneously with the superior cavopulmonary anastomosis or Fontan completion as well. Severe ventricular dysfunction and fixedly elevated PVR (>4 indexed Wood units), however, remain the most significant contraindications to Fontan completion in the modern era. The importance of preserved ventricular function cannot be overemphasized, and long-standing volume overload to an SV should be avoided. Similarly, severe afterload such as subaortic stenosis or residual/recurrent arch obstruction should be avoided.

Hemodynamic assessment of the pulmonary vascular bed can be challenging in the presence of accessory sources of pulmonary blood supply (such as collaterals and systemic to pulmonary shunts). Mean PA pressures need to be carefully considered relative to the amount of pulmonary blood flow not just as a single data point. We tend to rely not only on PA pressures but the size of the branch PAs and the presence or absence of distortion. Various methodologies have been described (*McGoon Ratio:* the sum of the diameter of the right and left PA [LPA] divided by the diameter of the aorta at the level of the diaphragm; and *Nakata index:* the sum of the cross-sectional area of the right and LPA divided by the body surface area) to assess branch PA size. The usefulness of these indices is variable from center to center because size alone does not account for the compliance of the vessel and the ability to augment the central PAs at the Fontan stage. Branch PA size and the lack of distortion, however, tend to be a logical and useful tool to predict Fontan candidacy.[3]

Pre-Fontan Staging

In SV patients the systemic and pulmonary outflows are mixed and in parallel. Mixing of saturated and unsaturated blood must occur within the heart before being divided between the two circuits. Only rarely does any form of SV anatomy lead to a balanced circulation. To reach the Fontan state (separated pulmonary and systemic circuits in series) many patients will need a preliminary operation to achieve a balanced circulation. The choice of operation to achieve a balanced circulation is dependent on the cardiac anatomy and PVR.

If additional pulmonary blood flow is needed early in life when the PVR is elevated, a systemic to PA shunt is performed. Most centers use either a modified Blalock-Taussig shunt or a central shunt to achieve a stable source of pulmonary blood supply. In patients in whom pulmonary blood flow is high, a PA band is used to restrict pulmonary blood flow and protect the pulmonary bed from irreversible vascular disease. Patients with obstructed systemic outflow will need a Damus-Kay-Stansel operation as well as a stable source of pulmonary blood supply. Details of a Norwood type of operation are discussed in other chapters of this text. Relief of obstructed pulmonary venous drainage, including atrial septectomy, or repair of coarctation of the aorta may also be required in preparation for Fontan circulation.

As the palliated child grows, the fixed diameter of a systemic to PA shunt or PA band becomes less effective, and further augmentation of the pulmonary blood supply is needed. Although there are some centers that will perform a single-stage Fontan procedure, most centers have evolved to a staged approach using a cavopulmonary anastomosis followed by total cavopulmonary connection or "Fontan circulation."

The history of cavopulmonary connection is rich with iconic surgical names dating back to the 1950s. It was not, however, until 1971 that the current era of SV palliation began with Fontan's report[4] of successful right heart bypass in a patient with tricuspid atresia. His original operation included a classic Glenn anastomosis, closure of the atrial septal defect, and an aortic homograft as a direct connection of the right atrium to the proximal end of the LPA. The main PA was ligated, and an additional homograft valve was placed in the inferior vena cava (IVC). Although this technique did not become the standard of care because the mortality rate was high, poor long-term results from other approaches encouraged continued application of "total right heart bypass." In 1973 Kreutzer and colleagues[5] reported the first Fontan procedure with a direct connection of the right atrium to the PA. Norwood and colleagues[6] reported the first successful Fontan operation in a patient with HLHS in 1983. Over the following decades many technical innovations collectively known as a *modified Fontan*, as well as other advancements in all areas of patient management, led to dramatically improved results in the Fontan procedure. These technical modifications include the total cavopulmonary connection (lateral tunnel)[7-9] extracardiac conduits,[7,10-12] and use of adjustable atrial defects[13] or fixed fenestrations in the intraatrial baffle.[14]

Interestingly, Dr. William Glenn was not the first to introduce the concept of the cavopulmonary (Glenn) shunt. Partial bypass of the right ventricle was achieved by Carlon and colleagues[15] in 1950 when they described the anastomosis of the superior vena cava (SVC) to the right PA. Cavopulmonary anastomoses were then performed and studied experimentally and clinically by several independent groups around the world. The classic cavopulmonary anastomosis, diverting SVC blood to only the right lung, was abandoned as the feasibility of an SVC to right PA end-to-side anastomosis became apparent. Azzolina et al.[16] performed a bidirectional cavopulmonary anastomosis in 1972, directing deoxygenated blood into both lungs. This bidirectional shunt, now referred to as a *bidirectional Glenn* (BDG), has become a definitive palliation in some and the preparation stage for Fontan completion in most patients with SV heart disease.

Achieving ideal Fontan physiology is the definitive, palliative goal for SV circulations. The Fontan operation, however, has continued to evolve from the initial use of the right atrium and venous valves to more efficient constructs of nonpulsatile flow. Experimental flow studies have demonstrated the inefficiency of the right atrium as a reservoir or pumping chamber. Valves within the circuit are obstructive, and atrial contraction can cause turbulence with significant energy loss. The venous system itself has been found to be an excellent reservoir for the pulmonary bed. With the energy loss associated with pulsations in nonvalved circuits, de Leval designed an atrial portioning technique known as a *lateral tunnel*. His technique essentially excludes the right heart and leads to a more energy-efficient total cavopulmonary connection. The lateral tunnel results in a direct pathway with little pulsation or turbulence and low atrial pressure, preventing distention, arrhythmias, and/or thrombus formation.[17,18] The lateral tunnel technique is still commonly used by some for almost all subtypes of SV patients. This technique avoids the use of conduits or valves and limits high systemic venous pressure in the majority of the right atrium.

In the current era the use of an extracardiac conduit between the transected IVC and right PA has gained popularity by avoiding atrial suture lines altogether and because of the ease of operation without the necessity for cardioplegically induced cardiac arrest. The elimination of atrial suture lines avoids potential disruption of intraatrial conduction and may decrease the incidence of sinus node dysfunction often seen in other Fontan variants. Atrial suture lines have been shown to participate in reentrant circuits and atrial flutter and fibrillation late after the Fontan operation.[17-20]

The early morbidity and mortality associated with various modifications of the Fontan operation remained high until the 1990s.[21,22] The incidence of prolonged effusions was higher in patients who did not have a superior cavopulmonary anastomosis several months or years before their Fontan completion.[23,24] The single-stage Fontan caused an acute decrease in SV end-systolic and diastolic volumes and a decrease in stroke volume index with no change in myocardial mass. These geometric changes caused an increase in the mass/volume ratio, ventricular wall thickness, and filling pressures with impaired diastolic function (compliance) leading to low cardiac output.[25,26] With these findings, most centers began intervening with a superior cavopulmonary connection at approximately 4 to 6 months of age between the neonatal palliation and the Fontan completion.[27-30]

A prolonged reliance on the increased volume load created by either an aortopulmonary shunt or banded PA constructed for neonatal palliation up until a time of single-stage Fontan completion results in an increased likelihood of ventricular hypertrophy and dilation. The use of an intervening superior cavopulmonary anastomosis reduces the shunt-induced volume load to the SV at a younger age. This benefit is most easily understood by recognizing that an SV that is pumping a circulation for the systemic output and another output to the lungs (via a shunt or across a banded PA) has an increased cardiac output requirement (at least two outputs if the pulmonary-to-systemic blood flow ratio [Q_p:Q_s] is 1:1, and more if the Q_p:Q_s is greater; each Q_p adds an additional cardiac output). All this volume returns to the heart (either through the pulmonary or systemic veins), so the volume and work load to the shunted or banded SV can be substantial. Once the cavopulmonary anastomosis is performed, the heart pumps only a single cardiac output—some of which returns through the SVC to PA connection via the pulmonary veins (oxygenated return) and some through the IVC into the SV. The improved volume status following a cavopulmonary connection on the SV encourages regression of ventricular hypertrophy and dilation, making the child a better candidate for ultimate Fontan completion.

Another contribution in the completion of Fontan circulation has been the use of a temporary communication or fenestration between the systemic venous and pulmonary venous pathways. This communication allows a "controlled" right-to-left shunt in the immediate postoperative period from the systemic venous return to the left (or pulmonary) atrium *without* the blood having to traverse the pulmonary circuit. This improves "filling or preload" of the systemic ventricle at a time when the resistance to flow across the pulmonary circuit might be high, thus maintaining cardiac output and improved systemic oxygen delivery at the cost of mild systemic desaturation. (Obviously, the fenestration needs to be small, or the right-to-left shunt might be too large, create intolerable oxygen desaturation, and impose a serious impairment to recovery). Several techniques have been used for fenestration, including an adjustable interatrial communication,[29,31] creation of a fixed fenestration by using a surgical punch to produce a small hole of precise size in the Fontan baffle,[32] or exclusion of a single hepatic vein, allowing drainage into the pulmonary venous atrium. Unfortunately, progressive increase in right-to-left shunting via intrahepatic collaterals occurring from hepatic vein exclusion has led to abandonment of this latter technique for creating a fenestration in the Fontan circuit.[33] The application of an interstage superior cavopulmonary connection and improved techniques of Fontan completion have dramatically reduced the early mortality and morbidity associated with the single-stage Fontan completion.

Indications for Surgery

Numerous advances in selection and preparation of children, cardiac catheter technology, operative techniques, and postoperative management have led to a broader application of the Fontan principle to a wide variety of patients with complex SV heart disease.[34] The optimal timing for all phases of SV palliation remain poorly defined. There is little argument that reduction of volume and/or pressure load on the immature ventricle is vital to Fontan success. Protection of the pulmonary bed and preventing central PA distortion is equally important in preparation for nonpulsatile pulmonary blood flow.

Following neonatal palliation, the second stage (stage II) of palliation creates a cavopulmonary connection either by a BDG anastomosis or a hemi-Fontan procedure. Each technique has its proponents, and outcomes are similar for these two techniques. Table 63.1 describes the advantages and disadvantage of the BDG and hemi-Fontan technique. We generally prefer to perform this palliative stage between 4 and 6 months of age. This serves to volume unload the SV (as described earlier) while providing a more effective and controlled source of low-pressure pulmonary blood flow.[35,36] Typically this operation allows for the correction of any anatomic or hemodynamic abnormality that may increase the risk of Fontan completion. PA stenosis and hemodynamically significant atrioventricular valve regurgitation can (and should) be addressed at the time of the BDG or Fontan completion. Likewise, it is valuable to perform a wide atrial septectomy at the time of BDG if this was not a part of the initial neonatal palliation. Progressive restriction to flow across the atrial septum can result in pulmonary venous or systemic venous obstruction, and even in cases in which there are two atrioventricular valves, potential for obstruction to flow at a subvalvar level dictates the wisdom of

TABLE 63.1	Summary of Advantages and Disadvantages of the Bidirectional Glenn and Hemi-Fontan Procedures	
Consideration	**Bidirectional Glenn**	**Hemi-Fontan**
Bypass technique	Normothermic, beating heart CPB, totally extracardiac repair; can be done without CPB in some cases	Cardioplegic arrest or total circulatory arrest for intracardiac work
Added material	Can be performed with no added prosthetic material	Requires patch material (usually allograft)
Cannulation	Usually SVC, RA, and Ao	RA and Ao only, if done with circulatory arrest
Prospects for PA enlargement	Requires additional PA plasty if enlargement is required	Excellent central PA enlargement is part of the operation
Fontan completion options	Extracardiac Fontan completion can be performed with normothermic beating heart CPB	Lateral tunnel TCPC is obligatory (barring takedown of the hemi-Fontan connection), with need for ischemia and/or circulatory arrest
Technique ease	Straightforward to learn and perform	More demanding technically
SA node blood supply	Untouched	Compromised, but may not be important for outcome
Risk of operation	Low	Low
Postoperative physiology	Equivalent	Equivalent
Eventual Fontan outcome	Very good in current era	Center dependent

Ao, Aorta; *BDG*, bidirectional Glenn; *CPB*, cardiopulmonary bypass; *PA*, pulmonary artery; *RA*, right atrium; *SA*, sinoatrial; *SVC*, superior vena cava; *TCPC*, total cavopulmonary connection.
From Karl TR: Staged reconstruction for hypoplastic left heart syndrome: the bi-directional cavopulmonary shunt. In: Rychik J, Wernovsky G, eds. *Hypoplastic Left Heart Syndrome*. Boston: Kluwer Academic Publishers; 2003:135; with permission.

performing an atrial septectomy in all patients being staged to Fontan. Likewise, it is also important to ensure not leaving a "blind" PA stump with a competent valve because this can create a nidus for thrombus and stroke. Thus if the patient is being converted from a banded PA to a BDG or hemi-Fontan circuit, and the PA is being divided, it is important to perform a pulmonary valvectomy in the proximal PA segment. Patients with discrete pulmonary vein stenosis are better Fontan candidates if corrected at the Glenn stage, though some may undergo Fontan completion and sutureless pulmonary vein repair simultaneously. In general, children completing stage II palliation have an 87% to 91% chance of survival to Fontan completion.[37]

Severe ventricular dysfunction (either systolic or diastolic) and fixedly elevated PVR (>4 indexed Wood units) remain the most significant contraindications to Fontan completion. Until recently, patients who were evaluated for Fontan completion typically underwent an echocardiogram and cardiac catheterization to assess anatomic and hemodynamic suitability for Fontan completion. Significant hemodynamic lesions were addressed either during the catheterization or at the time of the Fontan completion. Ro and associates[38] retrospectively assessed the utility of the pre-Fontan cardiac catheterization. Patients had a low incidence of unexpected additional lesions identified at cardiac catheterization if they had an arterial oxygen saturation (SaO_2) greater than 76% and a hemoglobin concentration less than 18 g/dL, unobstructed PALPA, absence of significant atrioventricular valve regurgitation, normal ventricular function, no neo–aortic arch obstruction, an unrestricted atrial communication, and no evidence of a decompressing vessel by echocardiography. The negative predictive value for the criteria was 93%, meaning that 93% of the time, no additional hemodynamically significant lesion would have been identified if the patient had had a preoperative cardiac catheterization.[38] If a cardiac catheterization before Fontan completion is not performed based on the Ro criteria, cardiac magnetic resonance imaging may be helpful to delineate further abnormalities of the PAs, systemic veins, and pulmonary veins that may not be fully appreciated on echocardiogram.

There is broad variability between centers regarding the timing of Fontan completion. Some centers advocate early intervention (as early as 18 months) to minimize the effects of persistent cyanosis and potential for paradoxical emboli, whereas others successfully wait until 5 to 6 years of age with no increased morbidity. Following the BDG we monitor patients to ensure the child is making satisfactory progress and not becoming excessively cyanotic. Although there are subtleties to every child undergoing staged palliation, we generally prefer to proceed with Fontan completion when the arterial oxygen saturations are consistently in the mid-70s. Once the child becomes more cyanotic, we typically perform a cardiac catheterization to evaluate pre-Fontan hemodynamics and address significant pulmonary venovenous collaterals with catheter intervention. Ideal hemodynamic measurements include a mean PA pressure of less than 20 mm Hg, PVR of less than 4 indexed Wood units, and an end-diastolic ventricular pressure of less than 10 to 12 mm Hg. Conversion to Fontan completion should be considered particularly in the setting of progressive cyanosis following the stage II procedure. Of particular importance is to rule out desaturation from venovenous collaterals (and to evaluate whether these have formed due to downstream resistance in the pulmonary circulation or to patency of the azygous vein—which is usually occluded at the time of stage II) or from arteriovenous malformations, which can occur if there is no "hepatic factor" getting into the pulmonary circulation.

Special Circumstances

The three-staged palliative strategy has significantly reduced the morbidity and mortality since the original descriptions of SV palliation.[39] Fontan completion provides improved systemic arterial saturation and increased pulmonary blood flow during a period of significant lung growth. Some institutions perform the Fontan completion with excellent results without an intervening cavopulmonary anastomosis, fenestration, or the use of CPB.[40,41] These case series are not typical at most contemporary centers and include few patients with HLHS. Although not common practice, if one were to consider a performing a single-stage Fontan on a selected patient, 12 to 18 months is generally considered the minimal age for a successful, single-stage Fontan procedure. Although the single-stage approach may expose the child to one less surgery, the delay exposes the SV to an additional 6 to 12 months of volume load.

Patients with SV and heterotaxy syndrome remain a high-risk population for Fontan physiology secondary to multiple associated abnormalities, including sinus node dysfunction, variability in systemic venous drainage, potential for pulmonary venous obstruction, atrioventricular valve regurgitation, and recurrent or persistent cyanosis in the presence of arteriovenous shunting. The presence of a common atrioventricular valve and the presence of an increased PA pressure are associated with an increased risk of early death. Venous anomalies may increase the risk of systemic or pulmonary venous pathway obstruction if a lateral tunnel completion is performed. Therefore a BDG shunt with an extracardiac Fontan completion is recommended for this subset of patients.

In patients with heterotaxy and an interrupted IVC, the Kawashima procedure can be used. This technique uses the SVC with azygous return (from the interrupted IVC) to be anastomosed to the PA. Following a Kawashima procedure, all the systemic venous blood is directed to the pulmonary circulation except for the hepatic venous effluent and coronary sinus blood, which enters the heart directly. This venous arrangement results in approximately 90% of systemic venous return directed to the lungs, and only 10% will bypass the pulmonary circulation, leading to mild desaturation. Patients with a Kawashima procedure can present with an early decline in oxygen saturations following second-stage palliation. Pulmonary arteriovenous malformations and abdominal venovenous collaterals cause a decline in systemic saturation in Kawashima patients.[42] It is our practice to follow similar staging principles when considering redirection of hepatic venous effluent (Fontan completion) in this subset of patients. Fontan completion is usually performed 1 to 3 years after the Kawashima procedure. This philosophy may prevent or allow regression of pulmonary arteriovenous malformations and abdominal venovenous collaterals without additional morbidity or mortality.

Surgical Technique

Lateral Tunnel Fontan Completion After the Hemi-Fontan Procedure. Children with HLHS who have undergone a previous hemi-Fontan procedure may have lateral tunnel Fontan completion, usually between 18 months and 6 years of age, depending on center-specific preference. The lateral tunnel modified Fontan completion requires limited mobilization of the neo-aorta and lateral aspect of the right atrium.

The lateral aspect of the right atrium is exposed and opened to the base of the hemi-Fontan baffle (Fig. 63.1A). This permits

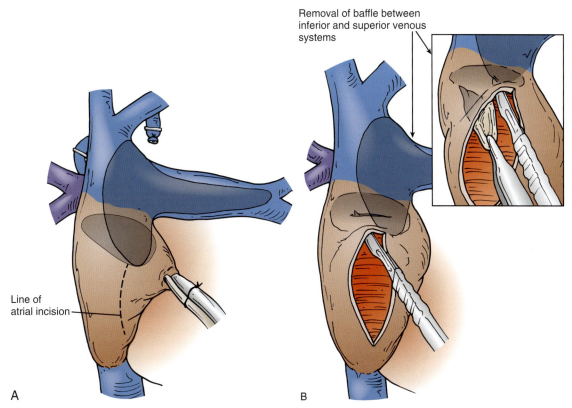

Removal of baffle between inferior and superior venous systems

Line of atrial incision

A   B

• **Figure 63.1** Lateral tunnel completion Fontan. (A) Working through the right atrial incision, the homograft dam between the superior vena cava and right atrium is readily identified. (B) This dam of tissue is excised under direct vision, creating an opening that is adequate in size for baffling of the inferior vena cava flow into the pulmonary arteries. This opening is created in such a way that a rim of tissue can be used for the suture line of the intracardiac lateral tunnel *(inset)*. (From Cox L, Sundt TM III, eds. *Operative Techniques in Cardiac & Thoracic Surgery*: *A Comparative Atlas*. Philadelphia: WB Saunders; 1997:247; with permission.)

access to the homograft dam that divides the right atrium and the SVC. The dam is then removed under direct vision. The resultant opening allows creation of a baffle to shunt IVC blood into the PAs (see Fig. 63.1B). A 10-mm polytetrafluoroethylene (PTFE) graft is used to create the intraatrial baffle. The graft is opened longitudinally so that a tunnel can be created that has a larger diameter than the diameter of the graft. Before placement a 4-mm punch-hole (fenestration) is typically made in the lower portion of the graft (Fig. 63.2). A suture line along the posterior aspect of the right atrium secures the baffle so that the right pulmonary veins are excluded from the systemic venous side of the baffle. The suture line is continued between the graft and the two walls of the right atrium to complete the lateral tunnel and close the atriotomy (Fig. 63.3). Transthoracic monitoring lines are placed in each side of the newly placed baffle in the PA and pulmonary venous atrium, respectively (Fig. 63.4).

This procedure requires cardiopulmonary bypass (CPB) and a short period of cardioplegic arrest. The inflammatory effects of CPB increase total body water and cause tissue edema and some degree of multisystem organ dysfunction. The myocardium and lung parenchyma are especially affected. Myocardial edema causes decreased SV compliance, elevated filling pressures, and decreased cardiac output. These myocardial changes are particularly problematic in the Fontan circuit, where the goal is to have the highest cardiac output at the lowest filling pressure possible. Edema of the lung parenchyma and pulmonary endothelium results in decreased

lung compliance and increased PVR, respectively. These pulmonary effects worsen with an increasing duration of exposure to CPB. The lateral tunnel completion after intervening hemi-Fontan reduces the time required on CPB, as well as the duration of aortic cross-clamping.

Extracardiac Fontan Completion After the Bidirectional Glenn. Children who have had an intervening BDG for their superior cavopulmonary anastomosis will generally undergo an extracardiac Fontan completion. Like the lateral tunnel Fontan completion, the extracardiac Fontan completion is typically performed between 18 months and 5 years of age, depending on center preference. An 18- to 20-mm extracardiac conduit is inserted between the IVC and the undersurface of the right PA slightly offset from the superior cavopulmonary anastomosis to complete the Fontan circuit. We have had equal success with both PTFE and Dacron tube grafts as conduit for this technique.

Some institutions complete the extracardiac Fontan procedure without the use of CPB or cardioplegic arrest, whereas others use CPB either with circulatory arrest or with bicaval cannulation and continuous CPB. After mobilization of the IVC to the level of the hepatic veins, the IVC is divided at the right atrial junction. Care is taken to identify and avoid the coronary sinus when oversewing the atrial end. An end-to-end anastomosis between the conduit and IVC is created (Fig. 63.5).

To complete the anastomosis of the conduit to the superior cavopulmonary anastomosis, the underside of the right PA is incised

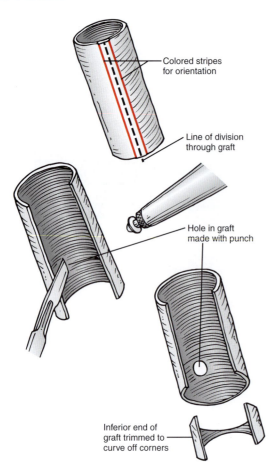

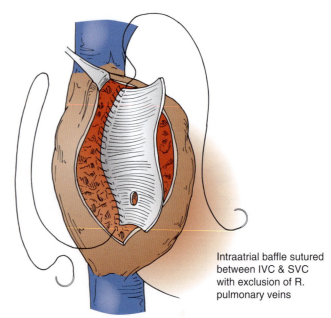

Intraatrial baffle sutured
between IVC & SVC
with exclusion of R.
pulmonary veins

• **Figure 63.3** Lateral tunnel completion Fontan. The opened polytetra-fluoroethylene graft with the previously created fenestration is secured in the right atrium, excluding the right *(R.)* pulmonary veins behind the baffle. The suture line along the posterior aspect of the right atrium directs inferior vena caval blood within the patch to the atriopulmonary anastomosis. Superiorly, the graft is sutured along the wall of the atrial septum up to the level of the excised dam in the cavoatrial junction. Then the graft is brought to the right and sewn to the margins of the previous excision of the homograft dam up to the level of the incision in the right atrium. The graft at this point can be trimmed if it is excessively wide and then the suture line continued, sandwiching the graft-free margin between the two walls of the right atrium to complete the lateral tunnel suture line. After completion of this suture line the atrium can be filled with saline solution and the venous cannula reinserted. *IVC,* Inferior vena cava; *SVC,* superior vena cava. (From Cox L, Sundt TM III, eds. *Operative Techniques in Cardiac & Thoracic Surgery: A Comparative Atlas*. Philadelphia: WB Saunders; 1997:249; with permission.)

• **Figure 63.2** Lateral tunnel completion Fontan. A polytetrafluoroethylene graft 10 mm in diameter is opened longitudinally so that a lateral tunnel can be created that is larger than the diameter of the graft used. Before implantation an incision is made in the left lower portion of the graft, and a 4-mm punch hole is made in the graft, which can be easily performed before implantation and avoids manipulating the graft after it is sewn in place. The inferior rim of the graft is then trimmed to a gentle curve and sewn into the lateral aspect of the right atrium. (From Cox L, Sundt TM III, eds. *Operative Techniques in Cardiac & Thoracic Surgery: A Comparative Atlas*. Philadelphia: WB Saunders; 1997:248; with permission.)

and sutured to the superior aspect of the conduit (Fig. 63.6). A pulmonary arterioplasty for pulmonary stenosis may be performed with a variety of patch material, or the extracardiac tube graft may be beveled to cross any stenotic areas at the PA end of the anastomosis. If the BDG has been directed slightly leftward toward the midline, this will allow offsetting of the superior and inferior cavopulmonary connections to minimize energy losses. With meticulous dissection, most central PAs can be exposed without transecting the aortic amalgamation. Only rarely is cardioplegic arrest and aortic transection needed to carry the Fontan under the aorta to address PA stenosis. If a fenestration is desired, a 4-mm punch-hole is created in the graft, as well as the right atrium. The anastomosis is sewn from the exterior of the graft to the right atrial free wall with a side-to-side anastomosis. Some centers prefer a 5- to 8-mm PTFE shunt placed between the conduit and the right atrium as a fenestration.

After the lateral tunnel or extracardiac Fontan completion, we try to avoid placing lines directly in the internal jugular vein, innominate vein, or SVC to reduce the risk of postoperative

thrombosis. In the circumstances in which these lines are placed, we recommend removing them as soon as clinically feasible and considering the use of low-dose anticoagulation during the time that they are in place. Given the incidence of postoperative arrhythmias after Fontan completion, temporary atrial and ventricular pacing wires are placed on the myocardium. After separation from CPB, modified ultrafiltration is performed to minimize the effects of CPB. A mediastinal chest tube is placed for bleeding, and bilateral pleural tubes are placed for effusions. Some centers have used intracardiac (common atrial) lines to help guide postoperative management, but we have found this to be more the exception than the rule.

Management of Associated Lesions

Left Pulmonary Artery Stenosis. Compression from the large neo-aorta or involution of the ductus arteriosus may lead to LPA stenosis after stage I reconstruction for HLHS.[43] Stenosis at the distal insertion of the Sano conduit is not uncommon following staged palliation for HLHS. The triangular baffle that is placed as part of the hemi-Fontan procedure generally augments the LPA

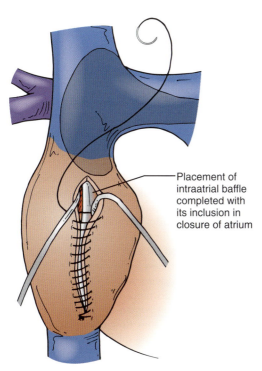

• **Figure 63.4** Lateral tunnel completion Fontan. An advantage of incorporating the wall of the lateral tunnel in the suture line is the ability to place lines easily for postoperative monitoring. Transthoracic atrial lines are positioned on either side of the polytetrafluoroethylene baffle, which places one line on the left atrial side of the baffle and the other on the pulmonary arterial side for measurement of pressures postoperatively. In this fashion, no lines must be placed directly in the internal jugular vein, innominate vein, or superior vena cava, reducing the risk of postoperative caval thrombosis. (From Cox L, Sundt TM III, eds. *Operative Techniques in Cardiac & Thoracic Surgery: A Comparative Atlas*. Philadelphia: WB Saunders; 1997:250; with permission.)

Placement of intraatrial baffle completed with its inclusion in closure of atrium

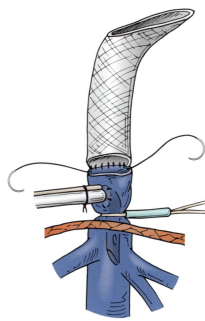

• **Figure 63.5** Extracardiac Fontan completion. After the institution of bypass the inferior vena cava (IVC) is clamped just inferior to the cavoatrial junction and transected between the clamp and the snared IVC cannula. The cardiac end of the transected IVC is doubly oversewn with running 4-0 or 5-0 nonabsorbable monofilament suture. The extracardiac conduit of polytetrafluoroethylene vascular tube graft is then tailored. The size of the conduit usually ranges from 20 to 25 mm in diameter. The cross-sectional diameter of the conduit is usually slightly oversized with respect to the diameter of the IVC. An end-to-end anastomosis between the conduit and the IVC is performed with 4-0 or 5-0 monofilament suture. After completion of the inferior anastomosis, the conduit is clamped at midlevel, and the IVC cannula snare is released, allowing the inferior half of the conduit to fill with blood. Any anastomotic suture-line bleeding can be repaired at this time. Cardiopulmonary bypass is continued with the cannula unsnared to allow more accurate approximation of conduit position in the mediastinum. The length of the conduit is then tailored to the undersurface of the right pulmonary artery. The superior orifice of the conduit is bevelled at an angle less than or equal to 45 degrees relative to the long axis of the conduit. This allows an oblique conduit to pulmonary artery anastomosis with a substantially greater anastomotic surface area rather than with direct end-to-side connection. In addition, this allows greater offsetting of the superior and inferior cavopulmonary connections, which has been shown by computational fluid dynamics to minimize energy losses at the cavopulmonary junction. Furthermore, this oblique anastomosis effectively serves as a central pulmonary arterioplasty, and the angle of the bevel can be adjusted to maximize this effect. At this point the superior vena cava is cannulated and snared, and full cardiopulmonary bypass is instituted. (From Cox L, Sundt TM III, eds. *Operative Techniques in Cardiac & Thoracic Surgery: A Comparative Atlas*. Philadelphia: WB Saunders; 1997:225; with permission.)

and addresses LPA stenosis if present. A separate patch augmentation of the LPA is necessary in patients who undergo BDG as the cavopulmonary anastomosis in situations where there is LPA stenosis. In some patients the LPA remains diffusely small despite augmentation during the cavopulmonary anastomosis. As mentioned previously, the use of extensive dissection behind the aortic amalgamation is helpful when augmenting the branch PAs. This technique provides excellent exposure and virtually eliminates the need to transect the aortic amalgamation. Balloon angioplasty with or without stent placement can be performed at the time of pre-Fontan cardiac catheterization or as hybrid technique at the time of Fontan completion.[44] Repeat pulmonary arterioplasty following Fontan completion is sometimes needed if branch PA stenosis persists. Stenting of the branch PAs, particularly the portion directly posterior to the large neo-aorta, may be required even following patch arterioplasty because mechanical compression is the likely cause.

Atrioventricular Valve Regurgitation. Atrioventricular valve performance in the systemic circulation is known to have important implications for survival following univentricular palliation. Significant atrioventricular valve insufficiency in patients with SV physiology can be problematic and associated with poor survival. Moderate tricuspid valve regurgitation is not an uncommon finding in patients with HLHS undergoing staged palliation. Regurgitation can result from either abnormal valve morphology and/or incomplete leaflet coaptation. Tricuspid regurgitation causes an additional volume load on the single right ventricle and frequently contributes to ventricular dysfunction. A concurrent valvuloplasty may be performed at the time of the Fontan completion for moderate to severe atrioventricular valve regurgitation. Although there is a small risk of heart block, tricuspid valvuloplasty at the time of Fontan completion improves the severity of regurgitation at a median follow-up of 24 months.[45] Other forms of valve and ventricular morphology such as a common atrioventricular valve with associated SV heart disease can lead to different regurgitant mechanisms further complicating the management.

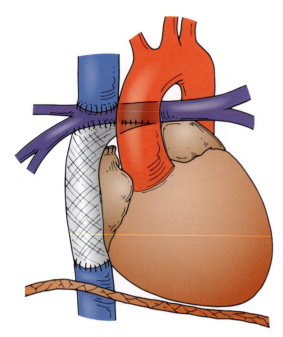

• **Figure 63.6** Extracardiac Fontan completion. The completed extracardiac conduit Fontan is shown. A fenestration is placed by performing a 4- to 5-mm side-to-side anastomosis between the conduit and the right atrial free wall. Another option for fenestration is to place a synthetic tube graft (5 to 8 mm) from the conduit to the free wall. (From Cox L, Sundt TM III, eds. *Operative Techniques in Cardiac & Thoracic Surgery: A Comparative Atlas.* Philadelphia: WB Saunders; 1997:227; with permission.)

Neo–Aortic Arch Obstruction. Neo–aortic arch obstruction may occur at either the proximal or distal end of the arch reconstruction. Distal obstruction at the end of the homograft patch augmentation near the ductal insertion site is common following arch reconstruction. Recoarctation is generally addressed by balloon dilation angioplasty at the time of the pre-Glenn/Fontan cardiac catheterization. In patients with significant proximal arch obstruction and/or persistent distal arch obstruction, patch augmentation at the time of the Glenn or Fontan completion is recommended.

Subaortic Obstruction. Subaortic or outflow tract obstruction is not uncommon in patients with double-inlet left ventricle or tricuspid atresia with transposed great vessels. A progressive restriction at the ventricular septal defect (VSD) is the most common site of systemic outflow obstruction in this subset of patients. Although not often used in the modern era, PA banding is known to promote outflow tract obstruction, particularly when aortic arch obstruction is present. Ventricular hypertrophy and diastolic dysfunction secondary to subaortic stenosis are significant risk factors for Fontan completion. Subaortic obstruction is considered significant when the size of the VSD is less than half the size of the aortic valve in end-systole. Surgical options to address subaortic stenosis include enlargement of the VSD and/or use of the subpulmonary outflow tract (Damus-Kaye-Stansel procedure). Although these strategies are sometimes inevitable, we feel that prevention of subaortic stenosis, particularly by recognizing the substrate that is likely to produce it, is paramount to the success of SV patients. When there is an anatomic risk for the development of aortic outflow obstruction, the use of a strategy to minimize this occurrence is paramount during the decision making for early palliation options.

Postoperative Physiology

After Fontan completion, patients may have both systolic and diastolic dysfunction, abnormal vascular hemodynamics, or a combination of these. Mahle and colleagues[46] demonstrated Fontan patients had diminished systolic and diastolic function based on a greater reliance on atrial contraction to achieve ventricular filling. The mean myocardial performance index in the single-right-ventricle patients also was significantly higher (worse) than that in controls, and the indexed ejection time was shorter, suggesting less efficient ventricular mechanics.

Postoperative Fontan patients frequently experience abnormal venous hemodynamics following cavopulmonary connection with elevated central venous pressure and a limited venous capacitance. Increased venous tone limits the ability to mobilize blood from the capacitance vessels, thereby impairing cardiac output. Hsia and colleagues[47] described the effects of respiration and gravity on infradiaphragmatic venous flow in patients with normal biventricular hearts compared with patients with a Fontan completion. Hsia's group described the importance of spontaneous inspiration in hepatic venous return. After Fontan completion, loss of the normal augmentation in portal venous flow takes place with expiration, resulting in elevated hepatic and splanchnic venous pressures. Hsia and colleagues[48] then showed that the fenestration moderates these findings. On the other hand, several reports have suggested that the effect of fenestration in the modern era has been less dramatic than it was in earlier eras.[49,50]

Early Complications After Fontan Completion

Management of patients with SV anatomy undergoing Fontan palliation has evolved significantly over the last four decades. To appreciate the dramatic improvement in the outcome after Fontan completion, it is useful to review results from earlier eras. The initial subset of patients undergoing Fontan completion had nonstaged, nonfenestrated, atriopulmonary Fontan completions.[22] In contrast, more recent patients had intervening superior cavopulmonary anastomosis and fenestrated lateral tunnel Fontan completion. The incidence of death or Fontan takedown decreased from 27.1% to 7.5% over the study period. HLHS was a risk factor for early failure in this study of Gentles and colleagues.[22] Throughout the 1990s, several other studies demonstrated improved outcomes after interstage superior cavopulmonary anastomosis.[28,30,51]

Improving early mortality over the years was not exclusive to patients with HLHS. Excellent outcomes are now observed with most forms of complex SV heart disease. Contemporary favorable results apply to both the intracardiac tunnel and extracardiac conduit Fontan techniques. Factors thought to have contributed to improved outcomes are multifactorial and include improved efficiency of the Fontan circuit and the reduction (or even elimination) of cross-clamp and bypass time. The beneficial effects of selective fenestration, the interstaging of bidirectional cavopulmonary shunt, and preoperative occlusion of collateral vessels is complex, patient specific, and remains a topic of discussion.[52]

The importance of *unobstructed surgical pathways* for functional SV physiology cannot be overemphasized. A gradient as low as 2 mm Hg within the cavopulmonary system can lead to significant energy loss and must be addressed either surgically or with catheter intervention. Some centers strictly monitor caval (or Fontan pressures) and common atrial pressure in the immediate postoperative

TABLE 63.2 Differential Diagnosis of Low Cardiac Output After Fontan

RA$_P$	LA$_P$	Cause(s)
Low	Low	Hypovolemia
High	Low	PVR, baffle obstruction, pulmonary artery hypoplasia or branch stenosis
High	High	Ventricular dysfunction, AV valve stenosis or regurgitation, arrhythmia, outflow obstruction, tamponade

AV, Atrioventricular; *PVR,* pulmonary vascular resistance.

period. Although the transpulmonary gradient may be elevated in the first 24 hours, failure to decrease following extubation and diuresis is ominous and typically a sign of impending Fontan failure. A low cardiac output state in the early postoperative period is concerning, and mechanical obstruction must be ruled out with echocardiography and/or cardiac catheterization. Table 63.2 describes the diagnostic algorithm in the immediate period following Fontan completion. Once obstructive surgical pathways have clearly been ruled out, mechanical circulatory support can be considered for severe myocardial dysfunction. If hemodynamic decline persists, failed Fontan circulation is inevitable, and the Fontan should be taken down to the Glenn stage.

Fontan physiology is particularly sensitive to *atrial-ventricular synchrony.* Proponents of the extracardiac conduit (ECC) Fontan suggest that this technique allows for optimal flow dynamics and preserves pulmonary and ventricular function. In addition, the ECC technique avoids sinus node manipulation, suture lines in the atrium, and atrial distention, theoretically minimizing the risk of postoperative atrial arrhythmias.[53] Patients with sinus node dysfunction must be paced with an epicardial lead system and typically have a worse prognosis.

Atrial and/or Fontan *thrombosis* has been described, although this is relatively uncommon. We typically do not anticoagulate patients with a normal coagulation profile immediately following Fontan completion but start aspirin therapy once enteral feedings are started. Our group also prefers to maintain all Fontan patients on aspirin unless contraindicated. Realizing the variability between patients with regard to laboratory test responses to aspirin, we typically do not monitor for aspirin resistance. Thrombus formation within the Fontan circuit is multifactorial and likely related to mechanical distortion, which should be ruled.

Pleural effusions and *ascites* are not uncommon following Fontan completion. We typically open both pleural spaces and leave chest tubes in place for at least 3 to 4 days. The pleural drainage is typically serous, though it can be chylous in the setting of systemic venous hypertension. If ongoing volume loss persists, Fontan hemodynamics should be evaluated and any pathway obstruction corrected. Ligation of the thoracic duct and use of sclerosing agents in the thoracic space should rarely be necessary. The risk of prolonged pleural effusions is increased in patients with HLHS. The use of a fenestrated Fontan has been exhaustibly debated and is center specific. There are no definitive data to support fenestration decreasing pleural effusions.[49] We have adopted the policy of nonfenestrated extracardiac Fontan irrespective of anatomic subtype and prefer to fenestrate only patients at highest risk. This subset typically includes

patients with atrioventricular valve regurgitation and those with high PVR.

Refinements in the surgical approach to Fontan completion as well as improvements in perioperative care have dramatically reduced the previously observed morbidity and mortality. Results for Fontan completion demonstrate a protocol of routine staging, addressing concomitant lesions, and selective use of fenestration results in very low morbidity and mortality. Institutional differences in technique, timing, and staging and variations in perioperative management make comparing studies on survival after Fontan completion difficult. Despite these confounding variables, analyses of Fontan completion over the past decade, from the original valveless atriopulmonary connection to the staged total pulmonary cavopulmonary connection (lateral tunnel versus extracardiac) with fenestration, have shown a progressive and dramatic improvement in operative survival.[54]

Late Complications After Fontan Completion

As the number of survivors after Fontan completion has increased, so too has the identification of challenging problems these patients face. The evolution of staged palliation allows for favorable ventricular compliance, PVR, and systemic venous connections for a potential lifetime of Fontan circulation.[55] Outcomes after SV staged palliation are equivalent for patients with systemic right ventricle (e.g., HLHS) and other forms of the univentricular heart.[34] Although early outcomes have improved, significant long-term complications are inevitable from a variety of causes. Abnormally high systemic venous pressure is needed to drive pulmonary perfusion and cardiac output within the Fontan circuit. Although the literature of long-term Fontan complications is predominantly older patients with atriopulmonary connections, the long-term effects of more contemporary reconstructions are not as clear.[52] The long-term circulatory state of Fontan physiology can lead to arrhythmias, reduced cardiac output and functional status, cyanosis, protein-losing enteropathy (PLE), hepatic and renal dysfunction, plastic bronchitis, cerebral emboli, and death.

Atrial arrhythmias are a common long-term morbidity and likely related to suture lines and distended atrial tissue in the lateral tunnel technique, particularly in the heterotaxy population. Atrial fibrillation and supraventricular reentry tachycardia can be difficult to control and can lead to ventricular failure. Use of extracardiac conduits in the Fontan modification result in much less atrial suturing, theoretically reducing the incidence of atrial arrhythmias. Fontan conversion to a total extracardiac, cavopulmonary connection with a concomitant atrial ablation procedure can be successful in controlling arrhythmias and should be considered if ventricular function is preserved. Optimally, atrial arrhythmias undergo transcatheter ablation procedures when such are indicated before the Fontan stage because transvenous access to the common atrium is most often obliterated with completion of the Fontan circulation.

Collateral circulations may develop in the palliated SV circulation. Systemic venous collaterals develop in many patients shortly after the cavopulmonary shunt. Pulmonary arteriovenous connections can occur following the cavopulmonary shunt or Fontan completion. Although the cause is debated, the lack of hepatic factor in the pulmonary circuit plays at least some role in the development of pulmonary arteriovenous malformations. These collateral vessels can result in a significant right-to-left shunt leading to cyanosis. Systemic to PA collaterals are also common and create a volume load on the SV. In patients with either volume load or cyanosis an aggressive search for collateral vessels should be made, and they should be occluded if possible.

Thromboembolic complications can occur at any time following the Fontan procedure. These events can involve conduit thrombosis, PA thrombosis, and cerebral embolic events. Many thromboembolic events probably go unrecognized, and the reported incidence of embolic events varies. The effectiveness of prophylactic anticoagulation following Fontan completion is debatable. At our institution we use only aspirin unless there are clinical reasons to alter this regimen. We typically treat patients who suffer from embolic events with long-term warfarin.

Protein-losing enteropathy (PLE) is an enigmatic problem with significant morbidity and mortality involving loss of protein from the gastrointestinal tract. Although the exact cause is unknown, elevated splanchnic pressures contribute to some degree. PLE can occur any time from weeks to years after surgery. The incidence is not insignificant, and mortality at 5 years following the diagnosis is notable. Nonselective protein loss results in varying degrees of peripheral edema, ascites, pleural effusions, immunodeficiency, and coagulopathies. The diagnosis is made by an elevated alpha-1 antitrypsin level in the stool. Medical treatment includes diuretics, good nutrition with protein supplementation, and optimizing Fontan hemodynamics. Interventional lymphatic catheterization is performed in a few centers. Little is known about why this ailment occurs, and, unfortunately, some patients persist with PLE despite drastic measures, including cardiac transplantation.

Problems with the surgical pathway can be seen following the Glenn or Fontan completion. Advancement in catheter technology has allowed nonoperative management for focal stenosis and/or baffle leaks. The extracardiac conduit technique can be problematic for smaller children because the prosthesis does not change with somatic growth and can lead to obstruction in the systemic venous pathway. We have consistently been successful at placing at least an 18-mm extracardiac conduit in all patients at the Fontan completion. We have not found the need to oversize conduits to allow for somatic growth and feel this strategy may lead to kinking and/or thrombosis. A potential consequence of the extracardiac conduit is pulmonary vein compression, which can occur if the conduit is too short. Some surgeons prefer to make the conduit a bit longer to allow for some growth. If right pulmonary vein obstruction is identified in a patient after an ECC Fontan, conduit compression should be considered and can be managed simply by tacking the conduit to the atrium to elevate it off the pulmonary veins.

Ventricular failure is an unfortunate problem in many patients with palliated SV heart disease, and the cause is frequently multifactorial. Intrinsic myocardial dysfunction can occur secondary to systemic outflow tract obstruction, volume overload, or chronic cyanosis. The acute changes placed on the myocardium at the time of Fontan palliation (acute loss of preload) lead to an increase in the mass/volume ratio and diastolic dysfunction. This change in end-diastolic function appears to have a major effect on the cardiac index in the HLHS Fontan circulation. Small changes in end-diastolic function result in dramatic changes in the cardiac index.[56] Simultaneously, there is an increase in afterload as the systemic and pulmonary circuits are now in series rather than parallel. This physiology results in the SV having to generate more cardiac output in the face of less reserve and limited preload.

Hepatic failure, although typically a late complication following Fontan completion, has been recognized as a potential pathology that must be prospectively evaluated and treated aggressively. In Fontan physiology the liver is wedged between the nonpulsatile pulmonary capillary bed and the splanchnic bed. The increased central venous pressure is transmitted directly to the liver through the hepatic veins and IVC. The clinical presentation of congestive hepatopathy is generally progressive and occurs over years. Chronic passive congestion can eventually lead to the development of cardiac cirrhosis. The exact incidence is unknown, and the clinical diagnosis is difficult because there are no conclusive studies correlating liver function test results and other serum markers to the disease process. We have increased our vigilance of this population with collaboration and follow-up from our hepatology colleagues every 5 years following Fontan completion and cardiac catheterization every 10 years.

Management of the Failing Fontan

The prevalence of "failing Fontan" physiology in contemporary congenital heart centers suggests a less than full understanding of the performance characteristics of this fragile circulatory arrangement. In patients with failing Fontan physiology from the early atriopulmonary connection era, significant improvement has been reported following conversion to a total cavopulmonary connection with associated arrhythmia surgery.[57] Specific selection criteria for Fontan conversion are not clearly defined, and transplant should be considered in the presence of significant ventricular dysfunction. Cardiac transplantation in the failing Fontan patient is often challenging in the setting of multiple previous interventions, the need for vascular reconstruction, and the high incidence of postoperative bleeding. Posttransplant RV failure secondary to elevated PVR is a very challenging problem with high mortality. Some patients, on the far end of the spectrum, with failing Fontan physiology will be considered for a heart/liver transplant once end-stage cirrhosis has occurred.

Neurodevelopmental Outcome

Neurodevelopmental outcome following Fontan completion is an active and important area of research. The category of complex congenital heart disease in which neurodevelopmental outcome is of the greatest concern is the univentricular heart. Patients with SV anatomy typically undergo a three-stage palliation during which their brains may experience inadequate blood flow. The initial palliative procedure frequently requires low-flow or even deep hypothermic circulatory arrest. The subsequent palliations usually require CPB and occasional aortic clamping. It is not uncommon for patients to experience inadequate cerebral blood flow secondary to hypotension in the perioperative period. Regardless of the timing of Fontan completion, patients live for some period of time in a state of relative hypoxia, which may contribute to late cognitive dysfunction and neurodevelopmental delays. Several studies have suggested palliated SV patients are within the low normal range for cognitive performance as well as other developmental domains.[58-60]

Gaynor and colleagues[61] have studied neurodevelopmental performance in multiple domains for children with various forms of SV physiology culminating in Fontan physiology. This unique analysis compares children palliated to Fontan physiology with other children with complex congenital heart disease with a two-ventricular repair. His group also evaluated the potential risk factors associated with adverse neurodevelopmental outcomes in the SV physiology cohort. Compared with patients with biventricular circulations, patients with SV performed worse in terms of processing speed, inattention, and impulsivity. Otherwise, there were no significant differences between the groups for any domain.

Patients with SV trended toward lower performance in visual motor integration as well. Outcomes of HLHS patients were not worse than other forms of SV heart disease.

Summary

The goal of staged reconstructive surgery for children with SV defects is ultimately to achieve a modified Fontan circulation. The modified Fontan circuit allows systemic venous blood from both the SVC and IVC to return to the PAs directly, thereby separating the systemic and pulmonary circulations. The Fontan circuit relieves cyanosis and volume load of the SV while permitting an adequate cardiac output at acceptable systemic venous pressures. The multiple technical modifications of the Fontan completion, combined with improved patient selection and postoperative management, have reduced the operative mortality to less than 2.5% in many centers, with acceptable perioperative and midterm morbidity. Despite improvements in mortality and perioperative morbidity, the long-term outcome in this high-risk population remains uncertain.[62]

Selected References

A complete list of references is available at ExpertConsult.com.

1. Jacobs JP, O'Brien SM, Pasquali SK, et al. Variation in outcomes for benchmark operations: an analysis of the Society of Thoracic Surgeon's Congenital Heart Surgery database. *Ann Thorac Surg.* 2011;92(6):2184–2191.

4. Fontan F, Baudet E. Surgical repair of tricuspid atresia. *Thorax.* 1971;26(3):240–248.

34. Tweddell JS, Nersesian M, Mussatto KA, et al. Fontan palliation in the modern era: factors impacting mortality and morbidity. *Ann Thorac Surg.* 2009;88(4):1291–1299.

39. Said S, Burkhart HM, Dearani JA. The Fontan connections: past, present, and future. *World J Pediatr Congenit Heart Surg.* 2012;3(2):171–182.

45. Kanter KR, Forbess JM, Fyfe DA, Mahle WT, et al. De Vega Tricuspid annuloplasty for systemic tricuspid regurgitation in children with univentricular physiology. *J Heart Valve Dis.* 2004;13(1):86–90.

50. Salazar JD, Zafar F, Siddiqui K, et al. Fenestration during Fontan palliation: now the exception instead of the rule. *J Thorac Cardiovasc Surg.* 2010;140(1):129–136.

52. D'Udekem Y, Iyengar AJ, Galati JC, et al. Redefining expectations of long-term survival after the Fontan procedure; twenty-five year follow-up from the entire population of Australia and New Zealand. *Circulation.* 2014;130:S32–S38.

54. Dabal RJ, Kirklin JK, Kukreja M, et al. The modern Fontan operation shows no increase in mortality out to 20 years: a new paradigm. *J Thorac Cardiovasc Surg.* 2014;148(6):2517–2523.e1.

55. Atz AM, Zak V, Mahony L, et al. Survival data and predictors of functional outcome an average of 15 years after Fontan procedure: the Pediatric Heart Network Fontan cohort. *Congenit Heart Dis.* 2015;10(1):E30–E42.

62. Dabal RJ, Kirklin JK, Kukreja M, et al. The modern Fontan operation shows no increase in mortality out to 20 years: a new paradigm. *J Thorac Cardiovasc Surg.* 2014;148(6):2517–2523.e1.

64

Ebstein Anomaly

T.K. SUSHEEL KUMAR, MD; CHRISTOPHER J. KNOTT-CRAIG, MD

Ebstein anomaly (EA) is a rare cardiac disease and accounts for less than 1% of all newly diagnosed congenital disorders. EA is not just a disorder of the tricuspid valve (TV) but also affects the right ventricle (RV) myocardium. It encompasses a wide anatomic spectrum, and the disorder can present itself either as cyanosis in the newborn or exercise intolerance in the older adult.[1-3] Symptomatic neonates present serious medical and surgical challenges and have uniformly dismal outcomes without timely intervention.[3,4]

Pathologic Anatomy

It is worth recapitulating the characteristic features of this disorder that are relevant to surgical management as described by Carpentier et al.[1]

1. There is a failure of delamination of the TV leaflets. The septal, posterior, and anterior leaflets are affected in order of severity. This effectively causes anterior and apical rotational displacement of the functional annulus. The downward displacement of the septal and posterior leaflets into the RV is the essence of EA.
2. The anterior leaflet is attached at the appropriate level but is large or sail-like. There are multiple chordal attachments to the ventricular wall. In neonates presenting with symptoms the anterior leaflet is often severely affected.[2]
3. The portion of the RV above the functional annulus ("atrialized right ventricle") is dilated and thin with variable hypertrophy. The true tricuspid annulus is almost always enlarged.
4. The cavity of the effective RV is reduced ("functional right ventricle").
5. The infundibulum of the RV is often obstructed by the redundant tissue of the anterior leaflet and its chordal attachments to the infundibulum.

   As mentioned earlier, EA is truly a disorder of both TV and RV. There is a variable degree of ventricular myocardial dysfunction. Morphometric histopathologic studies have demonstrated that there is an absolute decrease in the number of myocardial fibers in addition to thinning of the wall of the dilated RV in EA.[3]

   Carpentier et al.[1] also described four grades of EA.

Type A: The anterior leaflet has normal morphology, and the RV is adequate.

Type B: The anterior leaflet has abnormal chordae but normal mobility. The RV is reduced in volume but adequate.

Type C: The anterior leaflet is restricted in movement. The RV is small with a large atrialized component.

Type D: This is also called "tricuspide sac" because the leaflets form a complete sac of fibrous tissue adherent to the RV. The only functional part of the RV is the infundibulum.

Associated Anomalies

Cardiac

1. An atrial septal defect (ASD) is present in most of the cases.
2. There is a variable degree of RV outflow tract obstruction, and anatomic pulmonary atresia occurs in approximately half of the symptomatic neonates requiring surgical intervention.[4]
3. A patent ductus arteriosus (PDA) is present in EA with pulmonary atresia.
4. Wolff-Parkinson-White type of accessory pathway is present in approximately 10% of the cases.
5. Rarer associations include ventricular septal defect, transposition of great arteries, tetralogy of Fallot, and atrioventricular canal defect.

Noncardiac

Low-set ears, micrognathia, cleft lip and palate, absent left kidney, megacolon, undescended testes, and bilateral inguinal hernias are commonly associated anomalies.[5]

Pathophysiology

The pathophysiology and clinical presentation vary depending on the anatomic severity of the disorder. In fact there is a high rate of fetal demise for this disorder.[6] At its extreme end (type C and D) there is severe displacement of the TV, leading to an ineffective RV and severe valve regurgitation. This results in severe cardiomegaly with consequent lung hypoplasia and cyanosis because most of the systemic venous return is shunted across the ASD. Persistent elevation in pulmonary vascular resistance (PVR) is a major impediment to successful antegrade ejection from the smaller and less effective RV. The pulmonary blood flow is hence dependent upon the PDA because there is no effective flow generated by the small RV (physiologic pulmonary atresia). Often there can be true right ventricular outflow tract obstruction (anatomic pulmonary atresia). The left ventricle is often pancaked by the enlarged RV. When the disease is less severe (type A and B), the RV can establish effective antegrade flow as PVR decreases, and this is accompanied by clinical improvement in symptoms. Neonates with severe tricuspid regurgitation (TR) or gross cardiomegaly who are otherwise asymptomatic have an associated mortality of 45% within the first year of life without intervention.[7,8] The natural history of EA during infancy is thus gloomy.[5] However, those who survive early childhood can expect reasonable longevity. When the disease is mild, symptoms are not noticed until later in adult life. Symptoms are often related to exercise intolerance from progressive TR.

Diagnostic Studies

Chest X-Ray Examination

Results of the chest x-ray examination of a symptomatic EA patient are characteristic. There is significant cardiomegaly (box-like heart) with the cardiac silhouette almost filling the entire chest. It is not uncommon to have a cardiothoracic ratio of 1 on the chest x-ray examination results in a neonate presenting with severe symptoms.

Electrocardiogram

Results of electrocardiography are abnormal in most patients. Tall and broad P waves, bizarre morphologies of terminal QRS pattern, and first-degree heart block are all common. Between 6% and 36% have accessory pathways, with most of them located around the orifice of the malformed TV.[9]

Echocardiogram

This is confirmatory and provides sufficient anatomic and hemodynamic information. The principal echocardiographic characteristic that differentiates EA from other forms of congenital TR is the degree of apical displacement of the septal leaflet at the crux of the heart.[10] The echocardiogram also provides information on the degree of atrialization of the RV, size of the tricuspid annulus, severity of the TR, and degree of pulmonary stenosis. It may be difficult to differentiate physiologic from anatomic pulmonary atresia.

GOSE Scoring System

First reported by Celermajer et al.[8] from the United Kingdom, the Great Ormond Street Echocardiogram (GOSE) score has important prognostic value in stratifying risk of death and is based on the calculated ratio of the sum of the right atrium and atrialized RV areas to the sum of the remaining chambers derived from a four-chamber view on echocardiography (Fig. 64.1 and Table 64.1).

Cardiac Catheterization

A cardiac catheterization is unnecessary and often triggers fatal arrhythmias. The right ventricular and pulmonary pressures are usually normal, although the right ventricular end-diastolic pressure may be abnormal.

Treatment

Medical

Medical treatment of the symptomatic neonate depends on the degree of hemodynamic stability. Patients who are reasonably stable are treated with supplemental oxygen and prostaglandin infusion and closely observed for adequacy of cardiac output and oxygen saturations. Treatment of unstable patients involves intubation, deep sedation (fentanyl, 2 to 4 mcg/kg/h) and paralysis in addition to initiation of prostaglandins. Ventilation should be adjusted to

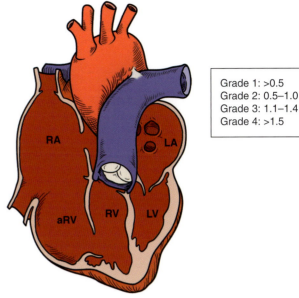

Grade 1: >0.5
Grade 2: 0.5–1.0
Grade 3: 1.1–1.4
Grade 4: >1.5

$$\frac{\text{Area of } (RA + aRV)}{\text{Area of } (RV + LV + LA)}$$

Figure 64.1 Great Ormond Street Echocardiogram (GOSE) score. *aRV*, Atrialized right ventricle; *LA*, left atrium; *LV*, left ventricle; *RA*, right atrium; *RV*, right ventricle.

TABLE 64.1	Mortality Risk by GOSE Score	
GOSE Score	Ratio	Mortality (%)
1-2	<1.0	8
3 (acyanotic)	1.1-1.4	10 early, 45 late
3 (cyanotic)	1.1-1.4	100
4	>1.5	100

GOSE 1 <0.5; GOSE 2 >0.5 and <1.0; GOSE 3 >1.0 and <1.5; GOSE 4 >1.5.
GOSE, Great Ormond Street Echocardiogram.

decrease PVR. We use large tidal volumes (12 to 15 mL/kg) to offset the effects of gross cardiomegaly on lung expansion. Inhaled nitric oxide may be invaluable in reducing PVR. A continuous infusion of bicarbonates and inotropes (usually dopamine, 5 to 10 mcg/kg/h) may be necessary. Following a confirmation of diagnosis by echocardiogram, the clinical progress should be monitored closely. Daily echocardiograms are obtained, looking specifically for enhanced antegrade pulmonary blood flow.[7] In our own experience, as well as others' experience, approximately half the neonates tend to stabilize and improve over a few days as PVR decreases.[4,6] Serial echocardiograms will document increasing pulmonary blood flow. Prostaglandin infusion and ventilation are weaned gradually as tolerated.

Surgical

Indications for Surgery

Neonates who continue to decline in spite of standard resuscitative measures need surgical intervention because death is certain

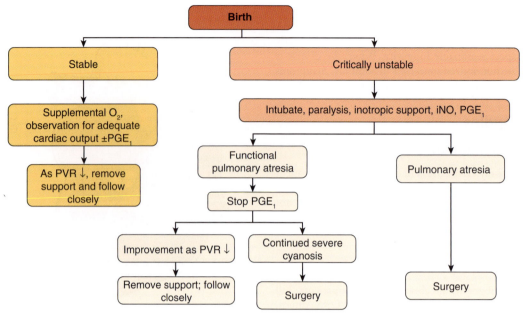

Figure 64.2 Algorithm for initial management of Ebstein anomaly in neonates. *iNO,* Inhaled nitric oxide; *O₂,* oxygen; *PGE₁,* prostaglandin E₁; *PVR,* pulmonary vascular resistance.

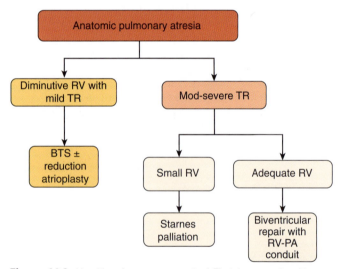

Figure 64.3 Algorithm for management of Ebstein anomaly with anatomic pulmonary atresia. *BTS,* Blalock-Taussig shunt; *RV,* right ventricle; *RV-PA,* right ventricle to pulmonary artery; *TR,* tricuspid regurgitation.

(Fig. 64.2). Those who respond to medical measures should be watched over a period of days to weeks. Prostaglandin should be weaned gradually as PVR drops and antegrade pulmonary blood flow increases. The child may be able to establish adequate RV output to be extubated and discharged home. If, however, the child does not tolerate weaning of prostaglandin (oxygen saturation below 80%) or positive pressure ventilation, surgical intervention will become necessary.[4,6] Those with anatomic pulmonary atresia will necessarily require surgery (see Fig. 64.3). Generally if the GOSE score is 3 or 4, the patients will require some form of surgical intervention in the neonatal period.[7] It is also worth noting that among those who somewhat respond to medical intervention the predominant symptom of right heart failure is difficulty in tolerating feedings secondary to mesenteric venous congestion.

Evolution of Principles of Surgical Management

Wilhelm Ebstein first described the anomaly named after him in 1866. However, it was not until 1958 that an attempt at total correction was made by Hunter and Lillehei.[11] They attempted to create a competent valve by repositioning the displaced leaflets with no success. Later Hardy and colleagues[12] modified the technique by placement of interrupted sutures over the spiral line of the displaced leaflets. Although the technique yielded moderate success, it was not effective in the more severe forms of the disease. In 1963 Bernard and Schrire described successful replacement of the TV using a mechanical prosthesis.[13] The anchoring sutures were placed cephalad to the coronary sinus and the atrioventricular node to avoid heart block. However, prosthetic valve replacement of the TV has yielded less than ideal results related to thrombosis of mechanical prosthesis in the tricuspid position and degradation of biologic valves.

Danielson et al.[14] described a new method of valve reconstruction in 1979. They described the importance of plication of the atrialized RV, posterior tricuspid annuloplasty, closure of ASD, and right reduction atrioplasty. In their series, all accessory pathways were mapped and divided. They described the first large series with satisfactory outcomes. Since then alternate techniques of repair have been described in adults and older children with variations in the theme of plication of the redundant atrialized RV and use of the sail-like anterior leaflet in construction of a competent monocuspid valve. Carpentier et al. described longitudinal plication of the RV to preserve the base to apex dimension of the RV. The anterior leaflet is detached and reattached to the new annulus after clockwise rotation. A prosthetic ring was inserted to reinforce repair.[1]

In 1997 Sebening described tricuspid valvuloplasty in EA using a single-stitch technique with satisfactory outcomes. This involved creation of a competent monocusp (the anterior leaflet) by transfer of anterior papillary muscle toward interventricular septum.[15]

The concept of cone reconstruction was conceived by da Silva and colleagues[16] and is based on the principles of the Carpentier techniques. In this operation the anterior and posterior leaflets of the TV are mobilized from their anomalous attachments in the RV, and the free edge of this complex is rotated clockwise to be sutured to the septal border of the anterior leaflet, thus creating a cone, the vertex of which remains fixed at the RV apex and the base of which is sutured to the true TV annulus. Whenever possible the septal leaflet is incorporated into the cone. The atrialized RV is longitudinally plicated, and the true TV annulus is plicated to match the proximal circumference of the already constructed cone-shaped valve. The ASD is closed in a valved fashion, and the redundant right atrium is excised. In comparison to the Carpentier technique, the new cone-shaped valve opens to a central blood flow and closes with full cooptation of leaflets (360 degrees of TV leaflet tissue guarding the right atrioventricular junction). Dr. Silva and his colleagues described their experience with this technique in 40 consecutive patients. Neonates were excluded from this study, although this procedure has been used in neonates by other groups.[4,6,17] Dearani et al.[17] at the Mayo Clinic have subsequently described the largest series of the cone procedure with good results.

In 1991 Starnes et al.[18] reported a single-ventricle palliation for severely ill neonates with good outcome. This involved pericardial patch closure of the TV orifice, atrial septectomy, and construction of a modified Blalock-Taussig (BT) shunt. Pulmonary regurgitation was addressed by ligation of the main pulmonary artery, thus creating pulmonary atresia. The patients eventually underwent a Fontan operation. Later Sano et al.[19] described a novel "RV exclusion" procedure based on single-ventricle physiology. The main difference between the Sano modification and the Starnes single-ventricle palliation is that in the former a large portion of the RV free wall is excised. This restores normal movement of the interventricular septum and LV function. In 2006 Starnes et al. updated their results of single-ventricle palliation on 12 neonates with 66% survival.[20] They also described two important modifications to their earlier technique. The coronary sinus was retained on the right atrial side of the TV patch to prevent drainage into the excluded RV. More importantly, the pericardial patch was fenestrated with a 4-mm opening to prevent distention of the RV, thereby preventing impingement of the left ventricle.

We first attempted a two-ventricle repair in three critically ill symptomatic neonates in 1994 and have subsequently applied this strategy to most neonates and young infants with EA requiring surgical intervention.[2,21-23]

Our Approach to Ebstein Anomaly in the Neonate

There continues to be considerable controversy over the choice of the right operation for a symptomatic neonate presenting with EA. As mentioned before, we are heavily biased toward a biventricular repair.[4] In general, patients who demonstrate antegrade pulmonary blood flow (with measures like inhaled NO) and have a reasonable-size RV are subjected to a biventricular repair.

Patients with pulmonary atresia seem to fall into two general groups. The first group consists of those with true anatomic obstruction of the main pulmonary artery (Fig. 64.3). These patients tend to be relatively stable on the ventilator, often with gross cardiomegaly, severe TR, and sometimes a dysplastic (rather than a true EA-like) valve. The choice of operation for patients with anatomic pulmonary atresia is dictated by the size of the RV. Those with a good-size RV receive a biventricular repair. A competent right ventricular outflow tract in the form of an RV to pulmonary artery conduit is used when the TV repair appears less than satisfactory. On the other hand, if the reconstructed TV appears good, we tend to do a transannular repair, sometimes with the addition of a monocusp valve. When the RV is small, patients undergo a Starnes repair with placement of a BT shunt followed subsequently by a Fontan or one-and-one-half ventricle repair.[4]

The second group consists of patients with functional pulmonary atresia (Fig. 64.4). They are often very unstable with ongoing metabolic acidosis and sometimes with retrograde flow back through the pulmonary valve. Such patients are best served with a Starnes repair and ligation of the main pulmonary artery. The strategy for stable patients depends once again on the size of the RV. If the RV is a decent size, a biventricular repair is performed. Rarely when the left ventricle is inadequate (non–apex forming), patients are listed for heart transplantation.[4]

Our approach to neonates with EA has evolved over time, and we continue to learn. The judgment whether a diminutive, poorly functional RV will be able to maintain circulation in the setting of a high PVR is still very subjective. Equally subjective is the question of the adequacy of a relatively small left ventricle compressed by the enlarged RV. When the branch pulmonary arteries are small, it may be better to place a BT shunt and delay definitive repair until they have grown. It is worthwhile remembering that an initial Starnes repair does not irrevocably place the patient on a one-ventricle pathway.[2] Conversion to a biventricular repair is certainly possible if the RV demonstrates interval growth.

Our Surgical Technique

The guiding principles of our approach have been as follows:
1. Creation of a competent TV based on the anterior leaflet
2. Right atrial volume reduction to reduce extrinsic compression of the lungs
3. Fenestrated patch closure of ASD
4. Simultaneous repair of all associated defects, including pulmonary atresia

A variety of techniques are used to create a competent monocuspid valve, including a Danielson type of repair, a De Vega annuloplasty, a Sebening stitch to approximate the free wall to the interventricular septum, septation, and augmentation of the anterior leaflet. Our techniques of valve repair have evolved over time, with the most recent emphasis being placed on the addition of a Sebening single-stitch approach to keep the anterior leaflet approximated to the interventricular septum to minimize TR during episodes of pulmonary hypertension.

The repair of EA is performed under cardiopulmonary bypass with bicaval cannulation, moderate hypothermia (rarely circulatory arrest), and antegrade cardioplegic arrest. The free wall of the right atrium is widely excised to enhance the mechanical efficiency of the remaining atrium and reduce the intrathoracic volume occupied by the heart. It is important to identify the course of the right coronary artery before excision of the right atrium to avoid inadvertent division.[2] A detailed inspection of the TV apparatus is made, paying attention to the size of the anterior leaflet of the TV and tethering of the anterior TV to the free wall of the RV. Specifically, the leading edge of the leaflet is assessed, which may be inserted directly into the free wall of the RV without discernible papillary muscles or chordae. The crux of the repair rests on creation of a monocuspid valve using a broad sheet of the anterior leaflet,

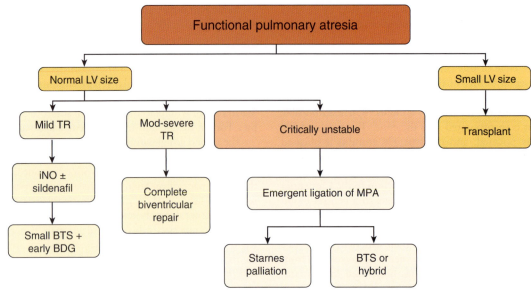

Figure 64.4 Algorithm for management of Ebstein anomaly with functional pulmonary atresia. *BDG,* Bidirectional Glenn; *BTS,* Blalock-Taussig shunt; *iNO,* inhaled nitric oxide; *LV,* left ventricle; *MPA,* main pulmonary artery; *TR,* tricuspid regurgitation.

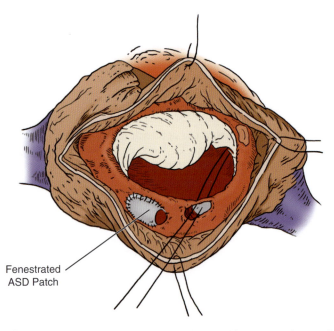

Fenestrated
ASD Patch

Figure 64.5 Tricuspid annuloplasty stitch placed in coronary sinus and at location of anteroposterior commissure. *ASD,* Atrial septal defect.

such that when the annular diameter is reduced with an annuloplasty, the edge of the anterior leaflet will coapt directly against its facing septal wall. The annuloplasty begins by placement of a pledgetted suture in the coronary sinus with its other end at the location of the commissure between the anterior and posterior leaflets (Fig. 64.5). Approximation of the annuloplasty stitch creates two openings, the "main" orifice and the "caudal" orifice (Fig. 64.6). Closure of the caudal opening plicates the atrialized RV. If the anterior leaflet is large, the annuloplasty should enable creation of a competent monocusp valve. A more complex repair is required if the anterior leaflet is tethered to the underlying myocardium. In such cases the leaflet is detached from its annulus, and the subvalvar attachments are mobilized (Fig. 64.7). The leaflet is then reattached to the reduced annulus (Fig. 64.8). If the leaflet is insufficient or dysplastic and does not reach the opposing wall, it can be detached and enlarged with an autologous pericardial patch (Fig. 64.9). The ASD is closed with a patch and is fenestrated with a 3- to 4-mm opening to serve as a vent to the right heart during the early postoperative period. Occasionally we have used the Sebening single-stitch valvuloplasty technique (Fig. 64.10).

The management of associated pulmonary atresia depends on the adequacy of TV repair. If the competency of TV appears satisfactory, a transannular patch is placed, perhaps including a monocusp valve. On the other hand, if the TV repair is not satisfactory or the branch pulmonary arteries are unusually small, a valved conduit should be used to construct the right ventricular outflow tract. Occasionally a small BT shunt may be needed to assist with pulmonary blood flow.

All associated cardiac defects should be corrected during the operation. A peritoneal dialysis catheter is placed at the conclusion of the operation to drain postoperative ascites.

Postoperative Care

Patients are kept well sedated and paralyzed on a ventilator during the early postoperative period. We tend to use large tidal volumes (12 to 15 mL/kg). Inhaled nitric oxide is of great value in reducing the PVR. Pulmonary hypertensive precautions are adopted. Continuous drainage of the ascites fluid minimizes pulmonary embarrassment from abdominal distention. Close attention is also paid to hemostasis and maintenance of adequate hematocrit (45 or higher). It is not unusual to continue inotropes (dopamine and a small dose of epinephrine) for a prolonged period. Frequently oxygen saturations will be low in the immediate postoperative period before returning to the normal range as PVR decreases.

Results of Our Approach

We first described our experience with two-ventricle repair in neonatal EA in 2000.[21] Since then we have successfully managed

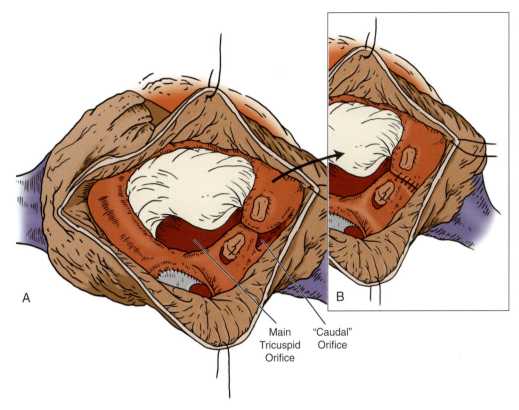

Main
Tricuspid
Orifice

"Caudal"
Orifice

Figure 64.6 (A) Approximation of annuloplasty stitch creates two openings, the "caudal" orifice containing the entrance to the atrialized right ventricle. (B) Closure of the caudal opening plicates the atrialized right ventricle and creates a competent monocuspid valve.

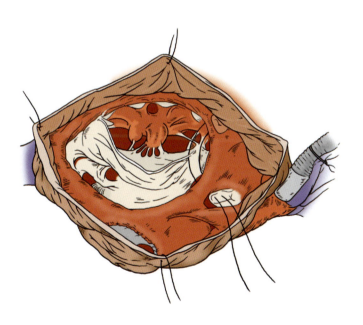

Figure 64.7 Detachment of anterior leaflet from tricuspid annulus. Subvalvular attachments are mobilized.

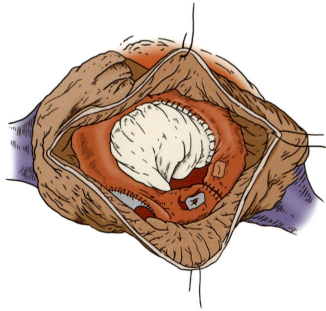

Figure 64.8 Annuloplasty stitch with reattachment of anterior leaflet.

EA with the same approach in a number of neonates.[2,22,23] Since 1994 we have operated on 26 neonates with EA; 23 of these (88%) underwent complete biventricular repair, whereas 1 patient had a Starnes repair and 2 others received a BT shunt. Of the 23 neonates with EA who underwent a biventricular repair, 13 had anatomic

pulmonary atresia. The mortality was significantly higher in this group (6 of 13) compared with those without anatomic pulmonary atresia (1 of 10). Thus overall survival to hospital discharge was 73%. We have also noted significantly higher mortality in patients with anatomic pulmonary atresia who received a transannular patch

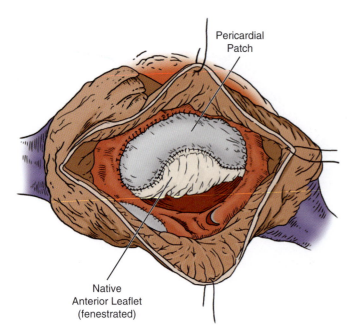

Figure 64.9 Augmentation of anterior leaflet with an autologous pericardial patch before annuloplasty.

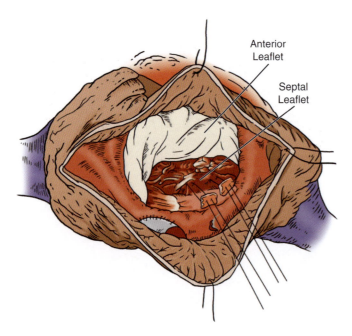

Figure 64.10 Sebening single-stitch valvuloplasty (papillary muscle of anterior leaflet through tethered septal leaflet).

compared with those who received a pulmonary homograft. A competent pulmonary valve seems critical to the survival of these neonates, who often have significant RV dysfunction in the immediate postoperative period. We have had no late deaths at follow-up, with most patients in New York Heart Association functional class I. Three patients required TV replacement during the follow-up period.

At present there is no uniform opinion regarding the approach and management of neonates with EA. Surgical techniques continue to be refined. The cone procedure has not yet found wide application in the neonatal population.[16] There is definitely a role for single-ventricle palliation, and multiple groups have reported favorable outcomes.[20,24] Multicenter studies are needed to establish the best modalities for surgical management. However, from our experience we believe that two-ventricle repair currently has similar early survival compared with single-ventricle palliation. The advantages of a better physiologic repair can be anticipated in the longer follow-up period.

Selected References

A complete list of references is available at ExpertConsult.com.

1. Carpentier A, Chauvaud S, Mace L, et al. A new reconstructive operation for Ebstein's anomaly of the tricuspid valve. *J Thorac Cardiovasc Surg.* 1988;96(1):92–101.
2. Knott-Craig CJ, Goldberg SP, Overholt ED, et al. Repair of neonates and young infants with Ebstein's anomaly and related disorders. *Ann Thorac Surg.* 2007;84(2):587–592, discussion 592–593.
3. Anderson KR, Lie JT. The right ventricular myocardium in Ebstein's anomaly: a morphometric histopathologic study. *Mayo Clin Proc.* 1979;54(3):181–184.
4. Knott-Craig CJ, Goldberg SP, Ballweg JA, et al. Surgical decision making in neonatal Ebstein's anomaly: An algorithmic approach based on 48 consecutive neonates. *World Journal for Pediatric and Congenital Heart Surgery.* 2012;3(1):16–20.
6. Bove EL, Jennifer CH, Ohye RG, et al. How I manage neonatal Ebstein's anomaly. *Semin Thorac Cardiovasc Surg Pediatr Card Surg Annu.* 2009;12(1):63–65.
7. Knott-Craig CJ, Goldberg SP. Management of neonatal Ebstein's anomaly. *Semin Thorac Cardiovasc Surg Pediatr Card Surg Annu.* 2007;112–116.
14. Danielson GK, Maloney JD, Devloo RA. Surgical repair of Ebstein's anomaly. *Mayo Clin Proc.* 1979;54(3):185–192.
16. da Silva JP, Baumgratz JF, da Fonseca L, et al. The cone reconstruction of the tricuspid valve in Ebstein's anomaly. The operation: early and midterm results. *J Thorac Cardiovasc Surg.* 2007;133(1):215–223.
18. Starnes VA, Pitlick PT, Bernstein D, et al. Ebstein's anomaly appearing in the neonate. A new surgical approach. *J Thorac Cardiovasc Surg.* 1991;101(6):1082–1087.
22. Knott-Craig CJ, Overholt ED, Ward KE, et al. Repair of Ebstein's anomaly in the symptomatic neonate: an evolution of technique with 7-year follow-up. *Ann Thorac Surg.* 2002;73(6):1786–1792, discussion 1792–1793.

65

Tricuspid Atresia

RAGHAV MURTHY, MD, DABS, FACS; JOHN NIGRO, MD; TARA KARAMLOU, MD, MSC

Definition

Tricuspid atresia (TA) is a type of cyanotic congenital heart defect (CCHD) characterized by complete obstruction of the atrioventricular (AV) valve associated with the morphologic right ventricle (RV). The floor of the right atrium is formed by muscular tissue or an imperforate vestigial remnant of the right AV valve. It is an archetypal lesion representing single-ventricle physiology.

Epidemiology

It is estimated that one in 10,000 babies born in the United States will have a diagnosis of TA.[1] It is the third most common CCHD, after transposition of the great arteries and tetralogy of Fallot. TA represents 1.6% and 2% of all diagnoses in neonates and infants, respectively, in the Society of Thoracic Surgeons Congenital Heart Surgery Database-2016. There is a male preponderance with this defect when associated with transposition of the great vessels. Without any intervention the lesion is associated with a 90% mortality by the end of the first year of life.

Embryology

The true embryologic basis for TA remains elusive, as is the case with many congenital heart defects. It appears to be related to a result of malalignment of the ventricular septum in relation to the atria and endocardial cushions.[2] The ultimate size of the bulbus cordis (RV) is determined by the extent to which the septum is shifted to the right and the size of the bulboventricular foramen (BVF). The series of abnormalities described earlier appears to occur during days 25 and 55 post conception.[2] The incidence of TA also appears to increase with maternal febrile illness.[3] Animal studies in mice associate *ZFPM2/FOG2* and *HEY2* genes in the pathogenesis of TA.[4]

Anatomy and Classification

The following are the anatomic characteristics of TA: (1) lack of communication between the right atrium (RA) and the morphologic RV, (2) the presence of an interatrial communication, (3) an enlarged left-sided AV valve, and (4) total absence of the inlet and varying degrees of deficiency of the trabecular portions of the RV (referred to as the *infundibular chamber*) because a "true" ventricle needs to have an inlet.[5] A communication (present 90% of the time) between the infundibular chamber and the left ventricle (LV) known as a *bulboventricular foramen* (BVF), commonly referred to as a

ventricular septal defect (VSD).[6] Twenty percent of patients with TA have other associated cardiac anomalies (such as transposition of the great vessels, coarctation of the aorta, aortic arch hypoplasia).

Kuhne (1906)[7] proposed a classification system for TA based on the interrelation of the great arteries. This has been further modified by Edwards and Burchell[8,9] and Rao[10] (Figs. 65.1 and 65.2). The principal groups based on the ventriculoarterial relations are depicted in Box 65.1.

A commonly associated anomaly with type 1 is a left superior vena cava (left SVC). Types 2 and 3 can be associated with varying degrees of obstruction at the level of the BVF and aortic arch.

Five variants of tricuspid valve morphology are found in TA.[2,11] The most common (76% to 84%) is muscular atresia. Dimpling of the muscular floor may be seen.[12] The membranous form accounts for 4% to 12%.[11] A valvar form (6%) is identified by a thin, imperforate membrane of tissue consisting of minute fused-valve leaflets.[11] This form may be associated with rudimentary chordae. The Ebstein form[13] (4% to 6%) and AV canal type (2%) account for the other types.[13]

Pathophysiology

Prenatal Circulation

Despite the clinically significant alterations in fetal circulation inherent in TA, these do not seem to be detrimental to fetal somatic development. The systemic venous return is forced across the foramen ovale into the left heart. As a consequence, the usual PO_2 differential present in a normally developing fetus is not present. The lowered PO_2 to the heart and brain and the elevated PO_2 to the lungs do not seem to produce any clinically significant anomalies. Almost all of the left ventricular output is ejected through the aorta in a fetus with type 1 defect; as a result the aorta is big and is rarely associated with arch obstruction. This is in contradistinction to type 2 defects, which predictably are associated with a higher prevalence of arch obstruction (30% to 50%).

Postnatal Circulation

An unrestrictive atrial septal defect (ASD) is crucial to allow mixing of the systemic and pulmonary venous blood and maintenance of cardiac output because there is a lack of communication between the RA and the RV. The pathophysiology of TA is dictated by the amount of pulmonary blood flow, which is determined by the anatomic obstruction to pulmonary blood flow (size of the BVF and degree of pulmonary stenosis [PS]), patency of the ductus

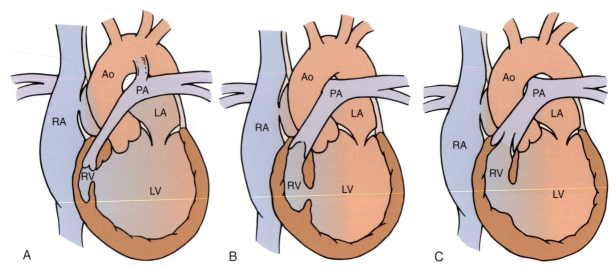

• **Figure 65.1** Native anatomy of tricuspid atresia (TA) with normally related great vessels. (A) Type 1A: TA with normally related great vessels and pulmonary atresia. (B) Type 1B: TA with normally related great vessels, restrictive ventricular septal defect (VSD), and pulmonic stenosis. (C) Type 1C: TA with normally related great vessels and a large VSD. *Ao,* Aorta; *LA,* left atrium; *LV,* left ventricle; *PA,* pulmonary artery; *RA,* right atrium; *RV,* right ventricle.

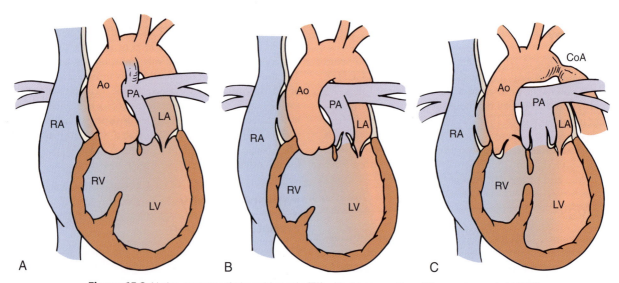

• **Figure 65.2** Native anatomy of tricuspid atresia (TA) with d-transposition of the great vessels (d-TGA). (A) TA with d-TGA, ventricular septal defect (VSD), and pulmonary atresia. (B) TA with d-TGA, VSD, and pulmonic stenosis. (C) TA with d-TGA, restrictive VSD, and coarctation of the aorta (CoA). Note the large pulmonary artery (PA) as the left ventricle (LV) ejects preferentially into the PA because of restrictive VSD (subaortic stenosis) and coarctation. The patent ductus arteriosus is omitted for clarity but may be required to supply systemic blood flow in this lesion. *Ao,* Aorta; *LA,* left atrium; *RA,* right atrium; *RV,* right ventricle.

• BOX **65.1** **Classification of Tricuspid Atresia**

Type 1: Normally related great vessels
Type 2: d-Transposition of the great arteries
Type 3: l-Transposition of the great arteries
   Each type is further subdivided based on the extent of restriction to pulmonary blood flow.
Subtype A: Pulmonary atresia
Subtype B: Pulmonary stenosis
Subtype C: No obstruction

---

arteriosus, and pulmonary vascular resistance (PVR). Patients may present with decreased pulmonary flow, increased pulmonary blood flow, or in the rare instance with a balanced circulation.

For patients with TA and normally related great vessels, blood from the LV enters the RV across the BVF to provide pulmonary blood flow. For those with concomitant PS or restriction at the BVF the pulmonary blood flow is provided via a patent ductus arteriosus (PDA). Patients may present with cyanosis due to reduced pulmonary blood flow or pulmonary overcirculation in the event that the BVF is nonrestrictive and there is not important PS. Cyanosis may worsen from progressive PS, narrowing of the BVF (there is a tendency for the BVF to decrease in size over the first 2 to 3 years of age), or closure of the PDA.

For patients with TA and transposed great vessels, systemic circulation is dependent on the size of the BVF, and the blood from the LV must traverse the BVF to reach the systemic great vessel. Systemic blood flow may become ductal dependent if there is severe subaortic stenosis, usually at the level of the BVF.[14-16] Most patients present with pulmonary overcirculation, especially in cases in which there is a degree of obstruction to systemic blood flow (either at the level of the aortic arch or at the subaortic region). Patients with l-transposition of the great vessels (l-TGA) have a higher incidence of subaortic stenosis.

Systemic arterial desaturation is present in all patients with TA secondary to an obligatory admixture of systemic, coronary, and pulmonary venous blood in the left atrium (LA). The degree of desaturation depends on the pulmonary blood flow. A pulmonary-to-systemic blood flow ratio ($Q_p:Q_s$) ratio of 1.5 to 2.5 : 1 usually results in adequate saturations, and higher shunt fractions will result in left ventricular volume loading, pulmonary overcirculation, and heart failure. Normal systemic ventricular function is one critical component of successful single-ventricle palliation, which eventuates in the Fontan operation.

Obstruction at the level of the interatrial communication is rare.[17,18] This is evident when there is a pressure gradient of more than 3 mm of Hg across the ASD or giant *a* waves. Spontaneous closure of the BVF has an estimated prevalence of 38% to 48%.[19,20] The mechanism involved is usually progressive muscular encroachment and fibrosis from endocardial proliferation. Echocardiographic studies have shown that a cross-sectional area of the BVF of less than 2 cm^2/m^2 may predict later restriction at the BVF or even indicate prescient obstruction.[21]

Diagnostic Assessment

Chest x-ray examination may demonstrate oligemic or plethoric lung fields based on the amount of pulmonary blood flow. Echocardiography provides definitive diagnosis (Fig. 65.3). The "tricuspid atresia" is seen as a hyperechoic shelf. Varying degrees of RV hypoplasia are seen. Attention must be directed to the relationship of the great arteries, arch obstruction, restrictiveness of the ASD and BVF, presence of and degree of PS, presence and size of the ductus, and identification of other associated anomalies. Electrocardiogram demonstrates RA enlargement, LV hypertrophy, and left axis deviation. The P wave duration is increased with a short PR segment. ST depression may be seen in the lateral leads, especially in patients with TGA (Fig. 65.4).

Cardiac catheterization is indicated for therapeutic interventions, such as enlargement of a restrictive ASD or ductal stenting,[22-24] which is becoming more common in lieu of aortopulmonary shunts. Pre-Glenn and pre-Fontan cardiac catheterizations are common. In patients undergoing a cavopulmonary shunt, the study provides important hemodynamic and anatomic details. These include the PVR, distortion of the pulmonary arteries, any arch obstruction if intervention on the arch was performed initially, and the location

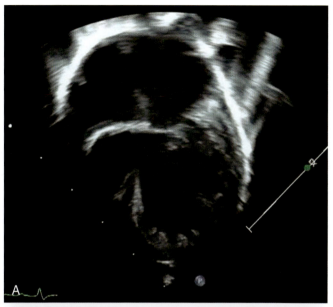

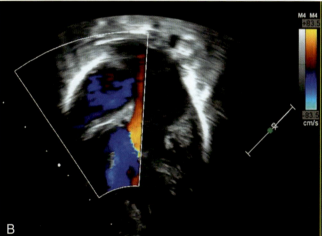

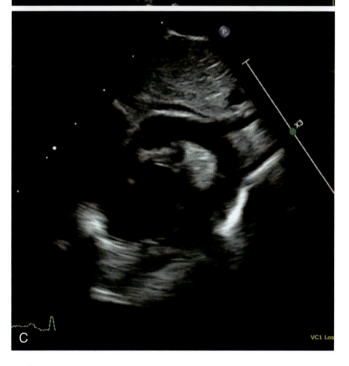

• **Figure 65.3** (A) Echocardiogram of a patient with tricuspid atresia type 1 showing an echogenic shelf in the region of the tricuspid valve, large nonrestrictive bulboventricular foramen (BVF), and a small hypoplastic right ventricle. (B) Color Doppler showing nonrestrictive flow across the BVF. (C) Echocardiogram demonstrating an unobstructed arch.

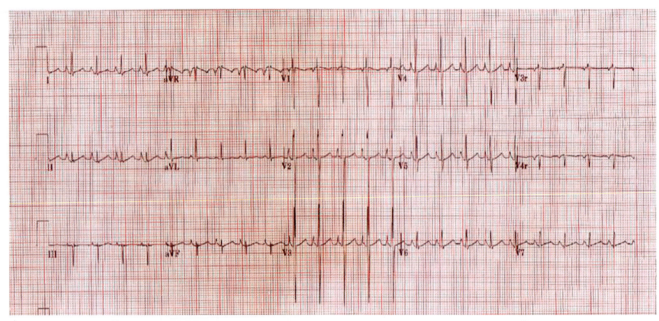

• **Figure 65.4** Electrocardiogram in a patient with tricuspid atresia demonstrating giant P waves, suggesting right atrial enlargement.

and size of the SVC. Pre-Fontan studies are aimed at obtaining hemodynamic data, including pulmonary artery (PA) pressure, transpulmonary gradient, PVR, left ventricular end-diastolic pressure (LVEDP), as well as anatomic data, including the presence of important PA stenosis, PA and bidirectional cavopulmonary shunt anatomy, presence and location of aortopulmonary and venovenous collaterals, and intervention on these collaterals as indicated. Recently magnetic resonance imaging (MRI) has been gaining popularity as a modality of anatomic and hemodynamic assessment before the Glenn or Fontan operation.[25-27] The lack of exposure to radiation and the noninvasive nature of the study are very appealing. Cardiac catheterization is reserved for patients in whom (1) noninvasive tests indicate the need for intervention, (2) ventricular function or hemodynamics appear poor, and (3) MRI is contraindicated (implants, pacemakers).[25,28]

Management of Tricuspid Atresia

TA was the first lesion successfully managed as a "single ventricle" and in fact was the lesion that was initially described in the so-called perfect Fontan. The treatment remains mainly surgical. The ultimate goal of the single-ventricle pathway is through a series of operations to convert parallel circulation of the systemic and pulmonary beds into an in-series circulation. The pulmonary circulation remains passive, whereas the single ventricle maintains systemic circulation. The transpulmonary gradient remains the driving force for the blood from the systemic venous side to the pumping ventricle. The classic stages include (1) providing a stable source of pulmonary blood flow with either an aortopulmonary shunt or ductal stent; (2) constructing passive flow of the upper-body venous blood to the pulmonary arteries with either a bidirectional cavopulmonary shunt (Glenn) or a hemi-Fontan; and (3) Fontan completion, which entails separation of the circulations by creating a pathway for the lower-body venous blood (inferior vena cava [IVC] and/or hepatic veins) to enter the passive pulmonary circulation.[29-31]

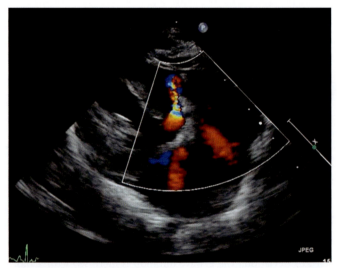

• **Figure 65.5** Echocardiogram demonstrating a patient with tricuspid atresia and a very restrictive bulboventricular foramen and decreased pulmonary blood flow requiring a shunt in the neonatal period.

Management of the Newborn With Decreased Pulmonary Blood Flow

The subgroups of neonates with decreased pulmonary blood flow (Fig. 65.5) require some form of a shunt to increase pulmonary blood flow. These patients are dependent on the PDA for their pulmonary blood flow. Ductal closure would lead to severe hypoxemia, metabolic acidosis, and death, therefore necessitating continuous infusion of prostaglandin E_1 (PGE_1) to maintain ductal patency.[32-34] Pulmonary overcirculation is a condition in which there is increased blood flow to the lungs compromising systemic perfusion and adequate tissue oxygen delivery. Arterial oxygen saturation, as measured by pulse oximetry, is surrogate to the Q_p:Q_s (shunt fraction). For example, an oxygen saturation of 75%

approximates a $Q_p:Q_s$ of 1:1, 85% of approximately 2:1, and 95% of 5:1. The serum lactate levels are a good indicator of the systemic cardiac output and systemic oxygen delivery. Lactate levels are elevated (>2) when the tissue perfusion is inadequate. Lactate levels are not a reflection of $Q_p:Q_s$ except that inadequate Q_p might result in significant hypoxemia, leading to inadequate tissue oxygen delivery, and excessive Q_p (in relation to Q_s) might correlate with inadequate Q_s (as more output is shunted toward the pulmonary circulation) and inability to sustain necessary systemic cardiac output. A $Q_p:Q_s$ of 1:1 requires a "double" cardiac output from the single ventricle (one output for the pulmonary circulation and one for the systemic circulation), and a $Q_p:Q_s$ of 3:1 requires a quadruple cardiac output! So it is understandable how the demands of increasing cardiac work from unlimited pulmonary blood flow can overwhelm the capability of the heart to provide essential systemic flow. Optimal $Q_p:Q_s$ is obtained by medical management with adjustments in pulmonary and systemic vascular resistance. This includes correction of acidosis, maintenance of normal blood glucose and calcium levels, normothermia, and manipulation of the blood PO_2 and CO_2 levels. Mechanical ventilation and sedation may be required to maintain physiologic $Q_p:Q_s$. The systemic vascular resistance can be altered by using vasodilators and vasoconstrictors. It is critical to realize that the $Q_p:Q_s$ is a *ratio* and not an absolute number for cardiac output. Lactic acidosis is an excellent parameter to reflect whether or not systemic oxygen delivery is adequate in the face of the $Q_p:Q_s$ presented by the patient. A patient with a systemic oxygen saturation of 95% and normal lactate levels may have a high $Q_p:Q_s$ but is clearly maintaining adequate systemic oxygen delivery (e.g., has a normal cardiac output). A patient with an oxygen saturation of 80% ($Q_p:Q_s$ 1.5:1) and a lactate level that is at 3 and rising may have less overall cardiac work but is also showing signs of inadequate cardiac output.

As mentioned previously, the first priority for management is to ensure a stable source of pulmonary blood flow. Flow generated across a BVF may be adequate initially, but the proclivity of the BVF to close mandates close follow-up of oxygen saturations and echocardiograms with willingness to place a shunt if the flow into the pulmonary arteries across the BVF becomes inadequate. If the baby is ductal dependent for pulmonary blood flow (common), then the initial management might require choosing between a ductal stent or a surgically placed aortopulmonary shunt.[35]

The Modified Blalock-Taussig Shunt

Creating an aortopulmonary shunt is used to provide a stable source of pulmonary blood flow. The classic Blalock-Taussig shunt (which entailed division of the subclavian artery and anastomosis of the subclavian artery to the PA), Potts shunt (direct connection between the left PA and the descending aorta), and Waterston shunt (direct connection between the posterior portion of the ascending aorta and the right PA where it courses behind the aorta) remain mostly of historical interest only.[36] At present the modified Blalock-Taussig shunt remains the choice for augmenting pulmonary blood flow in the neonate. Introduced by de Leval et al. in 1975, this aortopulmonary shunt[37] is a modification of the original description of the Blalock-Taussig shunt in 1944. It involves interposing an expanded polytetrafluoroethylene (ePTFE; Gore-Tex) graft between the innominate or subclavian artery and the ipsilateral PA (Fig. 65.6). The goal of the operation is to provide pulmonary blood flow to obtain a systemic oxygen saturation of approximately 75% to 85%. This provides a $Q_p:Q_s$ of 1 to 1.8:1. Depending on the size of the neonate and on whether there is an additional source

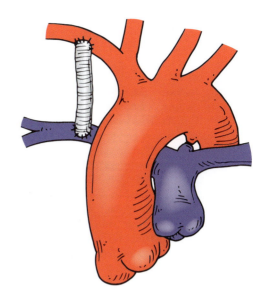

• **Figure 65.6** Right modified Blalock-Taussig shunt. In this illustration the patent ductus arteriosus has been ligated, but that is not always required.

of pulmonary blood flow (such as across a restrictive BVF), the most commonly used shunts are 3.5 mm or 4.0 mm in diameter. As shown by the Congenital Heart Surgeons Society study, an indexed shunt size of 0.8 to 1.0 results in more favorable outcomes (mortality and successfully transitioning to a cavopulmonary shunt).[38] The provision of a stable source of pulmonary blood flow allows for symmetric growth of the PAs without overcirculation, thus allowing favorable anatomic conditions for future cavopulmonary anastomosis.

The postoperative management of the newborn with an aortopulmonary shunt can be challenging. Optimum management requires meticulous attention to the $Q_p:Q_s$ and often involves titration of inotropic medications to ensure adequate systemic perfusion combined with ventilator management to minimize overcirculation. The goals are to maintain adequate shunt flow, arterial oxygen saturation (SaO_2) between 75% and 85%, and adequate ventricular function. If ventricular function is adequate to manage the increased cardiac output demands of increased $Q_p:Q_s$, many babies tolerate oxygen saturations of 85% to 90% quite well. Use of near-infrared spectroscopy (NIRS) has become standard with these neonates, and trends in both the cerebral and somatic NIRS may offer early warning signs of poor systemic perfusion.[39] The differential diagnosis for low SaO_2 includes hypotension, shunt stenosis (Fig. 65.7) or occlusion, lung disease (pulmonary venous desaturation), and impaired ventricular function (or low cardiac output). Although many surgeons favor subtherapeutic "low-dose" unfractionated heparin drip in the immediate postoperative course, which can be later transitioned to enteral aspirin to maintain shunt patency, there are no data to support the use of subtherapeutic heparin, and the efficacy of long-term use of aspirin may depend on platelet response to aspirin as measured by current assays. Some studies have shown that a significant number of neonates and infants are refractory to aspirin with respect to platelet effect. More recently, some surgeons have favored using ePTFE grafts that are infused with heparin, although the benefit of these grafts is also unproven.[40-42] Perhaps the most important factor for graft patency is the technical adequacy of the anastomosis and the quality of the vessels to which the graft is connected.

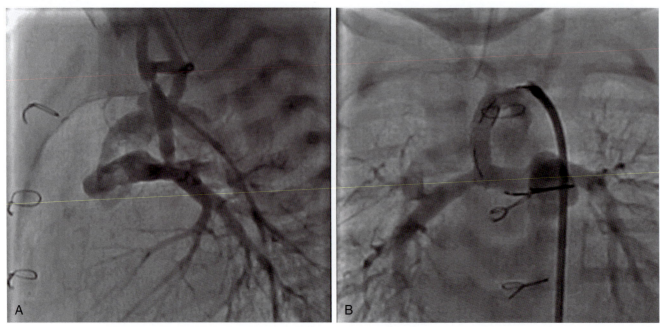

• **Figure 65.7** Angiogram performed after a modified right Blalock-Taussig shunt. (A) Proximal and distal shunt stenosis is demonstrated. (B) Appearance after stent placement.

Excessive pulmonary overcirculation may be manifested by high SaO_2 levels, pulmonary edema, and failure to wean from mechanical ventilation. This often requires manipulation of the PVR by judicious use of milrinone, permissive hypercapnia, and selective inotropic support to improve the ability of the heart to maintain the increased cardiac output demands of a high $Q_p:Q_s$. In extreme circumstances, persistent pulmonary overcirculation may also require operative revision to reduce shunt size (often by "clipping" or banding the shunt). An important factor in this type of circumstance is whether or not the ductus was left open at the time of shunt creation. Many surgeons leave the ductus alone and allow it to close by discontinuation of prostaglandin infusion. This has the advantage that if a shunt occludes in the postoperative period, the intensive care unit (ICU) team can reinstitute prostaglandin in hopes of restoring ductal patency. (The logic behind this is simply that in the era of classic BT shunts, performed via a thoracotomy, the PDA was never ligated). Occasionally, however, a PDA does not close after the cessation of prostaglandins and can create a significant additional source of pulmonary blood flow that may need surgical attention. Although this is unusual, it is important for the ICU team to know whether or not the ductus was ligated at the time of surgical shunt placement.

As mentioned earlier in this chapter, the management of patients with shunt physiology is potentially complex. Although the $Q_p:Q_s$ is an important determinant, it is merely a *ratio* and not an actual number. It is also important for the management team to assess the overall systemic oxygen delivery as a reflection of cardiac output. For example, if there is truly excessive pulmonary overcirculation, there may be a low systemic cardiac output, and this drives down the mixed venous O_2 saturation. If the mixed venous O_2 saturation is 40%, and there is a 5:1 shunt, but the pulmonary venous saturation is 90% due to pulmonary edema, then the O_2 saturation might be 81% (five parts 90 = 450 and one part 40 gives a mixing in the heart of 490, which divided by 6 provides a mixed saturation of 81). Although this may seem ideal, it clearly is not and will become manifest by rising lactate levels. Conversely, a patient may have a saturation of 93% and normal lactate levels. This would reflect that the heart is capable of maintaining excessive additional cardiac output (as much as six outputs to the lung for every output to the body), and, although this may not be a good long-term situation, if it is tolerable, it can be managed with systemic afterload reduction, permissive hypercapnia, and, if necessary, investigation into whether or not there is an additional source of pulmonary flow, such as across a patent ductus or BVF. The point to illustrate is that patients with shunts have *abnormal circulation,* and the astute management team takes into account a variety of factors beyond the $Q_p:Q_s$ in determining whether or not the patient is well palliated.

Hypoxemia in the immediate postoperative period represents an emergency. Absence of a "shunt murmur" (in a hypoxemic patient) represents shunt thrombosis until proven otherwise. Confirmation by echocardiography is important, and this usually requires emergent return to the operating room for revision or may even require institution of extracorporeal membrane oxygenation support if the operating room is not available. In instances in which the ductus was not ligated, rapid reinstitution of PGE_1 infusion may be lifesaving. Less acute and severe hypoxemia can sometimes be managed in the catheterization laboratory by balloon angioplasty or stenting of the shunt[43,44] (see Fig. 65.7). Other diagnoses in the differential of postoperative hypoxemia include low cardiac output, lung disease, atelectasis, and phrenic nerve paralysis.

Management of the Newborn With Increased Pulmonary Blood Flow

Infants with increased pulmonary blood flow who present with physiologically important "pulmonary overcirculation" will demonstrate significant clinical effects such as lactic acidosis, poor renal function with rising blood urea nitrogen or creatinine level, and even pulmonary edema—which may actually affect oxygenation leading to hypoxemia, despite the excessive pulmonary blood

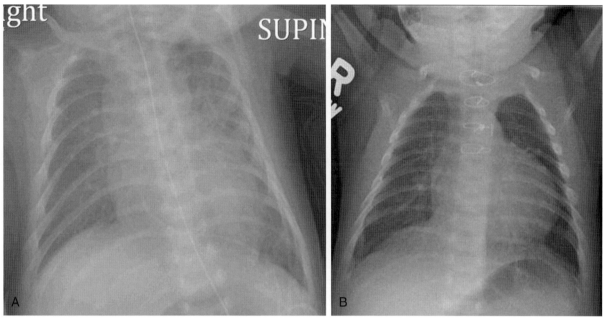

• **Figure 65.8** Infant with type 1 tricuspid atresia and increased pulmonary blood flow. (A) Before pulmonary artery (PA) bands, chest x-ray showing pulmonary edema. (B) After PA bands. Lung fields have cleared.

flow (which is why $Q_p:Q_s$ is a guideline to be used in conjunction with the overall clinical picture) (Fig. 65.8A). Patients with transposed great vessels and TA may actually have significant systemic outflow obstruction (either at the subaortic level or at the level of the aortic arch and isthmus or both).[14] This combination of defects creates the dual problem of decreased systemic perfusion and pulmonary overcirculation; and when there is aortic arch hypoplasia or a prominent coarctation, these infants may be ductal dependent for systemic perfusion and require, despite their "pulmonary overcirculation," the institution of PGE_1 for maintenance of ductal patency to perfuse the body (when the aorta is obstructed). These are complex circumstances. When pulmonary overcirculation is simply created by flow across a large BVF (VSD) into normal pulmonary arteries (without aortic obstruction), then consideration can be given to placing a PA band. Strict control of the pulmonary blood flow is required to protect the lung bed and prevent lung disease because the ultimate goal of palliation is a Fontan. PA banding was originally introduced by Muller in 1952.[7] Providers must be cognizant of the fact that PA banding may accelerate narrowing of the BVF over time with ensuing subaortic obstruction and cyanosis.[45] Further, PA distortion and ventricular hypertrophy represent additional risks inherent to PA banding. Patients who receive a PA band to control excessive pulmonary blood flow are at risk for developing rapidly progressive cyanosis that may necessitate further intervention in a short-term time frame.

Although PA banding can be performed through a thoracotomy, the sternotomy approach is currently most common because this allows superior access and ability to institute bypass and limits future incisions. The goal of the band, in patients being staged to Fontan, such as is the case for babies with TA, is to drop the pressure distal to the band to as low as possible (normal PA pressures) (Fig. 65.9). In a critically ill infant, adequate tightness of the band may be difficult to achieve initially (because this will create afterload to the heart), and in some cases, as the baby recovers, the band

may need to be tightened. It is important that ultimately the band is made tight enough to protect the pulmonary arteries from exposure to high flow and high pressure (see Fig. 65.8B).

In the patients described earlier who have the combination of pulmonary overcirculation and aortic obstruction with ductal dependency to maintain systemic perfusion, a PA band would be potentially deadly—because it would create afterload to both systemic *and* pulmonary outflow and not address the need for improved systemic perfusion. For these patients the Damus-Kaye-Stansel operation (main PA to aortic anastomosis) addresses the subaortic obstruction, and an additional shunt provides pulmonary blood flow (Fig. 65.10).

Bidirectional Glenn (Cavopulmonary Anastomosis)

The "classic Glenn" (as described by William Glenn[46] in 1958) involved end-to-end anastomosis of the divided right PA to the divided SVC with ligation of the proximal SVC. This operation is now rarely used secondary to the arteriovenous malformations that develop in the right lung secondary to lack of restoring (in the ultimate Fontan) the presence of "hepatic factor" into the right pulmonary circulation. The current approach involves a bidirectional Glenn (BDG) wherein the SVC supplies both the lungs, and that permits the ultimate Fontan connection to also perfuse both right and left lung circulation[47,48] (Fig. 65.11).

The BDG represents the next step of palliation. This follows the modified Blalock-Taussig shunt for newborns with decreased pulmonary blood flow (e.g., type 1A or 1B) or a PA band for newborns with pulmonary plethora (type 1C) or even the Damus-Kaye-Stansel for infants with transposition and TA who will ultimately require conversion from shunt physiology to cavopulmonary physiology. The BDG procedure converts the patient from an arterial shunt to a venous shunt. The goal is to perform the BDG when the PVR is at its nadir (usually at approximately 5

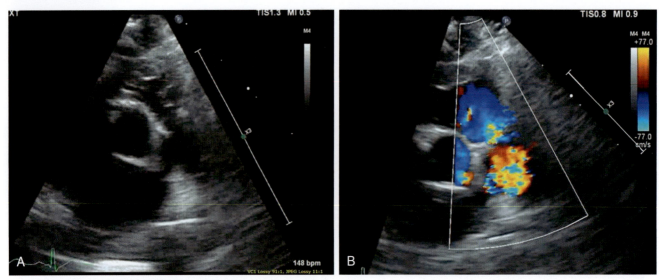

• **Figure 65.9** Echocardiography performed after pulmonary artery (PA) band placement. (A) Demonstrating the narrowing of the PA at the band site. (B) Peak gradient of 50 mm Hg measured across the PA band site.

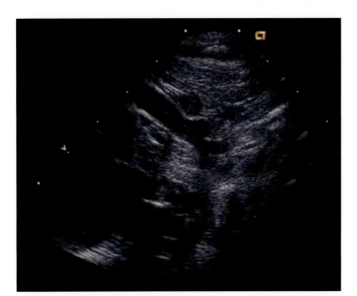

• **Figure 65.10** Tricuspid atresia with d-transposition of the great vessels, small bulboventricular foramen, hypoplastic aorta, and coarctation requiring Damus-Kaye-Stansel operation and shunt.

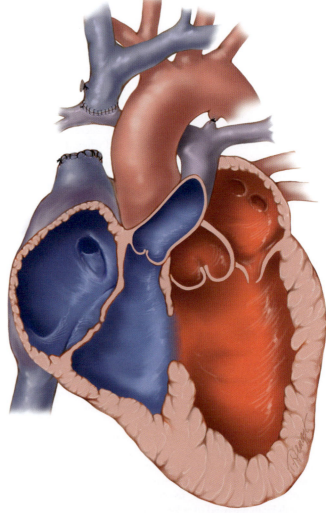

• **Figure 65.11** The bidirectional Glenn procedure.

months of age [from 3 to 6 months of age]). There are subgroups of patients with TA (type 1B or 2B) with balanced circulation who may undergo BDG as their first palliative operation.

The BDG is usually performed through a median sternotomy and uses cardiopulmonary bypass to facilitate careful takedown of the previous palliation (shunt or band), reconstruction of the PAs when needed, and accurate, carefully performed anastomosis of the delicate SVC to the PA. After the SVC is divided, the atrial end is oversewn. Some surgeons leave a small amount of antegrade pulmonary blood flow in hopes of decreasing arteriovenous malformation by allowing the "hepatic factor" to directly reach the pulmonary bed, allowing for better growth of the pulmonary arteries. This approach may lead to a "pulsatile" BDG, which is not well tolerated by some patients (manifested by pleural effusions and superior vena caval syndrome). However, leaving an additional source of pulmonary blood flow along with a BDG may allow this to be the final palliative operation. It is recommended that the azygous vein be ligated (or divided) at the time of BDG so that there is less likelihood for the higher venous pressures in the SVC following the construction of the BDG to create a venovenous "detour" from the SVC, via the azygous, to the IVC and thus reduce the pulmonary blood flow. (Ligation of the azygous should, of course, not be done in cases of IVC interruption—not typical in TA).

The hemi-Fontan is an alternative to the BDG. The operation is more extensive than a BDG but is felt by some to facilitate an intracardiac Fontan completion. This operation appears to be associated with an initial higher incidence of sinus node dysfunction but the dysfunction does not seem to be significant at the time of hospital discharge.[49]

Some patients with TA have bilateral SVCs (both a right and a left SVC, with the latter typically returning flow to the coronary sinus). In these cases, when there is no innominate (or "crossing") vein connecting the two SVCs, the patient will require bilateral, BDG procedures. The challenge with these patients lies in the small diameter of each SVC. Resistance to flow is related to the diameter of a tube, and when the tube (SVC) is smaller, there will be more natural resistance to flow (and in fact the resistance is increased to the fourth power given any change in diameter, so this influence of diameter on resistance is significant). For patients with bilateral SVC it is generally preferable to wait longer (often until a year of age, if possible) to convert the initial palliation to cavopulmonary flow, and this is a consideration when performing initial palliation in these patients.

Finally, at the time of the Glenn operation, it is prudent to consider performing an atrial septectomy. Although the intraatrial septum in TA is usually nonrestrictive, it can become restrictive as the child grows, and it is important that there be no obstruction to systemic venous return in order for the child to grow without this potential limitation to cardiac output.

Postoperative Management After a Bidirectional Glenn/Hemi-Fontan

Saturations of 80% to 85% are usually expected after BDG operations. To manage deviation from this result, such as significant hypoxemia, it is important for the provider to understand how these saturations are created. In the typical circumstance the SVC of a 5- to 6-month-old infant carries approximately one-third of the venous return, and the IVC carries approximately two-thirds of the venous return. There is an important physiologic advantage to BDG (or cavopulmonary physiology) compared with the physiology of the shunted or banded patient. As described earlier, the shunted or banded patient has an excess cardiac output. Even at a Q_p:Q_s of 1:1, the cardiac output demand on the heart is double (the heart has to pump one output to the lungs and one to the body). Once the BDG is performed, the heart simply pumps one single cardiac output, and this output is ejected into the aorta. When the flow returns to the heart, one-third of the return (from the upper body) is from the SVC, and this return now traverses the pulmonary bed and gets oxygenated and returns to the heart at 100% saturated—presuming the lungs are not impaired. The other two-thirds returns to the heart through the IVC (which includes renal vein return, which is generally not very desaturated because a lot of renal flow is for filtration and not simply to provide oxygen). We can presume that with normal cardiac output the IVC (mixed venous) saturation is 70%. So

in the typical case, two-thirds (two parts) of the return to the single ventricle is at 70% to mix with the one part, returning via the SVC and the lungs, at 100%. Two parts 70 = 140, plus one part 100 equals 240. Divide by 3, and you would expect a saturation of 80%! When patients present after BDG with a significant deviation from this expectation, it is important to work out the reason. A common reason is a lower than expected mixed venous saturation (from low cardiac output, high oxygen extraction [e.g., low hematocrit]). Suppose the mixed venous saturation is 60%. This would predict a systemic oxygen saturation, after mixing of two parts 60 with one part 100 in the heart of 73%. In this scenario the treatment has nothing to do with ventilation and everything to do with improving systemic oxygen delivery by increasing cardiac output. Of course, if there is significant atelectasis and the pulmonary venous return is at 85%, then one part 85 with two parts 60 would produce a reduction of the saturations to approximately 68%—usually a level that gets everyone concerned. The management of this is to BOTH treat the atelectasis *and* improve cardiac output. If obstruction of the Glenn (and imagine "pop off" into an untied azygous) creates a scenario in which Glenn flow is only 20% of venous return—even if the lungs are performing well; then one part 100 and four parts 70 might predict a saturation of 76%—not bad if simply following saturations, but not optimal for PA growth and long-term outcome. Glenn obstruction can be mechanical (from a suboptimal anastomosis), or it can be physiologic from pulmonary resistance abnormality, and the latter can be treated with oxygen and nitric oxide, whereas the former might need surgical intervention. Using this algorithm, it is possible for the intensive care team to troubleshoot and understand when the oxygen saturations deviate from expectations and require management. Although hypoxemia following BDG is one of the most common postoperative complications, it may be secondary to lung disease, pulmonary hypertension, ventricular dysfunction, or stenosis at the Glenn anastomosis (Fig. 65.12A). Measurement of pressures directly in the operating room avoids anatomic issues. However, identification of such anastomotic narrowing via echocardiography or computed tomography scan requires management in the catheterization laboratory or reoperation (see Fig. 65.12B). Elevation of PVR is suggested by a high transpulmonary gradient (SVC pressure − atrial pressure). Therapy should be directed toward lowering the PVR to promote pulmonary blood flow. This may entail inhaled nitric oxide or phosphodiesterase inhibitors. Mechanical ventilation parameters are set to maintain low mean airway pressures (low positive end-expiratory pressure, optimal inspiratory to expiratory times). Early extubation[50] is promoted to allow return of intrathoracic pressures to atmospheric levels and allows for cerebral autoregulation of blood flow. Elevation of the head end of the bed and permissive hypercarbia[51,52] (causes cerebral vasodilation) promote pulmonary blood flow and an increase in tissue oxygen delivery. Ventricular dysfunction is managed with inotropy.

The BDG allows for enough oxygen for growth of the young child. But as the child grows, the IVC blood assumes a greater proportion of ventricular preload, and the pulmonary venous return from the BDG assumes a lesser proportion. At this stage the next step of palliation is indicated.

The development of venous-venous collaterals over time may contribute to cyanosis with Glenn physiology. Elevated central venous pressure after a BDG promotes recanalization of some vestigial veins, and therefore intentional closure of these collaterals may improve saturations.[53]

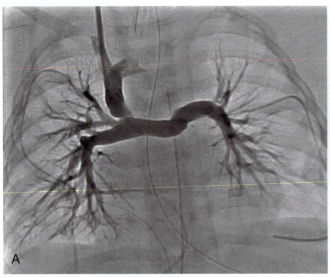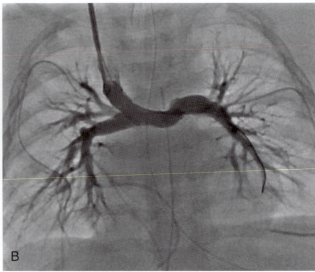

• **Figure 65.12** Cardiac catheterization after the bidirectional Glenn procedure with persistent hypoxia. (A) Moderate Glenn stenosis. (B) Stenosis adequately treated with a stent.

The Fontan Operation

The physiologic basis of this operation is to separate the pulmonary and systemic circulations. This is accomplished by directing all the systemic venous blood to the pulmonary blood directly and allowing the ventricle to support the systemic circulation. Thus this operation allows for better systemic saturations and reduced volume loading on the systemic ventricle and decreases the risk of paradoxical embolism from right-to-left shunts. The cost of this physiologic change is elevated systemic venous pressure, which remains the central cause of most of the long-term complications seen after this operation.

The original description of this operation by Fontan involved closing the ASD and establishing a connection between the RA and the PA. This was applied to a patient with TA in 1968.[54] It was initially believed that the RA would hypertrophy and act as a pumping chamber and that valves were essential in the circuit. However, both these assumptions proved to be wrong. The valves tend to get stuck in the open position and do not decrease the systemic venous pressure. The RA remains a passive conduit to blood flow to the lungs and dilates over time, contributing to energy loss and arrhythmias.[12,55] The classic Fontan as described originally is no longer performed. All subsequent modifications of this operation have been labelled *modified Fontan.*

The modified Fontan usually takes one of two forms, the lateral tunnel Fontan (introduced in 1988 by de Leval et al.[56]) or the extracardiac Fontan (described by Marcelleti et al.[57] in 1990). The former is achieved in combination with a BDG; the RA is then septated with a tube of prosthetic material to create a lateral tunnel allowing the IVC and SVC blood to be directed to the PAs. The alternative approach to achieving a total cavopulmonary connection is the extracardiac Fontan. This operation allows for placement of a prosthetic tube outside the atrium, connecting the IVC to the PAs at the level of the BDG (Fig. 65.13). The advantages and disadvantages of each of these options are still debatable. Theoretically the extracardiac approach limits the number of atrial suture lines and minimizes manipulation of the sinoatrial nodal area. Thrombogenicity and lack of growth remain long-term concerns with the extracardiac approach.[58-62]

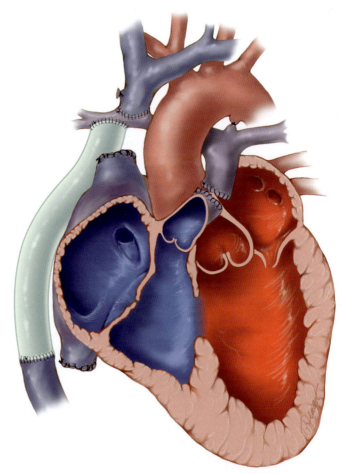

• **Figure 65.13** Extracardiac Fontan operation.

Fenestrated Fontan: Fenestration involves leaving a small communication between the Fontan pathway and the pulmonary venous atrium (Video 65.1). This was popularized by the Boston Children's Hospital group in 1990.[63] Sudden diversion of the entire systemic venous blood to the pulmonary circuit may result in low systemic blood flow and high systemic venous pressures. This can be addressed in the immediate perioperative period by fenestrating the Fontan. This allows for shunting of blood from the Fontan circuit to the pulmonary venous atrium. This augments the preload to the systemic (pumping) ventricle and decreases the systemic venous pressure (by allowing some of the blood on the systemic venous side to "pop off" into the systemic pumping side of the circulation without having to traverse the pathway through the lungs) at the expense of some obligatory desaturation. The fenestration allows a pathway for paradoxical embolization. Many fenestrations close spontaneously (25% to 30%),[64,65] but delayed closure can usually be performed in the catheterization laboratory. Some studies have demonstrated that fenestration is associated with decreased pleural drainage and decreased length of hospital stay, though at the expense of lower saturations, theoretical risk of paradoxical embolism, and need for potential future closure. These findings are consistent and reported by the Dallas group (prospectively studied)[66] and the Pediatric Heart Network-Fontan Study (retrospectively studied).[67] There does not seem to be any difference between the two groups in terms of exercise tolerance, growth, echocardiographic variables, or functional health status. Interestingly, the postoperative stroke rate remains the same in both the cohorts. Test closure of the fenestration can be performed before occluding the fenestration with a device, and hemodynamics measured before and after test occlusion before closure of the fenestration to assess the hemodynamics (and test tolerance) following closure. Fenestration closure usually provides improved saturations and decreased need for anticongestive therapy and improved somatic growth with a risk of developing new arrhythmias. The relative risks and benefits of routine fenestration are debated, with some surgeons using it selectively (i.e., in "high-risk" Fontan candidates) and others preferring routine fenestration.[66,68,69]

The ideal candidate for the Fontan operation is outlined in Box 65.2. These were the originally described "10 commandments." In the modern era most of these remain relative contraindications to performing a Fontan operation. Elevated PVR remains an important risk factor for perioperative death. Impaired ventricular function and decreased diastolic compliance are critical for the successful Fontan operation. Elevated LVEDP and LA pressure decrease the perfusion pressure gradient (SVC − LA pressure) for inflow into the LV. Greater than moderate AV valve regurgitation should generally be addressed before or at the time of the Fontan creation.

• BOX 65.2   **The "Ten Commandments"**

1. Minimum age of 4 years (not a requirement currently)
2. Sinus rhythm (not a requirement currently)
3. Normal caval drainage (not a requirement currently)
4. Right atrium of normal volume (not a requirement currently)
5. Mean PAP ≤15 mm Hg (relative contraindication currently)
6. Pulmonary artery resistance <4 Woods units × m²
   (relative contraindication currently)
7. Pulmonary artery to aorta diameter ratio ≥0.75 (not a requirement currently)
8. Normal ventricular function (EF >60%) (relative contraindication currently)
9. Competent left atrioventricular valve (relative contraindication currently)
10. No impairing effects of previous shunts (relative contraindication currently)

EF, *Ejection fraction*; PAP, *pulmonary artery pressure.*

Postoperative Problems After the Fontan Operation

Low cardiac output (early): After the Fontan operation the cardiac output is dependent on the pulmonary blood flow. As the single ventricle fills passively, blood return to the LA is dependent on the transpulmonary gradient (between the systemic venous pressure and LA pressure). In general this gradient needs to be approximately 7 mm Hg. Differential diagnosis for reduced pulmonary blood flow after the Fontan operation includes hypovolemia, increased PVR or systemic vascular resistance, obstruction to the Fontan circuit, pulmonary venous obstruction, distortion of the PAs, AV valve regurgitation, and ventricular dysfunction.

Elevation of the PA pressure with a normal LA pressure suggests increased PVR, which can be confirmed by cardiac catheterization. Pulmonary vasodilator administration and manipulation of the ventilator settings help manage this problem. Fenestration of the Fontan circuit helps maintain systemic output in this condition. Rarely, conversion back to a BDG or shunt physiology may be required.

Low cardiac output in the setting of high PA pressures and LA pressures suggest ventricular dysfunction, severe AV valve regurgitation, or systemic outflow obstruction.

Complications of Systemic Venous Hypertension

This remains the Achilles' heel of the Fontan operation. All patients with Fontan physiology have elevated systemic venous pressures. This leads to transudation of fluid into the interstitial compartment, leading to development of pleural effusions, ascites, peripheral edema, plastic bronchitis, and protein-losing enteropathy.

Pleural effusions (early) remain the most common complication after the Fontan operation. Fenestration may decrease the duration of chest tube drainage.[66,70] Other management strategies involve fluid restriction, minimal-fat diets, aggressive diuresis, and maintenance of sinus rhythm. Although once thought to be useful, duct ligation is no longer widely considered to be useful for the management of chylous effusions compared with more sophisticated lymphangiographic guided techniques.[71,72] Recently vasopressin has been advocated in the perioperative management of the Fontan patient in lieu of afterload reduction such as milrinone. This neurohypophysial hormone has been shown to decrease the need for fluid resuscitation and hence, secondarily, decrease the quantity and duration of chest tube output and reduce length of hospital stay.[73,74]

Passive venous congestion of the liver is common. Management of this requires decreasing the systemic venous pressure and maintaining adequate ventricular function. Chronic passive sinusoidal congestion of the liver leads to fibrosis. Modification of risk factors can ameliorate and possibly regress fibrosis but will not alleviate the problem completely. Progression to cirrhosis results in a "point of no return." It is important to know the functional state of the liver because this will determine the course and fate of the "failing Fontan." Liver biopsy has been the gold standard to determine the degree of fibrosis and cirrhosis in the liver, but noninvasive tools for assessing the liver in the Fontan population are emerging. Magnetic resonance (MR) elastography is very promising.[75] Low-amplitude acoustic waves are used to determine the stiffness of the liver while simultaneously imaging the liver using MR. Chronic systemic venous hypertension manifests as protein-losing enteropathy (PLE) (late). This represents a combination of gastrointestinal congestion, impaired absorption, and reduced

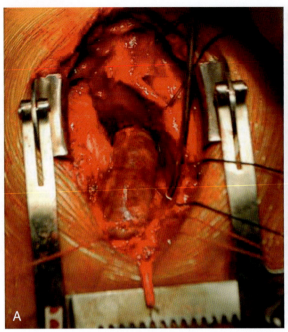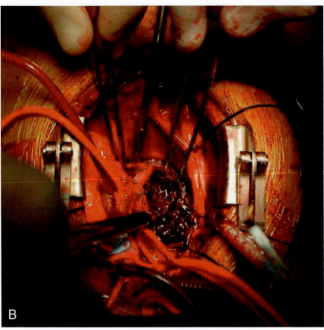

• **Figure 65.14** Thrombosis of the extracardiac Fontan circuit. (A) External appearance of a thrombosed extracardic Fontan circuit. (B) Unsuccessful salvage attempts perfomed in the catheterization laboratory followed by Fontan takedown. The picture shows the extensive thrombus in the extracardiac Fontan circuit. (Courtesy Dr. John Lamberti.)

lymphatic drainage. PLE carries a mortality of 50% at 5 years following diagnosis.[76-81]

Dysrhythmias (early and late): Atrial rhythm disturbances are common after the Fontan operation. Atrial pacing can improve cardiac output and systemic blood pressure, especially in the presence of junctional rhythm in the early postoperative period. Junctional ectopic tachycardia represents a serious rhythm disturbance after the Fontan operation. Therapy includes overdrive pacing, amiodarone, cooling, and discontinuation or reduction of catecholamine infusions. However, junctional rhythm and sinus node dysfunction remain the most common rhythm disturbance in the immediate postoperative period. Long-term, supraventricular arrhythmias are present in approximately 10% of the patients.[82-85] Fontan patients who are not predominantly in sinus rhythm should have permanent pacing systems placed to optimize the Fontan circulation.

Thrombosis (early): Thrombosis in the Fontan circuit is a risk because the flow is passive. Increased hematocrits and viscosity of the blood and slow flow rate contribute to this[83,86-90] (Fig. 65.14). Empiric anticoagulation, especially with extracardiac circuits, is usually administered. Thrombi may lead to paradoxical emboli in the presence of a fenestration. Antiplatelet therapy with aspirin and mild anticoagulation with warfarin to maintain an international normalized ratio of 1.5 is current general practice.

The incidence of Fontan takedown is 1% to 3%. This is usually believed to be secondary to poor patient selection or uncorrected anatomic abnormalities such as outflow tract obstruction or pulmonary/systemic venous obstruction. This, however, does not preclude performing a Fontan completion at a later age when the modifiable risk factors have been corrected.[91-94]

The failing Fontan can be of various phenotypes: reduced ejection fraction (systolic heart failure), preserved ejection fraction (diastolic heart failure), normal ventricle with portal venous congestion, ascites and cirrhosis or normal ventricle with PLE and plastic bronchitis. Heart transplantation offers a solution to the management of a patient with failing Fontan physiology. Survivors show uniform resolution of PLE. The mortality for transplantation in this high-risk group can be substantial. There is also a mortality risk while on the waiting list.[95,96]

There currently is limited experience using mechanical circulatory support to manage the failing single ventricle with durable mechanical devices. Several case reports of using traditional left ventricular assist devices after modifying the Fontan circuit have been reported.[97,98]

The Toronto group reported their outcomes in 2004 of a total of 137 patients with TA undergoing the Fontan operation between 1971 and 1999 with an 81% survival at 1 year and 70% at 10 years.[99] In a more contemporary series reported from Atlanta, 105 infants with TA were followed between 2002 and 2012. Seventy-four percent required neonatal palliation (44% shunt, 17% Damus-Kaye-Stansel, and 13% PA band), and 26% received a primary BDG. Overall 8-year survival was 84%. On multivariable analyses, risk factors for mortality included genetic/extracardiac anomalies and pulmonary atresia. The bulk of the mortality occurred in the interstage period between the first and second stages.[100]

Conclusion

TA is currently an uncommon single-ventricle diagnosis that can be managed with single-ventricle palliation and Fontan pathway. This interesting lesion represents a gamut of variations in anatomy and physiology, which require a variety of different surgical techniques and medical management strategies to obtain the goal of a successful Fontan completion. Because the systemic ventricle is the morphologic LV, most patients with TA, if prepared adequately, tend to have a good prognosis when compared with other single-ventricle lesions.

Selected References

A complete list of references is available at ExpertConsult.com.

4. Sarkozy A, Conti E, D'Agostino R, Digilio MC, Formigari R, Picchio F, et al. ZFPM2/FOG2 and HEY2 genes analysis in nonsyndromic tricuspid atresia. *Am J Med Genet A.* 2005;133A(2):68–70.

7. Rashkind WJ. Tricuspid atresia: A historical review. *Pediatr Cardiol.* 1982;2:85–88.

8. Edwards JE, Burchell HB. Congenital tricuspid atresia: A classification. *Med Clin North Am.* 1949;33:1117–1196.

10. Rao PS. A unified classification for tricuspid atresia. *Am Heart J.* 1980;99:799–804.

19. Rao PS. Further observations on the spontaneous closure of physiologically advantageous ventricular septal defects in tricuspid atresia: surgical implications. *Ann Thorac Surg.* 1983;35(2):121–131. Review.

54. Fontan F, Baudet E. Surgical repair of tricuspid atresia. *Thorax.* 1971;26:240–248.

66. Lemler MS, Scott WA, Leonard SR, et al. Fenestration improves clinical outcome of the Fontan procedure: A prospective, randomized study. *Circulation.* 2002;105:207–212.

68. Choussat A, Fontan F, Besse P, et al. Selection Criteria for Fontan's procedure. In: Anderson RH, Shinebourne EA, eds. *Pediatric Cardiology, 1977.* Edinburgh: Churchill Livingstone; 1978:559–566.

99. Sittiwangkul R, Azakie A, Van Arsdell GS, Williams WG, McCrindle BW. Outcomes of tricuspid atresia in the Fontan era. *Ann Thorac Surg.* 2004;77(3):889–894.

100. Alsoufi B, Schlosser B, Mori M, et al. Influence of Morphology and Initial Surgical Strategy on Survival of Infants With Tricuspid Atresia. *Ann Thorac Surg.* 2015;100(4):1403–1409, discussion 1409–14010.

66

Hypoplastic Left Heart Syndrome

JAMES QUINTESSENZA, MD; HOLLY C. DESENA, MD; LINDSEY JUSTICE, DNP, RN, CPNP-AC; MARSHALL L. JACOBS, MD

Definition

Hypoplastic left heart syndrome (HLHS) is the term used to describe a spectrum of congenital cardiac malformations that exhibit varying degrees of underdevelopment of the left-sided heart structures. Features of HLHS include mitral valve and aortic valve atresia or stenosis, with resultant hypoplasia or absence of the left ventricle and hypoplasia of the ascending aorta and aortic arch (Fig. 66.1). These anatomic defects result in single-ventricle physiology, which requires complete intracardiac mixing of pulmonary venous and systemic venous blood that is then supplied to parallel pulmonary and systemic circuits. Systemic blood flow is maintained by the right ventricle via the pulmonary artery (PA) and a patent ductus arteriosus (Fig. 66.2).

This chapter focuses on the initial stage of reconstructive surgery as a treatment modality for children born with HLHS. Beyond initial reconstruction these infants are managed in a manner analogous to the management of other univentricular heart malformations destined for a modified Fontan operation. Thus considerations relevant to subsequent stages of the reconstructive sequence culminating in Fontan circulation are discussed in Chapter 63. The other surgical option, cardiac transplantation, is discussed in detail in Chapter 73.

Epidemiology and Embryology

HLHS is the most common congenital cardiac malformation in which only one developed ventricle is found. The syndrome was described in 1952 by Lev[1] and later termed HLHS by Noonan and Nadas.[2] HLHS is estimated to occur in 2.3 per 10,000 live births in the United States each year.[3]

It accounts for 10.9% of mortalities from congenital heart disease, with a reported postoperative hospital mortality of 16% and interstage mortality of 8% to 12%.[4-8] The embryologic cause of HLHS is not fully understood, but the collection of lesions likely results from limitation of left ventricular inflow or outflow.

Risk Factors

HLHS occurs predominantly in males. It may be related to genetic abnormalities and is more likely to occur in infants with a family history of congenital heart disease. Additional modifiable risk factors that have been associated with HLHS are maternal prepregnancy overweight/obesity and periconceptional opioid use or fever.[9] Genetic syndromes in which HLHS has been seen include Turner syndrome, trisomy 13, trisomy 18, Holt-Oram, Smith-Lemli-Opitz, partial trisomy 9, and Jacobsen syndrome.[10]

Numerous risk factors for mortality in patients with HLHS have been reported, including low birth weight, prematurity, extracardiac anomalies, and genetic syndromes. Additionally, survival may be impacted by the specific HLHS subtype, smaller ascending aorta diameter, restrictive atrial septum, associated cardiac anomalies, right ventricular dysfunction, and severity of tricuspid regurgitation (TR).[5,11-18] Some series have reported a diminished stage I survival rate of only 79% for patients with mitral stenosis with aortic atresia, compared with the other subtypes.[19] Furthermore, HLHS with mitral stenosis and aortic atresia is associated with ventriculocoronary connections (sinusoids), which may negatively impact outcomes and survival.[19-21]

Prenatal diagnosis of patients with HLHS allows for better planning of perinatal care and is strongly associated with superior preoperative clinical status.[22,23] Although prenatal diagnosis may not have a significant impact on mortality, it is related to an improvement in morbidity, specifically with regard to neurodevelopmental outcomes.[10,17,24,25] Neonates who are not prenatally diagnosed are more likely to present in a shock state requiring resuscitation and inotropic support, which further increases their risk for right ventricular dysfunction and TR. Prenatal diagnosis also affords the opportunity to perform fetal interventions such as balloon dilation of the aortic valve or atrial septostomy, which may improve outcomes. Furthermore, if an intact or restrictive atrial septum is present, plans can be made for prompt balloon atrial septostomy immediately following delivery. HLHS with intact atrial septum or highly restrictive atrial septum without a decompressing vein, has significantly poorer outcomes with a survival rate of only approximately 70% to hospital discharge after the Norwood procedure.[26]

Pathophysiology

Overview

The left ventricle is a nonfunctional structure in the child with HLHS (Fig. 66.3). Pulmonary venous return must be routed to the right atrium through a stretched foramen ovale, an atrial septal defect, or rarely by total anomalous pulmonary venous connection. Systemic and pulmonary venous returns mix in the right atrium. The right ventricle supplies both the systemic and pulmonary circulations in a parallel fashion because the main PA (MPA) gives rise to the branch pulmonary arteries, as well as the systemic circulation via the ductus arteriosus. Blood flows retrograde from the

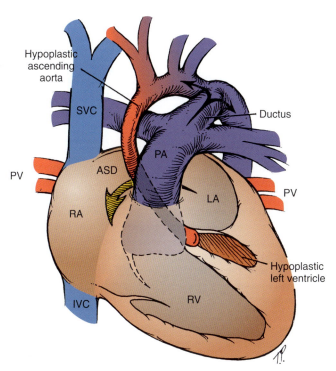

• **Figure 66.1** Native anatomy in hypoplastic left heart syndrome. Note hypoplastic left ventricle, aortic valve atresia, and hypoplastic ascending aorta. Systemic blood flow is propelled by the right ventricle *(RV)* via the pulmonary artery *(PA)* and ductus arteriosus. Pulmonary veins *(PV)* enter the left atrium *(LA)* and blood crosses the atrial septal defect *(ASD)* into the right atrium *(RA)*. Systemic venous flow returns normally from the inferior vena cava *(IVC)* and superior vena cava *(SVC)* to the RA.

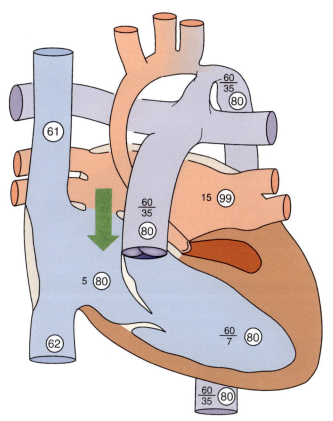

• **Figure 66.2** Schematic diagram of O₂ saturations *(circled values)* and pressures in native anatomy of hypoplastic left heart syndrome. Note increase in O₂ saturation due to mixing of systemic and pulmonary venous blood in the right atrium. The resultant systemic O₂ saturation of 80% represents balanced pulmonary and systemic blood flow (Q_p:Q_s = 1). Left atrial pressure (15 mm Hg) exceeds right atrial pressure (5 mm Hg), indicating restriction to left-to-right flow through the atrial communication.

ductus arteriosus through the transverse aortic arch to its branches and through the ascending aorta to the coronary arteries. Flow to the lower body is supplied antegrade from the ductus arteriosus to the descending aorta. Ductal closure results in inadequate systemic and coronary perfusion, leading to progressive metabolic acidosis, ischemia, and death. Based on this physiology, the clinical presenting signs of HLHS are (1) shock related to closure of the ductus arteriosus or (2) an imbalance in the ratio of pulmonary to systemic blood flow (Q_p:Q_s), resulting in signs of congestive heart failure (Chapter 72) or hypoxemia.

Changes in Pulmonary Vascular Resistance

With the pulmonary and systemic arteries connected in parallel the Q_p:Q_s depends on a delicate balance between the pulmonary and the systemic vascular resistances. The pulmonary vascular resistance (PVR) in any normal newborn is elevated at birth but then precipitously decreases with the first breaths and continues to fall over the first few weeks of life. The decrease in PVR results in increased, likely excessive, pulmonary blood flow. This increases the volume load of the right ventricle, and thus increased total cardiac output by the right ventricle is necessary to preserve adequate systemic output. By this mechanism, HLHS represents the most common cause of congestive heart failure in the first weeks of life. Unless other anatomic features act to limit pulmonary blood flow, the progressive imbalance in Q_p:Q_s will result in high-output failure, acidemia reflecting inadequate systemic perfusion, and potentially death.

Degree of Interatrial Communication

The character of the interatrial communication serves as the most common anatomic determinant of pulmonary blood flow. Because the left ventricle accepts minimal or no flow, the interatrial communication provides the only route for egress of pulmonary venous blood entering the left atrium. In neonates with HLHS and a foramen ovale as the only interatrial communication, left atrial pressure typically exceeds right atrial pressure, so blood will flow left to right at the foramen ovale (see Fig. 66.2). The resultant elevation in pulmonary venous pressure increases PVR and limits pulmonary blood flow. When the foramen ovale or an additional atrial septal defect permits unobstructed interatrial flow of blood from left to right, pulmonary blood flow increases dramatically as PVR decreases. Alternatively, excessive narrowing or obliteration of the foramen ovale imposes severe restriction on pulmonary blood flow. Therefore the systemic saturation reflects the mixture of systemic venous return with variable pulmonary venous return permitted by the interatrial communication (see Fig. 66.2).

Diagnostic Assessment

Physical Findings

Neonates with a nearly balanced Q_p:Q_s will have adequate systemic perfusion, as evidenced by a normal systemic arterial blood flow. Although this cohort may appear vigorous immediately after delivery, the deleterious cardiovascular and metabolic effects of profound hypoxemia, characterized by PaO₂ values of 20 mm Hg or lower in the most severe cases, ultimately become apparent. Myocardial performance deteriorates, and the infant will exhibit listlessness, diminished peripheral pulses, acidosis, and hypoglycemia.

Diagnostic Tests

The electrocardiogram (ECG) shows right atrial enlargement with peaked P waves in leads II, III, and aVF and right ventricular enlargement with a qR pattern in the right precordial leads. The chest radiograph reveals cardiomegaly because of right atrial, right ventricular, and proximal PA enlargement. The lung fields exhibit pulmonary congestion in the majority. In patients with severely obstructed interatrial communication the cardiomegaly is less prominent, and the pulmonary vascular markings vary from diminished to congested in a more reticular pattern, which reflects the pulmonary venous hypertension.

Two-dimensional echocardiography is sufficient to diagnose this lesion. Echocardiographic imaging determines the anatomic details. Pulse and continuous wave Doppler in conjunction with color flow analysis are then used to evaluate several aspects of the physiology. For example, the relative pulmonary and systemic resistances can be inferred from the direction of flow in the ductus arteriosus during diastole. Assessment of the tricuspid or common atrioventricular valve for regurgitation is particularly important, as well as identification of the insertion and drainage of the pulmonary veins.

Routine cardiac catheterization is not necessary in the evaluation of neonates with HLHS.

Preoperative Critical Care Management

All interventions in the preoperative period are directed toward two goals: (1) preserving ductal patency and (2) establishing or maintaining the Q$_p$:Q$_s$ ratio at unity.

Prostaglandin E₁ Infusion

Nearly all infants will have physiologic closure of the ductus arteriosus by the fourth day of life, but 20% of infants will demonstrate functional ductal closure during the first day of life, and more than 80% of infants demonstrate ductal closure during the second day of life.[27] A continuous infusion of prostaglandin E₁ (PGE₁) should be instituted once the diagnosis of HLHS has been made to preserve the infant's ductal dependent systemic circulation. Patients who were not diagnosed prenatally should receive PGE₁ infusion as soon as the diagnosis is suspected. Hence any newborn with unexplained shock is a candidate for PGE₁ infusion until HLHS or other forms of ductal dependent systemic circulation have been specifically excluded.

For patients who present in shock with suspected ductal closure or a restrictive ductus, initial prostaglandin dosing will range from 0.05 to 0.1 mcg/kg/min, and then once ductal patency is achieved, the infusion can be decreased to an effective dose of 0.01 to 0.02 mcg/kg/min.[28] It is important to maintain ductal patency with the lowest effective prostaglandin dose to minimize the most common dose-dependent side effects of the medication. Hypotension requiring volume resuscitation and respiratory depression requiring mechanical ventilator support may occur.

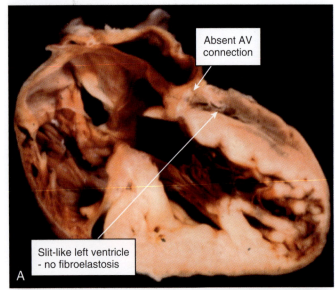

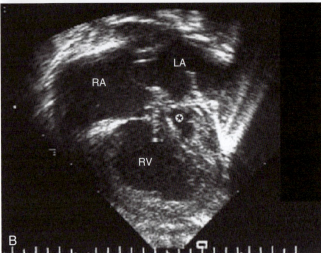

• **Figure 66.3** Morphologic specimen of hypoplastic left heart syndrome (A) with corresponding echocardiogram of hypoplastic left heart (B). *AV,* Atrioventricular. (This figure was prepared by Robert H. Anderson specifically for the use of Dr. Quintessenza. Dr. Anderson retains his intellectual copyright in the original images from which the figures were prepared.)

pressure, warm extremities with good peripheral pulses, and the absence of a metabolic acidemia. The skin color is usually dusky. Auscultation reveals a systolic ejection murmur and a single second heart sound.

Patients with widely patent atrial septal defects have a Q$_p$:Q$_s$ well in excess of 1:1. This can be tolerated as long as the right ventricle can maintain a compensatory increase in the total cardiac output (total Q). However, if total Q is inadequate, excessive pulmonary blood flow occurs at the expense of systemic blood flow, and systemic hypoperfusion develops. The physical findings in this cohort are dominated by evidence of shock and congestive heart failure. These infants appear listless and tachypneic with diminished pulses in all extremities. The liver is enlarged. Acidosis, hyperkalemia, and hypoglycemia signify metabolic decompensation.

Conversely, patients with little or no interatrial communication are deeply cyanotic because of inadequate pulmonary blood

Physiologic Assessment and Manipulation of the Ratio of Pulmonary Blood Flow to Systemic Output

Much of the preoperative management of neonates with HLHS entails optimizing the condition of the cardiovascular and other organ systems. Because the right ventricle must perfuse the pulmonary and systemic circulations in parallel, emphasis is placed on strategies that promote optimal systemic oxygen delivery with minimal overall volume work imposed on the ventricle. This goal is usually attained when pulmonary blood flow approximates systemic output (i.e., Q_p:Q_s is 1:1). Although HLHS is not unique in posing the need to balance Q_p:Q_s, there is a tendency for this cardiac malformation to exhibit high pulmonary blood flow and marginal systemic output. Perhaps the anatomic relation whereby the systemic flow must traverse the MPA on its way to the aorta contributes to this phenomenon. In addition, speculation persists as to whether the right ventricle is intrinsically less well suited to the excess volume work imposed by a high Q_p:Q_s state.

The key to management of HLHS perioperatively rests with the ability to assess systemic perfusion and Q_p:Q_s. These variables often cannot be quantified precisely under typical clinical circumstances, but clinicians can predict, measure, and manipulate this complex physiology by calculating Q_p:Q_s according to the Fick equation:

$$Q_p{:}Q_s = (Ao - SVC)/(PV - PA)$$

where Ao, SVC, PV, and PA all represent oxygen-content values at the aorta (Ao), superior vena cava (SVC), pulmonary vein (PV), and pulmonary artery (PA), respectively.

In patients with cardiac lesions that result in complete mixing and parallel systemic and pulmonary circulations, one can assume that content in the aorta and PA are equal, and the former is usually conveniently measured. When significant pulmonary disease does not complicate the clinical situation, clinicians typically assume that the PV is fully saturated with oxygen, or nearly so. That leaves the SVC content to be ascertained, and in the clinical environment, measurement of oxygen saturation usually replaces calculation of content because accurate measurement instruments are readily available, and the relation of the two values is reasonably constant. SVC saturation can be directly measured by obtaining a mixed venous saturation from a central line residing in the SVC or indirectly measured by near-infrared spectroscopy (NIRS) monitoring, a noninvasive way to continuously trend the patient's mixed venous oxygen saturation. NIRS values decrease as oxygen delivery decreases or demand increases and have been shown to assist with detection of hypoxic-ischemic conditions.[29,30]

Without a mixed venous oxygen saturation measurement, the clinical estimate of Q_p:Q_s is made on the basis of a single value, the systemic arterial saturation. However, it is problematic to assume that systemic venous saturation, as well as the difference between arterial oxygen saturation and mixed venous oxygen saturation (AVO_2 difference), is normal, especially given that the physiology of these infants makes it highly likely that systemic cardiac output may be inadequate.

For example, if the systemic oxygen saturation were 80%, and normal values are assumed for pulmonary venous saturation and AVO_2 difference, the calculation would result as follows:

$$Q_p{:}Q_s = (80 - 60)/(100 - 80) = 1$$

By using similar assumptions and a systemic oxygen saturation of 60%, the Q_p:Q_s calculation would result as follows:

$$Q_p{:}Q_s = (60 - 40)/(100 - 60) = 0.5$$

A systemic oxygen saturation of 90% might yield the following:

$$Q_p{:}Q_s = (90 - 70)/(100 - 90) = 2$$

However, these calculations can be highly inaccurate when such assumptions are made. The calculated values can be significantly altered by changing the underlying assumptions, even within normal boundaries.

For example, an infant with HLHS and excessive pulmonary blood flow at the expense of systemic perfusion could have a decreased mixed venous saturation. Using a directly or indirectly measured value for mixed venous saturation, the calculation might result as follows:

$$Q_p{:}Q_s = (90 - 50)/(100 - 90) = 4$$

On occasion these estimates can lead to serious misinterpretation and inappropriate therapy. For example, the conclusion that low systemic arterial saturation represents low Q_p:Q_s may lead to measures directed at reducing PVR. If, however, the systemic oxygen saturation reflected low cardiac output, as illustrated in the following equation, such measures would be counterproductive.

$$Q_p{:}Q_s = (70 - 35)/(95 - 70) = 1.4$$

Data from Rychik and colleagues[31] comparing the accuracy of various methods used to estimate Q_p:Q_s reveal a weak correlation between aortic oxygen saturation and measured Q_p:Q_s (Fig. 66.4). When available, the addition of data to quantify systemic output and Q_p:Q_s accurately, such as mixed venous oxygen saturation or Doppler aortic flow patterns, should be used. These measurements allow for more accurate and precise evaluation of Qp:Qs and substantially improve the assessment and appropriate intervention in patients with HLHS. This information assumes even greater importance in the context of volatile physiologic changes characteristic during the early postoperative period.

Management Strategies

Augmenting Systemic Output in the Setting of Excessive Pulmonary Blood Flow. In the preoperative period, neonates with HLHS who have been resuscitated and stabilized and who are not impaired by other vital organ system dysfunction are initially assumed to be able to maintain satisfactory balance in Q_p:Q_s or an increased total Q to compensate for a high Q_p. The most common imbalance of Q_p:Q_s typically manifests itself with signs of inadequate systemic output and relative excess in pulmonary blood flow. These signs might include hypotension, lactic acidosis, and diminished urine output in the context of relatively high systemic oxygen saturation.

In the past, clinicians administered inhaled gas mixtures to selectively constrict pulmonary vasculature and increase PVR. Infants were placed in a head hood supplemented with nitrogen to reduce alveolar PO_2 (P_AO_2) and promote hypoxic pulmonary vasoconstriction or with carbon dioxide to increase alveolar PCO_2 (P_ACO_2) to achieve constriction via local effects on pH or tissue CO_2. However, these interventions are not routinely performed in the current era. Mild hypoventilation can result in significant hypoxemia in neonates breathing a fraction of inspired oxygen

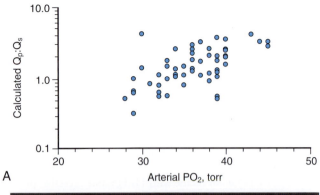

A

B

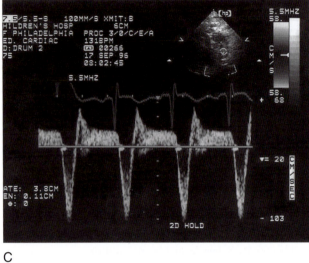

C

• **Figure 66.4** Comparison of methods used to estimate pulmonary-to-systemic blood flow ratio (Q_p:Q_s). (A) Although arterial PO_2 exhibited trend correlation with Fick determinations of Q_p:Q_s at any one value, a low correlation coefficient translates into a wide variation in Q_p:Q_s for any given arterial PO_2 ($P = .84$, $R^2 = 0.78$). (B) Conversely, estimates of Q_p:Q_s made using Doppler diastolic flow reversal exhibit a much higher coefficient of determination ($P < .001$, $R^2 = 0.94$). (C) Doppler flow pattern in the distal aortic arch. (Data and graphic from Rychik J, Bush DM, Spray TL, et al. Assessment of pulmonary/systemic blood flow ratio after first-stage palliation for hypoplastic left heart syndrome: development of a new index with the use of Doppler echocardiography. *J Thorac Cardiovasc Surg.* 102:81-87, 2000.)

(FiO_2) less than 0.21. This is illustrated by using a modification of the alveolar gas equation listed:

$$P_AO_2 = 713 \text{ mm Hg} \times FiO_2 - \frac{P_ACO_2}{0.8}$$

Under conditions of hypoxia (FiO_2 of 0.17), if the neonate hypoventilates or is apneic to the point that the P_ACO_2 reaches 70 mm Hg or both, this will result in a P_AO_2 of only 34 mm Hg. The systemic arterial PO_2 will be significantly lower because it represents a combination of the mixed venous and alveolar PO_2.

Therefore current management strategies for patients in whom Q_p:Q_s is elevated and systemic output is compromised are aimed at increasing total cardiac output, decreasing systemic vascular resistance (SVR), and augmenting intravascular volume and oxygen delivery. In the setting of low systemic perfusion the patient may likely be hypotensive, thus the addition of afterload-reducing medications is difficult. Low-dose epinephrine infusions can be used to increase contractility to augment total cardiac output. Because neonates have an immature sarcoplasmic reticulum, a calcium chloride infusion may be beneficial to improve hemodynamics because the myocardium is highly responsive to exogenous calcium.[32] Because these patients often have elevated heart rates as a consequence of low cardiac output, calcium chloride may be preferable over epinephrine because it will increase contractility without further provoking tachycardia. To maximize oxygen delivery in cyanotic patients, keeping the hemoglobin level in the range of 13 to 16 mg/dL increases mixed venous and arterial oxygen

saturations and decreases the ratio of pulmonary to systemic flow by increasing PVR.[33-35]

Respiratory Management. In current practice, mechanical ventilation is reserved only for patients with respiratory insufficiency or failure or as a means to decrease oxygen demand for patients with low systemic output.[36,37] Spontaneous breathing is preferable, but noninvasive ventilatory support may be used if necessary to reduce work of breathing and oxygen consumption.

When additional respiratory support is necessary, the use of supplemental oxygen should be avoided because oxygen decreases PVR and leads to pulmonary overcirculation. Noninvasive positive pressure ventilation or invasive positive end-expiratory pressure can be used to achieve lung volumes that exceed functional residual capacity. At higher lung volumes the pulmonary vasculature is compressed, thus increasing PVR and diminishing pulmonary blood flow.[33] Positive pressure ventilation decreases afterload on the ventricle by decreasing transmural wall stress. Therefore intubating a patient has two benefits: it decreases oxygen consumption by reducing work of breathing and decreases afterload, which subsequently increases cardiac output. The patient can benefit from these effects if intubation is necessary due to respiratory failure or low systemic output, but spontaneous breathing remains preferable in the absence of these conditions.[38]

Nutrition. Preoperative enteral nutrition has historically been avoided in patients with single–ventricle physiology and ductal dependent systemic blood flow due to the potential for systemic hypoperfusion.[38] However, preoperative trophic feedings before Norwood palliation have been shown to be safe and associated with shorter duration of mechanical ventilation, more stable postoperative hemodynamics, less fluid overload, and earlier postoperative feeding tolerance.[39] Despite this, allowance of enteral nutrition by clinicians remains variable. A survey of medical providers in the United States and Europe showed that routine preoperative feeding is prescribed by 56% of US providers and 93% of non-US providers.[40] Intestinal hypoperfusion was one of the primary concerns for withholding enteral feedings, but the relationship of enteral feeding to preoperative necrotizing enterocolitis (NEC) is unclear. Although the incidence of NEC is known to be far greater in the congenital heart disease population compared with the general population, a study evaluating the role of enteral feedings in the development of NEC in infants with congenital heart disease found that NEC developed in 3% of infants studied (45 of 1500 infants). Infants with congenital heart disease who are on high-dose prostaglandin therapy or who have experienced shock or low cardiac output are at highest risk.[41] If enteral nutrition is provided, close monitoring is required to evaluate systemic perfusion and signs of feeding intolerance, such as abdominal distention and bloody stools.

Hypoplastic Left Heart Syndrome With Severe Pulmonary Venous Obstruction

In rare circumstances, infants with elevated PVR related to pulmonary infection and those with obstruction of pulmonary venous egress due to pulmonary venous obstruction or restrictive atrial septum and no alternative decompressing vein have an extremely low Q_p:Q_s. Despite transient hemodynamic and metabolic stability that might ensue with aggressive therapeutic maneuvers designed to reduce PVR and promote pulmonary blood flow, these infants exhibit marked hypoxemia that requires urgent intervention (cardiac operation or cardiac catheterization intervention) to decompress pulmonary venous return to have any hope of survival.[42,43] Endotracheal intubation facilitated by neuromuscular blocking agents and anesthetic agents, as tolerated, is accompanied by hyperventilation with an FiO_2 of 1.0. Aggressive sedation should be administered to decrease metabolic demand. In addition, measures should be undertaken to augment the right ventricular pressure to promote pulmonary blood flow, including ensuring adequate intravascular volume and metabolic status, and in some infants, inotropic agents. Inducing systemic vasoconstriction with medications such as vasopressin or phenylephrine hydrochloride (Neo-Synephrine) may be helpful for increasing pulmonary blood flow.

The use of sodium bicarbonate to address a metabolic acidemia in the face of extremely limited pulmonary blood flow offers limited benefit and may even be hazardous. The elimination of carbon dioxide after bicarbonate hydrolysis is severely impaired. Hence bicarbonate administration will often result in a shift from metabolic to respiratory acidemia, with little change in pH, and the attendant prospect of a highly undesirable increase in PVR.

Historical Overview

Despite considerable progress in the surgical management of many forms of critical congenital heart disease in neonates and infants, the spectrum of congenital cardiac anomalies that we now refer to as HLHS continued to be considered fatal with or without surgery by most practitioners through the decades of the 1960s and 1970s. For the majority of babies no intervention was undertaken once that diagnosis was established. In rare instances, early attempts were made to prevent the seemingly inevitable death during the first weeks of life of babies born with severe hypoplasia or critical obstruction of one or more elements of the left heart-aorta complex. A very early attempt to provide surgical therapy to a patient with some features of HLHS was reported by Redo and colleagues[44] in 1961. A 2.5-month-old infant with mitral atresia underwent atrial septectomy under inflow occlusion through a right thoracotomy. This addressed the role of a restrictive interatrial communication as an impediment to the necessary flow of pulmonary venous return from left atrium to right atrium because the tricuspid valve constituted the only patent atrioventricular connection. Several theoretical approaches to surgical palliation of HLHS and related lesions were proposed as early as 1968, based on the findings at review of autopsy cases. Sinha and associates[45] analyzed 30 such cases and postulated that stabilization of the circulation in newborns with HLHS could be achieved by ensuring an unobstructed interatrial communication to allow for unimpeded left-to-right flow of pulmonary venous blood to the right side of the heart and providing a durable right-to-left shunt at the arterial level. They speculated that right-to-left ductal shunting might be sustained by high resistance to PA blood flow and suggested the possibility of surgical banding of both pulmonary arteries. Occasional case reports and small surgical series began to appear by about 1970.[46,47] However, most of the infants described in these reports did not actually have HLHS but rather had either aortic valve stenosis with mild left ventricular hypoplasia or aortic atresia with large ventricular septal defect and a well-developed left ventricle. In 1970 Cayler and associates[46] described placement of bilateral branch PA bands and construction of a proximal ascending aorta-to-MPA shunt (Waterston shunt) in an infant with critical aortic valve stenosis and left ventricular hypoplasia.

By the late 1970s and early 1980s there were several case reports describing operative survival after surgical palliation for classic aortic valve atresia, notably by Behrendt and Rocchini,[48] Doty and colleagues,[49] Levitsky and colleagues,[50] and Mohri and colleagues.[51] The surgical techniques described were characterized by complex but ingenious methods of directing flow from the proximal main pulmonary trunk to the aorta in combination with either intraluminal or external constrictors to limit flow into the branch pulmonary arteries. Some such techniques had their origins in palliative approaches to anomalies other than HLHS, such as a technique for palliation of interrupted aortic arch that had been proposed in 1972 by Litwin and colleagues.[52] That procedure included placement of a graft from the proximal main pulmonary trunk to the descending aorta in combination with placement of a band on the distal MPA beyond to the takeoff of the MPA-to-aorta graft. These early attempts to stabilize the circulation in infants with HLHS and related anomalies were conceived not so much as being preparatory with respect to some eventual durable surgical reconstruction, but rather as temporizing means of avoiding circulatory collapse, which was otherwise nearly universally unavoidable within the first few weeks of life.

Several attempts at initial palliation during the newborn period were followed by short-term survival, but none were successful in achieving long-term stability because the palliated state was characterized by a volume-loaded functionally single ventricle supporting both the systemic and the pulmonary circulations, together with a fragile and dynamic balance of pulmonary and systemic flow. Frustration with the failure of early attempts to achieve satisfactory palliation served as motivation for some to explore the seemingly radical concept of definitively separating the systemic and pulmonary circulations in a single early surgical intervention based on conversion to a Fontan type of circulation. In 1977 Doty and Knott[53] described a series of cases of primary reconstruction for HLHS, including "Fontan-style" connection of the right atrium to the pulmonary arteries. Under deep hypothermic circulatory arrest the patent ductus was ligated, and the atrial septum was excised. The main pulmonary trunk was connected to the aortic arch using a Dacron tube graft. The confluent right and left branch pulmonary arteries were directly connected to the right atrium (atriopulmonary connection). The atrium was then repartitioned with a pericardial baffle so that the pulmonary venous return was separated from the caval veins and atriopulmonary connection and was directed to the tricuspid valve and right ventricle, which functioned as the systemic ventricle. All of the infants died, with death being attributed to inadequate right ventricular performance or compromised coronary blood flow. It now appears obvious that failure was in fact related to the impracticality of establishing the Fontan circulation very early in infancy because of the prohibitively high PVR, which precluded "passive" flow of blood from the venous circulation through the lungs in the absence of a subpulmonary ventricle.

During the same period (1970–1980) it was observed that short-term survival without surgical intervention might occur under the rare condition of continued patency of the ductus arteriosus in an infant with HLHS. It became apparent, however, that although a reasonably balanced Q_p:Q_s might serendipitously be maintained for a period of weeks or even months under such circumstances, prolonged parallel arrangement of the pulmonary and systemic circulations inevitably resulted in either intractable congestive heart failure or development of pulmonary vascular obstructive disease. Thus it became apparent that both early intervention and planned, additional subsequent surgical reconstruction would be necessary to achieve long-term survival.

Development of the Staged Repair of Hypoplastic Left Heart Syndrome

By the early 1970s Fontan and Baudet[54] and Kreutzer and colleagues[55] had independently introduced operations to treat tricuspid atresia that resulted in nearly normal systemic arterial oxygen saturation and normal volume work for the single ventricle (see also Chapter 65 on tricuspid atresia). The "Fontan circulation" placed the pulmonary and systemic circulations in series, thus reducing the work of the single ventricle to the job of pumping fully saturated blood to the systemic circulation. The systemic venous return passes directly to the pulmonary vascular bed, through which it must pass without benefit of a separate subpulmonary ventricular pump. The pulmonary vascular bed must be well developed and characterized by low resistance to flow to maintain the pulmonary circulation. After initial success in patients with tricuspid atresia, the principle of the Fontan operation was applied to a variety of cardiac anomalies characterized as functionally univentricular hearts.

The evolution of approaches to initial surgical palliation of neonates with HLHS by William I. Norwood in Boston moved in a direction that was conceptually different from that of many others, whose principal objective had been simply to avert death from circulatory failure in early infancy. Norwood embraced the idea that the goal of eventual successful separation of the systemic and pulmonary circulations based on the principles demonstrated by Fontan and Kreutzer would require that an initial strategy of palliation be designed in such a way as to preserve ventricular function while also protecting the pulmonary vasculature from the changes that occur when subjected to high flow and high pressure. He argued that ideally it should also allow for growth of the surgically created pathway for flow from the right ventricle and proximal main pulmonary trunk into the aorta and systemic circulation. Early reports by Norwood and colleagues[56,57] in 1980 and 1981 described a variety of palliative operations, with several patients recovering fully and eventually being discharged from the hospital in satisfactory condition. Among these were patients whose initial palliation had included atrial septectomy, amalgamation of the proximal main pulmonary trunk with the diminutive ascending aorta and arch, in combination with a controlled source of pulmonary blood flow. Norwood had by this time explored various techniques of establishing and controlling pulmonary blood flow, including both systemic to PA shunts and right ventricle to PA conduits.[57] Also, he had encountered instances in which the arch reconstruction could be accomplished relying entirely on autologous tissue and other instances in which he used various patch materials to augment the hypoplastic aortic arch. The first successful physiologic repair of HLHS with aortic atresia was reported by Norwood, Lange, and Hansen in 1983.[58] This success was accomplished with two separate operations, one in the newborn period and the second (conversion to the Fontan circulation) approximately a year later. This approach established the principle of staged reconstruction. Through more than three decades of further evolution of the details of initial surgical palliation of HLHS, the basic principles of the initial palliative operation have remained unchanged:

- Unobstructed association of right ventricle with aorta, with potential for aortic growth
- Atrial septectomy to ensure unobstructed pulmonary venous return
- Systemic to pulmonary shunt to limit pulmonary blood flow and attenuate pulmonary vascular changes due to excessive flow or pressure

In 1989 Norwood introduced the hemi-Fontan procedure as a planned interval reconstruction between the initial neonatal stage I palliation and the eventual completion of the Fontan circulation. The hemi-Fontan procedure, which is typically performed at age 3 to 8 months, is essentially a superior cavopulmonary connection in combination with patch augmentation of the confluence of the right and left branch pulmonary arteries, which effectively addresses any areas of stenosis, hypoplasia, or distortion. The interposition of this operation between stage I and the Fontan completion addresses both the risk associated with the inherently unstable palliated state after stage I, and the adaptation of the ventricle to the period of increased volume work.[59] The basic principles underlying the decision to adopt a policy of performing the Fontan operation in two stages include the following:

- Shortened duration of the fragile palliated state of parallel circulations
- Earlier removal of volume load
- Allowance for remodeling of the systemic ventricle (normalization of mass/volume ratio) before completion of the Fontan circulation

Thus at most centers stage I palliation is undertaken during the first weeks of life, a superior cavopulmonary connection is generally performed at 3 to 6 months of age, and completion of the Fontan circulation is generally accomplished in a third-stage procedure between 2 and 4 years of age, depending on patient factors and institutional preference.[60]

With respect to fundamental aspects of the initial (stage I) palliative procedure, there has been relatively little that has changed over the past 30 years. Technical modifications have been proposed, including the use of a variety of cardiopulmonary bypass (CPB) perfusion strategies, in an effort to minimize the duration of periods of deep hypothermic circulatory arrest. These include either continuous antegrade selective cerebral perfusion or "whole body perfusion." The latter relies upon multiple sites of arterial cannulation, one of which is the descending aorta. For the surgical reconstruction itself, some surgeons have favored reliance entirely on autologous tissue, avoiding the use of either prosthetic material or vascular homograft patch material for reconstruction of the neo-aorta and aortic arch.[61] Throughout the decade of the 90s most practitioners followed the example of Norwood's practice at the time and used a polytetrafluoroethylene shunt from the innominate artery to the proximal portion of the ipsilateral branch PA (modified Blalock-Taussig shunt [MBTS]) as the source of pulmonary blood flow. Successful results reported by Sano and associates[62,63] led to a resurgence of interest in the use of a right ventricle to PA conduit as the source of pulmonary blood. The choice between these two strategies to control pulmonary blood flow has been perceived to be of sufficient importance as to have been the principal study intervention of a prospective randomized clinical trial sponsored by the US National Heart, Lung, and Blood Institute.[64]

It is now apparent that patients with HLHS may be expected to achieve early outcomes from the Fontan operation that are comparable to those with other functionally univentricular heart malformations.[65] The Fontan operation is discussed in Chapters 63 and 65.

Stage I Surgical Reconstruction

The physiologic goals of stage I reconstruction for hypoplastic left heart, as mentioned, have remained constant since the early conception of the surgical approach. The major goals include (1) adjoining of the aortic and pulmonary outlets associated with the reconstruction of the hypoplastic aortic arch using autologous tissue supplemented with patch material to provide unobstructed systemic perfusion, (2) replacement of the nonrestrictive patent ductus with a restrictive conduit (right ventricle [RV]-PA or aortopulmonary) to provide adequate but not excessive pulmonary blood flow, and (3) relief of any obstruction of the atrial septum/PVs to allow nonrestrictive pulmonary venous inflow to the systemic pumping chamber (RV). The physiologic consequence of this arrangement obligates the single ventricle to provide cardiac output to both the pulmonary and systemic circulations, with the end goal of optimizing systemic oxygen delivery. The workload of the single ventricle is therefore quite high until the separation of pulmonary and systemic circulations, which occurs at the second stage, cavopulmonary connection. As an example, with a $Q_p:Q_s$ of $1:2$ at rest, the single ventricle must provide three cardiac output equivalents to maintain hemodynamic stability. With any increased stress state or increased cardiac output demand, one can understand how tenuous the circulation becomes. The physiology is, however, more stable and resilient with a restrictive shunt in place compared with the preoperative state with a nonrestrictive ductus.

Surgical Reconstructive Techniques

Over the last 30 years there have been many modifications and variations on the technical details of the stage I reconstructive procedure. There are numerous patient-related variables and surgeon-specific modifiable variables, which result in a myriad of possible variations as to the precise technique that is employed. Boxes 66.1 and 66.2 list some examples of these variables.

• BOX 66.1 Examples of Patient-Related Variables (Nonmodifiable)

Age
Prematurity
Presence of genetic syndrome
Weight
Right ventricular function
Tricuspid valve function
Aortic/mitral valve atresia vs hypoplasia
Aortic arch morphology
Restrictive atrial septum
Presence of left ventricular cavity
Presence of coronary fistulas

• BOX 66.2 Examples of Surgical Variables (Modifiable)

Cannulation strategy
Circulatory arrest versus regional perfusion
Hypothermia/normothermia
Cardioplegic solution/frequency
Classic patch repair versus coarctation resection
CPB and cross-clamp time
RV-PA conduit versus aortopulmonary shunt
Use of modified ultrafiltration

CPB, Cardiopulmonary bypass; PA, pulmonary artery; RV, right ventricle.

The surgical techniques have been well described in numerous publications.[66-69] Figs. 66.5 to 66.15 depict the surgical steps using one method for stage I reconstruction, in this case with an RV-PA conduit

Once the surgical reconstruction is completed, the patient is rewarmed, and preparations to wean off CPB are initiated. Reliable central venous access is essential for fluid/drug administration, as well as central venous pressure monitoring. Our preferred vascular access for a neonatal cardiac patient going to the operating room is umbilical venous and arterial lines. Our preference is to place additional peripheral intravenous (IV) lines and radial arterial line access with induction. Before weaning bypass, a double-lumen right atrial line is placed for inotropes and central monitoring. The umbilical catheters are routinely removed in the first 1 to 3 postoperative days. We very much try to avoid upper compartment lines in neonates, especially those who will need a cavopulmonary connection. Femoral venous and arterial access can be a reasonable second choice at times.

Before the patient exits bypass, inotropic infusion is commenced. Our typical cocktail is milrinone at 0.25 to 0.5 mcg/kg/min, epinephrine at 0.03 to 0.05 mcg/kg/min, and CaCl 10 mg/kg/h. With the patient on bypass and warmed we can assess the need for further manipulation of SVR and need for adjustment or additional agents for SVR modulation (i.e., vasopressin or sodium nitroprusside [Nipride]). We prefer to exit bypass at a target central venous pressure of 6 to 8 mm/hg and assess the need for further volume or drug manipulation. Target values for hemodynamic parameters may be a systolic blood pressure of 65 to 75 mm Hg, heart rate of 135 to 150 beats/min, and a central venous pressure of 8 to 10 mm Hg. Despite a significant pump run and ischemic arrest, the neonatal heart should recover with the ability to

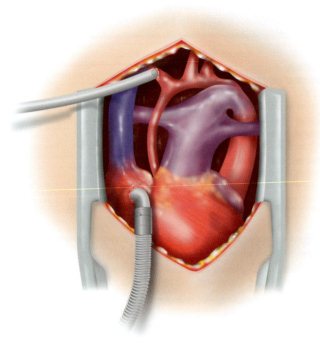

• **Figure 66.5** Stage I Norwood procedure. Cannulation for cardiopulmonary bypass. A Gore-Tex graft (3.0 to 3.5 mm) is sewn to the innominate artery and used for arterial inflow. A single venous cannula in the right atrium (12 to 14 Fr) is used for venous return.

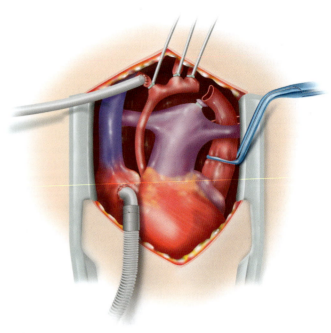

• **Figure 66.7** After diastolic arrest with Mg/lido cardioplegia, regional cerebral perfusion is initiated at a flow of 50 mL/kg/min and a radial artery pressure of 35 to 50 mm Hg. The distal arch and isthmus are divided and ductal tissue removed down to just proximal to the intercostal artery takeoff.

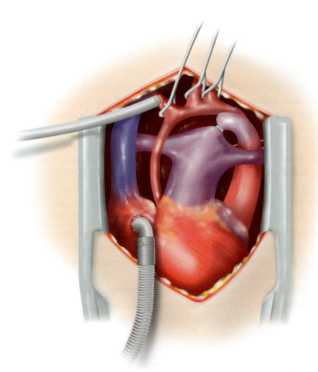

• **Figure 66.6** Cardiopulmonary bypass is initiated, and the patient is cooled to 18°C. The ductus is ligated. The head vessels, arch, descending aorta, and central pulmonary arteries are mobilized.

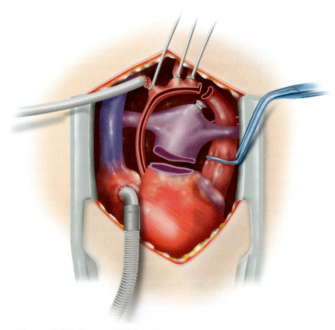

• **Figure 66.8** The underside of the arch and ascending aorta are filleted open down to the level of the transected pulmonary artery. A short cutback is made in the main pulmonary artery just to the left of the rightward posterior commissure.

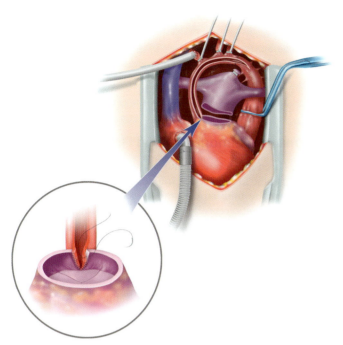

• **Figure 66.9** The aorta and pulmonary artey are sewn together at the cutback. The descending aorta is then anastomosed for 80% of its circumference to the distal aortic arch. The lesser curve of the descending aorta is cut back for 8 to 10 mm down to the intercostals.

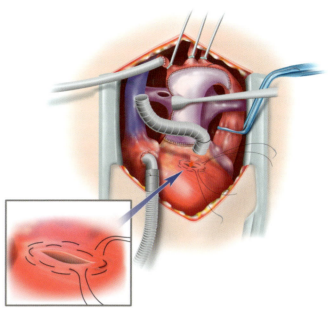

• **Figure 66.11** Construction of the Sano shunt. A ringed Gore-Tex graft (5 mm for <3.2 kg and 6 mm for >3.2 kg patient weight) is selected. The tube is cut nearly flush with a ring, and the third ring from the end is marked. The graft is fashioned into a 90-degree angle and inserted full thickness into the infundibulum and held in place with two concentric purse-strings of 5-0 polypropylene (Prolene).

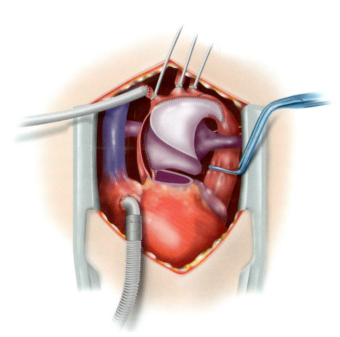

• **Figure 66.10** The underside of the arch is reconstructed with pulmonary homograft down to the level of the pulmonary trunk.

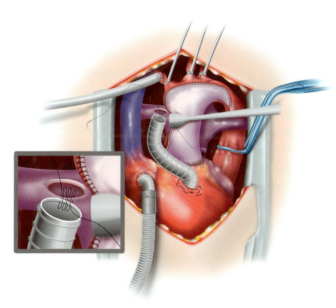

• **Figure 66.12** The Gore-Tex graft length is determined, and the distal end is cut 1 mm from the last ring. An anastomosis is made by sewing the ring of the graft to an opening in the pulmonary artery with 7-0 polypropylene (Prolene) ("distal dunk technique").[70] It is essential that the proximal and distal connections are widely patent to ensure optimal pulmonary blood flow and oxygenation.

generate a stable and adequate cardiac output for systemic oxygen delivery.

Considerable time and effort should be directed at optimizing the patient for transition to the cardiac intensive care unit (ICU) at this time. First and foremost should be an assessment of the adequacy of the repair based on the immediate hemodynamics and stability of the patient once off bypass. Additionally, intraoperative epicardial echocardiography is typically performed because we avoid transesophageal echocardiography in neonates undergoing arch reconstruction. Modified ultrafiltration is typically carried out. Meticulous hemostasis with correction of all surgical and coagulopathic hemorrhage is essential before leaving the operating room. Our goal is to reach a target hematocrit of 45% to optimize oxygen delivery. Pacing wires are placed. Sternal closure is typically delayed, although some units routinely close skin, if not the entire sternum, in selected patients. Appropriate monitoring is established,

and an efficient and expeditious transport of the patient to the cardiac ICU is carried out. Once the patient is in the cardiac ICU, a formal handoff procedure is used to transfer care from anesthesia to the intensive care team with the surgical team present and ready for any untoward events. Outcomes for stage I palliation continue to improve with current Society of Thoracic Surgeons database median participant operative mortality of 14.9%.[71]

Options for Pulmonary Blood Flow

There has been much interest and study to determine which type of shunt is best to use for the source of pulmonary blood flow. Unless there are unusual circumstances, both shunts allow for adequate, but limit excessive, pulmonary blood flow for the neonatal single ventricle. From a physiologic standpoint the RV-PA shunt avoids the continuous diastolic runoff of an aortopulmonary shunt and maintains higher diastolic pressure, which presumably provides better coronary perfusion. The obvious downside is the uncertainty of potential long-term effects of a ventriculotomy on the single ventricle necessary to create the RV-PA shunt.

The Single Ventricle Reconstruction Trial[72] was a prospective, randomized trial designed to study the differences between the

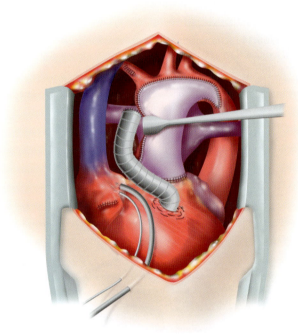

• **Figure 66.13** Completed stage I reconstruction with Sano right ventricle (RV) to pulmonary artery (PA) conduit and placement of double-lumen right atrial line and atrial pacing wire.

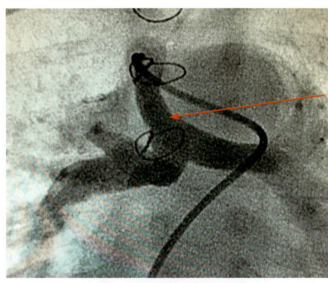

• **Figure 66.15** Anteroposterior angiogram of anastomotic site of graft to pulmonary confluence.

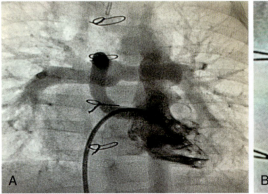
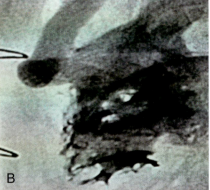

• **Figure 66.14** (A) Anteroposterior and (B) lateral angiogram of right ventricle (RV) to pulmonary artery (PA) (Sano) connection.

RV-PA shunt and MBTS in patients undergoing the Norwood stage I procedure. There was a significant difference in their primary end point of death or cardiac transplant at 12 months, 26.3% versus 36.4% (P = .01), favoring the RV-PA shunt patients. The difference was no longer significant by 32-month follow-up. Additionally, the RV-PA group had more unintended reinterventions (P = .003) and less need for cardiopulmonary resuscitation (P = .04) than the MBTS group. It is noteworthy that many surgeons at the time were not routinely performing the RV-PA shunt, so the effect of a "learning curve" was not accounted for, which may have imparted a negative bias for the RV-PA group.

Some recent data from the Congenital Heart Surgeons Society,[72] used propensity-matched methodology on a cohort of 454 patients undergoing the Norwood operation from 21 institutions. Overall 6-year survival was better after RV-PA shunt (70%) versus MBTS (55%; P < .001). Additionally, transplant-free survival during this time was better after RV-PA shunt (64%) versus MBTS (53%; P = .004). Overall prevalence of greater than moderate RV dysfunction reached 11% within 3 months post Norwood procedure. Right ventricular dysfunction after MBTS was 16% versus 6% after RV-PA shunt. For survivors, late RV dysfunction was less than 5% and was not different between groups (P = .36). Overall presence of greater than moderate TR reached 13% 2 years post Norwood procedure and was increased 16% after MBTS versus 11% after RV-PA shunt (P = .003). Late TR was similar between groups. They concluded that among propensity-scored matched neonates RV-PA shunt offers superior 6-year survival, with no greater prevalence of RV dysfunction or TR, over conventional MBTS operations[73] (Fig. 66.16).

Hybrid Therapy

Considerable effort by some groups has been directed at initial palliation of hypoplastic left heart patients with a hybrid approach consisting of ductal stenting and bilateral branch PA bands. Certain centers using hybrid therapy as their preferred approach realized outcomes comparable to standard reconstructive surgery of the time.[74] Recent findings from a large inception cohort study of critical neonates with left ventricular outflow tract obstruction (692 patients) reviewed outcomes of 110 patients that underwent hybrid therapy.[75] They concluded that although hybrid strategies were not a lower-risk strategy overall, the impact of low birth weight on survival (less than 2 kg) may be mitigated after hybrid procedures compared with Norwood operations (Fig. 66.17).

Transplantation

Based on the pioneering work of Leonard Bailey demonstrating successful transplantation for newborns with hypoplastic left heart syndrome, some centers focused on this therapy as their primary approach. What became clear was that 1-year survival in excess of 85% was possible with replacement therapy at a time when stage reconstruction was struggling to achieve 60% to 70% survival.[76-78] At the time the donor pool for neonates for heart transplantation was reasonable with relatively short waiting times. Primary transplantation began to become popular, the limited donor pool issue magnified, and wait times increased and continue today to be a major limitation of this therapy. Copeland et al.[76] recently reported their experience of late survivors among pediatric heart transplant patients and demonstrated neonatal transplant survival in excess of 85% at 25 years (Fig. 66.18).

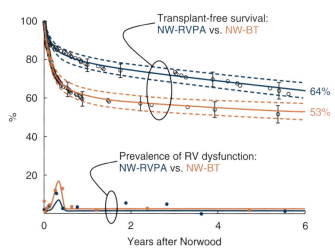

• **Figure 66.16** Transplant-free survival and prevalence of RV dysfunction for NW-RVPA and NW-BT. Transplant-free survival versus the prevalence of moderate postoperative RV dysfunction for patients who underwent NW-RVPA *(blue curve)* versus NW-BT *(red curve)*. The early prevalence of RV dysfunction coincides temporally with the early hazard for death, both of which were significantly better after NW-RVPA versus NW-BT. Open blue circles represent an event (death or transplant) after NW-RVPA, and open red circles are events after NW-BT positioned on the vertical axis by the Kaplan-Meier estimator. Vertical bars are confidence limits equivalent to ±1 SE. Solid black lines are parametric estimates enclosed within dashed 68% confidence bands equivalent to ±1 SE. The solid blue line shows the estimated probability for moderate RV dysfunction after NW-RVPA. The solid red line is the estimated probability for moderate RV dysfunction after NW-BT. Closed circles represent data grouped by associated operation (without regard to repeated measurements) within time frames to provide crude verification of model fit. *NW-BT,* Norwood operation with modified Blalock-Taussig shunt; *NW-RVPA,* Norwood operation with right ventricle to pulmonary artery conduit; *RV,* right ventricular; *SE,* standard error. (From Wilder TJ, McCrindle BW, Phillips AB, et al. Survival and right ventricular performance for matched children after stage-1 Norwood: modified Blalock-Taussig shunt versus right-ventricle-to-pulmonary-artery conduit. *J Thorac Cardiovasc Surg.* 2015;150[6]:1440-1450, 1452 e1441-1448; discussion 1450-1442.)

In summary, the selection of the specific treatment arm and/or shunt remains related to many objective and subjective variables. There continues to be variation from center to center as to what an actual patient might receive. The algorithm in Fig. 66.19 is an example of what may be an acceptable decision tree. Programs must use the existing as well as evolving data to determine what is best for their patients given their specific set of circumstances and skill set.

Postoperative Management

Optimization of Systemic Cardiac Output. Maximizing the ratio of oxygen delivery to extraction represents the underlying physiologic goal that dominates early postoperative management.[79] However, in a manner characteristic of many major cardiac interventions in neonates and young infants, myocardial performance may deteriorate appreciably in the first 6 to 12 postoperative hours before starting to improve.[80] As a result, reduction of metabolic demands should be accomplished by maintaining normothermia and with a continuous sedation infusion (e.g., morphine 0.04 to 0.1 mg/kg/h or fentanyl 1 to 5 mcg/kg/h if hemodynamic instability is noted with morphine administration). Scheduled IV acetaminophen can also be given for the first 48 hours to

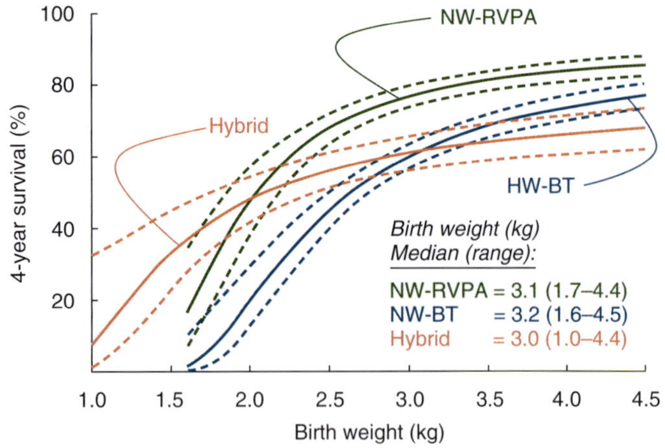

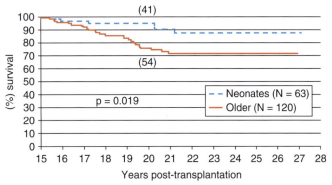

• **Figure 66.17** Impact of birth weight on survival overall and stratified by stage I procedure. Risk-adjusted nomogram depicting the overall impact of birth weight on survival (A) and the impact of birth weight on survival stratified by stage I procedure (B). Survival is censored at the time of transition to a Fontan operation, transplantation, or biventricular repair. The estimated 4-year survival (*vertical axis*) is plotted against birth weight (*horizontal axis*). A, For all patients, birth weight had a nonlinear association with survival, such that at birth weight of approximately 2.0 to 2.5 kg there was a substantial decline in survival (*solid black line*). B, The estimated 4-year survival plotted against birth weights, stratified by NW-BT (*n* = 232; *blue curve*), NW-RVPA (*n* = 222; *green curve*), and hybrid procedure (*n* = 110; *red curve*) truncated to fit the range of birth weights for each group. There was a significant interaction between birth weight and hybrid procedures, such that birth weight had a disproportionate impact on survival for hybrid relative to NW-BT and NW-RVPA. Solid lines are parametric estimate enclosed within dashed 68% confidence bands equivalent to ± 1 SE. Risk factors other than birth weight, and procedure for B, were held constant at their median or mean value. Risk factors (median value): hybrid, 0.2; NW-RVPA conduit, 0.39; ascending aorta index, 1.8 cm/m²; atretic aortic valve, 0.48; mitral valve z score, −15; years, 4. *NW-BT,* Norwood operation with modified Blalock-Taussig shunt; *NW-RVPA,* Norwood operation with right ventricle to pulmonary artery conduit; *SE,* standard error. (From Wilder TJ, McCrindle BW, Hickey EJ, et al. Is a hybrid strategy a lower-risk alternative to stage 1 Norwood operation? *J Thorac Cardiovasc Surg.* 2017;153[1]:163-172 e166.)

• **Figure 66.18** Survival after pediatric heart transplantation: neonates versus older recipients. (From Copeland H, Razzouk A, Chinnock R, et al. Pediatric recipient survival beyond 15 post-heart transplant years: a single-center experience. *Ann Thorac Surg.* 2014;98[6]:2145-2150; discussion 2150-2141.)

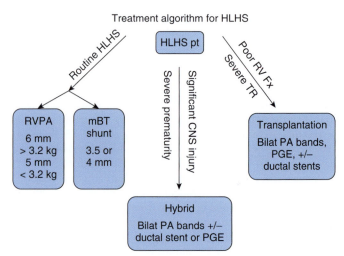

• **Figure 66.19** Hypoplastic left heart syndrome algorithm.

minimize the increase in metabolic demands associated with fever. Intravenous acetaminophen has the additional benefit of decreasing the need for opioids postoperatively.[81] Neuromuscular blockade is added only if there is significant hemodynamic instability or difficulty with ventilation due to patient-ventilator dyssynchrony and is not routinely used in the postoperative period because it may delay patient progression forward with fluid mobilization and subsequent weaning from the ventilator. The importance of adequate sedation in the early postoperative period has been shown by Murdison and associates.[82]

Examination of the clinical course and outcome after stage I reconstruction and before a modified Fontan operation in 200 neonates born with HLHS treated at The Children's Hospital of Philadelphia showed that 70% of the mortality of these patients occurred during their initial hospitalization, the majority of which was associated with an acute or unrelenting mismatch between pulmonary and systemic flow on the first postoperative night. Cardiovascular collapse appeared to be related to events associated with sudden increases in PVR, often temporally associated with early spontaneous motor activity or interventions such as endotracheal suctioning. Endotracheal suctioning might precipitate acute elevations in PVR, either by reduction in alveolar ventilation and oxygenation or by a reflex mechanism[83]; thus care should be taken to adequately sedate patients before noxious stimuli such as suctioning in the early postoperative period.

Low-dose inotrope infusions are used in the early postbypass period to augment oxygen delivery without the expense of increased oxygen consumption, which is typically seen at higher doses. Epinephrine (0.02 to 0.05 mcg/kg/min) is used in favor of dopamine given data showing increased oxygen consumption and the extraction ratio of oxygen, resulting in no net increase in cardiac output or oxygen delivery.[84] Calcium chloride infusion (5 to 10 mg/kg/h) can be particularly useful in neonates due to the neonatal myocardium's immature sarcoplasmic reticulum and therefore reliance on extracellular calcium for optimization of contractility.[85] In addition, the deleterious effects of beta-adrenergic stimulation with other inotropes are avoided while maintaining the beneficial effects of increased inotropy. The phosphodiesterase III-inhibitor milrinone (0.5 mcg/kg/min) or rarely, the long-acting alpha-antagonist phenoxybenzamine (0.25 mg/kg/d) is used to decrease SVR, increasing systemic blood flow relative to pulmonary blood flow and decreasing ventricular afterload, both resulting in an increase in systemic cardiac output.[86,87] If the systemic arterial pressure exceeds desired goals, further vasodilator therapy (e.g., nitroprusside) is added rather than reduction of inotropic support. This tactic emerges from the systematic observation of central venous oxygen saturation (SvO_2) values that regularly indicate marginal or low systemic cardiac output during this period of recovery.

Volume Status. In the immediate postoperative period, intravascular volume supplementation serves to replace blood and urine losses, as well as the changes in capacitance that occur with warming. Volume requirements are guided by heart rate, systemic arterial pressure, and physical examination of peripheral perfusion, including temperature and capillary refill in the distal extremities. Although a transthoracic catheter placed in the common atrium at the time of surgery provides some information with respect to the intravascular volume status, it also reflects the compliance of the ventricle. In the face of satisfactory hemodynamics, ventricular compliance usually improves in the early postoperative period; hence the atrial pressure at a given intravascular volume should decrease concomitantly. To avoid volume overload, the least amount of fluid necessary to produce satisfactory systemic hemodynamics and perfusion is administered, rather than rigidly adhering to a specific atrial pressure target. If the hemodynamic goals cannot be achieved despite a common atrial pressure consistently in excess of 10 mm Hg and no evidence of tamponade is found, consideration should be given to augmenting inotropic support.

There are few points of data on the optimum hemoglobin/hematocrit targets for postoperative single-ventricle patients; however, many intensivists target a hematocrit of 45% in clinical practice in the immediate postoperative period. It is known that in the setting of a left-to-right shunt, increasing hemoglobin concentration is associated with an increase in PVR and an increase in oxygen delivery.[88] However, some evidence suggests that targeting higher hematocrits can result in prolonged mechanical ventilation, with no improvement in outcomes following the Norwood procedure.[89,90] Therefore, once mediastinal hemorrhage has subsided and hemoglobin concentration exceeds 15 g/dL, any additional volume requirements should be met with colloid solutions.

Digoxin and furosemide are reinstituted expectantly in the postoperative period to ameliorate the impact of the obligatory increased volume load under which the single ventricle must operate. Because the systemic and pulmonary circulations remain connected in parallel at the arterial level, the volume work of the right ventricle continues to be equal to the sum of the systemic and pulmonary blood flow ($Q_p + Q_s$). A furosemide infusion (0.1 to 0.3 mg/kg/h) may be better tolerated than bolus dosing (1 mg/kg IV) because an infusion should produce a steady increase in urine output instead of a large one-time increase following the dose. If adequate hemodynamics are ensured and increased diuresis is still required, chlorothiazide (5 mg/kg IV or 10 mg/kg orally) can be added to augment urine output.

There is increasing use of peritoneal dialysis catheters among centers, with a recent study showing earlier achievement of a negative fluid balance, earlier extubation, improved inotrope scores, and fewer electrolyte abnormalities in patients treated with planned peritoneal dialysis catheter placement compared with those without catheter placement.[91]

Pulmonary Mechanics and Weaning From Mechanical Ventilation. Pulmonary mechanics are most commonly abnormal in these infants because of changes in airway resistance, lung compliance, or bellows function. Increased airway resistance usually results from luminal narrowing related either to intrinsic accumulation of secretions or to extrinsic compression from interstitial edema or dilated neighboring vessels or both in the bronchovascular pedicle

associated with pulmonary venous hypertension. Although many pathologic processes culminate in reduced lung compliance, the most common mechanism in these neonates is the perioperative accumulation of interstitial lung water.[92] DiCarlo and colleagues[93] demonstrated reduced mean lung compliance in all of 28 neonates (17 with HLHS) after cardiac surgical procedures. The subgroup in whom respiratory failure developed after initial withdrawal of mechanical ventilatory support also exhibited increased airway resistance. The routine use of modified ultrafiltration (MUF) has dramatically reduced the frequency and magnitude of these intrinsic problems with pulmonary mechanics. In patients who have had the benefit of MUF, abnormalities of pulmonary mechanics of sufficient magnitude to cause respiratory failure are limited almost entirely to the subset of patients with significant hemodynamic issues or infection. Apart from the residual effects of neuromuscular blockade, the most common cause of bellows dysfunction in these neonates is diaphragmatic paresis, presumably resulting from phrenic nerve injury.

Patients are commonly managed with pressure-regulated volume control ventilation to deliver a set tidal volume, limiting airway pressure below a selected high-pressure threshold. The ventilator is adjusted to maintain normal ventilation with the patient at functional residual capacity to minimize increases in PVR due to acidosis or alveolar collapse/distention. Because confirmation of sufficient cardiac reserve and manageable abnormalities in pulmonary mechanics is difficult to quantify in neonates, mechanical ventilatory support can be empirically tapered on the first or second postoperative day once hemodynamics are satisfactory. Minimal support is maintained to offset the resistance to breathing imposed by the endotracheal tube. The infant is evaluated at each step, with particular attention to the effort expended in spontaneous breaths and cardiovascular evidence of excessive sympathetic response to the increased metabolic demand (i.e., increased heart rate, systemic arterial pressure, atrial pressure).

Tracheal extubation is performed if the neonate exhibits minimal effort with spontaneous respiration and no evidence is noted of sympathetic response to the metabolic demand posed by the threshold level of support. When either of these criteria is not met, an attempt is made to identify and treat the underlying cause while continuing an appropriate level of ventilatory support. A decision to proceed with a trial of extubation may be made in the absence of a clearly identified cardiopulmonary cause (e.g., inadequate cardiac reserve, abnormal pulmonary mechanics, increased work imposed by spontaneous respiration through a tracheal tube), recognizing the potential for immediate respiratory failure.

Reintubation is as frequently based on cardiovascular signs as on blood gas–tension abnormalities. In a 1988 series of 56 neonates extubated after stage I, the 30% who were ultimately reintubated manifested significant increases in heart rate, systemic arterial pressure, and atrial pressure during the period of spontaneous ventilation.[94] These changes probably reflected sympathetic discharge and diminished ventricular compliance. Analysis of arterial blood in these infants before and after extubation demonstrated reduced arterial pH (diminished metabolic alkalemia), but gas tensions were no different compared with those in patients successfully weaned. Recent data indicate that the median duration of mechanical ventilation after stage I is approximately 5 days.[95]

Common Problems in the Early Postbypass Period

Hypoxemia. Excessive hypoxemia represents one of the more commonly encountered problems in the early postbypass period.

Although inadequate $Q_p:Q_s$ was usually the assumed cause, factors that impair systemic oxygen delivery, thereby reducing mixed venous oxygen saturation, are now known to be significantly more common than previously appreciated (see Fig. 66.1).[96-99] One typically observes a progressive increase in systemic oxygen saturation during MUF, for example, probably because of the impact that hemoconcentration and the resulting increased oxygen delivery have on mixed venous oxygen saturation. Thereafter, measures directed at maintaining hematocrit above 40% may alleviate excessive demands placed on the recovering heart to increase systemic output. The distinction between systemic hypoxemia due to low $Q_p:Q_s$, low pulmonary venous oxygen saturation, or low mixed venous saturation is a critical one because the therapies are diametrically different. Measures designed to reduce PVR will impose a further volume load on a heart already struggling to provide marginal systemic perfusion. Patients demonstrating low SvO_2 would be better served with therapies that promote systemic output, such as inotropic agents or vasodilators.

Those with low pulmonary venous oxygen saturation require a strategy of ventilatory support designed to reduce atelectasis and promote gas exchange in impaired alveoli. Unfortunately, the latter diagnosis is rarely made definitively in the operating room or postoperative ICU because blood sampling from the PVs presents logistic challenges. Intraoperatively, expectant measures directed at complete expansion of the lungs and maintenance of normal functional residual capacity usually suffice to avoid PV desaturation. Among the three causes of persistent systemic hypoxemia, this was believed to be the least common, but PV desaturation is found in as many as 30%.[100]

When systemic hypoxemia occurs because of low $Q_p:Q_s$, other manifestations provide supporting evidence. Trial opening of the shunt during the latter phases of rewarming on CPB typically fails to produce a significant decrease in systemic arterial pressure. The early postbypass hemodynamics reveal a relatively narrow systemic pulse pressure or diastolic pressure that exceeds expectations (i.e., normal). A substantial discrepancy often exists between arterial and end-tidal CO_2 measurements. These suggestive pieces of inferential evidence can be confirmed by aortic Doppler flow analysis or calculation of a Fick ratio by using oxygen saturation determinations. Most commonly, diminished pulmonary blood flow reflects a subtle technical aspect of the arch reconstruction, innominate artery dimension, Sano conduit, or the Blalock-Taussig (BT) shunt.

Acute shunt occlusion, the most life-threatening cause of diminished pulmonary blood flow, is manifested by profound hypoxemia and subsequent resultant loss of systemic cardiac output. In the intubated patient a decrease in end-tidal CO_2 measurement can be a clue to the source of hypoxemia. On physical examination, lack of a shunt murmur is diagnostic, as is lack of demonstrable flow across the shunt on echocardiogram. Treatment includes bolus administration of 100 U/kg of heparin, along with measures to increase SVR and potentially dislodge the forming thrombus (epinephrine bolus dose). Relief of shunt occlusion by either direct manipulation once the chest is open or in the cardiac catheterization laboratory is the ultimate treatment, though patients frequently have cardiac arrest necessitating extracorporeal membrane oxygenation with true shunt occlusion. Recent data suggest that outcomes of pediatric cardiac surgery patients, including both survival to discharge and neurologic outcome, may be better for these patients compared with other patient populations receiving extracorporeal cardiopulmonary resuscitation.[101]

Physiologic derangements may exacerbate PVR (e.g., hypoventilation, hypoxemia, acidosis, or hypothermia). However, certain patient subsets exhibit profound abnormalities in the pulmonary vasculature that cause excessive PVR elevations. Neonates with HLHS routinely demonstrate extremely high and volatile PVR when born with extreme pulmonary venous obstruction due to intact atrial septum without alternative decompressing veins. Even the typical HLHS anatomic constellation is associated with marked abnormalities in the number and muscularization of the pulmonary vasculature by pathologic examination.[102] Hypotheses attribute these changes to chronic fetal pulmonary venous obstruction.[103] Pathology studies confirm that these developmental abnormalities become more extreme in the context of the marked obstruction caused by HLHS with intact atrial septum.[104] Fetal echocardiography has demonstrated that alteration in pulmonary venous flow pattern correlates with the magnitude of restriction at the atrial septum.[105]

In the context of hypoxemia due to low $Q_p:Q_s$, interventions fall into three categories: technical, pulmonary vasodilators, and systemic vasoconstriction. For patients expected to have unusually elevated PVR, modifications in the surgical technique might entail placement of a larger shunt or interposition between a larger systemic vessel (e.g., aorta) and PA. Pulmonary vasodilator therapy includes the strategies one might use in any patient demonstrating elevated PVR, such as high FiO_2, normothermia, alkali, and nitric oxide.[106-108] Should those measures prove insufficient to result in adequate pulmonary blood flow, the focus might be expanded to include measures designed to increase the driving pressure across the shunt, by using increased inotropic stimulant infusions or even vasoconstrictors. The latter necessitates careful monitoring to avoid jeopardizing perfusion of other vital organs and should be used only as a temporizing measure until more definitive diagnostic and therapeutic interventions can occur.

Myocardial Dysfunction. Depressed myocardial performance represents another potential problem in the early postbypass period. As mentioned previously, some degree of myocardial dysfunction typically occurs after this operation because no hemodynamic benefit is achieved to offset the cost of CPB and an ischemic interval. When this dysfunction becomes more significant than usual, specific causes should be sought. Even in the context of the typical conduct of stage I reconstruction, the consequences of aortic atresia make routine myocardial protection measures challenging, such as the infusion of cardioplegia solutions. Thus inadequate myocardial preservation represents one potential cause for persisting or excessive myocardial depression.

Technical considerations represent the predominant cause of myocardial dysfunction after this extraordinarily complex operative intervention. One of the most intricate aspects of this procedure is the reconstruction of an aortic arch in such a way that the small ascending aorta, which serves principally to provide coronary flow, is not compromised. This subtle finding may not become evident until the cardiac volume is restored in anticipation of terminating CPB. Residual hemodynamic derangement represents another potential cause of myocardial dysfunction. Because the patient emerges from the Norwood operation with no appreciable hemodynamic benefit, one would expect a heart facing a newly imposed volume or pressure load to tolerate it poorly. Examples of such findings include residual aortic arch obstruction, atrioventricular valve dysfunction, and semilunar valve obstruction or regurgitation.

Metabolic disturbances also result in significant myocardial dysfunction. The fragile right ventricle struggling to cope with significantly increased volume output demands at systemic pressure is perhaps more susceptible to what might otherwise be modest metabolic disturbances. As such, one should meticulously track and address those variables that have some impact on myocardial performance, such as ionized calcium and lactic acidosis. The rapid administration of blood products, for example, which contain calcium-binding drugs, high levels of potassium and lactic acid, as well as other vasoactive mediators, can result in an acute, profound deterioration in cardiac performance in the early postoperative period. Myocardial performance has been observed to deteriorate during the early postoperative period in neonates with HLHS when the arterial pH falls below 7.3 and may contribute to further reduction in systemic perfusion. The administration of IV sodium bicarbonate, calculated to eliminate the base deficit completely, often exerts a beneficial effect on both myocardial performance and systemic perfusion. In addition to the inherent cardiac sensitivity, inescapable anatomic peculiarities accentuate this vulnerability. Blood carrying the transfused products from the systemic venous circulation enters the right ventricle and is directed immediately to the reconstructed aorta, whereby the first branch is the coronary circulation. Therefore any constituent of the transfused blood (e.g., citrate, potassium, lactate) infused into the venous circulation arrives at the coronary arteries with greater speed and concentration than might have occurred had it followed a normal circulatory pattern and been dissipated over the course of the pulmonary vasculature before entering the aorta. This effect is further accentuated if central venous catheters are used to infuse the blood product. As such, a protocol whereby washed packed red blood cells are used for transfusion via central catheters or rapidly through peripheral catheters is employed.

Arrhythmias. Arrhythmias most commonly occur as manifestations of the problems described previously. When they become manifest early in the process of rewarming on CPB, coronary insufficiency represents the most common cause, particularly if the arrhythmia is ventricular in origin. Metabolic disturbances produce the same qualitative rhythm changes seen in normal hearts, although the manifestations might be more extreme. Given the predominantly extracardiac nature of the Norwood procedure, acquired heart block rarely follows this operation, unless it existed preoperatively. On very rare occasions a patient has HLHS and a primary arrhythmia, such as Wolff-Parkinson-White syndrome.

Excessive Pulmonary Blood Flow. Excessive pulmonary blood flow may complicate the early postoperative period. This diagnosis should be entertained cautiously because the insertion of an RV-PA conduit or MBTS should act as a "resistor" to pulmonary blood flow compared to the preoperative condition of unrestricted ductal flow. In many instances the apparent excess pulmonary blood flow really reflects a relative imbalance with respect to significantly diminished systemic cardiac output. The latter should be specifically excluded and addressed before invoking extreme measures to restrict pulmonary blood flow. Of course, subtle technical differences in the conduct of the operation can result in an anatomic propensity to an excessive $Q_p:Q_s$, and this can, in turn, jeopardize systemic perfusion. Such patients typically exhibit an extremely wide pulse pressure or low diastolic pressure reflecting pulmonary "runoff." If myocardial performance otherwise appears robust, the specific measures used to increase PVR and decrease SVR preoperatively are appropriate in this circumstance. In most patients this condition dissipates as the infant recovers from surgery. Should the problem persist beyond the first postoperative day, a cardiac catheterization might be warranted to evaluate the need for further surgical intervention aimed at diminishing pulmonary blood flow.

Central Nervous System. After stage I the incidence of clinically evident neurologic abnormalities (seizure, coma, stroke,

developmental delay) is reported to be between 6% ($n = 120$) and 22% ($n = 216$).[109-111] Both congenital and acquired causes were included. Several opportunities occur throughout the perioperative course during which an acquired brain injury may occur in infants with HLHS. Shock occurring as the ductus arteriosus closes, or as a result of inappropriate early management of an infant who exhibits severely imbalanced $Q_p:Q_s$ before diagnosis, may produce ischemic injury of all vital organs, including the brain. Even after diagnosis, certain subsets of infants with HLHS, notably those at the extremes of $Q_p:Q_s$, may have ongoing injury from inadequate oxygen delivery. HLHS is increasingly being diagnosed in utero, allowing planned management at delivery, suggesting greater stability through more controlled circumstances. A study of patients with critical left heart obstructive lesions (including HLHS) showed greater hemodynamic stability and a lower incidence of preoperative neurologic events in those patients with prenatal diagnosis.[112] A lower incidence of postoperative seizures was found in the prenatal group when neurologic outcome after stage I was compared.

Little attention has been given to the potential contribution of postoperative states to neurologic issues. Hyperthermia after CPB in adults is associated with neurologic impairment.[113] The recent observation of cerebral hyperthermia occurring in a pediatric population during the immediate postoperative period is particularly worrisome, but its cause and impact have yet to be determined.[114] Patients frequently have low diastolic blood pressure and low arterial oxygen saturation after stage I reconstruction. The combination of these elements suggests the potential for adversely affecting brain function.

Gastrointestinal System. Three retrospective studies evaluated the rate of NEC in patients following the Norwood procedure with a range of 11% to 20%, and two of those series showed increased mortality in patients diagnosed with NEC.[115-117] The cause appears to be decreased splanchnic perfusion due to the runoff lesion created by a systemic to PA shunt because abnormalities of mesenteric artery blood flow have been found in this patient population.[118-120] One retrospective review of 32 patients reported an incidence of NEC of 31% in patients with a BT shunt compared with 9% in patients with a Sano conduit; however, this did not reach statistical significance in this small series.[121] Caution should be exercised in advancement in feedings in patients following the Norwood procedure with care to follow for clinical signs of NEC, including abdominal distention, hematochezia, or hemodynamic changes in the most severe cases.

Late Postoperative Issues

After discharge, regular cardiovascular evaluations enable prompt detection of hemodynamically significant complications that would impose further pressure or volume loads on the right ventricle or impede pulmonary blood flow (Table 66.1). Aortic arch obstruction occurs most commonly at the distal arch, although it can develop more proximally at the anastomoses joining the MPA, ascending aorta, and homograft gusset. Whereas some infants may show signs of congestive heart failure, many with arch obstruction are without symptoms. Immediate relief via balloon dilation or patch aortoplasty should be performed to prevent progressive right ventricular hypertrophy.[122] If obstruction occurs distal to the systemic to PA shunt, a maldistribution of $Q_p:Q_s$ may impose an added volume burden on the right ventricle.

Impediments to pulmonary blood flow causing progressive cyanosis usually occur as a result of either obstruction at the systemic

TABLE 66.1	Late Complications After Stage I Reconstruction	
Presenting Sign	**Pathophysiology**	**Therapy**
CHF	• AV valve regurgitation	• AV valve repair
	• Distal arch obstruction	• Balloon dilation or surgical aortoplasty
Right ventricular hypertrophy	• Arch obstruction	• Balloon dilation or surgical aortoplasty
Hypoxemia	• Shunt stenosis	• Shunt revision ± pulmonary arterioplasty
	• Pulmonary artery distortion	• Early bidirectional Glenn or hemi-Fontan
	• Restrictive IAC	• Balloon atrial septostomy or surgical atrial septectomy
	• Pulmonary vein stenosis	• Sutureless pulmonary vein repair or orthotopic heart transplantation
	• CHF	• See above for CHF therapy
	• Anemia	• Packed red cell transfusion

AV, Atrioventricular; *CHF*, congestive heart failure; *IAC*, interatrial communication.

to PA shunt or progressive restriction to flow at the interatrial communication. Timing of these complications dictates treatment. If the shunt or Sano conduit becomes stenotic before the child reaches 3 to 4 months of age, when the PVR is likely to still be elevated, it can frequently be dilated or stented in the cardiac catheterization laboratory. Likewise a restrictive interatrial communication is addressed by balloon dilation or repeated atrial septectomy at the time of cavopulmonary anastomosis. Similar problems occurring when the child is older than 4 months are most commonly handled by performing an SVC-PA anastomosis earlier than planned, presuming favorable maturation of PVR and other hemodynamic variables.

Interstage Outcome

General

The outcome after stage I reconstruction for HLHS has improved substantially since its introduction, with overall *interstage* mortality of 12% in the Single Ventricle Reconstruction Trial, including 6% mortality in the MBTS group and 18% mortality in the RV to PA conduit group.[123] The investigators in the Single Ventricle Reconstruction Trial conducted a multicenter randomized clinical trial to compare outcomes in patients undergoing a Norwood procedure with an MBTS or an RV to PA conduit,[124] and although the transplant-free survival in the RV to PA conduit group was better at 12 months than the MBTS group, the transplant-free survival beyond 12 months was no different between the groups.[95] The risk factors for interstage mortality included prematurity (<37 weeks' gestation), Hispanic ethnicity, aortic atresia/mitral atresia, post-Norwood complications, census block poverty level, and MBTS

in patients with no or mild atrioventricular valve regurgitation.[123] Other series have also identified extracardiac abnormalities as a risk factor for mortality.[125,126]

Due to morbidity and mortality related to simple childhood illnesses such as respiratory tract infections, gastroenteritis, and fever resulting in hypovolemia, hypoxia, or increased SVR, home monitoring systems in patients discharged home following a Norwood procedure have been implemented at the majority of institutions. Monitoring typically consists of supplying the family with an infant scale and pulse oximeter to detect changes in systemic oxygenation, dehydration, or growth failure. Parents record daily weights and oxygen saturations, along with recording enteral intake in a logbook, and are taught to notify the care team for predetermined criteria. The hope is that with early detection of the development of anatomic lesions (e.g., shunt or conduit narrowing) or intercurrent illnesses, lifesaving intervention can occur in these vulnerable patients. Implementation of home monitoring systems has resulted in improved interstage survival at multiple centers throughout the country.[127-130]

Two recent observational studies have shown decreased interstage mortality in patients with no history of arrhythmia treated with digoxin,[131,132] prompting further study as to the use of this drug in the interstage period. Because the majority of patients who die in the interstage period experience sudden, unexpected death or had unsuccessful resuscitation following witnessed arrest,[133] there is a potential mechanism of decreasing occult arrhythmia in patients discharged home on digoxin, though more investigation is needed.

Neurologic Outcome

Abnormal neurologic states exist to a notable degree in HLHS but may not be different from those in patients with major congenital heart malformations requiring similar treatment. Brain dysfunction results from congenital anomalies and the insults occurring in the fetal, immediate perioperative, and interval periods between surgical procedures. Assessment of neurologic function early in life is limited, but as patients grow older, testing methods become applicable and are being reported with increasing frequency. A high degree of selection bias is present in every study population that has been reported, and the application of findings to local populations should be undertaken with caution.

As survival of infants with HLHS improves, the focus has shifted to ensuring that these patients have optimal neurodevelopmental outcomes. The Single Ventricle Reconstruction Trial showed that the initial thought that neurodevelopmental outcomes were more likely associated with operative interventions was incorrect, and intrinsic patient factors such as lower birth weight (<2.5 kg), longer Norwood procedure hospitalization, complications and prolonged mechanical ventilation following the Norwood procedure, presence of a genetic syndrome, lower maternal education, and Norwood center were associated with worse developmental outcomes, suggesting that future interventions aimed at the preoperative and postoperative period may be more likely to result in improvement in neurodevelopmental outcomes.[134] Focus on early intervention remains important because there is increasing evidence that significant injury is present in many patients from birth. In a study by Dent et al., preoperative magnetic resonance imaging showed ischemic lesions in 23% of patients, with worsened or new lesions present in 73% of patients on postoperative imaging. This study found that cerebral NIRS (cNIRS) could be used as a predictor of new or worsening ischemic injury, with cNIRS of less than

45% for more than 180 minutes to be predictive.[135] In fact, several studies have shown a correlation between cNIRS and both mortality and neurodevelopmental outcomes, making cNIRS a target for goal-directed therapies.[136-138]

Conclusion

Over the past several decades, significant progress has been made in the treatment of HLHS. Infants with HLHS now survive medical and surgical management of their initial stage of palliation virtually indistinguishable from those with other forms of functional single ventricle.[139] Early and intermediate-term outcomes rival those of other serious congenital heart malformations.

Nevertheless, numerous opportunities remain to improve outcome at all stages. The factors that contribute to sudden death in the late postoperative period after stage I reconstruction demand more attention, and efforts to increase survival through interstage monitoring and early symptoms recognition are paramount. As early survival increases, future attention and research efforts will focus on improved neurodevelopmental outcomes, as well as various other morbidities, especially as our patients survive further into adulthood.

References

A complete list of references is available at ExpertConsult.com.

67

Heterotaxy

ROHIT S. LOOMBA, MD, MS; DAVID L.S. MORALES, MD; ANDREW REDINGTON, MD

Cardiac isomerism is a clinical entity that affects approximately 1 in every 10,000 live births.[1-4] Although many use the terms *isomerism* and *heterotaxy* interchangeably, the latter is best reserved for cases in which the other visceral organs are malpositioned because, when applied to the heart, *heterotaxy* fails to define any meaningful constellation of abnormalities. Similarly, the segregation of isomerism or heterotaxy on the basis of splenic morphology is illogical, not only because splenic morphology is usually unknown at the time of cardiac diagnosis, but even if it is, it correlates poorly with the highly variable cardiac constellations that are sometimes associated with *polysplenia* or *asplenia*. Indeed, the morphologic methods of Anderson and Van Praagh both instruct us to assign morphologic uniqueness of a structure based on its most constant feature. While remaining a topic of debate, it is now felt that segregation into the subsets of left and right isomerism should be based on the morphology of the atrial appendages, themselves defined by the disposition of pectinate muscles within the appendage (left) or extending beyond the appendage around the vestibule of the atrium (right).[5,6] The differentiation is important because right and left isomerism are associated with markedly different findings.[7-11] Isomerism reflects the duplication of one vertical half of the body in regard to the thoracic organs, with unusual arrangements of the abdominal organs (visceral heterotaxy). Thus those with left isomerism will have morphologically left atrial appendages bilaterally, along with bilateral presence of long acutely angled hyparterial bronchi and bilobed lungs. Those with right isomerism will have morphologically right atrial appendages bilaterally, in the presence of bilateral short obtusely angled eparterial bronchi and trilobed lungs.[7] Any organ system nonetheless can be impacted by isomerism, although the number of organ systems involved, and the extent to which a specific organ system is influenced, can be highly variable from patient to patient. The abnormalities can be anatomic and/or functional in any organ system. In this review the anatomic and functional consequences of isomerism for each specific organ system and their long-term impacts are discussed.

Cardiovascular System

Atrial Appendages

As discussed briefly earlier, the basis of segregating isomerism should be the morphology of the atrial appendages.[1] The morphology of the atrial appendages is the best guide to atrial arrangement not only in patients with isomerism, but also in the overall setting of the congenitally malformed heart. Whereas isomerism was historically segregated on the basis of splenic anatomy, with subsets described in terms of polysplenia or asplenia, it is now known that the morphology of the appendages is of greater utility in identifying more consistent and homogenous patient cohorts for whom care strategies can be directed. Additionally, these patient cohorts, based on atrial appendage morphology, appear to be more aligned with the molecular underpinnings of isomerism. This is based on studies done by Uemura and colleagues,[5,12] who demonstrated that the syndromic clustering of associated features is greater when assessed on the basis of appendage morphology. Additionally, studies of knockout mice demonstrate that similar genetic mutations result in consistent findings in regard to the morphology of the appendages, although these are not always consistent with splenic morphology.[13,14] The assignment of "leftness" or "rightness" of the appendages has also undergone an evolution in thinking. Until relatively recently the external features of the appendage were used to define its morphology. However, although the morphologically right atrial appendage is usually broad and pyramidal in shape in comparison with the left atrial appendage, which is narrower and tubular, these external characteristics can be influenced by hemodynamic conditions. Consequently, we now use the internal features, specifically the extent of the pectinate muscles, to define appendage morphology. The pectinate muscles of the right atrial appendage spill outside of the atrial appendage and extend around the entirety of the atrioventricular junction (Fig. 67.1). The pectinate muscles of the left atrial appendage, in contrast, are confined to its tubular component and do not extend around the atrioventricular junction so as to reach the cardiac crux.[5] It should be noted, however, that appendage isomerism is not equivalent to atrial isomerism. The overall atrial chambers, including the venoatrial connections, are not isomeric, although the arrangements have features suggestive of isomerism. The atrial appendages, in contrast, when assessed according to the extent of the pectinate muscles, unequivocally are.[6]

That said, there are some significant clinical challenges when atrial morphology is defined in this way. Definition of pectinate morphology in the working heart is all but impossible in everyday practice. For example, the atrial appendages are difficult to image using transthoracic echocardiography, and, although transesophageal echocardiography can usually describe appendage shape and size, it is rare that the extent of the pectinate muscles can be defined with clarity. Magnetic resonance and computed tomography imaging can allow for visualization of the pectinate muscles (Fig. 67.2), but these techniques are expensive and not used in day-to-day practice. Paradoxically, the simple chest radiograph may be the most reliable surrogate because there is remarkable concordance between bronchial and appendage morphology. Even so, there are many other features that align with either right or left isomerism

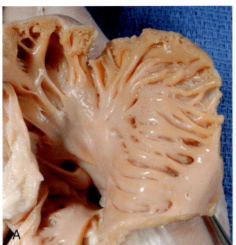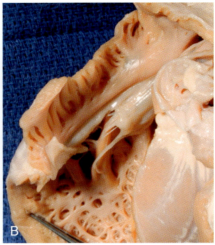

• **Figure 67.1** Images from a necroscopy specimen from a patient with right isomerism. (A) The right atrial appendage has been opened to demonstrate the pectinate muscles, which spill outside of the atrial appendage and extend to the atrioventricular junction. (B) The left-sided atrial appendage has been opened to demonstrate the pectinate muscles, which spill outside of the atrial appendage and extend around the atrioventricular junction as well.

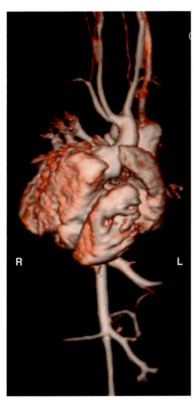

• **Figure 67.2** A three-dimensional magnetic resonance reconstruction from a 10-month-old with right isomerism demonstrating external visualization of the atrial appendages. Although external appendage morphology is not the gold standard to determine atrial appendage morphology, this patient has atrial appendages that both have a broad, pyramidal shape that is consistent with right isomerism. The extent of the pectinate muscles can be delineated by magnetic resonance imaging, although this can be quite difficult. Computed tomography reconstructions are easier to produce to demonstrate the extent of the pectinate muscles.

and that can be used to determine isomerism sidedness (Table 67.1), which will be discussed in detail later.

Cardiac Morphology

Outside of the atrial appendages, the remainder of the cardiac components also demonstrate characteristic findings. A right-sided superior caval vein is present in approximately 80% of those with either right or left isomerism. A left-sided superior caval vein is present in approximately 50% of those with either right or left isomerism. A left-sided superior caval vein may be present in isolation or concurrently in the presence of a right-sided superior caval vein. If a left superior caval vein is present, it may drain via the coronary sinus or directly to the roof of the left-sided atrium. This difference is of importance because the coronary sinus is uniquely a left-sided structure and so is always absent in the setting of right isomerism. Under such circumstances a left-sided superior caval vein, if present, will always connect directly to the atrial roof.[7,15] In the setting of right isomerism no coronary sinus will be present, and the cardiac veins will drain directly to the atrium.[12]

Defining the disposition of the inferior caval vein is the mainstay of echocardiographic diagnosis. In isomerism the abdominal great vessels are usually lateralized together on the right or left side of the spine. Interruption of the inferior caval vein is characteristic of left isomerism. When the inferior caval vein is interrupted, it will either drain into an azygos or hemiazygos vein, which then drains into the right- or left-sided superior caval vein, respectively. Consequently, the echocardiogram in left isomerism will show lateralized abdominal great vessels with the vein posterior to the aorta, whereas in right isomerism (where the inferior caval vein is usually uninterrupted) the vein will be anterior to the aorta. It should be remembered that there is an intact intrahepatic inferior vena cava in approximately 10% of patients with left isomerism, but even so, there is often a dominant azygous vein draining ipsilateral and posterior to the aorta. This has implications when it comes to staged palliation of those with functionally univentricular hearts, with regard to timing of the second-stage operation and postoperative physiology. In patients with left isomerism the

TABLE 67.1	Features Commonly Associated With Either Right or Left Isomerism[a]
Left Isomerism	**Right Isomerism**
• **Bilateral morphologically left atrial appendages with pectinate muscles confined to the appendages and not extending to the atrioventricular junction** • **Interruption of the inferior caval vein** • Left superior caval vein • **Absence of coronary sinus** • **Hepatic veins returning to right-sided atrium** • Common atrioventricular junction • **Two orifices to common atrioventricular junction** • **Concordant ventriculoarterial connections** • Double-outlet right ventricle • **Mirror-imaged spiraling of great arteries** • Pulmonary veins returning to left-sided atrium • **Atrioventricular block** • **Junctional rhythm** • **Long, hyparterial bronchi bilaterally** • **Bilaterally bilobed lungs** • Intestinal malrotation	• **Bilateral morphologically right atrial appendages with pectinate muscles spilling outside of the appendages and extending to the atrioventricular junction** • Inferior caval vein returning to right-sided atrium • Left superior caval vein • **Hepatic veins returning to inferior caval vein** • Common atrioventricular junction • Single orifice to common atrioventricular junction • **Discordant ventriculoarterial connections** • Double-outlet right ventricle • **No spiraling of great arteries** • **Extracardiac return of the pulmonary veins** • **Supraventricular tachycardia** • **Short, eparterial bronchi bilaterally** • **Bilaterally trilobed lungs** • Intestinal malrotation • Central nervous system anomalies

[a]Items in bold can help differentiate left and right isomerism.

bidirectional Glenn procedure, in which the superior caval vein or veins are anastomosed to the pulmonary arteries, will incorporate the return from the inferior caval vein when there is azygos or hemiazygous continuation. This second stage of palliation is known as the Kawashima operation and leaves only the hepatic veins to be redirected to the pulmonary arteries at the time of Fontan completion.[7,12,16]

The hepatic veins can return to the heart in a number of ways in those with isomerism. In left isomerism a little over half of patients will have all hepatic veins draining directly to the right-sided atrium. Approximately 20% of patients will have hepatic veins draining into the left-sided atrium, and another 20% will have hepatic veins draining in bilateral fashion to both the right- and left-sided atrial chamber. Only 10% will have hepatic venous drainage to the inferior caval vein.[7,12] In right isomerism the hepatic veins drain into the inferior caval vein in 75% of patients and directly to the right-sided atrium in 25% of patients.[7,12]

The pulmonary venous drainage and connection is also variable in those with isomerism. Necessarily, the pulmonary venous connections are always anomalous in right isomerism because there is no morphologic left atrium. The connections can be cardiac, infradiaphragmatic, supracardiac, or mixed, and defining the exact path of drainage of each pulmonary vein is crucial in these patients.

As is seen outside of the setting of isomerism, obstruction to the pulmonary venous return is anticipated when there is an infradiaphragmatic connection and also can be produced by the bronchopulmonary vice or a course under the bronchus itself when the connection is supracardiac. This can add to the complexity of surgical intervention, impact the need for reintervention, and influence mortality during long-term follow-up.[17-25]

In left isomerism, direct cardiac connections of the pulmonary veins to the atriums is expected, either bilateral or lateralized to one or the other left atrium. To the best of our knowledge, only a single case of extracardiac anomalous connection has been described in the setting of left isomerism.[7,25] Consequently, although it remains important to define exactly the mode of connection of the pulmonary veins, when planning septation of the atriums for example, their disposition has much less impact on outcomes than in patients with right isomerism.

At least four-fifths of those with either right or left isomerism will have a common atrioventricular junction, also referred to as an atrioventricular septal defect. This is more frequently observed in patients with right isomerism, who nearly always have a common atrioventricular junction. The presence of a tongue of tissue connecting the superior and inferior bridging leaflets in the setting of a common atrioventricular junction, thereby creating two separate orifices, is more frequent in those with left isomerism.[7,26] With respect to the ventriculoarterial connections, almost 75% of those with left isomerism will have concordant connections, albeit oftentimes with mirror-imaged spiraling of the aorta relative to the pulmonary trunk. Those with right isomerism most frequently have double-outlet right ventricle or discordant ventriculoarterial connections, typically with an anterior aorta, which may be right- or left-sided depending on the ventricular topology.[7]

Ventricular topology can be either left handed or right handed in either form of isomerism. Biventricular atrioventricular connections, however, are much more frequent in the setting of left isomerism, whereas double inlet through a common atrioventricular valve is more frequent in those with right isomerism. Those with right isomerism are more likely to have a true solitary ventricle, as evidenced by failure to identify a second slit-like incomplete ventricle at the time of necropsy.[7,27] Abnormal coronary arterial patterns are noted in approximately 20% of those with isomerism, with single coronary artery being the most frequent variant.[7,27]

Conduction System and Arrhythmias

The conduction system is expected to be malformed in those with isomerism. Twin sinus nodes are typically present in those with right isomerism, but de novo atrial arrhythmia is rare. The sinus node is universally hypoplastic in the setting of left isomerism. If found, it is abnormally located at a closer position relative to the atrioventricular junctions. Consequently, an abnormal P-wave axis is usual in left isomerism.[28]

Twinning of the atrioventricular nodes can also be found. Either or both of these nodes may connect to the ventricular conduction system, providing the possibility of a sling of conduction tissue to form between them, providing the substrate for a reentry type tachycardia. This is more frequent in those with right isomerism.[28] If one node does not connect to the ventricular conduction system, it is more frequently the anterior node. This has clinical consequences and may influence ablation plans. Discontinuity between both nodes and the ventricular system is more frequent in left isomerism, producing complete atrioventricular block.

A large proportion of children and adults with isomerism will have arrhythmias. Those with right isomerism are more likely to have supraventricular tachycardias during long-term follow-up, although whether this is related to intrinsic propensity or reflective of a greater extent of atrial surgery (e.g., repair of anomalous pulmonary venous connection, higher frequency of Fontan palliation) is not known. Nonetheless, electrophysiology studies and ablations can be effectively conducted in those with isomerism, particularly before Fontan completion.[29,30] Those with left isomerism are more likely to have atrioventricular block, and this is the commonest cause of fetal demise. Postnatally those with left isomerism and atrioventricular block may or may not require a pacemaker. Some patients tolerate a predominantly junctional rhythm without any significant clinical issues. However, all patients with left isomerism require careful and regular follow-up of their atrioventricular conduction, with annual evaluation by Holter monitoring.

Myocardial Fibrosis and Ischemia

Approximately 16% of hearts from those with isomerism will demonstrate some degree of myocardial fibrosis at the time of necropsy. Approximately 10% will demonstrate evidence of myocardial ischemia.[7] This early development of fibrosis and ischemia then leads to the question as to whether adults with isomerism are at an increased risk for myocardial infarction. Although the location of myocardial infarction differs slightly between those with and without isomerism, the age of myocardial infarction, ability to successfully stent the coronary lesions, and mortality from myocardial infarction do not differ in those with isomerism when compared to those without.[31]

Impact on Surgical Palliation

Approximately 85% of those with isomerism will require functionally univentricular palliation, whereas the remainder will require some form of biventricular repair. Functionally univentricular neonatal repairs may consist of either a Norwood procedure, pulmonary artery banding, or systemic to pulmonary shunt with or without pulmonary vein repair. Some patients require no intervention initially if pulmonary stenosis is present with an adequate balance of the ratio of pulmonary and systemic blood flow. Careful monitoring during the neonatal period and early infancy will obviously be required, particularly if there is associated anomalous pulmonary venous return. This is important because data from Toronto show that if pulmonary venous repair can be delayed beyond the third month of life, the outcomes are far superior compared with neonatal intervention.

The second and third stages of palliation can also be somewhat different in that the second stage could be a bidirectional Glenn procedure, a bilateral bidirectional Glenn procedure, or a Kawashima procedure with or without a contralateral Glenn procedure. For the latter, given that such surgery directs over 85% of the systemic venous return to the lungs, it may be advantageous to delay surgery beyond the usual 3- to 6-month window that is usually chosen for "traditional" bidirectional Glenn procedures, to allow for greater pulmonary artery growth and an optimally low pulmonary vascular resistance.

The third palliation is usually a Fontan completion or, in patients with left isomerism, a hepatic vein to pulmonary artery connection. Both procedures can be technically challenging. In right isomerism care must be taken to avoid the extracardiac conduit from impinging on the pulmonary veins, and in some cases an intraatrial tube graft

is preferred. Similarly, in left isomerism routing of the hepatic veins to the pulmonary artery can be technically challenging, especially if the hepatic veins come into different sides of the atrial septum, or "physiologically challenging" if the hepatic venous flow is directed predominantly to one pulmonary artery because this may increase the propensity to form pulmonary atrioventricular malformations on the contralateral side (see later).

One of the more challenging issues with single-ventricle palliation in these patients is the function of the common atrioventricular valve because few consistently effective techniques exist. A detailed discussion of the usually individualized approach to valve repair is beyond the scope of this chapter, but suffice it to say that both short- and long-term outcomes will be significantly impacted by the degree of residual regurgitation and/or stenosis, particularly in those pursuing a univentricular pathway, but also in those undergoing biventricular repair.

Biventricular repairs will often include atrioventricular septal defect repair, baffling of an intraventricular communication in the setting of double-outlet right ventricle and complex intraatrial tunnels. These procedures can be quite successful in carefully selected patients. The technical success of these repairs in the short term should rarely be an issue under those circumstances; however, the long-term problems associated with atrioventricular valve failure or stenosis of the frequently required complex surgical tunnels, be they intraatrial or intraventricular, needs to be kept in mind when deciding whether to pursue a two-ventricle repair.

It should come as no surprise, given the complexities discussed earlier, that there is a significant impact of isomerism on the outcomes of surgical palliation, particularly in the setting of functionally univentricular palliation. Hospitalization for stage I palliation is often longer in those with isomerism, and patients are more likely to either remain inpatient during the interstage period or have more interstage hospitalizations. Mortality before stage I palliation and during the interstage period is also greater in those with isomerism. However, length of stay, cost, frequency of extracorporeal oxygenation, and frequency of mortality does not differ for stage II palliation between those with and without isomerism.[32]

The outpatient trajectory after stage II palliation, however, can differ between those with and without isomerism. Those with left isomerism in particular are more likely to develop pulmonary arteriovenous malformations, leading to progressive hypoxia. Up to 33% of patients with left isomerism will develop such pulmonary arteriovenous malformations, believed to be due to the lack of hepatic factor reaching the lungs from the hepatic veins (Fig. 67.3).[33-35] In those patients who develop pulmonary arteriovenous malformations after the Kawashima procedure, completion of the Fontan circulation can lead to regression of these arteriovenous malformations by introducing hepatic factor to the lungs once again, a process that can take approximately 6 months.[36] Teams have to keep in mind the technical issues with trying to evenly distribute the hepatic factor when completing the Fontan, especially when there is a bilateral bidirectional Glenn or a Glenn and a Kawashima procedure.

Although there is limited published experience with the Y-graft Fontan, this approach to the Fontan has been demonstrated, by several studies based on computer modeling and small clinical cohorts, to provide a decrease in Fontan power loss and provide a more equal distribution of hepatic blood flow to both lungs. Pre-Fontan magnetic resonance imaging studies with four-dimensional flow analysis and computed flow dynamics are important to design the Y-graft properly, with limb size of the

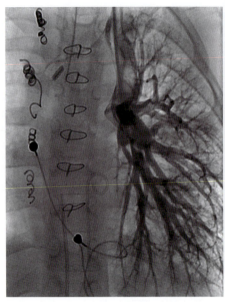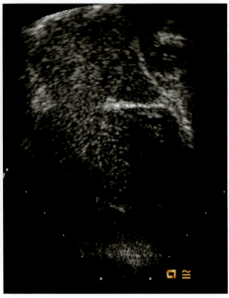

• **Figure 67.3** Left pulmonary angiography in a 5-year-old with left isomerism after stage II palliation *(left)*. The granularity in her left pulmonary vasculature was highly concerning for severe burden of pulmonary arteriovenous malformations, which were then confirmed by saline contrast echocardiography *(right)*. Similar findings were noted with the right lung as well.

Y-graft, caliber of the branch pulmonary arteries, pulmonary artery resistances, and superior caval flow dynamics being of great importance when planning a Y-graft. This as a practical approach for most programs may be limited. Alternative strategies to direct the hepatic veins towards the azygous vein, rather than directly into the pulmonary arteries, are also being explored.

After Fontan completion, isomerism has been demonstrated to be associated with increased length of hospital stay, cost of stay, and need for extracorporeal membrane oxygenation. Isomerism does not appear to be associated with increased inpatient mortality during the Fontan hospitalization.

There is minimal published data with regard to cardiac transplantation in the setting of isomerism, although anecdotally these children do tend to tolerate transplantation well. As is the case with any heart transplantation, success is based on the overall condition of the patient. Patients with isomerism, given their other associated pathologies, must be thoroughly evaluated for pulmonary arteriovenous malformations, hepatic dysfunction, renal dysfunction, immune issues, and severe neurodevelopmental delay. Although complex anatomy such as systemic venous abnormalities, pulmonary abnormalities, and rightward cardiac apex are relative contraindications to transplantation, at most congenital centers there are really no anatomies that would exclude these patients from cardiac transplantation.

Pulmonary System

Bronchopulmonary Isomerism

The pulmonary system is almost always affected in those with cardiac isomerism. The most apparent finding is that of bronchopulmonary isomerism. The bronchi in those with left isomerism are often long and hyparterial and have a tracheobronchial angle of less than 135 degrees bilaterally. Those with right isomerism have bronchi that are short and eparterial and have a tracheobronchial angle of greater than 135 degrees. These patterns are found in nearly all of those

with cardiac isomerism. In some infrequent instances, however, bronchial isomerism is not consistent with overall isomerism.[37-40] The lungs also demonstrate isomerism. Those with right isomerism typically have trilobed lungs bilaterally, whereas those with left isomerism have bilobed lungs bilaterally.[7] Bronchopulmonary morphology can be determined by chest radiography, computed tomography, or magnetic resonance imaging.[38]

Three examples of a bilaterally dual bronchial system have also been reported, two during necropsy studies and one in a living patient (Fig. 67.4). In this arrangement the trachea initially branches into two isomeric bronchi. The trachea then continues inferiorly after the initial bronchial bifurcation, with the trachea ultimately terminating with two additional isomeric bronchi bifurcating from it.[7]

Lung Function and Cardiopulmonary Exercise Testing

The presence of isomerism does have functional consequences. Approximately 33% of those with left isomerism experience recurrent upper respiratory infections. Nearly 40% of those with left isomerism are also more likely to require pulmonology follow-up, with 50% of those with left isomerism requiring home oxygen at some point.[41] The mechanism of this is unclear, although this could be due to ciliary dysfunction. Further studies regarding ciliary dysfunction will help further elucidate this.

With respect to cardiopulmonary exercise testing, those with isomerism tend to demonstrate components of both restrictive and obstructive lung disease. The restrictive lung disease is likely the consequence of repeat sternotomies, although the cause of the obstructive component is not entirely clear at this point. Although differences in pulmonary function testing may be present, those with isomerism do not tend to have impaired exercise tolerance as evaluated by the Bruce protocol during childhood and adolescence. These findings have not been evaluated in adults at this point. Interestingly, those with isomerism did not demonstrate

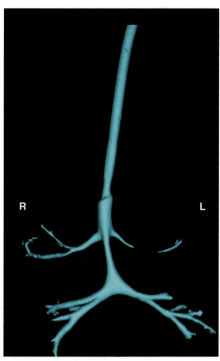

• **Figure 67.4** Computed tomographic reconstruction of the airway in a 1-year-old with left isomerism following bilateral bidirectional superior cavopulmonary anastomoses found to have a dual bronchial system. The superior bronchi are isomeric and are consistent with left isomerism with acute tracheobronchial angles. The left upper lobe bronchus is diffusely hypoplastic. The trachea then continues inferiorly with another set of bronchi arising bilaterally. These bronchi are also isomeric and have tracheobronchial angles that are consistent with left isomerism.

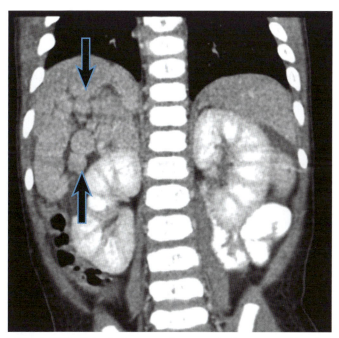

• **Figure 67.5** Abdominal computed tomography in a 1-year-old patient with left isomerism. Coronal imaging demonstrating multiple spleens *(arrows)* located in the right side of the abdomen.

similar cardiopulmonary exercise testing findings as those with primary ciliary dyskinesia.[42] It should be acknowledged that the data from children and adolescents may be the result of referral and survival bias.

Pulmonary Vascular Disease and Pulmonary Hypertension

Pulmonary vascular disease and pulmonary hypertension have been anecdotally noted to be increased in those with isomerism. Although data in children are not available at this point, isomerism has been demonstrated to be an independent risk factor for pulmonary hypertension in adults. Those with isomerism had an increase of almost 80% in the odds of pulmonary vascular disease or pulmonary hypertension. Factors predictive of such findings in adults with isomerism was increasing age, obesity, and a history of anomalous pulmonary venous connection.[43] The mechanism of pulmonary vascular disease or pulmonary hypertension in the setting of isomerism is not clear, and the efficacy of different medical therapies for pulmonary hypertension in the setting of isomerism has not been evaluated as of yet.

Immune System

Splenic and Thymic Morphology

The immune system is likely to be abnormal in those with isomerism. Splenic morphology has long been noted to be abnormal.

More importantly, splenic function may also be abnormal. This is to be anticipated when the spleen is absent but is also the case in those with multiple spleens or a solitary spleen (Fig. 67.5). Patients in either subset of isomerism, furthermore, may also have either a right-sided or left-sided solitary spleen, although solitary spleens are more frequently seen in those with right isomerism.[5,7,44,45] When there is a solitary spleen present, the location of it in the right or left abdomen does not seem to play a role in whether the spleen is functional or not. Abnormal thymic involution is also noted in patients with isomerism, being found in approximately 20% of those with isomerism.

Risk of Bacteremia

The anatomic anomalies impact the function of the spleen as well. Those with any splenic anatomy, including the presence of multiple spleens or solitary spleens, are often associated with impaired or absent splenic function.[46] In patients with multiple spleens, splenic function will be abnormal in at least 12% of patients, and in those with a solitary spleen, splenic function will be abnormal in at least 11% of patients. This subsequently leads to an increased risk of bacteremia. At least 25% of patients with isomerism will have documented bacteremia, a majority of these episodes being nosocomial and occurring under 2 years of age. Mortality in those with bacteremia is at least 10% but may be as high as 58%, with the average age of mortality from sepsis being approximately 21 months of age.[45,47-51] Both encapsulated and unencapsulated organisms have been documented to cause bacteremia in patients with isomerism, although approximately 66% of those reported are due to encapsulated organisms. Risk factors for bacteremia in patients include both absence of a spleen and presence of multiple spleens. A low number of immunoglobulin memory B cells also increases the risk of bacteremia in those with isomerism.[45,52] Episodes of bacteremia also tend to occur at an earlier age in those with absence of a spleen.[48,50,51]

Antibiotic Prophylaxis and Vaccination

The role of antibiotic prophylaxis is currently unclear. Splenic function testing in the first few years of life is not accurate and thus should not be used to guide whether or not prophylactic antibiotics should be initiated.[49] When data from the sickle cell population is considered (they have functional asplenia due to chronic ischemic damage), along with the limited data available from those with isomerism, it becomes apparent that the most reasonable strategy would be to use antibiotic prophylaxis in those with isomerism who are under 5 years of age.[53,54] Those with a diagnosis of isomerism and uncertain splenic functional status should be started on antibiotic prophylaxis as early as possible. For those who are not able to take oral medications, intravenous ampicillin should be used, whereas for those who are able to take oral medications, amoxicillin should be used. Amoxicillin should be dosed at 20 mg/kg/d and can be divided over one or two doses a day.

At 2 years of age, those with presence of a solitary spleen or multiple spleens should be evaluated for splenic function. If function is normal, then antibiotic prophylaxis may be discontinued. Pitted red blood cell testing is the preferred method of testing at this point, although Howell-Jolly body testing may be used when pitted red blood cell testing is not available. Pitted red blood cell testing is more sensitive and specific in detecting impaired splenic function when compared with Howell-Jolly body testing.[55-58] Technetium scintigraphy is no longer required with the advent of the newer techniques.

For all patients with isomerism in whom antibiotic prophylaxis was continued beyond 2 years of age, antibiotic prophylaxis may be discontinued at 5 years of age based on data from the sickle cell population.[53,54,59] This is supported by data from isomerism patients as well because these data have demonstrated that a majority of bacteremia occurs early in life.[45,60]

Vaccinations are also of utmost importance. The standard vaccination schedule, as set forth by the American Academy of Pediatrics, should be used for all patients. In addition to the vaccinations described in the standard schedule, those with isomerism should also receive a 23-valent polysaccharide pneumococcal vaccination after 2 years of age. This should be in addition to the standard 13-valent polysaccharide pneumococcal vaccination. Meningococcal vaccinations should also be started sooner in life.[61]

Febrile Episodes

Because of the increased risk of bacteremia and bacteremia-associated mortality in those with isomerism, parents and patients should be counseled that a fever of 38.5°C must prompt thorough evaluation and management. Those who are well appearing can then be given a single dose of intramuscular ceftriaxone and discharged home with appropriate follow-up. Those who are ill appearing should receive intravenous antibiotics and be admitted to the hospital.[60,62]

Gastrointestinal System

Anatomic Anomalies

Abnormal positioning of the abdominal organs should be anticipated, although no particular pattern has been found in the settings of right as opposed to left isomerism, although symptomatic malrotation of the gut appears to be more common in left isomerism. Some form of intestinal nonrotation or malrotation has been reported to occur in 33% to 90% of children with isomerism.[63,64] Although this is a large burden, only a very small proportion, approximately 1%, of those with such rotational anomalies experience volvulus.[64-67] Thus the question must be asked whether routine evaluation and a prophylactic Ladd's procedure is warranted in this population. With such a low frequency of volvulus in the setting of such a high frequency of intestinal rotational anomalies, intervention is not warranted unless the patient is symptomatic. It also becomes logical to defer routine evaluation of the upper gastrointestinal tract until patients become symptomatic and demonstrate concern for volvulus. There is now a growing body of literature supporting this approach, particular because the Ladd procedure in itself is associated with an increased risk for thrombosis of a Blalock-Taussig shunt if already present or if constructed shortly after the Ladd procedure.[63,68-71] Malposition of the solid abdominal organs is also expected, although the term *situs ambiguus* should be avoided because there is no true ambiguity in the positioning of the organs. Instead, the position of the organs should simply be described because this provides more valuable and helpful information. The basic arrangements include left-sided stomach with right-sided liver, right-sided stomach with left-sided liver, left-sided stomach with midline liver, or right-sided stomach with midline liver. The position of the gallbladder and pancreas may also be abnormal. Other malformations involving the gastrointestinal tract that may be present in the setting of isomerism include tracheoesophageal fistula, congenital diaphragmatic hernia, omphalocele, biliary atresia, duodenal atresia, agenesis of the dorsal pancreas, anal atresia, and Abernethy malformation.[72-83] Most of these abnormalities have a frequency of 10% or less in those with isomerism.

Growth and Feeding

Although growth has not been formally evaluated in children with isomerism, it can be impaired. This may be a result of impaired feeding, with nearly 25% of infants with isomerism requiring a nasogastric or gastrostomy tube. The nasogastric or gastrostomy tube can usually be removed by 1 year of age when oral intake improves.

Central Nervous System

Anatomic Anomalies

Up to a third of those with isomerism will demonstrate central nervous system anomalies at necropsy.[7] Manifestations of such anomalies include cerebral volume asymmetry, craniorachischisis, holoprosencephaly, abnormalities of the corpus callosum, aqueductal stenosis, and neural tube defects.[18,84-89] Several of these findings can be noted prenatally by ultrasonography or by magnetic resonance imaging.[10] Those with right isomerism are more likely to have central nervous system anomalies, with as many as half being documented to have such anomalies in one series.[7] Also of interest is the recent finding that mice with right isomerism lack normal right-left asymmetry of hippocampal synapses. They instead demonstrated isomerism of the hippocampal synapse distribution, thus demonstrating another region of the body in which isomerism may be noted.[90]

Neurodevelopmental Delay

The long-term impacts of these findings have yet to be delineated. Of particular interest are the neurodevelopmental findings. Because children with isomerism may spend increased periods of time in the hospital and require more and longer cardiac interventions, it is highly likely that those with isomerism may be at greater risk for neurodevelopmental delay, independent of any direct impact of isomerism within the brain. Furthermore, the high prevalence of ciliary dysfunction in those with isomerism and recent evidence linking ciliary dyskinesia to developmental delay makes this an increasing possibility.[91] Further research in this area is more than justified, given all of these associations.

Survival and Mortality

Survival of those with isomerism has improved in the recent era for both biventricular and functionally univentricular circulation patients.[92,93] This is likely the result of improvements in understanding of isomerism and general improvements in pediatric cardiothoracic surgery and pediatric cardiac critical care.[93] Mortality for all of those with isomerism appears to be highest in the first 3 years of life with 73% survival at 3 years of age. Survival at 10 years of age is 61%, and survival at 25 years of age is 35%.[93] If only those born after the year 2000 are analyzed, survival is 78% at 3 years of age and 70% at 13 years of age.[93] Those with left isomerism seem to have an early survival advantage when compared with those with right isomerism, although a reversal of this is seen at approximately 14 years of age. For those with left isomerism survival is 94% and 83% at 5 and 10 years of age, respectively. For right isomerism survival is 76% and 64% at 5 and 10 years of age, respectively.[93] For those with biventricular circulations, survival is much better than those with functionally univentricular hearts with 89% and 84% survival at 5 and 10 years of age, respectively.[93] Factors associated with increased risk of death include obstructed anomalous pulmonary venous connection, presence of congenital heart block, moderate or greater atrioventricular valve regurgitation, presence of a common atrioventricular junction, pulmonary atresia, and need for extracorporeal membrane oxygenation.[19-21,24,25,94-101]

Future Considerations

Despite huge advances in our knowledge during the past two decades, there is clearly much to be learned in regard to the underlying causes, pathobiology, and optimization of outcomes of isomerism. One major area of potential learning is in the field of cilia biology. The mechanism of the effects of isomerism remains unclear at this time, although there is an increasing body of evidence that points to cilia (both motor and sensory) playing a potentially large role in this. Motile cilia are present at the earliest stages of development on the embryonic node. The cilia at this point generate a flow of embryonic fluid that is believed to lead to left-right patterning and lateralization in the body. A lack of nodal cilia and, more importantly, ciliary dysfunction at the node can thus lead to abnormalities in lateralization as is seen in the setting of isomerism.

Beyond these early stages of embryology, cilia may also be implicated in mediating the effects of isomerism. At least a single sensory cilium is present on every cell of the body. In the brain, heart, liver, and spleen these are likely to play a role in the development of these organs and also their postnatal functioning. Ciliary dysfunction has been demonstrated to be associated with hydrocephalus and abnormal brain development, development of atrioventricular septal defect in the heart, hepatic dysfunction, and splenic dysfunction. All of these are noted in those with isomerism as well. The role of motile cilia is perhaps best appreciated in the airway. Here, ciliary dysfunction can lead to recurrent sinopulmonary infections, impaired mucociliary clearance, and abnormal respiratory mechanics. These, too, are found in increased frequency in patients with isomerism.

Ciliary dysfunction has been noted by investigating ciliary function from nasal epithelial cells in those with isomerism. Nearly half of those with isomerism were noted to have ciliary dysfunction. Sensory cilia have yet to be specifically investigated in those with isomerism. It appears, however, that both motile and sensory cilia are likely to mediate several findings of isomerism. It remains to be seen whether a better understanding of ciliary function and an ability to influence it positively will have any impact on outcomes, but it remains a rich area of research potential, both in terms of basic mechanisms and clinical impact.

Conclusion

Isomerism is a complex multisystem clinical entity. An understanding of the full spectrum of associated anatomic and functional findings is important in guiding a thorough evaluation, which can allow for early detection and management. An understanding of how the different aspects of isomerism impact long-term morbidity and mortality is also necessary to optimize management of these complex patients.

References

A complete list of references is available at ExpertConsult.com.

68

Arrhythmia Surgery

TIMOTHY S. LANCASTER, MD; PIROOZ EGHTESADY, MD, PHD;
RALPH J. DAMIANO JR., MD

The definitive treatment of arrhythmias began in the late 1960s with the development of surgical techniques for disruption of accessory atrioventricular (AV) connections in Wolff-Parkinson-White syndrome by Sealy, Wallace, and Boineau at Duke University.[1-3] From this foundation, extensive experimental work by Cox, Boineau, and colleagues at Duke and then at Washington University in St. Louis led to the development of surgical techniques for treatment of ventricular arrhythmias, AV and AV nodal reentry tachycardia, and the Maze procedure for atrial fibrillation.[4-8] Experimental and translational work in our laboratory has produced continued refinement of the original "cut-and-sew" Cox-Maze procedure, most notably through the application of energy sources for replacement of most of the suture lines with either radiofrequency (RF) or cryothermal ablation lines.[9-12] This has allowed for reduced complexity, reduced operative time, and greater reproducibility of the Maze procedure, as well as its completion through minimally invasive approaches.[13-16]

Techniques for catheter-based electrophysiologic mapping and arrhythmia ablation also developed alongside of, and were greatly informed by, the advances made in arrhythmia surgery over this time.[17-20] Catheter ablation has found wide adoption given its relatively low invasiveness and frequent effectiveness and today is usually the first treatment approach for patients requiring arrhythmia intervention. However, the long-term outcomes of catheter ablation can fall short of surgical ablation, especially for patients with long-standing arrhythmias or complex arrhythmia substrates.[21-23] Surgical ablation therefore remains an important method of arrhythmia therapy for patients who have experienced failure of catheter ablation, who are undergoing cardiac surgery for another reason, or who have specific anatomic or electrophysiologic reasons to suggest that catheter ablation may be unsuccessful.

With improved overall survival of patients with congenital heart disease, the common occurrence of late postoperative arrhythmias has been appreciated, along with their contributions to late morbidity and mortality in this population.[24-26] Arrhythmias remain a leading cause of death in adults with congenital heart disease,[25] and those who develop atrial arrhythmias have a 50% increase in mortality, a twofold increase in risk of stroke and/or heart failure, and a threefold increase in risk of needing reintervention.[27] Lesions such as Ebstein anomaly, single-ventricle lesions, tetralogy of Fallot, atrial repairs of transposition of the great arteries, truncus arteriosus, and atrial septal defects (ASDs) have the highest risk for late arrhythmia development. Frequently these patients have additional indications for reoperation at some point in their management (Table 68.1).[28] A variety of modifications to established surgical

ablation techniques have been developed and reported for such patients.

This chapter reviews indications, techniques, postoperative management, and expected outcomes of arrhythmia surgery for patients with congenital heart disease. We review the standard Cox-Maze IV lesion set and surgical technique that we apply for patients with normal anatomy undergoing atrial ablation. We also review published modifications to this lesion set based on the particular arrhythmia substrate or special anatomic considerations when being applied to patients with congenital heart disease. Because persistent arrhythmias are generally a late-developing burden of congenital heart disease, this review is most relevant to older children and adults with congenital heart disease.

Indications for Arrhythmia Surgery

Expert consensus guidelines have been recently developed by the Pediatric and Congenital Electrophysiology Society (PACES) and the Heart Rhythm Society (HRS) to provide indications for arrhythmia surgery in patients with congenital heart disease and to guide the selection of arrhythmia procedure type (Tables 68.2 to 68.4).[28] Indications for arrhythmia surgery are generally grouped into three main categories: (1) patients with arrhythmias who have experienced failure of catheter ablation, (2) patients with known arrhythmias who are undergoing concomitant surgery for congenital heart disease, and (3) prophylactic ablation in patients with high risk for future arrhythmia development who are undergoing concomitant surgery for congenital heart disease.

Although the most common role for arrhythmia surgery in patients with congenital heart disease is the completion of a Maze procedure for atrial fibrillation or atrial macro-reentry tachycardias, surgical ablation is also indicated in patients with accessory pathways, focal atrial tachycardias, or AV nodal reentry circuits who have experienced failure of catheter ablation.[28] In comparison with catheter ablation, especially in complex anatomy, surgical ablation techniques allow direct visualization of the anatomy, can be more efficient for performing complete lines of block between difficult-to-access anatomic structures, and can provide more complete lines of ablation.

Cox-Maze IV Procedure

The Cox-Maze procedure for atrial fibrillation went through several revisions throughout its development based on the results of extensive laboratory testing, with serial refinement of lesion sets and surgical technique.[8,10] The Cox-Maze IV procedure refers to

TABLE 68.1	Reoperation Rates and Estimated Prevalence of Arrhythmias in Adults With Congenital Heart Disease		
CHD Lesion	Reoperation	Atrial Arrhythmias	Ventricular Tachycardia
Ebstein anomaly	30%-50%	33%-60%	>2%
Single ventricle	>25%	40%-60%	>5%
Tetralogy of Fallot	26%-50%	15%-25%	10%-15%
Transposition of the great arteries, atrial switch	15%-27%	26%-50%	7%-9%
Transposition of the great arteries, arterial switch	12%-20%	<2%	1%-2%
Congenitally corrected transposition of the great arteries	25%-35%	>30%	>2%
Truncus arteriosus	55%-89%	>25%	>2%
Atrioventricular septal defect	19%-26%	5%-10%	<2%
Atrial septal defect	<2%	16%-28%	<2%

CHD, Congenital heart disease.
Reproduced with permission from Khairy P, Van Hare GF, Balaji S, et al. PACES/HRS Expert Consensus Statement on the Recognition and Management of Arrhythmias in Adult Congenital Heart Disease: developed in partnership between the Pediatric and Congenital Electrophysiology Society (PACES) and the Heart Rhythm Society (HRS). Endorsed by the governing bodies of PACES, HRS, the American College of Cardiology (ACC), the American Heart Association (AHA), the European Heart Rhythm Association (EHRA), the Canadian Heart Rhythm Society (CHRS), and the International Society for Adult Congenital Heart Disease (ISACHD). *Heart Rhythm.* 2014;11(10):e102-165.

TABLE 68.2	Recommendations for Concomitant Atrial Arrhythmia Surgery in Adults With Congenital Heart Disease Undergoing Open Cardiac Surgery
Class I	1. A modified right atrial Maze procedure is indicated in adults undergoing Fontan conversion with symptomatic right atrial reentry tachycardia (Level of evidence: B). 2. A modified right atrial Maze procedure in addition to a left atrial Cox-Maze procedure is indicated in patients undergoing Fontan conversion with documented atrial fibrillation (Level of evidence: B).
Class IIa	1. A left atrial Cox-Maze procedure with right atrial cavotricuspid isthmus ablation can be beneficial in adults with CHD and atrial fibrillation (Level of evidence: B). 2. A (modified) right atrial Maze procedure can be useful in adults with CHD and clinical episodes of sustained typical or atypical right atrial flutter (Level of evidence: B).
Class IIb	Adults with CHD and inducible typical or atypical right atrial flutter without documented clinical sustained atrial tachycardia may be considered for (modified) right atrial Maze surgery or cavotricuspid isthmus ablation (Level of evidence: B).

CHD, Congenital heart disease.
Reproduced with permission from Khairy P, Van Hare GF, Balaji S, et al. PACES/HRS Expert Consensus Statement on the Recognition and Management of Arrhythmias in Adult Congenital Heart Disease: developed in partnership between the Pediatric and Congenital Electrophysiology Society (PACES) and the Heart Rhythm Society (HRS). Endorsed by the governing bodies of PACES, HRS, the American College of Cardiology (ACC), the American Heart Association (AHA), the European Heart Rhythm Association (EHRA), the Canadian Heart Rhythm Society (CHRS), and the International Society for Adult Congenital Heart Disease (ISACHD). *Heart Rhythm.* 2014;11(10):e102-165.

the modern, ablation-assisted, biatrial technique performed by most arrhythmia surgeons today, in which many of the suture lines of previous versions are replaced by lines of ablation.[11,12,16] Many energy devices are commercially available for surgical cardiac ablation, but we advocate the primary use of bipolar RF ablation clamps because they safely create rapid, consistently transmural lesions in both animal and human studies.[29,30] Cryothermal energy is an important adjunct that is used for creating lesions close to valve tissue and the fibrous skeleton of the heart because it induces cell death while preserving tissue collagen and normal architecture.[31]

The following sections outline the surgical technique of the Cox-Maze IV procedure as performed in patients with normal atrial anatomy, which forms an important basis for understanding modifications to these techniques for patients with congenital heart disease.

Preparation

Although patients undergo transthoracic echocardiography during preoperative assessment, the left atrial appendage (LAA) is not well visualized with this modality, and thrombus cannot be excluded with certainty. The left atrium is therefore thoroughly examined with intraoperative transesophageal echocardiography (TEE) or epicardial ultrasonography, and in those rare patients with identified thrombus, care is taken to minimize manipulation of the heart until exclusion of the LAA has been performed. Coexisting congenital lesions and valvular disease are also assessed by TEE. At the conclusion of the procedure TEE is used to confirm successful exclusion of the LAA and to evaluate any additional repairs performed.

The Cox-Maze IV procedure can be broken down into three primary components: (1) pulmonary vein (PV) isolation, (2) creation of the right atrial lesion set, and (3) creation of the left atrial lesion set.

Pulmonary Vein Isolation

A median sternotomy is performed, and the pericardium is opened in standard fashion. Bicaval and aortic cannulas are placed, and normothermic cardiopulmonary bypass is initiated. The right and left PVs are bluntly dissected, with care taken to fully dissect the epicardial fat pad off the atrial surface, and are surrounded with umbilical tapes. If the patient is in atrial fibrillation and there is no thrombus on ultrasound evaluation, amiodarone is administered, and the patient is electrically cardioverted to normal sinus rhythm. Pacing thresholds are obtained from each PV using a bipolar pacing probe. The right and left PVs are each isolated using

TABLE 68.3	Recommendations for Concomitant Ventricular Arrhythmia Surgery in Adults With Congenital Heart Disease Undergoing Open Cardiac Surgery
Class IIa	Surgical ventricular tachycardia ablation guided by electrophysiologic mapping should be considered in adults with CHD and clinical sustained monomorphic ventricular tachycardia (Level of evidence: B).
Class IIb	1. Surgical ventricular tachycardia ablation guided by electrophysiologic mapping is reasonable in adults with CHD, no clinical sustained ventricular tachycardia, and inducible sustained monomorphic ventricular tachycardia with an identified critical isthmus (Level of evidence: C). 2. Adults with CHD and rapid ventricular tachycardia not mapped preoperatively but mapped intraoperatively may be considered for ventricular arrhythmia surgery (Level of evidence: C).

CHD, Congenital heart disease.
Reproduced with permission from Khairy P, Van Hare GF, Balaji S, et al. PACES/HRS Expert Consensus Statement on the Recognition and Management of Arrhythmias in Adult Congenital Heart Disease: developed in partnership between the Pediatric and Congenital Electrophysiology Society (PACES) and the Heart Rhythm Society (HRS). Endorsed by the governing bodies of PACES, HRS, the American College of Cardiology (ACC), the American Heart Association (AHA), the European Heart Rhythm Association (EHRA), the Canadian Heart Rhythm Society (CHRS), and the International Society for Adult Congenital Heart Disease (ISACHD). *Heart Rhythm.* 2014;11(10):e102-165.

TABLE 68.4	Recommendations for Prophylactic Atrial or Ventricular Arrhythmia Surgery in Adults With Congenital Heart Disease
Class IIa	1. A modified right atrial Maze procedure should be considered in adults undergoing Fontan conversion or revision surgery without documented atrial arrhythmias (Level of evidence: B). 2. Concomitant atrial arrhythmia surgery should be considered in adults with Ebstein anomaly undergoing cardiac surgery (Level of evidence: B).
Class IIb	1. Adults with CHD undergoing surgery to correct a structural heart defect associated with atrial dilatation may be considered for prophylactic atrial arrhythmia surgery (Level of evidence: C). 2. Adults with CHD and left-sided valvular heart disease with severe left atrial dilatation or limitations of venous access may be considered for left atrial Maze surgery in the absence of documented or inducible atrial tachycardia (Level of evidence: C). 3. Closure of the left atrial appendage may be considered in adults with CHD undergoing atrial arrhythmia surgery (Level of evidence: C).
Class III	1. Prophylactic arrhythmia surgery is not indicated in adults with CHD at increased risk of surgical mortality from ventricular dysfunction or major comorbidities, in whom prolongation of cardiopulmonary bypass or cross-clamp times due to arrhythmia surgery might negatively impact outcomes (Level of evidence: C). 2. Empiric ventricular arrhythmia surgery is not indicated in adults with CHD and no clinical or inducible sustained ventricular tachyarrhythmia (Level of evidence: C).

CHD, Congenital heart disease.
Reproduced with permission from Khairy P, Van Hare GF, Balaji S, et al. PACES/HRS Expert Consensus Statement on the Recognition and Management of Arrhythmias in Adult Congenital Heart Disease: developed in partnership between the Pediatric and Congenital Electrophysiology Society (PACES) and the Heart Rhythm Society (HRS). Endorsed by the governing bodies of PACES, HRS, the American College of Cardiology (ACC), the American Heart Association (AHA), the European Heart Rhythm Association (EHRA), the Canadian Heart Rhythm Society (CHRS), and the International Society for Adult Congenital Heart Disease (ISACHD). *Heart Rhythm.* 2014;11(10):e102-165.

a bipolar RF clamp, such that a circumferential line of ablation surrounds as large a cuff of atrial tissue as possible (Fig. 68.1). For these and all subsequent lines created using the bipolar RF clamp, three discrete ablations are performed with slight adjustments in clamp position, effectively forming three closely approximated concentric circles to ensure isolation. If the surgeon is using a nonirrigated bipolar clamp, the jaws must be cleaned of char every two to three ablations to ensure the creation of transmural lesions. PV isolation is confirmed by documenting exit block, or failure of atrial capture, with epicardial pacing from each of the PVs. Further ablations are performed as needed until exit block is obtained.

Right Atrial Lesion Set

The patient is cooled to 34°C, and the right atrial lesion set is performed on the beating heart. A small purse-string suture is placed at the base of the right atrial appendage, and a stab incision is made at its center, wide enough to accommodate one jaw of the bipolar RF ablation clamp. An ablation lesion is created with the clamp across the free wall of the right atrium down toward the superior vena cava, taking care to avoid the sinoatrial (SA) node (Fig. 68.2). A vertical atriotomy is then made from the interatrial septum up toward the AV groove near the free margin of the heart. When possible, this incision should be at least 2 cm from the first free wall ablation to avoid creating an area of slow conduction. A linear cryoprobe is used to create an endocardial cryoablation from the superior aspect of the atriotomy down to the tricuspid annulus at the 2 o'clock position. All cryoablations are performed for 3 minutes at −60°C. Cryoablation is preferable to RF ablation over annular tissues because it preserves the fibrous

skeleton of the heart, avoiding any potential compromise of valve competency. The linear cryoprobe is then inserted through the previously placed purse-string suture, and an endocardial cryoablation is created down to the tricuspid valve annulus at the 10 o'clock position (Fig. 68.3). The bipolar RF clamp is then used to create ablation lines running from the inferior aspect of the right atriotomy up along the lateral aspect of the SVC and down the inferior vena cava (IVC). The SVC ablation should be performed as lateral and posterior as possible to minimize the risk of injury to the SA node, and the IVC ablation line should travel as far as possible onto the IVC (Fig. 68.4). Finally, the right atriotomy is closed in standard fashion.

Left Atrial Lesion Set

The aorta is cross-clamped, and the heart is arrested with cold blood cardioplegia. The heart is retracted, and the LAA is amputated.

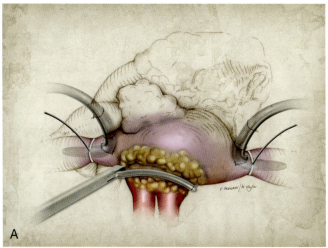

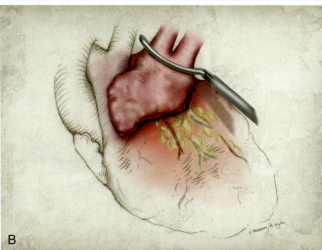

• **Figure 68.1** Right (A) and left (B) pulmonary vein isolation with the bipolar radiofrequency clamp after bicaval cannulation and initiation of cardiopulmonary bypass.

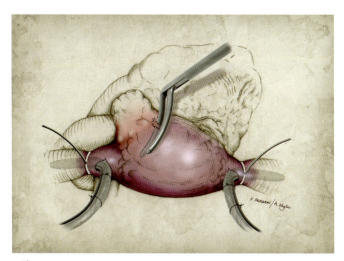

• **Figure 68.2** Right atrial free wall lesion with bipolar radiofrequency clamp.

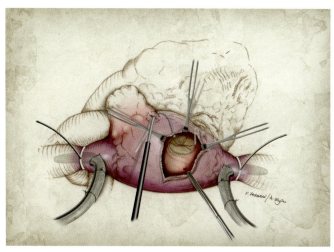

• **Figure 68.3** Right atriotomy with cryoablation lesions made to the 2 o'clock and 10 o'clock positions of the tricuspid valve annulus.

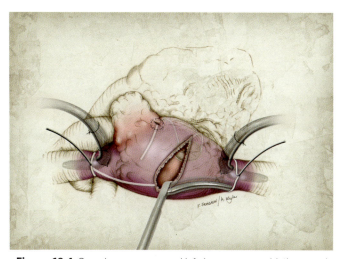

• **Figure 68.4** Superior vena cava and inferior vena cava ablations made with the bipolar radiofrequency clamp.

Through the amputated LAA the bipolar RF clamp is used to create an ablation line to either of the left PVs. The LAA is then oversewn in two layers with 4-0 polypropylene suture. The coronary sinus is marked with methylene blue at a position between the posterior descending artery and the terminal branch of the circumflex artery. A standard left atriotomy is performed, extending superiorly onto the dome of the left atrium (LA) and inferiorly to the previous right PV ablation.

Full isolation of the posterior LA is ensured by completion of a left atrial box lesion using the bipolar RF clamp. An inferior connecting ablation is made from the inferior aspect of the atriotomy across the floor of the LA and into the left inferior PV orifice, and a superior connecting ablation is similarly created from the superior aspect of the atriotomy across the roof of the LA and into the left superior PV orifice (Fig. 68.5).

A combination of bipolar RF and cryothermal energy is required to complete the mitral isthmus ablation because of the thickness of the AV groove near the mitral annulus. The mitral isthmus ablation is begun with the bipolar RF clamp from the inferior aspect of the atriotomy across the floor of the LA, directed toward the mitral valve annulus (Fig. 68.6). In patients with a

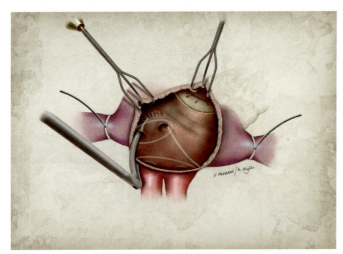

• **Figure 68.5** The left atrial appendage is amputated and oversewn after creation of an ablation through the appendage to the left superior pulmonary vein. A left atriotomy is made, and superior and inferior connecting lesions are made between the previously placed circumferential pulmonary vein ablations. This completes a full box isolation of the posterior left atrium.

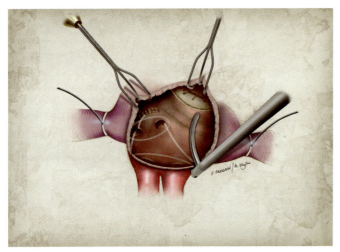

• **Figure 68.6** Mitral isthmus ablation with the bipolar radiofrequency clamp.

right-dominant coronary system, the isthmus line is generally directed toward the junction of the P2 and P3 scallops of the posterior mitral valve leaflet and should cross the coronary sinus at the area previously marked with methylene blue. Injury to the circumflex artery can be avoided in patients with a left-dominant system, however, by directing the ablation toward the posteromedial commissure between P3 and A3. The end of this RF ablation line is marked with methylene blue to serve as a starting point for a subsequent endocardial cryoablation, performed with a linear cryoprobe to connect the ablation line to the mitral valve annulus. To ensure that a full-thickness ablation is achieved, a simultaneous epicardial cryoablation is performed over the coronary sinus in line with the endocardial lesion (Fig. 68.7).

The left atriotomy is then closed, the heart is deaired, and the patient is subsequently weaned from cardiopulmonary bypass. Temporary atrial and ventricular epicardial pacing wires are routinely placed before sternal closure.

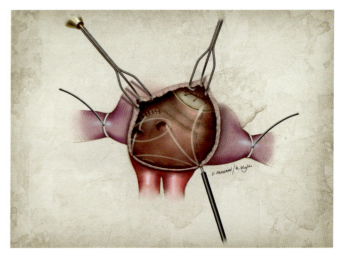

• **Figure 68.7** Mitral isthmus ablation is completed by extending the radiofrequency ablation line to the mitral valve annulus with the cryoprobe and then creating an epicardial cryoablation lesion overlying the coronary sinus.

Modified Surgical Techniques for Ablation in Congenital Heart Disease

Whereas we generally espouse completion of the full biatrial Cox-Maze IV lesion set for patients with atrial fibrillation, more limited or modified ablation techniques may be appropriate for patients with other arrhythmia types or with unique anatomic considerations relating to their congenital heart disease and prior operative interventions. It should be noted, however, that incomplete Maze lesion sets, including lone PV isolation and lesion sets that do not fully "box" isolate the posterior left atrium, are associated with higher recurrence rates of atrial fibrillation and therefore cannot be recommended for this arrhythmia type.[16,32,33]

Preoperative electrophysiologic evaluation is important and recommended for adults undergoing operation for congenital heart disease. Depending on patient symptoms, noninvasive testing, including electrocardiogram, exercise testing, and 24-hour ambulatory cardiac rhythm monitoring, should be obtained as part of the preoperative assessment. Based on these results, invasive electrophysiologic testing can be obtained to help distinguish the mechanisms, sustainability, and hemodynamic significance of identified arrhythmias. The specific arrhythmia substrate can be mapped to aid the surgeon in selecting an appropriate ablation strategy.[28] A fundamental distinction in the decision making about lesion set selection is to identify the mechanism of the arrhythmia, broadly as either a focal tachycardia (treated with localized ablation or resection) or a reentry circuit (treated with isolation by a Maze procedure or ablation of an accessory connection).[34] Table 68.5 summarizes the general ablation strategies that have been reported for patients with congenital heart disease based on arrhythmia type.[28,35]

Supraventricular Arrhythmias

Accessory connection–mediated arrhythmias, focal atrial tachycardias, and AV nodal reentry tachycardia are most often amenable to catheter ablation with excellent results, and this is usually the preferred approach even for patients who have another anatomic need for cardiac surgery. Catheter ablation before operative

TABLE 68.5	Operative Techniques for Arrhythmia Surgery
Type of Arrhythmia	**Surgical Techniques**
Supraventricular	
• Accessory connections	Endocardial or epicardial dissection and division, cryoablation
Focal atrial tachycardia	Map-guided resection, cryoablation
AV nodal reentry tachycardia	Slow pathway modification with cryoablation
Right atrial macro-reentry	
• Cavotricuspid isthmus dependent	Cavotricuspid isthmus ablation
• Multiple reentry circuits	Modified right atrial Maze
Left atrial macro-reentry	Left atrial Cox-Maze
Atrial fibrillation	Left atrial Cox-Maze; cavotricuspid isthmus ablation ± right atrial Maze ± left atrial appendectomy
Ventricular tachycardia	
• Scar related	Scar or endocardial fibrosis resection, focal ablation, lines of ablation between anatomic landmarks; map-guided resection or ablation

AV, Atrioventricular.
Reproduced with permission from Khairy P, Van Hare GF, Balaji S, et al. PACES/HRS Expert Consensus Statement on the Recognition and Management of Arrhythmias in Adult Congenital Heart Disease: developed in partnership between the Pediatric and Congenital Electrophysiology Society (PACES) and the Heart Rhythm Society (HRS). Endorsed by the governing bodies of PACES, HRS, the American College of Cardiology (ACC), the American Heart Association (AHA), the European Heart Rhythm Association (EHRA), the Canadian Heart Rhythm Society (CHRS), and the International Society for Adult Congenital Heart Disease (ISACHD). *Heart Rhythm.* 2014;11(10):e102-165.

intervention can reduce the risk of postoperative tachycardia and hemodynamic compromise. These arrhythmias may, however, be addressed surgically in rare circumstances of failed catheter ablation or special anatomic considerations. For example, patients with a right-to-left shunt may be at risk for embolic stroke during right atrial catheter ablation. Patients with Ebstein anomaly may be more likely to experience failure of catheter ablation for AV reentry tachycardia because of broad bands of accessory connections, which can be addressed surgically. Additionally, catheter access for ablation may be limited by patient anatomy or may interfere with surgical repairs, as with reconstructions of the tricuspid valve in patients with Ebstein anomaly.

Surgical technique for accessory connections and their resulting AV reentry tachycardia date to the original work of Sealy et al. and involve either an epicardial or endocardial approach to isolation and division of the accessory connections.[1] In modern times, cryoablation is frequently used to ablate the accessory connections, which normally reside in and can be mapped to the AV region of the left free wall, right free wall, or anterior or posterior septum.[36] Surgical treatment of focal atrial arrhythmias involves ablation or resection of the focal source, which can be based on preoperative or intraoperative electrophysiologic mapping.[35] Wider areas of automatic foci may require electrical isolation with connecting ablation lines.[34] Ablation of AV nodal reentry tachycardia is based on the anatomic approach of ablating the slow conducting pathway,

with a linear lesion created from the posterior inferior rim of the coronary sinus ostium to the IVC and, when a right-sided AV valve is present, from the tricuspid valve annulus to the posterior coronary sinus ostium.[18,37]

Modified Right Atrial Maze Lesions

Patients with congenital heart disease often have variant atrial anatomy and unique mechanisms of atrial reentry compared with those with normal cardiac anatomy, which has prompted modifications of the right atrial Maze lesion set for the treatment of both right atrial macro-reentry tachycardias and atrial fibrillation in this population. Although the potential lesion set variations are many, the principle of ablation in this setting is to terminate reentry circuits by connecting anatomic barriers with lines of ablation.[34]

The key role played by the right atrial cavotricuspid isthmus in perpetuating typical right atrial flutter (isthmus-dependent right atrial macro-reentry) has been appreciated through electrophysiology studies.[38,39] In fact, isthmus-dependent macro-reentry may be present in 30% to 60% of patients with repaired congenital heart disease.[40] Considered as the area between the tricuspid valve annulus, the coronary sinus, and the IVC, targeted ablation of the right atrial isthmus creates block that effectively terminates typical atrial flutter[41] (Fig. 68.8).

Additional right atrial macro-reentry circuits have been identified that contribute to non–isthmus-dependent reentry tachycardia, most importantly in patients with repaired congenital heart disease. These circuits involve reentry around prior incisions or prosthetic material such as ASD patches because scar tissue creates areas of slow conduction that can generate reentry. The approach to ablation of non–isthmus-dependent right atrial tachycardia, then, is elimination of the isthmus of slow conduction between these incisions, patches, or electrical scars.[42]

Anatomic variants in congenital heart disease complicate matters further, in that typical anatomic barriers may be absent or anomalous. Mavroudis and colleagues[34,36] have shared many potential modifications to the right atrial lesion set in these scenarios. For instance, because there is no tricuspid valve in tricuspid atresia, the lesions are placed as noted in Fig. 68.9A. Fig. 68.9B and C show the lesions used for functionally single right ventricle/mitral atresia and functionally single ventricle with unbalanced AV canal, respectively.[34,43]

When surgical ablation is performed for the treatment of atrial fibrillation in the congenital heart disease population, a full biatrial lesion set should be used, including cavotricuspid isthmus ablation and any needed modifications to the right atrial lesion set.

Ablation During Fontan Conversion

Mavroudis and colleagues have published widely on the Fontan conversion, which refers to replacement of an atriopulmonary Fontan anastomosis with an extracardiac total cavopulmonary connection. In their hands this operation normally involves surgical ablation as well, given the high risk of atrial macro-reentry tachycardias and atrial fibrillation in this population. A modified right atrial Maze lesion set is performed, along with a left atrial Maze lesion set for patients with left atrial macro-reentry or atrial fibrillation.[34-36,43-45]

Prophylactic Arrhythmia Surgery

Prophylactic arrhythmia surgery refers to surgical ablation in patients with congenital heart disease who do not yet have a diagnosed

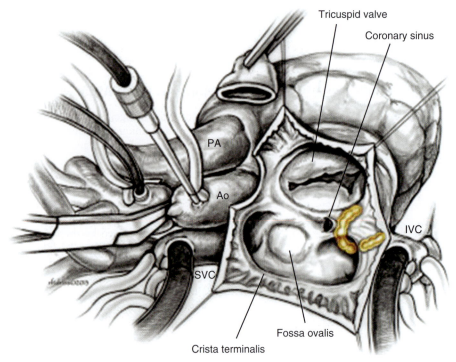

• **Figure 68.8** Right atrial cavotricuspid isthmus ablation. *Ao,* Aorta; *IVC,* inferior vena cava; *PA,* pulmonary artery; *SVC,* superior vena cava. (Reproduced with permission from Mavroudis C, Stulak JM, Ad N, et al. Prophylactic atrial arrhythmia surgical procedures with congenital heart operations: review and recommendations. *Ann Thorac Surg.* 2015;99[1]:352-359.)

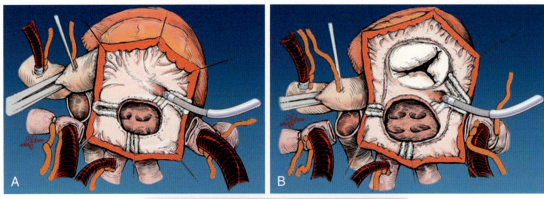

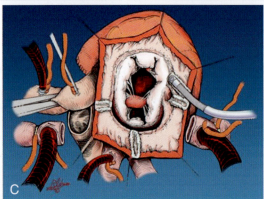

• **Figure 68.9** Illustration of modified right atrial Maze lesions in patients with tricuspid atresia (A), double-outlet right ventricle and mitral atresia (B), and unbalanced atrioventricular canal and single ventricle (C). (Reproduced with permission from Mavroudis C, Backer CL, Deal BJ, et al. Total cavopulmonary conversion and Maze procedure for patients with failure of the Fontan operation. *J Thorac Cardiovasc Surg.* 2001;122[5]:863-871.)

arrhythmia but are likely to develop one over time. Although guidelines are still not firmly established, the recent PACES/HRS consensus statement suggests that prophylactic arrhythmia surgery should consider those patients at highest risk for tachycardia development, should use standardized lesion sets, should carry minimal potential morbidity and minimal arrhythmogenicity, and should be performed with rigorous tracking of outcomes.[28]

Congenital heart disease lesions with the highest incidence of arrhythmias over time include univentricular hearts, Ebstein anomaly, transposition of the great arteries following atrial switch, congenitally corrected transposition, ASD, and tetralogy of Fallot.[46] In addition to those undergoing reoperation, approximately 20% of adults undergoing congenital heart surgery have primary repairs of proarrhythmic lesions, including ASDs, Ebstein anomaly, and mitral or aortic valve disease. Patients undergoing primary repair of ASDs beyond the age of 40 years, for example, have a 20% to 35% incidence of subsequent atrial arrhythmias, particularly atrial fibrillation.[47,48] Risk factors for atrial arrhythmia development include significant AV valve regurgitation, atrial dilation, elevated pulmonary artery pressure, decreased ventricular function, multiple prior surgeries, and age over 45 years.[49] Table 68.6 lists congenital heart lesions that might benefit from prophylactic ablation during concomitant surgery, as well as the appropriate ablation procedure (Fig. 68.10). Targeted populations to be considered for prophylactic right atrial arrhythmia surgery include patients with unrepaired ASDs presenting over 40 years of age, patients with Ebstein anomaly, patients with tetralogy of Fallot presenting for pulmonary valve insertion, and single-ventricle patients who present for Fontan operations.[41] Prophylactic surgery for atrial fibrillation can be considered in patients with significant left AV valve disease and severe left atrial dilation undergoing planned surgery.[38]

In all of these scenarios the decision to perform prophylactic arrhythmia surgery must balance the potential likelihood of future arrhythmia development with the added operative risks of an ablation procedure. The extent of dissection required for full atrial access and the additional cardiopulmonary bypass, cross-clamp, and overall operative times needed to perform ablation may be of little consequence for patients undergoing primary repair of simple lesions but may be prohibitive for patients undergoing a multiple reoperative sternotomy and extensive cardiac repair.

Postoperative Management

Rhythm management is the most unique postoperative consideration following the Cox-Maze procedure. Most patients have junctional rhythms immediately following the procedure, which have been attributed to denervation of the sinus node and usually resolve in the first several postoperative days. Before resolution, however, the atria should be paced at 80 to 100 beats/min to restore AV synchrony. AV sequential pacing (DDD mode) may be required if there is first- or second-degree AV block. Antiarrhythmic medications should not be initiated until sinus rhythm is achieved, particularly in patients with bradyarrhythmias. Five to ten percent of noncongenital heart disease patients will require a permanent pacemaker following the Cox-Maze IV procedure, usually due to failed recovery of sinus node function. Consideration should be given to placing permanent epicardial pacemaker leads in patients with limited postoperative access for transvenous device placement, such as is frequently done in Fontan conversion patients.[44]

Early atrial tachyarrhythmias affect almost half of patients after the Cox-Maze IV procedure, although they are usually transient and frequently resolve over the first postoperative month. The

TABLE 68.6	Prophylactic Arrhythmia Surgery in Adults With Congenital Heart Disease	
Congenital Heart Substrate	**Arrhythmia**	**Technique**
Fontan revision or conversion	IART, atrial fibrillation	Modified right atrial Maze ± left atrial Cox-Maze
Ebstein anomaly	Accessory connection	Dissection and division or ablation
	IART	Modified right atrial Maze
	Atrial fibrillation	Left atrial Cox-Maze with right-sided lesion set ± left atrial appendectomy or oversew orifice
Right heart conduit revisions, tricuspid valve repair or replacement, congenital lesions with atrial dilation	IART	Cavotricuspid isthmus ablation or modified right atrial Maze
Left-sided valve repair/replacement	Atrial fibrillation	Left atrial Cox-Maze with cavotricuspid isthmus ablation, ± left atrial appendectomy or oversew orifice
Atrial septal defect closure	IART	Cavotricuspid isthmus ablation, modified right atrial Maze
	Atrial fibrillation	Left atrial Cox-Maze with cavotricuspid isthmus ablation ± left atrial appendectomy or oversew orifice

IART, Intraatrial reentry tachycardia.

Reproduced with permission from Khairy P, Van Hare GF, Balaji S, et al. PACES/HRS Expert Consensus Statement on the Recognition and Management of Arrhythmias in Adult Congenital Heart Disease: developed in partnership between the Pediatric and Congenital Electrophysiology Society (PACES) and the Heart Rhythm Society (HRS). Endorsed by the governing bodies of PACES, HRS, the American College of Cardiology (ACC), the American Heart Association (AHA), the European Heart Rhythm Association (EHRA), the Canadian Heart Rhythm Society (CHRS), and the International Society for Adult Congenital Heart Disease (ISACHD). *Heart Rhythm.* 2014;11(10):e102-165.

atrial electrocardiogram can be helpful in diagnosing atrial arrhythmias because the P wave is often small and difficult to see after the procedure. Stable atrial arrhythmias are managed initially with pharmacologic rate control. If persistent, elective direct current cardioversion can be performed, but ideally this is postponed until 1 to 3 weeks after surgery to allow postoperative inflammation to subside and provide a greater chance of achieving sustained sinus rhythm. Amiodarone is usually continued for the first 2 postoperative months, and the QT interval is followed closely.

For patients with atrial fibrillation, warfarin is initiated postoperatively unless contraindicated and is continued for at least 3 months. We recommend discontinuation of warfarin after this period if the patient has no evidence of atrial arrhythmias, has

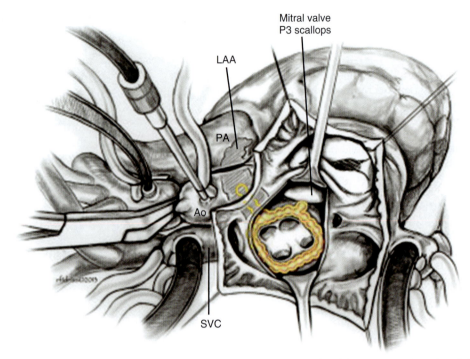

• **Figure 68.10** Potential prophylactic ablation lesions. Shown through atrial septum are circumferential isolation of the pulmonary vein confluence, connection of pulmonary vein confluence with P3 location of posterior mitral valve annulus, and connection of pulmonary vein confluence with base of left atrial appendage. *Ao,* Aorta; *LAA,* left atrial appendage; *PA,* pulmonary artery; *SVC,* superior vena cava. (Reproduced with permission from Mavroudis C, Stulak JM, Ad N, et al. Prophylactic atrial arrhythmia surgical procedures with congenital heart operations: review and recommendations. *Ann Thorac Surg.* 2015;99[1]:352-359.)

discontinued antiarrhythmic medications, and demonstrates no atrial stasis on echocardiogram.

Conclusion

Arrhythmias remain one of the leading causes of death for adults with congenital heart disease.[25] Although catheter ablation is often successful in this population, patients with complex arrhythmia mechanisms or complex cardiac anatomy stand to benefit from surgical ablation, often performed at the time of other indicated cardiac surgery. In the setting of atrial fibrillation in noncongenital heart disease patients, the full biatrial lesion set of the Cox-Maze IV procedure has produced excellent long-term results, with nearly 80% freedom from atrial tachycardias at 5 years,[16] as well as improved long-term survival.[50] A variety of modified lesion sets have been applied to congenital heart patients with success in expert hands. The largest report of surgical ablation outcomes in patients with congenital heart disease demonstrated 77% freedom from atrial tachycardias at 10 years in patients undergoing Fontan conversion with concomitant surgical ablation.[45] Efforts to establish guidelines for intervention and lesion set selection[28] should help to increase the provision of these therapies to the growing adult congenital heart population going forward.

Selected References

A complete list of references is available at ExpertConsult.com.

1. Cobb FR, Blumenschein SD, Sealy WC, Boineau JP, Wagner GS, Wallace AG. Successful surgical interruption of the bundle of Kent in a patient with Wolff-Parkinson-White syndrome. *Circulation.* 1968;38(6):1018–1029.

10. Cox JL, Jaquiss RD, Schuessler RB, Boineau JP. Modification of the Maze procedure for atrial flutter and atrial fibrillation. II. Surgical technique of the Maze III procedure. *J Thorac Cardiovasc Surg.* 1995;110(2):485–495.

16. Henn MC, Lancaster TS, Miller JR, et al. Late outcomes after the Cox Maze IV procedure for atrial fibrillation. *J Thorac Cardiovasc Surg.* 2015;150(5):1168–1176, 1178 e1161–1162.

28. Khairy P, Van Hare GF, Balaji S, et al. PACES/HRS Expert Consensus Statement on the Recognition and Management of Arrhythmias in Adult Congenital Heart Disease: developed in partnership between the Pediatric and Congenital Electrophysiology Society (PACES) and the Heart Rhythm Society (HRS). Endorsed by the governing bodies of PACES, HRS, the American College of Cardiology (ACC), the American Heart Association (AHA), the European Heart Rhythm Association (EHRA), the Canadian Heart Rhythm Society (CHRS), and the International Society for Adult Congenital Heart Disease (ISACHD). *Heart Rhythm.* 2014;11(10):e102–e165.

34. Mavroudis C, Deal B, Backer CL, Stewart RD. Operative techniques in association with arrhythmia surgery in patients with congenital heart disease. *World J Pediatr Congenit Heart Surg.* 2013;4(1):85–97.

35. Deal BJ, Mavroudis C. Arrhythmia Surgery for Adults with Congenital Heart Disease. *Card Electrophysiol Clin.* 2017;9(2):329–340.

45. Deal BJ, Costello JM, Webster G, Tsao S, Backer CL, Mavroudis C. Intermediate-Term Outcome of 140 Consecutive Fontan Conversions With Arrhythmia Operations. *Ann Thorac Surg.* 2016;101(2): 717–724.

69

Congenitally Corrected Transposition

DAVID J. BARRON, MD, FRCP, FRCS(CT)

This rare condition accounts for 0.5% of all congenital heart disease and is characterized by the combination of atrio-ventricular (AV) and ventriculoarterial (VA) discordance. This extraordinary and unique morphologic arrangement results in a physiologically "corrected" circulation in that the systemic venous blood passes into the lungs (but via a morphologic left ventricle [mLV]) and the pulmonary venous return is directed to the systemic circulation (via a morphologic right ventricle [mRV]). The condition was first described by Rokitansky in 1875 and is typified by *levo-* or l-transposition in which the transposed aorta sits anterior and to the left of the pulmonary artery (PA). In its pure form this is a corrected circulation and produces no symptoms, some patients living a completely normal life.

However, the condition is typified by the existence of associated defects such as ventricular septal defect (VSD) and outflow-tract obstruction (present in 85% of cases). Most cases require surgical treatment either to address these associated defects or due to the unpredictable performance of the mRV and the tricuspid valve within the systemic circulation.

Despite being a rare condition, there is a huge heterogeneity in the underlying morphology and the pattern of associated lesions, meaning that classification is complex and that there is a similar heterogeneity in terms of clinical presentation and symptoms.

Morphology and Anatomic Features

The full name of the condition is congenitally corrected transposition of the great arteries (ccTGA); there is AV and VA discordance, and the aorta is anterior and usually to the leftward side. There is usually normal atrial situs, and the equivalent Van Praagh classification is S, L, L. Although the majority have normal atrial situs, 5% to 8% of cases have situs inversus, which is much commoner than in most cardiac conditions.

Abnormal positioning of the heart is also common, with dextrocardia or mesocardia in 25% of cases. The AV valves always correspond to the ventricular morphology; thus the right atrium leads into the mLV through a mitral valve, and the left atrium leads into the mRV through a tricuspid valve. As a consequence, there is reverse offsetting of the AV valves on a four-chamber view because the tricuspid valve maintains its relationship of being slightly closer to the apex than the mitral valve. Furthermore, more exaggerated apical displacement of the septal leaflet of the tricuspid valve can be seen in ccTGA—so-called Ebsteinoid tricuspid valve (although not associated with the failed delamination or extreme leaflet anomalies seen in true Ebstein anomaly), which predisposes to tricuspid valve dysfunction.

The commonest associated defect is VSD, present in 85% of cases and usually perimembranous but variable in size. However, the most important classification is with respect to the presence or absence of left ventricular outflow tract obstruction (LVOTO)—either as pulmonary stenosis or atresia—which is almost always associated with a VSD. Approximately half of all cases will fall into this group and will therefore be cyanosed. There is considerable geographic variability in this feature, being much commoner in the Far East, whereas unobstructed LVOT is commoner in the Western hemisphere.

Coarctation and aortic arch hypoplasia occur in 10% of patients in the presence of VSD and unobstructed LVOT. A list of associated features is shown in Table 69.1.

The conduction system and AV node are very abnormal in ccTGA. The AV node is displaced anteriorly, away from the triangle of Koch and near the root of the right atrial appendage. The bundle then runs a long and circuitous course anterior to the root of the pulmonary valve (Fig. 69.1), usually running down the superior and lateral border of any perimembranous VSD. This long and abnormal course of the conduction system predisposes patients with ccTGA to heart block, some presenting with block at birth but up to 40% developing block as part of the natural history of the condition. Note, however, that in cases of situs inversus the morphology of the heart is now I, D, D, and the conduction system reverts to its normal position.

Physiology and Natural History

The broad spectrum of associated defects and the unpredictable performance of the systemic mRV means there is a wide range of ages and modes of presentation. It is best to consider patients in two groups, those with stenosis/atresia of the subpulmonary outflow and those with unobstructed pulmonary outflow.

Unobstructed Pulmonary Outflow

If there is no VSD, then these patients may be completely free of symptoms and may not require any intervention. However, most do have a VSD, and presentation is related to the size of the defect—large defects cause high-output congestive cardiac failure and usually present in infancy with respiratory distress and failure to thrive. Moderate-size defects may cause a lesser degree of heart failure. Up to 10% of these patients with VSD have associated coarctation and/or arch hypoplasia and present in the neonatal period with circulatory collapse when the ductus closes.

TABLE 69.1	Common Features Associated With Congenitally Corrected Transposition of the Great Arteries	
		Frequency (%)
Atrial situs		
Normal		80-85
Inversus		10-15
Isomeric		2-4
Position		
Levocardia		70-75
Mesocardia		10-15
Dextrocardia		15-20
VSD		70-80
LVOTO		40-80
Pulmonary atresia		3-8
Arch hypoplasia/CoA		5-15
Ebsteinoid tricuspid valve		10-20
Heart block		10-15
DORV		3-5

CoA, Coarctation of the aorta; *DORV,* double-outlet right ventricle; *LVOTO,* left ventricular outflow tract obstruction; *VSD,* ventricular septal defect.

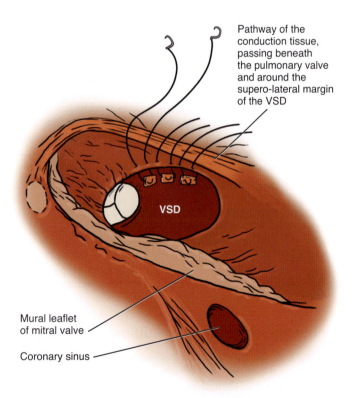

Pathway of the conduction tissue, passing beneath the pulmonary valve and around the supero-lateral margin of the VSD

VSD

Mural leaflet of mitral valve

Coronary sinus

• **Figure 69.1** Diagram showing the relationship of the conduction tissue to the ventricular septal defect (VSD) in congenitally corrected transposition of the great arteries.

Pulmonary Stenosis/Atresia

These patients usually have an associated large VSD, and presentation depends on the degree of obstruction. Mild obstruction can cause no early symptoms and patients can be well balanced, analogous to an acyanotic Fallot. More severe forms of obstruction will cause an increasing degree of cyanosis with cases of pulmonary atresia being duct dependent neonates.

In addition to these two categories, patients may present with congenital heart block, which can be present at birth or develop insidiously during childhood. The behavior of the systemic mRV is very unpredictable but usually is normal during infancy. Even patients with no associated defects may develop mRV dysfunction and tricuspid regurgitation (TR) during childhood at virtually any age, with some only presenting in adulthood with exercise intolerance and breathlessness on exertion.

In view of this great heterogeneity in both anatomy and mRV function, the natural history of the condition is difficult to define. Unrestricted VSDs and pulmonary atresia are fundamentally life-threatening lesions, need early intervention, and so skew the natural history. However, even accounting for these cases, the fundamental question in ccTGA is the natural history of the systemic mRV, which is unpredictable from one individual to another but is generally much worse than the normal population. Even with no other significant defects, over half the population with ccTGA will develop congestive heart failure by their late 30s. The cause is a complex combination of systemic mRV failure and increasing TR, which are closely interlinked, and is related to the fact that the right ventricle (RV) is not an efficient shape to function in the systemic circulation and has a different coronary blood supply and the tricuspid valve is equally not designed to work at such pressures with its septal attachments, meaning that it is more prone to dysfunction as the ventricle dilates and the septum moves away from the free wall.

Despite the fact that the vast majority of patients with ccTGA will need surgical intervention, there remains a small group (probably <5%) that remains well with preserved mRV function into old age.

Diagnosis

The condition and all the associated lesions can usually be established by detailed transthoracic echocardiography. Each component of the anatomy and physiology should be carefully assessed on echocardiography, paying particular attention to the position of the cardiac chambers and to the function and morphology of the AV valves. The position of the VSD should be carefully delineated together with the positioning of a PA band and the presence of any associated pulmonary root dilation and/or pulmonary incompetence. A chest x-ray examination may reveal an abnormal position of the heart in some cases and the narrow superior mediastinum typical of transposition but is not diagnostic. An electrocardiogram is essential to look for rhythm abnormalities because first- and second-degree heart block may be present even in patients thought to have normal rhythm, and they are predictors of subsequent complete block.

Cardiac catheterization is not usually required for diagnosis but may be essential in assessing patients for surgery, especially if they had required a PA band (see later). Magnetic resonance imaging (MRI) is not necessary in most patients except when there is concern regarding the relationship of the aorta to the VSD in consideration of a Rastelli type of repair. Because the position and size of the VSD can be variable, MRI reconstructions and even

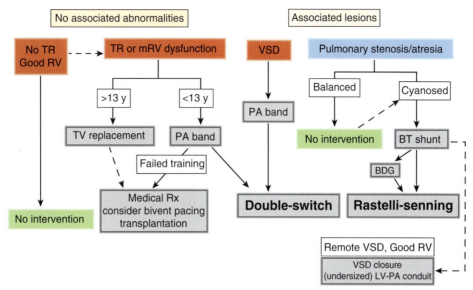

• **Figure 69.2** Decision tree for management of the spectrum of congenitally corrected transposition of the great arteries. *BDG,* Bidirectional Glenn; *BT,* Blalock-Taussig; *LV,* left ventricle; *mRV,* morphologic right ventricle; *PA,* pulmonary artery; *RV,* right ventricle; *TR,* tricuspid regurgitation; *TV,* tricuspid valve; *VSD,* ventricular septal defect.

three-dimensional modeling can be helpful to guide repair and surgical technique.

Indications for Surgery

Patients with pulmonary atresia or severe pulmonary stenosis require a systemic pulmonary shunt (usually a Blalock-Taussig shunt) as a neonate. Patients with a large VSD and unobstructed pulmonary blood flow may need PA banding to control heart failure. The central question in the management of ccTGA is the concept of "physiologic" verses "anatomic" repair. The former implies treating any associated lesions on their own merit but leaving the mRV as the systemic ventricle: this would include simple VSD closure or, in the setting of ccTGA/VSD/pulmonary stenosis (PS), closing the VSD and placing a valved conduit between the subpulmonary ventricle (the mLV) and the pulmonary arteries. Technically these are the simpler options, but they should be considered only if there is good mRV function and minimal TR. Anatomic repair involves repairing any associated lesions but also restoring the mLV to the systemic circulation—this requires an arterial switch (or Rastelli type of procedure in the setting of ccTGA/VSD/PS) together with an atrial switch (Senning or Mustard procedure).

Assessment and decision making become much more complicated in the scenario of a patient with ccTGA and intact septum (or small VSD) who develops mRV dysfunction and/or significant TR. These patients are likely to develop congestive cardiac failure within 5 years and need proactive intervention in the form of preemptive PA banding to retrain the mLV and splint the interventricular septum to preserve tricuspid valve function. If the mLV responds well to the band, then a double-switch procedure may be performed within the next 6 to 18 months. The age of these patients at presentation is crucial, and the younger the age, the more likely they are to respond to this retraining of the mLV. However, older children or adolescents may have lost the fundamental plasticity in ventricular remodeling to be able to respond to banding and may never be suitable for anatomic repair, being better diverted to management on a heart failure program and

consideration for transplantation if required. A small subset of adolescents with well-preserved mRV function and moderate or greater TR may benefit from isolated tricuspid valve replacement but need careful surveillance of mRV function. Tricuspid valve repair in this setting has been universally disappointing, and direct replacement is recommended.

The justification for intervention in symptomless patients is a cause for considerable debate, and if there is well-preserved mRV function, then they should be left well alone and managed expectantly. A summary of the treatment decisions is shown in Fig. 69.2.

Surgical Management

Systemic to Pulmonary Artery Shunt

Neonates or infants with severe cyanosis may require a systemic shunt. This is preferably performed through a midline sternotomy, and in the setting of normal situs we prefer to place a right modified Blalock-Taussig shunt because this is easy to access at subsequent surgery. If the arterial duct is still patent, then this is ligated at the same procedure to prevent competitive flow. A thin-walled expanded polytetrafluoroethylene (ePTFE [Gore-Tex]) tube is used as an end-to-side graft between the underside of the distal innominate artery and the superior surface of the right PA; a 3.5-mm shunt is usually used except in older children (>3 months), when a 4-mm shunt can be selected. The pericardium is loosely closed at the end of the procedure to aid with future resternotomy.

Physiologic Repair

Simple VSD closure can be performed in cases for which anatomic repair is not preferred, approaching the VSD through the right atrium and working through the mitral valve. Care has to be taken with suture placement to avoid the conduction tissue, which will run over the superior and around the lateral margin of the defect (see Fig. 69.1). Sutures in these areas should be placed from the right side of the defect (i.e., passing the needle holder inside the VSD with the needle placed in the mRV side) so as to avoid the bundle as it runs along the edge of the VSD on the mLV side of the septum. Physiologic repair can also be considered in cases of ccTGA/VSD/PS by simply closing the VSD and placing an mLV-PA conduit. Care has to be taken when performing the ventriculotomy on the mLV not to damage the papillary muscles of the mitral valve—this can be helped by looking first through the mitral valve to identify their position and so guide placement of the ventriculotomy.

Anatomic Repair

The surgery restores the mLV to the systemic circulation, which is established by switching over the atrial inflows (the Senning and Mustard procedures), switching over the arterial outflows (either arterial switch or Rastelli procedure, dependent on the LVOT anatomy), and repairing any associated defects. These anatomic repairs are much more complex procedures than the physiologic repair but have the advantage of repairing the circulation while also establishing the mLV as the systemic ventricle and therefore excluding the unpredictable function of the tricuspid valve and mRV from the systemic position.

The procedures can be considered in their two main groups, dependent on whether the LVOT is normally developed or is stenotic or atretic.

Double-Switch Procedure. The LVOT is of good size with a normal-size pulmonary valve. These patients have usually had a PA band placed previously, either to train the mLV or, in the presence of a large VSD, to prevent pulmonary overcirculation. Preoperative assessment must include careful assessment of the mLV to ensure it is fully prepared to support the systemic circulation (see under "Pulmonary Artery Banding"). Surgery combines atrial switch (the Senning is described here, but the Mustard can be used) with arterial switch and closing any associated VSD.

The ascending aorta is cannulated as high as possible, and bypass is established with bicaval cannulation, with very low inferior vena cava (IVC) cannulation to facilitate the atrial switch. The branch pulmonary arteries are fully mobilized and controlled with Silastic slings, and Waterston's groove is fully developed. With the cross-clamp applied and the heart arrested the initial incisions are made for the Senning (see later) before proceeding to the arterial switch. The principles of the arterial switch are exactly as they are in a neonatal switch, but the great vessels tend to be slightly more side-to-side than the typical anteroposterior relationship seen in the neonate with d-transposition of the great arteries (d-TGA). The aorta is transected well above the level of the sinotubular junction and the coronary buttons excised on as large a button of aortic tissue as possible. The buttons are then mobilized to ensure they transfer comfortably—the posterior coronary (equivalent of the right coronary artery) usually runs directly backward and transfers readily. The anterior coronary (equivalent of the left coronary artery) needs to be carefully mobilized because the circumflex branch runs close to the aortic wall (Fig. 69.3).

The defects in the aorta are repaired with suitable patch material—autologous pericardium is ideal but is not always easy to obtain in a redo-procedure, and pulmonary homograft or xenograft pericardial patch can be used. The main PA is then transected, usually at the site of any previous band to try and preserve as much height on the neo-aortic root as possible. Incisions are cut into the facing sinuses to receive the coronary buttons—a simple incision for the posterior coronary is usually sufficient, and

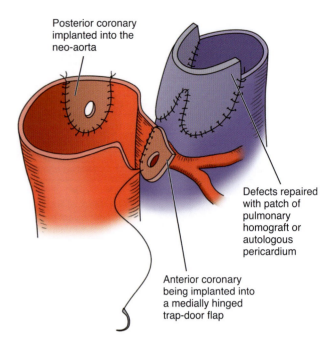

Posterior coronary implanted into the neo-aorta

Defects repaired with patch of pulmonary homograft or autologous pericardium

Anterior coronary being implanted into a medially hinged trap-door flap

• **Figure 69.3** Arterial switch in congenitally corrected transposition of the great arteries.

a medially hinged trapdoor incision for the anterior coronary helps to allow it to sit more comfortably (see Fig. 69.3).

The ductal ligament is then divided and the Lecompte maneuver performed so long as there is adequate elasticity to the branch pulmonary arteries—usually this is possible, but in older children it may be necessary to leave the arteries posteriorly, especially if the great vessels are more side-by-side. The neo-aorta is then reconstructed, and the main PA can be reconstructed at this point or left until after the cross-clamp is removed. Again, if the vessels are more side-by-side, it may be necessary to move the opening in the branch pulmonary arteries across to the left (i.e., close the original opening partially and then cut leftward to extend the opening) to avoid any torsion on the reconstructed vessels (Fig. 69.4).

Attention is then turned to the Senning. The procedure consists of three layers. The initial incisions are shown in Fig. 69.5, creating a septal flap of tissue and a separate opening through Waterston's groove that creates a wide channel into the left atrium. The first layer is created by taking the septal flap of tissue and sewing this into the back-wall of the left atrium so that only the pulmonary veins lie behind it. The suture line starts at the root of the left atrial appendage and runs across the floor of the heart toward the IVC inferiorly and up toward the root of the superior vena cava (SVC) superiorly, taking care to keep this suture line as posterior as possible so as to create space for the next layer (Fig. 69.6). The second layer will form the systemic venous pathway, folding the cut edge of the right atrium forward onto the remnant of the original atrial septum to create two "limbs" that direct the systemic venous return into the tricuspid valve. Note than the coronary sinus was traditionally excluded from the systemic venous pathway to ensure that the suture line avoided the AV node. However, in ccTGA the absence of the AV node from the triangle of Koch means that the coronary sinus can be safely incorporated into the inferior limb of the baffle if desired. Equally, the suture line must step back from the mitral annulus as it progresses more superiorly so as to avoid the anteriorly positioned AV node (Fig. 69.7).

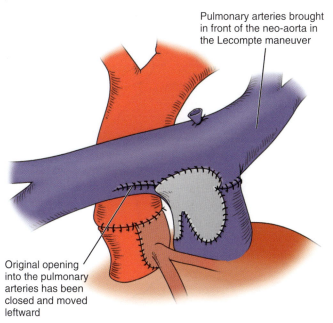

Pulmonary arteries brought in front of the neo-aorta in the Lecompte maneuver

Original opening into the pulmonary arteries has been closed and moved leftward

• **Figure 69.4** Completion of the arterial switch in congenitally corrected transposition of the great arteries.

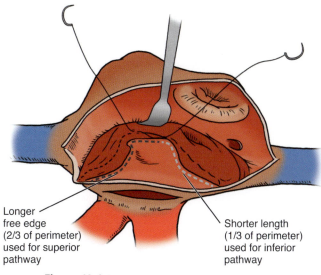

Longer free edge (2/3 of perimeter) used for superior pathway

Shorter length (1/3 of perimeter) used for inferior pathway

• **Figure 69.6** The first layer of the Senning procedure.

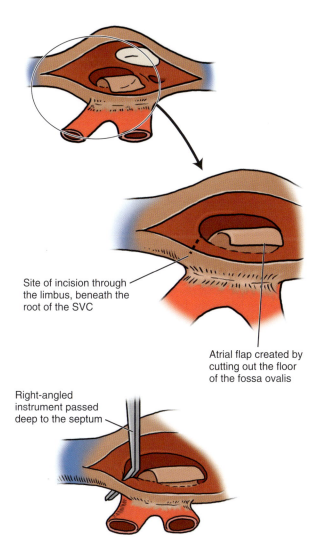

Site of incision through the limbus, beneath the root of the SVC

Atrial flap created by cutting out the floor of the fossa ovalis

Right-angled instrument passed deep to the septum

• **Figure 69.5** Creation of the initial septal flap in the Senning procedure. *SVC,* Superior vena cava.

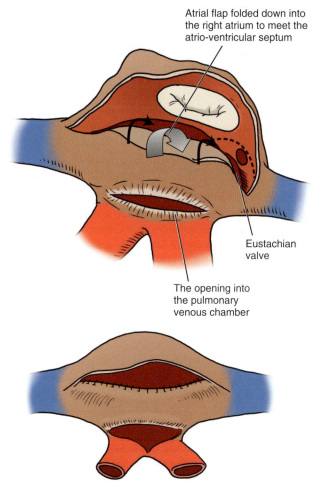

Atrial flap folded down into the right atrium to meet the atrio-ventricular septum

Eustachian valve

The opening into the pulmonary venous chamber

• **Figure 69.7** The second layer of the Senning procedure—creation of the systemic venous pathway.

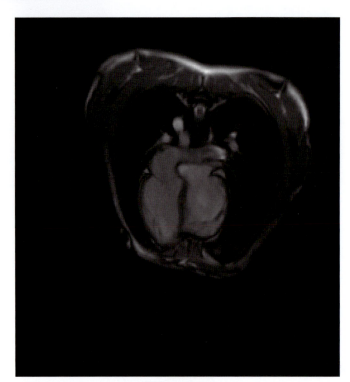

• **Figure 69.8** Magnetic resonance image showing the C-shaped pulmonary venous pathway of the Senning procedure.

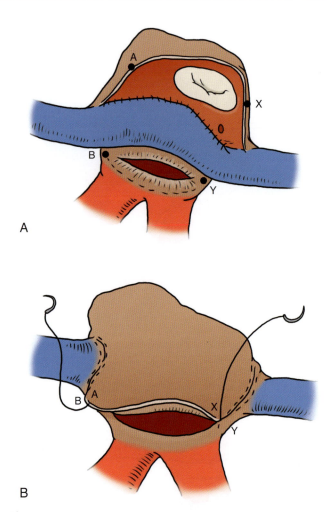

• **Figure 69.9** *A* and *B*, The third layer of the Senning procedure. Point *A* is brought to *B*, and point *X* is brought to *Y*.

The final layer of the Senning is now to connect the pulmonary veins through to the mitral valve with a C-shaped channel running laterally around the atrium (Fig. 69.8). This can be completed by bringing the superior cut edge of the free wall of the right atrium down to meet the opening created into the left atrium, through Waterston's groove—like shutting the lid of a suitcase (Fig. 69.9). There needs to be sufficient free edge to avoid "strangling" the limbs of the systemic venous pathway. If there is insufficient tissue, then this layer can be augmented with a patch of pulmonary homograft or of autologous pericardium if accessible (Fig. 69.10), or the free edges can be sewn to the in situ pericardium to create a pericardial well—known as the Schumacher technique.

Rastelli-Senning Procedure. In cases with subpulmonary stenosis (or atresia) and large VSD the arterial "switch" is achieved by performing a Rastelli procedure, committing the mLV through to the anteriorly positioned aorta. A longitudinal ventriculotomy is made into the body of the right ventricle, choosing a suitable site free from coronaries and starting well below the aortic valve. At this point the anatomy should be carefully assessed to confirm the position of the AV valves and VSD. Usually the VSD is large, but occasionally there may be some trabeculations to the leftward side beneath the aorta that can be resected to enlarge the pathway. The remnant of the outflow septum between the aorta and small pulmonary annulus should never be resected because the conduction tissue passes through here in ccTGA. The patch can be any strong material or can be fashioned from an ePTFE vascular graft, to give it a natural curve. It is fixed in place around the tricuspid valve with four or five pledgetted sutures before completing the suture line with a double layer of running suture. There is no risk to the conduction tissue inferiorly, and the sutures can pass close to the edge of the defect as the patch comes past the mitral valve. In cases of pulmonary stenosis (rather than atresia) the main PA must be ligated to exclude it from the mLV. If possible we also oversew the pulmonary valve leaflets from within the ventricle; this seals off what would otherwise be a small cul-de-sac of the PA stump, which can occasionally fill with thrombus postoperatively.

A valved conduit is then placed from the ventriculotomy to an opening created within the pulmonary arteries. This opening can be made either to the right or the leftward side of the aorta, wherever there is best access—however, if possible it is preferable to run the conduit to the leftward side because this helps avoid the conduit sitting up in the midline, directly behind the sternum (Fig. 69.11).

The Senning procedure is then completed exactly as for the double-switch.

Special Considerations

The great variability in the anatomy of ccTGA requires careful preoperative planning. It is important that the anesthetist is aware of the venous anatomy, and it may be helpful to be able to monitor both IVC and SVC pressure postoperatively because the dogleg shape of the SVC pathway often leads to a slightly higher SVC pressure in the early postoperative period. Patients with situs inversus will require the surgeon to operate from the left side of the operating table for components of the case. Intraoperative echocardiography has become routine now in most cardiac surgery, but it is absolutely essential in ccTGA to have intraoperative transesophageal

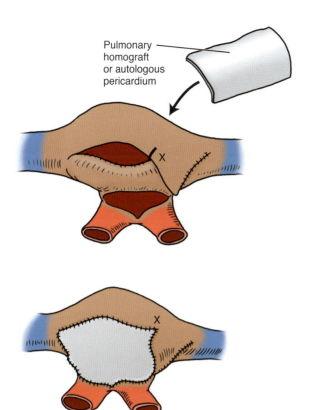

Pulmonary homograft or autologous pericardium

X

X

• **Figure 69.10** Augmentation of the third (outer) layer of the Senning procedure. An additional incision can be made at point X to further open out the pulmonary venous pathway.

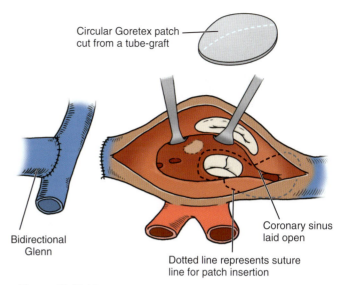

Circular Goretex patch cut from a tube-graft

Bidirectional Glenn

Coronary sinus laid open

Dotted line represents suture line for patch insertion

• **Figure 69.12** The one-and-one-half-ventricle repair as an alternative to the complete atrial switch. Also called the Hemi-Mustard procedure.

echocardiography (TEE) to assess the atrial pathways and the mLV function.

In cases with normal situs and mesocardia or dextrocardia, access to the atria is difficult because the ventricular mass is very much anterior. There tends to be smaller surface area to the free wall of the right atrium, and so it is commonly necessary to augment the outer layer of the Senning with a patch or to use a Schumacher technique.

Laying open of the coronary sinus is a useful way of giving more volume to the IVC pathway but should be avoided in situs inversus because the conduction reverts to its normal position in this morphology.

An alternative form of atrial switch is to perform a bidirectional Glenn for the SVC and then commit the IVC through to the tricuspid valve with a simple patch placed across the floor of the heart (so-called hemi-Mustard; Fig. 69.12). This simplifies the atrial switch component and is particularly useful if there is concern about the size/volume of the mRV (especially in the case of a Rastelli procedure, in which a long baffle may further reduce the volume of the mRV). The bidirectional Glenn could be performed as a palliative initial procedure in cases with pulmonary stenosis/atresia and so delay the need to progress to Rastelli. However, the PA pressures must be low to tolerate the Glenn, and the anatomy will deny access to the atrium should subsequent pacing or ablation procedures be required in the future.

Where there is a long tunnel from the VSD through to the aorta there is a concern that a Rastelli approach will create a subaortic stenosis. The Nikaidoh aortic translocation could be considered in this situation, but the position of the conduction tissue is such that there would be an extremely high risk of causing heart block with such an approach—although case reports have been published with no heart block. An alternative in borderline cases with PS (rather than atresia) is to add a Damus-Kaye-Stansel procedure to improve the flow through the LVOT.

Pulmonary Artery Banding

If banding for a large VSD, then the procedure is usually performed in a small infant, and the technique is as for any case with pulmonary

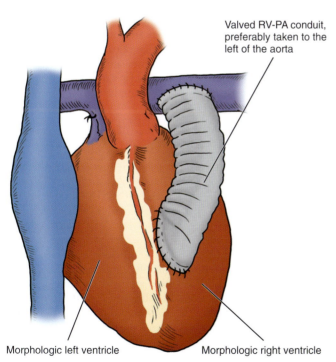

Valved RV-PA conduit, preferably taken to the left of the aorta

Morphologic left ventricle

Morphologic right ventricle

• **Figure 69.11** The Rastelli procedure in congenitally corrected transposition of the great arteries. *PA,* Pulmonary artery; *RV,* right ventricle.

overcirculation. However, in older children when banding is indicated for increasing TR or mRV dysfunction, then the situation is more unusual. A monitoring line can be placed into the mLV from the internal jugular to monitor pressures in the perioperative period. The band is then placed on the main PA in the usual position immediately above the sinotubular junction, and it may be easiest to start measuring the circumference of the main PA and placing the band at half-circumference. The aim is to increase mLV pressures to 60% to 70% systemic with preserved mLV function—so the band can then be adjusted until the right balance is found. Ideally, the banding will splint the position of the interventricular septum and help stabilize the tricuspid valve, often reducing the severity of the TR. The band is then fixed in place and secured to the adventitia to try to prevent migration.

Patients have to be monitored carefully for the next 24 to 48 hours because the mLV can show signs of strain or even failure, requiring loosening of the band. Conversely, if the pressures in the mLV fall during the first 24 hours, then it may be necessary to tighten the band.

Patients are then carefully followed up to assess the retraining of the mLV. The mLV free-wall thickness or left ventricular (LV) myocardial muscle mass can be helpful in judging response to the band, and careful echocardiography to demonstrate maintained mLV function and freedom from mitral regurgitation. Most studies suggest that 9 to 18 months are typically required before the mLV is satisfactory retrained. A cardiac catheter to measure mLV pressure and function with additional dobutamine stress is recommended to show that the heart is now suitable for a double-switch procedure.

Fontan Pathway

There is a small subgroup of patients with ccTGA/VSD/PS who have a remote VSD of only moderate size that is not easily committed to the aorta. Other cases may have borderline-size mRV with straddling of the tricuspid valve across the VSD. As long as the mRV function is well sustained, these cases are often better treated with a Fontan-strategy because attempting septation is too high risk and may create sequelae that are difficult to manage in the future.

Postoperative Critical Care Management

All these patients may have unusual anatomy and venous arrangements, and it is important to ensure that the intensive care team is fully aware of the position of indwelling monitoring lines and exactly what pressures they are recording. A left atrial line is commonly used to monitor the preload on the systemic ventricle.

In physiologic repairs the surgery itself is not usually particularly long or complex, but the systemic mRV may have variable degrees of dysfunction postoperatively, and use of inodilators and the importance of offloading the circulation should be emphasized.

An anatomic repair is usually a lengthy procedure with long cross-clamp time, and a degree of low cardiac output is not unusual. The chest may be left open for the first 24 hours. Monitoring of SVC and left atrial pressure is important—the dogleg SVC pathway of the Senning often leads to a slightly high SVC pressure, which tends to settle over the first 48 hours (probably partly due to decompression through the azygous system). It is important that the intensive care team is aware of this, and additional IVC pressure may be helpful to assess preload on the subpulmonary ventricle. Inodilators such as milrinone (0.5 to 0.7 mcg/kg/min)

TABLE 69.2	Transposition of the Great Arteries *Primary Diagnosis*		
		Number	Percentage of All Operations in STS CHSD
Congenitally corrected TGA		133	0.1%
Congenitally corrected TGA, IVS		85	0.1%
Congenitally corrected TGA, IVS-LVOTO		27	0.0%
Congenitally corrected TGA, VSD		228	0.2%
Congenitally corrected TGA, VSD-LVOTO		199	0.2%
TGA, IVS		2084	1.7%
TGA, IVS-LVOTO		30	0.0%
TGA, VSD		1391	1.2%
TGA, VSD-LVOTO		331	0.3%

IVS, Interventricular septum; *LVOTO*, left ventricular outflow tract obstruction; *STS CHSD*, Society of Thoracic Surgeons Congenital Heart Surgery Database; *TGA*, transposition of the great arteries; *VSD*, ventricular septal defect.
Data from Jacobs JP, Jacobs ML, Mavroudis C, et al. *Executive Summary: The Society of Thoracic Surgeons Congenital Heart Surgery Database—Twenty-fifth Harvest—(July 1, 2012–June 30, 2016)*. Durham, NC: The Society of Thoracic Surgeons (STS) and Duke Clinical Research Institute (DCRI), Duke University Medical Center; Fall 2016 Harvest.

are ideal. A small dose of adrenaline (0.05 to 0.1 mcg/kg/min) may also be necessary. Careful assessment of the venous baffles, outlet tracts and ventricular function on TEE is essential. TEE is helpful in postoperative assessment of the pathways, but unless obstruction is seen, these pathways do not usually need surgical revision. Ventilation and inotropes are continued until cardiac output has stabilized. Atrial tachycardias can occur in relation to the Senning but are rare in the early postoperative phase. Mechanical support (extracorporeal membrane oxygenation) has been used successfully for refractory low cardiac output state in a handful of reported cases.

Outcomes

Tables 69.2 and Table 69.3 present short-term mortality data from the Society of Thoracic Surgeons Congenital Heart Surgery Database (STS CHSD) about TGA and ccTGA. The STS CHSD contains 120,285 cardiac operations and 100,137 index cardiac operations during the 4-year analytic window of July 1, 2012, to June 30, 2016. Table 69.2 documents the number and percentage of operations with a primary diagnosis of TGA, including ccTGA, during this 4-year analytic window. Table 69.3 documents the number and percentage of operations with a primary procedure related to TGA, including ccTGA, during this 4-year analytic window. Operations for both concordant AV connections and discordant AV connections are included in these tables to provide perspective for the data about ccTGA.

The outcomes for physiologic repair have generally been disappointing and highlight the importance of case selection in that there must be good mRV function preoperatively. The early mortality has been 5% to 10% in such series but with larger series reporting high incidence of mRV failure over subsequent years with a 5-year survival of 75% and a 20-year survival of 50%. There is a suggestion

TABLE 69.3 Transposition of the Great Arteries *Primary Procedure*

	Number	Percentage of All Operations in STS CHSD	Operative Mortality
Congenitally corrected TGA repair, Atrial switch and ASO (double switch)	133	0.1%	4.9%
Congenitally corrected TGA repair, Atrial switch and Rastelli	60	0.1%	10.0%
Congenitally corrected TGA repair, VSD closure	4	0.0%	0.0%
Congenitally corrected TGA repair, VSD closure and LV to PA conduit	11	0.0%	9.1%
Congenitally corrected TGA repair, Other	0	0.0%	
Arterial switch operation (ASO)	1853	1.6%	2.3%
Arterial switch operation (ASO) and VSD repair	797	0.7%	5.1%
Arterial switch procedure + aortic arch repair	71	0.1%	5.6%
Arterial switch procedure and VSD repair + aortic arch repair	278	0.2%	13.3%
Senning	18	0.0%	0.0%
Mustard	18	0.0%	5.6%
Atrial baffle procedure, Mustard or Senning revision	31	0.0%	6.5%
Rastelli	200	0.2%	2.5%
REV	7	0.0%	14.3%
Aortic root translocation over left ventricle (including Nikaidoh procedure)	70	0.1%	4.3%
TGA, other procedures (Kawashima, LV-PA conduit, other)	6	0.0%	16.7%

LV, Left ventricle; *PA,* pulmonary artery; *STS CHSD,* Society of Thoracic Surgeons Congenital Heart Surgery Database; *TGA,* transposition of the great arteries; *VSD,* ventricular septal defect.
Data from Jacobs JP, Jacobs ML, Mavroudis C, et al. Executive Summary: The Society of Thoracic Surgeons Congenital Heart Surgery Database—Twenty-fifth Harvest—(July 1, 2012–June 30, 2016).
Durham, NC: The Society of Thoracic Surgeons (STS) and Duke Clinical Research Institute (DCRI), Duke University Medical Center; Fall 2016 Harvest.

that a physiologic repair that deliberately leaves slightly high pressures in the mLV (for example, placing a slightly small LV-PA conduit) may improve longer-term outcomes by splinting the interventricular septum and effectively supporting the mRV and tricuspid valve function.

Surgical outcomes for the anatomic repair in ccTGA-VSD are excellent with early mortality in the modern era of typically 2% to 4%. The outcomes can be stratified according to the nature and complexity of presentation: the highest-risk procedures tend to be in neonates and infants who are clinically unstable and in heart failure preoperatively, often requiring arch repair in addition to double switch, but in elective repairs in older children with well-preserved ventricular function the mortality approaches 0% to 2%. Most series report lower mortality among the Rastelli-Senning group compared with the double-switch because the former tend to be more elective procedures with no concerns over mLV function and no need for coronary transfer.

The commonest early complications are heart block (new pacemaker required in 5% to 10%) and low cardiac output—which is partly related to long bypass and cross-clamp times. Pleural effusions may occur in association with high SVC pressures. The one-and-one-half-ventricle repair (bidirectional Glenn) has gained some popularity with excellent early results and has the advantage in Rastelli-Senning that the conduit may last longer because it only has to carry the IVC blood flow. However, there is evidence that the functional capacity of the one-and-one-half-ventricle circulation is not as good as a full biventricular repair, and so critics would favor biventricular repair if the anatomy allows.

As longer-term follow-up is becoming available, it is clear that survival is considerably better than the natural history of symptomatic ccTGA managed conventionally (i.e., leaving the mRV as the systemic ventricle) with actuarial survival of 90% to 95% at 10 years. However, this comes at a cost, and the freedom from reintervention is lower, at 80% to 85% at 10 years—although some of this is conduit replacement in the Rastelli group, there is still significant incidence of reoperation for a mixture of other lesions, including Senning baffle obstruction, PA stenoses post switch, and aortic valve repair and replacement (most baffle stenoses can be successfully managed with balloon dilation or stenting). However, reoperations on the tricuspid valve are very rare, and simply removing the tricuspid valve from the systemic circulation universally improves function. A recent study from Boston emphasizes the importance of assessing the tricuspid valve at the time of surgery, and even simple repairs of anatomically abnormal valves further improve the late tricuspid valve performance. Baffle obstruction and late atrial tachycardias are commoner with the Mustard procedure than the Senning, which has contributed to the popularity of the Senning technique. In summary, the freedom from reintervention is strikingly similar in both the double-switch and Rastelli-Senning groups.

As longer follow-up results are reported, there is an emerging concern over the incidence of late mLV dysfunction, which occurs in 15% to 20% of patients at 20 years after surgery. This has been reported by several groups with similar findings and occurs in spite of what appears to be good mLV function early postoperatively. The etiology appears to be multifactorial, but late mLV dysfunction certainly appears to be commoner in the double-switch group than in the Rastelli-Senning group. Aortic regurgitation may be a factor because this is commoner in the double-switch group, in which the old pulmonary valve becomes the new aortic valve—but the relationship with mLV dysfunction is far from consistent. There is increasing interest in the fate of the mLV retrained by application of the PA band, and the interaction with late LV dysfunction. It seems that retraining of the mLV is unlikely to be possible beyond the age of 12 to 14 years, and that in general the younger the patient is at banding, the better the long-term outcome. However, although this relationship is also inconsistent, the Boston group has shown a greater risk of late mLV dysfunction in patients who were initially banded at above 2 years of age, whereas there was no incidence of late dysfunction in patients banded at less than 2 years of age. This group of retrained mLVs will certainly require careful follow-up, and these findings have fueled interest in the controversial concept of early "prophylactic" PA banding in symptomless infants, which might protect the mLV in these patients from late failure.

It has also been noted that this LV dysfunction is also associated with a high incidence of patients requiring pacing and of patients who have a prolonged QRS interval. There are several reported successes with resynchronization using biventricular LV and RV pacing improving the mLV function in these patients, with some individual cases of dramatic improvement. This may be of value in patients requiring pacemaker insertion after a double-switch procedure.

Overall the outcomes of the anatomic repair operations in ccTGA remain substantially better than the natural history of the condition and also superior to traditional "physiologic" repair, with more than 75% of patients sustaining good mLV function at 20 years. It is also important to note that the most challenging groups of patients who present with severe cardiac failure at a young age have done particularly well with no incidence of late mLV failure. Debate always returns to the few patients who remain free of symptoms into old age without ever requiring intervention; however, it must be remembered that these are a small minority of the whole population of patients with ccTGA and that the vast majority of patients with ccTGA will require intervention. The key is in identifying those patients who need intervention early such that a long-term plan is in place for future management and recognizing the vast heterogeneity within the ccTGA family, which means that the timing and nature of intervention has to be individualized to each case.

Bibliography

A complete bibliography is available at ExpertConsult.com.

70

Infective Endocarditis

MICHAEL J. WALSH, MD; AVINASH K. SHETTY, MD

The impact of infective endocarditis (IE) on the pediatric population continues to evolve. Since the last edition of this text, survival has continued to improve for infants and children with congenital heart disease (CHD), and advancements in echocardiographic techniques have enhanced diagnosis. At the same time the epidemiology and microbiology of IE have evolved, mandating novel therapeutic strategies. Accordingly, the recommendations for prevention and treatment of pediatric IE have been recently updated.[1,2]

Despite the advances in therapies and updated guidelines, IE remains a cause of considerable morbidity and mortality in children. Many patients require critical care for medical management of the hemodynamic effects of IE or for postoperative management when cardiac surgery is required. Cardiac surgery is a precedent for IE, but even intensive care unit (ICU) patients without structural heart disease can be at increased risk secondary to other invasive procedures and indwelling central venous catheters (CVCs). Given the complex nature of IE, collaboration between pediatric cardiologist, infectious disease specialist, primary care physician, ICU faculty and staff, and cardiothoracic surgery is essential for optimal outcome.

Definition

IE is an infection of the endothelium of the heart. Although the valves of the heart are most commonly affected, the infection can affect any endothelium-lined structures—including the great vessels, ductus arteriosus, or surgically placed shunts, patches, or prosthetics. Because bacteria are the primary microbial pathogens involved, the term *bacterial endocarditis* (BE) or *subacute bacterial endocarditis* (SBE) has been commonly used. However, a more inclusive term of *infective endocarditis* is preferred because it recognizes nonbacterial infections, such as those caused by fungus or virus. It should be noted that the term *nonbacterial thrombotic endocarditis* (NBTE) describes a spectrum of noninfectious lesions of the heart valves. Although this entity shares some features with IE, including echocardiographic appearance and risk for embolization, NBTE will not be discussed significantly in this chapter.

Epidemiology

IE is relatively uncommon, although incidence may be increasing over the last decade in adults[3,4] and children.[5-8] The increasing incidence of IE may be related to improved survival of patients with CHD and premature infants. Diagnostic value of echocardiography has improved, and advances in microbiologic techniques

have led to improved isolation of microorganisms and reduced frequency of culture-negative IE.[4]

Several large observational analyses have been recently published using national inpatient databases to evaluate the current incidence and risk factors of IE in the United States and Europe. A US database from 2000 to 2010 found an overall incidence of 0.43 per 100,000 children.[5] IE accounts for anywhere between 0.5 and 4.6 out of 10,000 hospital admissions.[6,7] Median length of stay for one series was 10 days.[5]

A bimodal age distribution is noted in pediatric IE, with peaks in infancy and late adolescence[9]; 15% to 46% of pediatric IE occurs in the first year of life.[5,6] Although many studies demonstrate rates of endocarditis being generally on the rise from year to year, there is particular interest in determining the impact of recently updated guidelines[1,10] for SBE prophylaxis on the incidence of IE. Three large pediatric database studies have suggested no important change[5-7] in IE rates during a study period that compared rates before and after the update, whereas two adult studies have noted a significant increase in IE incidence during the same time period.[3,4]

Before 1970, rheumatic heart disease (RHD) was the primary risk factor for IE in the United States, accounting for 30% to 50% of cases.[11] Since then the incidence of RHD (and therefore RHD-associated IE) in resource-rich countries has declined dramatically. However, RHD is a significant contributor to cardiac morbidity and mortality worldwide, specifically as it relates to IE. In a registry study in low- and middle-income African and Asian countries[12] an incidence of IE in RHD was noted to be 3.7 per 1000 patient-years.

In the current era, an underlying heart condition, specifically CHD, is a primary risk factor for IE, accounting for 34% to 68% of children with IE.[5-7] The changing epidemiology of IE has been comprehensively reviewed in children.[13]

Lesion-Specific Congenital Heart Defects

The most common reported CHD associated with IE (33% of all cases) is ventricular septal defect (VSD), which is not surprising because this is the most common form of CHD.[5] In 2013 a Canadian population-based study of 34,000 pediatric patients with CHD suggested that the cumulative risk of a CHD patient developing IE before the age of 18 was 6.1 first cases per 1000 patients (or 4.1 first cases per 10,000 patient-years). Table 70.1 shows incidence broken down by lesion—indicating that cyanotic CHD followed by endocardial cushion defects and left-sided lesions are the defects at the highest risk.[8]

TABLE 70.1	Lesion-Specific Incidence (per 1000 Children) and Incidence Rate (per 10,000 Patient-Years) of Infective Endocarditis in Children With Congenital Heart Disease			
CHD Lesion	Incidence 0-6 y	Incidence 0-12 y	Incidence 0-18 y	Incidence Rate
Cyanotic CHD	16.8	23.3	31.0	20.7
Atrioventricular septal defects	5.5	8.7	11.1	7.7
Left-sided lesions	2.7	4.8	7.9	4.4
Right-sided lesions	2.3	2.3	4.2	2.9
Ventricular septal defect	3.2	3.2	3.2	3.5
Patent ductus arteriosus	2.0	2.4	3.2	2.4
Atrial septal defect	1.9	2.2	3.0	2.3
Other CHD	2.9	3.7	5.5	3.7
Overall	3.2	4.2	6.1	4.1

CHD, Congenital heart disease.
Data from Rushani D, Kaufman JS, Ionescu-Ittu R, et al. Infective endocarditis in children with congenital heart disease: cumulative incidence and predictors. *Circulation.* 2013;128:1412-1419.

Postoperative Heart Disease

Although surgery to close shunt lesions and patent ductus arteriosus (PDA) can decrease the rate of IE over a lifetime, the CHD patient with recent surgical repair or palliation is at a particularly increased risk for IE. Patients with heart surgery within the prior 6 months are at a fivefold increase in the risk for development of IE.[8] With the common use of central venous catheters (CVC) and extended stays in ICU, and the long-term risk of residual heart defects (causing turbulent flow patterns in the heart) or prosthetic devices, the postsurgical risk for IE in the pediatric population must be appreciated. Postsurgical IE is most prevalent in valvar aortic stenosis,[14] can be acute or subacute, and can occur in the immediate postoperative period or years after the initial surgery.

Catheter-Based Interventions

The transcatheter approach to pulmonary valve replacement has gained widespread acceptance and usage as an alternative to open heart surgery. The largest review of adverse events from the Melody(R) transcatheter pulmonary valve (Medtronic Inc., Minneapolis, MN) suggests that IE is one of the most common.[16] McElhinney used data from prospective trials of the Melody valve to suggest an annualized risk of 2.4% per patient-year. The common pathogens (staphylococci and streptococci) closely mirror those seen in typical IE patients. The Melody valve has a significantly higher IE rate than surgically placed valves (7.5% to 11.6% versus 2% to 2.4%).[17,18] The exception was for the surgically placed Contegra conduit (Medtronic Inc., Minneapolis, MN)—which had an IE incidence of 20.4% with a median follow-up of 8.8 years. The

rate of IE with transcatheter occluders of atrial septal defect is very low. In a meta-analysis of over 28,000 patients with atrial septal defect or patent foramen ovale closed interventionally with a device, only 3 reports of IE were found.[19]

Children With Structurally Normal Hearts

In the absence of CHD, neonates, particularly premature infants in the ICU with indwelling vascular catheters are at risk for IE; a recent review showed 7% of all cases of pediatric IE occur in the first month of life.[9] Primary bacteremia due to *Staphylococcus aureus* can lead to IE in children with no structural cardiac disease or known risk factors.[20-21] Degenerative heart disease and intravenous drug abuse are well-described risk factors in adults but uncommon in children.

Microorganisms

Although many different microorganisms have been reported to cause IE, the vast majority of cases are caused by *Staphylococcus* and *Streptococcus* species.[9,21] The major causes of IE in four key pediatric series[9,21-23] are summarized in Table 70.2. In earlier studies, 32% to 43% of cases of pediatric IE are caused by viridans group streptococci (VGS), which are common commensals of the oral mucosa consisting of several species, including *Streptococcus mitis*, *Streptococcus sanguis*, *Streptococcus anginosus*, *Streptococcus salivarius*, and *Streptococcus mutans*.[21-23] In a recent large, national database study ($n = 1588$ admissions) a causative microorganism was found in 632 admissions. *S. aureus* was the most commonly isolated microorganism (57%), followed by the VGS (20%) and coagulase-negative staphylococcus (CONS) in 14%.[9]

IE due to VGS remains a primary cause of native valve IE in children with congenital or valvular heart disease without prior surgery. *S. aureus* and CONS are notable causes of acute IE following cardiac surgery (typically <60 days) and in the presence of prosthetic valves, endovascular materials, or indwelling vascular catheters. Both native and prosthetic valves can be infected by *S. aureus*. CONS are ubiquitous skin commensals that colonize CVCs and prosthetic devices, produce biofilms and abscess, and acquire multiantibiotic resistance.[24] IE due to *Enterococcus* species is less common in children than in adults and is characterized by a subacute presentation typically affecting native valves or occurring in patients more than 60 days after cardiac surgery.[2] The emergence of methicillin-resistant *S. aureus* (MRSA) strains and increasing resistance in *Enterococcus faecium* is a major concern.

Although catheter-related bacteremia due to gram-negative organisms such as enteric bacilli and *Pseudomonas aeruginosa* occurs frequently in hospital settings, these organisms are relatively uncommon as a cause of IE, likely due to their poor ability to adhere to endothelium.[2] A wide variety of fastidious bacteria, zoonotic bacteria, and fungi may rarely cause IE.[25] Infection caused by a fastidious group of gram-negative bacilli requiring special media for growth are the so-called HACEK organisms (*Haemophilus* spp., *Aggregatibacter* spp., *Cardiobacterium hominis*, *Eikenella corrodens*, and *Kingella* spp.).[25] HACEK are constituents of normal human oropharyngeal flora and remain susceptible to β-lactam agents. Fungal IE due to *Candida* or *Aspergillus* is unusual but may occur in neonates receiving parenteral nutrition with high glucose concentrations or immunocompromised children or following cardiac surgery, often involving prosthetic valves.[9]

Approximately 5% of IE patients have negative blood cultures, but recent studies have reported culture-negative endocarditis (CNE)

TABLE 70.2	Microorganisms Causing Infective Endocarditis in Children			
Study period	1933—1972	1958—1992	1978—1996	2000—2003
Total number of IE cases	*n* = 149	*n* = 76	*n* = 111	*n* = 632
Proportion of IE cases due to various microorganisms				
Staphylococci (%)				
Staphylococcus aureus	33	32	27	57
Coagulase-negative staphylococci	2	4	12	14
Streptococci and enterococci (%)				
Viridans group streptococci	43	38	32	20
Enterococcus species	N/A	7	4	N/A
Streptococcus pneumoniae	3	4	7	1
HACEK[a] (%)	N/A	5	4	N/A
Culture negative (%)	6	7	5	N/A

[a]*Haemophilus* spp., *Aggregatibacter* spp., *Cardiobacterium hominis*, *Eikenella corrodens*, *Kingella* spp.

IE, Infective endocarditis; *N/A*, not applicable.

Data from Baltimore RS, Gewitz M, Baddour LM. Infective endocarditis in childhood: 2015 update. A Scientific Statement from the American Heart Association. *Circulation.* 2015;132:1487-1515; Day MD, Gauvreau K, Shulman S, et al. Characteristics of children hospitalized with infective endocarditis. *Circulation.* 2009;119:865-870; Martin JM, Neches WH, Wald ER. Infective endocarditis: 35 years of experience at a children's hospital. *Clin Infect Dis.* 1997;24:669-675; Johnson DH, Rosenthal A, Nadas AS. A forty-year review of bacterial endocarditis in infancy and childhood. *Circulation.* 1975;51:581-588; and Stockheim JA, Chadwick EG, Kessler S, et al. Are the Duke criteria superior to the Beth Israel criteria for the diagnosis of infective endocarditis in children? *Clin Infect Dis.* 1998;27:1451-1456.

in 8% to 36% of IE cases.[26-28] Negative blood cultures in IE patients may result from (1) previous administration of antimicrobial therapy; (2) infection due to fastidious bacteria, such as HACEK; (3) inadequate microbiologic methods; (4) fungal IE; and (5) right-sided endocarditis. CNE may be rarely caused by zoonotic pathogens such as *Coxiella burnetii* and *Brucella* (from livestock), *Chlamydia psittaci* (from parrots and pigeons), and *Bartonella henselae* (from cats).[25]

Pathogenesis

Dating back to the 1970s, animal models have revealed a predictable pattern for the way that a pathogen can create IE in a host.[29,30] First, there should be predisposing structural damage to the endocardium, either from congenital or acquired heart disease or indwelling CVC. The damaged endocardium activates the coagulation system to generate a local thrombus, consisting of fibrin, platelets, and red blood cells (RBCs). This thrombus serves as a nidus for circulating bacteria or fungus in the bloodstream to adhere to the endocardial surface. Finally, the pathogen must be able to propagate, grow, and lead to inflammatory and/or embolic sequelae.[31]

The smooth endothelium of the heart and its valves is denuded primarily by mechanical stress from turbulent blood flow or direct trauma. Several cardiac lesions can create turbulent blood flow, including stenotic or regurgitant valves, shunt lesions, or abnormalities of the great vessels, like coarctation of the aorta. Endothelial damage typically occurs on the low-pressure side of a pressure gradient (e.g., the ventricular side of regurgitant semilunar valves, the atrial side of regurgitant atrioventricular valves, or the free wall of the right ventricle affected by a jet from a VSD). The integrity of the endothelium can also be interrupted by CVCs, pacemaker leads, and cardiac surgery.

Damaged endothelium induces thrombogenesis via local activation of the coagulation system. Platelets and fibrin adhere to injured endocardium and create a meshwork that may also involve leukocytes and RBCs. This sterile lesion is known as nonbacterial thrombotic endocarditis (NBTE). It can less commonly result from inflammation, rather than direct tissue injury. Thus even in the absence of direct endothelial damage, NBTE may develop in individuals with malignancies, burns, and systemic lupus erythematosus.

NBTE forms a nidus for infection by bacteria or fungus that may be present in the bloodstream. Activities of daily living (chewing, brushing, and flossing) incite transient bacteremia from oral flora. Noncardiac infections such as pneumonia or skin abscess can lead to bacteremia. Transient bacteremia is also noted when invasive procedures (like dental or genitourinary surgery, or the percutaneous introduction of a CVC) disrupt the integrity of mucosal surfaces that contain a dense microflora. When NBTE is caused by direct tissue damage from a CVC or pacemaker leads in the right ventricle, the nidus is typically right sided and prone to infection by introduction of pathogens through a percutaneous puncture site or through infected material passing through the catheter lumen itself. Right-sided endocarditis can alternatively be the result of intravenous drug use with contaminated needles.

Advances in molecular biologic techniques have resulted in greater understanding of virulence factors (adhesins) and complex host-pathogen interactions. Certain bacteria are more likely to adhere to NBTE and cause IE. The key pathogens for IE (VGS, *S. aureus,* and *Enterococcus* species) have a larger number of adhesins than other bacteria. These adhesins, known collectively as Microbial Surface Component Reacting with Adhesive Matrix Molecules (MSCRAMMs) mediate adherence to host proteins such as fibrin, fibronectin, and platelet proteins—whether they are part of NBTE or coating medical devices like pacemaker leads in the heart. Examples include clumping factor A and B, fibronectin-binding protein A and B, and Sdr (serine-aspartate repeat) protein from *S. aureus* and glucosyltransferases (GTFs), expressed by strains of VGS. In the case of clumping factor and GTF, an increased production of proinflammatory interleukins was noted when strains with these particular adhesins were involved.[32,33] Animal models of streptococcal IE suggest dextran as another important virulence factor.[34]

Biofilm production further facilitates bacterial persistence and contributes to antimicrobial tolerance.[35] Adhesion leads to the formation of an infective vegetation, which further provokes the coagulation cascade and inflammatory response. Thus the vegetation grows and engulfs the pathogen—providing an environment in which it can replicate and escape from host defenses. In VGS an organized mass of fibrin encases a proliferating pathogen and substantially limits the ability of the host's phagocytes or antimicrobial agents to penetrate it.

A growing infective vegetation can lead to local cardiac effects and systemic complications. Valve dysfunction can result from the mass effect of a primary vegetation or the destructive effects that a vegetation can have on a valve—namely loss of structural integrity, perforation of a valve leaflet, or aneurysmal changes leading to valvular regurgitation, and progression to heart failure in severe cases. Vegetations may less commonly obstruct inflow at the valve level, leading to valvar stenosis. IE can also spread locally within the heart—potentially invading the valve annulus, leading to an abscess, and/or into the myocardium. Alterations in heart function and cardiac conduction can be noted.[36]

The systemic complications of IE result from (1) metastatic infection, due to persistent bacteremia or fungemia; (2) embolization of vegetations or pieces thereof; and (3) immune stimulation and antigen-antibody complex formation. Metastatic infection can occur in any organ, but the brain, lung, kidney, spleen, bone, joint, skin, or eye are most often affected. These secondary foci may undergo suppuration and may present as focal infections. Septic emboli can also lead to ischemia in the brain and lung, and less commonly to other organs. Hemorrhage may result from rupture of a mycotic aneurysm, from septic arteritis without mycotic aneurysm formation, or as a complication of infarction. Pulmonary emboli can lead to pneumonia, lung abscess, empyema, and infarction. Risk factors for embolization in pediatric IE include large vegetation (>10 mm), failure of vegetation to get smaller with appropriate antibiotics, and right-sided lesions.[37]

In cases in which the infection lasts weeks to months (i.e., subacute presentation), there is a heightened immune response that results in two primary clinical features. Splenomegaly in IE is thought to be caused by chronic reticuloendothelial hyperplasia. Glomerulonephritis (focal, segmental, or diffuse) due to the deposition of circulating immune complexes in the glomerular basement membrane often presents with hematuria.

Clinical Features

The clinical manifestations of IE are highly variable depending on the causative agent, the primary site of infection, and host factors. Typically, IE is primarily classified by the way in which it presents—acute versus subacute. Acute IE is generally characterized by a toxic-appearing patient, with high fevers, and, often, hemodynamic instability. *S. aureus* is the most common pathogen associated with acute IE and can cause rapid destruction of valve tissue, abscess formation, and embolic phenomena. More commonly, IE has a subacute presentation, often caused by VGS or CONS. Subacute IE presents with a slowly progressive course of some combination of nonspecific symptoms such as low-grade fever, anorexia, myalgia, arthralgia, or fatigue.

Clinical findings associated with IE are typically due to one of the four major components of the disease process: (1) direct cardiac manifestations, (2) embolic phenomena, (3) immune-complex disease, and (4) systemic manifestations of bacteremia or fungemia. Valve damage from IE typically results in valve regurgitation, which is manifested clinically by new or changing murmurs—diastolic murmurs with semilunar insufficiency and holosystolic murmurs for atrioventricular valve insufficiency. Cardiac auscultation may reveal a gallop rhythm, in addition to a myriad of other extracardiac findings (i.e., crackles or diminished breath sounds, hepatomegaly, or peripheral edema). When valve damage is severe, congestive heart failure develops and leads to complaints of exercise intolerance, dyspnea, or swelling. If IE affects a systemic-pulmonary shunt in cyanotic or single-ventricle CHD, then the obstruction from the vegetation may cause cyanosis and/or diminution of the associated murmur.

Embolic phenomena may result from right-sided or left-sided IE, and clinical manifestations vary according to the site affected. Right-sided IE can lead to pulmonary embolism, which may not be clinically relevant unless the emboli are large. Left-sided emboli can cause metastatic infection, ischemia, infarction, and/or hemorrhage. Hematogenous spread of infection can also lead to the formation of mycotic aneurysms. Although the kidneys can be affected by septic emboli, glomerulonephritis in IE is commonly the result of immune complex disease. Hematuria, proteinuria, and pyuria can be demonstrated on urinalysis, although impaired renal function is infrequent in children, compared with adults.[36]

Several extracardiac manifestations of IE due to immune complexes and septic emboli have been classically described in adults but are relatively rare in children. Janeway lesions (Fig. 70.1A) are erythematous, macular, and tender lesions of the palms and soles that are due to septic emboli. Osler's nodes (see Fig. 70.1B) are raised, painful lesions on the pads of the fingers and toes and result from immune complex deposition. Roth spots (see Fig. 70.1C) are retinal hemorrhages with white centers noted on funduscopy. They are mediated by immune complex disease and not specific for IE. Splinter hemorrhages (see Fig. 70.1D) are seen to run vertically under the nails due to damage to small capillaries, likely from embolic phenomena.

Diagnosis

Diagnostic Criteria

With a variable presentation and no single test result that defines IE, specific diagnostic criteria were needed to facilitate research and epidemiologic efforts. These criteria are widely used in combination with good clinical acumen to make a clinical diagnosis. Published in 1994 by Durack and colleagues[38] and modified by Li and colleagues[39] in 2000, the Duke criteria provide a framework by which to evaluate a case based on clinical, pathologic, microbiologic, and echocardiographic findings (Table 70.3, Box 70.1). Although not specifically designed for use in children, these criteria have been validated in the pediatric population and have proven more sensitive than prior criteria.[40]

Compared with autopsy as a gold standard, the sensitivity and specificity of the Duke criteria are approximately 80% for native valve endocarditis.[41] Because many diagnoses hinge on positive echocardiographic findings, diagnostic sensitivity declines in patients with prosthetic valve endocarditis or cardiac device infection—where sensitivity of transthoracic echocardiography (TTE) is low, and additional imaging may be required.

The Duke criteria may overestimate the presence of IE in patients with CVCs because attempts to salvage a catheter colonized with *S. aureus* may lead to persistently positive blood cultures.[42] Thus

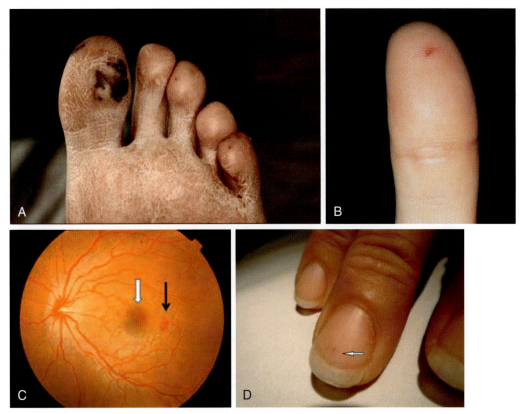

• **Figure 70.1** Clinical manifestations of infective endocarditis. (A) Janeway lesion. (B) Osler's node. (C) Roth spot *(black arrow)* along with cherry-red spot *(white arrow)*. (D) Splinter hemorrhage. ([A] from Beaulieu A, Rehman HU. Janeway lesions. *CMAJ.* 2010;182[10]:1075; [B] from Adams JG, Barton ED, Collings J, et al. *Emergency Medicine: Clinical Essentials.* 2nd ed. Philadelphia: Elsevier; 2013; [C] from Chang FP, Chien CY, Chaou CH, et al. Infective endocarditis with initial presentation of visual disturbances. *Am J Emerg Med.* 2016;34[10]:2052.e5-2052.e7; [D] from Chieng D, Janssen J, Benson S, et al. 18-FDG PET/CT scan in the diagnosis and follow-up of chronic Q fever aortic valve endocarditis. *Heart Lung Circ.* 2016;25[2]:e17-e20.)

debate continues on the application of Duke criteria in patients with CVCs and positive blood cultures, especially for *S. aureus.*

Blood Cultures

Because the hallmark of the disease is persistent bacteremia, the diagnosis of IE is confirmed by the demonstration of repeatedly positive blood cultures.[43] The bacteremia in IE is usually continuous and low grade (<100 organisms/mL of blood[43]); therefore adequate volumes of blood should be drawn. In adults at least 10 mL of blood should be drawn for each bottle.[43] Collection of large volumes of blood is not feasible in infants and young children. In general, 3 to 5 mL in infants and young children and 5 to 7 mL in older children should suffice.[2] At least three blood cultures via separate venipunctures should be drawn in the first 24 hours to (1) demonstrate persistent bacteremia, (2) increase the probability of a positive culture, and (3) increase the likelihood that the isolate is significant and not a contaminant (e.g., CONS and rarely viridans streptococci).[43] In adults, three sets of blood cultures would detect 96% to 98% of bacteremia when cultures are obtained before antibiotic therapy.[44] Cultures must be obtained with a meticulously aseptic technique and percutaneously, not through indwelling CVCs. When a small volume of blood is available for culture, preference must be given to inoculating blood into the aerobic bottle because IE due to anaerobic bacteria is very unusual.[2]

Automated blood culture systems and novel molecular diagnostic techniques can rapidly detect microorganisms and have superior sensitivity compared with traditional culture methods.[45,46] In ill-appearing patients with suspected IE, three sets of blood cultures should be drawn over a period of 1 to 2 hours, and appropriate antimicrobial therapy should be instituted. However, in patients with a more indolent course of illness or in whom the diagnosis is not clear—and especially if prior antimicrobial therapy has been given—one should not initiate antimicrobial therapy for at least 48 hours until the results of blood cultures become available. If the initial blood cultures are negative at 48 hours and the diagnosis of IE is still considered likely, two or three additional blood cultures should be obtained, and the various causes of CNE should be considered.[2,47] The optimal methods for identifying fastidious or unusual pathogens should be discussed with the clinical microbiologist.[47] Some experts recommend holding blood cultures for extended periods (≥ 14 days), but the yield may be low for the slow-growing HACEK bacteria.[2,48] In selected cases, serology for zoonotic pathogens (e.g., *Coxiella, Bartonella,* and *Brucella*) and urinary antigen testing for *Legionella pneumophilia* serogroup 1 may be helpful.[47]

Emboli or vegetations removed surgically should be submitted for (1) histologic analysis with tissue Gram stains, fungal stains (e.g., periodic acid–Schiff and silver impregnation stains), and mycobacterial stains and (2) cultures for aerobic, anaerobic, and

TABLE 70.3 Definitions of Terminology Used in the Modified Duke Criteria

Major Criteria

Positive blood culture for infective endocarditis	Typical microorganism for infective endocarditis from two separate blood cultures • Viridans streptococci,[a] *Streptococcus bovis*, HACEK group, OR • Community-acquired *Staphylococcus aureus* or enterococci in the absence of a primary focus Persistently positive blood culture for microorganisms consistent with IE • At least two blood cultures drawn more than 12 hours apart, OR • All of three or a majority of four or more separate blood cultures—with first and last drawn at least 1 h apart • Single positive blood culture for *Coxiella burnetii* or anti–phase-1 IgG antibody titer >1 : 800
Evidence of endocardial involvement	Positive echocardiogram for infective endocarditis • Oscillating intracardiac mass, on valve or supporting structures, or in the path of regurgitant jets or on implanted material, in the absence of an alternative anatomic explanation, OR • Abscess, OR • New partial dehiscence of prosthetic valve • New valvular regurgitation (increase or change in preexisting murmur not sufficient)

Minor Criteria

Predisposition	Predisposing heart condition or IV drug use
Fever	≥38.0°C (100.4°F)
Vascular phenomena	Major arterial emboli, septic pulmonary infarcts, mycotic aneurysm, intracranial hemorrhage, conjunctival hemorrhages, Janeway lesions
Immunologic phenomena	Glomerulonephritis, Osler's nodes, Roth spots, rheumatoid factor
Microbiologic evidence	Positive blood culture but not meeting major criterion as noted previously[b] or serologic evidence of active infection with organism consistent with infective endocarditis

[a]Including nutritional variant strains.
[b]Excluding single positive cultures for coagulase-negative staphylococci and organisms that do not cause endocarditis.
HACEK, *Haemophilus* spp., *Actinobacillus actinomycetemcomitans, Cardiobacterium hominis, Eikenella* spp., and *Kingella kingae; IgG*, immunoglobulin G; *IV*, intravenous.
From Durack DT, Lukes AS, Bright DK, et al. New criteria for diagnosis of infective endocarditis: utilization of specific echocardiographic findings. *Am J Med.* 96:200-209, 1994; and Li JS, Sexton DJ, Mick N, et al. Proposed modifications to the Duke criteria for the diagnosis of infective endocarditis. *Clin Infect Dis.* 2000;30(4):633-638.

• BOX 70.1 Diagnosis of Infective Endocarditis Using the Modified Duke Criteria

Definite Infective Endocarditis

Pathologic criteria
   Microorganisms: demonstrated by culture OR
   Histologic evaluation in a vegetation OR
   In a vegetation that has embolized OR
   In an intracardiac abscess
   Pathologic lesions: Vegetation or intracardiac abscess—confirmed by histology showing active endocarditis
Clinical criteria, using specific definitions listed in Table 70.3
   Two major criteria OR
   One major and three minor criteria OR
   Five minor criteria

Possible Infective Endocarditis

   One major criterion AND one minor criterion OR
   Three minor criteria

Rejected

   Firm alternate diagnosis for manifestations of endocarditis OR
   Resolution of manifestations of endocarditis, with antibiotic therapy for 4 days OR
   No pathologic evidence of infective endocarditis at surgery or autopsy, after antibiotic therapy for ≤4 days

From Durack DT, Lukes AS, Bright DK, et al. New criteria for diagnosis of infective endocarditis: utilization of specific echocardiographic findings. Am J Med. 1994;96:200-209; and Li JS, Sexton DJ, Mick N, et al. Proposed modifications to the Duke criteria for the diagnosis of infective endocarditis. Clin Infect Dis. 2000;30(4):633-638.

have received prior antimicrobial therapy, but false-positive results may still occur.[25] Broad-range sequencing of bacterial 16S ribosomal DNA on excised valve tissue represents an alternative approach for identifying the organism in both native and prosthetic valve IE.[50] Direct detection and characterization of bacteria from peripheral blood or heart valves in patients with IE using polymerase chain reaction–based technology combined with mass spectrometry is a novel approach warranting further investigation.[51]

Other Laboratory Findings

An elevated erythrocyte sedimentation rate, C-reactive protein, and normochromic-normocytic anemia are common nonspecific findings.[21,52] Anemia is often mild and related to chronic disease due to depression of the bone marrow and its failure to use iron. If anemia is severe, hemolysis due to intravascular damage to RBCs should be suspected; this occurs mainly in individuals with prosthetic valves.[2] Leukocytosis may be noted in acute IE. In neonates, thrombocytopenia is a frequent finding. Immunologic manifestations include positive rheumatoid factor, hematuria, RBC casts, and low serum complement reflecting immune complex glomerulonephritis. Electrocardiography may reveal ventricular ectopy or complete heart block in some cases, indicating severe course.[2]

Echocardiography

The modified Duke criteria include echocardiographic findings showing endocardial involvement as a major criteria for the diagnosis of IE. The classic echocardiographic finding is the oscillating, mobile intracardiac mass on heart valves, their support structures, or prosthetic material within the heart, including prosthetic valves.

fastidious bacteria, *Legionella* spp., mycobacteria, and fungi. However, conventional culture methods of excised surgical specimens are associated with very high false-positive rates (13% to 55%) compared with prior blood culture results or nucleic acid amplification tests (NAATs).[49]

NAAT-based molecular methods performed on surgical tissues are very helpful in establishing the diagnosis of IE in patients who

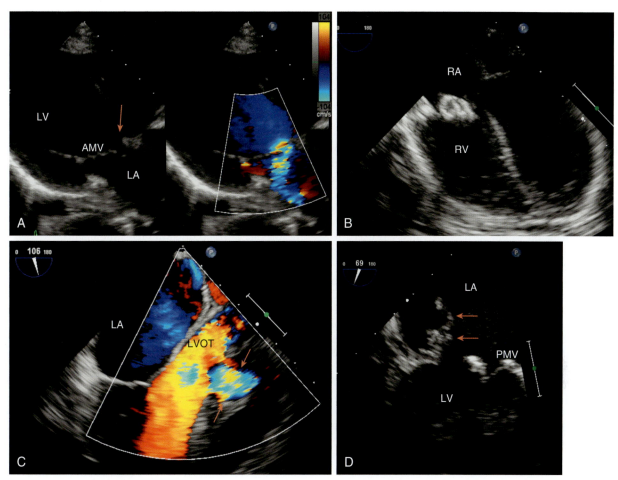

• **Figure 70.2** Echocardiographic manifestations of infective endocarditis. (A) Perforation *(red arrow)* of anterior mitral valve leaflet with regurgitation. (B) Tricuspid valve vegetation, immediately adjacent to ventricular septal defect. (C) Sinus of Valsalva aneurysm *(red arrows)*. (D) Mobile, strand-like vegetation *(red arrows)* on mitral valve. *AMV,* Anterior mitral valve leaflet; *LA,* left atrium; *LV,* left ventricle; *LVOT,* left ventricular outflow tract; *PMV,* posterior mitral valve leaflets; *RA,* right atrium; *RV,* right ventricle.

In the absence of this mobile mass, diagnostic criteria can also be met by an abscess of the valve ring, dehiscence of a prosthetic valve, or new or worsening valvular regurgitation. Vegetations typically occur in predictable locations, based on cardiac pathology. They are often seen (1) on the low-pressure side of a regurgitant valve (the atrial side of a regurgitant mitral valve, the ventricular side of a regurgitant aortic valve) or shunt lesion (the pulmonary side of a PDA, the right ventricular side of a VSD) or (2) at the site where turbulent flow strikes the endocardium (e.g., the anterior mitral leaflet with aortic insufficiency or the tricuspid valve in a VSD) (Fig. 70.2A). Although vegetations typically occur near the area of coaptation, they also may involve the cusps themselves, the chordae tendineae, or the sinuses of Valsalva.[53] Multiple lesions may be noted when one part of the heart is remotely affected by a primary source of infection.

In addition to aiding in diagnosis by revealing the location, size, and attachments of a vegetation, the echocardiogram can detail the degree of valvular insufficiency, the cardiac function, and whether remote valves are affected. As untreated or inadequately treated IE progresses, chamber dilation, alteration of ventricular performance with changes in loading conditions, and the development of pericardial effusions (especially with myocardial abscesses) can be seen. The echocardiogram can demonstrate the mechanism

for insufficiency, which will be important for surgical planning. An eccentric jet through a perforated valve leaflet (see Fig. 70.2B) can progress over time but often is amenable to primary repair in the operating room. Damage to the valve leaflets can also cause failure of coaptation of the valves—resulting in a prominent central jet of insufficiency. Damage to the support apparatus can cause prolapse of a valve leaflet or a flail valve leaflet (see Fig. 70.2C). Therapeutic decisions (e.g., the need for surgery) hinge on these and other echocardiographic findings. Echocardiography can suggest how likely a vegetation is to embolize, based on its attachment to the valve. Serial echocardiograms allow for assessment of vegetation size as a marker of response to antibiotic therapy. However, an echocardiogram is unable to differentiate an actively infected vegetation from a healing thrombus.

TTE is often the initial imaging modality in children and has very good spatial resolution in young children weighing less than 60 kg (up to 97% sensitivity).[54] However, transesophageal echocardiography (TEE) may be necessary in certain populations (e.g., obese or mechanically ventilated patients with poor acoustic windows, those with prosthetic valves, and those with *S. aureus* bacteremia) to improve sensitivity. In adults the sensitivity for TTE is 50% to 90% for native valve endocarditis and 36% to 69% in prosthetic valve endocarditis. In adults, TEE is recommended to follow the nondiagnostic TTE, but also is recommended in patients with typical complications of IE or in those in whom prosthetic leads are present. Published adult guidelines must be considered for children with the caveat that the detection rate for TEE often will not greatly exceed that of TTE. In larger children and adults, TEE is more sensitive for most cardiac lesions with the exception of the anterior aortic valve and pulmonary valve

The imaging specialist must also consider the use of cardiac computed tomography (CT), which has several advantages over echocardiography. Although it has a lower sensitivity for the evaluation of vegetation and valve regurgitation, it has a higher sensitivity for perivalvular abscesses and pseudoaneurysms and for understanding the spread of infection into the myocardium or pericardium. Cardiac CT can also optimally show the coronary anatomy in patients on whom aortic valve surgery is likely. It is also less susceptible to shadowing from prosthetic valve material compared with echocardiography. The 2014 American College of Cardiology (ACC)/American Heart Association (AHA) guidelines for valvular heart disease (not pediatric specific) now consider cardiac CT to be a class IIa recommendation for diagnosis when TTE/TEE is nondiagnostic for IE.[55] Intracardiac echocardiography has been proposed for the diagnosis of IE in percutaneous pulmonary valve replacement because sensitivity is limited with both TTE and TEE.[56]

Differential Diagnosis

A febrile child who recently underwent cardiac surgery can present a unique challenge because the child has risk factors for IE (recent cardiac surgery, prosthetic devices, and/or indwelling CVC) but can have fever for a multitude of other reasons—both infectious and noninfectious. Infectious causes include pneumonia, central line–associated bloodstream infection, surgical site infection, or urinary tract infection. Noninfectious causes of postoperative fever include atelectasis or inflammatory states resulting from surgical trauma, cardiopulmonary bypass, or blood transfusion.[57]

Postoperative cardiac patients can also demonstrate the postpericardiotomy syndrome (PPS)—an inflammatory state characterized by fever, pleuritic chest pain, pleural or pericardial effusions, and elevation of inflammatory markers. PPS typically develops 1 to 3 weeks postoperatively in approximately 1% to 40% of postoperative cardiac patients undergoing pericardiotomy.[58,59] PPS is uncommon in children less than 2 years of age. Despite the abundance of risk factors in those immediate postoperative patients, only 22% of cases in a large registry study of IE demonstrated acquisition of disease in the immediate postoperative period, compared with acquisition during long-term convalescence.[60]

To ensure timely treatment and prevent unnecessary exposure to long-term antibiotic use, the diagnosis of IE must be carefully considered as it relates to other diseases of childhood with common signs and symptoms (i.e., fever, heart failure, and other nonspecific symptoms). Although other inflammatory conditions of the heart share features with IE, viral myocarditis and pericarditis require the use of antiinflammatory agents as opposed to antibiotics. Vasculitides such as Kawasaki disease, with its ability to cause fever, new auscultatory findings on the cardiac examination, and heart failure must also be considered. In patients with CVCs, particularly neonates, IE must be distinguished from NBTE, in which injury from a catheter tip can lead to the development of a sterile thrombus.

Given the propensity for IE to cause embolic phenomena, infections at extracardiac sites (i.e., septic arthritis, brain abscess, or pneumonia) warrant consideration of a primary cardiac source of thromboembolism; in such patients, blood cultures and echocardiography should be obtained, especially in patients with risk factors for IE.

Neonatal Endocarditis

IE in the neonate has been recognized with increasing frequency during the past two decades.[9,60,61] This is probably due to increased use of CVCs in the management of babies, especially premature babies in the ICU, and improved survival of critically ill infants with complex CHD.[62] In a multicenter study of pediatric IE, neonatal IE accounted for 7.3% of cases; in this series 31% of deaths due to IE occurred in premature infants.[9]

The great majority of neonates with IE have no underlying heart disease.[9,60,61] NBTE in the neonate occurs mostly on the right side of the heart and follows hypoxia resulting from conditions such as persistent fetal circulation (PFC), hyaline membrane disease (HMD), and disseminated intravascular coagulation. This has been found in 8% to 10% of all neonatal autopsies.[63] PFC and HMD might result in IE by causing the release of vasoactive substances (e.g., thromboxane A_2 or other eicosanoids), which cause platelet aggregation.[64] Endothelial damage is caused by intravascular catheters, either percutaneous or umbilical venous catheters.[65]

Almost all cases of neonatal IE are nosocomial. The most common causative organisms are *S. aureus* (≈50% of all cases), CONS, streptococci (including group B streptococcus), and *Candida* spp.[62] The clinical features are nonspecific and may include temperature instability, respiratory distress, poor feeding, shock, and a new or changing heart murmur.[2,61,63] Thrombocytopenia is common. Septic emboli can result in focal infections such as pneumonia, osteomyelitis, and meningitis.[2]

Antimicrobial Therapy

The management of IE warrants a multidisciplinary approach with expertise in infectious diseases, cardiology, and cardiothoracic surgery. Management consists of four elements: (1) supportive care for severely ill patients, primarily treatment of heart failure, which is not discussed here; (2) antimicrobial therapy; (3) surgical therapy; and (4) management of complications.

General Principles of Antimicrobial Therapy

Antimicrobial treatment of IE can be challenging because the organism is buried within a fibrin-platelet vegetation where the bacterial cell division and metabolic rate is reduced, which hinders the penetration and activity of cell wall–active antibiotics. Therefore antimicrobial therapy must be microbicidal and administered intravenously (IV) at high dosage for 4 to 8 weeks (Table 70.7).[2,66,67] Administration of bacteriostatic antibiotics leads to treatment failures and relapses.[2] The choice of definitive antibiotic therapy is based on the causative organism and its antimicrobial susceptibility, disease severity, and whether the affected valve is native or prosthetic. Peak and trough serum levels of vancomycin and gentamicin should be measured once steady state has been attained and then weekly. Blood cultures should be repeated daily until they have become negative (often within several days after starting antimicrobial therapy, except for *S. aureus*). In such cases (e.g., prosthetic valve IE due to *S. aureus* complicated by persistent bacteremia), additional blood cultures may be obtained after cessation of therapy to demonstrate clearance of bacteremia and adequacy of treatment. Relapse is usually noted in the subsequent 4 weeks after completion of therapy.[2,68]

Empiric Treatment of Infective Endocarditis

In acutely ill patients with IE, antibiotics must be administered empirically as soon as blood cultures are obtained. In stable patients with subacute disease, withholding antibiotics for 48 hours or longer while awaiting the results of initial blood cultures is an option.[2] Table 70.4 depicts the initial empiric therapy for native valve and prosthetic valve endocarditis.[2]

Antimicrobial Therapy Against Specific Microorganisms

Tables 70.5 and 70.6 summarize AHA antimicrobial recommendations for IE caused by different microorganisms. The dosages, routes of administration, and dosing schedules of antimicrobial agents are shown in Table 70.7.[2]

Streptococci

Most streptococci causing IE belong to the viridans group. Although generally susceptible to penicillin, their degree of susceptibility

TABLE 70.4 Initial Empiric Antimicrobial Therapy of Infective Endocarditis

Organism (Unknown)/ Valve Type	Antimicrobial Agent of Choice	Alternative Agent
Native valve (community acquired) or "late" prosthetic valve (>1 y after surgery)	Ampicillin/sulbactam plus gentamicin With or without vancomycin Add rifampin for prosthetic valve endocarditis	Vancomycin (plus gentamicin)
Nosocomial IE associated with vascular cannulas or "early" prosthetic valve endocarditis (<1 y after surgery)	Vancomycin plus gentamicin (+ rifampin if prosthetic material present)	Unknown

IE, Infective endocarditis.
Data from Wilson W, Taubert KA, Gewitz M, et al. Prevention of infective endocarditis: guidelines from the American Heart Association: a guideline from the American Heart Association Rheumatic Fever, Endocarditis, and Kawasaki Disease Committee, Council on Cardiovascular Disease in the Young, and the Council on Clinical Cardiology, Council on Cardiovascular Surgery and Anesthesia, and the Quality of Care and Outcomes Research Interdisciplinary Working Group. *Circulation.* 2007;116:1736-1754; and Baltimore RS, Gewitz M, Baddour LM. Infective endocarditis in childhood: 2015 update. A Scientific Statement from the American Heart Association. *Circulation.* 2015;132:1487-1515.

TABLE 70.5 Antimicrobial Therapy of Native Valve Infective Endocarditis Caused by Gram-Positive Bacteria

Organism	Antimicrobial Agent of Choice (Duration)[a]	Alternative Agent
Streptococci, highly susceptible to penicillin[b]	Penicillin G or ceftriaxone for 4 wk[c]	Vancomycin or first-generation cephalosporin or ceftriaxone
Streptococci, relatively resistant to penicillin[d]	Penicillin G (or ampicillin) for 4 wk plus gentamicin (for first 2 wk) Penicillin G (or ampicillin) plus gentamicin for 4-6 wk for enterococci	Vancomycin plus gentamicin for enterococci (6 weeks' duration) Ampicillin plus ceftriaxone (for aminoglycoside-resistant enterococci or aminoglycoside-intolerant patient) Ceftriaxone plus gentamicin (not for enterococcal endocarditis)
Staphylococci (Staphylococcus aureus or CONS)[e]		
Susceptible to ≦1 mcg/mL penicillin G (unusual)	Penicillin G for 4-6 wk	Oxacillin or nafcillin or first-generation cephalosporin or vancomycin
Resistant to 0.1 mcg/mL penicillin G	Oxacillin or nafcillin for 4-6 wk ± gentamicin (for 3-5 d)	Vancomycin or a first-generation cephalosporin
Resistant to 4 mcg/mL oxacillin (MRSA)	Vancomycin for 6 wk	Daptomycin for right-sided IE, maybe for left-sided
Vancomycin resistant or intolerant	Daptomycin for at least 6 wk	Unknown

[a]Depending on susceptibilities; additional therapy may be necessary in complicated cases or recurrent IE.
[b]Minimal bactericidal concentration ≦0.1 mcg/mL to penicillin G; streptococci include most viridans streptococci, groups A, B, C, G nonenterococcal, group D streptococci (*Streptococcus bovis, Streptococcus equinus*).
[c]In adult patients, 2 weeks of therapy may suffice but is not recommended for children due to lack of effectiveness data.
[d]Minimal bactericidal concentration ≧0.2 mcg/mL to penicillin G; streptococci include enterococci and less-susceptible viridans streptococci.
[e]Add rifampin (at least 6 weeks) and gentamicin (for first 2 weeks) for prosthetic valve IE due to staphylococci.
CONS, Coagulase-negative staphylococcus; *IE*, infective endocarditis; *MRSA*, methicillin-resistant *Staphylococcus aureus*.
Data from Wilson W, Taubert KA, Gewitz M, et al. Prevention of infective endocarditis: guidelines from the American Heart Association: a guideline from the American Heart Association Rheumatic Fever, Endocarditis, and Kawasaki Disease Committee, Council on Cardiovascular Disease in the Young, and the Council on Clinical Cardiology, Council on Cardiovascular Surgery and Anesthesia, and the Quality of Care and Outcomes Research Interdisciplinary Working Group. *Circulation.* 2007;116:1736-1754; and Baltimore RS, Gewitz M, Baddour LM. Infective endocarditis in childhood: 2015 update. A Scientific Statement from the American Heart Association. *Circulation.* 2015;132:1487-1515.

TABLE 70.6 Antimicrobial Therapy of Infective Endocarditis Caused by Gram-Negative Bacteria and by Fungi

Organism	Antimicrobial Agent	Duration (wk)
HACEK organisms[a]	Third-generation cephalosporin (ceftriaxone or cefotaxime)	4
	or	
	Ampicillin-sulbactam[b]	4
Gram-negative enteric bacilli	Extended spectrum cephalosporin[c]	At least 6
	+ Aminoglycoside[d]	6
Pseudomonas aeruginosa[e]	Antipseudomonal penicillin (ceftazidime)[f]	6
	+ Aminoglycoside[d]	6
	or	
	Ceftazidime	6
	+ Aminoglycoside[d]	6
Fungi (Candida spp., Aspergillus spp.)	Amphotericin B	At least 6
	±	
	Flucytosine	At least 6
	(for infection with yeast) AND Surgical resection	Lifelong suppressive therapy if no surgery or relapse after surgery

[a]Haemophilus spp., Aggregatibacter spp., Cardiobacterium hominis, Eikenella corrodens, Kingella spp.
[b]Alternative antibiotic drug choice for HACEK group includes ampicillin (for susceptible organisms) plus aminoglycoside.
[c]Ceftazidime, cefepime, cefotaxime, or ceftriaxone.
[d]Gentamicin (or tobramycin or amikacin, depending on susceptibility).
[e]Depending on susceptibilities.
[f]Alternative antipseudomonal penicillins include piperacillin/tazobactam, depending on susceptibility.
Data from Wilson W, Taubert KA, Gewitz M, et al. Prevention of infective endocarditis: guidelines from the American Heart Association: a guideline from the American Heart Association Rheumatic Fever, Endocarditis, and Kawasaki Disease Committee, Council on Cardiovascular Disease in the Young, and the Council on Clinical Cardiology, Council on Cardiovascular Surgery and Anesthesia, and the Quality of Care and Outcomes Research Interdisciplinary Working Group. Circulation. 2007;116:1736-1754; and Baltimore RS, Gewitz M, Baddour LM. Infective endocarditis in childhood: 2015 update. A Scientific Statement from the American Heart Association. Circulation. 2015;132:1487-1515.

TABLE 70.7 Dosages, Routes, and Dosing Schedules for Antimicrobial Agents Used in the Treatment of Infective Endocarditis in Children

Drug	Pediatric Dosage and Route	Schedule
Amphotericin B[a]	1 mg/kg/24 h IV	q24 h
Amikacin	15 mg/kg/24 h IV	q8-12 h
Amphotericin liposomal/lipid-associated formulations	3-5 mg/kg/24 h IV	q24 h
Ampicillin	200-300 mg/kg/24 h IV	q4-6 h
Cefazolin	100 mg/kg/24 h IV	q8 h
Cefotaxime	200 mg/kg/24 h IV	q6 h
Ceftazidime	100-150 mg/kg/24 h IV	q8 h
Ceftriaxone	100 mg/kg/24 h IV	q12 h
Flucytosine	150 mg/kg/24 h PO	q6 h
Gentamicin	3-6 mg/kg/24 h IV	q8 h
Ampicillin-sulbactam	200-300 mg/kg/24 h IV	q4-6 h
Piperacillin/tazobactam	240 mg/kg/24 h IV	q8 h
Nafcillin	200 mg/kg/24 h IV	q4-6 h
Oxacillin	200 mg/kg/24 h IV	q4-6 h
Penicillin G high dosage	200,000-300,000 U/kg/24 h IV	q4 h
Rifampin	20 mg/kg/24 h PO	q12 h
Tobramycin	3-6 mg/kg/24 h IV	q8 h
Vancomycin	40 mg/kg/24 h IV	q8-12 h

[a]Administer over 3 to 4 hours.
IM, Intramuscular; IV, intravenous; PO, oral.
Data from Wilson W, Taubert KA, Gewitz M, et al. Prevention of infective endocarditis: guidelines from the American Heart Association: a guideline from the American Heart Association Rheumatic Fever, Endocarditis, and Kawasaki Disease Committee, Council on Cardiovascular Disease in the Young, and the Council on Clinical Cardiology, Council on Cardiovascular Surgery and Anesthesia, and the Quality of Care and Outcomes Research Interdisciplinary Working Group. Circulation. 2007;116:1736-1754; and Baltimore RS, Gewitz M, Baddour LM. Infective endocarditis in childhood: 2015 update. A Scientific Statement from the American Heart Association. Circulation. 2015;132:1487-1515.

varies. The duration of therapy and aminoglycoside requirement for treatment of streptococcal IE are based on the following penicillin susceptibility categories: highly susceptible to penicillin (minimal inhibitory concentration [MIC] ≤0.1 mcg/mL) and relatively resistant to penicillin (MIC >0.2 mcg/mL).[2] Treatment of highly penicillin-susceptible streptococcal IE with a 4-week regimen of IV penicillin G or ampicillin (if penicillin G is unavailable) results in high cure rates.[69] In cases of IE caused by resistant streptococci, bactericidal activity is achieved by using a 4-week regimen of penicillin, ampicillin, or ceftriaxone combined with gentamicin for the initial 2 weeks of treatment. Treatment of cases with resistant streptococci (MIC >0.5 mcg/mL) is the same as for those with

enterococci. Nutritionally variant streptococci (Abiotrophia and Granulicatella species) can demonstrate relative or high-level resistance to penicillin and must be treated with the combination antimicrobial therapy listed for enterococci.

In cases of prosthetic valve IE caused by penicillin-susceptible streptococci, the recommended treatment consists of a 6-week regimen of penicillin, ampicillin, or ceftriaxone combined with gentamicin for the initial 2 weeks of treatment. Prosthetic valve IE due to streptococci with an MIC of greater than 0.1 mcg/mL for penicillin or Abiotrophia and Granulicatella species must be treated with penicillin, ampicillin, or ceftriaxone combined with gentamicin for 6 weeks.[2]

Enterococci

Enterococci comprise *Enterococcus faecalis, E. faecium,* and several other species. Treatment of enterococcal endocarditis is complicated because they exhibit relative resistance to penicillin and ampicillin as the result of expression of low-affinity penicillin-binding proteins and a variable resistance to aminoglycosides and vancomycin.[70] Combination antimicrobial therapy is recommended for enterococcal endocarditis, whether it is a native or prosthetic valve.[2,71] Generally, ampicillin (for susceptible isolate) or vancomycin in combination with an aminoglycoside is required. Penicillin and vancomycin can achieve bactericidal activity only by the addition of gentamicin for synergy. Synergy cannot be achieved if high-level resistance to gentamicin is demonstrated by in vitro susceptibility testing in the laboratory. The emergence of high-level antimicrobial resistance among certain species of enterococci to vancomycin, ampicillin, and aminoglycoside is a major concern.[72]

Although enterococci are resistant to all cephalosporins, studies have found that a combination of ampicillin plus ceftriaxone is effective against aminoglycoside-nonsusceptible *E. faecalis* strains.[73,74] The most effective treatment of endocarditis due to vancomycin-resistant enterococci (VRE) is unclear given paucity of data. Quinupristin-dalfopristin, a novel antimicrobial agent that has activity against vancomycin-resistant *E. faecium* (but not *E. faecalis*), has been used successfully in combination with rifampin and doxycycline to treat *E. faecium* endocarditis.[75] Other agents active against VRE include linezolid, daptomycin, and tigecycline.[72] Infectious disease consultation is recommended in all cases of enterococcal IE.[2]

Staphylococci

Presently *S. aureus* and the various species of CONS (mainly *Staphylococcus epidermidis*) are almost always resistant to penicillin and ampicillin due to their production of a β-lactamase.[76] Semisynthetic penicillins (e.g., nafcillin, oxacillin) are active against most strains of *S. aureus* (methicillin-susceptible or MSSA) and some strains of CONS. In recent years the number of invasive MRSA infections have increased in children.[77] MRSA strains and many strains of CONS are resistant to semisynthetic penicillins due to alterations in their penicillin-binding proteins and also resistant to cephalosporins.[76,78]

Native Valve Staphylococcal IE. Semisynthetic, β-lactamase-resistant penicillin (nafcillin or oxacillin) administered IV for a minimum of 4 to 6 weeks is the recommended treatment regimen of choice for IE due to MSSA endocarditis.[2] In the treatment of *S. aureus* endocarditis the addition of gentamicin has been shown to shorten the duration of bacteremia but not to influence the ultimate outcome of the infection.[79] Based on experimental studies, gentamicin use may be considered for the first 3 to 5 days of therapy, but renal and otic toxicity can occur, warranting close monitoring of drug levels.[2]

Vancomycin is the mainstay of therapy of IE due to MRSA strains, with or without the addition of gentamicin for the initial 3 to 5 days.[2] MRSA strains with intermediate susceptibility to vancomycin (MIC of 4 to 8 mcg/mL) have been reported. Vancomycin-intermediate *S. aureus* (VISA) may emerge during vancomycin therapy.[80] Cases of IE caused by VISA strains are very difficult to treat and may require use of newer agents such as daptomycin.[2] Pediatric experience with other drugs (e.g., linezolid, quinupristin-dalfopristin, daptomycin, and tigecycline) is limited.[80]

Development of several novel anti-MRSA antibiotics is being pursued.[81]

Prosthetic Valve Staphylococcal IE. CONS are often the causative organism in prosthetic valve endocarditis, typically occurring less than 1 year after surgery.[71] *S. aureus* can also cause early prosthetic valve IE and is often associated with serious complications (e.g., root abscess formation, valve dehiscence) and very high mortality.[82,83] Prosthetic value IE due to staphylococci require the addition of rifampin and gentamicin (for the initial 2 weeks) for synergy.[2,71] Surgical removal of the infected valve or device is usually necessary and preferred, particularly with *S. aureus* infection.

Gram-Negative Bacteria (Including HACEK Organisms)

The HACEK group of organisms (most common cause of gram-negative IE) may produce β-lactamase, resulting in resistance to ampicillin. A third-generation cephalosporin (e.g., ceftriaxone) or ampicillin-sulbactam should be used unless susceptibility to ampicillin is demonstrated.[2,71] Treatment duration is 4 weeks for native valves and 6 weeks for prosthetic valves.

Treatment of gram-negative IE must be based on pathogen identification and antimicrobial susceptibilities. Treatment should consist of a third-generation cephalosporin (ceftazidime, ceftriaxone, or cefotaxime) and an aminoglycoside, and that of *P. aeruginosa* endocarditis should consist of ceftazidime plus an aminoglycoside or an antipseudomonal penicillin (e.g., piperacillin/tazobactam) plus an aminoglycoside. Carbapenems (e.g., imipenem/cilastatin or meropenem) may be indicated to treat IE caused by gram-negative bacteria with multidrug resistance (e.g., extended-spectrum β-lactamase production).

Fungal Endocarditis

Many patients with fungal IE will require surgery in addition to antifungal therapy, although medical treatment alone has been successful in neonates with mural endocarditis. Amphotericin B remains the drug of choice for IE due to *Candida* or *Aspergillus* species, but penetration of the drug into vegetations is limited. In patients with IE caused by *Candida* strains susceptible to flucytosine (5-FC), amphotericin in combination with 5-FC may be considered for additional benefit.[2]

Route of Administration and Duration of Therapy

Treatment should be administered IV in infants and children with IE. Intramuscular administration of antibiotics is not recommended due to small muscle mass compared to adults.[2] Intravenous antibiotics should be given for 4 to 6 weeks in native valve endocarditis, whereas therapy should be continued for 6 to 8 weeks in prosthetic valve infection (Table 70.7).[2,71] Additional therapy may be needed in complicated cases with persistent bacteremia or recurrent disease. In adults with uncomplicated native valve IE due to highly susceptible streptococci, a short 2-week course of IV penicillin, ampicillin, or ceftriaxone in combination with gentamicin is highly effective (cure rates of up to 98%); however, the shorter, 2-week combination therapy is not recommended for children due to lack of data and concerns of gentamicin toxicity.

Outpatient Therapy

After an initial treatment course in the hospital, selected patients with IE may be eligible for outpatient (home) IV treatment (e.g., those responding to treatment, afebrile and clinically stable with low risk for complications, and negative blood cultures).[2] Patient and family must adhere to the medical plan, including visitation by a home health nurse to monitor wellness, evaluate medication compliance and drug toxicity, and assess complications.[2] The necessary social environment, home care services, and follow-up medical care must be available.

Surgery

Surgery is indicated in patients with IE with progressive valve dysfunction leading to heart failure and persistent infection and for prevention of embolism.[2,25] Early surgery (within a week of diagnosis) has been shown to be associated with a low risk of postoperative septic emboli, recurrence, and mortality in a pediatric cohort.[84] In some patients the decision to proceed with surgery will be more difficult—weighing the risk of surgery against the risk of conservative care. Guidelines exist, but their utility is limited. First, they are often extensions of adult guidelines because pediatric data are limited. Second, there is a wide spectrum of interpretation for terms such as *heart failure* or *persistent bacteremia*. Finally, recommendations of "early surgery" do not specify a definitive time frame for such. Thus decisions about surgical management of IE should be individualized and made by a multispecialty team of intensivists, cardiologists, surgeons, and infectious disease specialists.[55]

Updated in 2014, the ACC/AHA valvular heart disease guidelines suggest the following as indications for surgery in IE: (1) valve dysfunction causing symptomatic heart failure, (2) resistant organisms such as *S. aureus* or fungus, (3) heart block or perivalvular abscess, (4) persistent fevers or bacteremia despite 5 to 7 days of appropriate treatment, and (5) recurrent emboli with persistence of vegetations (class IIa).[55] The most common reasons for surgical intervention in the pediatric population are congestive heart failure (typically as a result of valvular dysfunction) and embolic phenomena. Given the lifetime risk associated with valve replacement in children, surgery is not recommended for the prevention of a primary embolic event, although it may be considered in the presence of recurrent emboli.[2]

In the adult population a trend toward earlier surgery is noted. A retrospective study[85] of 239 patients diagnosed with IE secondary to CHD in Japan found that 26% of the patients with IE required surgery during the active phase of IE (while still receiving antibiotics). Other institutions reported a higher rate of surgical intervention—61% of IE cases (54% of which were within 3 days of diagnosis).[84] Independent risk factors associated with the need for surgery were heart failure, perivalvular abscesses, and the need for a change in antibiotics.[85]

Outcome

The overall mortality rate of IE in children is approximately 5%, although mortality may vary based on the virulence of the infecting organism and clinical setting.[9,86] Other studies have reported higher mortality rates varying from 10% to 24%.[87-89] There are several identifiable conditions that place IE patients at increased risk for complications[90] (Box 70.2). IE in children remains a significant cause of morbidity and resource use, especially in children with heart disease.[86]

• BOX 70.2   Clinical Situations Constituting High Risk for Complications of Infective Endocarditis

Cyanotic congenital heart disease
Systemic-to-pulmonary shunts
Staphylococcus aureus IE
Left-sided IE
Prosthetic cardiac valves
Fungal IE
Prolonged clinical symptoms (>3 mo)
Poor clinical response to antimicrobial therapy
Previous IE

IE, Infective endocarditis.
Reprinted with permission. Circulation. 1998;98:2936-2948. Copyright 1998 American Heart Association, Inc.

Prevention

For years, efforts to prevent IE in children primarily focused on ensuring that oral antibiotics were given before dental procedures—despite a lack of evidence that would suggest that antibiotic prophylaxis prevented IE. Gradually evidence began to mount that (1) exceedingly few cases of IE result from dental procedures, and (2) IE caused by typical oral flora were much more likely due to activities of daily living like brushing teeth, chewing food, or flossing—where the cumulative risk of frequent bacteremia was far greater than that of routine dental cleanings and minor procedures. Additionally, the risk of frequent antibiotic prophylaxis (anaphylaxis and increased antimicrobial resistance) led experts to reevaluate those practices.[91] A shift of focus began to take place that deemphasized antibiotic use before procedures and focused on optimizing oral health and hygiene for cardiac patients at risk for IE. This shift culminated in 2007 with a substantial revision of AHA guidelines regarding how and when to offer chemoprophylaxis.

The AHA guidelines from 2007 have been updated several times.[55] Other societies, including the European Society of Cardiology (ESC), have published similar recommendations.[10] The UK national guidelines have recommended complete cessation of routine antibiotic prophylaxis for IE.[92]

The ESC and AHA guidelines now recommend antibiotic prophylaxis for only those cardiac conditions that confer the highest rates of morbidity (often surgical intervention) and mortality with IE, including (1) previous IE, (2) prosthetic cardiac valves, (3) prosthetic material used as part of valve repair (recommended by ESC but not updated AHA guidelines), (4) cardiac valvulopathy after heart transplantation, (5) unrepaired cyanotic CHD including palliative shunts, (6) placement of a device or prosthetic material in the heart within the prior 6 months (allowing time for endothelialization), and (7) repaired CHD with residual defect adjacent to a prosthetic patch (in which endothelialization is inhibited).

The recommended antibiotic regimens are detailed in Table 70.8. Prophylaxis is indicated for invasive respiratory procedures (not routine bronchoscopy) and for procedures involving infected skin or musculoskeletal tissue. Antibiotics given for the sole purpose of preventing IE with gastrointestinal or genitourinary tract procedures are no longer recommended. Patients who take daily antibiotic prophylaxis for conditions such as asplenia or rheumatic fever will often be given a different antibiotic before a dental procedure.

TABLE 70.8	Regimens for Infective Endocarditis Prophylaxis in Appropriate Patients		
		REGIMEN: SINGLE DOSE 30-60 MIN BEFORE A DENTAL PROCEDURE	
Situation	Agent	Adults	Children
Oral	Amoxicillin	2 g	50 mg/kg
Unable to take oral medication	Ampicillin OR	2 g IM or IV	50 mg/kg IM or IV
	Cefazolin or Ceftriaxone	1 g IM or IV	50 mg/kg IM or IV
Allergic to penicillins or ampicillin—oral	Cephalexin OR[a]	2 g	50 mg/kg
	Clindamycin OR	600 mg	20 mg/kg
	Azithromycin or Clarithromycin	500 mg	15 mg/kg
Allergic to penicillins or ampicillin—cannot take oral	Cefazolin or Ceftriaxone[a] OR	1 g IM or IV	50 mg/kg IM or IV
	Clindamycin	600 mg IM or IV	20 mg/kg IM or IV

[a]Cephalosporins are to be avoided in patients with history of anaphylaxis, angioedema, or urticaria with penicillins or ampicillin.

IM, Intramuscular; *IV*, intravenous.

Data from Wilson W, Taubert KA, Gewitz M, et al. Prevention of infective endocarditis: guidelines from the American Heart Association: a guideline from the American Heart Association Rheumatic Fever, Endocarditis, and Kawasaki Disease Committee, Council on Cardiovascular Disease in the Young, and the Council on Clinical Cardiology, Council on Cardiovascular Surgery and Anesthesia, and the Quality of Care and Outcomes Research Interdisciplinary Working Group. *Circulation*. 2007;116:1736-1754.

Selected References

A complete list of references is available at ExpertConsult.com.

1. Wilson W, Taubert KA, Gewitz M, et al. Prevention of infective endo-carditis: guidelines from the American Heart Association: a guideline from the American Heart Association Rheumatic Fever, Endocarditis, and Kawasaki Disease Committee, Council on Cardiovascular Disease in the Young, and the Council on Clinical Cardiology, Council on Cardiovascular Surgery and Anesthesia, and the Quality of Care and Outcomes Research Interdisciplinary Working Group. *Circulation*. 2007;116:1736–1754.

2. Baltimore RS, Gewitz M, Baddour LM. Infective endocarditis in childhood: 2015 update. A Scientific Statement from the American Heart Association. *Circulation*. 2015;132:1487–1515.

9. Day MD, Gauvreau K, Shulman S, et al. Characteristics of children hospitalized with infective endocarditis. *Circulation*. 2009;119:865–870.

22. Johnson DH, Rosenthal A, Nadas AS. A forty-year review of bacterial endocarditis in infancy and childhood. *Circulation*. 1975;51:581–588.

32. Veloso TR, Chaouch A, Roger T, et al. Use of a human-like low-grade bacteremia model of experimental endocarditis to study the role of

Staphylococcus aureus adhesins and platelet aggregation in early endocarditis. *Infect Immun*. 2013;81:697–703.

39. Li JS, Sexton DJ, Mick N, et al. Proposed modifications to the Duke criteria for the diagnosis of infective endocarditis. *Clin Infect Dis*. 2000;30:633–638.

47. Fournier PE, Thuny F, Richet H, et al. Comprehensive diagnostic strategy for blood culture-negative endocarditis: a prospective study of 819 new cases. *Clin Infect Dis*. 2010;51:131–140.

54. Penk JS, Webb CL, Shulman ST, et al. Echocardiography in pediatric infective endocarditis. *Pediatr Infect Dis J*. 2011;30:1109–1111.

55. Nishimura RA, Otto CM, Bonow RO. 2014 AHA/ACC guideline for the management of patients with valvular heart disease: a report of the American College of Cardiology/American Heart Association Task Force on Practice Guidelines. *J Am Coll Cardiol*. 2014;63:e57–e185.

71. Baddour LM, Wilson WR, Bayer AS, et al. Infective endocarditis: diagnosis, antimicrobial therapy, and management of complications: a statement for healthcare professionals from the Committee on Rheumatic Fever, Endocarditis, and Kawasaki Disease, Council on Cardiovascular Disease in the Young, and the Councils on Clinical Cardiology, Stroke, and Cardiovascular Surgery and Anesthesia, American Heart Association: executive summary. *Circulation*. 2015;111:3167–3184.

71

Pulmonary Hypertension

RAJEEV S. WADIA, MD; PRIYA SEKAR, MD, MPH; CHINWE UNEGBU, MD;
EPHRAIM TROPP; PATRICIA L. KANE, MSN, CNS, CPNP; MEGHAN BERNIER, MD;
JOHN D. COULSON, MD; LEWIS H. ROMER, MD

Pulmonary Hypertension in Congenital Heart Disease

Epidemiology, Physiology, and Anatomy of Pulmonary Vascular Disease

Abnormally high pulmonary vascular tone has been known to be an adversary to optimal cardiac function in the perioperative period in premier pediatric cardiac surgical programs for decades.[1] This challenge has seemingly intensified recently, as the recognition and targeted care of pulmonary hypertension (PH) have skyrocketed in pediatric inpatients across the board—including those with congenital heart disease (CHD). This dynamic upswing in PH care in the United States is attested to by an increase in inflation-adjusted national inpatient hospital charges for care of this problem from $926 million to $3.12 billion between 1997 and 2012.[2]

Pulmonary arterial hypertension (PAH) is a clinical condition of precapillary PH defined in adults by a mean pulmonary artery pressure (mPAP) of 25 mm Hg or higher. PAP can be elevated either from increased pulmonary vascular resistance (PVR) or from increased blood flow. According to Ohm's law the voltage difference (i.e., pressure difference) is equal to the current (i.e., blood flow) multiplied by the resistance to flow (i.e., PVR).

$$Pressure = (Flow) \times (Resistance)$$

Although many children with PH in the setting of CHD have acquired this problem because of elevated PVR, two additional clinical scenarios are worth mentioning, and both may be understood based upon the relationships described by the previous equation. First, elevated PVR may exist when mPAP is normal (<25 mm Hg) if pulmonary blood flow is also low—such as in patients without a pulmonary ventricle who have undergone cavopulmonary anastomosis (bidirectional Glenn shunt).[3] Second, some children may have increased pulmonary blood flow (i.e., intraventricular shunt with left-to-right flow) resulting in an mPAP of 25 mm Hg or higher but not have increased PVR from pulmonary vascular disease (PVD).[3]

Deleterious histologic changes are often seen in pediatric patients with PH. Patients with PH may have a deficiency of vasodilator pathways as evidenced by less endogenous prostacyclin, reduced expression of nitrogen oxide synthase and vasoactive intestinal peptide in the lungs, and increased levels of circulating endothelin-1 and serotonin.[4-7] These conditions may ultimately result in migration of smooth muscle cells into peripheral arteries that are normally nonmuscularized, to medial hypertrophy in the muscular arteries, impaired microvascular growth, progressive loss of arterioles, and a decrease in arterial density. There is general consensus that the early changes in this evolution of pathophysiology may be remodeled toward normal microvascular infrastructure over time but that the later and more advanced vascular wall changes may become irreversible.

Challenges Specific to Congenital Heart Disease

PH may substantially contribute to morbidity and mortality in infants and children with CHD.[8] Pathogenesis of PH in many children with CHD may be linked to three types of aberrations of pulmonary circulatory dynamics: excessive pulmonary blood flow, fixed obstruction of the right ventricular (RV) outflow tract or the main or branch pulmonary arteries, or obstruction of pulmonary venous return (Table 71.1). Conditions involving either intracardiac (i.e., ventricular septal defect [VSD], complete atrioventricular [AV] canal) or extracardiac (i.e., aortopulmonary window, patent ductus arteriosus [PDA], truncus arteriosus) communication between the systemic and pulmonary circulation can result in increased blood flow in the developing pulmonary circulation. The expected response to this increase in pulmonary blood flow is a decrease in the vascular resistance, to maintain normal pulmonary pressure. In this situation it is considered abnormal when PVR remains normal or is increased. Thus when PVR does increase, this suggests that progressive pulmonary vascular remodeling has occurred with increased vascular smooth muscle. When PVR fails to appropriately decrease, it may be termed *hyperkinetic pulmonary hypertension.*[9] This is one reason that children with CHD should undergo repair early in life to reduce the occurrence of PVD.

In the fetus, PVR is very high, and pulmonary blood flow is approximately 30 to 40 mL/kg/min, or approximately 8% of combined ventricular output. With the initiation of breathing at birth, there is an initial rapid decrease in PVR, allowing pulmonary blood flow to increase to approximately 350 to 400 mL/kg/min.[10] This is followed by a slower, progressive decline in PVR (and therefore pulmonary pressure) over the next 6 to 8 weeks after birth. However, in some newborns high PVR persists after birth, and the expected increase in pulmonary blood flow is never observed. If no underlying congenital heart lesion is present, this is referred to as *persistent pulmonary hypertension of the newborn* (PPHN). Elevated PVR may cause right-to-left shunting of blood and

TABLE 71.1	Perioperative Management Priorities for Pulmonary Hypertension in Common Congenital Heart Disease Lesions	
Pathogenesis of RV Hypertension	Cardiac Lesion(s)	Perioperative Management Priorities
Excessive pulmonary blood flow	VSD ASD PDA Truncus arteriosus Aortopulmonary window TGA	1. Respiratory status may be tenuous due to excessive PBF, leading to pulmonary edema and poor lung compliance. 2. Heart failure with suboptimal systemic perfusion (metabolic acidosis, systemic hypotension, liver or kidney dysfunction). Afterload reduction may be necessary to augment systemic perfusion. 3. Optimize the balance of $Q_p:Q_s$ with interventions that modify PVR and SVR.
Fixed right ventricular outflow tract or pulmonary artery obstruction	TOF with or without hypoplastic PAs	1. Maintain RV function, and avoid agents that may depress ventricular performance. Inotropic agents may be necessary in cases of RV failure. 2. Maintain SVR to promote coronary perfusion of the RV. RVH will increase RVEDP; therefore blood pressure management is essential to maintain right coronary perfusion. Vasopressin may preferentially increase SVR without changing PVR. CPP = systemic DBP − ventricular EDP
Obstructed pulmonary venous return	Pulmonary vein obstruction with or without TAPVR Mitral stenosis/atresia LV diastolic dysfunction	1. Poor lung compliance may result from pulmonary edema that is secondary to increased pulmonary venous pressure from outlet obstruction. 2. Increased pulmonary venous congestion may result in a secondary increased PVR. Acute vasoreactivity testing in the cardiac catheterization laboratory is indicated to define the effects of pulmonary vasodilators. 3. Caution with interventions that may cause pulmonary vasodilation, and therefore increased PBF, in setting of an outlet obstruction (e.g., 100% FiO_2, pulmonary vasodilators).

ASD, Atrial septal defect; *CPP*, coronary perfusion pressure; *DBP*, diastolic blood pressure; *EDP*, end-diastolic pressure; *FiO₂*, fraction of inspired oxygen; *LV*, left ventricular; *PA*, pulmonary artery; *PBF*, pulmonary blood flow; *PDA*, patent ductus arteriosus; *PVR*, pulmonary vascular resistance; *Qₚ:Qₛ*, pulmonary-to-systemic blood flow ratio; *RV*, right ventricular; *RVEDP*, right ventricular end-diastolic pressure; *RVH*, right ventricular hypertrophy; *RVOT*, right ventricular outlet tract; *SVR*, systemic vascular resistance; *TAPVR*, total anomalous pulmonary venous return; *TGA*, transposition of the great arteries; *TOF*, tetralogy of Fallot; *VSD*, ventricular septal defect.

subsequent hypoxemia in the presence of a persistent foramen ovale and/or PDA.

In contrast to PPHN the development PVD in the presence of CHD is a usually a consequence of the underlying cardiac lesion, rather than the primary disorder. The evolution of PVD in CHD depends not only on the location and size of the shunt but also on the hemodynamic burden it imposes on the pulmonary vasculature.[11] Cardiac lesions that shunt left to right and result in hyperkinetic pulmonary circulation include septal defects, aortopulmonary connection, and PDA. When small, these lesions pose minimal risk for the development of PVD. Some patients do not develop symptoms of congestive heart failure or pulmonary vascular congestion even when the defect is large,[12] but this should not prevent a child with a large, unrestrictive defect from undergoing percutaneous or surgical closure early in life to subvert the development of PH. In the first 2 years of life, closure of a VSD (even in the presence of markedly elevated PVR) may result in normal or near-normal PVR following repair (despite a 50% risk of preoperative PH at 2 years of age), with the likelihood of favorable pulmonary vascular remodeling being even better if the operation is performed in the first year of life.[13-15] A PDA may also cause PVD, but the occurrence of irreversible PVD seldom occurs before 2 years of age. On the other hand, older children who undergo surgical repair may not have a substantial drop in PVR postoperatively. Thus the approach to the older patient with PH and CHD involves careful evaluation and perioperative planning. Factors that raise concern for elevated PVR include late presentation, lack of pulmonary congestion, bidirectional shunting, systemic oxygen desaturation, and presence of underlying genetic syndromes. (Down syndrome, DiGeorge syndrome, and Noonan syndrome are some more common examples.)

In contrast, prolonged exposure to increased pulmonary blood flow from an atrial septal defect (ASD) causes PVD in children less commonly,[16] although large ASDs may lead to moderate or severe PH in up to 59% of patients by adulthood[17-19] and may shorten the life expectancy by 50% if repaired beyond the fourth decade of life.[20]

If PH occurs in the presence of a small atrial-level shunt, investigation for a possible underlying genetic predisposition to developing PVD is needed. Genetics consultation has a growing and vital role in the management of PH in CHD. For example, transforming growth factor beta receptors have a pivotal role in cardiac embryogenesis and vascular development; therefore gene mutations in these receptors, especially *BMPR2* (bone morphogenetic protein receptor 2) and in *ALK-1* (activin A receptor-like kinase type 1—present in hereditary hemorrhagic telangiectasia), are of critical interest.[21,22]

Infants with transposition of the great arteries (TGA) with VSD who are not repaired within the early neonatal period may develop severe PVD during the first year of life.[23] This is likely is due to in utero preconditioning of the pulmonary vasculature.[24-26] Pulmonary arteries normally carry low oxygen content from the right ventricle, whereas the oxygen-rich blood from the placenta is preferentially shunted from the inferior vena cava across the foramen ovale to the left heart by the eustachian valve and then is ejected out the left ventricle into the aorta. In d-TGA, oxygen-rich blood from the placenta is instead delivered to the pulmonary arteries, and the pulmonary vessels dilate in utero, leading to stretch injury of the vascular intima with secondary vasoconstriction.[24,27,28] This may explain why some children with d-TGA (with or without a VSD) may develop PVD despite a successful early neonatal arterial switch operation.[29]

Truncus arteriosus, aortic origin of a pulmonary artery, complete AV canal defects, and double-outlet right ventricle with VSD may all be associated with rapid evolution of PVD.[30,31] These lesions all result in excessive pulmonary-to-systemic flow ratios ($Q_p{:}Q_s$) as PVR decreases after birth, and many of these infants are at risk of death in the first year without surgical correction.[32,33] These lesions therefore warrant consideration for complete repair in early infancy.[34-38]

In infants with unobstructed total anomalous pulmonary venous connection (TAPVC), the added pulmonary venous return to the right heart causes RV volume overload and increased pulmonary blood flow. This may induce muscularization of the pulmonary vascular bed and irreversible PH.[39] Partial anomalous pulmonary venous connection with more than half of the pulmonary veins draining anomalously and an associated ASD can also cause right heart failure with PH, but this usually evolves later in life.[40] If the anomalous veins are obstructed, elevation of pulmonary pressures occurs from pulmonary venous hypertension rather than from increased pulmonary blood flow.

Shunt-mediated PH is usually reversible if the surgical correction is performed early. In one study involving 280 autopsies in infants under 1 year of age with CHD, advanced degrees of pulmonary hypertensive arteriopathy (grade IV or more) occurred in only 6 infants.[41] Rabinovitch et al.[13] performed lung biopsy on 74 patients with congenital heart defects who had either PH or high-risk lesions, including VSD, d-TGA, and complete AV canal. One year after repair, mPAP and/or PVR were normal in all patients whose conditions were corrected surgically before 9 months of age, regardless of the severity of the pulmonary vascular changes on biopsy at the time of the operation. Furthermore, pulmonary arterial pressure and PVR were increased in all patients whose conditions were repaired after 2 years of age with grade C morphometric findings and severely elevated in children with Heath-Edwards grade III biopsy.

Elevated pulmonary arterial pressures may also occur secondary to postcapillary PH (i.e., secondary to left heart dysfunction and/or pulmonary venous obstruction). This occurs because the elevated left heart pressure (high left atrial pressure) is passively transmitted back toward the pulmonary veins and arteries, leading to reflex changes in pulmonary artery pressure. Hemodynamic measurements will initially show an elevated pulmonary capillary wedge pressure (PCWP) with normal PVR of less than 3 Wood units and transpulmonary gradient (mean PA pressure − PCWP) of approximately 12 mm Hg. In patients in whom pulmonary vascular remodeling has occurred, the PA pressure will increase to a much higher degree than the left atrial pressure (LAP), resulting in an elevated transpulmonary gradient above 12 mm Hg. In older children and adults, left heart lesions (i.e., mitral valve stenosis, aortic valve stenosis, cor triatriatum) and both systolic and diastolic ventricular dysfunction can cause PH.[42-46] In newborns, postcapillary PH is more commonly due to obstructed TAPVC, in which elevated LAP is absent because the obstruction is proximal to the left atrium. The pulmonary venous obstruction can quickly lead to subsequent pulmonary vascular changes.[39] Pulmonary artery vasoconstriction and alveolar capillary remodeling occur as a compensatory mechanism protecting against the development of pulmonary edema that occurs from transudation of fluid into the alveolar space in the setting of downstream obstruction. Prolonged, severe pulmonary venous hypertension promotes hypertrophy of the pulmonary arterioles and arterialization of the pulmonary venules.[47] Autopsies of infants with obstructed TAPVC demonstrated increased arterial medial thickness, intimal proliferation in periacinar veins, and

abnormally small and thick-walled extrapulmonary veins.[39] It is therefore no surprise that neonates with obstructed TAPVC are extraordinarily vulnerable to PAH in the perioperative period despite a successful repair.[48]

Perioperative Risk in Patients With PH

Children with PH have increased perioperative risk, and those with underlying congenital cardiac disease are more likely to have cardiac arrest.[49] Preoperative planning and risk assessment are guided by a child's preoperative functional status, current medical therapies, coexisting medical conditions, the type of procedure (e.g., emergency versus elective, open versus laparoscopic, intrathoracic versus intraabdominal), the planned anesthetic approach (sedation versus general anesthetic, use of a neuroaxial or regional nerve block), and postoperative disposition (need for postoperative mechanical ventilation).

Baseline perioperative risk assessment encompasses clinical symptoms, biomarker data, echocardiographic findings, and hemodynamic parameters from cardiac catheterization[50] (Fig. 71.1). The most substantial risk factors for adverse perioperative events include suprasystemic PA pressures,[49,51,52] decreased RV function,[50,51] young age,[52] home use of supplemental oxygen,[52] new PH diagnosis before therapy,[53] and lack of a stable therapeutic regimen.[53] Children with idiopathic or heritable PH may also be at higher perioperative risk.[51,52,54] Finally, patients with chronic or long-standing PH may develop RV hypertrophy and be at risk for RV ischemia due to increased resistance to coronary flow and lowered systemic vascular resistance (SVR) with general anesthesia.

One single-center retrospective study of 156 children undergoing noncardiac surgical procedures and cardiac catheterizations from 1999 to 2004 found that suprasystemic PA pressure was a predictor of major perioperative complications (odds ratio [OR], 9.1; $P = .02$), including cardiac arrest (with overall prevalence of 1.17%) and pulmonary hypertensive crisis.[54] Another study of 97 cardiac catheterization procedures in children with known PH, between 2009 and 2014, showed 3% incidence of systemic hypotension and zero incidence of cardiac arrest and death. All patients who had an adverse event had suprasystemic pulmonary artery pressures and moderate to severe RV dysfunction.[51] In yet another study of 284 non–cardiopulmonary bypass surgical cases, suprasystemic PAH, young age, and home oxygen use were significant risk factors for complications, whereas the cause of PAH was not associated with an increased risk.[52] Van der Griend et al. evaluated 101,885 anesthetics of pediatric patients and found that 50% of all deaths occurred in patients with PH. The deaths encompassed the entire perioperative period—induction of anesthesia, maintenance of anesthesia, and in the postoperative care unit.[49] Another large study evaluating 43,391 pediatric patients undergoing anesthesia for surgery in Spain showed that the presence of PAH made death more likely if a cardiac arrest occurred.[55]

Comorbid conditions augment perioperative risk for children with PH. Sleep-disordered breathing, reactive airway disease, chronic lung disease, chronic aspiration, obesity, sickle cell disease, neuromuscular disease, and congenital or acquired cardiac disease can each decrease cardiopulmonary or airway reserve and increase risk of decompensation.[53] In a retrospective multicenter study of infants with bronchopulmonary dysplasia who underwent surgical repair of CHD, 25% of the deaths were attributed to PH.[56] Chi and Krovetz[57] reported that children with Down syndrome, who may have underlying upper airway obstruction and pulmonary alveolar

AHA/ATS consensus pediatric PAH: disease severity

LOWER RISK	DETERMINANTS OF RISK	HIGHER RISK
No	Clinical evidence of RV failure	Yes
I,II	WHO class	III,IV
None	Syncope	Recurrent syncope
Minimal RV enlargement/dysfunction	Echocardiography	Significant RV enlargement/dysfunction Pericardial effusion
PVRI <10 WU • m^2 CI >3.0 L/min/m^2 PVR/SVR <0.5	Hemodynamics	PVRI >20 WU • m^2 CI <2.0 L/min/m^2 PVR/SVR >1.0
Minimally elevated	BNP / NTproBNP	Significantly elevated
Longer (>500 m)	6MWD	Shorter (<300 m)
Peak VO$_2$ >25 mL/kg/min	CPET	Peak VO$_2$ <15 mL/kg/min

• **Figure 71.1** 2015 American Heart Association and American Thoracic Society guidelines for determining pulmonary hypertension disease severity. *AHA,* American Heart Association; *ATS,* American Thoracic Society; *BNP,* brain natriuretic peptide; *CI,* cardiac index; *CPET,* cardiopulmonary exercise testing; *NTproBNP,* N-terminal pro-brain natriuretic peptide; *PAH,* pulmonary arterial hypertension; *PVR,* pulmonary vascular resistance; *PVRI,* pulmonary vascular resistance index; *RV,* right ventricle; *6MWD,* 6-minute walk distance; *SVR,* systemic vascular resistance; *VO$_2$,* oxygen consumption; *WHO,* World Health Organization; *WU,* Wood units. (Reprinted with permission. *Circulation.* 2015;132:2037-2099. Copyright 2015 American Heart Association, Inc.)

hypoplasia, have an unusually high PVR and a propensity for early development of severe PVD.

Finally, anesthetic and surgical factors can increase the risk for morbidity and mortality in patients with PH. These include emergency surgical procedure,[55,58,59] ASA III or poorer status,[58,60] presence of a difficult airway (which may potentially lead to hypoxemia or hypercarbia either while attempting to secure the airway or immediately after extubation), prolonged procedure times (which can cause atelectasis and necessitate increased fluid administration), intraoperative hemodynamic lability, procedures that can generate compressive forces on the heart and lung (intrathoracic and abdominal surgery), interventions that cause a systemic inflammatory response (e.g., abdominal washout for abscess, bowel resection), and surgery that may provoke major fluid shifts (e.g., exploratory laparotomy, orthopedic trauma).[53,61] Of special consideration are procedures in the cardiac catheterization laboratory because they are associated with high risk of cardiac arrest, especially during pulmonary angioplasty and stenting, in which direct stimuli to the pulmonary arterial tree is applied.[62,63]

Given the high-risk nature of this patient population, communication among all providers, including nurses, surgeons, anesthesiologists, intensive care unit (ICU) team, PH specialists, and the primary physician, must be standard of practice and must encompass the following checklist: (1) medical optimization before elective surgical cases without interruption in the administration of pulmonary vasodilators; (2) scheduling procedures early in the day to avoid prolonged fasting and dehydration; (3) assignment of an experienced pediatric anesthesiology team that is skilled in acute PH management; (4) availability of postoperative care in a pediatric intensive care unit as needed; (5) minimization of anesthetic exposure; and (6) immediate availability of pediatric subspecialists, nurses, and pharmacologists who are skilled in the care of children with PH.[53,61] Management priorities in specific subtypes of CHD are outlined in Table 71.1.

Noninvasive Assessment of Pulmonary Hypertension

Echocardiography for Pulmonary Hypertension

Echocardiography has been a first-line test in the evaluation of the intensive care patient with PH. The benefits include bedside availability, minimal coordination of staff, relatively low cost, and the fact that it is noninvasive. Although echocardiography is a very useful tool in the assessment and ongoing care of these patients, the child with PH presents unique challenges to echocardiographic assessment. These include limited acoustic windows due to hyperinflation accorded by often concomitant lung disease, ventilator modes such as high-frequency ventilator oscillation that challenge logistics and compromise image quality, and the risks inherent to sedating pediatric patients with PH. Additionally, the right ventricle is a major imaging target for PH, and its proximity to the airways as an anterior cardiac structure presents a challenge.

Quantification of right heart pressure can be achieved noninvasively in several ways but depends on the presence of right-sided valve regurgitation or cardiac shunts. Right ventricular systolic pressure (RVSP) is most often estimated by interrogating tricuspid

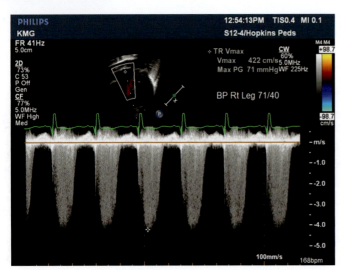

• **Figure 71.2** Tricuspid regurgitation in a newborn with pulmonary hypertension.

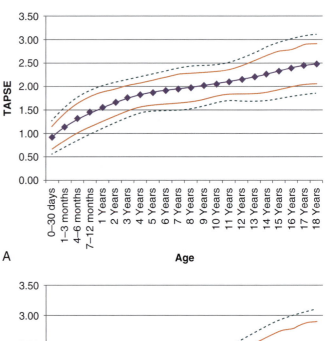

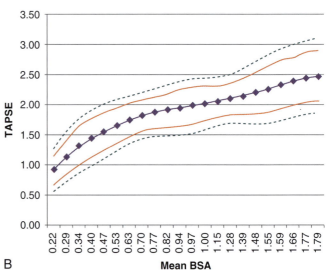

• **Figure 71.3** Tricuspid Annular Planar Systolic Excursion (TAPSE) values by age and mean body surface area (BSA). Echocardiographic data from 640 children were collected to determine the relationship for both age (A) and BSA (B) to mean value of TAPSE ± 2 and 3 z scores. The mean is indicated by the blue solid line with the squares. The z score ± 2 and z score ± 3 lines are indicated by the red solid line and green broken line, respectively. As the age and mean BSA of a child increase, so does the TAPSE, with the greatest increase occurring in neonates and infants compared with older children and adolescents. (From Koestenberger M, Ravekes W, Everett AD, et al. Right ventricular function in infants, children and adolescents: reference values of the tricuspid annular plane systolic excursion [TAPSE] in 640 healthy patients and calculation of z score values. *J Am Soc Echocardiogr.* 2009;22[6]:715-719. doi:10.1016/j.echo.2009.03.026.)

regurgitation (TR) velocity by continuous wave Doppler evaluation (Fig. 71.2; Video 71.1). RVSP is equivalent to pulmonary artery systolic pressure when pulmonary stenosis and RV outflow obstruction have both been excluded—determination that must be made on initial imaging. TR velocity (meters/s) estimates the RVSP (mm Hg) using the modified Bernoulli equation but requires either direct catheter measurement or estimation of right atrial (RA) pressure (mm Hg):

$$RVSP = 4 \times (TR \ velocity)^2 + RA \ pressure$$

Pulmonary regurgitation velocity should also be interrogated, when present, and this may provide an estimate of pulmonary artery end-diastolic pressure (PAEDP):

$$PAEDP = PR \ gradient \ at \ end \ diastole + RV \ diastolic \ pressure$$

RV diastolic pressure is approximated by RA pressure in the absence of tricuspid valve stenosis. When cardiac shunts exist, specifically a PDA (Video 71.2) or VSD, these velocities should be estimated, and the Bernoulli equation should be applied. Subtracting the resulting gradient from a simultaneous systemic systolic blood pressure will yield an estimate of pulmonary artery systolic pressure or an RV systolic pressure estimate—depending on the location of the shunt. When more than one of these shunts and tricuspid valve regurgitation are available, it is useful to use multiple methods to cross-reference the validity of the estimated right heart pressure.

Disappointingly, over 50% of patients do not have enough TR to estimate RV pressure and do not have any shunts. Indirect methods are then used to determine RV pressure. Specifically, this entails evaluation of the ventricular septal geometry in systole. When flattened (Fig. 71.3; Video 71.3) in systole, the RV pressure is greater than 50% systemic.

Serial assessment of RV function may also be necessary in the care of the ICU patient with PH. The RV function is known to be adversely affected (at rest) when more than 50% of the pulmonary resistance vessels are dysfunctional (Video 71.4), and preservation of RV function is a critical prognostic factor in management of PH in adults. Barriers to quantification of RV systolic function include RV geometry, as well as image quality. Several methods exist to assess RV function, but their use widely varies between

centers. Tricuspid Annular Planar Systolic Excursion (TAPSE) is perhaps the most widely used, and normal values exist for children, showing a positive correlation to age[64] (see Fig. 71.3). This method measures the longitudinal displacement of the tricuspid valve annulus in systole, recognizing that the RV fiber orientation is more longitudinal than that of the left ventricle. It is measured using the M-mode of echocardiography along the lateral aspect of the tricuspid annulus in the apical four-chamber view, evaluating the maximum movement of the annulus from high in the atrium during diastole to down into the right ventricle during systole.

Decreased values have been associated with poor prognosis in adults with PH and heart failure.[65,66] Limitations of this method include the fact that it is dependent upon load, angle, and orientation of the heart within the chest. Additionally, the focus is limited to a small part of the RV myocardium—the basolateral wall, and it is affected by the overall motion of the heart. RV shortening fraction is another method for assessment of RV systolic function but is dependent on loading conditions, and there are currently no reference values for RV shortening fraction in children. Pulmonary artery acceleration time is a relatively new method proposed for RV functional assessment that inversely correlates with right heart catheterization-based pulmonary hemodynamics, including mPAP and PVR.[67] However, this method is also dependent upon heart rate, and normal values are available only for older children.

Two other methods that bear mentioning include RV speckle tracking and RV Tei index (sum of RV isovolumetric contraction time + RV isovolumetric relaxation time, divided by the RV ejection time)[68] because both have been studied in adults with PH. Unfortunately, the RV Tei index has not been found to be helpful in assessing the RV function during the newborn transition period, which is often the age and stage of one of the most common pediatric ICU patient types with CDH and PH.

In summary, bedside echocardiography will continue to be the mainstay method for evaluation of right heart pressure and RV function in children with PH in the ICU, with some promising new techniques for its application on the horizon.

Biomarkers for Pulmonary Hypertension

Serum biomarkers of disease severity and response to treatment in PH are highly valued tools that are under active investigation and development.[69] The biomarker that is currently used for pediatric PH is the amino-terminal fragment of the pro-form of the brain natriuretic peptide (BNP)—NTproBNP. This is an inactive byproduct of enzymatic cleavage of BNP that is triggered by wall stretch in the right atrium and in the right ventricle. NTproBNP levels have been shown to correspond well to changes in PVR and to echocardiographic measurements of PH severity in CHD, and it is the current standard for periodic assessment of children with an active PH course.[70] More specific markers are under development due to a higher range of normal NTproBNP values in pediatrics and more variability in some clinical settings—particularly those with active noncardiac systemic disease. Promising candidates for development as additional biomarkers with potential for higher specificity include hepatoma-derived growth factor and microRNA's miR-208b and miR-199a.[71,72]

Cardiac Catheterization in Pulmonary Hypertension

Indications

Cardiac catheterization can provide definitive and extensive information about hemodynamics, responsiveness to pulmonary vasodilators, and cardiovascular anatomy in PH patients. Furthermore, cardiac catheterization allows interventions to be performed, which can alleviate or palliate PH or otherwise facilitate PH management.

Various recommendations have been made regarding which children with PH should undergo cardiac catheterization and when. In one series of formerly premature infants with bronchopulmonary dysplasia and PH, 31% underwent cardiac catheterization.[73] Mourani et al.[74] in 2008 emphasized the inability of echocardiography to reliably assess PH severity in a significant proportion of young patients. Bobhate et al.[51] in 2015 proposed catheterization for most children with PH with the exception of those in overt right heart failure or requiring mechanical ventilation and inotropic support. Guidelines from the American Heart Association and the American Thoracic Society recommend catheterization before initiation of therapy, except for critically ill patients requiring immediate treatment.[3] Guidelines recently published by the Pediatric and Congenital Heart Disease Task Forces of the Pulmonary Vascular Research Institute specify that nearly all children with PH should undergo diagnostic cardiac catheterization with acute vasoreactivity testing (AVT) at least once.[75] In general, catheterization should be undertaken when the cause, severity, and/or course of PH is to be assessed; when acute responsiveness to pulmonary vasodilators is to be determined; when severe PH is not satisfactorily responding to therapy; when transcatheter or surgical therapy may be indicated; to assess operability; and to evaluate candidacy for heart or heart-lung transplantation.[3]

Catheterization Procedure

Catheterization for pediatric patients with PH often requires general anesthesia. Some centers have developed strategies to avoid or minimize general anesthesia for selected patients. Anesthesia and catheter manipulations do entail risk. An earlier study reported resuscitation or death in as many as 6% of patients.[76] However, a later registry study showed that cardiac catheterization for pediatric patients with PH can be performed with few adverse events and zero mortality.[77] Zuckerman et al.[78] in 2013 reported a 5.7% complication rate, a 1.2% major complication rate, and a 0.2% mortality rate associated with cardiac catheterization for children and adults with PH. A recent study from another single center reported a 6% rate of complications but no deaths.[51] Due to potential for complications to occur during cardiac catheterization, pediatric patients with PH should undergo catheterization in tertiary care centers where cardiology and anesthesiology teams with requisite expertise and experience are available.[79] Comprehensive guidelines for cardiac catheterization of pediatric patients with PH have recently been published by the Pulmonary Vascular Research Institute, Pediatric and Congenital Heart Disease Task Forces.[75] Chest computed tomography angiography (CTA) should be considered in advance of catheterization to identify large airway, pulmonary parenchymal, and vascular anomalies and to guide catheterization planning. Furthermore, CTA may also identify patients with pulmonary venoocclusive disease or pulmonary vein stenosis in whom acute pulmonary vasoreactivity testing may lead to severe pulmonary edema (Fig. 71.4).

Diagnostic criteria for PH are mPAP of 25 mm Hg or higher, mean PCWP of less than 15 mm Hg, and PVR of 3 Wood units or higher.[80] Although these adult criteria are applied to children, it is necessary to be mindful that systemic blood pressure is typically lower in children, and therefore the adult criteria may be too strict for some children.

Cardiac catheterization allows informed decision making by quantitatively assessing acute responses to pulmonary vasodilators. Typically, baseline hemodynamic measurements (pressure, oxygen saturation, blood gas determinations, oxygen consumption measurements, and thermodilution measurements of cardiac output) are made while the patient is breathing room air or the patient's baseline fraction of inspired oxygen (FiO_2) with supplemental oxygen. The

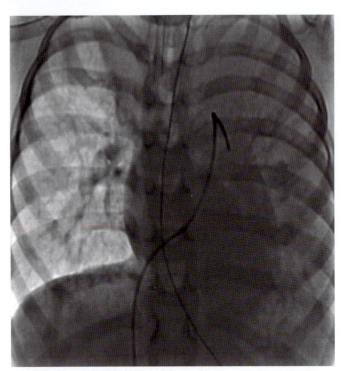

• **Figure 71.4** Unilateral pulmonary edema developed during acute pulmonary vasoreactivity testing performed in the catheterization laboratory for a child with severe pulmonary hypertension and unrecognized left common pulmonary vein stenosis. Vasoreactivity testing should be undertaken with great caution or avoided entirely in cases of pulmonary vein stenosis or pulmonary venoocclusive disease. In addition to painstaking echocardiography, meticulous computed tomographic angiography is invaluable in identifying pulmonary vein stenosis and raising suspicion for pulmonary venoocclusive disease (ground-glass opacities and interlobular septal thickening) before catheterization is undertaken. A catheter is present in the left pulmonary artery.

FiO_2 is then increased to between 0.4 and 1.0 (depending on a given practitioner or center's usual practice), and the hemodynamic measurements are repeated with this new condition. Nitric oxide in concentrations ranging between 20 and 80 ppm (depending on a given practitioner or center's practice) may then be added to the inspired oxygen, and hemodynamic measurements are repeated. Responses to other agents such as intravenous or inspired prostacyclin analogues or enteral sildenafil may be assessed in similar fashion. Important derived hemodynamic results include pulmonary and systemic blood flow indexed to body surface area and pulmonary and systemic vascular resistances also indexed to body surface area. Responsiveness to pulmonary vasodilators in pediatric patients has been defined as a decrease in mPAP of more than 20% in the setting of increased or unchanged cardiac output. In addition, responsiveness is defined as a decrease in the ratio between PVR and systemic vascular resistance. This measured responsiveness is used to identify patients who are likely to be successfully treated with calcium channel blockers (CCBs) or more selective pulmonary vasodilators.[81] Responsiveness has also been defined as decrease in mPAP by 10 to 40 mm Hg, together with an increase or no change in cardiac output.[82] These latter criteria, however, are not applicable to all children whose baseline mPAP is less than 40 mm Hg despite the presence of severe PH. Some investigators have found other measures such as pulmonary artery capacitance index to be useful in predicting survival.[83]

Beyond the assessment of the severity of PH and its responsiveness to pulmonary vasodilators, additional diagnostic information may be obtained from cardiac catheterization. First, contributions to PH by shunt lesions such as persistent foramen ovale or ASDs, VSDs, PDA, and aortopulmonary collateral arteries can be evaluated. Second, hemodynamic measurements and angiography can provide definitive information about the presence and significance of any pulmonary arterial and/or venous narrowings. Third, the presence and degree of left ventricular (LV) diastolic dysfunction can be assessed to guide further medical management. Fourth, inconclusive hemodynamic and angiographic findings can point to rare disorders such as alveolar-capillary dysplasia, pulmonary venoocclusive disease, or surfactant deficiency. Finally, serial cardiac catheterization enables assessment of progression of disease and response to therapy.

Catheter-Based Interventions for Pulmonary Hypertension

Balloon angioplasty and stent implantation are established procedures for treating pulmonary artery narrowings to improve distribution of pulmonary blood flow and reduce RSVP.[84] More daunting, however, is the management of pulmonary venous stenosis (Fig. 71.5). Although balloon angioplasty and stent implantation are regularly used as alternatives to open surgical intervention, outcomes have been mixed, with a significant proportion of patients experiencing disease progression and death despite intervention.[85,86]

A variety of shunting lesions contribute to increased pulmonary artery pressure and PVR. These include ASDs, VSDs, PDAs, and aortopulmonary collateral arteries. Many, although not all, of these lesions can be closed during cardiac catheterization procedures.

In patients in whom these shunt lesions are associated with severe PH, closure can potentially exacerbate the patient's clinical situation by removing an avenue for relief of suprasystemic pulmonary artery pressure via right-to-left shunting. Thus careful case selection of patients for intervention is necessary. For some shunts it is possible to perform temporary balloon occlusion by a balloon catheter, which then allows rapid assessment of the acute physiologic effects that closure may have before proceeding with permanent closure, either by transcatheter or surgical intervention.

Atrial septostomy is an established palliative intervention that can decompress the right ventricle and increase LV preload and cardiac output in the setting of elevated right heart pressure. Although systemic deoxygenation is a consequence of this intervention due to right-to-left shunting, the overall result may be favorable with improved clinical status, echocardiographic findings, 6-minute walk distance, functional class, and survival.[87-89]

Compared with atrial septostomy, which causes deoxygenation of blood within the left heart from the right-to-left shunt, a pulmonary artery-to-descending aorta shunt may be advantageous because it limits the supply of deoxygenated blood to the descending aorta. Thus, blood supplying the coronary and cerebral circulations typically remains well saturated. Surgical and more recently transcatheter creation of left pulmonary artery-to-descending aorta shunts (Potts shunts) has been used to decompress the pulmonary circulation. Although one small study showed a mortality of 25% to 50%,[90,91] outcomes in survivors are encouraging. In analogous fashion a small PDA may be enlarged with a stent to create a pulmonary artery-to-descending-aorta shunt.[92,93]

Some children with hemoptysis due to PH will benefit from cardiac catheterization to embolize pulmonary arterial or aortopulmonary collateral sources of bleeding. In addition, when children with PH undergo cardiac catheterization with general anesthesia

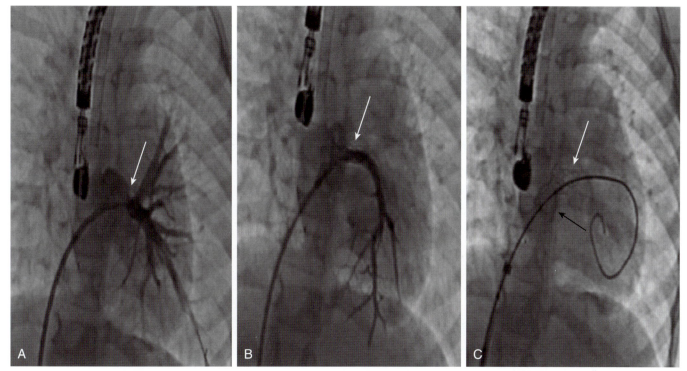

• **Figure 71.5** Stent placement in pulmonary vein stenosis. A, Contrast material introduced via a long vascular sheath filled all proximal branches of the left pulmonary venous tree and demonstrated discrete stenosis of the common vein at its junction with the left atrium *(arrow)*. The sheath was placed in the vein after a transseptal procedure was performed to enter the left atrium from the right. Extracorporeal membrane oxygenation cannulas and a transesophageal echocardiography probe are present. B, Angiography was performed in the lower left pulmonary vein after stent deployment. The caliber of the stenotic segment of the left common pulmonary vein was improved. Note that tissue from the wall of the stenotic venous segment immediately extruded through the sides of the stent to encroach upon the venous lumen *(arrow)*. C, A stent *(black arrow)* was placed in the atrial septal opening to provide a permanent route for atrial right-to-left shunting in case of persistent severe pulmonary hypertension, as well as to facilitate future interventions upon the pulmonary venous stent *(white arrow)*. The atrial septal stent was secured in position in the septum by creating in it a diabolo-like or hourglass-like shape. The guide wire is advanced across the mitral valve and curled in the left ventricle.

and remain hemodynamically stable, there can be an opportunity to perform procedures such as placement of a central venous catheter (percutaneous or tunneled); flexible bronchoscopy to evaluate for tracheobronchomalacia, look for signs of chronic aspiration, or remove mucous secretions; open lung biopsy for tissue diagnosis in suspected lung disease; or placement of a chest tube to drain a pleural effusion.

Emerging Interventions and Alternatives

Implantable hemodynamic monitoring devices that allow for ambulatory pulmonary pressure monitoring, such as the CardioMEMS HF System (St. Jude Medical, St. Paul, MN), require transcatheter placement. Such devices allow pulmonary artery pressures to be assessed in real time, and trends may be evaluated to guide management.[94]

It is recognized that sympathetic overactivation occurs in patients with PH and that increased pulmonary artery pressure is associated with pulmonary nerve stimulation. Limited experimental and clinical evidence has been published to suggest that transcatheter pulmonary artery denervation to treat PH may be beneficial.[95]

Electrical and mechanical ventricular dyssynchrony is common in pediatric patients with PH.[96] RV pacing in adult patients with

PH can lead to improved diastolic relaxation and increased stroke volume.[97] Resynchronization therapy for RV failure in PH has yet to become established as a standard strategy of treatment for PH.[98]

In conclusion, it is clear that cardiac catheterization remains an important diagnostic tool for the management of pediatric PH. It is often a valuable therapeutic tool as well. Emerging technologies will both modify the use of and increase the utility of cardiac catheterization in the care of children with PH.

Treating Children With Pulmonary Hypertension in the Intensive Care Unit

Pulmonary Hypertensive Crisis Management

Pulmonary hypertensive crisis may be defined as two or more of the following changes that occur acutely over a period of 10 minutes or less: a decline in systemic blood pressure by greater than 20% from baseline (the average blood pressure for the hour before the change); a decline in oxygen saturation to less than 90% in acyanotic patients or a decline of more than 10% in cyanotic patients in the absence of any other obvious cause; an increase in central

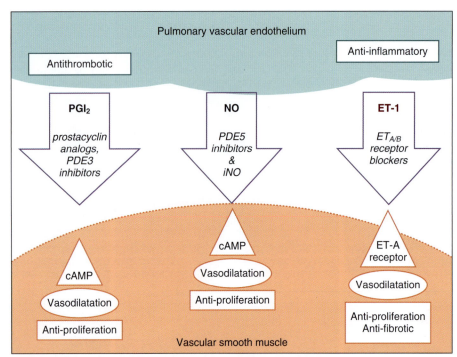

• **Figure 71.6** Targets for current therapies for PH. Schematic shows three major strategies *(arrows)* for both acute contraction state control and chronic remodeling of pulmonary vascular smooth muscle cells (SMCs). All three strategies are derived from natural products of the pulmonary endothelium cells (PECs) that are shown in bold at the tops of the arrows. Classes of therapeutic agents are shown in italics in each arrow. Principal molecular targets of each pharmacotherapeutic strategy are shown in triangles, and acute effects are shown in ellipses. Subacute and longer-term therapeutic consequences are shown in rectangles in either the vascular smooth muscle or pulmonary endothelial target tissues. PGI$_2$, or prostacyclin, is a natural PEC product that relaxes SMCs via increases in intracellular cAMP levels. Inhibitors of type 3 PDE, such as milrinone, stabilize the cAMP concentration. PECs also produce the gasotransmitter NO, which dilates SMCs by boosting cGMP levels, and these levels are buttressed by the PDE-5 inhibitors, including sildenafil. The third class of PEC products that has inspired pharmacotherapy for PH is the ET receptor antagonist group. ET-1 is a vasoconstrictor that is produced by PECs, and broad-spectrum blockers of both ET-A and ET-B type receptors, such as bosentan, decrease SMC tone. *cAMP*, Cyclic adenosine monophosphate; *cGMP*, cyclic guanosine monophosphate; *ET*, endothelin; *iNO*, inhaled nitric oxide; *NO*, nitric oxide; *NO$_2$*, nitrogen dioxide; *PDE3*, phosphodiesterase type 3A; *PDE5*, phosphodiesterase type 5A; *PEC*, pulmonary endothelium cell; *PH*, pulmonary hypertension; *sGC*, soluble guanylate cyclase. (From Collaco JM, Romer LH, Stuart BD, et al. Frontiers in pulmonary hypertension in infants and children with bronchopulmonary dysplasia. *Pediatr Pulmonol.* 2012;47[11]:1042-1053. doi:10.1002/ppul.22609.)

venous pressure (CVP) by more than 20%; and an increase or decrease in heart rate by 20% (excluding patients with epicardial pacing). Progressive worsening of PH crisis frequency and severity may be presaged by elevation of NTproBNP, but this may not be the case in an isolated episode.

The ICU management of a PH crisis requires an integrative approach that is focused on the treatment of increased PVR and its impact on RV function. Initial treatment should be the administration of oxygen due to its ease of administration, quick onset of action, and selective pulmonary vasodilation. In situations in which controlled ventilation can be performed, minute ventilation should be increased to reduce the effect of hypercarbia on PVR, while avoiding excessive positive end-expiratory pressure, high peak pressures, and long inspiratory times that may cause lung overdistention and reduce preload to a challenged RV. Furthermore, if the patient is ventilated, it is prudent to use sedation strategies to attenuate sympathetic outflow that can increase PVR. Bolus doses of sedatives are often helpful—narcotics and dexmedetomidine offer hemodynamic stability, whereas benzodiazepines and

barbiturates are more likely to have adverse effects. In addition, neuromuscular blockade can facilitate patient-ventilator synchrony and reduce PA pressure. Coexistent metabolic acidosis should be corrected because PVR is also directly related to H$^+$ concentration.[99] When such interventions do not result in resolution of the PH crisis, pharmaceutical interventions targeting PVR are necessary (Fig. 71.6).[100] As detailed earlier, agents such as prostacyclin analogues, nitric oxide (NO), and phosphodiesterase (PDE) inhibitors provide avenues for modulating PVR. When RV dysfunction persists during a PH crisis, low cardiac output may result due to decreased left heart filling and septal bowing to the left that reduces LV ejection. Ensuring adequate preload and administering inotropic support with either dopamine or epinephrine promotes forward flow of blood across the pulmonary vasculature to the left heart. Although milrinone is useful for patients with ventricular dysfunction due to PH, its long onset of action and propensity to cause hypotension limit its usefulness in an acute PH crisis. Furthermore, vasopressor support to maintain SVR and enhance coronary perfusion may be necessary to avoid RV ischemia. Vasopressin is often chosen because it increases SVR with a minimal effect on increasing PVR. If cardiac output continues to decline and/or hypoxemia persists, extracorporeal membrane oxygenation (ECMO) should be considered.

Directed Pharmacotherapy for Pulmonary Hypertension

Overall therapeutic goals in pediatric PH are to dilate and reverse the abnormal pulmonary vascular bed, restore endothelial function, and prevent PH crisis. The most common agents used to achieve this are directed at the NO, prostacyclin, and endothelin pathways. A summary of current pharmacotherapies for children with PH is shown in Table 71.2, and mechanisms of action are shown in Fig. 71.6. A discussion of each category of pulmonary vasodilators and other agents follows here.

A proposed treatment algorithm for the pharmacologic approach to pediatric PH is outlined in the 2015 American Heart Association (AHA)/American Thoracic Society (ATS) pediatric PH guidelines (Fig. 71.7).[3] Treatment options are largely extrapolated from adult data. In the algorithm, CCBs or other more specific pulmonary vasodilators may be considered in those who respond to AVT via cardiac catheterization, defined as a 20% decrease in mPAP, no change or improvement in cardiac output, or no change or decrease in PVR/SVR ratio. However, the higher potential for negative inotropic effects associated with CCBs, especially in children less than 1 year of age, limit their safety and utility in children. Furthermore, the majority of children are nonresponders to AVT, and therapy with other medications is usually required. Higher-risk patients who do not respond to AVT usually have RV dysfunction or functional limitations (see Fig. 71.7). Such patients likely need immediate parenteral prostacyclin analogue therapy with early consideration of combination therapy. On the other hand, those considered lower risk should be first started on oral agents (either a PDE-5 inhibitor or endothelin receptor antagonist). From there, additional agents should be administered to achieve specified goal-directed therapeutic targets. Atrial septostomy, palliative pulmonary-to-systemic shunts, or lung transplant should be reserved for patients with World Health Organization (WHO) functional class IV, who have progressive decline in clinical status despite maximal medical therapy.

Phosphodiesterase Type 5 Inhibitors (PDE-5 Inhibitors)

PH is often associated with disruption of endogenous NO production or activity. Normally, endothelium-derived NO activates soluble guanylate cyclase, which then stimulates production of cyclic guanosine monophosphate (cGMP) in PA smooth muscle cells, leading to vasodilation.[101-103] Within the pulmonary vascular bed, cGMP-specific PDE type 5 (PDE-5) degrades cGMP. In patients with PH this enzyme is upregulated, leading to impaired vasodilation and abnormal vascular growth and infrastructure.[103-105] PDE-5 inhibitors reduce the degradation of cGMP, preserve intracellular cGMP, augment cGMP-mediated vasodilation (via calcium uptake into the sarcoplasmic reticulum), and suppress pulmonary vascular smooth muscle proliferation.

Sildenafil is a potent and selective PDE-5 inhibitor that is most often given orally, but a parenteral formulation is available. It is approved by the US Food and Drug Administration (FDA) to treat PH in adults. All use in pediatric PH is off label. A 2012 FDA black box warning against sildenafil use in pediatric PH was

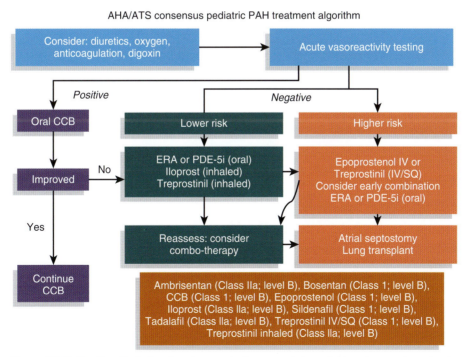

• **Figure 71.7** Algorithm illustrating the pharmacologic approach to pediatric pulmonary hypertension: *AHA,* American Heart Association; *ATS,* American Thoracic Society; *CCB,* calcium channel blocker; *ERA,* endothelin receptor antagonist; *IV,* intravenous; *PAH,* pulmonary arterial hypertension; *PDE-5i,* phosphodiesterase type 5 inhibitor; *SQ,* subcutaneous. (From Abman SH, Hansmann G, Archer SL, et al. Guidelines from the American Heart Association and American Thoracic Society. *Circulation.* 2015;132[21]:2037-2099. doi:10.1161/CIR.0000000000000329.)

TABLE 71.2 Therapeutic Agents in Pediatric Pulmonary Hypertension

Pharmacologic Pathway	Medication Class	Mechanism of Action	Therapeutic Agents	Route of Administration	Adverse Effects
	34	Mean (SD), 38.3 (1.7) weeks' GA	Comparator: MgSO$_4$ (serum level 7-11 mg/dl)	200 mg/kg IV LD then 20 mg/ kg/h to max 100 mg/kg/h; tapered and stopped in 1d when OI <15 and PAP <20	
cGMP augmentation	iNO	Via diffusion across the alveolar-capillary membrane →↑cGMP in pulmonary smooth muscle vasculature → smooth muscle relaxation	iNO	Inhaled	Methemoglobin Formation of NO$_2$
	L-Arginine	Increases endogenous NO synthesis	L-Arginine	Oral Intravenous	——
	PDE-5 inhibitors	Via PDE-5 inhibition →↑cGMP in pulmonary smooth muscle vasculature → pulmonary vasodilation and inhibition of vascular remodeling	Sildenafil

Tadalafil
Vardenafil | Oral Intravenous

Oral
Oral | Headache Flushing Dizziness Hypotension Priapism |
| cAMP augmentation | Prostacyclin analogues | Via cell-surface G-protein receptors on pulmonary endothelial cells, or platelets → ↑cAMP → pulmonary and systemic vasodilation, inhibition of vascular remodeling and inhibition of platelet aggregation | Epoprostenol

Treprostinil

Iloprost

Beraprost | Intravenous Inhaled

Intravenous
Oral
Subcutaneous

Intravenous
Inhaled

Oral | Flushing Headache Hypotension Jaw pain Thrombocytopenia Bronchospasm (Iloprost) |
	PDE-3 inhibitors	Via PDE-3 inhibition →↑cAMP in arterial smooth muscle cells and cardiac myocytes → pulmonary and systemic vasodilation and inotropy	Milrinone	Intravenous Inhaled	Hypotension Thrombocytopenia
Endothelin receptor blockade	ET-1 antagonists	Via specific competitive dual endothelin receptor A and B blockade → pulmonary vasodilation and inhibition of vascular remodeling	Bosentan	Oral	Liver toxicity Anemia Headache Flushing Nasal congestion Peripheral edema
	ET-A antagonists	Via selective endothelin receptor A blockade → pulmonary vasodilation, antiproliferation and ET-1 clearance	Ambrisentan Sitaxentan	Oral	Extremity pain Teratogenicity
	Vasoactive intestinal peptide	Blocks pulmonary vasoconstriction caused by ET-1	Vasoactive intestinal peptide	——	Does not cause increased airway resistance often seen with other ET-1 antagonists
Calcium channel blockers	Calcium channel antagonists	Reduce calcium influx into vascular smooth muscle and cardiac myocytes	Nifedipine Diltiazem Amlodipine	Oral Intravenous	Negative inotropic effect Caution <1 year of age
Anticoagulation	——	Varying depending on anticoagulant selected	Heparin Coumadin Lovenox	Oral Intravenous Subcutaneous	Bleeding Unclear indications

cAMP, Cyclic adenosine monophosphate; cGMP, cyclic guanosine monophosphate; ET, endothelin; iNO, inhaled nitric oxide; NO, nitric oxide; PDE, phosphodiesterase.

later modified by the FDA, partly due to acknowledgment that its use in children is reported to be safe and efficacious.[103,106-109]

Tadalafil (Adcirca) and vardenafil are two additional PDE-5 inhibitors used in the management of PH. Compliance is likely higher with tadalafil because it has a longer half-life than sildenafil (17 versus 4 hours) and can be taken once daily, whereas sildenafil requires three doses a day. Tadalafil is well tolerated by children and produces improvement in PVR index and mPAP when transitioning from sildenafil. Vardenafil is used in adults with PH, and pediatric literature is lacking.[109-111]

As with other pulmonary vasodilators discussed here, sildenafil and other PDE inhibitors may have a role in optimizing pulmonary blood flow and heart function in children with single ventricles.[112,113]

Prostacyclin Analogues

Prostacyclin is a metabolite of arachidonic acid that is endogenously produced by the pulmonary vascular endothelium, leading to pulmonary and systemic vasodilation. It also has antiplatelet, antithrombotic, and antiproliferative activity. Prostacyclin exerts these effects by increasing cyclic adenosine monophosphate (cAMP) through stimulation of adenylate cyclase. Children with PH show decreased expression of prostacyclin synthase in their lung vasculature.[114] Prostacyclin analogues include epoprostenol, treprostinil, and iloprost, and routes of their administration include intravenous, inhalation, and subcutaneous.

Epoprostenol is FDA approved for use in adults; however, studies show chronic therapy improves survival and functional status in both adults and children with PH.[115-120] Children have improved survival with long-term intravenous infusions, with a 4-year survival of over 90%, and 10-year freedom from death, transplantation, or atrial septostomy of 37%. Side effects of epoprostenol include hypotension, flushing, jaw pain, bone pain, headaches, rashes, and thrombocytopenia.[121] Epoprostenol has a short half-life of less than 6 minutes; therefore accidental interruption of a continuous infusion can potentially lead to a rapid increase in PVR and hemodynamic collapse. This makes treatment with intravenous epoprostenol challenging in children, often mandating an indwelling central venous catheter. Placement of central venous access in children with PH has risk, both the anesthetic risk and the inherent risks of indwelling catheters, such as local and systemic infection.[122,123] Continuous inhaled formulations of epoprostenol are used in the pediatric ICU. Administration of prostacyclin analogue therapy by the inhaled route circumvents the risk of bloodstream infection, optimizes ventilation-perfusion matching, and provides an acute intervention for sudden changes in PVR.[124,125] An annotated bibliography on experience with use of these agents by inhalation is included in the online content for this chapter as Appendix 71.1.

Treprostinil is a prostacyclin analogue that is FDA approved for adults with PH by intravenous, subcutaneous, oral, and inhaled routes, and it has a longer half-life than epoprostenol, thereby providing a higher margin of safety if discontinuation occurs. Transition of pediatric PH patients as young as 3 years of age from intravenous epoprostenol to treprostinil has been quite feasible, although a higher incidence of central line–associated bloodstream infections has been noted with treprostinil.[126] The ability to administer treprostinil via continuous subcutaneous infusion pump obviates the need for long-term central access and provides a delivery system for outpatient therapy.[127] Unfortunately, this route may be irritating, limiting its usefulness for some patients. Finally, inhaled treprostinil has been administered to children via standard ICU ventilators[128] and was effective and well tolerated for vasoreactivity testing in the adult cardiac catheterization laboratory, reducing both mPAP and PVR.[129]

Iloprost is an inhaled prostacyclin analogue that also has a long half-life (20 to 30 minutes), allowing for intermittent administration every 2 to 4 hours. Unfortunately, its use is limited by frequency of administration and its propensity to cause bronchospasm in infants and children with reactive airways.[130]

Endothelin Receptor Antagonists

Endothelin-1 is a potent vasoactive peptide produced by vascular endothelium that acts via endothelin type A (ET-A) and endothelin type B (ET-B) receptors to mediate vasoconstriction and promote proliferation of smooth muscle cells. When stimulated in isolation, ET-B receptors actually mediate vasodilation via the release of both NO and prostacyclin and are antiproliferative.[131,132] Patients with PH have increased levels of circulating endothelin-1 that likely contributes to a chronic state of vasoconstriction with cellular proliferation.[5,6,133,134]

Bosentan is an orally administered, nonselective ET-A and ET-B antagonist. It is an appropriate agent for subacute and chronic therapy. It has been shown to lower both PA pressure and PVR and to improve exercise capacity and long-term outcomes in children with PH.[135-138] A retrospective study[139] showed that bosentan (either alone or in combination with prostacyclin therapy) was safe and efficacious in children (including those with CHD) treated for a median exposure length of 14 months. One- and 2-year Kaplan-Meier survival estimates were 98% and 91%, respectively. Importantly, a decline in the beneficial effect of bosentan may occur after 1 year.[140] In a 16-week multicenter, randomized, double-blind, placebo-controlled study of patients above 12 years of age with Eisenmenger syndrome (Bosentan Randomized Trial of Endothelin Antagonist Therapy-5 [BREATHE-5]), those treated with bosentan had good tolerance, increased exercise capacity, reduced mPAP, and improved hemodynamics.[141] Furthermore, bosentan was well tolerated with improved PA pressures, ventricular systolic function, and functional class in both a child with elevated PVR following bidirectional cavopulmonary anastomosis and in adults with Fontan circulation and diminished exercise capacity.[142]

Bosentan may cause dose-dependent liver dysfunction. Elevation in levels of aminotransferases was found in 7.8% of children 12 years of age or older and in 2.7% of those younger than 12 years of age. Most abnormalities occurred within 5 months of starting therapy, and most were less than five times the upper limit of normal.[143] Fortunately, increases in levels of aminotransferases decrease in most patients without further sequelae after dose modification or discontinuation of bosentan. Many pediatric centers monitor liver function tests monthly in patients on endothelin receptor antagonists.

In September 2017, bosentan received US FDA approval for use in pediatric patients 3 years of age or older with idiopathic diseased or CHD associated PH. With this approval, bosentan became the first FDA-approved medicine for pediatric PH in the United States.

Selective oral ET-A receptor antagonists, such as ambrisentan (Letairis), block the vasoconstrictor effect of ET-A stimulation while maintaining the vasodilator benefits of ET-B. Compared with bosentan, ambrisentan causes less liver dysfunction and requires only once-daily dosing (versus twice daily for bosentan). In a single-center, retrospective study of children above 12 years of age with PH in the setting of CHD, ambrisentan therapy was associated with improvement in exercise capacity, arterial oxygen saturation, functional class, and hemoglobin level.[144] A more recent study of children (mean age of 11 years) taking ambrisentan showed improved mPAP, improved functional class, and minimal adverse effects (including an absence of aminotransferase abnormalities).[145] Ambrisentan has been shown to be safe when used in combination with sildenafil, and dose adjustment is not necessary for either drug when given in combination.[146]

Finally, for both bosentan and ambrisentan, concern exists regarding teratogenicity and reduction in the effectiveness of oral contraceptives. Therefore caution and full disclosure should be made when deciding to administer either drug to females of reproductive age.

Combination Therapy

Because PH may involve dysregulation of multiple molecular pathways, combination therapy has considerable appeal, as compared with monotherapy. Indeed, a recent study of 275 pediatric PH patients at centers in Denver, New York, and the Netherlands demonstrated improved 5-year survival with combination versus monotherapy.[147] Forty-two percent of these patients had CHD. Closer study and clearer definition of optimal combination PH for children with CHD is needed.[3,5] Drug interactions are important considerations when using combined therapy regimens. For example, sildenafil and bosentan may each affect the other's plasma concentration, and this necessitates close monitoring and appropriate dose adjustments.[147a] Further studies are needed to determine whether initial treatment of PH should begin with combination or monotherapy in order to achieve optimal outcomes.

Inhaled Nitric Oxide

When pulmonary vasodilators are administered acutely for PH, inhaled nitric oxide (iNO) is generally considered first line, especially in PPHN. iNO bypasses the pulmonary vascular endothelium and diffuses into pulmonary vascular smooth muscle cells, where it activates guanylate cyclase, increases cGMP concentrations in pulmonary smooth muscle cells, and increases calcium uptake by sarcoplasmic reticulum. This causes muscle relaxation, reduced PA pressure, and decreased PVR.[148] iNO that is absorbed from the lungs into the systemic circulation is quickly deactivated within the red blood cells, thereby minimizing systemic effects.[149-151]

Early use of iNO in newborns with PPHN may result in improvement in oxygenation and a reduced need for ECMO,[152] but this salutary effect may not be sustained. iNO has been used with or without oxygen to test pulmonary vascular reactivity during cardiac catheterization.[153] Nitric oxide may also be used to optimize the postanesthetic course in children following congenital heart surgery or ventricular assist device (VAD) placement[154] because elevated PAP may impair ventricular performance following cardiopulmonary bypass or VAD placement. The most recent Cochrane systematic review of iNO for postoperative management of PH in infants and children with CHD was published in 2014 and evaluated both physiologic changes and short-term clinical outcomes. As compared with control patients who received conventional therapy without iNO, no difference in mortality, mPAP, heart rate, or $PaO_2:FiO_2$ ratio was seen in the iNO group.[155] Methemoglobin did rise in the iNO treatment group. One randomized study of iNO versus standard care did not demonstrate differences in the incidence of PH crisis in the immediate postoperative period

following congenital heart surgery.[156] Therefore it is reasonable to use iNO on a case-by-case basis when RV dysfunction due to reactive PVR is suspected, and it should be discontinued if no beneficial effect is observed.

iNO is an inorganic gas, and there is no concern for bronchospasm with administration, unlike other inhaled pulmonary vasodilators, which are aerosolized solutions. INOmax (Mallinckrodt Pharmaceuticals, Dublin, Ireland) is the exclusive medical delivery system used. It allows administration either through an endotracheal tube or noninvasively by continuous positive pressure (i.e., continuous positive airway pressure, biphasic positive airway pressure [BiPAP], synchronized inspiratory positive airway pressure), standard nasal cannula, or heated humidified nasal cannula.

Clinically significant rebound PH can occur following withdrawal of iNO, resulting in hypoxemia and RV dysfunction that compromises cardiac output. This is believed to be due to negative feedback inhibition of endogenous NO synthase activity with iNO administration, leading to low levels of endogenous NO and cGMP and rebound PH with abrupt iNO withdrawal. Use of PDE-5 inhibitors (or perhaps endothelin receptor blockers) may reduce the incidence of this rebound PH.[103,106,157,158]

Phosphodiesterase Type 3 Inhibitor (PDE-3 Inhibitor)

Milrinone, a PDE-3 inhibitor, prevents the breakdown of cAMP in both cardiac and vascular smooth muscle cells. Its effects include ventricular inotropy and lusitropy, as well as pulmonary and systemic vasodilation. It is therefore useful for patients with ventricular dysfunction due to PH. Unfortunately, intravenous administration may cause hypotension that may persist for hours after cessation of its use, handicapping its utility. Alternatively, inhaled milrinone can selectivity dilate pulmonary vessels and improve ventilation/perfusion matching without unwanted effects on SVR.[159]

Anticoagulation

As stated in recently published consensus guidelines (AHA/ATS), the role of anticoagulation in primary PH therapy is not straightforward.[3] Implementation may therefore be limited to those scenarios that are complicated by secondary issues that warrant modulation of coagulation function, including chronic indwelling catheters in the setting of low cardiac output.

Transitions to Home Care With Pulmonary Hypertension

A multidisciplinary discharge planning process is needed for children with PH. Insights from nurses, pharmacists, social workers, and physicians must be integrated into a care plan that balances multiple priorities: the needs of the growing and developing infant or child; life-sustaining and expensive complex medical therapies; and the physical, psychologic, and financial well-being of the family. For some families the therapies will be too complex to incorporate into home life, and this may mean that the child needs to remain in a subacute care center for a prolonged stay. In any setting, developing a schedule that allows for sleep, playtime, and school time while complying with various therapies is challenging but essential.

Insurance companies and specialty pharmacies are the gatekeepers that control the availability of many PH medications. Case managers and nurse practitioners help the patient and health care team navigate the multiple prior authorization, enrollment, consent, and referral forms. WHO classification group,[3] WHO or NYHA functional classification, and diagnostic data are often required for requisite paperwork.[160] Restrictions to specific patient ages or categories of PH are common. Some medications can be filled at local pharmacies, but many PHTN medications are obtained exclusively through specialty pharmacies. Liquid suspensions may require extra time for preparation or procurement and may increase the cost. Despite the best planning, hospital discharge may be delayed by awaiting insurance authorization and by medication preparation and delivery. Experienced personnel may facilitate priority handling, anticipation of appeals for insurance denials with review boards or physician-to-physician peers, prior authorizations, and communications with pharmaceutical companies for assistance with unanticipated out-of-pocket copayments.

Sildenafil for PH therapy is available in 20-mg tablets or a powder that may be reconstituted into a 10 mg/mL suspension that may be quite costly. Cost and 60-day expiration date after reconstitution may prompt pharmacies to dispense large minimum volumes, causing increased cost and waste. Tadalafil is dosed once daily and may be a good option for adolescents. Common side effects of PDE-5 inhibitors include headache, nosebleeds, muscle pain, nausea, flushing, and stuffy nose and should be discussed with the health care team at routine clinic appointments. Sudden vision loss, hearing loss, priapism longer than 6 hours, and syncope are serious side effects that require immediate evaluation. Some institutions require patients or guardians to sign informed consent forms before dispensing sildenafil to children.

The recent approval of Tracleer (bosentan) for use in children from the age of 3 years and upward will have a positive impact on the formulation and availability of this medication for pediatric use.[161] Tracleer requires prior authorization from the insurance company, as well as completion of enrollment and consent forms. Due to the risk of hepatotoxicity, patients must agree to have monthly liver function testing. Teratogenicity risk dictates that women with reproductive potential must use contraception and have monthly pregnancy testing. Access to Tracleer may take as long as 1 week following insurance, enrollment, and consent procedures and also requires both a mail order specialty pharmacy that is certified in the Tracleer REMS Program and prescribers who are enrolled in this program. Each month's shipment is contingent upon availability of the requisite laboratory results. Tracleer is available in 62.5-mg and 125-mg sizes, and a new 32-mg "cloverleaf" design is intended to improve dosage accuracy for smaller patients. Macitentan (Opsumit) and ambrisentan are dosed daily and are useful for older teenagers and adults.

Compact, lightweight ambulatory infusion pumps are used for outpatient delivery of subcutaneous or intravenous prostacyclin analogues. These pumps are different from hospital infusion pumps. Specialty pharmacies often send nurses to the bedside to teach the health care team as well as the patient and family how to operate the pumps. Inhaled treprostinil modalities, including Tyvaso, and iloprost (Ventavis) may be options for the older child or adolescent.

At the time of discharge, many patients are on combination therapy, including supplemental oxygen, oral medications, and continuous infusions. Routine outpatient follow-up may be with interdisciplinary pediatric cardiology, pulmonary, and PH teams. Periodic monitoring will likely include serial echocardiograms to assess RV function and hypertrophy and to estimate pulmonary artery pressure, NTproBNP and serum chemistries, and sequential 6-minute walk and pulmonary function tests for older children.

Cardiac catheterizations may be done to assess the hemodynamic effects of the medical therapy and disease progression.

Continuity outpatient pediatric care is also essential for PH patients with CHD following hospital discharge. Patients with PH are at increased risk for adverse events with intercurrent viral respiratory infections, and yearly influenza vaccinations for the patient and immediate household members are needed. Infants with PH and CHD may also meet criteria to receive monthly palivizumab (Synagis) injections during RSV season.[162,163]

Working Toward the Future

An Acute Need for Change

Despite substantial progress in PH therapy for children with CHD, there is an urgent need for new therapeutic targets and strategies for patients of all ages and causes of PH.[164] Nearly exclusive focus on vasodilator development to date has contributed to an evolving crisis in this field due to high costs of medications, incomplete responses to treatment, and the persistent reality of refractory disease progression for many patients despite vasodilator medicines. These issues have prompted the PH community to focus on genetic and epigenetic control of inflammation, aberrant growth control, and other sources of cellular dysfunction in the pulmonary circulation.[165,166] Other environmental stressors have been implicated in the pathogenesis of PH, including altered estrogen metabolism, mitogen exposure, and oxidative stress.[167-171] This section focuses on strategic directions in the PH research agenda (Fig. 71.8).

Animal Models of Pulmonary Hypertension

Although animal models of PH have been sources of substantial insights into pathophysiology and potential therapeutics, no model is able to fully recapitulate the heterogeneity and nuances that are found in the spectrum of human PH.[172,173] Current animal models range from transgenic mice to large mammal ungulates, with each model generally recapitulating one of the main histologic or molecular features of PH. After early studies documented pulmonary vascular changes in large animals to chronic hypoxia at elevation, laboratory rats were observed to develop pulmonary vascular remodeling and RV hypertrophy after exposure to chronic hypoxia[174,175] and have become the preferred mammalian platform for PH disease modeling and for therapeutic trials.[176-180] Monocrotaline (a pyrrolizidine alkaloid that is damaging to pulmonary endothelial cells) or Sugen 5416 (a vascular endothelial growth factor receptor inhibitor causing occlusive neointimal lesions) have been used by themselves or in combination with hypoxia to recapitulate many histopathologic features of PH.[181-184]

Medium-size animals, like sheep and pigs, allow for anastomoses (such as subclavian artery to pulmonary artery connections) that mimic pulmonary overcirculation via systemic-to-pulmonary shunts with resultant medial hypertrophy, smooth muscle cell proliferation, and small artery obliteration in the lung microcirculation.[185,186] Pig and primate models of PH associated with chronic thromboembolic disease allow for the studies of clot resolution, hemodynamics, and cell signaling in obstructed and unobstructed regions of the lung.[187]

Pediatric-specific models of PH that are relevant to CHD include those with left-to-right shunting or developmental lung abnormalities. In utero aortopulmonary anastomoses have been accomplished in fetal lambs to induce shunting with evidence of increased pulmonary artery pressure and chronic vascular remodeling.[188,189] Models of congenital diaphragmatic hernia include surgical creation

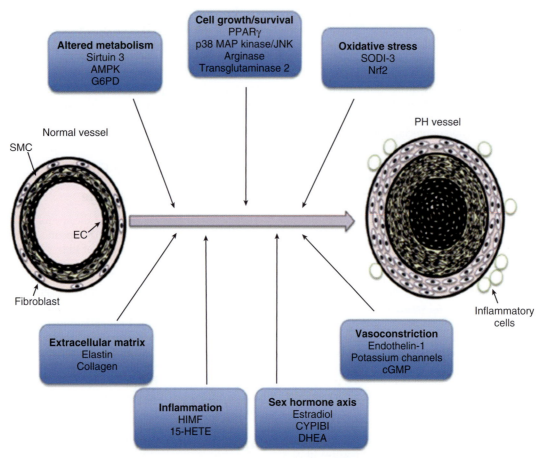

• **Figure 71.8** Overview of mechanisms contributing to pulmonary hypertension. Pulmonary hypertension is characterized by remodeling of all layers of the pulmonary vasculature, including endothelial cells (ECs), smooth muscle cells (SMCs), and fibroblasts, resulting in vascular wall thickening and occlusion of the lumen, which play roles of varied prominence depending on the cause of disease. In addition, recruitment of inflammatory cells contributes to the remodeling process. Included here are several of the pathogenic mechanisms that are highlighted in this review of recent progress in the field. *AMPK,* AMP-activated protein kinase; *cGMP,* cyclic guanosine monophosphate; *CYP1B1,* cytochrome P450 1B1; *DHEA,* dehydroepiandrosterone; *G6PD,* glucose-6-phosphate dehydrogenase; *15-HETE,* 15 hydroxyeicosatetraenoic acid; *HIMF,* hypoxia-induced mitogenic factor; *JNK,* c-Jun NH2-terminal kinase; *Nrf2,* nuclear factor E2-related factor 2; *PPARγ,* peroxisome proliferator-activated receptor-gamma; *SOD 1-3,* superoxide dismutase. (From Huetsch JC, Suresh K, Bernier M, et al. Update on novel targets and potential treatment avenues in pulmonary hypertension. *Am J Physiol Lung Cell Mol Physiol.* 2016;311[5]:L811-L31. doi:10.1152/ajplung.00302.2016.)

of diaphragmatic defects, genetic knockouts such as *Wt1, Slit3,* or *Lox,* and teratogens such as nitrofen and retinoids.[190-192] However, none of these provides an adequate model of the combination of pulmonary vascular and parenchymal hypoplasia that is seen in the clinical setting.[193] PPHN has been modeled in fetal and newborn sheep via surgical or pharmacologic constriction of the ductus arteriosus with increases in vascular smooth muscle density.[194,195] Mouse models of bronchopulmonary dysplasia are induced via short-term exposures to either neonatal hyperoxia or hypoxia, fetal hypoxia, or serial exposures to fetal hypoxia and then postnatal hyperoxia, with resultant changes in the vascular relaxation and rarefaction of the microvasculature with increases in smooth muscle cell markers.[171,196] Models of familial hereditary PH causes include *Bmpr2* knockout mice that allow for further study of molecular etiologic mechanisms of PH.[197,198]

Efforts continue to develop animal models that are conducive to trials of chronic therapies and better understanding of the reversibility of histologic changes in the microvascular.

Molecular Models

Understanding molecular pathways that lead to maladaptive remodeling of the pulmonary vasculature in the setting of inflammation, fibrosis, evolution of plexiform lesions, mitochondrial dysfunction, and altered endothelial proliferation with abnormal apoptosis may lead to new avenues for therapies that halt or even reverse disease.[171,199]

Several intriguing molecular targets have been targeted as triggers of these abnormal signaling cascades. The *BMPR2* pathway is known to involve altered angiogenesis, endothelial cell proliferation, and inflammatory cell recruitment.[200] Female sex hormone imbalances have been implicated in abnormal energy metabolism in the pulmonary vasculature.[200,201] Mitogen-activated protein kinase is integral to cell proliferation and motility, and abnormalities can lead to an oncologic-like phenotype of uncontrolled cell growth in the vascular wall. The renin-angiotensin-aldosterone system, Rho-kinase, transforming growth factor beta, platelet-derived growth factor, and peroxisome proliferator-activator receptors have each been implicated in the pathogenesis of PH.[202] Endothelial-to-mesenchymal transition is a process that involves loss of endothelial markers, expression of mesenchymal markers, loss of barrier function, and increased cell migration[203] and may contribute to microvasculopathy in childhood PH.

Biomimetic Models of the Pulmonary Vasculature

Tissue-engineered vascular models allow for the creation of bio-mimetic vessels in which tissue-level physiology and heterotypic cellular interactions between endothelium and vascular smooth muscle may be studied.[204,205] Some proposed vessel constructs incorporate microfluidics[206] and allow for study of relationships between cell form and function.[207] Some organ-on-a-chip devices simulate in vivo environments and allow manipulations of various environmental factors.[208] These three-dimensional systems may also serve for pharmaceutical development and toxicity testing[209] and provide great promise for new frontiers in PH therapeutics.

Summary

Pulmonary hypertension (PH) is a syndrome with formidable impact on both perioperative and longitudinal outcomes in CHD. Definition and control of PH have been important and lifesaving developments in the care of children with heart disease. This chapter encompasses some of the conceptual basis and practical guidelines for current approaches to this challenging problem, with a look at new developments that will redound to changes in bedside management.

The multidisciplinary author team for this chapter posit that concerted and well-coordinated interdisciplinary efforts are needed for the optimal care of these children. Communication and clinical pathway development are central to this effort and must integrate input from all of the following: pediatric cardiologists with longitudinal data on the patient's course, with noninvasive diagnostics, and with interventional skills; congenital heart surgeons; cardiology and ICU nursing; social services; pediatric cardiac anesthesiologists; and pediatric intensivists. Anticipated continued rapid changes and improvement in the diagnostic and therapeutic tools for children with CHD and PH will build on these foundations of multidisciplinary collaboration.

Acknowledgments

The authors of this chapter appreciate the efforts of Gabrielle Fink with manuscript preparation.

Selected References

A complete list of references is available at ExpertConsult.com.

3. Abman SH, Hansmann G, Archer SL, Ivy DD, Adatia I, Chung WK, et al. Pediatric pulmonary hypertension: guidelines from the American Heart Association and American Thoracic Society. *Circulation*. 2015;132(21):2037–2099. doi:10.1161/CIR.0000000000000329. PubMed PMID: 26534956.

12. Galie N, Torbicki A, Barst R, Dartevelle P, Haworth S, Higenbottam T, et al. Guidelines on diagnosis and treatment of pulmonary arterial hypertension. The Task Force on Diagnosis and Treatment of Pulmonary Arterial Hypertension of the European Society of Cardiology. *Eur Heart J*. 2004;25(24):2243–2278. doi:10.1016/j.ehj.2004.09.014. [Epub 2004/12/14]; PubMed PMID: 15589643.

23. Haworth SG. Pulmonary vascular disease in different types of congenital heart disease. Implications for interpretation of lung biopsy findings in early childhood. *Br Heart J*. 1984;52:557–571. doi:10.1136/hrt.52.5.557.

30. Landzberg MJ. Congenital heart disease associated pulmonary arterial hypertension. *Clin Chest Med*. 2007;28(1):243–253, x. doi:10.1016/j.ccm.2006.12.004. [Epub 2007/03/07]; PubMed PMID: 17338939.

47. Fang JC, DeMarco T, Givertz MM, Borlaug BA, Lewis GD, Rame JE, et al. World Health Organization Pulmonary Hypertension group 2: pulmonary hypertension due to left heart disease in the adult–a summary statement from the Pulmonary Hypertension Council of the International Society for Heart and Lung Transplantation. *J Heart Lung Transplant*. 2012;31(9):913–933. doi:10.1016/j.healun.2012.06.002. [Epub 2012/08/14]; PubMed PMID: 22884380.

50. Ivy DD, Abman SH, Barst RJ, Berger RM, Bonnet D, Fleming TR, et al. Pediatric pulmonary hypertension. *J Am Coll Cardiol*. 2013;62(suppl 25):D117–D126. doi:10.1016/j.jacc.2013.10.028. [Epub 2013/12/21]; PubMed PMID: 24355636.

51. Bobhate P, Guo L, Jain S, Haugen R, Coe JY, Cave D, et al. Cardiac catheterization in children with pulmonary hypertensive vascular disease. *Pediatr Cardiol*. 2015;36(4):873–879. doi:10.1007/s00246-015-1100-1. [Epub 2015/01/13]; PubMed PMID: 25577228.

53. Chau DF, Gangadharan M, Hartke LP, Twite MD. The post-anesthetic care of pediatric patients with pulmonary hypertension. *Semin Cardiothorac Vasc Anesth*. 2016;20(1):63–73. doi:10.1177/1089253215593179. [Epub 2015/07/03]; PubMed PMID: 26134177.

75. Del Cerro MJ, Moledina S, Haworth SG, Ivy D, Al Dabbagh M, Banjar H, et al. Cardiac catheterization in children with pulmonary hypertensive vascular disease: consensus statement from the Pulmonary Vascular Research Institute, Pediatric and Congenital Heart Disease Task Forces. *Pulm Circ*. 2016;6(1):118–125. doi:10.1086/685102. PubMed PMID: 27076908. PMCID: PMC4809667.

99. Chang AC, Zucker HA, Hickey PR, Wessel DL. Pulmonary vascular resistance in infants after cardiac surgery: role of carbon dioxide and hydrogen ion. *Crit Care Med*. 1995;23(3):568–574. [Epub 1995/03/01]; PubMed PMID: 7874911.

103. Unegbu C, Noje C, Coulson JD, Segal JB, Romer L. Pulmonary hypertension therapy and a systematic review of efficacy and safety of PDE-5 inhibitors. *Pediatrics*. 2017;139(3):doi:10.1542/peds.2016-1450. [Epub 2017/02/27]; PubMed PMID: 28235796.

115. Barst RJ, Maislin G, Fishman AP. Vasodilator therapy for primary pulmonary hypertension in children. *Circulation*. 1999;99(9):1197–1208. [Epub 1999/03/09]; PubMed PMID: 10069788.

135. Barst RJ, Ivy D, Dingemanse J, Widlitz A, Schmitt K, Doran A, et al. Pharmacokinetics, safety, and efficacy of bosentan in pediatric patients with pulmonary arterial hypertension. *Clin Pharmacol Ther*. 2003;73(4):372–382. [Epub 2003/04/24]; PubMed PMID: 12709727.

152. Roberts JD Jr, Fineman JR, Morin FC 3rd, Shaul PW, Rimar S, Schreiber MD, et al. Inhaled nitric oxide and persistent pulmonary hypertension of the newborn. The Inhaled Nitric Oxide Study Group. *N Engl J Med*. 1997;336(9):605–610. doi:10.1056/NEJM199702273360902. [Epub 1997/02/27]; PubMed PMID: 9032045.

160. Lammers AE, Adatia I, Cerro MJ, Diaz G, Freudenthal AH, Freudenthal F, et al. Functional classification of pulmonary hypertension in children: report from the PVRI pediatric taskforce, Panama 2011. *Pulm Circ*. 2011;1(2):280–285. doi:10.4103/2045-8932.83445. [Epub 2011/08/30]; PubMed PMID: 21874157. PMCID: PMC3161406.

72

Pediatric Heart Failure and Pediatric Cardiomyopathies

SCOTT I. AYDIN, MD; NIDA SIDDIQI, PHARMD; CHRISTOPHER M. JANSON, MD;
SARAH E. NORRIS, MD; GILES J. PEEK, MD; KIMBERLY D. BEDDOWS, NP;
JACQUELINE M. LAMOUR, MD; DAPHNE T. HSU, MD

Historical Perspective: Pediatric Heart Failure

The definition of heart failure has expanded over the millennia from a clinical syndrome of fluid retention and fatigue to include structural and physiologic disruptions of normal genetic, metabolic, and neurohormonal processes.[1] The Ebers Papyrus, dating from 1500 BC, contains one of the earliest descriptions of the symptoms of heart failure, including fluid retention in association with weakness of the heart, even distinguishing between pulmonary and hepatic congestion.[2] Histologic analysis performed on the lungs of a 3500-year-old Egyptian mummy showed evidence of massive intraalveolar displacement and siderosis consistent with acute decompensated heart failure with pulmonary edema and pulmonary hemorrhage.[3] A portrayal of a child with ascites and a dark discolored face can be found in a 1620 baroque painting by Giovanni Lanfranco of St. Luke, suggesting the presence of heart failure in association with a cyanotic heart lesion.[4] In 1882 John Keating[5] published an extensive description of the symptoms of dyspnea, dropsy, and palpitations in a child with ventricular dilation. Interestingly, Keating classified several distinct morphologic cardiac features associated with these symptoms as ventricular dilation, dilation with hypertrophy, or hypertrophy alone.

Causes of Pediatric Heart Failure

Currently heart failure is conceptualized as a clinical and pathophysiologic syndrome that begins with an event that causes disruption of normal myocardial function.[1,6] Although the clinical signs and symptoms of heart failure in children are similar to those seen in adults, the underlying cardiac diseases that lead to heart failure differ significantly. In an analysis of a large US database comparing pediatric and adult heart failure hospitalizations, the most common cause of heart failure in children was congenital heart disease (60% of patients), and a higher proportion of children underwent an interventional procedure to treat heart failure than in the adult cohort (60% versus 0.3%).[7] This highlights the fact that a large proportion of pediatric patients admitted with clinical heart failure have venous congestion secondary to ventricular volume overload from a left-to-right shunt or valvular regurgitation. Treatment strategies in the pediatric heart failure population with high cardiac output and normal ventricular function are directed toward surgical

or catheter intervention. The specific therapies depend on the underlying congenital heart defect and are addressed in other sections of this book. The remainder of this chapter will focus on the pediatric patient with heart failure due to primary or secondary myocardial dysfunction or a congenital heart lesion not amenable to surgical or interventional repair. Among children undergoing heart transplantation the causes of end-stage heart failure are split relatively evenly between cardiomyopathy and congenital heart disease; in the adult heart transplant population the causes of end-stage heart failure are ischemic cardiomyopathy in 35% and congenital heart disease in only 3%.[8,9] The most common underlying causes of heart failure in children are listed in Box 72.1.

Clinical Manifestations of Pediatric Heart Failure

Similar to adults, clinical heart failure in children with systolic ventricular dysfunction and a reduced ejection fraction, known as HFrEF, includes the signs and symptoms of venous congestion and/or poor perfusion and low cardiac output (Fig. 72.1). In 2003 Nohria and colleagues[10] proposed a simple algorithm to assess the clinical status of adult patients in decompensated heart failure that proved useful in directing therapy and predicting outcome. Patients were assigned to a category based on fluid status, "wet" or "dry," and peripheral perfusion, "warm" or "cold" (Fig. 72.2).

Recently there has been increasing recognition that the clinical syndrome of heart failure can also occur in the setting of a preserved ejection fraction, known as HFpEF. In heart failure with a preserved ejection fraction (HFpEF), symptoms of dyspnea and venous congestion are the result of elevated diastolic filling pressures and decreased ventricular compliance.[11] Decreased ventricular filling and a low stroke volume can lead to poor perfusion and a low cardiac output state, which manifests as poor growth and fatigue in children. In adults, HFpEF is more commonly found in older adults, patients with systemic hypertension, and in women.[12,13] HFpEF can occur in pediatric patients with hypertrophic, restrictive, or noncompaction cardiomyopathy or complex congenital heart disease such as left ventricular outflow tract obstruction.[14-22]

The management of children who successfully transition from acute decompensated heart failure to chronic compensated heart

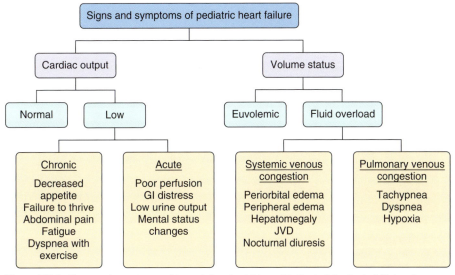

• **Figure 72.1** Signs and symptoms of heart failure in children. *GI,* Gastrointestinal; *JVD,* jugular venous distention.

• BOX 72.1   Causes of Heart Failure in Children

Systolic Heart Failure (HFrEF)

- Cardiomyopathy
  - Dilated
    Idiopathic/genetic
    Metabolic
    Ischemic
    Arrhythmogenic
    Infiltrative
    Infectious/inflammatory
    Endocrine
    Toxic (chemotherapy, cocaine)
  - Mixed cardiomyopathy
    Hypertrophic
    Restrictive
- Congenital heart disease
  - Postcardiopulmonary bypass
  - Valvular insufficiency or residual shunt
  - Outflow tract obstruction
  - Cyanosis

Diastolic Heart Failure (HFpEF)

- Cardiomyopathy
  - Hypertrophic
  - Restrictive
- Hypertension
- Congenital heart disease
  - Single-ventricle physiology
  - Shone's complex

HFrEF, Heart failure with reduced ejection fraction; HFpEF, heart failure with preserved ejection fraction.

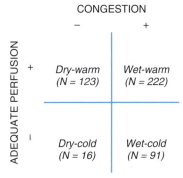

• **Figure 72.2** Classification system for heart failure symptoms. (Modified from Nohria A, Tsang SW, Fang JC, et al. Clinical assessment identifies hemodynamic profiles that predict outcomes in patients admitted with heart failure. *J Am Coll Cardiol.* 2003;41:1797-1804.)

• BOX 72.2   Ross Heart Failure Class

Ross Heart Failure Class

I   No limitations
II   Mild tachypnea or diaphoresis with feedings in infants, dyspnea at exertion in older children, no growth failure
III   Marked tachypnea or diaphoresis with feedings or exertion and prolonged feeding times with growth failure from CHF
IV   Symptomatic at rest with tachypnea, retractions, grunting, or diaphoresis

CHF, Congestive heart failure.
Modified from Ross RD, Daniels SR, Schwartz DC, et al. Plasma norepinephrine levels in infants and children with congestive heart failure. Am J Cardiol. 1987;59:911-914.

failure includes the use of tools to grade heart failure severity and quantify the impact of symptoms on the patient's health-related quality of life and functional status. In the adult heart failure population, New York Heart Association functional class or heart failure–specific quality of life questionnaires such as the Kansas City Cardiomyopathy or the Minnesota Living With Heart Failure questionnaires have been shown to be correlate with clinical outcomes.[23] Despite a lack of validation against mortality or worsening heart failure, the Ross Heart Failure Classification system (Box 72.2) has been adopted as a tool to serially monitor children less than 5 years of age[24,25] and has been used as an outcome measure in several clinical trials.[26,27]

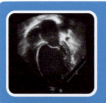

Dilated cardiomyopathy

- LV fractional shortening of EF > 2 SD below the normal mean for BSA
- LV end diastolic dimension or volume > 2 SD above normal for BSA
- Ratio of LV end-diastolic dimension to wall thickness < 0.12

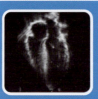

Hypertrophic cardiomyopathy

- LV posterior wall thickness at end-diastole > 2 SD above the normal mean for BSA
- Localized ventricular hypertrophy such as septal thickness > 1.5 times the LV posterior wall thickness with at least normal LV posterior wall thickness
- Concentric hypertrophy in the absence of hemodynamic cause

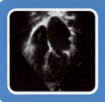

Restrictive cardiomyopathy

- One or both atria enlarged relative to ventricles of normal or small size with evidence of impaired diastolic filling and in the absence of significant valvar heart disease

• **Figure 72.3** Echocardiographic criteria used by the Pediatric Cardiomyopathy Registry to classify cardiomyopathy subtypes. *BSA,* Body surface area; *EF,* ejection fraction; *LV,* left ventricular; *SD,* standard deviation. (Modified from Grenier MA, Osganian SK, Cox GF, et al. Design and implementation of the North American Pediatric Cardiomyopathy Registry. *Am Heart J.* 2000;139:S86-S95.)

Neurohormonal Activation in Pediatric Heart Failure

In adults the recognition that chronic activation of the sympathetic nervous system and upregulation of the renin-angiotensin-aldosterone system (RAAS) in response to myocardial injury play a key role in ongoing myocardial damage revolutionized the treatment of heart failure in the early 1990s.[28-30] Neurohormonal and RAAS activation results in vasoconstriction, cardiac hypertrophy, and through alteration in collagen turnover by myofibroblasts, leads to the development of myocardial fibrosis.[31] The neurohormonal response to heart failure in children has not been as well characterized and may differ from adults, due to the difference in causes of heart failure in children. Small studies have demonstrated upregulation of the sympathetic nervous system and the RAAS in children with cardiomyopathy.[32,33] In children with dilated cardiomyopathy, serum brain natriuretic peptide (BNP) and N-terminal pro-brain natriuretic peptide (NTproBNP) levels have been shown to correlate well with the degree of heart failure, and a decrease in these levels may be a predictor of a positive response to medical therapy.[34-37] In the congenital heart disease population there has been more equivocal associations of heart failure with activation of the autonomic system and the RAAS.[38,39] Markers of neurohormonal activation and elevations in serum BNP level have been demonstrated to correlate with heart failure in patients with congenital heart disease, but the levels are often lower compared to patients with cardiomyopathy.[38,40] In children with single ventricle and heart failure, absolute BNP and NTproBNP levels were lower than those seen in adults and children with dilated cardiomyopathy; however, higher BNP and NTproBNP levels were associated with worse outcome.[40-42]

Pediatric Cardiomyopathies and Heart Failure

In 1980 the World Health Organization (WHO) classified cardiomyopathy subtypes largely based on morphology.[43] Since its inception in 1995 the National Institutes of Health (NIH)-funded Pediatric Cardiomyopathy Registry has used echocardiography for case definition for hypertrophic, dilated, noncompaction, and restrictive cardiomyopathy (Fig. 72.3).[44-49] More recently, revisions to the WHO classification system have been proposed by the European Society of Cardiology and the American Heart Association in an effort to formulate a more comprehensive approach designed to include genetic and pathophysiologic characteristics that span across the morphologic classes.[50-52] Although these efforts are broader in scope, a primarily morphologic classification continues to be the most commonly applied approach in the clinical setting.

Primary pediatric cardiomyopathy is a rare disease, occurring in 1.1 to 1.2 per 100,000 children.[45,53] The incidence of pediatric cardiomyopathy has been estimated by studies across the world to be 0.75 to 1.3 per 100,000 children.[45,53,54] Dilated and hypertrophic cardiomyopathy are the most common subtypes with annual incidences of 0.3 to 0.7 per 100,000 and 0.2 to 0.5 per 100,000, respectively.[45,53,54] Genetic testing has become more accepted in this population, and the importance of mutations in genes controlling the sarcomere, cytoskeleton, desmosome, and metabolic pathways is being increasingly recognized.[55-59]

Viral myocarditis is an important cause of pediatric cardiomyopathy and heart failure in children. Establishing the diagnosis of myocarditis is of great importance because the rate of recovery of normal function is high, even in patients who present with severe decompensated heart failure.[60-65] Acquired cardiomyopathies are also an important cause of heart failure in children (see Box 72.1). These include cardiomyopathy secondary to tachyarrhythmias, (e.g., ectopic atrial tachycardia), volume or pressure overload lesions such as left-to-right shunts or valvar stenosis or regurgitation, and coronary ischemic events due to Kawasaki disease or anomalous origin of the coronary arteries. Acquired cardiomyopathies can also occur due to an infectious, endocrinologic, or toxic insult. The most common example of a toxin-induced cardiomyopathy is the cardiomyopathy that can occur after the use of chemotherapeutic agents such as anthracycline.[66]

The incidence of heart failure differs significantly among the subtypes of cardiomyopathy. In children with dilated cardiomyopathy, heart failure is the presenting finding in 70% to 90%, whereas only 9% to 28% of hypertrophic cardiomyopathy patients present with heart failure.[45,53] Patients with hypertrophic or restrictive cardiomyopathy can present with HFpEF or HFrEF. In HFpEF cases, heart failure symptoms result from increased venous congestion due to decreased ventricular compliance and left atrial hypertension.[21,67-71] Patients with a mixed type of cardiomyopathy (hypertrophic/dilated, noncompaction/dilated, restrictive/dilated) may have symptoms of both HFrEF and HFpEF due to a higher ventricular filling pressure than expected in the presence of systolic dysfunction.[45]

Dilated Cardiomyopathy

Dilated cardiomyopathy typically affects the left ventricle but may be bilateral and is characterized by ventricular dilation and impaired systolic function (Fig. 72.3). Mitral insufficiency may be present secondary to dilation of the valve annulus.

Clinical Presentation. Infants and children with dilated cardiomyopathy most often present with signs of biventricular congestive heart failure. Manifestations of heart failure in infants include respiratory distress with tachypnea, retractions, and grunting. Poor feeding and failure to thrive by weight criteria with relative preservation of length often occurs. In the older child, clinical signs of pulmonary edema are often present, and gastrointestinal complaints are common.[72] Cardiomyopathies associated with an inborn error of metabolism can appear as congestive heart failure as metabolic demand outstrips supply or as toxic metabolites accumulate. Infants with these disorders can have associated hypoglycemia, metabolic acidosis, and/or encephalopathy.[73]

Physical Examination. On physical examination, signs of congestive heart failure include pulmonary edema, hepatomegaly, and poor peripheral perfusion. Cardiac findings include tachycardia, pulsus alternans, distant heart tones, an S_3 gallop, and often a murmur of mitral regurgitation. Jugular venous distention is uncommonly observed in the infant but is a useful indicator of central venous hypertension in the older child. Failure to thrive is common in patients with long-standing cardiomyopathy. Neurologic abnormalities, including hypotonia and generalized muscle weakness, are important findings leading to the diagnosis of cardiomyopathy associated with inborn errors of metabolism.

Cardiac Evaluation. Electrocardiography typically demonstrates increased left ventricular forces, flattening or inversion of the ST-T waves, and atrial enlargement. Low-voltage R waves and elevated ST-T segments are more characteristic of myocarditis .If there an anomalous left coronary artery originating from the pulmonary artery or another rare coronary obstructive lesion, the electrocardiogram may have evidence of myocardial ischemia. The electrocardiogram is an important diagnostic tool that can diagnose the presence of a tachyarrhythmia, such as permanent junctional reciprocating tachycardia, ectopic atrial tachycardia, or junctional tachycardia, that may result in ventricular dysfunction.

Chest radiography often shows pulmonary venous congestion and cardiomegaly. Congestive heart failure can be exacerbated by infectious respiratory disease, and the chest radiograph is essential in diagnosing these processes, including pneumonia. Atelectasis, particularly of the left lower lobe, is commonly seen in severe cardiomyopathy because of compression of the left bronchus.

Echocardiography allows the quantitative determination of ventricular volume and function, both systolic and diastolic. It is essential to rule out anatomic causes of ventricular dysfunction, such as left ventricular outflow tract obstruction, coarctation, primary valvular disease, or coronary artery anomalies. The severity of atrioventricular valve regurgitation can be determined by using color flow Doppler. If tricuspid regurgitation is present, continuous wave Doppler of the jet allows estimation of pulmonary artery pressure. Thrombi secondary to low cardiac flow may be seen most commonly in the left ventricular apex and in the left atrial appendage.

Cardiac magnetic resonance imaging (MRI) has been used in adult dilated cardiomyopathy to evaluate the degree of myocardial fibrosis.[74]

Exercise stress testing with determination of maximal oxygen consumption has been shown to be useful in the prediction of 1-year survival in adult patients with dilated cardiomyopathy. An oxygen consumption of less than 15 mL/kg/min is associated with a poorer 1-year survival.[75] Although these data have not been validated in children, exercise testing is recommended in the evaluation of the older child with dilated cardiomyopathy being considered for heart transplantation.[76]

Cardiac catheterization is not routinely performed to establish the diagnosis of dilated cardiomyopathy. If anatomic abnormalities such as anomalous left coronary artery or aortic coarctation cannot be reliably excluded with noninvasive imaging, coronary angiography and aortography should be performed. Hemodynamic measurements such as cardiac output, ventricular filling pressures, and pulmonary vascular resistance may be helpful in determining both the effectiveness of therapy and the long-term prognosis. When significant ventricular outflow tract obstruction or valvular insufficiency is found, hemodynamic measurements may help to determine the relative contribution of the associated lesions to the heart failure syndrome. Endomyocardial biopsy may show distinctive histologic or ultrastructural findings that may be helpful in diagnosing myocarditis or certain metabolic diseases. However, myocardial biopsy may have only 60% sensitivity in detecting myocarditis, even when multiple biopsy specimens are obtained, because of the focal nature of myocardial involvement. Demonstration of myocardial fibrosis may indicate a worse prognosis.[77]

Hypertrophic Cardiomyopathy

Hypertrophic cardiomyopathy is characterized by myocardial hypertrophy of the left and/or right ventricle (Fig. 72.3). Tremendous heterogeneity exists in morphology, natural history, and the functional course of hypertrophic cardiomyopathy. Hypertrophic cardiomyopathy may involve either ventricle alone or together. The most common form of hypertrophy is asymmetric, involving the interventricular septum; however, concentric hypertrophy also occurs. Disease severity and symptoms, in particular, obstruction to ventricular outflow and myocardial ischemia, are related, although not consistently, to the extent and location of the hypertrophy. Systolic ventricular function is normal or hyperdynamic until later phases of the disease. Obstruction to left or right ventricular outflow is common because of septal hypertrophy and the presence of systolic anterior motion of the mitral valve. The anterior mitral leaflet is pulled anteriorly by the Venturi effect during early systole, making contact with the septum and exacerbating subaortic obstruction. Repeated contact between the anterior leaflet and the septum may result in extensive leaflet fibrosis and further dysfunction.

Clinical Presentation. Significant heterogeneity exists in morphology, natural history, and the functional course of hypertrophic cardiomyopathy, and heart failure is rarely the presenting symptom in children with hypertrophic cardiomyopathy.[78] The presenting finding of hypertrophic cardiomyopathy in children may be a murmur of outflow tract obstruction or an electrocardiogram with abnormal findings. Diastolic dysfunction in hypertrophic cardiomyopathy results from decreased ventricular compliance because of increased wall tone, decreased chamber volume, and myocardial fibrosis. Diastolic ventricular pressure is increased, and the volume of filling is reduced, leading to symptoms of dyspnea, angina, presyncope or syncope on exertion due to systemic and pulmonary venous congestion, and low cardiac output.

Physical Examination. *Clinical findings* in children with hypertrophic cardiomyopathy can be subtle. Patients with no obstruction to outflow will have no murmur or faint systolic murmurs appreciated at the apex. Patients with latent obstruction have a grade I or II/VI systolic apical murmur that increases to grade III/VI with provocation (e.g., Valsalva maneuver, assuming the upright posture, systemic hypotension) Patients with obstruction at rest will have a grade III to IV/VI murmur that radiates to the left sternal border and the axilla, reflecting the obstruction to flow and mitral regurgitation. Right ventricular involvement in hypertrophic cardiomyopathy may be difficult to detect, especially in the infant or young child. In the older child a prominent A wave in the jugular venous pulse may be found.

Cardiac Evaluation. *Electrocardiography* often shows abnormal findings in patients with hypertrophic cardiomyopathy, with the most common finding being that of left ventricular hypertrophy with or without a strain pattern. Signs of right ventricular hypertrophy may be appreciated in patients with prominent right ventricular or septal involvement. The QRS axis may be abnormal. Abnormal Q waves mimicking myocardial infarction are sometimes present. These reflect the increased forces of the hypertrophied septum.

Holter monitoring is used routinely to determine the presence of associated dysrhythmias and to assess the risk for malignant arrhythmias.

Chest radiography results are often normal. Radiographic findings can include left ventricular, left atrial, or right atrial enlargement. Additional findings may include pulmonary vascular congestion and a bulge along the left heart border, reflecting anterior extension of septal hypertrophy.

Transthoracic echocardiography is the most common modality used to establish the diagnosis of hypertrophic cardiomyopathy (see Fig. 72.3). The echocardiogram can determine the extent and location of the hypertrophy, the pressure gradient across the outflow tracts, and the degree of systolic and diastolic dysfunction. In addition, the severity and direction of mitral regurgitation can be estimated, and associated mitral valve abnormalities can be detected. Other noninvasive modalities

such as cardiac MRI may be useful to identify patients at risk for sudden death.[79]

Cardiac catheterization and invasive studies are rarely necessary but may be indicated in selected cases to evaluate the degree of ventricular outflow obstruction. Catheterization also is performed in a therapeutic intervention such as alcohol septal ablation or for the investigation of end-stage disease as part of the evaluation for cardiac transplantation. Invasive electrophysiologic studies have been used to provoke malignant arrhythmias and to guide antiarrhythmic therapy.

Restrictive Cardiomyopathy

Restrictive cardiomyopathy is a rare form of pediatric cardiomyopathy characterized by diastolic ventricular dysfunction in the face of relatively preserved systolic function and normal wall thickness. Markedly elevated diastolic filling pressures and low cardiac output are the hemodynamic hallmarks of the disease. Atrial enlargement is often present along with elevated atrial and ventricular end-diastolic pressures. The differential diagnosis of restrictive physiology includes secondary causes of diastolic dysfunction, such as constrictive pericarditis, myocarditis with associated myocardial fibrosis, coronary artery disease, and conditions increasing left ventricular mass such as left ventricular outflow tract obstruction or systemic hypertension. Systemic diseases or treatments can cause a restrictive cardiac physiology because of infiltration or injury. These include amyloid heart disease, scleroderma, doxorubicin (Adriamycin) or radiation, infiltrating neoplasms, and hemochromatosis.

Clinical Presentation. The clinical presentation of the patient with restrictive cardiomyopathy is often subtle because of the indolent nature of diastolic dysfunction. In small children, low cardiac output is manifested by growth failure or exercise intolerance. Acute pulmonary edema is rare; however, evidence of chronic systemic or pulmonary venous congestion is common. Systemic venous hypertension leads to ascites, peripheral edema, and hepatomegaly. Resting tachypnea and dyspnea on exertion also are common; in addition, a dry cough may be described in older children. Syncope also may be a presenting sign and carries a higher risk of death than do other presenting signs and symptoms.[80]

Arrhythmias are a common presenting sign of restrictive cardiomyopathy. Marked atrial dilation occurs in association with the elevated ventricular filling pressures and can lead to atrial flutter or fibrillation or supraventricular tachycardia. Complete heart block has been described in patients with desmin cardiomyopathy.[81] Ventricular arrhythmias are less common but may occur, especially in the setting of depressed ventricular function. Atrial thrombi can form secondary to atrial dilation or atrial arrhythmias or both, and a thromboembolic event can be the presenting sign of restrictive cardiomyopathy.

Physical Examination. Findings on physical examination include generalized growth failure, often with short stature, in conjunction with poor weight gain. Evidence of "right heart failure" is common, including hepatomegaly, jugular venous distention, and ascites. Borderline systemic hypotension can be present in advanced disease. The cardiac examination results can be unremarkable. An S_3 or S_4 may be audible; the P_2 may be accentuated in the setting of significant pulmonary hypertension. A murmur of tricuspid insufficiency may be present. A prominent apical impulse can be felt.

Cardiac Evaluation. *Electrocardiography* is characterized by biatrial enlargement. Nonspecific ST-T wave changes may be noted. In the setting of pulmonary hypertension, right ventricular enlargement may be present. The electrocardiogram is essential to making the diagnosis of atrial arrhythmias or heart block associated with restrictive cardiomyopathy.

Echocardiography reveals prominent atrial enlargement with normal or even mildly reduced ventricular dimensions (see Fig. 72.3). The atrial four-chamber view is distinctive, and the appearance analogous to a "mushroom," with the ventricle reassembling the stalk and the atrium, the cap. The hepatic veins and inferior vena cava are frequently quite dilated, reflecting elevated venous pressures. Pericardial effusion may be seen. Systolic ventricular function is normal or mildly reduced, but atrioventricular inflow patterns are frequently abnormal, reflecting diastolic dysfunction and elevated filling pressures.

Chest radiography findings can be normal, although careful inspection often reveals the presence of atrial enlargement. Pulmonary venous congestion may be present.

Holter monitoring is important in the clinical management to evaluate for the presence of tachyarrhythmias or bradycardia.

Cardiac MRI may help to distinguish constrictive pericarditis from restrictive cardiomyopathy. MRI can reliably evaluate the pericardial thickness and can lead to the diagnosis of constrictive pericarditis, allowing prompt surgical intervention.

Cardiac catheterization also may help in differentiating constrictive from restrictive processes. In restrictive cardiomyopathy, markedly elevated ventricular diastolic pressures are present, and in contrast to constrictive pericarditis, the end-diastolic pressure on the left is often higher than that on the right. In constrictive pericarditis, equalization of ventricular end-diastolic, atrial, and pulmonary artery end-diastolic pressures may be found. Maneuvers such as volume infusion may be necessary to bring out differences in ventricular filling pressures. Cardiac catheterization also may yield important information on the prognosis of patients with restrictive cardiomyopathy. Pulmonary vascular resistance may be elevated at the time of diagnosis, secondary to left atrial hypertension. Low cardiac output or high pulmonary vascular resistance or both are important predictors of poor outcome and herald the need for cardiac transplantation.

Other Cardiomyopathies

Left ventricular noncompaction cardiomyopathy is a recently recognized, rare form of cardiomyopathy. Diagnosis is based purely on structural features seen on imaging. Two-dimensional transthoracic echocardiogram is most commonly used for diagnosis.[82] Characteristic echocardiographic findings of noncompaction are multiple, prominent myocardial trabeculations (minimum of four) and deep intertrabecular recesses communicating with the left ventricular cavity in the absence of any other cardiac lesions. Color Doppler imaging demonstrates blood flow through these deep recesses in continuity with the ventricular cavity. Its clinical manifestations are highly variable but in severe cases can be associated with left ventricular systolic impairment, cardiac arrhythmias, and systemic thromboembolism.[83] Diastolic dysfunction has been linked to abnormal relaxation and restrictive filling due to excessive trabeculation. An association with some form of neuromuscular disorder is common. Treatment and prognosis differs depending on clinical signs and symptoms.

Arrhythmogenic right ventricular cardiomyopathy is a heritable heart-muscle disorder that causes progressive replacement of right ventricular myocardium by fibrofatty tissue. Arrhythmogenic right ventricular cardiomyopathy is infrequently identified in children. It is characterized clinically by ventricular arrhythmias of right ventricular origin that may lead to sudden death, mostly in young adults and athletes.[84]

Genetic Basis for Pediatric Cardiomyopathy

Genetic syndromes, neuromuscular diseases, inborn errors of metabolism, mitochondrial disorders, and mutations in genes encoding structural components of the cardiomyocyte, including the sarcomere and cytoskeleton, have all been described in children with cardiomyopathies. There is significant overlap in the genetic mutations identified in phenotypically distinct cardiomyopathies. Mutations in genes controlling the sarcomere, beta-myosin heavy chain, and myosin-binding proteins have been described in pediatric dilated, hypertrophic, noncompaction and restrictive cardiomyopathies.[85] Hypertrophic cardiomyopathy has largely been considered a disease of the sarcomere, with mutations in beta-myosin heavy chain (*MYH7* gene) and myosin binding protein C3 (*MYBPC3* gene) combining to explain approximately 80% of mutation-positive cases.[86] Dilated cardiomyopathy is inherited in over 30% of cases, and patterns of inheritance can be autosomal dominant, X-linked, or recessive.[85,87] Inborn errors of metabolism and genetic syndromic causes are responsible for a significant number of dilated cardiomyopathy cases in infancy. In adolescence, neuromuscular disorders, including Duchenne muscular dystrophy, account for a large number of cases. Noncompaction cardiomyopathy is also commonly identified in patients with genetic syndromic conditions or inborn errors of metabolism, such as Barth syndrome, an X-linked disorder with mitochondrial dysfunction and abnormal cardiolipin metabolism.[88] Recent data indicate that mutations in sarcomeric genes were the most prevalent in patients with noncompaction.[89] Restrictive cardiomyopathy is the least common cardiomyopathy and has been associated with mutations in desmin and sarcomere genes.[81,90] A genetic abnormality for arrhythmogenic right ventricular cardiomyopathy has been demonstrated in nearly 50% of cases, with an autosomal dominant pattern of inheritance. Desmosomal protein abnormalities are often implicated in the pathogenesis of the disease. Electrocardiographic abnormalities are detected in up to 90% of arrhythmogenic right ventricular cardiomyopathy patients.[91]

Outcomes of Heart Failure in Children With Cardiomyopathy

Children with dilated cardiomyopathy who present with heart failure have a high risk of death or heart transplantation within the first year after presentation, in which in-hospital mortality is approximately 11% and survival at 1 year after presentation ranges between 25% and 30%.[92-94] The majority of events occur within 6 months of presentation. Long-term data demonstrate that improvement of ventricular function and stabilization of heart failure symptoms can occur in children with dilated cardiomyopathy and are more common in the infant and young child (Fig. 72.4).[95-98] Conditional 5-year survival in children with dilated cardiomyopathy who survive more than 1 year after presentation is excellent and ranges between 90% and 95%.[96,98] Although heart failure is uncommon as the presenting symptom in hypertrophic cardiomyopathy, when it occurs, it is associated with ventricular systolic dysfunction and is associated with worse outcome.[78,99] The prognosis of restrictive cardiomyopathy in children is grave, with reports of 34% to 53% 2-year transplant-free survival after presentation.[70] Heart failure is also significant risk factor for death or transplant in patients with restrictive or noncompaction cardiomyopathy.[70,83,100-102] In a study consisting of noncompaction cardiomyopathy in the

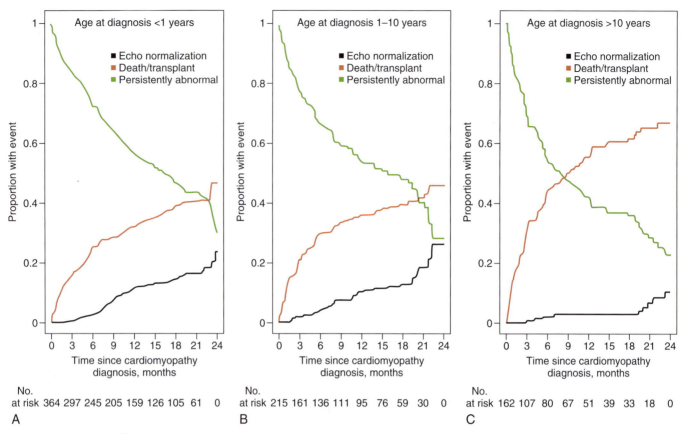

• **Figure 72.4** Outcomes after presentation with a dilated cardiomyopathy by age-group. (Reprinted with permission from Everitt MD, Sleeper LA, Lu M, et al. Recovery of echocardiographic function in children with idiopathic dilated cardiomyopathy: results from the pediatric cardiomyopathy registry. *J Am Coll Cardiol.* 2014;63:1405-1413.)

pediatric population the mortality rate associated was 12.8%. Cardiac arrhythmias and ventricular dysfunction were associated with highest risk of death.[83]

Congenital Heart Disease and Heart Failure

Survival in infants and children with congenital heart disease has vastly improved over the past 30 years, due to earlier detection of disease, better medical management, and improved results following cardiac surgical intervention.[103-105] As they age, patients with complex congenital heart disease are at risk for heart failure.[106-108] The etiology of heart failure in patients with congenital heart disease is multifactorial. Myocardial dysfunction secondary to ischemia, cyanosis, and fibrosis following cardiopulmonary bypass is an important component of heart failure in this population. Hemodynamic stresses from volume overload as a result of residual left-to-right shunt lesions or valvar insufficiency pressure overload resulting from valvular disease and other obstructive lesions such as coarctation of the aorta, pulmonary hypertension caused by chronic exposure to a left-to-right shunt, ventricular dysfunction or comorbidities such as obstructive sleep apnea, systemic arterial hypertension resulting from acquired renal disease or essential hypertension, and coronary artery disease related to congenital heart disease or the aging process can all play an important role in the development of heart failure.

The congenital heart disease lesions at highest risk for heart failure are shown in Fig. 72.5. The single-ventricle population

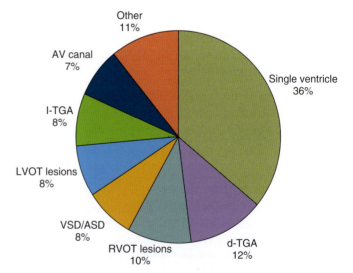

• **Figure 72.5** Congenital heart lesions present in adults and children undergoing heart transplantation. *ASD,* Atrial septal defect; *AV,* atrioventricular; *LVOT,* left ventricular outflow tract; *RVOT,* right ventricular outflow tract; *TGA,* transposition of the great arteries; *VSD,* ventricular septal defect. (Modified from Lamour JM, Kanter KR, Naftel DC, et al. The effect of age, diagnosis, and previous surgery in children and adults undergoing heart transplantation for congenital heart disease. *J Am Coll Cardiol.* 2009;54:160-165.)

constitutes the largest proportion of congenital heart disease patients who develop heart failure.[109] Heart failure can also be the consequence of failure of the subpulmonary ventricle, as is found in patients with tetralogy of Fallot, or as a result of failure of a systemic right ventricle, as is present following the Mustard or Senning procedure or in corrected transposition of the great arteries. HFpEF can occur because of diastolic dysfunction in complex left ventricular outflow tract obstruction (Shone's complex).

In Fontan patients, atrial arrhythmias and manifestations of low cardiac output such as progressive exercise intolerance, cyanosis, or poor somatic growth are common.[110-113] Heart failure in the Fontan patient can occur as a result of poor flow through the Fontan circuit in the setting of normal ventricular function and is known colloquially as the *failing Fontan*.[114] The heart failure syndrome associated with the failing Fontan is characterized by the effects of high venous pressures and includes ascites, protein-losing enteropathy, plastic bronchitis, and chronic effusions.[115-117] In this population heart failure symptoms are more insidious, with a gradual deterioration of exercise performance and a high incidence of growth failure.[115,118]

Outcomes of Heart Failure in Congenital Heart Disease Patients

Heart failure is a significant risk factor for late mortality and morbidity in the congenital heart disease population. It is the most common cause of hospitalization in adult patients with congenital heart disease, and mortality after the onset of heart failure is high.[119,120] In a large study of adults admitted to the hospital with heart failure and congenital heart disease, 2-year mortality was 35%.[119] Factors associated with worse outcome in children with congenital heart disease and heart failure include the presence of complex heart disease, arrhythmia, older age, shorter duration of heart failure and cyanosis.[121-123] In the Fontan population, increased morbidity at the time of the Fontan procedure and the presence of AV valve regurgitation predict increased risk of death and/or transplantation late after the Fontan.[118]

Comorbidities in Pediatric Heart Failure

Arrhythmias

Heart failure can be exacerbated by the presence of tachyarrhythmias (atrial or ventricular) or bradyarrhythmias (junctional rhythm or heart block) (Table 72.1).[58,124-129] Arrhythmias can arise in response to hemodynamic stress such as elevated intracardiac pressure or volume overload, as the result of an underlying cardiac injury such as ischemia or fibrosis, or can be due to a genetic mutation that disrupts the ion channels controlling electrical activation of the myocardium.

Tachyarrhythmias impair ventricular filling, leading to fluid retention and poor perfusion and in some cases sudden death. In cardiomyopathy patients, genetic mutations in arrhythmogenic genes such as *SCN5A* and *LMNA* have been described in patients with dilated cardiomyopathy and arrhythmias.[113,127,130-132] In congenital heart patients, atrial flutter and intraatrial reentrant tachycardias are common, particularly in patients with residual atrioventricular valve disease or the Fontan procedure.[133-135] Ventricular arrhythmias are relatively uncommon in patients with dilated cardiomyopathy, except in those with a history of cardiac ischemia, but have been described in up to 25% of patients with heart failure due to noncompaction or restrictive cardiomyopathy.[101,136-138]

Bradyarrhythmias can worsen heart failure by decreasing cardiac output due to a nonphysiologic slow rate or loss of atrioventricular synchrony. Junctional rhythm is a particular concern in the Fontan patient because of the increased dependence of cardiac output on atrioventricular synchrony.[133-135] Complete heart block has been described in cardiomyopathy patients with mutations in the desmin or *LMNA* gene and is not uncommon in patients following repair of congenital heart disease.[124] Mechanical dyssynchrony has been described with right ventricular pacing in complete heart block and is a risk factor for the development of ventricular dysfunction and heart failure in both cardiomyopathy and congenital heart disease patients.[139-143]

Pulmonary Hypertension

Elevated pulmonary vascular resistance is an important comorbidity in patients with end-stage heart failure due to the risk of right heart failure and increased morbidity after heart transplant.[144,145] Patients with restrictive cardiomyopathy and congenital heart disease are at risk for the development of pulmonary vascular disease.[145] In patients with the Fontan circulation, pulmonary vascular disease can be contributing factor to heart failure because pulmonary blood flow is highly dependent on the presence of low pulmonary artery pressures.[146]

Renal

The cardiorenal syndrome has been described for centuries as an important component of heart failure. The complex interaction between the heart and kidney has been identified as a risk factor for worse outcome and as a potential therapeutic target.[147] Renal dysfunction is common in children with decompensated heart failure and has been associated with a higher hazard ratio of death and the need for mechanical circulatory support.[148,149] Approximately 15% of children listed for heart transplant have evidence of worsening renal function and the incidence of renal dysfunction in children with end-stage heart failure undergoing ventricular assist device placement has been reported to be as high as 55%.[148,150,151] Renal dysfunction is a risk factor for death on the heart transplant waiting list and death early after transplantation.[151-153] Hyponatremia, which may be due to an increase in free water retention or disruption of the sodium-potassium exchange in the kidney, has been associated with worse outcome in pediatric heart failure patients.[154,155]

Hepatic

Chronically elevated central venous pressures can lead to hepatic fibrosis and cirrhosis in patients with right heart failure due to congenital heart disease, restrictive cardiomyopathy, or in patients with the Fontan circulation.[156,157] Fibrosis has been documented by liver histology early after the Fontan procedure, with evidence of cirrhosis increasing over time.[158-161] Cirrhosis is a risk factor for hepatocellular carcinoma and is an important consideration when assessing candidacy for heart transplantation.[162,163]

Cyanosis

Significant cyanosis can occur in patients with unrepaired or palliated congenital heart disease and a right-to-left shunt. Cyanosis impairs oxygen delivery and exacerbates the symptoms of fatigue and exercise intolerance. In patients with the Fontan procedure, oxygen saturation usually falls between 5% and 8% with maximal exercise.[164]

TABLE 72.1 Arrhythmias

	Predisposing Factors in Heart Failure	ECG Findings	Acute Treatment	Special Considerations in Heart Failure
Supraventricular Tachyarrhythmias				
Atrial flutter/ intraatrial reentry tachycardia	Atrial scar, prior surgical incisions (repaired CHD) Atrial enlargement Sinus node dysfunction (sick sinus syndrome)	• Sawtooth pattern for typical atrial flutter • Variable AV conduction (2:1, 3:1)	• Rate control • Diltiazem • Digoxin • Rhythm control • Amiodarone • Cardioversion (synchronized) • Anticoagulation	Class I antiarrhythmic agents are generally avoided in patients with ventricular dysfunction Consider pace-termination if pacemaker in situ
Atrial fibrillation (AF)	Left atrial pressure/volume overload; mitral valve disease	• Irregularly irregular • Absence of distinct P waves	• Rate control • Diltiazem • Digoxin • Rhythm control • Amiodarone • Cardioversion (synchronized) • Anticoagulation	Class I antiarrhythmic agents are generally avoided in patients with ventricular dysfunction
Ventricular Tachyarrhythmias				
Premature ventricular contractions (PVCs)	Sympathetic activation Electrolyte abnormalities	• Singles, couplets • Grouped beating: bigeminy, trigeminy • Monomorphic vs. polymorphic	• Observation • Correct electrolyte abnormalities • Beta-blocker for HF management	Rarely, high PVC burden can cause or worsen LV dysfunction—consider Rx or ablation
Nonsustained ventricular tachycardia (NSVT)	Ventricular scar; prior surgical incisions (repaired CHD)	≥3 consecutive PVCs, duration <30 s	• Beta-blocker for HF • Consider Rx for frequent or symptomatic NSVT (amiodarone)	Possible predictor of malignant ventricular arrhythmias, depending on underlying disease—consider EPS ± ICD
Ventricular tachycardia (VT)	Ventricular scar; prior surgical incisions (repaired CHD)	• Sustained >30 s • Wide QRS complex • VA dissociation • Monomorphic vs. polymorphic	• Antiarrhythmic agents • Amiodarone • Lidocaine • Cardioversion (synchronized)	ICD placement Polymorphic VT in the setting of prolonged QTc (torsades de pointes): Rx with magnesium, lidocaine, isoproterenol; consider overdrive pacing
Ventricular fibrillation (VF)	Ischemia; electrolyte abnormalities; scar	• Rapid, irregular deflections with varying amplitude • No distinct QRS complexes	• Defibrillation	ICD placement
Bradyarrhythmias				
Junctional bradycardia	Sinus node dysfunction (Fontan, atrial switch)	• Absence of P wave, bradycardia for age	• Temporary or permanent atrial pacing	Bradycardia and lack of AV synchrony can contribute to heart failure
Complete heart block	Post cardiac surgery; ischemia; genetic disease	• AV dissociation with atrial rate slower than ventricular rate	• Temporary ventricular pacing or permanent DDD pacemaker	Bradycardia and lack of AV synchrony can contribute to heart failure Pacemaker-induced ventricular dysfunction due to dyssynchronous ventricular pacing

AV, Atrioventricular; *CHD,* congenital heart disease; *DDD,* dual chamber; *ECG,* electrocardiogram; *EPS,* electrophysiology study; *HF,* heart failure; *ICD,* implantable cardiac defibrillator; *LV,* left ventricle; *QTc,* corrected QT interval; *Rx,* therapy; *VA,* ventriculoarterial.

Respiratory

Respiratory failure in children with cardiomyopathy and heart failure is largely secondary to the effects of pulmonary edema. Children with congenital heart disease often have underlying restrictive lung disease that contributes to poor exercise intolerance in patients with heart failure.[165,166] Scoliosis is also more common in congenital heart disease patients compared with normal children and may impair exercise performance and lung function.[167,168]

Infection

Congenital heart disease patients with prosthetic valve or conduit material or residual left-to-right shunts are at risk for endocarditis.[169-171] Endocarditis can cause or exacerbate heart failure symptoms. Consideration should always be given to the possibility of endocarditis in a patient with congenital heart disease presenting with new heart failure symptoms.[172-174]

Anemia

In adults with heart failure, anemia and iron deficiency has been identified as a common comorbidity that impacts outcome.[175] Anemia is common in children with heart failure and in adults with complex congenital heart disease.[176,177] There are no data in children correlating anemia with outcomes in heart failure.

Growth

Growth failure is common in children with heart failure due to increased metabolic demand and decreased intake.[178] Obesity occurs less commonly in children with heart failure, with 8% of children listed for heart transplantation classified as overweight. In patients with the Fontan physiology, obesity has been associated with heart failure and worse outcome.[179-181] At the time of listing for heart transplant between 23% and 43% of children are underweight.[180-182] Underweight and overweight have been identified as risk factors for waiting list mortality in children with cardiomyopathy.[183] In children less than 2 years of age, moderate to severe wasting was an independent risk factor for death on the transplant waiting list.[184]

Psychosocial Stress and Functional Status

Heart failure has a negative effect on quality of life and functional status in children. Decreased health-related quality of life in both the psychosocial and physical domains on the Child Health Questionnaire have been described in children with dilated cardiomyopathy, with young age and less ventricular dilation associated with better functional status.[185] Worse health-related quality of life has been associated with worse clinical outcomes in children with dilated cardiomyopathy.[186] Measures of parental well-being, including emotional state, have also been associated with worse outcome in children with dilated cardiomyopathy.[185,186]

In adolescents with a Fontan circulation, the Pediatric Quality of Life Inventory demonstrated significant physical impairment in 45% of patients and significant psychosocial impairment in 30% of patients, which worsened over time.[187] Impairment in the physical and psychosocial domain was associated with worse exercise performance and the outcomes of death or transplantation.[110]

Evaluation of Heart Failure in Children

The initial evaluation of the child with heart failure includes clinical assessment, laboratory testing, and imaging. The goals are to identify the clinical manifestations and severity of the heart failure, screen for important comorbidities, and identify underlying causes (Fig. 72.6).

Clinical

A careful history and physical is the cornerstone in the evaluation and management of the child with heart failure. This evaluation also includes gathering information that may help diagnose syndromic or genetic diseases. The signs and symptoms of fluid overload or low cardiac output can be characterized as described in

Fig. 72.2. Compared with the adult heart failure population, biventricular failure occurs more often in children, both in those with cardiomyopathy and those with congenital heart disease; thus the manifestations of fluid overload often include signs and symptoms of systemic venous congestion in addition to pulmonary edema.[72,188] The severity of heart failure can be graded using the Ross Heart Failure Class (see Box 72.2) in preschool children and the New York Heart Association class in older children. Assessment of functional status and quality of life are important metrics that can be used in serial monitoring.

Laboratory

Assessment of laboratory parameters that can aid in assessing the severity of heart failure should be performed in children presenting with heart failure. These include evaluation of end-organ function (renal, hepatic, pulmonary, neurologic) that will indicate the adequacy of cardiac output and natriuretic peptide levels, which can monitor the severity of heart failure. Laboratory testing can be diagnostic or highly suggestive of the underlying cause of the heart failure, particularly in the metabolic or genetic cardiomyopathies.

Imaging

Electrocardiography and continuous rhythm monitoring are used to identify conduction abnormalities and screen for tachyarrhythmias or bradyarrhythmias. Echocardiography is a mainstay in the assessment of systolic and diastolic ventricular size and function.[189] Echocardiographic evaluation is also fundamental to establishing an accurate diagnosis and evaluating the hemodynamic and structural pathophysiology underlying heart failure. Cardiac MRI or computed tomography may have utility in the diagnosis of myocarditis and is able to quantify the hemodynamic effects of residual lesions on ventricular function in congenital heart disease.[190-193] Diagnostic cardiac catheterization for hemodynamic assessment of heart failure due to cardiomyopathy is rarely performed, unless pulmonary hypertension is suspected.[144] In congenital heart disease patients, diagnostic and interventional cardiac catheterization have an important role in the evaluation and treatment of heart failure because relief of residual shunts or stenoses may improve symptoms and ventricular function.

Medical Management of Heart Failure in Children

The pathophysiology that produces the heart failure syndrome is an intersection of multiple models of physiologic derangements, with the burden of each model changing in an individual patient dependent on the nature of the event, patient-specific characteristics and other comorbidities. The goal of heart failure therapies is to treat the symptomatic manifestations and address the underlying causes.

Evidence to support heart failure therapies in children is lacking. The challenges of performing randomized controlled trials in children with heart failure are substantial. The heterogeneity of the underlying causes of heart failure and the rarity of the disease limits patient selection and the ability to measure meaningful outcomes. The scarcity of evidence to support treatment recommendations in children has led to a reliance on the adult heart failure experience. This approach should be undertaken with caution

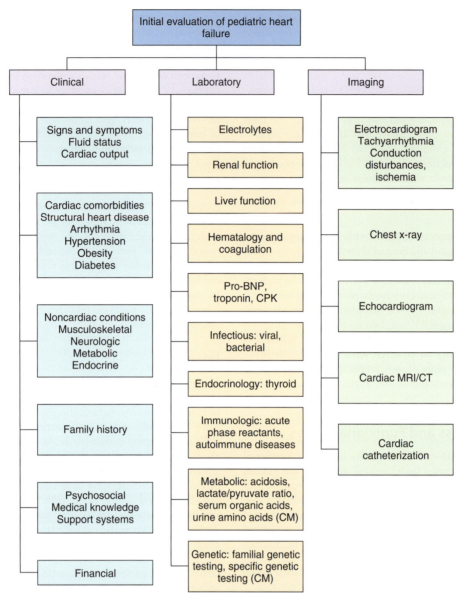

• **Figure 72.6** Initial evaluation of pediatric heart failure. *BNP,* Brain natriuretic peptide; *CM,* cardiomyopathy; *CPK,* creatine phosphokinase; *CT,* computed tomography; *MRI,* magnetic resonance imaging.

because composition of the adult and pediatric heart failure populations differs substantially.[194] In adults with heart failure, myocardial ischemia is the most common underlying cause; primary cardiomyopathies and congenital heart disease are the most common causes in children. Comorbidities such as hypertension, coronary artery disease, obesity, smoking, and diabetes are common in adults, whereas these comorbidities are exceedingly rare in children.[194] The efficacy of adult heart failure therapies may be related not only to beneficial effects on the myocardium and neurohormonal axis but also to treatment of hypertension and coronary artery disease; thus results of adult studies may not be relevant to the pediatric heart population. In 2014 the International Society for Heart and Lung Transplantation published an extensive monograph on pediatric heart failure that includes recommendations on heart failure management based largely on expert opinion.[25] A practical approach to the medical management of the child with heart failure that incorporates available data from children and adults is presented in this chapter.

Management of Acute Decompensated Heart Failure in Children

Even in the adult heart failure population there is a paucity of evidence demonstrating that acute decompensated heart failure therapies have a beneficial effect on morbidity or mortality.[195] Thus the medical management of the child in acute decompensated heart failure is directed toward optimizing fluid status and cardiac output to achieve symptom relief and prevent end-organ dysfunction (Fig. 72.7).

Fluid Management

If there is evidence of pulmonary edema and/or venous congestion, diuretics are the mainstay of therapy in an effort to reduce right and left ventricular end-diastolic pressures. In contrast, diuretics may be contraindicated in children with low cardiac output and

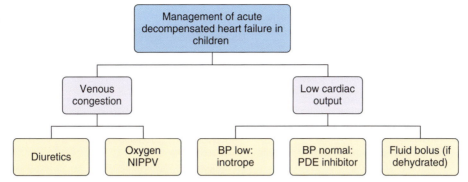

• **Figure 72.7** Management of acute decompensated heart failure in children. *BP,* Blood pressure; *NIPPV,* noninvasive positive pressure ventilation; *PDE,* phosphodiesterase.

no signs of venous congestion because hypovolemia will further decrease cardiac output and worsen end-organ perfusion. Studies in adult heart failure patients do not provide convincing data regarding the optimal mode, dose, and frequency of diuretic administration; thus decisions regarding their administration in children should be directed by response to therapy. In patients with very poor cardiac function, care should be taken to avoid rapid diuresis that may decrease preload and further reduce cardiac output. Continuous infusion of a loop diuretic may be particularly effective in providing sustained diuresis with smaller swings in filling pressures. The NIH-sponsored Diuretic Optimization Strategies Evaluation (DOSE) trial demonstrated that higher initial doses of diuretics in adults with heart failure resulted in a more rapid improvement in symptoms, but there was no difference in symptoms or renal dysfunction by 3 days.[196] The doses of commonly prescribed diuretics are shown in Table 72.2. In adults, diuretic therapy has been associated with the development of acute kidney injury and activation of the RAAS; thus careful monitoring of renal function should be performed.

Ventilatory Support

In patients with dyspnea due to pulmonary edema the use of oxygen and noninvasive as well as invasive positive pressure ventilation can relieve symptoms. Mechanical ventilation may also reduce the work of breathing; however, the stress of intubation carries a risk of cardiac arrest due to increased vagal tone and hemodynamic instability.[197]

Inotrope, Vasodilator, and Vasopressor Therapy

In adults with acute decompensated heart failure the long-term use of inotropic agents has been associated with worse outcomes compared with treatment with vasodilators or diuretics alone; thus this therapy is recommended only for the short-term stabilization of adult patients with hypotension and low cardiac output.[198,199] Although there are data demonstrating a beneficial effect of milrinone in the early postoperative period after congenital heart surgery, little data exist regarding the efficacy of long-term phosphodiesterase inhibitor therapy in children with heart failure.[200,201] Patients with end-stage cardiac dysfunction or vasodilatory shock from multiple organ system failure or sepsis may have systemic hypotension. The management of these patients is particularly challenging and requires infusions of vasopressors to maintain systemic blood pressure. In such situations, judicious use of alpha-adrenergic agents, such as epinephrine or dopamine, may be required, but they are proarrhythmic and must be carefully titrated. Avoidance

of initiation of beta-blockers (due to negative inotropy) during acute decompensated heart failure is recommended.

Comorbidities

Although there is scant evidence linking the treatment of comorbidities, such as optimizing nutritional status, treating associated infections, and managing electrolyte and hematologic abnormalities, with improved outcomes, logic argues that this approach should be beneficial in children with heart failure, and the risks are minimal. The prevention of thromboembolic complications is controversial in both the adult and pediatric heart failure literature. Currently the adult heart failure guidelines do not recommend the routine use of anticoagulation in patients with HFrEF in the absence of atrial arrhythmias, a prior thromboembolic event, or a cardioembolic source.[11]

Management of Chronic Heart Failure in Children

If medical therapy for acute decompensated heart failure achieves relief of symptoms and establishes an adequate cardiac output, then the focus shifts toward maintaining clinical stability and addressing the underlying pathophysiology of heart failure (Fig. 72.8). If medical therapy is not effective in the treatment of acute decompensated heart failure in children, advanced cardiac therapies such as mechanical support and transplantation must be considered (Box 72.3). Substantial evidence exists to support the use of neurohormonal modulation to decrease activation of the sympathetic adrenergic system and the RAAS in adults with HFrEF.[11] In pediatric dilated cardiomyopathy the evidence to support the use of angiotensin-converting enzyme inhibition and beta-blockade is not strong, but expert opinion is in favor of the use of these agents.[25] In patients with congenital heart disease and ventricular dysfunction, results of randomized trials of angiotensin-converting enzyme inhibition[26,202] and beta-blockade[27] have been negative and even suggest an adverse effect of these medications; thus they are not recommended for routine use.[25] There is no evidence to support the use of neurohormonal blockade in children with HFpEF. Diuretics should be used sparingly because of the dependence of cardiac output on higher filling pressures.

Hypertrophic Cardiomyopathy

For patients with hypertrophic cardiomyopathy, negative inotropic agents like beta-blockers and calcium channel blockers have, in some

| TABLE 72.2 | **Medications for Pediatric Heart Failure** | | |

Medication	Starting Dose	Common/Serious Side Effects	Comments
Loop Diuretics			
Note: All loop diuretics carry the risk of cross-reactivity in patients with sulfa allergy.			
Bumetanide (oral, IV)	*Term N:* 0.01-0.05 mg/kg/dose q24h-48h (*max:* 0.06 mg/kg/dose) *I/C:* 0.015-0.1 mg/kg/dose q24h-48h (*max:* 10 mg/d) *Note:* For infants 0-6 mo, no additional benefit seen at >0.05 mg/kg/dose	*Class effect:* hypokalemia, hypomagnesemia, hypocalcemia, hyponatremia, GI upset, hyperuricemia, hypotension, ototoxicity, renal failure *Furosemide only:* nephrolithiasis with long-term use in premature infants	• Due to presence of benzyl alcohol in IV formulation, do not use IV in neonates
Furosemide (oral, IV)	*N:* 1-2 mg/kg/dose IV/PO, given q12h-q24h, or 0.16 mg/kg/h continuously (*max:* 0.4 mg/kg/h) *I/C:* 1-2 mg/kg/dose q6h-q12h, or 0.05 mg/kg/h continuously *Note:* For adolescents and older, minimal benefit seen in doses greater than 200 mg/d		• PO and IV doses are not interchangeable • Continuous infusions should be titrated to clinical effect • Significantly absorbed in ECMO circuits—may require higher dosing
Thiazide Diuretics			
Note: All thiazide diuretics carry the risk of cross-reactivity in patients with sulfa allergy. Avoid use in patients with CrCl <40 mL/min/1.73 m^2.			
Chlorothiazide (oral, IV)	*N:* 20-40 mg/kg/d given q12h *I/C/A:* 10-40 mg/kg/d given twice daily *IV:* See comments section *Max I/C <2 y:* 375 mg/d *Max C 2-12 y:* 1000 mg/d *Max A:* 2000 mg/d	*Class effect (chlorothiazide[a]/HCTZ only):* hypokalemia, hypomagnesemia, hyponatremia, hypercalcemia, hyperglycemia, hyperuricemia, hypotension, vertigo, GI upset, pancreatitis, SLE exacerbation, photosensitivity, rash, alopecia, toxic epidermal necrolysis, muscle cramps, leukopenia, thrombocytopenia, pneumonitis, interstitial nephritis, renal failure, impotence	• Due to presence of benzyl alcohol in IV formulation, do not use IV in neonates • Clinicians recommend decreasing IV by 50%-75% of starting oral dose
Hydrochlorothiazide (HCTZ) (oral)	*N:* 1-2 mg/kg/dose q12 h *I/C/A:* 1-3 mg/kg/d given once or twice daily *Max:* *I/C <2 y:* 37.5 mg/d *C 2-12 y:* 100 mg/d *A:* 200 mg/d		• May interfere with parathyroid function tests
Metolazone (oral)	0.05-0.4 mg/kg/d *Max A:* 20 mg/d	*Chlorothiazide only:* hypercholesteremia and hypertriglyceridemia reported *Metolazone only:* hypophosphatemia	• Typically used in combination with loop diuretic
ACE Inhibitors			
Note: Initiate ACE-I dosing at lower than recommended starting dose for CrCl <50 mL/min/1.73 m^2.			
Captopril (oral)	*Premature and term N <7 d:* 0.01 mg/kg/dose q12h-q8h *Term N >7 days:* 0.05-0.1 mg/kg/dose q8-24h (*max:* 0.5 mg/kg/dose q6h-q24h) *I:* 0.3-2.5 mg/kg/d, divided q8-12 h *C/A:* 0.3-6 mg/kg/d divided q8-12 h (*max:* 150 mg/d)	*Class effect:* Hypotension, dry cough, Raynaud phenomenon, hyponatremia, hyperkalemia, proteinuria, angioedema, agranulocytosis, rash, anemia, transaminitis, cholestatic jaundice, elevated serum creatinine, dysgeusia	• To be taken on empty stomach • Zinc deficiency with long-term use
Enalapril (oral)	*N:* 0.04-0.1 mg/kg/d q24h *I/C/A:* 0.1 mg/kg/d divided once or twice daily *Max:* 0.5 mg/kg/d (40 mg)	*Captopril only:* impotence, gynecomastia, leukopenia, thrombocytopenia, neutropenia, pancreatitis	• Use in neonates with CrCl <30 mL/min/1.73 m^2 is not recommended • Conversion between oral enalapril and IV enalaprilat is not equivalent

TABLE 72.2	Medications for Pediatric Heart Failure—cont'd		
Medication	**Starting Dose**	**Common/Serious Side Effects**	**Comments**
ARBs			
Note: Primarily used if intolerant to ACE-I. Use in C/A with CrCl <30 mL/min/1.73 m^2 is not recommended.			
Candesartan	*C 1-6 y:* 0.2 mg/kg/d *Max:* 0.4 mg/kg/d *C 6-16 y:* 0.7 mg/kg (*max:* 32 mg) once daily	*Class effect:* Hypotension, hyperkalemia, angioedema, dry cough (incidence higher in those with cough on ACE-I), diarrhea, UTI *Candesartan only:* hypertriglyceridemia, hyperuricemia, hyperglycemia, depression, anxiety, vertigo, skin rash, gastroenteritis, increased CPK, UTI, epistaxis *Valsartan only:* vertigo, diarrhea, upper abdominal pain, neutropenia, viral infections, arthralgias	
Losartan	*C ≥6 y:* 0.7 mg/kg/d once daily (*max:* 50 mg/d) *A ≥17 y:* 25-50 mg once daily (*max:* 150 mg/d)		
Valsartan	*C 1-5 y weighing ≥8 kg:* 0.4-3.5 mg/kg/d once daily (*max:* 40 mg/d) *C 6-16 y:* 1.3-2.7 mg/kg/d once daily (*max:* 160 mg/day) *A ≥17 y:* 80-160 mg/d divided twice daily (*max:* 320 mg/d)		• In HTN clinical trial (*N* = 90) of C <6 y, 2 deaths and 3 cases of elevated liver enzymes reported—use not recommended
Spironolactone (aldosterone antagonist)	*N:* 1-3 mg/kg/d divided every 12-24 h *C:* 1-3.3 mg/kg/d divided every 6-12 h (*max:* 100 mg/d) *A/Ad:* on ACE-I, loop diuretic ± digoxin—12.5-25 mg/d (*max:* 50 mg/d)	Dizziness, lethargy, hyperkalemia, gynecomastia, amenorrhea, GI upset, impotence, urticaria, vasculitis, agranulocytosis, hepatotoxicity, DRESS syndrome, renal failure	• Food increases absorption • When initiating treatment in CHF, ensure CrCl >30 mL/min/1.73 m^2
Beta-Blockers			
Note: Do not discontinue chronic beta-blocker therapy abruptly to avoid rebound tachycardia. Use with caution in patients with history of bronchospasms. Can mask signs and symptoms of hypoglycemia and hypothyroidism.			
Carvedilol (oral)	0.075-0.08 mg/kg/dose twice daily, titrated to 0.2-0.4 mg/kg/dose twice daily (*max:* 50 mg/d)	Syncope, bradycardia, AV block, depression, vertigo, hyperkalemia, GI upset, arthralgias, dyspnea, nasal congestion, flu-like syndrome, exacerbation of psoriasis	• Highly protein bound (>98% to albumin) Faster elimination seen in C <3.5 y and may require TID dosing and/or higher mg/kg target
Metoprolol (oral)	Tartrate— *C/A:* 0.1-0.2 mg/kg/dose twice daily *Max:* 2 mg/kg/d (200 mg) Can consider extended-release (succinate formulation) in adolescents ≥50 kg: initial dose 50 mg once daily (*max:* 200 mg/d)	Syncope, bradycardia, AV block, claudication, cold extremities, depression, vertigo, skin photosensitivity, confusion, hallucinations, nightmares, temporary amnesia, heartburn, GI upset, musculoskeletal pain, tinnitus	
Digoxin (oral)	*N:* *Preterm:* 5-7.5 mcg/kg/d *Full-term:* 8-10 mcg/kg/d *C 1-24 mo:* 10-15 mcg/kg/d *2-5 y:* 8-10 mcg/kg/d *5-10 y:* 5-10 mcg/kg/d *>10 y:* 2.5-5 mcg/kg/d *Max:* 0.5 mg/d	Digoxin toxicity: anorexia, nausea, vomiting, visual changes, cardiac arrhythmias Confusion, delirium, depression, mental disturbances, rash, GI upset, hypokalemia	• Will require dose reduction for CrCl <50 mL/min/1.73 m^2 • Will require serum level monitoring, with goal serum concentrations of 0.5-0.9 ng/mL • Dose decreased 50% with concomitant amiodarone administration

A, Adolescent; *ACE-I,* angiotensin-converting enzyme inhibitor; *ARB,* angiotensin receptor blocker; *AV,* atrioventricular; *C,* child; *CPK,* creatine phosphokinase; *CrCl,* creatinine clearance; *DRESS,* drug reaction with eosinophilia and systemic symptoms; *ECMO,* extracorporeal membrane oxygenation; *GI,* gastrointestinal; *HTN,* hypertension; *I,* infant; *IV,* intravenous; *max,* maximum; *N,* neonate; *PO,* orally; *SLE,* systemic lupus erythematosus; *UTI,* urinary tract infection.

patients, brought relief of ventricular outflow tract obstruction and improvement of symptoms, particularly angina.[79,203] Surgical relief of left ventricular outflow tract obstruction through a transaortic myotomy or myectomy or both may be performed, with the goals of enlarging the ventricular outflow tract and thereby relieving obstruction. An additional benefit may be a reduction in mitral regurgitation by relief of mitral–septal wall contact. In patients with severe mitral disease, concomitant mitral valvuloplasty or mitral valve replacement may be required. Ideal surgical candidates are older children with obstructive hypertrophic cardiomyopathy for

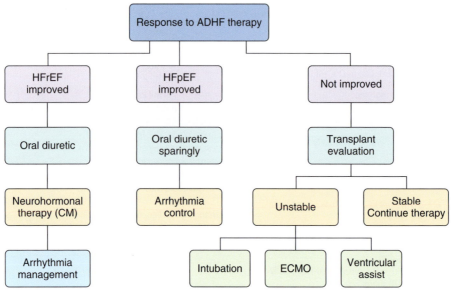

• **Figure 72.8** Management of chronic heart failure in children. *ADHF,* Acute decompensated heart failure; *CM,* cardiomyopathy; *ECMO,* extracorporeal membrane oxygenation; *HFpEF,* heart failure with preserved ejection fraction; *HFrEF,* heart failure with reduced ejection fraction.

• BOX 72.3 Evaluation for Mechanical Support or Transplant

- Body size (height, weight, body surface area)
- Cardiac
  - Left, right, or biventricular dysfunction
  - Pulmonary hypertension
  - Arrhythmia/sudden death risk
  - Ventricular dimensions
  - Valvar insufficiency
  - Patency of the foramen ovale
- Congenital heart disease
  - Surgical history
  - Residual lesions
  - Structural abnormalities (situs, great vessels, postsurgical)
- Vascular
  - Femoral and head and neck vessel anatomy
  - Vessel patency
- Noncardiac comorbidities
  - Renal
  - Hepatic
  - Coagulation
  - Neurologic
  - Infectious
- Psychosocial
  - Developmental
  - Family support
  - Medical knowledge
  - Cultural and religious beliefs
- Assess long-term benefits and risks

---

whom medical management fails. Other indications are significant mitral regurgitation and left atrial enlargement with arrhythmia.

Restrictive Cardiomyopathy

Medical therapy has not proven effective in reversing the diastolic dysfunction found in restrictive cardiomyopathy. Symptomatic treatment includes the cautious use of diuretics to relieve systemic and pulmonary venous congestion, with careful attention to maintaining adequate intravascular volume to optimize cardiac output. In the terminal stages of disease, inotropic support may improve cardiac output but carries the risks described earlier.

Arrhythmia Management

Management of tachyarrhythmias and bradyarrhythmias is an important component of heart failure management, particularly in children with congenital heart disease. Establishing a normal heart rate and atrioventricular synchrony is of particular importance in patients with the Fontan circulation and heart failure.[204] Table 72.1 details treatment options for arrhythmias commonly found in children with heart failure. The use of biventricular pacing in the pediatric cardiomyopathy population has not been shown to improve outcomes. In patients with congenital heart disease undergoing pacing for complete heart block, there is an increased risk for pacemaker-induced ventricular dysfunction that may be lessened by biventricular pacing.[205] Although sudden death is rare in the pediatric heart failure population, placement of an implantable cardioverter-defibrillator may be indicated in patients with hypertrophic cardiomyopathy, dilated cardiomyopathy, and a history of ischemia or in congenital heart patients with ventricular arrhythmias.[136,206]

Management of Psychosocial Stresses of Heart Failure in Children

Heart failure in children is often an unexpected diagnosis that carries an uncertain prognosis and requires lifelong medical care. Children with heart failure and their families should ideally be supported with early integration of palliative care.[207] Palliative care teams focus on integrating care of the body, mind, and spirit of a child while supporting the child's family as they live with illness. This is accomplished with a wide range of specialists who work together to alleviate all suffering, be it physical, spiritual, social, financial, or emotional.[208] Teams reflect a wide range of expertise, including physicians, nurses, psychologists, integrative therapists, chaplains, social workers, financial counselors, and child life specialists.[209] They work alongside the medical team to enhance the patient and family experience and help families clarify their goals of care through shared decision making that is reflective of their values and understanding of the current medical condition of their child.

Involvement of the palliative care team at the onset of heart failure management in children is particularly important because of the potential need for advanced heart therapies, which carry substantial risk to the health and well-being of the child. At present, waiting list mortality is 20%,[210] and many children are placed on mechanical circulatory support to improve end-organ function while awaiting transplant.[211] In the case of children who require mechanical circulatory support (MCS), the palliative care team can help patients, families, and the medical team with pre-MCS preparedness planning by allowing patients and families to express their wishes in the event of a devastating complication, device failure, decline in quality of life, or inability to remain/be listed for heart transplant.[212,213] Teams also help with deactivation checklists to ensure that pain-free, family-centered care is provided through the end of life, including circumstances of compassionate deactivation.[214] Children with advanced heart disease most frequently die in the intensive care setting.[215,216] Involvement of palliative care allows for earlier discussions regarding end-of-life wishes, improved pain management, and bereavement support.[217]

Heart Failure Team

The care of the child with heart failure is one of the most complex care processes found in pediatrics. The phases of care span from the critical care unit to the outpatient clinic. Patients may have multiple comorbidities and require the expertise of specialists that encompass all organ systems, ranging from intensive care to routine pediatric diseases. The importance of a multidisciplinary team in the care of patients with end-stage heart failure undergoing a program of heart transplantation has long been recognized and mandated by the Centers for Medicare and Medicaid Services and the United Network for Organ Sharing. Multidisciplinary care has been shown to improve heart failure outcomes in the outpatient care of the adult heart failure patient.[218] Little data exist regarding the use of a multidisciplinary team in the care of pediatric heart failure patients; however, given the complexity of the disease, it is logical to predict that achieving optimal outcomes children with heart failure requires a multidisciplinary patient-centered team. In addition, pediatric heart failure is a rare disease; thus concentrating knowledge and experience into a small team has the highest potential for the delivery of efficient and effective care.

This team must have expertise in medical and surgical therapies, pharmacology, arrhythmias, and critical and palliative care. Heart failure nurse practitioners play a unique and vital role in the care of the hospitalized pediatric heart failure patient. They are often the permanent fixture in patient care teams who can provide continuity of care in both the inpatient and outpatient settings and be used as a source of information for patient management. Nurse practitioners provide coordination of these complex patients by collaborating with multiple patient care team members, including intensive care unit medical and nursing staff, general cardiology floor medical and nursing staff, pharmacists, nutritionists, and social workers. Members of a pediatric heart failure team and their roles in the care of pediatric heart failure patients are summarized in Box 72.4. The patient and family are also integral members of

the team and in the highest sense of the word are the most important members of the team because the ultimate metric of success is improvement in patient-centered outcomes.

• **BOX 72.4** Heart Failure Team Members: Roles and Responsibilities

Heart failure cardiologist
- Team leader
- Evaluation for causes
- Clinical assessment and risk stratification
- Medical management of acute and chronic heart failure

Subspecialty cardiologist
- Noninvasive imaging
- Interventional cardiology
- Electrophysiology
- Pulmonary hypertension

Cardiac surgeon
- Evaluation and management of residual congenital heart disease
- Evaluation and management of advanced cardiac therapies

Critical care intensivist
- Management of acute decompensated heart failure
- Evaluation and management of ECMO and ventricular assist device therapies

Cardiac anesthesiologist
- Risk stratification for interventions and surgeries
- Management of cardiac performance during interventions and surgeries

Palliative care specialist
- Assessment of family medical competency
- Risk assessment and tolerance
- Involvement in decision making to ensure consideration of patient and medical perspectives

Heart failure nurse practitioner or physician assistant
- Evaluation
- Education
- Maintenance of regulatory compliance
- Maintenance of data, assess quality performance

Pharmacist
- Management of appropriate medication dose and administration
- Monitor for drug complications and interactions
- Education

Nutritionist
- Assessment of nutritional status
- Optimization of nutritional support

Social worker
- Assessment of patient and family psychologic health
- Identification of gaps in family support
- Coordination of long-term care

Child life specialist
- Maintenance of developmentally appropriate behavior as medical condition allows
- Provision of support to patient and family to ensure better compliance with therapies

Financial service advisor
- Assess insurance needs for medical and surgical interventions
- Advocate for patient with payers and providers

ECMO, Extracorporeal membrane oxygenation.

References

A complete list of references is available at ExpertConsult.com.

73

Heart and Lung Transplantation

THOMAS D. RYAN, MD, PHD; CLIFFORD CHIN, MD; ROOSEVELT BRYANT III, MD

For children with advanced acquired or congenital cardiopulmonary disease, heart and lung transplantation, alone or in combination, have become important treatment alternatives to medical or surgical thearpy.[1] Despite continued improvements in early outcomes following pediatric thoracic organ transplantation, the annual number of heart transplants and lung transplants has been relatively stable for the last decade, whereas heart and lung combined has significantly declined since a peak in the early 1990s.[2,3] Donor availability continues to limit the number of transplants performed in infants and children, with more than 15% of heart transplant candidates[4] and 20% to 25% of lung transplant candidates[5] dying on the waiting list. Medium- to long-term complications, including chronic rejection, coronary artery vasculopathy, bronchiolitis obliterans, and the side effects of chronic immunosuppression remain serious problems. Even with these concerns, however, heart and lung transplantation improve the length and quality of life for children with end-stage cardiopulmonary disease.

Indications

Heart Transplantation

The indication for heart transplantation in children is influenced by the age of the child. Approximately 55% of infants younger than 1 year of age who are listed for cardiac transplantation have complex congenital heart disease, whereas the 44% to 54% of older children (1 to 17 years of age) suffer from cardiomyopathy, with the percentage transplanted for congenital heart disease decreasing steadily as patients age (Fig. 73.1).[3] There has also been a shift in the type of lesions primarily palliated with transplantation. In the 1980s heart transplantation had better long-term survival than staged palliation for hypoplastic left heart syndrome (HLHS), which was the most frequent indication for neonatal heart transplantation with some centers using transplantation as the primary therapy for this disease.[6] However, with improved surgical techniques and alternate options such as the "hybrid procedure" and surveillance programs all leading to increased survival, HLHS is now less common as an indication for heart transplantation than non-HLHS congenital heart disease.[7] Other congenital malformations that can lead to consideration of heart transplantation include pulmonary atresia with intact ventricular septum and right ventricular dependent coronary circulation, the more complex forms of single ventricle, truncus arteriosus, double-outlet right ventricle, Ebstein anomaly, unbalanced atrioventricular canal, and transposition of the great arteries. Once palliative or corrective surgery has been undertaken, patients may develop heart failure requiring transplantation. This may be due to systemic ventricular dysfunction (systolic or diastolic), pulmonary ventricular dysfunction, cyanosis, intractable arrhythmias, or complications of single-ventricle palliation such as plastic bronchitis, protein-losing enteropathy, or chronic effusions.

Whereas cardiomyopathy is the second most common indication for transplantation in infants, it is the most frequent diagnosis of children requiring transplantation beyond infancy. Idiopathic dilated cardiomyopathy is the most common diagnosis followed by idiopathic restrictive cardiomyopathy, familial dilated cardiomyopathy, and myocarditis.[8] Unresectable cardiac tumors and chemotherapy-induced myocardial dysfunction are less common indications for transplantation in older children.

Lung Transplantation

Guidelines from the International Society for Heart and Lung Transplantation (ISHLT) recommend that lung transplantation should be considered in adult patients when predicted 2-year survival is less than 50%, whereas in children it is less specific and rather states "a short predicted life expectency."[9] As with heart transplantation, the indications for pediatric lung transplantation are related to the age of the child at presentation. Infants (<1 year of age) most commonly present with pulmonary hypertension of various causes, interstitial lung disease, and surfactant protein deficiency. Cystic fibrosis begins to play a role, albeit small, from ages 1 to 5 years and is responsible for half or more of the cases after age 6 years (Table 73.1).[2] Despite improvements in the treatment and prognosis of cystic fibrosis, some children develop early pulmonary dysfunction and should be considered for transplantation when they develop progressive hypercapnia or oxygen dependence, increasing frequency of hospitalizations, or poor weight gain despite adequate nutrition. Another problem that patients with cystic fibrosis face is the development of multidrug-resistant pseudomonal infections. Given the difficulties in treating infections with these organisms in immunocompromised patients, some consideration must be given to transplant listing before development of panresistant strains.

Patients with primary pulmonary hypertension typically do not present for lung transplantation until adulthood; however, some children can develop rapidly worsening symptoms. Children with pulmonary hypertension due to pulmonary vein stenosis are at increased risk for sudden death while waiting for transplantation. Children with secondary pulmonary hypertension due to cardiac disease (Eisenmenger syndrome) can be considered for bilateral lung transplantation with concomitant cardiac repair, if the cardiac defect is amenable to surgical correction, rather than combined heart-lung transplantation.[10,11]

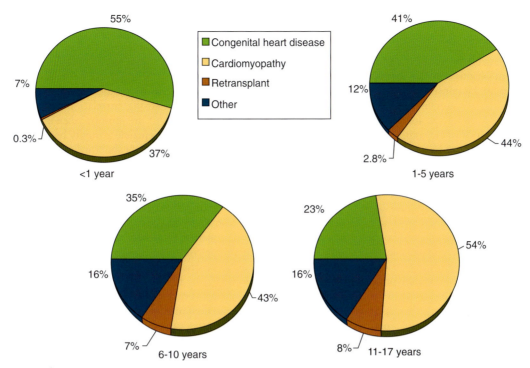

• **Figure 73.1** Indications for heart transplantation broken down by recipient age. (From Rossano JW, Cherikh WS, Chambers DC, et al. The Registry of the International Society for Heart and Lung Transplantation: Twentieth pediatric heart transplantation report-2017; focus theme: allograft ischemic time. *J Heart Lung Transplant.* 2017;36[10]:1060-1069.)

TABLE 73.1   Pediatric Lung Transplant Indications by Age-Group

Diagnosis	<1 Year No. (%)	1-5 Years No. (%)	6-10 Years No. (%)	11-17 Years No. (%)
Cystic fibrosis	0	4 (3.7)	116 (50.0)	814 (66.7)
Non–cystic fibrosis–bronchiectasis	0	0	2 (0.9)	23 (1.9)
ILD	5 (8.3)	9 (8.3)	6 (2.6)	37 (3.0)
ILD other	6 (10.0)	10 (9.3)	21 (9.1)	46 (3.8)
Pulmonary hypertension/pulmonary arterial hypertension	7 (11.7)	28 (25.9)	24 (10.3)	100 (8.2)
Pulmonary hypertension				
• Eisenmenger syndrome	0	1 (0.9)	2 (0.9)	6 (0.5)
• Other	15 (25.0)	21 (19.4)	8 (3.4)	20 (1.6)
Obliterative bronchiolitis (nonretransplant)	0	10 (9.3)	26 (11.2)	58 (4.8)
Bronchopulmonary dysplasia	4 (6.7)	4 (3.7)	3 (1.3)	3 (0.2)
ABCA3 transporter mutation	5 (8.3)	4 (3.7)	1 (0.4)	1 (0.1)
Surfactant protein B deficiency	13 (21.7)	4 (3.7)	1 (0.4)	0
Surfactant protein C deficiency	0	1 (0.9)	0	1 (0.1)
Retransplant				
• Obliterative bronchiolitis	0	4 (3.7)	8 (3.4)	41 (3.4)
• Not obliterative bronchiolitis	0	4 (3.7)	6 (2.6)	41 (3.4)
COPD, with or without A1ATD	2 (3.3)	1 (0.9)	3 (1.3)	10 (0.8)
Other	3 (5.0)	3 (2.8)	5 (2.2)	20 (1.6)

A1ATD, Alpha-1 antitrypsin deficiency; *COPD,* chronic obstructive pulmonary disease; *ILD,* interstitial lung disease.
Modified from Goldfarb SB, Levvey BJ, Cherikh WS, et al. Registry of the International Society for Heart and Lung Transplantation: Twentieth pediatric lung and heart-lung transplantation report-2017; focus theme: allograft ischemic time. *J Heart Lung Transplant.* 2017;36(10):1070-1079.

Heart-Lung Transplantation

Though some children with Eisenmenger syndrome have cardiac defects that are amenable to surgical repair, those with poor ventricular function, serious valvular disease, or uncorrectable cardiac anomalies must be considered for combined heart and lung transplantation. Heart-lung transplantation has been employed for patients with cystic fibrosis, occasionally with use of the recipient's heart for subsequent "domino" transplantation; however, the majority of institutions perform bilateral lung transplants in cystic fibrosis patients with normal cardiac function.

Contraindications

Contraindications to pediatric thoracic organ transplantation include any uncontrolled medical problem that cannot be directly attributed to the organ of interest. Where applicable, contraindications to heart and/or lung transplantation in pediatric patients are modified from adult criteria, but the population presents several unique challenges not faced in adults.[9,12] The charge for any given program is to be good stewards of the organs transplanted, which means recipients should be free from irreversible, noncardiac or nonpulmonary conditions that are expected to shorten life expectancy independent of the transplant. Patients with end-organ dysfunction involving other organ systems may be candidates for thoracic organ transplantation if circumstances permit multiple organ transplantation or if end-organ function can be improved with mechanical circulatory support (MCS). Multiple organ transplants such as heart/kidney, heart/liver, lung/kidney, and lung/liver have been performed in children. Importantly, once a patient is listed, there must be ongoing evaluation to determine whether any changes in medical status warrant either upgrading, downgrading, or delisting.

Current infection, apart from patients with MCS, should be resolved before exposure to the significant immunosuppression required after a heart transplant. Pulmonary infections, other than active *Mycobacterium tuberculosis,* are not considered contraindications to lung transplantation unless the organisms are resistant to all antibiotics. Prior viral illness is not a contraindication, but prophylactic therapy or increased monitoring may be warranted in the case of certain causes due to the risk of significant disease with reactivation (e.g., cytomegalovirus [CMV], Epstein-Barr virus [EBV]).[13,14] Infection with human immunodeficiency virus (HIV) is considered an absolute contraindication at many centers, but there is growing experience transplanting such patients particularly in the current era of antiretroviral therapy.[9,15]

Active neoplasm and ongoing chemotherapy and/or radiotherapy is a contraindication to transplantation at most centers. Transplantation can be considered if recurrence of the tumor is deemed to be low and there is a negative metastatic work-up; the tumor type and response to therapy are also considered.[12] No objective time after therapy is required before listing, although many centers require 2 years of remission before transplantation. With appropriately selected patients, there is no difference in long-term graft survival after heart transplantation in patients with anthracycline cardiomyopathy when compared to dilated cardiomyopathy.[16]

In adult patients when pulmonary artery pressure is 50 mm Hg or higher and either transpulmonary gradient is 15 mm Hg or higher or pulmonary vascular resistance (PVR) is greater than 3 Wood units (WU) • m^2, a vasodilator challenge is recommended. If the acute challenge is unsuccessful, then medical therapy is attempted to achieve reduction. Should medical and/or MCS

therapy fail to improve the PVR, then the pulmonary hypertension should be considered irreversible and serve as a contraindication to heart transplantation alone.[12] Older data in pediatric patients supported using PVR indexed to body surface area (PVRI) greater than 6 WU • m^2 as a cutoff value for listing, particularly when there was no reactivity to vasodilator testing.[17,18] More recent studies have not found a strong correlation between PVRI and posttransplant survival.[19] Care must be taken in interpreting PVR data in palliated single-ventricle patients because this value may be inaccurate due to structural abnormalities, collateral vessels, multiple sources of pulmonary blood flow, or differential blood flow patterns between lung segments.[20]

Several additional factors may serve as contraindications based on center preference, although most are considered relative. Down syndrome and other genetic syndromes are not contraindications to transplantation as long as the syndrome is not associated with any other contraindications and the patient's family support is capable of strict adherence to the posttransplant medical regimen. However, the benefit of transplantation in patients with severe cognitive or behavioral disabilities is highly controversial. Complex congenital anomalies, including pulmonary and systemic venous abnormalities, can present technical challenges during transplantation; however, these anomalies do not constitute a contraindication in and of themselves. Heart and lung transplant guidelines recommend weight loss before listing for any patient with body mass index above 35 kg/m^2,[9,12] although pediatric-specific studies have identified only borderline higher adjusted mortality after transplantation.[21] History of current illicit drug use or medical noncompliance may be of concern, but for juvenile patients the social setting must be considered and addressed if possible.

Preoperative Management

Recipient Evaluation

When a patient is referred for transplant evaluation, initial steps include determination of disease severity and whether there are any reversible or treatable factors responsible.[22] This is all highly dependent on the cause of heart or respiratory failure, which itself is variable by age-group (see Fig. 73.1 and Table 73.1). If there are no alternative treatment options, then a complete evaluation is undertaken, which includes medical, surgical, and psychosocial evaluation. The first, and possibly most important, step in the process is to have an in-depth discussion with the family/caregivers, and patient if appropriate, to fully inform them of the benefits, risks, and outcomes expected with transplantation. Only after they have provided their informed consent should the evaluation proceed.

Specific laboratory testing in patients is indicated to identify end-organ dysfunction, active infections, historical infectious exposures, coagulopathy, neoplasm, blood type, nutritional deficiencies, effects of chronic medications, and sensitization to human leukocyte antigens (HLAs) as represented by panel-reactive antibodies (PRAs). Based on initial testing, diagnosis, or other comorbid conditions, further diagnostic studies, particularly imaging, may be indicated to assess end-organ function, vascular access, surgical approach, or presence of neoplasm.

The ISHLT recommends right heart catheterization should be performed on all adult candidates for heart transplant listing and periodically thereafter until transplantation. In cases of suspected myocarditis, biopsy can help determine the extent of involvement and potential for reversibility[23]; however, recent advances in cardiac magnetic resonance imaging have led to less dependence on invasive studies.[24,25] The same may be said of determination of complex anatomy by computed tomography and cardiac magnetic resonance imaging, but data regarding hemodynamics remain the unique purview of catheterization, especially when a potential intervention is discovered. Determination of PVRI by catheterization is of particular importance in pediatric patients given the potential impact on outcomes after transplantation.[17]

The inclusion of cardiopulmonary exercise testing (CPET) in evaluation for transplantation in pediatric and adolescent patients is variable. For those in whom CPET can be performed, assessment of peak oxygen consumption (VO_2) may be useful in the decision to list for heart transplantation. Guidelines from ISHLT use VO_2 cutoff values of less than 14 mL/kg/min or 50% or less predicted as guides to consider listing for adult patients but offer no specific guidance on pediatric patients.[12] Pulmonary and musculoskeletal disease can negatively affect results. Normal values for pediatric patients are different than in adults,[26] and patients with palliated single-ventricle physiology may have a depressed baseline.[27] Other parameters, such as heart rate reserve, minute ventilation/carbon dioxide production, and peak systolic blood pressure during CPET have been shown to predict risk in patients with congenital heart disease.[28] Pulmonary function testing and 6-minute walk test may also be indicated, particularly for lung transplant evaluation.

The goal of the psychosocial evaluation is to assess whether there are sufficient social supports to achieve compliant care in the outpatient setting to maximize the chances for a successful outcome. This assessment includes the parents/caregivers and patient if appropriate and addresses home environment, extended support networks, history of compliance with medical management recommendations, and history of illicit drug use or social welfare concerns. It is important to stress to families that there is no bias based on race, ethnicity, socioeconomic status, or family structure.

Determination of pretransplant HLA sensitization by PRAs is necessary to assess risk of rejection and to identify donor HLA to avoid. A number of factors, including use of human homograft material in surgical palliation, frequent blood transfusions, MCS, and prior transplantation can contribute to antibody generation. These preformed, circulating antibodies can engage in cell- and antibody-mediated rejection and lead to graft loss or death. The current combination of flow cytometry using beads coated with single HLA antigens and a C1q complement-fixing assay allows detection of clinically significant antibodies, yielding the calculated PRA (cPRA).[29] In patients who are highly sensitized and can expect long wait times as a result of many identified antibodies to HLA, desensitization protocols have shown efficacy in reducing the cPRA.[30]

Recipient Management

Waiting list mortality in pediatric patients is higher for heart transplantation than any other solid organ. The most important factor in predicting mortality is the level of invasive hemodynamic support.[31] Management of patients on the waiting list can vary from standard heart failure therapy as an outpatient to MCS and mechanical ventilation and depends on a variety of factors, including severity of cardiac dysfunction, cardiac diagnosis, and end-organ dysfunction. The level of support required also factors into the listing status (Table 73.2). Overall, the goal is to maintain end-organ function, optimize nutrition, and deliver the patient to transplant with as few comorbidities as possible.

The goals of medical management are to reduce fluid overload, reduce afterload, and downregulate neurohormonal responses. When patients cannot be adequately managed with oral heart

TABLE 73.2	Criteria for Listing Status in Pediatric Heart Transplant
Status	**Criteria**
1A[a]	Candidate is <18 years of age at time of listing, and meets *one* of the following: • Requires continuous mechanical ventilation • Requires assistance of an intraaortic balloon pump • Has ductal dependent pulmonary or systemic circulation, with ductal patency maintained by stent or prostaglandin • Has hemodynamically significant congenital heart disease, requires infusion of a single high-inotrope dose or multiple intravenous inotropes • Requires assistance of mechanical circulatory support
1B	Candidate is <18 years of age at time of listing and meets one of the following: • Requires infusion of one or more inotropic agents but does not qualify for pediatric status 1A • Is <1 year of age at time of initial listing and has a diagnosis of hypertrophic or restrictive cardiomyopathy
2	Candidate is <18 years of age at time of listing and does not meet the criteria for status 1A or 1B but is suitable for transplant
7	Inactive

[a]Patient must be admitted to the hospital that listed the candidate.
Modified from Organ Procurement and Transplantation Network Policies document, effective date 2/5/2018.

failure medications, a number of inotropic and vasoactive agents are available. Milrinone, dopamine, dobutamine, and epinephrine are all options.

Certain patients will continue to deteriorate despite maximal medical therapy and ultimately may require mechanical ventilator support. Positive intrathoracic pressure benefits patients with left ventricular systolic and diastolic dysfunction by reducing afterload, as well as working to improve pulmonary edema and atelectatic lung segments. However, positive pressure can have mixed effects on the right heart if there is pulmonary distention beyond functional residual capacity. High intrathoracic pressures also increase systemic venous pressures and can worsen systemic edema, inhibit ventricular filling, and worsen secondary organ injury due to elevation of central venous pressure.

For decades the mainstay of MCS has been extracorporeal membrane oxygenation (ECMO). More recently a growing number of support devices have become available for patients in need of only circulatory support. Device selection depends on support goals, patient size, and native cardiac anatomy among other factors. For small children the primary option outside of ECMO has been the Berlin EXCOR pulsatile ventricular assist device. This pneumatically driven extracorporeal device is the only one approved in the United States by the Federal Drug Administration for use in children as a bridge to transplantation. The Berlin EXCOR comes in multiple pump sizes and is capable of supporting children as small as 3 to 4 kg. The device allows for reliable support of either or both ventricles. Overall success rate for bridge to transplant or explant and recovery is roughly 75%, with superior survival after heart transplant when compared with ECMO.[32,33] It should be noted that in children under 10 kg at implantation, survival was lower than that of the entire group, predominantly due to patients with congenital heart disease, weight less than 5 kg, and evidence of biventricular failure through elevated bilirubin level.[34] Further analysis has revealed that end-organ function at device implantation predicts adverse outcomes, and that neonates and infants with congenital heart disease, particularly those with prior heart surgery and ECMO support, may have poorer outcomes when considering bridge to transplant or weaning.[35] When analyzing patients who went on to transplantation, posttransplant survival at 30 days, 1 year, and 5 years was equivalent between patients bridged with EXCOR and those who underwent transplant without MCS.[36]

Beyond the EXCOR, several other MCS options exist for pediatric and adolescent patients, with the latter being eligible for most of the devices available to adult patients.[37,38] Determination of the needed duration of support, patient size, one or two ventricular support, and native cardiac anatomy all effect the choice. Options include short-term versus long-term, extracorporeal versus implanted versus catheter-based, pulsatile versus continuous flow, and even options for complete cardiac replacement with a total artificial heart. Once a device is selected, advanced imaging techniques can be used to perform a virtual "fit test" to anticipate any anatomic or mechanical complications.[37] Management after placement is contingent on the device selected, but major themes emerge based on the most common complications: bleeding, thrombus formation, infection, and right heart failure in the case of isolated left heart support.[38] A growing body of literature supports successful use of these devices in congenital heart disease.[39-44]

Children who are listed for lung transplantation are frequently critically ill with a significant percentage requiring hospitalization with or without mechanical ventilation and pressor support before donor organs become available. As a result, aggressive maneuvers may be necessary in an attempt to maintain end-organ viability and transplant candidacy for as long as possible. Over the past decade, advances in mechanical ventilation with jet and high-frequency ventilators, the availability of prostacyclin and nitric oxide, and artificial lung devices have broadened the armamentarium available for use in these children. Despite these measures, mortality on the waiting list remains in the range of 20% to 25% for infants and children.[5]

The use of ECMO before lung transplantation has been less common than for heart transplantation; however, there has been experience reported in both the adult and pediatric populations. A recent systematic review of published data from 14 studies with adult patients bridged to lung transplant by ECMO found mortality rate of patients before lung transplant and 1-year survival ranged from 10% to 50% and 50% to 90%, respectively.[45] In a single-center report of pediatric patients supported with ECMO, mechanical ventilation without ECMO, or neither, outcomes of transplanted patients were not statistically different regarding hospital discharge and 1-year survival.[46] Given the risks associated with ECMO, there has recently been interest in the use of paracorporeal lung assist devices as a bridge to lung transplantation in neonates and children, including reports of isolated successful cases.[47,48]

Donor Management

Initial donor evaluation must begin with determination of brain death. Involvement of an organ procurement agency should be initiated as soon as possible after brain death has been established to minimize the length of time between brain death and possible organ harvest. The hormonal and hemodynamic changes associated with brain death are detrimental to both cardiac and pulmonary

function, so special consideration must be given to maintenance of donor organ function in the physiologically abnormal state produced by brain death.[49] Treatment with thyroxine often results in decreased inotrope requirements with salvage of some organs that might otherwise not be considered for transplantation. Management of neurogenic shock requires volume resuscitation, but care must be employed in both the amount and type of volume administered. If possible, blood or colloids should be used, and volume status should be assessed using central venous or pulmonary capillary wedge pressures. Bronchoscopy can be useful both for diagnostic and therapeutic purposes such as removal of mucous plugs, which can decrease atelectasis and improve pulmonary gas exchange.[50] Transthoracic echocardiography is usually performed on potential heart donors to rule out any intracardiac abnormalities or regional wall motion abnormality. Arterial blood gas measurement performed on potential lung donors may determine the adequacy of gas exchange, and a chest x-ray is done to rule out the possibility of pulmonary contusion or infectious infiltrate. Blood should be obtained from the potential organ donor for serologic studies to determine if there are any transmissible diseases (e.g., HIV, hepatitis) and ABO blood typing. Preference for ABO blood group matching is the general rule, but in the last decade some centers are opting for protocols to offer ABO-incompatible transplantation, primarily in infants, with the goal of decreasing waiting time.[51]

Given the scarcity of pediatric organs available for transplantation, alternate strategies to increase the donor pool have been considered. Many patients are considered for organ donation even if organ function is initially borderline or unacceptable. Studies have shown that aggressive donor management can significantly improve donor organ function and early posttransplant results.[50,52] Additionally, it is clear that some organs turned down for pediatric patients based on concerns over donor quality may be acceptable, with similar outcomes between quality-refused hearts and those offered primarily[53,54] or hearts refused in pediatric patients that were successfully transplanted in adult recipients.[55] Because of the limited donor pool, neonatal transplant programs often accept organs from a wider geographic area, and thus with longer cold ischemic times, than an adult program would consider. Ischemic times as long as 9.5 hours have not been shown to adversely affect long-term outcomes for pediatric heart transplant recipients,[56] with greater tolerance for prolonged ischemic time in grafts from younger (<19 years) when compared with older (≥20 years) donors.[57] Finally, over the last decade there has been interest in accepting organs from donors after circulatory death (as opposed to after brain death), with long-term results in adult lung transplants,[58,59] and limited cases in pediatric heart transplants,[60] showing promising results.

The size range of donor organs that can be accepted for pediatric heart transplants is larger than for adults. Donors up to 2.5 times the weight of the recipient can be accepted with no evidence of ill effects in most cases. Evaluations of graft growth have shown that the velocity of cardiac growth is initially slow for these oversized organs with normal growth later in life, essentially allowing the recipient to grow into the larger organ.[61] Certain children with dilated cardiomyopathy and massive cardiomegaly can tolerate organs from donors as much as three times their weight, although care must be taken to prevent atelectasis from pulmonary compression. Contemporary data suggest use of imaging-measured cardiac volume could prove more useful in achieving an appropriate match.[62]

Another option that has increased donor lung availability for small recipients is the use of lobar transplants from adult donors into children. This technique can be applied for both brain-dead and living-related donors. Living-related lobar transplantation is a relatively new technique that provides organs for transplantation for a limited population of children. In the majority of cases children receive a lower lobe from each parent for bilateral lung transplantation. Donors have generally done well after the procedure, and early to midterm outcomes for recipients have been comparable to cadaveric transplant recipients. There have been reports that recipients of living-related lobar transplants have better pulmonary function at 2 years and experience bronchiolitis obliterans less frequently when compared to cadaveric donation,[63] and that these transplants may be a better option for patients in need of retransplantation.[64]

Operative Techniques

Donor Organ Retrieval

Successful thoracic organ transplantation begins with precise anatomic dissection and preservation of the donor organ. The process is complex and involves coordination between multiple teams from different locations and coordination between the retrieval team and recipient facility. There are many opportunities within this interaction for misadventure, but the coordinated effort of the surgical teams during anatomic dissection allows the organ-specific needs of each team to be met. Identification of the donor by a United Network for Organ Sharing–specific ID is a critical first responsibility of the retrieval team along with confirmation of ABO compatibility. All donor clinical information should be reviewed, including documentation for confirmation of brain death. This includes echocardiograms, chest x-ray, and results of laboratory work (including serology). Fiberoptic bronchoscopy is usually performed by the lung retrieval team as an adjunct to determine suitability for proceeding with transplantation.

Accurate hemodynamic monitoring should be guided by central venous pressure and an arterial catheter. Maintenance of a normal mean arterial blood pressure for the patient's age is the goal along with avoidance of fluid overload and dehydration. The central venous pressure should be kept less than 10 mm Hg. For management of the donor lungs, the tidal volume is maintained at 10 mL/kg or less. The fraction of inspired oxygen is kept at less than 50%. Airway heaters and heating blankets should be avoided. Vasoactive infusions may be necessary. This should be coordinated with the abdominal organ retrieval team. Interventions, special protocols, and any specific donor medications should be coordinated between the retrieval teams. If the lungs are to be retrieved, it is also critical to communicate to the anesthesiologist to maintain ventilation of the lungs after the heart is explanted.

A generous median sternotomy is made and usually will be in continuity inferiorly with the abdominal incision (Fig. 73.2). A double-bladed sternal retractor is ideal for exposure of the heart and access to both pleural spaces. The thymus should be excised completely. This will allow access to the trachea above the innominate vein and enhances exposure of the great vessels. The pericardium is incised, and pericardial sutures are secured to hemostats, which allows easy access to the pleural spaces if the lungs are to be harvested (Fig. 73.3). The heart is inspected to assess function and evidence of chamber distention, particularly the right ventricle. This initial visual assessment should be used to rule out undocumented injuries or evidence of congenital anomalies. The coronary vessels should be palpated as well for evidence of atherosclerosis. Palpation of the lungs should be carried out, if retrieval is planned, to assess for masses and to assess for air underneath the visceral pleura. Air

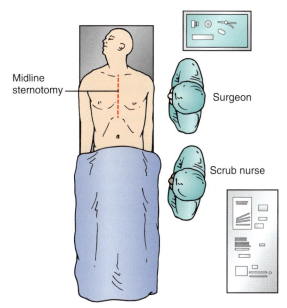

• **Figure 73.2** Donor procedure: median sternotomy. A generous median sternotomy is created in continuity with the abdominal midline incision. Care should be taken at the inferior aspect to protect the liver. (From Camp PC. Heart transplantation donor operation for heart and lung transplantation. *Oper Tech Thorac Cardiovasc Surg.* 2010;15[2]:125-137.)

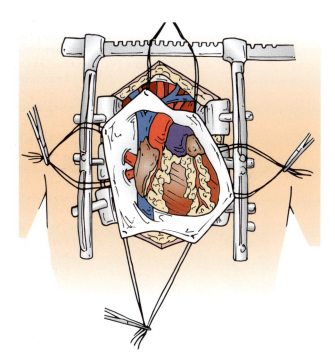

• **Figure 73.3** Exposure of the heart for explant. The pericardium is opened vertically from the diaphragm to its inflection at the ascending aorta. (From Camp PC. Heart transplantation donor operation for heart and lung transplantation. *Oper Tech Thorac Cardiovasc Surg.* 2010;15[2]:125-137.)

underneath the visceral pleura can be a subtle sign of undiagnosed injury to the airway. If the organs are felt to be acceptable, the implantation team is informed, so the recipient operation can be timed appropriately.[65,66]

The heart is prepared for explant at this time. The preference is to complete all necessary cardiac dissection as the abdominal dissection proceeds. The needs of the implanting team to achieve a successful recipient reconstruction should have been communicated. This may require additional segments of the aortic arch, descending aorta, and possibly the branch pulmonary arteries, particularly in patients with complex congenital heart disease. The innominate vein is mobilized from the anterior wall of the aortic arch. The aorta is dissected free of the main pulmonary artery with exposure of the proximal right pulmonary artery. The ascending aorta is dissected free from the main pulmonary artery to allow cross-clamp application. The superior vena cava (SVC) is circumferentially mobilized from surrounding tissues, exposing the azygous vein and the junction of the innominate and jugular veins. The azygous vein is ligated and divided. Next, the inferior vena cava (IVC) is dissected free from the diaphragm. For lung retrievals the trachea is circumferentially dissected free of surrounding structures above the innominate vein (Fig. 73.4). Another critical maneuver when the lungs are retrieved is the development of the interatrial groove (Fig. 73.5). Having this plane exposed before application of the aortic cross-clamp will allow accurate division of the atrial cuff for equal distribution to the heart and lung teams.[65,66]

Purse-string stitches are placed in the ascending aorta and the pulmonary artery just proximal to the pulmonary artery bifurcation. Cannulas are inserted in each vessel if the heart and lungs are retrieved. When the abdominal team is ready and if the lungs are being retrieved, prostacyclin is injected into the proximal main pulmonary artery to ensure equal distribution to both lungs. Inflow occlusion of the SVC and IVC occurs. The heart is allowed to empty for two to three beats, and the aorta is cross-clamped. The respective preservative solutions are instilled. It is critical to avoid distention of the heart at this time. The IVC is transected, and

the left side of the heart is decompressed via an incision in the left atrial appendage. When the lungs are not being retrieved, this incision can be made in the right upper pulmonary vein. As the preservation solutions are instilled, topical cooling of the organs is achieved by immersing the mediastinum and both pleural spaces in iced slush. Once the solutions are completed, the organs are explanted.[65,66]

Cardiac Explant. Once the cardioplegia solutions have been infused, the heart can be excised. The IVC is transected, and the apex of the heart is retracted superiorly, exposing the pulmonary veins, which are transected individually in an isolated cardiac retrieval. If the lungs are taken, the left atrium is divided halfway between the entry of the pulmonary veins and the coronary sinus/left atrial appendage insertion. The SVC, aorta, and pulmonary artery are divided at an appropriate level, depending on the recipient's needs. The heart is packed in iced preservative solution and bagged for transport. Ventilation of the lungs should be maintained at this point if the lungs are being retrieved (Fig. 73.6).[65]

Lung Explant. With the heart explanted and the lungs remaining in situ, each pulmonary vein is retrograde flushed individually. The effluent from each vein into the pulmonary artery is assessed. The goal is to achieve a clear effluent free of any blood clots. Each lung is mobilized by first dividing the inferior pulmonary ligament. The posterior mediastinal pleura is incised bilaterally. On the right, this incision is along the esophagus. On the left, it is along the descending thoracic aorta. The endotracheal tube is withdrawn slightly at this time, but ventilation is maintained. The trachea is stapled with a TA 30 stapler, paying particular attention not to overdistend the lungs. They are packed in iced preservative solution and bagged for transport (Fig. 73.7).[65]

Heart-Lung Block. In this instance, once the preservation solutions are completed, the procedure commences as described except for the incisions made for explanting the organs en bloc. Those incisions are aorta, IVC, SVC, and trachea. The block is packed in iced preservative solution for transport.

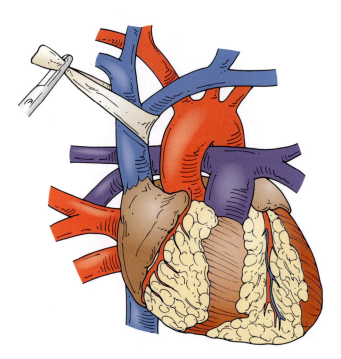

• **Figure 73.4** Preparation of the heart for explant. The aorta is mobilized from the main pulmonary artery. The innominate vein is mobilized off the arch to allow exposure of the great vessels. Once the arch is dissected, the pulmonary artery is mobilized at the point of bifurcation of the left and right side. (From Camp PC. Heart transplantation donor operation for heart and lung transplantation. *Oper Tech Thorac Cardiovasc Surg.* 2010;15[2]: 125-137.)

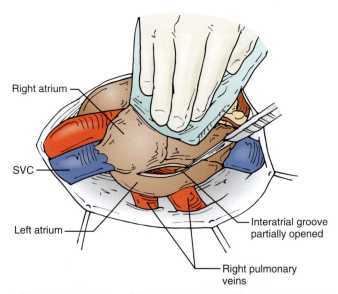

• **Figure 73.5** Exposure of the interatrial groove. The heart is retracted to the left, exposing the right pulmonary veins. The interface of the left and right atria is opened along its entire length to better define the interface of the left atria and right pulmonary veins. *SVC,* Superior vena cava. (From Camp PC. Heart transplantation donor operation for heart and lung transplantation. *Oper Tech Thorac Cardiovasc Surg.* 2010;15[2]:125-137.)

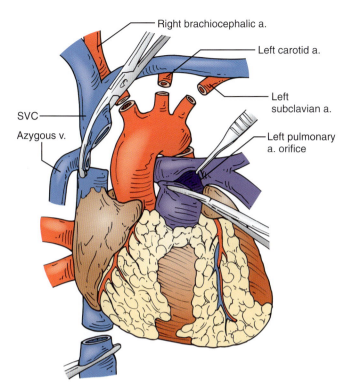

• **Figure 73.6** Cardiac explant. *a.,* Artery; *SVC,* superior vena cava; *v.,* vein. (From Camp PC. Heart transplantation donor operation for heart and lung transplantation. *Oper Tech Thorac Cardiovasc Surg.* 2010;15[2]: 125-137.)

Labels: Right brachiocephalic a.; Left carotid a.; Left subclavian a.; Left pulmonary a. orifice; SVC; Azygous v.

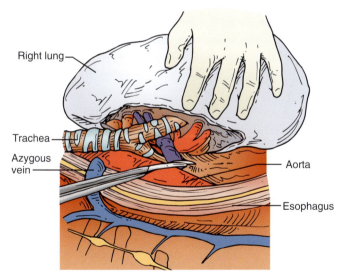

• **Figure 73.7** Lung explant. (From Camp PC. Heart transplantation donor operation for heart and lung transplantation. *Oper Tech Thorac Cardiovasc Surg.* 2010;15[2]:125-137.)

Labels: Right lung; Trachea; Azygous vein; Aorta; Esophagus

Heart Implantation

A median sternotomy is performed. After achieving adequate systemic heparinization, ascending aorta and direct caval cannulation are used to place the patient on cardiopulmonary bypass. The aorta is cross-clamped, and the heart is removed, leaving a generous cuff of aorta, pulmonary artery, left atrium around the pulmonary veins, and long lengths of IVC and SVC for a bicaval implant.

The atria are divided just above the atrioventricular groove for a biatrial implant, leaving each cava intact.[65]

The allograft is prepared by first ensuring the absence of any intraatrial communications. The aorta is dissected away from the pulmonary artery. A left atrial cuff is created by connecting the pulmonary venous ostia. The left-sided anastomoses are carried out starting with the left atrium and then the aorta. A vent can be left across the left atrial suture line as the aorta is reconstructed. At this time, if the ischemic time has been long, the aortic cross-clamp can be removed. To deair the left side of the heart, an active vent can be placed in the ascending aorta before allowing the heart to eject blood. The venous anastomoses can be completed with the heart beating. Those anastomoses include the IVC, main pulmonary artery, and SVC. Continuous monofilament suture is used for all anastomotic sites. The bicaval technique is the primary technique of the author for all patients undergoing orthotopic heart transplant regardless of age (Fig. 73.8). However, flexibility in the application of different implant techniques is valuable as different situations arise. That said, for a biatrial implant, the donor left atrium is then anastomosed to the recipient left atrium (Fig. 73.9). Before completion of the suture line, the left atrium is filled with cold saline to evacuate as much air as possible. The lateral wall of the donor right atrium is incised to create an appropriate opening for anastomosis to the recipient right atrial cuff. Once the atrial suture lines are completed, the pulmonary artery and aorta are trimmed and anastomosed with running sutures. At this point the left side of heart is deaired by ventilating the patient, agitating the heart, and using an active vent placed in the ascending aorta. The patient is then separated from cardiopulmonary bypass.[65,66]

Lung Implantation

A bilateral thoracosternotomy is made (Fig. 73.10). Cardiopulmonary bypass is established with right atrial and ascending aorta cannulation after systemic heparinization. However, if concomitant intracardiac repair is required, bicaval cannulation can be used, and the repair conducted under cardioplegic arrest after the recipient pneumonectomy is performed. The advantages of using cardiopulmonary bypass for bilateral sequential lung transplantation in children are as follows: the removal of the recipient's lungs is a relatively simple and safe matter, the airways can be irrigated with antibiotic solution after removal of both lungs in cases of septic lung disease, and the ischemic time for the second lung to be implanted is minimized. Each lung is excised by individually ligating and then dividing the pulmonary artery, vein, and main stem bronchus.

When the donor lungs arrive, the lung block is wrapped in cold pads, and the hilar structures are dissected. The bronchi are divided approximately two rings above the takeoff of the upper lobe bronchi. The pulmonary arteries are trimmed to appropriate length, and the pulmonary venous confluence is divided in the midline. Typically the left lung is implanted first, starting with the bronchial anastomosis, which is performed as close to the carina as possible. For the bronchial anastomosis, a continuous suture of polydioxanone (PDS) is used for the membranous segment of the airway. The cartilaginous segment is sewn with simple interrupted sutures. A partial occlusion clamp is placed on the recipient left atrium so as to include the upper and lower veins, which are connected to provide a large cuff of atrium for the anastomosis. This cuff is sewn to the donor pulmonary vein cuff using running absorbable suture. This clamp is left in place as the

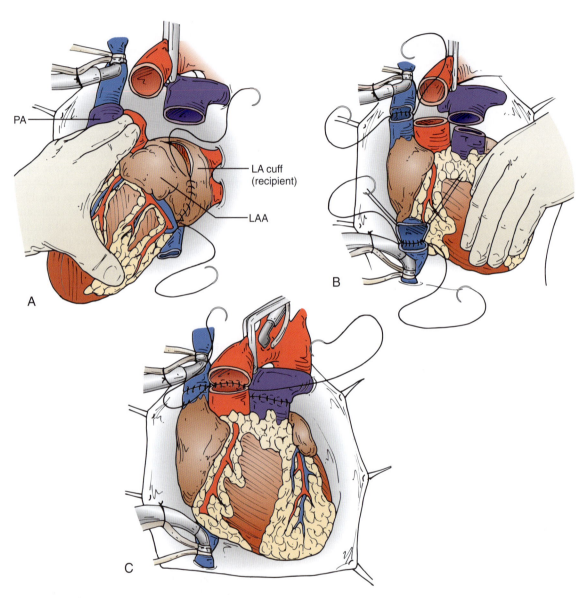

PA

LA cuff
(recipient)

LAA

A

B

C

• **Figure 73.8** Bicaval heart implant showing (A) left atrial anastomosis, (B) superior and inferior vena caval anastomosis, and (C) pulmonary artery and aortic anastomosis. *LA,* Left atrium; *LAA,* left atrial anastomosis; *PA,* pulmonary artery. (From John RJ, Liao K. Orthotopic heart transplantation. *Oper Tech Thorac Cardiovasc Surg.* 2010;15[2]:138-146.)

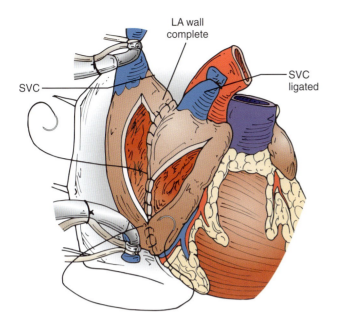

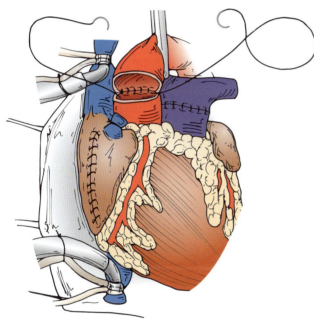

• **Figure 73.9** Biatrial heart implant. *LA,* Left atrium; *SVC,* superior vena cava. (From John RJ, Liao K. Orthotopic heart transplantation. *Oper Tech Thorac Cardiovasc Surg.* 2010;15[2]:138-146.)

arterial anastomosis is fashioned (Fig. 73.11A). The pulmonary artery is anastomosed with a continuous monofilament suture. The lung is deaired by partially unclamping the left atrium before completion of the pulmonary artery anastomosis, so as to back-bleed through the lung (see Fig. 73.11B). The right lung is implanted using a similar technique.

Heart-Lung Implantation

En bloc heart-lung transplantation is typically performed through a bilateral thoracosternotomy (clamshell incision) using the fourth intercostal spaces. Cardiopulmonary bypass is established as described but with bicaval venous cannulation. The lungs are mobilized bilaterally with care taken to protect the phrenic nerves, which are left intact on a pedicle of pericardium. The lungs are then excised as described previously. The heart is excised, leaving only a cuff of aorta and right atrium. Once the heart is removed, the trachea can be mobilized in the posterior mediastinum and divided just above the carina. Once this dissection is complete and adequate hemostasis has been achieved, the donor organs are placed in the mediastinum with the lungs passed behind the phrenic nerve pedicles. The trachea is anastomosed first using a combination of running suture for the membranous septum and interrupted sutures for the cartilaginous portion. The aorta, IVC, and SVC anastomosis complete the implant. However, right atrial implantation can be used in infants and very small children to avoid the risk of caval anastomotic stricture. The right atrium and aorta are anastomosed using running sutures, and the cross-clamp is removed after aggressive deairing. In most cases bicaval implantation is used rather than the atrial technique so as to improve the geometry of the right atrium and decrease tricuspid regurgitation.

Complications

Many complications that occur after cardiothoracic transplantation, particularly early, are similar to those encountered after nontransplant cardiothoracic surgical procedures. Other complications are unique to transplantation and the required postoperative management. Morbidities are influenced by the preoperative state, including neurologic, hematologic, infectious, immunologic, nephrologic, and the general state of health. Nutritional, muscular, and respiratory status, as well as the number of previous thoracic surgeries are of particular concern before cardiothoracic surgery, including transplantation. The peak hazard risk for mortality occurs in the first year following transplantation, with the greatest risk in the first 3 months (Fig. 73.12).[3] The leading causes of early mortality are graft failure, acute rejection, and non-CMV infection (Fig. 73.13).[67]

Graft Failure

Nonspecific graft failure typically relates to allograft failure that cannot be attributed to cellular or antibody-mediated rejection. Mortality within the first 30 days is largely due to acute graft failure, accounting for nearly 40% of deaths after heart transplantation according to the ISHLT[67]; the rate is lower for lung transplantation at 15%.[2] Primary graft failure is the leading cause of death (47%) among all listed causes that meet the definition of early graft failure in heart transplantation.[68] Causes of failure include ischemic time of the donor graft and ischemia-reperfusion injury. Acute right heart failure often can be predicted by the presence of pretransplant elevation in PVR. It is not uncommon that a recipient will be supported by agents that affect systemic vascular resistance (e.g., milrinone, beta-adrenergic agonists, angiotensin-converting enzyme inhibitors) and also by therapies that can affect PVR (e.g., nitroprusside, milrinone, inhaled nitric oxide). Need for MCS is uncommon but, when necessary, includes ECMO in situations of allograft dysfunction causing hemodynamic and/or respiratory insufficiency. Other forms of mechanical support include temporary right, left, and biventricular pulsatile or continuous flow devices.[69] (A detailed discussion of ECMO and other MCS options is found in Chapters 39 and 40.) Consideration for cardiac retransplantation for early, acute graft failure is controversial. A multi-institutional report from the Pediatric Heart Transplant Study (PHTS) database reviewed all pediatric recipients over a 10-year

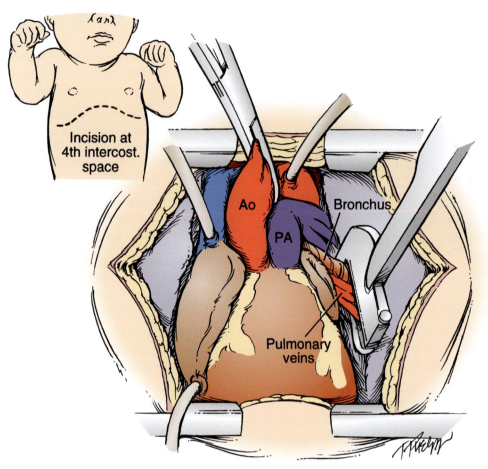

• **Figure 73.10** The thoracosternotomy (clamshell) incision through the fourth intercostal space is shown in the insert. Bicaval venous cannulation is used to initiate cardiopulmonary bypass. The lungs are removed by serially dividing and ligating the pulmonary artery branches and pulmonary veins. The main stem bronchi are stapled. *Ao,* Aorta; *PA,* pulmonary artery.

period between 1993 and 2004. The authors concluded that survival after pediatric retransplantation was inferior when compared with primary transplant outcomes, and the greatest risk for mortality was retransplantation for early, acute graft failure.[70] Retransplantation at any time after primary transplant is the highest risk factor for death in the first year, with a hazard ratio of 2.4.[68]

Acute Rejection

Acute rejection is a significant cause of mortality in the first 30 postoperative days (7% of all-cause mortality in cardiac, 3% in lung),[2,67] and the peak hazard risk for the first rejection episode occurs in the first 3 months (Fig. 73.14).[71] Rejection is not only a short-term complication but remains as a significant cause of long-term morbidity and mortality.[2,72] The majority of pediatric heart transplant patients experience at least one episode of rejection, with 31% having multiple episodes.[73] Eighteen percent of patients died during the rejection event when associated with hemodynamic compromise. Additionally, 55% died by 5 years after the rejection event.[74] In the current era (2009–2015), approximately 15% of patients will experience rejection requiring treatment beyond maintenance immunosuppression in the first year after transplantation. When comparing patients with rejection in the first year to those without, a significant decrease is seen in survival over the following 10 years.[3]

Historically, cellular-mediated rejection dominated clinical and academic practices with conventional therapies primarily targeting T-cell responses. B cell–mediated rejection, which is poorly responsive to standard immunosuppressive management, has gained wider appreciation over the last decade. This entity, also known as antibody-mediated rejection, can lead to the development of graft vasculopathy, cardiac dysfunction, and death.[75] Antibodies against human HLA target endothelial cells. The interplay between donor-specific HLA antibodies and antigens activates the complement cascade, ultimately leading to the formation of membrane attack complexes that create pores in the targeted cell membrane. Cell death ensues after the integrity of the membrane is disrupted, allowing the diffusion of molecules down their concentration gradients.[76]

Rejection of the graft has been recognized since the dawn of transplantation. Over many decades, various immunosuppressive therapies have been developed, primarily aimed at preventing cellular rejection. Since 2004, 60% to 70% of cardiac transplant recipients receive some form of induction therapy, with 40% to 50% commonly cytolytic agents in the form of polyclonal antibodies (antilymphocyte globulin and antithymocyte globulin). Another 20% of recipients receive an interleukin-2 receptor antagonist (e.g., basiliximab), and approximately 20% receive no induction therapy.[67] In similar fashion approximately 70% of lung transplant patients receive induction therapy; however, the majority are in the form

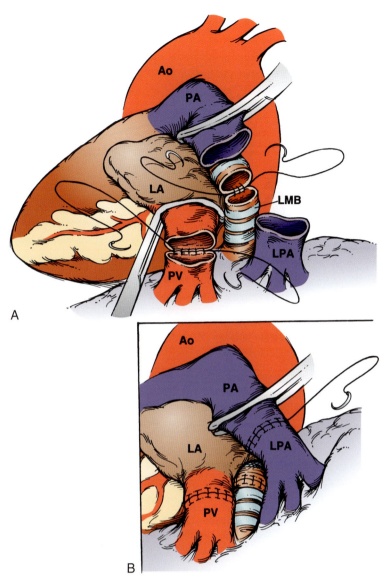

• **Figure 73.11** A, Lung implantation. Typically the bronchus is anastomosed first, followed by the left atrial/pulmonary venous connection. B, The implantation is completed with the left pulmonary artery anastomosis. *Ao,* Aorta; *LA,* left atrium; *LMB,* left main stem bronchus; *LPA,* left pulmonary artery; *PA,* pulmonary artery; *PV,* pulmonary vein.

of interleukin-2 receptor antagonists.[2] The goals of induction therapy include reduction of early rejection, delaying initiation of calcineurin inhibitors (cyclosporine and tacrolimus) that may lower the likelihood of renal insufficiency, and reduction of corticosteroid exposure. Choice of agent (or to defer induction) is dependent on center experience and goals. A large, multicenter PHTS report in 1999 demonstrated that pediatric cardiac recipients who received polyclonal antibodies had significantly lower cumulative rejection and higher freedom from mortality due to rejection compared with muromonab CD3 (OKT3) but not significantly different from those who received no induction.[77] The nonsuperior finding of rejection prevention by induction therapy is also noted in contemporary ISHLT reports.[68,78] Although use of induction therapy has increased since 2004, there is no statistical difference in survival compared to the cohort that did not receive induction therapy.[68] Notably, treated rejection has declined and is significantly lower today, compared with the incidence before 2009. Serious

complications related to cytolytic induction therapy include increased rate of infections[79] and the cytokine release syndrome. This is a serious, life-threatening reaction resulting from T-cell destruction with subsequent release of cytokines that can lead to high-grade fever, anaphylaxis, pulmonary edema, and death. Pretreatment with an antihistamine, a corticosteroid, and acetaminophen is recommended to reduce the likelihood of an adverse event. Aside from the cytokine release syndrome, more common adverse events include fever, chills, leukopenia, pain, headache, abdominal pain, diarrhea, hypertension, nausea, thrombocytopenia, edema, dyspnea, hyperkalemia, and tachycardia.[80]

Prevention of short- and long-term allograft rejection requires use of maintenance immunosuppression. Often this is a calcineurin inhibitor (e.g., cyclosporine, tacrolimus) in combination with an antiproliferative agent (e.g., azathioprine, mycophenolate mofetil) and corticosteroids. The goal of most transplant centers is to be free of corticosteroids within the first year following transplantation; however, some shorten

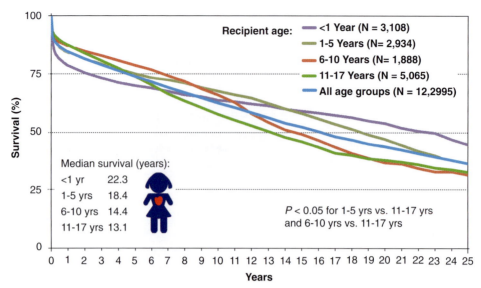

• **Figure 73.12** Pediatric heart transplantation Kaplan-Meier survival by age-group, January 1982 to June 2015. (From Rossano JW, Cherikh WS, Chambers DC, et al. The Registry of the International Society for Heart and Lung Transplantation: Twentieth pediatric heart transplantation report-2017; focus theme: allograft ischemic time. *J Heart Lung Transplant.* 2017;36[10]:1060-1069.)

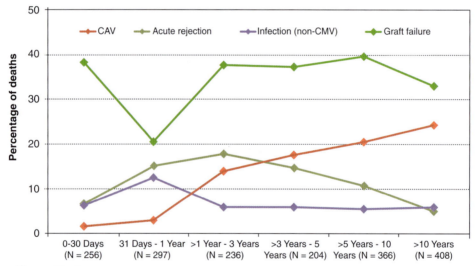

• **Figure 73.13** Relative incidence of causes of death in pediatric heart transplant recipients, January 2004 to June 2015. *CAV,* Cardiac allograft vasculopathy; *CMV,* cytomegalovirus. (From Rossano JW, Dipchand AI, Edwards LB, et al. The Registry of the International Society for Heart and Lung Transplantation: Nineteenth pediatric heart transplantation report-2016; focus theme: primary diagnostic indications for transplant. *J Heart Lung Transplant.* 2016;35[10]:1185-1195.)

that time to weeks, whereas still others do not use steroids outside of the immediate perioperative period. The most common immunosuppressant combination used currently is tacrolimus with mycophenolate mofetil.[67] In recent years, use of mammalian target of rapamycin (mTOR) inhibitors (e.g., everolimus, sirolimus), in combination with or in place of calcineurin inhibitors has gained favor in heart transplantation. This is primarily due to potential prevention of allograft vasculopathy and the allowance for lower target levels of calcineurin inhibitors when used in combination.[81-83] Use of mTOR inhibitors in lung transplantation is infrequent.[2]

The gold standard for diagnosis of allograft rejection is the invasive cardiac biopsy, allowing for histologic evaluation of the right ventricle, meant to represent the state of health of the entire graft. Diagnosis of rejection, however, is often made on clinical grounds in the absence of a biopsy or in the presence of negative biopsy samples. Regardless of how diagnosed, treatment of acute cellular rejection may be delivered in an intensive care setting, especially when associated with hemodynamic compromise. Treatment may consist of augmentation of immunosuppression, including a burst of high-dose steroids and/or administration of cytolytic therapy. Monitoring of hemodynamics, cardiac rhythm, and pulmonary status are paramount, especially when faced with high-grade allograft rejection. Unlike management to prevent or treat cellular rejection, antibody-mediated rejection is poorly responsive to standard acute and chronic immunosuppressive strategies.[84] Preemptive strategies are aimed at the reduction of

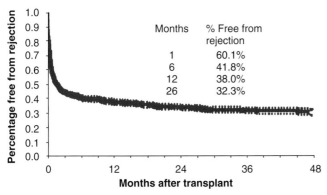

• **Figure 73.14** Time to first rejection after pediatric transplantation. (From Hsu DT, Naftel DC, Webber SA, et al. Lessons learned from the pediatric heart transplant study. *Congenit Heart Dis.* 2006;1[3]:54-62.)

circulating HLA antibodies before transplantation (desensitization) or during transplantation. There is a lack of consensus regarding the approach, but many centers have used preoperative and postoperative therapies that include plasmapheresis, intravenous immune globulin, rituximab, bortezomib, mycophenolate mofetil, and cyclophosphamide.[85-98] Not all HLA antibodies activate the complement cascade, however, and perhaps only those that fix complement yield a detrimental response. Assays that identify complement-fixing HLA antibodies (C1q) have been helpful to potentially reduce unnecessary anti-HLA antibody therapies.[99-101]

Infection

Infection of all forms is another leading cause of death (7%) in the first 30 postoperative days.[67] The greatest risk for a bacterial infection occurs in the first month after transplantation[102,103] with coagulase-negative staphylococci, *Enterobacter*, and *Pseudomonas* the most common pathogens identified. *Streptococcus pneumoniae* becomes a more frequently seen pathogen after the first year and typically is pulmonary or blood-borne. Antibacterial prophylaxis is recommended preoperatively, and, if the donor had a bacterial infection, appropriate antibiotics should be considered after implantation.[69] Pretransplant risk factors associated with infections include younger age, ventilator need, or ECMO at the time of transplantation. Posttransplant risk factors include use of potent immunosuppressive agents. Use of induction therapy, however, does not appear to affect the incidence or frequency of infections.[77] The PHTS analysis reported in 2017 identified an overall postinfection mortality of 33.8% with previous cardiac surgery and multiple sites of infection as independent risk factors.[102] Although CMV is an important pathogen to cardiothoracic transplantation and is a common infection in pediatric cardiothoracic transplant recipients, mortality directly related to this virus is low. The peak hazard risk for CMV viremia occurs within the first 2 months following transplant.[103] CMV-naïve recipients entering into transplant are at greatest risk for posttransplant infection. Prophylactic therapy is thus recommended for up to 3 months after transplantation.[69]

Fungal infections are less common, accounting for less than 7% of all posttransplant infections according to a contemporary PHTS study, with a peak hazard for infection in the first posttransplant month. *Candida* and *Aspergillus* species were the two most common fungal pathogens identified. Multivariate analysis

bore out history of previous surgery and MCS as risk factors for the subsequent development of fungal infections.[104] Prophylaxis is typically limited to preventing mucocutaneous candidiasis, although intravenous agents are recommended for antifungal prophylaxis for infants who have an open chest and/or required ECMO support in the perioperative period.[69] Although originally classified as a protozoan, *Pneumocystis* is more closely related to fungi. *Pneumocystis jiroveci* is generally an important pathogen in immunosuppressed patients, but the prevalence of infection in pediatric heart transplant patients is very low and rarely causes death.[105] Prophylaxis with trimethoprim/sulfamethoxazole, pentamidine, or other agents, however, is still recommended.[69]

Bronchiolitis Obliterans Syndrome

Bronchiolitis obliterans is diagnosed by histologic examination of lung biopsy specimen and includes peribronchial and endobronchial lymphocytic infiltration, fibromyxoid deposits, and fibrous replacement of the airways. Bronchiolitis obliterans syndrome (BOS) is a clinical diagnosis intended to serve as a surrogate for histologic diagnosis, is based on noninvasive testing, and is thought to be the clinical correlate of chronic allograft dysfunction.[106] BOS is the most common long-term complication after lung transplantation, occurring in more than 50% of surviving recipients by 5 years and accounting for more than 40% of deaths beyond 1 year after transplantation.[2] Risk factors for development of BOS may include acute rejection episodes, lymphocytic bronchiolitis, specific infections, medication noncompliance, air pollution, and genetic background. Intensification of immunosuppressive therapy does not appear to have success in treating BOS, and macrolide therapy (i.e., azithromycin) has become standard clinical practice.[107]

Hypertension and Renal Dysfunction

Hypertension is relatively common both early and late after transplantation. Early risk factors include use of calcineurin inhibitors and corticosteroids, especially when administered in high doses. Nearly half of pediatric recipients are hypertensive in the first posttransplant year with a 63.2% prevalence within 5 years.[108] Significant hypertension in the early posttransplant period should be treated to reduce the risk of associated seizures. Moderate to severe renal dysfunction is uncommon early after transplant and is typically related to the pretransplant state, time on cardiac bypass, and early initiation of calcineurin inhibitors, especially when the drug levels are elevated. After heart transplantation, survival free from severe renal dysfunction (serum creatinine >2.5 mg/dL, dialysis, or renal transplant) is variable by age at transplant, from 83% to 97% at 10 years, with patients younger than 5 years at transplant faring best.[3] Freedom from severe renal dysfunction after lung transplantation is approximately 70% at 10 years.[2] Although calcineurin inhibitors are associated with renal disease, the form of inhibitor (cyclosporine versus tacrolimus) is not associated with greater risk.[3]

Cardiac Rhythm

Cardiac output is a product of heart rate and stroke volume. Increases in output with exercise are largely due to progressive increases in heart rate with maximal changes in stroke volume occurring early. Recipients of cardiac transplantation lack innervation to the graft and thus respond solely to endogenous catecholamines and exogenously administered medications. Rhythm disturbances after pediatric heart transplantation include atrial tachyarrhythmias with flutter and fibrillation most commonly encountered. Notably atrial flutter is associated with allograft rejection, and atrial fibrillation is associated with higher mortality, whereas ectopic atrial tachycardia follows a relatively benign course.[109] Temporary pacing in the early time period after cardiac transplantation is not uncommon, but implantation of permanent pacemakers is rare.[110]

Cardiac Allograft Vasculopathy

Cardiac allograft vasculopathy (CAV) becomes the third major cause of death after the first year and surpasses acute rejection after 3 years following transplant (see Fig. 73.13).[3] Although the causes of CAV remain poorly understood, consensus is that the process is immune mediated, leading to significant structural changes within the coronary arteries. Most of the knowledge regarding CAV come from adult studies using intravascular ultrasonography (IVUS), and the hallmarks of the disease include negative remodeling, especially in the first year,[111] and intimal proliferation. Use of IVUS in the pediatric population is limited to older and larger patients, limiting our knowledge regarding the true incidence and prevalence of CAV. One single-center study noted a 74% prevalence of IVUS-evident disease within 5 years after transplant.[112] Angiographic disease, however, is well characterized in children, with a constant risk over time and 25% of patients having at least mild vasculopathy by 8 years following transplant. Notably in the PHTS study there is a 50% risk of death or retransplantation within 2 years for those with moderate to severe vasculopathy (Fig. 73.15).[113]

Prevention and mitigation of CAV are perhaps more successful than treatment of established disease. Therapies to prevent or reduce the rate of disease progression include the use of statins[114-117] and mTOR inhibitors. Despite the benefits demonstrated in adult studies, however, a large retrospective pediatric study did not show an association between mTOR inhibition with sirolimus and freedom from CAV.[118] Medical treatment of pediatric CAV with an mTOR inhibitor has yet to be demonstrated beyond small series. Interventional approaches using coronary angioplasty and stenting are generally unsuccessful because the disease process is often diffuse rather than focal. Intervention for targeted lesions, however, may have merit in selected cases, especially as a bridge to cardiac retransplantation.[119-122] Ultimately, cardiac retransplantation appears to be the only viable option in the vast majority of cases of advanced disease with retransplant survival outcomes for CAV statistically similar compared with survival after primary transplant.[70]

Malignancy

Posttransplant lymphoproliferative disorder (PTLD) accounts for the majority of oncologic disorders encountered in pediatric cardiothoracic transplantation.[3] EBV is a known factor for development of PTLD with transplantation of an EBV+ donor into a negative recipient the greatest risk, especially in young recipients.[14,123,124] There are inconsistent correlations between use of induction therapy in the peritransplant period and the development of PTLD; likely the risk is more associated with overall immunosuppression rather than specific therapies.[123]

Freedom from PTLD in pediatric heart transplant recipients is noted at 98.5% and 87% (1 and 15 years, respectively). The peak hazard occurs at 5.6 months after transplant with children (1 to <10 years of age at time of transplant) at greatest risk compared with infants and adolescents (Fig. 73.16).[14] After lung

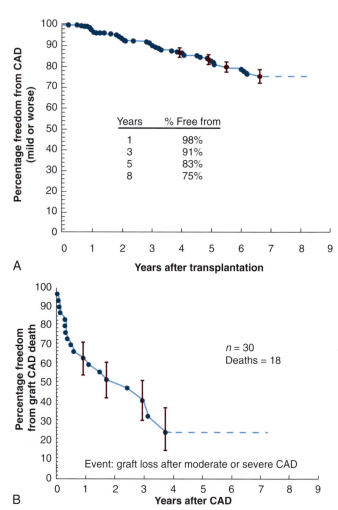

• **Figure 73.15** Freedom from presence of any coronary artery disease (CAD) (A), and freedom from death after diagnosis of moderate or severe CAD (B) in pediatric transplant recipients. (From Pahl E, Naftel DC, Kuhn MA, et al. The impact and outcome of transplant coronary artery disease in a pediatric population: a 9-year multi-institutional study. *J Heart Lung Transplant.* 2005;24:645-651.)

transplantation, survival free from malignancy is approximately 80% at 10 years.[2] Treatment of PTLD depends on the histology and includes reduction in maintenance immunosuppression (especially for polymorphic PTLD) but then places the patient at risk for the development of acute and chronic allograft rejection.[124] Reduction of immunosuppression, however, can lead to long-term remission in a majority of cases. Other therapies include antiviral agents, surgical debulking, and chemotherapy. Rituximab for lesions exhibiting the CD20 antigen appears effective, especially in combination with low-dose chemotherapy.[125]

Outcomes

Heart Transplantation

Through October 2016 the registry of the ISHLT included information on more than 12,500 isolated pediatric heart transplants (age <18 years at time of transplant) performed worldwide, with 500 to 600 new patients added per year. Overall median survival was 22.3 years for infants, 18.4 years for recipients 1 to 5 years of age,

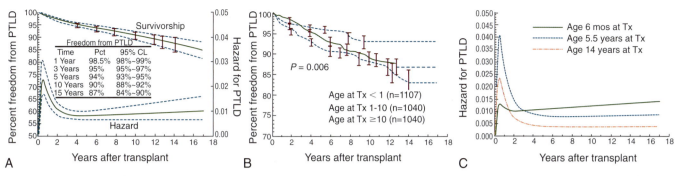

• **Figure 73.16** Kaplan-Meier estimate of freedom from posttransplant lymphoproliferative disorder (PTLD) and the hazard for PTLD as a function of time after transplant. (A) Decline in freedom from PTLD was observed over time, with peak hazard at 5.6 months. Dotted lines depict the 95% confidence limits. (B) Freedom from PTLD stratified by age at time of transplant. (C) Separate hazard functions for PTLD over time. Plots were generated from predictive equations for patients transplanted at ages 6 months (*solid line*), 5.5 years (*dotted line*), and 14 years (*dash-dotted line*). Each showed a peak hazard within the first year after transplant. (From Chinnock R, Webber SA, Dipchand AI, et al. A 16-year multi-institutional study of the role of age and EBV status on PTLD incidence among pediatric heart transplant recipients. *Am J Transplant.* 2012;12[11]:3061-3068.)

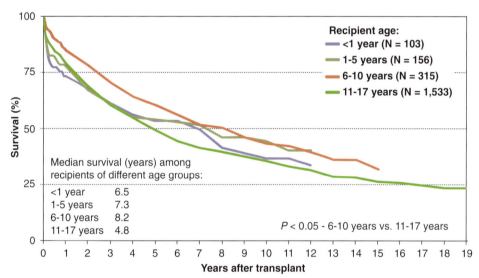

• **Figure 73.17** Pediatric lung transplantation Kaplan-Meier survival by age-group, January 1990 to June 2015. (From Goldfarb SB, Levvey BJ, Cherikh WS, et al. Registry of the International Society for Heart and Lung Transplantation: Twentieth pediatric lung and heart-lung transplantation report-2017; focus theme: allograft ischemic time. *J Heart Lung Transplant.* 2017;36[10]:1070-1079.)

14.4 years for those 6 to 10 years of age, and 13.1 years for those 11 to 17 years of age (see Fig. 73.12). Although these data represent all transplants in the registry since its inception, there have been significant improvements by era such that those patients transplanted in the last decade are expected to surpass these survival data as a group. Eight risk factors were associated with 1-year mortality in the registry data: congenital heart disease, diagnosis other than cardiomyopathy, retransplantation, preoperative mechanical ventilation, infection requiring intravenous drug therapy within 2 weeks of transplantation, recipient need for dialysis, donor cause of death cerebrovascular, and ECMO.[3]

Lung Transplantation

Since data recording by the ISHLT started in 1986, there have been 2229 isolated pediatric lung transplants and 701 pediatric heart-lung transplants, adding approximately 100 to 130 cases per year over the last decade (Fig. 73.17). In contrast to other organ systems, survival after lung transplantation is poor. Median survival after lung transplantation in the pediatric population was 5.4 years. This accounts for a lower median survival after single-lung transplant (2.2 years), which is less common, when compared to bilateral lung transplant (5.6 years).[2] In the first 30 days after transplant, graft failure, non-CMV infection, and multiple organ failure were the leading causes of death. Beyond the first 30 days, BOS and graft failure were the leading causes of death.[2]

Children who receive heart-lung transplants have long-term outcomes similar to those who receive lung transplants alone. As with the lung transplant patients, chronic rejection with BOS is the most common cause of death in the late posttransplant period.

Conclusion

Thoracic organ transplantation is now well established as an accepted therapy for children and infants with end-stage cardiopulmonary disease. Significant advances in critical care, anesthesia, immunosuppression, and postoperative management have improved outcomes for these children with 1-year survival over 90% in the case of heart transplantation; however, considerable problems remain to be solved. There continues to be an elusive balance point between rejection and infection/malignancy that is difficult to maintain. These early difficulties may then contribute to the long-term banes of thoracic organ transplantation: cardiac graft vasculopathy and bronchiolitis obliterans. Despite these difficulties, transplant waiting lists continue to grow, and mortality on the waiting list remains high because of the limited supply of donor organs. Heart and lung transplantation has matured over the last decade, but there are still ample avenues for further research and improvement, including improved support strategies with mechanical circulatory and respiratory support.

References

A complete list of references is available at ExpertConsult.com.

74

Pulmonary Embolism

KEVIN PATRICK SCHOOLER, MD, PHD

Key Points

- Pulmonary embolism (PE) carries a high risk of mortality and is underdiagnosed in children.
- PE is a complication of venous thromboembolism (VTE).
- The highest risk for VTE is the use of a central venous line, but congenital heart disease is also a significant, independent risk factor.
- The symptoms of PE in children are variable but unlikely if tachypnea and hypoxia are absent. Timely diagnosis requires a high degree of suspicion.
- Adult diagnostic algorithms for PE do not apply to children.
- Computed tomography pulmonary angiography is the most sensitive and specific diagnostic modality for PE in children.
- The treatment of PE requires anticoagulation at the minimum.
- If assays for anti-factor X_a are immediately available and surgery is not imminent, low-molecular-weight heparin is the first-line drug of choice in the treatment of PE.
- Systemic thrombolysis may be considered in an unstable child with an imminent risk to life, but bleeding complications are significant.
- When systemic thrombolysis is contraindicated, surgical or catheter-based embolectomy may be considered on a case-by-case basis in experienced centers.

Pathophysiology

Physiologic factors promoting the formation of venous thromboembolism (VTE) are well defined (Box 74.1). Virchow first described his famous "triad" over 100 years ago. His work suggested that a hypercoagulable state, venous stasis, and endothelial injury promoted both thrombus formation and clot growth. Although the quantitative degree to which each of Virchow's points contributes to thrombus formation will never be known, there is no denying that each increases the risk of VTE and therefore pulmonary embolism (PE).

The body's natural coagulation pathway begins with the exposure of tissue factor (TF) on the cell surface.[1] Even the most insignificant cellular damage exposes TF and initiates the coagulation cascade. When TF is uncovered, factors VII, V, and X are then activated locally. Their activation triggers a burst of thrombin activity and massive factor IX activation. Clot amplification then proceeds rapidly as thrombin and factor V_a activate platelets and factor VIII. At the terminal end of the cascade, fibrinogen is cleaved into fibrin, and the clot is stabilized by activated factor XIII.[1]

Unchecked, thrombus formation would be catastrophic. Fortunately, fibrinolysis begins in concert with coagulation. Fibrinolysis slows thrombus formation and keeps it localized.[1] Protein C, protein S, antithrombin (AT), and TF pathway inhibitor activation promote degradation of fibrin to fibrin degradation products simultaneously with clot formation. It is the balance of fibrinolysis and coagulation that determines the actual rate of clot formation as well as its terminal vascular extent.[1]

The repair of any congenital heart disease (CHD) creates the perfect conditions for clinically significant clot formation. The abnormal anatomy of the heart with CHD, by definition, decreases cardiac output and promotes abnormal flow dynamics even before repair. Cardiopulmonary bypass increases this low-flow status, dilutes both the procoagulation and anticoagulation factors, activates platelets, and initiates massive systemic inflammation.[2] Even myocardial and neurologic protective strategies, such as hypothermia and hypothermic arrest, promote a hypercoagulable state. The Virchow triad is completed by the cardiac surgery itself. By definition, cardiothoracic surgery causes direct vascular damage that exposes TF in both major vessels and the heart itself.

Following cardiac surgery, inflammation, myocardial stunning, and imperfect hemostasis further predispose the postoperative patient to thrombus formation in an unpredictable fashion. The postbypass low cardiac state increases venous stasis. Medical management using platelets, fresh frozen plasma, cryoprecipitate, and polycythemia further increase the hypercoagulable physiologic status to variable degrees. Combined with multiple central venous lines (CVLs) and direct atrial and/or ventricular access, the cardiac patient's postoperative physiologic state creates a perfect storm for VTE and therefore VTE complications.

Venous Thromboembolism

Because PE is considered a complication of VTE, clinicians should suspect a venous thrombus in any patient presenting with PE. Unlike adults, deep venous thrombosis (DVT) in children is rarely idiopathic (<4%) and, more often than not, is associated with CVL usage.[3] CHD, surgery, immobility, and hypovolemia are also significant risk factors for DVT formation. In the absence of a CVL, especially in patients with recurrent VTE, thrombophilia should also be considered. The most common thrombophilic disorders in children include protein S deficiency, protein C deficiency, factor V Leiden mutation, prothrombin G20210A mutation, hyperhomocysteinemia, and elevated lipoprotein A.[3]

• BOX 74.1 Risk Factors Associated With Pulmonary Embolism

Virchow Triad
1. Endothelium injury
   - Central venous catheters
   - Cardiopulmonary bypass (CPB)
   - Other surgery/trauma
   - Inflammation (e.g., lupus, inflammatory bowel disease, CPB)
   - Systemic infection
2. Vascular stasis (change in laminar blood flow)
   - Congenital or acquired heart disease
   - Heart failure
   - Local anatomic causes (e.g., congenital anomalies of pulmonary arteries or after corrective heart surgery [e.g., Fontan surgery])
   - Total parenteral nutrition
   - Immobilization/obesity
3. Thrombophilia
   a. Acquired
      - Nephrotic syndrome
      - Cancer
      - Medications (e.g., L-asparaginase therapy, oral contraceptive pills, erythropoietin)
      - Pregnancy or hormonal supplementation
      - Antiphospholipid antibodies
      - Elevated factor VIII
   b. Inherited
      - Deficiency of anticoagulants (e.g., protein S, protein C, and antithrombin III)
      - Factor V Leiden, prothrombin gene variant, and others
      - Elevated homocysteine

Venography is still considered the gold standard for locating DVTs, but ultrasonography (US) is not only rapid, but less invasive and quite sensitive.[4-6] In proximal DVTs, US has a sensitivity of 97% and a specificity of 94%.[7-9] In contrast to the lower extremities, US detection of clot in the upper limbs is difficult, especially when the clot occurs in the subclavian or deeper central veins. Upper extremity thrombus detection may still require venography for complete assessment.[4-6,8] Similarly, US may not allow visualization of the pelvic veins at all.[4] Echocardiography remains the modality of choice for visualization of intracardiac, central inferior vena cava, superior vena cava, and central pulmonary artery thrombi.[4,8] Because CVLs pose the greatest risk for VTE, any search for venous thrombus should initially focus in and around sites of CVL placement.

Incidence of Pulmonary Embolism

PE is a complication of VTE. Studies examining the incidence of PE in children report an incidence of 8.6 to 57 in 100,000 in hospitalized children.[10-14] This wide-ranging incidence in hospitalized children may be a manifestation of the "often clinically silent nature of PE, misdiagnosis, more comprehensive reporting, or a function of the biased population of a tertiary care center."[11] There appears to be a predilection for pediatric PE in infants and toddlers, with a second peak seen in teenagers. Black children are estimated to have an incidence 2.38 times higher than white children.[12] However, it is likely that these numbers are underestimated due to the frequent asymptomatic presentation of PE in children as noted earlier. Autopsy data show discordance

in the rate of actual PE presence in comparison with a clinical suspicion of PE. In one study the diagnosis of PE was considered in only 15% of patients with pathologically detected PE.[14] In contrast to adults, the time to diagnosis of PE in children is often longer, with a mean time to diagnosis as high as 7 days in some studies.[15] Therefore it is paramount that the clinician have a high index of suspicion for timely and effective care for children with PE.[15]

Almost 60% of pediatric patients with PE have a significant clot at another location.[3] In contrast to adults, most pediatric VTEs are found in an upper extremity rather than the lower.[3] When all pediatric hospital admissions are considered, the incidence of VTE is approximately 5 per 10,000 admissions.[7,16] The incidence is higher in the neonatal intensive care setting. One study found 24 individual thrombi in 10,000 admissions.[7,16]

Although any critical illness can promote VTE formation, only 3.6% of pediatric patients hospitalized for PE lacked identifiable risk factors for VTE.[17] In nearly every study of pediatric inpatients to date, the presence of a CVL posed the single greatest risk for thrombus development.[18] Not unexpectedly, bed rest for 3 or more days and recent surgery with general anesthesia also promote clot formation.[17] VTE risks in adults are similar to those of children, but, in that population, mechanical ventilation and hospital length of stay are also important.[18] Interestingly, for outpatient pediatric patients presenting with PE as their primary diagnosis, obesity appears to be the most significant risk factor.[19]

The incidence of PE in pediatric patients is unclear. In children with a high clinical suspicion of PE, a PE was present in only 15% of those patients.[20] A Canadian data registry study of children with VTE demonstrated PE in 0.86 children per 10,000 hospital admissions (0.14 to 0.9 events per 100,000 children).[7] When autopsy studies are considered, almost 4% of pediatric patients dying from any cause had gross or microscopic evidence of PE.[16,17,21-23]

Symptomatic PE in childhood is extremely rare and is underdiagnosed in pediatric patients for a number of reasons. First of all, because the symptoms of PE are extremely variable, without a high index of suspicion the diagnosis of PE will not be pursued. Following the development of rapid high-resolution computed tomography (CT) scans, diagnosis of PE in both adult and pediatric patients has become easier. The incidence of PE has risen concomitantly.[24-28] Unexpectedly, as the use of CT in the diagnosis of PE rises, mortality from PE in the adult population has been on the decline.[24-27] Although pediatric data are not available, a similar decrease in mortality in children would not be surprising. The decreased mortality likely stems from the fact that CT has made the diagnosis of asymptomatic PE possible. This allows for more intensive surveillance and, potentially, treatment in those children before they become symptomatic. In addition, the practice of earlier removal of CVLs and mandates for DVT prophylaxis in hospitalized adults has likely had a significant effect on the incidence of PE.

Children with CHD have an extremely high risk of thromboembolic complications, including PE. In infants presenting with strokes, nearly half of those children have some form of CHD.[29] After 6 months of age, children with CHD still account for one-third of patients with new-onset cerebral infarction.[29] Because children with right-to-left shunting at the cardiac level by definition have an elevated stroke risk compared with the general pediatric population, this finding is not unexpected. However, although the stroke studies mentioned previously did not examine the incidence of PE in their cohort, the extremely high incidence suggests these children may also be predisposed to other VTE-associated morbidities. In support of this supposition, bypass surgery for right heart defects is known to carry a high incidence of acute pulmonary artery obstruction.[4,30,31]

Signs and Symptoms of Pulmonary Embolism

The symptoms of PE are variable.[17,32-36] In adults the majority of patients with PE have pleuritis and difficulty breathing.[34] Only approximately one-third of adults have cough, wheezing, or orthopnea with PE. Very few patients (13%) present with hemoptysis. Not surprisingly, nearly half of those with PE have signs of deep venous thrombus such as calf or thigh pain.[34] Cardiovascular collapse, arrhythmia, and syncope are extremely rare presentations.[32-34]

The risk of PE in pediatric patients without rapid heart rate and hypoxia is very low (<1.5%).[28] In a single-center study of adolescents with PE, the most frequent presenting symptoms were chest pain, difficulty breathing, cough, and hemoptysis, but signs of DVT were also common.[3,17,19,34,37] Importantly, the incidence of PE in pediatric patients with documented VTE may be as high as 30% to 60%.[4,38,39]

Because younger children are unable to vocalize their symptoms, a high degree of clinical suspicion is required in any patient with risk factors for PE formation.[3,19,22,40] As in older children, rapid respiratory rates, pleuritic chest pain, cough, shortness of breath, and tachycardia are common but nonspecific symptoms. Sudden cardiac collapse in any pediatric patient requires immediate consideration of PE even though, as in adults, it is an extremely rare presentation.[19,22,40]

Diagnostic Workup for Pulmonary Embolism

In adults, specific, validated diagnostic prediction tools, such as the Wells criteria,[41] the Geneva score,[42] and the pulmonary embolism rule-out criteria,[43] exist for diagnosis of PE.[44,45] These models combine patient clinical signs and additional risk factors to assess pretest probability for the diagnosis of PE in adults. Similar models have not been validated in children.

Diagnostic algorithms for PE in adults immediately bifurcate based on the hemodynamic status of the patient at presentation.[3,46] If there is suspicion of PE in an unstable patient, the patient should be immediately stabilized, anticoagulated, and then sent for CT pulmonary angiography (CTPA). However, most patients are stable at presentation. Hemodynamically stable patients undergo a tiered diagnostic strategy based on clinical probability of PE. Based on symptoms, the risk of PE in adults can be determined by several different validated models. Patients with a high probability of PE undergo immediate CTPA. If the study is inconclusive, magnetic resonance pulmonary angiography or contrast pulmonary angiography may be required. In patients with a low probability of PE, an initial screening by quantitative D-dimer is initiated. If D-dimer is elevated, the patient again follows the high-probability algorithm (discussed previously). If the D-dimer level is low in patients with a low probability of PE, the diagnosis is excluded.[46]

Diagnosis of PE in children is more difficult than in adults.[4,17,47-50] Plain film chest x-ray findings are abnormal in the majority of children with PE, with cardiomegaly and pleural effusion being the most common findings.[8] The Westermark sign (oligemia), Hampton hump (pleura-based area of increased

opacification), and Fleischner sign (a prominent central pulmonary artery) are rarely seen.[8] Because risk models for clinical probability of PE have not been validated in children, nondefinitive test results are difficult to interpret regardless of the study used.[17,19,28,47] For instance, a low D-dimer in children does not rule out PE, but a high value lends support to the diagnosis.[3,28,47] Similarly, although a positive ventilation/perfusion (V/Q) scan may provide supportive evidence for PE, a negative scan will not rule it out because no probability model is available to guide interpretation. In addition, because participation in the youngest children is unreliable or impossible, needed radiographic V/Q views may not even be adequate.[4,8] More importantly for this discussion, CHD patients with left-to-right shunts have variable scan results due to uneven distribution of isotope.[3] Therefore, although V/Q scans have historically been used to test for diagnosis of PE in children, they are not guaranteed to provide a definitive diagnosis.

Due to its speed and reliability, CTPA has rapidly overtaken V/Q scans as a primary imaging technique for diagnosis of PE. The most significant disadvantages to this modality are the exposure to ionizing radiation and its insensitivity to small, subsegmental emboli. Pulmonary angiography has been the traditional gold standard for diagnosis of PE; it is both invasive and expensive, which limits its use in the pediatric population. When used in patients with CHD as part of a catheter-based evaluation and intervention, pulmonary angiography remains the modality of choice for diagnosis of PE.

Magnetic resonance imaging and magnetic resonance pulmonary angiography (MRI/MRPA) eliminates the effects of ionizing radiation and may be used in patients in whom CT is contraindicated. Although MRI/MRPA has become important in the diagnosis of childhood PE, the requirement for patient immobility during MRI and scan duration make it unlikely these will become the imaging modality of choice in unstable patients.[3,4,8] Most importantly, due to the absence of tests validating MRI in the detection of PE, a positive result may support the diagnosis of PE, but a negative MRI does not rule it out.[3]

Extrapolating from current algorithms for diagnosis of PE in adults, hemodynamically unstable pediatric patients with suspected PE should undergo immediate CTPA. Unfortunately, although CTPA has a 96% specificity, as noted previously, it may not reliably detect peripheral emboli in very small children.[3,4,17,47-51] CTPA with three-dimensional reconstruction appears to improve diagnostic resolution, but it has not yet been validated in children.[48]

Probability and prediction models for adults with PE stratify all patients into high risk (presentation with cardiovascular collapse), intermediate risk (patients who are normotensive but show evidence of right heart strain either on electrocardiogram (ECG) or echocardiography or by biomarkers), or low risk (symptomatic but absence of preceding features) categories.[52,53] Unfortunately, similar risk categorization is not validated in children. Therefore adjunctive testing, including ECG (right ventricular strain pattern), echocardiography, and biomarkers (brain natriuretic peptide, troponin), may aid in the diagnosis of pediatric PE.

When a substantial amount of pulmonary flow has been occluded, right ventricular heart strain invariably occurs.[8] Right axis deviation, ST segment elevation, and right bundle branch block on ECG can be useful in the verification of increased right heart work, but the findings are not specific for PE.[4] Similarly, echocardiographic data showing dyskinetic right ventricular motion compared with the apex has low sensitivity for PE but a positive predictive value and specificity of nearly 100%.[3,54,55]

Classification of Pulmonary Embolism

PE has numerous classification schemes. All are imprecise but can be important when assessing risk-benefit stratification before treatment.[50,54,56] A PE is considered acute if symptoms appear immediately after the pulmonary vasculature has been obstructed. If symptoms are delayed for several days after the initial obstruction occurs, the PE is classified as subacute. Chronic PE also occurs, but these patients present with pulmonary hypertension secondary to years of repeated obstruction.[50,54,56]

Although symptomatic patients will require immediate anticoagulation, the risk of systemic anticoagulation may outweigh potential benefits in the asymptomatic patient. Symptomatic patients can be broadly divided into two groups. If they are hypotensive at presentation, they are classified as hemodynamically unstable ("massive" PE).[50,54,56] In contrast, the majority of symptomatic patients are hemodynamically stable at diagnosis (submassive PE). This distinction is critical because unstable patients require not only immediate anticoagulation but also possible systemic thrombolysis or even surgical thombectomy.[50,54,56]

In the absence of preexisting cardiac or pulmonary disease, at least half of the total pulmonary flow must be obstructed before right heart strain occurs.[3,8] As emboli move beyond the pulmonary artery bifurcation, anatomic classification is determined by the total amount of vasculature obstructed.[24-27] The degree of occlusion ranges from an entire lobe (lobar) to individual segments (segmental) or only distal segments (subsegmental).[24-27] Although relatively new, the CT-derived vascular obstruction index may be helpful in quantifying the degree of arterial obstruction in PE and may even aid in treatment stratification. However, its utility in children is still unclear.[49,57]

Interestingly, the initial location of the PE at the time of diagnosis is less important in the determination of symptoms than previously believed. For instance, it is not surprising that subsegmental PEs usually cause localized infarction and pleuritis.[58,59] However, a saddle emboli, which obstructs both the left and right pulmonary arteries simultaneously, rarely terminates pulmonary flow completely.[24-27] In fact, recent studies have shown that saddle emboli cause death in only 5% of patients and promote hemodynamic instability in only 22%.[58,59]

Treatment of Pulmonary Embolism

The level of V/Q mismatch at any point in time is determined by the degree of pulmonary vein obstruction.[1] Cardiac output determines both hemodynamic stability and hypoxemia in the acute phase. When cardiac output is stabilized, the overall level of V\Q mismatch–induced hypoxemia becomes dependent on the existing intrapulmonary shunt.[1]

Treatment of patients presenting with PE begins with airway, breathing, and circulation. Oxygen will lessen hypoxemic vasoconstriction in all patients. Noninvasive positive pressure ventilation or mechanical ventilation may also be required to reduce atelectasis, maximize alveolar expansion, decrease hypercarbic vasoconstriction, and decrease afterload on an already strained heart.

Volume expansion will not only improve preload in patients with PE, it may also improve venous blood flow by reducing blood viscosity. In addition, because dehydration promotes thrombus expansion, adequate vascular expansion should be an immediate therapeutic goal. However, right heart failure and even impending failure requires cautious resuscitation to maximize the patient's position on the Starling curve without worsening the degree of cardiac dysfunction. For this reason, repeated small-volume boluses (5 to 10 mL/kg) should be used in place of large-volume loads (20 mL/kg). Similarly, early vasopressor and inotropic support should be considered in all patients with hemodynamically significant PE. Because increased heart rate may promote myocardial ischemia and worsen diastolic filling, agents that increase systemic vascular resistance without increasing heart rate (norepinephrine or vasopressin) are likely better first-line choices than vasoactive agents that increase chronotropy (epinephrine and dobutamine).

Along with initial stabilization, systemic anticoagulation forms the basis of treatment for both VTE and PE of any size. However, the clinician must weigh the risks for bleeding with presenting symptoms and the probability of progression on an individual basis. Although the mortality of children with PE may be as high as 10%, the bleeding risk during treatment varies with the anticoagulation compounds used.[3,28,60]

For years unfractionated heparin (UFH) has been the mainstay treatment for clots in any location.[3,4] By increasing the activity of AT, UFH inhibits clot formation by inhibiting thrombin and factor X activation. This tips the body's natural balance between coagulation and fibrinolysis in favor of clot dissolution.[3,60] In the presence of heparin, clot extension is halted and regression can begin. Although the risk of bleeding in children anticoagulated with UFH ranges from 2% to 18%, the primary benefit of heparin is its rapid reversibility with protamine sulfate. Unfortunately, UFH also carries a secondary bleeding risk of heparin-induced thrombocytopenia (HIT). If HIT develops, more exotic anticoagulants (such as direct thrombin inhibitors like bivalirudin or anti-X_a inhibitors such as fondaparinux) will be required.[3,60]

Low-molecular-weight heparin (LMWH) is gaining favor in pediatrics for treatment of PE.[61,62] Although both LMWH and UFH both inhibit AT, LMWH attenuates factor X activation much more than thrombin formation, whereas UFH attenuates them both equally.[3,60] The greatest advantage of LMWH over UFH is ease of use and its decreased monitoring requirements.[3,60] This is especially important in the outpatient setting. LMWH also carries a lower risk of bleeding, HIT, and osteoporosis in comparison to UFH.[3,4,60-62] It should be noted that, like UFH, LMWH may be reversed by protamine sulfate although less effectively.[3]

Warfarin and the Coumadin family of drugs all inhibit coagulation by blocking synthesis of vitamin K–dependent clotting factors (II, VII, IX, and X). In children, oral vitamin K antagonists require close monitoring of both international normalization ratio and diet. Although these drugs can be rapidly reversed with fresh frozen plasma, the variability of pediatric diets make this class of drugs highly undesirable. Most physicians now confine the use of these drugs to patients with mechanical heart valves and ventricular assist devices.

Current recommendations suggest treating PE for 7 to 10 days with LMWH or UFH followed by long-term anticoagulation with LMWH or vitamin K antagonists.[63] If there are no risk factors for PE, such as CVL use or recent surgery, anticoagulation should continue for 6 months. If risk factors exist, 3 months of treatment is likely sufficient.[63]

Progression from anticoagulation to systemic thrombolysis carries significant risk. It should be considered only in patients with hemodynamically unstable PE unresponsive to anticoagulation alone.[3,4,64] Current recommendations for systemic thrombolysis include intracardiac thrombi causing obstruction, unstable PE, and acute organ failure secondary to thrombus.[3,64] However, it should be remembered that the existence of right-to-left shunts in children with CHD is, by itself, a relative contraindication of systemic thrombolysis due to the risk of stroke. Brain surgery, active bleeding, and recent surgery are absolute contraindications.[4,64]

Although streptokinase, urokinase, and tissue plasminogen activator (t-PA) are all available for on- or off-label use, only t-PA is approved in children. All three agents convert plasminogen to plasmin and directly promote clot dissolution. For this reason, fresh frozen plasma is usually administered in parallel with systemic thrombolytics to ensure adequate levels of circulating plasminogen before infusion.[4,64]

The frequency of bleeding in patients treated with systemic thrombolytics is significant in all studies. In at least one small study, systemic t-PA therapy caused bleeding in almost 70% of patients.[3,65] Almost 40% of those patients required transfusion.[3,65] Another study reported resolution of PE in less than 12.5% with systemic thrombolysis but significant bleeding in nearly half of those treated.[17] Even in a study with the lowest reported bleeding rate, major bleeding occurred in approximately 40% of patients.[65] Low-dose t-PA protocols show promise in decreasing bleeding complications while still maintaining efficacy in clot resolution, but comparative trials are not yet available.[66,67]

Surgical or catheter-directed thrombectomy may be required in massive PE, especially when contraindications to thrombolytic therapy exist.[4,68] Unstable PE in the immediate postoperative period following surgical correction of CHD may be the most likely to benefit from surgical thrombectomy.[3] Catheter-based embolectomy is another intervention for massive PE, but published reports in children are scarce.[3,68]

In children over 10 kg, inferior vena cava (IVC) filters may be indicated. However, they carry the risk of significant complications.[4] One alternative is temporary placement of IVC filters in anticoagulated patients. This practice seems to have lower rates of complication and appear effective in small trials.[65] Thus the use of filters in children remains a viable though uncommon treatment option.[65]

Regardless of the treatment used, bleeding remains the most common complication. PE rarely occurs in isolation and almost always occurs due to another disease such as CHD or cancer. More likely than not, PE is a postsurgical complication.[65] Approximately 9% of patients treated for PE died of their embolic disease, whereas only approximately 4% died of bleeding complications after initiation of treatment. These data suggest that although treatment for PE has significant morbidity, compared with the mortality associated with massive PE, treatment risk is less than that of the thrombotic disease itself.[65] This has been demonstrated only for anticoagulation alone.[65]

In general for patients with asymptomatic thromboses, especially those associated with a CVL, treatment is probably not necessary.[64] The catheter should be removed if possible. Symptomatic patients require anticoagulation in addition to catheter removal. If the patient is at risk for surgery, UFH should be the first-choice agent due to its rapid reversibility. In the absence of surgical risk, provided anti–factor Xa monitoring is available, LMWH should be considered first-line therapy. However, UFH is an appropriate substitute, particularly if there is concern for renal dysfunction. Systemic anticoagulation should be considered only

if life, limbs, or vital organs are at risk. Surgical and catheter-based embolectomy can be considered on a case-by-case basis when systemic thrombolysis is contraindicated and even then, only when an experienced team is involved in the patient's care.[64] All anticoagulation treatments carry significant risk. One algorithm used for management of pediatric PE can be found in Fig. 74.1.[69]

Ancillary Diagnostic Evaluation

Several ancillary studies are usually performed as part of diagnostic and pretreatment workup for PE. These include complete blood count with differential, C-reactive protein, prothrombin time, activated partial thromboplastin time, fibrinogen level, and D-dimer. Renal and liver function tests should also be performed before initiating any anticoagulant therapy so that pharmacologic clearance mechanisms associated with individual compounds can be considered in determining bleeding risk. In addition, if thrombolytic therapy is being considered, a plasminogen level may be useful because neonates and children are often deficient and require supplementation with plasma to achieve therapeutic effect. Furthermore, clinicians should examine all extremities for signs of venous stasis or thromboembolism, and all four limbs should be evaluated with US to evaluate for any associated DVTs.[70] Chest radiography, although not helpful in the diagnosis of PE, may allow exclusion of lung pathology other than PE.

Thrombophilia Testing

The Subcommittee for Perinatal and Pediatric Thrombosis of the Scientific and Standardization Committee of the International Society on Thrombosis and Haemostasis recommends that all children with thrombosis be tested for thrombophilia.[71] However, the role of thrombophilia in categorization of risk, management, and outcomes has not been elucidated yet for pediatric PE. An initial workup for thrombophilic disorders in children should include the possibility of protein S deficiency, protein C deficiency, factor V Leiden mutation, prothrombin G20210A mutation, hyperhomocysteinemia, and elevated lipoprotein A.[3]

Conclusion

PE in children is a complication of VTE. Although likely underdiagnosed, PE is associated with significant mortality. The greatest risk of thromboembolism in childhood appears to be associated with the use of a CVL. Children with CHD have a high frequency of embolic complications, including PE, because of abnormal blood flow, hypercoagulability, and vascular injury following repair. The symptoms of PE are variable, but diagnosis is unlikely without tachypnea and hypoxia. Because diagnosis can be difficult, a high degree of suspicion is required to make a timely diagnosis. CTPA is the most reliable modality for diagnosing pediatric PE, especially in patients with hemodynamic instability, but other studies may be helpful. Once diagnosed, the risks of ongoing obstruction must be weighed against treatment complications, especially massive bleeding. All treatment regimens include anticoagulation. Research is needed in the development of both diagnostic and treatment algorithms for pediatric PE because the standards of care in the treatment of this vulnerable population are simply not known.

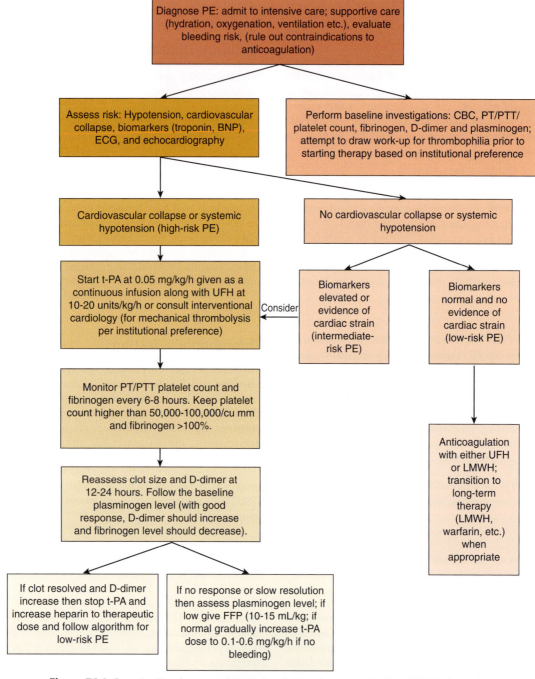

• **Figure 74.1** One algorithm for management of pediatric pulmonary embolism. *BNP,* Brain natriuretic peptide; *CBC,* complete blood cell count; *ECG,* electrocardiogram; *FFP,* fresh frozen plasma; *LMWH,* low-molecular-weight heparin; *PE,* pulmonary embolism; *PT,* prothrombin time; *PTT,* partial thromboplastin time; *t-PA,* tissue plasminogen activator; *UFH,* unfractionated heparin. (Modified from Zaidi AU, Hutchins KK, Rajpurkar M. Pulmonary embolism in children. *Front Pediatr.* 2017;5:170. doi:10.3389/fped.2017.00170.)

Selected References

A complete list of references is available at ExpertConsult.com.

1. Petruzzi MJF. Thromboembolism in pediatric critical care patients. In: Fuhrman BP, Zimmerman J, eds. *Pediatric Critical Care*. 3rd ed. Philadelphia: Mosby Elsevier; 2006:1156–1172.
3. Patocka C, Nemeth J. *J Emerg Med*. 2012;42:105–116.
4. Babyn PS, Gahunia HK, Massicotte P. *Pediatr Radiol*. 2005;35:258–274.
17. Biss TT, Brandao LR, Kahr WH, Chan AK, Williams S. *Br J Haematol*. 2008;142:808–818.
29. Monagle P. *Semin Thromb Hemost*. 2003;29:547–555.
47. Biss TT, Brandao LR, Kahr WH, Chan AK, Williams S. *J Thromb Haemost*. 2009;7:1633–1638.
50. Torbicki A, Perrier A, Konstantinides S, Agnelli G, Galie N, Pruszczyk P, et al. *Eur Heart J*. 2008;29:2276–2315.
53. Corrigan D, Prucnal C, Kabrhel C. Pulmonary embolism: the diagnosis, risk-stratification, treatment and disposition of emergency department patients. *Clin Exp Emerg Med*. 2016;3:117–125. doi:10.15441/ceem.16.146.
56. Pollack CV, Schreiber D, Goldhaber SZ, Slattery D, Fanikos J, O'Neil BJ, et al. *J Am Coll Cardiol*. 2011;57:700–706.
64. Monagle P, Chan AK, Goldenberg NA, Ichord RN, Journeycake JM, Nowak-Gottl U, et al. *Chest*. 2012;141:e737S–e801S.
67. Wang M, Hays T, Balasa V, Bagatell R, Gruppo R, Grabowski EF, et al. *J Pediatr Hematol Oncol*. 2003;25:379–386.
69. Zaidi AU, Hutchins KK, Rajpurkar M. Pulmonary embolism in children. *Front Pediatr*. 2017;5:170. doi:10.3389/fped.2017.00170.
71. Manco-Johnson MJ, Grabowski EF, Hellgreen M, Kemahli AS, Massicotte MP, Muntean W, et al. Laboratory testing for thrombophilia in pediatric patients. On behalf of the Subcommittee for Perinatal and Pediatric Thrombosis of the Scientific and Standardization Committee of the International Society of Thrombosis and Haemostasis (ISTH). *Thromb Haemost*. 2002;88:155–156.

75

Syndromes, Genetics, and Heritable Heart Disease

BENJAMIN J. LANDIS, MD; MATTHEW T. LISI, MD

The association between congenital cardiovascular malformations (CVMs) and genetic syndromes is well established.[1] Traditionally, a characteristic constellation of clinical features has defined a genetic syndrome. The list of syndromes associated with CVMs is expansive and includes disorders caused by different classes of genetic abnormalities. These include abnormality of chromosome number or large structural chromosomal defects. Down syndrome, which is caused by the presence of three copies of chromosome 21, is the most common aneuploidy syndrome among patients born with CVMs. Alternatively, syndromic CVMs may be caused by microdeletions or microduplications, which encompass smaller chromosomal regions. DiGeorge syndrome, which is caused by the presence of a deleted segment on the long arm of one of the copies of chromosome 22 (22q11.2 deletion), is a common example. A third mechanism known to cause syndromic CVMs is the alteration of DNA sequence at the nucleotide level, which includes single nucleotide variants (SNVs) and small insertions or deletions. Noonan syndrome, which is typically caused by pathogenic SNVs within genes involved in the RAS-MAP kinase signaling pathway (e.g., *PTPN11*), is an example. In addition to the genetic syndromes associated with CVMs, it is increasingly clear that many cases of isolated, or nonsyndromic, CVMs also have a primary genetic basis. For example, there are many reports of multigenerational families with isolated CVMs showing Mendelian inheritance patterns or complex inheritance patterns.[2,3] Furthermore, large epidemiologic studies confirm increased rates of familial recurrence of CVMs across the general population of patients with CVMs.[4]

The field of human genetics has grown expansively since the publication of the second edition of this textbook. Novel genetic testing technologies coupled with clinical insight have fundamentally changed the way clinicians approach the diagnosis of many diseases. The basic categorization of disease, including syndromic disease, continues to improve by combining the established constellations of clinical signs and symptoms with specific molecular diagnosis. As an example of one major shift in the genetic evaluation of patients with CVMs, chromosomal microarray analysis (CMA) is increasingly used in many pediatric cardiac intensive care units (ICUs) to identify small deletions and duplications of chromosomal material, termed copy number variants (CNVs), across the genome. In addition, next-generation sequencing (NGS) technology now facilitates interrogation of the genome for nucleotide sequence variants across multiple genes in parallel. "NGS panels" apply this

technology to test a defined set of genes that are known to be associated with the patient's clinical presentation (e.g., Noonan syndrome panels test for all the genes known to cause Noonan syndrome simultaneously). Alternatively, NGS technology can be leveraged to sequence all of the coding regions of the genome (exome) or the entire genome in an increasingly time- and cost-efficient manner. This rapid expansion of genetic testing technology and clinical implementation not only has led to the discovery of new genetic diseases, but has significantly advanced our understanding of the molecular basis of previously described clinical syndromes. The availability and increasing affordability of CMA, NGS panels, and exome sequencing tests have accelerated advancements made in the research setting and are being integrated into routine clinical management of CVMs and other forms of pediatric cardiovascular disease.

The clinical practitioner who cares for critically ill patients with CVMs will encounter many patients with genetic syndromes. The syndromic diagnosis may already be established either by prenatal or postnatal evaluations before arriving at the operating room or ICU, or, especially in neonates, the patient may not have a diagnosis yet established at the initial encounter. In either case, it is important not only to understand the genetic cause of these syndromes, but also to be familiar with the clinical features that are typically encountered. This allows providers to predict certain risks and preemptively intervene and may offer the patient and/or family information regarding prognosis, risk of familial recurrence, and identification of occult disease in relatives.

This chapter begins with an overview of the interaction between the most common genetic syndromes associated with CVMs and the management of cardiac disease in the ICU, including the important considerations of noncardiac factors. This will include some discussion of clinical outcomes data. A comprehensive review of the impact of genetic syndromes on perioperative outcomes is available to the interested reader.[5] Next, we explore our current understanding of the clinical utility of genetic testing in newborns with critical CVMs and highlight recent discoveries related to the genetic basis of syndromic and nonsyndromic CVMs using NGS technology. The chapter includes advisement for the routine involvement of genetics services within the pediatric cardiac ICU and surgical programs. The chapter focuses specifically on the genetic considerations for patients with CVMs, so readers should seek other resources for discussions of the genetics of other forms of pediatric cardiovascular disease, including cardiomyopathy, aortopathy, and channelopathy, for which the availability of comprehensive and affordable multigene panels using NGS techniques, has been a cornerstone of staggering growth in pediatric cardiology.

Syndromic Congenital Cardiovascular Malformations and the Factors Influencing Intensive Care

Large studies of pediatric patients with CVMs who require ICU care and/or cardiac surgery find that 10% to 30% of cases have a genetic diagnosis or noncardiac abnormalities.[6-10] The true burden of syndromic disease is not completely known due to differences in genetic testing and evaluation practices among studies. Other factors, such as selection of certain age ranges or type of CVMs, may differ between studies and lead to differences in the reported prevalence of disease. These factors notwithstanding, given the high burden of syndromic disease, an important question is whether having a syndromic diagnosis in general influences perioperative outcomes of pediatric patients undergoing cardiac surgery. This question has been assessed by several studies using large cohorts of patients treated over the past two to three decades. The most consistent conclusion among these studies is that a genetic diagnosis significantly increases the risk for postoperative morbidities such as increased risk for respiratory, infectious, and renal complications, resulting in prolonged hospitalization.[6,7,11,12] These complications may have long-standing, deleterious effects upon the child's health in addition to causing increased burden on the family and health care system.

Increased hospital mortality following a cardiac operation has been observed in some, but not all, studies. As one may expect, there is strong evidence to support that the risk for mortality is increased for syndromic patients requiring more complex operations. For example, data from the Society of Thoracic Surgeons (STS; years 2002 to 2006) and the Congenital Heart Surgeons' Society (years 1994 to 2001) showed increased postoperative mortality among patients with a genetic or noncardiac congenital anomaly following stage I palliation for left ventricular outflow tract lesions such as hypoplastic left heart syndrome (HLHS).[8] The design of this study highlights a common approach to batch groups of patients with a genetic syndrome together with those having a noncardiac congenital anomaly into one "syndromic" group.[9] Although this approach may increase the power to detect differences via study of larger groups of patients, understanding the risk for specific syndromes is more practically useful. Ideally outcomes data pertaining to specific syndromes will become increasingly available as the use of genetic evaluations for patients with CVMs expands, facilitating the study of larger syndrome-specific cohorts and more detailed classification of patients. Fortunately, modern outcomes data have become available for several of the most common syndromes associated with CVMs. We explore these syndromes in the remainder of this section.

Down Syndrome

Down syndrome, or trisomy 21, is the most frequent genetic syndrome among children born with a congenital CVM.[10] It is estimated to affect between 200,000 and 300,000 individuals in the United States and occurs in at least 1 in 1000 live births.[13] Congenital CVMs are present in 40% to 50% of affected children. Atrioventricular septal defect (AVSD) is the most common class

of CVM identified (50% to 60%), followed by ventricular septal defect (VSD), atrial septal defect (ASD), and tetralogy of Fallot.[10] Because of the high incidence of CVMs, all infants with known or suspected Down syndrome should have a comprehensive cardiac evaluation, including echocardiography, within the first few days to weeks of life. Many other organ systems are affected in Down syndrome (Fig. 75.1),[14] but the prominent characteristics include impaired cognition, delayed growth, and facial dysmorphism. Other problems of significant importance in the intensive care/surgical setting include upper airway obstruction, atlantoaxial instability, hypothyroidism, and immune deficiency. Congenital anomalies of the gastrointestinal system, including duodenal atresia, Hirschsprung disease, or tracheoesophageal fistula, occur at increased frequency.[15] In spite of these factors, the average life expectancy for individuals with Down syndrome now exceeds 50 years. However, these patients also face risks for the development of leukemia and early-onset Alzheimer's disease.[16,17]

The cytogenetic abnormality responsible for Down syndrome is the trisomy of chromosome 21 (47, +21) in 93% to 96% of cases or a translocation involving chromosome 21 in 2% to 5% of cases.[18] The diagnosis is typically established using the traditional karyotype. Approximately 2% to 4% of cases are associated with mosaicism due to postzygotic nondisjunction, in which case the clinical findings are usually milder. Although advanced maternal age is a risk factor, the majority of mothers bearing children with Down syndrome are between 18 and 35 years of age. If a balanced translocation is identified in a parent, genetic counseling should be performed to discuss that there is increased risk of recurrence in future offspring compared with the more typical cases caused by sporadic nondisjunction. At this time the precise pathogenetic mechanism by which trisomy of chromosome 21 leads to the Down syndrome phenotype remains incompletely understood.

A significant risk for patients with Down syndrome is the development of pulmonary vascular disease (PVD). This risk is particularly high among those with nonrestrictive interventricular communication such as complete AVSD or large VSD.[19] For example, some studies suggest that more than one-third of patients with trisomy 21 and a CVM have concomitant pulmonary artery hypertension.[20] Chronic hypoventilation secondary to upper airway obstruction and sleep apnea may significantly contribute to the development of pulmonary hypertension. This must be dutifully managed to avoid exacerbating what is likely an intrinsic predisposition to develop PVD (see Fig. 75.1).[21] The risk for early development of PVD has led to the practice of early repair of large left-to-right interventricular shunts, including complete AVSDs, usually by age 6 months. Airway and craniofacial anomalies may further complicate preoperative and postoperative management by creating difficulty with intubation, secretion clearance, atelectasis, and chylothorax, leading to risk for prolonged mechanical ventilation.[22] The palliation of single-ventricle lesions may be particularly precarious for patients with Down syndrome and PVD. Pulmonary hypertension and PVD may be major contributors to the increased mortality observed in patients with Down syndrome after stage I, II, and III palliations.[23,24] Preoperative evaluations and postoperative protocols may be useful for the management of patients with Down syndrome and pulmonary hypertension.

Other important noncardiac problems that may complicate intensive care include atlantoaxial instability, immune deficiency, and hypothyroidism. Atlantoaxial instability may pose a risk of neurologic injury during intubation, particularly for older children and young adults.[25] Dysfunction of the humoral or innate immune

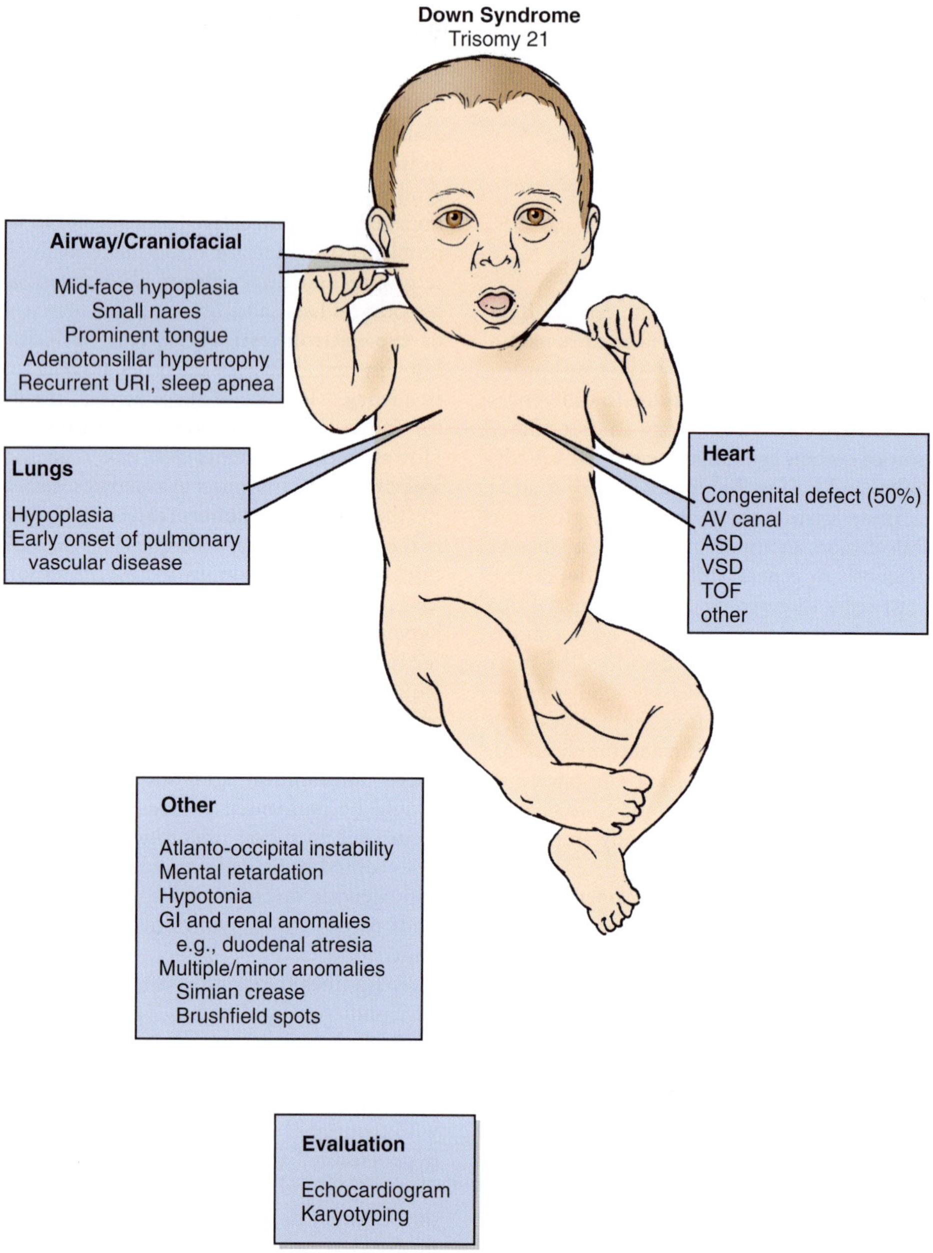

Down Syndrome
Trisomy 21

Airway/Craniofacial

Mid-face hypoplasia
Small nares
Prominent tongue
Adenotonsillar hypertrophy
Recurrent URI, sleep apnea

Lungs

Hypoplasia
Early onset of pulmonary
  vascular disease

Heart

Congenital defect (50%)
AV canal
ASD
VSD
TOF
other

Other

Atlanto-occipital instability
Mental retardation
Hypotonia
GI and renal anomalies
  e.g., duodenal atresia
Multiple/minor anomalies
  Simian crease
  Brushfield spots

Evaluation

Echocardiogram
Karyotyping

• **Figure 75.1** Associated defects of Down syndrome. *AV,* Atrioventricular; *ASD,* atrial septal defect; *VSD,* ventricular septal defect; *TOF,* tetralogy of Fallot.

systems may predispose to postoperative infections,[24,26] but whether this risk warrants alterations of typical postoperative antibiotic prophylaxis is not established. Hypothyroidism often develops in the first year of life. Because thyroid hormone contributes significantly to cardiovascular stability, it is good practice for all patients with Down syndrome to be screened for hypothyroidism in the time leading up to cardiac surgery and, if diagnosed, to receive adequate outpatient treatment before the operation. Despite the various health challenges associated with Down syndrome and established risk for postoperative complications, recent series including large numbers of patients indicate that hospital mortality after biventricular repairs, including complete AVSD, may be unchanged or even decreased compared with patients without Down syndrome.[23,24,27] For all patients with Down syndrome a planned approach to timing and coordination

of the health care team members involved is crucial for the child and family.

22q11.2 Deletion Syndrome

22q11.2 deletion syndrome occurs in approximately 1 in 4000 individuals and is the most common microdeletion syndrome associated with congenital CVMs. Nearly 75% of patients with 22q11.2 deletion syndrome have a CVM, which most commonly include conotruncal defects, abnormal patterning of the aortic arch and brachiocephalic arteries, and perimembranous VSD (Table 75.1).[28,29] The systemic features include facial dysmorphism (Box 75.1; Fig. 75.2) and cleft palate. Additional features likely to impact intensive care include hypoparathyroidism, immunodeficiency, congenital renal anomalies, and airway anomalies (Box 75.2). The

TABLE 75.1	Cardiac Defects Associated With 22q11.2 Deletion	
Defect		**Percentage**
No defect or clinically insignificant		22-25
Tetralogy of Fallot		17-20
Interrupted aortic arch		14-17
Ventricular septal defect (VSD)		14-16
Pulmonary atresia with VSD		10
Truncus arteriosus		9
Aortic arch anomaly		5
Vascular ring		3
Pulmonary valve stenosis		2
Other significant defect		4-5

Data from McDonald-McGinn DM, LaRossa D, Goldmuntz E, et al. The 22q11.2 deletion: screening, diagnostic workup, and outcome of results; report on 181 patients. *Genet Test.* 1997;1:99-108; and Ryan AK, Goodship JA, Wilson DI, et al. Spectrum of clinical features associated with interstitial chromosome 22q11 deletions: a European collaborative study. *J Med Genet.* 1997;34:798-804.

• BOX 75.1 Dysmorphic Features Associated With 22q11.2 Deletion Syndrome

Narrow palpebral fissures
Hooded eyelids
Hypertelorism
Small, rounded protuberant ears
Broad nasal bridge
Bulbous nose tip
Hypoplastic alae nasi
Small mouth
Retrognathia/micrognathia
Palatal abnormalities
Long thin digits

• BOX 75.2 Critical Care Considerations in 22q11.2 Deletion Syndrome

Difficult intubation
Laryngeal/tracheal abnormalities
Hypocalcemia
Seizures
Increased risk of infections
Possibility of transfusion-related graft-versus-host disease
Feeding difficulties

Deletion of Chromosome 22q11.2 Sndrome

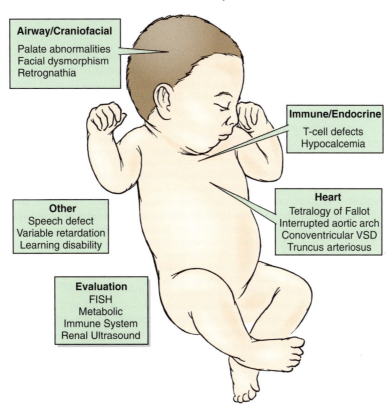

Airway/Craniofacial
Palate abnormalities
Facial dysmorphism
Retrognathia

Immune/Endocrine
T-cell defects
Hypocalcemia

Other
Speech defect
Variable retardation
Learning disability

Heart
Tetralogy of Fallot
Interrupted aortic arch
Conoventricular VSD
Truncus arteriosus

Evaluation
FISH
Metabolic
Immune System
Renal Ultrasound

• **Figure 75.2** Associated defects of 22q11.2 deletion syndrome.

long-term challenges associated with 22q11.2 deletion include developmental delay and neuropsychiatric disorders such as attention-deficit/hyperactivity disorder, autism spectrum disorders, and psychosis.[30-32]

The 22q11.2 deletion syndrome is caused by hemizygous deletion of a small region of variable length on the short arm of chromosome 22 and is associated with a range of clinical phenotypes. The deletion was initially discovered in patients with the clinical characteristics of DiGeorge syndrome, but it is now understood that the deletion also causes other clinically established syndromes, including velocardiofacial syndrome and conotruncal anomaly face syndrome.[33,34] The shift to combining these syndromes nominally into a single 22q11.2 deletion syndrome exemplifies the ongoing integration between syndromic diagnoses and their underlying genetic causes. The genetic test traditionally used to detect 22q11.2 deletion was fluorescence in situ hybridization (FISH), which uses a probe designed to target this chromosomal segment specifically. Practices are now turning toward use of CMA, which has higher diagnostic sensitivity because it is able to detect smaller deletions that may not be identified with FISH. When 22q11.2 deletion is not deleted, the CMA will potentially identify alternative pathogenic CNVs and therefore reach a diagnosis more efficiently. The length of the segment affected by this microdeletion is variable but typically contains between 30 and 40 individual genes. Hemizygous loss of the *TBX1* gene may play a major role in causing some features of this syndrome, including CVMs.[35]

Hypoplasia of the thymus is often present in patients with 22q11.2 deletion syndrome, typically leading to mild to moderate immunodeficiency. Rarely, the thymus is completely aplastic, resulting in severe immunodeficiency. Thymic hypoplasia leading to low T-lymphocyte counts and B-lymphocyte dysfunction may explain reports of increased infectious complications following cardiac surgery.[36,37] This may justify the use of broadened postoperative antibiotic regimens, including antifungal therapy,[38] although this approach has not been conclusively tested. Further, the immunocompromised status of the patients justifies use of cytomegalovirus-negative, irradiated blood products when transfusions are required to avoid the risk of iatrogenic infection and graft-versus-host disease. Airway management may be challenging due to retrognathia or a congenital airway anomaly, including laryngeal web.[39] Depending on the severity of the anomaly, the equipment and personnel necessary to establish an alternative airway should be readily available before the administration of hypnotics and neuromuscular blocking agents.[40] Postoperative vocal cord paralysis, particularly after operations involving the aortic arch, or diaphragmatic paralysis can have dramatic clinical consequences and should be investigated and treated. Overt cleft palate, submucous clefts, and velopharyngeal insufficiency may significantly impair swallow function. Hypocalcemia due to developmental hypoplasia of the parathyroid glands may be present, particularly in young infants, and tends to resolve or respond to calcium supplementation. Calcium level should be monitored preoperatively and postoperatively, especially given that patients with 22q11.2 deletion have increased seizure risk independent of the presence of hypocalcemia. Renal abnormalities detectable on ultrasonography, including absent, dysplastic, or multicystic kidneys, are another common finding.

The multiple noncardiac abnormalities associated with 22q11.2 deletion often complicate the postoperative course, leading to longer duration of postoperative intensive care.[41,42] Although few studies are sufficiently powered to examine patients with 22q11.2 deletion syndrome in terms of mortality, most data support that there is a

---

> **• BOX 75.3** **Evaluation for Patients With 22q11.2 Deletions**
>
> **Typical Subspecialty Evaluation**
> Genetics
> Cardiology
> Immunology
> Otolaryngology
> Plastic surgery
> Speech and audiology
> Neurodevelopmental
> Oral motor and swallowing
>
> **Additional Subspecialties as Necessary**
> Endocrinology
> Gastroenterology
> Orthopedics
> Urology
> Pediatric surgery
> Psychiatry
>
> **Laboratory Evaluation**
> Chromosomal microarray analysis
> Serum calcium level
> Complete blood count, T-cell studies, immunoglobulin concentrations
> Echocardiography
> Renal ultrasonography
>
> *Data from McDonald-McGinn DM, LaRossa D, Goldmuntz E, et al. The 22q11.2 deletion: screening, diagnostic workup, and outcome of results; report on 181 patients. Genet Test. 1997;1:99-108; and Ryan AK, Goodship JA, Wilson DI, et al. Spectrum of clinical features associated with interstitial chromosome 22q11 deletions: a European collaborative study. J Med Genet. 1997;34:798-804.*

---

slightly increased risk of death following a cardiac operation.[7,37,41,43] Mortality risk may be most significant for patients with pulmonary atresia, in which cases excessive bleeding may be a significant risk.[36,44] This bleeding risk may be secondary to increased anatomic complexity, but dysfunction of hemostatic pathways, including platelet function, may be contributory.[45] Altogether, the broad spectrum of noncardiac systemic anomalies in patients with 22q11.2 deletion syndrome highlights the importance of a multidisciplinary approach involving multiple pediatric specialists in the newborn, perioperative, and ambulatory setting. Box 75.3 lists the recommended specialties for the care team. These are ultimately tailored to match the spectrum of problems in an individual, once appropriate screening evaluations and testing have been completed.

Turner Syndrome

Approximately 1 in 2000 females is born with Turner syndrome, which is due to complete or partial absence of one of the two X chromosomes. Turner syndrome predisposes to left-sided CVMs such as bicuspid aortic valve and coarctation of the aorta. Many patients also manifest signs of arteriopathy, including thoracic aortic aneurysm and dissection (TAAD) and systemic hypertension. Venous anomalies, including partial anomalous pulmonary venous return and persistent left-sided superior vena cava, are also frequently encountered.[46] The noncardiac features providing clues to the diagnosis are short stature, ovarian dysgenesis, neck webbing, and widely spaced nipples. There is general consensus that patients with Turner syndrome have intrinsic dysfunction of lymphatics.[47] This may be one explanation for the high frequency of hydrops fetalis and spontaneous fetal loss. Peripheral lymphedema, which is typically present at birth and self-resolving by early childhood, may be another clue to early diagnosis. Most pertinent to intensive care is the risk for dysfunction of pulmonary lymphatics predisposing to chylothorax and pleural effusions. Congenital pulmonary lymphangiectasia may be the most drastic form of lymphatic dysfunction in Turner syndrome,[48] but there is likely a spectrum of lymphatic abnormality that may manifest clinically only when confronted with stressors such as mechanical injury and/or inflammation associated with cardiopulmonary bypass surgery. Congenital renal anomalies occur frequently enough to mandate screening with ultrasonography. There is a long-term risk for development of autoimmune hypothyroidism, so patients with Turner syndrome should undergo routine screening and be tested before cardiac surgery if over 4 years of age.[49]

Patients with Turner syndrome undergoing surgical repair of coarctation of the aorta have displayed good postoperative outcomes since the adoption of modern surgical techniques, which include careful manipulation of diseased aortic tissues to avoid postoperative hemorrhage.[50] In contrast, consistent with arteriopathy, there is evidence that treatment of coarctation with implanted stents may introduce a risk for development of aneurysm or dissection.[51-53] The most concerning outcomes data in Turner syndrome concern HLHS. For unknown reasons, patients with HLHS and Turner syndrome display very poor outcomes with mortality between

stage I and stage II palliations reported to be as high as 80% and only 25% survival to stage III palliation.[50,54] These poor outcomes may be related to underlying lymphatic disease, but there is a clear need for further study to understand the responsible mechanism.

To improve rates of early diagnosis, it is reasonable to perform a karyotype as a routine component of care for every female infant with coarctation. Recent data show testing yields approximately 5% to 12% in girls with coarctation,[55,56] and external features may be subtle in the neonatal period or in cases of mosaicism. All patients with Turner syndrome require long-term cardiac surveillance for development of hypertension and TAAD, even in the absence of bicuspid aortic valve. Routine screening with cardiac magnetic resonance imaging in late childhood may identify clinically silent features, including aortic dilation and anomalous pulmonary veins.[46] Thus an early diagnosis likely improves short- and long-term outcomes.

Noonan Syndrome

Noonan syndrome has a prevalence of 1 in 1000 to 2500 live births. Noonan syndrome is characterized by both cardiac and extracardiac defects (Fig. 75.3).[57-59] Noonan syndrome is genetically heterogeneous, but the currently known genes cluster within the RAS-MAP kinase signaling pathway, leading some to classify

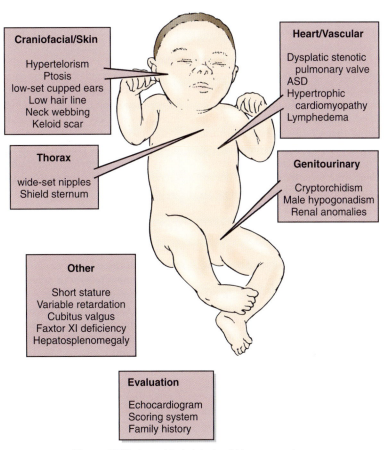

• **Figure 75.3** Associated defects of Noonan syndrome.

Noonan syndrome as a "RASopathy." The most commonly mutated gene in this syndrome is *PTPN11*.[60] Other causative genes in the pathway are *SOS1, RAF1, KRAS, NRAS, BRAF, SHOC2,* and *CBL.* Indeed, there are now several disorders related to Noonan syndrome with overlapping but clinically distinct phenotypes that are caused by mutations in the RAS-MAP kinase pathway. These include cardiofaciocutaneous syndrome *(BRAF, KRAS),* Costello syndrome *(HRAS),* and Noonan syndrome with multiple lentigines (formerly called LEOPARD syndrome; *PTPN11, RAF1*). There are important clinical considerations for each of these syndromes. The focus of this chapter will be the typical Noonan syndrome.

In Noonan syndrome CVMs are observed in at least 80% of cases.[61] Pulmonary valve stenosis, often with pulmonary valve dysplasia, is the most frequent cardiac anomaly, followed by hypertrophic cardiomyopathy (HCM). Secundum ASD is often associated with pulmonic stenosis, and a variety of other CVMs are reported.[61] The noncardiac features of this syndrome include facial dysmorphism, short stature, kyphoscoliosis, vertebral anomalies, winged scapula, pectus sternal deformity, neck webbing, and cryptorchidism in males. Most cases represent de novo (i.e., not inherited) mutations. However, autosomal dominant familial presentations are also frequently encountered. Currently patients suspected to have Noonan syndrome are tested using an NGS panel designed to sequence all of the genes known to be associated with the clinical phenotype. When a molecular diagnosis of Noonan syndrome is established, screening of parents for the mutation should be strongly considered to identify previously unrecognized carriers who may lack obvious physical features.

Whether involved in the perioperative management of cardiac or extracardiac anomalies, intensive care and surgical providers should be cognizant of several features of Noonan syndrome. Abnormalities in coagulation or platelet function are common and may predispose to bleeding complications. Some of the initial descriptions of platelet function deficit and neonatal amegakaryocytic thrombocytopenia have been corroborated by subsequent reports.[62,63] Although congenital thrombocytopenia is a rare occurrence,[64] comprehensive testing of platelet function has identified abnormalities in greater than 80% of patients.[65] In pioneering work Sharland and colleagues,[66] studied 72 affected individuals with a mean age of 11.4 years and found that 47 (65%) had a history of abnormal bruising or bleeding and 29 (40%) had a prolonged activated partial thromboplastin time with deficiencies of factors VIII, XI, and XII. These findings were recently replicated in an independent cohort of 39 patients.[65] Together these data suggest that preoperative assessment for coagulation-factor deficits and platelet dysfunction may be warranted. Providers should be alert to bleeding complications and exercise caution toward the use of antiplatelet medications.

Similar to Turner syndrome, Noonan syndrome may be complicated by disorders of the lymphatic system. Peripheral lymphedema is a common finding in neonates with Noonan syndrome that typically resolves early in life. However, lymphatic dysfunction may assume more severe forms, including lymphatic dysplasia or pulmonary lymphangiectasia.[67,68] Recurrent pleural effusion is a rare but troublesome postoperative complication. This appears to be due to a nonspecific effect of thoracotomy in exacerbating previously mild chronic low-grade pulmonary lymphangiectasia. Good response is generally obtained with a combination of thoracentesis, restriction from dietary long-chain fatty acids, fluid restriction, and/or diuretics. Prenatal evidence of lymphedema or fluid accumulation, including fetal hydrops, may be another clue to the diagnosis.[69]

In terms of the cardiovascular features of Noonan syndrome, the pulmonary valve is usually thickened and dysplastic. The short-term outcomes after balloon valvuloplasty do not appear significantly different from pulmonary valve stenosis in patients without Noonan syndrome, but long-term outcomes are unknown. HCM was originally described as developing late in childhood but has now been recognized in infancy and even prenatally.[70,71] The presence of HCM, which is particularly high among patients with mutations in *RAF1,* increases anesthetic and intraoperative risk. A recent echocardiogram should be available before anesthesia for cardiac or noncardiac surgery in infants or children with Noonan syndrome. There is evidence that some patients with HCM and Noonan syndrome experience worse outcomes compared to non–Noonan syndrome HCM.[72] A baseline preoperative electrocardiogram (ECG) is also recommended before surgery. ECG abnormalities, including negative forces in left precordial leads, left axis deviation, and abnormal Q waves, are often present and unrelated to the cardiovascular anatomic phenotype.[73] Characterizing the ECG appearance at baseline may help to discern whether abnormalities observed on cardiac monitors during or after surgery represent acute pathology. Although Noonan syndrome does not predispose to cardiac arrhythmia, patients with the related Costello syndrome *(HRAS* mutation) do have a significant risk for developing supraventricular tachycardia and multifocal atrial tachycardia in particular.

Most individuals with Noonan syndrome develop normal cognitive function. Indeed, most children are able to attend regular school. However, increased risk for long-term intellectual disability warrants close monitoring for early signs of developmental delay. In early reports there was concern for a possible association between Noonan syndrome and malignant hyperthermia, as postulated by Hunter and Pinsky.[74] Fortunately, this connection has not been supported over time, and risk for malignant hyperthermia is considered to be no different from the general population.[75]

With increased awareness and advances in genetic testing practices, including family screening, diagnoses are established earlier than in past series.[76] Nonetheless the phenotypic variability, including subtlety of features and the changes in facial pattern with growth, still contributes to missed diagnoses.[77] In the context of these diagnostic challenges, the pediatric intensivist confronted by a child with growth delay, pulmonary stenosis, and/or cardiomyopathy may be the first to recognize the syndrome in the child and in a parent.

Trisomy 18 (Edwards Syndrome)

Trisomy 18 is a severe genetic syndrome characterized by the presence of three copies of chromosome 18. Rarely this additional chromosome is present in only some cell lines, leading to a variable clinical presentation, referred to as mosaic trisomy 18. Trisomy 18 occurs in approximately 1 in 6000 live births and is the second most common trisomy syndrome after trisomy 21. Overall the clinical features of this syndrome are quite dramatic with a very high mortality (90% to 95% in the first year of life) coupled with severe cognitive impairment and diffuse multisystem anomalies among the approximately 50% who survive beyond the first week.[78] Congenital CVMs are very common with a prevalence between 80% and 100%. Common cardiac lesions include VSD, ASD, and patent ductus arteriosus (PDA). More complex lesions such as tetralogy of Fallot, double-outlet right ventricle, polyvalvular dysplasia, and AVSDs are also encountered.[79,80] Due to the severe

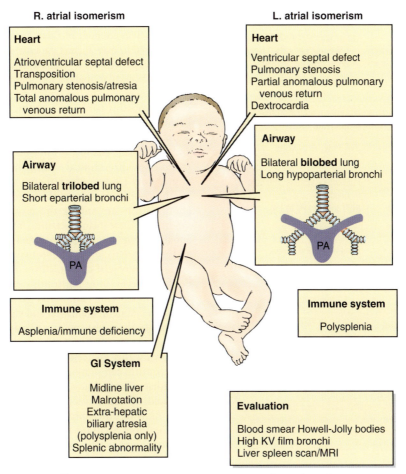

Ivemark Syndrome

R. atrial isomerism

Heart

Atrioventricular septal defect
Transposition
Pulmonary stenosis/atresia
Total anomalous pulmonary
 venous return

Airway

Bilateral **trilobed** lung
Short eparterial bronchi

PA

Immune system

Asplenia/immune deficiency

GI System

Midline liver
Malrotation
Extra-hepatic
 biliary atresia
 (polysplenia only)
Splenic abnormality

L. atrial isomerism

Heart

Ventricular septal defect
Pulmonary stenosis
Partial anomalous pulmonary
 venous return
Dextrocardia

Airway

Bilateral **bilobed** lung
Long hypoparterial bronchi

PA

Immune system

Polysplenia

Evaluation

Blood smear Howell-Jolly bodies
High KV film bronchi
Liver spleen scan/MRI

• **Figure 75.4** Associated defects of heterotaxy/Ivemark syndrome.

impact of this syndrome on expected outcomes, rapid testing may be considered when the diagnosis is suspected postnatally.

Given the grim overall prognosis, including profound neurodevelopmental impairment, the role of cardiac intervention for patients with trisomy 18 has been a significant topic of discussion, and there is little consensus among congenital heart programs at present. There is significant debate surrounding the role of cardiac intervention in modifying mortality and morbidity for these patients. Recent studies have stirred significant debate surrounding this issue by showing optimistic short-term survival rates (80% to 90%) among the few trisomy 18 patients who undergo cardiac surgery.[81,82] Others suggest that cardiac surgery and aggressive perioperative care may improve life expectancy and increase the likelihood of hospital discharge.[83] Despite these observations it is clear that patient selection was a key aspect of the improvements seen in those who received cardiac surgery. Patients with low birth weight, unstable initial hospital course, very early mortality, and a high burden of noncardiac congenital anomalies and medical complications were significantly less likely to be offered surgical intervention. The appropriateness and utility of cardiac intervention for patients with trisomy 18 remain unclear. Individualized approaches to clinical decision making with the family in partnership with specialists in palliative care are most likely to achieve the best possible outcome for patients with this severe disease.

Heterotaxy Syndrome

Heterotaxy syndrome is characterized by disruption of normal thoracoabdominal situs and includes a spectrum of CVMs and noncardiac organ problems (Fig. 75.4).[84] This condition is discussed in detail in Chapter 67 of this textbook. Relevant to this chapter, the understanding of the genetic basis of heterotaxy is rapidly advancing. Genes in the Nodal signaling pathway, including *DNAH5, ZIC3, CFC1, NODAL, ACVR2B, DNAI1,* and *LEFTY2,* are known to harbor mutations that cause heterotaxy. NGS panels testing for these genes and others are now available clinically. Overall, the risk of familial recurrence of heterotaxy is increased compared with other classes of CVMs.[4]

Postoperative outcomes for patients with heterotaxy are relatively poor. For example, the diagnosis of heterotaxy was associated with increased postoperative mortality among more than 70,000 total cases in the STS database from 1998 to 2009.[85] Mortality risk may be especially elevated in patients with heterotaxy and single-ventricle lesions, but these outcomes may be improving over time.[86,87] The presence of complex cardiac anatomy may explain some of these observations, including an increased risk for arrhythmia due to anatomic abnormalities of the cardiac conduction system. Frequent findings of asplenia and polysplenia, which are associated with decreased splenic function, increase the risk for postoperative bacterial infections and sepsis (Table 75.2).[88,160] Long-term antibiotic

TABLE 75.2	Anomalies in Heterotaxy Syndrome
Asplenia	**Polysplenia**
Common atrioventricular canal (85%) with DORV, transposed great arteries, and pulmonic outflow atresia or extreme stenosis	Ventricular septal defect with pulmonic stenosis, normal great arteries or DORV without subaortic conus
IVC intact: frequent anomalous drainage of hepatic vein	IVC interruption with azygos drainage
SVC bilateral, unroofed coronary sinus	SVC may be bilateral
Pulmonary veins often drain into systemic vein, obstructed	Pulmonary venous drainage divided (RPV to RA, LPV to LA)
Lungs: bilateral trilobed	Lungs: bilateral bilobed
Liver: symmetric	Liver: symmetric or normally lobulated, risk of extrahepatic biliary atresia
Viscera: heterotaxy with risk of obstruction due to malrotation	Viscera: heterotaxy with risk of obstruction due to malrotation

This table summarizes the most frequently encountered anomalies, recognizing that a frequent overlap occurs in the cardiosplenic variants.
DORV, Double-outlet right ventricle; *IVC,* inferior vena cava; *LA,* left atrium; *LPV,* left pulmonary vein; *RA,* right atrium; *RPV,* right pulmonary vein; *SVC,* superior vena cava.
Data from Applegate KE, Goske MJ, Pierce G, et al. Situs revisited: imaging of the heterotaxy syndrome. *Radiographics.* 1999;19:837-852.

25% of patients. Approximately 20% of patients have valvar abnormalities, including stenosis and dysplasia of semilunar or atrioventricular valves. Coarctation of the aorta and conotruncal defects such as tetralogy of Fallot are also reported. Cardiomyopathy is diagnosed in over 25% of patients, manifesting as noncompaction cardiomyopathy and/or dilated cardiomypathy.[93,94] Interestingly, detailed molecular analysis has mapped the clinical phenotype of CVM presentation to five critical regions within 1p36. Meanwhile, cardiomyopathy, particularly the noncompaction phenotype, has been mapped to two nonoverlapping critical regions.[95,96] This is an important consideration for the management of these patients and an excellent example of using genotype-phenotype relationships to individualize clinical management, risk stratification, and anticipatory guidance for patients and their families.

The systemic features of this syndrome vary widely. Neurologic abnormalities are among the most prominent features of this syndrome. These include seizures, infantile spasms, structural brain anomalies, hypotonia, developmental delay, behavioral abnormalities, and moderate to severe intellectual disability. Almost all patients exhibit craniofacial abnormalities, including midface hypoplasia, deeply set eyes, long philtrum, posteriorly rotated low-set ears, and a pointed chin. Limb and genitourinary anomalies are also common.[93] Careful evaluation and vigilant monitoring is important to identify these features in a timely manner. The extensive and severe features of this syndrome highlight the importance of identifying this microdeletion in the neonatal period. Many of these features can significantly impact perioperative management of cardiac disease. Furthermore, careful analysis of the genotype may guide clinical decisions targeting specific cardiac and noncardiac risks. Akin to other rare genetic syndromes, risk prediction will become more accurate as greater numbers of these patients are diagnosed and followed over time.

Diagnostic Considerations in Cardiovascular Genetics

Genetic testing adds an important dimension to the diagnosis and management of congenital CVMs. Establishing a genetic diagnosis often enhances the accuracy of information about prognosis available for patients and families. Genetic testing may facilitate individualized treatment decisions directed toward mitigating both short- and long-term risk factors and, in some cases, may determine the optimal timing and type of cardiac intervention or indication thereof. A genetic diagnosis enhances the accuracy of predicting recurrence risk, which, for example, may be as high as 50% for individuals with autosomal dominant disorders such as Noonan syndrome.

Many cardiac ICUs have begun to use genetic evaluation and testing in a systematic way for patients with congenital CVMs. In general, genetic testing decisions may be guided by the patient's specific type of CVM or may involve the combined consideration of CVM with the presence of specific noncardiac congenital anomalies. Initial testing may target a specific syndromic diagnosis, such as a karyotype when Down syndrome is suspected. In cases in which a specific syndrome is not suspected, broad testing with CMA may be the first consideration. Some congenital heart centers have developed algorithms to streamline the processes for genetic evaluation and testing in the ICU,[97] but at this time there is no standardized approach. There is strengthening evidence to support using the CMA as a first-line test for all infants with clinically significant CVMs admitted to the ICU. A systematic approach to testing, assisted by institutional protocols, can significantly enhance

prophylaxis is indicated in the presence of splenic dysfunction. Recent data indicate that ciliary dysfunction is frequent in heterotaxy[89] and may be a significant contributor to postoperative complications, including prolonged mechanical ventilation and increased need for tracheostomy.[90] Screening for ciliary dysfunction may be useful in patients with single-ventricle lesions or unexpectedly prolonged duration of respiratory support.

1p36 Deletion Syndrome

1p36 deletion syndrome is the most common terminal deletion syndrome, affecting nearly 1 in 5000 live births.[91] The syndrome is caused by deletion within a large 30-Mb region constituting the terminal portion of the short arm of chromosome 1. An important aspect of this syndrome is significant variation in the length and position of the deleted segment between affected individuals,[92] which likely contributes to phenotypic variability observed among cases. The significant majority of patients have de novo mutations. Less commonly, inheritance may occur via balanced translocation or germline mosaicism in an unaffected parent. Adequate genetic counseling and parental genetic testing is essential to delineating the inheritance pattern and providing information about recurrence risk of future pregnancies.

The cardiovascular features of this syndrome are diverse, occur in over 70% of patients, and can be divided into two general categories: congenital heart disease and cardiomyopathy. Congenital CVMs include ASD and VSD, each occurring in approximately

the accuracy and cost-effectiveness of genetic testing for cardiac patients.[98]

The overall yield for CMA testing varies between studies and partially depends on lesion type. Recent publications together estimate that approximately 10% of patients with significant CVMs harbor a CNV that is clinically actionable,[99-104] even when excluding known syndromic causes such as 22q11.2 deletion syndrome. This high yield of testing supports its routine use, recognizing that yields may vary between different classes of CVMs. Future studies are necessary to begin to define whether testing may be stratified clinically according to class of CVM. The CNVs that have been most frequently identified in large studies using CMA include 1q21.1 duplication or deletion, 8p23.1 deletion or duplication, and 15q11.2 deletion or duplication. Early screening with CMA can identify patients with rare syndromic conditions that would be challenging to diagnose by clinical assessment alone. Testing with CMA may drastically accelerate the timing of diagnosis for infants with subtle dysmorphic features or subclinical noncardiac congenital anomalies and before the onset of symptoms manifesting later in life such as developmental delay. Interestingly, recent studies have consistently identified CNVs that are typically associated with syndromic CVMs in patients lacking the typical noncardiac features, highlighting the variable expression of many genetic syndromes. Importantly, CMA has greater resolution than FISH to detect small duplications and deletions in patients with microdeletion or microduplication syndromes such as 22q11.2 deletion syndrome or Williams syndrome (7q23.11 deletion) and therefore may be considered a first-line test even when these specific diagnoses are suspected.

1q21.1 deletion syndrome is a rare condition associated with a spectrum of congenital CVMs, including left-sided obstructive lesions, ASD, VSD, and conotruncal defects.[105] Craniofacial anomalies such as frontal bossing, epicanthal folds, long philtrum, and/or highly arched palate occur in over 75% of individuals. Other risks include developmental delay, behavioral abnormalities, microcephaly, hypotonia, and seizures.[106-108] An early diagnosis of this rare condition facilitates the opportunity to screen for neurodevelopmental abnormalities and intervene early. 1q21.1 deletion is also characterized by reduced penetrance and variable phenotypic expression. For example, CVM is present in 10% to 25%, and inheritance of the deletion from an undiagnosed parent who apparently lacks CVM and has an overall mild phenotype may equal the rate of de novo occurrences.[106,107] This possibility highlights the importance of routinely testing the parents of genotype-positive children, independent of parental signs or symptoms for certain syndromes, including 22q11.2 deletion and Noonan syndrome. This enables counseling about recurrence risk for future pregnancies and identification of other family members who are at risk. Clearly, adequate genetic counseling and family testing are an essential part of the care plan.

Applying Genomic Testing to Cardiovascular Malformations

The advent of NGS technology and exome sequence analysis has facilitated major advances in the understanding of the genetic basis of CVMs.[109] Most strikingly, exome data from the Pediatric Cardiac Genomics Consortium (PCGC) support that de novo mutations at the nucleotide level may account for up to 10% of congenital CVMs.[110] At the same time, it is becoming clear that inherited variants with reduced penetrance also contribute to a significant proportion of CVMs, particularly among those patients with apparently isolated CVMs.[111,112] Another major finding that has emerged from the PCGC data is the significant overlap between genes that cause CVMs and the genes that cause neurodevelopmental disorders in patients without CVMs.[110] Thus early diagnosis of a pathogenic mutation in certain genes may indicate the need for closer neurodevelopmental monitoring and early intervention. As we better understand the effect of these genotypes on neurodevelopmental outcomes in patients with CVMs, genetic testing may increasingly guide surgical decisions, including the optimal timing for operation. There remains much to be learned in terms of the analysis and interpretation of the voluminous data generated by exome and whole genome sequencing. It is likely that expanded clinical use of these technologies, coupled with improved understanding of underlying mechanisms, will advance the care of pediatric cardiovascular disease in completely new directions.

Cardiovascular Genetics in a Multidisciplinary Team

Given the advantages and continual improvements of genetic testing, it may be tempting for programs to implement widespread use of testing without an adequate consideration of the risks and necessary counseling involved. The results of any genetic test can be confusing, equivocal, and difficult to explain to a patient or family. Tests may identify a previously documented genetic change that has a known association with the cardiac and noncardiac anomalies present in the patient. Conversely, tests may identify genetic changes that are novel, poorly understood, or difficult to associate with the patient's clinical finding. Results of this nature, frequently called variants of unknown/uncertain significance, are common and frustrating to both families and providers.[113] Adequate family counseling before genetic testing can make a significant difference in a family's ability to cope with unexpected or confusing results. For this reason, genetic counseling services must be a central part of any team considering a comprehensive genetic testing program. Providers trained in genetic medicine, including genetic counselors and medical geneticists, should function as part of the planning, development, and ongoing use of any genetic testing protocol. The involvement of genetic counseling services dramatically improves the efficacy, efficiency, and patient satisfaction of genetic testing, and a genetic counselor should be available for consultation to discuss testing options and results with patients and their families. Dedicated cardiovascular genetics services are optimally positioned to work collaboratively as part of multidisciplinary teams consisting of cardiothoracic surgeons, cardiologists, intensivists, medical geneticists, and genetic counselors. Constant changes in genetic testing technology, coupled with the variable availability of medical genetics professionals across centers, make this an ongoing challenge for congenital heart programs. An important step toward developing strong clinical programs will be to improve training in cardiovascular genetics.[114]

Additional Cardiac Syndromes

Alagille: Intrahepatic biliary cirrhosis due to bile duct paucity, dysmorphic facies, ocular anomalies, vertebral anomalies. Frequent cardiac defects are *branch pulmonary artery stenosis, tetralogy of Fallot, pulmonary valve stenosis.* Genetics: heterozygous mutation in *JAG1* (majority) or *NOTCH2* gene.[115,116]

CHARGE: Eye anomaly (*C*oloboma), *H*eart defect usually *conotruncal defects including tetralogy of Fallot and VSD,* (choanal *A*tresia), *R*etardation of growth and/or development, *G*enitourinary abnormality, and *E*ar anomalies/deafness, including cochlear dysplasia. Genetics: heterozygous mutation in *CHD7* (majority) or *SEMA3E* gene.[117,118]

Cornelia de Lange: Craniofacial anomalies, including cleft palate, intellectual disability, seizure, renal anomalies. Frequent cardiac defects include *pulmonary valve stenosis, peripheral pulmonary stenosis, septal defects, tetralogy of Fallot, and risk for progressive dysplasia of the atrioventricular valves.* Genetics: heterozygous mutation in genes important for cohesin complex (*NIPBL, SMC1A,* or *SMC3* gene).[119]

Cri du chat: Craniofacial anomalies, severe neurologic impairment, laryngeal anomalies likely contributing to characteristic high-pitched cry. Frequent cardiac defects are *septal defects, PDA, and TOF.* Genetics: hemizygous 5p15 deletion.[120]

Ellis–van Creveld: Short stature with polydactyly; dysplasia of nails, hair, and teeth; risk for thoracic dystrophy; normal cognitive development. Frequent cardiac defects are *common atrium, AVSD, and systemic or pulmonary venous anomalies.* Genetics: mutation of *EVC* or *EVC2* gene. Usually autosomal recessive: clusters noted among Amish communities.[121]

Fetal alcohol: Facial dysmorphism, intellectual disability, short fingers. A variety of heart defects with *VSD and ASD* as the most common.[122]

Goldenhar: Unilateral facial microsomia, microtia, preotic skin tag, coloboma of the eye, renal anomalies. Frequent heart defects include *tetralogy of Fallot and septal defects.* Also referred to as oculoauricular vertebral syndrome. Genetic cause unknown.[123,124]

Holt-Oram: Although originally described as an autosomal dominant syndrome with absent thumb and an ASD, considerable phenotypic heterogeneity exists, with "digitalized" (finger-like) thumb or rarely phocomelia. Cardiac defects are variable and usually involve septation defects with *ASD* as the most frequent.[125] Genetics: heterozygous mutation of the *TBX5* gene at chromosome 12q24.[126]

Jacobsen: Craniofacial anomalies including trigonocephaly, syndactyly, intellectual disability, platelet dysfunction, including Paris-Trousseau syndrome. Cardiac defects include *VSD and left-sided obstructive lesions including HLHS.* Genetics: hemizygous deletion on long arm of chromosome 11 (breakpoint at 11q23).[127]

Kabuki: Characteristic facial appearance, fetal finger pads, intellectual disability, cleft lip/palate, renal anomaly. Cardiac defects include *septal defects, coarctation of the aorta, and tetralogy of Fallot.* Genetics: heterozygous mutation in *KMT2D* (also known as *MLL2*).[128,129]

Marfan: see Chapter 53.

Duchenne muscular dystrophy: Progressive muscular weakness often complicated by *cardiomyopathy.*[130] Genetics: mutation in the dystrophin gene located at chromosome Xq22. X-linked recessive.

PHACE: *P*osterior fossa malformation, *H*emangioma, *A*rterial anomalies consisting of stenosis/aneurysm of cervicocranial arteries increasing risk for stroke, *C*ardiac defects, and *E*ye anomalies. Frequent cardiac defects are *coarctation of the aorta, VSD, and aberrant subclavian artery.* Genetics: unknown.[131]

Pompe: Most severe of the many forms of glycogen storage disease due to an inherited deficiency in α-1,4-glucosidase (acid maltase). *Cardiomyopathy with short PR interval.* Genetics: autosomal recessive.[132]

Rubella: Congenital deafness, cataracts, and sometimes intellectual disability and microcephaly may follow maternal rubella in early pregnancy. Cardiac sequelae usually *PDA and pulmonary arterial stenosis.*[133] An example of a preventable "environmental" syndrome.[134]

Smith-Lemli-Opitz: Intellectual disability, microcephaly, skeletal anomalies. Cardiac defects include *septal defects and tetralogy of Fallot.* Genetics: mutation in the *DHCR7* gene with autosomal recessive inheritance.[135,136]

Smith-Magenis: Craniofacial abnormalities, ocular abnormalities, developmental delay, sleep disturbance, seizures, hypercholesterolemia. Frequent cardiac defects are *septal defects, tetralogy of Fallot, and total anomalous pulmonary venous return.* Genetics: hemizygous deletion of 17p11.2.[137]

Trisomy 13 (Patau): Severe psychomotor delay, polydactyly, cleft lip/palate, holoprosencephaly. Frequent cardiac defects are *ASD, VSD, cardiac positional anomalies.*[138,139]

VACTERL association: *V*ertebral defects, *A*nal atresia, *C*ardiac defects, *T*racheo-esophageal fistula, *R*enal anomalies, and *L*imb defects. Frequent cardiac defects are *VSD (most cases) and tetralogy of Fallot.* Genetics: unknown.[140]

Williams: Characteristic facial features, intellectual disability, neonatal hypercalcemia (usually transient), hypothyroidism. Frequent cardiac defects are *supravalvar aortic and pulmonary stenosis, branch pulmonary stenosis, peripheral pulmonary stenosis, stenosis of thoracic aorta, bicuspid aortic valve.* Genetics: a contiguous gene deletion syndrome with hemizygosity at chromosome 7q11.23, including the locus for *ELN* (elastin). Nonsyndromic familial supravalvar aortic stenosis involves heterozygous mutation of *ELN.*[141-143]

Wolf-Hirschhorn: Characteristic facial features ("Greek warrior helmet"), cleft lip/palate, seizures, renal anomalies. Frequent cardiac defects are *septal defects, pulmonary stenosis, and patent ductus arteriosus.* Genetics: hemizygous deletion of 4p16.3.[144]

Ethical Considerations

Child-Parent–Health Care Team Triad

Ethics and cardiology are inseparable. When an infant or child with a heart problem needs intensive care, decisions involving life and death or possible long-term morbidity are made on a daily, even hourly basis. By necessity these decisions are being made by surrogates, the family (or legal guardian) and the health care team, not by the child. This triangular relationship of child, family, and health care team has been referred to as the *triangle of understanding.*[145] It is an error to infer that ethical issues arise for discussion only when a disorder is in its terminal stages or when a genetic syndrome associated with a poor prognosis is diagnosed. Ethical considerations are always with us, as in Fost's memorable phrase "Ethics, ethics everywhere."[146]

In this brief section we revisit an infant described in a previous edition who was treated in the pediatric ICU setting and review some of the ethical considerations. These considerations are affected not only by the rapid advances in technology, making previously lethal conditions treatable, but also by new genetic information and by rapid societal change.[147-150]

Illustrative Case. A young married woman, Mrs. M., had routine obstetric ultrasound imaging at 18 weeks. Previous obstetric history was significant for two previous uncomplicated pregnancies. The prenatal sonogram documented multiple congenital anomalies, including microcephaly and hydrocephalus, bilateral shortened arms, and congenital heart disease. The couple declined amniocentesis. Despite the high potential for in utero fetal death, they wished to maintain the pregnancy. The next several sonograms showed poor fetal growth.

Mrs. M. arrived at the labor and delivery suite at 39 weeks for elective induction and delivery. A viable baby girl weighing 1.6 kg was delivered without difficulty: The Apgar scores were 6 and 8. The infant was transferred to the neonatal intensive care unit for further evaluation. After multiple consultations it was confirmed that she had complex congenital heart disease with microcephaly, hydrocephalus, imperforate anus, limb and vertebral anomalies, diffuse tracheomalacia, and renal anomalies. Chromosomes were 46 XX. A diagnosis of VACTERL association was made. On the first day of life, the infant required intubation and mechanical ventilation.

Family meetings were arranged to review and discuss the infant's status. Based on examination and magnetic resonance imaging scans, pediatric neurology anticipated that Baby M would be severely impaired, cognitively and physically, and partially blind and deaf. Bronchoscopic findings of severe diffuse tracheomalacia led pediatric pulmonologists to conclude that long-term mechanical ventilation would most likely be needed. Pediatric cardiologists predicted that surgery to repair the infant's complex heart defect was possible, but the current weight of 1.6 kg was a complicating factor. Pediatric orthopedic specialists, after reviewing the arm anomalies, concluded that future surgical intervention might be able to make the arms functional. Despite the poor overall prognosis and recommendations of the medical team not to intervene, the family wished to proceed with the multiple palliative and corrective surgeries.

Current Concepts

This infant presented a dilemma, which allows a chance to review some of the concepts that are brought to bear on pediatric ethical dilemmas in general. Landwirth,[151] in discussing pediatric and neonatal resuscitation, emphasized the unique nature of pediatrics, including the standing of the parents as surrogate decision makers. Others have stressed that in caring for the critically ill infant, three long-term issues must be considered: benefit to the child, the parents, and society as a whole. Some of the concepts currently under active discussion are those of beneficence, societal good, quality of life years, and patient autonomy. How can these concepts be applied to the difficult problem of Baby M? If the family and health care team disagree, what help is available to bring about consensus?

Although each of us tries to bring both reason and moral thinking to these discussions, we are each influenced by our prior experiences, whether of an infant once deemed unsalvageable who grew to give happiness to all his family, or of some child who, after many years of care and support, died tragically after prolonged suffering.

Beneficence. Beneficence, and its corollary, lack of maleficence, is clearly a paramount concept. In simple terms, the infant should receive treatment focused on ensuring or restoring an active happy life, with the minimum of pain and distress involved in the treatment.[152,153] The pediatrician, in considering beneficence, has to imagine how he or she would wish to be treated if in the infant's place.[154] Achieving such a goal is very difficult in an infant like Baby M with a complex cardiac problem and many extracardiac anomalies. For example, often lack of knowledge of the true prognosis exists; less often, controversy occurs over the certainty and accuracy of the various diagnoses.

Most physicians would not find it beneficent to submit an infant to several cardiac operations, multiple invasive procedures, and 6 months in intensive care on ventilator support, if the outcome for that particular condition were known to be uniformly fatal by age 1 year. However, in the real world, the knowledge database is very rarely that conclusive. For example, although most infants with trisomy 18 and heart disease die very early, between 5% and 10% live for more than a year, and no certain way is known at present of identifying the potential survivors.[155] Some parents of such an infant, even when informed of the poor prognosis for intellectual development, do not feel justified in withholding cardiac or other surgical care. Room exists for much honest disagreement on the optimal course to pursue, but it is essential that the parents and health care team have the best available facts and be able to participate knowledgeably in the decision.

Societal Good. Societal good is clearly achieved by the restoration to health of a child with coarctation of the aorta or tetralogy of Fallot, who can be expected to reach adult life and become a full member of society; indeed, although this is often not mentioned, society benefits in uncounted ways from the joy and activity of a healthy growing child. However, when an infant such as Baby M has severe multisystem involvement with anticipated developmental disability of uncertain degree, the picture is intuitively less clear. A wide philosophic gulf stretches between those who think societal good means raising a child who will be a wage earner and those who think society benefits from seeing and helping the handicapped. Sometimes, as may have happened with Baby M, the family's religious or ethical beliefs hold that the sanctity of individual life transcends all other considerations. The health care team always must consider societal good, but in a broad context.

Quality-adjusted life-years. Quality-adjusted life-years (QALYs) is a concept discussed in medical ethics and also in medical economics. For the critically ill infant with successfully repaired coarctation of the aorta and no other anomalies, it is reasonable to estimate a future normal life expectancy of more than 70 years with an excellent quality of life. Any calculations of this kind are precarious in Baby M because of uncertainties surrounding the duration of time on ventilator support and the ultimate neurologic and cognitive outcome. Again, individual philosophic variations exist as to the definition of quality of life. Individual lives vary in intensity, duration, and beauty, and each can have its own essential value. Some authors use the term *slippery slope* to express the dangers of being judgmental and derogatory about the quality of life of others.

Autonomy. Autonomy implies the importance of the individual in making his or her own life decisions. Respect for individual autonomy, implying the need for truly informed consent, is a concept accepted for both adults and children. Vicarious decisions must necessarily be made for infants such as Baby M, who are not yet autonomous but are completely dependent on others for care, love, and decisions. In intensive care settings the triangle of understanding may become complex, particularly if care is prolonged. Instead of one physician, a health care team is present, whose chief may change on a weekly or other timed basis; the ICU nurse and cardiac nurse specialist often provide most of the vital sense of continuity. Instead of two involved parents, there may be a single teenage mother, often accompanied by varying family members with differing philosophies, or the parents may already be separated or divorced, each accompanied by a new partner. When confronted with the question of whose autonomy should be most considered, that of the health care team or the family, it can be helpful to remember that the family will be the long-term caregivers.

Informed Consent. Informed consent is integral to respect for the patient's or family's autonomy: in the absence of good knowledge of the medical facts and the probable prognosis, they cannot act autonomously. Some of the most public discussions of informed consent have involved gene therapy and other major advances involving the revolutionary upsurge in genetic knowledge.[156,157]

Other concepts discussed in the literature on medical ethics concern futility and wrongful life. The *concept of futility* implies that treatment may be discontinued or withheld if efforts to prolong life will be futile or result in a meaningless existence. Decisions involving this concept are made almost daily in active intensive care settings in the presence of irreversible brain damage from various causes. Like most ethical concepts, this one is easier in the more extreme situations. Now generally accepted objective criteria are known for a diagnosis of brain death. The presence of profound irreversible brain injury may be more difficult to determine with certainty. When doubt exists as to how long life may be prolonged or the implications of a cardiac syndrome for a "meaningful" life, unanimity may be hard to achieve.

Bringing Ethical Concepts to the Bedside, or How Can These Concepts Be Applied to Baby M and Others With Severe Syndromes?

First, the health care team, in helping the child and family, must avoid being overly directive. Although the team has an obligation to share with the family their medical and scientific knowledge of the child's status and prognosis, they must separate the facts from their own individual feelings and beliefs. Some of us believe that it also is important to share at least some of one's uncertainties: For example, with Baby M the degree of sight and hearing loss can probably be established with accuracy, but the cognitive function and need for ventilator support are less predictable.

The forceful projection of medical beliefs on others is often described as "paternalism." Conversely, it is almost impossible, if even supposing it to be desirable, to counsel without conveying some sense of one's own stance. Each member of the health care team must know and examine his or her own ethical and moral viewpoint. This helps in the control of bias and provides assurance in the decision-making process. The increasing use of formal teaching on ethics and moral reasoning in medical and nursing schools is a major advance, one that will help future generations caring for the critically ill child with cardiac disease.[158] Every physician, nurse, and health care team member involved in critical care knows how difficult the concept of beneficence can be in practice.

Second, if possible, the health care team should develop a consensus so that the family's great and overwhelming sense of grief, loss, and uncertainty should not be further exacerbated by conflicting opinions and prognoses. Divisions among the health care team tend to arise most often in three critical situations: (1) the medical *facts* are unknown or in dispute; a consensus can be built only on what all know to be the truth; (2) the concept of *meaningful life* cannot be agreed on for the individual child; and

(3) the moral, ethical, and philosophic *viewpoints* of the team and family either are unknown, at variance, or have not yet been properly discussed. After the medical facts are known with clarity, a consensus must be established. This involves much time and empathy. Discussion with an ethics committee may clarify the facts and cool some of the heated dialogue.[159] All the team members may be helped to realize that pediatrics, usually such a joyful field, may sometimes present severe ethical dilemmas.

It is very helpful to have seen older children and even adults who have survived long and arduous times in intensive care and are now leading healthy lives. The perspective of future possibilities is daily involved in the ethics of critical care. The child is and must remain the focus, the apex of the triangle of understanding.

Some of the ethical dilemmas faced today arise from technologic advances; some have always existed. The ethical challenge in an intensive care setting lies in providing skilled, compassionate, thoughtful, and well-informed care and information to the critically ill child and family. In most infants with heart defects and syndromes, societal good and many excellent individual QALYs can be achieved if the concepts of beneficence and autonomy accompany skilled and loving care. Even on the rare occasions when the goal of treatment and the assurance of a normal life fail, skilled care accompanied by compassion, love, and grace still avails much. The suffering of the child, the family, and the caregivers is, to some degree, allayed by ethical treatment. Each person reading this chapter should consider how he or she would have advised the family of Baby M or how an ethics committee consultation could bring light and consensus. Caring for the heart of a child remains forever inseparable from ethics.

Conclusion

The role of genetics in the evaluation and treatment of patients with congenital CVMs continues to grow. Cumulative experience in the intensive care of patients with syndromic disorders has led to improved perioperative outcomes for certain syndromes. Nonetheless, there is a need for collaboration between centers to delineate the perioperative risks and outcomes for patients with the less common syndromes. This includes the need to understand long-term outcomes. At the same time, technologic advances in genetic testing expand our ability to establish an early genetic diagnosis in patients with syndromic and nonsyndromic CVMs. These technologies are opening new avenues to investigate the etiology of CVMs. It will be important to define the clinical implications of newly discovered classes of genetic diagnoses. Genetics services interfacing directly with the cardiac ICU team will help to counsel families, guide testing choices, interpret results of testing, and supply insight about the implications of negative or positive testing results. We can safely project that genetics will have an increasingly prominent role in the care of patients with CVMs.

References

A complete list of references is available at ExpertConsult.com.

76

Adult Congenital Heart Disease

ABIGAIL MAY KHAN, MD; DANIEL R. SEDEHI, MD; CRAIG S. BROBERG, MD

Intensive care unit (ICU) admissions are not uncommon in adult congenital heart disease (ACHD) patients. Much of the growing population of individuals with congenital defects will require cardiac care throughout their adult lives, including a substantial portion who will need intensive cardiac care.[1] Consistent with the increase in the number of adults living with congenital heart disease (CHD), there has been a significant increase in the number of ACHD hospitalizations in the United States, including hospitalizations to the ICU.[2] In one population-based Canadian study, 16% of ACHD patients required ICU admission over a 4-year period.[3] Even patients considered to have undergone "complete repair" have a high rate of long-term cardiac complications, including arrhythmias, heart failure, and the need for reoperation. This is particularly true for those with moderate or complex disease, who require more interventions and have worse outcomes.[4]

It has been said that adults are not large children. Although adult and pediatric patients with CHD share common anatomy and physiology, there are also key differences between these two populations. Unique features of adults include the presence of medical comorbidities and a higher percentage of redo surgeries that pose greater risk. Adults with CHD also have different physiologic and social factors that set them apart from children with CHD. Providers often struggle to apply data obtained from pediatric CHD populations to their adult patients or to extrapolate from studies performed in adults with acquired heart disease as opposed to CHD.

Systems of care for hospitalized ACHD patients vary by city, with no agreement as to which model is best. Many young adults with CHD continue to receive their care, including ICU care, at pediatric hospitals. Alternatively, many adults are found in adult cardiac care, either through deliberate transition to an adult ACHD program or by establishing care with a non-ACHD adult cardiologist. Specialized ACHD care has been associated with decreased mortality,[5] and the location of care is especially important for ACHD patients in the ICU, who require a team that is experienced in the management of both CHD and non-CHD aspects of their care. Such combined expertise may be best found in either an adult or pediatric ICU, depending on the region.

Common Reasons for Intensive Care Unit Admission in Adult Congenital Heart Disease

The most common indications for ICU admission in ACHD patients are postoperative care,[4] followed by heart failure and arrhythmias. Many ACHD patients undergo cardiac reoperations, which are associated with a higher risk of morbidity and mortality than primary repairs.[6] A postoperative admission to the ICU may be as short as 24 hours in an uncomplicated postoperative patient or longer in patients who are slow to wean off the ventilator, have ongoing hemodynamic or respiratory compromise, or have significant bradyarrhythmias or tachyarrhythmias.

Published mortality rates for ACHD patients undergoing surgery are low; however, at least one in five patients has a major adverse event, including stroke, renal failure, and prolonged ventilation.[7,8] Arrhythmias are the most common type of postoperative cardiac complication. Our ability to predict which ACHD patients are at highest risk of postoperative complications is limited, although it is an area of active investigation. It seems that pediatric risk scores are of reasonable predictive value for assessing surgical risk in adults,[7] and existing ICU risk scores can also be used with some success.[4]

Heart failure is another common indication for ICU admission and is on the rise.[9] Although many ACHD patients with heart failure can be successfully managed on a medical floor or cardiac step-down unit, some will require ICU admission. At our institution the most common indications for ICU admission in a heart failure patient are the need for inotropes, unstable respiratory status (e.g., a patient requiring biphasic positive airway pressure or intubation), or unstable supraventricular or ventricular arrhythmias.

Less commonly, pregnant ACHD patients may be admitted to the ICU for labor and delivery (e.g., a woman with severe left ventricular outflow tract obstruction). These patients require complex, coordinated team-based care with input from high-risk obstetrics, ACHD, critical care, electrophysiology, and obstetric and cardiac anesthesia.

Adult Congenital Heart Disease Patient in the Intensive Care Unit: Systems Factors

Patients with moderate to complex ACHD require coordinated, multidisciplinary care when in the ICU. It is now clear that there are specific systems-level challenges facing providers and hospital systems caring for these patients. First, like many complex medical populations, patients with ACHD have a high rate of health resource utilization (HRU). ICU care is an important contributor to HRU and one that is anticipated to grow over time as the population ages. The costs and degree of HRU are higher for complex patients as opposed to those with simple lesions.[4] Several risk factors for HRU at either pediatric or adult hospitals have been identified in ACHD, including admissions with greater surgical complexity, emergency admissions, heart failure or renal failure, and patient factors such as government insurance, DiGeorge syndrome, and depression.[10,11]

As mentioned earlier, ACHD patients may receive care in a variety of locations, and whether ACHD patients are better cared for at an adult or a pediatric hospital is a source of ongoing controversy. Despite their age, ACHD patients constitute a small but not insignificant proportion of admissions at pediatric hospitals. This proportion has grown commensurately with the size of the ACHD population.[10] Adult cardiac surgeries are frequently performed at children's hospitals with good results.[12] Surgical mortality appears to be lower when ACHD surgery is performed by a congenital heart surgeon, although this may be at an adult or a pediatric hospital.[13,14] In either location it is essential that there is familiarity and experience with CHD at all levels of patient care. The surgical team, anesthesiologists, intensivists, subspecialists, and nurses all play an important role in caring for these patients. In addition, the ACHD provider, when available, has an essential role in following patients throughout the system and helping to guide their care.

Finally, loss to follow-up is a major issue in the ACHD population, and some patients who are lost to follow-up may represent to the medical system at the time of ICU admission. In these cases it is imperative that the ICU team attempt to identify a CHD provider who can assist in the patient's management and also help facilitate their long-term care, including transfer to the care of an appropriate outpatient ACHD provider.

Adult Congenital Heart Disease Patient in the Intensive Care Unit: Unique Physiologic Factors

Comorbidities Not Related to Congenital Heart Disease

There are several extracardiac features that make the ACHD patient unique in the ICU (Box 76.1) and more vulnerable to unforeseen complications. These noncardiac comorbidities are more prevalent in adults than in the pediatric CHD population and can jeopardize optimal management.[3,15] These include renal and hepatic problems, as well as acquired cardiac conditions and chronic lung disease. All should be seriously considered as potential risk factors by the intensivist.

Chronic renal dysfunction is more common in ACHD patients than in the general population,[16] presumably because of abnormal cardiac physiology and its impact on renal perfusion, as well as factors such as nephrotoxic medications, chronic hypoxia, and neurohormonal abnormalities.[16] One study found that significant renal dysfunction was 18 times higher in noncyanotic ACHD patients and 35 times higher in cyanotic ACHD patients than in the general population,[16] whereas another suggested that 30% to 50% of ACHD patients have significantly impaired renal function.[17] The presence of renal dysfunction, either subclinical or clinical, can complicate ICU management and is a predictor of adverse outcomes.[4] Additionally, cardiopulmonary bypass is associated with acute kidney injury and is a frequent contributing factor in renal dysfunction in ACHD patients in the ICU.[18] Providers caring for ACHD patients should be mindful of the impact of selected therapies on renal perfusion and take renal function into account when selecting medications and interventions.

Hepatic dysfunction is also common in ACHD patients, especially those with the Fontan circulation.[19] In addition to being

• BOX 76.1 Unique Risks to Consider in the Adult Congenital Heart Disease Patient in the Intensive Care Unit

Central Venous Access

Anatomic features can complicate central line placement (e.g., persistent left superior vena cava).

Placement of a central line across a Glenn anastomosis into the pulmonary arteries carries a risk of thrombosis and should be avoided when possible.

Positive Pressure Ventilation

The use of positive pressure ventilation may decrease preload, and therefore cardiac output, in patients with a Fontan circulation.

There is a high frequency of chronic lung disease, especially restrictive disease, in adults with repaired CHD.

Inotropes

Patients with systemic right ventricles or a Fontan repair may not have the expected response to inotropes. Attention should be paid to other factors, such as preload, pulmonary vascular resistance, and chronotropic response, which also have an important hemodynamic impact.

Thrombosis Risk

Some patients with ACHD, such as those with Fontan palliation or Eisenmenger syndrome, are at increased risk of thrombosis. Eisenmenger syndrome also carries an increased risk of bleeding, and therefore decisions about anticoagulation should be undertaken in consultation with a CHD specialist.

Hepatic Dysfunction

Hepatic dysfunction and even cirrhosis can develop in Fontan patients and in those with chronically elevated right heart pressures and resultant hepatic dysfunction. Providers should have a low threshold for screening for hepatic dysfunction and manage patients appropriately.

Renal Dysfunction

Thirty percent to 50% of ACHD patients have significantly impaired renal function, which may not always manifest as a significantly elevated serum creatinine level. Patients with cyanotic heart disease are at especially high risk.

ACHD, Adult congenital heart disease; CDH, congenital heart disease.

a risk factor for surgical mortality,[20] hepatic dysfunction can impact hemodynamics and the clearance of certain medications. All patients with Fontan physiology and those with passive venous congestion of the liver should be considered to be at high risk for liver disease and managed appropriately (e.g., Ebstein anomaly, repaired tetralogy of Fallot with pulmonic regurgitation).

Other common adult comorbidities with impact on ICU management include obstructive sleep apnea,[21] acquired heart disease such as coronary artery disease (CAD),[22] and chronic lung disease. Nearly half of ACHD patients have impaired lung function. Approximately 30% of ACHD patients have moderate to severe respiratory impairment.[23] Restrictive lung disease is particularly common in those with previous chest surgery.[24] This has important implications for ventilation strategies and for ventilator weaning.

Systemic Right Ventricle

Patients with a systemic right ventricle (RV) (congenitally corrected transposition of the great arteries or d-transposition of the great arteries after an atrial switch procedure) constitute a small but important part of the ACHD population. Patients with a hypoplastic left heart are another group of survivors with systemic RV, in whom many of these same issues may be faced.

Important anatomic and physiologic differences between the systemic morphologic RV and the systemic morphologic left ventricle (LV) have implications not only for the long-term risk of RV failure and arrhythmia but also for ICU management.[25] Due to differences in myocardial geometry, atrioventricular valve structure, and papillary muscles, the RV as a systemic pump is inferior to the morphologic LV.

Importantly, a systemic RV may not respond to inotropy in the same manner as a systemic LV, as evidenced by the fact that stroke volume fails to augment with dobutamine stress, particularly in those with an atrial switch palliation.[26] It has been hypothesized that this is due to the rigid atrial baffle that alters preload as opposed to some factor intrinsic to the systemic RV because a similar impairment is not seen in those with congenitally corrected transposition.[27] Theoretically, atrial switch patients can compensate for the inability to augment stroke volume by increasing heart rate, but this may also be limited in those with chronotropic incompetence or chronic pacing, both of which are common.[28]

Myocardial dysfunction leading to clinical heart failure is a common presentation in individuals with a systemic RV. Unfortunately, data are lacking regarding the efficacy of conventional heart failure therapy for the failing RV. In the absence of specific data, many providers use similar therapies for the failing RV as they do for the failing LV. This is discussed in further detail later.

Fontan Circulation

The Fontan pathways for single ventricle palliation have created a growing cohort of patients who are aging into adulthood and experiencing complications. These include Fontan pathway obstruction, single-ventricle dysfunction, atrioventricular valve regurgitation, arrhythmias, cyanosis, protein-losing enteropathy, and liver dysfunction, among others.[29] As this population ages, we anticipate that ICU admission will become increasingly common. Specific issues that are pertinent to the Fontan patient in the ICU include vascular access, the importance of preload and low pulmonary vascular resistance (PVR), and the response to inotropes.

Because the systemic venous return is directly anastomosed to the pulmonary arteries (bidirectional Glenn shunt), placement of a central line via the SVC into the Glenn shunt or pulmonary arteries should be avoided if possible given the theoretical risk of catheter-associated thrombosis and Fontan obstruction. Alternate forms of venous access, such as a midline catheter, are preferable in Fontan patients. In someone with a classic atriopulmonary Fontan connection, interpretation of a central venous waveform, measured pressure, or quantification of output should be done with the unique Fontan physiology in mind.

Mechanical ventilation also presents unique challenges in the Fontan patient. Normal negative intrathoracic pressure during spontaneous inhalation is a key contributor to pulmonary blood flow, and therefore to ventricular preload, in Fontan patients. The hemodynamic benefit of spontaneous breathing was first recognized by Fontan after his initial procedures.[30] As estimated by magnetic resonance blood tagging, 30% of systemic venous pathway flow is respiratory dependent, with inspiration being one of the highest periods of Fontan flow.[31] Therefore positive pressure ventilation may have a deleterious impact on lung perfusion, ventricular preload, and cardiac output. This is evidenced by the fact that the cardiac

index increases significantly when patients are extubated after the Fontan procedure.[32] Early extubation is now considered the optimal management strategy after initial Fontan palliation,[33] and avoidance of positive pressure ventilation is recommended whenever possible. Recognizing that mechanical ventilation is sometimes unavoidable, we recommend the use of low-pressure strategies, such as avoidance of positive end-expiratory pressure, as well as careful attention to preload and contractility during the period that the patient is ventilated.

Ventricular preload is an important determinant of cardiac output in Fontan patients. Preload is determined by the transpulmonary gradient and by flow through a Fontan fenestration, if present. PVR is also an important determinant of cardiac output in Fontan patients.[34] Even small increases in PVR can result in a decrease in ventricular preload and hence cardiac output.[35] Therefore ICU providers caring for Fontan patients should be attentive to PVR and avoid factors that cause it to increase when possible.

Inotropes fail to increase the stroke volume output of a Fontan patient to the same degree that they do in a patient with a two-ventricle circulation.[34,36] This finding is probably because preload is a more important determinant of cardiac output than contractility in the majority of Fontan patients. The exception to this is the patient with severely impaired ventricular function, who may benefit from inotropy. It is important to note that increasing heart rate may also not be an effective mechanism to increase cardiac output, at least not by atrial pacing.[37]

Common Management Concerns in Adult Congenital Heart Disease Patients

Central Venous Access

Central venous access is commonly used to guide management in ICU patients. ACHD patients may have abnormal venous anatomy, such as a left-sided SVC, which may necessitate the use of imaging guidance for line placement (e.g., persistent left SVC, present in approximately 1% of individuals with CHD).[38] Venous obstruction can be an issue in patients who have had prior invasive procedures. Finally, as mentioned earlier, patients with Glenn shunts (e.g., Fontan) have a direct connection between the SVC and the pulmonary arteries. Placing a catheter in the Glenn shunt or pulmonary arteries is generally not recommended due to the theoretical risk of thrombosis and Fontan obstruction in this relatively low-flow system.

Right Ventricular Dysfunction

RV dysfunction is common among ACHD patients and occurs in patients with a systemic LV as well as those with a systemic RV. Subpulmonic RV dysfunction is frequently seen postoperatively and can be associated with clinical RV failure in some patients.[39] RV failure can occur after either left- or right-sided congenital heart surgery and is associated with a high mortality in the ACHD population. Preoperative RV dysfunction, cardiopulmonary bypass time of longer than 150 minutes, and postoperative supraventricular tachycardia have been identified as important risk factors for RV failure in ACHD patients.[40] For example, a patient with Ebstein anomaly and seemingly normal preoperative RV systolic function may exhibit very poor systolic function postoperatively, even jeopardizing LV filling as a result.[41] Although subpulmonic right ventricular assistant devices are an enticing option for these patients, the data in ACHD are extremely limited at this time.

Acute Arrhythmias

Arrhythmias are the most common cause of hospital admission in ACHD.[2] ACHD patients are at risk of arrhythmias for a variety of reasons, including complex anatomy, surgical scars, and abnormal hemodynamics. Age is also an important factor. The prevalence of arrhythmias in tetralogy of Fallot, for example, increases sharply in older patients.[42] Hence the frequency of ICU admission for arrhythmias is likely to increase as the population ages.

Atrial arrhythmias commonly seen in the ACHD population include intraatrial reentrant tachycardia, atrial flutter, and atrial fibrillation. In general, CHD patients benefit from a rhythm control strategy for atrial arrhythmias, as opposed to the rate control strategy, which is widely employed in the management of adult atrial fibrillation. This can be performed with medications (most commonly amiodarone in the ICU) and/or cardioversion. In some cases adenosine may be useful to break atrial arrhythmias or determine cause. Providers using amiodarone should be mindful of the high frequency of liver dysfunction in CHD patients, especially those after Fontan palliation.

Some patients with atrial arrhythmias, particularly those after Fontan palliation, may deteriorate rapidly if sinus rhythm is not restored. Early cardioversion should be seriously considered, with a low threshold for transesophageal echocardiography beforehand. ACHD patients have a higher than expected risk for thromboembolic complications.[43] Transesophageal echocardiography may not be anatomically straightforward, particularly in a systemic RV or Fontan patient. Therefore in certain instances expeditious cardioversion in response to a new rhythm may be preferable to waiting. Ablation may be appropriate for the management of atrial arrhythmias in some patients, although it is generally performed in stable patients, as opposed to those requiring ICU care. Consultation with an electrophysiologist experienced in CHD is recommended to determine the optimal management strategy.

CHA_2DS_2-VASc score is not applicable in this population, and providers should not use it to predict risk of stroke in patients with moderate or complex CHD.[43] Additionally, providers should understand that there are CHD-specific factors that increase the risk of bleeding in this population, such as liver dysfunction, renal dysfunction, and cyanosis. Although vitamin K antagonist therapy is the traditional anticoagulant used in CHD patients, we anticipate that direct oral anticoagulants (DOACs) will be used with increasing frequency in the coming years. At the current time there is an overall lack of data about DOAC use in ACHD, although the preliminary data appear promising.[44]

Some patients with CHD are also at risk for bradyarrhythmias and heart block, such as those with l-transposition of the great arteries or atrioventricular septal defects. Dysfunction of the sinus and/or atrioventricular node is common in ACHD patients, particularly after surgery.[45] Patients may require temporary and/or permanent pacemaker implantation to maintain hemodynamic stability or alleviate symptoms. Consultation with an electrophysiologist experienced in CHD is recommended because some patients may have issues with access and/or physiology that necessitate the use of nonstandard protocols for pacemaker implantation. Examples include an atrial switch patient with superior venous baffle stenosis who requires concurrent baffle stenting or a single-ventricle patient who requires an epicardial device for ventricular pacing.

Although sudden death is a recognized feature of ACHD, new presentations of sustained ventricular tachycardia (VT) are uncommon.[46] Nonsustained VT occurs fairly frequently, however. Predisposing factors for VT in this population include prior ventriculotomy repair (such as the older patient with tetralogy of Fallot) and ventricular dysfunction. Scar-related VT may be amenable to catheter ablation, whereas VT related to underlying ventricular dysfunction is more challenging to treat.[47]

Heart Failure

The prevalence of heart failure in ACHD has risen dramatically over the last few decades, reflective of an aging and increasing complex ACHD population. Heart failure is one of the most common causes of death in ACHD patients, constituting approximately 25% of all deaths.[48,49] As discussed earlier, patients with a systemic RV and those with a single-ventricle circulation are at especially high risk of developing heart failure. Other ACHD patients, such as those with valvar disease, pulmonary hypertension, or ventricular dysfunction after repair of tetralogy of Fallot, may also commonly develop heart failure.

Manifestations of heart failure in the ACHD patient are often different than in the non-ACHD patient, leading to improper recognition and/or treatment.[50] A classic example is the Fontan patient, who may present with "heart failure" of a variety of clinical phenotypes. Some failing Fontan patients present with a reduced ejection fraction, elevated filling pressures, low cardiac output, and high systemic vascular resistance (SVR), similar to the typical adult patient with systolic heart failure. Yet other "failing" Fontan patients present with signs of right-sided heart failure in the setting of preserved ejection fraction and normal filling pressures.[51] These different phenotypes require markedly different treatment strategies.

The neurohormonal changes in ACHD heart failure are similar to those in non-ACHD heart failure, suggesting that similar treatment paradigms may apply.[52] Unfortunately, the use of traditional chronic heart failure treatment strategies, such as angiotensin-converting enzyme inhibitors, beta-blockers, and spironolactone, is currently limited by lack of data and/or efficacy in the ACHD population. Large heart failure trials have tended to exclude individuals with CHD, and CHD-specific studies have often been retrospective or underpowered or have failed to show a benefit.[53] Similarly, therapies for acute heart failure have not been validated in the ACHD population. In the absence of evidence-based therapies, providers caring for ACHD patients with heart failure typically use standard therapies that have been validated in non–CHD-associated heart failure while also trying to be mindful of unique aspects of the ACHD patient.

In contrast to patients with non–CHD-associated heart failure, ACHD-associated heart failure may be related to residual hemodynamic lesions, which can be treated with catheter-based therapy. Common examples include baffle leaks or stenosis in patients after an atrial switch procedure, pulmonary valve stenosis and/or regurgitation in a patient with repaired tetralogy of Fallot, or branch pulmonary artery stenosis in a patient with Fontan circulation (Table 76.1). Because of the unique hemodynamic factors in individuals with CHD, intensive care providers caring for ACHD patients with heart failure should obtain early consultation from a provider with specific training in CHD. Depending on the setting, this provider could be a trained ACHD provider, a pediatric cardiologist or CHD surgeon, or an interventional cardiologist with experience in CHD.

TABLE 76.1	Selected Hemodynamic Consequences of Complex Adult Congenital Heart Disease
Type of CHD	**Hemodynamic Consequence**
Tetralogy of Fallot	Valvar regurgitation: pulmonary or tricuspid Left or right ventricular systolic dysfunction Restrictive right ventricular physiology Pulmonic stenosis: prosthesis, main or branch pulmonary arteries Residual shunts
d-Transposition of the great arteries, atrial switch	Systemic ventricular dysfunction Tricuspid regurgitation Baffle leaks or stenosis Left ventricular outflow tract obstruction
l-Transposition of the great arteries	Systemic ventricular dysfunction Tricuspid regurgitation Left ventricular outflow tract obstruction
Ebstein anomaly	Right ventricular dysfunction Tricuspid regurgitation Atrial-level shunt Poor LV filling leading to LVOT obstruction
Single ventricle, Fontan palliation	Systemic ventricular dysfunction Atrioventricular valve regurgitation Semilunar valve regurgitation Outflow tract obstruction Fontan pathway obstruction Pulmonary artery stenosis Collateral flow: venovenous or aortopulmonary Shunting through Fontan fenestration

CDH, Congenital heart disease; *LV,* left ventricular; *LVOT,* left ventricular outflow tract.

As in the non-CHD population, diuretics can be used in standard doses to treat pulmonary edema and congestion. Care should be taken in those patients who are particularly preload dependent (e.g., after the Fontan palliation or those with outflow tract obstruction). Close monitoring of renal function is mandatory given the high prevalence of renal dysfunction in this cohort.[17] Although the ACHD data are limited, there is evidence to support the use of afterload reduction in non-ACHD heart failure, and by extension it is often used in ACHD patients unless there is a contraindication.[53] Inotropes are required in some patients with acute decompensated heart failure and are discussed in the next section.

Pulmonary Vascular Resistance

Some patients, most notably those after Fontan palliation or those with subpulmonary ventricular dysfunction, will experience increases in cardiac output when the PVR is lowered. Factors that can exacerbate pulmonary hypertension in ICU patients include hypercapnia, acidosis, hypoxemia, and pain. As mentioned previously, mechanical ventilation can also impact PVR and is especially problematic in Fontan patients. The management of pulmonary hypertension is discussed in further detail in Chapter 71.

Inotropes and Vasopressors

Inotropes and vasopressors have important roles to play in the management of hypotension and cardiogenic shock. Robust evidence in the ACHD population is lacking, but much can be inferred from studies of their use in non-ACHD patients. Important factors to consider include their proarrhythmic nature, vasodilatory or vasoconstrictive properties, and preferential effects on systemic versus pulmonary vasculature and how this applies to the exact cardiac anatomy of the patient. Appropriate vasoactive support for hemodynamic compromise is achievable with knowledge of the medications as well as the patient's physiology.

Inotropes. The exogenous catecholamines dopamine, dobutamine, and epinephrine, along with the phosphodiesterase type 3 inhibitor milrinone, exert inotropic and chronotropic effects on the heart. They carry a not insignificant risk of arrhythmias, both supraventricular and ventricular. None of these medications are pure inotropes, and recognizing their effects upon the systemic and pulmonary vasculature is of the utmost importance.

Dopamine exerts its effects upon the alpha- and beta-receptors and acts as an inotrope and vasopressor, a so-called inoconstrictor. Although classically viewed as the vasopressor of choice in cardiogenic shock, it is beginning to fall out of first-line favor with the publication of the Sepsis Occurrence in Acutely Ill Patients (SOAP) and SOAP 2 trials, indicating potential for harm and no superiority over norepinephrine in all varieties of shock.[54,55] Dobutamine is an alpha-antagonist and beta-agonist, and a rapid-on, rapid-off, easily titratable inodilator. It can increase blood pressure by increasing stroke volume, but in systemically vasodilated patients the decrease in SVR can worsen hypotension. Epinephrine is an aggressive agonist of alpha- and beta-receptors and acts similarly to dopamine as an inoconstrictor. Epinephrine provides a nonpreferential increase in both SVR and PVR.

As a phosphodiesterase type 3 inhibitor, milrinone serves an important role in the ACHD population. Data suggest that there is an oversaturation of beta-receptors in chronic heart failure patients. By using milrinone, one can continue to augment inotropy by bypassing the adrenergic receptor. Milrinone has been shown to decrease PVR in animal models and humans, particularly when related to hypoxic pulmonary vasoconstriction.[56,57] In patients with persistent shunting or Fontan physiology, maintenance of normal PVR is of vital importance for venous return to the systemic ventricle. It should also be recognized that milrinone is an inodilator, which can potentiate hypotension in low SVR states. In contrast to dobutamine, milrinone has a 4- to 6-hour half-life and is therefore less readily titratable.

Vasopressors. Norepinephrine and vasopressin are the primary vasoconstrictors of choice in patients with refractory hypotension. These are frequently used in addition to the aforementioned inotropes to augment vasoconstriction in patients with hypotension, whether from sepsis or hypovolemic or cardiogenic shock. Norepinephrine is a potent vasoconstrictor. It is predominantly an alpha-agonist but has a small amount of beta-agonism as well. It acts to increase SVR and PVR without preference for one over the other and is readily titratable. In a head-to-head comparison with dopamine, the SOAP 2 trial demonstrated there was no difference in mortality between norepinephrine and dopamine in either septic or cardiogenic shock, with dopamine resulting in an increased frequency of arrhythmias, primarily atrial fibrillation.[54] Vasopressin is a V1 agonist that has unique hemodynamic effects, mainly a preferential increase in SVR without increase in PVR within the normal dose range. In the Vasopressin and Septic Shock

Trial (VASST), vasopressin was found to be equivalent to norepinephrine for septic shock.[58] Its noninferiority to norepinephrine in shock and the preferential increase in SVR over PVR makes it a tempting choice for ACHD patients.

Emerging Considerations

Acquired Heart Disease

The ACHD patient with significant atherosclerotic CAD is still relatively rare in ACHD practice, but this is likely to change. CHD patients can develop coronary events related to congenital coronary anomalies or as a consequence of prior surgical repair.[59,60] In addition, they are at risk for atherosclerotic CAD. Although individuals with CAD constitute only a small minority of the ACHD population at the current time, the prevalence of CAD in ACHD is expected to rise as the ACHD population ages.[22,61] Risk factors for acquired heart disease, such as hyperlipidemia, hypertension, diabetes mellitus, smoking, and physical inactivity, are common in the ACHD population and will contribute to this growing issue.[62]

Mechanical Circulatory Support

The current evidence for the use of mechanical circulatory support devices in ACHD is mainly anecdotal.[63] However, this is likely to be an area of significant growth in the coming years. Anatomic abnormalities in ACHD patients present significant challenges in using mechanical support, but it has been described with some success.[64]

Conclusion

Adults with CHD constitute a large and growing population that is at high risk of long-term cardiac complications.[65-67] As the ACHD population ages, we expect to see a burgeoning need for ICU care, especially among those with moderate or complex CHD. Although ACHD patients can receive high-quality care in either pediatric or adult hospitals, the presence of a coordinated, experienced care team is essential for optimal outcomes.

Selected References

A complete list of references is available at ExpertConsult.com.

4. Price S, Jaggar SI, Jordan S, et al. Adult congenital heart disease: intensive care management and outcome prediction. *Intensive Care Med.* 2007;33(4):652–659.
13. Karamlou T, Diggs BS, Ungerleider RM, Welke KF. Adults or big kids: what is the ideal clinical environment for management of grown-up patients with congenital heart disease? *Ann Thorac Surg.* 2010;90(2):573–579.
14. Kogon BE, Plattner C, Leong T, et al. Adult congenital heart surgery: adult or pediatric facility? Adult or pediatric surgeon? *Ann Thorac Surg.* 2009;87(3):833–840.
16. Dimopoulos K, Diller GP, Koltsida E, et al. Prevalence, predictors, and prognostic value of renal dysfunction in adults with congenital heart disease. *Circulation.* 2008;117(18):2320–2328.
23. Alonso-Gonzalez R, Borgia F, Diller GP, et al. Abnormal lung function in adults with congenital heart disease: prevalence, relation to cardiac anatomy, and association with survival. *Circulation.* 2013;127(8):882–890.
39. Piran S, Veldtman G, Siu S, Webb GD, Liu PP. Heart failure and ventricular dysfunction in patients with single or systemic right ventricles. *Circulation.* 2002;105(10):1189–1194.
42. Khairy P, Aboulhosn J, Gurvitz MZ, et al. Arrhythmia burden in adults with surgically repaired tetralogy of Fallot: a multi-institutional study. *Circulation.* 2010;122(9):868–875.
43. Khairy P, Aboulhosn J, Broberg CS, et al. Thromboprophylaxis for atrial arrhythmias in congenital heart disease: a multicenter study. *Int J Cardiol.* 2016;223:729–735.

Index

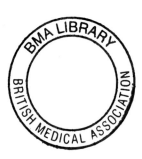

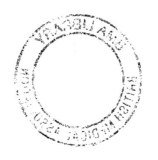

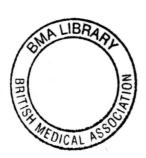